D1828125

Cancer Drug Discovery and Development

Series Editor: Beverly A. Teicher

For further volumes:
http://www.springer.com/series/7625

W. Meyer

Erwin G. Van Meir
Editor

CNS Cancer

Models, Markers, Prognostic Factors, Targets, and Therapeutic Approaches

Humana Press

Editor
Erwin G. Van Meir
Department of Neurosurgery
Hematology and Medical Oncology
and Winship Cancer Institute
Emory University School of Medicine
1365C Clifton Road NE
Atlanta, GA 30322
USA
evanmei@emory.edu

ISBN 978-1-60327-552-1 e-ISBN 978-1-60327-553-8
DOI 10.1007/978-1-60327-553-8
Springer Dordrecht Heidelberg London New York

Library of Congress Control Number: 2009920397

© Humana Press, a part of Springer Science+Business Media, LLC 2009
All rights reserved. This work may not be translated or copied in whole or in part without the written permission of the publisher (Humana Press, c/o Springer Science+Business Media, LLC, 233 Spring Street, New York, NY 10013, USA), except for brief excerpts in connection with reviews or scholarly analysis. Use in connection with any form of information storage and retrieval, electronic adaptation, computer software, or by similar or dissimilar methodology now known or hereafter developed is forbidden.
The use in this publication of trade names, trademarks, service marks, and similar terms, even if they are not identified as such, is not to be taken as an expression of opinion as to whether or not they are subject to proprietary rights.
While the advice and information in this book are believed to be true and accurate at the date of going to press, neither the authors nor the editors nor the publisher can accept any legal responsibility for any errors or omissions that may be made. The publisher makes no warranty, express or implied, with respect to the material contained herein.

Cover design: The cover art was designed by Acilino F. Vieira, Rita G. de Noronha and Erwin G. Van Meir.

Printed on acid-free paper

Springer is part of Springer Science+Business Media (www.springer.com)

This book is dedicated to my parents Annie and Eugene and my sister Veerle who are largely responsible for who I am, to my wife Erika and children Jessica and Gwendolyn who lovingly tolerate the long working days and always show support for what I am doing.

It is also dedicated to my scientific mentors, the late Riccardo Wittek who taught me careful experimentation, critical thinking and molecular virology, Nicolas de Tribolet who launched my interest in brain tumors and provided me with unique early career opportunities, and Webster Cavenee for giving me a great training environment in his laboratory. I also acknowledge the hard work and dedication of all my collaborators, several of them devoted their career to brain tumors and are authors in this book.

Finally, it is dedicated to the many patients and their families who have donated their tissue for experimentation and have helped raise funds to support brain tumor research.

Foreword

Cancers of the central nervous system are among the most lethal of human neoplasms. They are recalcitrant to even intensive multimodality therapies that include surgery, radiotherapy, and chemotherapy. Moreover, especially in children, the consequences of these therapies can itself be devastating and involve serious cognitive and developmental disorders. It is small wonder that such cancers have come under the intense scrutiny of each of the subspecialties of clinical care and investigation as well as attracting some of the best basic research scientists. Their joint efforts are gradually peeling away the mysteries surrounding the genesis and progression of these tumors and inroads are being steadily made into understanding why they resist therapies.

This makes it an especially opportune time to assemble some of the best investigators in the field to review the "state of the art" in the various arenas that comprise the assault on CNS tumors. The breadth of this effort by the clinical and basic neuro-oncology community is quite simply amazing. To a large extent, it evolves from the knowledge of the human genome and its regulation that has been hard won over the past two decades. This information makes it possible to rapidly identify genes that are likely to play causative roles in the initiation and malignant progression of the disease, to test this candidacy in cells and animals, to use validated targets to design and develop both markers for prognostication as well as therapeutic approaches—of a variety of kinds—aimed directly and specifically at the targets and to use experimental and clinical trials of these to test real hypotheses. While the lethality of these tumors has remained dismal over the past decades, there is finally real reason for optimism as our knowledge base grows exponentially larger.

Most of the major areas of this endeavor are displayed in *CNS Cancer Models, Markers, Prognostic Factors, Targets, and Therapeutic Approaches.* Each of the chapters in the book represents illustrative examples of the road from discovery through translation to clinical importance, although many begin the journey at different parts of this continuum. This includes several chapters on incredibly clever mouse models for deciphering the genetic wiring underlying the development of CNS tumors and how that wiring might be targeted for therapeutic benefit. This is an area of explosive growth and increasing sophistication that was unimaginable even a few years ago. Such approaches are complemented by other experimental systems including cell and tissue manipulation and transplantation, spontaneous tumor occurrence in other organisms such as dogs and flies. A great deal of attention has been paid in the book to the development of genetic prognostic factors and biomarkers that could be used for assessing individual responses to therapies and so could lead to truly personalized medicine. Other possible prognostic factors/biomarkers that arise from an understanding of CNS tumor pathophysiology are discussed in some detail and include tumor vascularization and hypoxia. Several of the new and rapidly developing methodologies that allow these rapid advances are detailed for the reader as well and include RNA expression profiling, proteomic analyses of both tumors and biological fluids as well as profiling small non-coding RNAs and DNA modification. Finally, several chapters explore aspects of therapeutic targeting employing small molecules and combinations thereof, various sorts of cells, viruses, and immune modulation. In sum, these treatises represent the cutting edge of research that is driven to be of benefit to patients with these dreaded diseases.

The audience that will benefit from the information contained in *CNS Cancer Models, Markers, Prognostic Factors, Targets, and Therapeutic Approaches* includes clinicians, brain tumor scientists, medical residents, postdoctoral researchers, and the informed patient. This is a wonderful compendium of the most timely information from leaders in the battle against CNS tumors and its timeliness fills a niche in a manner that is accessible and contemporary. The authors and especially the editor, Dr. Erwin Van Meir, are to be congratulated for providing this service to the community.

San Diego, CA Webster K. Cavenee, Ph.D.

Preface

These are exciting times in neuro-oncology. By the time this book is published I will have worked in this field for 20 years, giving me enough perspective to contemplate significant changes during these two decades. In 1989 little was known about brain tumors and the community of researchers was small. Pioneers such as Charles Wilson had the foresight to foster inter-disciplinary approaches to the brain tumor treatment and investigation. Treatment options were limited to surgery, radiotherapy, and a few modestly effective chemotherapeutic agents such as BCNU. Over the ensuing decades, the neuro-oncology field has expanded and traversed a number of "waves", each of which was expected to yield a rapid cure. The 1980s ushered in research that tapped into the power of the immune system and promised immunotherapies, whether antibody-based or cell-based. When I entered the field there was a strong interest in identifying autocrine growth factors that drive tumor growth and the early groundbreaking genetic studies were being performed. Amplification of the *EGFR* gene on chromosome 7 in glioblastoma had been identified as an important oncogenic event in 1984. In subsequent years, the application of karyotypic analyses and loss of heterozygosity studies pinpointed the location of tumor suppressor loci on chromosomes 9, 10, and 17. In 1989, the p53 gene was identified as the tumor suppressor lost from chromosome 17 in glioblastoma and other cancers. In 1993 the p16 cell cycle inhibitor was described and in 1997 the PTEN phosphatase was discovered as a critical gene product lost due to genetic alterations on chromosome 10. Genetic discoveries in glioma spearheaded the use of similar technology for the discovery of new signaling pathways in medulloblastoma, meningioma, ependymoma, and other brain tumors.

The 1990s witnessed the advent of cancer gene therapy and anti-angiogenic therapies. The remarkable results obtained in mouse glioma models with retroviral thymidine kinase/ganciclovir gene therapy systems were not reproduced in clinical trials, yet led to new generations of virotherapy through the use of oncolytic viruses. The definition of angiogenic mechanisms and the discovery of endogenous negative regulators of these processes have led directly to clinical applications in which tumoral blood vessels are targeted by anti-angiogenic therapies, a strategy which is bearing fruit with anti-VEGF antibodies.

Subsequent breakthroughs have included the sequencing of the human genome in 2003 and the use of new techniques that permit whole-genome analyses for gene expression and alterations. The impact of these discoveries is in full bloom for glioblastoma multiforme with The Cancer Genome Atlas (TCGA), an unprecedented, NIH-sponsored, effort to identify every possible genetic and epigenetic alteration and gene expression change in 500 glioblastoma specimens. The initial results of the TCGA Research Network as well as an independent effort to sequence all genes in 22 glioblastoma have just been published. These important studies have shown that, not surprisingly, this disease is complex, with up to 60 mutated genes per tumor. Fortunately, these genes can be distilled to a lesser number of pathways that make their study more palatable. Studying 60 genes, and even fewer pathways, is certainly easier than 30,000! We know that with enough effort and research teams focusing on all these new therapeutic targets, we will be able to fully comprehend the biological complexity of the disease and further accelerate the discovery of life-saving medicines. Novel targeted therapeutics and biomarker-based imaging will benefit in the near future from the emergence of nanotechnology.

Independently, the last decade has brought major discoveries on cell lineages in the central nervous system and the differentiation events that take place from stem cells to neurons, astrocytes, and oligodendrocytes. The application of markers identified in normal CNS development to the understanding of tumor heterogeneity gave birth to the "cancer stem cell hypothesis", a concept that has promoted a rethinking of the basic tenets in oncology and has blended the study of cancer and neuroscience. The speed of discovery summarized above is remarkable and gives no hint of slowing down. Many of these exciting developments are described within this book.

Today the prognosis of malignant brain tumors, such as glioblastoma, is still dismal, but what has changed is that there is real hope for a cure. The research efforts touched upon above and described in much more eloquent fashion by the authors in this book are bearing fruit. New biomarkers and therapeutic targets are being identified. We are seeing successful therapies emerge from the use of antibodies and cytotoxins, signaling pathway-targeted small molecules, anti-angiogenesis strategies, better use of "old-fashioned" alkylating drugs following increased knowledge of DNA repair pathways, and vaccination approaches targeting unique tumor epitopes uncovered by genetic approaches. Further development of novel therapies is advancing at rapid pace and there is an increased need for animal models to evaluate them. A full third of the book is devoted to present a comprehensive selection of the models currently available.

The light at the end of the tunnel is becoming visible. It is encouraging to witness, and exciting to participate in, the dramatic improvements in brain tumor treatment that are being made.

Atlanta, GA
March, 2009

Erwin G. Van Meir

Editor

Erwin G. Van Meir is Professor of Neurosurgery and Hematology & Medical Oncology in the School of Medicine at Emory University. A native of Belgium, he obtained Bachelor's degrees in Biology and Education at the University of Fribourg, Switzerland. He pursued graduate studies in Molecular Virology at the University of Lausanne, Switzerland where he obtained his PhD in 1989. He then became interested in cancer Research and completed postdoctoral work at the University Hospital in Lausanne and at the Ludwig Institute for Cancer Research in San Diego. In 1994 he was granted his first Faculty position as Director of the Laboratory of Brain Tumor Biology and Genetics in the Neurosurgery Department at the University of Lausanne. In 1998 he joined Emory University in Atlanta, where he now serves as the Leader of the Winship Cancer Institute Molecular Pathways and Biomarkers scientific program and is co-Director of the Brain Tumor Research Group.

For the past 20 years Dr. Van Meir's research has focused on defining the biological significance of specific genetic alterations for brain tumor development. He is particularly interested in how tumors divert extracellular signals regulating heterotypic cell communication for their own benefit such as occurs in tumor angiogenesis, and in translating this new knowledge into novel therapeutic approaches. His research is described in more than 140 peer-reviewed research papers and review articles in internationally recognized journals that have cumulated over 5,000 citations and received several awards. These contributions were presented in over 100 invited seminars worldwide and have furthered the understanding of cytokine expression for glioma biology, Turcot syndrome, the role of p53, HIF, IL-8, thrombospondin-1 and brain angiogenesis inhibitor-1 in brain tumor angiogenesis, hypoxia, and pseudopalisading necrosis formation. He also discovered biomarkers in the cerebrospinal fluid of brain tumor patients and developed novel therapeutic agents including oncolytic hypoxia-activated adenoviruses, pro-apoptotic galectin-3, anti-angiogenic vasculostatins, and small molecule HIF inhibitors that are covered by several US and foreign patents. Perhaps most importantly, over his 20-year independent career, Dr. Van Meir has mentored and trained over 60 postdoctoral fellows, students, and visiting scientists, many of which now hold independent leading positions in Academia or Industry.

Dr. Van Meir is an active member of the international neuro-oncology community and served on the Board of Directors of the Society for Neuro-Oncology from 2004 to 2008. He organized several international conferences on brain tumors, has served on the Scientific Committee of the European Association for Neuro-Oncology, the Scientific Advisory Board of the Southeastern Brain Tumor Foundation, and is a current or former member of several other international cancer societies including the American Association for Cancer Research, the European Association for Cancer Research, and the American Society for Investigative Pathology.

Dr. Van Meir currently serves on the Editorial Board of *Neuro-Oncology, Frontiers in Bioscience*, and *International Journal of Oncology,* and is a former Associate Editor of the *International Journal of Cancer*. He has served as a reviewer for over 30 international scientific journals and for grant proposals from public and private agencies including the US National Institutes of Health, the US Department of Defense, the European Commission, the Swiss National Science Foundation, the Swiss Cancer Society, the Wellcome Trust of the UK, Cancer Research UK, the Research Grants Council of Hong Kong, the Israel Science Foundation, the Belgian Fournier-Majoie, and King Baudouin Foundations, and the Italian Association for Cancer Research.

He acknowledges present and past support by multiple funding agencies for his scientific work, including the US National Institutes of Health, the Swiss National Science Foundation, the Goldhirsh Foundation, the Charlotte Geyer Foundation, the Southeastern and National Brain Tumor Foundations, The Brain Tumor Society, the Pediatric Brain Tumor Foundation of the US, the American Brain Tumor Association, the Brain Tumor Foundation for Children, the Al Musella, Wayne O Rollins and Frances Wood Wilson Foundations, the Brain Tumor Trust, the Emory University Research Council and EmTechBio, the Swiss Cancer League and Anti-Cancer Foundations, the San Salvatore, Tossizza, Ott and Chuard-Smith Foundations, and the European Institute of Oncology.

Contents

Contributors

Roger Abounader Department of Neurology and Microbiology, University of Virginia, Charlottesville, VA 22908, USA, ra6u@virginia.edu

Sameer Agnihotri Hospital for Sick Children, University of Toronto, Toronto, ON, Canada

Ken Aldape Department of Pathology and Radiation Oncology, The University of Texas M.D. Anderson Cancer Center, Houston, TX, USA, kaldape@mdanderson.org

Wadih Arap David H. Koch Center, The University of Texas M.D. Anderson Cancer Center, Houston, TX 77030, USA, warap@mdanderson.org

Marcela Assanah Department of Neurological Surgery, Columbia University Medical Center and the Columbia Brain Tumor Center, New York, NY 10032, USA

Jennifer M. Atkinson Department of Developmental Neurobiology, St Jude Children's Research Hospital, Memphis, TN 38105, USA

Joanne E. Ayriss Department of Pathology, Duke University Medical Center, 181A Medical Sciences Research Building, Durham, NC 27710, USA, joanne.ayriss@duke.edu

Rolf F. Barth Department of Pathology, The Ohio State University, 165 Hamilton Hall, Columbus, OH 43210, USA, rolf.barth@osumc.edu

Tracy T. Batchelor Division of Hematology and Oncology, Department of Neurology and Radiation Oncology, Massachusetts General Hospital Cancer Center and Harvard Medical School, Boston, MA, USA, tbatchelor@partners.org

Anita C. Bellail Department of Pathology & Laboratory Medicine, Winship Cancer Institute, Emory University School of Medicine, Atlanta, GA 30322, USA, abellai@emory.edu

Etty N. Benveniste Department of Cell Biology, University of Alabama, Birmingham, AL 35294-0004, USA, tika@uab.edu

Gabriele Bergers Department of Neurological Surgery, Brain Tumor Research Center and UCSF Helen Diller Family Comprehensive Cancer Center, University of California San Francisco, San Francisco, CA 94143-0520, USA, gabriele.bergers@ucsf.edu

Rameen Beroukhim Broad Institute, Massachusetts Institute of Technology and Harvard University, Cambridge, MA 02142; Department of Medicine, Harvard Medical School and Division of Medical Oncology, Dana–Farber Cancer Institute, Boston, MA 02115, rameen@broad.mit.edu

Darell D. Bigner Department of Pathology, 177 Medical Sciences Research Building, Duke University Medical Center, Box 3156, Durham, North Carolina 27710, bigne001@mc.duke.edu

Oliver Bogler Department of Neurosurgery and Department of Neuro-Oncology, Brain Tumor Center, University of Texas M.D. Anderson Cancer Center, Houston, TX 77030, USA, obogler@mdanderson.org

Jean-Louis Boulay Laboratory of Neuro-Oncology, Department of Biomedicine and Neurosurgery, University Hospital, CH-4031 Basel, Switzerland, jean-louis.boulay@unibas.ch

Susan T. Boulton Duke University Medical Center, Box 3624, The Preston Robert Tisch Brain Tumor Center, Department of Surgery/Neuro-oncology, Room 047 Baker House, Trent Drive Durham, North Carolina 27710, boult001@mc.duke.edu

Daniel J. Brat Department of Pathology and Laboratory Medicine, Winship Cancer Institute, Emory University School of Medicine, Atlanta, GA, USA, dbrat@emory.edu

Jeffrey N. Bruce Department of Neurological Surgery, Columbia University Medical Center and the Columbia Brain Tumor Center, New York, NY 10032, USA

Elizabeth Bullitt Division of Neurosurgery, Lineberger Comprehensive Cancer Center, University of North Carolina, Chapel Hill, NC, USA

Peter Canoll Department of Pathology and Cell Biology, Columbia University Medical Center, New York, NY, USA, pc561@columbia.edu

Clark C. Chen Division of Neurosurgery, Beth Israel Deaconess Medical Center, Harvard Medical School, Boston, MA, USA; Department of Radiation Oncology, Dana Farber Cancer Institute, Boston, MA, USA, cchen1@partners.org

Thomas C. Chen Department of Neurosurgery, University of Southern California Keck School of Medicine, Los Angeles, CA, USA, tchen68670@aol.com

Shi-Yuan Cheng Cancer Institute and Department of Pathology, University of Pittsburgh, Pittsburgh, PA 15213, USA, chengs@upmc.edu

Charles S. Cobbs Department of Neuroscience, California Pacific Medical Center Research Institute, San Francisco, CA 94107, USA; Department of Neurological Surgery, University of California, San Francisco, CA 94143, USA, Charles.Cobbs@gmail.com

Joseph F. Costello Brain Tumor Research Center, Department of Neurosurgery, University of California San Francisco, San Francisco, CA 94143, USA, jcostello@cc.ucsf.edu

Alan D'Andrea Department of Radiation Oncology, Dana Farber Cancer Institute, Boston, MA, USA, alan_dandrea@dfci.harvard.edu

Waldemar Debinski Brain Tumor Center of Excellence, Wake Forest University School of Medicine, Winston-Salem, NC 27157, USA, debinski@wfubmc.edu

Pierre-Yves Dietrich Centre of Oncology, Geneva University Hospitals and University of Geneva, rue Micheli-du-Crest 24, 1211 Geneva 14, Switzerland, Pierre-Yves.Dietrich@hcuge.ch

Terry Van Dyke Department of Genetics, Lineberger Comprehensive Cancer Center, University of North Carolina, Chapel Hill, NC, USA; Mouse Cancer Genetics Program, Centers for Cancer Research and Advanced Preclinical Research, National Cancer Institute, Frederick, MD, USA, vandyket@mail.nih.gov

Burt G. Feuerstein Barrow Neurological Institute, St. Joseph's Hospital and Medical Center, Phoenix, AZ, USA, burt.feuerstein@chw.edu

Gregory N. Fuller Department of Pathology, University of Texas M.D. Anderson Cancer Center, Houston, TX, USA, gfuller@mdanderson.org

Frank B. Furnari Ludwig Institute for Cancer Research, Department of Medicine, Cancer Center, University of California-San Diego, La Jolla, CA 92093-0660, USA, ffurnari@ucsd.edu

Elizabeth R. Gerstner Division of Hematology and Oncology, Department of Neurology, Massachusetts General Hospital Cancer Center and Harvard Medical School, Boston, MA, USA

Gaddy Getz Broad Institute, Massachusetts Institute of Technology and Harvard University, 7 Cambridge Center, Cambridge, MA 02142, USA

Richard J. Gilbertson Department of Developmental Neurobiology, and Oncology, St Jude Children's Research Hospital, Memphis, TN 38105, USA, Richard.Gilbertson@stjude.org

Marisol Guerrero Department of Pathology, The University of Texas M.D. Anderson Cancer Center, Houston, TX, USA

Abhijit Guha Hospital for Sick Children, University of Toronto, Toronto, ON, Canada, Abhijit.Guha@uhn.on.ca

Anupama Gururaj Department of Neurosurgery, Brain Tumor Center, University of Texas M.D. Anderson Cancer Center, Houston, TX 77030, USA

David H. Gutmann Department of Neurology, Washington University School of Medicine, St. Louis, MO 63110, gutmannd@wustl.edu

Costas G. Hadjipanayis Department of Neurological Surgery, Winship Cancer Institute, Emory University School of Medicine, Atlanta, GA 30322, USA, chadjip@emory.edu

Chunhai Hao Department of Pathology & Laboratory Medicine, Winship Cancer Institute, Emory University School of Medicine, Atlanta, GA 30322, USA, chao@emory.edu

Saikh Jaharul Haque Department of Cancer Biology, Lerner Research Institute; Brain Tumor and Neuro-Oncology Center, Division of Neurosciences, Cleveland Clinic, Cleveland, OH 44195, USA, haquej@ccf.org

Eric C. Holland Department of Neurosurgery, Neurology, Surgery and Cancer Biology and Genetics, Memorial Sloan Kettering Cancer Center, New York, NY 10021, USA, hollande@mskcc.org

Tod D. Holland Department of Neurosurgery, Neurology, Surgery and Cancer Biology and Genetics, Memorial Sloan Kettering Cancer Center, New York, NY 10021, USA

Bo Hu Cancer Institute and Department of Medicine, University of Pittsburgh, Pittsburgh, PA 15213, USA

Paul H. Huang Department of Biological Engineering, Massachusetts Institute of Technology, Cambridge, MA 02139, USA, phuang@mit.edu

YeoHyeon Hwang Department of Neurosurgery, Brain Tumor Center, University of Texas M.D. Anderson Cancer Center, Houston, TX 77030, USA

C. David James Department of Neurological Surgery and Brain Tumor Research Center, University of California, San Francisco, CA 94143, USA, david.james@ucsf.edu

Rongcai Jiang Department of Neurosurgery, Tianjin Medical University General Hospital, Tianjin 300052, China, jianghope@gmail.com

Kristopher T. Kahle Department of Neurosurgery, Massachusetts General Hospital, Boston, MA, USA

Natalie O. Karpinich Department of Genetics, Lineberger Comprehensive Cancer Center, University of North Carolina, Chapel Hill, NC, USA

Balveen Kaur Dardinger Laboratory of Neurosciences, Department of Neurological surgery, The Ohio State University, Columbus, OH 43210, USA, balveen.kaur@osumc.edu

Fatima W. Khwaja Laboratory of Molecular Neuro-Oncology, Department of Neurosurgery, Hematology and Medical Oncology, and Winship Cancer Institute, Emory University School of Medicine, Atlanta, GA 30322, USA; Basic Science Lab, Shaukat Khanum Memorial Cancer Hospital & Research Center, Lahore, Pakistan, fkhwaja@emory.edu

Andrea Kindler-Röhrborn Institute of Pathology and Neuropathology, University Hospital of Essen, University of Duisburg-Essen, Hufelandstr. 55, 45122 Essen, Germany, andrea.kindler@uk-essen.de

Bernd U. Koelsch Institute of Pathology and Neuropathology, University Hospital of Essen, University of Duisburg-Essen, Hufelandstr. 55, 45122 Essen, Germany, bernd.koelsch@uk-essen.de

Serguei Kozlov Mouse Cancer Genetics Program, Centers for Cancer Research and Advanced Preclinical Research, National Cancer Institute, Frederick, MD, USA, kozlovse@mail.nih.gov

Chien-Tsun Kuan Department of Pathology, 181C Medical Sciences Research Building, Duke University Medical Center, Box 3156, Durham, North Carolina 27710, kuan@duke.edu

Chang-Hyuk Kwon Department of Neurological Surgery, Tumor Microenvironment Program and Dardinger Center for Neuro-oncology and Neurosciences, James Comprehensive Cancer Center, The Ohio State University Medical Center, Columbus, OH 43210, USA, Chang-Hyuk.Kwon@osumc.edu

John Laterra Kennedy Krieger Research Institute and Johns Hopkins University School of Medicine, Baltimore, MD 21205, USA, laterra@kennedykrieger.org

Khatri Latha Department of Neurosurgery, Brain Tumor Center, University of Texas M.D. Anderson Cancer Center, Houston, TX 77030, USA

Travis Laver Department of Cell Biology, University of Alabama, Birmingham, AL 35294-0005, USA

Sean E. Lawler Dardinger Laboratory for NeuroOncology and Neurosciences, Department of Neurological Surgery, The Ohio State University Medical Center and James Comprehensive Cancer Center, Columbus, OH 43210, USA, sean.lawler@osumc.edu

Jian Yi Li Department of Pathology, Harvey Cushing Brain Tumor Institute, Feinstein Institute for Medical Research, North Shore-LIJ Health System, North Shore University Hospital, Manhasset, NY, USA, jli2@nshs.edu

Linda M. Liau UCLA Department of Neurosurgery, David Geffen School of Medicine at UCLA, 10833 Le Conte Avenue, CHS 74-145, Los Angeles, CA 90095-6901, USA, LLIAU@mednet.ucla.edu

Kim A. Lopez Department of Neurological Surgery, Columbia University Medical Center and the Columbia Brain Tumor Center, New York, NY 10032, USA

Ingo K. Mellinghoff Human Oncology and Pathogenesis Program and Department of Neurology, Memorial Sloan-Kettering Cancer Center, New York, NY 10065, USA, mellingi@mskcc.org

Adrian Merlo Laboratory of Neuro-Oncology, Departments of Biomedicine and Neurosurgery, University Hospital, CH-4031 Basel, Switzerland, adrian.merlo@gmx.ch

C. Ryan Miller Department of Pathology & Laboratory Medicine and Lineberger Comprehensive Cancer Center, University of North Carolina, Chapel Hill, NC, rmiller@med.unc.edu

Anjan Misra Barrow Neurological Institute, St. Joseph's Hospital and Medical Center, Phoenix, AZ, USA, anjan.misra@chw.edu

Patrick Mulligan Department of Pathology & Laboratory Medicine, Winship Cancer Institute, Emory University School of Medicine, Atlanta, GA 30322, USA, pmullig@learnlink.emory.edu

Diana Munoz Hospital for Sick Children, University of Toronto, Toronto, ON, Canada

Raman P. Nagarajan Brain Tumor Research Center, Department of Neurosurgery, University of California San Francisco, San Francisco, CA 94143, USA

Elizabeth W. Newcomb Department of Pathology, New York University Cancer Institute, New York University School of Medicine, New York, NY 10016, USA, newcoe01@med.nyu.edu

Kimberly Ng Department of Radiation Oncology, Dana Farber Cancer Institute, Boston, MA, USA

Masayuki Nitta Department of Radiation Oncology, Dana Farber Cancer Institute, Boston, MA, USA

Susan Nozell Department of Cell Biology, University of Alabama, Birmingham, AL 35294-0004, USA, snozell@uab.edu

Michael G. Ozawa David H. Koch Center, The University of Texas M.D. Anderson Cancer Center, Houston, TX 77030, USA

Tomoko Ozawa Department of Neurological Surgery and Brain Tumor Research Center, University of California, San Francisco, CA 94143, USA, tomoko.ozawa@ucsf.edu

Renata Pasqualini David H. Koch Center, The University of Texas M.D. Anderson Cancer Center, Houston, TX 77030, USA, rpasqual@mdanderson.org

Russell O. Pieper Brain Tumor Research Center, Department of Neurological Surgery, and The UCSF Cancer Center, University of California – San Francisco, San Francisco, CA 94115-0875, USA, rpieper@cc.ucsf.edu

Simon R. Platt Department of Small Animal Medicine & Surgery, College of Veterinary Medicine, University of Georgia, Athens, GA 30602, USA, srplatt@uga.edu

Dawn E. Post Departments of Neurosurgery and Microbiology & Immunology, State University of New York Upstate Medical University, Syracuse, NY, USA, postd@upstate.edu

Robert M. Prins UCLA Department of Neurosurgery, David Geffen School of Medicine at UCLA, 10833 Le Conte Avenue, CHS 74-145, Los Angeles, CA 90095, USA, RPrins@mednet.ucla.edu

James Provenzale Department of Radiology, Biomedical Engineering and Oncology, Emory University School of Medicine, Atlanta, GA 30322, USA; Department of Radiology, Duke University Medical Center, Durham, NC 27710, USA, jmprove@emory.edu

Benjamin Purow Neuro-Oncology Division, Neurology Department, University of Virginia, Charlottesville, VA 22908, USA, bwp5g@virginia.edu

Peter Pyrko Department of Neurosurgery, University of Southern California Keck School of Medicine, Los Angeles, CA, USA, ppyrko@yahoo.com

David A. Reardon Duke University Medical Center, Box 3624, The Preston Robert Tisch Brain Tumor Center, Department of Surgery, Department of Pediatrics, Room 047, Baker House, Trent Drive, Durham, North Carolina 27710, reard003@mc.duke.edu

Karlyne M. Reilly Mouse Cancer Genetics Program, National Cancer Institute, Frederick, MD 21702, USA, kreilly@ncifcrf.gov

Jeremy N. Rich Department of Stem Cell Biology and Regenerative Medicine, Cleveland Clinic, Cleveland, OH 44195, USA, richj@ccf.org

Marta Rojas Department of Neurosurgery, Brain Tumor Center, University of Texas M.D. Anderson Cancer Center, Houston, TX 77030, USA

Yuan Rong Department of Pathology and Laboratory Medicine, Winship Cancer Institute, Emory University School of Medicine, Atlanta, GA, USA, yrong@emory.edu

Axel H. Schönthal Department of Molecular Microbiology and Immunology, University of Southern California Keck School of Medicine, Los Angeles, California, USA

Pankaj Sharma Department of Cancer Biology, Lerner Research Institute, Cleveland Clinic, Cleveland OH 44195, USA, sharmap@ccf.org

Hyunsuk Shim Department of Radiology, Winship Cancer Institute, Emory University School of Medicine, Atlanta, GA 30322, USA, hshim@emory.edu

Richard L. Sidman Harvard Medical School and Department of Neurology, Beth Israel Deaconess Medical Center, Center for Life Science, Boston, MA 02215, USA

Liliana Soroceanu Department of Neuroscience, California Pacific Medical Center Research Institute, San Francisco, CA 94107, USA, Liliana_Soroceanu@yahoo.com

Fernanda I. Staquicini David H. Koch Center, The University of Texas M.D. Anderson Cancer Center, Houston, TX 77030, USA

David Stokoe Department of Molecular Biology, Genentech Inc., 1 DNA Way, South San Francisco, CA 94080, USA, stokoe.david@gene.com

Erik P. Sulman Department of Radiation Oncology, The University of Texas M.D. Anderson Cancer Center, Houston, TX, USA

Erwin G. Van Meir Department of Neurosurgery, Hematology and Medical Oncology, and Winship Cancer Institute, Emory University School of Medicine, Atlanta, GA, USA, evanmei@emory.edu

Mariano S. Viapiano Department of Neurological Surgery, Center for Molecular Neurobiology, The Ohio State University Medical Center and James Comprehensive Cancer Center, Columbus, OH 43210, USA, viapiano.1@osu.edu

Paul R. Walker Centre of Oncology, Geneva University Hospitals and University of Geneva, rue Micheli-du-Crest 24, 1211 Geneva 14, Switzerland, Paul.Walker@hcuge.ch

Forest M. White Department of Biological Engineering, Massachusetts Institute of Technology, Cambridge, MA 02139, USA, fwhite@mit.edu

Matthew J. Wortham Department of Pathology, Duke University Medical Center, 189 Medical Sciences Research Building, Durham, NC 27710, USA, matthew.wortham@duke.edu

Jill Wykosky Brain Tumor Center of Excellence, Wake Forest University School of Medicine, Winston-Salem, NC 27157, USA

Hai Yan Department of Pathology, Duke University Medical Center, 199B Medical Sciences Research Building, Durham, NC 27710, USA, hai.yan@duke.edu

Shaoman Yin Department of Neurosurgery, Emory University School of Medicine, Atlanta, GA, USA, syin4@emory.edu

David Zagzag Department of Pathology and Division of Neuropathology and Department of Neurosurgery, New York University Cancer Institute, New York University School of Medicine, New York, NY 10016, USA, dz4@nyu.edu

Qian Zhang Mouse Cancer Genetics Program, Centers for Cancer Research and Advanced Preclinical Research, National Cancer Institute, Frederick, MD, USA

Wei Zhang Department of Pathology, University of Texas M.D. Anderson Cancer Center, Houston, TX, USA, wzhang@mdanderson.org

Color Plates

Color Plate 1 GFP+ and GFP– tumor cells express markers of proliferative glial progenitor cells. Double-immunofluorescence analysis of tumors at 17 dpi with the PDGF-IRES-GFP retrovirus shows that GFP (*green*) is expressed in only a subset of tumor cells. However, nestin (A′, A″), NG2 (B′, B″), PDGFR-α (C′, C″), and olig2 (D′, D″), each stained red, are expressed in the vast majority of GFP+ and GFP– tumor cells. Ki67 proliferation marker is expressed in a significant number of both GFP+ and GFP– cells (E′, E″). GFAP+/GFP– reactive astrocytes (*red*) are seen scattered throughout the tumor (F′, F″). Rare GFAP+/GFP+ cells were seen (<3%) (Chapter 1, Fig. 2; *see* discussion on p.12).

Color Plate 2 GFP expression reveals the distribution of retrovirally infected cells (Chapter 1, Fig. 3; *see* complete caption on p. 15 and discussion on p. 16).

Color Plate 3 **A.** Adult rat glial progenitors infected in vitro with a pNIT-GFP retrovirus (*green*) do not proliferate, migrate, or form tumors when reinjected into subcortical white matter (diagram inset) (Chapter 1, Fig. 4; *see* complete caption and discussion on p. 18).

Color Plate 4 Retroviral virion (**A**) binds to the target cell via interaction of envelope protein with its receptor (**B**). The nucleocapsid enters the cytoplasm and RNA genome (**F**) is converted to double-stranded DNA (**C**), which is integrated into the genome as a provirus (**G**) and transcribed (**D, H**). The proviral transcripts are translated into viral proteins and full-length transcripts serve as the viral genome of the next generation of virus (**E**) (Chapter 2, Fig. 1; *see* discussion on p. 32).

Color Plate 5 RCAS/tv-a-based somatic cell gene transfer. RCAS vectors are engineered to encode a gene downstream of the *env* gene and will only infect mammalian cells if they express the RCAS receptor TVA (**A**) (Chapter 2, Fig. 2; *see* complete caption on p. 35 and discussion on p. 34).

Color Plate 6 Glioma formation with the RCAS/tv-a system. (**A**) Survival curves for mice of different genetic backgrounds infected with RCAS-PDGF demonstrating cooperativity between gain of function oncogenes and loss of tumor suppressors (Chapter 2, Fig. 3; *see* complete caption on p. 37 and discussion on p. 36).

Color Plate 7 RCAS/tv-a-mediated medulloblastoma and bioluminescence imaging. (**A**) MRI scan of human medulloblastoma. (**B**) MRI scan of RCAS–SHH-induced medulloblastoma (courtesy of Jason Koutcher MSKCC) with (**C**) H&E-stained whole mount. (**D**) Normal adult cerebellum. (**E**) Cluster of cells trapped in the region of the external granule cell layer by SHH autocrine signaling showing proliferation by Ki67 staining (**F**). Medulloblastoma bearing mouse in a gli-luciferase reporter background (**G**). Brain removed from mouse showing light production arising from the medulloblastoma (**H**) shown on whole mount (**I**) (Chapter 2, Fig. 4; *see* discussion on p. 39).

Color Plate 8 Histologic features of human pilocytic astrocytomas. (**A**) Biphasic pattern of regions with more compact cellularity alternating with regions with more loosely structured architecture (Chapter 3, Fig. 1; *see* complete caption and discussion on p. 46).

Color Plate 9 *Nf1*+/−^{GFAP}CKO mice develop optic gliomas similar to those observed in children with neurofibromatosis-1 (Chapter 3, Fig. 3; *see* complete caption and discussion on p. 51).

Color Plate 10 General principle of classical ES transgenesis. DNA Vector carrying gene of interest is transfected into cultured mouse ES cells. In our case we used a retrovirus carrying the ^{V12}Ha-Ras gene under the control of the astrocyte-specific human GFAP promoter and a neomycin selection marker expression cassette. Selection of ES cells with the transgene of interest is first accomplished by selecting for neomycin-resistant clones. Thereafter NeoR ES clones are tested for their ability to express the transgene by in vitro differentiation to astrocytes. This process confirms activation of the GFAP promoter expression and specificity. Positive ES cells undergo aggregations and are transferred to a pseudo-pregnant female mouse to create chimeric embryos (striped mouse in picture). The chimeric mice are bred to normal mice and those mice having incorporated the transgene in their germ-line will generate transgenic offspring (Chapter 4, Fig. 1; *see* discussion on p. 63).

Color Plate 11 RasB8-pathologocal/molecular progression. **A.** *RasB8 GEM-Pathological progression.* The hGFAP-regulated transgene is expressed as early as E13.5 where the mice are similar to normal littermates. For the first few weeks there are no astrocytomas, but diffuse astroglial hyperplasia. At 3–4 weeks LGA appear with p53 mutations, as demonstrated by microdissection. At 12 weeks and beyond one sees HGA with infiltrative and necrotic tumors. **B.** *RasB8-Molecular progression.* Astrocytes isolated at 1 week are not transformed, in contrast, astrocytoma cells from the HGA after 12 weeks show genetic alterations which are known to be associated with human GBMs: loss of p16, p19, PTEN, and overexpression of EGFR (Chapter 4, Fig. 3; *see* discussion on p. 66).

Color Plate 12 Inducible GEM astrocytomas. T mice developed diffuse astrocytomas, WHO grade II (**A**). Tumors were immunoreactive for GFAP (**B**). TR mice developed anaplastic astrocytomas, WHO grade III (**C**), characterized by numerous mitoses (*arrowheads*). $TRP^{+/-}$ (not shown) and $TRP^{-/-}$ mice (D) developed glioblastomas, WHO grade IV, characterized by numerous mitoses (*arrowhead*) and areas of pseudopalisading necrosis (*arrow*) (Chapter 7, Fig. 5; *see* discussion on p. 129).

Color Plate 13 Generation and characterization of cell lines derived from conditional GEM models of astrocytomas (Chapter 7, Fig. 10; *see* complete caption on p. 139 and discussion on p. 137).

Color Plate 14 Comparing the intracranial invasiveness of GBM cell lines propagated as monolayer cultures in serum-supplemented media (*upper panels*) vs. propagation as neurospheres in EGF + FGF supplemented media (*lower panels*). Upper panels show a well-circumscribed intracranial tumor established from U-87 MG monolayer culture (image shown to the right is an enlargement of the area indicated by the black rectangle in *left panel*). Note the well-delineated plane of separation between U-87 MG tumor and surrounding normal brain (*upper right panel*). In contrast, intracranial tumors established from GS2 cells propagated as a neurosphere culture (*bottom panels*) show diffuse infiltration, as highlighted by the enlargement image shown in the lower right section of the figure (Chapter 8, Fig. 1; *see* discussion on p. 151).

Color Plate 15 Approaches to establishing orthotopic brain tumor xenografts. Following the midline incision and separation of the skin covering the skull (panel **A**: *pen mark* shows location for injection of cells, approximately 2.5–3 mm right from the bregma and just behind the coronal suture), tumor cells can either be injected "freehand" (panel **B**), or by use of a small animal stereotactic frame (panel **C**), which provides increased stability and control of injection depth. The opening in the skull for injection can be created either with a small drill or by simply pricking the skull with a 25 gauge needle. For the freehand method, injection depth is limited by a pipette tip (shown) or rubber sleeve covering all but the exposed end of the needle. Once the hole has been created, tumor cells are injected 3 mm below the outer table of the skull for routine supratentorial tumor establishment. Following injection, the separated skin is closed by use of clip (panel **D**) that eventually dislodges as the skin closes (heals). Especially when injecting large series of mice (>50), we recommend the freehand method as it increases throughput 3–4× relative to use of the stereotactic frame. For example, as many as 50 mice can be injected in an hour when two investigators are working in tandem (i.e., one investigator exposing the skull and the other performing the injection), whereas 12–16 mice per hour is an achievable rate when using a stereotactic frame (Chapter 8, Fig. 3; *see* discussion on p. 153).

Color Plate 16 Histopathologic features of the C6, 9L, RG2, F98, CNS-1, and BT4C brain tumors. **A** (Chapter 10, Fig. 1; *see* complete caption on p. 187 and discussion on p. 186).

Color Plate 17 Histopathology: Comparison between high-grade human gliomas and the murine GL261 glioma (Chapter 12, Fig. 2; *see* complete caption on p. 233 and discussion on p. 231).

Color Plate 18 Homozygous and heterozygous losses and amplifications are better defined by aCGH than by conventional CGH (Chapter 17, Fig. 3; *see* complete caption on p. 382 and discussion on p. 379).

Color Plate 19 Identification of genetic subgroups in GBM. (**A**) The classification tree shows three sub groups (Chapter 17, Fig. 5; *see* complete caption on p. 383 and discussion on p. 379).

Color Plate 20 Map showing frequency of copy number aberrations in grade 4 (**A**) and grade 3 (**B**) astrocytoma. The ordinate marks the frequency of gain (positive) and loss (negative). The abscissa shows the genome in 1p to Yq direction (Chapter 17, Fig. 6; *see* discussion on p. 379).

Color Plate 21 Markers of survival in GBM. In an age-matched comparison of GBM patients with poor (>2 yr) survival and better (<2 yr) survival, frequent 7 gain, 10 loss, and 19 gain were found in those with poor survival. Global gene expression profiles of the same tumors separated the poor and better survivors into almost identical groups (Nigro et al., 2005) (Chapter 17, Fig. 7; *see* discussion on p. 379).

Color Plate 22 After undergoing surgery followed by radiation and chemotherapy, young patients with GBM do better than older patients (Chapter 17, Fig. 8; *see* complete caption on p. 386 and discussion on p. 379)

Color Plate 23 Supervised analysis to identify genetic differences between grade 3 and grade 4 astrocytomas (Chapter 17, Fig. 9; *see* complete caption on p. 387 and discussion on p. 384).

Color Plate 24 Three major affected pathways (a, b, c) in grade 4 astrocytoma that showed DNA copy number changes, mutation, and amplification of their member genes. More pathways are expected to be added to this list. (TCGA, 2008) (Chapter 17, Fig. 11; *see* discussion on p. 389).

Color Plate 25 "Driver" and "passenger" mutations in the cancer genome (Chapter 18, Fig. 1; *see* discussion on p. 396).

Color Plate 26 Overview of the GISTIC. After identifying the locations and magnitudes of chromosomal aberrations in multiple tumors (*left*), GISTIC scores each genomic marker with a *G*-score that is proportional to the total magnitude of aberrations at each location. By permuting the locations in each tumor, GISTIC determines the frequency with which a given score would be attained if the events were due to chance and randomly distributed (*center*). A significance threshold (*green line*) is determined such that significant scores are unlikely to occur by chance alone and alterations are considered significant if they occur in regions that surpass this threshold (*right*) (Chapter 18, Fig. 3; *see* discussion on p. 398).

Color Plate 27 Application of GISTIC to glioma. (**A**) Amplifications (*red*) and deletions (*blue*), determined by segmentation analysis of normalized signal intensities from 100 K SNP arrays are displayed across the genome (chromosome positions indicated along the *y*-axis) for 141 gliomas (*x*-axis, diagnosis is displayed on top). (**B**) GISTIC analysis with statistical significance of the aberrations displayed as FDR *q*-values to account for multiple hypothesis testing. Centromere positions are indicated for each chromosome by a dotted line. The locations of the peak regions and the known cancer-related genes within those peaks are indicated to the right of each panel (Chapter 18, Fig. 4; *see* discussion on p. 402).

Color Plate 28 GISTIC identifies cancer-specific patterns of gene copy-number alterations. (Chapter 18, Fig. 5; *see* complete caption on p. 407 and discussion on p. 405).

Color Plate 29 Primary GBM cells endogenously expressed HCMV IE1. Primary glioma-derived cultures were processed for IE1 immunofluorescence using MAB810 (Chemicon) and Alexa 488-labeled secondary antibody. Nuclei were counterstained using DAPI. Panel **A** shows nuclear localization of endogenous IE1 in one GBM culture; panels **C** and **D** illustrate IE1 perinuclear staining in a different GBM primary culture (Chapter 19, Fig. 1; *see* complete caption and discussion on p. 424).

Color Plate 30 Co-localization of PDGFRα and IE1 in primary human GBM samples. GBM primary cultures and tissues were examined for the presence of IE1 and PDGFRα using double immunofluorescence. Panels **A and D** represent immunofluorescence detection of PDGFRα in primary cultures, panels **B** and **E** show IE1 detection in the same cells. Panels **C** and **F** show examples of cells double positive for HCMV IE1 and PDGFRα.(superimposed single-staining photographs). Control stained sections were negative for both antigens (**G, H, I**). **J, K, L**. HMCV treatment induces recruitment of the αvβ3 integrin to focal adhesions in a PDGFRα-dependent manner (Chapter 19, Fig. 3; *see* complete caption and discussion on p. 431).

Color Plate 31 Adult human normal NPCs can be grown as neurospheres and are permissive to HCMV infection (Chapter 19, Fig. 4; *see* complete caption on p. 432 and discussion on p. 431).

Color Plate 32 Pathologic features of glioblastoma (Chapter 22, Fig. 2; *see* complete caption on p. 510 and discussion on p. 509).

Color Plate 33 Potential mechanism of pseudopalisade formation (Chapter 22, Fig. 3; *see* complete caption on p. 511 and discussion on p. 510).

Color Plate 34 Fluorescence in situ hybridization (FISH) analysis of *EGFR* gene status and IHC analysis of EGFR and TF protein in human GBM and AA specimens (Chapter 22, Fig. 5; *see* complete caption on p. 519 and discussion on p. 517).

Color Plate 35 Gene expression profiling in brain tumors. Tumor-specific, such as tumor imaging and histopathology, as well as patient-specific information, such as age and sex, is used to provide prognostic information. Tissue obtained at diagnosis, either from biopsy or from surgical resection, is utilized to develop a complex profile of gene expression in the tumor. Labeled (typically fluorescently) target samples are made from total RNA that is enzymatically processed into complementary DNA (or RNA) and represent relative messenger RNA (mRNA) abundance within the tumor for all expressed genes. This is hybridized to filter-, glass slide-, or silicon chip-based arrays of cDNA or oligonucleotide probes and the signals are measured and normalized. Clustering provides a means to identify sets of genes with similar expression and group tumors based on these clusters (unsupervised), thus identifying unique molecular signatures or group genes based on known characteristics of the tumors (supervised). Gene signatures identified may have prognostic significance. Tumors that appear similar on imaging and histologic examination may be shown to exhibit differing molecular profiles and therefore different clinical outcomes using microarray technologies (Chapter 23, Fig. 1; *see* discussion on p. 530).

Color Plate 36 A mesenchymal molecular signature in GBM is prognostic for poor survival. (**A**) Identification of distinct molecular subtypes of malignant gliomas from gene expression profiling consisting of proneural, mesenchymal, and proliferative phenotypes (Phillips et al. 2006). Genes with high expression are shown in *red*, while those with low expression are shown in *green*. The proneural, mesenchymal, and proliferative subtypes demonstrate statistically significant associations with patient outcome in both grade III and IV glioma (**B**) and in an independent data set consisting only of grade IV GBM with necrosis (**C**). Adapted with permission from Elsevier Limited (Chapter 23, Fig. 2; *see* discussion on p. 539).

Color Plate 37 Summary of the protein separation and the MS-based protein identification (Chapter 24, Fig. 1; *see* complete caption on p. 563 and discussion on p. 561).

Color Plate 38 Detection of IGFBP2 expression in a glioma TMA. GBM, glioblastoma; AA, anaplastic astrocytoma; LGA, low grade astrocytoma; AO, anaplastic oligodendroglioma; O, oligodendroglioma; MOA, mixed oligoastrocytoma; AMOA, anaplastic mixed oligoastrocytoma; GS, gliosarcoma; NB, normal brain; CL, cell lines (Chapter 24, Fig. 2; *see* discussion on p. 563).

Color Plate 39 Protein arrays. Antibody array (forward-phase protein array) is formatted by printing the selective antibodies on a slide, while the reverse-phase protein array is printed with the cellular lysate extracted from tissue, cerebral spinal fluid, or cell lines (Chapter 24, Fig. 3; *see* complete caption and discussion on p. 565).

Color Plate 40 Glioma protein lysate array. Protein was isolated from frozen glioma tissues and adjusted to 20 mg/mL with lysis buffer tissue. The serially diluted protein lysates were printed on PVDF-coated glass slides in triplicate using a robotic spotter (G3, Genomics Solutions). Detection was conducted with a DakoCytomation-catalyzed signal amplification system kit. Individual glass slide can be hybridized with antibodies against β-actin, pThr308 AKT, pSer473 AKT, total AKT, or other proteins; β-actin served as a positive control. The hybridized slides were scanned at an optical resolution of 1200 dpi and saved as uncompressed TIFF files (Chapter 24, Fig. 4; *see* discussion on p. 567).

Color Plate 41 Magnetic resonance imaging enables to noninvasively visualize whole brain structures and CSF at high resolution and sharp contrast (Chapter 25, Fig. 1; *see* complete caption on p. 581 and discussion on p. 579).

Color Plate 42 Blood–brain barrier and blood–CSF barrier. **A.** Simplified structure of normal blood vessel not present in the brain. In normal blood vessels, the endothelial cells (shown in *pink*) are surrounded by mural cells such as pericytes and smooth muscle cells. **B.** Blood–brain barrier: In normal brain, the endothelial cells of the capillaries contain tight junctions creating a strong barrier that prevents diffusion of hydrophilic substances from CNS capillaries into the surrounding tissues and vice versa. However, necessary nutrients and metabolites such as glucose are transported with the aid of specific transport mechanisms. **C.** Blood–CSF barrier: In the choroid plexus, the blood–brain barrier is absent as the capillary endothelial cells here are fenestrated. This allows substances to pass freely from the bloodstream into the brain tissue and also in the opposite direction. However, here, tight junctions are present in the overlying ependyma (choroid plexus epithelium), thus creating a two-way barrier between brain tissue and ventricular CSF (Chapter 25, Fig. 2; *see* discussion on p. 582).

Color Plate 43 **A.** Schematic illustration of the flow of CSF in the brain and the different cellular structures that create the blood–CSF barrier. This representation is not intended to be entirely anatomically correct and does not show many ultrastructural details. Incoming arterial blood flow from the heart connects to the choroid plexus, a cauliflower-shaped organ where blood is "filtered" through a double cellular layer, endothelial cells lining the arterial capillary and the choroid plexus epithelial cells that are connected through tight junctions. This constitutes the first component of the blood–CSF barrier. Note that the endothelial cells in the choroid plexus are not connected by tight junctions (Chapter 25, Fig. 3; *see* complete caption on p. 587 and discussion on p. 585).

Color Plate 44 Potential biomarker panels differentiate between astrocytoma grades using CSF. **A.** Panel of 32 proteins that can be used to differentiate between AII–IV patients, nontumoral controls, and other forms of brain tumors. *Black* = no expression, *yellow* = low expression, *orange* = moderate expression, and *red* = high expression level as determined from ImageMaster analysis of 2-DE gels. C = Biomarker class; *white* = control specific, *light blue* = AII, *green* = AIII, and *pink* = AIV biomarker. **B.** Restricted panel containing top 13 proteins from panel **A**. *White* = control, *light blue* = AII, *green* = AIII, and *purple* = AIV biomarkers. Vertical axis represents relative level (0–4) of each protein as estimated from 2-DE (Reproduced from Khwaja et al. Journal of Proteome Research 2007.) (Chapter 25, Fig. 6; *see* discussion on p. 596).

Color Plate 45 Possible future applications of CSF biomarkers. Protein markers found in the CSF through a spinal tap could be used individually or in combination in a biomarker panel to diagnose CNS malignancies. A protein or an antibody array developed using identified biomarkers would allow for personalized medicine based on the unique limited protein profile. These markers could also allow for early detection of original, residual, or recurrent disease in a minimally invasive procedure compared to biopsy or surgery (Chapter 25, Fig. 7; *see* complete caption on p. 597 and discussion on p. 596).

Color Plate 46 Role of DNA methylation and histone modifications at promoter CpG islands in normal cells and cancer. In normal cells, most promoter CpG islands do not exhibit DNA methylation. Thus the expression status of CpG island-containing genes is primarily determined by the presence or absence of transcription factors and by histone modifications around the promoters of such genes. **(A)** In general, transcriptionally active CpG island loci exhibit unmethylated DNA and high levels of histone H3 lysine 9 acetylation, which are accompanied by an open chromatin configuration. **(B)** Transcriptionally silent genes, however, are marked by histone H3 lysine 27 trimethylation, a modification catalyzed by EZH2 (enhancer of zeste 2), a member of the Polycomb repressor complex 2 (PRC2). Following H3 lysine 27 trimethylation, these promoters can be bound by members of the Polycomb repressor complex 1 (PRC1), which blocks transcription initiation by RNA polymerase II. This is also a mechanism of abnormal gene silencing in cancer, in the absence of aberrant DNA methylation. **(C)** In cancer, a large number of CpG islands are hypermethylated at their DNA, which generally correlates with transcriptional repression of the associated genes. These CpG islands generally exhibit a closed chromatin configuration, marked by histone H3 lysine 9 methylation, loss of acetylation, nucleosome occupancy around the transcription start site and various types of methyl-binding domain proteins. Altogether, these modifications render the chromatin non-permissive for transcription initiation (Chapter 26, Fig. 1; *see* discussion on p. 619).

Color Plate 47 HIF1 recruits bone marrow-derived cells (BMDC) to orthotopic glioblastomas (GBM) (Chapter 31, Fig. 1; *see* complete caption on p. 754 and discussion on p. 752).

Color Plate 48 Congruence of region of contrast enhancement and region of highest relative cerebral blood volume (rCBV), suggesting that contrast-enhancing region is the most aggressive portion of tumor, in a 37-year-old man with biopsy-proved World Health Organization grade III astrocytoma. (**a**) Axial contrast-enhanced T1-weighted image shows inhomogeneously enhancing mass in the right frontal lobe. Contrast enhancement is confined to the central portion of the mass. (**b**) rCBV map in which regions of high rCBV are depicted in *red* and *yellow* shows that the region of highest rCBV corresponds to the contrast-enhancing region shown in **a**. (Reprinted, with permission, from Provenzale et al. 2006) (Chapter 33, Fig. 2; *see* discussion on p. 793).

Color Plate 49 Elevation of rCBV despite the absence of contrast enhancement (i.e., no evidence of elevated permeability) in a 44-year-old woman with World Health Organization grade III astrocytoma. (**a**) Axial T2-weighted MR image shows hyperintense region (*arrow*) consistent with a neoplasm in the left frontal lobe. (**b**) Axial contrast-enhanced T1-weighted MR image does not show any regions of contrast enhancement. On the basis of the T2-weighted image and the contrast-enhanced T1-weighted image, one might have assumed that the lesion is a low-grade neoplasm with no areas of elevated rCBV. (**c**) rCBV map in which *red* and *yellow* colors indicate areas of elevated rCBV shows a region of high rCBV area (*arrow*) corresponding to the region of hyperintense abnormality on the T2-weighted image. At biopsy, this region was shown to represent high-grade glioma (Reprinted, with permission, from Wong et al. 2000) (Chapter 33, Fig. 3; *see* discussion on p. 793).

Color Plate 50 Lack of correlation of all regions of elevated permeability with elevated rCBV in a 51-year-old man with biopsy-proven glioblastoma multiforme. (**a**) Axial contrast-enhanced T1-weighted image shows large enhancing mass in the left temporal lobe. (**b**) Color-coded relative permeability map obtained using dynamic contrast-enhanced imaging superimposed on the image shown in (**a**). The color-coded map shows pixels having one of the three different colors. Left hemisphere regions that have peak signal intensity values in the range of 3–5 standard deviations (SD) above mean signal intensity in the normal right hemisphere are depicted in *blue*. The pixels that are in the range of 5–7 SD above baseline are shown in *yellow* color and the *red* pixels are those in which the increased signal intensity is greater than 7 SD above baseline. Thus, a large area of the tumor has pixels in the highest range of permeability values. (**c**) Axial rCBV map derived from T2*-weighted dynamic susceptibility imaging sequence shows that regions of elevated rCBV (seen in *red* and *yellow* color) are essentially confined to medial and anterior aspects of the tumor. (**d**) Superimposition of rCBV map shown in **c** on permeability map shown in **b** depicts the fact that large portions of the contrast-enhancing regions showing marked permeability in (**a**) and (**b**) do not have elevated rCBV values (*arrows*). (Reprinted, with permission, from Provenzale et al. 2006b) (Chapter 33, Fig. 4; *see* discussion on p. 793).

Color Plate 51 A 62-year-old man with glioblastoma multiforme. Illustration of changes in contrast material leakage (a reflection of degree of blood–brain barrier disruption) after administration of an antiangiogenesis agent. This case is an example of the fact that decreases in permeability after angiogenesis therapy may be greater than changes in tumor size. (**a**) Axial contrast-enhanced T1-weighted image prior to therapy shows large contrast-enhancing left temporal lobe tumor. (**b**) Color-coded map derived from dynamic contrast-enhanced imaging sequence before therapy (performed during the same MR examination as in **a**) shows relative degrees of permeability in each pixel. Pixels having signal intensity that are 120–149% of normal tissue are shown in *blue*, those with signal intensity of 140–159% of normal tissue are shown in *green*, and those having signal intensity ≥160% of normal tissue are in *red*. The majority of pixels are in the >160% category, consistent with marked leakage of contrast material throughout the tumor and indicating widespread disruption of the blood–brain barrier. (**c**) Repeat imaging was performed 30 days after beginning therapy with antiangiogenesis therapy. Axial contrast-enhanced T1-weighted image shows mild decrease in size of contrast-enhancing mass. (**d**) Color-coded map derived from dynamic contrast-enhanced imaging data on imaging at 30 days after beginning therapy (during same MR examination as **c**) shows marked decrease in number of pixels associated with the highest degree of permeability (i.e., *green* and *red* pixels). Reprinted, with permission, from Provenzale (2007) (Chapter 33, Fig. 5; *see* discussion on p. 798).

Color Plate 52 Dark-field mRNA expression of CXCR4 (*upper left*) and CXCL12 (*upper right*) and bright-field (H&E) picture (*lower panels*) of adjacent brain sections from 7-day-old mouse brain by in situ hybridization (*sagittal view*). (Chapter 34, Fig. 3; *see* complete caption and discussion on p. 819).

Color Plate 53 Complex regulation of angiogenesis by CXCR4/CXCL12 via VEGF-dependent manner (Chapter 34, Fig. 4; *see* complete caption and discussion on p. 824).

Color Plate 54 Simplified scheme of EphA2, IL-13Rα2 and also fos-related antigen 1 (Fra-1) regulation of expression and role in GBM progression. Mitogenic/oncogenic/growth-promoting factors, such as EGF, LIF, OSM, FGF-2, and HGF, are all highly upregulated in GBM. They all activate c-Fos transiently, but they appear to stimulate Fra-1 stably and in a sustained manner (Debinski and Gibo 2005). EGFRvIII is a receptor that is constitutively activated in GBM. EphA2, Fra-1, and IL-13Rα2 belong to a selected group of factors that are its gene targets. EphA2, Fra-1, and IL-13Rα2 collectively contribute to tumor neovasculature, tumor cell migration and invasiveness, and thus tumor progression (Chapter 35, Fig. 2; *see* discussion on p. 851).

Color Plate 55 Eph receptors and ephrin ligands. Each color represents a functionally or structurally distinct domain or motif. EphrinA ligands exist as GPI-anchored or soluble proteins, while ephrinB ligands are transmembrane proteins with a cytoplasmic domain. Tyrosine phosphorylation sites within Eph receptor are denoted by "P." SAM, sterile alpha motif (Chapter 35, Fig. 3; *see* discussion on p. 854).

Color Plate 56 EphA2 staining in GBM cells. Glioblastoma cell lines (U-251 MG, DBTRG-MG, G48a) were grown on sterile glass slides and fixed in acetone for 2 min at –20°C, washed in PBS, and either used immediately or stored at –80°C. Slides were blocked for 1 h in 10% normal goat serum (NGS) at RT. Primary EphA2 monoclonal antibody B208 (1:200; MedImmune) was diluted in 1.5× NGS and incubated overnight at 4°C. Slides were incubated with secondary antibody for 45 min at RT. The secondary antibody was a goat antimouse IgG Oregon Green (1:200) (Molecular Probes, Eugene, OR). Control slides without primary antibody were also used as negative controls for nonspecific binding of the secondary antibody. Confocal microscopy analysis of samples stained with monoclonal EphA2 antibody was performed using a Zeiss LSM 510

Laser Scanning Confocal Microscope with a 63× lens. Photomicrographs were taken with a 40× magnification objective lens in all cases with a Retiga EXi digital camera. Images were processed with Jasc Paint Shop Pro v6.0 (Chapter 35, Fig. 4; *see* discussion on p. 855).

Color Plate 57 HGF/c-Met deregulation and oncogenic effects (Chapter 39, Fig. 3; *see* discussion on p. 937).

Color Plate 58 Therapeutic targeting strategies of HGF/c-Met (Chapter 39, Fig. 4; *see* discussion on p. 943).

Color Plate 59 Oncogenic signaling networks in glioblastoma (Chapter 40, Fig. 1; *see* complete caption on p. 955 and discussion on p. 954).

Color Plate 60 Bench-to-bedside strategy for personalized therapeutic treatment of glioblastoma patients (Chapter 40, Fig. 4; *see* complete caption on p. 969 and discussion on p. 968).

Color Plate 61 HSV-1 productive infection. HSV-1 cell attachment and entry, gene expression, DNA replication, assembly, and release are shown (Chapter 46, Fig. 3; *see* discussion on p. 1108).

Color Plate 62 Diagram of DNA DSB production by IR and inhibition of NHEJ DNA repair pathway by ICP0 through degradation of DNA-PK_{CS}. IR, ionizing radiation; DSB, double-strand break; NHEJ, non-homologous end joining (Chapter 46, Fig. 4; *see* discussion on p. 1118).

Color Plate 63 Strategies used to target Ad replication specifically to tumor cells. (**A**) Targeting Ad replication to tumor cells by viral gene mutation. Specific mutations within the Ad *E1A*, *E1B*, or viral-associated RNA-coding sequences that abrogate protein function have been shown to result in the selective replication of the mutant Ad in tumor cells that contain dysfunctional pRb, p53, or Ras pathways, respectively (Chapter 47, Fig. 2; *see* complete caption on p. 1142 and discussion on p. 1140).

Part I
Animal Models for Central Nervous Tumors

Chapter 1
Modeling Gliomas Using PDGF-Expressing Retroviruses

Marcela Assanah, Kim A. Lopez, Jeffrey N. Bruce, and Peter Canoll

Abstract Despite decades of research, very modest advancements have been made in terms of improving outcomes in patients with gliomas. This highlights the need for preclinical animal models that more closely recapitulate the histopathology, molecular and cellular biology, and genetic heterogeneity of the human disease. Retroviral glioma models, particularly those driven by platelet-derived growth factor (PDGF), combine several of the desirable features of other model systems (i.e., xenografts and transgenic mice) yet avoid their limitations. They have proven to be powerful tools to address questions regarding cell of origin, genetic lesions necessary for tumor formation, tumor cell interactions with the brain's microenvironment, and testing of experimental therapeutic modalities. In this chapter, we compare and contrast the existing PDGF retrovirus models with other systems and discuss what lessons and insights these models have provided so far to the extremely challenging field of glioma research.

Contents

P. Canoll (✉)
Department of Pathology and Cell Biology, Columbia University Medical Center, New York, NY, USA
e-mail: pc561@columbia.edu

E.G. Van Meir (ed.), *CNS Cancer*, Cancer Drug Discovery and Development, DOI 10.1007/978-1-60327-553-8_1,
© Humana Press, a part of Springer Science+Business Media, LLC 2009

1.1 The Utility of Animal Glioma Models

Diffusely infiltrating gliomas, which include glioblastomas, astrocytomas, and oligodendrogliomas, are the most common type of primary brain tumors. Although gliomas are relatively rare (accounting for approximately 2% of all human tumors), they are notoriously aggressive and difficult to treat. Most patients with glioblastoma multiforme (GBM; the most common and most malignant form of glioma) die within 14 months of diagnosis. For several decades now, gliomas have been a major focus of both basic and clinical neuro-oncology research. While significant progress has been made, many important questions remain unanswered and improvements in the survival of glioma patients, particularly those with GBMs, have been modest. One area of research that has recently seen considerable advancement is the generation of new small-animal models that more accurately recapitulate the genetic and histological features of gliomas. These models are proving to be powerful tools to address basic biological and translational questions (see Chapters 1, 2, 3, 4, 5, 6, 7, 8, 9, 10, 11, 12, and 13).

Molecular and genetic analyses of human gliomas have identified a large (and growing) number of genetic alterations that may be responsible for gliomagenesis. However, the question of how these various alterations contribute to glioma growth and progression cannot be addressed solely through the study of human tumor tissue. Using animal models, one can directly test the tumorigenic effects of specific genetic alterations, both alone and in combination. The effects of certain types of genetic alterations may be cell-type specific; therefore experimental models that allow one to target discrete populations of cells provide a means to test the effect of genetic lesions in a cell-type-specific manner and to characterize the tumorigenic potential of defined cell populations in the neonatal and adult brain. Also, animal models that recapitulate the human pathology can be used to study aspects of glioma biology that involve interactions between tumor cells and their environment such as brain invasion, angiogenesis, and progenitor cell recruitment. Finally, animal models are essential tools to evaluate new treatments preclinically. In this chapter we will discuss the advantages of the retroviral glioma models, comparing them to other commonly used animal models of glioma (see Table 1.1). We will focus on the use of retroviruses that express platelet-derived growth factor (PDGF), which have proven to be robust experimental tools to study gliomagenesis. We will discuss in detail the theoretical underpinnings of PDGF-driven models and the biological and clinical questions that these models have addressed.

1.2 Comparing Retroviral Glioma Models to Other Model Systems

There is no "best" model to study brain tumors. The different models have advantages that make them well suited to address certain questions and disadvantages that make them less appropriate to address others. Below we discuss

Table 1.1 Comparison of commonly used glioma models

Model	Genetic lesions	Control of tumor initiation	Cell of origin	Pathology	Rate and frequency of tumor formation
Transplantation of glioma cell lines	Undefined	Can initiate tumor at specific place and time	Unknown	Does not resemble human gliomas	Rapid and consistent
Transplantaion of primary glioma cells or cancer stem cells	Undefined	Can initiate tumor at specific place and time	Unknown	Recapitulates some aspects of human gliomas	Variable
Transgenic models	Well defined	Cannot control when and where tumor forms	Target cells on basis of specific promoters	Closely resembles human tumors	Variable
Retroviral models	Well defined	Can initiate tumor at specific place and time	Target specific cells at specific time and place	Closely resembles human tumors	Rapid and consistent

some of the advantages and disadvantages of the different types of animal models, focusing our discussion on the many advantages offered by the retroviral approach. An in-depth discussion of the other models can be found in the succeeding chapters.

1.2.1 Transplantation of Glioma Cell-Lines

Historically, the most widely used brain tumor models have been generated through the transplantation of established glioma cell lines, either human cell lines generated from surgical specimens (Chapter 8) or rodent lines generated from chemical mutagen-induced brain tumors (Barth 1998) (Chapters 10, 11, and 12). These models allow for the manipulation of cells prior to implantation and provide control over tumor development (varying the number of cells will increase or decrease survival time, for example). Tumor formation is highly consistent and reproducible, with virtually 100% of the animals forming tumors within a relatively narrow time window. Also, the exact time and location of tumor initiation is experimentally determined which allows one to monitor tumor growth and start treatments at well-controlled time points. However, the histologic features of the tumors do not resemble that of human gliomas. In particular, in most instances the tumor cells do not diffusely infiltrate the brain, and when they do it is only over short distances. Invasion into surrounding brain tissue is limited to migration along the abluminal surface of host blood vessels (Farin et al. 2006, Nagano et al. 1993, Zagzag et al. 2000). Furthermore, tumor cells can contain numerous genetic lesions (including unidentified lesions), making it difficult to determine the contributions of each genetic lesion to the process of tumor formation. New genomic technologies should allow us to more fully characterize the genetic alterations in a given cell line but, even in that case, in vitro culture conditions may select for genetically distinct subpopulations after several passages (Giannini et al. 2005). Therefore, the genetic alterations of these cell lines may not resemble those of the tumors from which they were derived. Despite these limitations, these lines provide a convenient and reproducible model system and for this reason continue to be used extensively in the preclinical testing of new therapies.

1.2.2 Transplantation of Primary Glioma Cells or Cancer Stem Cells

More recent studies have used the transplantation of freshly isolated glioma cells that are serially passaged in nude mice (Giannini et al. 2005) or the so-called cancer stem cells that have been isolated from human glioma specimens (Lee et al. 2006, Singh et al. 2003). The major interest in these models comes from the idea that these tumors contain specific populations of bona fide glioma cells that represent highly relevant therapeutic targets. Also, these primary xenograft tumors recapitulate certain aspects of the pathology of human gliomas. They are highly infiltrative and a subset shows the robust vascular proliferation that is characteristic of GBMs (Bao et al. 2006, Giannini et al. 2005, Ogden et al. 2008) (see Chapters 21 and 22). They also maintain the amplification of the *EGFR* gene, a characteristic of human tumors which is lost in culture. However, the cell of origin and the genetic alterations that initiate tumor formation are undefined and will likely vary from one surgical specimen to the next. Furthermore, models using human cells must be performed in immunodeficient rodents and thus the immunological interactions between tumor and host are not recapitulated.

1.2.3 Glioma Models Using Genetically Engineered Mice (GEM)

Transgenic mice carrying germ line mutations have proven to be a powerful approach to dissect the role of specific molecular pathways in gliomagenesis.

A significant and ever-expanding number of transgenic mice have been engineered to carry a variety of genetic alterations, alone and in combinations, and these mice have been used to study the spontaneous formation of brain tumors. These transgenic models have included either conditional expression of oncogenes (such as mutant RAS or mutant forms of SV40 large T antigen) or conditional inactivation of tumor suppressor genes (such as *p53*, *PTEN*, *NF1*, and *INK4a*) (Bachoo et al. 2002, Bouvier et al. 2003, Ding et al. 2001, Farin et al. 2006, Gil-Perotin et al. 2006, Kwon et al. 2008, Zhu et al. 2005) (see Chapters 3, 4, 5, and 6). Interestingly, several studies have shown that single genetic lesions involving these tumor suppressors are not sufficient to induce glioma formation but will cooperate with other genetic lesions to facilitate gliomagenesis. Together, these transgenic models suggest that multiple genetic lesions cooperate in the initiation and progression of gliomas and that the histological type and grade of the tumors depends, at least in part, on the assortment of genetic lesions that a cell accumulates.

Several transgenic mouse models have used the cre-lox system to achieve cell-type-specific deletion of tumor suppressor genes. The bacterial cre recombinase recognizes a specific sequence of DNA referred to as a *loxP* site and will selectively excise a segment of DNA that is flanked by two *loxP* sites (referred to as a floxed sequence). There are a large variety of transgenic mice carrying floxed genes, including mice with floxed tumor suppressor genes such as $PTEN^{lox/lox}$ and $p53^{lox/lox}$. In the absence of cre, the *loxP* sites are genetically silent and the floxed mice have a normal phenotype. However, when the transgenic mice carrying the floxed gene(s) are crossed with mice that express cre off of a cell-type-specific promoter, the floxed gene is genetically deleted in a cell-type-specific manner as well. Recent studies have used mice driving cre expression off of the promoter of the genes encoding glial fibrillary acidic protein (GFAP) or nestin to selectively delete tumor suppressor genes in specific cell populations in the brain. However, it is important to note that both of these promoters drive expression in embryonic neural progenitor cells. As a result the genetic deletions are introduced at early stages of brain development and are widely distributed in neurons and glia throughout the brain. Therefore, most transgenic mouse models, even those using conditional systems, more closely recapitulate tumor formation associated with germ line cancer syndromes (such as Li–Fraumeni syndrome and neurofibromatosis) rather than somatic mutations associated with sporadically occurring gliomas. Recent advancements in inducible genetic systems (such as tamoxifen-inducible cre-ER) should allow for tighter temporal control of GEM models of brain tumors (Chow et al. 2008). However, these systems still carry the important technical caveat that the genetic lesions are introduced into widely distributed populations of cells. In *GFAP-creER* mice, for example, the tamoxifen-induced recombinations will occur in all GFAP+ cells throughout the brain and spinal cord. Thus, tumors could potentially arise anywhere in the CNS. In this regard it is interesting to note that several studies using GEM glioma models have reported that early lesions tend to occur in the subventricular zone (SVZ) of the lateral ventricle, suggesting that progenitor cells or neural stem cells in the SVZ may be acting as the cell of origin for these tumors (Gil-Perotin et al. 2006, Kwon et al. 2008, Zhu et al. 2005). However, formally testing this idea would require a means to selectively target the transforming genetic lesions to the adult SVZ. At present, transgenic models do not provide the spatial control needed for such experiments.

Advancements in transgenic mouse technology could theoretically allow for the generation of new models that explore many combinations of genetic alterations targeted to specific populations of brain cells in an inducible manner. In practice, however, generating transgenic mice that harbor numerous genetic alterations requires extensive breeding and is, therefore, expensive and time consuming. The tumors arising in GEMs closely resemble the pathology seen in human gliomas. However, in most transgenic mouse models to date, tumor formation has been relatively slow and inconsistent and it is not possible to predict when and where the tumors will arise. This inherent variability in the time and location of tumor formation makes it challenging to study early events in tumor formation. It also presents a significant disadvantage to using transgenic mouse models for preclinical studies.

1.2.4 Retroviral Glioma Models

Retroviral models combine several advantages of the transplantation models and the transgenic mouse models. One can deliver genetic lesions to discrete populations of cells at a specific time and place, the resulting tumors closely resemble human gliomas, and tumor formation is relatively rapid and consistent, making these models well suited for preclinical drug studies. Each of these points is discussed in detail below.

1.2.4.1 Using Retroviruses to Deliver Genetic Lesions to Discrete Cell Populations at a Specific Place and Time

As opposed to transgenic mice that carry germ line mutations, retroviruses introduce the transforming genetic lesions via somatic gene delivery. Retroviruses selectively infect dividing cells. The retroviral genome is inserted into the host cell genome, and therefore, the progeny of the infected cells inherit the retrovirally encoded genes. Effective entry of virus into host cells depends on interactions between the glycoprotein encoded by the virus envelope gene and the cell receptors expressed on host cells. Thus, the envelope protein can provide a high degree of selectivity with regard to the type of cells that a retrovirus will infect. For example, the avian leukosis virus (ALV) will only infect cells that express the avian retrovirus receptor tv-a. This receptor is normally not expressed by mammalian cells. However, mouse cells that are genetically engineered to express tv-a can be infected with ALV–RCAS (Replication Competent Avian Sarcoma Leukosis Virus with Splice acceptor) virus. Several glioma models have been developed using the RCAS virus in conjunction with transgenic mice that express tv-a off of either the *nestin* or the *GFAP* promoter. The major advantage of this approach is that it allows one to selectively target specific populations of neural progenitors and glial cells on the basis of cell-type-specific promoter expression. This system, referred to as RCAS/tv-a, is discussed briefly below and is described in detail in the next chapter.

Another commonly used type of viral envelope is the ecotropic class, which allows entry only into rat and mouse cells that express the ecotropic receptor. Ecotropic viruses will not infect human cells and are thus considered relatively safe. However, as is the case with the ALV-RCAS virus, ecotropic envelopes do not endure the physical stress of high-speed centrifugation used to concentrate virus. Nor do they endure freezing and thawing, making it difficult to generate stocks of high-titer virus. One approach to circumvent these limitations is viral pseudotyping. This refers to packaging a virus with an envelope protein from a different viral genome. This can be achieved by transfecting a producer cell line, such as 293T cells, with three separate plasmids: (1) the viral vector encoding LTR, the ψ packaging sequence, and the genes of interest (such as *PDGF*), (2) a second plasmid containing the *gag* (encodes the core protein) and *pol* genes (encodes the polymerase that mediates reverse transcriptase and integrase functions), and (3) a third plasmid containing the *env* gene (encodes the envelope protein). Using this approach, one will generate replication-incompetent viral particles that can infect cells without the use of helper virus. Vesicular stomatitis virus envelope protein (VSVg) has been widely used for pseudotyping because it recognizes membrane phospholipids as a minimal receptor, providing high affinity for a wide assortment of eukaryotic cells, including those of rats, mice, and humans. Thus, the pseudotyped viruses can be used to infect cells in a variety of different genetic backgrounds. Furthermore, like adenoviruses, VSVg-typed retroviruses can be concentrated to high titers by centrifugation and frozen and thawed with minimal loss of activity (Burns et al. 1993). This allows one to generate frozen stocks of high-titer virus, which not only is convenient but also greatly improves the reproducibility of the experimental system.

Stereotactic injection of retroviruses can be used to deliver genes to a small focus of cells at a specific place and time, which provides several important advantages. First, introducing the genetic lesion into a small, defined cell population approximates early stages of human gliomas, which also start as a point source and spread by cell migration and infiltration. Second, delivery into a defined area of the brain offers advantages when monitoring tumor growth and response to therapy since one knows exactly when and where the tumor starts. Third, one can easily target different regions of the CNS. Thus, retroviruses can be used to test the tumorigenic potential of discrete populations of cells in specific regions of the neonatal or adult nervous system. For example, stereotactic delivery of retrovirus has been used to induce the formation of tumors in the adult subcortical white matter (Assanah et al. 2006), the neonatal SVZ (Assanah et al., "submitted"), the brain stem (Suzuki et al., "unpublished results"), and the adult spinal cord (Ellis and Ogden, "unpublished results").

To date, the most robust (and extensively studied) retroviral glioma models have been those that use retroviruses that express PDGF. In the sections below, we will first discuss the biological relevance of PDGF in gliomagenesis and then provide a detailed review of the PDGF-driven glioma models.

1.2.4.2 PDGF as a Link Between Glial Progenitors and Gliomas

Several lines of evidence have implicated PDGF signaling in both normal glial development and gliomagenesis. During normal brain development, PDGF regulates the migration, proliferation, and differentiation of a subset of glial progenitors that express PDGF receptor-alpha (PDGFR-α) and that normally give rise to cells of the oligodendrocyte lineage. Transgenic mice that over-express PDGF from either the neuron-specific *enolase* promoter or the *GFAP* promoter show a marked increase in the number of PDGFR-α+ glial progenitors throughout the CNS (Calver et al. 1998, van Heyningen et al. 2001), suggesting that the numbers of progenitors are, in part, regulated by ambient levels of PDGF. This work also suggests that PDGFR-α+ progenitor cells will continue to proliferate as long as there is sufficient PDGF available. In vitro studies have shown that exogenously applied PDGF directly stimulates the migration and proliferation of neonatal glial progenitors (Armstrong et al. 1990, Noble et al. 1988). Furthermore, when neonatal glial progenitors are treated with a combination of PDGF and FGF in culture, they remain immature, migratory, and proliferative for an indefinite time (Bogler et al. 1990, Tang et al. 2000). These studies also demonstrate that glial progenitors possess a remarkable capacity to self-renew, an intrinsic feature of these cells which is highly relevant to their tumorigenic potential.

Human gliomas frequently co-express PDGF ligands and receptors, although they may be expressed in different populations of cells within the tumors, suggesting that both autocrine and paracrine signaling are at play (Hermanson et al. 1992, Hermansson et al. 1988). While PDGF expression is frequently seen across all grades (including low-grade astrocytomas and oligodendrogliomas), the highest levels of PDGF are found in GBMs (Guha et al. 1995, Ranza et al. 2007, Westermark et al. 1995), which suggests that PDGF signaling plays a role in both early stages of gliomagenesis and tumor progression. PDGF is a potent mitogen for glioma cells and stimulates their proliferation in a dose-dependent manner (Pollack et al. 1991, Westermark et al. 1995). Amplification and mutation of the *PDGFR*-α gene have been detected in some glioblastomas (Giannini et al. 2005, Kumabe et al. 1992a, b, TCGA, 2008). In most cases, however, genetic alterations in the *PDGFR*-α gene are not present, suggesting that the expression of PDGFR-α and robust responsiveness to PDGF that is frequently seen in human gliomas is an inherent property of the cells that give rise to these tumors.

Most gliomas occur in adults and, therefore, the cells that give rise to these tumors must reside in the adult brain. In fact, PDGFR-α expression is one of the defining features of adult glial progenitors. PDGFR-α+ glial progenitors are widely distributed throughout the adult white matter and represent one of the largest populations of cycling cells in the adult brain (Dawson et al. 2003, Gensert and Goldman 2001, Roy et al. 1999). Furthermore, PDGF will stimulate adult glial progenitors to proliferate more rapidly, to migrate significant distances, and to maintain an undifferentiated phenotype (Shi et al. 1998, Wolswijk and Noble 1992, Wolswijk et al. 1991). We propose that these robust effects on glial progenitor cell migration and proliferation underlie the potent tumorigenic effects of PDGF-expressing retroviruses.

1.2.4.3 PDGF Retroviruses Drive the Formation of Tumors That Closely Resemble Human Gliomas

The hypothesis that PDGF is playing an important role in glioma formation has been most definitively demonstrated using retroviral models. The first retroviral glioma model was established in marmosets via the use of simian sarcoma virus (SSV) and its helper virus simian sarcoma-associated virus (SSAV). The tumors that formed were reported to have the histopathologic features of GBM (Deinhardt 1980). The subsequent finding that the v-*sis* oncogene of SSV is a retroviral homologue of PDGF-B (Devare et al. 1983, Doolittle et al. 1983, Waterfield et al. 1983) provided the impetus for much of the subsequent work on PDGF and its role in gliomas.

The first mouse models used a Moloney murine leukemia virus (MMLV) carrying the *PDGF-B* gene (Uhrbom et al. 1998). The PDGF-B-expressing virus and a helper virus (in a volume of 10 μl) were co-injected into the right cerebral hemisphere of neonatal mice. Forty percent of the animals developed tumors between 14 and 29 weeks post-injection. In these studies some of the resultant tumors showed the histological features of GBM (infiltration, necrosis with pseudopalisading, and vascular proliferation), while others more closely resembled primitive neuroectodermal tumors. This variability may have resulted from the effects of additional genetic lesions that were acquired spontaneously during tumor formation, or as a result of insertional mutagenesis (Johansson et al. 2004, 2005). Alternatively, variability may have resulted from differences in the distribution and types of cells that were initially infected with the retrovirus. The neonatal rodent brain contains multiple populations of progenitor cells and the types of cells that will be infected depend on precisely when and where the virus is injected. It is important to note that in these early studies stereotactic procedures were not used to deliver the retroviruses and no analysis was performed to characterize the number, distribution, phenotype, or normal fate of the infected cells.

A second model using PDGF overexpression in the neonatal mouse utilized the aforementioned ALV-based RCAS vectors (Dai et al. 2001). For these experiments, transgenic mice expressing the ALV receptor tv-a were needed. The advantage of this system is that tv-a can be modified to be expressed by specific populations of cells if driven with different cell-specific promoters (such as *GFAP* or *nestin*). Injecting the PDGF-expressing RCAS virus into *GFAP/tv-a* mice led to the formation of gliomas in 40% of the animals by 12 weeks. These tumors resembled either oligodendrogliomas or mixed oligoastrocytomas. When the same virus was injected into *nestin/tv-a* mice, the rate of tumor formation was higher (60%) and their histology more consistently resembled low-grade oligodendrogliomas. Subsequent studies using the RCAS system with a construct that expressed higher PDGF levels showed that tumor formation was dose dependent (Shih et al. 2004). Ninety-seven percent of animals injected with this retrovirus formed tumors with shorter latency and the tumor histology resembled that of anaplastic oligodendrogliomas.

1.2.4.4 PDGF Drives Adult Glial Progenitors to form Malignant Gliomas

More recently, PDGF-expressing retroviruses have been used to test the tumorigenic potential of progenitor cells in the adult brain (Assanah et al. 2006). In this study, MMLV-based retroviruses pseudotyped with the VSVg envelope were used to infect glial progenitor cells in the subcortical white matter of *adult* rats. Injection with control retroviruses expressing a green fluorescent protein (GFP) reporter showed that approximately 90% of the infected cells expressed markers of the oligodendrocyte lineage (i.e., PDGFR-α+/olig2+/NG2+/GFAP–). Normally, these resident white matter progenitors are non-migratory, with the majority of retrovirally infected cells remaining within a few hundred microns of the injection site. However, when rats were injected with retroviruses expressing PDGF and GFP (coupled by an internal ribosomal entry site), 100% of the animals formed large brain tumors by 3 weeks post-injection. Histological analysis revealed that all tumors closely resembled human GBMs, showing extensive infiltration, marked vascular proliferation, and pseudopalisading necrosis (Fig. 1.1). The tumors were composed of cells that closely resembled glial progenitors morphologically and immunophenotypically with the vast majority of tumor cells expressing PDGFR-α, NG2, and olig2, but not GFAP (Fig. 1.2 and Color Plate 1).

Notably, *human* gliomas also contain an abundance of cells that closely resemble glial progenitors and express some of the same markers which identify glial progenitors including PDGFR-α (Hermanson et al. 1992), olig2 (Bouvier et al. 2003, Ligon et al. 2004, Lu et al. 2001), NG2 (Chekenya and Pilkington 2002, Shoshan et al. 1999), A2B5 (Colin et al. 2006, Ogden et al. 2008), and O4 (Rebetz et al. 2008). Taken together, these findings strongly suggest that the adult glial progenitor may be the cell of origin of gliomas.

In addition to the work discussed above, a recent study has provided intriguing evidence that GFAP+ neural stem cells (NSC) in the SVZ may also express PDGFR-α and that infusing exogenous PDGF into the lateral ventricles will induce the formation of glioma-like lesions (Jackson et al. 2006). This finding raises the interesting possibility that PDGF may be able to stimulate NSC to form tumors. However, three points must be kept in mind: (1) the vast majority of PDGFR-α+ cells in the adult brain are GFAP– and therefore distinct from the NSC of the SVZ, (2) retroviruses selectively infect actively proliferating cells and, therefore, relatively quiescent populations such as the

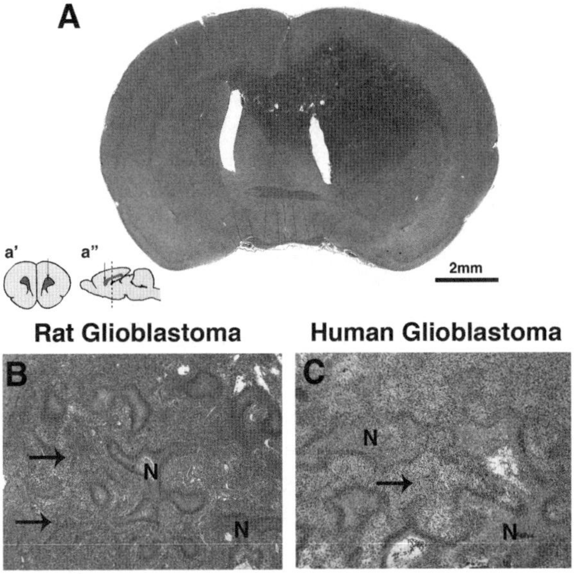

Adapted from Assanah M et al. (2006). J Neurosci 26(25):6781-6790.

Fig. 1.1 PDGF overexpression induces the formation of malignant gliomas that closely resemble human GBMs. **A.** Large infiltrative tumors with the histological features of human glioblastoma formed by 14 days post-injection (dpi) with PDGF-IRES-GFP retrovirus on H&E. This section shows the tumor extending across the corpus callosum into the contralateral hemisphere. Insets in A are coronal (a′) and sagittal (a″) schematic diagrams of the injection site (*arrow*) at the level of the *forceps minor corpus callosum* (fmcc) (*dotted line* in a" shows the level of the coronal section shown; scale bar = 2 mm). **B.** Higher magnification photomicrograph showing areas of glomeruloid vascular proliferation (*arrows*) and pseudopalisading necrosis (N). **C.** Same magnification photomicrographs of a human GBM specimen also showing areas of glomeruloid vascular proliferation (*arrows*) and pseudopalisading necrosis (N). Note the similarities between the rat and human tumors

mature astrocytes or GFAP+ NSC in the SVZ are not infected in significant numbers (after retroviral injection into the subcortical white matter of adult rats, less than 3% of infected cells expressed detectable levels of GFAP) (Assanah et al. 2006), and (3) immunohistochemical analysis of brains at early time points after injection with PDGF-expressing retrovirus into the subcortical white matter has revealed that the tumors begin as hypercellular lesions in the white matter around the injection site and are composed of proliferating glial progenitors (i.e., PDGFR-α+/NG2+/olig2+/GFAP–). Therefore, the preponderance of evidence points to PDGFR-α+ glial progenitors as the cells that give rise to the tumors in response to PDGF-expressing retrovirus. However, this does not rule out the possibility that NSC in the adult SVZ also have the capacity to form tumors and future studies should be aimed at directly addressing this question.

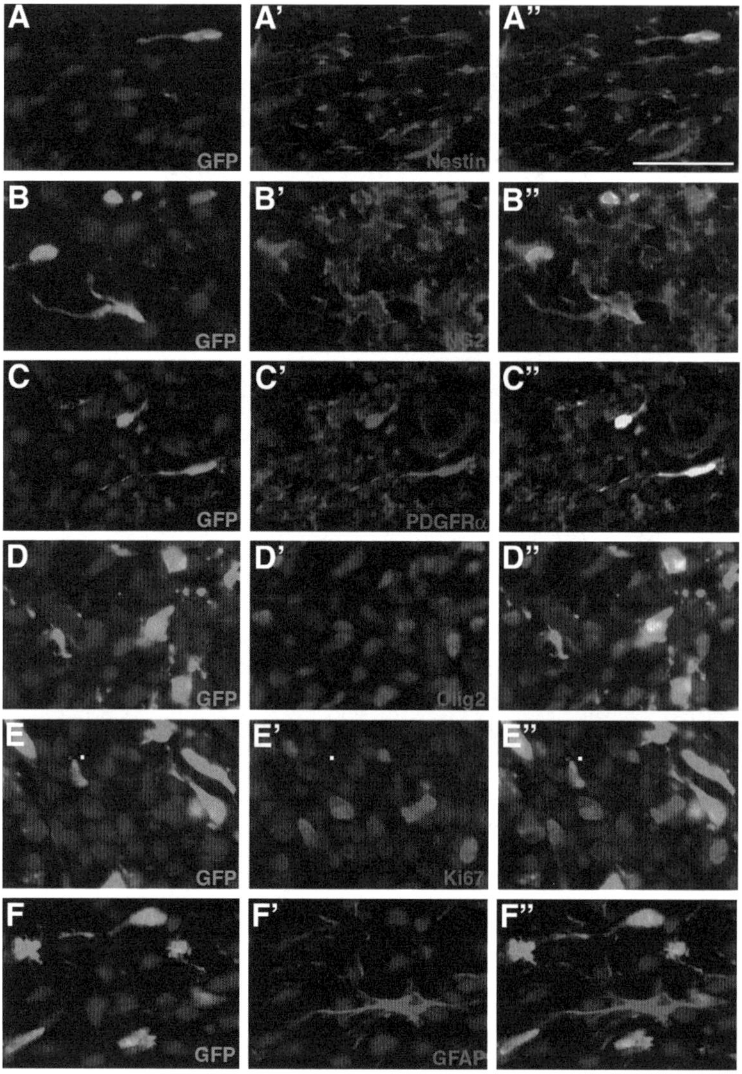

Adapted from Assanah M et al. (2006) J Neurosci 26(25):6781-6790

Fig. 1.2 GFP+ and GFP– tumor cells express markers of proliferative glial progenitor cells. Double-immunofluorescence analysis of tumors at 17 dpi with the PDGF-IRES-GFP retrovirus shows that GFP (*green*) is expressed in only a subset of tumor cells. However, nestin (A′, A″), NG2 (B′, B″), PDGFR-α (C′, C″), and olig2 (D′, D″), each stained red, are expressed in the vast majority of GFP+ and GFP– tumor cells. Ki67 proliferation marker is expressed in a significant number of both GFP+ and GFP– cells (E′, E″). GFAP+/GFP– reactive astrocytes (*red*) are seen scattered throughout the tumor (F′, F″). Rare GFAP+/GFP+ cells were seen (<3%) (*see* Color Plate 1)

1.2.4.5 Using Retroviruses to Test the Effects of Multiple Genetic Lesions

The findings discussed above demonstrate that retroviral delivery of a single growth factor (PDGF) is sufficient to induce the formation of brain tumors that closely resemble human gliomas. However, human gliomas typically harbor multiple genetic aberrations that contribute to malignant transformation (TCGA, 2008). Therefore, it is of great interest to develop models that will incorporate multiple genetic alterations. One approach to increasing the genetic complexity of these models is the injection of PDGF-expressing retroviruses into transgenic mice that carry genetic lesions, which are by themselves insufficient to induce tumor formation. Several studies in which PDGF-expressing viruses have been injected into a variety of transgenic strains have provided insight into how PDGF signaling interacts with other genetic alterations during gliomagenesis. PDGF overexpression in the background of *p53* or *INK4a-Arf* deletion, for example, causes tumors of higher grade, increased frequency, and decreased tumor latency, suggesting that deletion of these tumor suppressor genes can cooperate with PDGF signaling to facilitate in tumor formation (Dai et al. 2001, Hesselager et al. 2003, Tchougounova et al. 2007, Uhrbom et al. 2000).

Another way to increase the genetic complexity of retrovirus-induced tumor models is to co-inject multiple viruses, each encoding a separate set of genes. However, there are important technical caveats to this approach. We have shown that co-injecting two viruses with different reporters genes (GFP and DsRed) results in mixed populations of cells infected with either virus or both viruses. The relative abundance of the different populations depends on the titers of each viral vector, but in our experience co-infection with both viruses is a relatively rare event (Assanah et al. 2006). We have also co-injected viruses that express PDGF-IRES-DsRed and cre-GFP into $PTEN^{lox/lox}$ and $p53^{lox/lox}$ mice with floxed tumor suppressor genes (Ellis et al., "unpublished results"). This approach provides a unique way to generate tumors composed of heterogeneous populations of cells harboring different genetic lesions and also to monitor population dynamics and paracrine signaling between different cells within a tumor (as discussed below).

1.2.4.6 Using Retroviral Models to Study Glioma Infiltration

Glioma cells have a remarkable capacity to infiltrate the brain and migrate long distances, making complete surgical resection impossible (see Chapter 49). Thus glioma infiltration represents a major obstacle to effective treatment of brain tumors and there is great need for animal models that recapitulate glioma infiltration. The retrovirus-induced tumors have several features that make them well suited to study glioma migration and infiltration: (1) the tumors begin as a small focus of infected cells and grow by diffusely infiltrating into the surrounding brain tissue, (2) the patterns of invasion resemble those seen in human gliomas, with extensive migration through white matter and along blood vessels, and (3) the fluorescent reporters (GFP and DsRed) provide a means to map the distribution of retrovirus-infected cells and monitor their

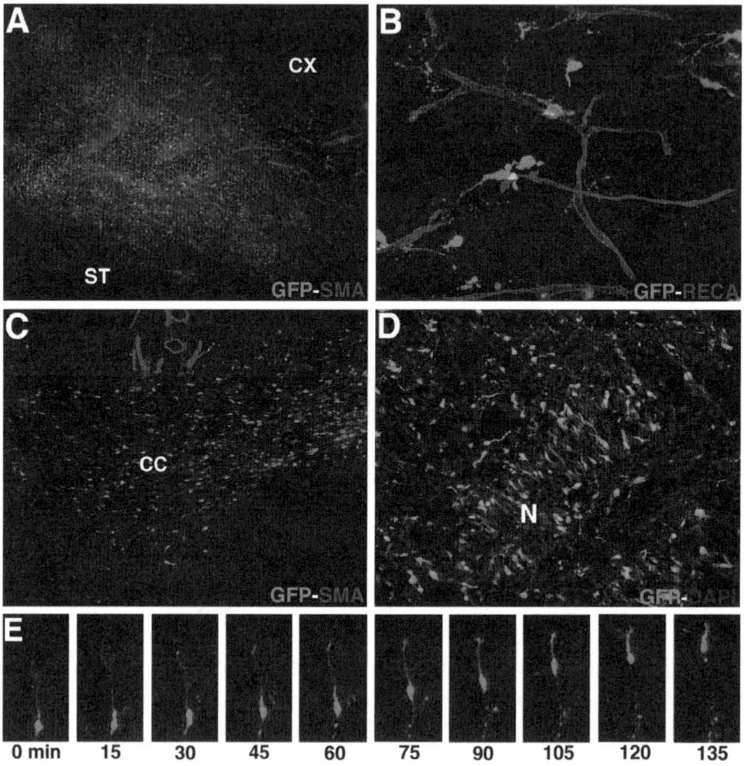

Fig. 1.3 GFP expression reveals the distribution of retrovirally infected cells. Immunofluorescence analysis for GFP and SMA was performed on sections of PDGF-IRES-GFP tumors. **A.** Low-magnification photomicrograph shows GFP+ cells (*green*) throughout the tumor, crossing the corpus callosum (CC) and invading the ipsilateral hemisphere. SMA immunofluorescence (*red*) shows marked vascular proliferation with recruitment of perivascular smooth muscle cells. **B.** Confocal micrograph of GFP and RECA (*red*) showing tumor cells migrating on blood vessels. **C.** Immunofluorescence micrograph (GFP: *green*; SMA: *red*) showing numerous tumor cells crossing the corpus callosum and invading the contralateral hemisphere. **D.** GFP+ and GFP– cells are seen intermingled throughout the tumor, including in areas of pseudopalisading necrosis (N). Note that only a subset of the cells is GFP+. **E.** Fluorescent time-lapse kymograph depicts the saltatory movement of a PDGF-IRES-GFP tumor cell showing that the leading cell process extends forward prior to movement of the cell body (Assanah et al., submitted) (*see* Color Plate 2)

migratory behavior in living slices of brain tissue using time-lapse fluorescence microscopy (Fig. 1.3 and Color Plate 2).

Results of time-lapse microscopy show that the migrating tumor cells proliferate en route, stopping for approximately an hour to divide before the daughter cells resume migrating (Assanah et al., "submitted", Beadle et al., 2007). The migratory behavior of PDGF-driven tumor cells resembles that of normal glial progenitors; the migratory cells have a bipolar morphology with a prominent leading process that extends and retracts while the nucleus and cell body move in a saltatory manner with bursts of forward movement separated by periods of little or no movement. As is the case with normal progenitors (Bellion et al. 2005, Schaar and McConnell 2005, Tsai et al. 2007), the forward movement of the cell body requires myosin II and treating tumor-bearing brain slices with myosin II inhibitors effectively blocked cell migration in slice culture (Beadle et al. 2008). Interestingly, the same inhibitors did not stop glioma cells from migrating on a coverslip, suggesting that migration in slice cultures was impeded because the tumor cells could not squeeze their cell bodies and nuclei through the mechanically restricted extracellular space of the brain. This study illustrates the importance of studying glioma migration within a physiologically relevant environment. It also demonstrates how the PDGF retrovirus model and the slice culture system can be used to test new anti-invasive therapies. The model provides a convenient way to treat the tumor cells with small molecule inhibitors and monitor the effects on migration and proliferation within the context of vital brain tissue.

1.2.4.7 Using Retroviral Models to Study Interactions Within the Brain Microenvironment

Because of their diffusely infiltrative growth pattern, gliomas are composed of a heterogeneous mixture of tumor cells intermingled with normal reactive brain parenchyma, including proliferating blood vessels, reactive astrocytes, and recruited glial progenitors. To date, very little is known about how glioma cells interact with the surrounding brain tissue. As described above, PDGF-driven gliomas recapitulate the key histological features of human gliomas, including marked vascular proliferation and diffuse infiltration, making this an ideal experimental system with which to study paracrine signaling between tumor cells and the microenvironment.

The initial characterization of PDGF ligands and their receptors in malignant glioma cell lines and in human surgical specimens led to the hypothesis that both autocrine and paracrine PDGF signaling pathways were at work in glioma growth. Since both ligand and receptor were co-localized on the same tumor cells, this finding was taken as evidence for the existence of autocrine PDGF loops (Maxwell et al. 1990, Nister et al. 1991, 1988). Hermanson et al. expanded on this when they observed in human tumor specimens that PDGF-A and PDGFR-α were primarily found on tumor cells while PDGF-B and PDGFR-β were found on hyperplastic capillaries (Hermanson et al. 1992). The authors concluded, therefore, that autocrine loops were found as tumor cell-to-tumor cell interactions while paracrine loops existed between tumor cells and the vasculature.

In both retroviral PDGF-driven glioma models (Assanah et al. 2006, Shih et al. 2004), vascular proliferation was a prominent feature. This is not particularly surprising since PDGF has been implicated as a pro-angiogenic factor both in normal development (Leveen et al. 1994, Lindahl et al. 1998, Soriano 1994) and in gliomas (Brockmann et al. 2003, Dunn et al. 2000, Guo et al. 2003). Pericytes and smooth muscle cells express PDGFR-β and PDGF-B facilitates the paracrine recruitment of these perivascular cells to augment the development of new tumor vessels. The retroviral PDGF glioma models, however, have not only demonstrated paracrine signaling via blood vessel recruitment but also provided evidence that paracrine signaling was occurring between PDGF-expressing tumor cells and PDGFR-α+ glial progenitors.

One of the most interesting findings from both these studies was the observation that the majority of proliferating cells in the PDGF-driven tumors were actually recruited progenitors that were *not* infected by retrovirus. In Shih et al., immunohistochemical staining for the hemagglutinin (HA) protein tag of their PDGF-B-HA construct revealed that tumor cells expressed varying levels of PDGF from very robust to undetectable. The authors concluded that, if levels of PDGF were high enough, uninfected progenitors could be stimulated to proliferate as well. In support of this hypothesis, Assanah et al. showed that PDGF-driven tumors in the adult rat contained large numbers of uninfected, recruited glial progenitors (Assanah et al. 2006). The recruited cells were highly proliferative based upon their Ki67 labeling index and were strongly positive for PDGFR-α as well as other glial progenitor markers such as olig2, NG2, and A2B5.

To further investigate the recruitment phenomenon, separate cultures of isolated adult glial progenitors were infected in vitro with a PDGF-IRES-DsRed retrovirus or a control pNIT-GFP retrovirus. Equal numbers of GFP+ progenitor cells were then injected into adult rats either alone or in combination with cells expressing PDGF-IRES-DsRed. When injected alone, the GFP+ progenitors stopped proliferating and differentiated into mature oligodendrocytes, and the rats never formed tumors. In contrast, co-injecting the PDGF-IRES-DSRED and control GFP cells generated large tumors that were composed of mixed populations of red cells (expressing PDGF) and green cells (recruited progenitors). Both populations were highly migratory and proliferative (Fig. 1.4 and Color Plate 3). These experiments provided strong evidence that paracrine PDGF signaling is sufficient to drive adult glial progenitors to proliferate massively and contribute to tumor growth.

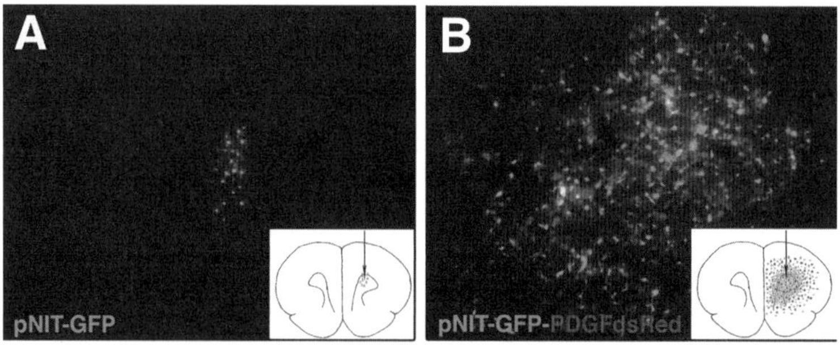

Adapted from Assanah M et al. (2006). J Neurosci 26(25):6781-6790

Fig. 1.4 **A.** Adult rat glial progenitors infected in vitro with a pNIT-GFP retrovirus (*green*) do not proliferate, migrate, or form tumors when reinjected into subcortical white matter (diagram inset). **B.** In contrast, when equal numbers of GFP-labeled cells are co-injected with PDGF-DsRed cells (*red*; also infected with retrovirus in vitro), GFP-labeled cells proliferate, migrate, and form tumors composed of a mixture of both cell populations (*see* Color Plate 3)

More recently, we have shown that human tumor cells freshly isolated from surgical glioblastoma specimens also have the capacity to recruit progenitor cells when transplanted into nude rats. Using species-specific antibodies, we observed that the xenograft tumors generated from most of these human glioma specimens contained massive numbers of rat-derived PDGFR-α+ progenitors that were induced to proliferate via paracrine growth factor stimulation and significantly contributed to tumor growth (Lopez et al., "submitted").

These findings provide novel insights into the basic mechanisms of gliomagenesis. The PDGF retroviral models reveal that the contributions of the different components of the tumor microenvironment to tumor growth and progression (i.e., growth factor-responsive endogenous glial progenitors and vascular cells) are more significant than previously appreciated. For example, while it is well established that genetic lesions are relevant to glioma formation (and that gliomas contain clonal expansions of mutated cells), these retroviral models raise the intriguing possibility that paracrine growth factor signaling alone can induce untransformed progenitors to behave malignantly. Additionally, recapitulation of vascular proliferation by these models (which is part and parcel of human glioma and is essentially another form of cell recruitment) makes them invaluable for further studying angiogenesis in an in vivo system. These models may allow us to analyze not only how tumor cells regulate vascular proliferation but also how blood vessels may reciprocally affect tumor growth both through vascular supply and the secretion of their own growth factors.

1.2.4.8 Using Retroviral Models for Preclinical Studies

The retroviral glioma models have several features that make them excellent tools for preclinical trials of new drugs and drug delivery methods for gliomas. As mentioned above, they combine the favorable characteristics of xenograft models (i.e., ease of use, efficiency of tumor formation, precise localization of the lesion, relatively short survival curves) with those of GEMs (i.e., well-defined relevant genetic lesions, histopathologic recapitulation). The RCAS/*tv-a* system, for example, has been extensively used to investigate the utility of several targeted inhibitors of signal transduction pathways presumed to be active in that particular model. These include inhibitors of PDGF and VEGF receptors (Shih et al. 2004), *Akt* (Momota et al. 2005), and mTOR (Hu et al. 2005).

In our own lab, we have been using the PDGF-driven glioma model to test the effects of intratumoral convection-enhanced delivery (CED) of various cytotoxic agents. Briefly, CED is the direct infusion of drug into the tumor at a slow constant rate using a positive-pressure catheter system, allowing drugs to bypass the blood–brain barrier and thus achieve a higher tissue concentration while avoiding dose-limiting toxicities of systemic administration (Lopez et al. 2006). Our experiments using the topoisomerase I-inhibitor topotecan (Lopez et al., "unpublished data") highlight the reproducibility of our retroviral model. As shown in Fig. 1.5A, three separate experiments with only two

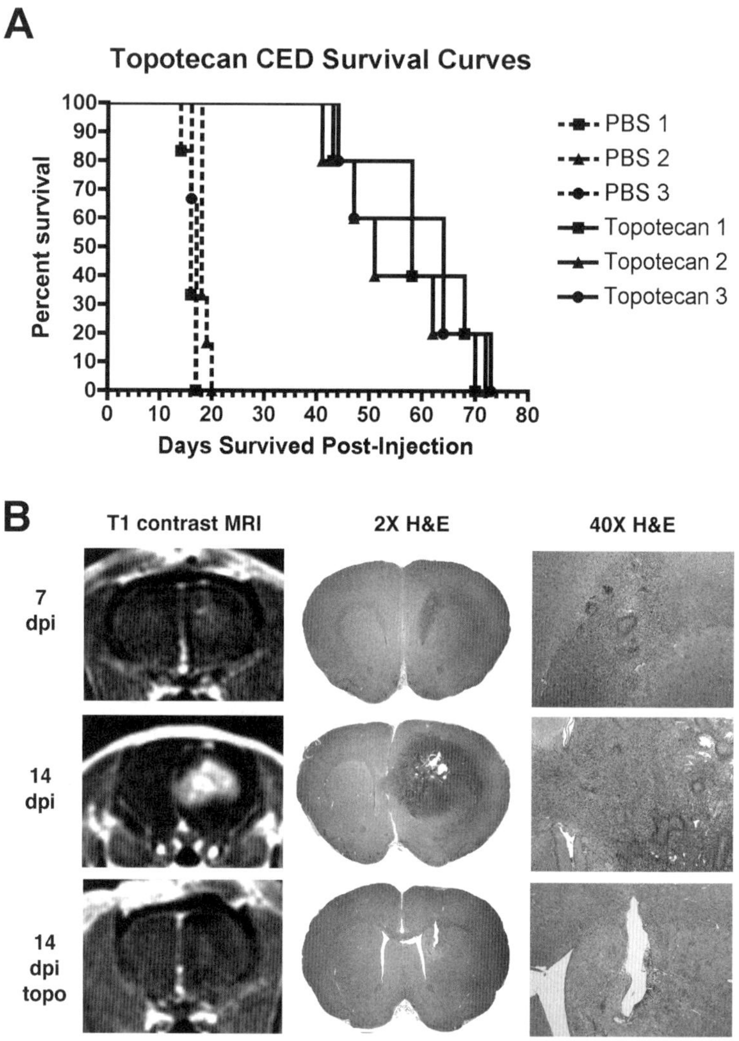

Fig. 1.5 A. Three separate survival experiments with highly consistent and similar Kaplan–Meier curves. Animals were given either PBS (*dashed lines*) or topotecan (*solid lines*) via intratumoral convection-enhanced delivery. **B.** First two rows show T1 contrast MRIs and H&E photomicrographs of PDGF retrovirus tumors at 7 and 14 dpi. The bottom row shows a tumor-bearing animal treated with topotecan via CED at 7 dpi and sacrificed at 14 dpi. H&E shows an absence of tumor cells post-treatment and the MRI shows a small contrast-enhancing region, which probably corresponds to treatment-related necrosis

small groups each (i.e., control vs. treated) yield remarkably similar survival curves. The precision and consistency with which we can run survival experiments such as these allow us to obtain dependable results very quickly. The number of animals used is kept to a minimum because truly significant effects and trends are easily determined. Because we have precisely determined where tumors start forming and when they become detectable on histology or magnetic resonance imaging (Fig. 1.5B), we can make rational decisions on when treatments are ideally started. The speed and reliability of the model (with 100% of the animals developing tumor morbidity between 16 and 21 days post-injection in every experiment) also let us use "historical" survival data from control experiments to rapidly screen drugs of interest for in vivo activity. In the case of CED studies, the fact that our tumors are highly invasive poses an additional challenge to achieving adequate treatment. Cell-line xenograft models, in contrast, are significantly easier to cure with loco-regional therapy because tumors grow as well-circumscribed lesions and can therefore be sufficiently covered even with small drug distribution volumes (Kaiser et al. 2000). The use of an invasive model such as the PDGF retrovirus tumors allows one to not only determine whether a drug has relevant biochemical activity but also ascertain the contribution of adequate drug delivery toward durable therapeutic effects. Histological and immunohistochemical analysis of brains after CED treatment with topotecan shows a near-complete eradication of tumor cells in proximity to the treatment site (Fig. 1.5B). However, viable retrovirus-infected tumor cells (detected by virtue of the GFP reporter) can be found at significant distances away from the treatment site, suggesting that these highly infiltrative cells have migrated outside the zone of effective treatment and contributed to tumor recurrence.

Tumor recurrence is, in fact, another unique aspect of our retroviral model. As shown above, treatment with topotecan via CED provides a significant survival advantage but tumors invariably recur and lead to animal mortality. Recurrence occurs just as reliably and consistently as initial tumor formation and is therefore amenable to experimentation and analysis. Furthermore, because recurrent tumors can be developed de novo after a specific treatment within the native brain environment, the study of recurrence mechanisms with the retroviral models may potentially lead to more clinically relevant insights and results.

Taking our experience together with that of other groups' preclinical therapeutic work using retroviral glioma models, it becomes clear that combination therapy will be necessary to eventually cure the human disease. Furthermore, these models have not only taught us that a multi-modal approach (e.g., signal transduction inhibitors, cytotoxic agents, and anti-angiogenics, some or all delivered via CED) will be necessary for therapeutic success but also provide us the means to actually perform relevant experiments using a wide variety of rational combinations.

In this chapter, we have broadly discussed the use of animal models to further our understanding of gliomas. In particular, we have focused on the advantages and disadvantages of using PDGF-driven retroviral models as well as the insights that we have learned from them. Other authors in the succeeding chapters will provide more specific information about the other models. We reiterate that there is no single model that is currently able to completely recapitulate the cellular and genetic pathophysiology of human gliomas. This is mostly due to the inherent heterogeneity of these tumors. As we continue to discern genetic and phenotypic patterns within gliomas that allow us to further divide tumors into clinically relevant subclasses (TCGA, 2008, Phillips et al. 2006), we must also continue to refine the models with which we study them. It will be of paramount importance in the future to be able to tailor models to fit these specific glioma subtypes.

References

Armstrong, RC Harvath, L and Dubois-Dalcq, ME (1990) Type 1 astrocytes and oligodendrocyte-type 2 astrocyte glial progenitors migrate toward distinct molecules. J Neurosci Res 27(3):400–407

Assanah, M Lochhead, R Ogden, A Bruce, J Goldman, J and Canoll, P (2006) Glial progenitors in adult white matter are driven to form malignant gliomas by platelet-derived growth factor-expressing retroviruses. J Neurosci 26(25):6781–6790

Bachoo, RM Maher, EA Ligon, KL Sharpless, NE Chan, SS You, MJ Tang, Y DeFrances, J Stover, E Weissleder, R Rowitch, DH Louis, DN and DePinho, RA (2002) Epidermal growth factor receptor and Ink4a/Arf: convergent mechanisms governing terminal differentiation and transformation along the neural stem cell to astrocyte axis. Cancer Cell 1(3):269–277

Bao, S Wu, Q Sathornsumetee, S Hao, Y Li, Z Hjelmeland, AB Shi, Q McLendon, RE Bigner, DD and Rich, JN (2006) Stem cell-like glioma cells promote tumor angiogenesis through vascular endothelial growth factor. Cancer Res 66(16):7843–7848

Barth, RF (1998) Rat brain tumor models in experimental neuro-oncology: the 9L, C6, T9, F98, RG2 (D74), RT-2 and CNS-1 gliomas. J Neurooncol 36(1):91–102

Beadle, C Assanah, MC Monzo, P Vallee, R Rosenfeld, SS and Canoll, P (2008) The role of myosin II in glioma invasion of the brain. Mol Biol Cell 19(8):3357–3368

Bellion, A Baudoin, JP Alvarez, C Bornens, M and Metin, C (2005) Nucleokinesis in tangentially migrating neurons comprises two alternating phases: forward migration of the Golgi/centrosome associated with centrosome splitting and myosin contraction at the rear. J Neurosci 25(24):5691–5699

Bogler, O Wren, D Barnett, SC Land, H and Noble, M (1990) Cooperation between two growth factors promotes extended self-renewal and inhibits differentiation of oligodendrocyte-type-2 astrocyte (O-2A) progenitor cells. Proc Natl Acad Sci USA 87(16):6368–6372

Bouvier, C Bartoli, C Aguirre-Cruz, L Virard, I Colin, C Fernandez, C Gouvernet, J and Figarella-Branger, D (2003) Shared oligodendrocyte lineage gene expression in gliomas and oligodendrocyte progenitor cells. J Neurosurg 99(2):344–350

Brockmann, MA Ulbricht, U Gruner, K Fillbrandt, R Westphal, M and Lamszus, K (2003) Glioblastoma and cerebral microvascular endothelial cell migration in response to tumor-associated growth factors. Neurosurgery 52(6):1391–1399; discussion 1399

Burns, JC Friedmann, T Driever, W Burrascano, M and Yee, JK (1993) Vesicular stomatitis virus G glycoprotein pseudotyped retroviral vectors: concentration to very high titer and efficient gene transfer into mammalian and nonmammalian cells. Proc Natl Acad Sci USA 90(17):8033–8037

Calver, AR Hall, AC Yu, WP Walsh, FS Heath, JK Betsholtz, C and Richardson, WD (1998) Oligodendrocyte population dynamics and the role of PDGF in vivo. Neuron 20(5):869–882

Chekenya, M and Pilkington, GJ (2002) NG2 precursor cells in neoplasia: functional, histogenesis and therapeutic implications for malignant brain tumours. J Neurocytol 31(6–7):507–521

Chow, LM Zhang, J and Baker, SJ (2008) Inducible Cre recombinase activity in mouse mature astrocytes and adult neural precursor cells. Transgenic Res 17(5):919–928

Colin, C Baeza, N Tong, S Bouvier, C Quilichini, B Durbec, P and Figarella-Branger, D (2006) In vitro identification and functional characterization of glial precursor cells in human gliomas. Neuropathol Appl Neurobiol 32(2):189–202

Dai, C Celestino, JC Okada, Y Louis, DN Fuller, GN and Holland, EC (2001) PDGF autocrine stimulation dedifferentiates cultured astrocytes and induces oligodendrogliomas and oligoastrocytomas from neural progenitors and astrocytes in vivo. Genes Dev 15(15):1913–1925

Dawson, MR Polito, A Levine, JM and Reynolds, R (2003) NG2-expressing glial progenitor cells: an abundant and widespread population of cycling cells in the adult rat CNS. Mol Cell Neurosci 24(2):476–488

Deinhardt, F (1980) Biology of primate retroviruses. In: Klein, G (ed) Viral Oncology. Raven Press, New York

Devare, SG Reddy, EP Law, JD Robbins, KC and Aaronson, SA (1983) Nucleotide sequence of the simian sarcoma virus genome: demonstration that its acquired cellular sequences encode the transforming gene product p28sis. Proc Natl Acad Sci USA 80(3):731–735

Ding, H Roncari, L Shannon, P Wu, X Lau, N Karaskova, J Gutmann, DH Squire, JA Nagy, A and Guha, A (2001) Astrocyte-specific expression of activated p21-ras results in malignant astrocytoma formation in a transgenic mouse model of human gliomas. Cancer Res 61(9):3826–3836

Doolittle, RF Hunkapiller, MW Hood, LE Devare, SG Robbins, KC Aaronson, SA and Antoniades, HN (1983) Simian sarcoma virus onc gene, v-sis, is derived from the gene (or genes) encoding a platelet-derived growth factor. Science 221(4607):275–277

Dunn, IF Heese, O and Black, PM (2000) Growth factors in glioma angiogenesis: FGFs, PDGF, EGF, and TGFs. J Neurooncol 50(1–2):121–137

Farin, A Suzuki, SO Weiker, M Goldman, JE Bruce, JN and Canoll, P (2006) Transplanted glioma cells migrate and proliferate on host brain vasculature: A dynamic analysis. Glia 53(8):799–808

Gensert, JM and Goldman, JE (2001) Heterogeneity of cycling glial progenitors in the adult mammalian cortex and white matter. J Neurobiol 48(2):75–86

Giannini, C Sarkaria, JN Saito, A Uhm, JH Galanis, E Carlson, BL Schroeder, MA and James, CD (2005) Patient tumor EGFR and PDGFRA gene amplifications retained in an invasive intracranial xenograft model of glioblastoma multiforme. Neuro Oncol 7(2):164–176

Gil-Perotin, S Marin-Husstege, M Li, J Soriano-Navarro, M Zindy, F Roussel, MF Garcia-Verdugo, JM and Casaccia-Bonnefil, P (2006) Loss of p53 induces changes in the behavior of subventricular zone cells: implication for the genesis of glial tumors. J Neurosci 26(4):1107–1116

Guha, A Dashner, K Black, PM Wagner, JA and Stiles, CD (1995) Expression of PDGF and PDGF receptors in human astrocytoma operation specimens supports the existence of an autocrine loop. Int J Cancer 60(2):168–173

Guo, P Hu, B Gu, W Xu, L Wang, D Huang, HJ Cavenee, WK and Cheng, SY (2003) Platelet-derived growth factor-B enhances glioma angiogenesis by stimulating vascular endothelial growth factor expression in tumor endothelia and by promoting pericyte recruitment. Am J Pathol 162(4):1083–1093

Hermanson, M Funa, K Hartman, M Claesson-Welsh, L Heldin, CH Westermark, B and Nister, M (1992) Platelet-derived growth factor and its receptors in human glioma tissue:

expression of messenger RNA and protein suggests the presence of autocrine and paracrine loops. Cancer Res 52(11):3213–3219

Hermansson, M Nister, M Betsholtz, C Heldin, CH Westermark, B and Funa, K (1988) Endothelial cell hyperplasia in human glioblastoma: coexpression of mRNA for platelet-derived growth factor (PDGF) B chain and PDGF receptor suggests autocrine growth stimulation. Proc Natl Acad Sci USA 85(20):7748–7752

Hesselager, G Uhrbom, L Westermark, B and Nister, M (2003) Complementary effects of platelet-derived growth factor autocrine stimulation and p53 or Ink4a-Arf deletion in a mouse glioma model. Cancer Res 63(15):4305–4309

Hu, X Pandolfi, PP Li, Y Koutcher, JA Rosenblum, M and Holland, EC (2005) mTOR promotes survival and astrocytic characteristics induced by Pten/AKT signaling in glioblastoma. Neoplasia 7(4):356–368

Jackson, EL Garcia-Verdugo, JM Gil-Perotin, S Roy, M Quinones-Hinojosa, A VandenBerg, S and Alvarez-Buylla, A (2006) PDGFR alpha-positive B cells are neural stem cells in the adult SVZ that form glioma-like growths in response to increased PDGF signaling. Neuron 51(2):187–199

Johansson, FK Brodd, J Eklof, C Ferletta, M Hesselager, G Tiger, CF Uhrbom, L and Westermark, B (2004) Identification of candidate cancer-causing genes in mouse brain tumors by retroviral tagging. Proc Natl Acad Sci USA 101(31):11334–11337

Johansson, FK Goransson, H and Westermark, B (2005) Expression analysis of genes involved in brain tumor progression driven by retroviral insertional mutagenesis in mice. Oncogene 24(24):3896–3905

Kaiser, MG Parsa, AT Fine, RL Hall, JS Chakrabarti, I and Bruce, JN (2000) Tissue distribution and antitumor activity of topotecan delivered by intracerebral clysis in a rat glioma model. Neurosurgery 47(6):1391–1398; discussion 1398–1399

Kumabe, T Sohma, Y Kayama, T Yoshimoto, T and Yamamoto, T (1992a) Amplification of alpha-platelet-derived growth factor receptor gene lacking an exon coding for a portion of the extracellular region in a primary brain tumor of glial origin. Oncogene 7(4):627–633

Kumabe, T Sohma, Y Kayama, T Yoshimoto, T and Yamamoto, T (1992b) Overexpression and amplification of alpha-PDGF receptor gene lacking exons coding for a portion of the extracellular region in a malignant glioma. Tohoku J Exp Med 168(2):265–269

Kwon, CH Zhao, D Chen, J Alcantara, S Li, Y Burns, DK Mason, RP Lee, EY Wu, H and Parada, LF (2008) Pten haploinsufficiency accelerates formation of high-grade astrocytomas. Cancer Res 68(9):3286–3294

Lee, J Kotliarova, S Kotliarov, Y Li, A Su, Q Donin, NM Pastorino, S Purow, BW Christopher, N Zhang, W Park, JK and Fine, HA (2006) Tumor stem cells derived from glioblastomas cultured in bFGF and EGF more closely mirror the phenotype and genotype of primary tumors than do serum-cultured cell lines. Cancer Cell 9(5):391–403

Leveen, P Pekny, M Gebre-Medhin, S Swolin, B Larsson, E and Betsholtz, C (1994) Mice deficient for PDGF B show renal, cardiovascular, and hematological abnormalities. Genes Dev 8(16):1875–1887

Ligon, KL Alberta, JA Kho, AT Weiss, J Kwaan, MR Nutt, CL Louis, DN Stiles, CD and Rowitch, DH (2004) The oligodendroglial lineage marker OLIG2 is universally expressed in diffuse gliomas. J Neuropathol Exp Neurol 63(5):499–509

Lindahl, P Hellstrom, M Kalen, M Karlsson, L Pekny, M Pekna, M Soriano, P and Betsholtz, C (1998) Paracrine PDGF-B/PDGF-Rbeta signaling controls mesangial cell development in kidney glomeruli. Development 125(17):3313–3322

Lopez, KA Waziri, AE Canoll, PD and Bruce, JN (2006) Convection-enhanced delivery in the treatment of malignant glioma. Neurol Res 28(5):542–548

Lu, QR Park, JK Noll, E Chan, JA Alberta, J Yuk, D Alzamora, MG Louis, DN Stiles, CD Rowitch, DH and Black, PM (2001) Oligodendrocyte lineage genes (OLIG) as molecular markers for human glial brain tumors. Proc Natl Acad Sci USA 98(19):10851–10856

Maxwell, M Naber, SP Wolfe, HJ Galanopoulos, T Hedley-Whyte, ET Black, PM and Antoniades, HN (1990) Coexpression of platelet-derived growth factor (PDGF) and PDGF-receptor genes by primary human astrocytomas may contribute to their development and maintenance. J Clin Invest 86(1):131–140

Momota, H Nerio, E and Holland, EC (2005) Perifosine inhibits multiple signaling pathways in glial progenitors and cooperates with temozolomide to arrest cell proliferation in gliomas in vivo. Cancer Res 65(16):7429–7435

Nagano, N Sasaki, H Aoyagi, M and Hirakawa, K (1993) Invasion of experimental rat brain tumor: early morphological changes following microinjection of C6 glioma cells. Acta Neuropathol 86(2):117–125

Nister, M Claesson-Welsh, L Eriksson, A Heldin, CH and Westermark, B (1991) Differential expression of platelet-derived growth factor receptors in human malignant glioma cell lines. J Biol Chem 266(25):16755–16763

Nister, M Libermann, TA Betsholtz, C Pettersson, M Claesson-Welsh, L Heldin, CH Schlessinger, J and Westermark, B (1988) Expression of messenger RNAs for platelet-derived growth factor and transforming growth factor-alpha and their receptors in human malignant glioma cell lines. Cancer Res 48(14):3910–3918

Noble, M Murray, K Stroobant, P Waterfield, MD and Riddle, P (1988) Platelet-derived growth factor promotes division and motility and inhibits premature differentiation of the oligodendrocyte/type-2 astrocyte progenitor cell. Nature 333(6173): 560–562

Ogden, AT Waziri, AE Lochhead, RA Fusco, D Lopez, K Ellis, JA Kang, J Assanah, M McKhann, GM Sisti, MB McCormick, PC Canoll, P and Bruce, JN (2008) Identification of A2B5+CD133- tumor-initiating cells in adult human gliomas. Neurosurgery 62(2):505–514; discussion 514–505

Phillips, HS Kharbanda, S Chen, R Forrest, WF Soriano, RH Wu, TD Misra, A Nigro, JM Colman, H Soroceanu, L Williams, PM Modrusan, Z Feuerstein, BG and Aldape, K (2006) Molecular subclasses of high-grade glioma predict prognosis, delineate a pattern of disease progression, and resemble stages in neurogenesis. Cancer Cell 9(3):157–173

Pollack, IF Randall, MS Kristofik, MP Kelly, RH Selker, RG and Vertosick, FT, Jr. (1991) Response of low-passage human malignant gliomas in vitro to stimulation and selective inhibition of growth factor-mediated pathways. J Neurosurg 75(2):284–293

Ranza, E Facoetti, A Morbini, P Benericetti, E and Nano, R (2007) Exogenous platelet-derived growth factor (PDGF) induces human astrocytoma cell line proliferation. Anticancer Res 27(4B):2161–2166

Rebetz, J Tian, D Persson, A Widegren, B Salford, LG Englund, E Gisselsson, D and Fan, X (2008) Glial progenitor-like phenotype in low-grade glioma and enhanced CD133-expression and neuronal lineage differentiation potential in high-grade glioma. PLoS ONE 3(4):e1936

Roy, NS Wang, S Harrison-Restelli, C Benraiss, A Fraser, RA Gravel, M Braun, PE and Goldman, SA (1999) Identification, isolation, and promoter-defined separation of mitotic oligodendrocyte progenitor cells from the adult human subcortical white matter. J Neurosci 19(22):9986–9995

Schaar, BT and McConnell, SK (2005) Cytoskeletal coordination during neuronal migration. Proc Natl Acad Sci USA 102(38):13652–13657

Shi, J Marinovich, A and Barres, BA (1998) Purification and characterization of adult oligodendrocyte precursor cells from the rat optic nerve. J Neurosci 18(12):4627–4636

Shih, AH Dai, C Hu, X Rosenblum, MK Koutcher, JA and Holland, EC (2004) Dose-dependent effects of platelet-derived growth factor-B on glial tumorigenesis. Cancer Res 64(14):4783–4789

Shoshan, Y Nishiyama, A Chang, A Mork, S Barnett, GH Cowell, JK Trapp, BD and Staugaitis, SM (1999) Expression of oligodendrocyte progenitor cell antigens by gliomas: implications for the histogenesis of brain tumors. Proc Natl Acad Sci USA 96(18):10361–10366

Singh, SK Clarke, ID Terasaki, M Bonn, VE Hawkins, C Squire, J and Dirks, PB (2003) Identification of a cancer stem cell in human brain tumors. Cancer Res 63(18):5821–5828

Soriano, P (1994) Abnormal kidney development and hematological disorders in PDGF beta-receptor mutant mice. Genes Dev 8(16):1888–1896

Tang, DG Tokumoto, YM and Raff, MC (2000) Long-term culture of purified postnatal oligodendrocyte precursor cells. Evidence for an intrinsic maturation program that plays out over months. J Cell Biol 148(5):971–984

Tchougounova, E Kastemar, M Brasater, D Holland, EC Westermark, B and Uhrbom, L (2007) Loss of Arf causes tumor progression of PDGFB-induced oligodendroglioma. Oncogene 26(43):6289–6296

The Cancer Genome Atlas Research Network, McLendon, R Friedman, A Bigner, D Van Meir, EG Brat, DJ Mastrogianakis, M Olson, JJ Mikkelsen, T Lehman, N Aldape, K Alfred Yung, WK Bogler, O Vandenberg, S Berger, M Prados, M Muzny, D Morgan, M Scherer, S Sabo, A Nazareth, L Lewis, L Hall, O Zhu, Y Ren, Y Alvi, O Yao, J Hawes, A Jhangiani, S Fowler, G San Lucas, A Kovar, C Cree, A Dinh, H Santibanez, J Joshi, V Gonzalez-Garay, ML Miller, CA Milosavljevic, A Donehower, L Wheeler, DA Gibbs, RA Cibulskis, K Sougnez, C Fennell, T Mahan, S Wilkinson, J Ziaugra, L Onofrio, R Bloom, T Nicol, R Ardlie, K Baldwin, J Gabriel, S Lander, ES Ding, L Fulton, RS McLellan, MD Wallis, J Larson, DE Shi, X Abbott, R Fulton, L Chen, K Koboldt, DC Wendl, MC Meyer, R Tang, Y Lin, L Osborne, JR Dunford-Shore, BH Miner, TL Delehaunty, K Markovic, C Swift, G Courtney, W Pohl, C Abbott, S Hawkins, A Leong, S Haipek, C Schmidt, H Wiechert, M Vickery, T Scott, S Dooling, DJ Chinwalla, A Weinstock, GM Mardis, ER Wilson, RK Getz, G Winckler, W Verhaak, RG Lawrence, MS O'Kelly, M Robinson, J Alexe, G Beroukhim, R Carter, S Chiang, D Gould, J Gupta, S Korn, J Mermel, C Mesirov, J Monti, S Nguyen, H Parkin, M Reich, M Stransky, N Weir, BA Garraway, L Golub, T Meyerson, M Chin, L Protopopov, A Zhang, J Perna, I Aronson, S Sathiamoorthy, N Ren, G Wiedemeyer, WR Kim, H Won Kong, S Xiao, Y Kohane, IS Seidman, J Park, PJ Kucherlapati, R Laird, PW Cope, L Herman, JG Weisenberger, DJ Pan, F Van Den Berg, D Van Neste, L Mi Yi, J Schuebel, KE Baylin, SB Absher, DM Li, JZ Southwick, A Brady, S Aggarwal, A Chung, T Sherlock, G Brooks, JD Myers, RM Spellman, PT Purdom, E Jakkula, LR Lapuk, AV Marr, H Dorton, S Gi Choi, Y Han, J Ray, A Wang, V Durinck, S Robinson, M Wang, NJ Vranizan, K Peng, V Van Name, E Fontenay, GV Ngai, J Conboy, JG Parvin, B Feiler, HS Speed, TP Gray, JW Brennan, C Socci, ND Olshen, A Taylor, BS Lash, A Schultz, N Reva, B Antipin, Y Stukalov, A Gross, B Cerami, E Qing Wang, W Qin, LX Seshan, VE Villafania, L Cavatore, M Borsu, L Viale, A Gerald, W Sander, C Ladanyi, M Perou, CM Neil Hayes, D Topal, MD Hoadley, KA Qi, Y Balu, S Shi, Y Wu, J Penny, R Bittner, M Shelton, T Lenkiewicz, E Morris, S Beasley, D Sanders, S Kahn, A Sfeir, R Chen, J Nassau, D Feng, L Hickey, E Weinstein, JN Barker, A Gerhard, DS Vockley, J Compton, C Vaught, J Fielding, P Ferguson, ML Schaefer, C Madhavan, S Buetow, KH Collins, F Good, P Guyer, M Ozenberger, B Peterson, J and Thomson, E (2008) Comprehensive genomic characterization defines human glioblastoma genes and core pathways. Nature 455:1061–1068

Tsai, JW Bremner, KH and Vallee, RB (2007) Dual subcellular roles for LIS1 and dynein in radial neuronal migration in live brain tissue. Nature Neurosci 10(8):970–979

Uhrbom, L Hesselager, G Nister, M and Westermark, B (1998) Induction of brain tumors in mice using a recombinant platelet-derived growth factor B-chain retrovirus. Cancer Res 58(23):5275–5279

Uhrbom, L Hesselager, G Ostman, A Nister, M and Westermark, B (2000) Dependence of autocrine growth factor stimulation in platelet-derived growth factor-B-induced mouse brain tumor cells. Int J Cancer 85(3):398–406

van Heyningen, P Calver, AR and Richardson, WD (2001) Control of progenitor cell number by mitogen supply and demand. Curr Biol 11(4):232–241

Waterfield, MD Scrace, GT Whittle, N Stroobant, P Johnsson, A Wasteson, A Westermark, B Heldin, CH Huang, JS and Deuel, TF (1983) Platelet-derived growth factor is structurally related to the putative transforming protein p28sis of simian sarcoma virus. Nature 304(5921):35–39

Westermark, B Heldin, CH and Nister, M (1995) Platelet-derived growth factor in human glioma. Glia 15(3):257–263

Wolswijk, G and Noble, M (1992) Cooperation between PDGF and FGF converts slowly dividing O-2Aadult progenitor cells to rapidly dividing cells with characteristics of O-2Aperinatal progenitor cells. J Cell Biol 118(4):889–900

Wolswijk, G Riddle, PN and Noble, M (1991) Platelet-derived growth factor is mitogenic for O-2Aadult progenitor cells. Glia 4(5):495–503

Zagzag, D Amirnovin, R Greco, MA Yee, H Holash, J Wiegand, SJ Zabski, S Yancopoulos, GD and Grumet, M (2000) Vascular apoptosis and involution in gliomas precede neovascularization: a novel concept for glioma growth and angiogenesis. Lab Invest 80(6):837–849

Zhu, Y Guignard, F Zhao, D Liu, L Burns, DK Mason, RP Messing, A and Parada, LF (2005) Early inactivation of p53 tumor suppressor gene cooperating with NF1 loss induces malignant astrocytoma. Cancer Cell 8(2):119–130

Chapter 2
Modeling Brain Tumors Using Avian Retroviral Gene Transfer

Tod D. Holland and Eric C. Holland

Abstract RCAS/tv-a is a system for postnatal cell-type-specific gene transfer. It is used for the modeling of gliomas and medulloblastomas. This system provides a combination of lineage tracing from the cell origin with oncogenesis induced by mis-expression of specific genes. The genes that are most potent at inducing tumors are those that encode components of signal transduction and undifferentiated cells are most capable of serving as the cell of origin. The system effectively generates tumors with the histologic characteristics of human disease. Mice bearing RCAS/tv-a-induced brain tumors are currently being used for preclinical trials to understand the biology of therapeutic response in the various cell types that make up gliomas and medulloblastomas.

Contents

E.C. Holland (✉)
Departments of Neurosurgery, Neurology, Surgery and Cancer Biology and Genetics, Memorial Sloan Kettering Cancer Center, 1275 York Avenue, New York, NY 10021, USA
e-mail: hollande@mskcc.org

E.G. Van Meir (ed.), *CNS Cancer*, Cancer Drug Discovery and Development, DOI 10.1007/978-1-60327-553-8_2,

© Humana Press, a part of Springer Science+Business Media, LLC 2009

2.1 History

The history of retroviruses and our understanding of cancer are intertwined and illuminated by some of the most important scientific breakthroughs in the last century. In 1908, Danish scientists Vilhelm Ellerman and Oluf Bang discovered an infectious pathogen that could be transmitted from one chicken to another, a non-cellular pathogen capable of causing cancer. The agent was able to pass through filters designed for cells and bacteria, leading them to the observation that a non-cellular pathogen was inducing cancer (Ellerman and Bang, 1908). A few years later, in 1911, Peyton Rous from Rockefeller University made a related observation by identifying a similar pathogen, naming it the Rous sarcoma virus (RSV). Peyton Rous was awarded the Nobel Prize for his discovery, the first identifiable retrovirus (Rous, 1911).

Between 1911 and 1960, many other cancer-causing viruses were identified and cataloged. The viruses were named after either the species that were their hosts or the tumor types that they caused. It became apparent, even before the mechanisms were understood, that these viruses were highly specific to the target hosts that they are able to infect. This newfound study of cancer-causing viruses brought about an understanding of this universal phenomenon that could be observed in mammalian and avian organisms. The concept that cancer was caused by an infectious agent was a natural thought process that followed the discoveries of multiple external agents responsible for disease throughout the eighteenth and nineteenth centuries, including the vaccination work against smallpox by Edward Jenner in 1796. The concept of cancer being caused by an infectious agent had the unwanted consequence of sending researchers on the wrong track, since we now know that most human cancers are not caused by viruses but rather from "within" (see below).

The structure and function of DNA, proposed by James Watson and Francis Crick in 1953, postulated that information flowed in a set pattern that would begin from DNA transcribed to RNA, which would be the blueprint to form proteins. This central dogma was widely accepted to be invariant in every organism and implied that something that changed a cell's phenotype (such as a virus) would necessarily require that its genetic information be stored in the form of DNA (Watson and Crick, 1953). However, in 1959, Howard Temin found the first exception to this rule while doing research for his PhD thesis on RSV and other viruses that would soon be compiled into a family known as Retroviridae. His viral stocks were absent of DNA and appeared to use RNA as their genome, implying that retroviruses did not replicate themselves in the set pattern described in the Central Dogma. As a graduate student, Temin had managed to prove that there were viruses that could replicate through a process he called reverse transcription. The reason it was called as such was due to the fact that replication seemed to occur in reverse, using a single strand of RNA to form double-stranded DNA (Temin and Rubin, 1958). Furthermore, before Temin's work, it was unclear whether a virus was a quantal unit or a solution with transforming potential. He proved that viruses were actually particles capable of transforming the phenotype of an infected cell and all of its progeny. Temin also proved the existence of the enzyme that was responsible for reverse transcription, which he called reverse transcriptase. This enzyme was isolated by David Baltimore, who shared the Nobel Prize with Howard Temin for this work (Temin, 1964).

The nature of the transforming potential of retroviruses became evident after the technology to identify the specific sequence of nucleic acids was invented. In the 1970s, Harold Varmus, Mike Bishop, and colleagues identified the general structure of retroviral genomes as having two repeated sequences on the ends and three viral genes, *gag*, *pol*, and *env*. However, in the case of the tumor-forming viruses, there was another gene downstream of *env* that turned out to be responsible for the induction of the transformed phenotype. In the case of RSV, the gene was called *Src* and referred to as an oncogene because it caused cancer (Stehelin et al., 1976). Further experiments showed that this fourth gene was different from virus to virus, and unlike the other viral genes, the oncogene was closely related to a cellular gene found in the cells of the host animal that the virus previously infected. These oncogenes appeared to be stolen from the host genome and then expressed either in the wrong cell type or in an unregulated manner by the virus leading to the formation of cancer (Kurth, 1983). The realization that our own genes caused cancer and that cancer was a product formed from within us changed the way we think about this disease and led to Varmus and Bishop being awarded the Nobel Prize for their work (Bishop, 1983).

The collection of genes expressed as oncogenes from the known retroviruses was then catalogued, and the functions of the normal cellular homologues (proto-oncogenes) were identified. These cellular proto-oncogenes were found to encode the components of signal transduction pathways involved in both the proliferation and the inhibition of apoptosis. These gene products cover the entire spectrum from overexpression of ligands such as PDGF (v-SIS) to mutant active receptors such as EGFR (v-erbB), to constitutively active downstream components such as Ras and Akt, and transcription factors such as Myc, Jun, and Fos (Pech et al., 1989). Because of their natural ability to function as tumor-inducing agents, retroviruses became prime candidates for the creation of genetically engineered tumorigenic vectors that could be designed to transfer any gene and test its ability to induce tumor formation. In the 1990s, RSV was turned into a viral vector by Steve Hughes. The *Src* gene was replaced by any gene of interest that was less than 2.5 kb (due to packaging constraints) and became known as the replication-competent ALV splice acceptor, or RCAS in short (Petropoulos and Hughes, 1991).

2.2 RCAS

The most commonly used version of RCAS is based on the subgroup A avian leukosis (ALV) viruses. The cell surface receptor that permits ALV-A subgroup infection of host cells is limited to birds (Coffin et al., 1997). The genetic locus that encodes the receptor for subgroup A viruses is referred to as tv-a, or tumor virus-a. This gene was cloned from quail cells by Bates, Young, and Varmus using expression cloning from quail DNA into mouse cells and identified by its ability to confer susceptibility to RCAS infection (Bates et al., 1993). When expressed in mammalian cells, this gene product, tv-a, allows the infection by RCAS vectors and subsequent expression of whatever gene is inserted downstream of the *env* gene. Furthermore, due to splicing differences between avian and mammalian cells, the mRNAs that encode the viral gene products *gag, pol*, and *env* are unstable and produce essentially no protein. The overall result is receptor-mediated gene targeting to mammalian cells engineered to express tv-a. Federspiel and Hughes were the first to demonstrate the specificity of this system in transgenic mice. They showed that RCAS vectors expressing the marker gene alkaline phosphatase would specifically infect myocytes of mice transgenic for expression of tv-a from a muscle-specific promoter (Federspiel et al., 1994).

2.3 Retroviral Life Cycle

The life cycle of a retrovirus is comprised of a series of steps through which the virus replicates itself and its genetic information (Figure 2.1 and Color Plate 4). Genetically engineered retroviruses are called "ecotropic" when they can only infect host cells of the same species as the natural hosts of the wild-type virus and "xenotropic" when they can only infect cells from species that differ from its natural host. "Amphotropic" viruses are capable of infecting both host cells and cells of other species (Katen et al., 2001). It is largely due to the polytropic characteristics of amphotropic viruses that diseases can transfer from one species to another. Two examples of cross-species disease transfer are seen in the HIV virus (monkey to human) and the virus that causes SARS (avian to human) (Marx et al., 2001). Retroviruses have two identical copies of single-stranded RNA, called a capsid and an outer envelope comprised of glycoproteins used in the docking of the virus to the host cell. The envelope glycoproteins interact in a highly specific manner, allowing them to dock only to a corresponding receptor protein on the membrane of the cell. For example, avian sarcoma and leucosis viruses and mouse mammary tumor virus infect in a species-specific manner (DeLarco and Todaro, 1976).

The binding of the virion to the cell membrane marks the first stage in viral replication. Following the binding stage, the viral glycoproteins fuse to the cell membrane without undergoing endocytosis. Upon successful completion of the envelope–membrane fusion, the nucleocapsid (the viral equivalent of a nucleus) makes its way into the cytoplasm of the host cell. Deoxynucleoside triphosphates (dNTPs) enter the nucleocapsid, where the process of reverse transcription is carried out by Temin and Baltimore's famous enzyme, reverse transcriptase. Reverse transcriptase, as well as several other proteins, begins the conversion from the virus' single-stranded RNA to a piece of double-stranded DNA copy (Baltimore, 1970).

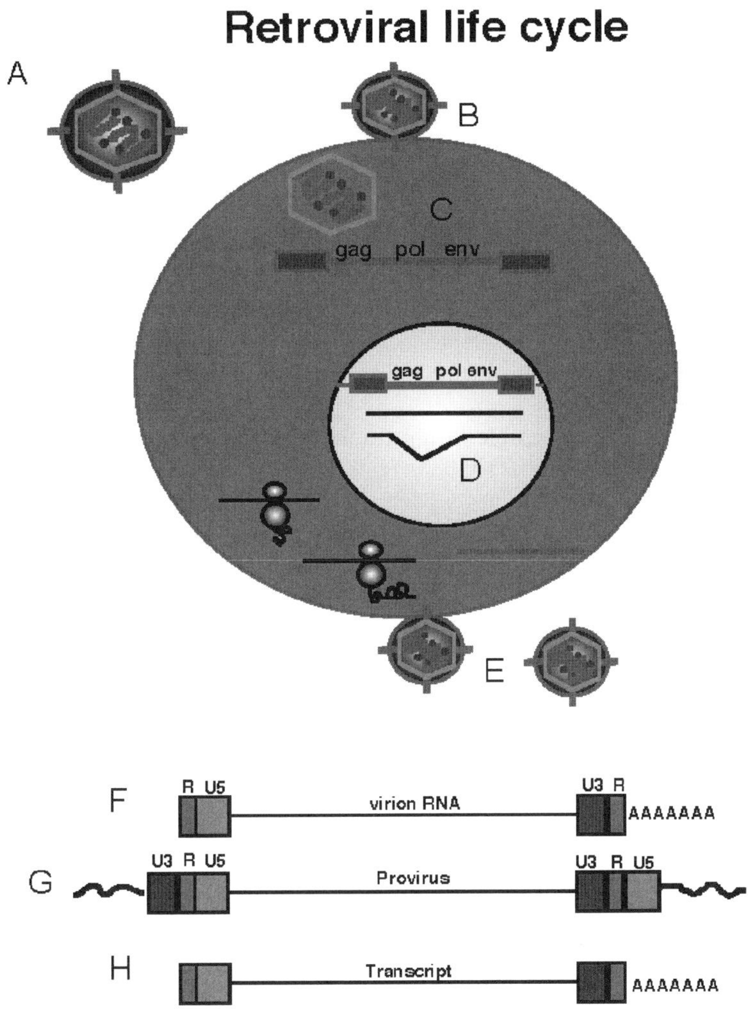

Fig. 2.1 Retroviral virion (**A**) binds to the target cell via interaction of envelope protein with its receptor (**B**). The nucleocapsid enters the cytoplasm and RNA genome (**F**) is converted to double-stranded DNA (**C**), which is integrated into the genome as a provirus (**G**) and transcribed (**D, H**). The proviral transcripts are translated into viral proteins and full-length transcripts serve as the viral genome of the next generation of virus (**E**) (*see* Color Plate 4)

The DNA is synthesized beginning at the U3 region of the strand, which holds the enhancer and promoter elements. The R region at the 5′ LTR contains the transcription start site, and the RNA processing signal lies at the 3′ end. Proviral transcription gives rise to a single primary transcript, some of which will be spliced in order to produce alternative subgenomic messenger RNAs (Coffin et al., 1997). The viral transcripts will be exported out of the nucleus and synthesized into proteins. These viral proteins will be transported along the secretory pathway to the packaging site and along with two copies of the DNA (Mulligan, 1993).

Upon synthesizing this DNA molecule, it is transported directly into the nucleus of the host cell. From this stage, integrase (coded by the *pol* gene) allows for the integration of the DNA into one of many possible sites. The extensive number of integration sites is directly related to the size of the host cell's genome. The newly integrated viral DNA, now called a provirus, is transcribed using the host cell's RNA polymerase, generating mRNA and genomic RNA molecules (Mikkers and Berns, 2003). It is at this stage that the machinery of the host cell translates the viral mRNA copied from the provirus to glycoproteins and nucleocapsid proteins, identical to that which initiated the procedure (Mulligan, 1993).

The nucleocapsids assemble with genomic RNA to generate several progeny nucleocapsids, also identical to the original retrovirus that catalyzed the infection. The new progeny nucleocapsids interact with membrane-bound viral glycoproteins, restoring the progeny to their full form. The host-cell membrane buds out and the progeny virions are expelled to begin the entire process again. The only difference between the initial infecting agent and its second-generation progeny is the sheer number of virions that can be produced from a single pathogen infecting a single cell (Mikkers and Berns, 2003).

2.4 Tv-a Transgenic Mice

In order for RCAS to be able to effectively infect mice cells, it is essential that they express the avian tv-a receptor (Federspeil et al., 1994). This is achieved by genetically altering the mouse cells so as to make them express the receptor used by the retrovirus, either by in vitro transfection or by creating a transgenic mouse. As noted above, the tv-a expression in mammals does not occur, so infection with RCAS vectors will only happen if the mammal is transgenically modified to express tv-a in order for susceptibility to RCAS to occur. Usually, there is no obvious phenotype expressed by tv-a expression, because its only effect is to force susceptibility to RCAS (Fisher et al., 1999). Several transgenic mice have been generated that express tv-a from a variety of tissue-specific promoters, including those from the *GFAP* (glial fibrillary acidic protein) and *nestin* genes which direct expression of tv-a in brain tissue (Holland and Varmus, 1998, Holland et al., 1998) (Figure 2.2 and Color Plate 5).

The cell type that is infectable is defined by the promoter that drives the tv-a gene. This gives the opportunity to control the cell of origin in RCAS/tv-a modeling experiments. For example, the first tv-a transgenic mice used for brain tumor modeling drove the tv-a gene from the *GFAP* promoter. The second line drove tv-a from the *nestin* promoter (Holland et al., 1998). Comparison between the two demonstrated that properties of the two cell populations in

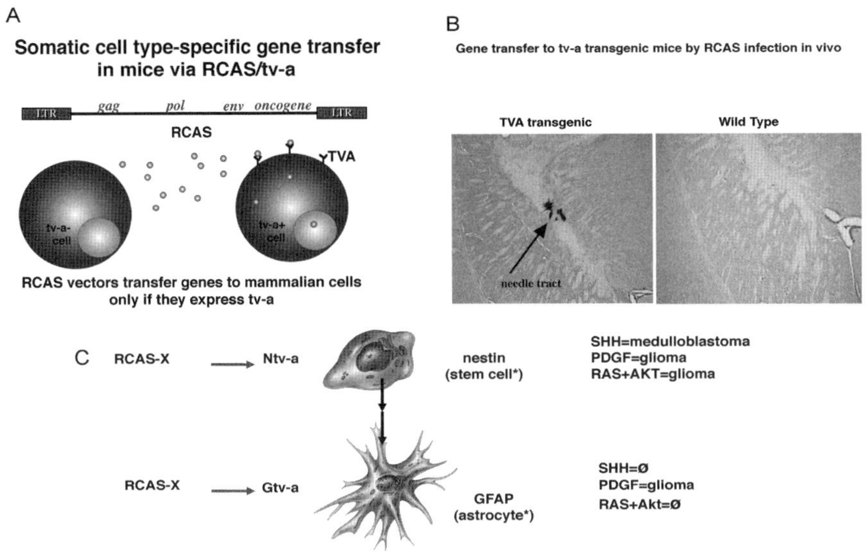

Fig. 2.2 RCAS/tv-a-based somatic cell gene transfer. RCAS vectors are engineered to encode a gene downstream of the *env* gene and will only infect mammalian cells if they express the RCAS receptor TVA (**A**). Mice are engineered to express tv-a as a transgene limiting gene transfer to specific cell types in a receptor-mediated gene transfer (**B**). Depending on the specificity of the promoter that drives tv-a expression, specific cell types or differentiation states can be targeted (**C**) (*see* Color Plate 5)

vivo controlled their ability to form tumors from one oncogenic stimulus or another. Generally speaking, less differentiated cells are more capable of serving as the cell of origin for gliomas in an otherwise wild-type background. Loss of tumor suppressor genes changes the spectrum of tumors that form and enables some cell types to form tumors that were otherwise not able to do so (see Section 2.5.2).

2.5 Modeling Brain Tumors with RCAS/tv-a

The main advantage of somatic cell gene transfer is modeling gain of function mutations as these are the genes that are typically carried on the RCAS vector. As noted above, the neutral experiment done by nature of identifying genes that cause cancer when carried on retroviruses identified a predominance of genes encoding signal transduction components. This is the case for experimental modeling of tumor formation with these vectors. Both gliomas (Dai and Holland, 2001) and medulloblastomas (Rao et al., 2004) are modeled effectively by gene transfer of genes encoding signaling components involved in cell–cell interaction and differentiation and development of the CNS.

2.5.1 Gliomas

There have been a significant amount of knowledge and information gained on the development of medulloblastomas and gliomas in recent years. Gliomas probably form from stem cells or progenitors and are driven by the signaling pathways that drive normal development in the CNS such as PDGF and downstream effectors such as RAS and Akt. The most potent oncogene in the formation of gliomas is the PDGFB ligand (Dai et al., 2001). Several systems including RCAS/tv-a have shown that the histology of glial tumors induced by PDGF is that of a diffuse glioma with oligodendroglioma characteristics, including oval-shaped cells with the "fried egg" white halo appearance and the full secondary structures of Scherer. There appears to be a correlation with the amount of PDGF expression and the grade of the tumors, ranging from either low-grade gliomas to those having anaplastic features such as pseudopalisading necrosis and microvascular proliferation (Shih et al., 2004). The bulk of the cells in these tumors shows low Akt activity and GFAP expression consistent with their counterparts in humans. The activation of Akt by infection with constitutively active Akt leads to the formation of cells with more astrocytic histology with irregular nuclei, cytoplasm staining for GFAP, and astrocytic morphology (Uhrbom et al., 2002).

The activation of the MAP Kinase pathway by constitutively active Ras in and of itself is not capable of forming gliomas from either GFAP- or nestin-expressing cells using the RCAS/tv-a system. However, coinfection of nestin but not GFAP-expressing cells with both constitutively active Ras and constitutively active Akt leads to astrocytic gliomas (Holland et al., 2000).

2.5.2 Loss of Function, Knockouts, and Cre/lox

Loss of tumor suppressor genes are common events in the progression of gliomas in humans. Although the RCAS system is designed for gain of function experiments, it can be adapted to additionally investigate the consequences of tumor suppressor loss as well. The easiest approach is to cross the tv-a transgenic mice to mice strains with germline deletion of the tumor suppressors in question and compare the tumor formation seen with RCAS vectors to mice wild type for that tumor suppressor.

Mice deficient in the tumor suppressor locus *INK4a/Arf* are particularly susceptible to brain tumor formation. Tv-a transgenic mice with an *ink4a/arf* −/− background form gliomas at a considerably higher frequency than wild-type mice upon RCAS-mediated *PDGF* gene transfer. Furthermore, the histology of the tumors that form in this background shows that they are of higher grade than if *INK4a/arf* is intact. The data indicate that loss of *ink4a/arf* in humans during glioma progression is likely to enhance the oncogenic effects of PDGF signaling and lead to malignant histology (Figure 2.3 and Color Plate 6).

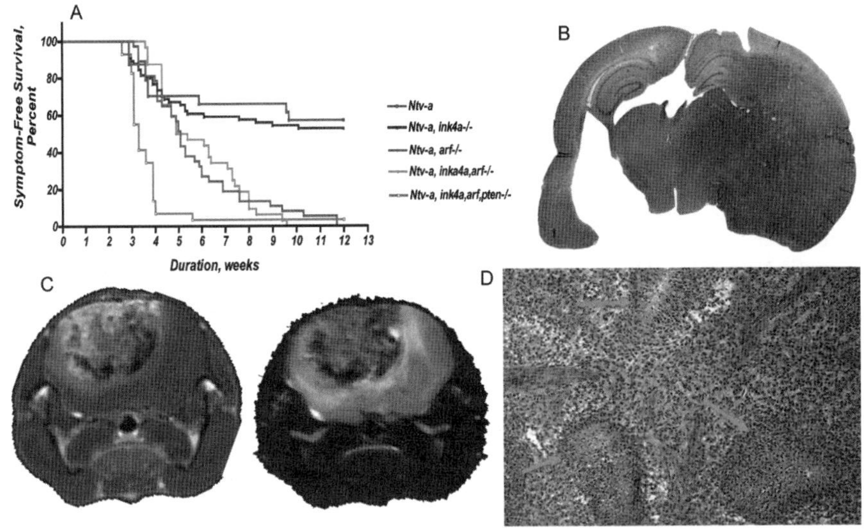

Fig. 2.3 Glioma formation with the RCAS/tv-a system. (**A**) Survival curves for mice of different genetic backgrounds infected with RCAS-PDGF demonstrating cooperativity between gain of function oncogenes and loss of tumor suppressors. (**B**) Whole mount H&E-stained section of mouse brain harboring large high-grade glioma. (**C**) T1 with contrast and T2-weighted MRI scans of a necrotic contrast enhancing high-grade glioma (courtesy of Brian Ross U. Mich.). (**D**) H&E section of high-grade tumor demonstrating microvascular proliferation and pseudopalisading necrosis (*green arrows*) (*see* Color Plate 6)

In the case of Ras-driven oncogenesis, loss of *ink4a/arf* enables Ras to form tumors that are similar to those obtained with the co-activation of the Akt and Ras pathways (Uhrbom et al., 2002).

In a similar way, the p53 tumor suppressor has been investigated by crossing tv-a transgenic mice to a p53-deficient background. Tumor protein 53, or p53, is important in multicellular eukaryotic organisms, and its main functions are cell cycle regulation and apoptosis control. Due to its role in maintaining the rate at which cells undergo mitosis, it functions as a tumor suppressor involved in the prevention of cancerous malignancies. p53 has been called the "guardian of the genome" for its role in conserving genetic stability by preventing genomic DNA damage (Lane, 1992). When this gene is knocked out, the mouse becomes susceptible to various types of gene mutations, thereby deactivating and removing the "guardian angel" effect that p53 has over the DNA (Xu et al., 2001). Loss of p53 results in increased penetrance and grade in RCAS/tv-a-induced gliomas. The effect is most pronounced in tumors derived from a nestin-expressing cell of origin.

Homozygous loss of some tumor suppressors, which are critical in glioma progression, such as PTEN, is embryonically lethal, rendering the above approach obsolete (Penninger and Woodgett, 2001). In this case, conditional knockout of the locus can be achieved with RCAS gene transfer. This process uses cre–lox recombination with the site-specific gene recombinase cre that catalyzes recombination between two specific and identical sites in the DNA, called the lox p sites. The core sequence flanked by the lox sites (or floxed) is then deleted when the two lox sites are recombined. The *PTEN* gene was floxed by knocking in a floxed version of PTEN to the endogenous locus resulting in a functional PTEN allele that could be deleted by cre expression. The RCAS vector has also been engineered to carry the cre recombinase, and cells from mice with the floxed PTEN allele that are infected with RCAS-cre subsequently delete PTEN (Hu et al., 2005). Loss of PTEN in this context enhances glioma formation in both PDGF- and Ras-driven gliomas derived from RCAS/tv-a technology.

2.5.3 Medulloblastomas – SHH Signaling

Medulloblastomas probably arise from stem cells in the rhombic lip and external granule cell layer of the brain, and at least some of these tumors are driven by the SHH signaling pathway that gives rise to formation of the normal cerebellum (Weiner et al., 2002). Mouse models of medulloblastomas have been generated by activating this pathway using several methods such as SHH overexpression, loss of PTC, and activation of SMO. In addition, loss of function of the DNA damage repair pathways contributes substantially to these SHH medulloblastomas such as loss of p53, Lig4, or Chk2.

Medulloblastomas are modeled using the RCAS/tv-a system. Originally, it was recognized that myc was insufficient to cause these tumors but that myc overexpression created nests of undifferentiated cells (Fults et al., 2002). Then SHH gene transfer with RCAS vectors into nestin-expressing cells of the rhombic lip created medulloblastomas in a minority of mice (Rao et al., 2004). This incidence of medulloblastoma formation was increased by several genes including Myc, Akt, and IGF2 (Rao et al., 2003). Although the incidence of tumors formed is increased by additional gene transfer, the incidence of medulloblastomas remains significantly below that seen with PDGF gene transfer to generate gliomas in this modeling system (Hambardzumyan et al., 2008).

It is possible that cell types other than nestin-expressing cells can serve as the cell of origin for these tumors. For example, math-1-expressing cells of the external granule cell layer can give rise to medulloblastomas using other genetic modification strategies (Yang et al., 2008). This is a good example of how various modeling strategies give different complementary results. It is likely that there are several cell types that can give rise to brain tumors and the development of further strains of transgenic mice with tv-a driven by other CNS cell population-specific promoters is expected to permit to derive models for any tumor type in the brain.

2.6 Imaging, Stem Cell Niches, and Preclinical Trials

The use of RCAS/tv-a-induced brain tumors in preclinical trials has been made possible by the development of several imaging technologies that allow each mouse to serve as its own control (Momota and Holland 2005). Bioluminescence imaging (BLI) has been developed in other systems to follow the fate of cells in vivo noninvasively. The most commonly used source of light production for BLI is the *firefly luciferase* gene that can be expressed from a tissue-specific promoter or a promoter that responds to a signaling pathway that is critical to the biology of the tumor. The mice are then injected with the substrate for luciferase, luciferin, and the enzyme cleaves luciferin in an ATP-dependent manner. The light is quantified by a CCD camera and is a direct and noninvasive readout of the activity of the promoter that drives luciferase expression (Momota et al., 2005).

BLI was used to generate a reporter mouse that would read out cell cycle proliferation using the *E2F1* gene promoter. This mouse emitted light from PDGF-driven gliomas allowing identification of mice with tumors and a non-invasive measure of therapeutic effect (Uhrbom et al., 2004). A second reporter line was generated that expressed luciferase from a Gli responsive promoter which is a downstream readout of SHH signaling. Not surprisingly, this background gives off light from SHH-driven medulloblastomas as well (Figure 2.4 and Color Plate 7). The strength of such reporter systems is in showing the activity of pathways not previously known to be activated in a given tumor type. In this case, PDGF-induced gliomas also produced light; the tumors produce the SHH ligand from trapped and reactive astrocytes (Becher et al., 2008).

Several trials have been performed with the mice harboring RCAS-induced gliomas and medulloblastomas. In PDGF-induced gliomas, the effect of PDGFR and mTOR inhibition was shown to result in cell cycle arrest but not death (Uhrbom et al., 2004). Temozolomide had a modest effect on survival of these tumors and proliferation, but little immediate effect on the histological appearance of the tumors (Momota et al., 2005, McConville et al., 2007). Similar to what is seen in human gliomas, a radiation dose of 2 Gy had little effect on any cell type in these tumors and increasing the dose to 10 Gy was needed to achieve an effect, which was mainly cell cycle arrest.

In contrast to the relative resistance of glioma to radiation, medulloblastomas in a wild-type p53 background show substantial killing with 2 Gy and cell cycle arrest only in the perivascular niche. These surviving cells activate Akt in the process of arresting and blockade of Akt prior to radiation sensitizes these cells resulting in fewer perivascular cells surviving radiation (Hambardzumyan et al., 2008).

Cells with stem cell properties have been shown to exist in the perivascular structures of both medulloblastomas and gliomas (Calabrese et al., 2007). In the RCAS/tv-a models of these tumors, resistant cells with stem-like properties also exist in the same region allowing these models to serve as excellent systems for understanding the importance of such cells in the biology of these tumors and

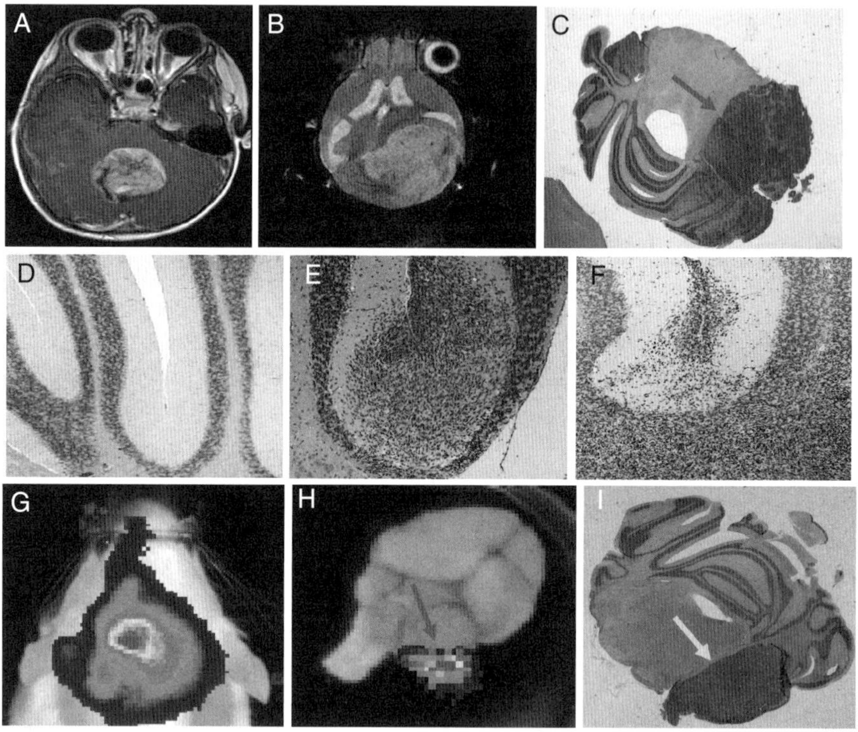

Fig. 2.4 RCAS/tv-a-mediated medulloblastoma and bioluminescence imaging. (**A**) MRI scan of human medulloblastoma. (**B**) MRI scan of RCAS–SHH-induced medulloblastoma (courtesy of Jason Koutcher MSKCC) with (**C**) H&E-stained whole mount. (**D**) Normal adult cerebellum. (**E**) Cluster of cells trapped in the region of the external granule cell layer by SHH autocrine signaling showing proliferation by Ki67 staining (**F**). Medulloblastoma bearing mouse in a gli-luciferase reporter background (**G**). Brain removed from mouse showing light production arising from the medulloblastoma (**H**) shown on whole mount (**I**) (*see* Color Plate 7)

their response to treatment. Furthermore, RCAS/tv-a models for brain tumors provide the ability to modulate the genetics of the specific cell types and treat the tumors with therapies that parallel the treatments given to humans (Hambardzumyan et al., 2007).

Acknowledgments The authors would like to thank Eletha Carbajal for help with editing the text and Dolores Hambardzumyan and Oren Becher for histology and imaging figures. We would also like to thank Peter Canoll for his careful reading of the manuscript.

References

Baltimore D. RNA-dependent DNA polymerase in virions of RNA tumour viruses. Nature. 1970, 226(252):1209–11.

Bates P, Young JA, Varmus HE. A receptor for subgroup A Rous sarcoma virus is related to the low density lipoprotein receptor. Cell. 1993 Sep 24; 74(6):1043–51.

Becher OJ, Hambardzumyan D, Fomchenko EI, Momota H, Mainwaring L, Bleau AM, Katz AM, Edgar M, Kenney AM, Cordon-Cardo C, Blasberg RG, Holland EC. Gli activity correlates with tumor grade in platelet-derived growth factor-induced gliomas. Cancer Res. 2008 Apr 1; 68(7):2241–9.

Bishop JM. Cellular oncogenes and retroviruses. Annu Rev Biochem. 1983, 52:301–54.

Calabrese C, Poppleton H, Kocak M, Hogg TL, Fuller C, Hamner B, Oh EY, Gaber MW, Finklestein D, Allen M, Frank A, Bayazitov IT, Zakharenko SS, Gajjar A, Davidoff A, Gilbertson RJ. A perivascular niche for brain tumor stem cells. Cancer Cell. 2007 Jan; 11(1):69–82.

Coffin JM, Hughes SH et al. *Retroviruses*. Plainview, N.Y., Cold Spring Harbor Laboratory Press, 1997.

DeLarco J, Todaro GJ. Membrane receptors for murine leukemia viruses: characterization using the purified viral envelope glycoprotein, gp71. Cell. 1976 Jul; 8(3):365–71.

Dai C, Holland EC. Glioma models. Biochim Biophys Acta. 2001 Aug 31; 1551(1):M19–27. Review.

Dai C, Celestino JC, Okada Y, Louis DN, Fuller GN, Holland EC. PDGF autocrine stimulation dedifferentiates cultured astrocytes and induces oligodendrogliomas and oligoastrocytomas from neural progenitors and astrocytes in vivo. Genes Dev. 2001 Aug 1; 15(15):1913–25.

Ellerman V, Bang O. Experimentelle Leukämie bei Hühnern. Zentralbl Bakteriol Parasitenkd Infectionskr Hyg. Abt Orig. 1908; 46:595.

Federspiel MJ, Bates P, Young JA, Varmus HE, Hughes SH. A system for tissue-specific gene targeting: transgenic mice susceptible to subgroup A avian leukosis virus-based retroviral vectors. Proc Natl Acad Sci USA. 1994 Nov 8; 91(23):11241–5.

Fisher GH, et al. Development of a flexible and specific gene delivery system for production of murine tumor models. Oncogene 1999; 18:5253–5260.

Fults D, Pedone C, Dai C, Holland EC. MYC expression promotes the proliferation of neural progenitor cells in culture and in vivo. Neoplasia. 2002 Jan–Feb; 4(1):32–9.

Hambardzumyan D, Lyustikman Y, Holland EC. An update on mouse brain tumor models in cancer drug discovery. Expert Opin Drug Discovery. 2007 Nov; 2(11) 1435–51.

Hambardzumyan D, Becher OJ, Rosenblum MK, Pandolfi PP, Manova-Todorova K, Holland EC. PI3K pathway regulates survival of cancer stem cells residing in the perivascular niche following radiation in medulloblastoma in vivo. Genes Dev. 2008 Feb 15; 22(4):436–48.

Holland EC, Varmus HE. Basic fibroblast growth factor induces cell migration and proliferation after glia-specific gene transfer in mice. Proc Natl Acad Sci USA. 1998 Feb 3; 95(3):1218–23.

Holland EC, Hively WP, DePinho RA, Varmus HE. A constitutively active epidermal growth factor receptor cooperates with disruption of G1 cell-cycle arrest pathways to induce glioma-like lesions in mice. Genes Dev. 1998 Dec 1; 12(23):3675–85.

Holland EC, Celestino J, Dai C, Schaefer L, Sawaya RE, Fuller GN. Combined activation of Ras and Akt in neural progenitors induces glioblastoma formation in mice. Nat Genet. 2000 May; 25(1):55–7.

Hu X, Pandolfi PP, Li Y, Koutcher JA, Rosenblum M, Holland EC. mTOR promotes survival and astrocytic characteristics induced by Pten/AKT signaling in glioblastoma. Neoplasia. 2005 Apr; 7(4):356–68.

Katen LJ, Januszeski MM, Anderson WF, Hasenkrug KJ, Evans LH. Infectious entry by amphotropic as well as ecotropic murine leukemia viruses occurs through an endocytic pathway. J Virol. 2001 Jun; 75(11):5018–26.

Kurth R. Oncogenes in retroviruses and cells. Naturwissenschaften. 1983 Sep; 70(9):439–50. Review.

Lane DP. Cancer. p53, guardian of the genome. Nature. 1992 Jul 2; 358(6381):15–6.

Marx PA, Alcabes PG, Drucker E. Serial human passage of simian immunodeficiency virus by unsterile injections and the emergence of epidemic human immunodeficiency virus in Africa. Philos Trans R Soc Lond B Biol Sci. 2001 Jun 29; 356(1410):911–20.

McConville P, Hambardzumyan D, Moody JB, Leopold WR, Kreger AR, Woolliscroft MJ, Rehemtulla A, Ross BD, Holland EC. Magnetic resonance imaging determination of tumor grade and early response to temozolomide in a genetically engineered mouse model of glioma.Clin Cancer Res. 2007 May 15; 13(10):2897–904.

Mikkers H, Berns A. Retroviral insertional mutagenesis: tagging cancer pathways. Adv Cancer Res. 2003; 88:53–99. Review.

Momota H, Holland EC. Bioluminescence technology for imaging cell proliferation. Curr Opin Biotechnol. 2005 Dec; 16(6):681–6.

Momota H, Nerio E, Holland EC. Perifosine inhibits multiple signaling pathways in glial progenitors and cooperates with temozolomide to arrest cell proliferation in gliomas in vivo. Cancer Res. 2005 Aug 15; 65(16):7429–35.

Mulligan RC. The basic science of gene therapy. Science. 1993 May 14; 260(5110):926–32. Review.

Pech M, Gazit A, Arnstein P, Aaronson SA. Generation of fibrosarcomas in vivo by a retrovirus that expresses the normal B chain of platelet-derived growth factor and mimics the alternative splice pattern of the v-sis oncogene. Proc Natl Acad Sci USA. 1989 Apr; 86(8):2693–7.

Penninger JM, Woodgett J. Stem cells. PTEN – coupling tumor suppression to stem cells? Science. 2001 Dec 7; 294(5549):2116–8.

Petropoulos CJ, Hughes SH. Replication-competent retrovirus vectors for the transfer and expression of gene cassettes in avian cells. J Virol. 1991 Jul; 65(7):3728–37.

Rao G, Pedone CA, Coffin CM, Holland EC, Fults DW. c-Myc enhances sonic hedgehog-induced medulloblastoma formation from nestin-expressing neural progenitors in mice. Neoplasia. 2003 May–Jun; 5(3):198–204.

Rao G, Pedone CA, Valle LD, Reiss K, Holland EC, Fults DW. Sonic hedgehog and insulin-like growth factor signaling synergize to induce medulloblastoma formation from nestin-expressing neural progenitors in mice. Oncogene. 2004; 23:6156–62.

Rous, P. A sarcoma of the fowl transmissible by an agent separable from the tumor cells. J Exp Med. 1911; 13:397–411.

Shih AH, Dai C, Hu X, Rosenblum MK, Koutcher JA, Holland EC. Dose-dependent effects of platelet-derived growth factor-B on glial tumorigenesis. Cancer Res. 2004 Jul 15; 64(14):4783–9.

Stehelin D, Varmus HE, Bishop JM, Vogt PK. DNA related to the transforming gene(s) of avian sarcoma viruses is present in normal avian DNA. Nature. 1976 Mar 11; 260(5547): 170–3.

Temin HM. Nature of the provirus of Rous sarcoma. Natl Cancer Inst Monogr. 1964; 17:557–70.

Temin HM, Rubin H. Characteristics of an assay for Rous sarcoma virus and Rous sarcoma cells in tissue culture. Virology. 1958 Dec; 6(3):669–88.

Uhrbom L, Dai C, Celestino JC, Rosenblum MK, Fuller GN, Holland EC. *Ink4a-Arf* loss cooperates with KRas activation in astrocytes and neural progenitors to generate glioblastomas of various morphologies depending on amount of Akt activity. Cancer Res. 2002 Oct 1; 62(19):5551–8.

Uhrbom L, Nerio E, Holland EC. Dissecting tumor maintenance requirements using bioluminescence imaging of cell proliferation in a mouse glioma model. Nat Med. 2004 Nov; 10(11):1257–60. Epub 2004 Oct 24.

Watson JD, Crick FHC. A structure for deoxyribose nucleic acid. Nature. 1953; 171:737–8.

Weiner HL, Bakst R, Hurlbert MS, Ruggiero J, Ahn E, Lee WS, Stephen D, Zagzag D, Joyner AL, Turnbull DH. Induction of medulloblastomas in mice by sonic hedgehog, independent of Gli1. Cancer Res. 2002 Nov 15; 62(22):6385–9.

Xu GW, Nutt CL, Zlatescu MC, Keeney M, Chin-Yee I, Cairncross JG. Inactivation of p53 sensitizes U87MG glioma cells to 1,3-bis(2-chloroethyl)-1-nitrosourea. Cancer Res. 2001 May 15; 61(10):4155–9.

Yang ZJ, Ellis T, Markant SL, Read TA, Kessler JD, Bourboulas M, Schüller U, Machold R, Fishell G, Rowitch DH, Wainwright BJ, Wechsler-Reya RJ. Medulloblastoma can be initiated by deletion of Patched in lineage-restricted progenitors or stem cells. Cancer Cell. 2008 Aug 12; 14(2):135–45.

Chapter 3
Using Neurofibromatosis Type 1 Mouse Models to Understand Human Pediatric Low-Grade Gliomas

David H. Gutmann

Abstract Neurofibromatosis type 1 (NF1) is the most common genetic cause for low-grade glioma in children and accounts for 15% of all reported cases of World Health Organization (WHO) grade I astrocytomas. Children with NF1 develop low-grade pilocytic astrocytomas most frequently along the anterior optic pathway with a mean age at diagnosis of 4.5 years. Recent advances in mouse genetic engineering have resulted in the generation of *Nf1* mutant mice that form low-grade glial tumors involving the optic nerve and chiasm. These genetically engineered mice have been instructive in identifying the key growth control pathways that regulate glial cell survival and proliferation as well as defining how the tumor microenvironment modulates tumor formation and growth in a temporally and spatially restricted pattern. Lastly, *Nf1* mutant mice are now being employed in preclinical therapeutic studies in which new therapies can be evaluated prior to testing in children.

Contents

D.H. Gutmann (✉)
Department of Neurology, Washington University School of Medicine,
Box 8111; 660 South Euclid Avenue, Saint Louis MO 63110, USA
e-mail: gutmannd@wustl.edu

E.G. Van Meir (ed.), *CNS Cancer*, Cancer Drug Discovery
and Development, DOI 10.1007/978-1-60327-553-8_3,
© Humana Press, a part of Springer Science+Business Media, LLC 2009

3.1 Pediatric Low-Grade Glioma

Unlike adults, children are most commonly affected by low-grade glial neoplasms (astrocytomas). The vast majority of these low-grade astrocytomas are classified by the World Health Organization (WHO) as grade I pilocytic astrocytomas (Louis et al. 2007). Pilocytic astrocytomas (PAs) are characterized by a biphasic histologic appearance in which bipolar cells and Rosenthal fibers alternate with more loosely packed areas composed of multipolar cells associated with microcysts and eosinophilic deposits (Fig. 3.1 and Color Plate 8). These astrocytic tumors are immunoreactive for glial fibrillary acidic protein (GFAP) expression and exhibit low to moderate cellularity. Macroscopically, these tumors may form intratumoral cysts which can be seen on magnetic resonance imaging (MRI).

Microscopically, PAs have rare mitotic figures and low mitotic (proliferative) indices, consistent with their relatively indolent growth rates. Despite their slow growth rates, these low-grade tumors are frequently highly vascular

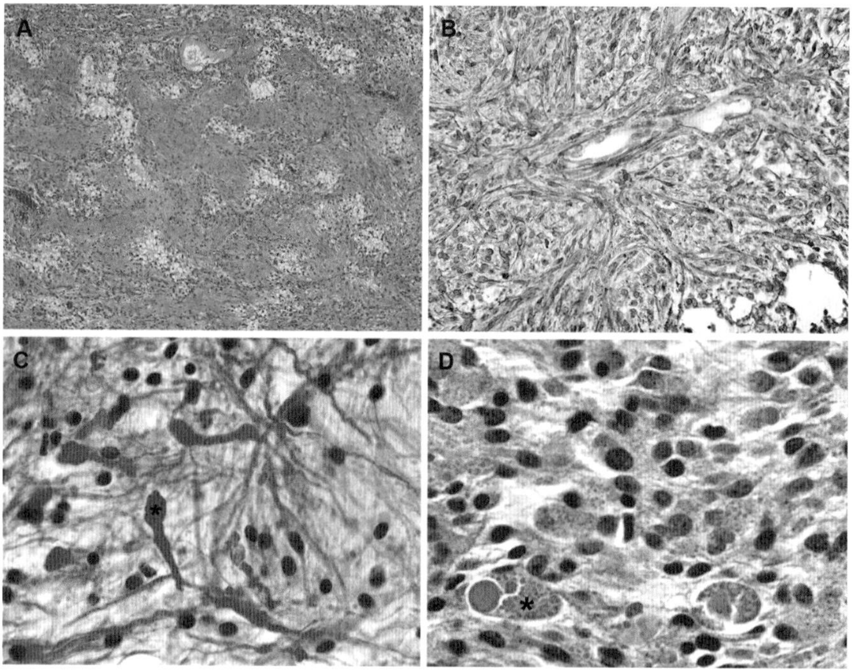

Fig. 3.1 Histologic features of human pilocytic astrocytomas. (**A**) Biphasic pattern of regions with more compact cellularity alternating with regions with more loosely structured architecture. (**B**) Pilocytic astrocytomas are GFAP-immunoreactive. Pilocytic astrocytomas characteristically contain Rosenthal fibers (**C**; asterisk) and eosinophilic granular bodies (**D**; asterisk). Photomicrographs were generously provided by Dr. Arie Perry (Division of Neuropathology, Washington University School of Medicine) (*see* Color Plate 8)

(Gesundheit et al. 2003) and exhibit robust contrast enhancement on MRI (Fulham et al. 1993). In addition, PAs often demonstrate microglial infiltration (Tanaka et al. 2008). The characteristic histologic features of these tumors include Rosenthal fibers and eosinophilic granular bodies. Rosenthal fibers are brightly eosinophilic corkscrew-shaped intracytoplasmic hyaline masses, while eosinophilic granular bodies are globular aggregates that form within astrocytic processes.

Pilocytic astrocytoma is typically considered a pediatric brain tumor, with the majority of cases reported in children less than 19 years of age. While they may arise anywhere along the neuraxis, the majority of sporadic cases arise in the cerebellum. Less commonly, sporadic PAs may develop along the optic pathway or in the brainstem. The genetic etiology for sporadic PA has only recently become clearer: Nearly two-thirds of PAs harbor alterations or mutations in the BRAF kinase gene (Bar et al. 2008, Jones et al. 2008, Pfister et al. 2008), while rare oncogenic KRAS mutations have been reported (Sharma et al. 2005, Janzarik et al. 2007). Lastly, 15% of PAs arise in children with the inherited cancer predisposition syndrome, neurofibromatosis type 1 (NF1) (Listernick et al. 1989, 1995).

3.2 Neurofibromatosis Type 1

3.2.1 NF1 Clinical Features

Neurofibromatosis type 1 (NF1) is one of the most common tumor predisposition syndromes affecting the nervous system. In this regard, NF1 affects 1:2500–3000 individuals worldwide (Friedman 1999). Individuals with NF1 are typically identified when they present with pigmentary abnormalities, including hyperpigmented skin macules (café-au-lait macules), skinfold (axillary or inguinal) freckling, and pigmented hamartomas of the iris (Lisch nodules). In addition, adults with NF1 develop the characteristic peripheral nerve sheath tumors for which the disorder is named (neurofibromas). Children are also prone to the development of distinctive bony abnormalities, learning disabilities, cardiovascular defects, and brain tumors (Friedman et al. 1999). The majority of the brain tumors that arise in children with NF1 are PAs (Listernick et al. 1997; Rodriguez et al. 2008).

3.2.2 Brain Tumors in NF1

Although histologically identical to their sporadic counterparts, NF1-associated PAs most frequently involve the anterior optic pathway (optic nerves and optic chiasm). These tumors commonly grow in early childhood, with a mean age at diagnosis of 4.5 years (Listernick et al. 1994). In contrast to sporadic optic gliomas, NF1-associated PAs usually cease growing by the second decade of life and only one-third of these tumors actually become symptomatic. When children with NF1-associated PA become symptomatic from their optic gliomas, they will usually present with decreased vision or hypothalamic dysfunction (Habiby et al. 1995, King et al. 2003).

3.3 Mouse Models of NF1-Associated Optic Glioma

Initial attempts to develop small-animal models of NF1 involved the generation of mice heterozygous for an inactivating mutation in the murine *Nf1* gene (Brannan et al. 1994, Jacks et al. 1994). These *Nf1*+/– mice were viable and fertile but failed to develop the tumors characteristic of patients with NF1. In order to accelerate tumor formation, *Nf1*+/– mice were intercrossed to produce *Nf1*–/– mice; however, these mice die during embryogenesis (E13.5) as a result of a cardiac neural crest-derived heart defect (Lakkis and Epstein 1998). To circumvent the embryonic lethality associated with biallelic *Nf1* loss, Parada and associates developed *Nf1* conditional knockout mice in which the *Nf1* gene could be inactivated in specific tissues or cell types using Cre-Lox technology (Zhu et al. 2001).

Using these *Nf1* conditional mice, we and others generated *Nf1* mutant mice specifically lacking *Nf1* gene expression in glial cells (Bajenaru et al. 2002, Zhu et al. 2005). This was achieved by GFAP promoter-driven expression of Cre recombinase to direct *Nf1* inactivation to glial cells (astrocytes). Efficient loss of *Nf1* protein (neurofibromin) expression was found in astrocytes, enabling a detailed examination of the mechanisms underlying neurofibromin growth regulation in astrocytes relevant to optic glioma growth. In addition, these *Nf1* mutant mice have begun to elucidate the contribution of the tumor microenvironment to glioma formation and growth as well as provide a robust preclinical model for therapeutic drug testing (Gutmann et al. 2006).

3.3.1 Growth Regulatory Pathways

One of the uses of genetically engineered mice is the identification of the critical intracellular signaling pathways deregulated in *Nf1*-deficient glial cells: The molecules in these growth control pathways represent potential targets for therapeutic drug design. Previous studies in other cell types have shown that neurofibromin is both a positive regulator of intracellular cyclic AMP (cAMP) generation and a negative regulator of Ras activity (Fig. 3.2). This latter function of neurofibromin has been mapped to a 300-residue domain that shares sequence homology with members of the GTPase-activating protein (GAP) family (Gutmann et al. 1993, Martin et al. 1990, Xu et al. 1990). The observation that neurofibromin inhibits Ras activation by accelerating the conversion of active, GTP-bound Ras to the inactive, GDP-bound form prompted clinical

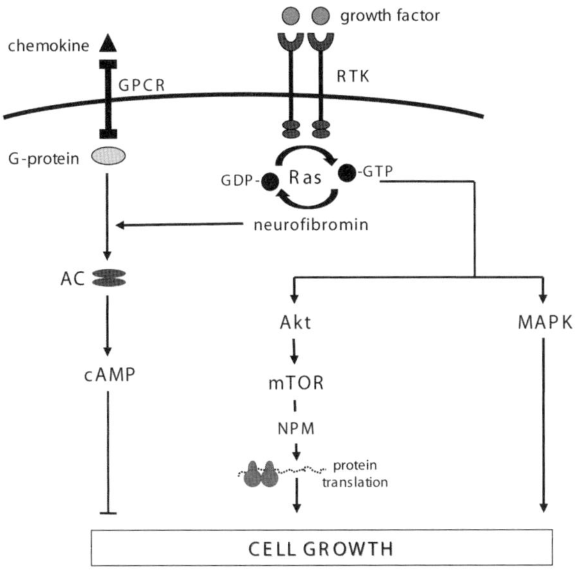

Fig. 3.2 Neurofibromin regulates both cAMP and RAS signaling in the brain. Chemokine-mediated activation of a G protein-coupled receptor (GPCR) leads to altered G-protein function which culminates in increased intracellular cAMP generation. Loss of neurofibromin is associated with reduced cAMP generation as a result of impaired adenylyl cyclase (AC) activity. In addition, growth factor activation of receptor tyrosine kinase (RTK) molecules leads to increased Ras activation (Ras-GTP), which results in increased MAPK and Akt signaling. Neurofibromin functions as a negative Ras regulator and converts GTP-bound Ras to its inactive GDP-bound form. Loss of neurofibromin leads to inappropriate Akt and MAPK activation. Akt activation results in increased mTOR signaling through nucleophosmin (NPM), which in turn dictates the translation of select transcripts at the level of the polysome. The net impact of neurofibromin loss is increased cell growth

trials aimed at inhibiting Ras function. Ras requires a secondary lipid modification (farnesylation) in order to insert into the plasma membrane and initiate Ras downstream signaling cascades. Farnesyltransferase inhibitors (FTIs) block Ras modification and interfere with Ras signaling (Konstantinopoulos et al. 2007). Unfortunately, FTI drug trials have not shown efficacy in treating NF1-associated tumors to date (Widemann et al. 2006).

In nervous system cells, there are three major Ras isoforms, K-Ras, Ha-Ras, and N-Ras, which differ from each other in terms of their sensitivity to FTI treatment. Whereas Ha-Ras is inhibited by FTI treatment, K-Ras and N-Ras are relatively resistant. To determine whether the unsatisfactory clinical trial results obtained using FTI drugs reflected neurofibromin differential Ras regulation, we analyzed Ras isoform expression and activation in wild-type and *Nf1*-deficient primary mouse astrocytes. While all three Ras isoforms are expressed in astrocytes, only K-Ras was hyperactivated in *Nf1*-deficient astrocytes (Dasgupta et al. 2005a). Moreover, K-Ras, but not Ha-Ras, activation in astrocytes in vivo was able to substitute for neurofibromin loss in the formation of murine optic glioma tumors. Similar observations have now been reported for other *NF1*-deficient cell types (Khalaf et al. 2007, Morgan et al. 2007). These findings in *Nf1* genetically engineered mice provide an explanation for the failure of FTIs in NF1 and suggest that future therapies may have to target K-Ras-dependent growth control pathways.

To identify K-Ras downstream signaling pathways, we initially employed an unbiased proteomic approach. When compared to wild-type primary mouse brain astrocytes, *Nf1–/–* astrocytes express high levels of proteins involved in ribosome biogenesis and protein translation control (Dasgupta et al. 2005b). This led to the discovery that neurofibromin regulates the mammalian target of rapamycin (mTOR) pathway in a Ras- and Akt-dependent manner in *NF1*-deficient mouse and human astrocytes as well as in human and mouse NF1-associated brain tumors. Comparable findings were subsequently reported for other *NF1*-deficient cell types and tumors (Johannessen et al. 2005). Importantly, mTOR is inhibited by a clinically available drug rapamycin. Treatment of *Nf1*-deficient astrocytes with rapamycin in vitro or in vivo results in decreased proliferation (Dasgupta et al. 2005b). These results raise the exciting possibility that rapamycin might be a suitable drug for human NF1-associated tumor clinical trials.

The observation that neurofibromin regulates ribosomal biogenesis and protein translation suggests that *Nf1* gene cell growth control might involve the selective production of specific proteins. Recent studies have shown that neurofibromin regulates the protein levels of a ribosome shuttling protein, nucleophosmin (NPM). NPM functions to transport newly synthesized ribosomes from the nucleolus into the cytoplasm to direct protein translation at the level of the polysome (Sandsmark et al. 2007).In this regard, inhibition of NPM function completely reverses the growth and actin cytoskeleton abnormalities seen in *Nf1–/–* astrocytes. Efforts are ongoing to identify the critical effector proteins regulated by neurofibromin at the level of the polysome, which may represent more refined targets for future therapeutic drug design.

In addition to neurofibromin Ras regulation, *Nf1* loss in astrocytes leads to reduced cAMP generation and cAMP-dependent intracellular signaling (Dasgupta et al. 2003, Tong et al. 2002). This decrease in intracellular cAMP levels in *Nf1–/–* astrocytes results in increased astrocyte survival (Warrington et al. 2007). Although the precise mechanism underlying neurofibromin control of cAMP generation remains unsolved (Hannan et al. 2006, Walker et al. 2006), it likely operates in a Ras-independent manner at the level of adenylyl cyclase (AC).

3.3.2 Tumor Microenvironment

Patients with NF1 start life with one mutated and one functional copy of the *NF1* gene in all cells of their body; however, tumors only form when the one remaining functional *NF1* allele undergoes somatic inactivation. Biallelic loss of *NF1* expression in tumors is consistent with the Knudson two-hit hypothesis for inherited cancer syndromes (Knudson 1971) and has been demonstrated for brain tumors arising in individuals with NF1 (Gutmann et al. 2000, Kluwe et al. 2001). To develop a mouse model for NF1-associated optic glioma, we and others inactivated the *Nf1* gene in glial cells using the human GFAP promoter (Bajenaru et al. 2002). These *Nf1* conditional knockout mice exhibited loss of neurofibromin in astrocytes associated with increased Ras pathway activation and increased glial cell numbers in vivo. However, *Nf1* loss in astrocytes was insufficient for glioma formation. These seemingly contradictory results suggest that other cellular or biochemical events are required for glioma formation in NF1.

To more accurately recapitulate the genetic makeup of individuals with NF1, mice heterozygous for a germline mutation in the *Nf1* gene were generated that also had complete neurofibromin loss in glial cells. These *Nf1*+/−^{GFAP}CKO mice were viable and healthy (Bajenaru et al. 2003, Zhu et al. 2005). Examination of their brains demonstrated that nearly 100% of the mice harbored low-grade glial neoplasms along the prechiasmatic optic nerves and optic chiasm (Fig. 3.3 and Color Plate 9). Similar to children with NF1, these GFAP+ tumors had low proliferative indices, significant microvascularity, and microglial infiltration (Bajenaru et al. 2005). *Nf1* mouse optic gliomas were first detected between

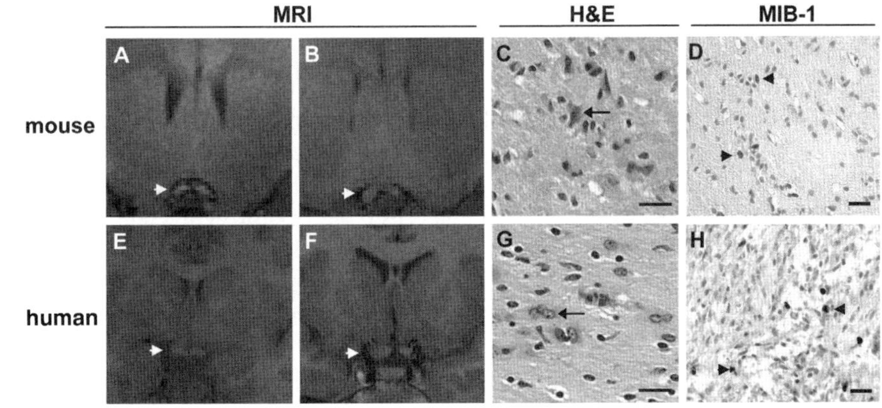

Fig. 3.3 *Nf1*+/−^{GFAP}CKO mice develop optic gliomas similar to those observed in children with neurofibromatosis-1. MR imaging (MEMRI) demonstrates asymmetrically enlarged optic nerves in one representative *Nf1*+/−^{GFAP}CKO mouse (**B**) compared to control animals (**A**). Mouse optic gliomas display limited hypercellularity with occasional nuclear atypia (**C**) and low mitotic activity (**D**). MR imaging demonstrates asymmetrically enlarged optic nerves in a child with NF1 (**F**) compared to MR imaging of the optic nerves from a healthy individual (**E**). Low cellularity and parenchymal infiltration (**G**) as well as low proliferation rate (**H**) are characteristic of the human tumors. *White arrowheads* point to the optic nerves. *Black arrowheads* indicate MIB-1-labeled cells. *Black arrows* point to atypical nuclei. **B–D**, representative mouse optic gliomas. **F–H**, optic gliomas from children with NF1. Scale bars = 30 μm. Reproduced from Hegedus et al. (2008) (*see* Color Plate 9)

8 and 12 weeks of age and did not proliferate beyond 6 months of age. Moreover, these murine tumors did not progress to higher grade glial malignancies.

The finding that *Nf1+/–* mice with complete loss of neurofibromin in astrocytes develop optic gliomas, whereas wild-type mice with identical astrocyte *Nf1* inactivation do not, supports the concept that cells and signals emanating from *Nf1+/–* cells (microenvironment) are essential for glioma formation and growth (Rubin and Gutmann 2005). To define the cellular and molecular signaling found in the tumor microenvironment necessary for glioma formation or growth, natural history studies were performed on *Nf1+/–*^{GFAP}CKO mice. During the earliest phases of optic nerve tumor development, infiltrating activated brain microglia were detected in the prechiasmatic optic nerve and chiasm (Bajenaru et al. 2005). Brain microglia are specialized immune system cells that populate the central nervous system during embryonic development, and, when activated, produce a variety of chemokines and growth factors (Badie and Schartner 2001, Graeber et al. 2002, Watters et al. 2005). Consistent with the hypothesis that *Nf1+/–* cells in the microenvironment produce growth-promoting signals that facilitate glioma growth, we showed that *Nf1+/–*, but not wild-type, microglia uniquely stimulate the growth of *Nf1–/–* astrocytes in vitro through the elaboration of soluble factors (Daginakatte and Gutmann 2007). One of the soluble factors identified was a member of the hyaluronidase family of enzymes known to degrade high molecular hyaluronic acid found in the extracellular matrix to smaller bioactive fragments that promote cell growth and motility. In this regard, purified hyaluronidase treatment increased the proliferation of *Nf1–/–* astrocytes in a Ras-/MAPK-dependent manner. The importance of microglia to mouse optic glioma growth is further underscored by the observation that pharmacologic inhibition of microglia activation and proliferation in vivo resulted in decreased optic glioma tumor cell proliferation. Collectively, these results demonstrate that microglia are key stromal cells which produce growth-promoting molecules that increase the proliferation of *Nf1–/–* glioma cells (Daginakatte et al. 2008).

In addition to growth factors, there are a host of other molecules that instruct cells to survive or migrate during specific stages of brain development (Klein and Rubin 2004, Lazarini et al. 2003). These spatially- and temporally restricted signals are critical for determining where and when cells will grow and differentiate during embryogenesis and early postnatal life. Chemokines comprise one such class of developmentally regulated signaling molecules that dictate patterning in the developing cerebellum (Klein et al. 2001). Recent work has shown that CXCL12 (stroma-derived growth factor-1α) is a chemokine which uniquely promotes *Nf1–/–* astrocyte survival in a cAMP-dependent fashion (Warrington et al. 2007). In contrast, CXCL12 has the opposite effect on wild-type astrocytes and instead leads to cell death. Detailed studies further revealed that CXCL12 expression is highest along the optic pathway in young animals and in this manner might provide both the spatial and temporal signal to facilitate NF1-associated glioma development along the optic pathway in young children.

Collectively, these findings suggest that optic glioma formation and continued growth requires biallelic *NF1* gene inactivation in astrocytes (glial cells) which must be coupled with specific cellular (e.g., microglia) and molecular signals (e.g., hyaluronidase, CXCL12) from the *NF1* + /– tumor microenvironment (Fig. 3.4).

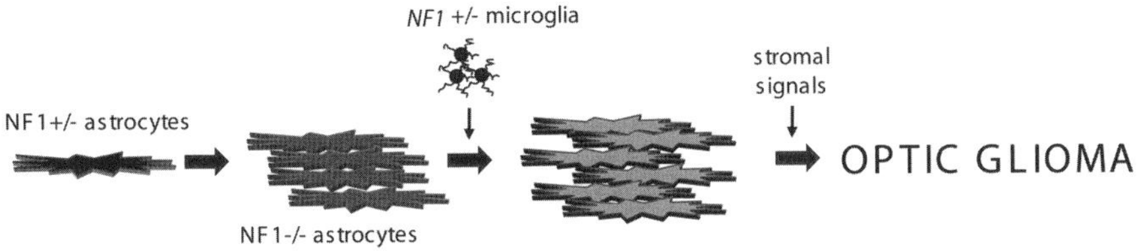

Fig. 3.4 Stromal influences on NF1-associated optic glioma development. Somatic inactivation of the one remaining functional *NF1* gene in *NF1* + /– astrocytes leads to complete neurofibromin loss, which by itself is insufficient for glioma formation. In concert with signals from microglia in the tumor microenvironment (e.g., hyaluronidase) as well as other stroma-derived signals (e.g., CXCL12), *NF1*–/– astrocyte growth is deregulated and results in optic glioma formation

3.3.3 Preclinical Therapeutic Studies

In addition to improving our understanding of the molecular and cellular pathogenesis of NF1-associated optic glioma formation and growth, *Nf1* genetically engineered mice can be used to improve the treatment of children with these low-grade tumors (Fig. 3.5). Advancements in small-animal MR

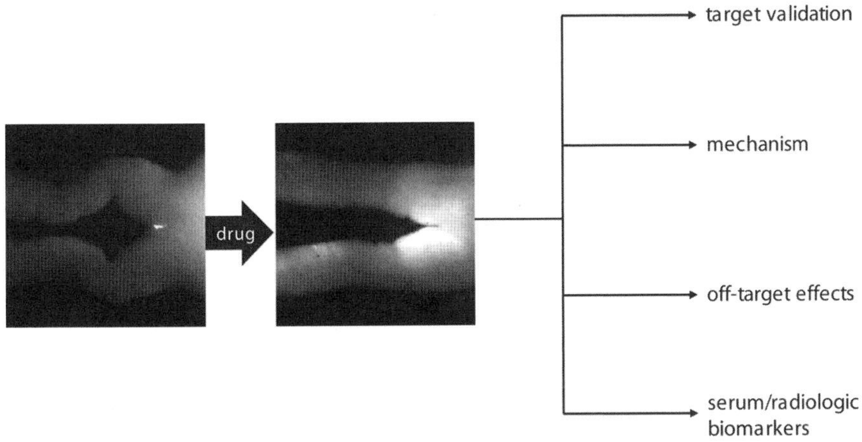

Fig. 3.5 Preclinical evaluation of novel therapies for pediatric low-grade glioma. Treatment of *Nf1* GEM optic glioma tumors with anti-cancer drugs provides unique opportunities to address important questions relevant to the success of future chemotherapeutic approaches. The first photomicrograph depicts a dissected mouse optic nerve containing swollen prechiasmatic optic nerves and chiasm (right side of image) compared with a dissected mouse optic nerve following treatment in which the nerves are no longer swollen or kinked

imaging have recently provided unparalleled opportunities to rapidly detect these small tumors in vivo and to monitor their growth during drug trials (Banerjee et al. 2007). We and others have begun to use these genetically engineered mouse strains to demonstrate that conventional chemotherapies used to treat children with NF1-associated optic gliomas are also effective as anti-cancer therapies in mice, further validating the use of these mouse models (Hegedus et al. 2008, Johannessen et al. 2008). In addition, these mice have been successfully employed to evaluate new biologically targeted agents that derive from basic science discoveries, such as rapamycin to block mTOR pathway activation or agents that restore cAMP levels in *Nf1–/–* glioma cells. The use of mouse low-grade glioma models as preclinical "filters" to select compounds most likely to be effective in clinical practice may accelerate the delivery of promising compounds to children with NF1.

Another opportunity that mouse low-grade glioma models afford is the ability to define the effect of anti-cancer drugs on the neoplastic cells within the tumor as well as in the normal brain. This is particularly important when treating children whose brains are continuing to develop. Mouse models provide tractable experimental platforms to determine whether the drug actually reached the tumor cells and had the intended effect on the signaling pathway which it was designed to inhibit. For example, demonstrating that rapamycin blocks mTOR signaling and astrocyte proliferation in glioma cells in a dose-dependent manner in vivo provides strong evidence that rapamycin is "hitting" its intended target and slowing glioma cell growth ("target validation"). Similarly, understanding how the drugs exert their effect on tumor growth is equally important. Does the anti-tumoral effect reflect suppression of cell growth or an increase in cell death? In the case of rapamycin, its ability to suppress mouse optic glioma growth did not cause programmed cell death but rather led to decreased tumor cell proliferation (Hegedus et al. 2008). In contrast, temozolomide, an alkylating agent, promoted programmed cell death and led to a more durable, long-lasting effect on tumor growth.

While most biologically targeted agents are selective, they may inhibit or increase signaling through unanticipated pathways and lead to deleterious consequences. In this regard, rapamycin inhibition of mTOR can lead to increased Akt activity by silencing a feedback loop operative in many cell types (Martin et al. 2007, O'Reilly et al. 2006, Zhang et al. 2006). Increased Akt signaling as a result of rapamycin treatment would then promote the growth of tumor cells, instead of attenuating glioma proliferation: Mouse tumor models can be used to determine whether such "off-target" effects exist following drug treatment in vivo. Finally, genetically engineered mice also provide unique opportunities to explore the effects of chemotherapies on normal developing brain tissue. This is especially germane to the treatment of brain tumors in young children.

Another potential use of mouse low-grade glioma models is the discovery of serum or radiographic biomarkers that predict or monitor the response to therapy. We and others have used GEM models to identify proteins secreted into the blood or cerebrospinal fluid (Dasgupta et al. 2005c). These secreted proteins may serve as potential biomarkers of tumor growth. Since tumor shrinkage, as assessed on conventional MRI, typically occurs months after the onset of tumor growth suppression, the availability of surrogate indicators of tumor growth would greatly improve our ability to make rapid decisions regarding the success of our treatments. Similarly, with the advancements in small-animal imaging, it becomes possible to consider using dynamic contrast enhancement (measures of tumor vascularity) and diffusion-based imaging methods (measures of tumor cellularity) to more rapidly determine whether MRI can detect changes in the tumor that reflect a positive response to chemotherapy.

3.4 Future Directions

As we move into an era of molecular medicine, it becomes increasingly important to develop efficient pipelines for drug discovery and preclinical evaluation. Recent advances in mouse genetic engineering have facilitated the generation of robust small-animal models for low-grade glioma based on known cancer-causing genetic changes. These mouse glioma models offer unprecedented tools to identify new targets for therapeutic drug design based on an improved understanding of the molecular and cellular basis for low-grade glioma formation and growth. In addition, they also provide invaluable reagents to assess the efficacy of new compounds and determine their effects on the intact animal in vivo prior to human clinical trials.

Lastly, although NF1 accounts for a minority of pediatric low-grade gliomas, it is highly likely that these NF1-based findings will provide critical insights into the pathogenesis and treatment of sporadic tumors arising outside of the context of NF1. Several recent studies have highlighted the translation of observations made initially by investigating NF1 glioma biology to sporadic pediatric low-grade glioma: First, there have been two reports of non-NF1-associated pilocytic astrocytomas with activating mutations in the *KRAS* gene (Janzarik et al. 2007, Sharma et al. 2005). Mutational activation of *KRAS* in glial cells should mimic many of the effects of neurofibromin loss. Second, sporadic low-grade gliomas harbor hyperactivation of the Ras signaling pathway, and most pilocytic astrocytomas exhibit Akt/mTOR hyperactivation (Sharma et al. 2005). This suggests that Akt/mTOR pathway deregulation is a central growth regulatory signature of low-grade glioma. Lastly, the stromal signals identified by examining *Nf1* mutant mice have revealed instructive growth cues provided by microglia and other cell types in the low-grade glioma tumor microenvironment. As sporadic low-grade gliomas also contain infiltrating microglia, similar stroma-derived growth factors may also be important for sporadic low-grade growth. Future studies on sporadic low-grade gliomas that springboard from studies originally focused on NF1 may yield new treatments for these common pediatric brain tumors.

Abbreviations

AC	adenylyl cyclase
Akt	protein kinase B
cAMP	cyclic adenosine monophosphate
GFAP	glial fibrillary acidic protein
LGG	low-grade glioma
MAPK	mitogen-activated protein kinase
MRI	magnetic resonance imaging
mTOR	mammalian target of rapamycin
NF1	neurofibromatosis type 1
NPM	nucleophosmin
OPG	optic pathway glioma
PA	pilocytic astrocytoma
WHO	World Health Organization

References

Badie B, Schartner J (2001) Role of microglia in glioma biology. Microsc Res Tech 54:106–113

Bajenaru ML, Zhu Y, Hedrick NM et al. (2002) Astrocyte-specific inactivation of the neurofibromatosis 1 gene (NF1) is insufficient for astrocytoma formation. Mol Cell Biol 22:5100–5113

Bajenaru ML, Hernandez MR, Perry A et al. (2003) Optic nerve glioma in mice requires astrocyte Nf1 gene inactivation and Nf1 brain heterozygosity. Cancer Res 63:8573–8577

Bajenaru ML, Garbow JR, Perry A et al. (2005) Natural history of neurofibromatosis 1-associated optic nerve glioma in mice. Ann Neurol 57:119–127

Banerjee D, Hegedus B, Gutmann DH et al. (2007) Detection and measurement of neurofibromatosis-1 mouse optic glioma in vivo. Neuroimage 35:1434–1437

Bar EE, Lin A, Tihan T et al. (2008) Frequent gains at chromosome 7q34 involving BRAF in pilocytic astrocytoma. J Neuropathol Exp Neurol 67:878–887

Brannan CI, Perkins AS, Vogel KS et al. (1994) Targeted disruption of the neurofibromatosis type-1 gene leads to developmental abnormalities in heart and various neural crest-derived tissues. Genes Dev 8:1019–1029

Daginakatte GC, Gutmann DH (2007) Neurofibromatosis-1 (Nf1) heterozygous brain microglia elaborate paracrine factors that promote Nf1-deficient astrocyte and glioma growth. Hum Mol Genet 16:1098–1112

Daginakatte GC, Gianino SM, Zhao NW et al. (2008) Increased JNK signaling in Neurofibromatosis-1 (*NF1*) heterozygous microglia drives microglia activation and promotes optic glioma proliferation. Cancer Res 68:10358–10366

Dasgupta B, Dugan LL, Gutmann DH (2003) The neurofibromatosis 1 gene product neurofibromin regulates pituitary adenylate cyclase-activating polypeptide-mediated signaling in astrocytes. J Neurosci 23:8949–8954

Dasgupta B, Li W, Perry A et al. (2005a) Glioma formation in neurofibromatosis 1 reflects preferential activation of K-RAS in astrocytes. Cancer Res 65:236–245

Dasgupta B, Yi Y, Chen DY et al. (2005b) Proteomic analysis reveals hyperactivation of the mammalian target of rapamycin pathway in neurofibromatosis 1-associated human and mouse brain tumors. Cancer Res 65:2755–2760

Dasgupta B, Yi Y, Hegedus B et al. (2005c) Cerebrospinal fluid proteomic analysis reveals dysregulation of methionine aminopeptidase-2 expression in human and mouse neurofibromatosis 1-associated glioma. Cancer Res 65:9843–9850
Friedman JM (1999) Epidemiology of neurofibromatosis type 1. Am J Med Genet 89:1–6
Friedman JM, Gutmann DH, MacCollin M et al. (1999) Neurofibromatosis: Phenotype, Natural History, and Pathogenesis Johns Hopkins Press, Baltimore
Fulham MJ, Melisi JW, Nishimiya J et al. (1993) Neuroimaging of juvenile pilocytic astrocytomas: an enigma. Radiology 189:221–225
Gesundheit B, Klement G, Senger C et al. (2003) Differences in vasculature between pilocytic and anaplastic astrocytomas of childhood. Med Pediatr Oncol 41:516–526
Graeber MB, Scheithauer BW, Kreutzberg GW (2002) Microglia in brain tumors. Glia 40:252–259
Gutmann D, Boguski M, Marchuk D et al. (1993) Analysis of the neurofibromatosis type 1 (NF1) GAP-related domain by site directed mutagenesis. Oncogene 8:761–769
Gutmann DH, Donahoe J, Brown T et al. (2000) Loss of neurofibromatosis 1 (NF1) gene expression in NF1-associated pilocytic astrocytomas. Neuropathol Appl Neurobiol 26:361–367
Gutmann D, Hunter-Schaedle, K, Shannon, K (2006) Harnessing preclinical mouse models to inform human clinical cancer trials. J Clin Invest 116:847–852
Habiby R, Silverman B, Listernick R et al. (1995) Precocious puberty in children with neurofibromatosis type 1. J Pediatr 126:364–367
Hannan F, Ho I, Tong JJ et al. (2006) Effect of neurofibromatosis type I mutations on a novel pathway for adenylyl cyclase activation requiring neurofibromin and Ras. Hum Mol Genet 15:1087–1098
Hegedus B, Banerjee D, Yeh TH et al. (2008) Preclinical cancer therapy in a mouse model of neurofibromatosis-1 optic glioma. Cancer Res 68:1520–1528
Jacks T, Shih TS, Schmitt EM et al. (1994) Tumour predisposition in mice heterozygous for a targeted mutation in NF1. Nat Genet 7:353–361
Janzarik WG, Kratz CP, Loges NT et al. (2007) Further evidence for a somatic KRAS mutation in a pilocytic astrocytoma. Neuropediatrics 38:61–63
Johannessen CM, Reczek EE, James MF et al. (2005) The NF1 tumor suppressor critically regulates TSC2 and mTOR. Proc Natl Acad Sci USA 102:8573–8578
Johannessen CM, Johnson BW, Williams SM et al. (2008) TORC1 is essential for NF1-associated malignancies. Curr Biol 18:56–62
Jones DT, Kocialkowski S, Liu L et al. (2008) Tandem duplication producing a novel oncogenic BRAF fusion gene defines the majority of pilocytic astrocytomas. Cancer Res 68:8673–8677
Khalaf WF, Yang FC, Chen S et al. (2007) K-ras is critical for modulating multiple c-kit-mediated cellular functions in wild-type and Nf1 +/– mast cells. J Immunol 178:2527–2534
King A, Listernick R, Charrow J et al. (2003) Optic pathway gliomas in neurofibromatosis type 1: The effect of presenting symptoms on outcome. Am J Med Genet 122:95–99
Klein RS, Rubin JB (2004) Immune and nervous system CXCL12 and CXCR4: parallel roles in patterning and plasticity. Trends Immunol 25:306–314
Klein RS, Rubin JB, Gibson HD et al. (2001) SDF-1 alpha induces chemotaxis and enhances Sonic hedgehog-induced proliferation of cerebellar granule cells. Development 128:1971–1981
Kluwe L, Hagel C, Tatagiba M et al. (2001) Loss of NF1 alleles distinguish sporadic from NF1-associated pilocytic astrocytomas. J Neuropathol Exp Neurol 60:917–920
Konstantinopoulos PA, Karamouzis MV, Papavassiliou AG (2007) Post-translational modifications and regulation of the RAS superfamily of GTPases as anticancer targets. Nat Rev Drug Discov 6:541–555
Knudson AG, Jr. (1971) Mutation and cancer: statistical study of retinoblastoma. Proc Natl Acad Sci USA 68:820–823

Lakkis MM, Epstein JA (1998) Neurofibromin modulation of ras activity is required for normal endocardial–mesenchymal transformation in the developing heart. Development 125:4359–4367
Lazarini F, Tham TN, Casanova P et al. (2003) Role of the alpha-chemokine stromal cell-derived factor (SDF-1) in the developing and mature central nervous system. Glia 42:139–148
Listernick R, Charrow J, Greenwald MJ et al. (1989) Optic gliomas in children with neurofibromatosis type 1. J Pediatr 114:788–792
Listernick R, Charrow J, Greenwald M et al. (1994) Natural history of optic pathway tumors in children with neurofibromatosis type 1: a longitudinal study. J Pediatr 125:63–66
Listernick R, Darling C, Greenwald M et al. (1995) Optic pathway tumors in children: the effect of neurofibromatosis type 1 on clinical manifestations and natural history. J Pediatr 127:718–722
Listernick R, Louis DN, Packer RJ et al. (1997) Optic pathway gliomas in children with neurofibromatosis 1: consensus statement from the NF1 Optic Pathway Glioma Task Force. Ann Neurol 41:143–149
Louis DN, Ohgaki H, Wiester OD et al. (2007) WHO Classification of Tumours of the Central Nervous System. WHO Press, Geneva
Martin GA, Viskochil D, Bollag G et al. (1990) The GAP-related domain of the neurofibromatosis type 1 gene product interacts with ras p21. Cell 63:843–849
Martin KA, Merenick BL, Ding M et al (2007) Rapamycin promotes vascular smooth muscle cell differentiation through insulin receptor substrate-1/phosphatidylinositol 3-kinase/Akt2 feedback signaling. J Biol Chem 282:36112–36120
Morgan KJ, Rowley MA, Wiesner SM et al. (2007) The GAP-related domain of neurofibromin attenuates proliferation and downregulates N- and K-Ras activation in Nf1-negative AML cells. Leuk Res 31:1107–1113
O'Reilly KE, Rojo F, She QB et al. (2006) mTOR inhibition induces upstream receptor tyrosine kinase signaling and activates Akt. Cancer Res 66:1500–1508
Pfister S, Janzarik WG, Remke M et al. BRAF gene duplication constitutes a mechanism of MAPK pathway activation in low-grade astrocytomas. J Clin Invest 2008 118:1739–1749
Rodriguez FJ, Perry A, Gutmann DH et al. (2008) Gliomas in neurofibromatosis type 1: a clinicopathologic study of 100 patients. J Neuropath Exp Neurol 67:240–249
Rubin JB, Gutmann DH (2005) Neurofibromatosis type 1 – a model for nervous system tumour formation? Nat Rev Cancer 5:557–564
Sandsmark DK, Zhang H, Hegedus B et al. (2007) Nucleophosmin mediates mammalian target of rapamycin-dependent actin cytoskeleton dynamics and proliferation in neurofibromin-deficient astrocytes. Cancer Res 67:4790–4799
Sharma MK, Zehnbauer BA, Watson MA et al. (2005) RAS pathway activation and an oncogenic RAS mutation in sporadic pilocytic astrocytoma. Neurology 65:1335–1336
Tanaka Y, Sasaki A, Ishiuchi S et al. (2008) Diversity of glial cell components in pilocytic astrocytoma. Neuropathology doi: 10111/j1440-1789200800896x
Tong J, Hannan F, Zhu Y et al. (2002) Neurofibromin regulates G protein-stimulated adenylyl cyclase activity. Nat Neurosci 5:95–96
Walker JA, Tchoudakova AV, McKenney PT et al. (2006) Reduced growth of Drosophila neurofibromatosis 1 mutants reflects a non-cell-autonomous requirement for GTPase-Activating Protein activity in larval neurons. Genes Dev 20:3311–3323
Warrington NM, Woerner BM, Daginakatte GC et al. (2007) Spatiotemporal differences in CXCL12 expression and cyclic AMP underlie the unique pattern of optic glioma growth in neurofibromatosis type 1. Cancer Res 67:8588–8595
Watters JJ, Schartner JM, Badie B (2005) Microglia function in brain tumors. J Neurosci Res 81:447–455

Widemann BC, Salzer WL, Arceci RJ et al. (2006) Phase I trial and pharmacokinetic study of the farnesyltransferase inhibitor tipifarnib in children with refractory solid tumors or neurofibromatosis type I and plexiform neurofibromas. J Clin Oncol 24:507–516

Xu GF, Lin B, Tanaka K et al. (1990) The catalytic domain of the neurofibromatosis type 1 gene product stimulates ras GTPase and complements ira mutants of S. cerevisiae. Cell 63:835–841

Zhang HH, Lipovsky AI, Dibble CC et al. (2006) S6K1 regulates GSK3 under conditions of mTOR-dependent feedback inhibition of Akt. Mol Cell 24:185–197

Zhu Y, Romero MI, Ghosh P et al. (2001) Ablation of NF1 function in neurons induces abnormal development of cerebral cortex and reactive gliosis in the brain. Genes Dev 15:859–876

Zhu Y, Harada T, Liu L et al. (2005) Inactivation of NF1 in CNS causes increased glial progenitor proliferation and optic glioma formation. Development 132:5577–5588

Chapter 4
Transgenic Mouse Models of CNS Tumors: Using Genetically Engineered Murine Models to Study the Role of p21-Ras in Glioblastoma Multiforme

Diana Munoz, Sameer Agnihotri, and Abhijit Guha

Abstract Robust animal models have come to the forefront of understanding GBM biology and cancer biology in general. Specifically, genetically engineered murine models or GEMs have provided a great deal of understanding in investigating the role of p21-Ras in GBM. Elevation of Ras activity is a molecular hallmark of GBM and is under intense investigation. Several animal models have been engineered to express mutant forms of Ras or aberrantly express receptors, which modulate Ras activity. Embryonic stem cell transgenesis is a key methodology in engineering these mice models and so is tissue-specific targeting. We highlight several advantages of using ES-cell mediated transgenesis to generate mouse models expressing activated Ras. These animal models have been crucial in studying GBM formation, identifying novel GBM tumor suppressor genes using retroviral gene-trapping and how Ras synergizes with other signaling pathways to give rise to GBM. Lastly these models can be useful in identifying the potential cell of origin in GBM.

Contents

A. Guha (✉)
Transgenic mouse models of CNS Tumors, Hospital for Sick Children, University of Toronto, Toronto, Canada
e-mail: Abhijit.Guha@uhn.on.ca

E.G. Van Meir (ed.), *CNS Cancer*, Cancer Drug Discovery and Development, DOI 10.1007/978-1-60327-553-8_4,
© Humana Press, a part of Springer Science+Business Media, LLC 2009

4.1 Introduction

Glioblastoma multiforme (GBM) is the most common and lethal of all gliomas and is defined by several hallmark features such as hyper-cellular proliferation, resistance to apoptosis, genomic instability, necrosis, and robust invasion. GBM is a highly heterogeneous tumor broadly characterized by several gain-of-function and loss–of-function alterations, epigenetic reprogramming, and somatic mutations. Emerging biologically relevant targeted therapies depend on an enhanced understanding of the underlying mechanisms that contribute to the malignant phenotype. Amongst these targets is p21-Ras, and it has attracted much attention due to its central role in normal and cancer cell intracellular signaling pathways. Primary activating mutations of p21-Ras are seen in 30% of cancers, but not in GBM. Higher levels of Ras can also arise through secondary activation of p21-Ras-regulated pathways through aberrant receptor expression as seen in breast cancer and gliomas.

To further the understanding of GBM aberrancies including p21-Ras, robust animal models such as genetically engineered mouse models (GEMs) have come to the forefront. These GEMs are based on known human genetic alterations with the hope that they will recapitulate the histological and molecular pathogenesis of astrocytomas including GBM. GEMs serve as excellent tools to better understand the biology of GBM by understanding the biological consequences of known GBM genetic alterations, identifying novel GBM modifier genes, used in pre-clinical studies, and serve as a model for identifying the cell of origin. We highlight how GEMs provide an invaluable tool to study GBM and p21-Ras signaling.

4.2 Embryonic Stem Cell Transgenesis to Generate Mouse Models

As previously mentioned, p21-Ras is a key aberration of GBM and as our knowledge of the molecular pathogenesis of GBM increases with new effective biological therapies, there is a need to develop better pre-clinical models. The mouse is the model organism most closely related to humans. Human and mouse genomes are approximately the same size, contain the similar number of genes, and have high synteny (conserved gene order). Most human genes have mouse counterparts with similar function. Mutations or alterations that cause diseases in humans often cause similar diseases in mice. Mouse models can be generated by somatic gene transfer, germ line transmission, and human cell and tissue transplantations. The valuable features of a robust GBM model include but are not limited to (1) tumors arise from the cell of origin/astrocytes; (2) tumors in the animal model have similar molecular pathogenesis as human GBM such as proliferation, necrosis, invasion, and angiogenesis; (3) tumors are responsive to known therapeutics; (4), tumors develop at a high incidence and are predictable; (4) tumors share molecular profiles similar to human GBM; (5) tumor induction is short to allow for therapeutic intervention. Here we focus on germ line or embryonic stem cell (ES) transgenesis. See relevant chapters for more information on somatic gene transfer such as the RCAS system and tissue transplantation or xenograft mouse models. ES cells are derived from pre-implantation embryos, specifically from the inner cell mass (ICM) of the blastocyst stage (Evans and Kaufman, 1981). ES cells can be established under in vitro conditions with complete medium and leukemia inhibitory factor (LIF), which keeps the ES cells undifferentiated and maintains their potential to develop into tissues of all lineages. When injected into a host blastocyst or aggregated with the blastomere stage of mouse embryos, the donor ES cells can integrate into host ICM and give rise to cells of all tissue types resulting in a chimeric mouse, Fig. 4.1 and Color Plate 10 (Evans and Kaufman, 1981; Nagy et al., 1990). Since ES cells can contribute to germ cells of the chimeric mouse, the ES cell genome is transferred to progeny leading to stable germ line transmission.

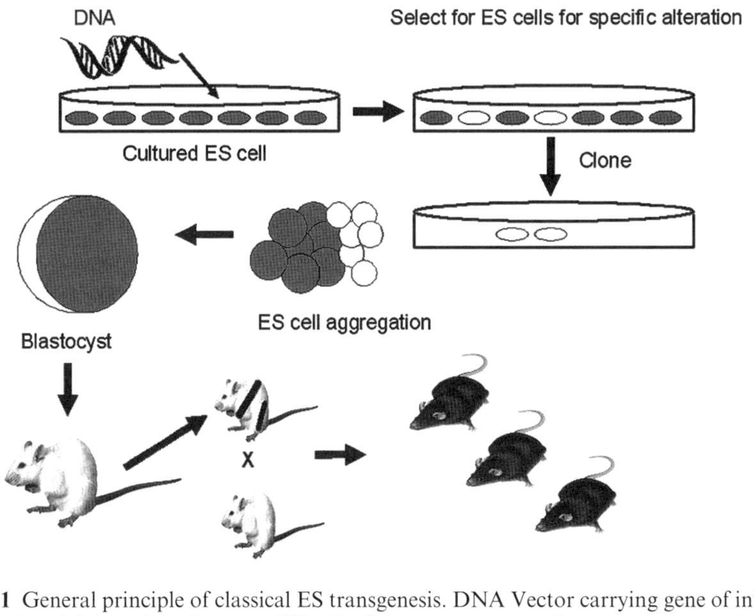

Fig. 4.1 General principle of classical ES transgenesis. DNA Vector carrying gene of interest is transfected into cultured mouse ES cells. In our case we used a retrovirus carrying the ^{V12}Ha-Ras gene under the control of the astrocyte-specific human GFAP promoter and a neomycin selection marker expression cassette. Selection of ES cells with the transgene of interest is first accomplished by selecting for neomycin-resistant clones. Thereafter NeoR ES clones are tested for their ability to express the transgene by in vitro differentiation to astrocytes. This process confirms activation of the GFAP promoter expression and specificity. Positive ES cells undergo aggregations and are transferred to a pseudo-pregnant female mouse to create chimeric embryos (striped mouse in picture). The chimeric mice are bred to normal mice and those mice having incorporated the transgene in their germ-line will generate transgenic offspring (*see* Color Plate 10)

A powerful feature of transgenics that involves ES cells is based on homologous recombination, which allows specific mutagenesis of any gene or genomic locus (Capecchi, 1989). This has been advantageous in cancer research since this technique can allow for targeting and disruption of tumor suppressor genes (TSGs) such as PTEN and P53. Classical transgenesis involves to introduction of an exogenous gene expression construct to create genomic alterations (DePrimo et al., 1996). This procedure involves targeting the transgenic vector into ES cells that are then injected into a host blastocyst or aggregated within a morula stage embryo to give rise to chimeric mice that are then bred to give rise to transgenic mice of the desired genotype. ES cell transgenesis has several advantages over standard pro-nuclear injection methods. Conventional pro-nuclear injection results in multiple-copy integrations which can result in variation or even inhibition of transgene expression (Garrick et al., 1998). ES cell transgenesis provides higher frequency of low-copy transgene integration including single-copy integration, which is often desirable. Second, ES cell transgenesis allows for testing of cells in vitro. Therefore, using in vitro assays you can select for cells that express the transgene of interest and test tissue specificity of the transgene using differentiation assays if the transgene is under a tissue-specific promoter (TSP). These tests are less expensive and labor intensive compared to pro-nuclear injections since you do not have to invest in making the actual mice yet. ES-cell transgenesis also has the possible advantage of avoiding embryonic lethality due to tissue-specific transgene expression. The chimeric mice do not have transgene expression in every cell, which may circumvent the lethality seen in many pro-nuclear injections. In addition to ES-cell transgenesis, conditional inducible transgenics can be employed such as the Cre/LoxP or the Flp/FRT systems in which the transgene expression can be induced or silenced at times deemed necessary for experimental investigation.

4.3 Genetically Engineered Murine Mouse Models (GEMs) of GBM

Several efforts have been employed to create a transgenic mouse model that can recapitulate the GBM phenotype using the astrocyte-specific promoter. The GFAP promoter which is activated by embryonic day 16.5 has been widely used to target differentiated astrocytes. The rational being that GBMs were believed to be derived from astrocytes or an astrocytic lineage. Expression of oncogenes using the astrocyte-specific glial fibrillary acidic protein (GFAP) promoter, such as the SV40 large T antigen (Danks et al., 1995) and *v-src* (Weissenberger et al., 1997), has led to some glioma models, though with unpredictable and low frequency and pathology. For example, GFAP-SV40 large T transgenic mice develop aggressive non-astrocytic brain tumors with hyperplasia of the choroid plexus. GFAP-*v-src* transgenics form abnormal nests of proliferating astrocytes perinatally, which later evolves into overt malignant astrocytomas in the brain and spinal cord in 14% of mice by 65 weeks (Weissenberger et al., 1997; Danks et al., 1995). Our lab has developed a transgenic mouse astrocytoma model, based on our findings of increased p21-Ras activation in malignant human astrocytomas, in which the 12VHa-*ras* Transgene is driven by the human GFAP promoter (Ding et al., 2001). This mouse model reproduces many but not all of the pathological and molecular characteristics found in human tumors including a high mitotic index, nuclear pleomorphism, infiltration, necrosis, and increased vascularity.

4.4 GFAP:12 V-HaRas Astrocytoma Model: Characterization of RasD7, RasB8

We and others have demonstrated that activation of p21-Ras from aberrantly expressed/activated RPTKs such as mutant EGFRs promotes growth of GBMs (Guha et al., 1997; Feldkamp et al., 2001). This led us to develop a transgenic mouse using embryonic stem (ES) cell transgenesis, with the GFAP promoter-regulating oncogenic 12VHa-*ras*. We chose a 2.2 Kb human GFAP promoter which contains the essential transcription regulatory elements directing the expression of the GFAP gene: AP-1, ets-1, RAR, etc. Because ES transgenesis was used, we were able to perform in vitro differentiation screens to identify ES clones which had incorporated the transgene and maintained the regulation conferred by the GFAP promoter. Retinoic acid (RA) treatment, which turns on the GFAP promoter (Fraichard et al., 1995), allowed selection of ES cells that expressed 12VHa-*ras* and the accompanying IRES-LacZ construct, before blastocyst introduction.

Several transgenic GFAP-Ras lines were created from selected ES clones, which demonstrated a dose-dependent increase in the incidence and grade of astrocytomas (Ding et al., 2001). The RasD7 line was found to contain several 12 V-HaRas transgene integration sites and high levels of activated p21-Ras expression, and mice died from multifocal malignant astrocytomas within 2 weeks as chimeras (Fig. 4.2). Examination of the brains of these mice demonstrate diffuse glial hyperplasia with multiple foci of astrocytoma with regions of necrosis, hemorrhage, and hypervascularity (Shannon et al., 2005), features associated with malignant astrocytomas (Kleihues and Cavanee, 2000). In contrast, mice from the RasB8 line had a single 12 V-HaRas integration site, displayed moderate levels of p21-Ras transgene expression, and achieved germ line transmission (Fig. 4.2). RasB8 are phenotypically identical to normal littermates at E16.5, with expression of the hGFAP regulated $^{12\,\mathrm{V}}$H-Ras transgene as early as E13.5, but without any significant increase in GFAP+ astrocytes or any other detectable histological central nervous system abnormalities. In the next 3 weeks RasB8 differ from littermates by harboring increased numbers of GFAP+/Nestin- astrocytes diffusely in the brain. Astrocyte isolates from this early hyperplasia stage (RasB8-P0) are not transformed as they fail to form

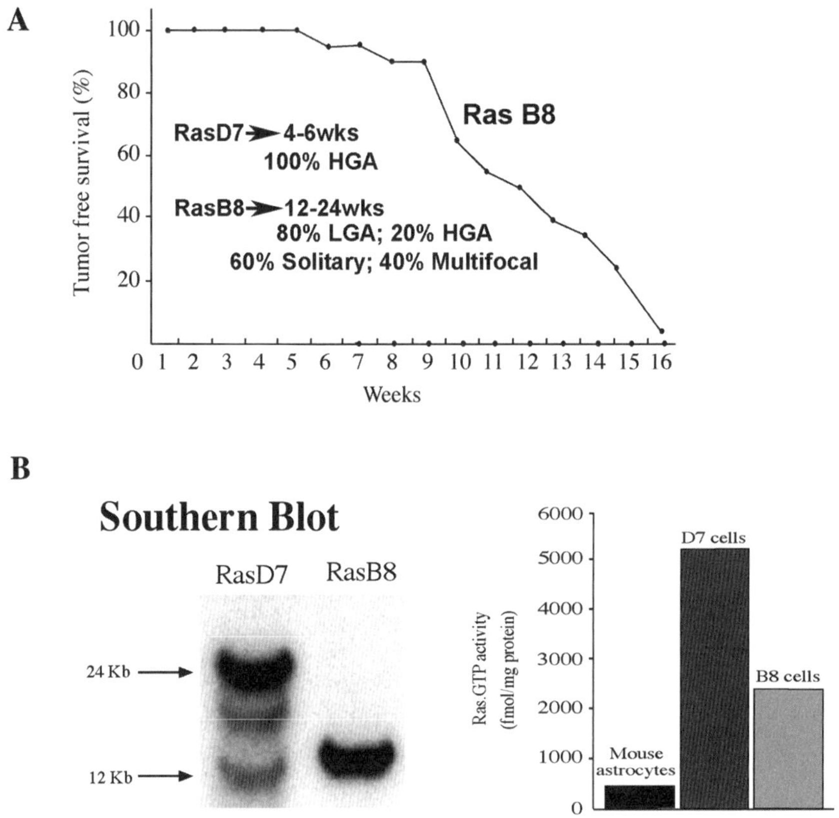

Fig. 4.2 ***RasD7, RasB8 GEMs.*** **A.** Survival curve of the RasB8 GEM. Pups are born normally and can go on to breeding with germ line transmission. Fifty percent of the RasB8 mice are dead at ~12 weeks and show an assortment of uni- and multifocal low (LGA) and high-grade astrocytomas (HGA). **B**. Southern blot analysis of transgenic integration in GFAP-V12Ha-Ras transgenic mice with LacZ cDNA probe (*Left panel*). P21-Ras-GTP levels (fmol/mg of protein) in the RasD7 and RasB8 astrocytoma cell lines (*Right panel*)

tumors when re-introduced into a syngeneic host. At 3–4 weeks multiple foci of invasive GFAP+/Nestin+ astrocytes develop, which upon micro-isolation harbor *Tp53* mutations and aberrant EGFR expression similar to low grade astrocytomas (LGA) in humans (Fig. 4.3a and Color Plate 11). At 12 weeks highly invasive and angiogenic GFAP+/ Nestin+ high-grade astrocytomas are observed. This progression from low-grade to high-grade astrocytomas is accompanied by additional genetic changes, including loss of PTEN and p16 cell cycle inhibitor expression.

Further Cytogenetic analysis of astrocytes isolated from RasB8 mice at 3 months and not post natal day 0 (P0) demonstrated several clonal aberrations such as trisomy of mouse chromosome 10, which is syntenic to a region on chromosome 12q commonly amplified in human malignant astrocytomas

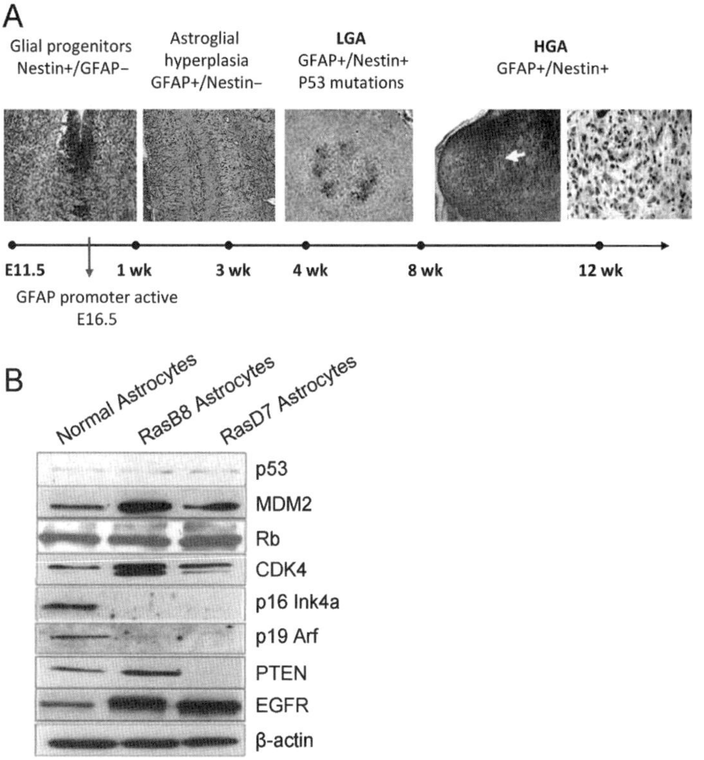

Fig. 4.3 RasB8-pathologocal/molecular progression. **A.** *RasB8 GEM-Pathological progression.* The hGFAP-regulated transgene is expressed as early as E13.5 where the mice are similar to normal littermates. For the first few weeks there are no astrocytomas, but diffuse astroglial hyperplasia. At 3–4 weeks LGA appear with p53 mutations, as demonstrated by microdissection. At 12 weeks and beyond one sees HGA with infiltrative and necrotic tumors. **B.** *RasB8-Molecular progression.* Astrocytes isolated at 1 week are not transformed, in contrast, astrocytoma cells from the HGA after 12 weeks show genetic alterations which are known to be associated with human GBMs: loss of p16, p19, PTEN, and overexpression of EGFR (*see* Color Plate 11)

which contain well-known oncogenes such as CDK4 and MDM2. At the protein level, these cells harbor many genetic alterations seen in human GBMs (Fig. 4.3b), including loss of cell cycle growth regulators (p16, p19, and tp53) expression, over expression of MDM2 or cyclin-dependent kinase (CDK4), increased expression of the epidermal growth factor receptor (EGFR), loss of *PTEN/MMAC1* tumor suppressor gene, and increased expression of pro-angiogenic molecules such as vascular endothelial growth factor and several angiopoietins.

In addition to this cytogenetic and molecular changes, cell lines derived from the GFAP:12VHa-*ras* GBMs grow in culture, soft agar and make tumors in Nod-Scid mice. However, astrocytes derived from ~2- to 3-week-old animals are not transformed, do not grow in soft agar or Nod-Scids. These results imply that activated Ras by itself does not induce gliomas, but may result in chromosomal and genetic instability (Denko et al., 1994) in astrocytes or CNS progenitors, which leads to the acquisition of additional genetic alterations and subsequent tumor development. These results suggest that the RasB8 GEM resembles the progressive "Secondary" pathogenic model of GBM.

The astrocytoma progression observed in the RasB8 model could be employed to identify additional gene expression changes associated in the formation and progression of human GBMs. For this purpose, we used high density oligonucleotide arrays to perform gene expression profiling on cultured wild-type mouse astrocytes, non-neoplastic B8 transgenic astrocytes, and neoplastic astrocytes derived from three independently generated Ras transgenic mouse lines, B8, D7, and B8/B5 (Gutmann et al., 2002). We identified several unique groups of genes, whose expression is specifically altered upon neoplastic transformation, which also demonstrated differential expression in malignant human astrocytomas cell lines. Genes previously associated with growth regulatory processes such as decorin, gadd45, and STAT6 were differentially expressed between pre malignant and malignant astrocyte cultures. Over expression of decorin in C6 rat glioma cells results in tumor regression in vivo (Stander et al., 1998), perhaps by modulating p21-WAF1/CIP1 expression. Therefore, the reduced expression of decorin in the B8 astrocytoma tumors may contribute to the increased growth of these cells. We also observed lower expression of the growth-arrest protein, gadd45, suggesting that astrocyte transformation might be associated with reduced growth-arrest signaling. STAT6 is a signaling molecule that specifically transduces proliferative signals from interleukin-4 and -12 receptors through the Janus family of kinases (Wurster et al., 2000) (see also Chapter 38) Although its role in glioma pathogenesis has not been explored, increased STAT6 expression might also augment mitogenic signaling and increase astrocytoma proliferation.

One feature of astrocytomas cells is their ability to display enhanced motility in vitro and in vivo (Chicoine and Silbergeld, 1995). Therefore, it is not surprising that we identified a number of differentially expressed transcripts involved in astrocyte cytoskeleton remodeling (gem, GAP43, and F52). To further examine the functional significance of these differentially expressed genes we analyzed the effects of the re-introduction of the downregulated astrocytomas associated protein GAP43. The re-expression of GAP43 into GAP43-deficient C6 glioma cells resulted in cell growth suppression; however, additional studies will be required to determine the mechanisms underlying GAP43 growth regulation.

As detailed above, we have exploited the RasB8 transgenic mouse model of high-grade astrocytomas to identify genes that might underlie the pathogenesis of human GBMs.

The power of this approach lies in its ability to detect gene expression changes that reflect both the non-neoplastic and neoplastic states.

4.5 Study of Cooperative Interactions Between Ras Overexpression and Other Known Genetic Alterations in Human Astrocytomas

Using the Ras B8 model we have undertaken a series of experiments to understand the role of Ras overexpression and its cooperative interactions with other known genetic alterations in human astrocytomas, based on transgenic models. We created transgenics with hGFAP-regulated expression of EGFRwt and mutant EGFRvIII, the most common gain-of-function alterations in human GBMs (Ding et al., 2003). Neither of these mice formed gliomas by themselves, leading us to conclude that aberrant EGFR signaling does not induce gliomas per se. To determine if aberrant EGFR signaling can promote progression, we made double transgenics with our RasB8 GEM. Mutant EGFRvIII, but not EGFRwt, double transgenics exhibited dramatic reduction in survival with 50% of these mice dying with gliomas at 2–4 weeks of age (Fig. 4.4a). In addition to an effect on tumor latency, EGFRvIII; GFAP-V12Ha-Ras transgenic mice developed tumors with histopathological features of oligodendrogliomas, with a small subset resembling mixed oligoastrocytomas (Fig. 4.4b). This was unexpected since EGFRvIII is linked to human adult GBMs and not high-grade oligodendrogliomas. However, consistent with our results, oligodendrogliomas also arise with EGFRvIII transduction into astrocyte progenitor pools, such as Ink4aArf –/– NSC (Bachoo et al., 2002) or Nestin-tva mice (Dunn et al., 2000). To determine if the subtype of glioma was a reflection of embryonic vs adult expression of the EGFRvIII and ^{12V}H-Ras transgenes, Ad:EGFRvIII was injection into the frontal subcortical white matter of adult RasB8 mice. These animals developed high-grade astrocytomas (HGA), as detected by MRI and pathological examination (Fig. 4.5), suggesting that the subtype, grade, and incidence of gliomas are not only dependent on the specific transforming genetic alterations, but also on their state of differentiation.

A second group of experiments investigated the role of loss of Pten in gliomagenesis (Wei et al., 2006), the most common loss-of-function alteration in human GBMs. Since *Pten* knockout is embryonically lethal, we utilized transgenic mice which have a *PTEN* gene flanked by LoxP sites (*Pten*$^{f/f}$ mice), so that it can be excised upon Cre recombinase expression. We used different strategies for Cre-excision. First we generated double transgenics, in which *Pten* was conditionally inactivated in astrocytes by crossing *Ptenf/f* transgenics to mice that express Cre recombinase under the control of the *GFAP* promoter (hGFAP-Cre). The resultant *Pten* conditional knockout mice were indistinguishable from their control littermates at birth. However, offspring died within a few weeks after birth, with enlarged brains containing increased numbers of proliferating, but not transformed, astrocytes (Fig. 4.6) (Wei et al., 2006). These data indicate that although absence of PTEN expression in astrocytes increases their proliferation and promotes an overall increase in brain size, it is insufficient for glioma formation. To more closely mimic a situation where only a focus of cells loses expression of PTEN in the brain, we developed and utilized

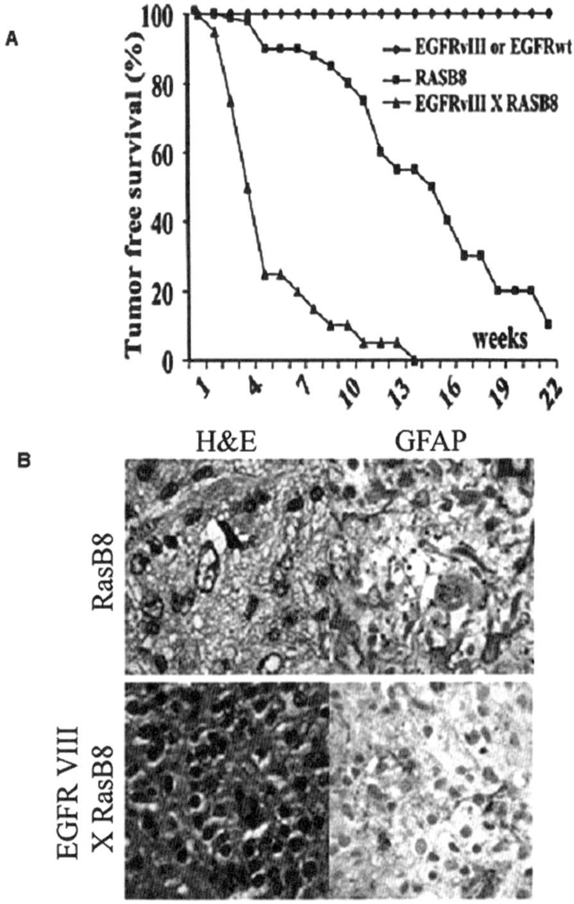

Fig. 4.4 ***RasB8 X EGFRvIII X double transgenics.*** **A.** hGFAP:EGFRvIII or EGFRwt single transgenics did not induce gliomas. Double transgenics with RasB8 X EGFRvIII (not EGFRwt) led to increased incidence and death from gliomas compared to RasB8. **B.** However, unlike RasB8 GFAP+ astrocytomas, the double RasB8 X EGFRvIII gliomas were mainly GFAP-negative oligodendrogliomas

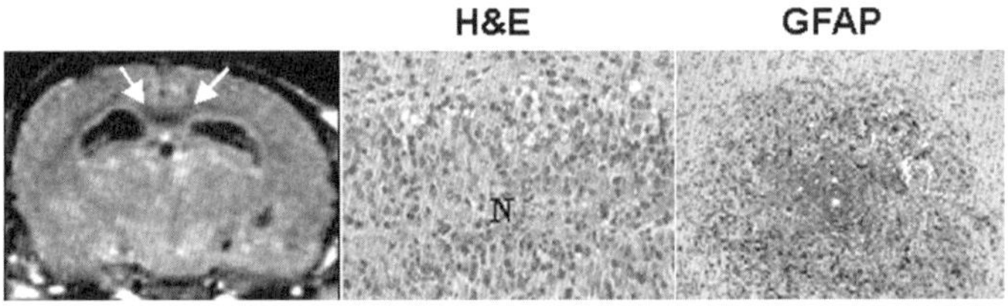

Fig. 4.5 ***4 Week-RasB8 + AdEGFRvIII.*** Adenoviral:EGFRvIII injected to RasB8 mice injection at 4 weeks of age. The left panel shows gliomas as dark lesions (white arrows), detected by small animal MRI after $MnCl_2$ contrast enhancement. The middle and right panels show sections corresponding to MRI lesions with regions of necrosis (**N**) and increased number of GFAP+ high-grade invasive astrocytomas (HGA)

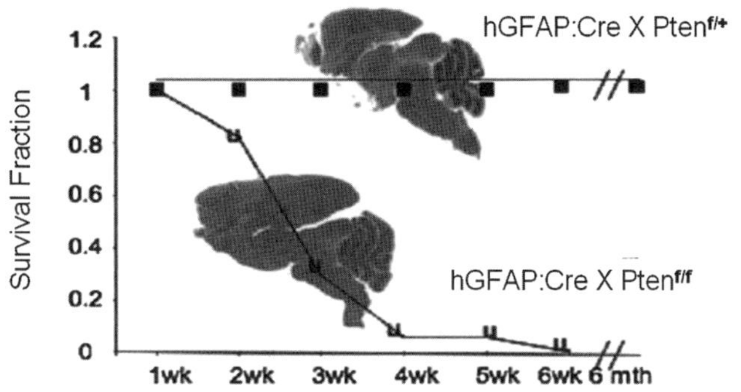

Fig. 4.6 Genetic interactions pten. Brains of hGFAP:Cre X *Pten*$^{f/f}$ double transgenics with glial-specific excision of *Pten* alleles showed progressive increase in mass relative to body size, although no gliomas were observed. By 4 weeks of age the brains of these double transgenics weighted ~ 30% more than those of control littermates

Ad:Cre intracranial injections to excise *Pten* in adult mice. Excision of *Pten* by itself did not form gliomas, but in the background of RasB8, there was increased number of high-grade GBM-like tumors (Table 4.1) supporting the role for *Pten* in glioma progression but not initiation.

Table 4.1 Excision of both *Pten*$^{f/f}$ alleles by adenoviral (Ad):Cre in 4 weeks RasB8 X *Pten*$^{f/f}$ mice led to increased number of HGA formation compared to RasB8 X *Pten*$^{f/wt}$ controls. Excision of *Pten*$^{f/f}$ by itself did not lead to any gliomas

	Low-Grade	High-Grade	No Tumour
Ras B8 + Pten$^{f/f}$ (n = 14)	2	11 (10: HGA) (1: LGA)	1
Ras B8 + Pten$^{f/wt}$ (n = 9)	4	2	3
Pten$^{f/f}$ (n = 11)	0	0	11
Pten$^{f/wt}$ (n = 10)	0	0	10

4.6 Identifying Novel GBM Modifier Genes Using the RasB8 GEM and Gene-Trapping

GEMs such as our RasB8 mouse model may also shed light on novel genetic alterations in human cancers that were previously unknown. One such approach is using a random mutagenesis technique known as retroviral gene-trapping (Stanford et al., 2001). This non-biased strategy uses a retroviral cassette that integrates into the genome randomly. Disruption of a critical gene in these tumor prone astrocytes may accelerate transformation and tumor grade (Fig. 4.7). Identification of the gene can be carried out using inverse PCR or 5′RACE PCR. Using in vitro retroviral gene-trapping on newborn (P0) transgenic

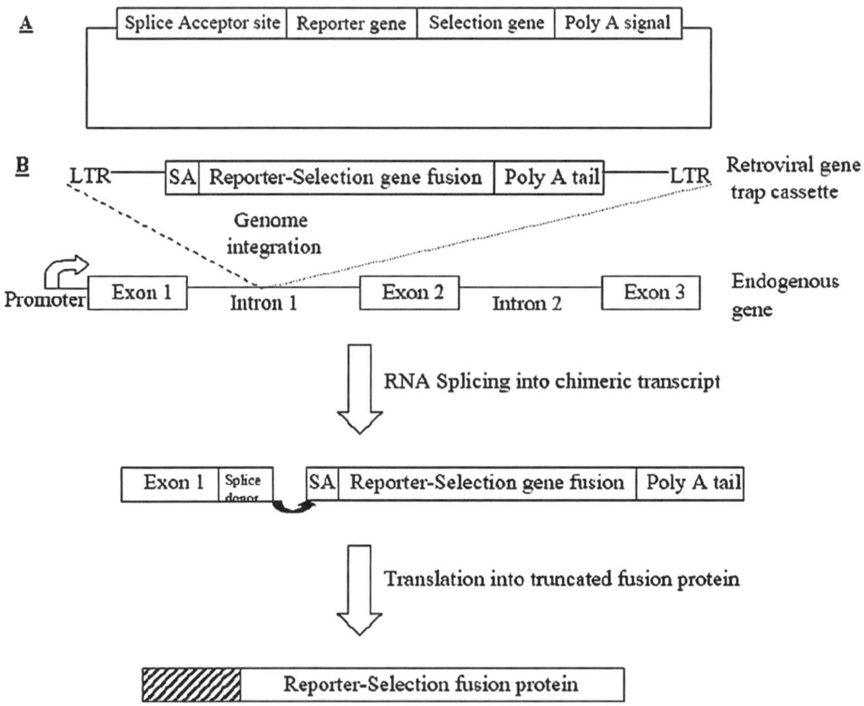

Fig. 4.7 General principle of gene-trapping. A. A retroviral gene-trap consists of a splice acceptor, a reporter gene, and a selection marker flanked by retroviral (long terminal repeats) LTRs that facilitate integration into the genome. **B.** Upon stable integration into the genome the gene-trap will disrupt native gene transcription with the splice acceptor leading to a novel transcript. This novel transcript encodes a reporter-selection fusion protein and will allow for monitoring and cloning the site of integration through inverse PCR or 5′RACE PCR. Finally to test if the site of integration and the disruption of the endogenous gene are sufficient to induce transformation, a soft agar transformation assay can be employed

astrocytes, established from a GFAP:^{V12}HaRas GEM astrocytoma model, we identified *Gata6* as a transforming modifier with ^{V12}*HaRas* in astrocytes (Kamnasaran et al., 2007). Expression, mutational, and functional analyses all demonstrate that *GATA6* is a novel tumor suppressor gene not only in the GEM model, but also more importantly in human GBM. This novel discovery showed the power of using gene-trapping and demonstrated the role of a new transcription factor in GBM progression. GATA6 is one of six members of the mammalian GATA family of transcription factors, all containing two highly conserved zinc-finger DNA-binding domains that interact with a canonical DNA motif (G/A)GATA(A/T) (Molkentin, 2000). GATA6 is located on human chromosome 18q and is an important transcription factor for differentiation and organogenesis. GATA6 and its close family member are highly expressed in cardiac tissue. We and others have recently demonstrated GATA6 expression in a variety of adult murine and human cells of the nervous system, such as the choroid plexus epithelium, neurons, astrocytes, and endothelial cells (Kamnasaran and Guha, 2005). Several compelling pieces of evidence show GATA6 as a novel tumor suppressor in GBM: (1) GATA6 protein expression was absent in several established human GBM lines and explant xenografts; (2) *GATA6* mRNA expression was absent in 20/22 ($\approx$90%) human GBM operative specimens; (3) GATA6 protein expression by IHC was absent in the majority ($\approx$85%) of human GBM specimens and a much lower number ($\approx$10%) of LGA compared to normal brain. In a patient demonstrating a secondary GBM, GATA6 expression was absent in the GBM lesion but present in the LGA lesion, similar to what we found with the B8 GEM. These findings collectively suggest loss of GATA6 to play a role in astrocytoma progression rather than initiation. (4) Nonpolymorphic *GATA6* mutations were found in all five GBMs sequenced, with resultant loss of GATA6 transcriptional activity. These mutations were associated with LOH. (5) Stable reduction of GATA6 expression by two shRNA in nontransformed ^{V12}*Ha-Ras* immortalized mouse and human astrocytes resulted in in vitro and in vivo transformation. (6) Replacement of wild-type *GATA6* into human GBM cell lines lacking GATA6 expression reverted in vitro and in vivo growth potentiation, as a consequence of increasing the number of cells arresting in G_1 and decreasing VEGF expression (Kamnasaran and Guha, 2005). GATA4, a close family member of GATA6 is also expressed in human and murine CNS but is lost in human GBM and several other CNS tumors (unpublished findings). In a broader perspective, random mutagenesis approaches on GBM GEMs or other cancer GEMs are a robust technology to identify novel cancer oncogenes and tumor suppressor genes.

4.7 Ontogeny of Astrocytomas

One of the reasons for the lack of clinical advances in our treatment of human GBMs is insufficient understanding of the cell of origin of this disease. For several decades it was widely assumed that differentiated glia were the only cells capable of transformation, as the adult brain was thought to be mitotically inactive. However, demonstration of functional neurogenesis (Smart and i, 1961; Kaplan and Bell, 1983) and the isolation of brain tumor stem cells (BTSCs) from human GBM specimens underscores the need to consider the role of normal stem/progenitor cells in brain tumor biology.

Currently, controversy exists on whether the initial transformed cell is a differentiated astrocyte, progenitor, or neural stem cell. Putative cancer stem cells (CSCs) have features of normal stem cells (self-renewal, multi-potent differentiation) plus the ability to recapitulate the tumor phenotype in vivo, these cells have been identified from a variety of solid human cancers including GBMs (Singh et al., 2004), lending support to the possibility that brain tumors might arise from the malignant transformation of neural stem cells. However, it is also possible that some brain cancer stem cells arise from differentiated cells, which acquired stem cell properties as a consequence of secondary mutations and subsequent de-differentiation. For example, retroviral transduction of INK4a/Arf$^{-/-}$ astrocytes with the constitutively active mutant EGFRvIII induced astrocyte de-differentiation (Bachoo et al., 2002), as these cells gave rise to tumors with a mixed glial composition. This phenomenon is also observed when GFAP positive cells are infected with a platelet-derived growth factor (PDGF) expressing retrovirus using the RCAS/tva system (Dai et al., 2001). Hence, the nature of the cell of origin in gliomas being a stem cell or a differentiated glial cell remains controversial, with potential biological and therapeutic implications.

Several reasons exist why direct testing of the glioma-CSC hypothesis has proven difficult. First, there is a lack of distinct cell surface markers to delineate and select astroglial progenitor pools and their corresponding differentiated progeny. Commonly used glioma-CSC markers such as CD133 and Nestin are also present in reactive but nontransformed mature astrocytes (Tamagno and Schiffer, 2006). Second, GBMs are well recognized to express markers of non-differentiated cells and lose mature astrocyte markers such as GFAP and express progenitor markers such as Nestin and those of other cell lineages such as Olig2, NeuN. More importantly there are inherent difficulties in the in vitro approaches used to determine the stem cell properties of tumor-derived cell types. Neurosphere formation assays, used to determine the number of cancer stem cells within sorted tumor populations, do not select for quiescent stem-like cells within the tumor but rather for highly proliferating cells such as transit amplifying progenitors (Doetsch et al., 2002). As a result the use of in vivo models will help to make distinctions between these two cell types. Using GEMs where transgenes such as ^{12V}H-Ras are expressed in a cell-specific and inducible manner by Cre-mediated excision and tetracycline-regulated expression might present a better way of addressing questions on the cell of origin of gliomas.

4.8 Conclusions

Animal models provide an indispensable genetic tool in cancer research. Their ability to recapitulate the disease phenotype and genetic background provide much needed insight into cancer biology. GEMs have come to the forefront of GBM biology and GBM GEMs are an invaluable tool providing landmark discoveries that would otherwise be impossible to obtain. GEMs have been an invaluable tool to decipher the neoplastic role pf p21-Ras in GBM in terms of the molecular pathogenesis of this tumor. Also, GEMs based on activated Ras can be employed as gene discovery reagents and thus identify GBM modifier genes such as novel oncogenes and TSGs. In addition, GEMs based on activated Ras can be crossed to other GBM predisposed GEMs to study cancer gene interactions, relationships, and possibly shed light into the cell of origin. Ultimately, a better understanding of p21-Ras complexity and the use of animal models will lead to novel, enhanced, and more effective therapeutic strategies.

References

Bachoo, R.M., Maher, E.A., Ligon, K.L., Sharpless, N.E., Chan, S.S., You, M.J., Tang, Y., DeFrances, J., Stover, E., Weissleder, R., Rowitch, D.H., Louis, D.N., and DePinho, R.A. (2002). Epidermal growth factor receptor and Ink4a/Arf: convergent mechanisms governing terminal differentiation and transformation along the neural stem cell to astrocyte axis. Cancer Cell *1*, 269–277.

Capecchi, M.R. (1989). Altering the genome by homologous recombination. Science *244*, 1288–1292.

Chicoine, M.R. and Silbergeld, D.L. (1995). The in vitro motility of human gliomas increases with increasing grade of malignancy. Cancer *75*, 2904–2909.

Dai, C., Celestino, J.C., Okada, Y., Louis, D.N., Fuller, G.N., and Holland, E.C. (2001). PDGF autocrine stimulation dedifferentiates cultured astrocytes and induces oligodendrogliomas and oligoastrocytomas from neural progenitors and astrocytes in vivo. Genes Dev. *15*, 1913–1925.

Danks, R.A., Orian, J.M., Gonzales, M.F., Tan, S.S., Alexander, B., Mikoshiba, K., and Kaye, A.H. (1995). Transformation of astrocytes in transgenic mice expressing SV40 T antigen under the transcriptional control of the glial fibrillary acidic protein promoter. Cancer Res. *55*, 4302–4310.

Denko, N.C., Giaccia, A.J., Stringer, J.R., and Stambrook, P.J. (1994). The human Ha-ras oncogene induces genomic instability in murine fibroblasts within one cell cycle. Proc. Natl. Acad. Sci. USA *91*, 5124–5128.

DePrimo, S.E., Stambrook, P.J., and Stringer, J.R. (1996). Human placental alkaline phosphatase as a histochemical marker of gene expression in transgenic mice. Transgenic Res. *5*, 459–466.

Ding, H., Roncari, L., Shannon, P., Wu, X., Lau, N., Karaskova, J., Gutmann, D.H., Squire, J.A., Nagy, A., and Guha, A (2001). Astrocyte-specific expression of activated p21-ras results in malignant astrocytoma formation in a transgenic mouse model of human gliomas. Cancer Res. *61*, 3826–3836.

Ding, H., Shannon, P., Lau, N., Wu, X., Roncari, L., Baldwin, R.L., Takebayashi, H., Nagy, A., Gutmann, D.H., and Guha, A (2003). Oligodendrogliomas result from the expression of an activated mutant epidermal growth factor receptor in a RAS transgenic mouse astrocytoma model. Cancer Res. *63*, 1106–1113.

Doetsch, F., Petreanu, L., Caille, I., Garcia-Verdugo, J.M., and Alvarez-Buylla, A (2002). EGF converts transit-amplifying neurogenic precursors in the adult brain into multipotent stem cells. Neuron *36*, 1021–1034.

Dunn, K.J., Williams, B.O., Li, Y., and Pavan, W.J. (2000). Neural crest-directed gene transfer demonstrates Wnt1 role in melanocyte expansion and differentiation during mouse development. Proc. Natl. Acad. Sci. USA *97*, 10050–10055.

Evans, M.J. and Kaufman, M.H. (1981). Establishment in culture of pluripotential cells from mouse embryos. Nature *292*, 154–156.

Feldkamp, M.M., Lau, N., Roncari, L., and Guha, A (2001). Isotype-specific Ras. GTP-levels predict the efficacy of farnesyl transferase inhibitors against human astrocytomas regardless of Ras mutational status. Cancer Res. *61*, 4425–4431.

Fraichard, A., Chassande, O., Bilbaut, G., Dehay, C., Savatier, P., and Samarut, J (1995). In vitro differentiation of embryonic stem cells into glial cells and functional neurons. J. Cell Sci. *108 (Pt 10)*, 3181–3188.

Garrick, D., Fiering, S., Martin, D.I., and Whitelaw, E (1998). Repeat-induced gene silencing in mammals. Nat. Genet. *18*, 56–59.

Guha, A., Feldkamp, M.M., Lau, N., Boss, G., and Pawson, A (1997). Proliferation of human malignant astrocytomas is dependent on Ras activation. Oncogene *15*, 2755–2765.

Gutmann, D.H., Huang, Z.Y., Hedrick, N.M., Ding, H., Guha, A., and Watson, M.A. (2002). Mouse glioma gene expression profiling identifies novel human glioma-associated genes. Ann. Neurol. *51*, 393–405.

Kamnasaran, D and Guha, A (2005). Expression of GATA6 in the human and mouse central nervous system. Brain Res. Dev. Brain Res. *160*, 90–95.

Kamnasaran, D., Qian, B., Hawkins, C., Stanford, W.L., and Guha, A (2007). GATA6 is an astrocytoma tumor suppressor gene identified by gene trapping of mouse glioma model. Proc. Natl. Acad. Sci. USA *104*, 8053–8058.

Kaplan, M.S. and Bell, D.H. (1983). Neuronal proliferation in the 9-month-old rodent-radioautographic study of granule cells in the hippocampus. Exp. Brain Res. *52*, 1–5.

Kleihues, P and Cavanee, W.K. World Health Organization Classification of Tumors: Pathology and Genetic: Tumors of the Nervous System. 2000. IARC, Press. Ref Type: Generic

Molkentin, J.D. (2000). The zinc finger-containing transcription factors GATA-4, -5, and -6. Ubiquitously expressed regulators of tissue-specific gene expression. J. Biol. Chem. *275*, 38949–38952.

Nagy, A., Gocza, E., Diaz, E.M., Prideaux, V.R., Ivanyi, E., Markkula, M., and Rossant, J (1990). Embryonic stem cells alone are able to support fetal development in the mouse. Development *110*, 815–821.

Shannon, P., Sabha, N., Lau, N., Kamnasaran, D., Gutmann, D.H., and Guha, A (2005). Pathological and molecular progression of astrocytomas in a GFAP:12 V-Ha-Ras mouse astrocytoma model. Am. J. Pathol. *167*, 859–867.

Singh, S.K., Hawkins, C., Clarke, I.D., Squire, J.A., Bayani, J., Hide, T., Henkelman, R.M., Cusimano, M.D., and Dirks, P.B. (2004). Identification of human brain tumour initiating cells. Nature *432*, 396–401.

Smart, I. The subependymal layer of the mouse brain and its cell production as shown by autoradiography after [H3]-thymidine injection. J. Comp. Neurol. 116, 325. 1961. Ref Type: Generic

Stander, M., Naumann, U., Dumitrescu, L., Heneka, M., Loschmann, P., Gulbins, E., Dichgans, J., and Weller, M (1998). Decorin gene transfer-mediated suppression of TGF-beta synthesis abrogates experimental malignant glioma growth in vivo. Gene Ther. *5*, 1187–1194.

Stanford, W.L., Cohn, J.B., and Cordes, S.P. (2001). Gene-trap mutagenesis: past, present and beyond. Nat. Rev. Genet. *2*, 756–768.

Tamagno, I and Schiffer, D (2006). Nestin expression in reactive astrocytes of human pathology. J. Neurooncol. *80*, 227–233.

Wei, Q., Clarke, L., Scheidenhelm, D.K., Qian, B., Tong, A., Sabha, N., Karim, Z., Bock, N.A., Reti, R., Swoboda, R., Purev, E., Lavoie, J.F., Bajenaru, M.L., Shannon, P., Herlyn, D., Kaplan, D., Henkelman, R.M., Gutmann, D.H., and Guha, A (2006). High-grade glioma formation results from postnatal pten loss or mutant epidermal growth factor receptor expression in a transgenic mouse glioma model. Cancer Res. *66*, 7429–7437.

Weissenberger, J., Steinbach, J.P., Malin, G., Spada, S., Rulicke, T., and Aguzzi, A (1997). Development and malignant progression of astrocytomas in GFAP-v-src transgenic mice. Oncogene *14*, 2005–2013.

Wurster, A.L., Tanaka, T., and Grusby, M.J. (2000). The biology of Stat4 and Stat6. Oncogene *19*, 2577–2584.

Chapter 5
Pten-Deficient Mouse Models for High-Grade Astrocytomas

Chang-Hyuk Kwon

Abstract Despite vigorous efforts in clinics and laboratories, the overall prognosis for patients with glioblastoma multiforme (GBM), the most common and aggressive glioma, has not greatly improved over the last few decades. Innovative new therapies based on detailed molecular mechanisms of glioma biology are highly desired. Mutation or loss of PTEN (phosphatase tensin homolog deleted on chromosome ten), a key phosphatase that antagonizes the PI3K/AKT pathway, is one of the most frequent abnormalities found in high-grade astrocytomas. Whether this genetic alteration is causal or consequential to the tumorigenic process has begun to be elucidated through tumor genetics and new mouse models. This chapter describes the key findings from mouse astrocytoma models involving *Pten* deficiency or Akt activation, with specific emphasis on the recently reported *Pten*-heterozygous mouse models. In addition, future directions to inform the design of novel therapeutics for this devastating disease are discussed.

Contents

C.-H. Kwon (✉)
Department of Neurological Surgery, Tumor Microenvironment Program, Dardinger Center for Neuro-oncology and Neurosciences, James Comprehensive Cancer Center, The Ohio State University Medical Center, Room 820 Biomedical Research Tower, 460 W. 12th Ave., Columbus, OH 43210, USA
e-mail: Chang-Hyuk.Kwon@osumc.edu

E.G. Van Meir (ed.), *CNS Cancer*, Cancer Drug Discovery and Development, DOI 10.1007/978-1-60327-553-8_5,

© Humana Press, a part of Springer Science+Business Media, LLC 2009

5.1 Introduction

The phosphatidyl inositol 3′ kinase (PI3K) family is a group of intracellular lipid kinases that phosphorylate the 3′-hydroxyl group of phosphatidyl inositol substrates (Cantley, 2002; Engelman et al., 2006). One key substrate is phosphatidyl inositol 3,4,5-triphosphate (PIP3), which can bind to the pleckstrin homology domain of Ser/Thr kinase AKT (see also Chapter 15). PIP3 binding effectively translocates AKT to the cellular membrane where it is subsequently activated by the PDK1 and mTORC2 kinases (Guertin and Sabatini, 2007; Manning and Cantley, 2007). PTEN negatively regulates the PI3K/AKT pathway through its lipid phosphatase activity against the 3′ position of phosphatidyl inositol substrates (Cantley and Neel, 1999; Maehama and Dixon, 1998) (Fig. 5.1), and loss of PTEN function results in AKT activation in a majority of experimental and pathological conditions (Li and Ross, 2007). In turn, activated AKT phosphorylates a diverse spectrum of substrates, including MDM2, FOXO, BAD, GSK3β, and TSC, ultimately leading to increases in cell survival, proliferation, growth, and/or migration (Manning and Cantley, 2007) (also see Fig. 15.2a). The PI3K/PTEN/AKT pathway controls many developmental processes as well as normal homeostasis. In many experimental systems, activation of this pathway results in hypertrophy, hyperplasia, ectopia, or a combination of these, depending on the affected cell type (Goberdhan and Wilson, 2003). In both humans and mice, perturbation of this pathway is associated with brain disorders, such as macrocephaly, ataxia, seizure, Lhermitte–Duclos disease, autism, schizophrenia, and

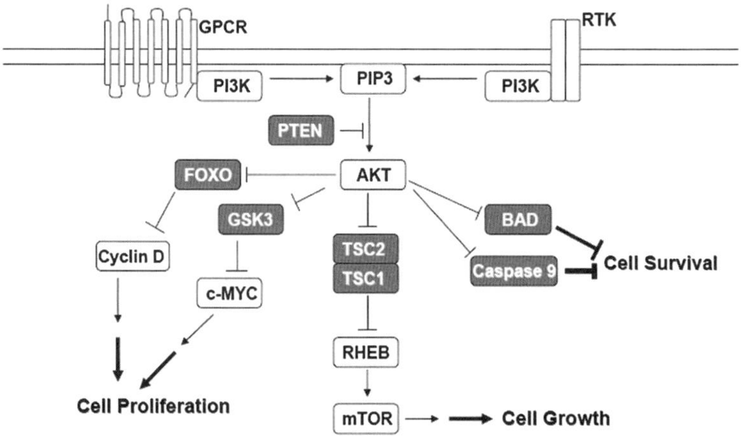

Fig. 5.1 The PI3K/PTEN/AKT pathway. PI3K activated by RTK or GPCR increases PIP3 levels. PIP3 binds to the pleckstrin homology domain of AKT, which leads to the translocation of AKT to the membrane where it is activated. Activated AKT can phosphorylate a large number of substrates, including FOXO, GSK3, BAD, caspase 9, and the TSC2 gene product tuberin, which results in increased cell proliferation, growth, or survival. PTEN antagonizes the PI3K/AKT pathway by dephosphorylating PIP3, thus decreasing PIP3 levels

high-grade astrocytomas (Ali et al., 1999; Butler et al., 2005; Emamian et al., 2004; Eng, 2003; Kwon et al., 2006; Kwon et al., 2001).

Astrocytoma is a type of glioma with a predominantly astrocyte-like morphology. This tumor type constitutes approximately 75% of all gliomas and 30% of all brain tumors (CBTRUS, 2005). Frequent genetic abnormalities found in high-grade astrocytomas include mutation or loss of tumor suppressor genes, such as *TP53*, *PTEN*, *INK4A*, *ARF*, and *RB*, and amplification, activating mutation, or overexpression of proto-oncogenes, including *EGFR*, *PDGFR*, and *CDK4* (Maher et al., 2001; Zhu and Parada, 2002). According to a recent report from The Cancer Genome Atlas, *PTEN* mutation is one of the most frequent genetic abnormalities found in astrocytomas (Kaiser, 2008). As in many other cancer types, *PTEN* mutation is more frequent in higher grade astrocytomas than in lower grade counterparts (Baker and McKinnon, 2004). Therefore, PTEN inactivation has been thought to be crucial for astrocytoma progression, but not for initiation. Although *PTEN* mutation is more frequent in primary GBMs (also called de novo GBMs, 25%), which arise without clinical evidence of a prior low-grade tumor, than in secondary GBMs (also called progressive GBMs, 4%) that occur through progression from a grade II or III astrocytoma, loss of heterozygosity (LOH) of chromosome 10q where *PTEN* is located is a common feature in both GBM types (70 and 63%, respectively) (Ohgaki et al., 2004) (also see Fig. 15.3). Additionally, decreased PTEN expression correlates with AKT activation and has been shown to be a poor prognosis marker for high-grade astrocytomas (Phillips et al., 2006).

5.2 *Pten*-Null or Akt-Activated Mouse Models of High-Grade Astrocytoma

A genetic abnormality frequently observed in a cancer type can provide crucial clues for investigating the disease. However, such information is not always sufficient to distinguish causal versus consequential relationship of the abnormality to the cancer type. This is especially true for high-grade astrocytomas where diverse genetic abnormalities are present. A mouse model with precise temporal and/or spatial manipulation of such a genetic abnormality can provide insights into cancer etiology. Transgenic technology, delivery of oncogenic viruses, and germline or *cre/loxP*-mediated conditional gene targeting have been used to model high-grade astrocytomas in mice. To understand the role of *PTEN* inactivation in human astrocytomas, several groups have generated mouse astrocytoma models with *Pten* deficiency or Akt activation (summarized in Table 5.1). Since other chapters detail many of these models, this chapter will focus on a brief description of the mouse models and the major insights gleaned from them.

The first mouse astrocytoma model with constitutive Akt activation employed the delivery of avian retroviruses to express Akt as well as Kras in nestin-expressing neural progenitors or GFAP-expressing glial progenitors of

Table 5.1 Summary of *Pten*-deficient or Akt-activated mouse models of astrocytoma[a]

Name	Description	Tumor penetrance	Tumor grade	Mean survival	Reference
Ntv-a + Akt and Kras	Retroviral injection of activated Akt and Kras into neural progenitors of P0 mice	22% ($n = 74$) by 12 weeks	IV	ND[b]	Holland et al. (2000)
Ntv-a or *Gtv-a* in *Ink4a-Arf*$^{-/-}$ + Akt and Kras	Retroviral injection of activated Akt and Kras into neural (*Ntv-a*) or glial (*Gtv-a*) progenitors of P0 *Ink4a-Arf* double null mice	*Ntv-a*: 49% ($n = 43$) *Gtv-a*: 42% ($n = 31$) by 12 weeks	IV?	ND	Uhrbom et al. (2002)
GFAP-V^{12}*-Ras* (B8) + *Pten* cKO[c]	Transgenic expression of activated *Ras* under human *GFAP* promoter + conditional *Pten* deletion by injection of adenovirus-cre	Almost complete?	B8 only: II (80%) or III; higher grade by *Pten* cKO	B8/+: 3 months; this was shortened by deletion of *Pten*	Ding et al. (2001); Wei et al. (2006)
$TgG(\Delta Z)T_{121}$ (with *Pten*$^{+/-}$)	Inactivation of Rb family proteins under human *GFAP* promoter (+ *Pten* germline heterozygosity)	Complete	II or III	5–6 months (4–6 weeks?)	Xiao et al. (2002)
$TgG(\Delta Z)T_{121}$ + *Pten* cKO	Inactivation of Rb family proteins under human *GFAP* promoter + conditional *Pten* deletion by cre-expressing retrovirus in adult brain	Complete?	ND	ND	Xiao et al. (2005)
Mut4	*GFAP-cre*; *Nf1*$^{loxP/+}$; *p53*$^{-/+}$; *Pten*$^{loxP/+}$	Complete	III or IV	Mut4: 18 weeks Mut6: 16 weeks	Kwon et al. (2008)
Mut6	*GFAP-cre*; *Nf1*$^{loxP/+}$; *p53*$^{-/loxP}$; *Pten*$^{loxP/+}$				

[a]This table excludes xenograft or orthotopic models. Also excluded are genetic models with insufficient mouse numbers or insufficient tumor information.
[b]Not determined.
[c]Conditional knockout.

neonatal mouse brain (Holland et al., 2000). Constitutive activation of both Akt and Kras was able to induce GBM in neural progenitors but not in the glial progenitors, in which a third genetic alteration, *Ink4a/Arf* double loss, was required for GBM induction (Uhrbom et al., 2002). Thus, in neonatal mouse brain, both neural and glial progenitors can become transformed depending on defined combinations of oncogenic activation and tumor suppressor inactivation (for more details, see Chapter 2).

$TgG(\Delta Z)T_{121}$ is a transgenic mouse line with inactivation of Rb family proteins by transgenic expression of T_{121}, a truncated SV40 large T antigen, under the human *GFAP* promoter (Xiao et al., 2002). This line develops grade II or III astrocytomas with complete penetrance. To examine the effect of Pten loss in the tumor cells, the $TgG(\Delta Z)T_{121}$ mice were crossed to contain $Pten^{loxP/loxP}$ alleles and a cre-expressing retrovirus was stereotactically injected into the adult frontal cortex where the tumor cells are frequently present (Xiao et al., 2005). All cells locally infected with the virus will constitutively express cre recombinase, which in turn excises the engineered *loxP*-flanked *Pten* gene. Dense neoplastic cell clusters with Akt activation signals (phospho-Akt at Ser473) were observed 5 weeks after the cre-mediated *Pten* deletion. The *Pten*-inactivated tumor cells showed reduced apoptosis and increased invasiveness and angiogenesis, thus indicating that *Pten* loss in tumor cells with Rb family protein inactivation results in tumor progression.

$GFAP\text{-}V^{12}\text{-}Ras$ is a transgenic mouse line expressing activated V12-Ras under the human *GFAP* (*hGFAP*) promoter (Ding et al., 2001). The B8 line of $GFAP\text{-}V^{12}\text{-}Ras$ mice develops grade II (80%) or III astrocytomas. Effect of *Pten* loss was examined by deleting both *Pten* alleles in $GFAP\text{-}V^{12}\text{-}Ras;$ $Pten^{loxP/loxP}$ mice through stereotactic adenovirus injection into the frontal lobe of 4-week-old mouse brain (Wei et al., 2006). This resulted in the formation of higher grade tumors, demonstrating that *Pten* inactivation plays a pivotal role in astrocytoma progression in $GFAP\text{-}V^{12}\text{-}Ras$ mice.

Although neither *Pten* deficiency nor Akt activation was a part of the design of their genotypes, other mouse models also showed evidence of Akt activation in high-grade astrocytomas. Mice heterozygous for both *Nf1* and *p53* on the same chromosome (*Nf1*; *p53 cis* mice) spontaneously develop astrocytomas of varying grade and penetrance depending on the mouse strain (Reilly et al., 2000) (see Chapter 6 for details). Since the *Nf1*; *p53 cis* mice also develop soft tissue sarcomas (Vogel et al., 1999), the model was further improved through conditional deletion of the *loxP-Nf1* allele (Zhu et al., 2002) in neural cells by *hGFAP-cre* mice (Zhuo et al., 2001). Both Mut1 (*hGFAP-cre*; $Nf1^{loxP/loxP}$; $p53^{-/-}$) mice with homozygous deletion and Mut3 (*hGFAP-cre*; $Nf1^{loxP/+}$; $p53^{-/+}$) mice with heterozygous deletion spontaneously developed grade II-IV astrocytomas with full penetrance (Zhu et al., 2005). In the mouse astrocytomas, higher phospho-Akt signal was detected in higher grade tumors. An additional mouse astrocytoma model is FIG–ROS mice (Charest et al., 2006). It has been reported that an orphan RTK ROS is ectopically expressed in 30% of glioma cell lines and tumors (Birchmeier et al., 1987; Watkins et al., 1994). To verify the role of the ectopic

ROS expression, adenovirus expressing constitutively activated ROS (a FIG–ROS fusion form) was stereotactically delivered into the striatum of adult mice (Charest et al., 2006). Forty percent of the mice developed malignant astrocytomas between 33 and 55 weeks after the stereotactic injection, and an *Ink4a/Arf* null background increased penetrance (to 80%) and shortened latency (within 15 weeks postinjection). In this mouse model as well, Akt activation was observed in higher grade tumors and tumor-derived cell lines. Taken together, in several mouse astrocytoma models tested, Akt activation was detected in higher grade tumors, but not (or to a lesser extent) in lower grade tumors, reminiscent of the frequent *PTEN* mutation in higher grade human astrocytomas.

5.3 *Pten*-Heterozygous Mouse Models of High-Grade Astrocytoma

The above-mentioned *Pten*-null or Akt-activated mouse models have provided crucial insights into the cellular origin of malignant astrocytomas and supported the view that *PTEN* inactivation plays a crucial role in tumor progression. However, intriguingly, a majority of human astrocytomas with *PTEN* mutations still harbor an intact *PTEN* allele or a different type of *PTEN* mutation. Similarly, in prostate tumors and breast cancers, monoallelic *PTEN* mutation is predominant over biallelic loss (Ali et al., 1999; Gray et al., 1998; Salmena et al., 2008; Whang et al., 1998). These findings suggest successive loss of *PTEN* alleles and a potential role for *PTEN* heterozygosity in tumorigenicity, at least in some cancer types. Additionally, acute loss of both *Pten* alleles specifically in the mouse brain results in hypertrophy, hyperplasia, or both depending on cell types, but not tumor formation (Backman et al., 2001; Fraser et al., 2004; Groszer et al., 2001; Kwon et al., 2006, 2001; Marino et al., 2002). Interestingly, acute loss of both *Pten* alleles in mouse prostate resulted in p53-mediated cellular senescence rather than increased proliferation (Chen et al., 2005), suggesting that *Pten*-heterozygous tumor models might have more physiological relevance than models with either acute loss of both *Pten* alleles or Akt activation.

The first *Pten*-heterozygous mouse model for astrocytoma was the $TgG(\Delta Z)T_{121}$; $Pten^{+/-}$ mice (Xiao et al., 2002). Intriguingly, the introduction of germline *Pten* heterozygosity into the $TgG(\Delta Z)T_{121}$ background shortened tumor latency but did not affect tumor grade. This suggests that *Pten* heterozygosity may contribute to astrocytoma initiation. However, the status of Akt activation or *Pten* LOH in the *Pten*-heterozygous tumors has not been reported. In a second model (Mut4 mice), conditional *Pten* heterozygosity was introduced into the Mut3 mice (*hGFAP-cre*; $Nf1^{loxP/+}$; $p53^{-/+}$, Table 5.2) (Kwon et al., 2008). Mut6 mice have an additional *loxP-p53* allele replacing the *trans wt p53* allele of Mut4 mice. Unlike many other reported mouse models that succumb to developmental defects, Mut3-Mut6 mice are indistinguishable from

Table 5.2 Genotype and median survival of Mut3-Mut6 mice (Kwon et al., 2008)

Mouse line	Genotype[a] *Nf1*	*p53*	*Pten*	Median survival (weeks)[c]	Astrocytoma grade[d]	Tumor penetrance[e]	Tumor growth[f]
Mut3	*loxP*/+	–/+[b]	+/+	27.5	III (72.7%) or IV	91.4%	22.4%
Mut4	*loxP*/+	–/+	*loxP*/+	18.0	III (80.0%) or IV	100%	99.6%
Mut5	*loxP*/+	–/*loxP*	+/+	24.4	III (33.3%) or IV	91.3%	ND[g]
Mut6	*loxP*/+	–/*loxP*	*loxP*/+	15.6	III (12.5%) or IV	100%	ND[g]

[a]*hGFAP-cre* (Zhuo et al., 2001) was used for all genotypes to conditionally delete *loxP* allele(s) in neural cells.
[b]*Cis* mutation on the same chromosome with *loxP-Nf1*.
[c]From analysis on 23 or more mice per line.
[d]From symptomatic mice analyzed ($n = 6$–11 per line). Younger, asymptomatic Mut3 mice also develop grade II tumor.
[e]When analyzed up to 9 months of age. In an independent study (Zhu et al., 2005), Mut3 mice showed full penetrance of astrocytoma onset when analyzed up to 50 weeks of age.
[f]Median tumor growth per week when equivalent size of grade III tumors was compared by MRI.
[g]Not determined.

littermate controls until adult ages when they spontaneously form high-grade astrocytomas with complete or near-complete penetrance (Table 5.2 and Fig. 5.2). The *Pten*-heterozygous Mut4 and Mut6 mice show interesting features as follows.

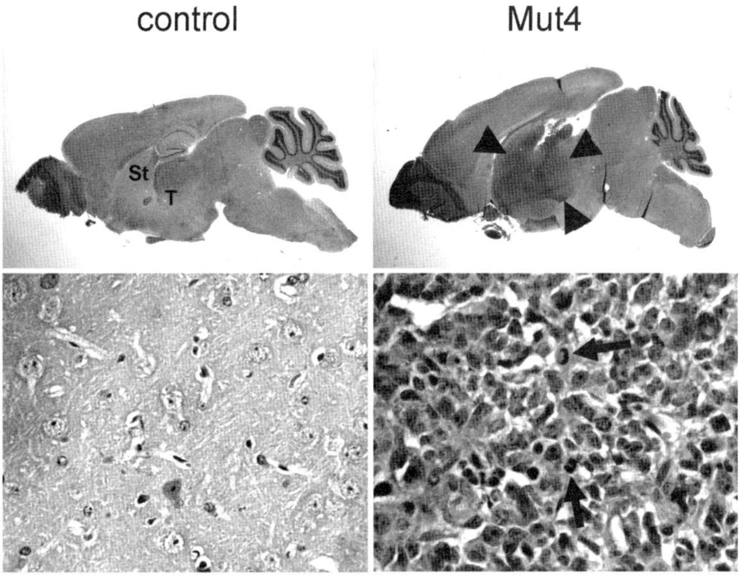

Fig. 5.2 A representative high-grade astrocytoma from *Pten*-heterozygous Mut4 mice. *Upper panels*, a diffusely infiltrating brain tumor (arrow heads) encompassing the striatum (St) and thalamus (T) spontaneously developed in adult Mut4 brain. Such a neoplasm is not present in control brain. *Lower panels*, a higher magnification image shows characteristic morphology of diffusely infiltrating astrocytomas, including mitotic index (arrows, for example), which is absent in a matched area of control

In contrast to the view that *PTEN* inactivation is mainly important for tumor progression, introduction of conditional *Pten* heterozygosity into Mut3 mice does not change final tumor grade (Kwon et al., 2008). Instead, it results in earlier onset of more malignant astrocytomas in asymptomatic mice. Unlike in *Pten-wt* Mut3 mice, grade II tumors have never been detected in *Pten*-heterozygous Mut4 or Mut6 genotype at any ages. Evidence of *Pten* LOH was detected in grade IV tumors or cultured tumor cells with signals of Akt activation, but not in the majority of *in situ* grade III tumors with absence of Akt activation. In cultured *Pten-wt* Mut3 tumors, decreased Pten expression was detectable, but increased Akt activation was not observed. These data, together with previous reports, suggest that although *Pten* heterozygosity alone is insufficient to induce astrocytoma, it can cooperate with inactivation of other tumor suppressors to initiate astrocytomas, perhaps through an Akt-independent mechanism. It is only upon losing the second *Pten* allele that progression to grade IV GBM is observed, suggesting that the first allelic loss contributes to tumor initiation, whereas loss of the second allele drives tumor progression. In addition, MRI and subsequent histological analysis revealed that the *Pten*-heterozygous Mut4 tumors grow approximately five times faster than *Pten wt* Mut3 tumors at the same grade and equivalent sizes. These data, and previous reports that *PTEN* mutation is more frequent in primary than secondary GBMs (Ohgaki et al., 2004), suggest that the faster tumor growth resulting from *PTEN* deficiency may underlie the sudden onset of primary GBMs.

Kaplan–Meier survival curves and histological analyses indicate that a majority of Mut4 and Mut6 mice die of high-grade astrocytomas within a narrow window of time (Kwon et al., 2008). This provides a good opportunity to investigate earlier cellular events before tumor initiation. Indeed, it was found that at 6-8 weeks of age, ectopic migration of neural stem/progenitor populations precedes tumor initiation in the *Pten*-deficient Mut4 and Mut6 mice as analyzed by marker staining and BrdU chasing. Even at a younger age (4 weeks), Mut3 or Mut4 subventricular zone (SVZ) cells cultured as neurospheres showed abnormal features, including hypertrophic neurospheres, increases in proliferation and self-renewal, and decreases in cell death and astrocyte differentiation (Alcantara-Llaguno et al., 2009). Yet, these young abnormal cells do not show evidence of loss of heterozygosity (LOH) at *Nf1*, *p53*, or *Pten*, indicating that combined heterozygosity of the tumor suppressors is responsible for these tumor-prone properties. These data also suggest that the SVZ stem/progenitor population is likely the cellular origin of astrocytomas, at least in the mouse models.

5.4 Discussion

As suggested from the diverse types of genetic abnormalities found in human astrocytomas and the findings in mouse models, the formation of malignant astrocytoma appears to require at least two mutations. Thus, it is likely that cooperation of multiple oncogenic stimuli is mandatory for tumorigenicity.

Although many combinations of human astrocytoma signature mutations have generated a true phenocopy in mice, not all of them have been successful. For example, Akt activation or *Pten* deletion plus *Ink4a/Arf* null mutation in neonatal progenitors did not induce brain tumor formation in mice (Hu et al., 2005; Uhrbom et al., 2002). This indicates that there are multiple, yet to be defined, genetic combinations initiating astrocytomas. For example, *NF1* mutation occurs in concert with *TP53* mutation (Kaiser, 2008), indicating the same tumorigenic pathway. *TP53* mutation and *EGFR* amplification are usually mutually exclusive in human GBMs (Watanabe et al., 1996), suggesting different oncogenic pathways. These observations are important for the design of rational therapies based on molecular pathways leading to astrocytoma formation. If such multiple initiation pathways are present and converge into a single progression pathway, this would be the consensus molecular target for astrocytoma treatment. On the other hand, if each initiation pathway employs a different progression pathway, the tumor treatment should be altered, depending on tumor genotype. Further genomic analysis of multiple genotypes of human astrocytomas and equivalent mouse astrocytoma models would enlighten this issue.

The high frequency of combined *PTEN* mutation and 10q LOH in both primary and secondary GBMs (Ohgaki et al., 2004) indicates that *PTEN* inactivation plays a pivotal role in the most aggressive gliomas. The *Pten*-heterozygous mouse models of astrocytomas (Kwon et al., 2008; Xiao et al., 2002) strongly suggest that *PTEN* haploinsufficiency plays an important role in tumorigenicity. The absence of Akt activation or *Pten* LOH in a majority of grade III Mut4 tumors implies that an Akt-independent mechanism accounts for the contribution of *Pten* heterozygosity in astrocytoma formation. Similarly, Akt-independent contribution of *PTEN* deficiency to tumor formation has been reported in other tumor types as well (Blanco-Aparicio et al., 2007; Freeman et al., 2003; Yoo et al., 2006). Comparative analysis of *Pten* wt, heterozygous, and null cells during tumor development would provide insights into the underlying molecular mechanisms.

The mechanism by which primary GBMs develop so suddenly without medical evidence of previous low-grade tumors has remained an enigma. *Pten*-heterozygous Mut4 tumors grow approximately five times faster than *Pten*-wt Mut3 tumors when equivalent size of grade III tumors was compared (Kwon et al., 2008). Histology data revealed that Mut4 astrocytomas contain higher density of mitotic index and signals of Ki67, a proliferation marker, than those of Mut3 tumors. In addition, *PTEN* mutation is more frequent in primary GBMs (25%) than in secondary GBMs (4%) (Ohgaki et al., 2004). Primary GBMs occur suddenly and rapidly, while progressive GBMs evolve from lower grade astrocytomas over time. Therefore, the sudden onset of primary GBMs may result from faster tumor growth due to *PTEN* deficiency. Since *PTEN* mutation is also present with mutations other than *NF1* and *TP53* in human GBMs, additional *Pten*-heterozygous mouse models are needed to test this hypothesis.

It is also intriguing that the SVZ cultures from presymptomatic Mut3 or Mut4 mice already display tumor-prone cellular phenotypes without evidence of tumor suppressor LOH (Alcantara-Llaguno et al., 2009). This suggests that the tumor suppressor heterozygosity generates a synergistic mechanism initiating astrocytomas. Further functional analysis of the role of tumor suppressor heterozygosity could reveal the molecular mechanisms for astrocytoma initiation. The SVZ culture data and the ectopic migration of neural stem/progenitors prior to tumor formation in the *Pten*-heterozygous Mut4 and Mut6 mice (Kwon et al., 2008) support the neural stem/progenitor origin of astrocytomas (Hemmati et al., 2003; Ignatova et al., 2002; Singh et al., 2003; Zhu et al., 2005). Similarly, the first abnormal cell population was also observed in the SVZ of $TgG(\Delta Z)T_{121}$ mice (Xiao et al., 2002). Determining the tumor cell of origin will require more accurate gene targeting in mice and in cultured cells. Comparison of the "origin" cells with cells isolated from various stages of mouse astrocytomas should reveal key molecular and cellular mechanisms responsible for initiation and progression of high-grade astrocytomas. Also, comparative analysis with human tumors should provide therapeutic clues to attack this devastating disease.

Careful analysis of a causal versus a consequential role for a particular genetic alteration is crucial: pursuing consequential changes may not improve cancer treatment. For example, activation of the mTOR pathway has been detected in a majority of high-grade astrocytomas (Choe et al., 2003; Kondo et al., 2004). However, a clinical trial using an mTOR inhibitor did not improve overall survival of astrocytoma patients, although the treatment efficiently blocked the molecular pathway (Galanis et al., 2005). In a mouse model, blocking the pathway indeed suppressed astrocytoma but paradoxically increased oligodendroglioma formation, resulting in no changes in overall prognosis (Hu et al., 2005). These examples emphasize the importance of functional studies on the causal versus consequential role of genetic abnormalities found in a tumor type. It is not necessary that all astrocytoma signature mutations contribute to the tumor biology. Activation of the mTOR pathway could be a by-product of AKT activation during GBM progression or mainly required for maintenance of the astrocytoma lineage. Therefore, pinpointing cancer etiology-specific changes, by comparison with an origin cell type, would be a key step in finding therapeutic targets for high-grade astrocytomas.

The study of cancer stem cells is another approach to investigate this problem. CD133-positive cells from human GBMs or medulloblastomas have been shown to be much more tumorigenic than CD133-negative cells from the same tumor type (Singh et al., 2003, 2004). In addition, the CD133-positive GBM cells were more angiogenic and resistant to radiation therapy (Bao et al., 2006a, b), possibly explaining why GBMs do not respond to conventional cancer therapies. These putative cancer stem cells have been isolated from other human cancer types as well (Al-Hajj et al., 2003; Bonnet and Dick, 1997; Collins et al., 2005; Eramo et al., 2007; Lapidot et al., 1994; Li et al., 2007; O'Brien et al., 2007;

Prince et al., 2007). Since putative origin cells (neural stem cells, astrocytes, or both) can be isolated from mouse brain and cultured *in vitro*, cancer stem cell-specific genomic changes could be identified through comparison with the putative origin cells in mice, providing more promising therapeutic clues for cancer treatment. However, purification of the putative cancer stem cell population has not been reported in mouse cancer models. CD133 is an embryonic neural stem cell marker, with expression restricted to ependymal cells, and not observed in neurogenic astrocytes present in the stem cell niches of adult mouse brain (Pfenninger et al., 2007). The functional significance of CD133 expression has not yet been reported. This puzzling discrepancy of CD133 reactivity between human and mouse cancer cells needs to be resolved if cancer stem cells are to be compared with cell(s) of origin in mouse brain tumor models. Alternatively, other markers that are conserved and play a role in both human and mouse cancers need to be identified.

Candidate therapies derived from the above-mentioned schemes can be tested by using the diverse mouse models with different combinations of oncogenic stimuli, assuming that the high-grade astrocytomas can be generated by multiple pathways. An ideal mouse model of high-grade astrocytoma for such translational studies should meet several criteria as follows. The model should be a phenocopy, that is, tumor properties should recapitulate those of human astrocytomas. Higher penetrance, narrower window of time for tumor development, and minimal side phenotypes, such as developmental defects or formation of other tumor types, will help the design of translational studies. Mouse models with oncogenic targeting or loss of both tumor suppressor alleles early in development tend to have developmental defects. Mouse models with germline hetero- or nullizygosity of tumor suppressor gene(s) tend to eventually develop non-brain tumors as well. Some models involving stereotactic injection are labor intensive and can produce variable phenotypes. Since the functional role of many astrocytoma signature mutations still remains unclear, a model with the same mutation (genocopy) would be better than a pathway-targeted model (phenocopy).

Recent advances in cancer genetics, tumor biology, and mouse models have provided many crucial insights into where and how high-grade astrocytomas are generated. However, a successful therapy for this deadly disease is not in sight yet. Innovative strategies for identifying possible therapeutic targets are sorely needed. As our knowledge of brain tumorigenesis increases, so will the challenges we face in this field. This stems from the complicated nature of brain neoplasms, due to diverse tumorigenic pathways, potentially with multiple cellular origins. Therefore, thorough and careful investigation is required in trying to understand the mechanisms by which these tumors are initiated and progress. As many of the reported mouse models have provided crucial insights into astrocytoma biology and etiology, additional new models with precise genetic manipulations might unveil the remaining mysteries of this devastating disease.

Abbreviations

AKT	v-akt murine *t*hymoma viral oncogene homolog
ARF	alternate open reading frame
BAD	BCL2 antagonist of cell death
CDK4	cyclin-dependent kinase 4
Cre	causes recombination
EGFR	epidermal growth factor receptor
FIG	a fusion transcript isolated from a glioblastoma cell line
FOXO	forkhead box
GBM	glioblastoma multiforme
GPCR	G-protein-coupled receptor
GSK3β	glycogen synthase kinase 3 beta
hGFAP	human glial fibrillary acidic protein
INK4A	inhibits CDK4
Kras	V-Ki-ras2 Kirsten rat sarcoma viral oncogene homolog
LOH	loss of heterozygosity
loxP	locus of crossing over
MDM2	mouse double minute 2
mTORC2	mammalian target of rapamycin kinase complex 2
NF1	neurofibromatosis type 1
PDGFR	platelet-derived growth factor receptor
PDK1	3-phosphoinositide-dependent kinase-1
PI3K	phosphatidyl inositol 3′ kinase
PIP3	phosphatidyl inositol 3,4,5-triphosphate
PTEN	phosphatase tensin homolog deleted on chromosome ten
RB	retinoblastoma
RHEB	Ras homolog enriched in brain
ROS	Ros proto-oncogene
RTK	receptor tyrosine kinase
SVZ	subventricular zone
TSC	tuberous sclerosis complex

Acknowledgments The author thanks Luis Parada for support and guidance and Jian Chen, Sheila Alcantara Llaguno, Yanjiao Li, Dennis Burns, Dan Zhu, and Renee McKay for helpful suggestions and discussion. This work is supported in part by Basic Research Fellowships from the American Brain Tumor Association (in memory of Daniel J. Martinelli and Geoffrey J. Cunningham).

References

Al-Hajj, M., Wicha, M. S., Benito-Hernandez, A., Morrison, S. J., and Clarke, M. F. (2003). Prospective identification of tumorigenic breast cancer cells. Proc Natl Acad Sci USA *100*, 3983–3988.

Alcantara-Llaguno, S., Chen, J., Kwon, C. H., Jackson, E. L., Li, Y., Burns, D. K., Alvarez-Buylla, A., and Parada, L. F. (2009). Malignant astrocytomas originate from neural stem/progenitor cells in a somatic tumor suppressor mouse model. Cancer Cell *15*, 45–56.

Ali, I. U., Schriml, L. M., and Dean, M. (1999). Mutational spectra of PTEN/MMAC1 gene: a tumor suppressor with lipid phosphatase activity. J Natl Cancer Inst *91*, 1922–1932.

Backman, S. A., Stambolic, V., Suzuki, A., Haight, J., Elia, A., Pretorius, J., Tsao, M. S., Shannon, P., Bolon, B., Ivy, G. O., and Mak, T. W. (2001). Deletion of Pten in mouse brain causes seizures, ataxia and defects in soma size resembling Lhermitte-Duclos disease. Nat Genet *29*, 396–403.

Baker, S. J., and McKinnon, P. J. (2004). Tumour-suppressor function in the nervous system. Nat Rev Cancer *4*, 184–196.

Bao, S., Wu, Q., McLendon, R. E., Hao, Y., Shi, Q., Hjelmeland, A. B., Dewhirst, M. W., Bigner, D. D., and Rich, J. N. (2006a). Glioma stem cells promote radioresistance by preferential activation of the DNA damage response. Nature *444*, 756–760.

Bao, S., Wu, Q., Sathornsumetee, S., Hao, Y., Li, Z., Hjelmeland, A. B., Shi, Q., McLendon, R. E., Bigner, D. D., and Rich, J. N. (2006b). Stem cell-like glioma cells promote tumor angiogenesis through vascular endothelial growth factor. Cancer Res *66*, 7843–7848.

Birchmeier, C., Sharma, S., and Wigler, M. (1987). Expression and rearrangement of the ROS1 gene in human glioblastoma cells. Proc Natl Acad Sci USA *84*, 9270–9274.

Blanco-Aparicio, C., Renner, O., Leal, J. F., and Carnero, A. (2007). PTEN, more than the AKT pathway. Carcinogenesis *28*, 1379–1386.

Bonnet, D., and Dick, J. E. (1997). Human acute myeloid leukemia is organized as a hierarchy that originates from a primitive hematopoietic cell. Nat Med *3*, 730–737.

Butler, M. G., Dasouki, M. J., Zhou, X. P., Talebizadeh, Z., Brown, M., Takahashi, T. N., Miles, J. H., Wang, C. H., Stratton, R., Pilarski, R., and Eng, C. (2005). Subset of individuals with autism spectrum disorders and extreme macrocephaly associated with germline PTEN tumour suppressor gene mutations. J Med Genet *42*, 318–321.

Cantley, L. C. (2002). The phosphoinositide 3-kinase pathway. Science *296*, 1655–1657.

Cantley, L. C., and Neel, B. G. (1999). New insights into tumor suppression: PTEN suppresses tumor formation by restraining the phosphoinositide 3-kinase/AKT pathway. Proc Natl Acad Sci USA *96*, 4240–4245.

CBTRUS (2005). Statistical Report: Primary Brain Tumors in the United States, 1998–2002: Central Brain Tumor Registry of the United States.

Charest, A., Wilker, E. W., McLaughlin, M. E., Lane, K., Gowda, R., Coven, S., McMahon, K., Kovach, S., Feng, Y., Yaffe, M. B., et al. (2006). ROS fusion tyrosine kinase activates a SH2 domain-containing phosphatase-2/phosphatidylinositol 3-kinase/mammalian target of rapamycin signaling axis to form glioblastoma in mice. Cancer Res *66*, 7473–7481.

Chen, Z., Trotman, L. C., Shaffer, D., Lin, H. K., Dotan, Z. A., Niki, M., Koutcher, J. A., Scher, H. I., Ludwig, T., Gerald, W., et al. (2005). Crucial role of p53-dependent cellular senescence in suppression of Pten-deficient tumorigenesis. Nature *436*, 725–730.

Choe, G., Horvath, S., Cloughesy, T. F., Crosby, K., Seligson, D., Palotie, A., Inge, L., Smith, B. L., Sawyers, C. L., and Mischel, P. S. (2003). Analysis of the phosphatidylinositol 3′-kinase signaling pathway in glioblastoma patients in vivo. Cancer Res *63*, 2742–2746.

Collins, A. T., Berry, P. A., Hyde, C., Stower, M. J., and Maitland, N. J. (2005). Prospective identification of tumorigenic prostate cancer stem cells. Cancer Res *65*, 10946–10951.

Ding, H., Roncari, L., Shannon, P., Wu, X., Lau, N., Karaskova, J., Gutmann, D. H., Squire, J. A., Nagy, A., and Guha, A. (2001). Astrocyte-specific expression of activated p21-ras results in malignant astrocytoma formation in a transgenic mouse model of human gliomas. Cancer Res *61*, 3826–3836.

Emamian, E. S., Hall, D., Birnbaum, M. J., Karayiorgou, M., and Gogos, J. A. (2004). Convergent evidence for impaired AKT1-GSK3beta signaling in schizophrenia. Nat Genet *36*, 131–137.

Eng, C. (2003). PTEN: one gene, many syndromes. Hum Mutat *22*, 183–198.

Engelman, J. A., Luo, J., and Cantley, L. C. (2006). The evolution of phosphatidylinositol 3-kinases as regulators of growth and metabolism. Nat Rev Genet *7*, 606–619.

Eramo, A., Lotti, F., Sette, G., Pilozzi, E., Biffoni, M., Di Virgilio, A., Conticello, C., Ruco, L., Peschle, C., and De Maria, R. (2007). Identification and expansion of the tumorigenic lung cancer stem cell population. Cell Death Differ *15*, 504–514.

Fraser, M. M., Zhu, X., Kwon, C. H., Uhlmann, E. J., Gutmann, D. H., and Baker, S. J. (2004). Pten loss causes hypertrophy and increased proliferation of astrocytes in vivo. Cancer Res *64*, 7773–7779.

Freeman, D. J., Li, A. G., Wei, G., Li, H. H., Kertesz, N., Lesche, R., Whale, A. D., Martinez-Diaz, H., Rozengurt, N., Cardiff, R. D., et al. (2003). PTEN tumor suppressor regulates p53 protein levels and activity through phosphatase-dependent and -independent mechanisms. Cancer Cell *3*, 117–130.

Galanis, E., Buckner, J. C., Maurer, M. J., Kreisberg, J. I., Ballman, K., Boni, J., Peralba, J. M., Jenkins, R. B., Dakhil, S. R., Morton, R. F., et al. (2005). Phase II trial of temsirolimus (CCI-779) in recurrent glioblastoma multiforme: a North Central Cancer Treatment Group Study. J Clin Oncol *23*, 5294–5304.

Goberdhan, D. C., and Wilson, C. (2003). PTEN: tumour suppressor, multifunctional growth regulator and more. Hum Mol Genet *12 Spec No 2*, R239–248.

Gray, I. C., Stewart, L. M., Phillips, S. M., Hamilton, J. A., Gray, N. E., Watson, G. J., Spurr, N. K., and Snary, D. (1998). Mutation and expression analysis of the putative prostate tumour-suppressor gene PTEN. Br J Cancer *78*, 1296–1300.

Groszer, M., Erickson, R., Scripture-Adams, D. D., Lesche, R., Trumpp, A., Zack, J. A., Kornblum, H. I., Liu, X., and Wu, H. (2001). Negative regulation of neural stem/progenitor cell proliferation by the Pten tumor suppressor gene in vivo. Science *294*, 2186–2189.

Guertin, D. A., and Sabatini, D. M. (2007). Defining the role of mTOR in cancer. Cancer Cell *12*, 9–22.

Hemmati, H. D., Nakano, I., Lazareff, J. A., Masterman-Smith, M., Geschwind, D. H., Bronner-Fraser, M., and Kornblum, H. I. (2003). Cancerous stem cells can arise from pediatric brain tumors. Proc Natl Acad Sci USA *100*, 15178–15183.

Holland, E. C., Celestino, J., Dai, C., Schaefer, L., Sawaya, R. E., and Fuller, G. N. (2000). Combined activation of Ras and Akt in neural progenitors induces glioblastoma formation in mice. Nat Genet *25*, 55–57.

Hu, X., Pandolfi, P. P., Li, Y., Koutcher, J. A., Rosenblum, M., and Holland, E. C. (2005). mTOR promotes survival and astrocytic characteristics induced by Pten/AKT signaling in glioblastoma. Neoplasia *7*, 356–368.

Ignatova, T. N., Kukekov, V. G., Laywell, E. D., Suslov, O. N., Vrionis, F. D., and Steindler, D. A. (2002). Human cortical glial tumors contain neural stem-like cells expressing astroglial and neuronal markers in vitro. Glia *39*, 193–206.

Kaiser, J. (2008). GENOMICS: Billion-Dollar Cancer Mapping Project Steps Forward. Science *321*, 26–27.

Kondo, Y., Hollingsworth, E. F., and Kondo, S. (2004). Molecular targeting for malignant gliomas (Review). Int J Oncol *24*, 1101–1109.

Kwon, C. H., Zhu, X., Zhang, J., Knoop, L. L., Tharp, R., Smeyne, R. J., Eberhart, C. G., Burger, P. C., and Baker, S. J. (2001). Pten regulates neuronal soma size: a mouse model of Lhermitte-Duclos disease. Nat Genet *29*, 404–411.

Kwon, C. H., Luikart, B. W., Powell, C. M., Zhou, J., Matheny, S. A., Zhang, W., Li, Y., Baker, S. J., and Parada, L. F. (2006). Pten regulates neuronal arborization and social interaction in mice. Neuron *50*, 377–388.

Kwon, C.-H., Zhao, D., Chen, J., Alcantara, S., Li, Y., Burns, D. K., Mason, R. P., Lee, E. Y.-H. P., Wu, H., and Parada, L. F. (2008). Pten haploinsufficiency accelerates formation of high grade astrocytomas. Cancer Res *68*, 1–9.

Lapidot, T., Sirard, C., Vormoor, J., Murdoch, B., Hoang, T., Caceres-Cortes, J., Minden, M., Paterson, B., Caligiuri, M. A., and Dick, J. E. (1994). A cell initiating human acute myeloid leukaemia after transplantation into SCID mice. Nature *367*, 645–648.

Li, L., and Ross, A. H. (2007). Why is PTEN an important tumor suppressor? J Cell Biochem *102*, 1368–1374.

Li, C., Heidt, D. G., Dalerba, P., Burant, C. F., Zhang, L., Adsay, V., Wicha, M., Clarke, M. F., and Simeone, D. M. (2007). Identification of pancreatic cancer stem cells. Cancer Res *67*, 1030–1037.

Maehama, T., and Dixon, J. E. (1998). The tumor suppressor, PTEN/MMAC1, dephosphorylates the lipid second messenger, phosphatidylinositol 3,4,5-trisphosphate. J Biol Chem *273*, 13375–13378.

Maher, E. A., Furnari, F. B., Bachoo, R. M., Rowitch, D. H., Louis, D. N., Cavenee, W. K., and DePinho, R. A. (2001). Malignant glioma: genetics and biology of a grave matter. Genes Dev *15*, 1311–1333.

Manning, B. D., and Cantley, L. C. (2007). AKT/PKB signaling: navigating downstream. Cell *129*, 1261–1274.

Marino, S., Krimpenfort, P., Leung, C., van der Korput, H. A., Trapman, J., Camenisch, I., Berns, A., and Brandner, S. (2002). PTEN is essential for cell migration but not for fate determination and tumourigenesis in the cerebellum. Development *129*, 3513–3522.

O'Brien, C. A., Pollett, A., Gallinger, S., and Dick, J. E. (2007). A human colon cancer cell capable of initiating tumour growth in immunodeficient mice. Nature *445*, 106–110.

Ohgaki, H., Dessen, P., Jourde, B., Horstmann, S., Nishikawa, T., Di Patre, P. L., Burkhard, C., Schuler, D., Probst-Hensch, N. M., Maiorka, P. C., et al. (2004). Genetic pathways to glioblastoma: a population-based study. Cancer Res *64*, 6892–6899.

Pfenninger, C. V., Roschupkina, T., Hertwig, F., Kottwitz, D., Englund, E., Bengzon, J., Jacobsen, S. E., and Nuber, U. A. (2007). CD133 is not present on neurogenic astrocytes in the adult subventricular zone, but on embryonic neural stem cells, ependymal cells, and glioblastoma cells. Cancer Res *67*, 5727–5736.

Phillips, H. S., Kharbanda, S., Chen, R., Forrest, W. F., Soriano, R. H., Wu, T. D., Misra, A., Nigro, J. M., Colman, H., Soroceanu, L., et al. (2006). Molecular subclasses of high-grade glioma predict prognosis, delineate a pattern of disease progression, and resemble stages in neurogenesis. Cancer Cell *9*, 157–173.

Prince, M. E., Sivanandan, R., Kaczorowski, A., Wolf, G. T., Kaplan, M. J., Dalerba, P., Weissman, I. L., Clarke, M. F., and Ailles, L. E. (2007). Identification of a subpopulation of cells with cancer stem cell properties in head and neck squamous cell carcinoma. Proc Natl Acad Sci USA *104*, 973–978.

Reilly, K. M., Loisel, D. A., Bronson, R. T., McLaughlin, M. E., and Jacks, T. (2000). Nf1;Trp53 mutant mice develop glioblastoma with evidence of strain-specific effects. Nat Genet *26*, 109–113.

Salmena, L., Carracedo, A., and Pandolfi, P. P. (2008). Tenets of PTEN tumor suppression. Cell *133*, 403–414.

Singh, S. K., Clarke, I. D., Terasaki, M., Bonn, V. E., Hawkins, C., Squire, J., and Dirks, P. B. (2003). Identification of a cancer stem cell in human brain tumors. Cancer Res *63*, 5821–5828.

Singh, S. K., Hawkins, C., Clarke, I. D., Squire, J. A., Bayani, J., Hide, T., Henkelman, R. M., Cusimano, M. D., and Dirks, P. B. (2004). Identification of human brain tumour initiating cells. Nature *432*, 396–401.

Uhrbom, L., Dai, C., Celestino, J. C., Rosenblum, M. K., Fuller, G. N., and Holland, E. C. (2002). Ink4a-Arf loss cooperates with KRas activation in astrocytes and neural progenitors to generate glioblastomas of various morphologies depending on activated Akt. Cancer Res *62*, 5551–5558.

Vogel, K. S., Klesse, L. J., Velasco-Miguel, S., Meyers, K., Rushing, E. J., and Parada, L. F. (1999). Mouse tumor model for neurofibromatosis type 1. Science *286*, 2176–2179.

Watanabe, K., Tachibana, O., Sata, K., Yonekawa, Y., Kleihues, P., and Ohgaki, H. (1996). Overexpression of the EGF receptor and p53 mutations are mutually exclusive in the evolution of primary and secondary glioblastomas. Brain Pathol *6*, 217–223; discussion 223–214.

Watkins, D., Dion, F., Poisson, M., Delattre, J. Y., and Rouleau, G. A. (1994). Analysis of oncogene expression in primary human gliomas: evidence for increased expression of the ros oncogene. Cancer Genet Cytogenet *72*, 130–136.

Wei, Q., Clarke, L., Scheidenhelm, D. K., Qian, B., Tong, A., Sabha, N., Karim, Z., Bock, N. A., Reti, R., Swoboda, R., et al. (2006). High-grade glioma formation results from postnatal pten loss or mutant epidermal growth factor receptor expression in a transgenic mouse glioma model. Cancer Res *66*, 7429–7437.

Whang, Y. E., Wu, X., Suzuki, H., Reiter, R. E., Tran, C., Vessella, R. L., Said, J. W., Isaacs, W. B., and Sawyers, C. L. (1998). Inactivation of the tumor suppressor PTEN/MMAC1 in advanced human prostate cancer through loss of expression. Proc Natl Acad Sci USA *95*, 5246–5250.

Xiao, A., Wu, H., Pandolfi, P. P., Louis, D. N., and Van Dyke, T. (2002). Astrocyte inactivation of the pRb pathway predisposes mice to malignant astrocytoma development that is accelerated by PTEN mutation. Cancer Cell *1*, 157–168.

Xiao, A., Yin, C., Yang, C., Di Cristofano, A., Pandolfi, P. P., and Van Dyke, T. (2005). Somatic induction of Pten loss in a preclinical astrocytoma model reveals major roles in disease progression and avenues for target discovery and validation. Cancer Res *65*, 5172–5180.

Yoo, L. I., Liu, D. W., Le Vu, S., Bronson, R. T., Wu, H., and Yuan, J. (2006). Pten deficiency activates distinct downstream signaling pathways in a tissue-specific manner. Cancer Res *66*, 1929–1939.

Zhu, Y., and Parada, L. F. (2002). The molecular and genetic basis of neurological tumours. Nat Rev Cancer *2*, 616–626.

Zhu, Y., Ghosh, P., Charnay, P., Burns, D. K., and Parada, L. F. (2002). Neurofibromas in NF1: Schwann cell origin and role of tumor environment. Science *296*, 920–922.

Zhu, Y., Guignard, F., Zhao, D., Liu, L., Burns, D. K., Mason, R. P., Messing, A., and Parada, L. F. (2005). Early inactivation of p53 tumor suppressor gene cooperating with NF1 loss induces malignant astrocytoma. Cancer Cell *8*, 119–130.

Zhuo, L., Theis, M., Alvarez-Maya, I., Brenner, M., Willecke, K., and Messing, A. (2001). hGFAP-cre transgenic mice for manipulation of glial and neuronal function in vivo. Genesis *31*, 85–94.

Chapter 6
The *Nf1–/+; Trp53–/+cis* Mouse Model of Anaplastic Astrocytoma and Secondary Glioblastoma: Dissecting Genetic Susceptibility to Brain Cancer

Karlyne M. Reilly

Abstract Astrocytic gliomas are the most common primary brain tumors. They include diffuse astrocytomas, mixed oligoastrocytoma, anaplastic astrocytomas, and a subset of glioblastoma multiforme (GBM). Studies on human GBM have shown that upregulation of the Ras signaling pathway and disruption of the p53 checkpoint pathway are central to the formation of these tumors. Although much is now known about the molecular pathways altered in these tumors, they remain largely incurable, primarily due to their diffuse infiltration of the brain and lack of response to chemotherapeutics. The *Nf1–/+; Trp53–/+cis* mouse model develops diffuse anaplastic astrocytoma and GBM with histology that closely resembles the tumors seen in patients. The incidence of astrocytic gliomas varies in the model depending on the inheritance of mutations from the mother or father and on genetic background. Males and females show different effects, suggesting that sex influences the genetic and epigenetic factors that determine the susceptibility of an individual animal to astrocytic gliomas. This model system, including both genetically engineered mice and derivative cell lines, is useful for understanding the basic biological mechanisms underlying the formation of astrocytic gliomas and for preclinical testing of experimental therapeutics.

Contents

The author is supported by the Intramural Research Program of the NIH.

K.M. Reilly (✉)
Mouse Cancer Genetics Program, National Cancer Institute at Frederick, West 7th Street at Fort Detrick, PO Box B, Frederick, MD 21702, USA
e-mail: kreilly@ncifcrf.gov

E.G. Van Meir (ed.), *CNS Cancer*, Cancer Drug Discovery and Development, DOI 10.1007/978-1-60327-553-8_6,
© Humana Press, a part of Springer Science+Business Media, LLC 2009

6.1 Introduction

As described throughout this book, much work is currently being done to identify targets for new avenues of brain tumor therapy. Mouse models of astrocytoma provide controlled and malleable systems for understanding the biological mechanisms underlying the formation of these tumors. Several of these models are being presented in different chapters of this book, using different initiating events, and providing insights into the types of brain tumors observed in patients. Here I present the *Nf1–/+; Trp53–/+ cis* mouse model, discuss its value as a model mimicking the histopathology of human astrocytomas with p53 mutations and Ras overactivation for the discovery of novel biological mechanisms underlying the formation of these tumors and as a tool for the testing of novel therapeutics.

6.2 Clinical History, Pathology, and Genetics of Astrocytomas

Brain tumors are classified according to their appearance and their relationship to the hypothesized line of neurobiological differentiation. To understand the origins of these neoplasms and develop effective therapies, we must understand the cells from which they originate and the respective genetic programs that drive differentiation, cell survival, and migration. An open question in the field is whether tumors originate from the cells they resemble or whether they undergo independent differentiation or dedifferentiation of the initiating cell type to give rise to the final appearance of the tumor. Classification of gliomas is based on the type of normal cell the tumor most resembles, which has led to the designations of astrocytoma, oligodendroglioma, oligoastrocytoma, and ependymoma. Astrocytomas are central nervous system neoplasms containing tumor cells with characteristics of astrocytes, such as staining for glial fibrillary acidic protein (GFAP) (Tascos et al. 1982, Marsden et al. 1983). GBMs are believed to be grade IV forms of either astrocytoma or oligodendrogliomas, based on clinical history (such as a preexisting lower grade tumor) or on histology (such as more well-differentiated regions of tumor). However, many GBMs are very undifferentiated, making it difficult to assign these tumors to a specific line of neurobiological differentiation.

Astrocytomas are graded according to histological criteria (Kleihues and Cavenee 2000). They include benign pilocytic astrocytomas, discussed in Chapter 3, diffuse astrocytomas (grade II according to the World Health Organization classification; Kleihues and Cavenee 2000; WHO II), anaplastic astrocytoma (WHO grade III), and GBM (WHO grade IV), in addition to other rarer astrocytic tumors. Diffusely infiltrating astrocytomas (WHO II–IV) are the most common primary tumors of the brain, accounting for 30% of all primary central nervous system (CNS) tumors and 75% of all gliomas (CBTRUS 2006). WHO II diffuse astrocytomas have dysplastic astrocyte-like cells with nuclear atypia. WHO III anaplastic astrocytomas show increased cellularity and mitotic activity when compared to WHO II astrocytomas. WHO IV GBM is defined by the presence of necrosis or microvascular proliferation in the tumor. Giant cell glioblastoma is a specialized form of glioblastoma in which many multinucleated giant cells are present.

The average survival rate for patients with grade II astrocytomas is about 10 years, for grade III 3–5 years, and for grade IV 1–2 years. Very little improvement has been achieved in the survival of patients with diffusely infiltrating astrocytomas and GBM in the past 50 years (Oertel et al. 2005), with neurosurgery, pioneered at the turn of the 20th century, still being the primary focus of treatment. The failure of neurosurgery to provide a cure for these tumors is largely because it is difficult or impossible to completely resect astrocytomas and GBMs due to their pervasive ability to migrate and invade the surrounding normal brain. More recently, a combination of temozolomide and radiation has offered some benefit to a subset of patients, but better understanding of the molecular mechanisms driving these tumors is important to design more targeted therapies.

GBMs are divided into different clinical and molecular subtypes (von Deimling et al. 1993, Collins 1999, Kleihues and Cavenee 2000, Colman and Aldape 2008). Clinically, primary GBMs appear to arise de novo in older patients, whereas secondary GBMs progress from lower grades of astrocytoma and arise in younger adults. These two different subtypes are associated with different molecular characteristics (Fig. 6.1), although the tendency toward differences in individual genes between the two types of GBMs is not specific enough to be diagnostic. A common theme in the molecular alterations in GBMs is the alteration of the receptor tyrosine kinase (RTK) signaling pathways and pathways controlling cell cycle and cell survival (Fig. 6.2) (Furnari et al. 2007). Primary glioblastomas more frequently carry mutations and amplifications of the epidermal growth factor receptor gene (*EGFR*) (Libermann et al. 1985, Ekstrand et al. 1991, Lang et al. 1994, Watanabe et al. 1996) (see Chapter 20 for more details), combined with loss of the *INK4a/ARF* locus (Schmidt et al. 1994, Ichimura et al. 1996, Fulci et al. 2000) or amplification of the *MDM2/CDK4* locus (Reifenberger et al. 1993, 1996). Both ARF and MDM2 are upstream of the p53 pathway such that loss of ARF or amplification of

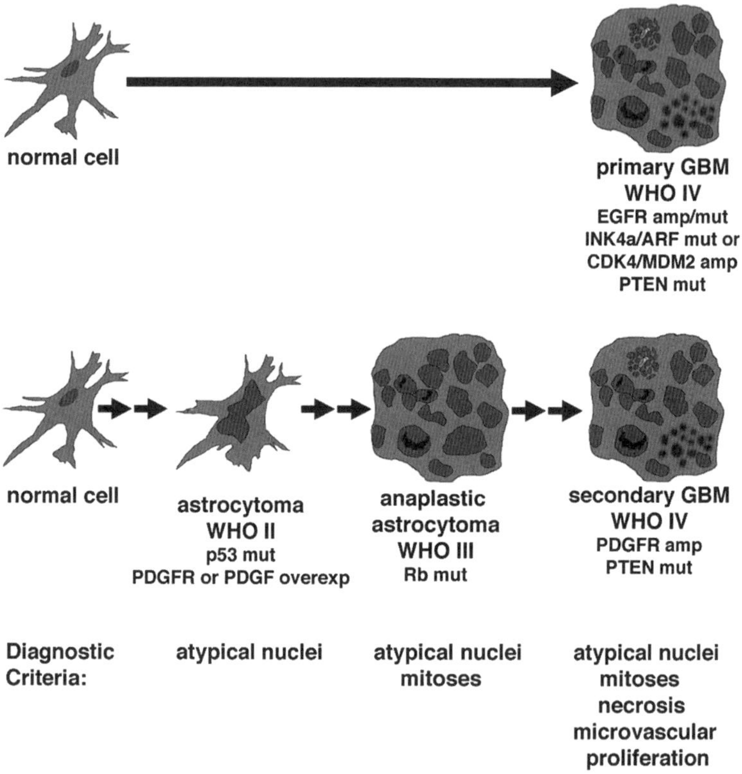

Fig. 6.1 Molecular alterations and diagnostic criteria in different grades of astrocytoma and GBM. Primary GBM (*top*) is observed de novo without the presence of a preexisting lower grade tumor, whereas secondary GBM (*bottom*) progresses from lower grades of astrocytoma. The diagnostic criteria for the different grades are listed at the bottom, and a simplified list of molecular changes characteristic of the different grades and primary vs. secondary GBM is listed below each tumor grade. For a more detailed description, see Furnari et al. (2007)

MDM2 leads to downregulation of p53 function (Sherr and Weber 2000). Both INK4a and CDK4 are upstream of the RB pathway such that loss of INK4a or amplification of CDK4 leads to downregulation of the RB pathway (Sherr 1996). Because INK4a and ARF are transcribed from the same locus, and MDM2 and CDK4 are closely linked, these alterations cause loss of the p53 and RB pathways in a single chromosomal event and may explain why primary glioblastomas progress so rapidly to WHO grade IV. In contrast, secondary glioblastomas arise from lower grades of astrocytoma (WHO grades II and III) with sequential loss of p53 (von Deimling et al. 1992, Lang et al. 1994, Rasheed et al. 1994, van Meyel et al. 1994, Watanabe et al. 1997, Ishii et al. 1999, Ichimura et al. 2000) (see Chapter 14 for details) and RB signaling pathways (Ichimura et al. 1996). The lower grades of astrocytoma tend to have overexpression of the platelet-derived growth factor receptor alpha (PDGFRα)

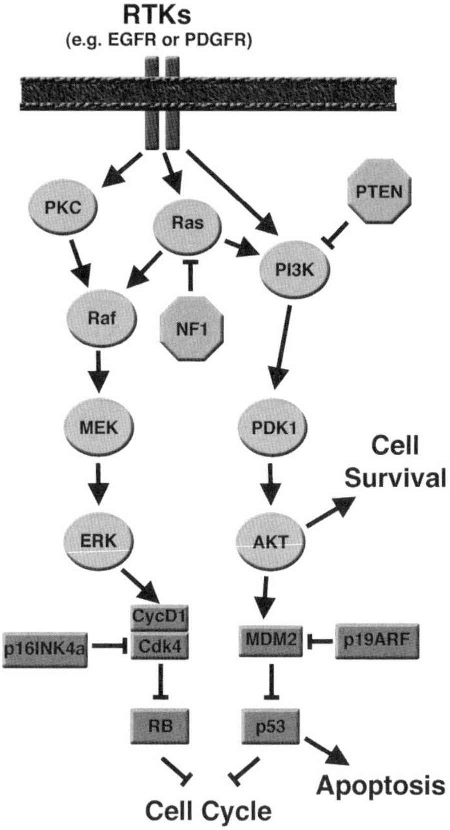

Fig. 6.2 Molecular pathways altered in GBM. Simplified version of some of the positive and negative molecular interactions believed to be important in astrocytoma and GBM tumorigenesis. As described in the text, proteins that block cell cycle progression or cell survival, such as RB, p53, p16INK4a, p19ARF, NF1, and PTEN, tend to be lost in GBMs, whereas proteins that activate cell cycle progression or cell survival, such as RTKs, CDK4, and MDM2, tend to be amplified or overexpressed in GBMs. For a more detailed description, see Furnari et al. (2007)

(Fleming et al. 1992, Hermanson et al. 1992) and loss or mutation of p53. As tumors progress from diffuse astrocytoma to anaplastic astrocytoma to secondary GBM, they tend to lose RB in addition to p53 and amplify the *PDGFRα* gene (Fig. 6.1). The amplification or overexpression of *EGFR* or *PDGFRα* in primary and secondary glioblastoma demonstrates the importance of receptor tyrosine kinase signaling in astrocytoma and glioblastoma and suggests that a combination of upregulation of Ras (Guha et al. 1997) (see Chapter 38 for details) and loss of p53 and RB is critical for these tumors to form.

With the advent of genome-wide approaches to characterize the molecular profiles of brain tumors, it has become possible to generate molecular signatures that correlate with patient survival (see Chapters 17 and 23 for details). These data have demonstrated further molecular subsets of GBMs, in addition to the primary and secondary subtypes that are based on clinical presentation. Analysis of genomic alterations using array comparative genomic hybridization (aCGH) demonstrated that within the secondary GBMs there are two subclasses with different prognoses (Maher et al. 2006). Analysis of gene expression profiles in WHO III and WHO IV tumors has demonstrated that WHO III tumors tend to cluster together and WHO III and WHO IV tumors cluster into three or four different groups depending on the study (Freije et al. 2004, Phillips et al. 2006). The differentially expressed genes associated with each group fell into the categories proneural, proliferative, and mesenchymal, with a fourth group associated with synaptic transmission found in one of the studies (Freije et al. 2004). With new initiatives to integrate DNA alterations and gene expression over larger sample numbers, a clearer picture of the similarities and differences between subtypes of astrocytoma and GBM is expected to emerge in the near future (TCGA, 2008, Parsons et al. 2008).

In addition to astrocytomas occurring spontaneously in patients, they are also associated with several inherited genetic disorders. These include Li–Fraumeni syndrome (Malkin 1994), associated with mutations in *TP53*, and neurofibromatosis type 1 (Blatt et al. 1986, Sorensen et al. 1986, Huson and Hughes 1994), associated with mutations in *NF1*, as well as other genetic disorders. Patients with Li–Fraumeni syndrome develop a wide variety of cancers due to the central role of the p53 protein in tumor suppression (Kleihues et al. 1997). Neurofibromatosis type 1 (NF1) is one of the most common genetic diseases affecting the nervous system, with an incidence of 1 in 3500. Patients with NF1 are at an increased risk for benign WHO grade I astrocytomas, particularly along the optic tract (see Chapter 3 for more details) (Huson and Hughes 1994), and also develop malignant WHO grade II–IV astrocytomas (Blatt et al. 1986, Sorensen et al. 1986), albeit with lower frequency. The product of the *NF1* gene, neurofibromin, acts as a RasGAP protein to downregulate active Ras signaling (Martin et al. 1990, Xu et al. 1990a, b, Gutmann et al. 1991, Hattori et al. 1992) (see Chapter 38). Mutations in *NF1* lead to upregulation of Ras and may give rise to similar cellular phenotypes as the overexpression of receptor tyrosine kinases seen in spontaneous astrocytomas and glioblastomas.

6.3 The *NPcis* Mouse Model of Astrocytoma/Glioblastoma

While the *NF1* gene encoding neurofibromin and *Tp53* gene encoding the p53 protein are on separate arms of chromosome 17 in humans, the mouse genes (*Nf1* and *Trp53*) are tightly linked on chromosome 11, separated by only 10 Mb. In an effort to model the malignancies associated with neurofibromatosis type 1, two groups generated mice with combined mutations in *Nf1* and *Trp53* on the same mouse chromosome (Cichowski et al. 1999, Vogel et al. 1999). *Nf1* mutant mice (Brannan et al. 1994, Jacks et al. 1994b) were crossed to *Trp53* mutant mice (Donehower et al. 1992, Jacks et al. 1994a), and double mutants were identified in which the mutations were on opposite chromosome 11 homologues. These *Nf1–/+;Trp53–/+ trans* double mutants were bred to wild-type mice, and rare germline recombination events were identified in the progeny such that the *Nf1* and *Trp53* mutations were located on the same chromosome (*Nf1–/+;Trp53–/+ cis* mice, abbreviated *NPcis*) (Fig. 6.3). Because the two

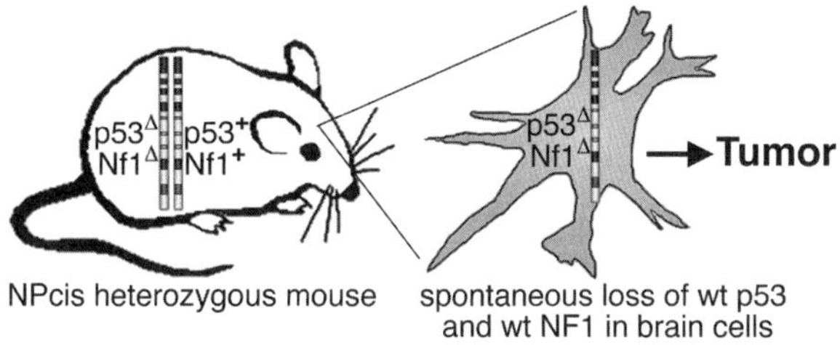

Fig. 6.3 *NPcis* mouse model of astrocytic glioma. *NPcis* mice carry a knockout mutation (Δ) in the *Trp53* (p53) and *Nf1* gene on the same chromosome copy of mouse chromosome 11 (in "cis"). The other copy of *Trp53* and *Nf1*on the opposite chromosome 11 is wild type (+). The wild-type copy of both *Trp53* and *Nf1* is spontaneously lost in brain cells as the mouse ages, initiating tumorigenesis and giving rise to malignant astrocytoma and glioblastoma

mutations are so tightly linked, they only very rarely become unlinked through germline recombination, and thus the two mutations are inherited as a single mutation with near Mendelian inheritance ratios in genetic crosses. Because all cells of the *NPcis* animal are mutant for one copy of *Nf1* and *Trp53*, there is a higher probability of spontaneous loss of the wild-type copies of both genes and the mice are highly tumor prone (Fig. 6.3) (Cichowski et al. 1999, Vogel et al. 1999, Reilly et al. 2000).

Studies of the *NPcis* mouse model have demonstrated the importance of genetic background on tumor susceptibility (Reilly et al. 2000, 2004, 2006). The original *Nf1* and *Trp53* mutations were made in 129S4/SvJae (129S4) embryonic stem cells such that the congenic genomic region surrounding the mutations is selectively maintained as the 129S4 strain with maintenance of the mutations in mouse crosses. The *Nf1* and *Trp53* mice were then maintained in parallel on an inbred 129S4 strain background or a mixed 129S4, C57BL6/J (B6) strain background. The original characterization of the *NPcis* mice was performed on the 129S4, B6 mixed strain background. These mice developed peripheral nerve sheath tumors similar to those seen in NF1 patients with high frequency (Cichowski et al. 1999, Vogel et al. 1999). Because tumor development in NF1 patients is subject to the effects of genetic background (Easton et al. 1993), the highly penetrant *NPcis* model is a potentially powerful system to study the influence of genetic background on the susceptibility to cancer driven by combined *Trp53* and *Nf1* loss. To isolate the effects of strain background on the tumor phenotype, the *NPcis* mouse model was regenerated on two different inbred strain backgrounds. In the first, *Nf1* and *Trp53* mutants were inbred onto the B6 background such that their genomes were on the order of 99.98% B6, and the *NPcis* chromosome was regenerated by crossing these mice together as described above to give *NPcis*-B6 congenic mice. In the second case, *Nf1* and *Trp53* mice maintained on the inbred 129S4 background were crossed to regenerate the *NPcis* chromosome to give *NPcis*-129S4 inbred mice. On the B6 background, the *NPcis* mutant chromosome led to the development of astrocytomas with high penetrance (Reilly et al. 2000), whereas the *NPcis*-129S4 mice were resistant to astrocytomas (Reilly et al. 2004).

6.3.1 Histology of NPcis *Astrocytomas*

The astrocytomas and GBMs observed in the *NPcis* mouse model have been characterized relative to the histologies observed in human brain tumors. About 50% of *NPcis* mouse brain tumors are classified as anaplastic astrocytoma (WHO grade III), depending on the genetic background, as described below. The *NPcis* brain tumors contain hyperchromatic cells with oblong nuclei that often appear contorted. These lesions can range from very low-density, infiltrative tumors to high-density tumor masses. The tumors also show a broad range of mitotic activity. A low percentage of tumors (up to 10% of observed brain tumors depending on genetic background) show characteristics of WHO IV tumors, primarily necrosis. These WHO IV tumors are often highly vascularized, with large regions of hemorrhage, and pseudopalisading tumor cells around the regions of necrosis. Although the WHO IV show evidence of neovascularization, the blood vessel walls do not over-proliferate as is seen in human GBM but remain of single-cell thickness. The remaining 40% of the observed tumors show very little to no mitotic activity and are classified as WHO II.

In addition to the human WHO grading criteria, *NPcis* murine astrocytomas show other characteristics of patient astrocytomas. The *NPcis* astrocytomas are very diffusely infiltrative (Fig. 6.4), and isolated tumor cells can often be observed in the spinal cord in mice with brain masses. Up to 15% of *NPcis* astrocytomas have a distinctive multinucleated giant cell phenotype, and this includes most of the GBM observed. Secondary structures of glioma cells have been described (Scherer 1940) in which tumor cells cluster around blood vessels (perivascular secondary structures) and neurons (satellitosis) and spread along the subpial zone of the brain. All three of these types of secondary structures are seen in the *NPcis* astrocytomas (Reilly et al. 2000, Reilly and Jacks 2001). Specifically, up to 7% of the observed astrocytomas have a distinctive satellitosis pattern. Gliomatosis cerebri is a specialized form of glioma in which there is no apparent focal point of tumor origin, and tumor cells are broadly and diffusely distributed throughout the central nervous system (Kleihues and Cavenee 2000). Because gliomatosis cerebri is so rare in human populations, little is known about its origins or relationship to other gliomas. Gliomatosis cerebri histology occurs in up to 2% of *NPcis* astrocytomas, suggesting a mechanism of initiation related to other diffuse astrocytomas. Gliomas of the brain stem are particularly difficult to treat in patients, because surgery at this site is often not possible. The *NPcis* model develops brain stem tumors in up to 20% of the observed astrocytomas, with many being clearly localized to the brain stem. In addition, up to 40% of the observed astrocytomas involve the spinal cord, with many clearly suggestive of the primary tumor initiating in

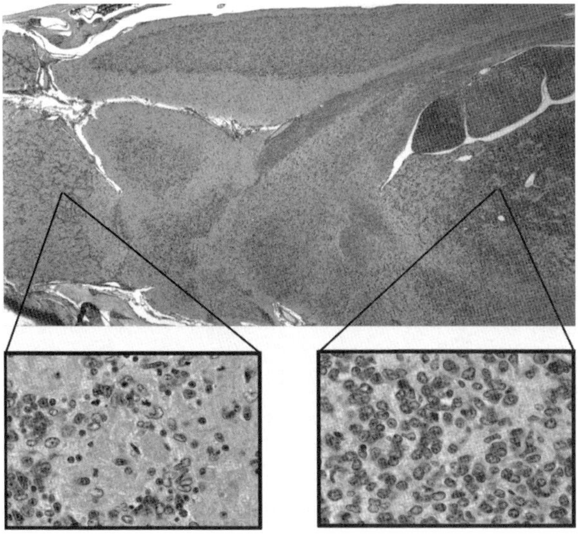

Fig. 6.4 Diffuse infiltration of *NPcis* astrocytomas. Top panel shows a low-magnification field of an astrocytoma in the thalamus of a *NPcis* mouse. The densely cellular region at the right edge of the photograph is the primary tumor mass. The olfactory bulb at the left edge of the top panel appears histologically normal at low magnification. The bottom two panels show high-magnification views of the indicated parts of the tumors. Diffuse infiltrative tumor cells are observed in the olfactory bulb (*lower left panel*) at a distance from the tumor mass (*lower right panel*)

the spinal cord itself, as opposed to migration of tumor cells from a primary brain tumor. It has been suggested that astrocytomas initiate in the subventricular zone (SVZ) within a neural stem cell niche and migrate out into the brain (Zhu et al. 2005). Although there is not evidence for involvement of the SVZ in all *NPcis* astrocytomas, the rostral migratory stream and SVZ is involved in up to 36% of observed astrocytomas (Fig. 6.5).

6.3.2 Molecular Biology of NPcis *Astrocytomas*

The astrocytomas from *NPcis* mice have been characterized molecularly to compare them to patient astrocytomas. They show variable expression of the astrocyte marker glial fibrillary acidic protein (GFAP) (Marsden et al. 1983, Reilly et al. 2000) and the neural/glial precursor marker nestin (Reilly, unpublished data), but no expression of the neural marker synaptophysin (Gould et al. 1986, Reilly et al. 2000), consistent with a glial tumor type. Similar to anaplastic astrocytomas and secondary GBMs, overexpression of Pdgfrα is frequently seen by immunohistochemistry in these tumors, while overexpression of Egfr is seen less frequently in a subset of tumors (Reilly, unpublished data). It is not yet known whether the *Egfr* gene is amplified or mutated in these tumors. These

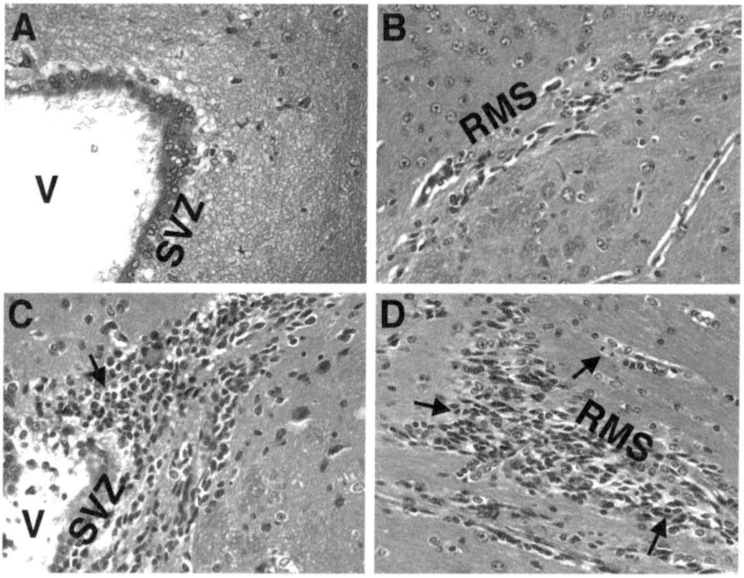

Fig. 6.5 Tumor involvement in the subventricular zone (SVZ) and rostral migratory stream (RMS). Panel A shows the SVZ in a normal *Nf1* wild-type and *Trp53* wild-type B6 animal. The ventricle is indicated by **V**. Panel B shows the RMS in a normal *Nf1* wild-type and *Trp53* wild-type B6 animal. Panel C shows tumor involvement of the SVZ in a *NPcis*, B6 mouse. Panel D shows tumor involvement of the RMS in an independent *NPcis*, B6 mouse. Arrows indicate mitotic figures visible on the section, supporting the presence of tumor at this location. Involvement of the SVZ or the RMS is observed in up to 36% of astrocytomas in *NPcis* mice

data are consistent with the *NPcis* mouse model encompassing the spectrum of low-grade astrocytoma, anaplastic astrocytoma, and secondary GBM. It is quite interesting to note that although the Ras signaling pathway is altered in these mice through mutation of *Nf1*, these tumors still evolve to overexpress tyrosine kinase receptors, particularly Pdgfrα. This suggests a unique requirement for Pdgfrα in astrocytoma tumorigenesis that is conserved between species. Furthermore, it indicates that the Ras signaling pathway must be actively driven and that mutation of the pathway that physiologically downregulates Ras is not sufficient to drive full development of these tumors. Alternatively, both receptor tyrosine kinases and neurofibromin may be involved in additional signaling pathways, such that their role in tumorigenesis is non-redundant, despite the common effects on ras signaling.

6.3.3 Tumor Cell Lines Derived from NPcis *Astrocytomas*

One of the central advantages of the *NPcis* mouse model of astrocytoma is the well-defined genetic background. This allows for controlled comparisons of genetic background, sex, and tumor grade on the biological behavior of the tumors. Tumor cell lines have been generated from 14 independent *NPcis* astrocytomas representing these different factors, allowing for controlled comparisons to be made. These cell lines represent WHO II and WHO III astrocytomas, with one cell line generated from a WHO IV GBM (Reilly et al. 2000) (Tuskan and Reilly, unpublished data). In addition to representing different tumors grades, genetic backgrounds, and sexes, these tumor lines have been developed from multiple brain regions of each tumor such that a single tumor is represented by multiple cell lines. This allows for comparison of different parts of the same tumor such that more dense regions can be compared to more diffuse regions. Many of the tumor lines have been tested in subcutaneous transplant models and show a growth rate that reflects the WHO grade of the original tumor, with WHO II tumor lines growing more slowly than WHO III lines (Gürsel and Reilly, unpublished data). Many of the tumor lines were established from asymptomatic mice and represent earlier stages of tumorigenesis.

The best characterized of these tumor lines is the KR158 anaplastic astrocytoma line, derived from an aggressive tumor in the thalamus of a female progeny from a *NPcis* mutant mother (Reilly et al. 2000). Derivative lines of KR158 have been made to express luciferase for following tumor growth in intracranial transplants using bioluminescent imaging (Tuskan, Hollingshead, and Reilly, unpublished data) and a two-color luciferase dual reporter system for use in high-throughput screening of anti-astrocytoma therapeutics (Hawes et al. 2008).

6.4 Factors Affecting Astrocytoma Susceptibility in *NPcis* Mice

6.4.1 The Effect of Parental Origin and Offspring Sex on NPcis *Astrocytomas*

NPcis progeny differ in the susceptibility to astrocytoma depending on whether they inherit the *NPcis* mutant chromosome from their mother or their father (Reilly 2004, Reilly et al. 2004) (Fig. 6.6). On the inbred B6 background, the progeny of fathers carrying the mutant *NPcis* allele develop astrocytomas in approximately 50% of the population, regardless of the sex of the individual, with approximately 30% of the mice developing a WHO II astrocytoma, 20% developing a WHO III anaplastic astrocytoma, and 2% developing WHO IV GBM (Fig. 6.6). The progeny of mutant mothers on the B6 background develop more astrocytomas of higher grades, with sex-specific differences in the effect. The male progeny of mutant mothers develop exclusively grade II and III astrocytomas in 70% of the population. In contrast, about 50% of females develop astrocytoma, but there is an increase in the percentage of WHO IV tumors to 13% compared to 2% in the progeny of mutant fathers.

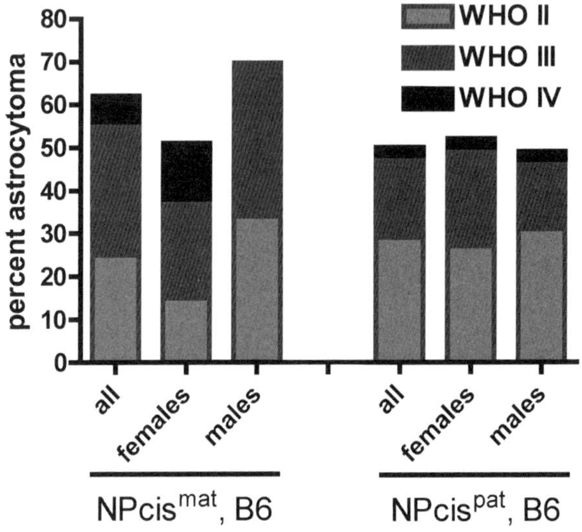

Fig. 6.6 The incidence and grade of astrocytoma in *NPcis* mice depending on parental inheritance of the mutation. *NPcis* mice that inherit the mutant chromosome 11 from their mother ($NPcis^{mat}$) develop more astrocytomas and higher grade astrocytomas compared to *NPcis* mice that inherit the mutant chromosome 11 from their father ($NPcis^{pat}$). (For $NPcis^{mat}$ progeny, data set includes 39 females and 48 males; for $NPcis^{pat}$ progeny, data set includes 48 females and 45 males)

To explain the differences in astrocytoma susceptibility in progeny of mutant mothers and mutant fathers, we hypothesize that an imprinted gene on mouse chromosome 11 may modify astrocytoma susceptibility (Reilly 2004). Imprinted genes are genes that are marked in the germline of the mother and the father to be expressed only from one parent's allele. The expression levels of these genes are tightly controlled and changes in gene dosage can give rise to mutant phenotypes in mammals (Wood and Oakey 2006). Because the difference in astrocytoma susceptibility is observed within an inbred strain background (B6) (Fig. 6.6), the difference in susceptibility is unlikely to be due to inheritance of polymorphic maternal factors such as mitochondria, because these should not vary within the inbred strain. Tissue from primary *NPcis* astrocytomas and derived cell lines show loss of the wild-type copies of *Nf1* and *Trp53* (Reilly et al. 2000), supporting the model that the astrocytomas initiate through full or partial loss of the wild-type chromosome 11. In the progeny of mutant fathers, the lost wild-type chromosome is from the mother, while in the progeny of mutant mothers it originated from the father. Because chromosome 11 carries imprinted genes (http://www.geneimprint.com/site/genes-by-species.Mus+musculus), the chromosome lost differs in imprinted marks between the two types of progeny, and therefore expression of an imprinted gene will be either lost or maintained, depending on the type of progeny (Fig. 6.7).

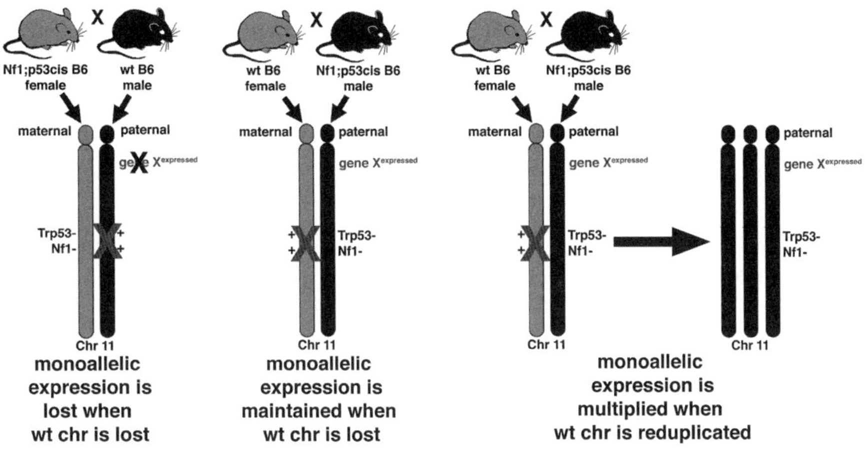

Fig. 6.7 Model for the potential effects of *NPcis* parental inheritance on tumor susceptibility. Imprinted genes are expressed from only one parental chromosome (in this example, the paternal chromosome). When the wild-type chromosome carries the expressed copy of the gene (*far left*), gene expression may be lost when tumorigenesis is initiated through loss of the wild-type chromosome. When the expressed copy of the gene is on the *NPcis* mutant chromosome, expression of the imprinted gene is expected to be maintained (*middle left*). Once the wild-type copy of the chromosome is lost, the *NPcis* mutant chromosome may be reduplicated (*right*) leading to amplification of the expressed copy of the imprinted gene (*far right*). Depending on whether gene expression has a tumor-promoting or tumor-inhibiting function, tumor growth will be differentially affected in each of these cases. This "allelic phasing" could explain why tumor susceptibility varies in the progeny of mutant mothers and the progeny of mutant fathers

This result is compatible with the expression of an imprinted gene that influences the rate of malignant progression of astrocytoma, i.e., a paternally expressed gene that enhances progression or a maternally expressed gene that suppresses progression. Furthermore, karyotypes of astrocytoma cell lines derived from the *NPcis* mice are hyperploid, often with at least three copies of chromosome 11 (Kumar and Reilly, unpublished data), suggesting that reduplication of the mutant chromosome may also occur in these tumors, leading to multiple copies of either the maternal or the paternal chromosome 11 depending on the cross (Fig. 6.7). Alternatively, it is also possible that the extra copies of chromosome 11 are an artifact of culturing the tumors in vitro; therefore future experiments will need to confirm the reduplication of chromosome 11 in primary tumors. These observations have led to the working hypothesis that changes in gene dosage of an imprinted gene on chromosome 11, either through loss of monoallelic expression on the wild-type chromosome or through amplification of monoallelic expression from reduplication of the mutant chromosome, give rise to changes in susceptibility to astrocytoma.

The effect of sex on astrocytoma susceptibility is cross dependent (Fig. 6.6), suggesting that the imprinted modifier may act in a sex-specific manner.

Females develop higher grade tumors in the progeny of mutant mothers, and the average age at death of mice with astrocytomas is longer (8.3 months in progeny of mutant mothers vs. 7.2 months in progeny of mutant fathers). This suggests that the astrocytomas do not necessarily grow faster in the female progeny of mutant mothers but that the females live longer for the tumors to progress further. This could be due to an absence of other tumors developing in these females (see Section 6.5.2) or to differences between females of different crosses in their ability to tolerate higher grade tumors before succumbing to neurological symptoms. Male progeny of mutant mothers develop more astrocytomas than the progeny of mutant fathers, with no significant difference in the average age of death of affected mice. This could be due to a greater rate of astrocytoma initiation in male progeny of mutant mothers compared to progeny of mutant fathers. The mechanism by which an imprinted gene could give rise to these differential effects remains to be determined.

In this context it is interesting to note that there is an increased incidence of astrocytoma in male patients for both WHO grade II and III tumors, with a male to female ratio of 1.18:1 (Kleihues and Cavenee 2000). Although the incidence of astrocytoma in *NPcis* mice is not consistently higher in males than in females (Figs. 6.6 and 6.8), it is higher in males of a particular subpopulation, with a male to female ratio of 1.38:1 in the progeny of mutant mothers. This suggests that the male predominance seen in the patient population could be due to a more significant increased risk in a subpopulation of males that averages over the entire population to give the 1.18:1 male to female ratio. Being able to identify subpopulations of individuals at higher risk and understanding the mechanisms underlying that increased risk could lead to methods for early detection or prevention of astrocytoma.

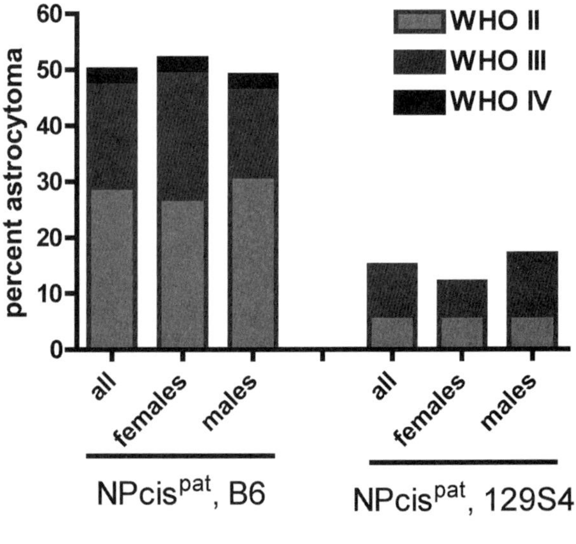

Fig. 6.8 The incidence and grade of astrocytoma in *NPcis*^{pat} progeny on B6 and 129S4 strain backgrounds. *NPcis* mice on the 129S4 strain background develop fewer astrocytomas of lower grade compared to *NPcis* mice on the B6 strain background. (For *NPcis*^{pat}, B6 progeny, data set includes 48 females and 45 males; for *NPcis*^{pat}, 129S4 progeny, data set includes 17 females and 18 males)

6.4.2 *The Effect of Background Polymorphisms on* NPcis *Astrocytomas*

In addition to the effects of parental origin of mutant chromosome 11 and the sex of the individual, susceptibility to astrocytoma in *NPcis* mice also depends on genetic background. The *NPcis* model on a B6 background has been crossed to seven different inbred strains, including 129S4, to examine dominant effects of strain background on the astrocytoma phenotype (Reilly et al. 2004). The 129S4 strain and the CBA/J strain both showed resistance to astrocytomas in F_1 progeny, indicating that polymorphisms between B6 and 129S4 and between B6 and CBA/J can affect resistance. There is no significant difference in the effect of the 129S4 strain background on males and females in *NPcis* 129S4 inbred progeny of mutant fathers, similar to what is observed on the B6 background (Fig. 6.8). The analysis of F_1 hybrids of B6 and 129S4 in *NPcis* mice showed codominance of the B6 and 129S4 strain phenotypes (Reilly et al. 2004) that could be separated from the inheritance of mutant chromosome 11 from the mother or the father. The data suggest that the inheritance of the *NPcis* mutant chromosome from the B6 background as opposed to the 129S4 background can also affect astrocytoma susceptibility. Because the knockout mutations in *Nf1* and *Trp53* were made in 129S4 embryonic stem cells, the strain of the congenic region of DNA around the mutations remains 129S4, even after inbreeding onto the B6 background for many generations. When F_1 hybrids are made from *NPcis* 129S4 mice crossed to wild-type B6 mice, the congenic region surrounding the mutations is heterozygous for B6 and 129S4 polymorphisms. When F_1 hybrids are made from *NPcis* B6 mice crossed to wild-type 129S4 mice, the congenic region surrounding the mutations is homozygous for 129S4. These two different types of F_1 hybrids are expected to be genetically identical across the genome with the exception of the congenic regions, and they show differences in susceptibility to astrocytoma. Analysis of heterozygosity across this region in F_1 hybrids suggests that a polymorphic allele between B6 and 129S4 in a 30 Mb region around *Nf1* and *Trp53* affects susceptibility to astrocytoma (Reilly et al. 2004).

These data on differences in susceptibility due to an imprinted effect, sex, and polymorphic alleles demonstrate the complexity of genetic and epigenetic effects controlling susceptibility to astrocytoma in mice. The combination of factors together can give rise to a very high incidence of astrocytoma in some mouse populations (up to 90% in progeny of *NPcis* mothers on certain strain backgrounds) or a very low incidence in other populations (as low as 14% in progeny of *NPcis* fathers on inbred 129S4). These combinatorial effects act as a barcode for the individual's susceptibility to astrocytoma, with each genetic or epigenetic factor specifying susceptibility in the context of all the other factors. Although astrocytoma is a relatively rare cancer, with an incidence rate of 1 per 100,000 person years (CBTRUS 2006), it is not clear whether the entire population has the same low risk of developing astrocytoma, or whether a small subset of the population has a significantly higher risk, due to the combination of genetic and epigenetic factors in their individual "barcode." This distinction has important implications for personalized medicine in the future, for although it may not be practical to screen a large number of low-risk individuals for early detection of brain cancer, it may be extremely effective to screen a high-risk subpopulation for early detection or prevention of brain cancer. A greater understanding of the mechanisms of susceptibility is necessary to address these issues.

6.5 Application of the *NPcis* Model of Astrocytoma

The *NPcis* model of astrocytoma is being used for multiple applications to better understand the biology of astrocytoma and to develop new therapeutic approaches. The model is being crossed to other genetically engineered mice to look at the ability of different oncogenes or tumor suppressor candidates to accelerate or block astrocytoma tumorigenesis. The model is being crossed to different genetic backgrounds, as described in detail in Section 6.4.2, to identify modifiers of susceptibility or resistance to astrocytoma. Tumor cell lines from this model described in Section 6.3.3 are being used to better understand the cell-autonomous signal transduction pathways important for tumorigenesis. The tumor lines are furthermore being used for high-throughput screening of candidate anti-astrocytoma therapeutics both in vitro and in syngeneic transplant models in vivo. Finally, the *NPcis* mice are being used to test candidate anti-astrocytoma therapies in vivo. In order to make the best use of this astrocytoma model system, it is important to understand the strengths and limitations of the model system.

6.5.1 Advantages of the NPcis *Astrocytoma Model*

Astrocytoma, as with all cancer, is a complex disease. Because it is a relatively rare disease that is highly variable, it is difficult to study the genetic factors that control susceptibility in human populations. Efforts to identify genetic risk factors for gliomas have had limited success thus far and have often shown conflicting results (see Fisher et al. 2007, for review). Due to the rareness of GBMs and the requirement for large cohorts to identify significant genetic risk factors, a consortium effort, GLIOGENE (Malmer et al. 2007), has been initiated to begin genome-wide association studies (GWAS) to better understand genetic risk factors for gliomas; however, GWAS studies are unlikely to be able to identify complex epistatic interactions described in Section 6.3. In addition, there is strong evidence that heterogeneity of genetic background and molecular characteristics of the tumor affects the response to therapies (Haas-Kogan et al. 2005a, b, Mellinghoff et al. 2005). One of the challenges in studying the biology of astrocytoma is to balance the need to isolate different variables, such as sex, genetic background, diet, and environment, with the need to model the complexity of the disease accurately (Reilly et al. 2008). Mouse models of brain tumors allow easy control of diet and environmental variables, as well as the ability to generate large numbers of tumor-bearing animals for better statistical comparisons.

The *NPcis* model of astrocytoma offers some additional advantages due to its simple genetics and inbred background. Because the *Nf1* mutation and *Trp53* mutation are so tightly linked on mouse chromosome 11, they are inherited as a single mutation with a near Mendelian ratio in genetic crosses. The mutations do become unlinked in rare cases of germline recombination in 1–2% of progeny, accounting for the slightly less than Mendelian ratio of double mutant to wild type in genetic crosses. The effect of this simple genetic system is that in crosses of *NPcis* mutant to wild-type mice, close to 50% of the progeny carry the *NPcis* mutation and can be included in cohorts for study. This is in contrast to models that involve combinations of many independent mutant loci, in which the number of available progeny carrying all mutations drops by half with each additional locus in the genetic cross. Because of this practical consideration, one is able to generate cohorts of hundreds of animals (Fig. 6.6) (Reilly et al. 2006) for increased statistical power. Because these mice are on inbred backgrounds, the progeny of a cross are genetically identical, essentially providing an extensive supply of the mouse equivalent of monozygotic twins. Given the importance of genetic heterogeneity in cancer in humans, it is very important to study astrocytoma on multiple genetic backgrounds and in the situation of heterozygosity, as well as homozygosity. The *NPcis* model offers the advantage that this can be done in a controlled manner, with heterogeneity being added to the system in a well-defined way. New tools being developed in the mouse systems genetics community (see Hunter and Crawford, 2008, for review), such as genetic reference panels (Chesler et al. 2003), chromosome substitution strains (Nadeau et al. 2000), the Collaborative Cross (Churchill et al. 2004), and heterogenous stocks (Mott and Flint 2002), will allow us to query this model in a controlled way with a level of heterogeneity to rival or exceed that found in the human population (Roberts et al. 2007).

The penetrance of astrocytomas in *NPcis* mice can be controlled by adjusting the cross design and genetic background, as described above, such that one can generate cohorts in which most of the mice or few of the mice will develop astrocytoma, using the same *NPcis* initiating mutation. This makes it straightforward to study treatments or genetic factors that reduce astrocytoma, by looking at the effects of tumor reduction in high-incidence cohorts. For example, by taking the progeny of *NPcis* mutant mothers on the B6 background and crossing them to a mutant of interest (such as overexpression of a tumor suppressor or a dominant-negative oncogene) or treating them with a candidate chemotherapy, one can look at whether the normally high penetrance of astrocytomas in these progeny is effectively reduced. Likewise, it is possible to test the effects of tumor-promoting agents or oncogenic gene mutations in cohorts of *NPcis* mice that develop low numbers of astrocytomas. By choosing the appropriate background, the differences between "treated" and "untreated" cohorts can be amplified, providing more statistical power to the experiment.

It is becoming clear that coevolution of tumors with their microenvironment is an important part of tumorigenesis (Reilly et al. 2008). Tumor stroma and vasculature supports tumor growth and the tumor in turn alters the surrounding microenvironment; thus a complete understanding of tumorigenesis requires accurate modeling of microenvironment interactions. In transplant-based models, such as xenografts, a mature tumor is put into the context of a naïve microenvironment. In contrast, in spontaneous models, such as the *NPcis* mouse model, tumors coevolve with their microenvironment. This is likely to be a more accurate representation of the situation found in human brain tumor patients facing treatment. For example, early in tumor development, tumor cells may be more dependent on their microenvironment before excessive mutations accumulate through selective pressures. As a tumor grows, it may reshape its microenvironment, such as the surrounding vasculature, by secreting factors and establishing a symbiotic, coevolutionary relationship between microenvironment and tumor cells. In the case of transplant models, this symbiosis would be absent, as the tumor cells are in the end state, but the microenvironment is in the naïve state. It is possible that the tumor cells in the context of the naïve environment are at a disadvantage, lacking the support of a truly evolved tumor microenvironment. This could explain why candidate therapies may be effective in xenograft models but fail in the context of clinical trials. It is striking that the *NPcis* model recapitulates many of the diverse secondary structures found in patient gliomas, such as satellitosis and perivascular structures. These structures suggest that the tumor cells are interacting with non-tumor structures in the brain and the tumor–microenvironment coevolution in the animal may be conserved across species. Testing experimental therapeutics in a spontaneous model such as the *NPcis* model takes advantage of the role of the immune system, integrated vascular system, and other stromal elements in enhancing or antagonizing candidate therapies. Although it remains to be tested rigorously, it is envisioned that these spontaneous models will be more predictive of patient response to therapies (Van Dyke and Jacks 2002, Reilly et al. 2008).

6.5.2 Limitations of the NPcis *Astrocytoma Model*

When working with mouse models of human cancer, there is always concern over whether the pathways necessary for cancer development are conserved between the two species. It is clear that the p53 protein is mutated or lost in astrocytomas and in secondary GBMs that arise from progression of an astrocytoma. Evidence for a role of neurofibromin mutation in human astrocytoma is less clear. Neurofibromin acts, at least in part, through its RasGAP domain to downregulate active Ras signaling. Tyrosine kinase receptors PDGFRα and EGFR are amplified frequently, overexpressed, or mutated to be constitutively active in astrocytomas and GBMs, suggesting that Ras signaling pathways play a key role in astrocytoma, and this is supported by data showing that inhibition of Ras signaling blocks the proliferation of astrocytoma cells (Guha et al. 1997) (see Chapter 38). In addition, as described in Chapter 4, overexpression of Ras can induce gliomas in mice (Ding et al. 2001). It is therefore possible that the loss of neurofibromin in the *NPcis* model of astrocytoma mimics the upregulation of Ras found in human astrocytomas and GBMs. Because of the large size of the *NF1* gene, it has been difficult until very recently to identify somatic mutations in *NF1* in GBMs (Li et al. 1992). Advances in genomic technologies coupled with a new initiative to completely sequence genes in human GBMs through The Cancer Genome Atlas project have now led to a revision in our understanding of the frequency of *NF1* mutation in GBM. Two independent studies recently found an *NF1* mutation frequency of 15–23% in GBMs (TCGA, 2008, Parsons et al. 2008). This may be an underestimation of the percentage of GBMs with inactivation of neurofibromin, as neurofibromin has been shown to be actively regulated through post-translational degradation (Cichowski et al. 2003), and the stability of neurofibromin levels in GBMs has not been fully explored yet. These findings combined with the astrocytoma predisposition in *NPcis* mice and human *NF1* syndrome patients show that neurofibromin plays a critical role in the formation of at least a subset of astrocytoma grades II–IV in humans. Because *NF1* mutations may be specific to a subset of GBMs, care must be taken in interpreting results in the model. While *pathways* identified as being important in this model are likely to be widely relevant to astrocytomas and GBMs, specific *molecules* will need to be validated across a broad range of astrocytomas and GBMs to determine whether they are important in these tumors generally or are specific for *NF1* mutant and/or *TP53* mutant astrocytomas and GBMs. This is likely to be the case for every genetically engineered mouse model of brain tumors and highlights the importance of the variety of models described in this book to examine brain tumors in the context of different initiating mutations.

The spontaneous coevolution of tumors with the microenvironment and the progression of WHO II to WHO IV tumors are major strengths of the *NPcis* model. However, this spontaneous and progressive growth occurs over a period of many months. Astrocytomas and GBMs are observed as early as 2 months and as late as 11 months, with average ages of 6–8 months depending on the cross. This relatively long latency and lack of control over the timing of tumor onset can pose difficulties in using these mice for preclinical trials. In this regard, these mice more closely mimic patient tumors, and need to be studied akin to clinical trials, with mice entered into preclinical trials as tumors develop. In vivo imaging, using magnetic resonance imaging or bioluminescence (Momota and Holland 2005), to identify tumors makes preclinical testing with this model more feasible. The incidence of astrocytoma is higher in older mice, approaching 100% in certain crosses, particularly in progeny of mutant mothers on strain backgrounds that suppress other tumor types in the model (see below) (Reilly et al. 2006). Mice older than 6 months can be used for preclinical studies such that the vast majority of the age-selected mice will develop astrocytoma between 6 and 9 months of age.

In addition to astrocytomas and GBMs, the *NPcis* mice develop other malignancies associated with neurofibromatosis type 1, as well as tumors associated with *Trp53* mutation in mice. These tumors include malignant peripheral nerve sheath tumors (Cichowski et al. 1999, Vogel et al. 1999, Reilly et al. 2006), pheochromocytomas (Tischler et al. 1995), and lymphomas (Jacks et al. 1994a), as well as other tumors in the brain, specifically pituitary carcinoma and ethesioneuroblastoma. These tumors are also subject to background effects, similar to the resistance of 129S4 mice to astrocytomas (see above), but they differ in the strains that modify them (Reilly et al. 2004, 2006). This allows one to choose strain backgrounds that maximize astrocytomas and minimize other tumor types. Many of the confounding tumor types occur in less than 20% of progeny. The only tumor type that occurs in a large percentage of the population is malignant peripheral nerve sheath tumor (MPNST), occurring in as low as 20% of the population and as high as 80% of the population, depending on the strain background and parental inheritance of *NPcis*. The modifier loci responsible for resistance or susceptibility to MPNSTs are currently being mapped and it will be interesting to compare them to modifiers identified in related systems, such as the rat schwannomas described in Chapter 11. In contrast to astrocytomas, MPNSTs are suppressed in progeny of *NPcis* mutant mothers and increased in progeny of mutant fathers (Table 6.1). MPNSTs

Table 6.1 Variation in astrocytoma and PNSTs in *NPcis*, B6 mice

	$NPcis^{mat}$, B6		$NPcis^{pat}$, B6	
Cross Tumor	Females (%)	Males (%)	Females (%)	Males (%)
Astrocytoma	51	71	52	49
PNST	34	46	60	82

appear in younger mice than do astrocytomas or GBMs. For this reason, mice that survive longer are less likely to develop MPNSTs and more likely to develop astrocytoma. By using *NPcis* mice for astrocytoma studies that have survived up to 6 months of age, are progeny of *NPcis* mutant mothers, and are on a strain background that suppresses MPNSTs, such as B6XA/J or B6XDBA/2 J F_1 backgrounds (Reilly et al. 2006), one can generate cohorts of *NPcis* progeny that will develop astrocytoma or GBM in close to 100% of the cohort over a 3-month period.

6.6 Summary

The development of astrocytoma and secondary GBM in mice carrying mutations in *Trp53* and *Nf1* demonstrates the causal role of the p53 and Ras pathways in astrocytic gliomas. These tumors display a broad range of histologies suggesting common underlying mechanisms of tumor development for different patient astrocytomas. The overexpression of PDGFRα in this model suggests that the role of this tyrosine kinase receptor in astrocytoma tumorigenesis is conserved across species. This model has revealed the complex interaction of sex of offspring and maternal/paternal inheritance in controlling susceptibility to astrocytoma and may lead to the identification of modifier genes controlling these processes. As a spontaneous model of astrocytoma, the *NPcis* model has the advantages of easily manipulated genetics, coevolution of the tumor with its microenvironment, and controlled genetic background, with the limitations that tumors initiate at different times over the course of many months. This model and the tumor lines derived from it can be used to better understand the basic biology underlying astrocytoma and to screen candidate therapeutics for potential efficacy against astrocytoma.

Acknowledgments I thank Carmen Sapienza and Erwin Van Meir for proofreading the manuscript and providing thoughtful comments.

References

Blatt J, Jaffe R, Deutsch M and Adkins JC (1986) Neurofibromatosis and childhood tumors. Cancer 57:1225–1229

Brannan C, Perkins A, Vogel K, Ratner N, Nordlund M, Reid S, Buchberg A, Jenkins N, Parada L and Copeland N (1994) Targeted disruption of the neurofibromatosis type 1 gene leads to developmental abnormalities in heart and various neural crest-derived tissues. Genes Dev 8:1019–1029

CBTRUS: 2005–2006 Primary brain tumors in the United States-Statistical report. (2006) Central Brain Tumor Registry of the United States, Chicago

Chesler EJ, Wang J, Lu L, Qu Y, Manly KF and Williams RW (2003) Genetic correlates of gene expression in recombinant inbred strains: A relational model system to explore neurobehavioral phenotypes. Neuroinformatics 1:343–357

Churchill GA, Airey DC, Allayee H, Angel JM, Attie AD, Beatty J, Beavis WD, Belknap JK, Bennett B, Berrettini W, Bleich A, Bogue M, Broman KW, Buck KJ, Buckler E, Burmeister M, Chesler EJ, Cheverud JM, Clapcote S, Cook MN, Cox RD, Crabbe JC, Crusio WE, Darvasi A, Deschepper CF, Doerge RW, Farber CR, Forejt J, Gaile D, Garlow SJ, Geiger H, Gershenfeld H, Gordon T, Gu J, Gu W, de Haan G, Hayes NL, Heller C, Himmelbauer H, Hitzemann R, Hunter K, Hsu HC, Iraqi FA, Ivandic B, Jacob HJ, Jansen RC, Jepsen KJ, Johnson DK, Johnson TE, Kempermann G, Kendziorski C, Kotb M, Kooy RF, Llamas B, Lammert F, Lassalle JM, Lowenstein PR, Lu L, Lusis A, Manly KF, Marcucio R, Matthews D, Medrano JF, Miller DR, Mittleman G, Mock BA, Mogil JS, Montagutelli X, Morahan G, Morris DG, Mott R, Nadeau JH, Nagase H, Nowakowski RS, O'Hara BF, Osadchuk AV, Page GP, Paigen B, Paigen K, Palmer AA, Pan HJ, Peltonen-Palotie L, Peirce J, Pomp D, Pravenec M, Prows DR, Qi Z, Reeves RH, Roder J, Rosen GD, Schadt EE, Schalkwyk LC, Seltzer Z, Shimomura K, Shou S, Sillanpaa MJ, Siracusa LD, Snoeck HW, Spearow JL, Svenson K, Tarantino LM, Threadgill D, Toth LA, Valdar W, de Villena FP, Warden C, Whatley S, Williams RW, Wiltshire T, Yi N, Zhang D, Zhang M and Zou F (2004) The Collaborative Cross, a community resource for the genetic analysis of complex traits. Nat Genet 36:1133–1137

Cichowski K, Santiago S, Jardim M, Johnson BW and Jacks T (2003) Dynamic regulation of the Ras pathway via proteolysis of the NF1 tumor suppressor. Genes Dev 17:449–454

Cichowski K, Shih T, Schmitt E, Santiago S, Reilly K, McLaughlin M, Bronson R and Jacks T (1999) Mouse models of tumor development in neurofibromatosis type 1. Science 286:2172–2176

Collins VP (1999) Progression as exemplified by human astrocytic tumors. Semin Cancer Biol 9:267–276

Colman H and Aldape K (2008) Molecular predictors in glioblastoma: Toward personalized therapy. Arch Neurol 65:877–883

Ding H, Roncari L, Shannon P, Wu X, Lau N, Karaskova J, Gutmann DH, Squire JA, Nagy A and Guha A (2001) Astrocyte-specific expression of activated p21-ras results in malignant astrocytoma formation in a transgenic mouse model of human gliomas. Cancer Res 61:3826–3836

Donehower L, Harvey M, Slagle B, McArthur M, Montgomery Jr C, Butel J and Bradley A (1992) Mice deficient for p53 are developmentally normal but susceptible to spontaneous tumors. Nature 356:215–221

Easton D, Ponder M, Huson S and Ponder B (1993) An analysis of variation in expression of neurofibromatosis (NF) type 1 (NF1): Evidence for modifying genes. Am J Hum Genet 53:305–313

Ekstrand AJ, James CD, Cavenee WK, Seliger B, Pettersson RF and Collins VP (1991) Genes for epidermal growth factor receptor, transforming growth factor alpha, and epidermal growth factor and their expression in human gliomas in vivo. Cancer Res 51:2164–2172

Fisher JL, Schwartzbaum JA, Wrensch M and Wiemels JL (2007) Epidemiology of brain tumors. Neurol Clin 25:867–890, vii

Fleming TP, Saxena A, Clark WC, Robertson JT, Oldfield EH, Aaronson SA and Ali IU (1992) Amplification and/or overexpression of platelet-derived growth factor receptors and epidermal growth factor receptor in human glial tumors. Cancer Res 52:4550–4553

Freije WA, Castro-Vargas FE, Fang Z, Horvath S, Cloughesy T, Liau LM, Mischel PS and Nelson SF (2004) Gene expression profiling of gliomas strongly predicts survival. Cancer Res 64:6503–6510

Fulci G, Labuhn M, Maier D, Lachat Y, Hausmann O, Hegi ME, Janzer RC, Merlo A and Van Meir EG (2000) p53 gene mutation and ink4a-arf deletion appear to be two mutually exclusive events in human glioblastoma. Oncogene 19:3816–3822

Furnari FB, Fenton T, Bachoo RM, Mukasa A, Stommel JM, Stegh A, Hahn WC, Ligon KL, Louis DN, Brennan C, Chin L, DePinho RA and Cavenee WK (2007) Malignant astrocytic glioma: Genetics, biology, and paths to treatment. Genes Dev 21:2683–2710

Gould VE, Lee I, Wiedenmann B, Moll R, Chejfec G and Franke WW (1986) Synaptophysin: A novel marker for neurons, certain neuroendocrine cells, and their neoplasms. Hum Pathol 17:979–983

Guha A, Feldkamp MM, Lau N, Boss G and Pawson A (1997) Proliferation of human malignant astrocytomas is dependent on ras activation. Oncogene 15:2755–2765

Gutmann D, Wood D and Collins F (1991) Identification of the neurofibromatosis type 1 gene product. PNAS 88:9658–9662

Haas-Kogan DA, Prados MD, Lamborn KR, Tihan T, Berger MS and Stokoe D (2005a) Biomarkers to predict response to epidermal growth factor receptor inhibitors. Cell Cycle 4:1369–1372

Haas-Kogan DA, Prados MD, Tihan T, Eberhard DA, Jelluma N, Arvold ND, Baumber R, Lamborn KR, Kapadia A, Malec M, Berger MS and Stokoe D (2005b) Epidermal growth factor receptor, protein kinase B/AKT, and glioma response to erlotinib. J Natl Cancer Inst 97:880–887

Hattori S, Maekawa M and Nakamura S (1992) Identification of neurofibromatosis type 1 gene product as an insoluble GTPase-activating protein toward ras p21. Oncogene 7:481–485

Hawes JJ, Nerva JD and Reilly KM (2008) Novel dual-reporter preclinical screen for anti-astrocytoma agents identifies cytostatic and cytotoxic compounds. J Biomol Screen 13:795–803

Hermanson M, Funa K, Hartman M, Claesson-Welsh L, Heldin CH, Westermark B and Nister M (1992) Platelet-derived growth factor and its receptors in human glioma tissue: Expression of messenger RNA and protein suggests the presence of autocrine and paracrine loops. Cancer Res 52:3213–3219

Hunter KW and Crawford NP (2008) The future of qtl mapping to diagnose disease in mice in the age of whole-genome association studies. Annu Rev Genet 42:131–141

Huson S and Hughes R (1994) The neurofibromatoses: A pathogenetic and clinical overview. Chapman & Hall Medical, London

Ichimura K, Bolin MB, Goike HM, Schmidt EE, Moshref A and Collins VP (2000) Deregulation of the p14ARF/MDM2/p53 pathway is a prerequisite for human astrocytic gliomas with G1-S transition control gene abnormalities. Cancer Res 60:417–424

Ichimura K, Schmidt EE, Goike HM and Collins VP (1996) Human glioblastomas with no alterations of the CDKN2A (p16INK4A, MTS1) and CDK4 genes have frequent mutations of the retinoblastoma gene. Oncogene 13:1065–1072

Ishii N, Tada M, Hamou MF, Janzer RC, Meagher-Villemure K, Wiestler OD, Tribolet N and Van Meir EG (1999) Cells with TP53 mutations in low grade astrocytic tumors evolve clonally to malignancy and are an unfavorable prognostic factor. Oncogene 18:5870–5878

Jacks T, Remington L, Williams BO, Schmitt EM, Halachmi S, Bronson RT and Weinberg RA (1994a) Tumor spectrum analysis in *p53*-mutant mice. Current Biol 4:1–7

Jacks T, Shih TS, Schmitt EM, Bronson RT, Bernards A and Weinberg RA (1994b) Tumour predisposition in mice heterozygous for a targeted mutation in Nf1. Nature Genet 7:353–361

Kleihues P and Cavenee W (2000) Pathology and genetics of tumours of the nervous system. International Agency for Research on Cancer, Lyon

Kleihues P, Schauble B, zur Hausen A, Esteve J and Ohgaki H (1997) Tumors associated with p53 germline mutations: A synopsis of 91 families. Am J Pathol 150:1–13

Lang FF, Miller DC, Koslow M and Newcomb EW (1994) Pathways leading to glioblastoma multiforme: A molecular analysis of genetic alterations in 65 astrocytic tumors. J Neurosurg 81:427–436

Li Y, Bollag G, Clark R, Stevens J, Conroy L, Fults D, Ward K, Friedman E, Samowitz W, McCormick F, White R and Cawthorn R (1992) Somatic mutations in the neurofibromatosis 1 gene in human tumors. Cell 69:275–281

Libermann TA, Nusbaum HR, Razon N, Kris R, Lax I, Soreq H, Whittle N, Waterfield MD, Ullrich A and Schlessinger J (1985) Amplification, enhanced expression and possible rearrangement of EGF receptor gene in primary human brain tumours of glial origin. Nature 313:144–147

Maher EA, Brennan C, Wen PY, Durso L, Ligon KL, Richardson A, Khatry D, Feng B, Sinha R, Louis DN, Quackenbush J, Black PM, Chin L and DePinho RA (2006) Marked genomic differences characterize primary and secondary glioblastoma subtypes and identify two distinct molecular and clinical secondary glioblastoma entities. Cancer Res 66:11502–11513

Malkin D (1994) *p53* and the Li–Fraumeni syndrome. Biochemica et Biophysica Acta 1198:197–213

Malmer B, Adatto P, Armstrong G, Barnholtz-Sloan J, Bernstein JL, Claus E, Davis F, Houlston R, Il'yasova D, Jenkins R, Johansen C, Lai R, Lau C, McCarthy B, Nielsen H, Olson SH, Sadetzki S, Shete S, Wiklund F, Wrensch M, Yang P and Bondy M (2007) GLIOGENE an international consortium to understand familial glioma. Cancer Epidemiol Biomarkers Prev 16:1730–1734

Marsden HB, Kumar S, Kahn J and Anderton BJ (1983) A study of glial fibrillary acidic protein (GFAP) in childhood brain tumours. Int J Cancer 31:439–445

Martin G, Viskochil D, Bollag G, McCabe P, Crosier W, Conroy L, Clark R, O'Connell P, Cawthorn R, Innis M and McCormick F (1990) The gap-related domain of the neurofibromatosis type 1 gene product interacts with *ras* p21. Cell 63:843–849

Mellinghoff IK, Wang MY, Vivanco I, Haas-Kogan DA, Zhu S, Dia EQ, Lu KV, Yoshimoto K, Huang JH, Chute DJ, Riggs BL, Horvath S, Liau LM, Cavenee WK, Rao PN, Beroukhim R, Peck TC, Lee JC, Sellers WR, Stokoe D, Prados M, Cloughesy TF, Sawyers CL and Mischel PS (2005) Molecular determinants of the response of glioblastomas to EGFR kinase inhibitors. N Engl J Med 353:2012–2024

Momota H and Holland EC (2005) Bioluminescence technology for imaging cell proliferation. Curr Opin Biotechnol 16:681–686

Mott R and Flint J (2002) Simultaneous detection and fine mapping of quantitative trait loci in mice using heterogeneous stocks. Genetics 160:1609–1618

Nadeau JH, Singer JB, Matin A and Lander ES (2000) Analysing complex genetic traits with chromosome substitution strains [published erratum appears in nat genet 2000 may;25(1):125]. Nat Genet 24:221–225

Oertel J, von Buttlar E, Schroeder HW and Gaab MR (2005) Prognosis of gliomas in the 1970s and today. Neurosurg Focus 18:e12

Parsons DW, Jones S, Zhang X, Lin JC, Leary RJ, Angenendt P, Mankoo P, Carter H, Siu IM, Gallia GL, Olivi A, McLendon R, Rasheed BA, Keir S, Nikolskaya T, Nikolsky Y, Busam DA, Tekleab H, Diaz LA, Jr., Hartigan J, Smith DR, Strausberg RL, Marie SK, Shinjo SM, Yan H, Riggins GJ, Bigner DD, Karchin R, Papadopoulos N, Parmigiani G, Vogelstein B, Velculescu VE and Kinzler KW (2008) An integrated genomic analysis of human glioblastoma multiforme. Science 321:1807–1812

Phillips HS, Kharbanda S, Chen R, Forrest WF, Soriano RH, Wu TD, Misra A, Nigro JM, Colman H, Soroceanu L, Williams PM, Modrusan Z, Feuerstein BG and Aldape K (2006) Molecular subclasses of high-grade glioma predict prognosis, delineate a pattern of disease progression, and resemble stages in neurogenesis. Cancer Cell 9:157–173

Rasheed BK, McLendon RE, Herndon JE, Friedman HS, Friedman AH, Bigner DD and Bigner SH (1994) Alterations of the *TP53* gene in human gliomas. Cancer Res 54: 1324–1330

Reifenberger G, Ichimura K, Reifenberger J, Elkahloun AG, Meltzer PS and Collins VP (1996) Refined mapping of 12q13–q15 amplicons in human malignant gliomas suggests CDK4/SAS and MDM2 as independent amplification targets. Cancer Res 56:5141–5145

Reifenberger G, Liu L, Ichimura K, Schmidt EE and Collins VP (1993) Amplification and overexpression of the MDM2 gene in a subset of human malignant gliomas without p53 mutations. Cancer Res 53:2736–2739

Reilly KM (2004) The importance of genome architecture in cancer susceptibility: Location, location, location. Cell Cycle 3:1378–1382

Reilly KM, Broman KW, Bronson RT, Tsang S, Loisel DA, Christy ES, Sun Z, Diehl J, Munroe DJ and Tuskan RG (2006) An imprinted locus epistatically influences Nstr1 and Nstr2 to control resistance to nerve sheath tumors in a neurofibromatosis type 1 mouse model. Cancer Res 66:62–68

Reilly KM and Jacks T (2001) Genetically engineered mouse models of astrocytoma: GEMs in the rough? Semin Cancer Biol 11:177–191

Reilly KM, Loisel DA, Bronson RT, McLaughlin ME and Jacks T (2000) Nf1;Trp53 mutant mice develop glioblastoma with evidence of strain-specific effects. Nat Genet 26:109–113

Reilly KM, Rubin JB, Gilbertson RJ, Garbow JR, Roussel MF and Gutmann DH (2008) Rethinking brain tumors: The fourth mouse models of human cancers consortium nervous system tumors workshop. Cancer Res 68:5508–5511

Reilly KM, Tuskan RG, Christy E, Loisel DA, Ledger J, Bronson RT, Smith CD, Tsang S, Munroe DJ and Jacks T (2004) Susceptibility to astrocytoma in mice mutant for *Nf1* and *Trp53* is linked to chromosome 11 and subject to epigenetic effects. Proc Natl Acad Sci USA 101:13008–13013

Roberts A, Pardo-Manuel de Villena F, Wang W, McMillan L and Threadgill DW (2007) The polymorphism architecture of mouse genetic resources elucidated using genome-wide resequencing data: Implications for qtl discovery and systems genetics. Mamm Genome 18:473–481

Scherer H (1940) The forms of growth in gliomas and their practical significance. Brain 63:1–35

Schmidt EE, Ichimura K, Reifenberger G and Collins VP (1994) CDKN2 (p16/MTS1) gene deletion or CDK4 amplification occurs in the majority of glioblastomas. Cancer Res 54:6321–6324

Sherr CJ (1996) Cancer cell cycles. Science 274:1672–1677

Sherr CJ and Weber JD (2000) The ARF/p53 pathway. Curr Opin Genet Dev 10:94–99

Sorensen SA, Mulvihill JJ and Nielsen A (1986) Long-term follow-up of von recklinghausen neurofibromatosis. Survival and malignant neoplasms. N Engl J Med 314:1010–1015

Tascos NA, Parr J and Gonatas NK (1982) Immunocytochemical study of the glial fibrillary acidic protein in human neoplasms of the central nervous system. Hum Pathol 13:454–458

The Cancer Genome Atlas Research Network, McLendon R, Friedman A, Bigner D, Van Meir EG, Brat DJ, Mastrogianakis M, Olson JJ, Mikkelsen T, Lehman N, Aldape K, Alfred Yung WK, Bogler O, Vandenberg S, Berger M, Prados M, Muzny D, Morgan M, Scherer S, Sabo A, Nazareth L, Lewis L, Hall O, Zhu Y, Ren Y, Alvi O, Yao J, Hawes A, Jhangiani S, Fowler G, San Lucas A, Kovar C, Cree A, Dinh H, Santibanez J, Joshi V, Gonzalez-Garay ML, Miller CA, Milosavljevic A, Donehower L, Wheeler DA, Gibbs RA, Cibulskis K, Sougnez C, Fennell T, Mahan S, Wilkinson J, Ziaugra L, Onofrio R, Bloom T, Nicol R, Ardlie K, Baldwin J, Gabriel S, Lander ES, Ding L, Fulton RS, McLellan MD, Wallis J, Larson DE, Shi X, Abbott R, Fulton L, Chen K, Koboldt DC, Wendl MC, Meyer R, Tang Y, Lin L, Osborne JR, Dunford-Shore BH, Miner TL, Delehaunty K, Markovic C, Swift G, Courtney W, Pohl C, Abbott S, Hawkins A, Leong S, Haipek C, Schmidt H, Wiechert M, Vickery T, Scott S, Dooling DJ, Chinwalla A, Weinstock GM, Mardis ER, Wilson RK, Getz G, Winckler W, Verhaak RG, Lawrence MS, O'Kelly M, Robinson J, Alexe G, Beroukhim R, Carter S, Chiang D, Gould J, Gupta S, Korn J, Mermel C, Mesirov J, Monti S, Nguyen H, Parkin M, Reich M, Stransky N, Weir BA, Garraway L, Golub T, Meyerson M, Chin L, Protopopov A, Zhang J, Perna I, Aronson S, Sathiamoorthy N, Ren G, Yao J, Wiedemeyer WR, Kim H, Won Kong S, Xiao Y, Kohane IS, Seidman J, Park PJ, Kucherlapati R, Laird PW, Cope L, Herman JG, Weisenberger DJ, Pan F, Van Den Berg D, Van Neste L, Mi Yi J, Schuebel KE, Baylin SB, Absher DM, Li JZ, Southwick A, Brady S, Aggarwal A, Chung T, Sherlock G, Brooks JD, Myers RM, Spellman PT, Purdom E, Jakkula LR, Lapuk AV, Marr H, Dorton S, Gi Choi Y, Han J, Ray A, Wang V, Durinck S, Robinson M, Wang NJ, Vranizan K, Peng V, Van Name E, Fontenay GV, Ngai J, Conboy JG, Parvin B, Feiler HS, Speed TP, Gray JW, Brennan C, Socci ND, Olshen A, Taylor BS, Lash A, Schultz N, Reva B, Antipin Y, Stukalov A, Gross B, Cerami E, Qing Wang W, Qin LX, Seshan VE, Villafania L, Cavatore M, Borsu L, Viale A, Gerald W, Sander C, Ladanyi M, Perou CM, Neil Hayes D, Topal MD, Hoadley KA, Qi Y, Balu S, Shi Y, Wu J, Penny R, Bittner M, Shelton T, Lenkiewicz E, Morris S, Beasley D, Sanders S, Kahn A, Sfeir R, Chen J, Nassau D, Feng L, Hickey E, Zhang J, Weinstein JN, Barker A, Gerhard DS, Vockley J, Compton C, Vaught J, Fielding P, Ferguson ML, Schaefer C, Madhavan S, Buetow KH, Collins F, Good P, Guyer M, Ozenberger B, Peterson J and Thomson E (2008) Comprehensive genomic characterization defines human glioblastoma genes and core pathways. Nature 455:1061–1068

Tischler A, Shih T, Williams B and Jacks T (1995) Characterization of pheochromocytomas in a mouse strain with a targeted disruptive mutation of the neurofibromatosis gene *Nf1*. Endocrine Pathol 6:5323–335

Van Dyke T and Jacks T (2002) Cancer modeling in the modern era: Progress and challenges. Cell 108:135–144

van Meyel DJ, Ramsay DA, Casson AG, Keeney M, Chambers AF and Cairncross JG (1994) *p53* mutation, expression, and DNA ploidy in evolving gliomas: Evidence for two pathways of progression. J Natl Cancer Inst 86:1011–1017

Vogel K, Klesse L, Velasco-Miguel S, Meyers K, Rushing E and Parada L (1999) Mouse tumor model for neurofibromatosis type 1. Science 286:2176–2179
von Deimling A, Eibl RH, Ohgaki H, Louis DN, von Ammon K, Petersen I, Kleihues P, Chung RY, Wiestler OD and Seizinger BR (1992) *p53* mutations are associated with 17p allelic loss in grade II and grade III astrocytoma. Cancer Res 52:2987–2990
von Deimling A, von Ammon K, Schoenfeld D, Wiestler OD, Seizinger BR and Louis DN (1993) Subsets of glioblastoma multiforme defined by molecular genetic analysis. Brain Pathol 3:19–26
Watanabe K, Sato K, Biernat W, Tachibana O, von Ammon K, Ogata N, Yonekawa Y, Kleihues P and Ohgaki H (1997) Incidence and timing of *p53* mutations during astrocytoma progression in patients with multiple biopsies. Clin Cancer Res 3:523–530
Watanabe K, Tachibana O, Sata K, Yonekawa Y, Kleihues P and Ohgaki H (1996) Overexpression of the EGF receptor and *p53* mutations are mutually exclusive in the evolution of primary and secondary glioblastomas. Brain Pathol 6:217–223; discussion 223–214
Wood AJ and Oakey RJ (2006) Genomic imprinting in mammals: Emerging themes and established theories. PLoS Genet 2:e147
Xu G, Lin b, Tanaka K, Dunn D, Wood D, Gesteland R, White R, Weiss R and Tamanoi F (1990a) The catalytic domain of the neurofibromatosis type 1 gene product stimulates *ras* GTPase and complements *ira* mutants of S. cerevisiae. Cell 63:835–841
Xu G, O'Connell P, Viskochil D, Cawthorn R, Robertson M, Culver M, Dunn D, Stevens J, Gesteland R, White R and Weiss R (1990b) The neurofibromatosis type 1 gene encodes a protein related to GAP. Cell 62:599–608
Zhu Y, Guignard F, Zhao D, Liu L, Burns DK, Mason RP, Messing A and Parada LF (2005) Early inactivation of p53 tumor suppressor gene cooperating with Nf1 loss induces malignant astrocytoma. Cancer Cell 8:119–130

Chapter 7
Modeling Astrocytomas in a Family of Inducible Genetically Engineered Mice: Implications for Preclinical Cancer Drug Development

C. Ryan Miller, Natalie O. Karpinich, Qian Zhang, Elizabeth Bullitt, Serguei Kozlov, and Terry Van Dyke

Abstract Astrocytomas, the most common intracranial malignancies, are a morphologically and molecularly heterogeneous group of brain tumors with potentially dismal patient outcomes for which few effective drugs are available. Genetically engineered mouse (GEM) models of astrocytoma represent a powerful technique for defining the molecular and genetic abnormalities that contribute to tumorigenesis. Based on the genetic aberrations observed in human astrocytomas, we have generated a series of conditional, inducible GEM models of astrocytomas that recapitulate the spectrum of morphological phenotypes of human astrocytomas. However, the extent to which any given GEM model recapitulates the molecular alterations in human tumors must be determined to validate its usefulness in preclinical studies. We are currently pursuing comparative evaluation of primary astrocytomas as formed in GEM and in patients to (1) examine the signaling pathway abnormalities caused by defined genetic lesions in GEM astrocytomas and (2) identify protein biomarkers that can define human astrocytomas that most closely resemble their murine counterparts. To utilize these GEM for combined preclinical evaluation of targeted therapeutic agents and biomarkers predictive of response, we have developed a panel of cell-based assays (CBA) and an orthotopic allograft model of high-grade astrocytomas using primary astrocytes derived from GEM. These tools should prove useful for preclinical drug development studies and provide a link between preclinical drug development in GEM astrocytoma models and rational design of human clinical trials involving only those patients with tumors having similar signaling pathway abnormalities.

C.R. Miller (✉)
Department of Pathology & Laboratory Medicine and Lineberger Comprehensive Cancer Center, University of North Carolina, Chapel Hill, NC
e-mail: rmiller@med.unc.edu

E.G. Van Meir (ed.), *CNS Cancer*, Cancer Drug Discovery and Development, DOI 10.1007/978-1-60327-553-8_7,
© Humana Press, a part of Springer Science+Business Media, LLC 2009

Contents

7.1 Introduction

Diffusely infiltrating gliomas are the most common primary intracranial neoplasms. They account for 36% of all primary and 81% of all malignant CNS tumors (CBTRUS 2008). Over 80% of these tumors are considered high grade (grades III and IV) when diagnosed according to the current World Health Organization (WHO) classification, a system based upon morphological evidence of differentiation along astrocytic, oligodendroglial, or mixed lineages (Louis 2007). Astrocytomas, which together constitute the vast majority (75%) of diffuse gliomas, are further stratified into WHO grades II–IV based upon the presence of histopathological features that correlate with patient outcomes. Specifically, mitotic activity is utilized to distinguish WHO grade III anaplastic astrocytoma (AIII) from its lower grade counterpart, diffuse astrocytoma, WHO grade II (AII). Median overall survival (OS) for patients with AII is greater than 10 years, whereas that with AIII is 3–5 years. Microvascular proliferation (MVP) and/or necrosis are distinguishing features of WHO grade IV astrocytoma, the latter being synonymous to glioblastoma (GBM) in the current WHO scheme (Louis 2007). The median OS of patients diagnosed with GBM remains approximately 12 months and has changed little over the last 40 years. Standard-of-care multimodal therapy, which currently includes surgical debulking, external beam radiotherapy, and/or alkylating agent-based chemotherapy, remains largely palliative (Louis 2007, Miller and Perry 2007).

Two distinct molecular pathways of neoplastic progression of astrocytomas to GBM have been described. GBMs that arise subsequent to diagnosed lower grade (II or III) astrocytomas, termed secondary or type 1 tumors, typically arise in younger individuals (fifth to sixth decade), progress from lower grade lesions over months to decades, and display both well- and poorly differentiated areas. In contrast, primary, type 2 GBMs develop in older individuals (sixth to seventh decade), have short clinical histories (often times less than 3 months), and thus have been proposed to arise de novo without any evidence of a lower grade precursor. Primary GBMs represent over 95% of GBM and are characterized by relatively high frequencies of *EGFR* amplification and *PTEN* mutation (Ohgaki 2004, Louis 2007). In contrast, secondary GBMs constitute a minority of GBM and have relatively high incidences of *TP53* mutation or *MDM2* gene amplification. Both GBM subtypes frequently harbor DNA copy number and sequence abnormalities in G1 cell cycle checkpoint pathway genes

(64% in Parsons et al. 2008 and 87% in Cancer Genome Atlas Research Network 2008), including RB, CDK4, cyclin D1, and CDKN2A (p16^{INK4A}), and PI3K/PTEN/AKT pathway genes (50% in Parsons et al. 2008 and 53% in Cancer Genome Atlas Research Network 2008), including *PTEN* loss of heterozygosity and *PIK3CA* mutation (Cancer Genome Atlas Research Network 2008, Parsons et al. 2008).

7.2 In Vivo Modeling of Astrocytomas in Genetically Engineered Mice

7.2.1 Overview of Genetic Modeling of Diffuse Gliomas

GEM models represent a powerful approach for examining molecular pathogenesis of neoplasia (e.g., Holland 2001, Van Dyke and Jacks 2002) and may become particularly useful in preclinical evaluation of targeted therapeutic agents (Holland 2004, Hu and Holland 2005). A variety of GEM models of diffuse gliomas have been described to date (Tables 7.1 and 7.2; see also Chapters 1–6). Data from these models have demonstrated that three main factors influence development of diffuse gliomas in GEM: (1) the GEM model design; (2) the putative cell of origin and its differentiation state; and (3) the specific genetic modification(s) and the pathways they target.

Six general model designs have been employed (Fig. 7.1): (A) traditional transgenic models in which expression of an oncogene is achieved in specific cell types through use of a cell type-specific promoter; (B) traditional knockout models in which a tumor suppressor gene is deleted; (C) conditional models in which genetic events are induced through cell-specific expression of a recombinase using cell type-specific promoters; (D) spatially restricted induction models that employ localized viral delivery to effect cell type-specific expression of a transgene in animals engineered to express (design A) a viral receptor under control of a cell type-specific promoter; (E) spatially restricted induction of conditional genetic events through viral vector delivery of a recombinase; and (F) conditional, systemic induction models that employ cell type-specific expression of a drug-inducible recombinase. Choice of model design influences experimental tractability, i.e., how easily the model system is manipulated in labs with variable technical capabilities, which in turn influences model dissemination through the research community and the utility of GEM for preclinical studies. We have chosen to focus on conditional, inducible models (F) in order to explore the effect of genetic lesions on tumorigenesis in adult murine astrocytes, based upon the hypothesis that genetic tumor induction in these cells may more closely mimic those that develop in adult humans. Use of these models should also foster their dissemination to laboratories of all technical capabilities and facilitate future preclinical studies. This model system may also be utilized to effect somatic genetic events at different stages of development, including prenatal, neonatal, and adult (Van Dyke and Jacks 2002).

Table 7.1 GEM models of astrocytomas

Tumor	Cell of origin	Model	Genetic modifications: RB	RTK	PI3K	TP53	Other	Penetrance (%)	Ref(s)
A2	GFAP+	C	RB_f (T_{121})					100	Xiao et al. (2002)
	GFAP+	B, C	RB_f (T_{121}) (C)			$TP53^{+/-}$ (B)		100	Xiao et al. (2002)
	GFAP+	A		v-src				10–20	Weissenberger et al. (1997) and Theurillat et al. (1999)
	GFAP+	A		^{12}V-Ha-Ras				70–100	Ding et al. (2001), Shannon et al. (2005), and Wei et al. (2006)
	Nestin+	D (RCAS)		$KRAS^{G12D}$			IGFBP2	17	Dunlap et al. (2007)
	GFAP+	F	RB_f (T_{121})					100	This chapter
AA	GFAP+	B, C	RB_f (T_{121}) (C)		$PTEN^{+/-}$ (B)			100	Xiao et al. (2002)
	GFAP+	F	RB_f (T_{121})	± $KRAS^{G12D}$				100	This chapter
	GFAP+	B, C		$NF1^{-/-}$(C)		$TP53^{-/-}$ (B)		100	Zhu et al. (2005)
GBM	All	B		$NF1^{+/-}$		$TP53^{+/-}$		92–100	Reilly et al. (2000, 2004)
	GFAP+	B, C		$NF1^{+/-}$(C)		$TP53^{+/-}$ (B)		100	Zhu et al. (2005)
	GFAP+	C		$NF1^{+/-}$(C)	$PTEN^{+/-}$	$TP53^{+/-}$		100	Kwon et al. (2008)
	GFAP+	C→E (MSCV)	RB_f (T_{121}) (C)		$PTEN^{+/-}$(E)			75	Xiao et al. (2005)
	GFAP+	F	RB_f (T_{121})	$KRAS^{G12D}$	$PTEN^{+/-}$ or $PTEN^{-/-}$			100	This chapter
	Nestin+ or GFAP+	D (RCAS)		$KRAS^{G12D}$	Akt-Myr-Δ11–60			22–30	Holland et al. (2000), Dai et al. (2001), Uhrbom et al. (2002), and Lassman et al. (2004)
	Nestin+ or GFAP+	D (RCAS)		$KRAS^{G12D}$	± Akt-Myr-Δ11–60		MYC	4–26	Lassman et al. (2004)
	Nestin+	D→E (RCAS)		$KRAS^{G12D}$(D)	$PTEN^{-/-}$ (E) ± Akt-Myr-Δ11–60 (D)			49–62	Hu et al. (2005)
	All	B→D (Ad)	INK4A/ARF^{-} (B)	FIG-ROS (D)				100	Charest et al. (2006)
	GFAP+	A→D (Ad)		^{12}V-Ha-Ras (A); EGFRvIII (D)				70	Wei et al. (2006)
	GFAP+	A→E (Ad)		^{12}V-Ha-Ras (A)	$PTEN^{+/-}$or $PTEN^{-/-}$(E)			79	Wei et al. (2006)

Table 7.1 (continued)

Tumor	Cell of origin	Model	Genetic modifications					Penetrance (%)	Ref(s)
			RB	RTK	PI3K	TP53	Other		
NOS	Nestin+ or GFAP+	B→D (RCAS)	INK4A/ARF$^{+/-}$ or $^{-/-}$ (B)	EGFRvIII (D)				6–52	Holland et al. (1998)
	Nestin+	B→D (RCAS)	INK4A/ARF^{-} (B); CDK4 (D)	EGFRvIII (D) ± bFGF		TP53$^{+/-}$ (B)		10–59	Holland et al. (1998)
	Nestin+ or GFAP+	B→D (RCAS)	INK4A/ARF^{-}(B)	KRAS^{G12D} (D)	± Akt-Myr-Δ11–60 (D)			30–49	Uhrbom et al. (2002)
	Nestin+ or GFAP+	B→D (RCAS)	INK4A^{-} or ARF^{-} (B)	KRAS^{G12D} (D)	± Akt-Myr-Δ11–60 (D)			5–83	Uhrbom et al. (2005)

Abbreviations: A2, WHO grade II astrocytoma; AA, anaplastic astrocytoma; GBM, glioblastoma; GFAP, glial fibrillary acidic protein; MSCV, murine stem cell virus; NOS, astrocytoma, not otherwise specified; RCAS, replication-competent avian leukemia virus. Model types, as illustrated in Fig. 7.1, include A (transgenic), B (knockout), C (conditional), D (somatic, viral transgene delivery), E (somatic conditional with viral recombinase delivery), and F (conditional, inducible).

Table 7.2 GEM models of oligodendroglial neoplasms (oligodendrogliomas and oligoastrocytomas)

Cell of origin	Model	Genetic modifications RB	RTK	PI3K	TP53	Other	Penetrance (%)	Ref(s)
S100β+	A		v-erbB				63	Weiss et al. (2003)
S100β+	A, B	INK4A/ ARF$^{+/-}$(B)	v-erbB (A)				90	Weiss et al. (2003)
S100β+	A, B		v-erbB (A)		TP53$^{+/-}$(B)		80	Weiss et al. (2003)
GFAP+	A		^{12}V-Ha-Ras; EGFRvIII				95–100	Ding et al. (2003)
Nestin+ or GFAP+	D (RCAS)		PDGFβ				16–60	Dai et al. (2001), Shih et al. (2004), Dunlap et al. (2007), and Tchougounova et al. (2007)
Nestin+ or GFAP+	B→D (RCAS)	INK4A$^{-/-}$(B)	PDGFβ (D)				79–82	Tchougounova et al. (2007)
Nestin+ or GFAP+	B→D (RCAS)	ARF$^{-/-}$(B)	PDGFβ (D)				63–77	Tchougounova et al. (2007)
Nestin+ or GFAP+	B→D (RCAS)	INK4A/ ARF$^{-/-}$(B)	PDGFβ (D)				68–85	Tchougounova et al. (2007)
Nestin+	D (RCAS)		PDGFβ			IGFBP2	97	Dunlap et al. (2007)
Nestin+	D (RCAS)		PDGFβ	Akt-Myr-Δ11–60			45	Dai et al. (2005)
GFAP+	D (RCAS)	Polyoma virus middle T antigen			Polyoma virus middle T antigen		27	Holland et al. (2000)
GFAP+	A→D (Ad)		^{12}V-Ha-Ras (A); EGFRvIII (D)				95	Wei et al. (2006)

Abbreviations: GFAP, glial fibrillary acidic protein; RCAS, replication-competent avian leukemia virus. See Table 7.1 for model type abbreviations.

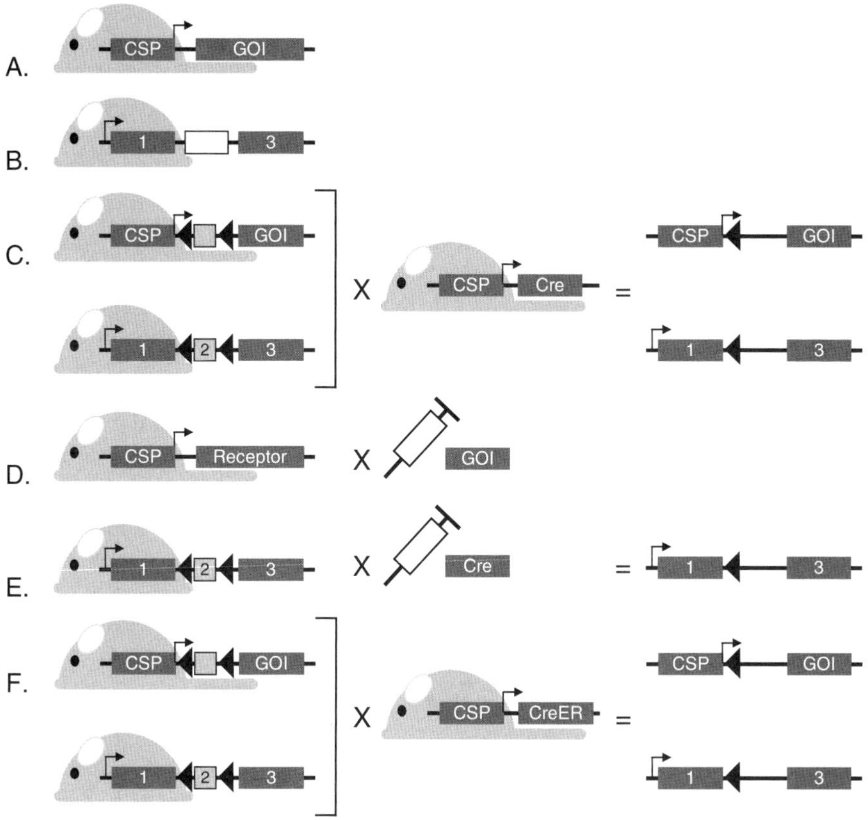

Fig. 7.1 Strategies to model cancer in genetically engineered mice (GEM). Traditional transgenic mice with random gene insertions or mice with targeted mutations of endogenous genes are produced usually by pronuclear DNA injection or via embryonic stem (ES) cell manipulation, respectively (diagrammed as mice with long and short tails, respectively). In traditional transgenic models (**A**), a gene of interest (GOI), typically an oncogene, is randomly integrated into the mouse genome, is transmitted through the germline, and is expressed in specific cell types of a transgenic mouse using a cell-specific promoter (CSP). Traditional knockout/knock-in models employ ES cell targeting strategies to create null (a knockout is shown in (B)) or specific mutated alleles (knock-in, not shown) at the endogenous gene locus in every cell of the GEM. Strategies C, E, and F offer conditional control of either transgene expression or endogenous gene mutation. Conditional models (**C**) utilize a recombinase, such as Cre, and its cognate binding sites (triangles) to induce deletions resulting in expression of a transgene, an endogenous gene, or mutated endogenous gene (not shown). The recombinase is typically introduced by crosses with transgenic mice expressing the recombinase under control of a CSP (**C**) or via injection of a vector encoding the recombinase (**E**) to achieve spatial restriction of gene induction. In the latter case, viral vectors have typically been used to effect recombinase expression. A subset of these strategies has been used in combination. For example, a traditional transgenic mouse engineered to express a viral receptor under control of a cell type-specific promoter (**D**) has been utilized to facilitate localized expression of virally encoded transgenes in a limited number of cells so as to model the stochastic nature of events that produce cancer in humans. Finally, in conditional, inducible models, a recombinase is fused to a ligand-regulated protein domain. For example, a mutated estrogen receptor

GEM glioma model design has benefited greatly from developmental neurobiology studies focused on cellular fate mapping and cellular ontogeny within the CNS (Shih and Holland 2004, Read et al. 2006). In an effort to determine whether specific genetic events are critical for glioma initiation and progression, several groups have employed mouse transgenic approaches to express dominant oncogenes or knockout tumor suppressor genes specifically in glial cells by using the same cell type-restricted promoter elements employed in developmental studies (Fig. 7.2). Use of these promoters has, therefore, permitted analysis of the putative cell of origin of gliomas (Fomchenko and Holland 2005, 2006a, b). Promoters used in GEM glioma studies have included those from the genes encoding the intermediate filament proteins nestin and GFAP, as well as S100β. Nestin (dark) is expressed in neural stem cells (NSC) and progenitors during embryonic development and after birth (Tohyama et al. 1992). GFAP is expressed in astrocyte precursors (radial glia or glial-restricted precursors, RG/GRP) and well-differentiated astrocytes (Brenner et al. 1994). S100β (gray) is expressed in glial precursors, astrocytes, and oligodendrocytes during embryonic development and after birth (Marenholz et al. 2004).

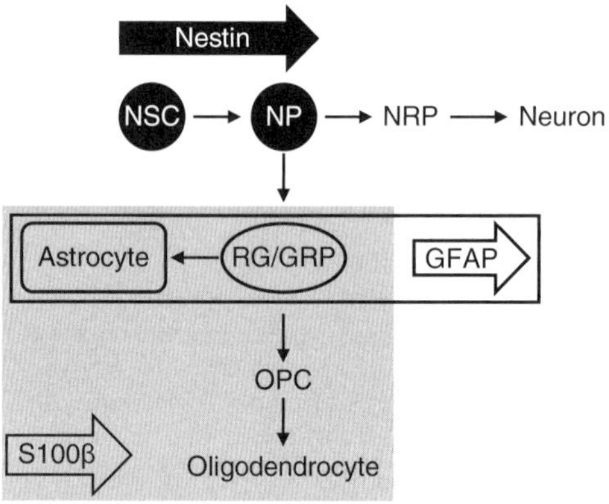

Fig. 7. 2 Neural ontogeny. A highly simplified view of the hierarchical relationship between neurons and glia in the *developing* nervous system is shown. Fate-mapping studies in GEM have employed promoters (*arrows*) that are active in the indicated cellular compartments. GFAP, glial fibrillary acidic protein; GRP, glial-restricted precursors; NSC, neural stem cells; NP, neural progenitors; NRP, neural-restricted precursors; OPC, oligodendroglial progenitor cell; RG, radial glia. In the adult CNS, NSCs are much less abundant and lie within defined niches. GFAP expression is restricted to these cells and to fully differentiated astrocytes

Fig. 7.1 (continued) ligand-binding domain responsive only to synthetic estrogen analogs, but not endogenous estrogens, has been used effectively to regulate Cre recombinase activity after systemic delivery of, for example, the estrogen analog tamoxifen. Adapted from Van Dyke and Jacks (2002)

GEM models have, in general, utilized genetic modifications that correspond to the frequently observed aberrations observed in human gliomas (Van Dyke and Jacks 2002). All GEM glioma models described to date have utilized genetic modifications that target one or more members of four intracellular signaling pathways common to both types of diffuse human gliomas: cell cycle (RB), mitogenic (RTK-RAS), pro-survival (PI3K-PTEN), and TP53 pathways (Fig. 7.3). Although model design, cellular targets (promoters), and specific genetic modifications vary considerably, the entire morphological spectrum of diffuse gliomas has been recapitulated in one or more models (Table 7.1). Most models have yielded tumors that morphologically resemble human astrocytomas. Guha and associates generated transgenic mice expressing an activated ^{12}V-Ha-Ras allele in GFAP+ astrocytes, resulting in mice that develop astrocytoma between 3 and 6 months of age (Ding et al. 2001, Shannon et al. 2005) (see Chapter 4). Holland and colleagues have utilized the Tva/RCAS system, which employs a combination of mouse transgenesis and avian leukemia retrovirus delivery to analyze the effects of distinct genetic events in astrocytes and progenitor cells (Holland et al. 1998, 2000) (see Chapter 2). Mouse GBM were obtained when constitutively active Akt and KRAS^{G12D} alleles were co-expressed in cells expressing a nestin promoter-driven Tva transgene but not in cells expressing GFAP-Tva, suggesting that the differentiation state of the cell of origin is a critical determinant of glioma formation (Holland et al. 2000). In some

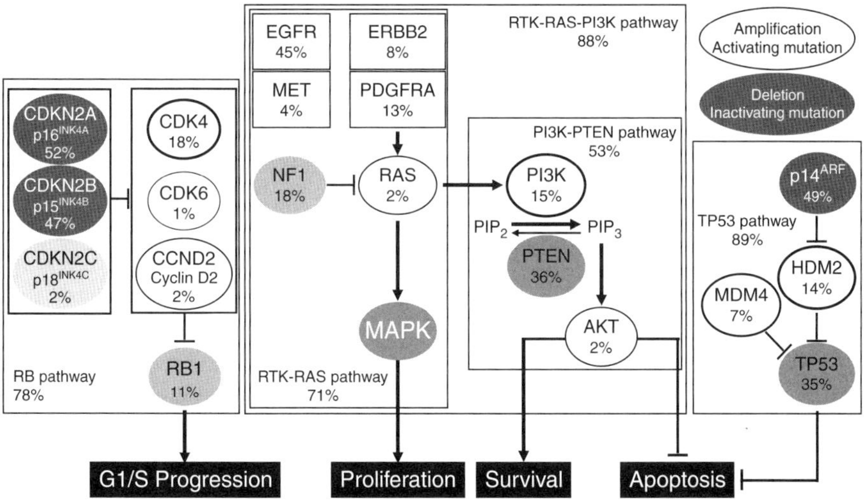

Fig. 7. 3 Molecular and genetic abnormalities in human glioblastomas. Frequencies for copy number and DNA sequence abnormalities at each locus are shown. Oncogenic alterations include gene amplifications and activating mutations (*outlined circles*). Tumor suppressor gene alterations include deletion/LOH and inactivating mutations (*filled circles*). Higher frequencies are indicated by thicker borders and darker shades. Abbreviations: RTK, receptor tyrosine kinase. Data adapted from Cancer Genome Atlas Research Network (2008)

cases, gene transfer into nestin+ cells resulted in the generation of more biologically aggressive gliomas and with a higher frequency than when the identical genes were transferred to more differentiated GFAP+ glial cells. DePinho and associates expressed an activated allele of the epidermal growth factor receptor (EGFR) in isolated INK4A/ARF-deficient neurospheres or neurosphere-derived astrocytes prior to implantation into naïve recipient mice. Mice receiving both types of cells developed high-grade astrocytoma (Bachoo et al. 2002). Individuals with several inherited cancer syndromes develop astrocytomas, including Li-Fraumeni (germline *TP53* mutation) and neurofibromatosis type 1 (germline *NF1* mutation). Mice lacking p53 are viable, but do not develop astrocytomas; NF1-deficient mice die during mid-embryogenesis of a cardiac vessel defect (Brannan et al. 1994, Jacks et al. 1994, Jacks et al. 1994, Donehower et al. 1995). Mice doubly heterozygous for targeted mutations in *NF1* and *TP53* develop high-grade gliomas when maintained on specific genetic backgrounds (Reilly et al. 2000) (Chapter 6).

To overcome the embryonic lethality associated with bi-allelic inactivation of some tumor suppressor genes implicated in glioma development, several groups have employed tissue-specific gene inactivation using Cre/Lox conditionality. This system employs transgenic expression of bacteriophage P1 site-specific Cre recombinase (Sauer 1998), typically under control of cell-specific promoter elements, to catalyze DNA recombination (excision) between directly repeated (oriented in the same direction) pairs of 34 bp *lox*P sites engineered into the gene of interest (Fig. 7.1C). For example, Gutmann and colleagues have developed transgenic mice expressing Cre recombinase in GFAP+ astrocytes and demonstrated that *NF1* gene inactivation by itself is not sufficient for (optic) glioma initiation (Bajenaru et al. 2002) (Chapter 3). Over the past several years, we have made a series of GEM astrocytoma models using three different Cre/Lox strategies (Table 7.1): (1) traditional transgenic, astrocyte-specific models with a human GFAP promoter-driven Cre recombinase to induce genetic abnormalities specifically in astrocytes of the developing embryo (Xiao et al. 2002); (2) somatic, spatially restricted induction models that employ localized retroviral (Xiao et al. 2005) or lentiviral (unpublished) Cre recombinase delivery; and (3) somatic, systemic induction models using a tamoxifen-inducible, GFAP-driven Cre cassette (CreER) (Casper et al. 2007), the latter two of which induce genetic events in adult astrocytes. The developmental astrocytoma model was generated by expressing an N-terminal fragment of the SV40 large T antigen (T_{121}) in GFAP+ cells to selectively inactivate all RB family (Rb_f) members, including RB, p107, and p130. This model showed that Rb_f inactivation was sufficient for astrocytoma initiation, but *PTEN* heterozygosity accelerated disease (Xiao et al. 2002) and homozygous deletion of a *PTEN* conditional allele via stereotaxic injection of Cre retrovirus facilitated disease dissemination (Xiao et al. 2005).

A minority of GEM models have yielded tumors that morphologically resemble human oligodendrogliomas. Guha and colleagues generated transgenic mice expressing a constitutively activated *EGFR* allele (EGFRvIII extracellular domain truncation mutant) in GFAP+ cells and demonstrated that EGFRvIII alone is insufficient for tumor initiation, but its combination with oncogenic ^{12}V-Ha-Ras resulted in tumors with oligodendroglial morphology (Ding et al. 2003) (Chapter 4). Similarly, Weiss and co-workers directed the expression of an activated *EGFR* allele (v-erbB) in S100β+ cells and found that mice develop oligodendroglioma (Weiss et al. 2003). Holland and colleagues found that overexpression of the platelet-derived growth factor (PDGF) in nestin+ progenitors was sufficient to induce oligodendrogliomas (Dai et al. 2001, Shih et al. 2004), with increased frequency and tumor grade in the presence of *INK4A/ARF* deficiency (Tchougounova et al. 2007). These results suggest that a subset of genetic modifications targeted to nestin+ progenitors or GFAP+/S100β+ glia may yield oligodendrogliomas. Yet to date, no GEM glioma models have been constructed that target genetic modifications specifically in terminally differentiated oligodendrocytes. Therefore, it remains unclear whether these cells are susceptible to genetically induced tumorigenesis.

7.2.2 Conditional, Inducible GEM of Astrocytomas

A series of inducible GEM models of astrocytoma were generated by genetically targeting RB, KRAS, and PTEN functions (Fig. 7.4 and Table 7.2). Alterations were induced specifically in adult GEM astrocytes by selective breeding of mice harboring Cre-conditional GFAP-T_{121}, $KRAS^{G12D}$, and *PTEN* deletion alleles, respectively, to a mouse with a tamoxifen-inducible, human GFAP promoter-driven CreER transgenic allele. Use of Cre recombinase genetically fused to a mutated estrogen receptor ligand-binding domain ($CreER^{T2}$) permits spatiotemporally controlled somatic mutagenesis in the mouse (Metzger and Chambon 2001) after systemic administration (intraperitoneal injection) of the synthetic estrogen receptor antagonist 4-hydroxy-tamoxifen (4OH-TAM or 4OHT), but remains unresponsive to endogenous estrogens such as estradiol (Feil et al. 1997). The effects on tumor initiation and progression of all possible combinations of four alleles were tested among RB deletion, KRAS activation, and both heterozygous and homozygous *PTEN* deletions (Table 7.2) in 3-month old adult mice after intraperitoneal injection of 1 mg 4OHT daily for 5 consecutive days. These GEM models represent technically advanced and biologically relevant models and yet require minimal technical expertise for disease induction.

GEM with RB inactivation alone developed the murine equivalent of WHO grade II astrocytomas (Fig. 7.5A and Color Plate 12), and tumor cells were immunoreactive for GFAP (Fig. 7.5B). Neither constitutive KRAS activation nor *PTEN* inactivation alone produced detectable brain pathology, even after 18 months of follow-up (data not shown). In fact, no tumors developed in the absence of RB cell cycle dysregulation. These findings contrast with those obtained using an independently derived GFAP-Cre GEM to

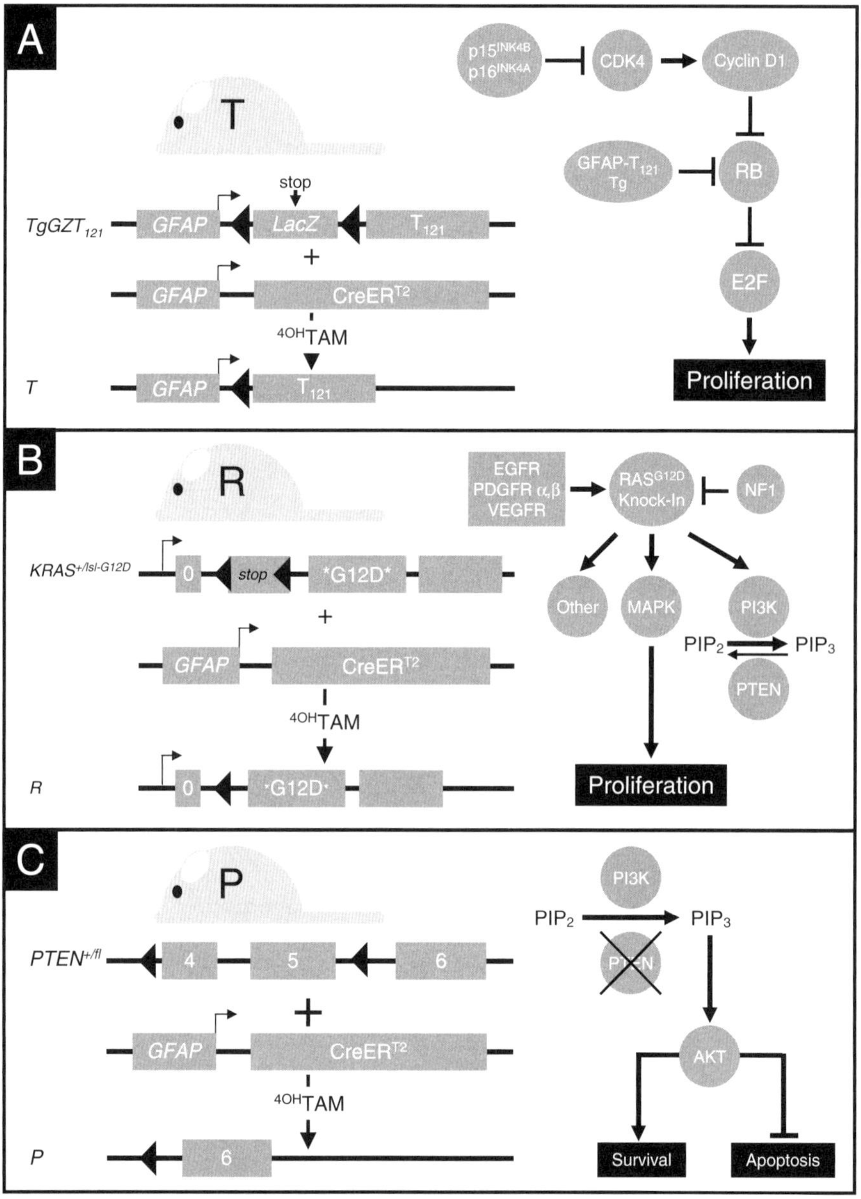

Fig. 7. 4 Conditional, inducible astrocytoma GEM models. T_{121} targets functional deletion of RB_f members specifically in astrocytes in *$TgGZT_{121}$* mice after breeding with GFAP-CreER^{T2} mice and systemic 4-hydroxy-tamoxifen (4OH-TAM) (**A**). Constitutive activation of KRAS^{G12D} and heterozygous deletion of PTEN, both of which are expressed from their endogenous loci, are similarly achieved using KRAS$^{+/lsl\text{-}G12D}$ (**B**) and PTEN$^{+/fl}$ mice (**C**). A homozygous PTEN deletion (PTEN$^{fl/fl}$) GEM was also generated (not shown). Genotypes are abbreviated as T, R, and P, as shown on the corresponding mouse in each panel

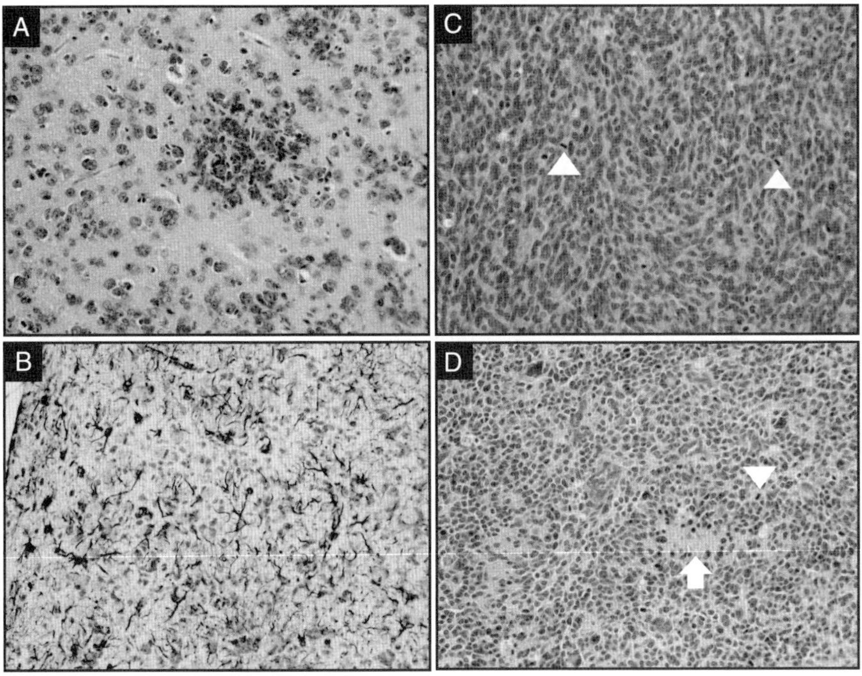

Fig. 7.5 Inducible GEM astrocytomas. T mice developed diffuse astrocytomas, WHO grade II (**A**). Tumors were immunoreactive for GFAP (**B**). TR mice developed anaplastic astrocytomas, WHO grade III (**C**), characterized by numerous mitoses (*arrowheads*). TRP$^{+/-}$ (not shown) and TRP$^{-/-}$ mice (D) developed glioblastomas, WHO grade IV, characterized by numerous mitoses (*arrowhead*) and areas of pseudopalisading necrosis (*arrow*) (*see* Color Plate 12)

facilitate conditional *PTEN* inactivation in the developing mouse embryo (Kwon et al. 2001, 2006). Although these mice also failed to develop gliomas, dysplastic neurons with increased soma size were evident in the cerebellar granular layer and hippocampal dentate gyrus. No such cytological abnormalities were evident in our conditional, inducible GEM harboring *PTEN* deletion. In addition to the different developmental contexts in which PTEN inactivation was achieved (developing embryo [Kwon et al. 2001, 2006] versus adult mice in the conditional, inducible system), GFAP-Cre GEM harboring different GFAP promoter constructs that showed distinct patterns of Cre-mediated recombination when bred to *ROSA26* Cre reporter mice were utilized. Cre activity was restricted to NeuN^{+} granule neurons of the cerebellum and dentate gyrus in postnatal day 5–14 mice, with infrequent activity in S100b+ or GFAP+ glial cells, with the GFAP Cre GEM utilized by the Baker group (Kwon et al. 2001). In contrast, Cre activity was evident in GFAP+ astrocytes throughout the neuroaxis with the GFAP-CreER^{T2} GEM described above; no activity was detected in non-astrocytic cell populations (Casper et al. 2007).

Tumor cells in T_{121}-expressing mice were evident by 2 weeks post-4OHT, progressed significantly by 4 months, and showed the histopathological features of human astrocytomas, including perineuronal and perivascular satellitosis. GEM harboring both inactivated RB and constitutively active KRAS (Fig. 7.5C) developed anaplastic astrocytomas (AIII, WHO grade III); addition of astrocyte-specific *PTEN* heterozygous or homozygous gene inactivation (Fig. 7.5D) produced tumors with histopathological features of GBM (WHO grade IV). All six models that involved RB inactivation were fully penetrant (100% of animals developed tumors). Those models with both RB deletion and KRAS activation (TR, $TRP^{+/-}$, and $TRP^{-/-}$) showed increased incidence of GBM (Fig. 7.6) relative to those without both of these abnormalities (T and TP). The frequency of GBM was dramatically increased in the triple transgenic mice containing abnormalities at all three loci ($TRP^{+/-}$ and $TRP^{-/-}$). The time-to-tumor development (latency) was dramatically decreased in TR double and TRP triple transgenic compared to T single or TP double transgenic

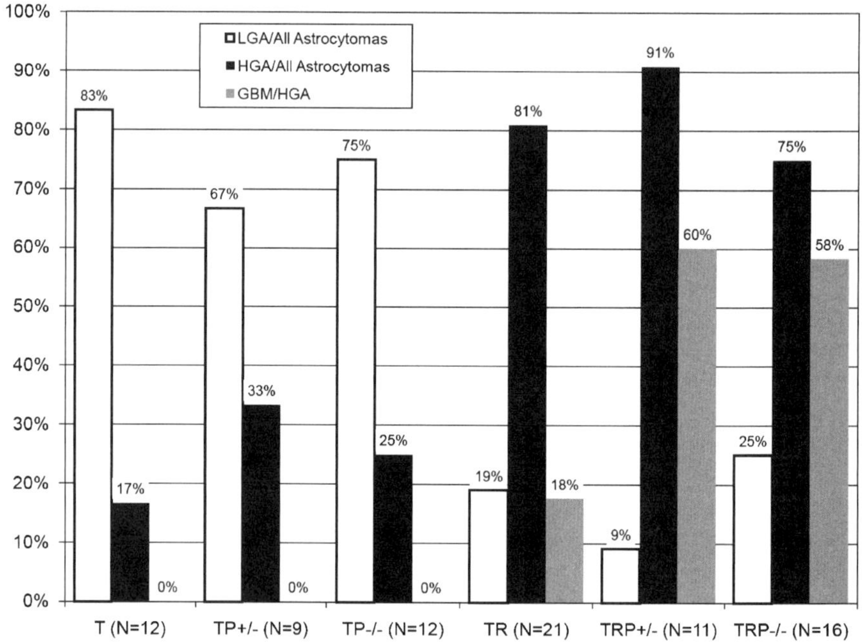

Fig. 7. 6 Incidence and grade of astrocytomas that develop in conditional, inducible GEM after 4OHT. Mice were sacrificed at signs of morbidity and their brains harvested for histopathological evaluation. Data show the percentages of LGA (*white*) and HGA (*black*) relative to all mice examined for each genotype. Note that all mice for the genotypes shown developed astrocytomas (100% penetrance). The percentage of HGA with GBM features (GBM/HGA) is shown in *gray*. Abbreviations: LGA, low-grade astrocytoma (WHO grade II); GBM, glioblastoma; HGA, high-grade astrocytoma (WHO grades III and IV). See Fig. 7.4 for genotype abbreviations

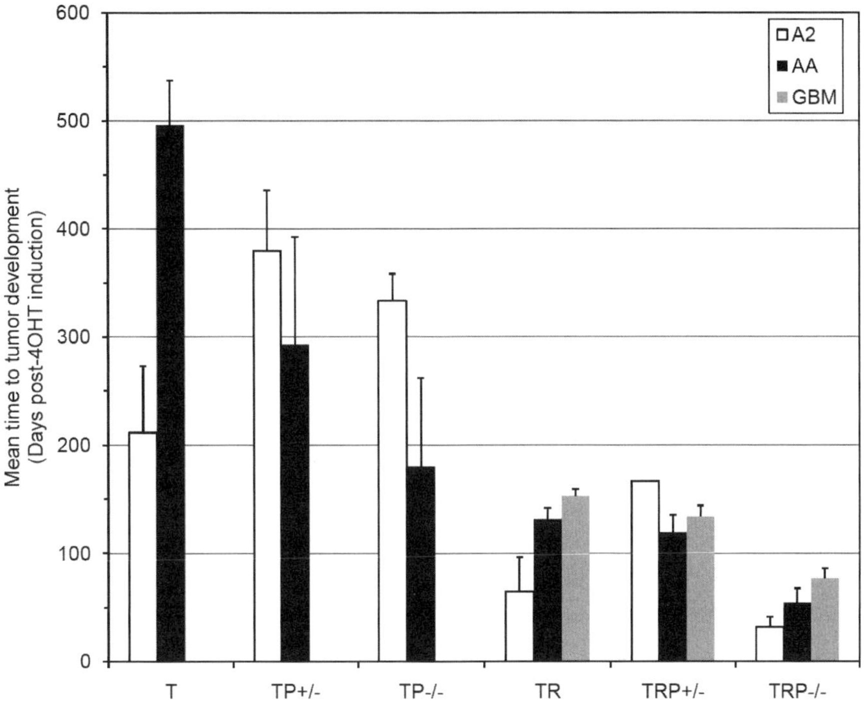

Fig. 7.7 Latency and grade of astrocytomas that develop in conditional, inducible GEM after 4OHT. Mice were sacrificed at signs of morbidity and their brains harvested for histopathological evaluation. Data show the mean time-to-tumor development (± SEM) for each genotype. See Fig. 7.4 for genotype abbreviations

animals (Figs. 7.7 and 7.8). These results suggest that adult murine astrocytes are susceptible to genetically induced tumorigenesis and can thus serve as "tumor-initiating cells." However, GFAP is also expressed in adult NSCs and whether these cells represent a target for the observed high-grade astrocytomas is not yet clear. These results demonstrate roles for RB and KRAS-PTEN pathways in astrocytoma initiation and progression, respectively.

We found that RB inactivation alone in GFAP+ adult murine astrocytes (T mice) is associated with marked increases in both proliferation and apoptosis, as measured by immunohistochemical staining for Ki67 and DNA fragmentation (TUNEL), respectively (data not shown). Similar results were obtained with PCNA and TUNEL staining, respectively, when RB function alone was inactivated in both astrocytes and GFAP+ cells in the developing mouse embryo (Xiao et al. 2002). In the adult inducible models, proliferation was further increased, albeit minimally, and apoptosis significantly decreased, through addition of a constitutively active $KRAS^{G12D}$ alone (TR) or in combination with *PTEN* inactivation ($TRP^{-/-}$). These results suggest the following: (1) RB-mediated cell cycle dysregulation causes a concomitant increase in both astrocyte proliferation and apoptosis during development of low-grade astrocytomas

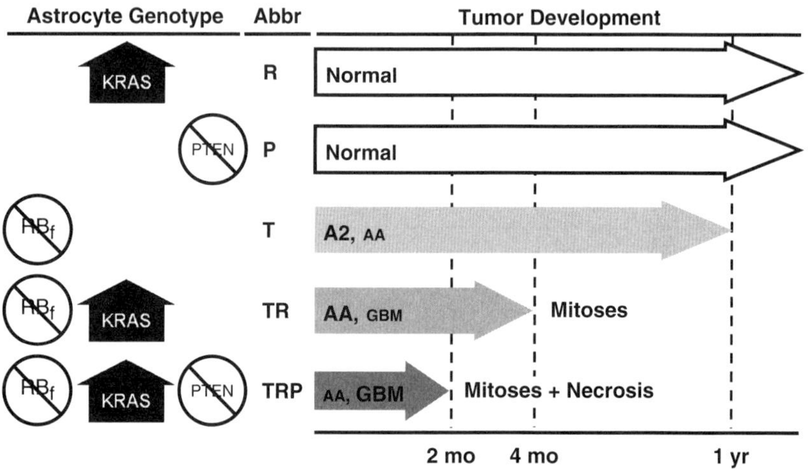

Fig. 7.8 Summary of the histopathological grade and latency for conditional, inducible GEM astrocytomas. Genotypes and their abbreviations are shown on the *left*. R and P mice failed to develop tumors. T mice developed low-grade astrocytomas (A2) over the course of approximately 1 year. The latency was decreased to 4 and 2 months and the grades increased to WHO grades III (AA) and IV (GBM) for TR and TRP mice, respectively

and (2) activation of KRAS, alone or in combination with *PTEN* deletion, potentiates the proliferative response while blunting the apoptotic response during high-grade astrocytoma development.

Although the signaling pathways involving RB, RAS, and PTEN are well defined, significant variation exists among different cell types in the involvement of specific downstream effectors and in the extent of pathway crosstalk. Preliminary immunohistochemical analyses of GEM astrocytomas show that RB-mediated cell cycle dysregulation induces activation of the MAPK ERK, as measured by phospho-ERK immunostaining, in both the presence (TR mice) and absence (T mice) of activated $KRAS^{G12D}$. However, no significant difference in the induction of phospho-ERK was evident between T and TR mice (data not shown). This result may in part reflect technical limitations inherent in quantification of chromogen-based immunohistochemical staining by light microscopy. However, the clear activation of the MAPK pathway by RB functional loss alone indicates that distinct KRAS-regulated pathway(s) drive(s) progression to AA.

7.2.3 The Future of GEM Astrocytoma Models

Cancer is an acquired disease of somatic genetic/epigenetic alterations (Vogelstein and Kinzler 2002) that is currently classified by microscopic morphology (Foucar 2001). Sophisticated tumor classification systems exist for all solid tumor types based on their tissue of origin and the microscopic features of the tumor, such as degree of differentiation, nuclear grade, and microscopic extent of spread. Tumors are treated empirically based on these classification schemes, traditionally with cytotoxic chemotherapy drugs, but increasingly with drugs targeted to specific dysregulated pathways within tumor cells (targeted chemotherapy). Neither the current classification schemes nor treatment with cytotoxic chemotherapy is based on an understanding of the underlying genetic/epigenetic alterations responsible for tumorigenesis. Major efforts are underway to transition from morphological classification and empirically derived treatment paradigms to a systematic approach based on underlying molecular pathogenesis.

In 1999, the Director of the National Cancer Institute issued a challenge to the cancer research community to develop cancer classification systems based on pathogenetic alterations (molecular classification). To date, thousands of peer-reviewed manuscripts have been published on the systematic, genome-wide quantification (profiling) of DNA copy number and gene (mRNA) expression in cancer using high-throughput, microarray-based genomics techniques such as aCGH and oligonucleotide microarrays. Through sophisticated bioinformatics approaches, these "omics" scale studies have identified sets of genes (signatures) with coordinated patterns of DNA copy number or mRNA expression abnormalities that (1) identify novel tumor subclasses (class discovery) (Golub et al. 1999, Phillips et al. 2006); (2) permit objective assignment of tumors to known classes (class prediction) (Golub et al. 1999, Nutt et al. 2003); (3) identify sets of differentially expressed genes (candidate genes for classification) (Golub et al. 1999, Tusher et al. 2001, Phillips et al. 2006); (4) relate to specific oncogenes and signaling pathways (Huang et al. 2003, Subramanian et al. 2005); and (5) correlate with biological features [tumor progression (Rickman et al. 2001, Phillips et al. 2006), invasion and metastasis (Hoelzinger et al. 2005), necrosis (Raza et al. 2004), chemotherapy response (Potti et al. 2006)] or patient outcomes [response to adjuvant therapy (Gianni et al. 2005, Oh et al. 2006), disease-free (van de Vijver et al. 2002), and overall survival (OS) (van de Vijver et al. 2002, Nutt et al. 2003, Rich et al. 2005, Phillips et al. 2006)]. The recent publication of large-scale omics profiling efforts of human GBM by the NCI, The Cancer Genome Atlas (TCGA) Consortium, and investigators at Johns Hopkins University promise to dramatically accelerate progress toward these goals (Cancer Genome Atlas Research Network 2008, Parsons et al. 2008). Preliminary analyses of these data have confirmed the importance of the G1 cell cycle progression (RB), RTK-MAPK, and PI3K-PTEN in human GBM.

In this regard, we have shown that conditional, inducible GEM models of astrocytomas recapitulate the histological progression (grades II–IV) of human astrocytomas. Furthermore, results demonstrate that genetic dysregulation of the RB, RTK-MAPK, and PI3K-PTEN pathways is sufficient for neoplastic initiation (RB_f) and progression (KRAS and PTEN) in the GFAP+ cell population in adult mice. These findings extend those of the large-scale human astrocytoma profiling efforts and illustrate how such data may be utilized to further improve GEM astrocytoma modeling efforts in the future.

However, the extent to which GEM models recapitulate the molecular alterations in human tumors must be determined to validate their usefulness in preclinical studies. Integrated evaluation of both GEM and human gliomas may be utilized to (1) examine the signaling pathway abnormalities caused by defined genetic lesions in GEM gliomas, (2) develop biomarkers that can define the human gliomas that most closely resemble their murine counterparts, and (3) co-develop predictive biomarkers and targeted chemotherapy drugs for future molecularly stratified clinical trials in humans. Genomics studies that have simultaneously evaluated mRNA expression profiles in both GEM and human tumors have recently been published (Ellwood-Yen et al. 2003, Bonner et al. 2004, Lee et al. 2004, Sweet-Cordero et al. 2005, Deeb et al. 2007, Herschkowitz et al. 2007, Kaiser et al. 2007). These studies have proven useful in defining the extent to which GEM models recapitulate the molecular alterations in human tumors, thus validating their usefulness in preclinical studies (Graeber and Sawyers 2005). Multigene signatures (metagenes) have been identified that define the initiating oncogenic event in GEM tumors (Desai et al. 2002, Sweet-Cordero et al. 2005) and the corresponding "best-fit" subgroup in their human counterparts (Desai et al. 2002, Lee et al. 2004, Herschkowitz et al. 2007). However, systematic genomics-level analyses of GEM gliomas are yet to be published.

7.3 Astrocytoma GEM Application in Translational and Preclinical Research

Preclinical cancer drug development has relied upon immunodeficient mouse xenograft models with human tumor cell lines as the principal model system for preclinical drug trials since the 1950s. However, this system is poorly predictive of drug efficacy in most cancer subtypes (Burchill 2006). Although much has been written about the promise of GEM models as alternative platforms for preclinical cancer drug development (Salpietro and Holland 2005, Becher and Holland 2006, Fomchenko and Holland 2006a, b, Gutmann et al. 2006, Sharpless and Depinho 2006), GEM remain experimentally less amenable to such studies than conventional xenograft models (Burchill 2006). Progress toward moving GEM from essential basic science tools to viable preclinical drug development platforms has been hampered by the following:

1. variable penetrance and latency of spontaneous tumor development in GEM in vivo;
2. the lack of uniform, temporal, and spatial control over growth in vivo; hence
3. the need to monitor tumor development and measure growth kinetics using small animal imaging techniques such as microCT, MRI, or light-based imaging prior to trial enrollment; and
4. the lack of genetically tractable GEM tumor cell culture systems for in vitro drug screening.

Because of these limitations, drug trials in GEM cancer models have largely been limited to proof-of-principle studies to validate the underlying genetic hypothesis using agents targeted to the oncogenic molecular abnormalities utilized in their construction.

The conditional, inducible GEM astrocytoma models described herein that involve all three genes ($TRP^{+/-}$ and $TRP^{-/-}$) may overcome the first two limitations outlined above and permit systematic examination of their utility in prioritizing drug candidates for human clinical trials. Although systemic 4OHT induces oncogenic genetic events in GFAP+ cells throughout the entire neuroaxis, these models develop high-grade astrocytomas (HGA) with 100% penetrance and short, relatively uniform periods of latency. To address the third issue above, we have defined the temporal and spatial characteristics of tumor growth in these mice using contrast-enhanced magnetic resonance imaging (Fig. 7.9) and computer-assisted vascular reconstruction techniques (Brubaker et al. 2005).

To address the fourth issue, we have derived continuous cell lines from cultured primary GEM astrocytes by adenoviral-mediated Cre recombination (Fig. 7.10 and Color Plate 13). These cells recapitulate the migratory and invasive phenotypes of human HGA in in vitro migration assays, including time-lapse video microscopy and wound closure (Liang et al. 2007), and collagen invasion assays (Demuth et al. 2007), respectively (Table 7.3). Proliferation assays showed that these cells were as sensitive to targeted and conventional cytotoxic chemotherapies as human glioma cell lines in culture (Table 7.3 and data not shown). Furthermore, stereotactic injection of 10^6 cells into the frontal cortex of syngeneic C57Bl/6 mice formed diffusely infiltrative tumors in vivo (Fig. 7.10). Preliminary experiments showed that T_{121}-immunoreactive astrocytomas developed in 100% of injected animals, approximately 30% of which were WHO grade III astrocytomas characterized

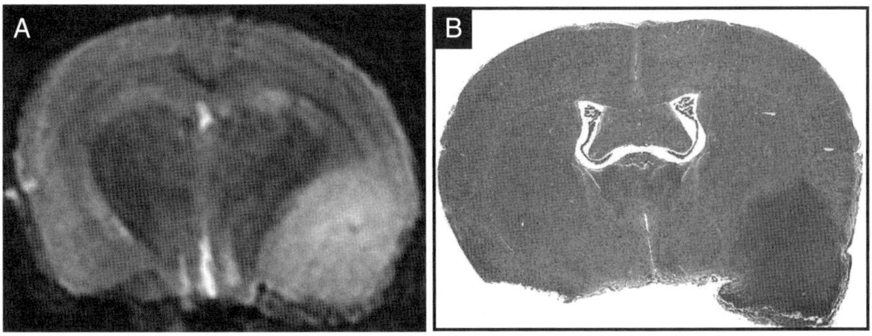

Fig. 7.9 Contrast-enhanced magnetic resonance imaging of astrocytoma development in $TRP^{-/-}$ GEM. Mice were serially imaged biweekly starting at 3 months post-4OHT and followed until moribund. A representative coronal post-gadolinium T1-weighted image (**A**) and the corresponding histological brain section (H&E stain, **B**) are shown

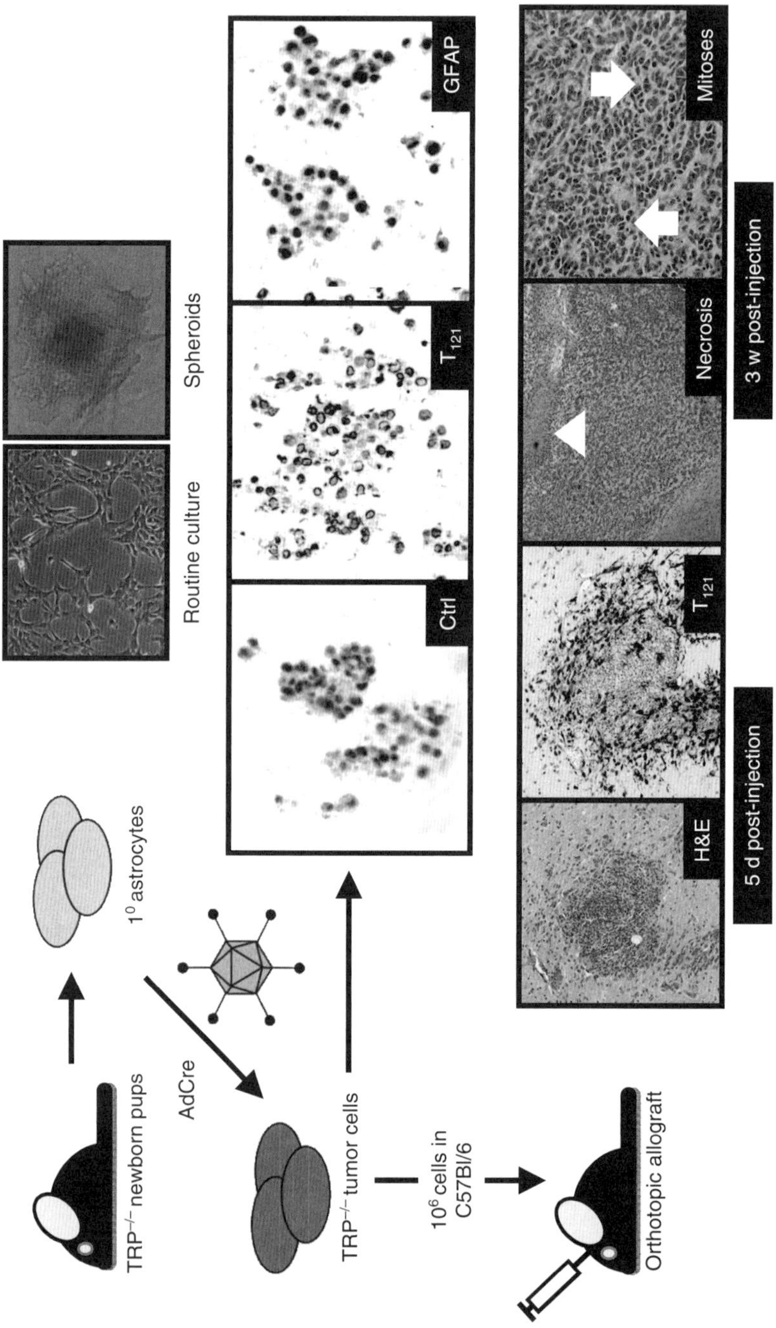
TRP−/− newborn pups
1⁰ astrocytes
Routine culture
Spheroids
AdCre
TRP−/− tumor cells
Ctrl
T121
GFAP
10⁶ cells in C57Bl/6
Orthotopic allograft
H&E
T121
Necrosis
Mitoses
5 d post-injection
3 w post-injection

Table 7.3 Phenotypic characterization of drug-treated TRP$^{-/-}$ GEM astrocytoma cells in vitro

			Extent of inhibition			
Inhibitor	Target	ToxicityIC_{50} (μM)	μM	Migration	Invasion	Proliferation
TMZ	DNA	190	300	ND	None*	65%↓
Rapamycin	mTOR	227	0.01	+	25%↓	20%↓
LY 294,002	PI3K	299	50	+ + +	30%↓	20%↓
U0126	MEK	215	10	+ + +	45%↓	0

The anti-proliferative effects of temozolomide (TMZ), rapamycin, LY294002, and U0126 were examined by MTS assay and IC_{50} calculated. Migration, invasion, and proliferation of TRP$^{-/-}$ were assessed by wound healing, collagen invasion, and MTS assays, respectively, without and with drugs at the indicated concentration (μM).Anti-invasive capabilities of TMZ (none*) could not be determined due to extensive cytotoxicity.

by increased mitoses (arrows) and 70% of which were WHO grade IV GBM characterized by the presence of pseudopalisading necrosis (arrowhead). The median overall survival was 3 weeks. These cells will therefore be useful for both in vitro and in vivo drug development using orthotopic allograft models of HGA, a model system more amenable to preclinical drug trials than inducible, conditional GEM models because of their uniform, temporospatially controlled growth in vivo.

Phenotypic drug response and signaling protein expression in cultured GEM cells often fails to recapitulate that found in vivo, emphasizing that microenvironmental factors are important. Therefore, combined in vitro and in vivo analyses *in the same system* are critical to draw biologically meaningful conclusions from these studies and use this information in prioritizing drug/biomarker combinations for further development. Concordant response/biomarker data between these models would indicate that this drug development paradigm warrants further testing of additional compounds, particularly in the spontaneous 4OHT-induced conditional, inducible models outlined above, as well as

Fig. 7. 10 Generation and characterization of cell lines derived from conditional GEM models of astrocytomas. Primary astrocytes were harvested from GEM, such as TRP$^{-/-}$ mice illustrated here, that had not been bred with mice harboring Cre recombinase genetic events were induced in vitro using an adenovirus vector encoding Cre recombinase. Continuous routine culture of infected astrocytes on tissue cultureware generated an immortalized cell line that may be utilized for in vitro analyses, either as adherent monolayers (routine culture) or as spheroids when cultured on semisolid media. These cells may be utilized to construct cell line microarrays (CLA) for analysis by immunohistochemistry (IHC). IHC staining showed that TRP$^{-/-}$ cells were immunoreactive for T_{121} and GFAP. Moreover, these cells formed tumors upon stereotaxic injection into the right frontal lobes of syngeneic, immunocompetent C57Bl/6 mice. Preliminary experiments showed that T_{121}-immunoreactive astrocytomas develop in 100% of injected animals, approximately 30% of which were WHO grade III astrocytomas characterized by increased mitoses (*arrows*) and 70% of which were WHO grade IV GBM characterized by the presence of pseudopalisading necrosis (*arrowhead*). The median overall survival was 3 weeks when 10^6 cells were injected (*see* Color Plate 13) investigation of the mechanism and molecular correlates of drug response/resistance and follow-up biomarker studies with archived human tumor TMA. Discordant data would aid identification of important microenvironmental factors and suggest novel in vivo pathways that could then be queried in an unbiased fashion, with expression profiling or RNAi libraries for example, to identify novel candidate genes for further investigation. Iterations of this process should facilitate integration of preclinical GEM drug/biomarker co-development with rationally designed clinical trials of targeted therapies in molecularly defined cancer patients.

In addition, data from GEM-derived cell-based assays will inevitably stimulate the subsequent refining of existing animal models to better recapitulate the course of human malignancies. More precise models will permit not only the careful dissection of molecular pathways impacting tumorigenesis, but also understanding the efficacy and mechanism of action of therapeutic compounds. Possible model improvements may include (1) utilization of alternative transcription regulatory elements to target genetic events to alternative cell types within the brain (Fig. 7.3) or improve the specificity and/or spatiotemporal activity of genetic event induction given that in humans the tumor likely originates from a single cell; (2) application of more versatile gene regulation tools, such as tet/dox-dependent inducible system as an alternative to the permanent "all-or-nothing" type of event based on the loxP/Cre system; and (3) development of genetic tools for sequential, as opposed to simultaneous, induction of genetic events to closer mimic the temporal occurrence of genetic abnormalities and the malignant progression seen in human astrocytomas.

References

Bachoo RM, Maher EA, Ligon KL, Sharpless NE, Chan SS, You MJ, Tang Y, DeFrances J, Stover E, Weissleder R, Rowitch DH, Louis DN, DePinho RA. Epidermal growth factor receptor and Ink4a/Arf: convergent mechanisms governing terminal differentiation and transformation along the neural stem cell to astrocyte axis. Cancer Cell 2002; 1: 269–77.

Bajenaru ML, Zhu Y, Hedrick NM, Donahoe J, Parada LF, Gutmann DH. Astrocyte-specific inactivation of the neurofibromatosis 1 gene (NF1) is insufficient for astrocytoma formation. Mol Cell Biol 2002; 22: 5100–13.

Becher OJ, Holland EC. Genetically engineered models have advantages over xenografts for preclinical studies. Cancer Res 2006; 66: 3355–8, discussion 8–9.

Bonner AE, Lemon WJ, Devereux TR, Lubet RA, You M. Molecular profiling of mouse lung tumors: association with tumor progression, lung development, and human lung adenocarcinomas. Oncogene 2004; 23: 1166–76.

Brannan CI, Perkins AS, Vogel KS, Ratner N, Nordlund ML, Reid SW, Buchberg AM, Jenkins NA, Parada LF, Copeland NG. Targeted disruption of the neurofibromatosis type-1 gene leads to developmental abnormalities in heart and various neural crest-derived tissues. Genes Dev 1994; 8: 1019–29.

Brenner M, Kisseberth WC, Su Y, Besnard F, Messing A. GFAP promoter directs astrocyte-specific expression in transgenic mice. J Neurosci 1994; 14: 1030–7.

Brubaker LM, Bullitt E, Yin C, Van Dyke T, Lin W. Magnetic resonance angiography visualization of abnormal tumor vasculature in genetically engineered mice. Cancer Res 2005; 65: 8218–23.
Burchill SA. What do, can and should we learn from models to evaluate potential anticancer agents? Future Oncol 2006; 2: 201–11.
Cancer Genome Atlas Research Network. Comprehensive genomic characterization defines human glioblastoma genes and core pathways. Nature 2008; 455: 1061–8.
Casper KB, Jones K, McCarthy KD. Characterization of astrocyte-specific conditional knockouts. Genesis 2007; 45: 292–9.
CBTRUS. Central Brain Tumor Registry of the United States: Statistical Report: Primary Brain Tumors in the United States, 2000–2004. Hinsdale, IL: Central Brain Tumor Registry of the United States; 2008.
Charest A, Wilker EW, McLaughlin ME, Lane K, Gowda R, Coven S, McMahon K, Kovach S, Feng Y, Yaffe MB, Jacks T, Housman D. ROS fusion tyrosine kinase activates a SH2 domain-containing phosphatase-2/phosphatidylinositol 3-kinase/mammalian target of rapamycin signaling axis to form glioblastoma in mice. Cancer Res 2006; 66: 7473–81.
Dai C, Celestino JC, Okada Y, Louis DN, Fuller GN, Holland EC. PDGF autocrine stimulation dedifferentiates cultured astrocytes and induces oligodendrogliomas and oligoastrocytomas from neural progenitors and astrocytes in vivo. Genes Dev 2001; 15: 1913–25.
Dai C, Lyustikman Y, Shih A, Hu X, Fuller GN, Rosenblum M, Holland EC. The characteristics of astrocytomas and oligodendrogliomas are caused by two distinct and interchangeable signaling formats. Neoplasia 2005; 7: 397–406.
Deeb KK, Michalowska AM, Yoon CY, Krummey SM, Hoenerhoff MJ, Kavanaugh C, Li MC, Demayo FJ, Linnoila I, Deng CX, Lee EY, Medina D, Shih JH, Green JE. Identification of an Integrated SV40 T/t-Antigen Cancer Signature in Aggressive Human Breast, Prostate, and Lung Carcinomas with Poor Prognosis. Cancer Res 2007; 67: 8065–80.
Demuth T, Reavie LB, Rennert JL, Nakada M, Nakada S, Hoelzinger DB, Beaudry CE, Henrichs AN, Anderson EM, Berens ME. MAP-ing glioma invasion: mitogen-activated protein kinase 3 and p38 drive glioma invasion and progression and predict patient survival. Mol Cancer Ther 2007; 6: 1212–22.
Desai KV, Xiao N, Wang W, Gangi L, Greene J, Powell JI, Dickson R, Furth P, Hunter K, Kucherlapati R, Simon R, Liu ET, Green JE. Initiating oncogenic event determines gene-expression patterns of human breast cancer models. Proc Natl Acad Sci U S A 2002; 99: 6967–72.
Ding H, Roncari L, Shannon P, Wu X, Lau N, Karaskova J, Gutmann DH, Squire JA, Nagy A, Guha A. Astrocyte-specific expression of activated p21-ras results in malignant astrocytoma formation in a transgenic mouse model of human gliomas. Cancer Res 2001; 61: 3826–36.
Ding H, Shannon P, Lau N, Wu X, Roncari L, Baldwin RL, Takebayashi H, Nagy A, Gutmann DH, Guha A. Oligodendrogliomas result from the expression of an activated mutant epidermal growth factor receptor in a RAS transgenic mouse astrocytoma model. Cancer Res 2003; 63: 1106–13.
Donehower LA, Harvey M, Vogel H, McArthur MJ, Montgomery CA, Jr., Park SH, Thompson T, Ford RJ, Bradley A. Effects of genetic background on tumorigenesis in p53-deficient mice. Mol Carcinog 1995; 14: 16–22.
Dunlap SM, Celestino J, Wang H, Jiang R, Holland EC, Fuller GN, Zhang W. Insulin-like growth factor binding protein 2 promotes glioma development and progression. Proc Natl Acad Sci U S A 2007.
Ellwood-Yen K, Graeber TG, Wongvipat J, Iruela-Arispe ML, Zhang J, Matusik R, Thomas GV, Sawyers CL. Myc-driven murine prostate cancer shares molecular features with human prostate tumors. Cancer Cell 2003; 4: 223–38.

Feil R, Wagner J, Metzger D, Chambon P. Regulation of Cre recombinase activity by mutated estrogen receptor ligand-binding domains. Biochem Biophys Res Commun 1997; 237: 752–7.

Fomchenko EI, Holland EC. Stem cells and brain cancer. Exp Cell Res 2005; 306: 323–9.

Fomchenko EI, Holland EC. Mouse models of brain tumors and their applications in preclinical trials. Clin Cancer Res 2006a; 12: 5288–97.

Fomchenko EI, Holland EC. Origins of brain tumors – a disease of stem cells? Nat Clin Pract Neurol 2006b; 2: 288–9.

Foucar E. Classification in anatomic pathology. Am J Clin Pathol 2001; 116 Suppl: S5–20.

Gianni L, Zambetti M, Clark K, Baker J, Cronin M, Wu J, Mariani G, Rodriguez J, Carcangiu M, Watson D, Valagussa P, Rouzier R, Symmans WF, Ross JS, Hortobagyi GN, Pusztai L, Shak S. Gene expression profiles in paraffin-embedded core biopsy tissue predict response to chemotherapy in women with locally advanced breast cancer. J Clin Oncol 2005; 23: 7265–77.

Golub TR, Slonim DK, Tamayo P, Huard C, Gaasenbeek M, Mesirov JP, Coller H, Loh ML, Downing JR, Caligiuri MA, Bloomfield CD, Lander ES. Molecular classification of cancer: class discovery and class prediction by gene expression monitoring. Science 1999; 286: 531–7.

Graeber TG, Sawyers CL. Cross-species comparisons of cancer signaling. Nat Genet 2005; 37: 7–8.

Gutmann DH, Hunter-Schaedle K, Shannon KM. Harnessing preclinical mouse models to inform human clinical cancer trials. J Clin Invest 2006; 116: 847–52.

Herschkowitz JI, Simin K, Weigman VJ, Mikaelian I, Usary J, Hu Z, Rasmussen KE, Jones LP, Assefnia S, Chandrasekharan S, Backlund MG, Yin Y, Khramtsov AI, Bastein R, Quackenbush J, Glazer RI, Brown PH, Green JE, Kopelovich L, Furth PA, Palazzo JP, Olopade OI, Bernard PS, Churchill GA, Van Dyke T, Perou CM. Identification of conserved gene expression features between murine mammary carcinoma models and human breast tumors. Genome Biol 2007; 8: R76.

Hoelzinger DB, Mariani L, Weis J, Woyke T, Berens TJ, McDonough WS, Sloan A, Coons SW, Berens ME. Gene expression profile of glioblastoma multiforme invasive phenotype points to new therapeutic targets. Neoplasia 2005; 7: 7–16.

Holland EC. Gliomagenesis: genetic alterations and mouse models. Nat Rev Genet 2001; 2: 120–9.

Holland EC. Mouse models of human cancer as tools in drug development. Cancer Cell 2004; 6: 197–8.

Holland EC, Celestino J, Dai C, Schaefer L, Sawaya RE, Fuller GN. Combined activation of Ras and Akt in neural progenitors induces glioblastoma formation in mice. Nat Genet 2000; 25: 55–7.

Holland EC, Hively WP, DePinho RA, Varmus HE. A constitutively active epidermal growth factor receptor cooperates with disruption of G1 cell-cycle arrest pathways to induce glioma-like lesions in mice. Genes Dev 1998; 12: 3675–85.

Holland EC, Li Y, Celestino J, Dai C, Schaefer L, Sawaya RA, Fuller GN. Astrocytes give rise to oligodendrogliomas and astrocytomas after gene transfer of polyoma virus middle T antigen in vivo. Am J Pathol 2000; 157: 1031–7.

Hu X, Holland EC. Applications of mouse glioma models in preclinical trials. Mutat Res 2005; 576: 54–65.

Hu X, Pandolfi PP, Li Y, Koutcher JA, Rosenblum M, Holland EC. mTOR promotes survival and astrocytic characteristics induced by Pten/AKT signaling in glioblastoma. Neoplasia 2005; 7: 356–68.

Huang E, Ishida S, Pittman J, Dressman H, Bild A, Kloos M, D'Amico M, Pestell RG, West M, Nevins JR. Gene expression phenotypic models that predict the activity of oncogenic pathways. Nat Genet 2003; 34: 226–30.

Jacks T, Remington L, Williams BO, Schmitt EM, Halachmi S, Bronson RT, Weinberg RA. Tumor spectrum analysis in p53-mutant mice. Curr Biol 1994; 4: 1–7.
Jacks T, Shih TS, Schmitt EM, Bronson RT, Bernards A, Weinberg RA. Tumour predisposition in mice heterozygous for a targeted mutation in Nf1. Nat Genet 1994; 7: 353–61.
Kaiser S, Park YK, Franklin JL, Halberg RB, Yu M, Jessen WJ, Freudenberg J, Chen X, Haigis K, Jegga AG, Kong S, Sakthivel B, Xu H, Reichling T, Azhar M, Boivin GP, Roberts RB, Bissahoyo AC, Gonzales F, Bloom GC, Eschrich S, Carter SL, Aronow JE, Kleimeyer J, Kleimeyer M, Ramaswamy V, Settle SH, Boone B, Levy S, Graff JM, Doetschman T, Groden J, Dove WF, Threadgill DW, Yeatman TJ, Coffey RJ, Jr., Aronow BJ. Transcriptional recapitulation and subversion of embryonic colon development by mouse colon tumor models and human colon cancer. Genome Biol 2007; 8: R131.
Kwon CH, Luikart BW, Powell CM, Zhou J, Matheny SA, Zhang W, Li Y, Baker SJ, Parada LF. Pten regulates neuronal arborization and social interaction in mice. Neuron 2006; 50: 377–88.
Kwon CH, Zhao D, Chen J, Alcantara S, Li Y, Burns DK, Mason RP, Lee EY, Wu H, Parada LF. Pten haploinsufficiency accelerates formation of high-grade astrocytomas. Cancer Res 2008; 68: 3286–94.
Kwon CH, Zhu X, Zhang J, Knoop LL, Tharp R, Smeyne RJ, Eberhart CG, Burger PC, Baker SJ. Pten regulates neuronal soma size: a mouse model of Lhermitte-Duclos disease. Nat Genet 2001; 29: 404–11.
Lassman AB, Dai C, Fuller GN, Vickers AJ, Holland EC. Overexpression of c-MYC promotes an undifferentiated phenotype in cultured astrocytes and allows elevated Ras and Akt signaling to induce gliomas from GFAP-expressing cells in mice. Neuron Glia Biol 2004; 1: 157–63.
Lee JS, Chu IS, Mikaelyan A, Calvisi DF, Heo J, Reddy JK, Thorgeirsson SS. Application of comparative functional genomics to identify best-fit mouse models to study human cancer. Nat Genet 2004; 36: 1306–11.
Liang CC, Park AY, Guan JL. In vitro scratch assay: a convenient and inexpensive method for analysis of cell migration in vitro. Nat Protoc 2007; 2: 329–33.
Louis DN, Ohgaki H, Wiestler OD, Cavenee WK, editors. WHO classification of tumours of the central nervous system. 4th ed. Lyon: IARC; 2007.
Marenholz I, Heizmann CW, Fritz G. S100 proteins in mouse and man: from evolution to function and pathology (including an update of the nomenclature). Biochem Biophys Res Commun 2004; 322: 1111–22.
Metzger D, Chambon P. Site- and time-specific gene targeting in the mouse. Methods 2001; 24: 71–80.
Miller CR, Perry A. Glioblastoma: Morphological and molecular genetic diversity. Arch Pathol Lab Med 2007; 131: 397–406.
Nutt CL, Mani DR, Betensky RA, Tamayo P, Cairncross JG, Ladd C, Pohl U, Hartmann C, McLaughlin ME, Batchelor TT, Black PM, von Deimling A, Pomeroy SL, Golub TR, Louis DN. Gene expression-based classification of malignant gliomas correlates better with survival than histological classification. Cancer Res 2003; 63: 1602–7.
Oh DS, Troester MA, Usary J, Hu Z, He X, Fan C, Wu J, Carey LA, Perou CM. Estrogen-regulated genes predict survival in hormone receptor-positive breast cancers. J Clin Oncol 2006; 24: 1656–64.
Ohgaki H, Dessen P, Jourde B, Horstmann S, Nishikawa T, Di Patre PL, Burkhard C, Schuler D, Probst-Hensch NM, Maiorka PC, Baeza N, Pisani P, Yonekawa Y, Yasargil MG, Lutolf UM, Kleihues P. Genetic pathways to glioblastoma: a population-based study. Cancer Res 2004; 64: 6892–9.
Parsons DW, Jones S, Zhang X, Lin JC, Leary RJ, Angenendt P, Mankoo P, Carter H, Siu IM, Gallia GL, Olivi A, McLendon R, Rasheed BA, Keir S, Nikolskaya T,

Nikolsky Y, Busam DA, Tekleab H, Diaz LA, Jr., Hartigan J, Smith DR, Strausberg RL, Marie SK, Shinjo SM, Yan H, Riggins GJ, Bigner DD, Karchin R, Papadopoulos N, Parmigiani G, Vogelstein B, Velculescu VE, Kinzler KW. An integrated genomic analysis of human glioblastoma multiforme. Science 2008; 321: 1807–12.

Phillips HS, Kharbanda S, Chen R, Forrest WF, Soriano RH, Wu TD, Misra A, Nigro JM, Colman H, Soroceanu L, Williams PM, Modrusan Z, Feuerstein BG, Aldape K. Molecular subclasses of high-grade glioma predict prognosis, delineate a pattern of disease progression, and resemble stages in neurogenesis. Cancer Cell 2006; 9: 157–73.

Potti A, Dressman HK, Bild A, Riedel RF, Chan G, Sayer R, Cragun J, Cottrill H, Kelley MJ, Petersen R, Harpole D, Marks J, Berchuck A, Ginsburg GS, Febbo P, Lancaster J, Nevins JR. Genomic signatures to guide the use of chemotherapeutics. Nat Med 2006; 12: 1294–300.

Raza SM, Fuller GN, Rhee CH, Huang S, Hess K, Zhang W, Sawaya R. Identification of necrosis-associated genes in glioblastoma by cDNA microarray analysis. Clin Cancer Res 2004; 10: 212–21.

Read TA, Hegedus B, Wechsler-Reya R, Gutmann DH. The neurobiology of neurooncology. Ann Neurol 2006; 60: 3–11.

Reilly KM, Loisel DA, Bronson RT, McLaughlin ME, Jacks T. Nf1;Trp53 mutant mice develop glioblastoma with evidence of strain-specific effects. Nat Genet 2000; 26: 109–13.

Reilly KM, Tuskan RG, Christy E, Loisel DA, Ledger J, Bronson RT, Smith CD, Tsang S, Munroe DJ, Jacks T. Susceptibility to astrocytoma in mice mutant for Nf1 and Trp53 is linked to chromosome 11 and subject to epigenetic effects. Proc Natl Acad Sci U S A 2004; 101: 13008–13.

Rich JN, Hans C, Jones B, Iversen ES, McLendon RE, Rasheed BK, Dobra A, Dressman HK, Bigner DD, Nevins JR, West M. Gene expression profiling and genetic markers in glioblastoma survival. Cancer Res 2005; 65: 4051–8.

Rickman DS, Bobek MP, Misek DE, Kuick R, Blaivas M, Kurnit DM, Taylor J, Hanash SM. Distinctive molecular profiles of high-grade and low-grade gliomas based on oligonucleotide microarray analysis. Cancer Res 2001; 61: 6885–91.

Salpietro M, Holland EC. Modeling and preclinical trials for gliomas. Clin Neurosurg 2005; 52: 104–11.

Sauer B. Inducible gene targeting in mice using the Cre/lox system. Methods 1998; 14: 381–92.

Shannon P, Sabha N, Lau N, Kamnasaran D, Gutmann DH, Guha A. Pathological and molecular progression of astrocytomas in a GFAP:12 V-Ha-Ras mouse astrocytoma model. Am J Pathol 2005; 167: 859–67.

Sharpless NE, Depinho RA. The mighty mouse: genetically engineered mouse models in cancer drug development. Nat Rev Drug Discov 2006; 5: 741–54.

Shih AH, Dai C, Hu X, Rosenblum MK, Koutcher JA, Holland EC. Dose-dependent effects of platelet-derived growth factor-B on glial tumorigenesis. Cancer Res 2004; 64: 4783–9.

Shih AH, Holland EC. Developmental neurobiology and the origin of brain tumors. J Neurooncol 2004; 70: 125–36.

Subramanian A, Tamayo P, Mootha VK, Mukherjee S, Ebert BL, Gillette MA, Paulovich A, Pomeroy SL, Golub TR, Lander ES, Mesirov JP. Gene set enrichment analysis: a knowledge-based approach for interpreting genome-wide expression profiles. Proc Natl Acad Sci U S A 2005; 102: 15545–50.

Sweet-Cordero A, Mukherjee S, Subramanian A, You H, Roix JJ, Ladd-Acosta C, Mesirov J, Golub TR, Jacks T. An oncogenic KRAS2 expression signature identified by cross-species gene-expression analysis. Nat Genet 2005; 37: 48–55.

Tchougounova E, Kastemar M, Brasater D, Holland EC, Westermark B, Uhrbom L. Loss of Arf causes tumor progression of PDGFB-induced oligodendroglioma. Oncogene 2007; 26: 6289–96.

Theurillat JP, Hainfellner J, Maddalena A, Weissenberger J, Aguzzi A. Early induction of angiogenetic signals in gliomas of GFAP-v-src transgenic mice. Am J Pathol 1999; 154: 581–90.
Tohyama T, Lee VM, Rorke LB, Marvin M, McKay RD, Trojanowski JQ. Nestin expression in embryonic human neuroepithelium and in human neuroepithelial tumor cells. Lab Invest 1992; 66: 303–13.
Tusher VG, Tibshirani R, Chu G. Significance analysis of microarrays applied to the ionizing radiation response. Proc Natl Acad Sci U S A 2001; 98: 5116–21.
Uhrbom L, Dai C, Celestino JC, Rosenblum MK, Fuller GN, Holland EC. Ink4a-Arf loss cooperates with KRas activation in astrocytes and neural progenitors to generate glioblastomas of various morphologies depending on activated Akt. Cancer Res 2002; 62: 5551–8.
Uhrbom L, Kastemar M, Johansson FK, Westermark B, Holland EC. Cell type-specific tumor suppression by Ink4a and Arf in Kras-induced mouse gliomagenesis. Cancer Res 2005; 65: 2065–9.
van de Vijver MJ, He YD, van't Veer LJ, Dai H, Hart AA, Voskuil DW, Schreiber GJ, Peterse JL, Roberts C, Marton MJ, Parrish M, Atsma D, Witteveen A, Glas A, Delahaye L, van der Velde T, Bartelink H, Rodenhuis S, Rutgers ET, Friend SH, Bernards R. A gene-expression signature as a predictor of survival in breast cancer. N Engl J Med 2002; 347: 1999–2009.
Van Dyke T, Jacks T. Cancer modeling in the modern era: progress and challenges. Cell 2002; 108: 135–44.
Vogelstein B, Kinzler KW. The genetic basis of human cancer. 2nd ed. New York: McGraw-Hill; 2002.
Wei Q, Clarke L, Scheidenhelm DK, Qian B, Tong A, Sabha N, Karim Z, Bock NA, Reti R, Swoboda R, Purev E, Lavoie JF, Bajenaru ML, Shannon P, Herlyn D, Kaplan D, Henkelman RM, Gutmann DH, Guha A. High-grade glioma formation results from postnatal pten loss or mutant epidermal growth factor receptor expression in a transgenic mouse glioma model. Cancer Res 2006; 66: 7429–37.
Weiss WA, Burns MJ, Hackett C, Aldape K, Hill JR, Kuriyama H, Kuriyama N, Milshteyn N, Roberts T, Wendland MF, DePinho R, Israel MA. Genetic determinants of malignancy in a mouse model for oligodendroglioma. Cancer Res 2003; 63: 1589–95.
Weissenberger J, Steinbach JP, Malin G, Spada S, Rulicke T, Aguzzi A. Development and malignant progression of astrocytomas in GFAP-v-src transgenic mice. Oncogene 1997; 14: 2005–13.
Xiao A, Wu H, Pandolfi PP, Louis DN, Van Dyke T. Astrocyte inactivation of the pRb pathway predisposes mice to malignant astrocytoma development that is accelerated by PTEN mutation. Cancer Cell 2002; 1: 157–68.
Xiao A, Yin C, Yang C, Di Cristofano A, Pandolfi PP, Van Dyke T. Somatic induction of Pten loss in a preclinical astrocytoma model reveals major roles in disease progression and avenues for target discovery and validation. Cancer Res 2005; 65: 5172–80.
Zhu Y, Guignard F, Zhao D, Liu L, Burns DK, Mason RP, Messing A, Parada LF. Early inactivation of p53 tumor suppressor gene cooperating with NF1 loss induces malignant astrocytoma. Cancer Cell 2005; 8: 119–30.

Chapter 8
Human Brain Tumor Cell and Tumor Tissue Transplantation Models

Tomoko Ozawa and C. David James

Abstract Transplantation models using human glioma cells, or cells from chemically induced rodent gliomas, have served an essential function in neuro-oncology research for many years. A major potential limitation of using the latter as a source for establishing tumor grafts is that the therapeutic response of rodent-derived cell lines can be different from those of human glioma cells, and such differences are certainly of importance to the translational researchers who depend upon tumor engraftment models for their studies. Consequently, the majority of neuro-oncology investigators use human brain tumor cells, and in most instances the procedure of human tumor xenograft establishment consists of the collection of cells from culture flasks, followed by the subcutaneous injection of the collected cells in immunocompromised mice. While this represents the most commonly used method for establishing a tumor graft, new tissue graft methods have emerged and gained popularity in neuro-oncology research. Over the past decade there has been increasing diversity and sophistication of approach in the use of human tumor cell transplantation models and these will be compared to the prior conventional methods.

Contents

T. Ozawa (✉)
Department of Neurological Surgery and Brain Tumor Research Center,
513 Parnassus Avenue, University of California, San Francisco, 94143, CA, USA
e-mail: tomoko.ozawa@ucsf.edu

E.G. Van Meir (ed.), *CNS Cancer*, Cancer Drug Discovery and Development, DOI 10.1007/978-1-60327-553-8_8,
© Humana Press, a part of Springer Science+Business Media, LLC 2009

8.1 Cell Culture-Based Approaches

The establishment of xenografts from permanent human tumor cell lines represents one of the most widely used procedures in support of cancer research. With respect to human gliomas, more specifically glioblastomas (GBMs), several series of permanent cell lines have been developed and have seen extensive use for in vivo as well as in vitro study. The first such series was established by Ponten and colleagues at the University of Uppsala, Sweden (Beckman et al. 1971), and use of the corresponding "U" series of GBM, especially the U-87 MG line, abstract references for which number more than 1000, has significantly influenced, and perhaps unduly biased, our current and collective understanding of GBM. Other widely distributed and utilized series of GBM cell lines include the "D" series from Duke University in North Carolina, USA (Bigner et al. 1981), the "SF" series from University of California San Francisco, USA (Rutka et al. 1987), and the "LN" series established by Diserens at the University of Lausanne, Switzerland (Diserens et al. 1981; de Muralt et al. 1985). Aside from adult GBM, medulloblastoma is one of only a few other types of brain tumor for which series of cell lines have been described (Bigner et al. 1990a; Keles et al. 1995; see also Chapter 45), suggesting that (1) grade IV malignancy may be required for permanent CNS tumor cell line establishment and that (2) tumor incidence is important for developing cell lines from a specific type of tumor (i.e., GBM and medulloblastoma are the most common grade IV malignancy CNS tumors of adults and children, respectively). Grade IV malignancy as a requirement for establishing permanent cell lines is speculative, however, and it is possible that the more commonplace use of defined medias supplemented with growth factors, rather than sera, and the propagation of tumor cells as spheroids (see below), rather than as monolayer cultures, may promote the sustained growth and establishment of cell lines from additional subtypes, and lesser malignancy grades of CNS tumors.

With respect to the different series of established GBM cell lines, it is important to note that there are cases among each that are non-tumorigenic in immunocompromised rodents (Ishii et al. 1999), and consequently a careful review of existing literature is necessary to form a basis for selecting specific cell lines to be used for in vivo experimentation. As concerns examining the tumorigenicity of primary cultures established from newly acquired surgical specimens, one should consider enriching for tumor-initiating cells prior to engraftment (Singh et al. 2004); the site of tumor engraftment (i.e., subcutaneous vs. intracranial: Shapiro et al. 1979); the type of immunodeficient mouse strain being used (Taghian et al. 1993); and the age of the mouse being used as a host (Sharkey and Fogh 1984). Each of these factors (Table 8.1) is likely to influence the frequency of successful xenograft establishment. Unfortunately, none have yet to be thoroughly and systemically investigated for the purpose of developing guidelines to be used in support of research for establishing CNS tumor xenografts, or more generally for investigating the heterotransplant

Table 8.1 Factors influencing tumor engraftment success and growth rate

Factor	Relationship	Recommendation
Age of mouse	Decreasing engraftment success with increasing age	Use mice $\leq$ 6 weeks of age
Extent of host immunodeficiency	Increasing engraftment success with increasing immunodeficiency (e.g., superior engraftment success using SCID rather than nude mice)	Choice based on malignancy of tumor of interest. When grafting a non-grade IV tumor, improved likelihood of success may result from using increasingly immunodeficient hosts
Location of tumor cell injection	Orthotopic injection potentially increases success rate	If sufficient cells/tissue, both intracranial and subcutaneous injections are recommended
Tumor initiating cell enrichment (e.g., CD133+ cell sorting)	Allows for smaller inoculum of cells to initiate xenograft	May be useful for selecting tumorigenic cells from large specimens that would fail to engraft if injected unsorted
Matrigel	May increase tumor engraftment success rate as well as growth rate of successfully engrafted tumors	1:1 (volume) tumor:matrigel injections is recommended

tumorigenicity of human brain tumor cells. In addition to these considerations, the mixing of Matrigel with tumor cells, prior to injection, for increasing tumor engraftment success rate as well as for increasing the in vivo growth rate of tumorigenic cells (Fridman et al. 1991; Wyrick et al. 1997; Rubenstein et al. 1999), is widely practiced, but even here the consistency of benefit from using this combination of extracellular matrix proteins and growth factors is mostly unclear.

In addition to effect on tumorigenicity, the lengthy in vitro propagation of CNS tumor cells, using conventional cell culture conditions, contributes to the loss of or suppression of other biologic properties that are manifested in patient tumors. This is perhaps most evident with respect to the orthotopic (intracranial) growth pattern of tumorigenic cell lines, which is often well circumscribed (Bullard et al. 1981; Finkelstein et al. 1994), rather than diffusely infiltrative, as is often the case in patients. Alterations in tumor biologic properties that are caused by extended cell culturing likely reflect changes in tumor cell transcriptional programs that are induced by the vastly different microenvironment associated with in vitro propagation (Camphausen et al. 2004; Lee et al. 2006), a specific example of which is the cell culture-associated suppression of GFAP expression in astrocytoma cells (Westphal et al. 1990).

Because of changes in tumor cell properties that result from extended in vitro propagation, when using conventional serum-supplemented medias, alternative cell culture approaches have been described in recent years for promoting tumor cell retention of biologic properties important for recapitulating human brain tumor intracranial growth patterns following intracranial injection in immunocompromised rodents. The so-called “stem cell” or “neurosphere” medias, that are supplemented with growth factors rather than fetal calf serum, and that are used in association with culture conditions that promote the propagation of unattached cellular aggregates (Engebraaten et al. 1999; Chaichana et al. 2006), rather than attached cell monolayers, have gained increasing

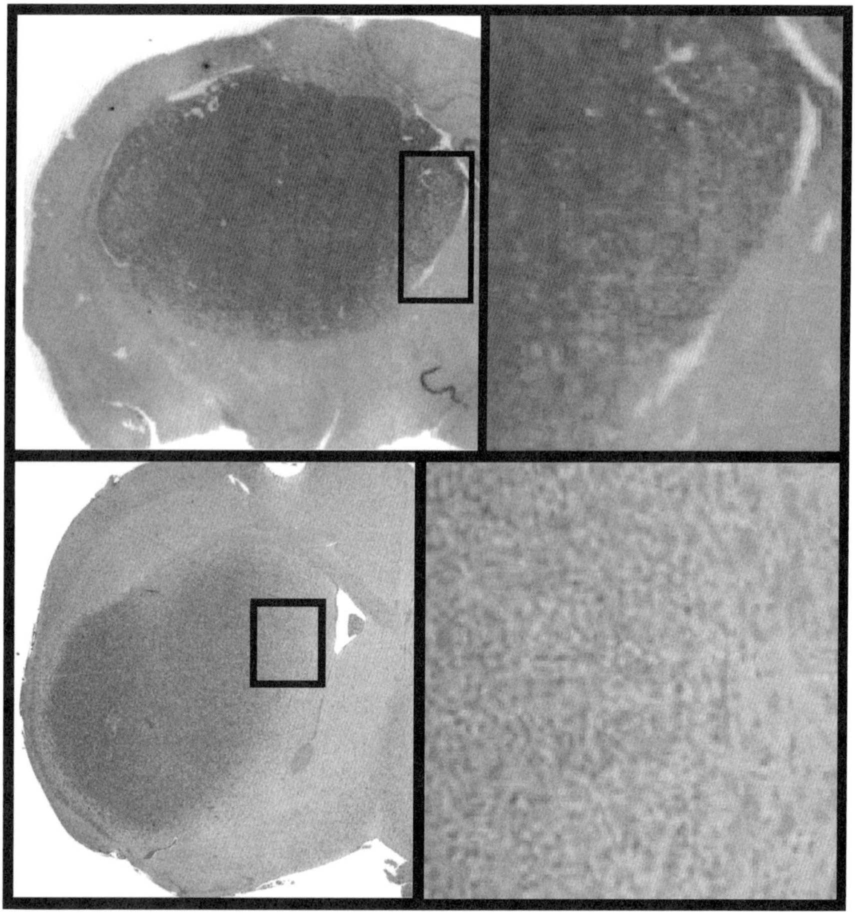

Fig. 8.1 Comparing the intracranial invasiveness of GBM cell lines propagated as monolayer cultures in serum-supplemented media (*upper panels*) vs. propagation as neurospheres in EGF + FGF supplemented media (*lower panels*). Upper panels show a well-circumscribed intracranial tumor established from U-87 MG monolayer culture (image shown to the right is an enlargement of the area indicated by the black rectangle in *left panel*). Note the well-delineated plane of separation between U-87 MG tumor and surrounding normal brain (*upper right panel*). In contrast, intracranial tumors established from GS2 cells propagated as a neurosphere culture (*bottom panels*) show diffuse infiltration, as highlighted by the enlargement image shown in the lower right section of the figure (*see* Color Plate 14)

acceptance and utilization in neuro-oncology research. It deserves mentioning that the complete neurosphere medias (i.e., including growth factors) are considerably more expensive than the conventional, serum-supplemented medias (as much as 10×). In spite of the issue of cost, the orthotopic growth pattern of GBM xenografts established from cells propagated in neurosphere media (Fig. 8.1 and Color Plate 14), and as contrasted with the circumscribed growth pattern of intracranial tumors produced by GBM cells cultured as a monolayer in serum-supplemented media, has helped to establish neurosphere culturing as the preferred way in which to maintain GBM cells in vitro.

Unfortunately, and in spite of the perceived importance of neurosphere culturing in neuro-oncology research, standardized protocols have yet to be established that would facilitate comparison of results between groups of investigators, and review of related literature shows significant variation in the composition of complete medias that are used (Chaichana et al. 2006). This variability involves the starting base media (e.g., DMEM, RPMI 1640, etc.), as well as the growth factor supplements, which have included different combinations of EGF, FGF, PDGF, LIF, NSF, and insulin (EGF and FGF are most commonly used). Each of these components is likely to have different as well as significant effects on neurosphere development and propagation and on the interpretation of data.

8.2 Xenograft-Based Tumor Propagation

Though less commonly used than cell culture methods of propagation, sustaining growth of GBM surgical specimens as subcutaneous xenografts has been described and used by a few groups (Humphrey et al. 1988; Leuraud et al. 2003; Pandita et al. 2004). At least one advantage of this approach is readily apparent: any specimen maintained as a xenograft is, by definition, tumorigenic, and therefore useful in association with in vivo studies. Less obvious, but nonetheless apparent in association with information reported by investigators using this approach, is that subcutaneous tumor tissue, or cells dispersed from resected subcutaneous tumors, often produce highly infiltrative tumors upon intracranial injection in immunocompromised mice (Antunes et al. 2000; Giannini et al. 2005). Whether the intracranial invasiveness of GBM tumor cells, from resected subcutaneous tumors, is effected overtime is uncertain, though one group has recently shown that two such xenografts, maintained for >10 years as subcutaneous growths, produced circumscribed tumors when injected in the brains of nude mice (Claes et al. 2008). In contrast, tumors that had been propagated through intracranial tumor passaging, in as many as 16 successive mice over a 3-year period, continued to show highly invasive character, suggesting that orthotopic (i.e., intracranial) vs. heterotopic (i.e., subcutaneous) propagation is a further consideration for investigations requiring the most faithful in vivo recapitulation of patient tumor properties by patient tumor cells.

GBM propagation, either as subcutaneous or intracranial xenografts, also promotes retention of patient tumor molecular characteristics, including EGFR amplification (Bigner et al. 1990b; Pandita et al. 2004; Claes et al. 2008), a key gene alteration observed in approximately one-third of patient GBMs. In fact, xenografts established from patient tumors have been shown to promote the retention of all genetic signature alterations identified in corresponding patient tumors (Leuraud et al. 2003; Pandita et al. 2004).

Disadvantages to the xenograft-based approach for tumor propagation include the need for an appropriate facility to house animals as well as for performing animal procedures, the need for appropriately trained animal technical staff, and the increased difficulty, relative to working with cell cultures, in manipulating and/or modifying tumor cells to investigate gene–protein function relationships (i.e., the development of isogenic derivatives). In addition, there is decreased convenience regarding the execution of experiments, since the availability of tumor cells is dependent on having ready access to specific and appropriately sized subcutaneous tumors. These problems are exacerbated in association with intracranial tumor propagation, since tumor growth and size cannot be checked by visual inspection or caliper measurement, and animals with intracranial tumor can undergo rapid demise due to the suddenness with which neurologic compromise, due to increasing tumor burden, often occurs. As additional studies are conducted regarding the benefits as well as shortcomings of tumor cell propagation in growth factor supplemented medias vs. propagation as xenografts, it is anticipated that a clearer picture will emerge regarding the most appropriate circumstances for using each method. Relative benefit and liability considerations that are associated with the various approaches for propagating human tumor cells are summarized in Fig. 8.2.

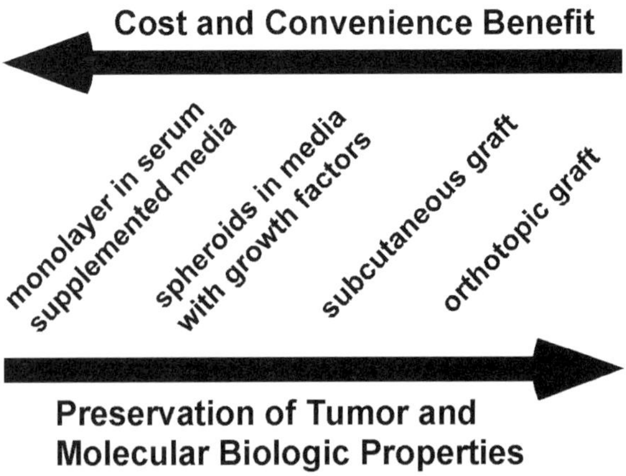

Fig. 8.2 Opposing benefit-to-liability summary for various means of propagating human CNS tumor cells. In essence, preserving patient tumor characteristics has its price, both with respect to time and financial considerations: i.e., approaches that best preserve patient tumor characteristics are the most expensive and least convenient (*arrows* are in the direction of lowest to highest)

8.3 Intracranial vs. Subcutaneous Tumor Therapy Response Experiments

Initial therapeutic testing is most commonly conducted by treating tumor cells grown as monolayers in culture. Alternative in vitro approaches have been used for preliminary assessment of therapeutic efficacy and include neurosphere culturing (Madsen et al. 2002) and culturing in semi-solid matrices (Ono et al. 2007). In attempt to more accurately model in vivo conditions, ex vivo models, such as the tumor cell:brain slice co-culture method, have also been utilized (Schichor et al. 2005).

Regardless of the merits of these approaches, xenograft-enabled research has served and will likely continue to serve as the "gold standard" as well as the final step of pre-clinical evaluation of cancer therapies. Routinely used methods for assessing in vivo tumor cell response to treatment with experimental therapies have been largely based on the following approaches, used either singularly or in different combinations:

- Determination of control vs. treatment group volume differences through caliper-based measurements of subcutaneous tumors.
- Determination of control vs. treatment group differences in tumor size at arbitrary, albeit identical time points in animals sacrificed subsequent to orthotopic tumor implantation.
- Determination of control vs. treatment group differences in survival time in animals receiving orthotopic tumor implants.

For CNS tumors, the basis for concern over the first approach is primarily associated with the assumption that subcutaneous tumor response to therapy is indicative of intracranial tumor response. Because of the different growth patterns of heterotopic vs. orthotopic tumors (Giannini et al. 2005), one would more likely anticipate different therapeutic responses between circumscribed (subcutaneous) and infiltrative (intracranial) growths, with therapeutic response of the latter type being more subject to properties of the normal tissue microenvironment within which the tumor cells disseminate. In addition, testing the efficacy of a systemically administered therapeutic, against a subcutaneous tumor, does not address blood–brain barrier permeability of the agent in question. Finally, for localized treatment of cancer, by focal beam radiation (Ozawa et al. 2006) or convection-enhanced delivery (Saito et al. 2004), intracranial tumor establishment is required.

At one time, the method for intracranial tumor injection may have presented a formidable technical barrier for many laboratories. Now, however, this procedure, especially for supratentorial injections in the caudate putamen, has been reasonably well detailed and is being used in many laboratories, with a success rate of orthotopic brain tumor establishment, using rodent stereotactic injection frames or freehand injection (Fig. 8.3 and Color Plate 15), that is quite good, and which has minimal procedure-related animal

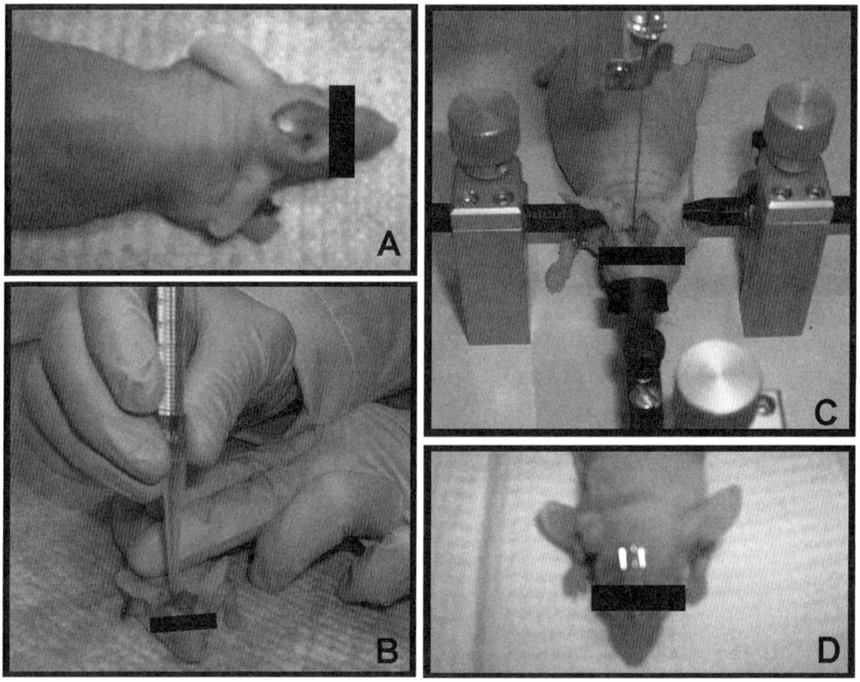

Fig. 8.3 Approaches to establishing orthotopic brain tumor xenografts. Following the midline incision and separation of the skin covering the skull (panel **A**: *pen mark* shows location for injection of cells, approximately 2.5–3 mm right from the bregma and just behind the coronal suture), tumor cells can either be injected "freehand" (panel **B**), or by use of a small animal stereotactic frame (panel **C**), which provides increased stability and control of injection depth. The opening in the skull for injection can be created either with a small drill or by simply pricking the skull with a 25 gauge needle. For the freehand method, injection depth is limited by a pipette tip (shown) or rubber sleeve covering all but the exposed end of the needle. Once the hole has been created, tumor cells are injected 3 mm below the outer table of the skull for routine supratentorial tumor establishment. Following injection, the separated skin is closed by use of clip (panel **D**) that eventually dislodges as the skin closes (heals). Especially when injecting large series of mice (>50), we recommend the freehand method as it increases throughput 3–4× relative to use of the stereotactic frame. For example, as many as 50 mice can be injected in an hour when two investigators are working in tandem (i.e., one investigator exposing the skull and the other performing the injection), whereas 12–16 mice per hour is an achievable rate when using a stereotactic frame (*see* Color Plate 15)

death. Tumor cell injections in other neuroanatomical locations have also been described (Wu et al. 2002; Shu et al. 2006; Baia et al. 2008) but are perhaps more subject to technical error causing animal morbidity.

Rodent species selection is an important consideration for intracranial xenograft experiments, with rats sometimes presenting advantages over mice due to their larger brain volume. For instance, if it is intended to dissect tumor from rodent brain, the use of rats will facilitate acquisition of larger quantity, and probably higher purity of tumor. In addition, for experiments involving convection-enhanced delivery, the increased size and thickness of the rat skull helps with proper positioning of the infusion cannula (Saito et al. 2004). The major advantage for mice, of course, is their decreased cost, both initial purchase as well as cages costs, since a single cage can be used to accommodate more mice (usually five) than rats (usually three).

There are, of course, not-so-obvious pitfalls for establishing intracranial xenografts, among which is avoiding large injection volumes that force tumor cells into the ventricles, with subsequent neuroaxis dissemination of tumor. With regard to this point, the nude rat brain is more accommodating. In our laboratory, when working with mice, we limit injections to 3 ml volumes, with cell concentrations at 105 cells/ml, and delivering cells into the caudate putamen. Armed with knowledge of this type, and a minimal amount of experience, one could envision the near-obligate use of orthotopic therapy response models among neuro-oncology researchers. Still, a shortcoming of this approach has persisted, in relation to the use of subcutaneous therapy response models, as indicated by the latter two points listed above: i.e., an investigator only being allowed a single observation per experimental animal.

8.4 The Impact of Bioluminescence Imaging

It is reasonable to speculate that much of the resistance to using orthotopic brain tumor transplantation models has stemmed from the inability to continuously monitor intracranial tumor growth and response to therapeutic testing. In recent years, however, bioluminescence imaging (BLI) has provided researchers with the ability to perform non-invasive, longitudinal studies for continuous monitoring of tumor biological processes such as growth rate during initial establishment and response to therapy (Gross and Piwnica-Worms 2005). In contrast to survival as an indication of agent activity, BLI is not limited to a single observation per animal used in an experiment.

Certainly there are other small animal imaging modalities being used in neuro-oncology research, including MRI and microPET. However, none currently compare with BLI with respect to combined considerations of cost, speed, and sensitivity. In addition to non-invasive serial monitoring of tumor growth and response to therapy, BLI facilitates more relevant timing of treatment initiation by allowing investigators to determine when injected tumor cells have achieved log phase growth. In many therapy response experiments, treatments are initiated shortly after intracranial tumor cell injection, such that efficacy evaluations are conducted under conditions which favor interpretation of significant anti-tumor activity, thereby contributing to unrealistic expectations of successful outcomes for human clinical trial results. Results from our laboratory, using BLI to monitor tumor growth, have shown that following the

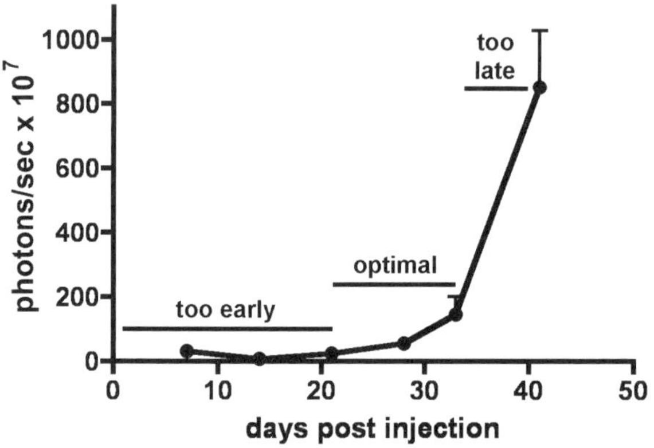

Fig. 8.4 Results from bioluminescence monitoring of intracranial U-87 MG xenograft growth, with graph showing mean luminescence of three mice subsequent to injection of 300,000 luciferase-modified cells in each (standard error of mean indicated at each time point). Note that progressive growth of the tumor is not indicated until imaging beyond day 21, with exponential growth not evident until day 33 imaging. Initiation of therapy prior to indication of progressive growth would yield results less meaningful for assessing efficacy, and clinical translation, than would initiation of therapy after indication of progressive growth being achieved. Optimal therapy administration, for efficacy evaluation, is after indication of progressive growth, but prior to the mouse experiencing a level of tumor burden that is too extensive for therapeutic response to be evident (indicated as "too late")

injection of GBM cells, propagated via conventional cell culture conditions, such as is used for the U-87 MG cell line, no net increase in cell number is evident for as many as 3 weeks following injection (Fig. 8.4); this is also the case for subcutaneous cell injections, where tumor cells appear to be latent for several weeks before showing measurable growth. Treating prior to tumor cells achieving log growth may result in tumor growth delay that could be erroneously interpreted as agent anti-tumor activity in the absence of bioluminescence monitoring and assessing agent activity by survival analysis only.

In addition to monitoring tumor response to therapy in a context meant to mimic that used for the treatment of patients with newly diagnosed GBM, a related and additional application of BLI is for conducting experiments to test the efficacy of salvage therapies against recurrent tumor (Dinca et al. 2007). Continuous bioluminescence monitoring permits the determination of intracranial tumor regrowth following initial therapeutic response (Fig. 8.5) and provides opportunity to treat mice in a context analogous to that of a patient whose cancer has relapsed. Because most novel therapies are initially tested in a setting of recurrent cancer, this approach provides a therapy evaluation paradigm that should, in principle, more closely resemble the clinical scenario in which the therapy would first be evaluated in patients. In addition to creating a salvage therapy evaluation model, treatment of recurrent tumor in association

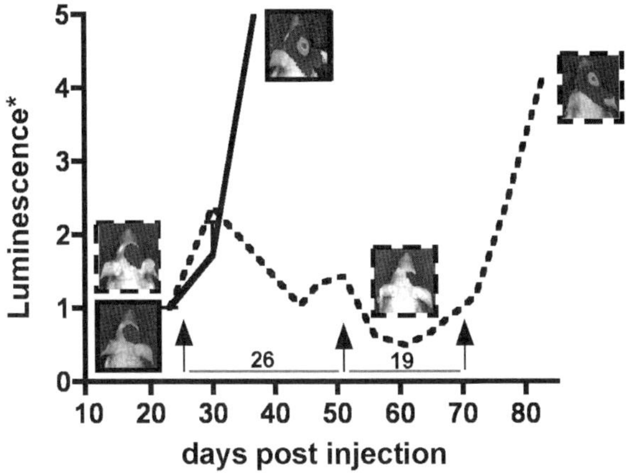

Fig. 8.5 Intracranial xenograft bioluminescence signal variation associated with repeated 100 mg/kg temozolomide treatments at days 25, 51, and 70 (indicated by arrows); *solid black line* represents the luminescence plot for an untreated mouse and shows rapid, log phase tumor growth beyond day 22 post tumor cell injection. First and second temozolomide treatments cause decreasing luminescence. However, note the decreasing benefit of temozolomide therapy i.e., the length of anti-tumor effect from the second treatment is less than that associated with the initial treatment (19 days vs. 26 days), and the third treatment has essentially no anti-tumor effect. Because serial luminescence monitoring permits detection of tumor regrowth, this technique creates opportunity to test novel therapies in a manner analogous to that in which patients with recurrent tumor are treated. In addition, by comparing molecular characteristics of tumors obtained from untreated vs. once-treated vs. twice-treated animals, candidate genes and corresponding proteins associated with acquired resistance to therapy can be identified

with BLI monitoring should be useful for studying the molecular biology associated with cancer acquisition of resistance to therapy, by comparing molecular profiles of untreated tumors vs. once-treated tumor vs. tumors subjected to multiple cycles of therapy (Fig. 8.5).

It is important to note that although bioluminescence is highly correlated with tumor volume (Dinca et al. 2007), it does not provide data that allow determination of tumor volume, in contrast to the results of magnetic resonance imaging. In addition, bioluminescence signal is affected by depth of tumor cell injection and growth, such that comparing the intracranial bioluminescence of any two animals cannot be interpreted as indicating relative tumor burden between those animals. A consequence of the attenuation of luminescence signal with increasing depth of tumor cell injection/growth is that BLI would not be useful in larger animals. With rodents, however, luminescence signal is easily detected in mice (over a range of 10^5 photons/sec) and is sufficiently penetrating to allow longitudinal monitoring of tumor growth in rats that have received tumor cell injection in the brain stem at 1 cm depth (Fig. 8.6).

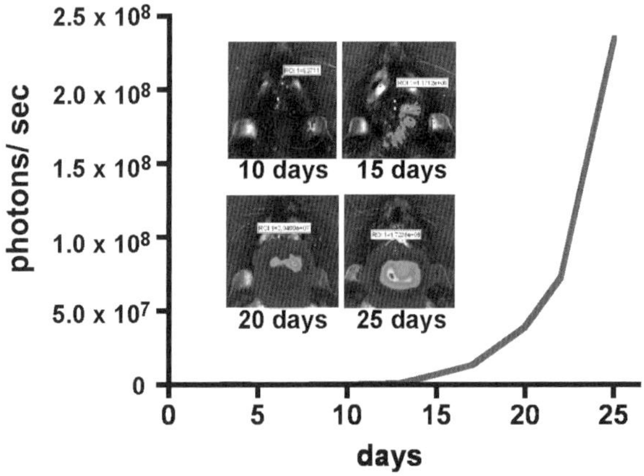

Fig. 8.6 Bioluminescence monitoring of luciferase-modified U-87 MG cells following brainstem injection in a nude rat. For rodent orthotopic studies this presents a stringent test of the ability to use BLI for monitoring tumor growth due to the depth of the injection (1 cm) and the relatively small tumor volume that can be tolerated in this neuroanatomic location. Results shown here indicate an ability to monitor tumor growth from day 10 onward. In this experiment, rats succumbed to tumor burden prior to day 30 imaging, thereby indicating a 2–3-week interval from time of initial tumor detection to required euthanasia for administering therapy, which is quite adequate for assessing efficacy or lack thereof for novel agents

8.5 Human Tumor Panels and Pre-Clinical Therapeutic Testing of Multiple Tumors

By using BLI monitoring with panels of specific types of CNS cancer, either maintained as cell cultures or as subcutaneous grafts, the concept of conducting high throughput and relevant pre-clinical trials for testing experimental therapies is making progress toward becoming reality. Recent demonstrations in support of a panel approach for investigating therapeutic efficacy have included the analysis of a large series of GBM xenografts for radiation sensitivity (Sarkaria et al. 2006), as well as for response to the EGFR kinase inhibitor erlotinib (Sarkaria et al. 2007). Given the vast number of existing therapeutics, the steady supply of additional novel therapeutics from industry, and the importance of testing therapies in combinations, it is clear that there are more therapeutic options to evaluate than there are patients to support evaluations through clinical trial activity. Consequently, the need for high throughput and relevant animal model pre-clinical testing is urgent. It seems likely that advances in approaches to propagating CNS tumor cells, combined with advances in monitoring orthotopic growth of CNS tumors in animal models, will help address this need.

References

Antunes L, Angioi-Duprez KS, Bracard SR et al. (2000) Analysis of tissue chimerism in nude mouse brain and abdominal xenograft models of human glioblastoma multiforme: what does it tell us about the models and about glioblastoma biology and therapy? J Histochem Cytochem 48:847–858.

Baia GS, Dinca EB, Ozawa T, Kimura ET, McDermott MW, James CD, VandenBerg SR, Lal A (2008) An orthotopic skull base model of malignant meningioma. Brain Pathol 18:172–179.

Beckman G, Beckman L, Ponten J et al. (1971) G-6-PD and PGM phenotypes of 16 continuous human tumor cell lines. Evidence against cross-contamination and contamination by HeLa cells. Hum Hered 21:238–241.

Bigner DD, Bigner SH, Pontén J et al. (1981) Heterogeneity of Genotypic and phenotypic characteristics of fifteen permanent cell lines derived from human gliomas. J Neuropathol Exp Neurol 40:201–229.

Bigner SH, Friedman HS, Vogelstein B et al. (1990a) Amplification of the c-myc gene in human medulloblastoma cell lines and xenografts. Cancer Res 50:2347–2350.

Bigner SH, Humphrey PA, Wong AJ et al. (1990b) Characterization of the epidermal growth factor receptor in human glioma cell lines and xenografts. Cancer Res 50:8017–8022.

Bullard DE, Schold SC Jr, Bigner SH et al. (1981) Growth and chemotherapeutic response in athymic mice of tumors arising from human glioma-derived cell lines. J Neuropathol Exp Neurol 40:410–427.

Camphausen K, Purow B, Sproull M et al. (2004) Influence of in vivo growth on human glioma cell line gene expression: convergent profiles under orthotopic conditions. Proc Natl Acad Sci USA 102:8287–8292.

Chaichana K, Zamora-Berridi G, Camara-Quintana J, et al. (2006) Neurosphere assays: growth factors and hormone differences in tumor and nontumor studies. Stem Cells 24:2851–2857.

Claes A, Schuuring J, Boots-Sprenger S et al. (2008) Phenotypic and genotypic characterization of orthotopic human glioma models and its relevance for the study of anti-glioma therapy. Brain Pathol 18:423–433.

de Muralt B, de Tribolet N, Diserens AC et al. (1985) Phenotyping of 60 cultured human gliomas and 34 other neuroectodermal tumors by means of monoclonal antibodies against glioma, melanoma and HLA-DR antigens. Eur J Cancer Clin Oncol 21:207–216.

Dinca EB, Sarkaria JN, Schroeder MA, Carlson BL, Voicu R, Gupta N, Berger MS, James CD. (2007) Bioluminescence monitoring of intracranial glioblastoma xenograft: response to primary and salvage temozolomide therapy. J Neurosurg 107:610–616.

Diserens AC, de Tribolet N, Martin-Achard A et al. (1981) Characterization of an established human malignant glioma cell line: LN-18. Acta Neuropathol 53:21–28.

Engebraaten O, Hjortland GO, Hirschberg H et al. (1999) Growth of precultured human glioma specimens in nude rat brain. J Neurosurg 90:125–132.

Finkelstein SD, Black P, Nowak TP et al. (1994) Histological characteristics and expression of acidic and basic fibroblast growth factor genes in intracerebral xenogeneic transplants of human glioma cells. Neurosurgery 34:136–143.

Fridman R, Kibbey MC, Royce LS et al. (1991) Enhanced tumor growth of both primary and established human and murine tumor cells in athymic mice after coinjection with Matrigel. J Natl Cancer Inst 83:769–774.

Giannini C, Sarkaria JN, Saito A et al. (2005) Patient tumor EGFR and PDGFRA gene amplifications retained in an invasive intracranial xenograft model of glioblastoma multiforme. Neuro-Oncol 7:164–176.

Gross S, Piwnica-Worms D (2005) Spying on cancer: molecular imaging in vivo with genetically encoded reporters. Cancer Cell 7:5–15.

Humphrey PA, Wong AJ, Vogelstein B et al. (1988) Amplification and expression of the epidermal growth factor receptor gene in human glioma xenografts. Cancer Res 48:2231–2238.

Ishii N, Maier D, Merlo A et al. (1999) Frequent co-alterations of TP53, p16/CDKN2A, p14ARF, PTEN tumor suppressor genes in human glioma cell lines. Brain Pathol 9:469–479.

Keles GE, Berger MS, Srinivasan J et al. (1995) Establishment and characterization of four human medulloblastoma-derived cell lines. Oncol Res 7:493–503.

Lee J, Kotliarova S, Kotliarov Y et al. (2006) Tumor stem cells derived from glioblastomas cultured in bFGF and EGF more closely mirror the phenotype and genotype of primary tumors than do serum-cultured cell lines. Cancer Cell 9:391–403.

Leuraud P, Taillandier T, Aguirre-Cruz L (2003) Correlation between genetic alterations and growth of human malignant glioma xenografted in nude mice. Br J Cancer 89:2327–2332.

Madsen SJ, Sun CH, Tromberg BJ et al. (2002) Effects of combined photodynamic therapy and ionizing radiation on human glioma spheroids. Photochem Photobiol 76:411–416.

Ono A, Kanno H, Hayashi A, et al. (2007) Collagen gel matrix assay as an in vitro chemosensitivity test for malignant astrocytic tumors. Int J Clin Oncol 12:125–130.

Ozawa T, Faddegon BA, Hu LJ, Bollen AW, Lamborn KR, Deen DF (2006) Response of intracerebral human glioblastoma xenografts to multifraction radiation exposures. Int J Radiat Oncol Biol Phys 66:263–270.

Pandita A, Aldape KD, Zadeh G et al. (2004) Contrasting in vivo and in vitro fates of glioblastoma cell subpopulations with amplified EGFR. Genes Chromosomes Cancer 39:29–36.

Rubenstein M, Shaw M, Mirochnik Y et al. (1999) In vivo establishment of T98G human glioblastoma. Methods Find Exp Clin Pharmacol 21:391–393.

Rutka JT, Giblin JR, Dougherty DY et al. (1987) Establishment and characterization of five cell lines derived from human malignant gliomas. Acta Neuropathol 75:92–103.

Saito R, Bringas JR, McKnight TR et al. (2004) Distribution of liposomes into brain and rat brain tumor models by convection-enhanced delivery monitored with magnetic resonance imaging. Cancer Res 64:2572–2579.

Sarkaria JN, Carlson BL, Schroeder MA et al. (2006) Use of an orthotopic xenograft model for assessing the effect of epidermal growth factor receptor amplification on glioblastoma radiation response. Clin Cancer Res 12:2264–2271.

Sarkaria JN, Yang L, Grogan PT et al. (2007) Identification of molecular characteristics correlated with glioblastoma sensitivity to EGFR kinase inhibition through use of an intracranial xenograft test panel. Mol Cancer Ther 6:1167–1174.

Schichor C, Kerkau S, Visted T et al. (2005) The brain slice chamber, a novel variation of the Boyden Chamber Assay, allows time-dependent quantification of glioma invasion into mammalian brain in vitro. J Neurooncol 73:9–18.

Shapiro WR, Basler GA, Chernik NL et al. (1979) Human brain tumor transplantation into nude mice. J Natl Cancer Inst 62:447–453.

Sharkey FE, Fogh J (1984) Considerations in the use of nude mice for cancer research. Cancer Metastasis Rev 3:341–360.

Shu Q, Antalffy B, Su JM, et al. (2006) Valproic Acid prolongs survival time of severe combined immunodeficient mice bearing intracerebellar orthotopic medulloblastoma xenografts. Clin Cancer Res 12:4687–4694.

Singh SK, Hawkins C, Clarke ID et al. (2004) Identification of human brain tumour initiating cells. Nature 432:396–401.

Taghian A, Budach W, Zietman A et al. (1993) Quantitative comparison between the transplantability of human and murine tumors into the subcutaneous tissue of NCr/Sed-nu/nu nude and severe combined immunodeficient mice. Cancer Res 53:5012–5017.

Westphal M, Nausch H, Herrmann HD (1990) Antigenic staining patterns of human glioma cultures: primary cultures, long-term cultures and cell lines. J Neurocytol 19:466–477.
Wyrick BJ, Ozawa T, Lamborn KR (1997) Effects of Matrigel on the SF-767 malignant glioma athymic mouse tumor model. Anticancer Res 17:2419–2425.

Chapter 9
Transformed Human Brain Cells in Culture as a Model for Brain Tumors

Russell O. Pieper

Abstract Brain tumor tissue provides a wealth of information as to the genetic and epigenetic alterations associated with the disease. The information provided, however, is by nature correlative, and as a result, investigators have turned to manipulable systems in which defined genetic alterations can be sequentially introduced and monitored for effect. While much of this work involves the use of animal models, a significant and growing number of investigators are turning to the use of cultured human brain cell systems. This review summarizes the benefits and limitations of such an approach, describes important recent findings derived from the use of defined human cells in the study of gliomagenesis, and highlights some new and innovative approaches that may ultimately help link gliomagenesis to normal differentiation and stem cell biology.

Contents

R.O. Pieper (✉)
Department of Neurological Surgery, Brain Tumor Research Center, The UCSF Cancer Center, University of California – San Francisco, San Francisco, CA 94115-0875, USA
e-mail: rpieper@cc.ucsf.edu

E.G. Van Meir (ed.), *CNS Cancer*, Cancer Drug Discovery and Development, DOI 10.1007/978-1-60327-553-8_9,
© Humana Press, a part of Springer Science+Business Media, LLC 2009

9.1 Introduction

The genetic events that lead to the formation of gliomas are carried in every tumor. Over many years, teams of investigators have used the most current technologies available to interrogate glioma tissue in the hope of identifying common genetic and epigenetic alterations carried in the tumor. The attempts to categorize the full range of genetic and epigenetic alterations in glioblastoma (GBM) have recently culminated in the most comprehensive set of genetic analyses of GBM to date, collectively called The Cancer Genome Atlas (Chin and Gray 2008). These findings appear to agree with the consensus that has emerged as to which lesions are most common, and therefore perhaps most important, in the genesis of the disease. The consensus reached by The Cancer Genome Atlas investigators and other investigators in the field is that there are three major pathways implicated in gliomagenesis: receptor tyrosine kinases, p53, and pRb (Furnari et al. 2007, Ichimura et al. 2000, Ichimura et al. 2004). Alterations in receptor tyrosine kinase signaling, including mutation and amplification of epidermal growth factor receptor (EGFR), are thought to drive Ras signaling, via MEK and p16, to ultimately drive the proliferative response, particularly in those cells in which the PTEN tumor suppressor protein has been eliminated by mutation or gene deletion (Furnari et al. 2007). Alterations in the Rb pathway are thought to result in cell cycle disregulation and loss of ability of cells to arrest in response to aberrant growth signaling, while alterations in the p53 pathway may limit the ability of cells to undergo apoptosis and terminate the aberrant growth signals generated by the other alterations (Furnari et al. 2007) (Fig. 9.1). While alterations in EGFR, pRb, and p53 are among the most common in GBM, additional novel alterations also seem to cluster along the growth factor receptor, p53, and pRb pathways, and alterations or disruptions in at least one of the three major pathways appear to occur in the vast majority of GBM (Ichimura et al. 2000). While these studies provide an excellent framework by which we can begin to understand the process of gliomagenesis, they cannot by nature address questions of whether these alterations actually do lead to glioma formation, which alterations are most critical, the timing of these alterations in the disease process, or how best to address these alterations therapeutically. These types of complicated questions cannot be addressed by simple correlative studies, but rather rely on the use of models in which suspected alterations can be introduced into cells and in which the consequences of these alterations can be monitored.

The search for an optimal model in which to study the events critical for brain tumor formation is a long and ongoing quest. Ideally one would like to begin with the cell of origin of gliomas and introduce into this cell the genetic alterations commonly found in the established tumor of interest. The limitation of this statement should be obvious. First, the cell of origin of gliomas has not been identified and may in fact represent any of several types of cells. Second, while various human brain cells can be isolated, many can be difficult to culture,

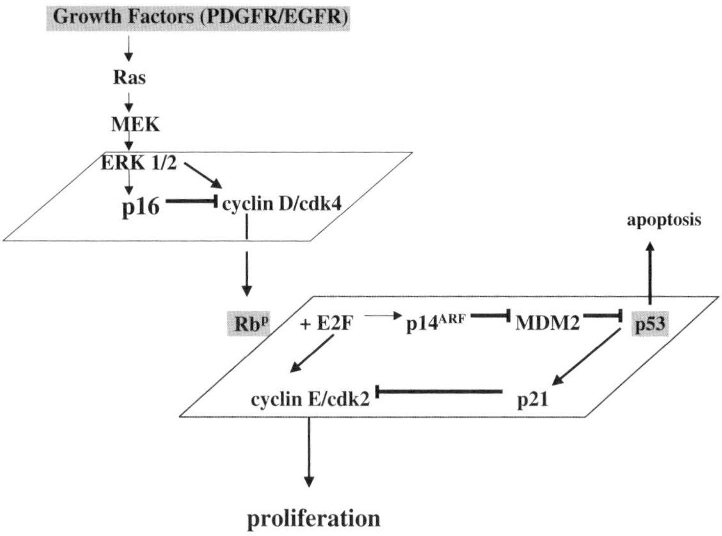

Fig. 9.1 Pathways thought to be critical in the development of GBM. Growth stimulation, by either growth factor receptor mutation or loss of control of Ras signaling, favors pRb phosphorylation and cell cycle progression. Loss of pRb or components that regulate pRb further favors cell cycle progression and in connection with loss of p53 promotes tumor growth and cell survival

and culturing runs the risk of destroying features potentially critical in the transformation process. Finally, even if appropriate human cells can be isolated and manipulated, there is no simple way to put modified human brain cells back into the appropriate human brain microenvironment, and as such no simple way to monitor consequences of the alterations induced. In the face of these problems, two solutions have been attempted, with varying degrees of success. Beginning in the 1920s and more rigorously in the 1940s, investigators interested in carcinogenesis treated animals with mixtures of carcinogenic compounds to induce the formation of tumors (Berenblum and Shubik 1949, Rous and Friedewald 1941). In the early 1970s, investigators showed that treatment of pregnant rats with the carcinogen ethyl nitrosourea led to the formation of a wide range of nervous system tumors including oligodendrogliomas, meningiomas, and astrocytomas (Koestner et al. 1971). While these studies strongly suggested that brain tumors were the result of genetic mutation and indirectly that cells of the fetal brain might be more susceptible than those of the adult brain, they were also limited in that the exact genetic alterations created could not be controlled. What was necessary was a system in which exact genetic alterations could be introduced at exact times in exact cells of the nervous system. The advent of embryonic stem cell technology less than 10 years later (Evans and Kaufman 1981, Martin 1981) provided researchers just this opportunity and ultimately allowed for the creation of animals that contained specific genetic alterations in specific cells of the brain. These more sophisticated animal models of gliomagenesis have been extremely successful in generating animals that develop tumors with many of the characteristics of human gliomas and with some of the same genetic alterations found in human GBM and also in beginning to help identify the cells of origin in these tumors (reviewed in Fomchenko and Holland 2006).Despite the success of these studies, however, they fall short in the ultimate goal of understanding human gliomagenesis in that the pathways and events that control the cell cycle, cell life span, and cell survival in short-lived rodents do not always match those in longer lived human. As an example, while human cells appear to be dependent on telomerase activity to maintain telomere length and sustain proliferation, rodent cells have longer telomeres and are less dependent on telomerase activity (Kipling 1997). Furthermore, studies have suggested that rodent cells use different aspects of Ras signaling to control growth than do human cells (Hamad et al. 2002). Thus, although mouse models have proven very useful, they alone may not be sufficient to fully understand the process of human gliomagenesis.

As a complement to mouse carcinogenesis studies and to mouse models, a limited group of investigators have begun to ask about genetic events that are important in gliomagenesis not in mouse cells but in human cells. In concept, these studies are relatively straightforward. The starting material, in most cases normal human astrocytes, is genetically modified by sequential introduction of genes encoding proteins that alter the function of pathways suspected of being important in gliomagenesis. The ability of the given genetic alteration to induce cellular transformation and tumorigenesis is then measured by determining if the cells gain the ability to grow in soft agar and intracranially in animals, both measures of cellular transformation. The results of these studies, their limitations, and the future directions of this work will be discussed in this review.

9.2 Early Developments

The use of normal human cells as the basis for studies of gliomagenesis, while simple in concept, is relatively new. For a number of years, investigators interested in the genetic alterations that lead to cancer used a standard set of cultured cells, typically NIH 3T3 cells, established by Todaro and Green (1963). These cells were derived from primary mouse embryo fibroblasts that underwent spontaneous immortalization and as such were a reliable and renewable source of cells for study. Many of the most important early studies of cellular transformation were performed in NIH3T3 cells, and their ease of use and reliability made them workhorses of early studies of oncogenesis. The results derived from NIH 3T3 cells, however, were somewhat misleading in the sense that because of their already immortalized status, 3T3 were considerably more susceptible to transformation than other “normal” cells. This ultimately became apparent in the late 1980s when several studies clearly showed that the genetic alterations that led to the transformation of NIH3T3 cells were insufficient to transform cultured human cells and in many cases actually led to growth suppression and cellular senescence (Fanton et al. 2001, Stevenson and Volsky 1986). The differing requirements for the transformation of normal human cells and NIH3T3 cells remained a puzzle for several years, although the observation itself made two clear points: one, there are differences between mouse cells and human cells with regard to the pathways and mechanisms that regulate the growth and survival of the cells, and two, the cellular transformation process is multistep and involves more than simple growth stimulation.

The seemingly increased complexity in transforming human cells remained largely unresolved until the late 1990s when Hahn and Weinberg made a landmark discovery (Hahn et al. 1999). These investigators, using normal human fibroblasts, reasoned that human cells required not only alterations that stimulated growth but also events that allowed cells to evade the normal control of life span. Because it was becoming increasingly clear that telomere length and the activity of the enzyme that regulated telomere length (the catalytic component of telomerase, hTERT) played a role in human cell life span (Greider and Blackburn 1985, 1996, Zhu et al. 1999), these investigators first introduced hTERT and assessed the effect on normal human cell life span, after which genetic alterations suspected of driving proliferation were introduced. In initial studies, the alteration studied included the introduction of a mutant form of H-ras (V12) shown to be sufficient for transformation of mouse fibroblasts, and SV40 large T antigen, a complex protein known to inactivate both p53 and pRb and to also be sufficient to transform NIH 3T3 cells (Brockman 1978) (summarized in Fig. 9.2). The results of these studies showed that while hTERT alone could extend the life span of the cells, additional alterations induced by

	Normal human fibroblasts	*Normal human astrocytes*	*Normal mouse fibroblasts*
hTERT + Tag + V12 Ras	**trans**	**trans**	trans
+ E6	not trans	not trans	trans
+E7	not trans	not trans	trans
+E6/E7	**trans**	**trans**	trans
+Ral	**trans**	**trans**	not trans
+Raf	not trans	not trans	trans
+PI3K	not trans	not trans	trans
+rapamycin		not trans	

Fig. 9.2 Fundamental difference in the genetic alterations required to transform normal human astrocytes, normal human fibroblasts, and mouse fibroblasts

large T antigen and mutant H-Ras were both required for transformation. Furthermore, in the absence of hTERT, the introduction of large T antigen and mutant H-Ras did not induce transformation but rather resulted in growth arrest and senescence of the cultured normal cells. These studies were the first to demonstrate that normal human cells could be turned into tumor cells by the introduction of a limited number of defined genetic alterations and in turn launched an investigation as to whether cells of different origin were similarly regulated with regard to tumorigenesis.

The first studies related to brain tumors followed relatively shortly after the studies of Hahn and Weinberg. Two groups published their work nearly simultaneously, both showing that as with fibroblasts, the transformation of normal human astrocytes could be accomplished by the introduction of a limited number of defined genetic alterations. The work of Rich et al. showed that the introduction of hTERT, mutant V12 H-Ras, and T antigen was sufficient to induce glial transformation (Rich et al. 2001), while that of Sonoda et al. further showed that the function of large T antigen in transformation could be replaced with p53- and pRb-disabling proteins HPV16 E6 and E7, directly suggesting that p53 and pRb played a key role in controlling the transformation of normal human astrocytes (Sonoda et al. 2001b) (Fig. 9.2). There was also great interest as to whether these in vitro transformed cells could, following intracranial implantation in animals, form tumors that in any way recapitulated the features seen in primary human glioma. The tumors that arose upon intracranial implantation of the transformed human astrocytes did in fact resemble primary human gliomas, and follow-up studies showed that while they exhibited a high proliferative index, the tumors did not exhibit the endothelial cell proliferation or necrosis that defines GBM. They were, however, consistent with the diagnosis of glioma and perhaps grade III astrocytoma, and as such these studies represented the first creation of glioma cells by the introduction of defined genetic alterations.

A number of subsequent studies have focused specifically on how alterations in Ras signaling, the p53 pathway, and the pRb pathway contribute to glial cell transformation. The first of these studies dealt with the contribution of mutant H-Ras to glioma cell transformation and showed that only a part of the signaling milieu induced by mutant H-Ras was necessary. In these studies, normal human embryonic kidney cells immortalized by the expression of hTERT and sent along the path to transformation by the expression of large and small T antigen were also subsequently engineered to express forms of mutant H-Ras that would selectively signal down one of the three pathways activated by mutant V12 H-Ras [the phosphoinositol 3 kinase (PI3K), Raf, or Ral pathways] (Hamad et al. 2002, Lim et al. 2005, 2006). The results of these studies showed that while the transformation of rodent cells was dependent only on the ability of Ras to activate the Raf-MEK-Erk signaling pathway, normal human cells could be transformed by specific activation of the Ras–Ral pathway, and specifically by the activation of RalA (Lim et al. 2005). The results of these studies were subsequently confirmed in normal human astrocytes where it was shown that activated RalA could substitute for mutant V12 H-Ras in hTERT/E6/E7-mediated transformation (Panner et al. 2006) (Fig. 9.2). Recently published studies, however, have also raised the possibility that while the PI3K pathway is not in and of itself sufficient to mediate transformation, it may contribute to the maintenance of the transformed state. In these studies, normal human astrocytes transformed by the expression of hTERT, E6, E7, and mutant V12 H-Ras were incubated with rapamycin, a selective inhibitor of mammalian target of rapamycin (mTOR) (and thereby at least part of the downstream PI3K arm of the Ras pathway), and monitored for growth in soft agar (Nakamura et al. 2008). Surprisingly, these studies showed that mTOR inhibition effectively blocked the growth of the transformed astrocytes. Further studies suggested that it was the effects of rapamycin on the S6K arm of the mTOR signaling pathway and not the eIF4E arm that was critical in blocking cell growth. These studies, combined with those defining the contribution of Ral signaling, raise several interesting questions. First, if the Ral signaling pathway plays such a critical role in glial cell transformation, is this pathway activated in gliomas, and is this pathway a reasonable therapeutic target? Second, although considerable effort has gone into the therapeutic targeting of PI3K and mTOR, is targeting the PI3K pathway further downstream a rational approach? And finally, what are the key effectors of transformation downstream of Ral? In addressing the mechanism by which normal human astrocytes can be converted into glioma, the above described studies have not only laid a path for our understanding of gliomagenesis in human cells but also pointed out several interesting and perhaps clinically relevant approaches to therapy.

9.3 Modifiers of Transformation and Tumor Behavior

The early studies of effectors of glial cell transformation confirmed that the p53, pRb, and growth factor receptor pathways via Ras were all important in gliomagenesis just as they appeared to be by analysis of genetic alterations in primary human GBM. And yet the tumors that were derived from intracranially implanted transformed human astrocytes were markedly different from GBM. The tumors derived from transformed human astrocytes were not invasive as were primary human gliomas of all varieties but rather grew as a well-demarcated mass more similar to that noted for most intracranially implanted cultured GBM cell lines (Lee et al. 2006, Sonoda et al. 2001b). Furthermore, the tumors derived from transformed human astrocytes, while variable with regard to vasculature, did not exhibit the microvascular proliferation common to primary human GBM (Rich et al. 2001, Sonoda et al. 2003, 2001a, b). The tumors formed by intracranially implanted transformed human astrocytes also seemed to most resemble grade III astrocytomas and did not resemble grade II or grade IV tumors (Sonoda et al. 2001b). While these points were viewed as weaknesses of the system, they were also viewed as an opportunity to identify additional genetic alterations that might be critical in generating the complete GBM phenotype and which might also therefore be important in the behavior of primary GBM.

The identification of the factors that contribute to the differences between a grade II low-grade glioma, a grade III astrocytoma, and a grade IV GBM is critical not only for understanding gliomagenesis but also for the prognosis and therapy of patients. The greatest need in this regard appears to be the creation of a reliable model of low-grade glioma (LGG). Patients with low-grade glioma have a much lower progression to disease than patients with high-grade glioma and a more variable progression (Gilbert and Lang 2007), and as such this tumor presents opportunities for therapeutic intervention. Furthermore, no cell lines have been established from LGG, no xenografts of LGG have been created, and no mouse models exist for the disease. Because LGG exhibits a more limited range of genetic alterations than GBM (Arjona et al. 2006), and because these alterations include p53 alterations and hTERT activation (Lang et al. 1994, Le et al. 1998), normal human astrocytes exhibiting these alterations might be hoped to form tumors that resemble LGG. This, however, does not seem to be the case as normal human astrocytes immortalized by the introduction of hTERT did not prove to be tumorigenic, nor did hTERT-immortalized astrocytes in which p53 function was eliminated by introduction of human papilloma virus E6 (Sonoda et al. 2001b). These findings suggest that LGG may not simply be a less-aggressive, less genetically altered version of GBM but rather perhaps a distinctly different tumor. A confounding factor however is that the growth fraction of LGG in situ can be extremely low (Burger et al. 1986), and these tumors are often suspected of taking years to form and years to grow and further accumulate lesions. As such the limited amount of time the minimally genetically altered normal human astrocytes spent in animals without tumor formation (6 months) may not accurately reflect their inability to form LGG.

As noted, the intracranially injected transformed human astrocytes also did not form tumors resembling GBM and as such may lack genetic alterations critical for the GBM phenotype. GBM frequently have alterations in PTEN that result in downstream Akt activation, and indeed the majority of GBM have elevated levels of pAkt (Holland et al. 2000). Because the transformed human astrocytes created contain wild-type PTEN, introduction of a constitutively active Akt might be expected to mimic the PTEN inactivation noted in most GBM and might allow the altered cells to assume the GBM phenotype in vivo. Human astrocytes transformed by hTERT, E6, E7, and H-Ras were therefore infected with a construct encoding constitutively active Akt and monitored for growth in vitro and in vivo (Sonoda et al. 2001a). While the cells infected with activated Akt showed elevated levels of pAkt, in culture these cells were identical to those expressing a blank construct. In vivo, however, Akt-driven differences were more apparent. The Akt over-expressing cells formed tumors that were larger, grew faster, and exhibited increased vascular density and regions of necrosis. The characteristics of the tumors formed by the intracranially injected

Akt-expressing cells most resembled those of GBM, suggesting that signaling down the PI3K pathway played a critical role in the progression from grade III to grade IV GBM (Sonoda et al. 2001a). The observation that Akt only provided a growth advantage in vivo and not in vitro also suggested that the GBM-driven effects of Akt were a result of the brain and/or tumor microenvironment. These suggestions were subsequently borne out by studies in which it was shown that accelerated growth of the intracranially injected Akt-expressing cells was coincident with the onset of hypoxia in the tumor (unpublished observation, R. Pieper). Furthermore, in separate studies, it was shown that activation of secreted protein acidic, rich in cysteine (SPARC), a secreted extracellular glycoprotein, also led to the activation of Akt and an enhanced survival of transformed human astrocytes under stress conditions (Shi et al. 2004). This is of particular interest as SPARC is expressed at the invading edges of GBM and is suggested to play a key role in glioma invasion. These results suggest that transformed astrocytes that can stimulate the Akt pathway, either directly or by loss of PTEN, may have a selective survival advantage under the hypoxic and/or nutrient-limiting conditions that accompany tumor growth, and as such may be able to grow even in the face of limiting nutrients, much as is seen in primary GBM.

Another puzzling aspect of the tumors formed following intracranial injection of transformed human astrocytes was that these tumors also did not form vasculature or areas of necrosis that matched those of GBM and as such appeared to lack the genetic alterations critical for these GBM features. Because vascular endothelial growth factor (VEGF) is a key regulator of vascular formation in tumors and because its upregulation is correlated with glioma grade, the effects of VEGF over-expression on tumorigenicity of transformed human astrocytes were also measured. The results of these studies showed that over-expression of VEGF drove the formation of vessels in the resultant intracranially implanted cells and also stimulated the growth of the resultant tumors as might be expected for a contributor to the GBM phenotype (Sonoda et al. 2003). The resultant VEGF-driven tumors were, however, better oxygenated than control tumors and similarly exhibited no regions of hypoxia or necrosis, inconsistent with the GBM phenotype (Sonoda et al. 2003). These results suggest that while VEGF over-expression is also commonly seen in GBM, the over-expression of VEGF in and of itself does not drive the generation of GBM and that the necrosis seen in GBM is not simply due to enhanced growth or VEGF over-expression but a more complex series of factors.

The well-circumscribed nature of the tumors generated from the intracranially implanted transformed human astrocytes also created the opportunity to examine the factors that might regulate tumor invasiveness, a key feature of all glioma. A variety of molecules that are known to play a role in cell motility and invasion have been identified, and many are upregulated at or near the invading edges of gliomas. These include SPARC, matrix metalloproteases, and integrins. With regard to the integrins, the $\alpha V\beta 3$ complex appears to be of particular importance because this complex is specifically upregulated in invasive tumors

(Bello et al. 2001), and because agents selectively targeting the αVβ3 complex lead to tumor regression in some models (Chatterjee et al. 2000). The issue of invasion, however, is quite complex. The ability of cells to migrate and invade is highly dependent on the microenvironment, and a number of components of the extracellular matrix including angiostatin, tumstatin, and collagen type IV have been suggested to alter the ability of cells to move through their surroundings (Hamano et al. 2003, Maeshima et al. 2000, O'Reilly et al. 1994). Furthermore, the factors that influence the ability of cells to degrade the extracellular matrix are often also the same factors that participate in the ability of endothelial cells to form new vessels (Ghajar et al. 2008, Hamano et al. 2003), and as such the issue of migration is closely related to the issues of angiogenesis and tumor growth. One study has begun to address this issue and has examined the role of the αVβ3 integrin complex in the invasion and angiogenesis of tumors formed following intracranial implantation of transformed human astrocytes. In these studies, the ability of transformed human astrocytes over-expressing αVβ3 to form invasive, angiogenic tumors was compared to that of cells not over-expressing αVβ3. While the growth of these two cell groups was identical in vitro, intracranially injected cells that over-expressed αVβ3 formed tumors that while still well circumscribed were also smaller and more hypoxic than those in control groups (Kanamori et al. 2004). These results were somewhat surprising, given that αVβ3 is over-expressed at the invading edges of most GBM and is considered to be involved in GBM growth and invasion. Subsequent studies, however, suggested that the growth-suppressive effect of αVβ3 over-expression was bypassed in cells in which Akt was activated or in which VEGF levels were high, as is the case in most GBM (Kanamori et al. 2006, 2004, Kawaguchi et al. 2006). As such these studies suggest that while αVβ3 appears to be growth-suppressive under certain conditions, GBM may override the growth-suppressive actions of αVβ3 over-expression and yet preserve other less defined functions, including those perhaps related to invasion.

9.4 Answers and More Questions

Studies with transformed human astrocytes have proven valuable in verifying the role of suspected genetic alteration in gliomagenesis, in clarifying the role of these genetic lesions, and in beginning to understand how these alterations cooperate to bring about cellular transformation. The studies have also, however, raised questions related to the cell of origin of gliomas, the invasive nature of gliomas, and the differences between mouse and human cells.

Gliomas have long been suspected of initiating in a limited number of cells that, having undergone genetic alteration, gain properties that allow for unlimited growth and/or loss of differentiation potential. The cell of origin of gliomas was initially assumed to be the mature astrocyte as most gliomas have an astrocytic appearance (hence the astrocytoma definition). This concept, however, is being re-examined with the identification of brain tumor stem cells (Galli et al. 2004, Hemmati et al. 2003, Ignatova et al. 2002, Singh et al. 2004). The stem cell hypothesis of gliomagenesis, rather than assuming that gliomas form as a result of an accumulation of genetic alterations in a clonally expanded pool of altered astrocytes, suggests that genetic alteration in a limited number of neural stem cells locks these cells into a state in which self-renewal continues and in which these cells alone retain indefinite/unlimited growth potential against a background of cells that have a more finite capacity (Stiles and Rowitch 2008). Rather than requiring a re-entry into the cell cycle and a dedifferentiation of mature astrocytes, therefore, gliomagenesis in the stem cell hypothesis begins with a cell at or very near the neural stem cell or early along the differentiation pathway. While these two seemingly different concepts seem mutually exclusive, there may be room to accommodate both ideas. Clearly GBMs contain cells, marked by expression of CD133 and other cell surface proteins, that have brain tumor stem cell-like properties including self-renewal and pluripotency and potential for long-term propagation and/or tumor formation (Ogden et al. 2008, Singh et al. 2004). Although the assumption is that the brain tumor stem cells are derived from neural stem cells, it is equally possible (although not yet proven) that self-renewing cells can result from dedifferentiation of fully mature astrocytes. Previously described work with transformed human astrocytes suggests that this might be possible, and further support for the idea has been generated by recent studies suggesting that the expression of a limited number of proteins in fully mature human cells can revert these cells not just back to neural stem cells but all the way back to totipotent stem cells capable of generating any tissue (Park et al. 2008a, b, Takahashi et al. 2007, Yu et al. 2007). It is worth noting, however, that in studies of the transformation of normal human astrocytes, the pool of normal human astrocytes used as starting material may not be as well defined as previously thought. In most cases, the cells used to study events necessary for transformation are human fetal astrocytes grown for a limited amount of time in culture (Rich et al. 2001, Sonoda et al. 2001b). While this starting culture certainly contains mature astrocytes, it also may contain less differentiated cells, and perhaps even a small percentage of cells more closely resembling stem cells. Since the frequency of transformation of human astrocytes following expression of hTERT and inactivation of the p53 and pRb pathways is very low (typically one in a million cells) (Sonoda et al. 2001b), there may also be good reason to think that a very small subset of specialized cells, and not the mature astrocytes, undergo transformation. As such the studies published to date may in fact be studies of the factors necessary to transform stem/progenitor-like cell rather than the factors needed to transform mature astrocytes. Furthermore, while there may in fact be a defined cell or cells of origin for some gliomas, the heterogeneity of the disease suggests that the tumor may arise from multiple starting points. As such the issue of cell of origin remains open and is the focus of intensive study.

A second question raised by the studies of human astrocyte transformation is the basis for the lack of invasive properties of the resultant tumors. As noted, transformed human astrocytes, upon intracranial injection, form encapsulated tumors with well-defined borders, very unlike the invasive gliomas noted in patients. A possible explanation for this difference may be that because of species differences, human cells in general might be incapable of expressing the right set of proteins required for migration through the mouse brain following intracranial implantation. While this idea is supported by the finding that many human GBM cell lines also form encapsulated tumors intracranially, more recent studies suggest that human tumors grown as xenografts in animals without selection in culture do form invasive tumors, as do cells derived from primary tumors and grown as neurospheres (Lee et al. 2006, Sarkaria et al. 2006). These results suggest that human cells can form invasive tumors in rodent brains if they have the correct genetic composition. A related problem, however, is that in studying the factors that control the ability of human cells to move through the mouse brain, one might in fact be studying factors that have little relevance to movement through the human brain. Nonetheless, all cells derived to date from transformation of normal human astrocytes form encapsulated tumors, suggesting either that the alterations necessary for invasion have not been introduced or that the culturing of the starting material has erased the ability of these cells to be invasive. The transformed human astrocytes system therefore may prove very useful in finding the factors required for the ability of transformed cells to move through the brain, although this process may in the end turn out to be more complicated than transformation itself.

A final question raised by transformed astrocyte studies is that of the difference between human and rodent cells with regard to the alterations that result in transformation. In studying the question of gliomagenesis, a primary assumption is the equivalency of mouse and human cells, and the idea that the lesions that drive tumorigenesis in mice are likely to be the same as those that drive transformation in human cells. The studies in human astrocytes however point out that while this in general may be true, there are important differences as well. In what is considered to be mature human astrocytes (with the caveats noted), the genetic alterations necessary for transformation are far fewer and somewhat different than those noted in normal rodent astrocytes. While human astrocytes require hTERT activation and alteration in p53, pRb, and Ras signaling, mouse astrocytes require only Ras alteration and either p53 or pRb alterations (O'Hayer and Counter 2006). Furthermore, while the transformation of normal human astrocytes depends on activation of the Ral arm of the Ras pathway, transformation of mouse astrocytes depends on Raf/MAPK and/or PI3K signaling (Lim et al. 2006, O'Hayer and Counter 2006). While these differences are subtle, they may have significant implications for therapy. As an example, while agents targeting PI3K may be effective in mouse models, they may be less so in human cells. Conversely, agents targeting Ral might make more theoretical sense in the human setting. Many of these issues, however, remain to be rigorously tested, and a more careful examination of Ras signaling pathway requirements in human cells might provide answers as well as new therapeutically relevant ideas.

9.5 New Approaches

While studies in human astrocytes have been extremely informative in our understanding of the events necessary for normal cell transformation, there are as noted some concerns as to the direct relevance of these studies to gliomas and whether normal human astrocytes are a reasonable starting material for the study of gliomagenesis. Fortunately, for the brain tumor field, novel alternative systems have been recently developed that may prove complementary to the systems already used and may help provide more in-depth and potentially more relevant answers to the question of what lesions are most critical in the formation of human brain tumors.

The most exciting of these new systems employs cells which have been designated iPS, or induced pluripotent stem cells. The seminal study in this field was published only last year and showed that fully differentiated mouse fibroblasts could be reverted, or dedifferentiated, into cells that in most ways resembled the pluripotent cells of the early embryo and that have the capability of differentiating into the cell types of the three germ cell layers under the appropriate conditions (Takahashi et al. 2007). These studies identified four factors, Oct4, Sox2, Klf4, and Myc, all previously suggested to be involved in differentiation, which if introduced by viral infection into mouse fibroblasts caused dedifferentiation. These studies were subsequently followed in short order by comparable work from three other groups which showed that the same trick could be accomplished in human cells as well (Park et al. 2008a, b, Yu et al. 2007). Furthermore, the results of these studies were remarkably similar to those in the mouse cells. In each case, Oct4 and Sox2 were required, while in one study Klf4 and MYC could be replaced by NANOG and LIN28, the latter subsequently shown not to be absolutely required (Yu et al. 2007). The simplicity and elegance of the system, as well as the magic number of four alterations needed to create a cell of unlimited growth potential, harkens back to the transformation studies of Hahn and Weinberg nearly a decade earlier (Hahn et al. 1999). The key difference, however, and the difference that could prove most interesting in the long run, is that the iPS cells derived are apparently devoid of lineage and under proper conditions can be pushed down any lineage, including those presumably most relevant for brain development. Early brain development requires an ordered series of proliferation and differentiation events, and the iPS system, combined with the vast amount of knowledge concerning differentiation of neural stem cells, suggests that in the near future it may be possible to recapitulate the path from stem cell to glia in vitro. As an example, the involvement of the leukemia inhibitory factor-STAT signaling axis in the astrocytic differentiation of neural stem cells has recently been the focus of several investigations (Lee et al. 2008, Singh et al. 2008), and it is possible to envision an in vitro system in which disruption of any of several components of this pathway could result in the lack of ability of the neural stem cell to differentiate down the glial lineage and to rather be stuck in a poorly regulated self-renewing loop. The connection of these stalled stem cells to cancer is obvious, and the demonstration that such cells were tumorigenic in the right set of circumstances could bring the debate about the origin of gliomas full circle. The dedifferentiation of normal cells (including possibly astrocytes) could result in self-renewing cells which if altered in specific ways could give rise to a range of brain tumors. There are of course limitations to this system as well. First, while normal human cells can be dedifferentiated, multiple alterations are necessary and the frequency of dedifferentiation is nearly as small as transformation (Sonoda et al. 2001b, Yu et al. 2007). Additionally the generation of iPS cells still relies on the use of viral delivery of agents, raising the possibility that integration-induced alterations, in addition to transcription factors, are necessary. The potentially large number of alterations necessary for dedifferentiation in combination with the large numbers of lesions necessary for transformation suggests that nature may employ a simpler means to the same end, and as such it remains to be seen if the cell of origin of glioma is the mature astrocyte or the neural stem cells (Fig. 9.3). The elegant iPS systems that are evolving should, however, be able to shine new light on this question and on the issue of gliomagenesis.

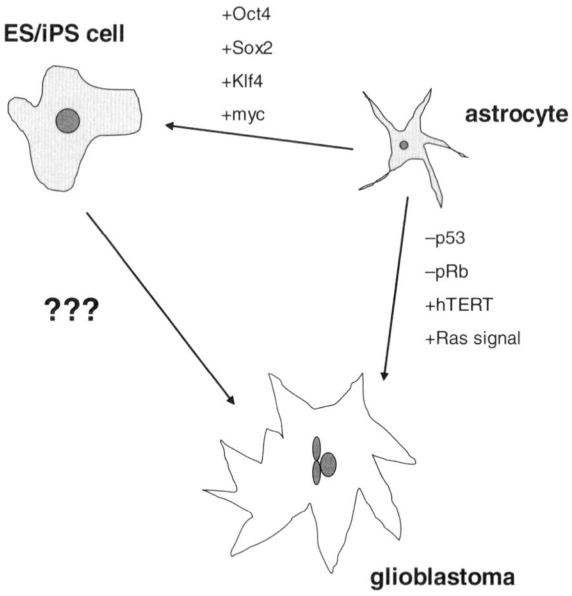

Fig. 9.3 Multiple possible routes to the development of GBM. Defined factors have been identified that can convert normal human cells into GBM or stem cells with unlimited self-renewal and differentiation potential. The factors that may influence the ability of stem cells to normally differentiate and self-renew (and which may be involved in aberrant self-renewal and gliomagenesis) are only beginning to be identified

9.6 Conclusions

Our knowledge of gliomagenesis has grown dramatically over the past 10 years, and in combination with new and powerful techniques to characterize and identify ever smaller genetic alterations, new techniques have also been developed to study the relevance of these lesions to the process. While elegant mouse models which can target genetic alterations in time and space have replaced coarser approaches, the need to connect findings to the human condition is as great as ever. The use of defined human cells systems to study the alterations and pathways required for human cell transformation has nicely complemented work in other systems and has not only verified the importance of pathways suggested to be involved in gliomagenesis but also implicated other novel human-specific pathways that if targeted appropriately may improve therapy for glioma. The advent of even more powerful human cell systems promises to not only provide new starting material to investigators but also allow investigators to seamlessly take cells of varying degrees of differentiation through the presumed steps of gliomagenesis, at each stage testing their ideas in a rigorous, elegant, and therapeutically important manner. The study of the factors contributing to human cell transformation and gliomagenesis therefore seems poised for a new round of discovery.

Abbreviations

GBM	glioblastoma multiforme
EGFR	epidermal growth factor receptor
hTERT	the catalytic component of human telomerase
PI3K	phosphoinositol-3 kinase
mTOR	mammalian target of rapamycin
LGG	low-grade glioma
SPARC	secreted protein acidic, rich in cysteine
VEGF	vascular endothelial growth factor
iPS	induced pluripotent stem cells

Acknowledgments I thank Yukihiko Sonoda, Masayuki Kanamori, and Jean Nakamura for their contributions to this work. This work was supported in part by NIH grants CA CA097257, CA100011, and CA115638.

References

Arjona D, Rey JA, and Taylor SM (2006) Early genetic changes involved in low-grade astrocytic tumor development. Curr Mol Med 6(6):645–50.

Bello L, Francolini M, Marthyn P, et al. (2001) Alpha(v)beta3 and alpha(v)beta5 integrin expression in glioma periphery. Neurosurgery 49(2):380–9; discussion 390.

Berenblum I and Shubik P (1949) The persistence of latent tumour cells induced in the mouse's skin by a single application of 9:10-dimethyl-1:2-benzanthracene. Br J Cancer 3(3):384–6.

Brockman WW (1978) Transformation of BALB/c-3T3 cells by tsA mutants of simian virus 40: temperature sensitivity of the transformed phenotype and retransformation by wild-type virus. J Virol 25(3):860–70.

Burger PC, Shibata T, and Kleihues P (1986) The use of the monoclonal antibody Ki-67 in the identification of proliferating cells: application to surgical neuropathology. Am J Surg Pathol 10(9):611–7.

Chatterjee S, Matsumura A, Schradermeier J, et al. (2000) Human malignant glioma therapy using anti-alpha(v)beta3 integrin agents. J Neurooncol 46(2):135–44.
Chin L and Gray JW (2008) Translating insights from the cancer genome into clinical practice. Nature 452(7187):553–63.
Evans MJ and Kaufman MH (1981) Establishment in culture of pluripotential cells from mouse embryos. Nature 292(5819):154–6.
Fanton CP,McMahon M, and Pieper RO (2001) Dual growth arrest pathways in astrocytes and astrocytic tumors in response to Raf-1 activation. J Biol Chem 276(22):18871–7.
Fomchenko EI and Holland EC (2006) Mouse models of brain tumors and their applications in preclinical trials. Clin Cancer Res 12(18):5288–97.
Furnari FB, Fenton T, Bachoo RM, et al. (2007) Malignant astrocytic glioma: genetics, biology, and paths to treatment. Genes Dev 21(21):2683–710.
Galli R, Binda E, Orfanelli U, et al. (2004) Isolation and characterization of tumorigenic, stem-like neural precursors from human glioblastoma. Cancer Res 64(19):7011–21.
Ghajar CM, George SC, and Putnam AJ (2008) Matrix metalloproteinase control of capillary morphogenesis. Crit Rev Eukaryot Gene Expr 18(3):251–78.
Gilbert MR and Lang FF (2007) Management of patients with low-grade gliomas.Neurol Clin 25(4):1073–88, ix.
Greider CW and Blackburn EH (1985) Identification of a specific telomere terminal transferase activity in Tetrahymena extracts. Cell 43(2 Pt 1):405–13.
Greider CW and Blackburn EH (1996) Telomeres, telomerase and cancer. Sci Am 274(2):92–7.
Hahn WC, Counter CM, Lundberg AS, et al. (1999) Creation of human tumour cells with defined genetic elements. Nature 400(6743):464–8.
Hamad NM, Elconin JH, Karnoub AE, et al. (2002) Distinct requirements for Ras oncogenesis in human versus mouse cells. Genes Dev 16(16):2045–57.
Hamano Y, Zeisberg M, Sugimoto H, et al. (2003) Physiological levels of tumstatin, a fragment of collagen IV alpha3 chain, are generated by MMP-9 proteolysis and suppress angiogenesis via alphaV beta3 integrin. Cancer Cell 3(6):589–601.
Hemmati HD, Nakano I, Lazareff JA, et al. (2003) Cancerous stem cells can arise from pediatric brain tumors. Proc Natl Acad Sci USA 100(25):15178–83.
Holland EC, Celestino J, Dai C, et al. (2000) Combined activation of Ras and Akt in neural progenitors induces glioblastoma formation in mice. Nat Genet 25(1):55–7.
Ichimura K, Bolin MB, Goike HM, et al. (2000) Deregulation of the p14ARF/MDM2/p53 pathway is a prerequisite for human astrocytic gliomas with G1-S transition control gene abnormalities. Cancer Res 60(2):417–24.
Ichimura K, Ohgaki H, Kleihues P, et al. (2004) Molecular pathogenesis of astrocytic tumours. J Neurooncol 70(2):137–60.
Ignatova TN, Kukekov VG, Laywell ED, et al. (2002) Human cortical glial tumors contain neural stem-like cells expressing astroglial and neuronal markers in vitro. Glia 39(3):193–206.
Kanamori M, Vanden Berg SR, Bergers G, et al. (2004) Integrin beta3 overexpression suppresses tumor growth in a human model of gliomagenesis: implications for the role of beta3 overexpression in glioblastoma multiforme. Cancer Res 64(8):2751–8.
Kanamori M, Kawaguchi T, Berger MS, et al. (2006) Intracranial microenvironment reveals independent opposing functions of host alphaVbeta3 expression on glioma growth and angiogenesis. J Biol Chem 281(48):37256–64.
Kawaguchi T, Yamashita Y, Kanamori M, et al. (2006) The PTEN/Akt pathway dictates the direct alphaVbeta3-dependent growth-inhibitory action of an active fragment of tumstatin in glioma cells in vitro and in vivo. Cancer Res 66(23):11331–40.
Kipling D (1997) Telomere structure and telomerase expression during mouse development and tumorigenesis. Eur J Cancer 33(5):792–800.
Koestner A, Swenberg JA, and Wechsler W (1971) Transplacental production with ethylnitrosourea of neoplasms of the nervous system in Sprague–Dawley rats. Am J Pathol 63(1):37–56.

Lang FF, Miller DC, Koslow M, et al. (1994) Pathways leading to glioblastoma multiforme: a molecular analysis of genetic alterations in 65 astrocytic tumors. J Neurosurg 81(3):427–36.
Le S, Zhu JJ, Anthony DC, et al. (1998) Telomerase activity in human gliomas. Neurosurgery 42(5):1120–4; discussion 1124–5.
Lee J, Kotliarova S, Kotliarov Y, et al. (2006) Tumor stem cells derived from glioblastomas cultured in bFGF and EGF more closely mirror the phenotype and genotype of primary tumors than do serum-cultured cell lines. Cancer Cell 9(5):391–403.
Lee J, Son MJ, Woolard K, et al. (2008) Epigenetic-mediated dysfunction of the bone morphogenetic protein pathway inhibits differentiation of glioblastoma-initiating cells. Cancer Cell 13(1):69–80.
Lim KH, Baines AT, Fiordalisi JJ, et al. (2005) Activation of RalA is critical for Ras-induced tumorigenesis of human cells. Cancer Cell 7(6):533–45.
Lim KH, O'Hayer K, Adam SJ, et al. (2006) Divergent roles for RalA and RalB in malignant growth of human pancreatic carcinoma cells. Curr Biol 16(24):2385–94.
Maeshima Y, Colorado PC, Torre A, et al. (2000) Distinct antitumor properties of a type IV collagen domain derived from basement membrane. J Biol Chem 275(28):21340–8.
Martin GR (1981) Isolation of a pluripotent cell line from early mouse embryos cultured in medium conditioned by teratocarcinoma stem cells. Proc Natl Acad Sci USA 78(12):7634–8.
Nakamura JL, Garcia E, and Pieper RO (2008) S6K1 plays a key role in glial transformation. Cancer Res 68(16):6516–23.
O'Hayer KM and Counter CM (2006) A genetically defined normal human somatic cell system to study ras oncogenesis in vivo and in vitro. Methods Enzymol 407:637–47.
O'Reilly MS, Holmgren L, Shing Y, et al. (1994) Angiostatin: a novel angiogenesis inhibitor that mediates the suppression of metastases by a Lewis lung carcinoma. Cell 79(2):315–28.
Ogden AT, Waziri AE, Lochhead RA, et al. (2008) Identification of A2B5 + CD133- tumor-initiating cells in adult human gliomas. Neurosurgery 62(2):505–14; discussion 514–5.
Panner A, Nakamura JL, Parsa AT, et al. (2006) mTOR-independent translational control of the extrinsic cell death pathway by RalA. Mol Cell Biol 26(20):7345–57.
Park IH, Arora N, Huo H, et al. (2008a) Disease-specific induced pluripotent stem cells. Cell.
Park IH, Zhao R, West JA, et al. (2008b) Reprogramming of human somatic cells to pluripotency with defined factors. Nature 451(7175):141–6.
Rich JN, Guo C, McLendon RE, et al. (2001) A genetically tractable model of human glioma formation. Cancer Res 61(9):3556–60.
Rous P and Friedewald WF (1941) The carcinogenic effect of methylcholanthrene and of tar on rabbit papillomas due to a virus. Science 94(2447):495–6.
Sarkaria JN, Carlson BL, Schroeder MA, et al. (2006) Use of an orthotopic xenograft model for assessing the effect of epidermal growth factor receptor amplification on glioblastoma radiation response. Clin Cancer Res 12(7 Pt 1):2264–71.
Shi Q, Bao S, Maxwell JA, et al. (2004) Secreted protein acidic, rich in cysteine (SPARC), mediates cellular survival of gliomas through AKT activation. J Biol Chem 279(50):52200–9.
Singh SK, Hawkins C, Clarke ID, et al. (2004) Identification of human brain tumour initiating cells. Nature 432(7015):396–401.
Singh SK, Kagalwala MN, Parker-Thornburg J, et al. (2008) REST maintains self-renewal and pluripotency of embryonic stem cells. Nature 453(7192):223–7.
Sonoda Y, Ozawa T, Aldape KD, et al. (2001a) Akt pathway activation converts anaplastic astrocytoma to glioblastoma multiforme in a human astrocyte model of glioma. Cancer Res 61(18):6674–8.
Sonoda Y, Ozawa T, Hirose Y, et al. (2001b) Formation of intracranial tumors by genetically modified human astrocytes defines four pathways critical in the development of human anaplastic astrocytoma. Cancer Res 61(13):4956–60.
Sonoda Y, Kanamori M, Deen DF, et al. (2003) Overexpression of vascular endothelial growth factor isoforms drives oxygenation and growth but not progression to glioblastoma multiforme in a human model of gliomagenesis. Cancer Res 63(8):1962–8.

Stevenson M and Volsky DJ (1986) Activated v-myc and v-ras oncogenes do not transform normal human lymphocytes. Mol Cell Biol 6(10):3410–7.
Stiles CD and Rowitch DH (2008) Glioma stem cells: a midterm exam. Neuron 58(6):832–46.
Takahashi K, Tanabe K, Ohnuki M, et al. (2007) Induction of pluripotent stem cells from adult human fibroblasts by defined factors. Cell 131(5):861–72.
Todaro GJ and Green H (1963) Quantitative studies of the growth of mouse embryo cells in culture and their development into established lines. J Cell Biol 17:299–313.
Yu J, Vodyanik MA, Smuga-Otto K, et al. (2007) Induced pluripotent stem cell lines derived from human somatic cells. Science 318(5858):1917–20.
Zhu J, Wang H, Bishop JM, et al. (1999) Telomerase extends the lifespan of virus-transformed human cells without net telomere lengthening. Proc Natl Acad Sci USA 96(7):3723–8.

Chapter 10
Rat Glioma Models for Preclinical Evaluation of Novel Therapeutic and Diagnostic Modalities

Balveen Kaur and Rolf F. Barth

Abstract In this chapter we review eight commonly used rat brain tumor models and their application for the development of novel therapeutic and diagnostic modalities. The first three tumors that we will discuss were induced by repeated injections of methylnitrosourea (MNU) to adult rats. The 9L gliosarcoma has been widely used and has provided important information relating to brain tumor biology and therapy. The T9 glioma, although not generally recognized, was and probably still is the same as 9L. Both of these tumors arose in Fischer rats and can be immunogenic in syngeneic rats. This must be taken into consideration when used in therapy studies, especially if survival is the endpoint. The C6 glioma has been used extensively for a variety of studies, but since it arose in an outbred Wistar rat, it is not syngeneic to any inbred strain, and its potential to evoke an alloimmune response is a serious limitation. The F98 and RG2 (D74) gliomas were both chemically induced by administering ethylnitrosourea (ENU) to pregnant rats, the progeny of which developed brain tumors. They are either weakly immunogenic or non-immunogenic and have an invasive pattern of growth and uniform lethality. This makes them particularly attractive models to test new therapeutic modalities. The avian sarcoma virus-induced tumors, and a continuous cell line derived from one of them designated RT-2, have been useful for studies in which de novo tumor induction is an important requirement. These tumors are also immunogenic and this limits their usefulness for therapy studies. The CNS-1 was induced by administering MNU to a Lewis rat. It has an infiltrative pattern of growth and is weakly immunogenic, which should make it useful in experimental neuro-oncology. Finally, the BT4C was induced by administering ENU to a BDIX rat, following which brain cells were propagated in vitro until a tumorigenic clone was isolated. This tumor has been used for a variety of studies to evaluate new therapeutic modalities. It is essential to recognize,

---

R.F. Barth (✉)
Department of Pathology, The Ohio State University, 165 Hamilton Hall, 1645 Neil Avenue, Columbus, OH 43210, USA
e-mail: rolf.barth@osumc.edu

E.G. Van Meir (ed.), *CNS Cancer*, Cancer Drug Discovery and Development, DOI 10.1007/978-1-60327-553-8_10,
© Humana Press, a part of Springer Science+Business Media, LLC 2009

however, the limitations of each of the models that have been described, and depending upon the nature of the study to be conducted, it is important that the appropriate model be selected.

Contents

10.1 Introduction

There is a major need in experimental neuro-oncology for animal models that can be used to assess the efficacy of innovative approaches for the diagnosis and treatment of brain tumors. The rat has been one of the most widely used experimental animals, and rat brain tumor models have been used extensively since the mid-1970s. This chapter will selectively focus on rat brain tumor models and their utility in evaluating the efficacy of various therapeutic modalities. Murine, feline, and canine models have been used less frequently (Gutmann 2009, Fomchenko and Holland 2006, Kimmelman and Nalbantoglu 2007, Krushelnycky et al. 1991) and are discussed in other chapters. It was first reported in the early 1970s that central nervous system tumors could be induced reproducibly and selectively in adult rats that had been given repeated weekly intravenous injections of *N*-methylnitrosourea (MNU) or a single dose of *N*-ethyl-*N*-nitrosourea (ENU) (Barth 1998) (see also Chapter 11). These studies led to the development of a number of rat brain tumor models that were highly reproducible and did not require the topical application of a chemical carcinogen to the brain. In this chapter, we will summarize some general principles relating to the use of brain tumor models. Xenograft models based on the intracerebral (i.c.) transplantation of human brain tumors into immunologically deficient rodents are discussed separately (see Chapters 8 and 9). However, it is most important to recognize that no currently available animal tumor model exactly simulates human high-grade brain tumors such as glioblastoma multiforme (GBM) or anaplastic astrocytomas (WHO grade III).

The cellular signaling pathways important for the genesis of brain tumor are multiple, with feedback mechanisms that can dramatically affect the efficacy of molecularly targeted therapeutic strategies. The heterogeneous composition of human high-grade gliomas, which consists of tumor stem cells and differentiated tumor cells with varying characteristics, further complicates their susceptibility to treatment. Brain tumors can also evolve within their microenvironment, adapting to changes that produce epigenetic effects, thereby altering their biology, but concomitantly providing additional targets for therapeutic intervention. Finally, genetic variations between individuals can dictate how tumors initiate, progress, and respond to treatment. Rat brain tumor models have provided a wealth of information on the in vitro and in vivo responses to various therapeutic modalities (see Table 10.1 for a comparison of utility of mouse glioma models with rat models of glioma). The larger rat brain compared to that of the mouse facilitates more precise tumor cell implantation and allows for relatively larger volume (15 μl) that can be injected versus mice (5 μl) (Table 10.1). They have allowed researchers to rigorously test hypotheses developed from examining human tumors by genetically manipulating them

Table 10.1 Advantages and disadvantages of rat brain tumor models compared to mouse models

Advantages	Disadvantages
1. Larger size of the rat brain permits more precise stereotactic implantation than in mice, a longer interval of time until death and a thicker skull essentially eliminates osseous invasion and subcutaneous (s.c.) growth	1. Rat brain tumor models cannot be as easily genetically engineered and manipulated as mouse models in order to elucidate the importance of genetic factors, signaling pathways, cell types, and stroma in tumor growth and invasion
2. Larger tumor size prior to death permits better in vivo localization and imaging by a variety of diagnostic modalities in the rat	2. The potential to produce genetically engineered tumor cell lines is less in the rat than in the mouse
3. Larger tumor size permits the administration of larger amounts of various therapeutic agents, especially if administered intracerebrally (i.c.) by convection enhanced delivery (CED), and more critical evaluation of their effectiveness	3. There are a smaller number of mAbs directed against rat surface antigens and chemokines compared to the mouse
4. More extensive literature on in vitro and in vivo studies of rat brain tumors compared to mouse tumors	4. Rats are more expensive to purchase and maintain than mice

and controlling specific variables such as environmental influences, in order to better understand the roles of different pathways, cell types, stromal factors, and genetic variation (Reilly et al. 2008). Mouse tumor models have also allowed researchers to test hypotheses derived from examining human tumors, in a controlled environment with specific genetic alterations and controlled environmental influences (Reilly et al. 2008).

There is a general consensus that valid brain tumor models should fulfill the following criteria: (1) they should be derived from glial cells; (2) it should be possible to grow and clone them in vitro as continuous cell lines and propagate them in vivo by serial transplantation; (3) tumor growth rates should be

Table 10.2 Comparison of various rat tumor models

Tumor	Strain of origin/ Haplotype*	Mode of tumor induction†	Minimum i.c. inoculum	Immuno genicity	Pattern of growth	Molecular markers	Original reference
9L	Fischer/ $RT1^{lvl}$	MNU	10^4	Strong	Circumscribed	Mutant *p53*, increased expression of *TGFα* and *EGFR*; decreased expression of *FGF-2*, *FGF-9*, *FGFR-1*, and *PDGFRβ*	Benda et al. (1971)
T9	Fischer/ $RT1^{lvl}$	MNU	10^4	Strong	Circumscribed	Presumably similar to 9L	Benda et al. (1971)
C6**	Outbred Wistar	MNU	10^4	Strong	Circumscribed	Deletion of *p16/CDkn2a/ Ink4a;* no expression of *p16* and *p19ARF* mRNAs or of wildtype *p53*; increased expression of *PDGFβ*, *IGF-1*, *EGFR*, and *ErbB3/HER3* precursor proteins, decreased expression of *EGF-9* and *10, and IGF-II* genes	Benda et al. (1971)
F98	Fischer/ $RT1^{lvl}$	ENU	10^1–10^2	Weak	Infiltrative	Deletion of p16/Cdkn2a/Ink4a gene; increased expression of *PDGFβ*, *Ras*, *EGFR*, *cyclin D1*, and *cyclin D2*	Ko et al. (1980)
RG2 (D74)	Fischer/ $RT1^{lvl}$	ENU	10^1–10^2	Weak	Infiltrative	Deletion of p16/Cdkn2a/Ink4a gene; increased expression of *PDGFβ*, *IGF-1*, *Ras*, and *Erb3/HER3* precursor mRNA, and *cyclin D2*	Ko et al. (1980)
CNS-1	Lewis/$RT1^{lvl}$	MNU	5 x 10^3	Weak	Infiltrative	Expression of vimentin	Kruse et al. (1994)
BT4C	BDIX/$RT1^{dvl}$	ENU	10^4	Weak	Infiltrative	Expression of VEGF, tPA, uPA and MVD	Laerum et al. (1975)

*The haplotype information was kindly provided by Dr. Carol Kruse, Sidney Kimmel Cancer Center, San Diego, CA.
**C6 cells express $RT1^u$, a haplotype of inbred Wistar-Furth rats (Beutler AS et al., Human Gene Ther 10:95–101, 1999).
†Abbreviations: MNU: methylnitrosourea; ENU: N-ethyl-N-nitrosourea.

predictable and reproducible; (4) the tumors should have glioma-like growth characteristics within the brain, including neovascularization, alteration of the blood–brain barrier (BBB), an invasive pattern of growth, and lack of encapsulation; (5) host survival time following i.c. tumor implantation should be of sufficient duration to permit therapy and determination of efficacy; (6) for therapy studies, the tumors should be either non- or weakly immunogenic in syngeneic hosts; (7) they should not grow into the epidural space or extend beyond the brain; and finally, (8) their response or lack thereof to conventional treatment should be predictive of the response in human brain tumors.

In studies carried out prior to the 1970s, either cells or tumor fragments were injected i.c. using a free hand approach, which generally lacked reproducibility and precision. A stereotactic implantation procedure using suspensions of tissue culture-derived brain tumor cells was more successful (Barker et al. 1973). This procedure was further improved by the use of concentrated cell suspensions in small volumes, improved injection needles, better stereotactic localization to structures deeper in the white matter such as the caudate nucleus, the use of slower injection rates (Kobayashi et al. 1980), 0.5–1.0% low gelling agarose to prevent backflow of tumor cells through the injection track (Kobayashi et al. 1980), and cleansing of the operative field with a solution of Betadine. Finally, rinsing the surface of the brain with sterile water, which destroys extravasated tumor cells, by osmosis prior to closure of the skull with bone wax has also been recommended (Landen et al. 2004). This implantation procedure results in high success rates of i.c. tumor growth with the elimination of spinal and extra cranial dissemination. The implantation of plastic (Kobayashi et al. 1980) or metallic screws (Lal et al. 2000) with an entry port, which are permanently implanted in the skull to inject tumor cells, has been very useful (Lal et al. 2000, Saini et al. 2004). Such devices can be left in place either at the time of or after tumor cell implantation in order to facilitate future administration of therapeutic agents at the same location without further stereotactic surgery. These are well tolerated and non-irritating in rats, but they cannot be used as easily in mice due to the thinness of their skulls (Saini et al. 2004). Keeping these general principles of tumor cell implantation in mind, we will now discuss the currently available rat glioma models that have been used in immunocompetent animals.

10.2 9L Gliosarcoma

The 9L gliosarcoma has been the most widely used experimental rat brain tumor model. It was produced by the intravenous injection of 5 mg/kg of MNU for 26 weeks in Fisher 344 rats (Benda et al. 1971, Schmidek et al. 1971). The original tumor was designated as tumor #9, which subsequently was cloned at the Brain Tumor Research Center, University of California, San Francisco, and was then designated "9L" (Barker et al. 1973, Benda et al. 1971)

(Schmidek et al. 1971). These tumor cells could be propagated in vitro, which made them very useful for in vivo studies to investigate the effects of various therapeutic modalities on brain tumors. The 9L cells can be implanted i.c. into syngeneic Fischer rats, following which they give rise to rapidly growing tumors. These are composed of spindle-shaped cells with a sarcomatoid appearance. The tumor margins are sharply delineated with little obvious invasion into the contiguous normal brain (Fig. 10.1A and Color Plate 16). The 9L gliosarcoma has a mutant *p53* gene (Asai et al. 1994), but there is normal expression of

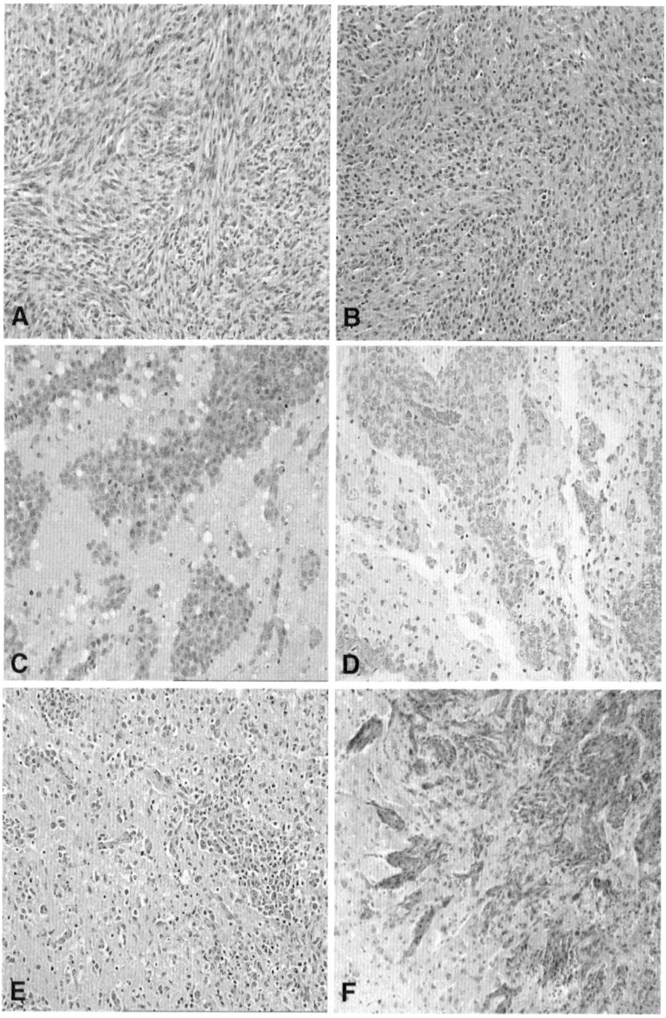

Fig. 10.1 Histopathologic features of the C6, 9L, RG2, F98, CNS-1, and BT4C brain tumors. **A.** The C6 glioma is composed of a pleomorphic population of cells with nuclei ranging from round to oblong. A herringbone pattern of growth is seen in some areas and there is focal

p16 and *p19ARF* mRNAs, indicating that there is a wildtype *p16/Cdkn2a/Ink4α* locus (Schlegel et al. 1999). Molecular characterization of the 9L, relative to rat stem cell-derived astrocytes, revealed an increased expression of the genes encoding TGFα and its receptor, EGFR (Sibenaller et al. 2005). Interestingly, decreased expression of *FGF-2, FGF-9*, *FGFR-1*, and *PDGFRβ* was also noted (Sibenaller et al. 2005). Recently, cancer stem-like cells (CSLCs) have been demonstrated in the 9L cell line. These CSLCs grow as neurospheres in chemically defined medium and express the neural stem cell markers Nestin and Sox2. They are self-renewable and differentiate in vitro into neuron- and glial-like cells (Ghods et al. 2007). The neurospheres have a lower proliferation rate and express several anti-apoptotic and drug-related genes. Furthermore, these cells form tumors that are more aggressive than the parental 9L tumor (Ghods et al. 2007), which could be an important property in future studies.

The 9L gliosarcoma model has been used extensively to investigate mechanisms and development of drug resistance (Barcellos-Hoff et al. 1992, Schepkin et al. 2006), transport of drugs across the blood–brain and blood–tumor barriers (Black et al. 2008, Fross et al. 1991, Khan et al. 2005, Warnke et al. 1987), imaging of brain tumors including radiological techniques such as magnetic resonance imaging (MRI) and positron emission tomography (PET) and imaging to evaluate tumor hypoxia and metabolism (Bansal et al. 2008, Yuan et al. 2006), pharmacokinetic studies of nitrosourea (Warnke et al. 1987),

Fig. 10.1 (continued) invasion of contiguous normal brain. There are scattered foci of necrosis with pseudo-palisading of tumor cells at the periphery. **B.** The 9L gliosarcoma is composed of spindle-shaped cells with a sarcomatoid appearance. A whorled pattern of growth is seen with sharp delineation of the margins of the tumor with little invasion of contiguous normal brain. **C.** The RG2 glioma is very similar in appearance to the F98 glioma and also has a highly invasive pattern of growth. **D.** The F98 glioma is composed of a mixed population of spindle-shaped cells with fusiform nuclei, frequently forming a whorled pattern of growth, and a smaller subpopulation of polygonal cells with round to oval nuclei. There is extensive invasion of contiguous normal brain with islands of tumor cells at varying distances from the main tumor mass, which form perivascular clusters. Usually, there is a central area of necrosis filled with tumor cell ghosts. **E.** The CNS-1 glioma is composed of a pleomorphic population of cells that show great variation in size and shape. There is extensive invasion of contiguous normal brain with dense infiltrates in some areas and in others, more circumscribed clusters of tumor cells. Small foci of hemorrhage are scattered through the tumor. **F.** The BT4C glioma is composed of a pleomorphic population of tumor cells with a sarcomatous pattern of growth. Scattered tumor giant cells are seen and mitotic figures are frequent. The tumor grows expansively and invades the surrounding normal brain along perivascular tracts and occasional tumor cell nests are seen in the surrounding normal brain. There is neo-vascularization, especially in the tumor periphery, where microhemorrhages are frequent. Central necrosis is usually not present but occasionally scattered areas of necrosis may be seen in larger tumors. (Photomicrograph of the BT4C was kindly provided by M. Sandström and description by M. Johansson and representative microscopic slides of the CNS-1 glioma were kindly provided by Dr. Carol Kruse.) All photomicrographs are at a magnification of 200×, except for F. (*see* Color Plate 16) mechanisms and effects of anti-angiogenic drugs (Wolff et al. 1997, Yang et al. 2007), effects of radiation (Regnard et al. 2008), chemotherapy (Bencokova et al. 2008, Donawho et al. 2007), gene therapy (Barba et al. 1993, Iwadate et al. 2005, Kumar et al. 2008, Miletic et al. 2007), cancer stem cells (Ghods et al. 2007), immunotoxin treatment (Chignola et al. 1995), immunotherapy and cytokine therapy (Iwadate et al. 2005, Liu et al. 2007), and oncolytic viral therapy (Aghi et al. 1999, Madara et al. 2005).

A number of these studies have yielded impressive therapeutic results, including apparent cures of tumor-bearing animals. *However, it must be noted that this tumor has been shown to be highly immunogenic.* Animals immunized with X-irradiated 9L cells were resistant to both s.c. and i.c. tumor challenges, compared to 100% tumor takes in immunologically naïve animals (Blume et al. 1974). This report was first published in the proceedings of a meeting, which did not receive wide circulation, but subsequent studies have confirmed the immunogenicity of this model (Denlinger et al. 1975, Morantz et al. 1979). Expression of the *s-Myc* gene under the control of a CMV promotor resulted in complete suppression of 9L tumor growth as well as rejection of subsequent challenges of tumor cells. Histological examination of tumors after s-*Myc* therapy revealed massive mononuclear cell infiltration with CD8+ T lymphocytes, which accounted for >70% of these infiltrating cells. These observations suggested that tumor rejection was due to a potent T-cell-mediated anti-tumor immune response (Asai et al. 1994). This and several more recent studies have underscored the significance of the anti-tumor immune response following gene therapy-induced tumor eradication observed with 9L model. It is now recognized that the in vivo bystander cell killing (Chen et al. 1995), which has been observed with the 9L gliosarcoma following delivery of the Herpes simplex virus thymidine kinase gene (HSV-TK) (Aghi et al. 1999, Moolten 1986), followed by treatment with ganciclovir was due in part to an anti-tumor immune response. The highly immunogenic nature of 9L glioma must be kept in perspective when utilizing this model to evaluate therapeutic efficacy of novel therapeutic agents. Early studies employing radiation or chemotherapy alone were largely unsuccessful in curing the 9L tumor. However, the success obtained by boron neutron capture therapy and gene therapy highlights the significance of utilizing anti-tumor treatments that can destroy individual cancer cells and simultaneously spare the host immune cells to evoke a successful anti-tumor immune response (Coderre et al. 1994, Moriuchi et al. 2002, Namba et al. 2000, Smilowitz et al. 2000).

Despite the fact that the 9L arose in a Fischer rat, 9L gliosarcoma cells can also form i.c. tumors in allogeneic Wistar rats (Stojiljkovic et al. 2003). Histopathological evaluation revealed these tumors formed circumscribed masses that were not infiltrative and did not spread into the subarachnoid space or ventricles (Stojiljkovic et al. 2003). Immunostaining of the tumors revealed the presence of glial fibrillary acidic protein (GFAP) positive infiltrating astrocytic cells, and activated ED1 immunoreactive macrophages/microglia (Stojiljkovic et al. 2003). Higher numbers of K(ATP) and K(Ca) channels have been observed in 9L tumors grown in allogeneic Wistar rats compared to those grown in syngeneic Fischer rats. Furthermore, the allogeneic tumors showed a greater increase in brain tumor permeability upon treatment with potassium channel agonists, compared to those grown in syngeneic hosts (Black et al. 2008). The 9L tumor model has also been used following treatment to study the effect of blood brain barrier (BBB) disruption (Black et al. 2008), implantation of devices for repeated intratumoral delivery (Saini et al. 2004), and imaging (Bhattacharya et al. 2007). *Due to its potential to evoke a strong anti-tumor immune response, even in syngeneic Fischer rats, caution must be exercised in interpreting therapeutic efficacy when the 9L model is used.*

The 9L glioma–sarcoma model has also been used to develop a model for brainstem tumors (Jallo et al. 2006). Progression to hemiparesis with the onset of symptoms occurred 17 days post-implantation into the brainstem. This model was also used to evaluate the efficacy of CED of carboplatin to the brainstem (Jallo et al. 2006) and to study the response of recurrent, chemo-resistant gliomas. Two bis-chloroethyl nitrosourea (BCNU)-resistant cell lines were derived from 9L cells by treating them with BCNU in vitro or in vivo. Both of these cell lines formed tumors in a 100% of the animals following i.c. implantation, and were much more invasive than the parental 9L cells (Saito et al. 2004). The 9L gliosarcoma has also been used as a model to evaluate drug-resistant and -invasive recurrent gliomas (Schepkin et al. 2006), but as indicated above, caution must be used in evaluating results obtained with such a highly immunogenic tumor.

10.3 T9 Glioma

Although not fully appreciated, the T9 glioma was at one time, and may still be, the same as the 9L gliosarcoma (Barth 1998). The original stock of T9 cells was obtained from Sweet's laboratory at the Massachusetts General Hospital (MGH) by Denlinger and Koestner, and it was renamed T9 by them (Denlinger et al. 1975). Similar to the immunogenicity of the 9L gliosarcoma (Blume et al. 1974), the T9 glioma was also found to be highly immunogenic (Denlinger et al. 1975). Kida et al. found that immunization of rats with irradiated T9 cells or T9 cells mixed with *Cryptosporidium parvum* rejected subsequent s.c. implants of T9 glioma cells (Kida et al. 1983). However, in order to immunize against intracranial tumors, rats initially had to reject intradermal T9 cells (Kida et al. 1983). As might have been predicted, these results indicated that, similar to the 9L gliosarcoma, the T9 glioma was also immunogenic. The T9 cell line subsequently has been shared among numerous investigators and has been used for many studies, including the evaluation of anti-angiogenic (Jeffes et al. 2005) and chemotherapeutic agents (Pietronigro et al. 2003), immunotherapy (Shibuya et al. 1984), and gene therapy with interferon-β (Harada et al. 1995). Although tumor-specific or tumor-associated antigens have yet to be identified, for the 9L gliosarcoma and T9 glioma, it is only a matter of time before they are identified.

10.4 C6 Glioma

The C6 glioma was another tumor produced by Benda et al. (1971) and Schmidek et al. (1971), in Sweet's laboratory at the MGH by repetitively administering MNU to outbred Wistar rats over a period of approximately 8 months. When animals developed neurological signs, they were euthanized, and the tumors were excised and explanted into tissue culture. Among these was a tumor designated as "#6", which subsequently was cloned by Benda et al. (1968) and was shown to produce S-100 protein. Following cloning, it was re-designated "C6" (Pfeiffer et al. 1970). The C6 glioma is composed of a pleomorphic population of cells with variably shaped nuclei. There is focal invasion into contiguous normal brain (Fig. 10.1B). The tumor initially was histopathologically classified as an astrocytoma, and eventually it was accessioned by the American Type Culture Collection, Rockville, MD (ATCC# CCL-107). The cells have been reported to have a mutant *p16/Cdkn2a/Ink4a* locus (Schlegel et al. 1999) with no expression of *p16* and *p19ARF* mRNAs, and a wildtype *p53* (Asai et al. 1994). More recent molecular characterization, which compared changes in gene expression between the C6 glioma and rat stem cell-derived astrocytes, revealed that the changes in gene expression observed in the C6 cell line were the most similar to those reported in human brain tumors (Sibenaller et al. 2005). Compared to astrocytes, they also had increased expression of the *PDGFβ*, *IGF-1*, *EGFR*, and *Erb3/HER3* genes, which are frequently overexpressed in human gliomas (Guo et al. 2003, Heimberger et al. 2005, Morford et al. 1997). In a recent study, the significance of PDGF in gliomagenesis in adult rats was established by infecting white matter with a retrovirus encoding for PDGF and GFP. Within 2 weeks 100% of the animals had tumors derived from both infected and uninfected glial progenitors, thereby implicating PDGF in both autocrine and paracrine stimulation of glial progenitor cells (Assanah et al. 2006). Although, *IGF-1* was overexpressed in C6 glioma cells, there was reduced expression of *IGF-2*, *FGF-9*, and *FGF-10* relative to astrocytes. Similar to the increased activity of the *Ras* pathway observed in human gliomas (Nakada et al. 2005), C6 cells also had an increase in both *Ras* expression and *Ras* guanine triphosphate activator protein (Sibenaller et al. 2005). However, contrary to what is known about human GBM, there was an increase in the expression of Rb in these cells (Sibenaller et al. 2005). A subclone of C6 cells, stably expressing β-galactosidase, was subsequently described (Lampson et al. 1993) and this permits immunohistochemical analysis of these tumors in the brain. This clone is available through the ATCC (# CRL-2303). However, it must be noted that the β-galactosidase marker protein itself can serve as a tumor antigen, and immunization of rats against the reporter gene protected the animals against tumor growth (Lampson et al. 1993). The C6 rat glioma model has been widely used in experimental neuro-oncology to evaluate the therapeutic efficacy of a variety of modalities, including chemotherapy (Doblas et al. 2008), anti-angiogenic therapy (Solly et al. 2008), proteasome inhibitors

(Ahmed et al. 2008), treatment with toxins (Zhao et al. 2008), radiation therapy (Sheehan et al. 2008), photodynamic therapy (Mannino et al. 2008), oncolytic viral therapy (Yang et al. 2004), and gene therapy (Tanriover et al. 2008). Since this tumor arose in an outbred Wistar rat, however, there is no syngeneic host in which it can be propagated. *This is a very serious limitation that diminishes its usefulness for survival studies since the tumor is immunogenic, even in Wistar rats.* The C6 glioma has also been demonstrated to be immunogenic in BDX rats (Parsa et al. 2000), and it is therefore not useful for evaluating the efficacy of immunotherapy. This problem is exemplified by prior studies in which C6 glioma cells were transfected with an anti-sense cDNA expression vector that downregulated the constitutive production of IGF-1 in these cells (Johnson et al. 1993, Trojan et al. 1993). The authors unfortunately used BDX rats, which they thought were syngeneic due to some ambiguity in the literature. Subsequently, it was reported that BDX rats, which had been immunized with the C6 anti-sense IGF-1-transfected cells, were resistant to both s.c and i.c challenges of the C6 glioma. Similarly, Wistar rats with C6 tumors (s.c. or i.c.) developed potent humoral and cellular immune responses; and rats, challenged simultaneously with s.c. and i.c. tumors, had a survival rate of 100% (Parsa et al. 2000). Since C6 glioma cells are allogeneic in all inbred strains, this should provide a strong cautionary note for future studies employing this tumor model in therapy studies, and especially immunotherapy studies. Despite this limitation, the C6 glioma model continues to be used for a variety of studies related to brain tumor biology (Karmakar et al. 2007). These have included studies on tumor growth, invasion, migration, BBB disruption, neovascularization, growth factor regulation and production, and biochemical studies (Assadian et al. 2008, Valable et al. 2008a, b). Finally, single-cell clonal analysis has revealed that C6 cells also have cancer stem cell-like characteristics, including self-renewal, the potential for multilineage differentiation in vitro, and tumor formation in vivo (Shen et al. 2008).

10.5 F98 Gliomas

The F98 glioma (ATCC # CRL-2397) was produced by Wechsler in Koestner's laboratory at The Ohio State University by the i.v. administration of ENU (50 mg/kg body weight) to a pregnant Fischer 344 rat on the 20th day of gestation. Subsequently, the in vitro growth and morphology of the F98 glioma was described in detail (Ko et al. 1980), and based on its histopathology it was classified as an anaplastic or undifferentiated glioma (Kobayashi et al. 1980). The F98 glioma is composed of a mixed population of spindle-shaped cells, the majority of which have fusiform nuclei, and a smaller number of polygonal cells with round to oval nuclei. There is extensive invasion of contiguous normal brain with islands of tumor cells at varying distances from the tumor mass, many of which form perivascular clusters (Fig. 10.1C). Similar to human GBM, these cells overexpress *PDGFβ* and *Ras* along with an increase in *EGFR, cyclin D1* and *cyclin D2* expression relative to rat astrocytes (Sibenaller et al. 2005), and like the C6 glioma, they also have increased expression of Rb relative to rat astrocytes (Sibenaller et al. 2005). Immunofluorescence studies of F98 cells also revealed low expression of BRCA1, and a lack of radiation and cisplatin induced BRCA1 foci in these cells (Bencokova et al. 2008). Usually, there is a necrotic core, scattered mitotic cells, and non-glomeruloid neovascular proliferation (Mathieu et al. 2007). The tumor is GFAP and vimentin positive with negligible staining for CD3+ T cells (Mathieu et al. 2007).

Since it simulates the behavior of human GBMs in a number of important ways, such as its highly invasive pattern of growth and low immunogenicity, it has been used to evaluate the efficacy of a variety of experimental therapeutic agents. It is refractory to a number of therapeutic modalities, including chemotherapy with paclitaxel, and carboplatin (von Eckardstein et al. 2005), and is poorly responsive to photon irradiation alone (Barth 1998), which in part may be related to its functionally impaired BRCA1 status which can favor genomic instability and impaired DNA repair (Bencokova et al. 2008). Recently, it has been shown to be responsive to a combination of synchrotron radiation with *cis*-diamminedichloroplatinum(II) (CDDP) (Biston et al. 2004), and to convection-enhanced delivery (CED) of carboplatin in combination with 6 MV photon irradiation in rats bearing i.c. tumors (Rousseau et al. 2007, Rousseau et al. 2009). This model has been used extensively to evaluate the efficacy of boron neutron capture therapy (BNCT) (Barth et al. 2003, Yang et al. 2008), radioiodine therapy (Cho et al. 2002), and iodine-enhanced synchrotron stereotactic radiotherapy (Adam et al. 2006). It has also been used to evaluate non-invasive MRI to visualize tumor growth (Blanchard et al. 2006), diffusion tensor imaging (Zhang et al. 2007), tumor angiogenesis (Zhang et al. 2008), and the tumor tropism of mesenchymal stem cells (Wu et al. 2008).

The F98 glioma is very weakly immunogenic (Tzeng et al. 1991) and transfection with the gene encoding B7.1 co-stimulatory molecule (Paul et al. 2000), or syngeneic cellular vaccination combination with GM-CSF, did not enhance its immunogenicity (Clavreul et al. 2006, Paul et al. 2000). This makes it a very attractive model to investigate the mechanisms underlying glioma resistance to immunotherapy. It has also been used to study the molecular genetic alterations in GBMs (Hanissian et al. 2005), effects of infusion rates on drug distribution in i.c. tumors (Khan et al. 2005), and for suicide gene therapy with Herpes simplex virus-1 thymidine kinase (HSV-TK) (von Eckardstein et al. 2001).

Like the 9L gliosarcoma, F98 cells have also been injected into the pontine tegmentum of the brainstem of Fischer rats to produce a model for brainstem tumors (Jallo et al. 2006). The histopathological and radiobiological characteristics of these tumors were comparable to aggressive, primary human brainstem tumors, which could facilitate preclinical testing of therapeutics to treat these lethal tumors. F98 cells have been stably transfected with expression vectors encoding for wildtype EGFR and EGFRvIII, and the resulting cell lines have been designated $F98_{EGFR}$ (ATCC# CRL-2948) and $F98_{npEGFRvIII}$ (ATCC#

CRL-2949). They each express ~10^5 non-functional (i.e., non-phosphorylatable) receptor sites per cell, which is below the threshold number of 10^6 sites per cell that can evoke a xenoimmune response against human EGFR in Fischer rats. These cell lines have been used in Fischer rats for studies on molecular targeting of EGFR (Yang et al. 2005) to evaluate the therapeutic efficacy of boronated mAbs and EGF for neutron capture therapy (NCT) (Wu et al. 2007, Yang et al. 2008). The boronated mAb, L8A4, which is specific for EGFRvIII, and cetuximab, which recognizes wildtype EGFR, specifically targeted their respective receptor-positive i.c. tumors after CED and they were therapeutically effective following NCT (Yang et al. 2005) (Wu et al. 2006, 2007, Yang et al. 2008). A bioluminescent F98 cell line recently was constructed by stably transfecting F98 cells with the luciferase gene. When implanted i.c. into the brains of Fischer rats, tumor size could be monitored by measuring luminescence. This model should permit rapid, non-invasive imaging of i.c. tumor growth to evaluate novel therapeutic modalities (Bryant et al. 2008). Finally F98 cells are also capable of growing as i.c. xenografts in cats (Ernestus et al. 1992), but since these cells can evoke a xenoimmune response, this model is of limited usefulness. As with all rat brain tumor models, however, what may be therapeutically effective in the rat, may not be in the human. However, it is probably safe to say that if a particular therapeutic approach is ineffective in a rat model, it is even more unlikely to be so in humans.

10.6 RG2 (or D74) Glioma

The RG2 glioma (ATCC #CRL-2433) also was produced in Koestner's laboratory at the same time as the F98 glioma, using the same procedure described above for the F98 glioma (Ko et al. 1980). The progeny of ENU-injected rats subsequently developed tumors, and following cloning by Wechsler in Germany, one of these clones was designated as "RG2" (rat glioma 2). The same clone was called the "D74-RG2" or "D74" in Koestner's laboratory at The Ohio State University. The RG2 glioma is similar in microscopic appearance to the F98 glioma, and has also a highly invasive pattern of growth (Fig. 10.1D), which has made it a good representative model for GBM (Weizsacker et al. 1982). Gene expression profiling of these cells established that they had increased gene expression of *PDGFβ*, *IGF-1*, *Ras*, *Erb3/HER3* precursor mRNA, and *cyclin D2* (Sibenaller et al. 2005). They express a wildtype *p53* and a concurrent loss in the expression of the *p16/Cdkn2a/Ink4* gene locus (Schlegel et al. 1999). It has been used for a variety of preclinical studies to evaluate changes in vascular permeability (Ferrier et al. 2007), disruption of the BBB (Hashizume and Black 2002, Ningaraj et al. 2002), anti-angiogenic therapy (Zagorac et al. 2008), gene therapy (Wang et al. 2006), chemotherapy (Miknyoczki et al. 2007, Tsai et al. 2005), and radionuclide therapy (Shen et al. 2004).

The RG2 glioma is non-immunogenic in syngeneic Fischer rats (Weizsacker et al. 1982) and has low levels of MHC-1 expression compared to the C6 and 9L gliomas (Oshiro et al. 2001). However, in vitro treatment with IFN-γ upregulated MHC class I antigen expression and also resulted in a significant in vivo anti-tumor immune response with increased survival of treated animals (Oshiro et al. 2001). More recently, the RG2 glioma has been stably transfected with human Herpes virus entry mediator C (HveC) to facilitate HSV infection and has been used to study the therapeutic effects of oncolytic Herpes simplex virus-1 treatment (Kurozumi et al. 2007). The transfected cells retained their tumorigenicity following i.c. implantation in Fischer rats, and transfection of the HveC gene did not affect i.c. tumor growth (Wakimoto et al. 2004). However, it has not been determined if HveC may confer any immunogenicity to these cells, and therefore, this must be taken into account when using the RG2-HveC for immunotherapy studies.

10.7 Avian Sarcoma Virus-Induced and RT-2 Gliomas

The induction of experimental brain tumors by the injection of Rous sarcoma virus has been described in canines, rats, and monkeys (Barth 1998). Tumors were induced by inoculating neonatal Fischer rats i.c. with purified avian sarcoma virus (ASV) suspensions (Copeland et al. 1976). All of the animals developed tumors within 2 weeks following ASV injection, 94% of which were anaplastic astrocytomas, and the remainder were low-grade gliomas or sarcomas (Copeland et al. 1976). This model has been used to study the effects of chemo- and radiotherapy, BBB disruption, and tumor permeability (reviewed by Barth (1998)). The response to immunotherapy indicated that these tumors were immunogenic, and expressed a variety of virally encoded tumor-specific antigens. A continuous cell line, designated "RT-2," was derived from an ASV-induced Fischer rat tumor, and this has been used to study tumor growth (Prabhu et al. 2000), photochemotherapy (Beckman et al. 1987), cytotoxic gene therapy (Valerie et al. 2001), and radiosensitization (Valerie et al. 2000). The RT-2 tumor appears to be immunogenic, as evidenced by its ability to evoke a CD8+ T-cell-mediated anti-tumor immune response (Shah and Ramsey 2003), and this must be taken into account if it is used for immunotherapy studies. RT-2 cells expressing GFP have been used for quantitative assessment of glioma invasion in the rat brain (Mourad et al. 2003). RT-2 cells have also been used to evaluate the therapeutic efficacy of oncolytic adenoviruses (see Chapter 47). Although they can be efficiently infected, they do not permit efficient replication of E1-attenuated adenoviruses (Madara et al. 2005). These cells have also been transfected with cDNA encoding heat shock protein 72 (HSP72), which was thought to be necessary for replication of E1-deleted adenoviruses (Madara et al. 2005). These transfectants have been found to be permissive for replication of E1-deleted, conditionally replication-competent adenoviruses (Madara et al. 2005). The inherent immunogenicity of the RT-2 glioma may limit its usefulness for survival studies, but nevertheless it still may be a useful model for other types of studies.

10.8 CNS-1 Glioma

The CNS-1 glioma was derived from an inbred Lewis rat that had received weekly i.v. injections of MNU for 6 months (Kruse et al. 1994). Following i.c. implantation into Lewis rats, it demonstrated an infiltrative pattern of growth with leptomeningeal, perivascular, and periventricular spread and extension of the tumor into the choroid plexus (Kruse et al. 1994). Histologically, these tumors exhibited hypercellularity, nuclear atypia, and pleomorphisim, and had necrotic foci that were surrounded by glioma cells arranged in a pseudo-palisading pattern (Fig. 10.1E), although to a lesser extent than that seen in human GBM (Candolfi et al. 2007). Like human GBMs, these tumors were also infiltrated with macrophages and T cells, but did not have extensive glomeruloid endothelial/microvascular proliferation (Candolfi et al. 2007). Kielian et al. identified the constitutive expression of monocyte chemotactic factor 1 (MCP-1) by CNS-1 cells (Kielian et al. 2002). In vivo, CNS-1 tumors also showed extensive infiltration by macrophages, which might confer a growth advantage (Platten et al. 2003). This model has been useful to study glioma invasion (Owens et al. 1998), changes in the biology of glioma cells and their extracellular matrix (Lapointe et al. 2005, Matthews et al. 2000, Nutt et al. 2001), and gene therapy (Biglari et al. 2004). It has also been used to study the efficacy of immunotherapy as a potential treatment for human GBM (Ali et al. 2004) although its immunogenicity has not been studied in great detail.

10.9 BT4C Glioma

The BT4C glioma was derived by giving a single transplacental pulse of *N*-ethyl-*N*-nitrosourea (ENU) to pregnant BDIX rats. Dissociated brain tumor cells from these animals were propagated in vitro and after 200 days in culture they became tumorigenic (Laerum and Rajewsky 1975). The cells subsequently were implanted s.c. into BDIX rats and the resulting tumors contained a mixture of multipolar glia-like cells and flattened cells with fewer and shorter cytoplasmic processes and occasional giant cells (Laerum et al. 1977). The BT4C glioma-derived tumors show high cellularity and has pleomorphic nuclei and numerous mitotic figures, and the tumor blood vessels are irregular, dilated and show areas of proliferation (Fig. 10.1F) (Stuhr et al. 2007). At the molecular level, BT4C cells express VEGF, tPA, uPA, and MVD in the periphery of the growing tumor and are S100 positive by immunohistochemistry (M. Johansson, Personal communication). This model has been useful to test novel chemotherapeutic targeting strategies (Pulkkinen et al. 2008), anti-tumor effects of gene therapy (Raty et al. 2004), anti-angiogenic agents alone (Huszthy et al. 2006), and in combination with radiation and temozolomide (Sandstrom et al. 2008). BT4C gliomas have also been used to investigate the impact of hyperoxia on tumor-bearing rats. This resulted in slower growth accompanied by increased apoptosis of tumor cells and reduced microvessel density (MVD). Apart from studies to evaluate therapeutic efficacy, the BT4C glioma model has also been used to study the molecular and biological changes induced by chemotherapy (Vallbo et al. 2002, Yoshida et al. 2001), radiation therapy (Andersson et al. 2002), and suicide gene therapy (Griffin et al. 2003). BT4C cells, stably transfected with cDNA encoding β-galactosidase, have been used to evaluate the migration of single migrating tumor cell glioma spheroids and fetal brain aggregate coculture systems in vitro and in rat brains in vivo (Garcia-Cabrera et al. 1996, Pedersen et al. 1995).

10.10 Concluding Comments

Rat brain tumor models have provided a wealth of information on the biology, biochemistry, imaging, and experimental therapeutics of brain tumors in experimental neuro-oncology, and there is every reason to believe that they will continue to do so. However, it is essential to recognize the limitations of each of the models that have been described, and depending on the nature of the study to be conducted, it is important that the appropriate model be selected (Table 10.2). It has now become clear that immunogenic tumors such as C6 and 9L are not good choices for studies in immunocompetent rats, if the endpoint is prolongation of survival time or cure of the tumor. Destruction of tumor cells in these models, which have tumor-infiltrating host of immune effector cells within the tumor, can lead to significant amplification of an anti-tumor response. This may be the single most important in vivo contributor to the bystander effect that has been observed with gene therapy of the C6 and 9L gliomas following transfection with the HSV-TK gene and the lack of such immune amplification with the weakly immunogenic RG2 (D74) glioma. Anti-tumor immune response following transfection with suicide genes such as HSV-TK initially was unanticipated, but it is an important effect associated with both gene therapy and boron neutron capture therapy, but not with conventional chemo- and radiotherapy of the 9L gliosarcoma. Since human high-grade brain tumors generally are regarded as being either non- or weakly immunogenic, therapeutic exploitation of this using modalities that spare tumor-infiltrating host immune effector cells could have important therapeutic implications. Undoubtedly other rat brain tumor models will be developed, especially cell lines derived from genetically engineered rats that will expand the types of studies that can be carried out in this very important laboratory animal.

References

Adam, J F, Joubert, A, Biston, M C, Charvet, A M, Peoc'h, M, Le Bas, J F, Balosso, J, Esteve, F, Elleaume, H (2006) Prolonged survival of Fischer rats bearing F98 glioma after iodine-enhanced synchrotron stereotactic radiotherapy. Int J Radiat Oncol Biol Phys 64:603–611

Aghi, M, Chou, T C, Suling, K, Breakefield, X O, Chiocca, E A (1999) Multimodal cancer treatment mediated by a replicating oncolytic virus that delivers the oxazaphosphorine/rat cytochrome P450 2B1 and ganciclovir/herpes simplex virus thymidine kinase gene therapies. Cancer Res 59:3861–3865

Ahmed, A E, Jacob, S, Nagy, A A, Abdel-Naim, A B (2008) Dibromoacetonitrile-induced protein oxidation and inhibition of proteasomal activity in rat glioma cells. Toxicol Lett 179:29–33

Ali, S, Curtin, J F, Zirger, J M, Xiong, W, King, G D, Barcia, C, Liu, C, Puntel, M, Goverdhana, S, Lowenstein, P R, Castro, M G (2004) Inflammatory and anti-glioma effects of an adenovirus expressing human soluble Fms-like tyrosine kinase 3 ligand (hsFlt3L): treatment with hsFlt3L inhibits intracranial glioma progression. Mol Ther 10:1071–1084

Andersson, U, Grankvist, K, Bergenheim, A T, Behnam-Motlagh, P, Hedman, H, Henriksson, R (2002) Rapid induction of long-lasting drug efflux activity in brain vascular endothelial cells but not malignant glioma following irradiation. Med Oncol 19:1–9

Asai, A, Miyagi, Y, Sugiyama, A, Gamanuma, M, Hong, S H, Takamoto, S, Nomura, K, Matsutani, M, Takakura, K, Kuchino, Y (1994) Negative effects of wild-type p53 and s-Myc on cellular growth and tumorigenicity of glioma cells. Implication of the tumor suppressor genes for gene therapy. J Neurooncol 19:259–268

Assadian, S, Aliaga, A, Del Maestro, R F, Evans, A C, Bedell, B J (2008) FDG-PET imaging for the evaluation of antiglioma agents in a rat model. Neuro Oncol 10:292–299

Assanah, M, Lochhead, R, Ogden, A, Bruce, J, Goldman, J,Canoll, P (2006) Glial progenitors in adult white matter are driven to form malignant gliomas by platelet-derived growth factor-expressing retroviruses. J Neurosci 26:6781–6790

Bansal, A, Shuyan, W, Hara, T, Harris, R A, Degrado, T R (2008) Biodisposition and metabolism of [(18)F]fluorocholine in 9L glioma cells and 9L glioma-bearing fisher rats. Eur J Nucl Med Mol Imaging 35:1192–1203

Barba, D, Hardin, J, Ray, J, Gage, F H (1993) Thymidine kinase-mediated killing of rat brain tumors. J Neurosurg 79:729–735

Barcellos-Hoff, M H, Linfoot, P A, Marton, L J, Deen, D F (1992) Production of stable phenotypes from 9L rat brain tumor multicellular spheroids treated with 1,3-bis(2-chloroethyl)-1-nitrosourea. Int J Cancer 52:409–413

Barker, M, Hoshino, T, Gurcay, O, Wilson, C B, Nielsen, S L, Downie, R, Eliason, J (1973) Development of an animal brain tumor model and its response to therapy with 1,3-bis(2-chloroethyl)-1-nitrosourea. Cancer Res 33:976–986

Barth, R F (1998) Rat brain tumor models in experimental neuro-oncology: the 9L, C6, T9, F98, RG2 (D74), RT-2 and CNS-1 gliomas. J Neurooncol 36:91–102

Barth, R F, Yang, W, Coderre, J A (2003) Rat brain tumor models to assess the efficacy of boron neutron capture therapy: a critical evaluation. J Neurooncol 62:61–74

Beckman, W C, Jr., Powers, S K, Brown, J T, Gillespie, G Y, Bigner, D D, Camps, J L, Jr. (1987) Differential retention of rhodamine 123 by avian sarcoma virus-induced glioma and normal brain tissue of the rat in vivo. Cancer 59:266–270

Bencokova, Z, Pauron, L, Devic, C, Joubert, A, Gastaldo, J, Massart, C, Balosso, J, Foray, N (2008) Molecular and cellular response of the most extensively used rodent glioma models to radiation and/or cisplatin. J Neurooncol 86:13–21

Benda, P, Lightbody, J, Sato, G, Levine, L, Sweet, W (1968) Differentiated rat glial cell strain in tissue culture. Science 161: 370–371

Benda, P, Someda, K, Messer, J, Sweet, W H (1971) Morphological and immunochemical studies of rat glial tumors and clonal strains propagated in culture. J Neurosurg 34:310–323

Bhattacharya, P, Chekmenev, E Y, Perman, W H, Harris, K C, Lin, A P, Norton, V A, Tan, C T, Ross, B D, Weitekamp, D P (2007) Towards hyperpolarized (13)C-succinate imaging of brain cancer. J Magn Reson 186:150–155

Biglari, A, Bataille, D, Naumann, U, Weller, M, Zirger, J, Castro, M G, Lowenstein, P R (2004) Effects of ectopic decorin in modulating intracranial glioma progression in vivo, in a rat syngeneic model. Cancer Gene Ther 11:721–732

Biston, M C, Joubert, A, Adam, J F, Elleaume, H, Bohic, S, Charvet, A M, Esteve, F, Foray, N, Balosso, J (2004) Cure of Fischer rats bearing radioresistant F98 glioma treated with cis-platinum and irradiated with monochromatic synchrotron X-rays. Cancer Res 64:2317–2323

Black, K L, Yin, D, Konda, B M, Wang, X, Hu, J, Ko, M K, Bayan, J A, Sacapano, M R, Espinoza, A J, Ong, J M, Irvin, D, Shu, Y (2008) Different effects of K(Ca) and K(ATP) agonists on brain tumor permeability between syngeneic and allogeneic rat models. Brain Res 1227:198–206

Blanchard, J, Mathieu, D, Patenaude, Y, Fortin, D (2006) MR-pathological comparison in F98-Fischer glioma model using a human gantry. Can J Neurol Sci 33:86–91

Blume, M R, Wilson, C P, Vasquez, D A. (1974) Immune response to a transplantable intracerebral glioma in rats. In: Sane, K, Ishi, S,Le Vey, D Recent progress in neurological surgery, Excerpta Medica, Amsterdam

Bryant, M J, Chuah, T L, Luff, J, Lavin, M F, Walker, D G (2008) A novel rat model for glioblastoma multiforme using a bioluminescent F98 cell line. J Clin Neurosci 15:545–551

Candolfi, M, Curtin, J F, Nichols, W S, Muhammad, A G, King, G D, Pluhar, G E, McNiel, E A, Ohlfest, J R, Freese, A B, Moore, P F, Lerner, J, Lowenstein, P R, Castro, M G (2007) Intracranial glioblastoma models in preclinical neuro-oncology: neuropathological characterization and tumor progression. J Neurooncol 85:133–148

Chen, C Y, Chang, Y N, Ryan, P, Linscott, M, McGarrity, G J, Chiang, Y L (1995) Effect of herpes simplex virus thymidine kinase expression levels on ganciclovir-mediated cytotoxicity and the "bystander effect". Hum Gene Ther 6:1467–1476

Chignola, R, Foroni, R, Franceschi, A, Pasti, M, Candiani, C, Anselmi, C, Fracasso, G, Tridente, G, Colombatti, M (1995) Heterogeneous response of individual multicellular tumour spheroids to immunotoxins and ricin toxin. Br J Cancer 72:607–614

Cho, J Y, Shen, D H, Yang, W, Williams, B, Buckwalter, T L, La Perle, K M, Hinkle, G, Pozderac, R, Kloos, R, Nagaraja, H N, Barth, R F, Jhiang, S M (2002) In vivo imaging and radioiodine therapy following sodium iodide symporter gene transfer in animal model of intracerebral gliomas. Gene Ther 9:1139–1145

Clavreul, A, Delhaye, M, Jadaud, E, Menei, P (2006) Effects of syngeneic cellular vaccinations alone or in combination with GM-CSF on the weakly immunogenic F98 glioma model. J Neurooncol 79:9–17

Coderre, J, Rubin, P, Freedman, A, Hansen, J, Wooding, T S, Jr., Joel, D, Gash, D (1994) Selective ablation of rat brain tumors by boron neutron capture therapy. Int J Radiat Oncol Biol Phys 28:1067–1077

Copeland, D D, Talley, F A, Bigner, D D (1976) The fine structure of intracranial neoplasms induced by the inoculation of avian sarcoma virus in neonatal and adult rats. Am J Pathol 83:149–176

Denlinger, R H, Axler, D A, Koestner, A, Liss, L (1975) Tumor-specific transplantation immunity to intracerebral challenge with cells from a methylnitrosourea- induced brain tumor. J Med 6:249–259

Doblas, S, Saunders, D, Kshirsagar, P, Pye, Q, Oblander, J, Gordon, B, Kosanke, S, Floyd, R A, Towner, R A (2008) Phenyl-tert-butylnitrone induces tumor regression and decreases angiogenesis in a C6 rat glioma model. Free Radic Biol Med 44:63–72

Donawho, C K, Luo, Y, Luo, Y, Penning, T D, Bauch, J L, Bouska, J J, Bontcheva-Diaz, V D, Cox, B F, DeWeese, T L, Dillehay, L E, Ferguson, D C, Ghoreishi-Haack, N S, Grimm, D R, Guan, R, Han, E K, Holley-Shanks, R R, Hristov, B, Idler, K B, Jarvis, K, Johnson, E F, Kleinberg, L R, Klinghofer, V, Lasko, L M, Liu, X, Marsh, K C, McGonigal, T P, Meulbroek, J A, Olson, A M, Palma, J P, Rodriguez, L E, Shi, Y, Stavropoulos, J A, Tsurutani, A C, Zhu, G D, Rosenberg, S H, Giranda, V L, Frost, D J (2007) ABT-888, an orally active poly(ADP-ribose) polymerase inhibitor that potentiates DNA-damaging agents in preclinical tumor models. Clin Cancer Res 13:2728–2737

Ernestus, R I, Wilmes, L J, Hoehn-Berlage, M (1992) Identification of intracranial liqor metastases of experimental stereotactically implanted brain tumors by the tumor-selective MRI contrast agent MnTPPS. Clin Exp Metastasis 10:345–350

Ferrier, M C, Sarin, H, Fung, S H, Schatlo, B, Pluta, R M, Gupta, S N, Choyke, P L, Oldfield, E H, Thomasson, D, Butman, J A (2007) Validation of dynamic contrast-enhanced magnetic resonance imaging-derived vascular permeability measurements using quantitative autoradiography in the RG2 rat brain tumor model. Neoplasia 9:546–555

Fomchenko, E I, Holland, E C (2006) Mouse models of brain tumors and their applications in preclinical trials. Clin Cancer Res 12:5288–5297

Fross, R D, Warnke, P C, Groothuis, D R (1991) Blood flow and blood-to-tissue transport in 9L gliosarcomas: the role of the brain tumor model in drug delivery research. J Neurooncol 11:185–197

Garcia-Cabrera, I, Edvardsen, K, Tysnes, B B, Read, T, Bjerkvig, R (1996) The lac-Z reporter gene: a tool for in vitro studies of malignant glioma cell invasion. Invasion Metastasis 16:107–115

Ghods, A J, Irvin, D, Liu, G, Yuan, X, Abdulkadir, I R, Tunici, P, Konda, B, Wachsmann-Hogiu, S, Black, K L,Yu, J S (2007) Spheres isolated from 9L gliosarcoma rat cell line possess chemoresistant and aggressive cancer stem-like cells. Stem Cells 25:1645–1653

Griffin, J L, Lehtimaki, K K, Valonen, P K, Grohn, O H, Kettunen, M I, Yla-Herttuala, S, Pitkanen, A, Nicholson, J K, Kauppinen, R A (2003) Assignment of 1H nuclear magnetic resonance visible polyunsaturated fatty acids in BT4C gliomas undergoing ganciclovir-thymidine kinase gene therapy-induced programmed cell death. Cancer Res 63: 3195–3201

Guo, P, Hu, B, Gu, W, Xu, L, Wang, D, Huang, H J, Cavenee, W K, Cheng, S Y (2003) Platelet-derived growth factor-B enhances glioma angiogenesis by stimulating vascular endothelial growth factor expression in tumor endothelia and by promoting pericyte recruitment. Am J Pathol 162:1083–1093

Gutman, DH (2009) Modeling human brain tumors in mice, Brain Pathol 19:108–111

Hanissian, S H, Teng, B, Akbar, U, Janjetovic, Z, Zhou, Q, Duntsch, C, Robertson, J H (2005) Regulation of myeloid leukemia factor-1 interacting protein (MLF1IP) expression in glioblastoma. Brain Res 1047:56–64

Harada, K, Yoshida, J, Mizuno, M, Kurisu, K, Uozumi, T (1995) Growth inhibition of intracerebral rat glioma by transfection-induced human interferon-beta. J Surg Oncol 59:105–109

Hashizume, K, Black, K L (2002) Increased endothelial vesicular transport correlates with increased blood-tumor barrier permeability induced by bradykinin and leukotriene C4. J Neuropathol Exp Neurol 61:725–735

Heimberger, A B, Suki, D, Yang, D, Shi, W, Aldape, K (2005) The natural history of EGFR and EGFRvIII in glioblastoma patients. J Transl Med 3:38

Huszthy, P C, Brekken, C, Pedersen, T B, Thorsen, F, Sakariassen, P O, Skaftnesmo, K O, Haraldseth, O, Lonning, P E, Bjerkvig, R, Enger, P O (2006) Antitumor efficacy improved by local delivery of species-specific endostatin. J Neurosurg 104:118–128

Iwadate, Y, Inoue, M, Saegusa, T, Tokusumi, Y, Kinoh, H, Hasegawa, M, Tagawa, M, Yamaura, A, Shimada, H (2005) Recombinant Sendai virus vector induces complete remission of established brain tumors through efficient interleukin-2 gene transfer in vaccinated rats. Clin Cancer Res 11:3821–3827

Jallo, G I, Volkov, A, Wong, C, Carson, B S, Sr., Penno, M B (2006) A novel brainstem tumor model: functional and histopathological characterization. Childs Nerv Syst 22:1519–1525

Jeffes, E W, Zhang, J G, Hoa, N, Petkar, A, Delgado, C, Chong, S, Obenaus, A, Sanchez, R, Khalaghizadeh, S, Khomenko, T, Knight, B A, Alipanah, R, Nguyen, T V, Shah, C, Vohra, S, Zhuang, J L, Liu, J, Wepsic, H T, Jadus, M R (2005) Antiangiogenic drugs synergize with a membrane macrophage colony-stimulating factor-based tumor vaccine to therapeutically treat rats with an established malignant intracranial glioma. J Immunol 174:2533–2543

Johnson, T R, Trojan, J, Rudin, S D, Ilan, J, Tykocinski, M L, Ilan, J. (1993) Evoking an immune response to glioblastoma cells transfected with episome-based plasmid expressing insulin-like growth factor I. In: Levine, AJ,Schmidek, HH Molecular genetics of nervous System tumors, Wiley-Liss, Inc., New York

Karmakar, S, Olive, M F, Banik, N L, Ray, S K (2007) Intracranial stereotaxic cannulation for development of orthotopic glioblastoma allograft in Sprague-Dawley rats and histoimmunopathological characterization of the brain tumor. Neurochem Res 32: 2235–2242

Khan, A, Jallo, G I, Liu, Y J, Carson, B S, Sr., Guarnieri, M (2005) Infusion rates and drug distribution in brain tumor models in rats. J Neurosurg 102:53–58

Kida, Y, Cravioto, H, Hochwald, G M, Hochgeschwender, U, Ransohoff, J (1983) Immunity to transplantable nitrosourea-induced neurogenic tumors. II. Immunoprophylaxis of tumors of the brain. J Neuropathol Exp Neurol 42:122–135

Kielian, T, van Rooijen, N, Hickey, W F (2002) MCP-1 expression in CNS-1 astrocytoma cells: implications for macrophage infiltration into tumors in vivo. J Neurooncol 56:1–12

Kimmelman, J,Nalbantoglu, J (2007) Faithful companions: a proposal for neurooncology trials in pet dogs. Cancer Res 67:4541–4544

Ko, L, Koestner, A, Wechsler, W (1980) Morphological characterization of nitrosourea-induced glioma cell lines and clones. Acta Neuropathol 51:23–31

Kobayashi, N, Allen, N, Clendenon, N R, Ko, L W (1980) An improved rat brain-tumor model. J Neurosurg 53:808–815

Kruse, C A, Molleston, M C, Parks, E P, Schiltz, P M, Kleinschmidt-DeMasters, B K, Hickey, W F (1994) A rat glioma model, CNS-1, with invasive characteristics similar to those of human gliomas: a comparison to 9L gliosarcoma. J Neurooncol 22:191–200

Krushelnycky, B W, Farr-Jones, M A, Mielke, B, McKean, J D, Weir, B K, Petruk, K C (1991) Development of a large-animal human brain tumor xenograft model in immuno-suppressed cats. Cancer Res 51:2430–2437

Kumar, S, Brown, S L, Kolozsvary, A, Freytag, S O, Kim, J H (2008) Efficacy of suicide gene therapy in hypoxic rat 9L glioma cells. J Neurooncol 90:19–24

Kurozumi, K, Hardcastle, J, Thakur, R, Yang, M, Christoforidis, G, Fulci, G, Hochberg, F H, Weissleder, R, Carson, W, Chiocca, E A, Kaur, B (2007) Effect of tumor microenvironment modulation on the efficacy of oncolytic virus therapy. J Natl Cancer Inst 99:1768–1781

Laerum, O D, Rajewsky, M F (1975) Neoplastic transformation of fetal rat brain cells in culture after exposure to ethylnitrosourea in vivo. J Natl Cancer Inst 55:1177–1187

Laerum, O D, Rajewsky, M F, Schachner, M, Stavrou, D, Haglid, K G, Haugen, A (1977) Phenotypic properties of neoplastic cell lines developed from fetal rat brain cells in culture after exposure to ethylnitrosourea in vivo. Z Krebsforsch Klin Onkol Cancer Res Clin Oncol 89:273–295

Lal, S, Lacroix, M, Tofilon, P, Fuller, G N, Sawaya, R, Lang, F F (2000) An implantable guide-screw system for brain tumor studies in small animals. J Neurosurg 92:326–333

Lampson, L A, Lampson, M A, Dunne, A D (1993) Exploiting the lacZ reporter gene for quantitative analysis of disseminated tumor growth within the brain: use of the lacZ gene product as a tumor antigen, for evaluation of antigenic modulation, and to facilitate image analysis of tumor growth in situ. Cancer Res 53:176–182

Landen, J W, Hau, V, Wang, M, Davis, T, Ciliax, B, Wainer, B H, Van Meir, E G, Glass, J D, Joshi, H C, Archer, D R (2004) Noscapine crosses the blood-brain barrier and inhibits glioblastoma growth. Clin Cancer Res 10:5187–5201

Lapointe, M, Lanthier, J, Moumdjian, R, Regina, A, Desrosiers, R R (2005) Expression and activity of l-isoaspartyl methyltransferase decrease in stage progression of human astrocytic tumors. Brain Res Mol Brain Res 135:93–103

Liu, Y, Wang, Q, Kleinschmidt-DeMasters, B K, Franzusoff, A, Ng, K Y, Lillehei, K O (2007) TGF-beta2 inhibition augments the effect of tumor vaccine and improves the survival of animals with pre-established brain tumors. J Neurooncol 81:149–162

Madara, J, Krewet, J A, Shah, M (2005) Heat shock protein 72 expression allows permissive replication of oncolytic adenovirus dl1520 (ONYX-015) in rat glioblastoma cells. Mol Cancer 4:12

Mannino, S, Molinari, A, Sabatino, G, Ciafre, S A, Colone, M, Maira, G, Anile, C, Arancia, G, Mangiola, A (2008) Intratumoral vs systemic administration of meta-tetrahydroxyphenylchlorin for photodynamic therapy of malignant gliomas: assessment of uptake and spatial distribution in C6 rat glioma model. Int J Immunopathol Pharmacol 21:227–231

Mathieu, D, Lecomte, R, Tsanaclis, A M, Larouche, A, Fortin, D (2007) Standardization and detailed characterization of the syngeneic Fischer/F98 glioma model. Can J Neurol Sci 34:296–306

Matthews, R T, Gary, S C, Zerillo, C, Pratta, M, Solomon, K, Arner, E C, Hockfield, S (2000) Brain-enriched hyaluronan binding (BEHAB)/brevican cleavage in a glioma cell line is mediated by a disintegrin and metalloproteinase with thrombospondin motifs (ADAMTS) family member. J Biol Chem 275:22695–22703

Miknyoczki, S, Chang, H, Grobelny, J, Pritchard, S, Worrell, C, McGann, N, Ator, M, Husten, J, Deibold, J, Hudkins, R, Zulli, A, Parchment, R, Ruggeri, B (2007) The selective poly(ADP-ribose) polymerase-1(2) inhibitor, CEP-8983, increases the sensitivity of chemoresistant tumor cells to temozolomide and irinotecan but does not potentiate myelotoxicity. Mol Cancer Ther 6:2290–2302

Miletic, H, Fischer, Y, Litwak, S, Giroglou, T, Waerzeggers, Y, Winkeler, A, Li, H, Himmelreich, U, Lange, C, Stenzel, W, Deckert, M, Neumann, H, Jacobs, A H, von Laer, D (2007) Bystander killing of malignant glioma by bone marrow-derived tumor-infiltrating progenitor cells expressing a suicide gene. Mol Ther 15:1373–1381

Moolten, F L (1986) Tumor chemosensitivity conferred by inserted herpes thymidine kinase genes: paradigm for a prospective cancer control strategy. Cancer Res 46:5276–5281

Morantz, R A, Wood, G W, Foster, M, Clark, M, Gollahon, K (1979) Macrophages in experimental and human brain tumors. Part 1: Studies of the macrophage content of experimental rat brain tumors of varying immunogenicity. J Neurosurg 50:298–304

Morford, L A, Boghaert, E R, Brooks, W H, Roszman, T L (1997) Insulin-like growth factors (IGF) enhance three-dimensional (3D) growth of human glioblastomas. Cancer Lett 115:81–90

Moriuchi, S, Wolfe, D, Tamura, M, Yoshimine, T, Miura, F, Cohen, J B, Glorioso, J C (2002) Double suicide gene therapy using a replication defective herpes simplex virus vector reveals reciprocal interference in a malignant glioma model. Gene Ther 9:584–591

Mourad, P D, Farrell, L, Stamps, L D, Santiago, P, Fillmore, H L, Broaddus, W C, Silbergeld, D L (2003) Quantitative assessment of glioblastoma invasion in vivo. Cancer Lett 192:97–107

Nakada, M, Niska, J A, Tran, N L, McDonough, W S, Berens, M E (2005) EphB2/R-Ras signaling regulates glioma cell adhesion, growth, and invasion. Am J Pathol 167:565–576

Namba, H, Tagawa, M, Miyagawa, T, Iwadate, Y, Sakiyama, S (2000) Treatment of rat experimental brain tumors by herpes simplex virus thymidine kinase gene-transduced allogeneic tumor cells and ganciclovir. Cancer Gene Ther 7:947–953

Ningaraj, N S, Rao, M, Hashizume, K, Asotra, K, Black, K L (2002) Regulation of blood-brain tumor barrier permeability by calcium-activated potassium channels. J Pharmacol Exp Ther 301:838–851

Nutt, C L, Zerillo, C A, Kelly, G M, Hockfield, S (2001) Brain enriched hyaluronan binding (BEHAB)/brevican increases aggressiveness of CNS-1 gliomas in Lewis rats. Cancer Res 61:7056–7059

Oshiro, S, Liu, Y, Fukushima, T, Asotra, K, Black, K L (2001) Modified immunoregulation associated with interferon-gamma treatment of rat glioma. Neurol Res 23:359–366

Owens, G C, Orr, E A, DeMasters, B K, Muschel, R J, Berens, M E, Kruse, C A (1998) Overexpression of a transmembrane isoform of neural cell adhesion molecule alters the invasiveness of rat CNS-1 glioma. Cancer Res 58:2020–2028

Parsa, A T, Chakrabarti, I, Hurley, P T, Chi, J H, Hall, J S, Kaiser, M G, Bruce, J N (2000) Limitations of the C6/Wistar rat intracerebral glioma model: implications for evaluating immunotherapy. Neurosurgery 47:993–999; discussion 999–1000

Paul, D B, Barth, R F, Yang, W, Shen, G H, Kim, J, Triozzi, P L (2000) B7.1 expression by the weakly immunogenic F98 rat glioma does not enhance immunogenicity. Gene Ther 7:993–999

Pedersen, P H, Edvardsen, K, Garcia-Cabrera, I, Mahesparan, R, Thorsen, J, Mathisen, B, Rosenblum, M L, Bjerkvig, R (1995) Migratory patterns of lac-Z transfected human glioma cells in the rat brain. Int J Cancer 62:767–771

Pfeiffer, S E, Herschman, H R, Lightbody, J, Sato, G (1970) Synthesis by a clonal line of rat glial cells of a protein unique to the nervous system. J Cell Physiol 75:329–339

Pietronigro, D, Drnovsky, F, Cravioto, H, Ransohoff, J (2003) DTI-015 produces cures in T9 gliosarcoma. Neoplasia 5:17–22

Platten, M, Kretz, A, Naumann, U, Aulwurm, S, Egashira, K, Isenmann, S, Weller, M (2003) Monocyte chemoattractant protein-1 increases microglial infiltration and aggressiveness of gliomas. Ann Neurol 54:388–392

Prabhu, S S, Broaddus, W C, Oveissi, C, Berr, S S, Gillies, G T (2000) Determination of intracranial tumor volumes in a rodent brain using magnetic resonance imaging, Evans blue, and histology: a comparative study. IEEE Trans Biomed Eng 47:259–265

Pulkkinen, M, Pikkarainen, J, Wirth, T, Tarvainen, T, Haapa-Aho, V, Korhonen, H, Seppala, J, Jarvinen, K (2008) Three-step tumor targeting of paclitaxel using biotinylated PLA-PEG nanoparticles and avidin-biotin technology: Formulation development and in vitro anticancer activity. Eur J Pharm Biopharm 70:66–74

Raty, J K, Airenne, K J, Marttila, A T, Marjomaki, V, Hytonen, V P, Lehtolainen, P, Laitinen, O H, Mahonen, A J, Kulomaa, M S, Yla-Herttuala, S (2004) Enhanced gene delivery by avidin-displaying baculovirus. Mol Ther 9:282–291

Regnard, P, Brauer-Krisch, E, Tropres, I, Keyrilainen, J, Bravin, A, Le Duc, G (2008) Enhancement of survival of 9L gliosarcoma bearing rats following intracerebral delivery of drugs in combination with microbeam radiation therapy. European Journal of Rad 68:S151–S155

Reilly, K M, Rubin, J B, Gilbertson, R J, Garbow, J R, Roussel, M F, Gutmann, D H (2008) Rethinking brain tumors: the fourth Mouse Models of Human Cancers Consortium nervous system tumors workshop. Cancer Res 68:5508–5511

Rousseau, J, Boudou, C, Barth, R F, Balosso, J, Esteve, F, Elleaume, H (2007) Enhanced survival and cure of F98 glioma-bearing rats following intracerebral delivery of carboplatin in combination with photon irradiation. Clin Cancer Res 13:5195–5201

Rousseau, R, Barth, R F, Moeschberger, M L, Elleaume, H (2009) Efficacy of intracerebral delivery of carboplatin in combination with photon irradiation for treatment of F98 glioma bearing rats. Int J Radiat Oncol 73:530–536

Saini, M, Roser, F, Samii, M, Bellinzona, M (2004) A model for intratumoural chemotherapy in the rat brain. Acta Neurochir (Wien) 146:731–734

Saito, R, Bringas, J, Mirek, H, Berger, M S, Bankiewicz, K S (2004) Invasive phenotype observed in 1,3-bis(2-chloroethyl)-1-nitrosourea-resistant sublines of 9L rat glioma cells: a tumor model mimicking a recurrent malignant glioma. J Neurosurg 101:826–831

Sandstrom, M, Johansson, M, Bergstrom, P, Bergenheim, A T, Henriksson, R (2008) Effects of the VEGFR inhibitor ZD6474 in combination with radiotherapy and temozolomide in an orthotopic glioma model. J Neurooncol 88:1–9

Schepkin, V D, Lee, K C, Kuszpit, K, Muthuswami, M, Johnson, T D, Chenevert, T L, Rehemtulla, A, Ross, B D (2006) Proton and sodium MRI assessment of emerging tumor chemotherapeutic resistance. NMR Biomed 19:1035–1042

Schlegel, J, Piontek, G, Kersting, M, Schuermann, M, Kappler, R, Scherthan, H, Weghorst, C, Buzard, G, Mennel, H (1999) The p16/Cdkn2a/Ink4a gene is frequently deleted in nitrosourea-induced rat glial tumors. Pathobiology 67:202–206

Schmidek, H H, Nielsen, S L, Schiller, A L, Messer, J (1971) Morphological studies of rat brain tumors induced by N-nitrosomethylurea. J Neurosurg 34:335–340

Shah, M R, Ramsey, W J (2003) CD8 + T-cell mediated anti-tumor responses cross-reacting against 9L and RT2 rat glioma cell lines. Cell Immunol 225:113–121

Sheehan, J, Ionescu, A, Pouratian, N, Hamilton, D K, Schlesinger, D, Oskouian, R J, Jr., Sansur, C (2008) Use of trans sodium crocetinate for sensitizing glioblastoma multiforme to radiation: laboratory investigation. J Neurosurg 108:972–978

Shen, D H, Marsee, D K, Schaap, J, Yang, W, Cho, J Y, Hinkle, G, Nagaraja, H N, Kloos, R T, Barth, R F, Jhiang, S M (2004) Effects of dose, intervention time, and radionuclide on sodium iodide symporter (NIS)-targeted radionuclide therapy. Gene Ther 11:161–169

Shen, G, Shen, F, Shi, Z, Liu, W, Hu, W, Zheng, X, Wen, L, Yang, X (2008) Identification of cancer stem-like cells in the C6 glioma cell line and the limitation of current identification methods. In vitro Cell Dev Biol Anim 44:280–289

Shibuya, N, Hochgeschwender, U, Kida, Y, Hochwald, G M, Thorbecke, G J, Cravioto, H (1984) Immunity to transplantable nitrosourea-induced neurogenic tumors. III. Systemic adoptive transfer of immunity. J Neuropathol Exp Neurol 43:426–438

Sibenaller, Z A, Etame, A B, Ali, M M, Barua, M, Braun, T A, Casavant, T L, Ryken, T C (2005) Genetic characterization of commonly used glioma cell lines in the rat animal model system. Neurosurg Focus 19:E1

Smilowitz, H M, Micca, P L, Nawrocky, M M, Slatkin, D N, Tu, W, Coderre, J A (2000) The combination of boron neutron-capture therapy and immunoprophylaxis for advanced intracerebral gliosarcomas in rats. J Neurooncol 46:231–240

Solly, F, Fish, R, Simard, B, Bolle, N, Kruithof, E, Polack, B, Pernod, G (2008) Tissue-type plasminogen activator has antiangiogenic properties without effect on tumor growth in a rat C6 glioma model. Cancer Gene Ther 15:685–692

Stojiljkovic, M, Piper ski, V, Dacevic, M, Rakish, L, Ruzdijic, S, Kanazir, S (2003) Characterization of 9L glioma model of the Wistar rat. J Neurooncol 63:1–7

Stuhr, L E, Raa, A, Oyan, A M, Kalland, K H, Sakariassen, P O, Petersen, K, Bjerkvig, R, Reed, R K (2007) Hyperoxia retards growth and induces apoptosis, changes in vascular density and gene expression in transplanted gliomas in nude rats. J Neurooncol 85:191–202

Tanriover, N, Ulu, M O, Sanus, G Z, Bilir, A, Canbeyli, R, Oz, B, Akar, Z, Kuday, C (2008) The effects of systemic and intratumoral interleukin-12 treatment in C6 rat glioma model. Neurol Res 30:511–517

Trojan, J, Johnson, T R, Rudin, S D, Ilan, J, Tykocinski, M L, Ilan, J (1993) Treatment and prevention of rat glioblastoma by immunogenic C6 cells expressing antisense insulin-like growth factor I RNA. Science 259:94–97

Tsai, N M, Lin, S Z, Lee, C C, Chen, S P, Su, H C, Chang, W L, Harn, H J (2005) The antitumor effects of Angelica sinensis on malignant brain tumors in vitro and in vivo. Clin Cancer Res 11:3475–3484

Tzeng, J J, Barth, R F, Orosz, C G, James, S M (1991) Phenotype and functional activity of tumor-infiltrating lymphocytes isolated from immunogenic and nonimmunogenic rat brain tumors. Cancer Res 51:2373–2378

Valable, S, Lemasson, B, Farion, R, Beaumont, M, Segebarth, C, Remy, C, Barbier, E L (2008a) Assessment of blood volume, vessel size, and the expression of angiogenic factors in two rat glioma models: a longitudinal in vivo and ex vivo study. NMR Biomed 21:1043–1056

Valable, S, Barbier, E L, Bernaudin, M, Roussel, S, Segebarth, C, Petit, E, Remy, C (2008b) In vivo MRI tracking of exogenous monocytes/macrophages targeting brain tumors in a rat model of glioma. Neuroimage 40:973–983

Valerie, K, Brust, D, Farnsworth, J, Amir, C, Taher, M M, Hershey, C, Feden, J (2000) Improved radiosensitization of rat glioma cells with adenovirus-expressed mutant herpes simplex virus-thymidine kinase in combination with acyclovir. Cancer Gene Ther 7:879–884

Valerie, K, Hawkins, W, Farnsworth, J, Schmidt-Ullrich, R, Lin, P S, Amir, C, Feden, J (2001) Substantially improved in vivo radiosensitization of rat glioma with mutant HSV-TK and acyclovir. Cancer Gene Ther 8:3–8

Vallbo, C, Bergenheim, T, Hedman, H, Henriksson, R (2002) The antimicrotubule drug estramustine but not irradiation induces apoptosis in malignant glioma involving AKT and caspase pathways. J Neurooncol 56:143–148

von Eckardstein, K L, Patt, S, Kratzel, C, Kiwit, J C, Reszka, R (2005) Local chemotherapy of F98 rat glioblastoma with paclitaxel and carboplatin embedded in liquid crystalline cubic phases. J Neurooncol 72:209–215

von Eckardstein, K L, Patt, S, Zhu, J, Zhang, L, Cervos-Navarro, J, Reszka, R (2001) Short-term neuropathological aspects of in vivo suicide gene transfer to the F98 rat glioblastoma using liposomal and viral vectors. Histol Histopathol 16:735–744

Wakimoto, H, Fulci, G, Tyminski, E, Chiocca, E A (2004) Altered expression of antiviral cytokine mRNAs associated with cyclophosphamide's enhancement of viral oncolysis. Gene Ther 11:214–223

Wang, W, Tai, C K, Kershaw, A D, Solly, S K, Klatzmann, D, Kasahara, N, Chen, T C (2006) Use of replication-competent retroviral vectors in an immunocompetent intracranial glioma model. Neurosurg Focus 20:E25

Warnke, P C, Blasberg, R G, Groothuis, D R (1987) The effect of hyperosmotic blood-brain barrier disruption on blood-to-tissue transport in ENU-induced gliomas. Ann Neurol 22:300–305

Weizsacker, M, Nagamune, A, Winkelstroter, R, Vieten, H, Wechsler, W (1982) Radiation and drug response of the rat glioma RG2. Eur J Cancer Clin Oncol 18:891–895

Wolff, J E, Molenkamp, G, Hotfilder, M, Laterra, J (1997) Dexamethasone inhibits glioma-induced formation of capillary like structures in vitro and angiogenesis in vivo. Klin Padiatr 209:275–277

Wu, G, Barth, R F, Yang, W, Kawabata, S, Zhang, L, Green-Church, K (2006) Targeted delivery of methotrexate to epidermal growth factor receptor-positive brain tumors by means of cetuximab (IMC-C225) dendrimer bioconjugates. Mol Cancer Ther 5:52–59

Wu, G, Yang, W, Barth, R F, Kawabata, S, Swindall, M, Bandyopadhyaya, A K, Tjarks, W, Khorsandi, B, Blue, T E, Ferketich, A K, Yang, M, Christoforidis, G A, Sferra, T J, Binns, P J, Riley, K J, Ciesielski, M J, Fenstermaker, R A (2007) Molecular targeting and treatment of an epidermal growth factor receptor-positive glioma using boronated cetuximab. Clin Cancer Res 13:1260–1268

Wu, X, Hu, J, Zhou, L, Mao, Y, Yang, B, Gao, L, Xie, R, Xu, F, Zhang, D, Liu, J, Zhu, J (2008) In vivo tracking of superparamagnetic iron oxide nanoparticle-labeled mesenchymal stem cell tropism to malignant gliomas using magnetic resonance imaging. Laboratory investigation. J Neurosurg 108:320–329

Yang, H, Chopp, M, Zhang, X, Jiang, F, Zhang, Z, Kalkanis, S, Schallert, T (2007) Using behavioral measurement to assess tumor progression and functional outcome after anti-angiogenic treatment in mouse glioma models. Behav Brain Res 182:42–50

Yang, W, Barth, R F, Wu, G, Ciesielski, M J, Fenstermaker, R A, Moffat, B A, Ross, B D, Wikstrand, C J (2005) Development of a syngeneic rat brain tumor model expressing

EGFRvIII and its use for molecular targeting studies with monoclonal antibody L8A4. Clin Cancer Res 11:341–350

Yang, W, Wu, G, Barth, R F, Swindall, M R, Bandyopadhyaya, A K, Tjarks, W, Tordoff, K, Moeschberger, M, Sferra, T J, Binns, P J, Riley, K J, Ciesielski, M J, Fenstermaker, R A, Wikstrand, C J (2008) Molecular targeting and treatment of composite EGFR and EGFRvIII-positive gliomas using boronated monoclonal antibodies. Clin Cancer Res 14:883–891

Yang, W Q, Lun, X, Palmer, C A, Wilcox, M E, Muzik, H, Shi, Z Q, Dyck, R, Coffey, M, Thompson, B, Hamilton, M, Nishikawa, S G, Brasher, P M, Fonseca, K, George, D, Rewcastle, N B, Johnston, R N, Stewart, D, Lee, P W, Senger, D L, Forsyth, P A (2004) Efficacy and safety evaluation of human reovirus type 3 in immunocompetent animals: racine and nonhuman primates. Clin Cancer Res 10:8561–8576

Yoshida, D, Noha, M, Watanabe, K, Bergenheim, T, Henriksson, R, Teramoto, A (2001) The bleb formation of the extracellular pseudopodia; early evidence of microtubule depolymerization by estramustine phosphate in glioma cell; in vitro study. J Neurooncol 52:37–47

Yuan, H, Schroeder, T, Bowsher, J E, Hedlund, L W, Wong, T, Dewhirst, M W (2006) Intertumoral differences in hypoxia selectivity of the PET imaging agent 64Cu(II)-diacetyl-bis(N4-methylthiosemicarbazone). J Nucl Med 47:989–998

Zagorac, D, Jakovcevic, D, Gebremedhin, D, Harder, D R (2008) Antiangiogenic effect of inhibitors of cytochrome P450 on rats with glioblastoma multiforme. J Cereb Blood Flow Metab 28:1431–1439

Zhang, D, Feng, X Y, Henning, T D, Wen, L, Lu, W Y, Pan, H, Wu, X, Zou, L G (2008) MR imaging of tumor angiogenesis using sterically stabilized Gd-DTPA liposomes targeted to CD105. European Journal of Radiology doi:10.1016/j.ejrad.2008.04.022

Zhang, J, van Zijl, P C, Laterra, J, Salhotra, A, Lal, B, Mori, S, Zhou, J (2007) Unique patterns of diffusion directionality in rat brain tumors revealed by high-resolution diffusion tensor MRI. Magn Reson Med 58:454–462

Zhao, S, Zhang, X, Zhang, J, Zhang, J, Zou, H, Liu, Y, Dong, X, Sun, X (2008) Intravenous administration of arsenic trioxide encapsulated in liposomes inhibits the growth of C6 gliomas in rat brains. J Chemother 20:253–262

Chapter 11
Neuro-oncogenesis Induced by Nitroso Compounds in Rodents and Strain-Specific Genetic Modifiers of Predisposition

Bernd U. Koelsch and Andrea Kindler-Röhrborn

Abstract The alkylating substances *N*-ethyl-*N*-nitrosourea (ENU) and *N*-methyl-*N*-nitrosourea (MNU) are the most potent systemically acting neurocarcinogens in rodents. They induce tumors of the central (CNS) and peripheral nervous system (PNS), which are similar to their human counterparts. The neuro-oncogenic effect of both chemicals depends on the dose, the rodent species, the strain, and the developmental stage at exposure. Neuro-oncogenesis induced by MNU and ENU has been widely used as a model system including studies of molecular mechanisms of malignant transformation, screening of therapeutics, and lately, the genetics of predisposition toward the development of these tumors. The induction of malignant tumors in the PNS of differentially susceptible rat strains made it possible to identify gene loci influencing tumor risk in an allele- and sex-specific way and to gain insight into molecular and cellular mechanisms underlying tumor susceptibility and resistance.

Contents

A. Kindler-Röhrborn (✉)
Institute of Pathology and Neuropathology, University Hospital of Essen, University of Duisburg-Essen, Hufelandstr. 55, 45122 Essen, Germany
e-mail: andrea.kindler@uk-essen.de

E.G. Van Meir (ed.), *CNS Cancer*, Cancer Drug Discovery and Development, DOI 10.1007/978-1-60327-553-8_11,
© Humana Press, a part of Springer Science+Business Media, LLC 2009

11.1 Introduction

While considerable progress has been made elucidating the molecular pathogenesis of human brain tumors; (TCGA, 2008), their etiology is largely unknown. Epidemiological studies trying to associate brain tumor incidence with environmental, occupational, and lifestyle factors have not been successful (Wrensch et al. 1993). Modeling malignant disease in inbred rodent strains provides the researcher with large numbers of identical individuals as test subjects and with the option to control tumor induction, promotion, and progression. These conditions are essential for analyzing biological mechanisms underlying the process of oncogenesis as a basis for prevention measures and the development of specific therapies. This is particularly important in the case of malignant disease responding poorly to conventional therapies as seen in tumors of the central and peripheral nervous systems.

In early experiments the chemical induction of brain tumors in rodents was achieved by intracerebral administration of crystalline polycyclic aromatic hydrocarbons (Bigner and Swenberg 1977; Zimmerman 1955). Subsequently over 40 compounds have been found to induce nervous system tumors in rodents when administered systemically. Some of them are directly acting carcinogens while others need metabolic activation. Among them the directly acting alkylating *N*-nitroso compounds *N*-ethyl-*N*-nitrosourea (ENU) and *N*-methyl-*N*-nitrosourea (MNU) are the most powerful neurocarcinogens in rodents also inducing neurogenic tumors in other mammalian species. Although there are no epidemiological studies available, it is assumed that ENU and MNU display carcinogenic effects in humans, too (IARC 1978). Neuro-oncogenesis induced by these substances in rodents has been frequently used as a model for the study of basic molecular mechanisms of malignant transformation, the contribution of environmental mutagens to brain tumor etiology, screening of potential therapeutics, the influence of host factors, and the genetics of predisposition toward the development of neurogenic tumors. The latter became possible when different rodent strains were discovered to display a broad spectrum of differential reactivity to the neuro-oncogenic effect of ENU ranging from high susceptibility to entire resistance and with the advent of polymorphic genetic markers for mice and rats.

11.2 The Neuro-Oncogenic Effect of ENU and MNU

The neuro-oncogenic effects of MNU und ENU were first detected by Druckrey and collaborators (Druckrey et al. 1966, 1965). They showed that a single dose of ENU administered to pregnant rats during the fetal stage of gestation led to 100% incidence of tumors in the central (CNS) and peripheral nervous systems (PNS) of the progeny. MNU was demonstrated to induce neurogenic tumors upon repeated administration in adult rats.

Malignant transformation by alkylating agents is thought to result from the interaction of the ultimate carcinogen, i.e., a methyl or ethyl diazonium ion, with cellular DNA (Kleihues and Rajewsky 1984). Nucleophilic substitution results in the alkylation of N and O atoms at various base positions and of the P atom in the DNA backbone (see Fig. 11.1). Although the alkyl adducts at guanine-O^6, thymine-O^2 and -O^4, and cytosine-O^2 together represent only a minor fraction (<15%; Beranek 1990), these lesions exhibit by far the highest

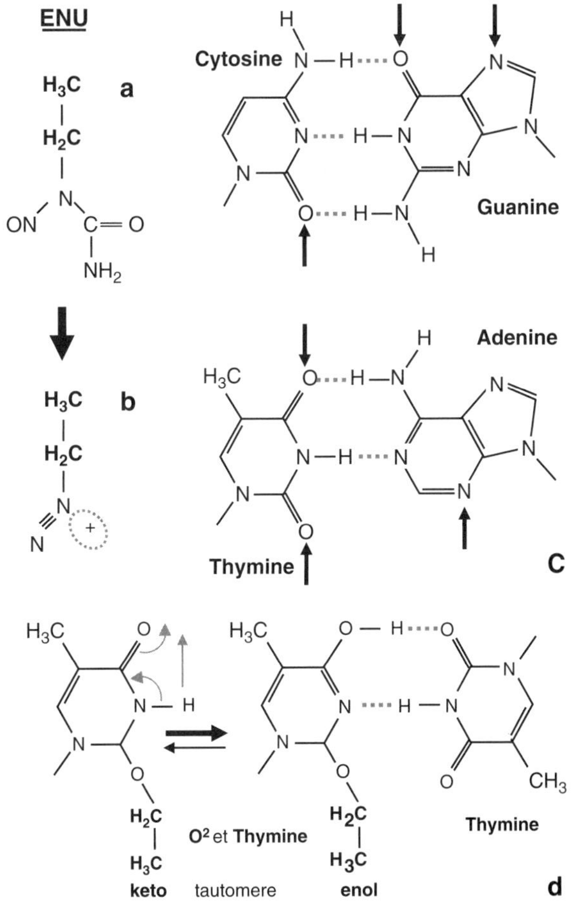

Fig. 11.1 ENU (**a**) reacts through an intermediate cation (**b**) with several N and O atoms (**c**) of the four DNA bases transferring the ethyl group. In contrast to thymine O^2-ethylthymine preferably exists as an enol favoring mispairing with thymine at replication (**d**)

mutagenic efficiency of all ENU- or MNU-induced DNA alkylation products. This is due to their mispairing character during DNA replication and correlates well with the carcinogenic potential of the respective chemicals (Singer 1983). Under in vivo conditions, ENU undergoes non-enzymatic heterolytic decomposition with a half-life $t_{1/2}$ of ≥ 8 min (Goth and Rajewsky 1972). The ethyl cation is thus produced in all tissues, yet the development of tumors occurs exclusively in the central and peripheral nervous systems. Insufficient cellular repair capacity for mutagenic DNA alkylation products may contribute to the tissue-specific carcinogenic effect of ENU. Accordingly, it was shown that the two most abundant O-alkylation products, O^6-ethylguanine causing G–C to A–T mutations and O^2-ethylthymine (T–A to AT), are highly persistent in neural cells in comparison to other cell types of ENU-exposed rats (Den Engelse et al. 1987; Engelbergs et al. 1998; Goth and Rajewsky 1974). Similar findings were described for O^6-methylguanine (Margison and Kleihues 1975). This notion is further supported by the particularly low activity of the DNA repair protein O^6-methylguanine-DNA methyltransferase (MGMT) in rodent and human brain cells (Gerson et al. 1986), a circumstance which has proved to be favorable for temozolomide therapy of human glioblastoma multiforme (Hegi et al. 2005). The selective persistence of such mutagenic lesions together with the high rate of DNA replication and cell division in the glial cells of the developing rat nervous system could be responsible for an increased probability of malignant transformation in this tissue and could thus provide an explanation for the nervous system specificity of the carcinogenic effect of ENU. However, while investigations in mice and gerbils showed a similar repair deficiency of the nervous system, these species did not display susceptibility to ENU-induced neuro-oncogenesis (Bamborschke et al. 1983; Kleihues and Rajewsky 1984). The organ and species specificity of the carcinogenic effect of ENU and MNU should, therefore, be determined by additional factors.

11.3 Characteristics of ENU- and MNU-Induced Nervous System Tumors

11.3.1 Histological Classification

ENU induces tumors of the brain, the spinal cord, and the PNS including the cranial nerves of rats with the proportion of tumors in different organ sites varying according to the time point of ENU exposure (see Fig. 11.2). In the CNS of Sprague–Dawley rats exposed to ENU on the 20th day of gestation moderately differentiated mixed gliomas and oligodendrogliomas prevail, while astrocytomas occur relatively rarely (Koestner 1990). These findings were largely confirmed in a study of brain tumors induced in 480 Sprague–Dawley rats by ENU on gestational day 15 (Zook et al. 2000). Notably, in this study 7.3% of untreated control rats have been reported to develop spontaneous

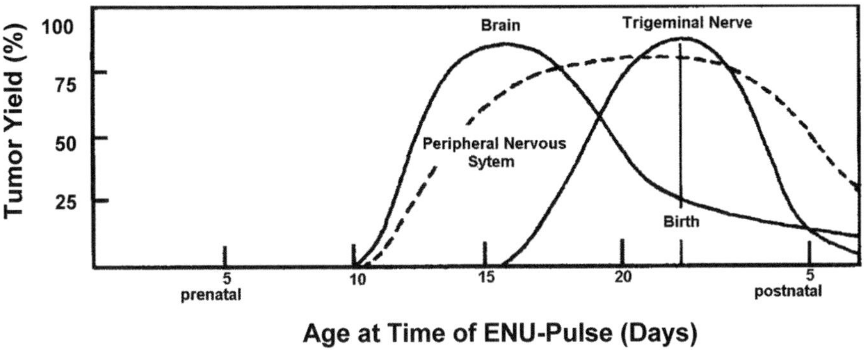

Fig. 11.2 (adapted from Druckrey 1973) The CNS and PNS display sensitivity to the effects of directly acting carcinogens during different time intervals of pre- and postnatal development

brain tumors most of them representing astrocytomas. In contrast, there are only anecdotal reports on spontaneous neuro-oncogenesis in the BD rat strains.

The great majority of PNS tumors induced by ENU on gestational day 20 in rats represent anaplastic neurinomas (Koestner 1990) corresponding to malignant peripheral nerve sheath tumors (MPNST) according to the WHO classification of nervous system tumors (Woodruff et al. 2000). Rats exposed to repeated doses of MNU during adulthood display primarily anaplastic gliomas and mixed gliomas and few differentiated oligodendrogliomas and astrocytomas (Koestner 1990), while tumors of the PNS are less frequent and more differentiated than ENU-induced MPNST. A detailed review of the morphological properties of ENU-/MNU-induced gliomas is provided by Bilzer and collaborators. The authors conclude that *N*-nitrosourea-induced neurogenic tumors can be considered a representative model for human tumors of the nervous system (Bilzer et al. 1989).

11.3.2 Genetic Alterations

Genetic alterations in oncogenes and tumor suppressor genes known to be involved in the development of human brain tumors do not appear to play a role in central nervous system oncogenesis induced by ENU and MNU. In a subset of brain tumors of BDIV × BDIX rat hybrids exposed to ENU neonatally, losses of heterozygosity (LOH) on rat chromosomes 1 and 17 were observed which occurred with a preference for the BDIV allele (Kindler-Rohrborn et al. 1999a). Notably, part of the segment on chromosome 1 representing the minimal region of overlap of the LOH corresponds to a portion of human chromosome 10 harboring the *PTEN* gene known to be frequently deleted in human high-grade glial tumors (Rasheed et al. 1997; TCGA, 2008).

ENU-induced MPNST display a T:A transversion mutation at nucleotide 2012 in the transmembrane region of the *Neu/ErbB-2* gene, presumably the initial event in MPNST development (Nikitin et al. 1991; Perantoni et al. 1987) (see below). Mutational events of the *Neu/ErbB-2* gene have also been shown to contribute to the development of human glioblastomas (TCGA, 2008). The transient expression of the *Neu/ErbB-2* gene plays an important role during Schwann cell maturation (Jessen and Mirsky 2005). The mutation is diagnostic of ENU-induced rat MPNST with a frequency of >98% as determined in 139 tumors of 4 different rat strains (M.F. Rajewsky, unpublished results). This genetic alteration may arise during DNA replication either from O^2-ethylthymidine which predominantly exists as an enol and mispairs with thymidine (Bhanot et al. 1992) (Fig. 11.1d) or from the preferential insertion of adenine at apurinic sites formed upon the spontaneous or repair-induced loss of an *N*-alkylated base (Huang and Greenberg 2008). During peripheral neuro-oncogenesis the wild-type allele of *Neu/ErbB*-2 is mostly lost through an LOH on rat chromosome 10 (Kindler-Rohrborn et al. 1999b). Interestingly, it was observed that in (BDIV × BDIX) F_1 hybrid tumors the LOH occurred with a strong bias toward the BDIV allele. With the coding sequence of the *ErbB-2* gene being identical between both strains (Holz, Koelsch, Kindler-Röhrborn; unpublished results), this pointed to the additional existence of strain-specific gene variants in this region negatively regulating tumor development. During further progression a second LOH on rat chromosome 5 is seen in the majority of cases (Koelsch et al. 2002).

11.4 Determinants of ENU- and MNU-Induced Neuro-oncogenesis

The yield of tumors induced by ENU/MNU and the organ site (CNS vs. PNS), respectively, as well as the length of the latency period is determined by the developmental stage of the animal at exposure, the dose, the way of administration, the rodent species, and the strain.

11.4.1 Developmental Stage of the Nervous System at ENU Exposure

A single exposure of pregnant rats to ENU results in up to 100% incidence of nervous system tumors in the offspring, depending on the time point chosen and the dose of the carcinogen. Susceptibility of the fetus starts at gestational day 12 and reaches a maximum at birth after which it gradually declines (Ivankovic and Druckrey 1968). The sensitivity of the nervous system to the carcinogen judged by tumor yield and latency time is 50-fold greater in the prenatal period than in adulthood (Druckrey et al. 1970b) with CNS and PNS displaying maximum sensitivity at different time intervals during perinatal development (Druckrey 1973) (see Fig. 11.2). It can be assumed that the developmental stage-specific carcinogenic effect of ENU depends on the transient presence of progenitor cells, which are especially vulnerable to malignant transformation due to their proliferative capacity and gene expression pattern.

Regarding the induction of nervous system tumors MNU is less efficient when administered transplacentally, but induces a similarly high number of tumors after repeated weekly doses in adult rats (Druckrey et al. 1965; Koestner 1990).

11.4.2 Doses and Route of Administration

In BDIX rats either treated with a single intravenous application of ENU on the 15th gestational day or with a subcutaneous injection during the early postnatal period, the dose was shown to be directly proportional to the incidence of nervous system tumors and inversely related to latency time, respectively (Ivankovic and Druckrey 1968). Similar experiments with MNU in BDIX rats showed a linear correlation between the total carcinogen dose administered in weekly fractions and tumor incidence as well as an inverse correlation to latency time (Druckrey et al. 1965). Additionally, the route of application of MNU appears to be important with the neurogenic tumor incidence being highest after intravenous administration (Swenberg et al. 1975).

11.4.3 Rodent Species and Strain

Different rodent strains exhibit differential sensitivity toward chemical induction of neurogenic tumors. While many rat strains show a high susceptibility to the development of nervous system tumors upon exposure to MNU or ENU, mice are in general more resistant, mostly developing neural tumors in single animals only of a given strain (Diwan and Meier 1974). However, the developmental stage at treatment and the genetic background of mice are, too, very important. Perinatal exposure of different mouse strains to ENU resulted in an overall incidence of neurogenic tumors of 6% (Wechsler et al. 1979), while postnatal treatment yielded neurogenic tumors in 0.33% of mice, only. Strains C2Hf/HeN and DBA/2 N were particularly susceptible (23% and 15%, respectively, rate of neurogenic tumors after transplacental ENU exposure), while strains C57BL/6 N and Swiss–Webster were resistant. In comparison to rats, mice display on average a 2-fold longer latency time. A tumor rate of 10% was reported for C3HeB/FeJ mice exposed to several intravenous doses of MNU during adulthood (Denlinger et al. 1974; Diwan and Meier 1974). It was suggested that the resistance of mice compared with rats is due to higher physiological levels of nerve growth factor in the former species (Vinores and Perez-Polo 1980). Resistance to ENU-induced brain tumor development was abrogated in $p53^{-/-}$ mice (C57 BL × CBA background; 70% incidence) indicating that p53 may play a role in protecting the fetus from DNA damage induced by transplacental carcinogen exposure (Oda et al. 1997).

Different inbred rat strains have also been reported to respond differently to exposure to alkylating agents. After neonatal ENU application, rats of the strains Wistar/Furth (WF), Long-Evans (LE), and Fischer 344 (F344) developed tumors of the CNS with similarly high incidences, while the rate of PNS tumors, including neoplasms of the cranial nerves and the spinal root, respectively, differed by strain. In contrast to WF and F344 rats, which were relatively resistant to the tumorigenic effects of ENU in the PNS, LE rats had a high susceptibility (Naito et al. 1982).

Intermediate incidences of trigeminal schwannomas in (LE × WF) $F_1$and F_2 rats, and high and low incidences, respectively, were found in backcrosses of both orientations. It was therefore concluded that susceptibility to the development of ENU-induced PNS tumors is likely to be a polygenic trait (Naito et al. 1985).

Of note, female F_1 rats had a lower tumor rate than males, which increased in ovariectomized females and decreased upon estrogen replacement suggesting that the hormone negatively regulated tumor development (Aoyama et al. 1989).

The 10 closely related inbred BD rat strains (Druckrey 1971) exhibit a broad spectrum of strain-specific sensitivity regarding ENU-induced development of neural tumors ranging from highest susceptibility in BDIX and BDVI rats to resistance in BDIV and BDVIII rats (Druckrey et al. 1970a; Kindler-Rohrborn et al. 1999b). According to Druckrey and collaborators the median time (T_{50}) until death from neuroectodermal neoplasms after ENU exposure on the 15th gestational day was approximately 3-fold longer in BDIV than in BDIX rats, with the average rate of neurogenic tumors/animal being 0.8 and 1.8, respectively (Druckrey et al. 1970a). After ENU exposure on postnatal day 1, the differences in malignant peripheral nerve sheath tumor (MPNST) development are even more pronounced (BDIX tumor incidence is >85% with a median latency time of 187 days vs. 0% in the BDIV rat) (Kindler-Rohrborn et al. 1999b).

11.5 Genetics of Susceptibility and Resistance to ENU-Induced Neuro-oncogenesis and Analyses of the Underlying Phenotypes

ENU-induced MPNST development in the trigeminal nerves of BD rats constitutes a model system for the genetic analysis of predisposition to the development of neurogenic tumors. For the identification of gene loci modifying tumor risk, BDIX and BDIV rats are well suited because their susceptibility to ENU-induced MPNST development varies extremely and the genetic difference of both strains suffices for linkage/association analyses. Although both strains are closely related, comparative genotyping of single nucleotide polymorphisms (SNP; http:snplotyper.mcw.edu) showed that appoximately 50% of their genomes are covered by SNP-containing regions >2 Mb (Saar et al. 2008). Moreover, the lower cellular complexity of the cranial nerves compared with the brain faciltates investigations addressing the cellular mechanisms underlying differential cancer risk in the nervous system. These analyses are an important prerequisite for the selection of functionally meaningful candidate genes. Once genes modifying the risk of ENU-induced MPNST development are identified using this model system, it will be comparatively easy to evaluate their function in human predisposition to CNS tumors as well.

After ENU application on postnatal day 1 *Neu*-mutant Schwann progenitor cells appear as early as day 7 at the predilection site of tumor development, the brain–nerve junction, and can be unequivocally identified: Knowing precisely the prospective location of the future tumor and being able to recognize and pursue premalignant cells on the basis of the diagnostic mutation and immunohistochemistry with antibodies against low affinity nerve growth factor receptor (Ngfr) provides us with the possibility of analysing early and intermediate stages of carcinogenesis in susceptible and resistant rats (see Fig. 11.3).

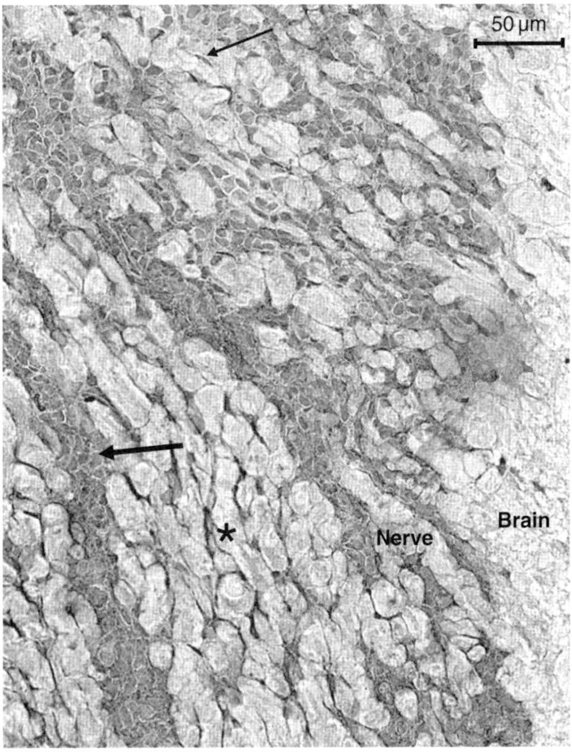

Fig. 11.3 Trigeminal nerve of a female BDIX rat, 70 days after ENU exposure on postnatal day 1, immunohistochemically stained with anti-nerve growth factor receptor antibodies. Note that small round *ErbB-2*-mutated premalignant Schwann cells with large nuclei only are stained (*thick arrow*), while regular Schwann cells (*asterisk*) with spindle-shaped nuclei (*thin arrow*) are devoid of stain

11.5.1 Inheritance of Susceptibility to ENU-Induced MPNST Development

(BDIV × BDIX) F_1 hybrids and F_2 animals from segregating inter- and backcrosses between BDIV and BDIX rats served to investigate the mode of inheritance of susceptibility and to localize genes determining the strain-specific risk to develop ENU-induced MPNST by association analysis (see below). Therefore, (BDIV × BDIX) hybrids were subcutaneously injected with 80 mg ENU/kg body weight on postnatal day 1. The development of MPNST was strongly suppressed in the (BDIV × BDIX) F_1 generation, see Table 11.1. (BDIV × BDIX) F_2intercross and (BDIV × BDIX) F_1 × BDIX backcross hybrids displayed intermediate MPNST incidences and latency times (Kindler-Rohrborn et al. 1999b). These data support the notion that predisposition to developing ENU-induced MPNST is likely to be a polygenic trait (Aoyama et al. 1989).

Table 11.1 Incidences and latency times of ENU-induced MPNST in BDIV and BDIX rats, F_1 and F_2 hybrids

	Number of animals	MPNST incidence (%)	Median latency time (days)
BDIV	24	0	–
BDIX	21	88	187
(BDIV × BDIX) F_1	55	20	298
(BDIV × BDIX) F_2	268	30	260
Males	122	39	316
Females	146	21	>425
(BDIV × BDIX) F_1 × BDIX	134	48	258
Males	60	50	272
Females	74	46	258

As previously shown for (LE × WF) F_1 females (see above), female (BDIV × BDIX) F_2 intercross rats had a considerably lower tumor risk than males and a longer survival time. In contrast, similar tumor rates and survival times were recorded for males and females in backcross hybrids. Therefore, female resistance is likely to be determined by recessively acting gene variants. Incidences and survival times are summarized in Table 11.1.

11.5.2 Identification and Characterization of Gene Loci Involved in Susceptibility or Resistance to ENU-Induced MPNST Development

The locus *Mss1 (mediating schwannoma susceptibility)* modifying susceptibility toward ENU-induced oncogenesis in the PNS had been identified on the basis of targeted linkage mapping in the region on chromosome 10, prone to BDIV allele biased LOH (Kindler-Rohrborn et al. 1999b). For this purpose 268 (BDIV × BDIX) F_2 intercross rats and 140 (BDIV × BDIX) × BDIX backcross rats had been genotyped for microsatellite markers on chromosome 10, only. Looking at the recombination events occurring in the core region of *Mss1* it was likely that additional loci contributed to susceptibility toward ENU-induced MPNST development. To detect further loci determining MPNST risk by association analysis, a whole genome scan was carried out on 268 (BDIV × BDIX) F_2 hybrids with an average microsatellite distance of 22 Mb. Six further loci residing on chromosomes 1 (*Mss2*), 3 (*Mss3*), 6, (*Mss4*), 13 (*Mss5*), 15 (*Mss6*), and 10 (*Mss7*) were found to control tumor incidence and/or survival time (Koelsch et al. 2006). Interestingly, most of these loci mediate allele- and sex-specific effects of variable strength ranging from minor influences on tumor development to complete tumor resistance. *Mss2, Mss3, Mss5,* and *Mss6* preferentially mediate tumor susceptibility to male individuals with *Mss3* having the strongest effects. Although in all other regions MPNST susceptibility is conferred by alleles of the susceptible BDIX strain, in the case of the loci *Mss3* and *Mss5* the alleles of the tumor-resistant BDIV strain mediate sensitivity to tumor induction by ENU. In contrast BDIV alleles at the loci *Mss4* and *Mss7* independently effect almost complete resistance to the development of ENU-induced MPNST in females. *Mss1* is the only locus not having an unequivocal sex-specific effect. The chromosomal location of all loci is depicted in Fig. 11.4. A sex-specific linkage signal on an autosome might mean that the interaction of transcription factors and/or sex hormones with DNA is affected by genetic polymorphisms. As most of the loci detected still exeed 20 Mb each one corresponds to several portions of human chromosomes not allowing conclusions on the human fragment actually harboring the causative gene.

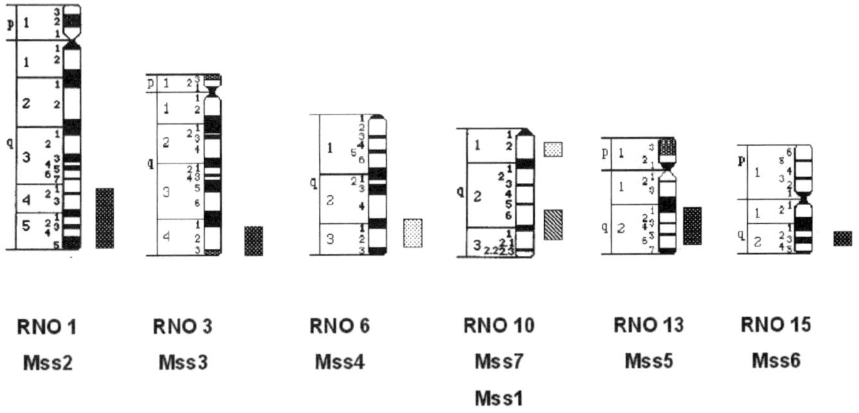

Fig. 11.4 Seven gene loci associated with susceptibility/resistance to ENU-induced PNS oncogenesis reside on six different rat chromosomes (*Rattus norvegicus*; RNO). *Black bars* represent loci which mediate tumor-modifying allele-specific effects in male animals only; *dotted bars* point to female-specific loci; the striped bar indicates no sex-specific effects

To visualize the sex-specific effect the numbers of tumor-affected male and female animals with the genotypes IX/IX, IV/IX, or IV/IV for microsatellite markers residing in the *Mss4* locus on chromosome 6 were compared and the relative risks of these animals of developing MPNST were calculated. As shown in Table 11.2A (BDIV × BDIX) F_2 females with a IV/IV genotype for *D6Mit1* appear to be almost entirely resistant. The relative risk of females heterozygous for *D6Mit1* is 12.3-fold that of IV/IV homozygotes, while the risk of female IX/IX homozygotes is increased 9.9-fold.

Table 11.2 Frequencies of tumor-bearing F_2 animals and relative risk of MPNST development dependent on sex and genotype for markers on chromosome 6 (A) and on chromosome 10 (B)

A						
Sex		Male animals			Female animals	
Marker		Genotype			Genotype	
location (Mb)	IV/IV	IV/IX	IX/IX	IV/IV	IV/IX	IX/IX
D6Mit1	11 (31)[1]	22 (58)[1]	14 (33)	1 (42)	19 (65)	9 (38)
98.8	35%[2]	38%[2]	42%	2%	29%	24%
		1.1[3]	1.2		12.3	9.9
		0.6–1.9[4]	0.6–2.2		1.7–88.3	1.3–74.9

B						
Sex		Male animals			Female animals	
Marker		Genotype			Genotype	
location (Mb)	IV/IV	IV/IX	IX/IX	IV/IV	IV/IX	IX/IX
D10Mgh12	10 (33)[1]	23 (61)[1]	14 (28)	1 (23)	22 (80)	8 (40)
19,1	30%[2]	38%[2]	50%	4%	28%	20%
		1.24[3]	1.65		6.33	4.6
		0.68–2.29[4]	0.87–3.12		0.9–44.44	0.61–34.49

[1] Frequencies of tumor-bearing F_2 animals and of all F_2 animals of identical sex and genotype.
[2] Percentage of tumor-bearing animals.
[3,4] Relative risk of developing MPNSTs compared to genotype IV/IV and confidence intervals.

In contrast the risk of male animals with IV/IV, IV/IX, or IX/IX genotypes for *D6Mit1*, respectively, did not significantly differ (Table 11.2A). Using the same model framework, a similar effect was detected in females for BDIV alleles on chromosome 10 (*Mss7*; see Table 11.2B). Females with heterozygous IV/IX or homozygous IX/IX alleles for *D10Mgh12* had, respectively, a 6.33- and 4.6-fold increased tumor risk compared with females carrying homozygous IV/IV alleles. Male animals show only a weak dependence of tumor incidence on the genotype for *D10Mgh12* (tumor risks of heterozygotes) and animals with IX/IX alleles increase to 1.2- and 1.6-fold, respectively.

We could show that BDIV alleles at either *Mss4* or *Mss7* are sufficient to cause female tumor resistance regardless of the genotype for the other (Winzen et al. 2006).

Remarkable gender preference has been observed for several types of human nervous system tumors, e.g., for glioblastoma multiforme and for medulloblastoma with a 1.5- and 2.7-fold incidence, respectively, in males compared to females (Giangaspero et al. 2000; Kleihues et al. 2000), and for meningiomas and acoustic nerve schwannomas with male:female ratios of 1:2 (Louis et al. 2000; Woodruff et al. 2000). The degree of individual genetic predisposition being definitely gender-dependent, genes and signal transduction pathways discovered to be responsible for genetic susceptibility and resistance toward chemically induced schwannomas in the rat might well turn out to be relevant to human nervous system tumor risk as well and provide target molecules for sex-specific prevention measures and early diagnosis.

Due to the main effects they exert, the loci *Mss4* and *Mss7* could be narrowed down by haplotype analysis to 20 and 13 Mb, respectively. *Mss4* corresponds to the fragments encompassing 48–51 Mb and 58–77 Mb on human chromosome 14, while *Mss7* is orthologous to the first 5 Mb of human chromosome 16, followed by a fragment of human chromosome 5 (174–165 Mb), both in inverse orientation. *Mss4* and *Mss7* harbor: 286 and 240 respectively, positional candidate genes. Considering functional aspects and sex specificity of tumor resistance and susceptibility, candidate genes located in *Mss4* are transforming growth factor beta 3 (*Tgfb3*), latent transforming growth factor beta-binding protein 2(*Ltbp2*), estrogen receptor beta (*Esr2*), and estrogen-related receptor beta (*Esrrb*). While Tgfb3 has been shown to act as an immunosuppressant thereby promoting malignant schwannoma growth in BDIX rats (Altenschmidt et al. 1997), *Esr2* and possibly *Esrrb* should be able to mediate sex-specific effects.

To confirm the *Mss* loci and to further narrow them down, congenic strains were bred carrying a fragment of the resistant BDIV rat encompassing the respective *Mss* locus on a BDIX genetic background. By treating (BDIX.(*Mss4*) BDIV congenic animals) with 80 mg ENU/kg body weight on postnatal day 1, we were able to confirm the female-specific tumor-suppressive effect of the *Mss4* locus (B. Koelsch and A. Kindler-Röhrborn, unpublished results). Subcongenic strains harboring fragments of the BDIV chromosomal segment originally integrated into the BDIX genome have also been treated with ENU. This way we will be able to assign the tumor-suppressive effect to a smaller BDIV fragment harboring less positional candidate genes.

11.5.3 Phenotypic Analyses of Effector Mechanisms Underlying Differential MPNST Risk

Even if only a small number of genes reside in a chromosomal fragment having been shown to cause tumor resistance, information about the putative function of the causative gene(s) is necessary for its identification. Therefore, a detailed analysis of the effector mechanisms underlying tumor susceptibility and resistance in which the candidate modifier genes are involved was performed. Potential biological mechanisms underlying differential tumor risk could include a smaller population of target cells in the resistant strain due to a different timing of trigeminal development, strain-specific differential frequency of mutational initiation, different rates of DNA repair, or a different fate of the mutant Schwann cells. As described above, the initial event during ENU-induced MPNST development is a T:A transversion mutation at nucleotide 2012 located in the transmembrane region of the *Neu/ErbB-2* gene . In the process of oncogenesis it characterizes a subset of immature Schwann cells that are mainly located near the nerve–brain junction and exhibit unrestrained proliferative activity in contrast to their differentiating wild-type counterpart cells. *Neu*-mutant Schwann cells are therefore at high risk of progressing toward the expression of fully malignant phenotypes (Nikitin et al. 1991).

In an attempt to differentiate between tumor resistance mechanisms coming into effect in BDIV rats early during ENU-induced oncogenesis or at later stages, we have previously quantified *Neu*-mutant Schwann cells in the trigeminal nerves of BDIV and BDIX rats as a function of time after ENU exposure on postnatal day 1 (Kindler-Rohrborn et al. 2000). Similar amounts of *Neu*-mutant cells were detected in the nerves of both strains during the first 80 days (see Fig. 11.5). This result excluded all potential resistance mechanisms coming into effect shortly after ENU application like numerical differences in target cells, different mutation frequencies, or more effective DNA repair.

Remarkably, in contrast to the progressive multiplication of *Neu*-mutant cells in BDIX trigeminal nerves during the intermediary phase of carcinogenesis, their numbers gradually decreased in BDIV rats. After 250 days, all BDIX rats had succumbed to their trigeminal tumors, while BDIV rats survived with their trigeminal nerves devoid of *Neu*-mutant cells. Tumor resistance in the BDIV rat was thus considered to be at least in part due to mechanisms effecting the disappearance of premalignant *Neu*-mutant schwannoma precursor cells from trigeminal nerves. The mutant cells were no longer detectable at the brain–nerve junction and in the more distal part of the nerve, excluding that premalignant cells could have differentiated and/or migrated as part of a tissue remodeling process as has been suggested for preneoplastic rat mammary and liver tissue (Wood et al. 2002). It was considered that these cells die through tissue intrinsic mechanisms or by host factors such as the immune system (Kindler-Rohrborn et al. 2000). The involvement of a cellular immune response was investigated using immunohistochemistry on sections of trigeminal nerves of both strains at different times after carcinogen exposure and controls. An inflammatory reaction involving sequentially $CD4^+$ macrophages and T helper cells, $CD8^+$ cytotoxic T cells, $ED1^+$, and $ED2^+$ macrophages, was detected in trigeminal nerve tissue of ENU-treated rats as early as postnatal day 40, briefly after the emergence of premalignant *Neu*-mutant Schwann cells (Gering et al. 2006). It persisted at all time points investigated (postnatal days 40–250). Interestingly, however, there were no gross differences in immune cell counts between tumor-susceptible and tumor-resistant rats. This suggested that either functional differences of immune

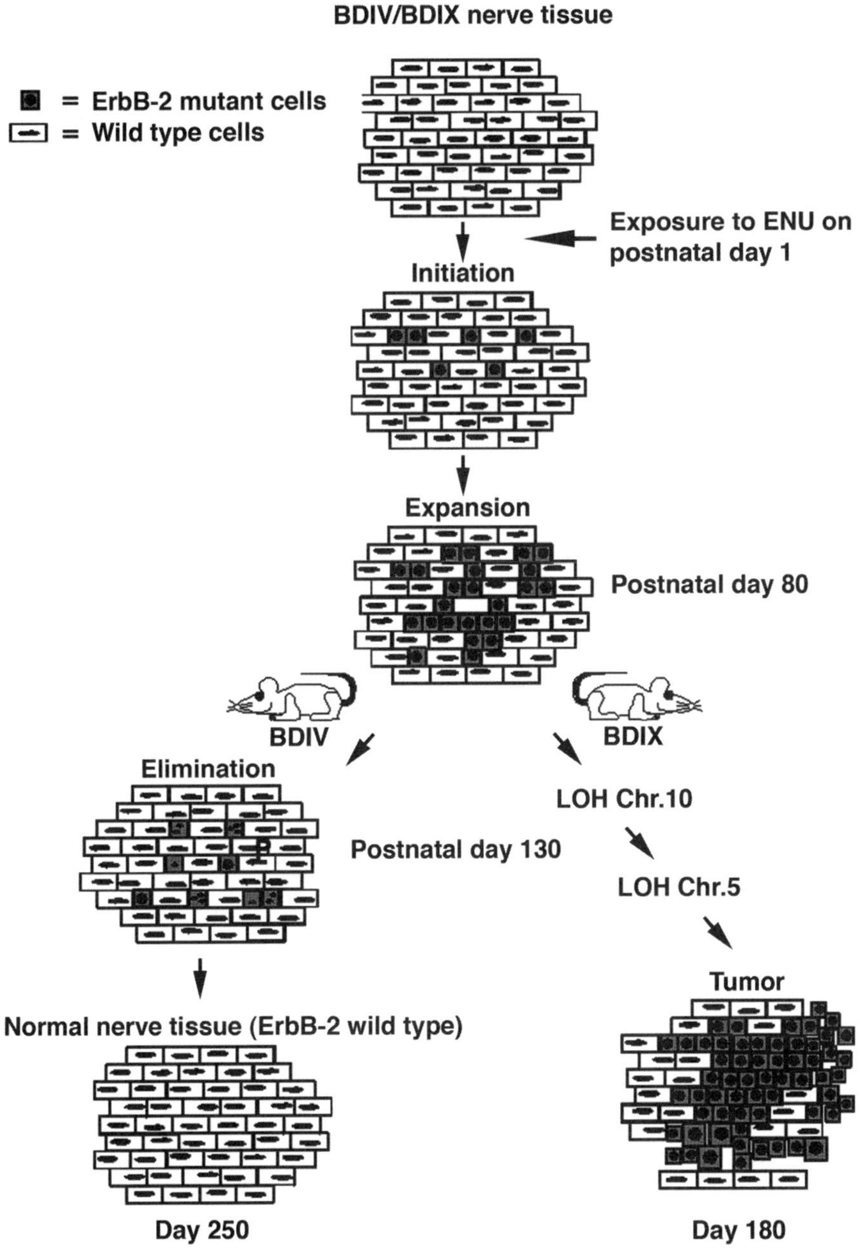

Fig. 11.5 Different fates of *Neu*/*ErbB-2*-mutant Schwann cells in trigeminal nerves of BDIV and BDIX rats during the post-initiation period of ENU-induced oncogenesis. During the first 80 days after ENU exposure on postnatal day 1 equal amounts of *Neu*-mutant premalignant Schwann cells are present in tumor-susceptible BDIX rats and tumor-resistant BDIV rats. While these cells are eliminated in BDIV rats they acquire further genetic alterations and progress to full malignancy in BDIV animals

effector cells exist between the two strains or that premalignant Schwann cells from different strains possess a differential capability to escape or counteract the immune response. Alternatively, the presence of immune effector cells in trigeminal nerve tissue might be of no functional consequence for the elimination of premalignant Schwann precursor cells.

To differentiate between these possible mechanisms, we prevented T cell maturation by neonatal thymectomy following ENU exposure. Thymectomy significantly decreased resistance against MPNST development in BDIV rats, while MPNST incidence and survival time remained unaltered in thymectomized BDIX rats (Marx et al. 2009). This suggests that T cells play a major role in BDIV rat resistance to MPNST formation supporting the immunosurveillance hypothesis originally postulated by Burnet (Burnet 1970).

In contrast to euthymic animals, a number of both thymectomized BDIV and BDIX rats developed MPNST lacking the *Neu/ErbB-2* mutation. This suggests that Schwann cells initiated by other genetic alterations can progress to full malignancy in immune-compromised rats only. T cell-dependent resistance against tumorigenesis originating from non-*Neu/ErbB-2*-mutant Schwann precursors might thus be shared by both strains while in the BDIV rat development of *Neu/ErbB-2*-mutant MPNST can additionally be prevented. Rat strain-specific differences in the interaction of T lymphocytes with (pre)-malignant *Neu*-mutant cells may thus critically contribute to susceptibility and resistance toward ENU-induced MPNST development. As the resistance mechanism against ENU-induced PNS tumors comes into effect during later steps of carcinogenesis, relevant candidate genes influencing tumor risk should exert their actions during the post-initiation period. This and the persistent immune response observed in the trigeminal nerves of ENU-treated animals of both strains with differential results in terms of tumor rejection invites the idea that in ENU-induced PNS carcinogenesis, genes encoding immune modifiers might be crucial for cancer susceptibility and resistance.

11.6 Conclusions

ENU-induced development of trigeminal MPNST in tumor-susceptible BDIX and tumor-resistant BDIV rat strains proved to be a well-suited model system for identifying molecular and cellular processes underlying differential risk of developing nervous system tumors. As the use of inbred animals reduces the genetic complexity found in humans, seven gene loci controlling MPNST incidence and latency time could be identified by association studies using segregating crosses of both rat strains. However, only a detailed analysis of the effector mechanisms underlying tumor susceptibility and resistance in which the genes to be identified are involved facilitates their selection on the basis of gene function. With the trigeminal nerve representing a relatively simple-structured target tissue, mechanisms modulating the strain-specific tumor risk were shown to include the elimination of premalignant *Neu/ErbB-2*-mutant cells in resistant BDIV rats, a process which is T lymphocyte dependent. Genes found to mediate predisposition or resistance to the development of ENU-induced MPNST in the rat will likely be part of networks of signal transduction pathways underlying human cancer risk with a variety of targets for the prevention and early diagnosis of human nervous system cancer.

Abbreviations

CNS	central nervous system
ENU	*N*-ethyl-*N*-nitrosourea
Mb	megabase
MNU	*N*-methyl-*N*-nitrosourea
LOH	loss of heterozygosity
MPNST	malignant peripheral nerve sheath tumor
PNS	peripheral nervous system
SNP	single nucleotide polymorphism

Acknowledgments The authors wish to thank Dr. Jürgen Thomale, Institute for Cell Biology, University Hospital of Essen, University of Duisburg-Essen, Germany for critically reading the manuscript and for helpful comments on the section on ENU–DNA interactions and on Fig. 11.1.

Glossary

allele: alternative forms of the same gene; one of the different forms of a gene that can exist at a single locus

association: a tendency of two characters (diseases, marker alleles, etc.) to occur together at non-random frequencies

congenic: nearly identical strains of an organism; they vary at only a single locus

genotype: the genetic constitution of an individual either overall or at a specific locus

haplotype: a series of alleles found at linked loci on a single chromosome

linkage: the tendency of characters (phenotypes, marker alleles, etc.) to cosegregate in a pedigree because their determinants lie close together on a particular chromosome

locus: a unique chromosomal location defining the position of an individual gene or DNA sequence

polygenic: a character determined by the combined action of a number of genetic loci

References

Altenschmidt U, Kahl R, Klundt E, et al. (1997) Schwannoma cells induce a tumor-cell-specific cytotoxic-T-cell response upon transplantation into syngeneic rats but escape elimination through the secretion of immunosuppressive factors. Int J Cancer 70:542–550

Aoyama H, Naito M, Fujimoto N, et al. (1989) Effects of sex difference, gonadectomy and estradiol on N-ethyl-N-nitrosourea-induced trigeminal nerve tumors in rats. Carcinogenesis 10:1505–1509

Bamborschke S, O'Connor PJ, Margison GP, et al. (1983) DNA methylation by dimethylnitrosamine in the Mongolian gerbil (Meriones unguiculatus): indications of a deficient, noninducible hepatic repair system for O6-methylguanine. Cancer Res 43:1306–1311

Beranek DT (1990) Distribution of methyl and ethyl adducts following alkylation with monofunctional alkylating agents. Mutat Res 231:11–30

Bhanot OS, Grevatt PC, Donahue JM, et al. (1992) In vitro DNA replication implicates O2-ethyldeoxythymidine in transversion mutagenesis by ethylating agents. Nucleic Acids Res 20:587–594

Bigner D, Swenberg J (1977) Experimental tumors of the central nervous system. Upjohn Company, Kalamazoo

Bilzer T, Reifenberger G, Wechsler W (1989) Chemical induction of brain tumors in rats by nitrosoureas: molecular biology and neuropathology. Neurotoxicol Teratol 11:551–556

Burnet FM (1970) The concept of immunological surveillance. Prog Exp Tumor Res 13:1–27

Den Engelse L, De Graaf A, De Brij RJ, et al. (1987) O2- and O4-ethylthymine and the ethylphosphotriester dTp(Et)dT are highly persistent DNA modifications in slowly dividing tissues of the ethylnitrosourea-treated rat. Carcinogenesis 8:751–757

Denlinger RH, Koestner A, Wechsler W (1974) Induction of neurogenic tumors in C3HeB-FeJ mice by nitrosourea derivatives: observations by light microscopy, tissue culture, and electron microscopy. Int J Cancer 13:559–571

Diwan BA, Meier H (1974) Strain- and age-dependent transplacental carcinogenesis by 1-ethyl-1-nitrosourea in inbred strains of mice. Cancer Res 34:764–770

Druckrey H (1971) Genotypes and phenotypes of ten inbred strains of BD-rats. Arzneimittelforschung 21:1274–1278

Druckrey H (1973) Specific carcinogenic and teratogenic effects of indirect alkylating methyl and ethyl compounds and their dependency on stages of ontogenic developments. Xenobiotica 3:271–303

Druckrey H, Ivankovic S, Preussmann R (1965) Selective Induction of Malignant Tumors in the Brain and Spinal Cord of Rats by N-Methyl-N-Nitrosourea. Z Krebsforsch 66:389–408

Druckrey H, Ivankovic S, Preussmann R (1966) Teratogenic and carcinogenic effects in the offspring after single injection of ethylnitrosourea to pregnant rats. Nature 210:1378–1379

Druckrey H, Landschutz C, Ivankovic S (1970a) Transplacental induction of malignant tumours of the nervous system. II. Ethyl-nitrosurea in 10 genetically defined strains of rats. Z Krebsforsch 73:371–386

Druckrey H, Schagen B, Ivankovic S (1970b) Induction of neurogenic malignancies by one single dose of ethyl-nitrosourea (ENU) given to newborn and juvenile BD IX-strain rats. Z Krebsforsch 74:141–161

Engelbergs J, Thomale J, Galhoff A, et al. (1998) Fast repair of O6-ethylguanine, but not O6-methylguanine, in transcribed genes prevents mutation of H-ras in rat mammary tumorigenesis induced by ethylnitrosourea in place of methylnitrosourea. Proc Natl Acad Sci USA 95:1635–1640

Gering KM, Marx JA, Lennartz K, et al. (2006) The interaction mode of premalignant Schwann and immune effector cells during chemically induced carcinogenesis in the rat peripheral nervous system is strongly influenced by genetic background. Cancer Res 66:4708–4714

Gerson SL, Trey JE, Miller K, et al. (1986) Comparison of O6-alkylguanine-DNA alkyltransferase activity based on cellular DNA content in human, rat and mouse tissues. Carcinogenesis 7:745–749
Giangaspero F, Bigner SH, Kleihues P, et al. (2000) Medulloblastoma. In: Kleihues P, Cavenee WK (eds) Pathology and Genetics of Tumors of the Nervous System, 2nd edn. IARC Press, Lyon
Goth R, Rajewsky MF (1972) Ethylation of nucleic acids by ethylnitrosourea-1- 14 C in the fetal and adult rat. Cancer Res 32:1501–1505
Goth R, Rajewsky MF (1974) Persistence of O6-ethylguanine in rat-brain DNA: correlation with nervous system-specific carcinogenesis by ethylnitrosourea. Proc Natl Acad Sci USA 71:639–643
Hegi ME, Diserens AC, Gorlia T, et al. (2005) MGMT gene silencing and benefit from temozolomide in glioblastoma. N Engl J Med 352:997–1003
Huang H, Greenberg MM (2008) Synthesis and analysis of oligonucleotides containing a basic site analogues. J Org Chem 73:2695–2703
IARC (1978) Some N-Nitroso Compounds IARC Press, Lyon
Ivankovic S, Druckrey H (1968) Transplacental induction of malignant tumors of the nervous system. I. Ethyl-nitroso-urea (ENU) in BD IX rats. Z Krebsforsch 71:320–360
Jessen KR, Mirsky R (2005) The origin and development of glial cells in peripheral nerves. Nat Rev Neurosci 6:671–682
Kindler-Rohrborn A, Koelsch BU, Buslei R, et al. (1999a) Allele-specific losses of heterozygosity on chromosomes 1 and 17 revealed by whole genome scan of ethylnitrosourea-induced BDIX x BDIV hybrid rat gliomas. Mol Carcinog 26:163–171
Kindler-Rohrborn A, Kolsch BU, Fischer C, et al. (1999b) Ethylnitrosourea-induced development of malignant schwannomas in the rat: two distinct loci on chromosome of 10 involved in tumor susceptibility and oncogenesis. Cancer Res 59:1109–1114
Kindler-Rohrborn A, Kind AB, Koelsch BU, et al. (2000) Suppression of ethylnitrosourea-induced schwannoma development involves elimination of neu/erbB-2 mutant premalignant cells in the resistant BDIV rat strain. Cancer Res 60:4756–4760
Kleihues P, Rajewsky MF (1984) Chemical neuro-oncogenesis: role of structural DNA modifications, DNA repair and neural target cell population. Prog Exp Tumor Res 27:1–16
Kleihues P, Burger PC, Collins VP, et al. (2000) Glioblastoma. In: Kleihues P, Cavenee WK (eds) Pathology and Genetics of Tumours of the Nervous System, 2nd edn. IARC Press, Lyon
Koelsch BU, Kindler-Rohrborn A, Held S, et al. (2002) Loss of heterozygosity in malignant rat schwannomas chemically induced in hybrids of inbred rat strains with differential tumor susceptibility. Carcinogenesis 23:1033–1037
Koelsch BU, Fischer C, Neibecker M, et al. (2006) Gender-specific polygenic control of ethylnitrosourea-induced oncogenesis in the rat peripheral nervous system. Int J Cancer 118:108–114
Koestner A (1990) Characterization of N-nitrosourea-induced tumors of the nervous system; their prospective value for studies of neurocarcinogenesis and brain tumor therapy. Toxicol Pathol 18:186–192
Louis DN, Scheithauer BW, Budka H, et al. (2000) Meningioma. In: Kleihues P, Cavenee WK (eds) Pathology and Genetics of Nervous System Tumors, 2nd edn. IARC Press, Lyon
Margison GP, Kleihues P (1975) Chemical carcinogenesis in the nervous system. Preferential accumulation of O6-methylguanine in rat brain deoxyribonucleic acid during repetitive administration of N-methyl-N-nitrosourea. Biochem J 148:521–525
Marx JA, Rohrborn AJ, Koelsch BU, et al. (2009) Ablation of T cell immunity differentially influences tumor risk in inbred BD rat strains. Cancer Immunol Immunotherapy; Jan 13. [Epub ahead of print]
Naito M, Naito Y, Ito A (1982) Strain differences of tumorigenic effect of neonatally administered N-ethyl-N-nitrosourea in rats. Gann 73:323–331

Naito M, Ito A, Aoyama H (1985) Genetics of susceptibility of rats to trigeminal schwannomas induced by neonatal administration of N-ethyl-N-nitrosourea. J Natl Cancer Inst 74:241–245
Nikitin A, Ballering LA, Lyons J, et al. (1991) Early mutation of the neu (erbB-2) gene during ethylnitrosourea-induced oncogenesis in the rat Schwann cell lineage. Proc Natl Acad Sci USA 88:9939–9943
Oda H, Zhang S, Tsurutani N, et al. (1997) Loss of p53 is an early event in induction of brain tumors in mice by transplacental carcinogen exposure. Cancer Res 57:646–650
Perantoni AO, Rice JM, Reed CD, et al. (1987) Activated neu oncogene sequences in primary tumors of the peripheral nervous system induced in rats by transplacental exposure to ethylnitrosourea. Proc Natl Acad Sci USA 84:6317–6321
Rasheed BK, Stenzel TT, McLendon RE, et al. (1997) PTEN gene mutations are seen in high-grade but not in low-grade gliomas. Cancer Res 57:4187–4190
Saar K, Beck A, Bihoreau MT, et al. (2008) SNP and haplotype mapping for genetic analysis in the rat. Nat Genet 40:560–566
Singer B (1983) Molecular biology of mutagens and carcinogens. Plenum Press, New York
Swenberg JA, Koestner A, Wechsler W, et al. (1975) Differential oncogenic effects of methylnitrosourea. J Natl Cancer Inst 54:89–96
The Cancer Genome Atlas Research Network, (2008) Comprehensive genomic characterization defines human glioblastoma genes and core pathways. Nature 455:1061–1068
Vinores SA, Perez-Polo JR (1980) The effect of nerve growth factor and antibodies to nerve growth factor on ethylnitrosourea carcinogenesis in mice. J Cancer Res Clin Oncol 98:59–63
Wechsler W, Rice JM, Vesselinovitch SD (1979) Transplacental and neonatal induction of neurogenic tumors in mice: comparison with related species and with human pediatric neoplasms. Natl Cancer Inst Monogr:219–226
Winzen B, Koelsch B, Fischer C, et al. (2006) Gender-specific Oligogenic Control of Resistance to Ethylnitrosourea-Induced Oncogenesis in the Rat Peripheral Nervous System. In: Regitz-Zagrosek V, Fuchs J (eds) Geschlechterforschung in der Medizin, Peter Lang, Europäischer Verlag derWissenschaften, Frankfurt
Wood GA, Korkola JE, Archer MC (2002) Tissue-specific resistance to cancer development in the rat: phenotypes of tumor-modifier genes. Carcinogenesis 23:1–9
Woodruff JM, Kourea HP, Louis DN, et al. (2000) Schwannoma. In: Kleihues P, Cavenee WK (eds) Pathology and Genetics of Tumours of the Nervous System, 2nd edn. IARC Press, Lyon
Wrensch M, Bondy ML, Wiencke J, et al. (1993) Environmental risk factors for primary malignant brain tumors: a review. J Neurooncol 17:47–64
Zimmerman HM (1955) The nature of gliomas as revealed by animal experimentation. Am J Pathol 31:1–29
Zook BC, Simmens SJ, Jones RV (2000) Evaluation of ENU-induced gliomas in rats: nomenclature, immunochemistry, and malignancy. Toxicol Pathol 28:193–201

Chapter 12
The Murine GL261 Glioma Experimental Model to Assess Novel Brain Tumor Treatments

Elizabeth W. Newcomb and David Zagzag

Abstract The GL261 glioma is representative of a carcinogen-induced mouse syngeneic glioma model. This model represents one of the very few brain tumor models developed in immunocompetent animals that has growth characteristics similar to human GBM. The ideal animal model should share the invasive properties that the human GBM displays, since this is a major reason for the failure of current treatment strategies. Here we demonstrate, through a detailed comparison with human GBM, that the murine GL261 glioma closely mimics its human counterpart in a number of significant ways, but most importantly in its invasive and angiogenic properties representing the relevant biology of human GBMs. Therefore, it should prove to be a valuable preclinical model for testing novel drugs and therapeutic strategies that inhibit glioma invasion and angiogenesis.

Contents

E.W. Newcomb (✉)
Department of Pathology, New York University Cancer Institute, New York University School of Medicine, New York, NY 10016
e-mail: newcoe01@med.nyu.edu

E.G. Van Meir (ed.), *CNS Cancer*, Cancer Drug Discovery and Development, DOI 10.1007/978-1-60327-553-8_12,
© Humana Press, a part of Springer Science+Business Media, LLC 2009

12.1 The Murine GL261 Glioma Experimental Model

Glioblastoma multiforme (GBM) is the most common form of primary malignant brain tumors occurring in adults. Due to the highly aggressive nature of these tumors, the prognosis remains poor, with a median survival time of approximately 1 year following diagnosis. New treatment options, as well as a better understanding of how GBMs develop, are essential to improve the clinical outcome of patients with GBM.

Animal models are frequently used to study tumor development and test therapeutic alternatives in the preclinical setting (Schold and Bigner, 1983; Peterson et al., 1994). The ideal animal model should imitate the human tumor in as many aspects as possible, such as histopathology, tumor biology, and genetics. The ideal animal model should share the invasive properties that the human GBM displays, since this is a major reason for the failure of current treatment strategies.

Three main categories of murine models are currently used for the study of GBM: transplantation of murine glioma cells into syngeneic mice, transplantation of human glioma cells into immunocompromised mice, and transgenic models (Peterson et al., 1994). Transplant models are useful because their growth rate is predictable and reproducible and the tumor is injected in a known location. Syngeneic models are particularly valuable to study tumor growth in vivo because, unlike the human xenograft models, the syngeneic models do not require a deficient immune system and may mimic more closely the interaction between tumor and immune system taking place in human GBM patients.

Several transgenic models have been developed that target specific genetic events recapitulating some of those known to occur during the development of GBM (Weissenberger et al., 1997; Holland et al., 2000; Reilly et al., 2000; Xiao et al., 2002). Some of these transgenic models were reviewed recently by a panel of neuropathologists and found to have histopathologic characteristics that resemble human GBM (Weiss et al., 2002). However, spontaneous tumor formation in the transgenic models is much less predictable than that seen in the transplant models. Often a mixture of tumor types develop, ranging from low-grade astrocytomas to high-grade glioblastomas, and penetrance can be low, typically with fewer than half of the mice developing tumors that display characteristics of GBM (Reilly and Jacks, 2001). In addition, there is a longer latency time for tumors to develop, making these models more costly and more time intensive to produce and study. Although transgenic models are useful for studying the underlying tumor biology predisposing to GBM development, they are less practical for large-scale screening of potential new drugs and novel treatment therapies.

The GL261 glioma is representative of a carcinogen-induced mouse glioma model. It was induced by Seligman and Shear (1939) through intracranial implantation of 20 methylcholanthrene pellets into brains of mice, out of which 11 developed gliomas. One of these gliomas was designated GL261 and was next reported by Ausman et al. (1970). In this study, the GL261 glioma was described as having characteristics of ependymoblastoma, with histopathologic features similar to three other gliomas: ependymoblastoma, glioma 26 (G-26), and ependymoblastoma A (Ausman et al., 1970). Since that initial report, both GL261 and G-26 have been described instead as containing poorly differentiated cells and exhibiting features more consistent with GBM (Schold and Bigner, 1983; Wiranowska et al., 1998; Zagzag et al., 2000a).

There are several syngeneic transplant models including CT-2A, another methylcholanthrene carcinogen-induced brain tumor in C57BL/6 strain mice (Zimmerman and Arnold, 1941). The CT-2A tumor has been recently characterized and proposed as suitable for preclinical studies (Martinez-Murillo and Martinez, 2007). Two other transplant models involve rare spontaneous development of glioma-like tumors. The 4C8 tumor arose in a transgenic mouse and is transplanted into F1 strain (C57BL/6 X DBA/2) mice (Weiner et al., 1999) and has been used in preclinical studies (Hellums et al., 2005). The spontaneous murine astrocytoma (SMA) arose in the VM/Dk mouse strain (Serano et al., 1980). The SMA-560 cell line, one clone derived from this tumor, has also been characterized (Sampson et al., 1997) and used in preclinical studies (Heimberger et al., 2000; Learn et al., 2007).

Among these syngeneic transplant models the glioma 261 (GL261) has been used frequently for preclinical testing (Miyatake et al., 1997; Plautz et al., 1997; Glick et al., 1999; Yu et al., 1997; Kjaergaard et al., 2000; Lumniczky et al., 2002; Newcomb et al., 2004). Although several studies have suggested that GL261 shares features similar to human GBM (Zagzag et al., 2000a, b), a more comprehensive demonstration of its histopathologic and biologic characteristics in comparison to human GBM was needed to verify its validity as a suitable preclinical model.

Here we demonstrate, through a detailed comparison with human GBM, that the murine GL261 glioma closely mimics its human counterpart in a number of significant ways, but most importantly in its invasive and angiogenic properties. Therefore, it should prove to be a valuable preclinical model for testing novel drugs and therapeutic strategies that inhibit invasion and angiogenesis.

12.2 The Murine GL261 Glioma Experimental Model: Validation Studies for a Predictive Preclinical Model

The Mouse Models for Human Cancer Consortium (MMHCC) was initiated by the NCI in 1999 to promote the development and characterization of genetically engineered murine (GEM) models that would recapitulate the initiation and progression of human malignancy. A meeting of neuropathologists was held in 2000 to review the existing GEM models for tumors of the central nervous system (Weiss et al., 2002). Recommendations were made how to characterize the model for pathology, for tumor biology, for neuroimaging, and for preclinical validation in screening and evaluating response to anti-tumor treatments. Although the GL261 glioma intracranial model is not a GEM model giving rise to "spontaneous" brain tumors as expected for transgenic mice engineered to overexpress a given transgene or have engineered mutations in specific tumor suppressors, it represents an important syngeneic transplant animal model that uses engraftment of murine GL261 glioma cells into the brain of an immunocompetent animal. Traditionally, mouse models for glioma have used primarily human U87MG glioma cells, xenografted into immunosuppressed mice (Eshleman et al., 2002; Heimberger et al., 2002; Miller et al., 2002; Mohanam et al., 2002; Abe et al., 2003; Hu et al., 2003). The consensus report committee felt that "as a group, this type of xenograft model fails to recapitulate the genetic heterogeneity and infiltrating neuropathology characteristic of the human tumor from which they were derived. As a result, xenograft models have generally been poorly predictive in preclinical trials of anti-tumor agents."

We suggest that one major reason for this discrepancy for being "poorly predictive" is the fact that U87MG tumors growing in the brains of immunosuppressed mice do not show an "invasive phenotype" characteristic of human GBM (Fig. 12.1). Tumors formed by human U87MG glioma cells (Fig. 12.1A) are spheroid and the leading edge of the tumor remains sharply demarcated from the brain adjacent to the tumor as described previously (Hu et al., 2003). No invading tumor cells, alone or in groups, were observed near to the tumor borders. In sharp contrast, tumors formed by the murine GL261 glioma cells (Fig. 12.1B) have irregularly shaped borders with clearly visible invading tongues of tumor cells advancing into the brain adjacent to the tumor as we and others have described (Wiranowska et al., 1998; Zagzag et al., 2003; Cha et al., 2003). Individual tumor cells invading into the brain adjacent to the tumor several millimeters away from the tumor margins are easily detected.

Below we describe in more detail the features of the GL261 glioma animal model that make it an attractive preclinical model for human GBM. As a guide,

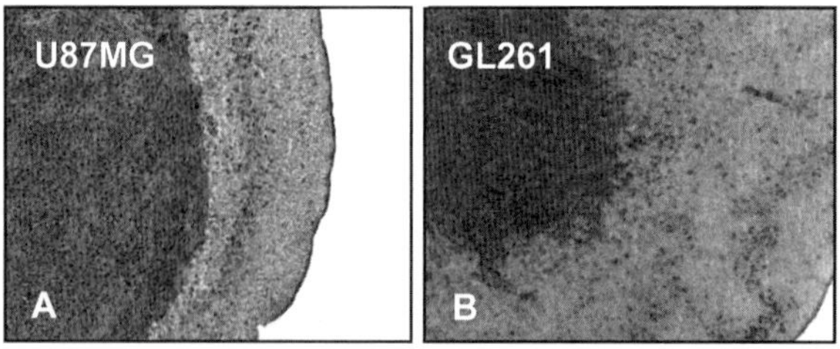

Fig. 12.1 Growth patterns of human U87MG glioma cells versus murine GL261 glioma cells in nude mice. Mice were injected with (**A**) human U87MG glioma cells or (**B**) murine GL261 glioma cells. The brains were harvested at day 15 following implantation. Experimental data and H&E-stained slides were kindly provided by Dr. Cheng, University of Pittsburg Cancer Institute. $\times$ 40

we have followed the recommendations of the consensus report from the neuropathology working group (Weiss et al., 2000). Characterization of any brain tumor model requires extensive pathological examination noting features that are hallmarks of the human glioma; immunohistochemistry for appropriate differentiation markers; an understanding of its tumor biology, e.g., signaling pathways relevant to the known biology of the human GBM; and non-invasive imaging techniques that can be used for the serial investigation of a single animal to follow response to a particular anti-tumor therapy.

12.3 Neuropathology

In vivo animal models of primary brain tumors are necessary to advance knowledge related to the complex interactions between glioma cells and the brain adjacent to the tumor. A cardinal feature of human GBMs, and a major reason why neurosurgical and adjunctive therapies ultimately fail, is their invasive properties. We have previously reported the invasive growth pattern of GL261 glioma cells in the brains of syngeneic C57BL/6 mice by both light and electron microscopy (Zagzag et al., 2000a, b, 2003). The GL261 glioma animal model recapitulates many of the histopathological features of human GBM (Fig. 12.2 and Color Plate 17).

To demonstrate the similarity of GL261 gliomas to human GBM, we examined H&E sections from patients who were diagnosed with GBM and immunostained tumor sections from human and murine tumors with a similar panel of primary antibodies. As shown in Fig. 12.2, GL261 gliomas clearly exhibit features that meet the criteria of GBM and closely resemble their human GBM counterpart. Numerous poorly differentiated, pleomorphic cells with atypical nuclei were observable throughout the tumors, including multinucleated cells and cells with hyperchromatic nuclei (Fig. 12.2B). Mitotic activity was particularly evident, as shown by several mitotic figures per field (Fig. 12.2D). Multiple necrotic areas were visible in irregularly shaped, band-like patterns of eosinophilic material consisting of non-viable or necrotic cells (Fig. 12.2F). Although not as prominent as in human GBM, densely packed, viable cells lined the necrotic zones in a pseudopalisading pattern characteristic of GBM. An increase in microvascular density was also observed throughout the tumor (Fig. 12.2H) and confirmed by immunostaining for CD31 antigen in the endothelial cells (Fig. 12.2 J).

To confirm its glial lineage, we performed immunohistochemistry using two glial differentiation markers, glial fibrillary acidic protein (GFAP) and S-100 protein. The fibrillary staining of astrocytic processes was displayed through GFAP staining (Fig. 12.2L) while a majority of tumor cells were found to be positive for S-100 protein (Fig. 12.2N). Proliferative activity was further analyzed using MIB-1 antibody in human and BrdU antibody in mouse tumors (Fig. 12.2O and P). MIB-1 antibody binds to the nuclear cell proliferation

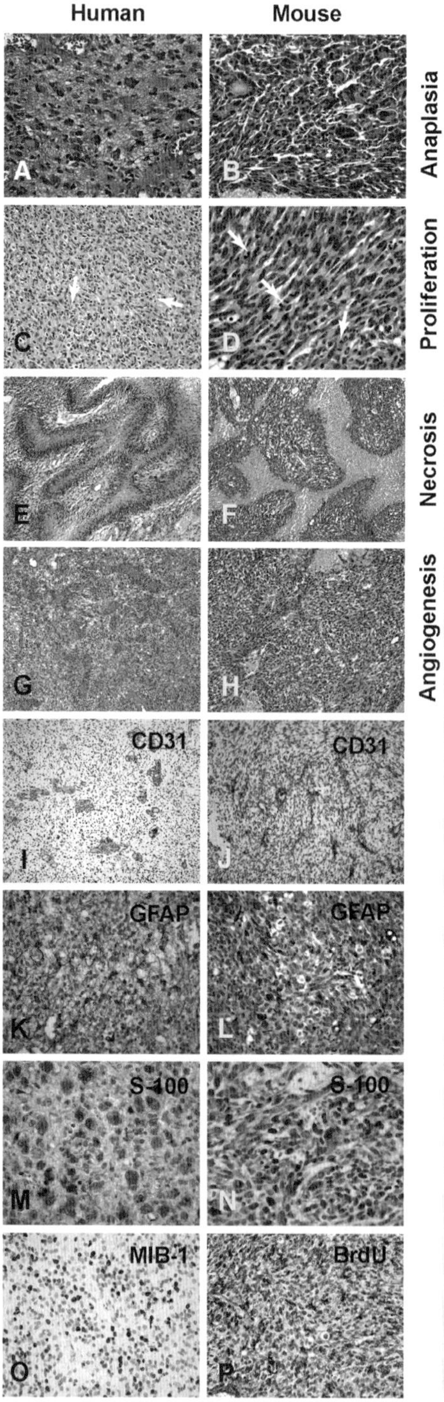

Fig. 12.2 Histopathology: Comparison between high-grade human gliomas and the murine GL261 glioma. Tumor sections from paraffin blocks were prepared for H&E stains or immunostained

marker Ki-67, which is found throughout the cell cycle in proliferating cells but is absent in G_0 resting cells. BrdU is a thymidine analogue that labels cells in S-phase. Both human and GL261 gliomas demonstrated a significant portion of proliferative cells within the tumor.

12.4 Tumor Biology

12.4.1 Invasion, Angiogenesis, and Hypoxia

To show similarities between the human and murine tumors, sections were immunostained with the appropriate antibodies to demonstrate invasion (p53/GFP), angiogenesis (VEGF), and tumor hypoxia (HIF-1α) (Fig. 12.3). Invading GL261 tumor cells were detected by immunostaining the murine tumor sections for green fluorescence protein (GFP) (Fig. 12.3B, Zagzag et al., 2003). As a comparison, we used an immunostain for p53 to visualize invading human tumor cells (Fig. 12.3A). Like the human counterpart, GL261 gliomas showed tumor cells diffusely invading into the normal brain adjacent to the tumor at some distance from the main tumor core. Cells invaded as single cells or as groups of cells along the vasculature.

VEGF has been shown to be an important factor in the process of angiogenesis during tumor development and its expression has been shown to be upregulated in human GBM (Shweiki et al., 1992; Plate et al., 1992). The endothelial cells in the blood vessels of GL261 gliomas, like the human counterpart, are positive for VEGF protein expression (Fig. 12.3C, D).

HIF-1α has also been implicated as playing a role in invasion and angiogenesis through its activation of many genes, including VEGF (Forsythe et al., 1996; Zagzag et al., 2000a). In Fig. 12.3 we demonstrate a similar pattern of HIF-1α expression in human GBM and GL261 gliomas. HIF-1α immunostaining was especially prominent in the pseudopalisading cells lining areas of

Fig. 12.2 (continued) with an appropriate antibody. The diagnosis of GBM is based on the presence of highly anaplastic glial cells, mitotic activity, vascular proliferation, and necrosis. Both the human and murine malignant glioma tumors are composed of poorly differentiated, pleomorphic tumor cells (**A, B,** $\times$ 400); and show high proliferation rates (arrows denote mitoses in **C, D,** $\times$ 400). One histological hallmark of GBM is cells in a pseudopalisading pattern (**E, F,** $\times$ 100). Tumors show large areas of necrosis in the center with viable tumor cells in the periphery with foci of densely packed, small fusiform tumor cells around necrotic zones known as pseudopalisading cells. Prominent vascular proliferation is also a histological hallmark of GBM (**G, H,** $\times$ 200). Tumors were immunostained with the vascular endothelial marker CD31 to highlight the vascularity (**I,** $\times$ 100; **J,** $\times$ 200). Two important differentiation markers are associated with glial tumors: GFAP (**K, L,** $\times$ 400) and S-100 (**M, N,** $\times$ 400). The GL261 tumors are representative of gliomas as shown by their positive immunostaining for the glial differentiation markers GFAP and S-100. High proliferation rates are associated with poor prognosis. Proliferation rates can be estimated from MIB-1 labeling (**O,** $\times$ 400) or BrdU incorporation into S-phase cells (**P,** $\times$ 400) (*see* Color Plate 17)

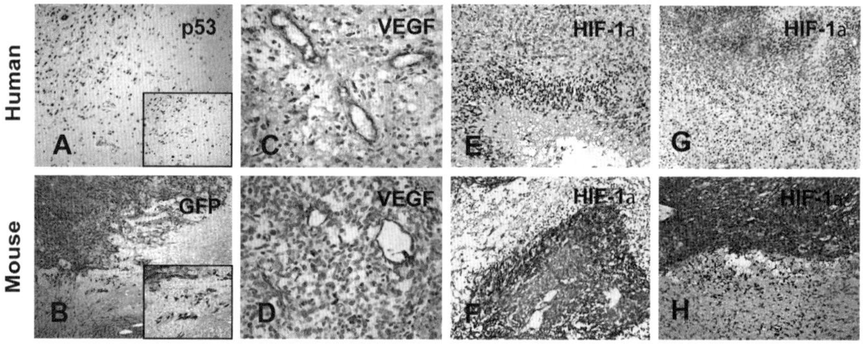

Fig. 12.3 Tumor invasion, angiogenesis, and hypoxia. Human GBM (**A, C, E, G**) and the murine GL261 glioma (**B, D, F, H**) were immunostained with the appropriate antibodies to demonstrate invasion into the brain adjacent to tumor and upregulation of markers for angiogenesis (VEGF) and hypoxia (HIF-1α). A human GBM shows p53-positive tumor cells detected at some distance away from the tumor margin (**A,** $\times$ 200; **inset** $\times$ 400). The murine GL261 tumor shows GFP-positive infiltrating cells (**B,** $\times$ 100; **inset** $\times$ 400). Here we show VEGF-positive endothelial cells within the blood vessels (**C, D,** $\times$ 400). HIF-1α is upregulated in response to hypoxia and regulates the expression of many genes important for cell survival adaptation. The upregulation of HIF-1α expression occurs in areas next to necrosis (**E, F,** $\times$ 200) and is observed in tumor cells at the invading edge of both human and murine GL261 glioma tumors (**G,** $\times$ 40; **H,** $\times$ 200)

necrosis (Fig. 12.3E, F). HIF-1α was commonly observed at the invading margins of human and murine gliomas (Fig. 12.3G, H) (Zhong et al., 1999; Zagzag et al., 2000a). For example, GFP labeling of GL261 glioma cells identified most HIF-1α-expressing cells as those invading into the surrounding brain. HIF-1 upregulates a variety of genes whose products play a well-established role in glioma invasion (Krishnamachary et al., 2003; Brat et al., 2004; Zagzag et al., 2006). These include CXCR4, SDF-1α, VEGF, MMP-2, and MMP-9 (Krishnamachary et al., 2003; Ehtesham et al., 2006). Previous studies by our group and others suggest that hypoxia stimulates glioma cell migration in vitro and invasion in orthotopic glioma models and human GBMs (Brat et al., 2004; Zagzag et al., 2000a, 2006).

In the GL261 model, as in other experimental glioma models, tumor growth in the brain goes through two vascular phases (Holash et al., 1999; Zagzag, 2000b). The native cerebral vessels are first co-opted by tumor cells followed by true neovascularization arising from existing vessels. In between these two phases, vascular apoptosis and regression followed by necrosis occur (Holash et al., 1999; Zagzag et al., 2000b). Angiopoietin-2 (Ang-2), one of the Tie2 receptor ligands, is detected prior to the onset of apoptosis in vascular cells as early as 1 week after tumor implantation, in vessels surrounded by tumor cells and in vascular cells at the edge of the tumors in the invaded brain (Holash et al., 1999; Zagzag et al., 2000b). Interestingly, Ang-2 is upregulated by hypoxia but independently of HIF-1α (Pichiule et al., 2004). More recently,

Ang-2 was also shown to promote glioma invasion by stimulating matrix metalloproteinase (MMP)-2 expression (Hu et al., 2006). Overall, the GL261 model has been shown to be a valuable tool for the study of several important molecules implicated in glioma invasion and angiogenesis. These include HIF-1, VEGF, Ang-2, CXCR4, and SDF-1α (Zagzag et al., 2000a, b, 2003, 2008).

12.4.2 Signaling Pathways

There is now considerable evidence that PI3K (phosphatidylinositol 3′kinase), a lipid kinase involved in diverse biological functions, plays a significant role in oncogenic transformation and tumor progression of many human tumors (Vivanco and Sawyers, 2002; Scheid and Woodgett, 2003). PI3K is an important signaling mediator of cell proliferation, survival, metabolism, and migration. One substrate activated by PI3K is a serine/threonine kinase, Akt, that once phosphorylated (p-Akt) regulates many biological processes including proliferation, apoptosis, and motility. Since deregulated PI3K signaling is a common denominator in human cancer, it provides an attractive target for therapy (Vivanco and Sawyers, 2002).

Human GBMs contain mutations and deletions of the PTEN (phosphatase and tensin homologue) tumor suppressor gene, a negative regulator of PI3K signaling (Ermoian et al., 2002; Davies et al., 1998). A recent study analyzed the PI3K signaling pathway in human GBM using immunohistochemistry for PTEN, p-Akt, and EGFR (epidermal growth factor receptor) to look for correlations with deregulated PI3K signaling (Choe et al., 2003). The loss of PTEN was correlated with activation of Akt as assessed by positive immunostaining of the tumors for phosphorylated Akt (p-Akt). In this context, it is important to note that some GEM models of glioma that have been studied recently demonstrate activation of the PI3K signaling pathway (Xiao et al., 2002; Hesselager et al., 2003). In one model with inactivation of the Rb tumor suppressor pathway, the presence of PTEN mutations accelerated glioma development (Xiao et al., 2002). Tumors arising in these mice showed regions in the brain of reduced apoptosis and these same areas expressed activated p-Akt by immunohistochemistry. In another brain tumor model using PDGF-B (platelet-derived growth factor) to induce gliomas, loss of either p53 or INK4a-ARF tumor suppressors accelerated tumor formation (Hesselager et al., 2003). Decreased expression of PTEN in tumor cells was associated with activation of Akt demonstrated on western blot analysis with detection of p-Akt (Hesselager et al., 2003). Thus, deregulation of the PI3K pathway, measured by detection of p-Akt, is an important signaling pathway driving human as well as murine gliomagenesis. As shown in Fig. 12.4, using western blotting and immunostains of tumors for p-Akt, we have shown that GL261 glioma, similar to their human counterpart, demonstrate activation of the PI3K pathway as demonstrated by the detection of p-Akt in vitro and in vivo.

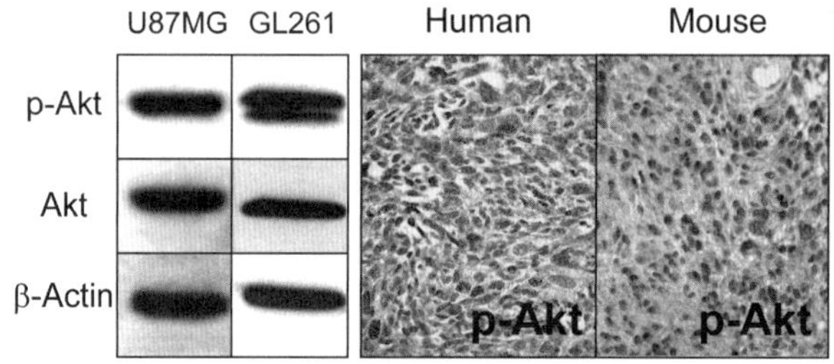

Fig. 12.4 Activation of the PI3K pathway: comparison between high-grade human and mouse gliomas. The human U87 and murine GL261 glioma cell lines were assessed for levels of expression of p-Akt by western blotting. Both glioma cell lines showed the presence of p-Akt, indicating activation of the PI3K signaling pathway. Similarly, p-Akt could be detected in paraffin-embedded tumor samples from a representative human GBM and a murine GL261 glioma by immunohistochemistry. × 100

12.5 Neuroimaging and Neuroradiology

Neuroimaging has proven to be a valuable technique for clinically monitoring tumor growth and estimating a response to therapy in human GBM (Nelson and Cha, 2003). Likewise, imaging can be used in the GL261 model to view the tumor during its in vivo progression and detect its response to different treatments. As shown in Fig. 12.5, a representative MR image of a patient diagnosed with GBM (Fig. 12.5A) is shown next to an MR image of a GL261 glioma (Fig. 12.5B). Like human GBM, the GL261 glioma on post-contrast T1-weighted images demonstrates a heterogeneous mass. The tumors are irregularly shaped with an enhanced border and display central hypointensity that marks the necrotic zones.

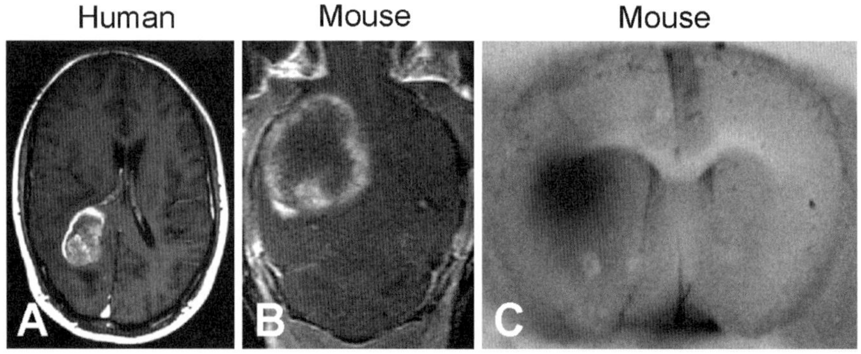

Fig. 12.5 Neuroimaging of gliomas. MRI images are shown for (**A**) a human GBM and (**B**) a GL261 glioma at 4 weeks post-implantation of GL261 cells. MRI is used clinically to monitor tumor growth and aid in diagnosis. Typically GBMs present as an irregular lesion with a peripheral, ring-like zone of contrast enhancement around a dark central area of necrosis. (**C**) Disruption of the blood–brain barrier is demonstrated in the murine GL261 glioma by Evans blue extravasation

We have established the use of MRI in the early detection of GL261 tumors following implantation (Fig. 12.5). We have used both conventional T1- and T2-weighted imaging and dynamic, contrast-enhanced T2*-weighted imaging. MRI measurements of relative cerebral blood volume (rCBV) were compared with histological measurements of microvascular density (MVD) and showed a good correlation for the same tumors (Cha et al., 2003). In addition, enhancement on post-contrast T1-weighted images was compared with histological assessment of Evans blue extravasation (Fig. 12.5C). We conclude that the blood–brain barrier (BBB) is disrupted early during the course of GL261 tumor growth, which ensures enhanced delivery of anti-tumor agents into the tumor bed.

In addition to MRI, we have developed non-invasive CT imaging to follow tumor growth and response to a novel immunotherapy approach (Newcomb et al., 2006). This imaging technique is well suited for imaging large numbers of mice in a timely fashion (e.g., imaging acquisition for 12 mice takes approximately 90 min) and is extremely time- and cost-effective in comparison with MR imaging which requires approximately one afternoon to image two live mice per afternoon session. As shown in Fig. 12.6, mice bearing established GL261 gliomas, detected on day 17 by CT scanning, received fractionated doses of radiation (2 Gy per fraction up to a total of 10 treatments for a total of 20 Gy) on days 17–21 and 23–28. The response to treatment was monitored by serial CT scanning. Representative CT scans are shown for a control and an irradiated animal on days 17 and 28 (Fig. 12.6A). Because fractionated radiotherapy is a standard care for GBM patients, the results show (Fig. 12.6B) that the GL261 glioma is radioresistant, similar to the human counterpart. Radiotherapy extended survival of GL261 brain tumor-bearing mice but was not curative, similar to the response observed in human GBM patients.

12.6 Significance of GL261 Glioma Animal Model for Use as a Predictive Preclinical Model

There are several advantages of a syngeneic transplant tumor model over GEM animal models with respect to predictive preclinical trials testing new and novel anti-tumor therapies for human GBM. First, we have characterized the five distinct stages of GL261 tumor growth occurring over a 4-week interval (Zagzag et al., 2000b). Stage I – implantation, where tumor cells are dispersed within the neuropil; Stage II –week 1: perivascular organization of tumor cells around native blood vessels; Stage III –week 2: a proliferative phase, where tumor cells actively proliferate around viable blood vessels; Stage IV – week 3: apoptosis combined with involution of host vascular cells resulting in degeneration of host blood vessels leading to hypoxia, which in turn promotes VEGF expression leading to angiogenesis; Stage V – week 4: angiogenesis, where neovascularization occurs as blood vessels grow toward and vascularize the now necrosing tumor. Second, knowing the changes that occur over the 4-week

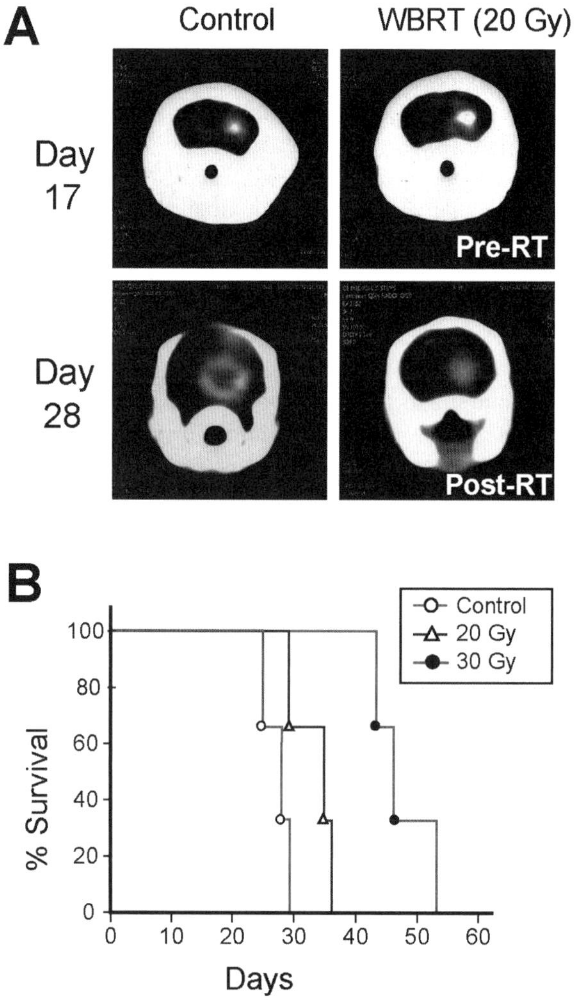

Fig. 12.6 Neuroradiology of gliomas. On day 17 after implantation, mice were anesthetized, injected with contrast agent (iothalamate meglamine, 100 μl intraorbitally) and axial images of the brain were acquired using the GE CT scanner within 10 min of contrast injection to detect the presence of tumors. Mice with established tumors were divided into control and radiation treatment (RT) groups. Following CT scanning, the mice were irradiated using a ^{60}Co source (Theratron 780-C, AECL Medical, Canada) for whole brain irradiation (WBRT) using a 3 cm size portal to a total dose of 20 Gy, in 10 daily fractions of 2 Gy over 2 weeks (days 17–21 and 24–28). (**A**) **CT imaging.** Control and treated animals were serially imaged on days 17, 24, and 28. A representative CT scan on day 28 from the brain of an untreated (*left*) or irradiated (*right*) animal is shown. Whereas the tumor volumes on day 17 appear similar in size, by day 28 after receiving a total of 20 Gy, the treated animal (*right*) clearly has a smaller tumor than that observed in the untreated control animal (*left*). (**B**) **Survival curves.** Animals were given WBRT in 10 daily fractions (2–3 Gy fraction every weekday for 2 weeks) starting on day 17 after tumor implantation. Animals receiving a total of 20 or 30 Gy had median survivals of 33 and 47 days, respectively, compared with 27 days in the control group

growth interval will allow the introduction of treatments at different stages of tumor cell growth, proliferation, and different phases of angiogenesis. Third, knowing the site of tumor cell implantation facilitates imaging studies used to evaluate response of the tumor to a given treatment. Lastly, the transplant model is very cost-effective since tumor latency is of short duration, usually 5 weeks compared to GEM models which may take months to develop tumors, and thus the transplant model can facilitate screening of potential therapies in a timely fashion. Based on the extensive characterization of the GL261 glioma model detailed above, we feel that it accurately represents the relevant biology of human GBMs as mandated by the NCI Brain Tumor Progress Review Group, with respect to its histopathology, especially its invasive phenotype, shown in the brains of both immunosuppressed and immunocompetent mice (Figs. 12.1 and 12.3). The tumor biology of GL261 closely parallels that of human GBM with respect to the markers that we have tested (Figs. 12.2–12.4). Moreover, we have demonstrated that different non-invasive imaging techniques (Figs. 12.5 and 12.6) can be used to effectively screen the response of the GL261 gliomas to different anti-tumor therapies relevant to the treatment of human GBM.

References

Abe T, Terada K, Wakimoto H, et al. (2003) PTEN decreases in vivo vascularization of experimental gliomas in spite of proangiogenic stimuli. Cancer Res 63:2300–2305

Ausman JI, Shapiro WR, Rall DP (1970) Studies on the chemotherapy of experimental brain tumors: development of an experimental model. Cancer Res 30:2394–2400

Brat DJ, Castellano-Sanchez AA, Hunter SB, et al. (2004) Pseudopalisades in glioblastoma are hypoxic, express extracellular matrix proteases, and are formed by an actively migrating cell population. Cancer Res 64:920–927

Cha S, Johnson G, Wadghiri YZ, et al. (2003) Dynamic, contrast-enhanced perfusion MRI in mouse gliomas: correlation with histopathology. Magn Reson Med 49:848–855

Choe G, Horvath S, Cloughesy TF, et al. (2003) Analysis of the phosphatidylinositol 3'-kinase signaling pathway in glioblastoma patients in vivo. Cancer Res 63:2742–2746

Davies MA, Lu Y, Sano T, et al. (1998) Adenoviral transgene expression of MMAC/PTEN in human glioma cells inhibits Akt activation and induces anoikis. Cancer Res 58:5285–5290

Ermoian RP, Furnis CS, Lamborn KR, et al. (2002) Dysregulation of PTEN and protein kinase B is associated with glioma histology and patient survival. Clin Cancer Res 8:1100–1106

Eshleman JS, Carlson BL, Mladek AC, et al. (2002) Inhibition of the mammalian target of rapamycin sensitizes U87 xenografts to fractionated radiation therapy. Cancer Res 62:7291–7297

Ehtesham M, Winston JA, Kabos P, et al. (2006). CXCR4 expression mediates glioma cell invasiveness. Oncogene 25:2801–2806

Forsythe JA, Jiang BH, Iyer NV, et al. (1996) Activation of vascular endothelial growth factor gene transcription by hypoxia-inducible factor 1. Mol Cell Biol 16:4604–4613

Glick RP, Lichtor T, de Zoeten E, et al. (1999) Prolongation of survival of mice with glioma treated with semiallogeneic fibroblasts secreting interleukin-2. Neurosurgery 45:867–874

Heimberger AB, Crotty LE, Archer GE, et al. (2000) Bone marrow-derived dendritic cells pulsed with tumor homogenate induce immunity against syngeneic intracerebral glioma. J Neuroimmunol 103:16–25

Heimberger AB, Learn CA, Archer GE, et al. (2002) Brain tumors in mice are susceptible to blockade of epidermal growth factor receptor (EGFR) with the oral, specific, EGFR-tyrosine kinase inhibitor ZD1839 (iressa). Clin Cancer Res 8:3496–3502
Hellums EK, Markert JM, Parker JN, et al. (2005) Increased efficacy of an interleukin-12 secreting herpes simplex virus in a syngeneic intracranial murine glioma model. Neuro-Oncol 7:213–224
Hesselager G, Uhrbom L, Westermark B, et al. (2003) Complementary effects of platelet-derived growth factor autocrine stimulation and p53 or Ink4a-Arf deletion in a mouse glioma model. Cancer Res 63:4305–4309
Holash J, Maisonpierre PC, Compton D, et al. (1999) Vessel cooption, regression, and growth in tumors mediated by angiopoietins and VEGF. Science 284:1994–1998
Holland EC, Celestino J, Dai C, et al. (2000) Combined activation of Ras and Akt in neural progenitors induces glioblastoma formation in mice. Nat Genet 25:55–57
Hu B, Guo P, Fang Q, et al. (2003) Angiopoietin-2 induces human glioma invasion through the activation of matrix metalloprotease-2. Proc Natl Acad Sci 100:8904–8909
Hu B, Jarzynka MJ, Guo P, et al. (2006) Angiopoietin 2 induces glioma cell invasion by stimulating matrix metalloprotease 2 expression through the alphavbeta1 integrin and focal adhesion kinase signaling pathway. Cancer Res 66:775–783
Kjaergaard J, Tanaka J, Kim JA, et al. (2000) Therapeutic efficacy of OX-40 receptor antibody depends on tumor immunogenicity and anatomic site of tumor growth. Cancer Res 60:5514–5521
Krishnamachary B, Berg-Dixon S, Kelly B, et al. (2003) Regulation of colon carcinoma cell invasion by hypoxia-inducible factor 1. Cancer Res 63:1138–1143
Learn CA, Grossi PM, Schmittling RJ, et al. (2007) Genetic analysis of intracranial tumors in a murine model of glioma demonstrate a shift in gene expression in response to host immunity. J Neuroimmunol 182:63–72
Lumniczky K, Desaknai S, Mangel L, et al. (2002) Local tumor irradiation augments the antitumor effect of cytokine-producing autologous cancer cell vaccines in a murine glioma model. Cancer Gene Ther 9:44–52
Martinez-Murillo R and Martinez A. (2007) Standardization of an orthotopic mouse brain tumor model following transplantation of CT-2A astrocytoma cells. Histol Histopathol 22:1309–1326
Miller CR, Williams CR, Buchsbaum DJ, et al. (2002) Intratumoral 5-fluorouracil produced by cytosine deaminase/5-flurocytosine gene therapy is effective for experimental human glioblastomas. Cancer Res 62:773–780
Miyatake S, Martuza RL, Rabkin SD (1997) Defective herpes simplex virus vectors expressing thymidine kinase for the treatment of malignant glioma. Cancer Gene Ther 4:222–228
Mohanam S, Cvhandrasekar N, Yanamandra N, et al. (2002) Modulation of invasive properties of human glioblastoma cells stably expressing amino-terminal fragment of urokinase-type plasminogen activator. Oncogene 21:7824–7830
Nelson SJ, Cha S (2003) Imaging Glioblastoma Multiforme. Cancer J 9:134–145
Newcomb EW, Tamasdan C, Entzminger Y, et al. (2004) Flavopiridol inhibits the growth of GL261 gliomas in vivo: Implications for malignant glioma therapy. Cell Cycle 3:230–234
Newcomb EW, Demaria S, Lukyanov Y, et al. (2006) The combination of ionizing radiation and peripheral vaccination produces long-term survival of mice bearing established invasive GL261 tumors. Clin Cancer Res 12:4730–4737
Peterson DL, Sheridan PJ, Brown WE, Jr. (1994) Animal models for brain tumors: historical perspectives and future directions. J Neurosurg 80:865–876
Pichiule P, Chavez JC, LaManna JC. (2004) Hypoxic regulation of angiopoietin-2 expression in endothelial cells. J Biol Chem 279:12171–12180
Plate KH, Breier G, Weich HA, et al. (1992) Vascular endothelial growth factor is a potential tumour angiogenesis factor in human gliomas in vivo. Nature 359:845–848

Plautz GE, Touhalisky JE, Shu S. (1997) Treatment of murine gliomas by adoptive transfer ex vivo activated tumor-draining lymph node cells. Cell Immunol 178:101–107
Reilly KM, Loisel DA, Bronson RT, et al. (2000) Nf1;Trp53 mutant mice develop glioblastoma with evidence of strain-specific effects. Nat Genet 26:109–113
Reilly KM, Jacks T (2001) Genetically engineered mouse models of astrocytoma: GEMs in the rough? Semin Cancer Biol 11:177–190
Sampson JN, Ashley DM, Archer GE, et al. (1997) Characterization of a spontaneous murine astrocytoma and abrogation of its tumorigenicity by cytokine secretion. Neurosurgery 41:1365–1372
Scheid MN, Woodgett Jr (2003) Unraveling the activation mechanisms of protein kinase B/Akt. FEBS Letts 546:108–112
Schold SC, Jr., Bigner DD (1983) A review of animal brain tumor models that have been used for therapeutic studies. In Walker MD ed. Oncology of the Nervous System. Boston: Nijhoff. p.31–63
Seligman AM, Shear MJ (1939) Studies in carcinogenesis. VIII. Experimental production of brain tumors in mice with methylcholanthrene. Am J Cancer 37:364–395
Serano RD, Pegram CN, Bigner DD. (1980) Tumorigenic cell culture lines from a spontaneous VM/Dk murine astrocytoma (SMA). Acta Neuropathol 51:53–64
Shweiki D, Itin A, Soffer D, et al. (1992) Vasular endothelial growth factor induced by hypoxia may mediate hypoxia-initiated angiogenesis. Nature 359:843–845
Vivanco I, Sawyers CL (2002) The phosphatidylinositol 3-kinase-Akt pathway in human cancer. Nature Rev Cancer 2:489–501
Weiner NE, Pyles RB, Chalk CL, et al. (1999) A syngeneic mouse glioma model for study of glioblastoma therapy. J Neuropathol Exp Neurol 58:54–60
Weiss WA, Israel M, Cobbs C, et al. (2002) Neuropathology of genetically engineered mice: consensus report and recommendations from an international forum. Oncogene 21: 7453–7463
Weissenberger J, Steinbach JP, Malin G, et al. (1997) Development and malignant progression of astrocytomas in GFAP-v-src transgenic mice. Oncogene 14:2005–2013
Wiranowska M, Tresser N, Saporta S (1998) The effect of interferon and anti-CD44 antibody on mouse glioma invasiveness in vitro. Anticancer Res 18:3331–3338
Xiao A, Wu H, Pandolfi PP, et al. (2002) Astrocyte inactivation of the pRb pathway predisposes mice to malignant astrocytoma development that is accelerated by PTEN mutation. Cancer Cell 1:157–168
Yu JS, Burwick JA, Dranoff G, et al. (1997) Gene therapy for metastatic brain tumors by vaccination with granulocyte-macrophage colony-stimulating factor-transduced tumor cells. Hum Gene Ther 8:1065–1072
Zagzag D, Zhong H, Scalzitti JM, et al. (2000a) Expression of hypoxia-inducible factor 1α in human brain tumors: Association with angiogenesis, invasion and progression. Cancer 88:2606–2618
Zagzag D, Amirnovin R, Greco MA, et al. (2000b) Vascular apoptosis and involution in gliomas precede neovascularization: A novel concept for glioma growth and angiogenesis. Lab Invest 80:837–849
Zagzag D, Miller DC, Chiriboga L, Yee H, et al. (2003) Green fluorescent protein immunohistochemistry as a novel experimental tool for the detection of glioma cell invasion in vivo. Brain Pathol 13:34–37
Zagzag D, Lukyanov Y, Lan L, et al. (2006) Hypoxia-inducible factor-1 and VEGF upregulate CXCR4 in glioblastoma: implications for angiogenesis and glioma cell invasion. Lab Invest 86:1221–1232
Zagzag D, Esencay M, Mendez O, et al. (2008) Hypoxia- and vascular endothelial growth factor-induced stromal cell-derived factor-1alpha/CXCR4 expression in glioblastomas: one plausible explanation of Scherer's structures. Am J Pathol 173:545–560
Zimmerman H, Arnold H. (1941) Experimental brain tumors. I. Tumors produced with methylcholanthrene. Cancer Res 1:919–938

Chapter 13
Spontaneous Occurrence of Brain Tumors in Animals: Opportunities as Preclinical Model Systems

Simon R. Platt

Abstract Naturally occurring neoplasia of the nervous system has been documented in many species in addition to humans, which include dogs, cats, mice, and even zebrafish. Some of the tumors in these species share many features including histopathological appearance, neuroimaging characteristics, tumor genetics, molecular targets, and biological behavior. Based on such similarities, studying the CNS tumors of dogs and mice and the genetics of neuronal neoplasia in *Drosophila* and zebrafish has been suggested as a valuable pursuit in the field of cancer research which can aid in the following areas: identification of cancer-associated genes, environmental risk factors, tumor biology, and progression and the development of novel therapeutics. This chapter reviews the current knowledge on the types of neoplasia documented to spontaneously affect the nervous system in dogs, mice, *Drosophila*, and zebrafish and demonstrates the potential utility of these naturally occurring models in cancer research.

Contents

S.R. Platt (✉)
Department of Small Animal Medicine & Surgery, College of Veterinary Medicine, University of Georgia, 501 DW Brooks Drive, Athens GA 30602, USA
e-mail: srplatt@uga.edu

E.G. Van Meir (ed.), *CNS Cancer*, Cancer Drug Discovery and Development, DOI 10.1007/978-1-60327-553-8_13,
© Humana Press, a part of Springer Science+Business Media, LLC 2009

13.1 Introduction

One of the most significant scientific and ethical hurdles in advancing novel diagnostic and therapeutic approaches for central nervous system (CNS) neoplasia is in deciding when preclinical evidence is sufficiently compelling to warrant introduction to human beings (Kimmelman and Nalbantoglu, 2007). A major component of this decision is an assessment of how well data collected in tumor-bearing models predict the actuality in the clinical setting. Unfortunately, many CNS tumor treatment trials have often been justified on the basis of models that involve numerous discontinuities with the human disease (Kimmelman and Nalbantoglu, 2007). The ideal animal model for human CNS malignant neoplasia has been suggested to be spontaneously arising, capable of intraparenchymal growth, uniformly fatal within a reasonable time period, capable of in vitro growth, transplantable both intracranially and subcutaneously in syngeneic animals, and to correlate with the therapeutic sensitivities of its human counterparts (Bradford et al., 1986).

The murine brain tumor models are well documented and some, such as the transgenic glioma models, reflect many of the structural and histological features of human tumors (Begemann et al., 2002). However, murine tumors may respond differently to cancer treatments than human cancers and additionally are inappropriate models to evaluate novel treatments in conjunction with standard surgical resection, which is not easily performed in mice.

Advances in molecular biology and genetics have rapidly improved our understanding of cancer. However, the concurrent application of this information to the human condition has been relatively slow, on account in large part to the unavailability of relevant in vivo cancer models. Lacking from most preclinical approaches is the use of models that are characterized by spontaneous cancer development in immune-competent and syngeneic hosts. The Mouse Models of Human Cancers Consortium has proposed criteria for the ideal cancer model (Weiss et al., 2002). It was recommended that all new models should be created under the supervision of a suitably qualified and experienced neuropathologist, histopathologically classified and graded based on the World Health Organization scheme and should range from low to high grade to ensure all stages of malignancy are represented. Additionally, all models should ideally be based on existing genetic information of corresponding human tumors (Weiss et al., 2002).

Spontaneous cancer models offer an opportunity to apply a 'comparative' perspective to the discovery and development of new drugs that is based on a diverse group of well-defined and well-characterized animal models (Hansen and

Khanna, 2004). Spontaneous brain tumors, including astrocytomas, glioblastoma multiforme, and ependymoma, have been documented infrequently in non-human primates (Herring et al., 1990; Long et al., 1998; Nichols and Dias, 1995; Yanai et al., 1992). Such rarity and the logistical issues associated with working with these species count against using them as models for brain tumor investigation. Even so, monkeys have been used to establish a brain tumor model using Rous sarcoma virus, as has been described in dogs and rats (Tabuchi et al., 1985). Several 'companion' (pet) or farm animal species have successfully contributed to investigations of cancer biology and drug development, including rabbits, cats, horses, ferrets, and dogs (Ernestus et al., 1992; Frank et al., 1987a, b; Paoloni and Khanna, 2008). Some of these, including the cat (Tomek et al., 2006; Troxel et al., 2003), horse (Covington et al., 2004; Paradis, 1998), and cow (Hoenerhoff et al., 2006), have been documented with spontaneously occurring central nervous system tumors, some of which have been investigated for translational purposes (Canfield and Doughty, 1980; Stoica et al., 2001); however, this disease seems to be more common in dogs making it a more satisfactory model.

Brain tumors have been detailed in all organisms from invertebrates to humans. This chapter will first focus on the review of CNS neoplasia in simple organisms like *Drosophila* and zebrafish, which are amenable to easy genetic manipulation. Next spontaneous occurrence of brain tumors in mice and their limitations are discussed. Finally, I review what is currently known about canine brain tumors, defining their similarities with their human counterparts based on their histologic, molecular and cytogenetic pathologies, and response to treatment characteristics.

13.2 *Drosophila* and Cancer Research

Despite very promising beginnings in the last century, the fly has not received much attention as a model system for cancer research for numerous reasons (Potter et al., 2000). However, a significant number of genes that have been studied in flies have turned out to be homologs of human oncogenes and tumor suppressors (Miklos and Rubin, 1996; Potter et al., 2000). Studies of these *Drosophila* homologs of known mammalian cancer genes have contributed tremendously toward the understanding of the developmental functions of these genes, their actions at the molecular level, and the genetic pathways in which the genes are involved.

The sacs of specialized epithelial cells, or imaginal discs, which give rise to most of the structures of the adult fly are single cell layer structures which have provided researchers with an excellent opportunity to study the development of cells whose biological properties are similar to those of mammalian cells that are susceptible to cancer (Bryant and Schmidt, 1990). The similarity between *Drosophila* and human cell cycle regulations suggests that *Drosophila* can serve as a model to study the process of proliferation and cell fate determination during tumorigenesis (Basler and Hafen, 1991).

As a model genetic organism, the entire genome of the fly can be screened systemically to identify any gene that, when mutated, affects the molecular mechanism of tumorigenesis. The fly can therefore be used as an excellent system for rapidly learning more about the genes involved in tumor development. Mutations and gene expression alterations in brain tumors have been extensively investigated; however, the causes of brain tumorigenesis are largely unknown. Animal models are necessary to correlate altered transcriptional activity and tumor phenotype and to better understand how these alterations cause malignant growth. Studies in flies, together with similar work in other model genetic organisms, can provide information regarding the conserved molecular and biochemical properties of the cancer-causing molecules. For example, characterization of the fly homolog of phosphatase and tensin (PTEN) confirmed the results from mammals that PTEN functions in the insulin pathway and also revealed its role in the regulation of cell size (Huang et al., 1999).

13.2.1 Drosophila *Brain Tumor (brat) Gene*

Over the last 10 years, a genetic abnormality associated with the production of a tumor-like neoplasm in the larval brain and lethality in the larval third instar and pupal stages of the *Drosophila* has been documented and given rise to investigations into the fly's 'brain tumor gene' (Arama et al., 2000). The *Drosophila* brain tumor gene (*brat*) encodes for a 1037 amino acid protein with an *N*-terminal B-boxl zinc finger followed by a B-box2 zinc finger, a coiled coil domain, and a *C*-terminal beta-propeller domain with six blades (Fig. 13.1) (Arama et al., 2000). All of these motifs are known to mediate protein–protein interactions. Sequence analysis of four *brat* alleles in the flies with brain tumors revealed that all of them are mutated at the beta-propeller domain (Arama et al., 2000). The clustering of mutations in this domain strongly suggests that it has a crucial role in the normal function of *brat*, and defines a novel protein motif involved in translational repression and tumor suppression activity (Arama et al., 2000; Sonoda and Wharton, 2001). The *brat* gene is expressed in the embryonic central and peripheral nervous systems including the embryonic brain. In third instar larva *brat* expression was detected in the larval central nervous system including the brain and the ventral ganglion, in two glands – the ring gland and the salivary gland, and in parts of the foregut – the gastric cecae and the proventriculus (Arama et al., 2000). A second *brat-like* gene was also found (AF145661), and homologs were identified in the nematode (*Caernorhabditis elegans* Ncl-1), mouse (HAC-1), rat (BERP), and human (Trim3, KIAA0517, BERP, and HT-2A) (Arama et al., 2000). Recent work has concluded that *brat* suppresses neuroblast stem cell self-renewal and promotes neuronal differentiation (Betschinger et al., 2006; Lee et al., 2006; Wodarz and Gonzalez, 2006), a function which warrants examining if it plays a role in the transformation of human brain stem cells. *brat* negatively regulates cell proliferation during larval central brain development of *Drosophila*, but how Prospero interacts as an effector of *brat* in cell fate specification and proliferation control is still uncertain (Fig. 13.2) (Bello et al., 2006; Betschinger et al., 2006; Lee et al., 2006). Accumulated data suggest that *brat* may regulate proliferation and

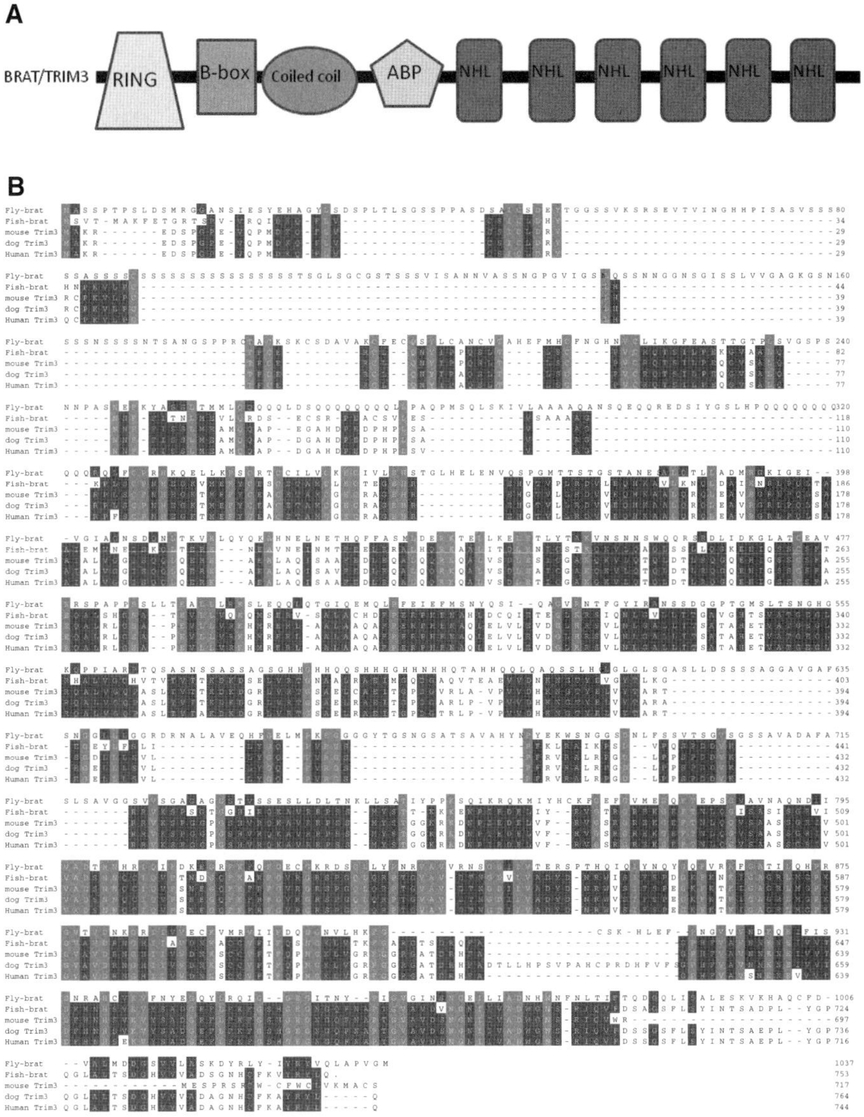

Fig. 13.1 **A**. Structure of *brat*/Trim3 gene showing the RING, B box, coiled coil, ABP domains, and the *C*-terminal NHL repeat region. **B**. Alignment of *Drosophila*'s *brat* gene with homologous genes from zebrafish, mouse, dog, and human. The alignment was done by using the MegAlign software from DNA Star. Database ID numbers were as follows: fly-*brat* GenBank ID: AAN11027 (fly base ID: FBpp0080702), Human Trim3 NM_033278, Mouse Trim3 NM_018880, Dog Trim3 XM_857596, Zebrafish *brat* is the blast search in zebrafish genome against human Trim3 NP_001073637.1. Trim3 is likely the human homolog of the *Drosophila*'s *brat* gene and its expression is brain-specific

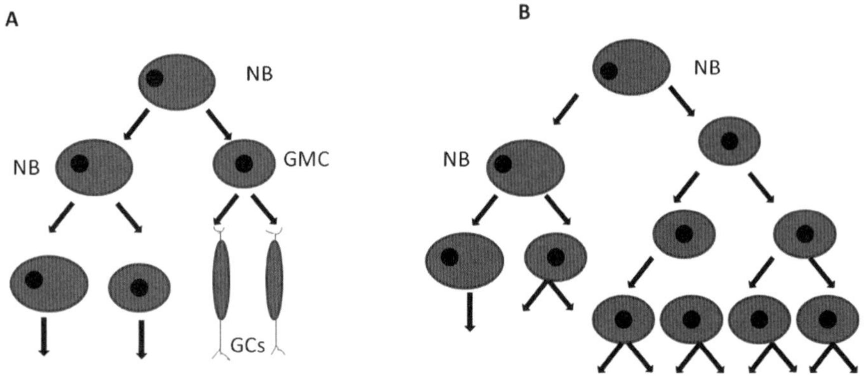

Fig 13.2 Neural lineage formation in larval central brain of the wild-type, *brat* and *pros* mutant clones. (**A**) In wild-type *Drosophila*, neural progenitor cells are required for lineage formation: neuroblasts (NB) self-renew by dividing asymmetrically producing series of ganglion mother cells (GMCs). Ganglion mother cells undergo a single terminal division that produces two post-mitotic ganglions cells (GCs), which send out axons contributing to fiber tracts. (**B**) Somatic mutation of *brat*, the tumor suppressor, and loss of function of the cell fate determinant *pros* in the NBs impede differentiation of the progenitor cells into GCs. The mutant cells retain progenitor cell-like characteristics and self-renew indefinitely, generating clonally derived brain tumors. Modified with permission (Bello et al., 2006)

differentiation by secretion/transport-mediated processes, controlling growth through repression of RNA synthesis (Frank et al., 2002). Current investigation using *Drosophila* as a model for neurogenesis and the role of neural stem cells are highlighting the role of *brat* gene in normal development and it is likely that work in this area will be extensive in the next few years (Bowman et al., 2008).

A homozygous mutation of *brat* results in the phenotype which is primarily due to the expansion of the optic neuroblasts (Kurzik-Dumke et al., 1992). Clonal analysis of the first larval instar indicates that the *brat* mutation affects cell proliferation in a cell-autonomous manner, and cell cycle marker expression shows that cells of *brat* mutant clones show uncontrolled proliferation, which persists into adulthood (Bello et al., 2006). Analysis of the expression of molecular markers, which characterize cell types in wild-type neural lineages, indicates that *brat* mutant clones comprise an excessive number of cells, which have molecular features of undifferentiated progenitor cells that lack nuclear transcription factor Prospero (Pros) (Bello et al., 2006). These findings provide an attractive model of how defects in the process of asymmetric cell divisions are involved in tumorigenesis.

Imaginal discs from third instar *brat* mutant larva, although appearing normal in situ, as well as the adult tumor cells are able to metastasize and form secondary tumors when injected into the abdomen of a wild-type host fly (Woodhouse et al., 1998); however, the metastatic cells have quite different properties than the original cells (Beaucher et al., 2007a). The metastatic ability of these tumors is determined by matrix metalloproteinases (MMPs), specifically MMP1 (Beaucher et al., 2007b).

Table 13.1 Selected cancerrelated genes in *Drosophila melanogaster*

Oncogenes		Tumor suppressor genes		Tumor growth or over-proliferation genes	
Fly	Mammalian gene or product	Fly	Mammalian gene or product	Fly	Mammalian gene or product
D. Abl	*c-abl*	*D-APC*	*APC*	*air8*	*S6 ribosomal protein*
D. Akt	*Akt*	*Caudal*	*CDX2*	*Cactus*	*IKB*
D. Jun	*c-jun*	*Gigas*	*TSC2*	*Discs large*	*hDlg, NE-Dlg*
Kayak	*c-fos*	*Medea*	*DPC4*	*Fat*	*FAT*
D. myb	*Myb*	*Merlin*	*NF2*	*Hyperplastic discs/ l(3)c43*	*UBE3A*
Diminutive	*c-Myc*	*D.NF1*	*NF1*	*Lats*	*Lats1, Lats2*
Notch	*hNotch1/TAN1*	*D. PTEN*	*PTEN/MMAC*	*l(2) giant larvae*	*LLGL1, LLGL2*
Ras	*Ras*	*D.p16*	*P16(INK4a)/MTS1*	*l(3) malignant blood neoplasm-1*	*Loricrin*
Src42A, Src64B	*c-src*			*l(3) discs overgrown*	*CSNK1D*
D. TCF	*TCF*			*L(3) malignant brain tumor*	Unknown
				brat	TRIM3

One-fifth of the genes identified by a genome-wide microarray expression analysis of an adult brain tumor in *Drosophila* show homology to known mammalian genes involved in cancer formation (Loop et al., 2004; Potter et al., 2000). This finding itself is likely to promote this model as potential for genetic therapeutic targeting of brain tumors (Table 13.1).

Recently, a glioma model in Drosophila was created; constitutive coactivation of EGFR-Ras and PI3K pathways in Drosophila glia and glial precursors was found to give rise to neoplastic, invasive glial cells that create transplantable tumor-like growths, mimicking human glioma. This model represents a robust organotypic and cell-type-specific Drosophila cancer model in which malignant cells are created by mutations in signature genes and pathways thought to be driving forces in a homologous human cancer. Genetic analyses demonstrated that EGFR and PI3K initiate malignant neoplastic transformation via a combinatorial genetic network composed primarily of other pathways commonly mutated or activated in human glioma, including the Tor, Myc, G1 Cyclins-Cdks, and Rb-E2F pathways. Further investigation may reveal that this model has great utility in the investigation of therapeutic targets in human glioma (Read et al., 2009).

13.3 Zebrafish: A New Model of Nervous System Tumorigenesis?

The zebrafish has recently become a model for studying the genetics and molecular biology of cancer. Short generation times, ease of mutagenesis, and large clutches per mating help make it an outstanding model system for genetics research. Several highly homozygous strains of zebrafish are available, and general methods for obtaining new strains have been established, largely due to the ability to artificially create and identify mutants in a single generation, to identify isogenic stocks, to cryopreserve gametes, and to generate transgenic fish.

Three tumor suppressor mutants in zebrafish have been generated by reverse genetics, all of which develop tumors (Berghmans et al., 2005; Faucherre et al., 2008). Recent work has described the isolation of zebrafish mutants for the mismatch repair (MMR) genes *mlh1*, *msh2*, and *msh6* and shown that homozygous mutants of all three lines develop brain neoplasms with a frequency of 6–45% (Feitsma et al., 2008). Most frequently, neurofibromas/malignant peripheral nerve sheath tumors in the eye and abdomen were observed in addition to PNETs of the brain (Feitsma et al., 2008). In humans, germline mismatch repair mutations are found in Turcot syndrome, an association of brain tumors and colonic polyps (Paraf et al., 1997), and more recently somatic mutations in the same genes were reported as being associated with tumor recurrence after temozolomide chemotherapy (TCGA, 2008). From this early work, it appears that the zebrafish is a useful cancer model that provides new insights and experimental possibilities, complementing studies in mice and humans.

13.4 Mouse and Rat Models of Brain Tumors

Mouse models of human cancer have proved to be excellent tools for dissecting the biology and biochemistry of particular pathways involved in cancer development and progression. However, they are limited in their representation of some of the features that define human cancer, including growth over long periods of time, genomic instability, and significant heterogeneity in both tumor cells and tumor microenvironment and stroma (Paoloni and Khanna, 2008).

Simplistically rodent brain tumor models are often classified as xenograft tumor models or models of spontaneous tumor formation in genetically engineered mice (GEM) (see Chapters 1, 2, 3, 4, 5, 6, 7, 8, 9, 10, 11, and 12) (Gutmann et al., 2006). Both models can help with anti-cancer drug development in terms of both toxicity and in vivo anti-tumor effectiveness. In principle, strains of mice forming spontaneous tumors due to mutations in the genes characteristic of a human malignancy are appealing due to the predictability of the tumor-initiating lesion, immunocompetence, and tumor development at the appropriate site (Fomchenko and Holland, 2006). However, in brain tumor modeling, the use of mouse models forming spontaneous tumors is complicated by poor reproducibility, low tumor penetrance, prolonged tumor formation latency, and a need for advanced in vivo imaging techniques. More complications arise from the fact that mutant alleles are often expressed or deleted from the whole animal or tissue, compared with human tumors that are thought to arise from a single mutant cell or a small mutant population. In this respect, GEMs are more representative of human cancer predisposition syndromes rather than random tumorigenesis (Van Dyke and Jacks, 2002; Hu and Holland, 2005). For further information on transgenic mouse models, see Chapters 2, 3, 4, 5, and 6.

13.4.1 The 4C8 Mouse Glioma Syngeneic Graft Model

Recently, various permutations of transgenic mice have been generated, and malignant gliomas arising as a consequence of transgene expression have been isolated and partially characterized. One of these is the MOCH-1 malignant glioma that arose in a mouse transgenic for the *neu*oncogene driven by the myelin basic protein promoter (Dyer and Philibotte, 1995). The 4C8 cell line was cloned from the MOCH-1 mouse tumor and grows as astrocyte-like or oligodendroglia-like cells in tissue culture, the phenotype depending on culture conditions. In the presence of >4% serum, it assumes the phenotype of an astrocytoma and develops into malignant gliomas when transplanted into brains of syngeneic B6D2F$_1$ mice (Hellums et al., 2005). The 4C8 cells grow with the invasion of normal brain parenchyma and develop into a highly vascularized tumor-expressing GFAP, with areas of necrosis and pseudopalisading, which are characteristic histopathological features of human glioblastoma multiforme (Dyer and Philibotte, 1995; Weiner et al., 1999). The average neurological endpoint following intracranial injection into immunocompetent mice was 51 days but the tumor cells were also noted to proliferate following flank inoculation, retaining histological features seen in intracranial tumors (Weiner et al., 1999). This tumor has been suggested to be an excellent model for therapeutic investigations in an orthotopic, immunocompetent mouse model of glioma (Hellums et al., 2005). It has been used for the preclinical evaluation of virus- and liposomal-encapsulated-mediated therapies (Harding et al., 2006a, b; Hellums et al., 2005; Higgins et al., 2004). Other syngeneic mouse graft models (including GL261 and CT-2A) are described in Chapter 12.

13.4.2 The Spontaneous VM/Dk Murine Astrocytoma

A solitary and single spontaneous murine astrocytoma (SMA) has been documented arising in the inbred VM/Dk strain of mice (Bradford et al., 1986; Serano et al., 1980). This is an immunocompetent model with a tumor suggested to more accurately represent the intrinsic qualities of spontaneously arising human tumors. From the SMA, three permanent cell lines with astrocytic nature have been derived (SMA-P497, -P540, and -P560), which are tumorigenic both intracranially and subcutaneously (Pilkington et al., 1983, 1985, 1982; Pires et al., 1987; Serano et al., 1980), extending the use of the SMA model by allowing quantitative in vivo and in vitro experiments.

13.4.2.1 Cytological Characteristics

Although the P560 cell line possesses the most astrocytic features, and has been used most extensively for quantitative assessment studies, it was the least differentiated P497 cell line which was originally used to give rise to six clones with dissimilar morphological, antigenic, kinetic, and chromosomal properties (Koppel et al., 1986; Serano et al., 1980). When these clones were evaluated following intracerebral injection into syngeneic hosts, five of the six clones produced tumors with incidences ranging from 25 to 100% and mean latencies of 43–100 days, according to the clone injected (Koppel et al., 1988). Histological, immunocytochemical, and electron microscopical examination of the resulting tumors revealed differences in the degree of invasiveness, but otherwise only slight variations in phenotype between the clones (Koppel et al., 1988). Generally, the tumors were considered glioblastoma-like, showing a pleomorphic histo-architectural pattern.

13.4.2.2 Biological Characteristics

In vitro correlation has been demonstrated between the therapeutic sensitivity of the VM/Dk cell lines and human glioma cultures (Bradford et al., 1986). The sensitivity to a given agent was expressed differentially by the three VM/Dk cell lines, with P497 being the least sensitive to most drugs tested which is consistent with it being the least well-differentiated cell line; the precise mechanism responsible for this difference in sensitivity is unknown (Bradford et al., 1986). However, many inconsistencies have arisen between in vitro drug studies using these cell lines, making interpretation of data difficult.

The P560 cell line was found to secrete a biologically active form of the immunosuppressive cytokine TGF-β, which contributes to the profound immunosuppression in human patients with glioblastoma multiforme (Ashley et al., 1998a; Sampson et al., 1997). For this reason, the P560 cell line has been utilized to demonstrate that cytokine production by glial tumors can abrogate their tumorigenicity in vivo; this work gave rise to the prediction that treatment in humans focused on cytokine production within astrocytomas might be an efficacious pursuit despite the notion that the CNS is 'immunologically privileged' (Ashley et al., 1998b; Sampson et al., 1997). Therefore, unlike chemically induced tumor models that cannot mirror the antigenic properties of human tumors arising 'spontaneously', syngeneic murine glioma models using cell lines derived from the VM/Dk SMA can be utilized in immunotherapy investigations. Dendritic cell-based therapy using the P560 cell line induced an anti-tumor response against a syngeneic murine glioma, further confirming the role of this model in immunotherapy investigations (Heimberger et al., 2000). Similar models using the SMA 560 cells and an MT539MG glioma cell line, also established from the VM/Dk mouse, have been used to investigate genetically engineered viral-mediated treatments for brain tumors (Chambers et al., 1995; Friese et al., 2003).

Recent work using the SMA 560 cell lines has supported the suggestion that brain tumor cells grown in vitro undergo selection away from their in vivo characteristics, responding specifically to their environment and therefore may not accurately represent the in vivo phenotype (Learn et al., 2007). Gene expression, evaluated using DNA microarray analysis, was noted to be significantly different between the P560 cell line in vitro and the tumor cells retrieved 17 days post-intracerebral implantation of P560 cells into immunocompetent VM/Dk mice (Learn et al., 2007). This finding supports the premise that such model systems need to be critically evaluated in the context of the result they produce.

13.4.3 Rat Brain Tumor Models

Rat brain tumor models, (including the 9L gliosarcoma, the C6 glioma, the F98 glioma, the RG2 glioma, the RT-2 gliomas, and the CNS-1 glioma) have been widely used in experimental neuro-oncology for almost four decades (Barth, 1998). Rat brain tumor models were first described occurring reproducibly and selectively in adult rats that had been given repeated, weekly, intravenous injections of *N*-methylnitrosourea (Schmidek et al., 1971). Subsequent to work in canines (Grove et al., 1967), the avian sarcoma virus was also shown to induce brain tumors in rats, which has additionally proven to be a useful model (Copeland et al., 1976; Lee et al., 1986). Further information on chemically induced tumor models in rats and mice can be found in Chapters 10, 11, and 12. A major limitation of some of these rat models is that they elicit an anti-immune response, in part because they were generated on an outbred strain (for example, C6) or because the mutagenic load might have created new epitopes (discussed in detail in Chapter 10).

Brain tumors have been induced in pregnant rats that were given a single intravenous injection of *N*-ethyl-*N*-nitrosourea (ENU) (Swenberg et al., 1972). The rats developed mixed gliomas, oligodendrogliomas, and a few astrocytomas (Zook et al., 2000). The F98 glioma cell line, an anaplastic glioma, was derived from the ENU research and its in vitro growth and in vivo morphology have been described in detail (Kobayashi et al., 1980). This cell line's characteristics closely resemble those of human glioblastoma multiforme and anaplastic astrocytomas, and it is now established as a particularly good model to evaluate experimental therapies where prolongation in survival time is the endpoint (Barth, 1998; Barth et al., 2003; Zook et al., 2000). During the evaluation of ENU-induced gliomas in rats, it was noted that approximately 7% of control rats developed spontaneous astrocytomas or oligodendrogliomas, most of which were found incidentally at necropsy when most rats were of 2-years old (Zook et al., 2000). Further investigation of the rat as a spontaneous model of brain tumors is warranted.

13.5 Spontaneous Brain Tumors in Dogs

Beyond the advantages of working with large animal models, provided by pet dog cancers, the similarities in tumor biology seen between specific human and canine cancers further contribute to their value as models of human cancer (Fig. 13.3) (Hansen and Khanna, 2004). The characteristics and similarities of canine brain tumors to the human counterpart are detailed below.

Investigations of cancer in dogs are not novel and have been documented for over 40 years (Paoloni and Khanna, 2008), but to date they represent an underutilized cancer model, which are more genetically outbred than laboratory animals and have an intact immune system. The recent deciphering of the canine genome provides evidence of strong similarities with humans, particularly with respect to the gene families associated with cancer which are significantly closer than the relationship between a mouse and a human (Lindblad-Toh et al., 2005; O'Brien and Murphy, 2003; Paoloni and Khanna, 2008).

Although canine models of viral-induced brain tumors have been utilized in experimental neuro-oncology (Bigner et al., 1972, 1969; Britt et al., 1987; Warnke et al., 1995; Whelan et al., 1988), it is the spontaneous tumors which are described in more detail in this chapter. Many of the naturally occurring canine brain tumors exhibit the same pathologic subtypes, molecular abnormalities, cytogenetic expressions, and neuroimaging characteristics as their human counterparts (Dickinson et al., 2008b; Lipsitz et al., 2003; Stoica et al., 2004; Sturges et al., 2008; Thomson et al., 2005). Chemo- and radio-sensitivity similarities are less well documented but conventional radiation therapy and stereotactic radiosurgery can prolong survival for a few months when compared to palliative treatment or surgery alone (Axlund et al., 2002; Heidner et al., 1991; Lester et al., 2001; Spugnini et al., 2000; Theon et al., 2000). The size of dogs makes multimodality protocols feasible

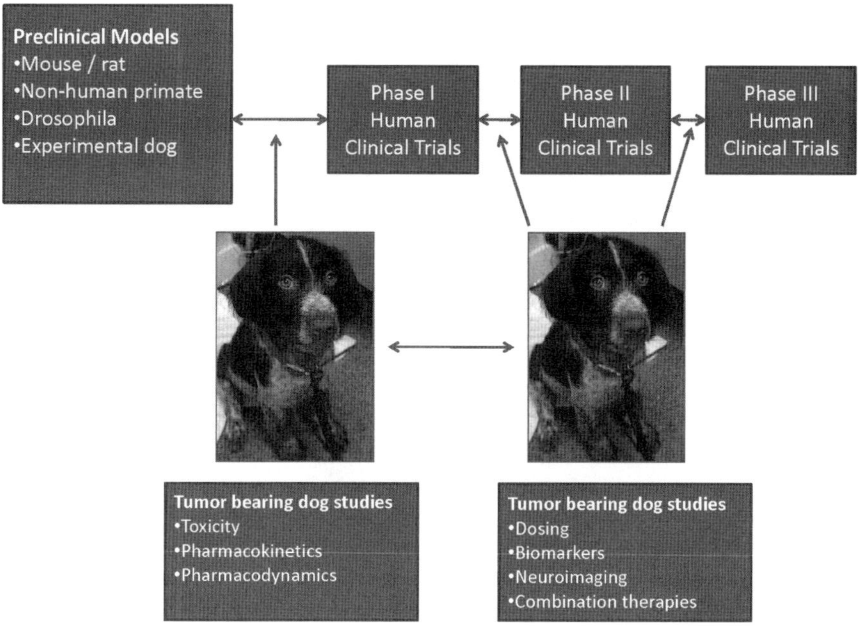

Fig. 13.3 An integrated approach is necessary to improve preclinical and clinical trial design utilizing dogs as preclinical models, similar to mice and non-human primate work, and as 'bridges' between the different phases of clinical trials. Modified with permission (Paoloni and Khanna, 2008)

and furthermore, the lack of 'gold standard' treatments permits early and humane testing of novel therapies.

The long history of dogs in biomedical research, their strong anatomical and physiological similarities to humans, and the sheer number of pet dogs that are diagnosed and managed with cancer each year have focused attention on this species. Importantly, pet dog owners are highly motivated to seek out new options for the management of cancer in their pets and have interest in receiving care that is provided as part of clinical trials when conventionally available treatments do not meet their goals.

13.5.1 Epidemiology and Pathology

Intracranial neoplasms in dogs may have an incidence rate of approximately 14–20 per 100,000 (Dobson et al., 2002; Moore et al., 1996), e.g., comparable to that in humans. Commonly reported primary brain tumors in dogs are meningiomas, gliomas (astrocytomas, oligodendrogliomas), undifferentiated sarcomas, pituitary tumors, and ventricular tumors (choroid plexus papillomas and ependymomas) (Koestner et al., 1999; Snyder et al., 2006) (Fig. 13.4). Other primary

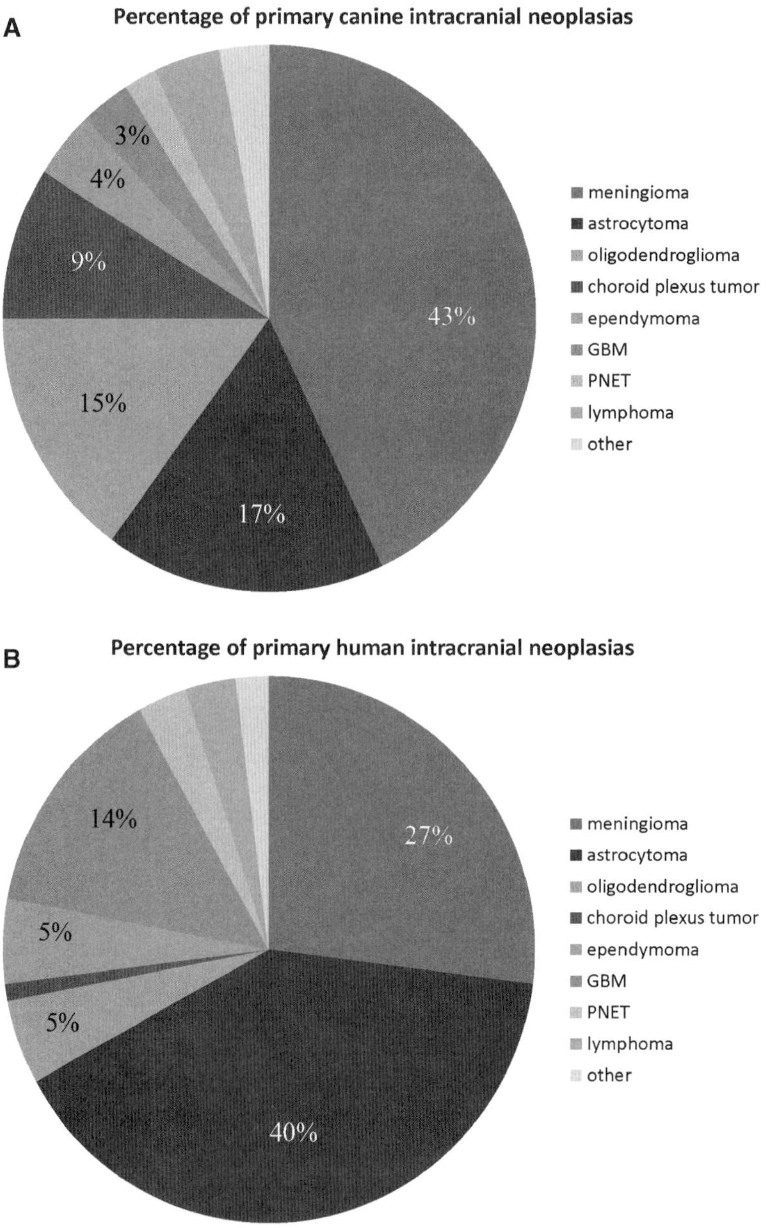

Fig. 13.4 **A.** A pie chart representation of the relative frequency of individual canine primary brain tumor types. **B.** A pie chart representation of the relative frequency of individual human primary brain tumor types

brain tumors, such as tumors of nerve cells (e.g., gangliocytomas, neuroblastomas), pinealomas, craniopharyngiomas (a suprasellar ectodermal tumor that may destroy the pituitary gland), spongioblastoma (or 'embryonal glioma', often with a periventricular orientation), and medulloblastomas (usually in the cerebellum), are less commonly described (Koestner et al., 1999; Snyder et al., 2006). Dogs over 7 years of age have the highest incidence of brain tumors among domestic animals, and of these, the meningiomas are the most frequent (Snyder et al., 2006; Sturges et al., 2008). Secondary brain tumors are also frequently documented in dogs. Hemangiosarcoma has been reported as the most frequent metastatic neoplasia of the CNS, accounting for 28% of all secondary brain tumors (Snyder et al., 2008).

13.5.1.1 Canine Meningiomas

Canine meningiomas are extra-axial tumors that arise from the arachnoid cap cells of the dura within the cranial and spinal spaces. These tumors comprise approximately 30–45% of all primary spontaneous tumors in dogs (Fig. 13.4) (Hayes et al., 1975; Heidner et al., 1991; Snyder et al., 2006; Sturges et al., 2008). In most reports, meningiomas occur in dogs over 7 years of age with median age ranging from 10 to 11 years (Snyder et al., 2006; Sturges et al., 2008); however, meningiomas have also been observed in young dogs less than 6 months of age (Keller and Madewell, 1992). These tumors most commonly occur in dolicocephalic breeds, especially German Shepherds and Golden Retrievers, but are also common in Boxers and in some studies there is a female prevalence (Snyder et al., 2006; Sturges et al., 2008).

Meningiomas in dogs share striking similarities to human meningiomas in neuroimaging characteristics, gross and histological appearance (Fig. 13.5), expression of growth factors and receptors, treatment responses (Fig. 13.6) as well as their initial cytogenetic expressions (Tables 13.2 and 13.3) (Adamo et al., 2003; Dickinson et al., 2008b., 2006; Koestner et al., 1999; Long et al., 2006; Mandara et al., 2002; Mandrioli et al., 2007; Platt et al., 2006c; Sturges et al., 2008; Theon et al., 2000; Thomson et al., 2005).

Gene expression patterns of canine meningiomas have recently been evaluated using a canine brain-specific cDNA microarray; up- and down-regulation of ribosomal proteins and CREG was documented, respectively (Thomson et al., 2005). A more recent study demonstrated that canine meningioma genome deletions spanned the chromosomal regions syntenic to those most often deleted in human meningiomas (Table 13.4) (Courtay-Cahan et al., 2008). Although a small study, the quantitative loss of DNA was associated with the shortest progression-free survival. The level of NF-2 gene expression has been evaluated in canine meningiomas but no significant difference was noted relative to normal canine tissues and no specific pattern of transcript expression was seen relative to tumor grade or subtype, even though several of the tumor samples had decreased expression of NF-2 protein based on western blotting (Campbell et al., 2006).

The neurochemical features of canine meningiomas have been evaluated through cerebrospinal fluid analysis of uric acid and glutamate levels (Platt et al., 2006a, b). These analytes could serve as molecular markers for future therapeutic investigations.

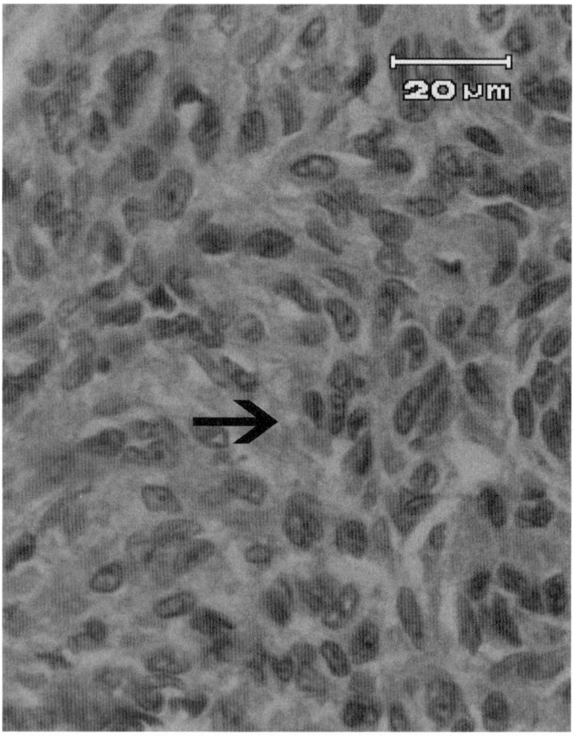

Fig. 13.5 A high-power magnification view of a canine grade I transitional meningioma with typically swirling accumulations of cells with ill-defined boundaries (*arrow*). The most current World Health Organization histological classification system of canine meningiomas, published in 1999 (Koestner et al., 1999), categorizes them into two major groups: benign, slow-growing tumors of various subtypes (meningothelial, fibroblastic, transitional, psammomatous, angiomatous, papillary, granular, myxoid) and anaplastic tumors. Since this time, the microcystic and the chordoid subtypes have been described independently and a new classification system mirroring the human scheme has been suggested to be more appropriate (Montoliu et al., 2006; Sturges et al., 2008). Using this system, approximately 56% of canine intracranial meningiomas are benign (Grade I), 43% are atypical (Grade II), and 1% are malignant (Grade III) (Sturges et al., 2008). This is compatible with an earlier study which demonstrated direct invasion of the brain in 27% (6/22) of meningiomas (Patnaik et al., 1986)

13.5.1.2 Canine Astrocytomas

Astrocytomas are the most common neuroectodermal brain tumors in dogs, representing 17% of all canine primary intracranial neoplasia (Figs. 13.4 and 13.7) (Snyder et al., 2006; Vandevelde et al., 1985). The mean age of dogs at the time of onset is 8.6 years, although the tumors have been documented in dogs less than 6 months of age (Keller and Madewell, 1992); the tumor is more common in brachycephalic dogs with Boxers and Border terriers seemingly over-represented (Snyder et al., 2006).

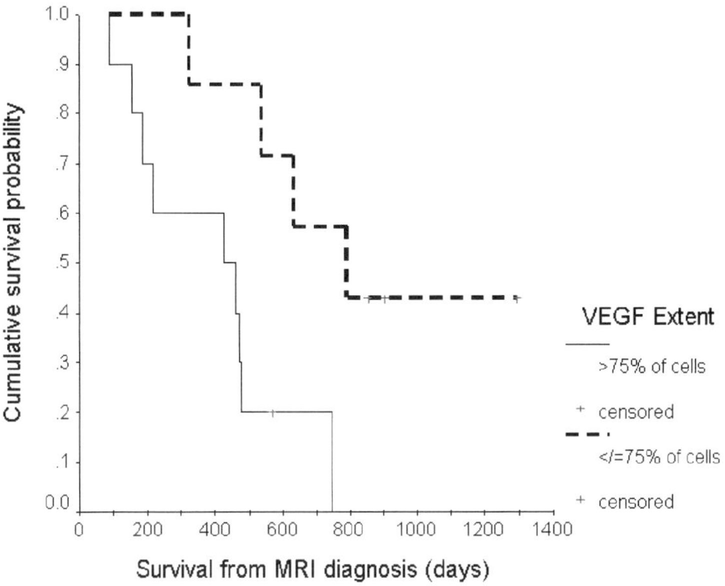

Fig. 13.6 A Kaplan–Meier curve demonstrating the association of meningioma vascular endothelial growth factor (VEGF) staining with survival in dogs. Reproduced with permission (Platt et al., 2006c)

In one study, approximately 35% of canine astrocytomas over-expressed p53 and 23% over-expressed EGFR based on immunohistochemistry, with the latter over-expressed in the malignant forms of astrocytomas (Table 13.3) (Stoica et al., 2004). Even though a point mutation of p53 has been documented in the canine astrocytoma, comparison of immunostaining and DNA sequence alterations of p53 have not shown a significant association between over-expression and genetic mutations (Stoica et al., 2004).

13.5.1.3 Canine Glioblastoma Multiforme

In contrast to humans, glioblastoma multiforme (GBM) represent only 3% of all primary CNS tumors in the dog and 12% of all neuroglial tumors (Snyder et al., 2006). As in humans, these tumors are considered to be 'high-grade' gliomas, of diverse origin, including astroglial, oligodendroglial, and ependymal tissue, with histopathological characteristics very similar to those seen in humans (Koestner et al., 1999; Lipsitz et al., 2003). Similar to canine astrocytomas, initial microarray analysis of these tumors reveals down-regulation for proteolipid protein, neuroblastoma protein, stathmin-like 2, nuclear receptor coactivator 4, synaptosomal-associated protein, apo-lipoprotein D, and NDRG family member 4 (Thomson et al., 2005).

Table 13.2 Immunohistochemical characteristics of canine primary brain tumors

	Vimentin	S100	Pancytokeratin	Neuron-specific enolase	Glial fibrillary acidic protein	Myelin-associated glycoprotein	Synpatophysin
Meningioma	+ + +	+ + +	+ +	+ +	+	–	–
Oligodendroglioma	+	+ +	–	–	+ +	+ +	+ +
Astrocytoma	+	+ +	+	+ +	+ + +	–	–
Glioblastoma multiforme	+	+ +	–	–	+ + +	–	–
Choroid plexus tumors	+ +	–	+ +	–	–	–	–

+ + +, common and extensive positive staining; + +, variable staining; +, infrequent staining; –, no staining reported.

Table 13. 3 Molecular marker expression and documented biological associations in canine primary brain tumors (Adamo et al., 2003; Dickinson et al., 2006; Long et al., 2006; Platt et al., 2006c; Rossmeisl et al., 2007)

	Progesterone receptors	VEGF	VEGFRs	EGFR-1	PDGFα	h-tert	Ki-67
Meningioma	+ + +/ associated with tumor proliferation rate	+ +/associated with malignancy and patient prognosis following treatment	+ +/associated with cell proliferation and malignancy	As for VEGFRs	As for VEGFRs	+/associated with malignancy	0–41%
Oligodendroglioma	–	+ +/associated with malignancy	+ + +/not associated with malignancy	As for VEGFRs	As for VEGFRs	+ +/associated with malignancy	0–38%
Astrocytoma	–	+ + +/ associated with malignancy	+ +/associated with malignancy	As for VEGFRs	As for VEGFRs	+/associated with malignancy	3–14%
Glioblastoma multiforme	–	+ + +	+ + +	+ + +	+ + +	+/associated with malignancy	6–26%

+ + +, extensive expression; + +, moderate expression; +, minimal expression; –, no expression reported;
VEGF, vascular endothelial growth factor;
VEGFRs, vascular endothelial growth factor receptors;
EGFR, endothelial-derived growth factor;
PDGF, platelet-derived growth factor;
h-tert, h-telomerase reverse transcriptase

Table 13.4 Genes located on chromosomal regions affected by aneuploidy in both canine and human meningioma. Modified with permission (Courtay-Cahan et al., 2008)

CFA[a]	Case[b]	HSA[c]	HSA aneuploidies[d]	Gene name	Biological process(es)[e]
7q23–q26	B	18q11.1–q21.1	d: II, III	Rho-associated protein kinase 1	Apoptosis (negative regulation)
		18p11.32–p11.21	d: II, III > I	Clusterin-like 1 (retinal)	Cell death
				Pituitary adenylate cyclase activating polypeptide precursor	Cell cycle (negative regulation)
10q22–q27.2	A	22q12.3–q13.33	d: I, II, III	Bcl-2-interacting killer	Apoptosis
				Histone acetyltransferase p300	Apoptosis, cell cycle
				Platelet-derived growth factor beta polypeptide	Cell cycle, cell proliferation
		12q23.3	a: II, III > I	Adapter protein containing PH domain, PTB domain and leucine zipper motif 2	Cell cycle, cell proliferation
		2p21–p13.3	a: II, III	Fanconi anemia, complementation group L	DNA repair, cell proliferation
				Transcriptional regulator interacting with the PHD-bromodomain 2	Cell growth (negative regulation)
17q13–q21	C	2q13–q14.1	d: II, III	T-cell differentiation protein	Apoptosis
				Interleukin 1, alpha	Apoptosis, cell cycle, cell proliferation
				Interleukin 1, beta	Apoptosis, cell cycle, cell proliferation

Table 13.4 (continued)

CFA[a]	Case[b]	HSA[c]	HSA aneuploidies[d]	Gene name	Biological process(es)[e]
		2p13.3–p11.2	a: II, III	HtrA serine peptidase 2	Apoptosis
		1p13.2–p12	d: II, III	Homeodomain interacting protein kinase 1	DNA damage response (apoptosis)
17q22–q24	B	1p13.2–p12	d: II, III	DEAD (Asp–Glu–Ala–Asp) box polypeptide 20	Apoptosis (positive regulation)
				Notch homolog 2 (*Drosophila*)	Apoptosis
27q11–q13	C	12p13.33–q13.2	d: III > I, II	Extra spindle pole bodies homolog 1	Cell cycle, apoptosis
				Nuclear receptor subfamily 4, group A, member 1	Apoptosis
				Serine/threonine–protein kinase receptor R3 precursor	Cell proliferation
32q14–q15.2	B	4q21.1–q27	d: III > II	Calcium/calmodulin-dependent protein kinase type II delta chain	G1/S transition of mitotic cell cycle

The genes listed are among those that are annotated (in the NCBI 36 and the CanFam 2.0 assemblies of the human and canine genome sequences, respectively) as being located on syntenic chromosomal segments that are affected by copy number abnormalities in both canine and human meningiomas. The basis for the selection of the genes listed here is the GO Consortium[37] 'Biological Process' annotation(s) assigned to each gene.
[a]The cytogenetic co-ordinates of the deleted chromosomal regions in the canine meningioma. [b]Cases are identified from the ideograms generated by the SmartCapture 2 software on the basis of the DAPI banded karyotype of the canine genome[35].
[c]The syntenic regions of the human genome were identified by reference to the 'Synteny View' application of the Ensembl Dog Genome Browser[38] and subsequently to the 'Map View' application of the Ensembl Human Genome Browser.
[d]The chromosomal copy number abnormalities in human meningiomas[18–21,23,25,34,53,54,55] are denoted by 'abnormality type: meningioma grade(s) affected by abnormality', where d = deletion, a = amplification, I = grade I, II = grade II and III = grade III.
[e]The only biological process(es) among those assigned to each gene that are listed here are those that correspond to the potentially biologically significant processes identified by EASE analysis.

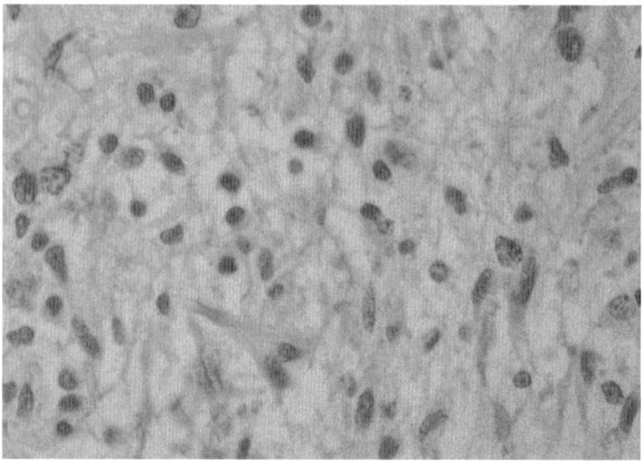

Fig. 13.7 A high-power magnification view of a canine protoplasmic astrocytoma. Astrocytomas consist of relatively large, protoplasmic-rich cells, or smaller cells with many processes. In most astrocytomas, there is a tendency for the cells to be arranged around blood vessels. Several variants have been described, e.g., fibrillary, protoplasmic, pilocytic, anaplastic, and gemistocytic

13.5.1.4 Canine Oligodendrogliomas

Oligodendrogliomas are relatively common tumors in dogs, especially affecting brachycephalic breeds, comprising 28% of neuroectodermal tumors and 14% of primary CNS tumors overall (Fig. 13.4) (Snyder et al., 2006). Many canine oligodendrogliomas are mixed tumors with areas of astrocytic, and sometimes ependymal, differentiation, with similar clinical neuroimaging (Fig. 13.8) and molecular expression characteristics to astrocytomas (Tables 13.2 and 13.3) (Koestner et al., 1999).

13.5.1.5 Canine Choroid Plexus Papillomas

Choroid plexus papillomas are relatively common tumors in dogs (Fig. 13.4), with a reported frequency similar to that of glioblastomas (about 12% of neuroglial tumors). The median age of dogs with these tumors is 6 years (Snyder et al., 2006). The majority (>50%) of these tumors in dogs are located in the fourth ventricle, with the lateral and third ventricles also being affected (Cantile et al., 2002; Ribas et al., 1989; Thankey et al., 2006; Westworth et al., 2008, 2006). Immunohistochemistry differs from some of the other canine neuroectodermal tumors (Tables 13.2 and 13.3).

13.5.2 Prognosis and Treatment for Canine CNS Tumors

In general, the prognosis of animals with tumors of the nervous system is guarded to poor, but depends on tumor location, surgical accessibility, rate of tumor growth, and degree of damage to the nervous tissue. There are many confounding factors present in the veterinary medical literature, often based on the fact that these animals are pets, which make interpretation of results difficult. These factors would always need to be considered when using the

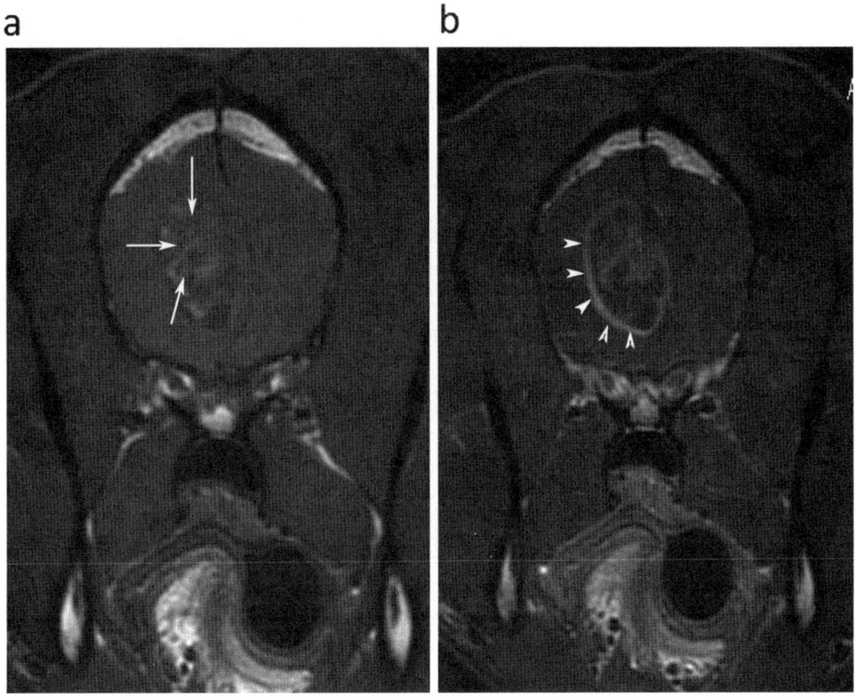

Fig. 13.8 A transverse T1-weighted pre-contrast **(a)** and post-contrast **(b)** MR scan of a dog with an oligodendroglioma (*arrows*). There is peripheral lesion (*ring*) contrast enhancement noted in this lesion (*arrowhead*) which is highly suggestive of a neuroectodermal tumor but neuroimaging is not specific for the tumor classification in dogs

dog as a natural tumor model. Such factors include (i) currently all data are retrospective; (ii) measures of outcome are poor: survival is often erroneously used as a marker of outcome but this is frequently determined by a owner's decision to euthanize their pet and is therefore susceptible to marked variability; (iii) many studies lack histological confirmation which often requires a surgical procedure that may not be an acceptable option for some owners. Where histological confirmation has existed, it has rarely been stratified by grade and molecular composition of the tumor; (iv) case recruitment is low and is often hampered by the financial aspects of treatment; (v) surgery and radiation protocols are extremely variable; (vi) inclusion of cases with marked variation in clinical signs; and (vii) lack of control data. Although this is frustrating, the end result is the lack of a 'gold standard' therapy for these cases, which means that enrollment in a well-designed trial evaluating a novel treatment is still very attractive for veterinary clinicians and animal owners alike. The size of dogs has been of value in the assessment of several therapeutic methods that would have been difficult to translate from murine models alone. Such approaches have included surgery, radiation and hyperthermia, photodynamic therapy, gene therapy, and novel imaging (Hansen and Khanna, 2004).

Standard management of canine brain tumors has tended to be similar to the human scenario, involving surgical resection, radiation therapy, and chemotherapy. Identification and characterization of tumors from tissue biopsies at the time of surgery or using stereotactic-guided biopsy devices is obviously beneficial in establishing the most appropriate therapeutic regimens (Koblik et al., 1999a, b; Long et al., 2002; Platt et al., 2002; Vernau et al., 2001). However, many dogs with brain tumors have been irradiated without a prior histopathological diagnosis, one of the several factors confounding the canine brain tumor survival data (Brearley et al., 1999; Evans et al., 1993; Heidner et al., 1991; Spugnini et al., 2000; Turrel et al., 1984). Clinical factors that have been shown to improve prognosis for dogs with brain tumors include a solitary site of involvement, mild-to-moderate neurologic signs, and normal cerebrospinal fluid findings (Heidner et al., 1991). More recently, the proliferation fraction of the tumor, the extent of VEGF expression within the tumor, and the quantitative DNA abnormalities present have been purported as having influence on outcome (Courtay-Cahan et al., 2008; Platt et al., 2006c; Theon et al., 2000).

Surgery is considered the primary therapeutic modality for meningioma in dogs. In several reports of canine meningiomas treated with surgery alone, mean survival times range from 138 to 1254 days (Axlund et al., 2002; Greco et al., 2006; Kostolich and Dulisch, 1987; Niebauer et al., 1991). No study stratified the tumors by grade or malignancy. The marked variability appears to relate at least to the extent of surgery performed, with radical total resection using ultrasonic aspirators achieving the best outcome (Greco et al., 2006). No significant data exist for the treatment of neuroectodermal tumors with surgery alone.

Several studies have shown that radiation therapy appears to significantly extend survival for a variety of canine intracranial tumors (Bley et al., 2005; Brearley et al., 1999; Heidner et al., 1991; Spugnini et al., 2000); mean survival in these studies ranges from 140 to 370 days. Radiation therapy protocols described for canine intracranial neoplasia include both hyperfractionated and hypofractionated weekly to daily doses, generally with a maximum total dose in the current literature of 38 Gy (Axlund et al., 2002; Brearley et al., 1999; Spugnini et al., 2000). The variability in the radiation regimens used in veterinary medicine has made interpretation of the literature in this area complicated; however, tolerance of the canine CNS to radiotherapy has been evaluated and more optimal treatment protocols have become customary (Gavin et al., 1997). Radiosurgery using a stereotactic head frame system has been documented in a small number of dogs; survival data cannot be interpreted but it was demonstrated to be a feasible and safe technique (Lester et al., 2001). Boron neutron capture therapy has also been evaluated in dogs in a phase I trial with safety demonstrated (Kraft et al., 1994); initial clinical results similar to that achieved with conventional radiation have been seen (Gavin et al., 1989; Kraft et al., 1992).

Dogs have also been used in radiation treatment trials evaluating hyperthermia and photodynamic therapy (Kangasniemi et al., 2004; Thrall et al., 1999; Whelan et al., 1993). Twenty-five dogs received radiation therapy and 20 the combination of radiation and whole body hyperthermia (WBH) (Thrall et al., 1999). Total radiation dose was randomly assigned and were 44, 48, 52, 56, or 60 Gy. Because of WBH toxicity, or tumor progression, 7 of the 45 dogs received less than the prescribed radiation dose. For WBH, the target rectal temperature was 42°C for 2 h and three treatments were planned. In 5 of the 20 dogs randomized to receive WBH, only one WBH treatment was given because of toxicity. WBH toxicity was severe in six dogs, and resulted in death or interruption in treatment. Most tumors did not undergo a complete response, making it impossible to differentiate tumor recurrence from brain necrosis as a cause of progressive neuropathy. Therefore, survival was the major study endpoint. There was no survival difference between groups. One-year survival probability (95% CI) for dogs receiving radiation therapy alone was 0.44 (0.25, 0.63) versus 0.40 (0.19, 0.63) for dogs receiving radiation and WBH. There was no difference in the incidence of brain necrosis in the two treatment groups. Results suggested that use of WBH alone to increase the temperature of intracranial tumors as a means to improve radiation therapy outcome is not a successful strategy (Thrall et al., 1999).

Photodynamic therapy was studied in dogs with posterior fossa glioblastomas (Whelan et al., 1993). This mode of therapy consisted of intravenous administration of Photofrin-II at doses ranging from 0.75 to 4 mg/kg 24 h prior to laser light irradiation in the posterior fossa. Tissue levels of Photofrin-II were four times greater in the tumor than in the surrounding normal brain. Irradiation was performed using 1 h of 500 mW laser light at a wavelength of 630 nm delivered through a fiberoptic catheter directly into the tumor bed via a burr hole. All animals receiving a high dose (4 or 2 mg/kg) of Photofrin-II developed serious brain stem neurotoxicity resulting in death or significant residual neurological deficits. A lower dose (0.75 mg/kg) of Photofrin-II produced tumor kill without significant permanent brain stem toxicity in either the control animals or the animals with cerebellar brain tumors receiving photodynamic therapy (Whelan et al., 1993).

Postoperative radiation therapy appears to further extend survival times in dogs with brain tumors (Axlund et al., 2002). Mean survival in dogs with meningiomas following surgery and radiation ranges from 441 to 1150 days (Axlund et al., 2002; Brearley et al., 1999; Theon et al., 2000). However, the same findings have not been shown with canine gliomas, in which there has only been a trend toward adjunctive radiotherapy being beneficial; when this literature is critiqued, it is most likely that this results from too few cases being evaluated and poor histological inclusion criteria.

The data documenting long-term control of canine brain tumors using cytotoxic chemotherapy with or without surgery and/or radiation are poor (Fulton and Steinberg, 1990). Both hydroxyurea and lomustine have been evaluated but interpretation of the results is not possible.

13.5.3 Canine Brain Tumor Experimental Treatment Trials

Several small-scale preclinical treatment trials have utilized the dog as a naturally occurring model. These include immunotherapy, gene therapy, convection-enhanced delivery, and cell-encapsulated anti-angiogenic therapy. These will be briefly highlighted here.

13.5.3.1 Immunotherapy

Cell-mediated immunity against spontaneous gliomas in five dogs was mobilized by culturing and stimulating autologous lymphocytes then returning them to the postoperative tumor bed (Ingram et al., 1990). Clinical improvement and reduction of tumor size were seen in all dogs.

13.5.3.2 Gene Therapy

The ideal use for the dog with spontaneous CNS neoplasia with regard to gene therapy has been for the investigation of delivery methods. Intra-arterial vector administration has been evaluated in dogs. Recombinant adenovirus vector bearing the *Escherichia coli* beta-galactosidase reporter gene was selectively injected into the vascular supply of a spontaneously occurring canine olfactory groove meningioma (Chauvet et al., 1998). The tumor and a small amount of peritumoral brain tissue were removed 5 days after viral injection and stained to assess gene delivery. The authors noted significant beta-galactosidase gene expression by the tumor, but not by surrounding brain tissue; no obvious viral-related cytotoxicity was noted (Chauvet et al., 1998).

13.5.3.3 Convection-Enhanced Delivery

Convection-enhanced delivery (CED), also referred to as high flow microinfusion, is a promising local delivery technique utilizing the bulk flow of molecules of varying sizes to specific areas within the central nervous system (Dickinson et al., 2008a; Fiandaca et al., 2008). The use of this delivery technique aids passage of significant volumes of drug past the blood–brain barrier, reaching the target with minimal toxicity. The technique has been documented in normal dogs (Dickinson et al., 2008a), with real time MR monitoring of the drug delivery for optimization of the infusion. Currently, a pilot clinical trial is underway by the same group, investigating intratumoral CED of liposomal CPT-11 (irinotecan), in canine spontaneous gliomas. Irinotecan, which is a topoisomerase 1 inhibitor, delivered in this manner has been well tolerated and resulted in improved clinical examinations and decreased MR-assessed tumor volumes (Dickinson, 2007).

13.5.4 Canine Glioma Cell Lines

Prior to the use of novel therapies in the dog with spontaneous intracranial neoplasia, animal use authorities and the dog's owners need to be convinced of safety. Therefore, prior in vitro and mice studies evaluating the proposed drug are preferable. For the in vitro and mice studies to be as representative as possible, it would be ideal to use brain tumor cell lines from a spontaneously occurring neoplasia in the dog. Tumor cells from a spontaneously arising canine astrocytoma have been isolated and cloned (Berens et al., 1993). The cell lines were tumorigenic as subcutaneous xenografts or as intracranial implants in athymic mice, or both (Berens et al., 1993). The histology of both the initial spontaneously occurring tumor in the dog and the intracranial astrocytoma in athymic mice demonstrated features of diffuse infiltration into normal brain. These canine glioma cell lines were proven to be karyotypically stable for 1 year in culture and carry the same marker chromosomes as the parental lines (Berens et al., 1993).

The same group subsequently induced long-term immune tolerance to an allogeneic cell line derived from a spontaneous canine astrocytoma in dogs (Berens et al., 1999). Allogeneic astrocytoma cells were implanted endoscopically into the subcutaneous space of fetal dogs before the onset of immune competency (<40th gestational day). At adulthood, the dogs rendered tolerant were proposed to successfully serve as recipients of intracranial transplants of their growing allogeneic, subcutaneous tumor (Berens et al., 1999). Transplanted dogs subsequently developed a solid brain tumor with histological features similar to the original astrocytoma. This model showed promise for the development and evaluation of new therapies for brain tumors; however, the ethics of this procedure were brought into question and it has not been further used. With these problems in mind, the established canine cell line, J3T, has since served as an in vitro model or used in vivo in mice.

It has been demonstrated that cultured J3T cells can be efficiently infected by adenovirus, herpes-simplex type I, or retrovirus vectors, as well as by non-virus vectors such as cationic liposome/DNA complexes (Rainov et al., 2000). Thus, in terms of infectability and transfectability, J3T cells seem to be closer to human glioma than the 9L rat gliosarcoma. Further, it was proven that J3T cells are tumorigenic and may grow heterotopically and orthotopically in a xenogeneic immunodeficient host, the SCID mouse, although morphology and growth pattern of these xenogeneic tumors differ from the demonstrated invasive phenotype in the Beagle dog (Rainov et al., 2000).

The J3T cells have also been efficiently transduced by HC-Ads expressing mCMV-driven HSV1-TK, which induced 90% reduction in cell viability in the presence of ganciclovir (Candolfi et al., 2007b). Additionally, adenoviral-mediated gene transfer of HSV1-TK, Flt3L, and betaGal was detected in J3T cells in vitro with 45% transduction efficiency (Candolfi et al., 2007a).

13.5.5 Problems and Challenges with the Use of Spontaneous Canine Brain Tumors

Companion animal models cannot be used in all translational settings. The progression of cancer in dogs, although faster than in humans, is slower than in most murine models, so it may take some time for large-animal trials to provide informative data (Hansen and Khanna, 2004). A randomized clinical trial of a new agent in companion animal cancer may require over a year for completion. The cost of clinical trials in companion animals is significantly greater than for most murine studies. In the development of new drugs, these costs are primarily associated with the production of sufficient quantities of drug to treat large animals. However, in general, clinical trials on veterinary patients can be completed at significantly less expense than similar human trials. Professional services, clinical pathology, and diagnostic imaging, although of high quality, are comparatively of low cost (Vail and MacEwen, 2000).

There are several further issues that challenge the use of dogs with spontaneously occurring intracranial tumors as preclinical experimental models. Case recruitment for trials will be hampered by (i) the relatively low number of cases diagnosed at a point which is too late for treatment; (ii) the potential financial obligations of the pet owner to obtain a diagnosis prior to inclusion; and (iii) the emotive nature of treatment trials on pet animals. Problems occurring during the treatment trial will potentially include (i) compliance and follow-up by the pet owner; (ii) the financial burden of addressing complications arising from the treatment; (iii) a practical, time-efficient yet objective surrogate measure of outcome; and (iv) difficulty obtaining the body for postmortem should the animal die at home.

Many of these issues are not insurmountable but overcoming them will require an extensive and organized collaboration between veterinary teams, pharmaceutical companies, basic scientists, and human medical neuro-oncology experts. The enthusiasm for this model already exists within many of these groups and the preclinical trial context has received some institutional support through the National Cancer Institute Comparative Oncology Program (Kimmelman and Nalbantoglu, 2007). The goals of this program are to facilitate companion animal cancers in cancer research through the characterization of these models and the design and implementation of preclinical translational trials (Hansen and Khanna, 2004).

13.6 Summary

The strong clinical, biologic, molecular, and genomic similarities between canine and human brain tumors suggest that studying dogs with cancer is likely to provide a valuable additional perspective to human and murine studies. The value of this opportunity is being increasingly recognized in the field of cancer research for further understanding of tumorigenesis and the evaluation of novel treatments. Provided well-designed humane guidelines are adhered to, clinical trials involving companion animals are more acceptable to the public at large than many laboratory animal investigations. Veterinary institutions involved in clinical trials consistently use informed client consent, and institutional review boards ensure proper study design, and ethical standards are maintained. However, because the 'standard of care' has not been established for canine brain tumors, more latitude in prospective clinical trials is allowable, and it is easier to instigate trials that attempt new and innovative treatment strategies. Most pet owners are highly committed and actively seek innovative and promising new therapies to treat their animal's cancer, with the potential for improving our ability to treat cancer in other companion animals and people being seen as an additional benefit. It is reasonable to believe then that the neuro-oncology field will view dogs and other animals with naturally occurring cancers as common, valued and necessary parts of tumorigenesis research and the drug development process.

Acknowledgments The author would like to thank Dr. Erwin Van Meir and Dr. Gang Chen of Emory University School of Medicine, Atlanta for assistance in the preparation of this chapter.

References

Adamo, P.F., Cantile, C., Steinberg, H., 2003. Evaluation of progesterone and estrogen receptor expression in 15 meningiomas of dogs and cats. Am J Vet Res 64, 1310–1318.

Arama, E., Dickman, D., Kimchie, Z., Shearn, A., Lev, Z., 2000. Mutations in the beta-propeller domain of the Drosophila brain tumor (brat) protein induce neoplasm in the larval brain. Oncogene 19, 3706–3716.

Ashley, D.M., Kong, F.M., Bigner, D.D., Hale, L.P., 1998a. Endogenous expression of transforming growth factor beta1 inhibits growth and tumorigenicity and enhances Fas-mediated apoptosis in a murine high-grade glioma model. Cancer Res 58, 302–309.

Ashley, D.M., Sampson, J.H., Archer, G.E., Hale, L.P., Bigner, D.D., 1998b. Local production of TGF beta1 inhibits cerebral edema, enhances TNF-alpha induced apoptosis and improves survival in a murine glioma model. J Neuroimmunol 86, 46–52.

Axlund, T.W., McGlasson, M.L., Smith, A.N., 2002. Surgery alone or in combination with radiation therapy for treatment of intracranial meningiomas in dogs: 31 cases (1989–2002). J Am Vet Med Assoc 221, 1597–1600.

Barth, R.F., 1998. Rat brain tumor models in experimental neuro-oncology: the 9L, C6, T9, F98, RG2 (D74), RT-2 and CNS-1 gliomas. J Neurooncol 36, 91–102.

Barth, R.F., Yang, W., Coderre, J.A., 2003. Rat brain tumor models to assess the efficacy of boron neutron capture therapy: a critical evaluation. J Neurooncol 62, 61–74.

Basler, K., Hafen, E., 1991. Specification of cell fate in the developing eye of Drosophila. Bioessays 13, 621–631.

Beaucher, M., Goodliffe, J., Hersperger, E., Trunova, S., Frydman, H., Shearn, A., 2007a. Drosophila brain tumor metastases express both neuronal and glial cell type markers. Dev Biol 301, 287–297.

Beaucher, M., Hersperger, E., Page-McCaw, A., Shearn, A., 2007b. Metastatic ability of Drosophila tumors depends on MMP activity. Dev Biol 303, 625–634.

Begemann, M., Fuller, G.N., Holland, E.C., 2002. Genetic modeling of glioma formation in mice. Brain Pathol 12, 117–132.
Bello, B., Reichert, H., Hirth, F., 2006. The brain tumor gene negatively regulates neural progenitor cell proliferation in the larval central brain of Drosophila. Development 133, 2639–2648.
Berens, M.E., Bjotvedt, G., Levesque, D.C., Rief, M.D., Shapiro, J.R., Coons, S.W., 1993. Tumorigenic, invasive, karyotypic, and immunocytochemical characteristics of clonal cell lines derived from a spontaneous canine anaplastic astrocytoma. In Vitro Cell Dev Biol Anim 29A, 310–318.
Berens, M.E., Giese, A., Shapiro, J.R., Coons, S.W., 1999. Allogeneic astrocytoma in immune competent dogs. Neoplasia 1, 107–112.
Berghmans, S., Murphey, R.D., Wienholds, E., Neuberg, D., Kutok, J.L., Fletcher, C.D., Morris, J.P., Liu, T.X., Schulte-Merker, S., Kanki, J.P., Plasterk, R., Zon, L.I., Look, A.T., 2005. tp53 mutant zebrafish develop malignant peripheral nerve sheath tumors. Proc Natl Acad Sci USA 102, 407–412.
Betschinger, J., Mechtler, K., Knoblich, J.A., 2006. Asymmetric segregation of the tumor suppressor brat regulates self-renewal in Drosophila neural stem cells. Cell 124, 1241–1253.
Bigner, D.D., Kvedar, J.P., Thomas, B.A., Shaffer, C., Vick, N.A., Engel, W.K., Day, E.D., 1972. Factors influencing the cell type of brain tumors induced in dogs by Schmidt-Ruppin Rous sarcoma virus. J Neuropathol Exp Neurol 31, 583–595.
Bigner, D.D., Odom, G.L., Mahaley, M.S., Jr., Day, E.D., 1969. Brain tumors induced in dogs by the Schmidt-Ruppin strain of Rous sarcoma virus. Neuropathological and immunological observations. J Neuropathol Exp Neurol 28, 648–680.
Bley, C.R., Sumova, A., Roos, M., Kaser-Hotz, B., 2005. Irradiation of brain tumors in dogs with neurologic disease. J Vet Intern Med 19, 849–854.
Bowman, S.K., Rolland, V., Betschinger, J., Kinsey, K.A., Emery, G., Knoblich, J.A., 2008. The tumor suppressors Brat and Numb regulate transit-amplifying neuroblast lineages in Drosophila. Dev Cell 14, 535–546.
Bradford, R., Darling, J.L., Thomas, D.G., 1986. The in-vitro chemosensitivity of three cell lines derived from the VM/DK spontaneous murine astrocytoma. J Neurol Neurosurg Psychiatry 49, 1361–1366.
Brearley, M.J., Jeffery, N.D., Phillips, S.M., Dennis, R., 1999. Hypofractionated radiation therapy of brain masses in dogs: a retrospective analysis of survival of 83 cases (1991–1996). J Vet Intern Med 13, 408–412.
Britt, R.H., Lyons, B.E., Enzmann, D.R., Saxer, E.L., Bigner, S.H., Bigner, D.D., 1987. Correlation of neuropathologic findings, computerized tomographic and high-resolution ultrasound scans of canine avian sarcoma virus-induced brain tumors. J Neurooncol 4, 243–268.
Bryant, P.J., Schmidt, O., 1990. The genetic control of cell proliferation in Drosophila imaginal discs. J Cell Sci Suppl 13, 169–189.
Campbell, M., Dickinson, P., Roberts, B., Leutenegger, C.M., LeCouteur, R.A., 2006. NF-2 Expression in canine meningiomas. J Vet Intern Med 20, 734–735.
Candolfi, M., Kroeger, K.M., Pluhar, G.E., Bergeron, J., Puntel, M., Curtin, J.F., McNiel, E.A., Freese, A.B., Ohlfest, J.R., Moore, P., Lowenstein, P.R., Castro, M.G., 2007a. Adenoviral-mediated gene transfer into the canine brain in vivo. Neurosurgery 60, 167–177; discussion 178.
Candolfi, M., Pluhar, G.E., Kroeger, K., Puntel, M., Curtin, J., Barcia, C., Muhammad, A.K., Xiong, W., Liu, C., Mondkar, S., Kuoy, W., Kang, T., McNeil, E.A., Freese, A.B., Ohlfest, J.R., Moore, P., Palmer, D., Ng, P., Young, J.D., Lowenstein, P.R., Castro, M.G., 2007b. Optimization of adenoviral vector-mediated transgene expression in the canine brain in vivo, and in canine glioma cells in vitro. Neuro Oncol 9, 245–258.

Canfield, P.J., Doughty, F.R., 1980. A study of virus-like particles present in bovine nerve sheath tumours. Aust Vet J 56, 257–261.
Cantile, C., Campani, D., Menicagli, M., Arispici, M., 2002. Pathological and immunohistochemical studies of choroid plexus carcinoma of the dog. J Comp Pathol 126, 183–193.
Chambers, R., Gillespie, G.Y., Soroceanu, L., Andreansky, S., Chatterjee, S., Chou, J., Roizman, B., Whitley, R.J., 1995. Comparison of genetically engineered herpes simplex viruses for the treatment of brain tumors in a scid mouse model of human malignant glioma. Proc Natl Acad Sci USA 92, 1411–1415.
Chauvet, A.E., Kesava, P.P., Goh, C.S., Badie, B., 1998. Selective intraarterial gene delivery into a canine meningioma. J Neurosurg 88, 870–873.
Copeland, D.D., Talley, F.A., Bigner, D.D., 1976. The fine structure of intracranial neoplasms induced by the inoculation of avian sarcoma virus in neonatal and adult rats. Am J Pathol 83, 149–176.
Courtay-Cahan, C., Platt, S. R., De Risio, L., Starkey, M., 2008. Preliminary analysis of genomic abnormalities in canine meningiomas. Vet Comp Oncol 6, 182–192.
Covington, A.L., Magdesian, K.G., Madigan, J.E., Maleski, K., Gray, L.C., Smith, P.A., Wisner, E.R., 2004. Recurrent esophageal obstruction and dysphagia due to a brainstem melanoma in a horse. J Vet Intern Med 18, 245–247.
Dickinson, P.J., 2007. Convection-enhanced delivery of drugs to the brain: Clinical applications. In: American College of Veterinary Internal Medicine (ACVIM) Annual Forum, Seattle, WA.
Dickinson, P.J., LeCouteur, R.A., Higgins, R.J., Bringas, J.R., Roberts, B., Larson, R.F., Yamashita, Y., Krauze, M., Noble, C.O., Drummond, D., Kirpotin, D.B., Park, J.W., Berger, M.S., Bankiewicz, K.S., 2008a. Canine model of convection-enhanced delivery of liposomes containing CPT-11 monitored with real-time magnetic resonance imaging: laboratory investigation. J Neurosurg 108, 989–998.
Dickinson, P.J., Roberts, B., Higgins, R.J., Leutenegger, C.M., Bollen, A.W., Kass, P.H., LeCouteur, R.A., 2006. Expression of receptor tyrosine kinases VEGFR-1 (FLT-1), VEGFR-2 (KDR), EGFR-1, PDGFRα and c-Met in canine primary brain tumours. Vet Comp Oncol 4, 132–140.
Dickinson, P.J., Sturges, B.K., Higgins, R.J., Roberts, B.N., Leutenegger, C.M., Bollen, A.W., LeCouteur, R.A., 2008b. Vascular endothelial growth factor mRNA expression and peritumoral edema in canine primary central nervous system tumors. Vet Pathol 45, 131–139.
Dobson, J.M., Samuel, S., Milstein, H., Rogers, K., Wood, J.L., 2002. Canine neoplasia in the UK: estimates of incidence rates from a population of insured dogs. J Small Anim Pract 43, 240–246.
Dyer, C.A., Philibotte, T., 1995. A clone of the MOCH-1 glial tumor in culture: multiple phenotypes expressed under different environmental conditions. J Neuropathol Exp Neurol 54, 852–863.
Ernestus, R.I., Wilmes, L.J., Hoehn-Berlage, M., 1992. Identification of intracranial liqor metastases of experimental stereotactically implanted brain tumors by the tumor-selective MRI contrast agent MnTPPS. Clin Exp Metastasis 10, 345–350.
Evans, S.M., Dayrell-Hart, B., Powlis, W., Christy, G., VanWinkle, T., 1993. Radiation therapy of canine brain masses. J Vet Intern Med 7, 216–219.
Faucherre, A., Taylor, G.S., Overvoorde, J., Dixon, J.E., Hertog, J., 2008. Zebrafish pten genes have overlapping and non-redundant functions in tumorigenesis and embryonic development. Oncogene 27, 1079–1086.
Feitsma, H., Kuiper, R.V., Korving, J., Nijman, I.J., Cuppen, E., 2008. Zebrafish with mutations in mismatch repair genes develop neurofibromas and other tumors. Cancer Res 68, 5059–5066.
Fiandaca, M.S., Forsayeth, J.R., Dickinson, P.J., Bankiewicz, K.S., 2008. Image-guided convection-enhanced delivery platform in the treatment of neurological diseases. Neurotherapeutics 5, 123–127.

Fomchenko, E.I., Holland, E.C., 2006. Mouse models of brain tumors and their applications in preclinical trials. Clin Cancer Res 12, 5288–5297.
Frank, D.J., Edgar, B.A., Roth, M.B., 2002. The Drosophila melanogaster gene brain tumor negatively regulates cell growth and ribosomal RNA synthesis. Development 129, 399–407.
Frank, J.A., Girton, M., Dwyer, A.J., Cohen, P.J., Knop, R.H., Diggs, R., Cobb, J., Doppman, J.L., 1987a. A reproducible model of metastatic brain and ocular tumor by hematogenous inoculation of the VX2 tumor in rabbits. J Neurosurg 67, 106–109.
Frank, J.A., Girton, M., Dwyer, A.J., Cohen, P.J., Lightman, S., Gansow, O.A., Brechbiel, M.W., Doppman, J.L., 1987b. Ocular and cerebral metastases in the VX2 rabbit tumor model: contrast-enhanced MR imaging. Radiology 164, 527–530.
Friese, M.A., Platten, M., Lutz, S.Z., Naumann, U., Aulwurm, S., Bischof, F., Buhring, H.J., Dichgans, J., Rammensee, H.G., Steinle, A., Weller, M., 2003. MICA/NKG2D-mediated immunogene therapy of experimental gliomas. Cancer Res 63, 8996–9006.
Fulton, L.M., Steinberg, H.S., 1990. Preliminary study of lomustine in the treatment of intracranial masses in dogs following localization by imaging techniques. Semin Vet Med Surg (Small Anim) 5, 241–245.
Gavin, P.R., Kraft, S.L., Huiskamp, R., Coderre, J.A., 1997. A review: CNS effects and normal tissue tolerance in dogs. J Neurooncol 33, 71–80.
Gavin, P.R., Kraft, S.L., Wendling, L.R., Miller, D.L., 1989. Canine spontaneous brain tumors – a large animal model for BNCT. Strahlenther Onkol 165, 225–228.
Greco, J.J., Aiken, S.A., Berg, J.M., Monette, S., Bergman, P.J., 2006. Evaluation of intracranial meningioma resection with a surgical aspirator in dogs: 17 cases (1996–2004). J Am Vet Med Assoc 229, 394–400.
Grove, A.S., Jr., Di Chiro, G., Rabotti, G.F., 1967. Experimental brain tumors, with a report of those induced in dogs by Rous sarcoma virus. J Neurosurg 26, 465–477.
Gutmann, D.H., Maher, E.A., Van Dyke, T., 2006. Mouse Models of Human Cancers Consortium Workshop on Nervous System Tumors. Cancer Res 66, 10–13.
Hansen, K., Khanna, C., 2004. Spontaneous and genetically engineered animal models; use in preclinical cancer drug development. Eur J Cancer 40, 858–880.
Harding, T.C., Dickinson, P.J., Roberts, B.N., Yendluri, S., Gonzalez-Edick, M., Lecouteur, R.A., Jooss, K.U., 2006a. Enhanced gene transfer efficiency in the murine striatum and an orthotopic glioblastoma tumor model, using AAV-7- and AAV-8-pseudotyped vectors. Hum Gene Ther 17, 807–820.
Harding, T.C., Lalani, A.S., Roberts, B.N., Yendluri, S., Luan, B., Koprivnikar, K.E., Gonzalez-Edick, M., Huan-Tu, G., Musterer, R., VanRoey, M.J., Ozawa, T., LeCouter, R.A., Deen, D., Dickinson, P.J., Jooss, K., 2006b. AAV serotype 8-mediated gene delivery of a soluble VEGF receptor to the CNS for the treatment of glioblastoma. Mol Ther 13, 956–966.
Hayes, H.M., Priester, W.A., Jr., Pendergrass, T.W., 1975. Occurrence of nervous-tissue tumors in cattle, horses, cats and dogs. Int J Cancer 15, 39–47.
Heidner, G.L., Kornegay, J.N., Page, R.L., Dodge, R.K., Thrall, D.E., 1991. Analysis of survival in a retrospective study of 86 dogs with brain tumors. J Vet Intern Med 5, 219–226.
Heimberger, A.B., Crotty, L.E., Archer, G.E., McLendon, R.E., Friedman, A., Dranoff, G., Bigner, D.D., Sampson, J.H., 2000. Bone marrow-derived dendritic cells pulsed with tumor homogenate induce immunity against syngeneic intracerebral glioma. J Neuroimmunol 103, 16–25.
Hellums, E.K., Markert, J.M., Parker, J.N., He, B., Perbal, B., Roizman, B., Whitley, R.J., Langford, C.P., Bharara, S., Gillespie, G.Y., 2005. Increased efficacy of an interleukin-12-secreting herpes simplex virus in a syngeneic intracranial murine glioma model. Neuro Oncol 7, 213–224.
Herring, J.M., Reyes, M., Dochterman, L.W., Bennett, B.T., 1990. Glioblastoma multiforme in a baboon. Lab Anim Sci 40, 645–647.

Higgins, R.J., McKisic, M., Dickinson, P.J., Jimenez, D.F., Dow, S.W., Tripp, L.D., LeCouteur, R.A., 2004. Growth inhibition of an orthotopic glioblastoma in immunocompetent mice by cationic lipid-DNA complexes. Cancer Immunol Immunother 53, 338–344.
Hoenerhoff, M.J., Janovitz, E., Ramos-Vara, J., Kiupel, M., 2006. Choroid plexus papilloma in a Scottish highland cow. J Comp Pathol 135, 146–149.
Hu, X., Holland, E.C., 2005. Applications of mouse glioma models in preclinical trials. Mutat Res 576, 54–65.
Huang, H., Potter, C.J., Tao, W., Li, D.M., Brogiolo, W., Hafen, E., Sun, H., Xu, T., 1999. PTEN affects cell size, cell proliferation and apoptosis during Drosophila eye development. Development 126, 5365–5372.
Ingram, M., Jacques D., Freshwater, D.B., 1990. Adoptive immunotherapy of brain tumors in dogs. Vet Med Rep 2, 398–401.
Kangasniemi, M., McNichols, R.J., Bankson, J.A., Gowda, A., Price, R.E., Hazle, J.D., 2004. Thermal therapy of canine cerebral tumors using a 980 nm diode laser with MR temperature-sensitive imaging feedback. Lasers Surg Med 35, 41–50.
Keller, E.T., Madewell, B.R., 1992. Locations and types of neoplasms in immature dogs: 69 cases (1964–1989). J Am Vet Med Assoc 200, 1530–1532.
Kimmelman, J., Nalbantoglu, J., 2007. Faithful companions: a proposal for neurooncology trials in pet dogs. Cancer Res 67, 4541–4544.
Kobayashi, N., Allen, N., Clendenon, N.R., Ko, L.W., 1980. An improved rat brain-tumor model. J Neurosurg 53, 808–815.
Koblik, P.D., LeCouteur, R.A., Higgins, R.J., Bollen, A.W., Vernau, K.M., Kortz, G.D., Ilkiw, J.E., 1999a. CT-guided brain biopsy using a modified Pelorus Mark III stereotactic system: experience with 50 dogs. Vet Radiol Ultrasound 40, 434–440.
Koblik, P.D., LeCouteur, R.A., Higgins, R.J., Fick, J., Kortz, G.D., Sturges, B.K., Pascoe, P. J., 1999b. Modification and application of a Pelorus Mark III stereotactic system for CT-guided brain biopsy in 50 dogs. Vet Radiol Ultrasound 40, 424–433.
Koestner, A., Bilzer, T., Fatzer, R., Schulman, F.Y., Summers, B.A., Van Winkle, T.J., 1999. Histological classification of tumors of the nervous system of domestic animals. In: WHO (Ed.), Vol. V. The Armed Forces Institute of Pathology, City.
Koppel, H., Martin, J.M., Pilkington, G.J., Lantos, P.L., 1986. Heterogeneity of a cultured neoplastic glial line. Establishment and characterisation of six clones. J Neurol Sci 76, 295–315.
Koppel, H., Pilkington, G.J., Lantos, P.L., 1988. Tumorigenicity of six clones of a cultured neoplastic cell line derived from a spontaneous murine astrocytoma: morphology and immunocytochemistry of tumours. J Neurol Sci 83, 227–242.
Kostolich, M., Dulisch, M.L., 1987. A surgical approach to the canine olfactory bulb for meningioma removal. Vet Surg 16, 273–277.
Kraft, S.L., Gavin, P.R., DeHaan, C.E., Leathers, C.W., Bauer, W.F., Miller, D.L., Dorn, R.V., 3rd, 1992. Borocaptate sodium: a potential boron delivery compound for boron neutron capture therapy evaluated in dogs with spontaneous intracranial tumors. Proc Natl Acad Sci USA 89, 11973–11977.
Kraft, S.L., Gavin, P.R., Leathers, C.W., DeHaan, C.E., Bauer, W.F., Miller, D.L., Dorn, R. V., 3rd, Griebenow, M.L., 1994. Biodistribution of boron in dogs with spontaneous intracranial tumors following borocaptate sodium administration. Cancer Res 54, 1259–1263.
Kurzik-Dumke, U., Phannavong, B., Gundacker, D., Gateff, E., 1992. Genetic, cytogenetic and developmental analysis of the Drosophila melanogaster tumor suppressor gene lethal(2)tumorous imaginal discs (1(2)tid). Differentiation 51, 91–104.
Learn, C.A., Grossi, P.M., Schmittling, R.J., Xie, W., Mitchell, D.A., Karikari, I., Wei, Z., Dressman, H., Sampson, J.H., 2007. Genetic analysis of intracranial tumors in a murine model of glioma demonstrate a shift in gene expression in response to host immunity. J Neuroimmunol 182, 63–72.

Lee, C.Y., Wilkinson, B.D., Siegrist, S.E., Wharton, R.P., Doe, C.Q., 2006. Brat is a Miranda cargo protein that promotes neuronal differentiation and inhibits neuroblast self-renewal. Dev Cell 10, 441–449.

Lee, Y.S., Bigner, S.H., Eng, L.F., Molnar, P., Kuruvilla, A., Groothuis, D.R., Bigner, D.D., 1986. A glial fibrillary acidic protein-expressing and tumorigenic cell line derived from an avian sarcoma virus-induced rat astrocytoma. J Neuropathol Exp Neurol 45, 704–720.

Lester, N.V., Hopkins, A.L., Bova, F.J., Friedman, W.A., Buatti, J.M., Meeks, S.L., Chrisman, C.L., 2001. Radiosurgery using a stereotactic headframe system for irradiation of brain tumors in dogs. J Am Vet Med Assoc 219, 1562–1567,1550.

Lindblad-Toh, K., Wade, C.M., Mikkelsen, T.S., Karlsson, E.K., Jaffe, D.B., Kamal, M., Clamp, M., Chang, J.L., Kulbokas, E.J., 3rd, Zody, M.C., Mauceli, E., Xie, X., Breen, M., Wayne, R.K., Ostrander, E.A., Ponting, C.P., Galibert, F., Smith, D.R., DeJong, P.J., Kirkness, E., Alvarez, P., Biagi, T., Brockman, W., Butler, J., Chin, C.W., Cook, A., Cuff, J., Daly, M.J., DeCaprio, D., Gnerre, S., Grabherr, M., Kellis, M., Kleber, M., Bardeleben, C., Goodstadt, L., Heger, A., Hitte, C., Kim, L., Koepfli, K.P., Parker, H.G., Pollinger, J.P., Searle, S.M., Sutter, N.B., Thomas, R., Webber, C., Baldwin, J., Abebe, A., Abouelleil, A., Aftuck, L., Ait-Zahra, M., Aldredge, T., Allen, N., An, P., Anderson, S., Antoine, C., Arachchi, H., Aslam, A., Ayotte, L., Bachantsang, P., Barry, A., Bayul, T., Benamara, M., Berlin, A., Bessette, D., Blitshteyn, B., Bloom, T., Blye, J., Boguslavskiy, L., Bonnet, C., Boukhgalter, B., Brown, A., Cahill, P., Calixte, N., Camarata, J., Cheshatsang, Y., Chu, J., Citroen, M., Collymore, A., Cooke, P., Dawoe, T., Daza, R., Decktor, K., DeGray, S., Dhargay, N., Dooley, K., Dorje, P., Dorjee, K., Dorris, L., Duffey, N., Dupes, A., Egbiremolen, O., Elong, R., Falk, J., Farina, A., Faro, S., Ferguson, D., Ferreira, P., Fisher, S., FitzGerald, M., Foley, K., Foley, C., Franke, A., Friedrich, D., Gage, D., Garber, M., Gearin, G., Giannoukos, G., Goode, T., Goyette, A., Graham, J., Grandbois, E., Gyaltsen, K., Hafez, N., Hagopian, D., Hagos, B., Hall, J., Healy, C., Hegarty, R., Honan, T., Horn, A., Houde, N., Hughes, L., Hunnicutt, L., Husby, M., Jester, B., Jones, C., Kamat, A., Kanga, B., Kells, C., Khazanovich, D., Kieu, A.C., Kisner, P., Kumar, M., Lance, K., Landers, T., Lara, M., Lee, W., Leger, J.P., Lennon, N., Leuper, L., LeVine, S., Liu, J., Liu, X., Lokyitsang, Y., Lokyitsang, T., Lui, A., Macdonald, J., Major, J., Marabella, R., Maru, K., Matthews, C., McDonough, S., Mehta, T., Meldrim, J., Melnikov, A., Meneus, L., Mihalev, A., Mihova, T., Miller, K., Mittelman, R., Mlenga, V., Mulrain, L., Munson, G., Navidi, A., Naylor, J., Nguyen, T., Nguyen, N., Nguyen, C., Nicol, R., Norbu, N., Norbu, C., Novod, N., Nyima, T., Olandt, P., O'Neill, B., O'Neill, K., Osman, S., Oyono, L., Patti, C., Perrin, D., Phunkhang, P., Pierre, F., Priest, M., Rachupka, A., Raghuraman, S., Rameau, R., Ray, V., Raymond, C., Rege, F., Rise, C., Rogers, J., Rogov, P., Sahalie, J., Settipalli, S., Sharpe, T., Shea, T., Sheehan, M., Sherpa, N., Shi, J., Shih, D., Sloan, J., Smith, C., Sparrow, T., Stalker, J., Stange-Thomann, N., Stavropoulos, S., Stone, C., Stone, S., Sykes, S., Tchuinga, P., Tenzing, P., Tesfaye, S., Thoulutsang, D., Thoulutsang, Y., Topham, K., Topping, I., Tsamla, T., Vassiliev, H., Venkataraman, V., Vo, A., Wangchuk, T., Wangdi, T., Weiand, M., Wilkinson, J., Wilson, A., Yadav, S., Yang, S., Yang, X., Young, G., Yu, Q., Zainoun, J., Zembek, L., Zimmer, A., Lander, E.S., 2005. Genome sequence, comparative analysis and haplotype structure of the domestic dog. Nature 438, 803–819.

Lipsitz, D., Higgins, R.J., Kortz, G.D., Dickinson, P.J., Bollen, A.W., Naydan, D.K., LeCouteur, R.A., 2003. Glioblastoma multiforme: clinical findings, magnetic resonance imaging, and pathology in five dogs. Vet Pathol 40, 659–669.

Long, P.H., Schulman, F.Y., Koestner, A., Fix, A.S., Campbell, M.K., Cameron, K.N., 1998. Primitive neuroectodermal tumor in a two-month-old black and white Colobus monkey. Vet Pathol 35, 64–67.

Long, S., Argyle, D.J., Nixon, C., Nicholson, I., Botteron, C., Olby, N., Platt, S., Smith, K., Rutteman, G.R., Grinwis, G.C., Nasir, L., 2006. Telomerase reverse transcriptase (TERT)

expression and proliferation in canine brain tumours. Neuropathol Appl Neurobiol 32, 662–673.
Long, S.N., Anderson, T.J., Long, F.H., Johnston, P.E., 2002. Evaluation of rapid staining techniques for cytologic diagnosis of intracranial lesions. Am J Vet Res 63, 381–386.
Loop, T., Leemans, R., Stiefel, U., Hermida, L., Egger, B., Xie, F., Primig, M., Certa, U., Fischbach, K.F., Reichert, H., Hirth, F., 2004. Transcriptional signature of an adult brain tumor in Drosophila. BMC Genomics 5, 24.
Mandara, M.T., Ricci, G., Rinaldi, L., Sarli, G., Vitellozzi, G., 2002. Immunohistochemical identification and image analysis quantification of oestrogen and progesterone receptors in canine and feline meningioma. J Comp Pathol 127, 214–218.
Mandrioli, L., Panarese, S., Cesari, A., Mandara, M.T., Marcato, P.S., Bettini, G., 2007. Immunohistochemical expression of h-telomerase reverse transcriptase in canine and feline meningiomas. J Vet Sci 8, 111–115.
Miklos, G.L., Rubin, G.M., 1996. The role of the genome project in determining gene function: insights from model organisms. Cell 86, 521–529.
Montoliu, P., Anor, S., Vidal, E., Pumarola, M., 2006. Histological and immunohistochemical study of 30 cases of canine meningioma. J Comp Pathol 135, 200–207.
Moore, M.P., Bagley, R.S., Harrington, M.L., Gavin, P.R., 1996. Intracranial tumors. Vet Clin North Am Small Anim Pract 26, 759–777.
Nichols, D.K., Dias, J.L., 1995. Melanotic ependymoma in a Goeldi's marmoset (Callimico goeldii). J Med Primatol 24, 49–51.
Niebauer, G.W., Dayrell-Hart, B.L., Speciale, J., 1991. Evaluation of craniotomy in dogs and cats. J Am Vet Med Assoc 198, 89–95.
O'Brien, S.J., Murphy, W.J., 2003. Genomics. A dog's breakfast? Science 301, 1854–1855.
Paoloni, M., Khanna, C., 2008. Translation of new cancer treatments from pet dogs to humans. Nat Rev Cancer 8, 147–156.
Paradis, M.R., 1998. Tumors of the central nervous system. Vet Clin North Am Equine Pract 14, 543–561, vii.
Paraf, F., Jothy, S., Van Meir, E.G., 1997. Brain tumor-polyopsis syndrome: two genetic diseases? J Clin Oncol 15, 2744–2758.
Patnaik, A.K., Kay, W.J., Hurvitz, A.I., 1986. Intracranial meningioma: a comparative pathologic study of 28 dogs. Vet Pathol 23, 369–373.
Pilkington, G.J., Darling, J.L., Lantos, P.L., Thomas, D.G., 1983. Cell lines (VMDk) derived from a spontaneous murine astrocytoma. Morphological and immunocytochemical characterization. J Neurol Sci 62, 115–139.
Pilkington, G.J., Darling, J.L., Lantos, P.L., Thomas, D.G., 1985. Tumorigenicity of cell lines (VMDk) derived from a spontaneous murine astrocytoma. Histology, fine structure and immunocytochemistry of tumours. J Neurol Sci 71, 145–164.
Pilkington, G.J., Lantos, P.L., Darling, J.L., Thomas, D.G., 1982. Three cell lines from a spontaneous murine astrocytoma show variation in astrocytic differentiation. Neurosci Lett 34, 315–320.
Pires, M.M., Pilkington, G.J., Lantos, P.L., 1987. Vascular permeability in transplantable murine gliomas: morphological correlation with tracer studies. Neuropathol Appl Neurobiol 13, 251–262.
Platt, S.R., Alleman, A.R., Lanz, O.I., Chrisman, C.L., 2002. Comparison of fine-needle aspiration and surgical-tissue biopsy in the diagnosis of canine brain tumors. Vet Surg 31, 65–69.
Platt, S.R., Marlin, D., Smith, N., Adams, V., 2006a. Increased cerebrospinal fluid uric acid concentrations in dogs with intracranial meningioma. Vet Rec 158, 830.
Platt, S.R., Marlin, D., Smith, N., Flack, D., De Stefani, A., Wieczorek, L., Adams, V., 2006b. Cerebrospinal fluid glutamate levels in dogs with intracranial neoplasia. J Vet Intern Med 20, 736.

Platt, S.R., Scase, T.J., Adams, V., Wieczorek, L., Miller, J., Adamo, F., Long, S., 2006c. Vascular endothelial growth factor expression in canine intracranial meningiomas and association with patient survival. J Vet Intern Med 20, 663–668.
Potter, C.J., Turenchalk, G.S., Xu, T., 2000. Drosophila in cancer research. An expanding role. Trends Genet 16, 33–39.
Rainov, N.G., Koch, S., Sena-Esteves, M., Berens, M.E., 2000. Characterization of a canine glioma cell line as related to established experimental brain tumor models. J Neuropathol Exp Neurol 59, 607–613.
Read, R.D., Cavenee, W.K., Furnari, F.B., Thomas, J.B., (2009). A drosophila model for EGFR-Ras and PI3K-dependent human glioma. PLoS Genet 5(2), e1000374. Epub 2009 Feb 13.
Ribas, J.L., Mena, H., Braund, K.G., Sesterhenn, I.A., Toivio-Kinnucan, M., 1989. A histologic and immunocytochemical study of choroid plexus tumors of the dog. Vet Pathol 26, 55–64.
Rossmeisl, J.H., Duncan, R.B., Huckle, W.R., Troy, G.C., 2007. Expression of vascular endothelial growth factor in tumors and plasma from dogs with primary intracranial neoplasms. Am J Vet Res 68, 1239–1245.
Sampson, J.H., Ashley, D.M., Archer, G.E., Fuchs, H.E., Dranoff, G., Hale, L.P., Bigner, D.D., 1997. Characterization of a spontaneous murine astrocytoma and abrogation of its tumorigenicity by cytokine secretion. Neurosurgery 41, 1365–1372; discussion 1372–1363.
Schmidek, H.H., Nielsen, S.L., Schiller, A.L., Messer, J., 1971. Morphological studies of rat brain tumors induced by N-nitrosomethylurea. J Neurosurg 34, 335–340.
Serano, R.D., Pegram, C.N., Bigner, D.D., 1980. Tumorigenic cell culture lines from a spontaneous VM/Dk murine astrocytoma (SMA). Acta Neuropathol 51, 53–64.
Snyder, J.M., Lipitz, L., Skorupski, K.A., Shofer, F.S., Van Winkle, T.J., 2008. Secondary intracranial neoplasia in the dog: 177 cases (1986–2003). J Vet Intern Med 22, 172–177.
Snyder, J.M., Shofer, F.S., Van Winkle, T.J., Massicotte, C., 2006. Canine intracranial primary neoplasia: 173 cases (1986–2003). J Vet Intern Med 20, 669–675.
Sonoda, J., Wharton, R.P., 2001. Drosophila Brain Tumor is a translational repressor. Genes Dev 15, 762–773.
Spugnini, E.P., Thrall, D.E., Price, G.S., Sharp, N.J., Munana, K., Page, R.L., 2000. Primary irradiation of canine intracranial masses. Vet Radiol Ultrasound 41, 377–380.
Stoica, G., Kim, H.T., Hall, D.G., Coates, J.R., 2004. Morphology, immunohistochemistry, and genetic alterations in dog astrocytomas. Vet Pathol 41, 10–19.
Stoica, G., Tasca, S.I., Kim, H.T., 2001. Point mutation of neu oncogene in animal peripheral nerve sheath tumors. Vet Pathol 38, 679–688.
Sturges, B.K., Dickinson, P.J., Bollen, A.W., Koblik, P.D., Kass, P.H., Kortz, G.D., Vernau, K.M., Knipe, M.F., Lecouteur, R.A., Higgins, R.J., 2008. Magnetic resonance imaging and histological classification of intracranial meningiomas in 112 dogs. J Vet Intern Med 22, 586–595.
Swenberg, J.A., Koestner, A., Wechsler, W., Denlinger, R.H., 1972. Quantitative aspects of transplacental tumor induction with ethylnitrosourea in rats. Cancer Res 32, 2656–2660.
Tabuchi, K., Nishimoto, A., Matsumoto, K., Satoh, T., Nakasone, S., Fujiwara, T., Ogura, H., 1985. Establishment of a brain-tumor model in adult monkeys. J Neurosurg 63, 912–916.
Thankey, K., Faissler, D., Kavirayani, A., Keating, J.H., McDonnell, J.J., 2006. Clinical presentation and outcome in dogs with histologically confirmed choroid plexus papillomas. J Vet Intern Med 20, 782–783.
The Cancer Genome Atlas Research Network, McLendon, R., Friedman, A., Bigner, D., Van Meir, E.G., Brat, D.J., Mastrogianakis, M., Olson, J.J., Mikkelsen, T., Lehman, N., Aldape, K., Alfred Yung, W.K., Bogler, O., Vandenberg, S., Berger, M., Prados, M., Muzny, D., Morgan, M., Scherer, S., Sabo, A., Nazareth, L., Lewis, L., Hall, O., Zhu, Y., Ren, Y., Alvi, O., Yao, J., Hawes, A., Jhangiani, S., Fowler, G., San Lucas, A., Kovar, C., Cree, A., Dinh, H., Santibanez, J., Joshi, V., Gonzalez-Garay, M.L., Miller, C.A., Milosavljevic, A., Donehower, L., Wheeler, D.A., Gibbs, R.A., Cibulskis, K., Sougnez, C., Fennell, T., Mahan, S., Wilkinson, J., Ziaugra, L., Onofrio, R., Bloom, T., Nicol, R., Ardlie, K., Baldwin, J., Gabriel, S., Lander, E.S., Ding, L., Fulton, R.S., McLellan, M.D.,

Wallis, J., Larson, D.E., Shi, X., Abbott, R., Fulton, L., Chen, K., Koboldt, D.C., Wendl, M.C., Meyer, R., Tang, Y., Lin, L., Osborne, J.R., Dunford-Shore, B.H., Miner, T.L., Delehaunty, K., Markovic, C., Swift, G., Courtney, W., Pohl, C., Abbott, S., Hawkins, A., Leong, S., Haipek, C., Schmidt, H., Wiechert, M., Vickery, T., Scott, S., Dooling, D.J., Chinwalla, A., Weinstock, G.M., Mardis, E.R., Wilson, R.K., Getz, G., Winckler, W., Verhaak, R.G., Lawrence, M.S., O'Kelly, M., Robinson, J., Alexe, G., Beroukhim, R., Carter, S., Chiang, D., Gould, J., Gupta, S., Korn, J., Mermel, C., Mesirov, J., Monti, S., Nguyen, H., Parkin, M., Reich, M., Stransky, N., Weir, B.A., Garraway, L., Golub, T., Meyerson, M., Chin, L., Protopopov, A., Zhang, J., Perna, I., Aronson, S., Sathiamoorthy, N., Ren, G., Wiedemeyer, W.R., Kim, H., Won Kong, S., Xiao, Y., Kohane, I.S., Seidman, J., Park, P.J., Kucherlapati, R., Laird, P.W., Cope, L., Herman, J.G., Weisenberger, D.J., Pan, F., Van Den Berg, D., Van Neste, L., Mi Yi, J., Schuebel, K.E. , Baylin, S.B., Absher, D.M., Li, J.Z., Southwick, A., Brady, S., Aggarwal, A., Chung, T., Sherlock, G., Brooks, J.D., Myers, R.M., Spellman, P.T., Purdom, E., Jakkula, L.R., Lapuk, A.V., Marr, H., Dorton, S., Gi Choi, Y., Han, J., Ray, A., Wang, V., Durinck, S., Robinson, M., Wang, N.J., Vranizan, K., Peng, V., Van Name, E., Fontenay, G.V., Ngai, J., Conboy, J.G., Parvin, B., Feiler, H.S., Speed, T.P., Gray, J.W., Brennan, C., Socci, N. D., Olshen, A., Taylor, B.S., Lash, A., Schultz, N., Reva, B., Antipin, Y., Stukalov, A., Gross, B., Cerami, E., Qing Wang, W., Qin, L.X., Seshan, V.E., Villafania, L., Cavatore, M., Borsu, L., Viale, A., Gerald, W., Sander, C., Ladanyi, M., Perou, C.M., Neil Hayes, D., Topal, M.D., Hoadley, K.A., Qi, Y., Balu, S., Shi, Y., Wu, J., Penny, R., Bittner, M., Shelton, T., Lenkiewicz, E., Morris, S., Beasley, D., Sanders, S., Kahn, A., Sfeir, R., Chen, J., Nassau, D., Feng, L., Hickey, E., Weinstein, J.N., Barker, A., Gerhard, D.S., Vockley, J., Compton, C., Vaught, J., Fielding, P., Ferguson, M.L., Schaefer, C., Madhavan, S., Buetow, K.H., Collins, F., Good, P., Guyer, M., Ozenberger, B., Peterson, J., Thomson, E., 2008. Comprehensive genomic characterization defines human glioblastoma genes and core pathways. Nature 455(7216), 1061–1068.

Theon, A.P., Lecouteur, R.A., Carr, E.A., Griffey, S.M., 2000. Influence of tumor cell proliferation and sex-hormone receptors on effectiveness of radiation therapy for dogs with incompletely resected meningiomas. J Am Vet Med Assoc 216, 701–707, 684–705.

Thomson, S.A., Kennerly, E., Olby, N., Mickelson, J.R., Hoffmann, D.E., Dickinson, P.J., Gibson, G., Breen, M., 2005. Microarray analysis of differentially expressed genes of primary tumors in the canine central nervous system. Vet Pathol 42, 550–558.

Thrall, D.E., Larue, S.M., Powers, B.E., Page, R.L., Johnson, J., George, S.L., Kornegay, J.N., McEntee, M.C., Levesque, D.C., Smith, M., Case, B.C., Dewhirst, M.W., Gillette, E.L., 1999. Use of whole body hyperthermia as a method to heat inaccessible tumours uniformly: a phase III trial in canine brain masses. Int J Hyperthermia 15, 383–398.

Tomek, A., Cizinauskas, S., Doherr, M., Gandini, G., Jaggy, A., 2006. Intracranial neoplasia in 61 cats: localisation, tumour types and seizure patterns. J Feline Med Surg 8, 243–253.

Troxel, M.T., Vite, C.H., Van Winkle, T.J., Newton, A.L., Tiches, D., Dayrell-Hart, B., Kapatkin, A.S., Shofer, F.S., Steinberg, S.A., 2003. Feline intracranial neoplasia: retrospective review of 160 cases (1985–2001). J Vet Intern Med 17, 850–859.

Turrel, J.M., Fike, J.R., LeCouteur, R.A., Pflugfelder, C.M., Borcich, J.K., 1984. Radiotherapy of brain tumors in dogs. J Am Vet Med Assoc 184, 82–86.

Vail, D.M., MacEwen, E.G., 2000. Spontaneously occurring tumors of companion animals as models for human cancer. Cancer Invest 18, 781–792.

Van Dyke, T., Jacks, T., 2002. Cancer modeling in the modern era: progress and challenges. Cell 108, 135–144.

Vandevelde, M., Fankhauser, R., Luginbuhl, H., 1985. Immunocytochemical studies in canine neuroectodermal brain tumors. Acta Neuropathol 66, 111–116.

Vernau, K.M., Higgins, R.J., Bollen, A.W., Jimenez, D.F., Anderson, J.V., Koblik, P.D., LeCouteur, R.A., 2001. Primary canine and feline nervous system tumors: intraoperative diagnosis using the smear technique. Vet Pathol 38, 47–57.

Warnke, P.C., Molnar, P., Lapin, G.D., Kuruvilla, A., Groothuis, D.R., 1995. The effects of dexamethasone on transcapillary transport in experimental brain tumors: II. Canine brain tumors. J Neurooncol 25, 29–38.

Weiner, N.E., Pyles, R.B., Chalk, C.L., Balko, M.G., Miller, M.A., Dyer, C.A., Warnick, R.E., Parysek, L.M., 1999. A syngeneic mouse glioma model for study of glioblastoma therapy. J Neuropathol Exp Neurol 58, 54–60.

Weiss, W.A., Israel, M., Cobbs, C., Holland, E., James, C.D., Louis, D.N., Marks, C., McClatchey, A.I., Roberts, T., Van Dyke, T., Wetmore, C., Chiu, I.M., Giovannini, M., Guha, A., Higgins, R.J., Marino, S., Radovanovic, I., Reilly, K., Aldape, K., 2002. Neuropathology of genetically engineered mice: consensus report and recommendations from an international forum. Oncogene 21, 7453–7463.

Westworth, D.R., Dickinson, P., Sturges, B.K., Vernau, K.M., Knipe, M.F., LeCouteur, R. A., 2006. Clinicopathological features of choroid plexus tumors in dogs:44 cases. J Vet Intern Med 20, 735.

Westworth, D.R., Dickinson, P.J., Vernau, W., Johnson, E.G., Bollen, A.W., Kass, P.H., Sturges, B.K., Vernau, K.M., Lecouteur, R.A., Higgins, R.J., 2008. Choroid Plexus Tumors in 56 Dogs (1985–2007). J Vet Intern Med 22(5), 1157–1165.

Whelan, H.T., Clanton, J.A., Wilson, R.E., Tulipan, N.B., 1988. Comparison of CT and MRI brain tumor imaging using a canine glioma model. Pediatr Neurol 4, 279–283.

Whelan, H.T., Schmidt, M.H., Segura, A.D., McAuliffe, T.L., Bajic, D.M., Murray, K.J., Moulder, J.E., Strother, D.R., Thomas, J.P., Meyer, G.A., 1993. The role of photodynamic therapy in posterior fossa brain tumors. A preclinical study in a canine glioma model. J Neurosurg 79, 562–568.

Wodarz, A., Gonzalez, C., 2006. Connecting cancer to the asymmetric division of stem cells. Cell 124, 1121–1123.

Woodhouse, E., Hersperger, E., Shearn, A., 1998. Growth, metastasis, and invasiveness of Drosophila tumors caused by mutations in specific tumor suppressor genes. Dev Genes Evol 207, 542–550.

Yanai, T., Teranishi, M., Manabe, S., Takaoka, M., Yamoto, T., Matsunuma, N., Goto, N., 1992. Astrocytoma in a cynomolgus monkey (*Macaca fascicularis*). Vet Pathol 29, 569–571.

Zook, B.C., Simmens, S.J., Jones, R.V., 2000. Evaluation of ENU-induced gliomas in rats: nomenclature, immunochemistry, and malignancy. Toxicol Pathol 28, 193–201.

Part II
Prognostic Factors and Biomarkers

Chapter 14
p53 Pathway Alterations in Brain Tumors

Shaoman Yin and Erwin G. Van Meir

Abstract Mutations in the *TP53* gene or the p53 pathway are required for the formation of many human cancers, including brain tumors. The p53 protein is a multi-modal tumor suppressor that controls many processes that are disrupted during tumor formation, in large part by functioning as a transcription factor. p53 regulates the expression of many target genes, including those encoding anti-proliferative, pro-apoptotic, and anti-angiogenic proteins that mediate many of its intracellular tumor-suppressive activities. The p53 protein can also directly induce apoptosis by associating with mitochondrial proteins in a transcription-independent fashion. Furthermore, p53 exerts oncosuppressive effects through cell-extrinsic mechanisms that rely heavily on its ability to control exosome-mediated protein secretion. Here we provide an overview of p53 functions in tumor suppression and review its involvement in the formation of brain tumors.

Keywords Cancer · p53 · p14ARF · MDM2 · MDM4 · Brain tumor · Tumor suppressor · Gliomas · Signaling · Apoptosis · Cell growth

Contents

E.G. Van Meir (✉)
Department of Neurosurgery, Hematology and Medical Oncology, and Winship Cancer Instititute, Emory University School of Medicine, 1365C Clifton Rd, N.E., Atlanta, GA, 30322, USA
e-mail: evanmei@emory.edu

E.G. Van Meir (ed.), *CNS Cancer*, Cancer Drug Discovery and Development, DOI 10.1007/978-1-60327-553-8_14,
© Humana Press, a part of Springer Science+Business Media, LLC 2009

14.1 Introduction

The p53 protein, co-discovered in 1979 by several groups (DeLeo et al., 1979; Kress et al., 1979; Lane & Crawford, 1979; Linzer & Levine, 1979; Melero et al., 1979), is a 53 kDa sequence-specific transcription factor. p53 prevents the development and progression of tumors by exerting important regulatory control over cell-intrinsic and extrinsic signaling. One of the main tumor-suppressive functions of p53 is to detect cellular damage and respond by triggering a protective response that can lead to cell cycle arrest and activation of repair mechanisms, or to the elimination of the damaged cell through apoptosis or senescence. This cell "policing" function of p53 earned it the title of "the guardian of the genome." Recent research shows that p53 also plays a role in angiogenesis, glycolysis, cell differentiation, development, and aging (Efeyan & Serrano, 2007; Joerger & Fersht, 2008; Ko & Prives, 1996; Levine, 1997; Strano et al., 2007a).

The p53 protein is a transcription factor that can directly activate the expression of many target genes, which influence multiple biological processes in the cell including apoptosis, cell proliferation, senescence, DNA repair, and others. The multiple biological pathways in which p53 is involved may explain in part why *TP53* is the most frequently inactivated gene in cancer. Here, we review the molecular and biological functions of p53 and examine how their loss may contribute to brain tumor development. These findings emphasize the importance of p53 in the formation of astrocytomas and allowed the development of therapies for cancers with disrupted p53 tumor suppressor pathways.

14.2 The p53 Family

The p53 protein family consists of three transcription factors: p53, p63, and p73. These proteins share significant structural and functional similarities. The p63 and p73 proteins share 63% identity with p53 in the DNA-binding domain and can bind to canonical p53-DNA-binding sites, transactivate the promoters of known p53 target genes and suppress growth and induce apoptosis (Jost et al., 1997; Kaghad et al., 1997). Other evidence shows that p63 and p73 play a role in the regulation of normal development (Mills et al., 1999; Yang et al., 1999, 2000). Nevertheless, it rapidly became clear that p53, p63, and p73 have overlapping but distinct functions (Levrero et al., 2000).

Both p63 and p73 have a variety of isoforms through both alternative gene splicing and the use of internal promoters. The human *p63* gene can be transcribed into six different mRNA splice variants, encoding six different p63 protein isoforms (Yang et al., 1998). The human *p73* gene can be transcribed into 35 different mRNAs, which can generate 28 different p73 protein isoforms (Ikawa et al., 1999). These isoforms not only exert dominant-negative effects (Benard et al., 2003; Melino et al., 2003), but also activate specific target genes (Dohn et al., 2001; Wu et al., 2003). The functions of each p73 or p63 isoform are still under investigation, and it seems that each of them may have specific and distinct activities (Harms & Chen, 2006). p73 is less frequently mutated in human cancers (Nimura et al., 1998; Shishikura et al., 1999), although a high rate of gene loss has been noted in advanced stage neuroblastoma. This suggests a possible role of p73 in the progression of neuroblastoma (Ichimiya et al., 1999; Ichimiya et al., 2001). Mutation in p63 is found in carcinomas at low frequency as well (Akahoshi et al., 2003; Kato et al., 1999).

Recently, human p53 itself was reported to have six different isoforms (Bourdon et al., 2005). Each p53 isoform may play different roles in the regulation of p53 function. The p53β isoform enhanced p53 target gene expression by binding p53-responsive elements, while another isoform (133p53) inhibits wt p53-mediated apoptosis when co-expressed in H1299 lung cancer cells. The interplay mechanisms between p53 isoforms remain unclear. It was found that the mRNA expression levels of p53 variants in human breast cancer were different than in normal breast tissue. This adds more complexity in linking p53 status to cancer drug sensitivity and biological characterization (Bourdon et al., 2005). The identification of p53 family members and their variant isoforms has enriched but also challenged our understandings of the basis of p53 regulation and mechanisms of activation. Clearly, further studies are needed in this area.

14.3 p53 Functions: Intracellular Effects

The major function assigned to p53 in cells of most human tissues is the maintenance of DNA integrity and genome stability, hence its designation as the "guardian of the genome." The p53 protein accomplishes this in two ways:

either by directly participating in the mechanisms of repairing DNA damage or by indirectly inducing cell cycle arrest, senescence, or apoptosis to prevent the propagation of DNA mutations in cells.

The p53 protein is a key regulator of transcription and it can directly activate the expression of many target genes containing a p53-responsive element with a consensus sequence formed of two PuPuPuC(A/T) motifs separated by 0–13 bp (el-Deiry et al., 1992). The p53 protein also indirectly influences gene transcription by interacting with other DNA-binding proteins, such as CBF (CCAAT binding factor)/CBP (CCACT binding protein) and TBP (TATA-binding protein), which inhibit the transactivation of genes containing CCAAT and TATA regulatory elements (Fulci et al., 1998; Fulci & Van Meir, 1999).

14.3.1 p53 and Cell Cycle Arrest

The p53 protein exerts its negative regulatory action on the cell cycle at the G1 or G2/M phases when the cell is exposed to DNA damage (Iliakis et al., 2003; Kastan et al., 1995). Induction of a reversible G1 cell cycle arrest was first studied in fibroblast cell lines (Nilausen & Green, 1965) and it was conceptualized that this mechanism was in place to provide the cell time to repair its damaged DNA before proceeding with cytokinesis. In other cell types, the p53 cell cycle arrest was found to be more profound and lead to an irreversible senescent-like process (Marusyk et al., 2007). In human glioma cells, p53-induced growth arrest has been found to be reversible in some cell lines (Mercer et al., 1990), whereas in others *TP53* transfer induced morphological changes reminiscent of a quiescent or senescent cellular state (Van Meir et al., 1995) or induced apoptosis (Cirielli et al., 1999).

The main molecular mechanism by which p53 induces cell growth arrest is by acting as a transcription factor. Many genes involved in cell cycle regulation are induced by p53, but the best characterized is *CDKN1A*. This gene encodes the p21 cell cycle inhibitor that binds and inhibits cyclin-dependent kinases, thus leading to cell cycle arrest (Fig. 14.1). A second important transcriptional target of p53 that regulates the cell cycle is the *14-3-3σ* gene. The 14-3-3σ protein can regulate cell cycle arrest by promoting cytoplasmic sequestration of the phosphatase cdc25c that is essential for G1-S phase cell cycle progression (Kumagai & Dunphy, 1999; Yang et al., 2003). The role of p53 in mediating cell cycle arrest at the G2/M transition appears to involve a separate set of p53 transcriptional targets including Reprimo, B99, and mcg10 (Ohki et al., 2000; Utrera et al., 1998; Zhu & Chen, 2000).

In summary, upon cellular DNA damage, activation of p53 can stop the progression of the cell cycle at both the G1/S and G2/M phases through distinct downstream targets. When DNA damage is successfully repaired, p53 signaling disappears and cell cycle progression can resume. Absence of p53 function in cancer allows multiplication of cells with increased mutation load and contributes to the accumulation of genetic defects which lead to cancer progression.

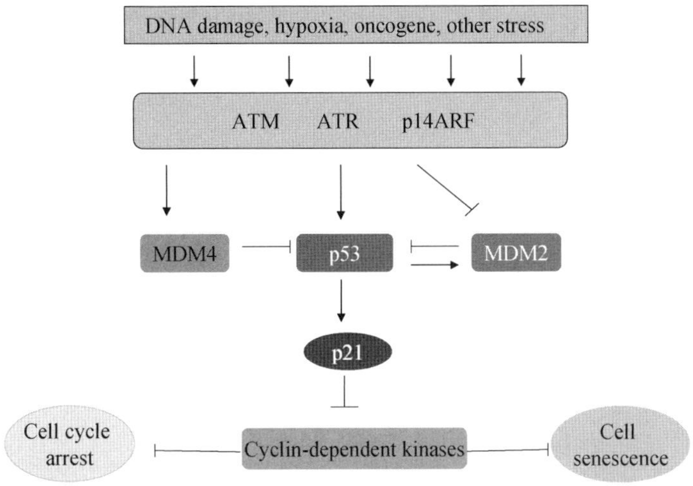

Fig. 14.1 Simplified representation of the p53 pathway. See text for details

14.3.2 p53 and Apoptosis

One of the main biological outcomes of p53 activation in cells is the induction of programmed cell death. Transfer of exogenous *TP53* can induce apoptosis in different cell types, including human brain tumor cells. Evasion of p53-mediated pro-apoptotic pathways is a key step in tumor development and can occur at different stages of tumor formation depending on organ type. Restoration of p53-mediated apoptosis via therapeutic agents is a sought-after strategy for the development of novel clinical treatments.

The mechanisms through which p53 can induce apoptosis are incompletely understood. It is now clearly established that p53 activates pro-apoptotic signaling through transcription-dependent and independent pathways. The most intensively investigated mechanism is the transcriptional activation of genes whose products are direct mediators of apoptosis signaling. A majority of studies have focused on a cell-intrinsic mechanism of apoptosis control and there is a long list of pro-apoptotic target genes of p53. Over 20 pro-apoptotic mediators have been documented to be direct transcriptional targets of p53 (Table 14.1). p53 can also influence apoptosis through transcriptional repression of genes involved in cell survival. A typical example is the *BCL-2* gene that is inhibited by p53 and blocks apoptosis (Miyashita et al., 1994).

In addition to the role of p53 in transcriptional activation of apoptosis-inducing genes and repression of apoptosis-suppressing genes, there is a growing appreciation for an apoptotic role of p53 separate from its nuclear transcription activity. Recent studies show that p53 participates in mitochondrial-mediated apoptosis. Upon stress stimuli, stabilized p53 is translocated to the mitochondria, where it forms complexes with BCLXL and BCL2, thereby activating BAX and other

Table 14.1 p53 target genes involved in apoptosis

Genes	References
APAF-1 (apoptotic protease-activating factor 1)	Robles et al. (2001)
Bax	Miyashita & Reed (1995)
BID	Sax et al. (2002)
BOK	Yakovlev et al. (2004)
CDIP (cell death-involved p53 target)	Brown et al. (2007)
DR4	Guan et al. (2001)
DR5/KILLER	Wu et al. (1997)
ei24/PIG8	Gu et al. (2000)
PERP	Attardi et al. (2000)
P53AIP1 (p53-regulated apoptosis-inducing protein 1)	Oda et al. (2000b)
P53DINP1 (p53-dependent damage-inducible nuclear protein 1)	Okamura et al. (2001)
PUMA	Nakano & Vousden (2001)
POX (proline oxidase)	Liu et al. (2008)
PIDD	Lin et al. (2000)
PIG (p53-inducible genes)	Polyak et al. (1997)
Scotin	Bourdon et al. (2002)
TSAP6 (tumor suppressor-activated pathway-6)	Passer et al. (2003)
TRAF4	Sax & El-Deiry (2003)
Fas	Tamura et al. (1995)
MCG10	Zhu & Chen (2000)
Noxa	Oda et al. (2000a)
NDRG1 (N-myc downregulated gene 1)	Stein et al. (2004)

pro-apoptotic BH3-only proteins. These changes result in cytochrome c release, caspase activation, and programmed cell death. Moreover, cytoplasmic p53 was found to be both necessary and sufficient to induce this process that is independent of new protein synthesis, consistent with a non-transcriptional mechanism (Chipuk et al., 2004; Erster & Moll, 2005).

14.3.3 p53 Regulation of Cellular Senescence

p53 activation plays an essential role in both replicative senescence and non-replicative senescence (Itahana et al., 2001). Normal human cells have a finite proliferative lifespan, ending in replicative senescence, known as the Hayflick limit. This process is largely controlled by the length of the telomeres, cap structures at the end of chromosomes that erode over cycles of DNA replication. Cancer cells need to overcome cellular senescence by reactivating telomerase, the enzyme responsible for rebuilding eroded telomeres. This leads to the process of telomere regeneration and cell immortalization and is critical to cell transformation. In human cancers this process is associated with inactivation of the *TP53* and *RB1* genes, and activation of hTERT and oncogene signaling (Hiyama et al., 1995; Ohki et al., 2003). Experimental transformation of fibroblasts illustrates the need for inactivation of the pro-senescence response of p53. Expression of oncogenic ras in murine fibroblasts can convert p53 into a senescence inducer, resulting in permanent cell cycle arrest (Ferbeyre G et al., 2002). Inactivation of p53 by SV40 virus T antigen extends the replicative lifespan in human-cultured primary fibroblasts (Lin & Simmons, 1991). Another senescence pathway is controlled by p16/RB. Like p21, the activation of p16 inhibits cyclin-dependent kinases, making them unavailable for pRb phosphorylation. As phosphorylation of pRb is an important step in cell cycle progression, this signaling also contributes to the occurrence of senescence. The relationships between the p53 and Rb-mediated pathways in cellular senescence are still unclear (Zhang, 2007), but the transformation of brain tumor cells usually requires the inactivation of both pathways. This usually occurs by p53 mutation and loss of the *p16* gene.

A tumor cell's ability to escape the control of senescence by alterations in the p53 signaling pathway is consistent with the tumor-suppressive roles of p53 (Vogelstein et al., 2000). However, it is unclear how activation of p53 results in variable outcomes, such as senescence, cell growth arrest, and apoptosis. There are two basic models to explain the different events after p53 activation. In the quantitative model, p53 expression level and its variant affinity to different downstream targets are sufficient to determine the outcome. Low protein levels of p53 may induce reversible cell growth arrest, while high levels of p53 may be responsible for senescence or apoptosis. In the qualitative model, p53 signaling is influenced by tissue origins, cell types, and different kinds of stress (Ruiz et al., 2008). Understanding what controls the downstream response switch of p53 is critically important for therapy. Ideally tumor cells should be driven toward apoptosis, while normal cells would undergo temporary cell cycle arrest.

14.3.4 p53 and the Mechanisms Maintaining Genomic Integrity

The p53 protein exerts its safeguarding functions on the genome through different mechanisms: (i) wt p53 represses DNA homologous recombinaion (HR) on both extrachromosomal and intrachromosomal DNA substrates. The regulation of HR is independent of p53's classic tumor suppressor function (Sengupta & Harris, 2005). (ii) the C-terminal domain of p53 binds to transcription-repair TFIIH-associated factors including ERCC2 and ERCC3, which are involved in strand-specific DNA repair (Wang et al., 1995). (iii) p53 activates target genes like CDKN1A, Msh2, and p48 to give time for repair and to directly promote removal of alkyl adducts, mismatch repair, and nucleotide excision repair (Gatz & Wiesmuller, 2006). (iv) p53 prevents the occurrence of multiple rounds of DNA replication before mitosis, thus preventing polyploidy, a hallmark of cancer cells (Duursma & Agami, 2005). (v) p53 also plays an important role in the monitoring of proper spindle polarity and spindle microtubule assembly so as to ensure balanced chromosome segregation during cell division (Kramer et al., 2002).

14.3.5 p53 and MicroRNA

Recent reports have found that wt p53 can induce the generation of active microRNAs, such as miR-34a and miR-34b/c. MicroRNAs are 20–23 base pair RNAs that bind to an RNA-induced silencing complex (RISC) which can bind to the 3′ untranslated regions of mRNAs and prevents their translation (see Chapter 27). The targets of miR-34a, including cyclin D1 (CCND1), CDK6, Bcl2, and c-met, contribute to cell survival and proliferation. Activation of miR-34a downregulates translation of these targets leading to the induction of apoptosis, cell cycle arrest, and senescence (Chang et al., 2007; Corney et al., 2007; He et al., 2007; Raver-Shapira et al., 2007). The most recent results show that another kind of microRNA, miR-21, activates p53-related signaling in glioblastoma cells, thereby inhibiting cell growth and promoting apoptosis (Papagiannakopoulos et al., 2008). Recent works also suggest that both microRNAs and p53 are important regulators in cancer stem cells (Jerry & yan, 2008; Papagiannakopoulos & Kosik, 2008; Zhang et al., 2008). As these different microRNAs regulate hundreds of different proteins, these findings add a new, challenging layer of complexity to the p53 network.

14.3.6 p53 and Invasion/Motility

Given the invasive nature of diffusely infiltrating astrocytomas of all grades and the presence of p53 mutations early in tumor progression, studies examining a potential role for p53 in cell motility are warranted. Initial studies have highlighted that the combination of activated H-ras and inactivated p53 promotes the migratory behavior of glioma cells. However, restoration of wt p53 alone is not sufficient to inhibit the invasion process (Gunther et al., 2003). In a mouse embryonic model, overexpression of CDC42 resulted in the formation of filopodia, and this process could be reversed by wt p53, suggesting that p53 regulates CDC42-mediated motility effects (Gadea et al., 2002). Recent experiments suggest that p53 coordinates an anti-invasive response by downregulating the CXCL12/CXCR4 signaling axis (Mehta et al., 2007; Moskovits et al., 2006). Whether the aforementioned mechanisms of p53 regulation of cellular invasion/motility are linked to the invasive properties of astrocytomas and other brain tumors remains to be determined.

14.3.7 p53 in Differentiation, Development, and Aging

The expression of p53 in several undifferentiated cell types results in progression to a more differentiated state (Porrello et al., 2000; Shaulsky et al., 1991; Soddu et al., 1996). For example, endogenous p53 was shown to induce the differentiation of mouse embryonic stem cells by suppressing *Nanog* expression (Xu, 2005). Conversely, astrocytes derived from $p53^{-/-}$ mice are more readily transformed to malignant gliomas through in vitro passaging (Yahanda et al., 1995). p53-Mediated apoptosis is also a necessary step in spermatogenesis (Shetty et al., 2008). Similarly, other p53 family members p63 and p73 have been implicated in the specification and differentiation of squamous epithelial cells (Candi et al., 2006; Koster et al., 2004), and neuron cells (Ozaki et al., 2005). The increased pro-apoptosis activity of p53 in the CNS may contribute to the development of several neurodegenerative diseases (Miller et al., 2000).

The p53 protein also regulates the aging process, which can be viewed as the senescence of the whole organism. However, the physiological role of p53 in aging seems to be controversial. Increased expression of p14ARF and p53 in mice induced strong resistance to tumor development and lowered levels of aging-related damage (Matheu et al., 2007). The authors hypothesized that p53 might activate some antioxidant-related genes, which might account for the decrease of aging-related damage. However, in another mouse model, the $p53^{+/m}$ mice had an increased p53 activity with better tumor resistance, yet a 20–30% shorter life span. It was suggested that p53-mediated apoptosis or senescence might deplete renewable tissues of proliferation-competent stem cells (Tyner et al., 2002). These seemingly conflicting results could be unified in a model, in which the expression level or regulation of p53/p14ARF determines how the aging process is affected. Constitutive expression of p53 is detrimental to aging because of uncontrolled cellular death or senescence, while mildly increased p53/p14ARF activity has anti-aging effects due to the elimination of damaged cells (Matheu et al., 2008).

14.3.8 p53 and Aerobic Respiration and Glycolysis

The p53 protein regulates mitochondrial respiration through SCO2 (synthesis of cytochrome c oxidase 2) with associated changes in glycolytic activity (Assaily & Benchimol, 2006; Kruse & Gu, 2006; Matoba et al., 2006). In the HCT116 human colon cancer line, the targeted disruption of p53 results in reduced cytochrome oxidase (COX) enzymatic activity and COX subunit II protein levels. The oxygen consumption is also decreased in $p53^{-/-}$ mice because of lower activity of COX (Matoba et al., 2006). In glial tumors, the glycolysis process is elevated and the content of mitochondria is lowered (La Schiazza et al., 2008; Oudard et al., 1997). Further work is warranted to determine whether these alterations in energy metabolism may be relevant to the high incidence of p53 loss in brain tumors.

14.4 p53 Function: Effects on the Tumor Microenvironment (p53 Extracellular Effects)

While the vast majority of studies have focused on p53's role in intracellular functions, a number of reports have found evidence that p53 can also exert extracellular effects. The mechanisms are largely unknown, but one possibility is that p53 loss in tumors disrupts cell–cell regulatory functions that control tissue homeostasis. One potential mechanism is that p53 directly activates the transcription of secreted products or cell surface molecules involved in tissue homeostasis (Buckbinder et al., 1995; Komarova et al., 1998). Most interestingly, p53 was recently shown to induce the secretion of proteins through the exosome-mediated non-classical secretion pathway (Yu et al., 2006). This new function of p53 is regulated by p53-induced transcription of *TSAP6* encoding a key regulator of exosome formation (Amzallag et al., 2004). The p53-regulated secretome contains proteins involved in various biological functions including extracellular matrix remodeling important for cell invasion and metastasis, release of cytokines and immune modulators, and signaling molecules affecting endothelial cells (Khwaja et al., 2006). These findings have important therapeutic implications, as p53 restoration in tumors through p53 gene therapy or other means might have therapeutic effects beyond the transduced cells and induce bystander effects in surrounding tumor cells (McCormick, 2001; Roth et al., 1996; Swisher et al., 1999). Here we will briefly discuss the emerging evidence for p53 involvement in two processes that involve heterotypic cell–cell communication, angiogenesis, and the immune response.

14.4.1 p53 and Angiogenesis

The formation of a tumor is a complex process and requires the de novo development of a vascular network to irrigate the tumor tissue. In the process of tumor angiogenesis, the tumor induces the formation of new blood vessels by sprouting of preexisting vessels or through recruitment of endothelial progenitors from the bone marrow. In the absence of neovascularization tumors remain small, limited in their growth and expansion, in a dormant state characterized by a balanced proliferation and cell death. Tumor expansion, growth, and metastasis proceed exponentially once the tumors switch to the angiogenesis phenotype. Loss of p53 function is one of the genetic switches for the activation of the angiogenic phenotype.

The p53 protein inhibits angiogenesis through both activation of angiogenesis inhibitors and repression of pro-angiogenesis factors (Teodoro et al., 2007). In cultured fibroblasts from patients with Li–Fraumeni syndrome, loss of the wild-type *TP53* allele results in decreased expression of thrombospondin-1 (TSP1), a potent inhibitor of angiogenesis (Dameron et al., 1994). Restoration of *TP53* alleles in these cells stimulates the endogenous *THBS1* gene and reactivates TSP1 expression. The p53 protein has been shown to regulate the secretion of an angiogenesis inhibitor in the conditioned media of human glioma cells (Van Meir et al., 1994). Several reports have suggested candidates for this glioblastoma-derived angiogenesis inhibitory factor (GD-AIF). A G-protein-coupled receptor called brain angiogenesis factor 1 (BAI1) has been proposed as a target of p53 regulation (Nishimori et al., 1997), although subsequent work has not confirmed the activation of *BAI1* by p53 in human glioma cells (Kaur et al., 2003). More recently p53 has been shown to activate the alpha-2 collagen prolyl-4-hydroxylase (*P4HA1*) gene, resulting in the extracellular release of anti-angiogenic fragments of collagen types IV and XVIII. Conditioned media containing these fragments selectively inhibited growth of primary human endothelial cells. When expressed intracellularly or exogenously delivered, P4HA1 significantly inhibited tumor growth in mice (Teodoro et al., 2006). The p53 protein can transcriptionally activate the expression of maspin, a mammary serin proteinase inhibitor (Zou et al., 2000). Maspin restricts a cell's ability to invade through basement membrane, a function required for cell invasion and metastasis as well as angiogenesis. Finally, p53 can also antagonize the expression of pro-angiogenic factors, including IL-8 (Khwaja et al., 2006), but the mechanisms underlying such inhibitory functions have not been investigated. In summary, through its transcriptional activity, p53 can block angiogenesis by inducing the expression of genes that block remodeling of the extracellular matrix and by inducing signals that directly block angiogenesis signaling.

14.4.2 p53 and the Immune Response

In addition to p53's active role in suppressing angiogenesis, p53 may play a more passive role in activating the immune system against tumors. The accumulation of either wt or mutated p53 protein in most human cancers suggests that p53 might be useful as an antigen to induce immune responses that could be exploited for immunotherapy (Bueter et al., 2006). The presence of p53 antibodies in sera of tumor patients suggests that B cells respond to p53 accumulation by initiating p53 antibody production (Lubin et al., 1993; Schlichtholz et al., 1992). These antibodies were mostly IgG type, consistent with a T-cell-dependent response. Compared to wt p53, mutant p53 is usually more stable in cancer cells and some "cryptic regions" may become tumor-specific antigens that could elicit an immune response and contribute to tumor elimination (Fedoseyeva et al., 2000). One of the strategies for tumor immunotherapy is to develop p53-specific cytotoxic T lymphocytes. Both wt and mutant p53-derived peptides can induce cytotoxic lymphocyte responses and some clinical trials have been performed with favorable results (Carbone et al., 2005; Eura et al., 2000; McArdle et al., 2000). More recently, it was found that p53-specific CTLs were not affected by self-tolerance in animal models, suggesting their potential for broad applications in cancer immunotherapy (Lauwen et al., 2008). However, much is still unknown about how wt and mutant p53 behave differently in immune response and which determinants are decisive in antigen presentation.

14.5 p53 Regulation

p53 plays an important role in tumor suppression, but requires strong negative regulation to allow for normal growth and development. Not surprisingly, this regulation has many different facets, including the regulation of expression, protein stability, and protein activity. Many post-translational modifications of p53 have been described including phosphorylation, acetylation, methylation, glycosylation, ribosylation, neddylation, and, most recently, O-GlcNAcylation (Bode & Dong, 2004) (Fig. 14.2). However, in vivo models have suggested that these modifications play only very subtle, modulatory roles in regulating p53 function (Toledo & Wahl, 2006).

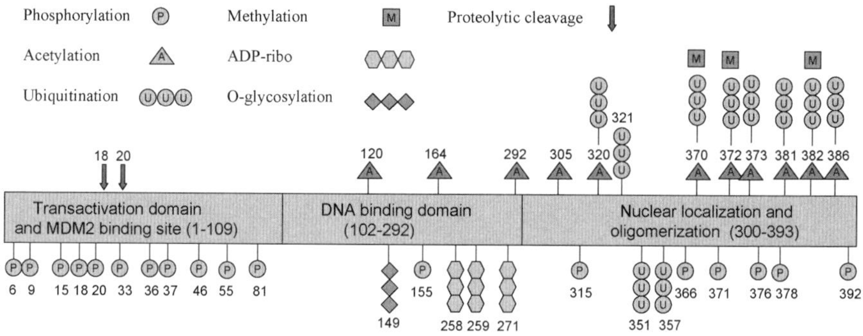

Fig. 14.2 Schematic representation of the p53 protein primary structure and the location and types of post-translational modifications

14.5.1 The p14ARF/MDM2/p53 Pathway

Under normal conditions, p53 is unstable and rapidly degraded following binding by the E3 ubiquitin ligase MDM2. MDM2 binding abrogates p53 transcriptional activity and leads to its ubiquitination and degradation by the proteasome. However, upon cellular stress or damage, p53 is post-translationally modified and the association of MDM2 with p53 is disrupted. The stabilized p53 gains full function by post-transcriptional modifications and activates its downstream effectors. Several proteins have been identified to increase p53 degradation by promoting the interaction between p53 and MDM2, such as YY1 (Gronroos et al., 2004) and gankyrin (Higashitsuji et al., 2005), or by promoting the poly-ubiquitination of p53, such as p300/CBP (Grossman et al., 2003). In contrast, the 14-3-3σ protein positively stabilizes p53 by directly binding and inhibiting MDM2-mediated degradation (Yang et al., 2003).

The p53/MDM2 circuit is well controlled by both positive and negative feedback loops. There are two major routes for the activation of p53 after DNA damage. In the ARF pathway, oncogenic signaling activates p14ARF, which binds MDM2 and inhibits its E3 ubiquitin ligase function. p53 is released from MDM2, stabilized, and restored to its transcriptional activity. p14ARF is an upstream regulator of the MDM2/p53 signaling axis. It binds MDM2 and negatively regulates its function either by promoting its degradation or by sequestering it into the nucleolus, or both (Gallagher et al., 2006; Sharpless, 2005).

Overexpression of MDM2 through *MDM2* gene amplification or the absence of p14ARF through gene loss both lead to increased availability of MDM2 for p53 downregulation, and favor cellular transformation. Another key regulator of p53 is MDM4 (MDMX), a structural relative of MDM2. Like MDM2, MDM4 contains an N-terminal p53-binding domain and a RING domain at its C-terminus (Momand et al., 2000). However, MDM4 does not show E3 ubiquitin ligase activity (Jackson & Berberich, 2000) and functions predominantly by directly inhibiting p53's transcriptional activity (Francoz et al., 2006) (Marine et al., 2007; Toledo & Wahl, 2007). The rates of alterations in the p55/mdm2/ARF pathway in glioblastoma are presented below.

In the ATM (ataxia telangiectasia-*m*utated) and ATR (*a*taxia *t*elangiectasia and *R*ad-3-related) pathways, DNA damage induces the activation of ATM or ATR kinases that lead to p53 phosphorylation and disruption of the p53–MDM2 association. ATM also modifies MDM2 by phosphorylation and increases its degradation, which further contributes to p53 stabilization. To prevent excessive p53 activation, a homeostatic negative feedback loop is activated in the cell. This physiological regulatory mechanism is directly coupled to the levels of active p53 in the cell and is based upon p53 activation of *MDM2* transcription, returning p53 to background levels (Harris & Levine, 2005; Proctor & Gray, 2008).

14.5.2 Phosphorylation

p53 has multiple phosphorylation sites both in its N- and C-termini (Fig. 14.2) and phosphorylation regulates p53 activity in vivo (Appella & Anderson, 2000; Giaccia & Kastan, 1998; Kruse & Gu, 2008). Two important kinases that regulate p53 in response to DNA damage are ATM and ATR. ATM is activated by gamma irradiation and phosphorylates p53 on Ser15 and Chk2 (checkpoint kinase 2) on Thr68 (Banin et al., 1998; Canman et al., 1998). In response to UV damage, ATR is activated and phosphorylates p53 on Ser15/17 and Chk1 on Ser317/345 (Appella & Anderson, 2001; Tibbetts et al., 1999). The phosphorylated p53 and Chk1/2 lead to further downstream events for cell checkpoint control. In addition, N-terminal phosphorylations of p53 can recruit histone acetyltransferases, such as p300/CBP and PCAF, to induce acetylation in the C-terminal domain that block the non-specific DNA-binding sites on p53 (Bode & Dong, 2004; Sakaguchi et al., 1998).

The phosphorylation sites on p53 include Ser6, Ser15, Ser20, Ser37, Ser392 (Kulkarni & Das, 2008), and Thr55 (Cai & Liu, 2008). Nevertheless, despite extensive studies, the role of the different kinases in affecting p53 biological functions remains controversial. Mutations in single p53 phosphorylation sites have not shown any dramatic effects on p53 transcription activity or ability to suppress cell growth in vivo (Toledo & Wahl, 2006). In contrast, in some cases simultaneous phosphorylation at two or more sites significantly lessens p53 transactivation potential and/or DNA binding (Milczarek et al., 1997). Therefore, phosphorylation is likely to be a complex regulatory system for p53 function, and additional experiments are needed to better understand the importance of phosphorylation in p53 regulation and function.

14.5.3 Acetylation

Another mechanism that may play a critical role in p53 activation is acetylation (Gu et al., 2004). Multiple lysine (Lys) residues in p53 are candidate sites for acetylation. In vitro, Lys320 can be acetylated by P/CAF (p300/CBP-associated factor), while Lys373 and Lys382 are acetylated by p300 and CBP (Sakaguchi et al., 1998). In vivo studies show that some of these sites are acetylated in response to DNA-damaging agents, demonstrating that acetylation is a bona fide modification for p53 (Liu et al., 1999; Sakaguchi et al., 1998; Wang et al., 2008). However, despite the observation that acetylation can stimulate p53 DNA-binding activity in vitro (Gu & Roeder, 1997; Liu et al., 1999), the exact function of p53 acetylation and the identities of the acetylases that modify these sites in vivo remain to be established.

14.5.4 Subcellular Localization

As might be expected for a protein with nuclear, cytoplasmic, and mitochondrial functions, the subcellular localization of p53 can also play an important role in regulating its activity. MDM2 can promote the nuclear export of p53 in an ubiquitin ligase-dependent manner (Boyd et al., 2000; Li et al., 2004; Lohrum et al., 2001). Deubiquitination of p53 by HAUSP, a ubiquitin hydrolase, leads to its stabilization (Li et al., 2004). MDM2 and p53 do not leave the nucleus together; rather it seems that mono-ubiquitination of p53 by MDM2 leads to an unmasking of the nuclear export sequence within the C-terminus of p53 (Gu & Roeder, 1997). Three other ubiquitin ligases, Cullin 7 (CUL7), WWP1 (Andrews et al., 2006), and Parc (Nikolaev & Gu, 2003; Nikolaev et al., 2003), also promote the cytoplasmic localization of p53. None of these E3 ligases target p53 for degradation, but result in the accumulation of transcriptionally inactive p53 in the cytoplasm. Similarly, regulation of p53 ubiquitination by the E2 ubiquitin-conjugating enzyme Ubc13 has been shown to drive nuclear export of p53 (Laine et al., 2006). Recent findings suggest that phosphorylation at Thr55 prevents p53 interaction with CRM1, a nuclear export factor (Cai & Liu, 2008). The cytoplasmic sequestration of p53 is used as a mechanism to inactivate p53 in some breast cancers and neuroblastomas (Moll et al., 1995, 1992). It is unknown whether this mechanism also plays a role in p53 inactivation in brain tumors.

14.6 *TP53* Mutations in Brain Tumors

14.6.1 p53 Mutation Spectrum in Brain Tumors

The *TP53* gene is the most commonly mutated gene in human cancer, affecting more than 50% of all tumors. Analysis of *TP53* status and overexpression of p53 have been well documented in primary central nervous system (CNS) tumors. Mutation frequencies for *TP53* are highest in tumors of astrocytic origin, with 67% in anaplastic astrocytoma (WHO grade III) and 41% in glioblastoma (GBM, WHO grade IV) (Tada et al., 1997). Mutation frequencies are much lower in oligodendroglioma (13%), medulloblastoma (11%), and pilocytic astrocytoma (<5%) and virtually absent in other CNS tumors. In GBM, the most frequent and malignant primary human brain tumor, *TP53* mutations are mainly found in the secondary GBM, accounting for about 67% of glioblastoma, while the mutation frequency in primary GBM is lower (11%). Recently, The Cancer Genome Atlas (TCGA) pilot project has confirmed that three critical pathways are altered in GBM formation: activation of receptor tyrosine kinase (RTK) signaling and inactivation of the p53 and retinoblastoma (Rb) tumor suppressor pathways. p53 signaling was found altered in 87% of 206 primary untreated human GBM samples (Fig. 14.3). Inactivation of the p53 pathway occurred in the form of *ARF* deletions (55%), amplification of *MDM2*

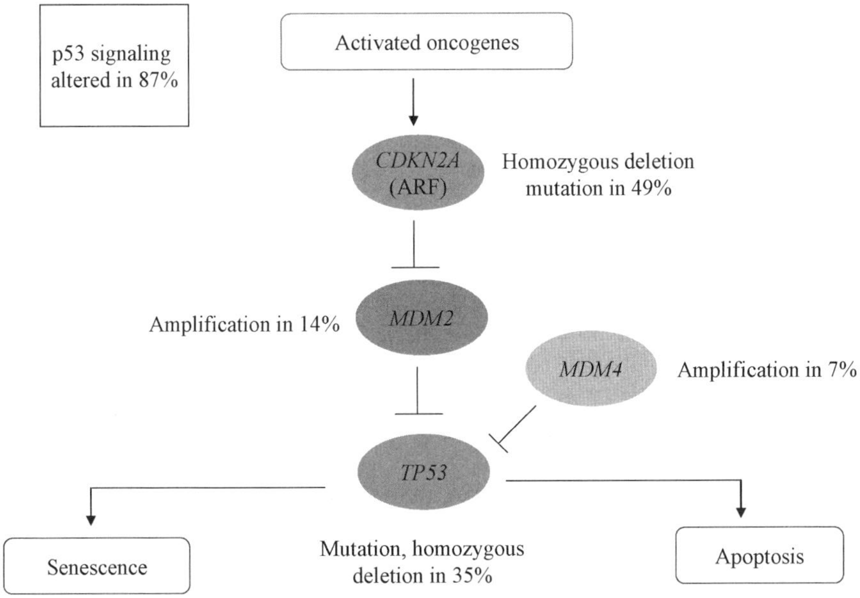

Fig. 14.3 Schematic representation of the frequency and types of genetic alterations in the p53 signaling pathway in human glioblastoma. Reproduced from The Cancer Genome Atlas Research Network (TCGA, 2008)

(11%) and *MDM4* (4%), in addition to mutations of p53 itself. Among 91 sequenced samples, genetic lesions in *TP53* were mutually exclusive of those in *MDM2* or *MDM4*, but not of those in *CDKN2A* (TCGA, 2008). The latter finding was independently confirmed by another research group, who sequenced these genes in 22 GBM (Parsons et al., 2008). Combined analysis of these data shows that the mutations of both *TP53* and *CDKN2A* have relatively higher co-occurrence (10.6%), while *TP53* mutation has no co-occurrence with *MDM2* or low frequency with *MDM4* (6%) (Fig. 14.4). The reasons for the mutation overlap between *TP53* and *CDKN2A* remain unclear. It may represent a need to eliminate the Rb pathway through the loss of the p16 cell cycle inhibitor or the function of p14ARF, which may have roles beyond MDM2/p53 regulation.

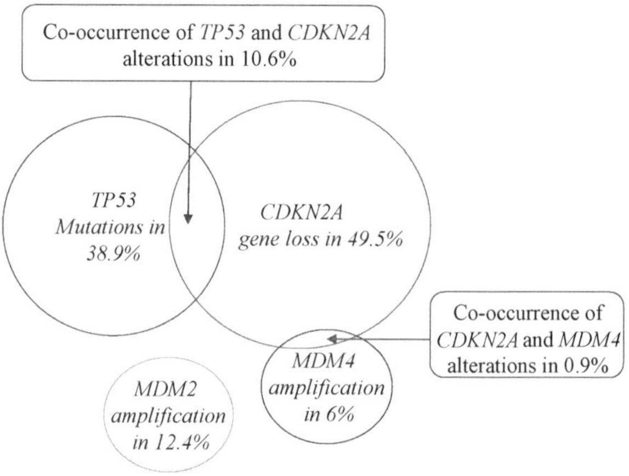

Fig. 14.4 Frequency of genetic alterations in the p53 pathway reported in 113 glioblastoma tumor samples (TCGA, 2008; Parsons et al., 2008). The co-occurrence of mutations among *CDKN2A, TP53, MDM2,* and *MDM4* is shown

In contrast to carcinomas where *TP53* gene mutations occur late during tumor progression, in astrocytomas they are an early event (Baker, 2003). *TP53* mutations occur roughly at similar frequencies in the astrocytomas that show progression from WHO grade II to IV. Analysis of low-/high-grade tumor pairs of patients with malignant recurrence showed that the percent of tumor cells carrying mutated *TP53* in the recurrent tumors increased with progression (Fulci et al., 2002; Ishii et al., 1999). These studies supported that tumor progression occurred by expansion of cells with *TP53* mutations through clonal evolution, likely accompanied by acquisition of additional mutations. Only a fraction of the cells in the original low-grade tumors were found to harbor *TP53* mutations, a finding that suggests that either *TP53* mutation is an early progression event rather than "the" initiation event in somatic astrocytoma formation or that early tumor development is associated with significant stromal cell recruitment. Clearly, the constitutive loss of p53 expression predisposes to brain tumors as seen in *Trp53* knockout mice and in patients with Li–Fraumeni syndrome, who are heterozygous for *TP53* mutant alleles (Donehower et al., 1992; Jacks et al., 1994; Varley, 2003). However, transgenic mouse models show that efficient brain tumorigenesis requires additional events such as activation of either the ras pathway through *NF1* gene loss (Reilly et al., 2000; TCGA, 2008) or the PI3 kinase pathway through loss of the *PTEN* gene (Zheng et al., 2008) (discussed further in Chapters 5, 6, and 15).

14.6.2 Mutation Sites

Most *TP53* gene alterations are spontaneous G:C→A:T transitions by 5′ methylcytosine deamination at CpG sites (Fig 14.5A). The mutations of p53 that occur in cancer generally cause three structural consequences: loss of DNA interaction, perturbation in the local conformation of the core domain, or unfolding of the entire core domain. The three most commonly mutated codons in cancer are 175, 248, and 249, and there are no brain tumor-specific mutations (Fig 14.5B). Mutation at codon 175 triggers local or global conformational changes in p53, resulting in altered binding properties of the mutated p53 to other important partners. Mutations in codons 248 and 249 directly disrupt the binding of p53 to p53 response elements in target genes, leading to loss of transcriptional function (Fulci et al., 1998; Joerger & Fersht, 2008).

14.6.3 Mechanism of Action of p53 Mutants

p53 mutants are usually stable, show nuclear accumulation, and correlate with poor prognosis in some cancer patients. The selection for mutant *TP53* genes in cancer had raised the hypothesis that mutated p53 might confer pro-tumorigenic advantages to the tumor cell beyond mere loss of wt p53 tumor suppressor function. Accumulated evidence supports this contention and it has become clear that p53 mutants contribute in multiple ways to the transformed phenotype and the mechanism of action is variable according to the location of the mutation within the protein. These functions include (i) dominant-negative effects of oncogenic core domain mutants on wt p53; by forming mixed tetramers, p53 mutants effectively reduce the cellular levels of wt homo-tetramers in a heterozygous cell (Blagosklonny, 2000). (ii) Gain of function of some p53 mutants, through activation or repression of a number of genes, such as *bFGF, EGFR, HSP70, C-myc*, and *VEGFR*. These gene products can promote transformation, cellular proliferation, and angiogenesis (van Oijen & Slootweg, 2000). (iii) A potentially more common mechanism underlying the gain of function is through protein–protein interaction between mutant p53 and other proteins (Strano et al., 2007a, b). (iv) Tight association with the nuclear matrix in vivo, suggesting that mutant p53 may disturb nuclear structure and function (Deppert et al., 2000). The plethora of effects of p53 gain-of-function mutants are being studied in

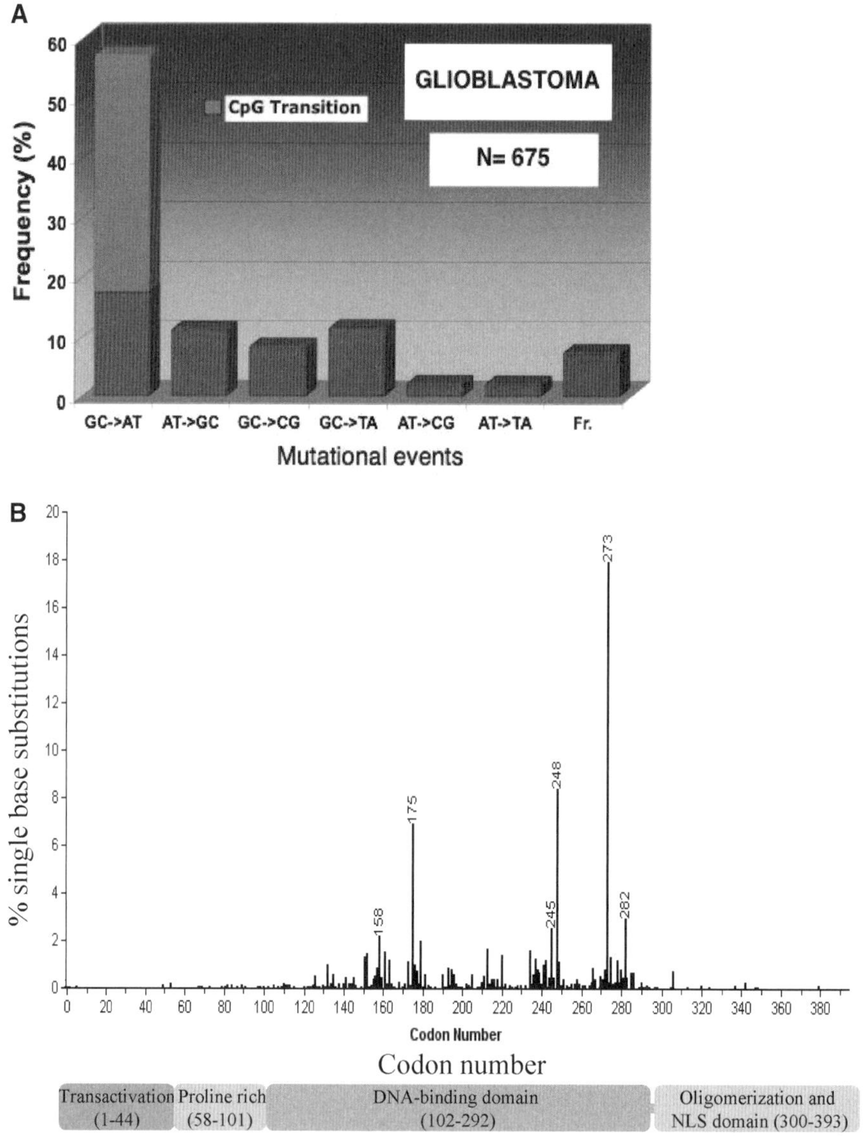

Fig. 14.5 (**A**) Type and frequency of mutations in the p53 gene in 675 glioblastoma according to the 2008 R2 release from the UMD p53 database (Linn Hjortsberg and Thierry Soussi, 2008; http://www.p53 free.fr). (**B**) Overall frequency of types of p53 mutations in brain tumors reported by the IARC database: http://www.iarc.fr, Release R12, 2006. Regions of functional domains in p53 are indicated

transgenic mouse models (Caulin et al., 2007; de Vries et al., 2002; Jackson et al., 2005; Olive et al., 2004; Wijnhoven et al., 2007). Of note, due to the heterogeneity of p53 mutations, the triggered biochemical pathways are expected to be diverse and complex (Song & Xu, 2007; Soussi & Lozano, 2005; Soussi & Wiman, 2007).

14.7 Mutant p53 as a Therapeutic Target

Because of the high frequency of p53 mutations in human cancer, any therapeutic strategy aiming at restoring p53 activity is of high clinical interest. Unlike many other tumor suppressors inactivated in cancer, *TP53* mutation usually preserves gene integrity overall and results in full-length protein expression. While genetic inactivation of other tumor suppressor genes often results in truncated proteins or missense mutations that abort protein translation, p53 is inactivated by point mutations, which occur mainly in the DNA-binding domain. The expression of an intact mutant p53 protein provides the opportunity to develop therapeutic strategies that could restore wt p53 function.

14.7.1 Reactivation of Mutant p53 by Structural Manipulations and Peptides

The DNA-binding activity of some mutant p53 proteins, such as R273H, R273C, R248Q, R282W, and G245S, can be restored by modifications to the C-terminus of the protein. For example, binding of the PAb421 antibody, truncation, or phosphorylation of the C-terminus modify mutant protein DNA binding (Abarzua et al., 1995; Hupp et al., 1993; Selivanova, 2001). A synthetic peptide derived from the p53 C-terminal domain (residues 361–382) can rescue the function of endogenous mutant p53 proteins, resulting in cell growth inhibition and apoptosis both in vitro (Selivanova et al., 1999) and in vivo (Senatus et al., 2006).

14.7.2 Small Molecules That Target Mutant p53

Screening for small molecule compounds that can reactivate mutant p53 has been carried out using either protein or cellular assays. Several structurally unrelated compounds have been found with the capacity to reactivate mutant p53; these include ellipticine, CP-31398, WR1065, PRIMA-1 (and PRIMA-1 MET), and MIRA (Beretta et al., 2008; Bykov et al., 2003; Staples et al., 2008; Vassilev, 2005). The lack of a precise mechanism of action for these compounds is one of the major limitations for their application, as knowledge of the compounds' target would significantly help their pharmacological development. Given the central role of MDM2 in p53 regulation, some drug screening has also been performed toward inhibiting MDM2 function (Fotouhi & Graves, 2005). One of the most successful attempts has been the discovery of the Nutlin family of compounds (Arva et al., 2008). On the other hand, small molecule inhibitors of p53 (cyclic pifithrin-α *p*-nitro) are reported to significantly increase the cytotoxic activity of temozolomide against glioblastomas in the presence of wt p53 (Dinca et al., 2008), which provides another promising application for p53-targeted drugs.

14.7.3 Gene Delivery of wt p53

The cell autonomous roles of p53 in cell cycle arrest, apoptosis, or senescence, and its ability to induce secretion of anti-angiogenic molecules, justify therapeutic approaches aiming at restoring p53 function in tumor cells, including brain tumors. Reintroduction of wt p53 using a virus-based gene-therapy approach was examined by several groups both in vitro and in vivo using retroviral and adenoviral gene-therapy constructs (Badie et al., 1995; Nakamizo et al., 2008; Shono et al., 2002; Van Meir et al., 1995). These studies showed that transfer and expression of exogenous wt p53 or a modified form with site-specific phosphorylations in glioblastoma cells lead to cell cycle arrest, morphological changes, or apoptosis.

Adenovirus-mediated wt p53 gene therapy is being actively tested in clinical trials. In patients with recurrent malignant glioma, the injected virus resulted in the expression of wt p53, which activated p21 and induced apoptosis around the injected sites. However, the newly expressed wt p53 had limited distribution and some side effects of gene therapy occurred (Lang et al., 2003). Combination of p53 gene therapy with radiotherapy or chemotherapy could result in improved anti-tumor effects (Chen et al., 2003). A genetically modified virus for p53 gene therapy (H101) has obtained significant results in a phase III clinical trial and was approved in China as the world's first gene-therapy virus for cancer patient treatment (Guo & Xin, 2006).

14.7.4 Viral Therapy Specific for Tumor Cells with Mutant p53

In the process of cellular infection by adenovirus, expression of the viral E1A protein stabilizes p53. The virus is equipped to overcome the deleterious effect of p53-mediated cell cycle arrest or apoptosis on its replication and has evolved a mechanism that circumvents this potential problem by expressing E1B 55 kDa, a viral protein whose function includes binding and inactivation of p53. In tumor cells containing mutant p53, this viral E1B function is not necessary and these cells can theoretically sustain the replication of a conditionally replicative adenovirus lacking *E1B*. This feature has been applied into the design of the adenovirus dl1520 (ONYX-015) specific for tumor cells with inactive p53. This virus was found to be 100-fold more toxic to *TP53* mutant tumor cells of a variety of tissues than to normal cells. In clinical trials, ONYX-015 showed promising effects in slowing the progression of tumors, especially when combined with classic chemotherapy. However, its further clinical development was limited due to the poor efficiency of virus replication and spread; E1A-induced apoptosis; and patient immunity reactions (Vecil & Lang, 2003). Further discussion of this oncolytic vector and other adenoviral vectors is found in Chapter 47.

14.8 Summary

Since the discovery of p53 in 1979, a wealth of knowledge on its function and regulation has been garnered. Our understanding of p53's role in a wide range of functions has greatly expanded and more proteins are being identified that are involved in its regulation or its effector functions. The spectrum of genetic alterations in the p53 pathway in brain tumors, especially glioblastomas, is now clearly defined and has been evaluated on an unprecedented scale by recent genome-wide analysis. All these developments have confirmed the central role played by p53 mutation in the genesis of brain and other tumors. New strategies to restore normal p53 function with a variety of novel therapeutic agents are being experimentally tested, but none have reached clinical validation. An acceleration of translating the vast knowledge acquired over the last 30 years to the clinic is critically needed, so that patients can begin to benefit from this exciting scientific progress.

Acknowledgments We thank Drs Karlyne Reilly and Abdessamad Zerrouqi for proofreading and providing comments to the manuscript.

References

Abarzua P, LoSardo JE, Gubler ML, Neri A (1995) Microinjection of monoclonal antibody PAb421 into human SW480 colorectal carcinoma cells restores the transcription activation function to mutant p53. *Cancer Res* **55**(16): 3490–3494

Akahoshi K, Sakazume S, Kosaki K, Ohashi H, Fukushima Y (2003) EEC syndrome type 3 with a heterozygous germline mutation in the P63 gene and B cell lymphoma. *Am J Med Genet A* **120A**(3): 370–373

Amzallag N, Passer BJ, Allanic D, Segura E, Thery C, Goud B, Amson R, Telerman A (2004) TSAP6 facilitates the secretion of translationally controlled tumor protein/histamine-releasing factor via a nonclassical pathway. *J Biol Chem* **279**(44): 46104–46112

Andrews P, He YJ, Xiong Y (2006) Cytoplasmic localized ubiquitin ligase cullin 7 binds to p53 and promotes cell growth by antagonizing p53 function. *Oncogene* **25**(33): 4534–4548

Appella E, Anderson CW (2000) Signaling to p53: breaking the posttranslational modification code. *Pathol Biol (Paris)* **48**(3): 227–245

Appella E, Anderson CW (2001) Post-translational modifications and activation of p53 by genotoxic stresses. *Eur J Biochem* **268**(10): 2764–2772

Arva NC, Talbott KE, Okoro DR, Brekman A, Qiu WG, Bargonetti J (2008) Disruption of the p53-Mdm2 complex by Nutlin-3 reveals different cancer cell phenotypes. *Ethn Dis* **18**(2 Suppl 2): S2-1-8

Assaily W, Benchimol S (2006) Differential utilization of two ATP-generating pathways is regulated by p53. *Cancer Cell* **10**(1): 4–6

Attardi LD, Reczek EE, Cosmas C, Demicco EG, McCurrach ME, Lowe SW, Jacks T (2000) PERP, an apoptosis-associated target of p53, is a novel member of the PMP-22/gas3 family. *Genes Dev* **14**(6): 704–718

Badie B, Drazan KE, Kramar MH, Shaked A, Black KL (1995) Adenovirus-mediated p53 gene delivery inhibits 9L glioma growth in rats. *Neurol Res* **17**(3): 209–216

Baker SJ (2003) Redefining p53 – entering the tumor suppressor era. *Cell Cycle* **2**(1): 7–8

Banin S, Moyal L, Shieh S, Taya Y, Anderson CW, Chessa L, Smorodinsky NI, Prives C, Reiss Y, Shiloh Y, Ziv Y (1998) Enhanced phosphorylation of p53 by ATM in response to DNA damage. *Science* **281**(5383): 1674–1677

Benard J, Douc-Rasy S, Ahomadegbe JC (2003) TP53 family members and human cancers. *Hum Mutat* **21**(3): 182–191

Beretta GL, Gatti L, Benedetti V, Perego P, Zunino F (2008) Small molecules targeting p53 to improve antitumor therapy. *Mini Rev Med Chem* **8**(9): 856–868

Blagosklonny MV (2000) p53 from complexity to simplicity: mutant p53 stabilization, gain-of-function, and dominant-negative effect. *FASEB J* **14**(13): 1901–1907

Bode AM, Dong Z (2004) Post-translational modification of p53 in tumorigenesis. *Nat Rev Cancer* **4**(10): 793–805

Bourdon JC, Fernandes K, Murray-Zmijewski F, Liu G, Diot A, Xirodimas DP, Saville MK, Lane DP (2005) p53 isoforms can regulate p53 transcriptional activity. *Genes Dev* **19**(18): 2122–2137

Bourdon JC, Renzing J, Robertson PL, Fernandes KN, Lane DP (2002) Scotin, a novel p53-inducible proapoptotic protein located in the ER and the nuclear membrane. *J Cell Biol* **158**(2): 235–246

Boyd SD, Tsai KY, Jacks T (2000) An intact HDM2 RING-finger domain is required for nuclear exclusion of p53. *Nat Cell Biol* **2**(9): 563–568

Brown L, Ongusaha PP, Kim HG, Nuti S, Mandinova A, Lee JW, Khosravi-Far R, Aaronson SA, Lee SW (2007) CDIP, a novel pro-apoptotic gene, regulates TNFalpha-mediated apoptosis in a p53-dependent manner. *Embo J* **26**(14): 3410–3422

Buckbinder L, Talbott R, Velasco-Miguel S, Takenaka I, Faha B, Seizinger BR, Kley N (1995) Induction of the growth inhibitor IGF-binding protein 3 by p53. *Nature* **377**(6550): 646–649

Bueter M, Gasser M, Lebedeva T, Benichou G, Waaga-Gasser AM (2006) Influence of p53 on anti-tumor immunity (review). *Int J Oncol* **28**(2): 519–525

Bykov VJ, Selivanova G, Wiman KG (2003) Small molecules that reactivate mutant p53. *Eur J Cancer* **39**(13): 1828–1834

Cai X, Liu X (2008) Inhibition of Thr-55 phosphorylation restores p53 nuclear localization and sensitizes cancer cells to DNA damage. *Proc Natl Acad Sci USA* **105**(44): 16958–16963

Candi E, Rufini A, Terrinoni A, Dinsdale D, Ranalli M, Paradisi A, De Laurenzi V, Spagnoli LG, Catani MV, Ramadan S, Knight RA, Melino G (2006) Differential roles of p63 isoforms in epidermal development: selective genetic complementation in p63 null mice. *Cell Death Differ* **13**(6): 1037–1047

Canman CE, Lim DS, Cimprich KA, Taya Y, Tamai K, Sakaguchi K, Appella E, Kastan MB, Siliciano JD (1998) Activation of the ATM kinase by ionizing radiation and phosphorylation of p53. *Science* **281**(5383): 1677–1679

Carbone DP, Ciernik IF, Kelley MJ, Smith MC, Nadaf S, Kavanaugh D, Maher VE, Stipanov M, Contois D, Johnson BE, Pendleton CD, Seifert B, Carter C, Read EJ, Greenblatt J, Top LE, Kelsey MI, Minna JD, Berzofsky JA (2005) Immunization with

mutant p53- and K-ras-derived peptides in cancer patients: immune response and clinical outcome. *J Clin Oncol* **23**(22): 5099–5107
Caulin C, Nguyen T, Lang GA, Goepfert TM, Brinkley BR, Cai WW, Lozano G, Roop DR (2007) An inducible mouse model for skin cancer reveals distinct roles for gain- and loss-of-function p53 mutations. *J Clin Invest* **117**(7): 1893–1901
Chang TC, Wentzel EA, Kent OA, Ramachandran K, Mullendore M, Lee KH, Feldmann G, Yamakuchi M, Ferlito M, Lowenstein CJ, Arking DE, Beer MA, Maitra A, Mendell JT (2007) Transactivation of miR-34a by p53 broadly influences gene expression and promotes apoptosis. *Mol Cell* **26**(5): 745–752
Chen CB, Pan JJ, Xu LY (2003) [Recombinant adenovirus p53 agent injection combined with radiotherapy in treatment of nasopharyngeal carcinoma: a phase II clinical trial]. *Zhonghua Yi Xue Za Zhi* **83**(23): 2033–2035
Chipuk JE, Kuwana T, Bouchier-Hayes L, Droin NM, Newmeyer DD, Schuler M, Green DR (2004) Direct activation of Bax by p53 mediates mitochondrial membrane permeabilization and apoptosis. *Science* **303**(5660): 1010–1014
Cirielli C, Inyaku K, Capogrossi MC, Yuan X, Williams JA (1999) Adenovirus-mediated wild-type p53 expression induces apoptosis and suppresses tumorigenesis of experimental intracranial human malignant glioma. *J Neurooncol* **43**(2): 99–108
Corney DC, Flesken-Nikitin A, Godwin AK, Wang W, Nikitin AY (2007) MicroRNA-34b and MicroRNA-34c are targets of p53 and cooperate in control of cell proliferation and adhesion-independent growth. *Cancer Res* **67**(18): 8433–8438
Dameron KM, Volpert OV, Tainsky MA, Bouck N (1994) Control of angiogenesis in fibroblasts by p53 regulation of thrombospondin-1. *Science* **265**(5178): 1582–1584
de Vries A, Flores ER, Miranda B, Hsieh HM, van Oostrom CT, Sage J, Jacks T (2002) Targeted point mutations of p53 lead to dominant-negative inhibition of wild-type p53 function. *Proc Natl Acad Sci USA* **99**(5): 2948–2953
DeLeo AB, Jay G, Appella E, Dubois GC, Law LW, Old LJ (1979) Detection of a transformation-related antigen in chemically induced sarcomas and other transformed cells of the mouse. *Proc Natl Acad Sci USA* **76**(5): 2420–2424
Deppert W, Gohler T, Koga H, Kim E (2000) Mutant p53: "gain of function" through perturbation of nuclear structure and function? *J Cell Biochem Suppl* **Suppl 35:** 115–122
Dinca EB, Lu KV, Sarkaria JN, Pieper RO, Prados MD, Hass-Kogan DA, VandenBerg SR, Berger MS, James CD (2008) p53 small molecule inhibitor enhances temozolomide cytotoxic activity against intracranial glioblastoma xenografts. *Cancer Res* **68**(24): 10034–10039
Dohn M, Jiang J, Chen X (2001) Receptor tyrosine kinase EphA2 is regulated by p53-family proteins and induces apoptosis. *Oncogene* **20**(45): 6503–6515
Donehower LA, Harvey M, Slagle BL, McArthur MJ, Montgomery CA, Jr., Butel JS, Bradley A (1992) Mice deficient for p53 are developmentally normal but susceptible to spontaneous tumours. *Nature* **356**(6366): 215–221
Duursma A, Agami R (2005) p53-Dependent regulation of Cdc6 protein stability controls cellular proliferation. *Mol Cell Biol* **25**(16): 6937–6947
Efeyan A, Serrano M (2007) p53: guardian of the genome and policeman of the oncogenes. *Cell Cycle* **6**(9): 1006–1010
el-Deiry WS, Kern SE, Pietenpol JA, Kinzler KW, Vogelstein B (1992) Definition of a consensus binding site for p53. *Nat Genet* **1**(1): 45–49
Erster S, Moll UM (2005) Stress-induced p53 runs a transcription-independent death program. *Biochem Biophys Res Commun* **331**(3): 843–850
Eura M, Chikamatsu K, Katsura F, Obata A, Sobao Y, Takiguchi M, Song Y, Appella E, Whiteside TL, DeLeo AB (2000) A wild-type sequence p53 peptide presented by HLA-A24 induces cytotoxic T lymphocytes that recognize squamous cell carcinomas of the head and neck. *Clin Cancer Res* **6**(3): 979–986

Fedoseyeva EV, Boisgerault F, Anosova NG, Wollish WS, Arlotta P, Jensen PE, Ono SJ, Benichou G (2000) CD4+ T cell responses to self- and mutated p53 determinants during tumorigenesis in mice. *J Immunol* **164**(11): 5641–5651

Fotouhi N, Graves B (2005) Small molecule inhibitors of p53/MDM2 interaction. *Curr Top Med Chem* **5**(2): 159–165

Francoz S, Froment P, Bogaerts S, De Clercq S, Maetens M, Doumont G, Bellefroid E, Marine JC (2006) Mdm4 and Mdm2 cooperate to inhibit p53 activity in proliferating and quiescent cells in vivo. *Proc Natl Acad Sci USA* **103**(9): 3232–3237

Fulci G, Ishii N, Maurici D, Gernert KM, Hainaut P, Kaur B, Van Meir EG (2002) Initiation of human astrocytoma by clonal evolution of cells with progressive loss of p53 functions in a patient with a 283H TP53 germ-line mutation: evidence for a precursor lesion. *Cancer Res* **62**(10): 2897–2905

Fulci G, Ishii N, Van Meir EG (1998) p53 and brain tumors: from gene mutations to gene therapy. *Brain Pathol* **8**(4): 599–613

Fulci G, Van Meir EG (1999) p53 and the CNS: tumors and developmental abnormalities. *Mol Neurobiol* **19**(1): 61–77

Gadea G, Lapasset L, Gauthier-Rouviere C, Roux P (2002) Regulation of Cdc42-mediated morphological effects: a novel function for p53. *EMBO J* **21**(10): 2373–2382

Gallagher SJ, Kefford RF, Rizos H (2006) The ARF tumour suppressor. *Int J Biochem Cell Biol* **38**(10): 1637–1641

Gatz SA, Wiesmuller L (2006) p53 in recombination and repair. *Cell Death Differ* **13**(6): 1003–1016

Giaccia AJ, Kastan MB (1998) The complexity of p53 modulation: emerging patterns from divergent signals. *Genes Dev* **12**(19): 2973–2983

Gronroos E, Terentiev AA, Punga T, Ericsson J (2004) YY1 inhibits the activation of the p53 tumor suppressor in response to genotoxic stress. *Proc Natl Acad Sci USA* **101**(33): 12165–12170

Grossman SR, Deato ME, Brignone C, Chan HM, Kung AL, Tagami H, Nakatani Y, Livingston DM (2003) Polyubiquitination of p53 by a ubiquitin ligase activity of p300. *Science* **300**(5617): 342–344

Gu W, Luo J, Brooks CL, Nikolaev AY, Li M (2004) Dynamics of the p53 acetylation pathway. *Novartis Found Symp* **259**: 197–205; discussion 205–197, 223–195

Gu W, Roeder RG (1997) Activation of p53 sequence-specific DNA binding by acetylation of the p53 C-terminal domain. *Cell* **90**(4): 595–606

Gu Z, Flemington C, Chittenden T, Zambetti GP (2000) ei24, a p53 response gene involved in growth suppression and apoptosis. *Mol Cell Biol* **20**(1): 233–241

Guan B, Yue P, Clayman GL, Sun SY (2001) Evidence that the death receptor DR4 is a DNA damage-inducible, p53-regulated gene. *J Cell Physiol* **188**(1): 98–105

Gunther W, Skaftnesmo KO, Arnold H, Terzis AJ (2003) Molecular approaches to brain tumour invasion. *Acta Neurochir (Wien)* **145**(12): 1029–1036

Guo J, Xin H (2006) Chinese gene therapy. Splicing out the West? *Science* **314**(5803): 1232–1235

Harms KL, Chen X (2006) The functional domains in p53 family proteins exhibit both common and distinct properties. *Cell Death Differ* **13**(6): 890–897

Harris SL, Levine AJ (2005) The p53 pathway: positive and negative feedback loops. *Oncogene* **24**(17): 2899–2908

He L, He X, Lim LP, de Stanchina E, Xuan Z, Liang Y, Xue W, Zender L, Magnus J, Ridzon D, Jackson AL, Linsley PS, Chen C, Lowe SW, Cleary MA, Hannon GJ (2007) A microRNA component of the p53 tumour suppressor network. *Nature* **447**(7148): 1130–1134

Higashitsuji H, Higashitsuji H, Itoh K, Sakurai T, Nagao T, Sumitomo Y, Masuda T, Dawson S, Shimada Y, Mayer RJ, Fujita J (2005) The oncoprotein gankyrin binds to MDM2/HDM2, enhancing ubiquitylation and degradation of p53. *Cancer Cell* **8**(1): 75–87

Hiyama K, Ishioka S, Shirotani Y, Inai K, Hiyama E, Murakami I, Isobe T, Inamizu T, Yamakido M (1995) Alterations in telomeric repeat length in lung cancer are associated with loss of heterozygosity in p53 and Rb. *Oncogene* **10**(5): 937–944

Hupp TR, Meek DW, Midgley CA, Lane DP (1993) Activation of the cryptic DNA binding function of mutant forms of p53. *Nucleic Acids Res* **21**(14): 3167–3174

Ichimiya S, Nimura Y, Kageyama H, Takada N, Sunahara M, Shishikura T, Nakamura Y, Sakiyama S, Seki N, Ohira M, Kaneko Y, McKeon F, Caput D, Nakagawara A (1999) p73 at chromosome 1p36.3 is lost in advanced stage neuroblastoma but its mutation is infrequent. *Oncogene* **18**(4): 1061–1066

Ichimiya S, Nimura Y, Kageyama H, Takada N, Sunahara M, Shishikura T, Nakamura Y, Sakiyama S, Seki N, Ohira M, Kaneko Y, McKeon F, Caput D, Nakagawara A (2001) Genetic analysis of p73 localized at chromosome 1p36.3 in primary neuroblastomas. *Med Pediatr Oncol* **36**(1): 42–44

Ikawa S, Nakagawara A, Ikawa Y (1999) p53 family genes: structural comparison, expression and mutation. *Cell Death Differ* **6**(12): 1154–1161

Iliakis G, Wang Y, Guan J, Wang H (2003) DNA damage checkpoint control in cells exposed to ionizing radiation. *Oncogene* **22**(37): 5834–5847

Ishii N, Tada M, Hamou MF, Janzer RC, Meagher-Villemure K, Wiestler OD, Tribolet N, Van Meir EG (1999) Cells with TP53 mutations in low grade astrocytic tumors evolve clonally to malignancy and are an unfavorable prognostic factor. *Oncogene* **18**(43): 5870–5878

Itahana K, Dimri G, Campisi J (2001) Regulation of cellular senescence by p53. *Eur J Biochem* **268**(10): 2784–2791

Jacks T, Remington L, Williams BO, Schmitt EM, Halachmi S, Bronson RT, Weinberg RA (1994) Tumor spectrum analysis in p53-mutant mice. *Curr Biol* **4**(1): 1–7

Jackson EL, Olive KP, Tuveson DA, Bronson R, Crowley D, Brown M, Jacks T (2005) The differential effects of mutant p53 alleles on advanced murine lung cancer. *Cancer Res* **65**(22): 10280–10288

Jackson MW, Berberich SJ (2000) MdmX protects p53 from Mdm2-mediated degradation. *Mol Cell Biol* **20**(3): 1001–1007

Jerry DJ TL, Yan H. (2008) Regulation of cancer stem cells by p53. *Breast Cancer Res* **10**(4): 304

Joerger AC, Fersht AR (2008) Structural biology of the tumor suppressor p53. *Annu Rev Biochem* **77**: 557–582

Jost CA, Marin MC, Kaelin WG, Jr. (1997) p73 is a simian [correction of human] p53-related protein that can induce apoptosis. *Nature* **389**(6647): 191–194

Kaghad M, Bonnet H, Yang A, Creancier L, Biscan JC, Valent A, Minty A, Chalon P, Lelias JM, Dumont X, Ferrara P, McKeon F, Caput D (1997) Monoallelically expressed gene related to p53 at 1p36, a region frequently deleted in neuroblastoma and other human cancers. *Cell* **90**(4): 809–819

Kastan MB, Canman CE, Leonard CJ (1995) P53, cell cycle control and apoptosis: implications for cancer. *Cancer Metastasis Rev* **14**(1): 3–15

Kato S, Shimada A, Osada M, Ikawa S, Obinata M, Nakagawara A, Kanamaru R, Ishioka C (1999) Effects of p51/p63 missense mutations on transcriptional activities of p53 downstream gene promoters. *Cancer Res* **59**(23): 5908–5911

Kaur B, Brat DJ, Calkins CC, Van Meir EG (2003) Brain angiogenesis inhibitor 1 is differentially expressed in normal brain and glioblastoma independently of p53 expression. *Am J Pathol* **162**(1): 19–27

Khwaja FW, Svoboda P, Reed M, Pohl J, Pyrzynska B, Van Meir EG (2006) Proteomic identification of the wt-p53-regulated tumor cell secretome. *Oncogene* **25**(58): 7650–7661

Ko LJ, Prives C (1996) p53: puzzle and paradigm. *Genes Dev* **10**(9): 1054–1072

Komarova EA, Diatchenko L, Rokhlin OW, Hill JE, Wang ZJ, Krivokrysenko VI, Feinstein E, Gudkov AV (1998) Stress-induced secretion of growth inhibitors: a novel tumor suppressor function of p53. *Oncogene* **17**(9): 1089–1096

Koster MI, Kim S, Mills AA, DeMayo FJ, Roop DR (2004) p63 is the molecular switch for initiation of an epithelial stratification program. *Genes Dev* **18**(2): 126–131
Kramer A, Neben K, Ho AD (2002) Centrosome replication, genomic instability and cancer. *Leukemia* **16**(5): 767–775
Kress M, May E, Cassingena R, May P (1979) Simian virus 40-transformed cells express new species of proteins precipitable by anti-simian virus 40 tumor serum. *J Virol* **31**(2): 472–483
Kruse JP, Gu W (2006) p53 aerobics: the major tumor suppressor fuels your workout. *Cell Metab* **4**(1): 1–3
Kruse JP, Gu W (2008) SnapShot: p53 posttranslational modifications. *Cell* **133**(5): 930–930 e931
Kulkarni A, Das KC (2008) Differential roles of ATR and ATM in p53, Chk1, and histone H2AX phosphorylation in response to hyperoxia: ATR-dependent ATM activation. *Am J Physiol Lung Cell Mol Physiol* **294**(5): L998–L1006
Kumagai A, Dunphy WG (1999) Binding of 14-3-3 proteins and nuclear export control the intracellular localization of the mitotic inducer Cdc25. *Genes Dev* **13**(9): 1067–1072
La Schiazza R, Lamari F, Foglietti MJ, Hainque B, Bernard M, Beaudeux JL (2008) Cellular energetic metabolism of cerebral tissue: metabolic characteristics of glial tumours. *Ann Biol Clin (Paris)* **66**(2): 131–141
Laine A, Topisirovic I, Zhai D, Reed JC, Borden KL, Ronai Z (2006) Regulation of p53 localization and activity by Ubc13. *Mol Cell Biol* **26**(23): 8901–8913
Lane DP, Crawford LV (1979) T antigen is bound to a host protein in SV40-transformed cells. *Nature* **278**(5701): 261–263
Lang FF, Bruner JM, Fuller GN, Aldape K, Prados MD, Chang S, Berger MS, McDermott MW, Kunwar SM, Junck LR, Chandler W, Zwiebel JA, Kaplan RS, Yung WK (2003) Phase I trial of adenovirus-mediated p53 gene therapy for recurrent glioma: biological and clinical results. *J Clin Oncol* **21**(13): 2508–2518
Lauwen MM, Zwaveling S, de Quartel L, Ferreira Mota SC, Grashorn JA, Melief CJ, van der Burg SH, Offringa R (2008) Self-tolerance does not restrict the CD4+ T-helper response against the p53 tumor antigen. *Cancer Res* **68**(3): 893–900
Levine A (1997) p53, the cellular gatekeeper for growth and division. *cell* **88**(3): 323–331
Levrero M, De Laurenzi V, Costanzo A, Gong J, Wang JY, Melino G (2000) The p53/p63/p73 family of transcription factors: overlapping and distinct functions. *J Cell Sci* **113 (Pt 10):** 1661–1670
Li M, Brooks CL, Kon N, Gu W (2004) A dynamic role of HAUSP in the p53-Mdm2 pathway. *Mol Cell* **13**(6): 879–886
Lin JY, Simmons DT (1991) The ability of large T antigen to complex with p53 is necessary for the increased life span and partial transformation of human cells by simian virus 40. *J Virol* **65**(12): 6447–6453
Lin Y, Ma W, Benchimol S (2000) Pidd, a new death-domain-containing protein, is induced by p53 and promotes apoptosis. *Nat Genet* **26**(1): 122–127
Linzer DI, Levine AJ (1979) Characterization of a 54 K dalton cellular SV40 tumor antigen present in SV40-transformed cells and uninfected embryonal carcinoma cells. *Cell* **17**(1): 43–52
Liu L, Scolnick DM, Trievel RC, Zhang HB, Marmorstein R, Halazonetis TD, Berger SL (1999) p53 sites acetylated in vitro by PCAF and p300 are acetylated in vivo in response to DNA damage. *Mol Cell Biol* **19**(2): 1202–1209
Liu Y, Borchert GL, Surazynski A, Phang JM (2008) Proline oxidase, a p53-induced gene, targets COX-2/PGE (2) signaling to induce apoptosis and inhibit tumor growth in colorectal cancers. *Oncogene* **27**(53): 6729–6737
Lohrum MA, Woods DB, Ludwig RL, Balint E, Vousden KH (2001) C-terminal ubiquitination of p53 contributes to nuclear export. *Mol Cell Biol* **21**(24): 8521–8532
Lubin R, Schlichtholz B, Bengoufa D, Zalcman G, Tredaniel J, Hirsch A, de Fromentel CC, Preudhomme C, Fenaux P, Fournier G, Mangin P, Laurent-Puig P, Pelletier G,

Schlumberger M, Desgrandchamps F, Le Duc A, Peyrat JP, Janin N, Bressac B, Soussi T, et al. (1993) Analysis of p53 antibodies in patients with various cancers define B-cell epitopes of human p53: distribution on primary structure and exposure on protein surface. *Cancer Res* **53**(24): 5872–5876

Marine JC, Dyer MA, Jochemsen AG (2007) MDMX: from bench to bedside. *J Cell Sci* **120**(Pt 3): 371–378

Marusyk A, Wheeler LJ, Mathews CK, DeGregori J (2007) p53 mediates senescence-like arrest induced by chronic replicational stress. *Mol Cell Biol* **27**(15): 5336–5351

Matheu A, Maraver A, Klatt P, Flores I, Garcia-Cao I, Borras C, Flores JM, Vina J, Blasco MA, Serrano M (2007) Delayed ageing through damage protection by the Arf/p53 pathway. *Nature* **448**(7151): 375–379

Matheu A, Maraver A, Serrano M (2008) The Arf/p53 pathway in cancer and aging. *Cancer Res* **68**(15): 6031–6034

Matoba S, Kang JG, Patino WD, Wragg A, Boehm M, Gavrilova O, Hurley PJ, Bunz F, Hwang PM (2006) p53 regulates mitochondrial respiration. *Science* **312**(5780): 1650–1653

McArdle SE, Rees RC, Mulcahy KA, Saba J, McIntyre CA, Murray AK (2000) Induction of human cytotoxic T lymphocytes that preferentially recognise tumour cells bearing a conformational p53 mutant. *Cancer Immunol Immunother* **49**(8): 417–425

McCormick F (2001) Cancer gene therapy: fringe or cutting edge? *Nat Rev Cancer* **1**(2): 130–141

Mehta SA, Christopherson KW, Bhat-Nakshatri P, Goulet RJ, Jr., Broxmeyer HE, Kopelovich L, Nakshatri H (2007) Negative regulation of chemokine receptor CXCR4 by tumor suppressor p53 in breast cancer cells: implications of p53 mutation or isoform expression on breast cancer cell invasion. *Oncogene* **26**(23): 3329–3337

Melero JA, Stitt DT, Mangel WF, Carroll RB (1979) Identification of new polypeptide species (48–55 K) immunoprecipitable by antiserum to purified large T antigen and present in SV40-infected and -transformed cells. *Virology* **93**(2): 466–480

Melino G, Lu X, Gasco M, Crook T, Knight RA (2003) Functional regulation of p73 and p63: development and cancer. *Trends Biochem Sci* **28**(12): 663–670

Mercer WE, Shields MT, Amin M, Sauve GJ, Appella E, Romano JW, Ullrich SJ (1990) Negative growth regulation in a glioblastoma tumor cell line that conditionally expresses human wild-type p53. *Proc Natl Acad Sci USA* **87**(16): 6166–6170

Milczarek GJ, Martinez J, Bowden GT (1997) p53 Phosphorylation: biochemical and functional consequences. *Life Sci* **60**(1): 1–11

Miller FD, Pozniak CD, Walsh GS (2000) Neuronal life and death: an essential role for the p53 family. *Cell Death Differ* **7**(10): 880–888

Mills AA, Zheng B, Wang XJ, Vogel H, Roop DR, Bradley A (1999) p63 is a p53 homologue required for limb and epidermal morphogenesis. *Nature* **398**(6729): 708–713

Miyashita T, Harigai M, Hanada M, Reed JC (1994) Identification of a p53-dependent negative response element in the bcl-2 gene. *Cancer Res* **54**(12): 3131–3135

Miyashita T, Reed JC (1995) Tumor suppressor p53 is a direct transcriptional activator of the human bax gene. *Cell* **80**(2): 293–299

Moll UM, LaQuaglia M, Benard J, Riou G (1995) Wild-type p53 protein undergoes cytoplasmic sequestration in undifferentiated neuroblastomas but not in differentiated tumors. *Proc Natl Acad Sci USA* **92**(10): 4407–4411

Moll UM, Riou G, Levine AJ (1992) Two distinct mechanisms alter p53 in breast cancer: mutation and nuclear exclusion. *Proc Natl Acad Sci USA* **89**(15): 7262–7266

Momand J, Wu HH, Dasgupta G (2000) MDM2 – master regulator of the p53 tumor suppressor protein. *Gene* **242**(1–2): 15–29

Moskovits N, Kalinkovich A, Bar J, Lapidot T, Oren M (2006) p53 Attenuates cancer cell migration and invasion through repression of SDF-1/CXCL12 expression in stromal fibroblasts. *Cancer Res* **66**(22): 10671–10676

Nakamizo A, Amano T, Zhang W, Zhang XQ, Ramdas L, Liu TJ, Bekele BN, Shono T, Sasaki T, Benedict WF, Sawaya R, Lang FF (2008) Phosphorylation of Thr18 and Ser20 of p53 in Ad-p53-induced apoptosis. *Neuro Oncol* **10**(3): 275–291
Nakano K, Vousden KH (2001) PUMA, a novel proapoptotic gene, is induced by p53. *Mol Cell* **7**(3): 683–694
Nikolaev AY, Gu W (2003) PARC: a potential target for cancer therapy. *Cell Cycle* **2**(3): 169–171
Nikolaev AY, Li M, Puskas N, Qin J, Gu W (2003) Parc: a cytoplasmic anchor for p53. *Cell* **112**(1): 29–40
Nilausen K, Green H (1965) Reversible arrest of growth in G1 of an established fibroblast line (3T3). *Exp Cell Res* **40**(1): 166–168
Nimura Y, Mihara M, Ichimiya S, Sakiyama S, Seki N, Ohira M, Nomura N, Fujimori M, Adachi W, Amano J, He M, Ping YM, Nakagawara A (1998) p73, a gene related to p53, is not mutated in esophageal carcinomas. *Int J Cancer* **78**(4): 437–440
Nishimori H, Shiratsuchi T, Urano T, Kimura Y, Kiyono K, Tatsumi K, Yoshida S, Ono M, Kuwano M, Nakamura Y, Tokino T (1997) A novel brain-specific p53-target gene, BAI1, containing thrombospondin type 1 repeats inhibits experimental angiogenesis. *Oncogene* **15**(18): 2145–2150
Oda E, Ohki R, Murasawa H, Nemoto J, Shibue T, Yamashita T, Tokino T, Taniguchi T, Tanaka N (2000a) Noxa, a BH3-only member of the Bcl-2 family and candidate mediator of p53-induced apoptosis. *Science* **288**(5468): 1053–1058
Oda K, Arakawa H, Tanaka T, Matsuda K, Tanikawa C, Mori T, Nishimori H, Tamai K, Tokino T, Nakamura Y, Taya Y (2000b) p53AIP1, a potential mediator of p53-dependent apoptosis, and its regulation by Ser-46-phosphorylated p53. *Cell* **102**(6): 849–862
Ohki R, Nemoto J, Murasawa H, Oda E, Inazawa J, Tanaka N, Taniguchi T (2000) Reprimo, a new candidate mediator of the p53-mediated cell cycle arrest at the G2 phase. *J Biol Chem* **275**(30): 22627–22630
Ohki S, Onda M, Fukushima T, Takita K, Suzuki S, Hoshino M, Tsuchiya A, Abe R, Takenoshita S (2003) Telomeric repeat-length alterations in colorectal carcinoma are associated with loss of heterozygosity and point mutation in p53 gene. *Int J Mol Med* **11**(4): 485–490
Okamura S, Arakawa H, Tanaka T, Nakanishi H, Ng CC, Taya Y, Monden M, Nakamura Y (2001) p53DINP1, a p53-inducible gene, regulates p53-dependent apoptosis. *Mol Cell* **8**(1): 85–94
Olive KP, Tuveson DA, Ruhe ZC, Yin B, Willis NA, Bronson RT, Crowley D, Jacks T (2004) Mutant p53 gain of function in two mouse models of Li-Fraumeni syndrome. *Cell* **119**(6): 847–860
Oudard S, Boitier E, Miccoli L, Rousset S, Dutrillaux B, Poupon MF (1997) Gliomas are driven by glycolysis: putative roles of hexokinase, oxidative phosphorylation and mitochondrial ultrastructure. *Anticancer Res* **17**(3C): 1903–1911
Ozaki T, Hosoda M, Miyazaki K, Hayashi S, Watanabe K, Nakagawa T, Nakagawara A (2005) Functional implication of p73 protein stability in neuronal cell survival and death. *Cancer Lett* **228**(1–2): 29–35
Papagiannakopoulos T, Kosik K (2008) MicroRNAs: regulators of oncogenesis and stemness. *BMC Med* **6**(15)
Papagiannakopoulos T, Shapiro A, Kosik KS (2008) MicroRNA-21 targets a network of key tumor-suppressive pathways in glioblastoma cells. *Cancer Res* **68**(19): 8164–8172
Parsons DW, Jones S, Zhang X, Lin JC, Leary RJ, Angenendt P, Mankoo P, Carter H, Siu IM, Gallia GL, Olivi A, McLendon R, Rasheed BA, Keir S, Nikolskaya T, Nikolsky Y, Busam DA, Tekleab H, Diaz LA, Jr., Hartigan J, Smith DR, Strausberg RL, Marie SK, Shinjo SM, Yan H, Riggins GJ, Bigner DD, Karchin R, Papadopoulos N, Parmigiani G, Vogelstein B, Velculescu VE, Kinzler KW (2008) An integrated genomic analysis of human glioblastoma multiforme. *Science* **321**(5897): 1807–1812

Passer BJ, Nancy-Portebois V, Amzallag N, Prieur S, Cans C, Roborel de Climens A, Fiucci G, Bouvard V, Tuynder M, Susini L, Morchoisne S, Crible V, Lespagnol A, Dausset J, Oren M, Amson R, Telerman A (2003) The p53-inducible TSAP6 gene product regulates apoptosis and the cell cycle and interacts with Nix and the Myt1 kinase. *Proc Natl Acad Sci USA* **100**(5): 2284–2289

Porrello A, Cerone MA, Coen S, Gurtner A, Fontemaggi G, Cimino L, Piaggio G, Sacchi A, Soddu S (2000) p53 regulates myogenesis by triggering the differentiation activity of pRb. *J Cell Biol* **151**(6): 1295–1304

Proctor CJ, Gray DA (2008) Explaining oscillations and variability in the p53-Mdm2 system. *BMC Syst Biol* **2**(1): 75

Raver-Shapira N, Marciano E, Meiri E, Spector Y, Rosenfeld N, Moskovits N, Bentwich Z, Oren M (2007) Transcriptional activation of miR-34a contributes to p53-mediated apoptosis. *Mol Cell* **26**(5): 731–743

Reilly KM, Loisel DA, Bronson RT, McLaughlin ME, Jacks T (2000) Nf1;Trp53 mutant mice develop glioblastoma with evidence of strain-specific effects. *Nat Genet* **26**(1): 109–113

Robles AI, Bemmels NA, Foraker AB, Harris CC (2001) APAF-1 is a transcriptional target of p53 in DNA damage-induced apoptosis. *Cancer Res* **61**(18): 6660–6664

Roth JA, Nguyen D, Lawrence DD, Kemp BL, Carrasco CH, Ferson DZ, Hong WK, Komaki R, Lee JJ, Nesbitt JC, Pisters KM, Putnam JB, Schea R, Shin DM, Walsh GL, Dolormente MM, Han CI, Martin FD, Yen N, Xu K, Stephens LC, McDonnell TJ, Mukhopadhyay T, Cai D (1996) Retrovirus-mediated wild-type p53 gene transfer to tumors of patients with lung cancer. *Nat Med* **2**(9): 985–991

Ruiz L, Traskine M, Ferrer I, Castro E, Leal JF, Kaufman M, Carnero A (2008) Characterization of the p53 Response to Oncogene-Induced Senescence. *PLoS ONE* **3**(9): e3230

Sakaguchi K, Herrera JE, Saito S, Miki T, Bustin M, Vassilev A, Anderson CW, Appella E (1998) DNA damage activates p53 through a phosphorylation-acetylation cascade. *Genes Dev* **12**(18): 2831–2841

Sax JK, El-Deiry WS (2003) Identification and characterization of the cytoplasmic protein TRAF4 as a p53-regulated proapoptotic gene. *J Biol Chem* **278**(38): 36435–36444

Sax JK, Fei P, Murphy ME, Bernhard E, Korsmeyer SJ, El-Deiry WS (2002) BID regulation by p53 contributes to chemosensitivity. *Nat Cell Biol* **4**(11): 842–849

Schlichtholz B, Legros Y, Gillet D, Gaillard C, Marty M, Lane D, Calvo F, Soussi T (1992) The immune response to p53 in breast cancer patients is directed against immunodominant epitopes unrelated to the mutational hot spot. *Cancer Res* **52**(22): 6380–6384

Selivanova G (2001) Mutant p53: the loaded gun. *Curr Opin Investig Drugs* **2**(8): 1136–1141

Selivanova G, Ryabchenko L, Jansson E, Iotsova V, Wiman KG (1999) Reactivation of mutant p53 through interaction of a C-terminal peptide with the core domain. *Mol Cell Biol* **19**(5): 3395–3402

Senatus PB, Li Y, Mandigo C, Nichols G, Moise G, Mao Y, Brown MD, Anderson RC, Parsa AT, Brandt-Rauf PW, Bruce JN, Fine RL (2006) Restoration of p53 function for selective Fas-mediated apoptosis in human and rat glioma cells in vitro and in vivo by a p53 COOH-terminal peptide. *Mol Cancer Ther* **5**(1): 20–28

Sengupta S, Harris CC (2005) p53: traffic cop at the crossroads of DNA repair and recombination. *Nat Rev Mol Cell Biol* **6**(1): 44–55

Sharpless NE (2005) INK4a/ARF: a multifunctional tumor suppressor locus. *Mutat Res* **576**(1–2): 22–38

Shaulsky G, Goldfinger N, Peled A, Rotter V (1991) Involvement of wild-type p53 in pre-B-cell differentiation in vitro. *Proc Natl Acad Sci USA* **88**(20): 8982–8986

Shetty G, Shao SH, Weng CC (2008) p53-dependent apoptosis in the inhibition of spermatogonial differentiation in juvenile spermatogonial depletion (Utp14bjsd) mice. *Endocrinology* **149**(6): 2773–2781

Shishikura T, Ichimiya S, Ozaki T, Nimura Y, Kageyama H, Nakamura Y, Sakiyama S, Miyauchi M, Yamamoto N, Suzuki M, Nakajima N, Nakagawara A (1999) Mutational analysis of the p73 gene in human breast cancers. *Int J Cancer* **84**(3): 321–325

Shono T, Tofilon PJ, Schaefer TS, Parikh D, Liu TJ, Lang FF (2002) Apoptosis induced by adenovirus-mediated p53 gene transfer in human glioma correlates with site-specific phosphorylation. *Cancer Res* **62**(4): 1069–1076

Soddu S, Blandino G, Scardigli R, Coen S, Marchetti A, Rizzo MG, Bossi G, Cimino L, Crescenzi M, Sacchi A (1996) Interference with p53 protein inhibits hematopoietic and muscle differentiation. *J Cell Biol* **134**(1): 193–204

Song H, Xu Y (2007) Gain of function of p53 cancer mutants in disrupting critical DNA damage response pathways. *Cell Cycle* **6**(13): 1570–1573

Soussi T, Lozano G (2005) p53 mutation heterogeneity in cancer. *Biochem Biophys Res Commun* **331**(3): 834–842

Soussi T, Wiman KG (2007) Shaping genetic alterations in human cancer: the p53 mutation paradigm. *Cancer Cell* **12**(4): 303–312

Staples OD, Steele RJ, Lain S (2008) p53 as a therapeutic target. *Surgeon* **6**(4): 240–243

Stein S, Thomas EK, Herzog B, Westfall MD, Rocheleau JV, Jackson RS, 2nd, Wang M, Liang P (2004) NDRG1 is necessary for p53-dependent apoptosis. *J Biol Chem* **279**(47): 48930–48940

Strano S, Dell'Orso S, Di Agostino S, Fontemaggi G, Sacchi A, Blandino G (2007a) Mutant p53: an oncogenic transcription factor. *Oncogene* **26**(15): 2212–2219

Strano S, Dell'Orso S, Mongiovi AM, Monti O, Lapi E, Di Agostino S, Fontemaggi G, Blandino G (2007b) Mutant p53 proteins: between loss and gain of function. *Head Neck* **29**(5): 488–496

Swisher SG, Roth JA, Nemunaitis J, Lawrence DD, Kemp BL, Carrasco CH, Connors DG, El-Naggar AK, Fossella F, Glisson BS, Hong WK, Khuri FR, Kurie JM, Lee JJ, Lee JS, Mack M, Merritt JA, Nguyen DM, Nesbitt JC, Perez-Soler R, Pisters KM, Putnam JB, Jr. , Richli WR, Savin M, Schrump DS, Shin DM, Shulkin A, Walsh GL, Wait J, Weill D, Waugh MK (1999) Adenovirus-mediated p53 gene transfer in advanced non-small-cell lung cancer. *J Natl Cancer Inst* **91**(9): 763–771

Tada M, Iggo RD, Waridel F, Nozaki M, Matsumoto R, Sawamura Y, Shinohe Y, Ikeda J, Abe H (1997) Reappraisal of p53 mutations in human malignant astrocytic neoplasms by p53 functional assay: comparison with conventional structural analyses. *Mol Carcinog* **18**(3): 171–176

Tamura T, Aoyama N, Saya H, Haga H, Futami S, Miyamoto M, Koh T, Ariyasu T, Tachi M, Kasuga M, et al. (1995) Induction of Fas-mediated apoptosis in p53-transfected human colon carcinoma cells. *Oncogene* **11**(10): 1939–1946

Teodoro JG, Evans SK, Green MR (2007) Inhibition of tumor angiogenesis by p53: a new role for the guardian of the genome. *J Mol Med* **85**(11): 1175–1186

Teodoro JG, Parker AE, Zhu X, Green MR (2006) p53-mediated inhibition of angiogenesis through up-regulation of a collagen prolyl hydroxylase. *Science* **313**(5789): 968–971

The Cancer Genome Atlas Research Network, McLendon R, Friedman A, Bigner D, Van Meir EG, Brat DJ, Mastrogianakis GM, Olson JJ, Mikkelsen T, Lehman N, Aldape K, Yung WK, Bogler O, Weinstein JN, VandenBerg S, Berger M, Prados M, Muzny D, Morgan M, Scherer S, Sabo A, Nazareth L, Lewis L, Hall O, Zhu Y, Ren Y, Alvi O, Yao J, Hawes A, Jhangiani S, Fowler G, San Lucas A, Kovar C, Cree A, Dinh H, Santibanez J, Joshi V, Gonzalez-Garay ML, Miller CA, Milosavljevic A, Donehower L, Wheeler DA, Gibbs RA, Cibulskis K, Sougnez C, Fennell T, Mahan S, Wilkinson J, Ziaugra L, Onofrio R, Bloom T, Nicol R, Ardlie K, Baldwin J, Gabriel S, Lander ES, Ding L, Fulton RS, McLellan MD, Wallis J, Larson DE, Shi X, Abbott R, Fulton L, Chen K, Koboldt DC, Wendl MC, Meyer R, Tang Y, Lin L, Osborne JR, Dunford-Shore BH, Miner TL, Delehaunty K, Markovic C, Swift G, Courtney W, Pohl C, Abbott S, Hawkins A, Leong S, Haipek C, Schmidt H, Wiechert M, Vickery T, Scott S, Dooling DJ, Chinwalla

A, Weinstock GM, Mardis ER, Wilson RK, Getz G, Winckler W, Verhaak RG, Lawrence MS, O'Kelly M, Robinson J, Alexe G, Beroukhim R, Carter S, Chiang D, Gould J, Gupta S, Korn J, Mermel C, Mesirov J, Monti S, Nguyen H, Parkin M, Reich M, Stransky N, Weir BA, Garraway L, Golub T, Meyerson M, Chin L, Protopopov A, Zhang J, Perna I, Aronson S, Sathiamoorthy N, Ren G, Yao J, Wiedemeyer WR, Kim H, Kong SW, Xiao Y, Kohane IS, Seidman J, Park P, Kucherlapati R, Laird PW, Cope L, Herman JG, Weisenberger DJ, Pan F, Van den Berg D, Van Neste L, Yi JM, Schuebel KE, Baylin SB, Absher DM, Li JZ, Southwick A, Brady S, Aggarwal A, Chung T, Sherlock G, Brooks JD, Myers RM, Spellman PT, Purdom E, Jakkula LR, Lapuk AV, Marr H, Dorton S, Choi YG, Han J, Ray A, Wang V, Durinck S, Robinson M, Wang NJ, Vranizan K, Peng V, Van Name E, Fontenay GV, Ngai J, Conboy JG, Parvin B, Feiler HS, Speed TP, Gray JW, Brennan C, Socci ND, Olshen A, Taylor BS, Lash A, Schultz N, Reva B, Antipin Y, Stukalov A, Gross B, Cerami E, Wang WQ, Qin LX, Seshan VE, Villafania L, Cavatore M, Borsu L, Viale A, Gerald W, Sander C, Ladanyi M, Perou CM, Hayes DN, Topal MD, Hoadley KA, Qi Y, Balu S, Shi Y, Wu J, Penny R, Bittner M, Shelton T, Lenkiewicz E, Morris S, Beasley D, Sanders S, Kahn A, Sfeir R, Chen J, Nassau D, Feng L, Hickey E, Barker A, Gerhard DS, Vockley J, Compton C, Vaught J, Fielding P, Ferguson ML, Schaefer C, Zhang J, Madhavan S, Buetow KH, Collins F, Good P, Guyer M, Ozenberger B, Peterson J, Thomson E (2008) Comprehensive genomic characterization defines human glioblastoma genes and core pathways. *Nature* **455**(7216): 1061–1068

Tibbetts RS, Brumbaugh KM, Williams JM, Sarkaria JN, Cliby WA, Shieh SY, Taya Y, Prives C, Abraham RT (1999) A role for ATR in the DNA damage-induced phosphorylation of p53. *Genes Dev* **13**(2): 152–157

Toledo F, Wahl GM (2006) Regulating the p53 pathway: in vitro hypotheses, in vivo veritas. *Nat Rev Cancer* **6**(12): 909–923

Toledo F, Wahl GM (2007) MDM2 and MDM4: p53 regulators as targets in anticancer therapy. *Int J Biochem Cell Biol* **39**(7–8): 1476–1482

Tyner SD, Venkatachalam S, Choi J, Jones S, Ghebranious N, Igelmann H, Lu X, Soron G, Cooper B, Brayton C, Hee Park S, Thompson T, Karsenty G, Bradley A, Donehower LA (2002) p53 mutant mice that display early ageing-associated phenotypes. *Nature* **415**(6867): 45–53

Utrera R, Collavin L, Lazarevic D, Delia D, Schneider C (1998) A novel p53-inducible gene coding for a microtubule-localized protein with G2-phase-specific expression. *EMBO J* **17**(17): 5015–5025

Van Meir EG, Polverini PJ, Chazin VR, Su Huang HJ, de Tribolet N, Cavenee WK (1994) Release of an inhibitor of angiogenesis upon induction of wild type p53 expression in glioblastoma cells. *Nat Genet* **8**(2): 171–176

Van Meir EG, Roemer K, Diserens AC, Kikuchi T, Rempel SA, Haas M, Huang HJ, Friedmann T, de Tribolet N, Cavenee WK (1995) Single cell monitoring of growth arrest and morphological changes induced by transfer of wild-type p53 alleles to glioblastoma cells. *Proc Natl Acad Sci USA* **92**(4): 1008–1012

van Oijen MG, Slootweg PJ (2000) Gain-of-function mutations in the tumor suppressor gene p53. *Clin Cancer Res* **6**(6): 2138–2145

Varley JM (2003) Germline TP53 mutations and Li-Fraumeni syndrome. *Hum Mutat* **21**(3): 313–320

Vassilev LT (2005) p53 Activation by small molecules: application in oncology. *J Med Chem* **48**(14): 4491–4499

Vecil GG, Lang FF (2003) Clinical trials of adenoviruses in brain tumors: a review of Ad-p53 and oncolytic adenoviruses. *J Neurooncol* **65**(3): 237–246

Vogelstein B, Lane D, Levine AJ (2000) Surfing the p53 network. *Nature* **408**(6810): 307–310

Wang H, Zhao Y, Li L, McNutt MA, Wu L, Lu S, Yu Y, Zhou W, Feng J, Chai G, Yang Y, Zhu WG (2008) An ATM- and Rad3-related (ATR) signaling pathway and a phosphorylation-acetylation cascade are involved in activation of p53/p21Waf1/Cip1 in response to 5-aza-2'-deoxycytidine treatment. *J Biol Chem* **283**(5): 2564–2574

Wang XW, Yeh H, Schaeffer L, Roy R, Moncollin V, Egly JM, Wang Z, Freidberg EC, Evans MK, Taffe BG, et al. (1995) p53 modulation of TFIIH-associated nucleotide excision repair activity. *Nat Genet* **10**(2): 188–195

Wijnhoven SW, Speksnijder EN, Liu X, Zwart E, vanOostrom CT, Beems RB, Hoogervorst EM, Schaap MM, Attardi LD, Jacks T, van Steeg H, Jonkers J, de Vries A (2007) Dominant-negative but not gain-of-function effects of a p53.R270H mutation in mouse epithelium tissue after DNA damage. *Cancer Res* **67**(10): 4648–4656

Wu G, Nomoto S, Hoque MO, Dracheva T, Osada M, Lee CC, Dong SM, Guo Z, Benoit N, Cohen Y, Rechthand P, Califano J, Moon CS, Ratovitski E, Jen J, Sidransky D, Trink B (2003) DeltaNp63alpha and TAp63alpha regulate transcription of genes with distinct biological functions in cancer and development. *Cancer Res* **63**(10): 2351–2357

Wu GS, Burns TF, McDonald ER, 3rd, Jiang W, Meng R, Krantz ID, Kao G, Gan DD, Zhou JY, Muschel R, Hamilton SR, Spinner NB, Markowitz S, Wu G, el-Deiry WS (1997) KILLER/DR5 is a DNA damage-inducible p53-regulated death receptor gene. *Nat Genet* **17**(2): 141–143

Xu Y (2005) A new role for p53 in maintaining genetic stability in embryonic stem cells. *Cell Cycle* **4**(3): 363–364

Yahanda AM, Bruner JM, Donehower LA, Morrison RS (1995) Astrocytes derived from p53-deficient mice provide a multistep in vitro model for development of malignant gliomas. *Mol Cell Biol* **15**(8): 4249–4259

Yakovlev AG, Di Giovanni S, Wang G, Liu W, Stoica B, Faden AI (2004) BOK and NOXA are essential mediators of p53-dependent apoptosis. *J Biol Chem* **279**(27): 28367–28374

Yang A, Kaghad M, Wang Y, Gillett E, Fleming MD, Dotsch V, Andrews NC, Caput D, McKeon F (1998) p63, a p53 homolog at 3q27–29, encodes multiple products with transactivating, death-inducing, and dominant-negative activities. *Mol Cell* **2**(3): 305–316

Yang A, Schweitzer R, Sun D, Kaghad M, Walker N, Bronson RT, Tabin C, Sharpe A, Caput D, Crum C, McKeon F (1999) p63 is essential for regenerative proliferation in limb, craniofacial and epithelial development. *Nature* **398**(6729): 714–718

Yang A, Walker N, Bronson R, Kaghad M, Oosterwegel M, Bonnin J, Vagner C, Bonnet H, Dikkes P, Sharpe A, McKeon F, Caput D (2000) p73-deficient mice have neurological, pheromonal and inflammatory defects but lack spontaneous tumours. *Nature* **404**(6773): 99–103

Yang HY, Wen YY, Chen CH, Lozano G, Lee MH (2003) 14-3-3 sigma positively regulates p53 and suppresses tumor growth. *Mol Cell Biol* **23**(20): 7096–7107

Yu X, Harris SL, Levine AJ (2006) The regulation of exosome secretion: a novel function of the p53 protein. *Cancer Res* **66**(9): 4795–4801

Zhang H (2007) Molecular signaling and genetic pathways of senescence: Its role in tumorigenesis and aging. *J Cell Physiol* **210**(3): 567–574

Zhang M, Behbod F, Atkinson RL, Landis MD, Kittrell F, Edwards D, Medina D, Tsimelzon A, Hilsenbeck S, Green JE, Michalowska AM, Rosen JM. (2008) Identification of tumor-initiating cells in a p53-null mouse model of breast cancer. *Cancer Res* **68**(12): 4674–4682

Zheng H, Ying H, Yan H, Kimmelman AC, Hiller DJ, Chen AJ, Perry SR, Tonon G, Chu GC, Ding Z, Stommel JM, Dunn KL, Wiedemeyer R, You MJ, Brennan C, Wang YA, Ligon KL, Wong WH, Chin L, DePinho RA (2008) p53 and Pten control neural and glioma stem/progenitor cell renewal and differentiation. *Nature* **455**(7216): 1129–1133

Zhu J, Chen X (2000) MCG10, a novel p53 target gene that encodes a KH domain RNA-binding protein, is capable of inducing apoptosis and cell cycle arrest in G(2)-M. *Mol Cell Biol* **20**(15): 5602–5618

Zou Z, Gao C, Nagaich AK, Connell T, Saito S, Moul JW, Seth P, Appella E, Srivastava S (2000) p53 regulates the expression of the tumor suppressor gene maspin. *J Biol Chem* **275**(9): 6051–6054

Chapter 15
The PTEN/PI3 Kinase Pathway in Human Glioma

David Stokoe and Frank B. Furnari

Abstract Phosphoinositide 3-kinase (PI3K) was discovered over 20 years ago as an enzyme that was active in growth factor-stimulated and oncogene-transformed cells. Ten years later, the *PTEN* gene was isolated by its deletion in a large proportion of human cancers, including glioblastoma. These two areas of research converged when it was shown that PTEN dephosphorylated the lipid product of PI3K activity, phosphatidylinositol (3,4,5) trisphosphate, or PIP3. Furthermore, it has since become clear that PTEN has tumor-suppressive activities that are independent of its lipid phosphatase activity. This chapter reviews the importance of PI3K activity in the development of glioblastoma, by describing the different genetic and epigenetic alterations that occur to deregulate the activity of this pathway. It will also describe the regulation of PTEN expression and activity, by transcriptional and posttranslational processes. Recent results implicating PI3K activity and PTEN in the cells that are thought to initiate early brain tumor development (brain tumor stem cells) are also reviewed. Finally, the possibilities of using this pathway both as a direct therapeutic target and as a way of predicting response to recently developed drugs are discussed.

Contents

F.B. Furnari (✉)
Ludwig Institute for Cancer Research, University of California-San Diego School of Medicine, 9500 Gilman Drive CMM-East Rm. 3020, 92093-0660, La Jolla, CA, USA
e-mail: ffurnari@ucsd.edu

E.G. Van Meir (ed.), *CNS Cancer*, Cancer Drug Discovery and Development, DOI 10.1007/978-1-60327-553-8_15,
© Humana Press, a part of Springer Science+Business Media, LLC 2009

15.1 Introduction

Neoplasms of glial cells, especially those derived from the astrocytic lineage, comprise 40–50% of the tumors that arise in the central nervous system. The most aggressive and deadly of these neoplasms is glioblastoma (WHO grade IV, GBM). Many biological processes contribute to the aggressive nature of glioblastoma; among these, the most prevalent are uncontrolled cellular proliferation, deregulated apoptosis, diffuse infiltration of brain parenchyma, and angiogenesis. Despite knowledge of the genetic alterations that underlie these tumor phenotypes and decades of technological advances in neurosurgery, radiation therapy, and clinical trials of conventional and novel therapies, little improvement in median survival has been achieved for glioblastoma patients. This lack of clinical progress has stimulated the development of more targeted therapeutic approaches. An important signaling pathway that is invariably activated in glioma cells and contributes to the recalcitrant nature of these tumors is that of the class 1 PI3Ks (phosphoinositide 3-kinase) and its major downstream effector serine/threonine kinase, PKB/Akt. The actions of these kinases are directly antagonized by the PIP3 3-phosphatase encoded by the *PTEN* (phosphatase and tensin homolog deleted on chromosome 10) gene. Together, the opposing functions of PI3K and PTEN maintain normal cellular physiology and proper response to growth-promoting signals; however, when dysregulated by oncogenic mutation, as in the case of PI3K, or inactivated by mutation, as in the case of PTEN, pathogenesis can ensue. This chapter focuses on the central role of this pathway in the gliomagenic process, in particular those findings and model systems that shed light on the regulation of these key enzymes and that broaden our understanding of therapeutic resistance.

15.2 Pathway Activation: PI3K Signaling and Downstream Effectors

15.2.1 Class 1 PI3Ks

PI3Ks are a family of enzymes that catalyze the phosphorylation of inositol-containing phospholipids at the 3 position of the inositol ring (for a detailed review, see Vanhaesebroeck et al. 2001). Typically, these enzymes are made of two heterodimeric subunits, a catalytic subunit that carries the kinase domain and a regulatory subunit that modulates its function and localization in the cell. PI3Ks are subdivided into three classes based on substrate specificity, regulation, and differences in associated regulatory subunits (Fig. 15.1). There are four members of the class 1 enzymes, which are able to phosphorylate PI, PI(4)P, and PI(4,5)P2 in vitro, with PI(4,5)P2 the likely preferred in vivo

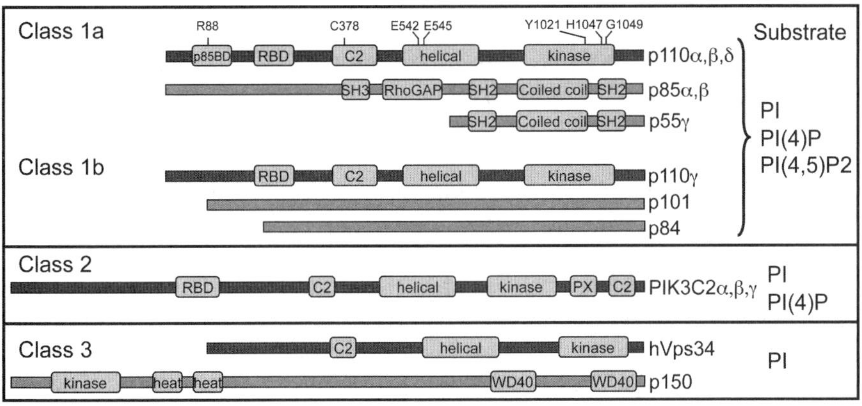

Fig. 15.1 PI3K subclasses and regulatory subunits. This figure illustrates how PI3Ks are divided into three subclasses, based on their structural features, their association with different regulatory subunits, and the types of phospholipid substrates they phosphorylate. Catalytic subunits are shown in dark gray, and regulatory subunits are shown in light gray. Class 1a enzymes are generally activated by receptor tyrosine kinases through binding of the SH2 domains of their regulatory subunits to phosphotyrosines. Class 1b subunits are generally activated by G-protein-coupled receptors. Some of the most frequent mutations in p110α found in glioblastoma are shown above the p110α catalytic subunit. Abbreviations: p85BD (p85-binding domain), RBD (Ras-binding domain), C2 (C2 domain), helical (helical domain, also referred to as PIK (PI kinase) domain), WD40 (trp-asp 40 amino acid domain), SH (src homology), PX (Phox homology domain), heat (Huntington, Elongation Factor-3, PR65/A, TOR)

substrate of these kinases. Class 1 enzymes are further subdivided into class 1a and class 1b based on their associated regulatory subunits: class 1a enzymes (p110α, β, and δ) associate with one of three subunits p85α, p85β, or p55γ, whereas the single class 1b enzyme (p110γ) forms a heterodimeric complex with one of two distinct regulatory subunits termed p101 (Stephens et al. 1997) or p84 (Suire et al. 2005). Three members of the class 2 PI3K family exist in mammalian cells, termed PI3K-C2α, β, and γ, which primarily phosphorylate PI and PI(4)P in vitro, although it is unclear which is the relevant substrate in vivo. Unlike class 1 and class 3 members, class 2 enzymes do not associate with a regulatory subunit and are thought to act as monomers. Class 3 enzymes phosphorylate phosphatidylinositol (PI) exclusively. There is a single 101 kDa member of this family in mammalian cells (hVps34), which associates with a 150 kDa regulatory subunit termed p150.

PI3Ks are also distinguished by their regulation in response to upstream signals. Class 3 PI3K (also known as hVps34) was initially thought to be a constitutively active kinase involved in endosomal trafficking, but more recently has been shown to play a signaling role in the response to intracellular amino acids (Nobukuni et al. 2005; Byfield, Murray, and Backer 2005) and Ca2+ (Gulati et al. 2008), through a conserved Ca/CaM-binding domain. The regulation of class 2 enzymes is also poorly understood, although there are reports that these proteins are activated by growth factors such as EGF, PDGF (Arcaro et al. 2000), and insulin (Falasca et al. 2007), and PI3K-C2α may be important in the insulin-induced production of PI(3)P and the subsequent translocation of GLUT4 glucose transporter to the plasma membrane (Falasca et al. 2007). The best understood regulation of PI3Ks is of the class 1 enzymes, which occur through receptor tyrosine kinases, G-protein-coupled receptors (GPCRs), and the small GTPase Ras (see below). Class 1 enzymes are also strongly implicated in tumor initiation and progression, and the remainder of this review will focus on the dysregulation of this pathway in gliomagenesis.

The most clearly demonstrated activation of PI3K that occurs in human tumors is through somatic mutations in p110α itself. Initially discovered in 2004 (Samuels et al. 2004), p110α mutations are now among the most prevalent in all human cancers, especially in breast (Oda et al. 2005), endometrial (Saal et al. 2005), and colon (Ikenoue et al. 2005) tumors. The most common mutations (E542, E545, and H1047) cluster in two regions of the *PIK3CA* gene on chromosome 3q26 and have been shown to confer increased catalytic activity, activation of downstream effectors, and increased transformation properties in experimental models (Isakoff et al. 2005). A number of studies have shown that p110α mutations are present in human gliomas, with a frequency of approximately 5% in glioblastoma (Knobbe et al. 2005; Broderick et al. 2004). Where examined, the frequency between primary and secondary glioblastoma was similar (Kita et al. 2007). Grade III oligodendroglioma and astrocytoma were also shown to harbor similar frequencies of p110α mutations, but mutations have not been found in grade II tumors (Hartmann et al. 2006; Broderick et al. 2004). In addition to point mutations, DNA amplification of the p110α gene is an additional mechanism underlying increased PI3K signaling. Initially shown for ovarian (Shayesteh et al. 1999) and non-small-cell lung (Massion et al. 2002) cancers, increased copy number of p110α has also been shown for primary and secondary glioblastoma. Gene amplification was found to be generally mutually exclusive with p110α mutations (Kita et al. 2007); therefore, mutation and amplification of the p110α catalytic subunit represent independent mechanisms to activate PI3K directly in brain tumors. Mutations in the regulatory subunits of class 1 PI3Ks have also recently been found in human breast and colorectal tumors (Wood et al. 2007). Although large numbers of glioma samples have not been analyzed for alterations in the corresponding genes, one report documented a 9 bp deletion that would lead to a truncated form of p85α (Mizoguchi et al. 2004), consistent with the inhibitory function of p85 seen in mouse knockout studies described below.

Loss of the phosphatase that antagonizes PI3K activity (PTEN) represents another frequent mechanism for increased PI3K signaling and will be discussed later. In addition, upstream regulators of PI3K are also frequently dysregulated in human gliomas, which are described in the following section.

15.3 Upstream Activation of PI3K by RTK Signaling

A major mechanism of PI3K activation occurs via ligand stimulation of receptor tyrosine kinases (RTKs), resulting in receptor auto/transphosphorylation on tyrosine residues, and utilization of these residues as docking sites for various signaling relay molecules. This process initiates a variety of intracellular signaling cascades including, in addition to PI3K/Akt, Ras/Raf/MEK/MAPK, PLC-γ, and the STAT transcription factors. Specifically, in the case of class 1a PI3Ks, recruitment to the activated RTK is achieved by association with their regulatory subunits (p85α, p85β, their splice variants p55 and p50, and p55γ) that dock to the receptor by their SH2 domains, thus placing the catalytic subunit in close proximity to PI(4,5)P2 substrate (Engelman et al. 2006). In contrast, the regulatory subunits of the class 1b kinase, p110γ, do not have SH2 domains (Stoyanov et al. 1995), but instead link p110γ to GPCRs for activation. GPCRs represent a large family of receptor proteins that bind a diverse repertoire of peptide and non-peptide ligands. GPCR agonists lead to the activation of heterotrimeric G$\alpha\beta\gamma$ proteins by exchanging the GDP molecule bound to the Gα subunit for GTP, which leads to the dissociation of the GTP-bound Gα subunits from the G$\beta\gamma$ subunits. The free G$\beta\gamma$ subunit also binds and activates p110γ by a mechanism that is stimulated by the regulatory p101 protein and thus plays a similar role in the recruitment (but not necessarily activation) of p110γ, as p85 does for p110α, p110β, and p110δ. Evidence has also been presented for the coupling of class 1a p110β to GPCRs (Kurosu et al. 1997; Guillermet-Guibert et al. 2008). Given that p110β has a much broader tissue distribution than leukocyte-restricted p110γ, p110β may provide the conduit for GPCR-linked PI3K signaling in many diverse cell types.

Epidermal growth factor (EGF) receptor (EGFR) and platelet-derived growth factor receptor (PDGFR) are prominent receptor tyrosine kinase pathways in gliomagenesis and in addition to PI3K, signal through several effector arms, including Ras/MAPK, PLC-γ, and JAK-STAT which regulate cellular proliferation, cell scatter and migration, and cytokine stimulation (reviewed in Heldin 1996). While these receptor-driven pathways can be activated in glioma by overexpression of both ligands and receptors, thus resulting in an autocrine loop, the most common activating alteration is genomic amplification, and/or mutation of a receptor leading to constitutive activation in the absence of ligand (Fig. 15.3).

15.3.1 Epidermal Growth Factor Receptor

The *EGFR* locus on chromosome 7 is the most frequently amplified genetic lesion in glioma, occurring in more than 50% of de novo glioblastomas and a few grade III anaplastic astrocytomas (Kleihues et al. 2002; Furnari et al. 2007), and is typically present as double-minute extrachromosomal elements. From a clinical perspective, the presence of this amplification has been shown to correlate with a shorter interval to relapse and poorer survival (Hurtt et al. 1992; Jaros et al. 1992; Schlegel et al. 1994). In about half of the cases with amplification, the event is coupled with gene rearrangement, and the majority encode truncated, constitutively active EGFR mutants (see also Chapter 20). Genomic alterations leading to deletion of exons 2–7 in the EGFR mRNA (de2-7, EGFR*, ΔEGFR; referred to here as EGFRvIII), which results in an in-frame truncation of a portion of the extracellular domain, are the most common of the rearrangements. Ectopic expression of EGFRvIII in glioblastoma cells causes constitutive self-phosphorylation, constitutive association with and activation of the Shc- Grb2-Ras and PI3K signaling pathways (Narita et al. 2002), enhanced tumorigenicity, reduced apoptosis (Nagane et al. 2001), and increased cellular proliferation (Narita et al. 2002). Resistance to apoptosis induced by chemotherapeutic drugs such as cisplatin is promoted by EGFRvIII through upregulation of Bcl-XL expression (Nagane et al. 1998). Furthermore, expression of EGFRvIII in mouse neural stem cells or astrocytes bearing a disrupted Ink4a/Arf locus induces transformation and glioma-like lesions in the brain (Bachoo et al. 2002; Holland et al. 1998), a phenotype that is not conferred by wt EGFR.

15.3.2 Platelet-Derived Growth Factor Receptor

In addition to the EGFR signaling axis, PDGFRα and its ligands, PDGF-A and PDGF-B, are expressed in gliomas, particularly in high-grade tumors (see also Chapter 19). In contrast, strong expression of PDGFRβ occurs in proliferating endothelial cells in glioblastoma (Plate et al. 1992; Hermanson et al. 1992; Di Rocco et al. 1998; Westermark, Heldin, and Nister 1995). In addition, PDGF-C and PDGF-D, which require proteolytic cleavage for activity, are frequently expressed in glioma cell lines and in glioblastoma tissues (Lokker et al. 2002). In contrast to EGFR, amplification or rearrangement of *PDGFRα* is much less common; however, a relatively rare oncogenic deletion mutation of PDGFRα (loss of exons 8 and 9) that is similar to EGFRvIII in activity has been described (Clarke and Dirks 2003). Given the tumoral co-expression of PDGF and PDGFR, autocrine and paracrine loops may be the primary means by which this growth factor axis exerts its effects. Interestingly, mice transgenic for neural progenitor-restricted PDGF-B expression result in the formation of oligodendrogliomas and forced elevation of PDGF-B levels increased overall tumor incidence (Shih et al. 2004; Dai et al. 2001; Assanah et al. 2006) (see Chapter 1), suggesting that targeted therapy against PDGFR could have therapeutic potential (Shih and Holland 2006). To this end, an orally active kinase inhibitor of STI571 (imatinib mesylate, Gleevec) that demonstrates specificity for PDGFR as well as c-Abl kinase has been shown to be a potent inhibitor of the PDGFR/PDGF oncogenic loops (Kilic et al. 2000; Hagerstrand et al. 2006) and when combined with hydroxyurea in a phase II study has been shown to achieve durable antitumor activity in some patients with recurrent glioblastoma (Reardon et al. 2005). In contrast, when used alone, STI571 has demonstrated minimal activity in malignant glioma (Wen et al. 2006), perhaps indicating that cooperating genetic lesions could convey resistance to PDGFR-directed therapeutics.

15.3.3 Receptor Co-activation as a Mechanism of Therapeutic Resistance in Glioma

One explanation for the failure of EGFR and PDGFR inhibitors to elicit significant clinical outcomes for glioma patients is that additional RTKs may cooperate to provide a signaling threshold that prevents the inhibition of mitogenic and survival signals through the inactivation of any single RTK (see also Chapter 40). In support of this hypothesis, recent work has demonstrated that multiple RTKs in addition to EGFR and PDGFR are simultaneously activated in primary glioblastomas and treatment of glioma cell lines with pharmacological agents or siRNAs targeting at least three of these different receptors were necessary to abrogate oncogenic signaling, survival, and anchorage-independent growth (Stommel et al. 2007). An independent study showed that glioma cells engineered to overexpress EGFRvIII caused increased c-MET phosphorylation (Huang et al. 2007). Similar to above, cross talk between the EGFRvIII and c-Met could be targeted with specific inhibitors to both, resulting in enhanced cytotoxicity in EGFRvIII-expressing cells compared with either compound alone. Taken together, these studies indicate that tumor RTK profiling may be an important step in the development of a personalized glioblastoma therapeutic regimen and that perhaps the initial disappointing clinical trials using RTK-targeted agents in glioblastoma should be reassessed with respect to the RTK activation profiles of responders and non-responders.

15.3.4 Ras

Ras comprises a family of small-molecular-weight proteins that bind and hydrolyze GTP (see also Chapters 4 and 38). Three members of this family, KRas, NRas, and HRas, are mutated in approximately 30% of all human tumors. Mutations abolish both the intrinsic GTPase activity and the ability to be stimulated by GTPase-activating proteins, or GAPs, resulting in constitutive association with effector proteins, including protein kinases such as Raf and exchange factors for the Ral family of GTPases. Although mutations in Ras proteins are infrequent in brain tumors (Knobbe et al. 2004b), copy number gains in all three isoforms were recently found in 13% of GBM (Jeuken et al. 2007), which may provide an additional mechanism for their previously described activation in GBM (Guha 1998). The notion that Ras might be involved in regulating PI3K activity was initially suggested by the presence of PI3K activity in anti-Ras immune precipitates (Sjolander and Lapetina 1992; Sjolander et al. 1991). Soon after, it was confirmed that p110α bound directly to HRas in a GTP-dependent manner and that activated Ras mutants were sufficient to elevate the levels of 3 phosphorylated phosphoinositides when transfected into cells (Rodriguez-Viciana et al. 1994). Moreover, purified processed HRas has been shown to directly stimulate the catalytic activity of p110α in vitro, alone, and in combination with phosphopeptides based on the p85α binding site of PDGFR (Rodriguez-Viciana et al. 1996). Similarly, processed but not unprocessed forms of HRas, NRas, and KRas are able to stimulate the activity of purified p110γ in a GTP-dependent manner (Pacold et al. 2000; Suire, Hawkins, and Stephens 2002). Ras increases PI3K activity, not by causing recruitment of PI3K to the plasma membrane, but by decreasing the Km for its substrate phospholipids, as well as possibly increasing Vmax (Suire et al. 2002).

Interestingly, significant differences exist between the ability of different Ras isoforms to activate different PI3K isoforms. While p110α and p110γ can be activated equally by H, N, and KRas, as well as by the related GTPases RRas, TC21, and RRas3, p110δ is only able to be stimulated by RRas and TC21, and p110β is unable to be stimulated by any Ras family member tested (Rodriguez-Viciana et al. 2004).

15.4 Regulation of Downstream PI3K Effectors

The best characterized mechanism for activation of PI3K effectors such as Akt and PDK1 is by their recruitment to the sites of lipid generation at the plasma membrane, through the engagement of phospholipid-binding domains such as pleckstrin homology (PH) domains. Such PIP3-binding PH domain-containing proteins include protein serine/threonine kinases (such as protein kinase B/Akt and phosphoinositide-dependent kinase-1 (PDK1)), protein tyrosine kinases (such as Brutons tyrosine kinase (Btk), tyrosine kinase expressed in hepatocellular carcinoma (TEK), and inducible T-cell kinase (Itk)) and exchange factors for the Rac family of GTPases (such as Tiam-1, Vav1, and P-Rex1). A large body of literature supports the notion that PI3K acts as a central node in polarized cell movement such as chemotaxis, as well as in the invasion that occurs in cancer metastasis (Barber and Welch 2006). The activation of Rac by PI3K via the PH domain-containing exchange factors mentioned above is likely to play an important role in this process, as well as in the local invasion of brain parenchyma by gliomas. In contrast, the role of PH domain-containing tyrosine kinases downstream of PI3K activity is likely limited to hematopoietic cells, as the expression of these protein kinases is generally restricted to these tissues. For example, mice lacking either p85α (Suzuki et al. 1999; Fruman et al. 1999) or Btk (Khan et al. 1995) or both display a block in the development of B cells, showing a genetic interaction between these proteins.

Activation of PKB/Akt by PI3K is thought to be one of the major consequences of PI3K activity in human cancer initiation and progression and has been extensively studied and discussed. PKB/Akt requires phosphorylation of two residues for activation: Thr-308 (numbering for PKBα/Akt1) in the activation loop and Ser-473 in the hydrophobic motif (Alessi et al. 1996). Thr-308 phosphorylation, like the equivalent site in many other protein kinases, is absolutely required for activity (Yang et al. 2002). However, monophosphorylated PKB/Akt remains disordered in critical activation domains and requires phosphorylation of the hydrophobic motif site Ser-473 to stabilize the active conformation (Yang, Cron, Thompson et al. 2002; Yang et al. 2002). PDK1 was isolated as the protein kinase responsible for phosphorylation of Thr-308 (Stokoe et al. 1997; Alessi et al. 1997). PDK1 also possesses a PH domain at its C-terminus, and it is likely that the generation of PIP3 at the plasma membrane results in co-localization of these two proteins, as well as a conformational change in PKB/Akt that exposes the Thr-308 site (Calleja et al. 2007). Ser-473 is phosphorylated by a complex of proteins that includes mammalian target of rapamycin (mTOR), Rictor, mSin1, and mLST8, collectively termed mTOR complex-2 (mTORC2). Although Ser-473 phosphorylation is regulated by growth factors, and mTORC2 activity toward Ser-473 is stimulated by growth factor treatment (Sarbassov dos et al. 2005), it is still not clear exactly how mTORC2 activity is regulated. mTORC2 also phosphorylates the turn motif phosphorylation site of PKB/Akt (Ser-450), a site that is not responsive to growth factors (Facchinetti et al. 2008), suggesting that mTORC2, like PDK1, could be a constitutively active kinase, whose regulated activity against substrates could be a result of factor-dependent changes in substrate conformation. PKB/Akt Ser-473 can also be phosphorylated by DNA-dependent protein kinase following DNA damage (Bozulic et al. 2008), as well as through autophosphorylation (Facchinetti et al. 2008), although it is not clear whether autophosphorylation occurs physiologically. The phosphorylation of various substrates of PKB/Akt and the consequences for cell proliferation and survival have recently been reviewed (Manning and Cantley 2007; Parcellier et al. 2008) and are summarized in Fig. 15.2 A. Somatic genetic alterations in downstream

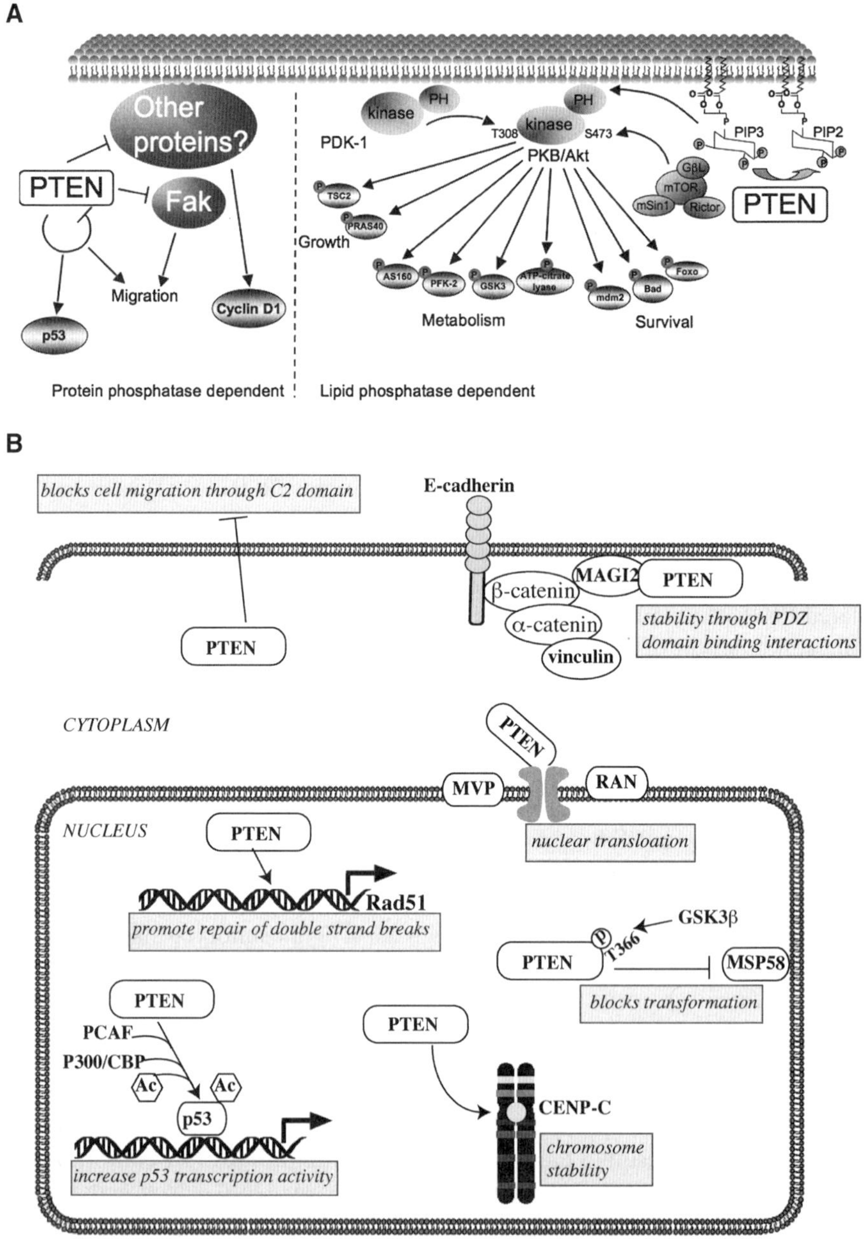

Fig. 15.2 (continued)

components of the PI3K signaling pathway in human tumors are quite infrequent, although mTOR has been found to be mutated in a small percentage of tumors, including 1/30 glioblastomas examined (Greenman et al. 2007).

15.5 Mouse Models Defining the Function of Class 1 PI3Ks

Constitutive and conditional mouse knockouts, as well as "knockins", for most of the regulatory and catalytic subunits of the class 1 PI3Ks have been generated, shedding light on the important role these enzymes play during development and tumorigenesis. Constitutive deletion of regulatory subunit p85α, including its two splice variants p55α and p50α, results in perinatal lethality (Fruman et al. 1999), which is rescued by maintaining expression of the truncated splice forms (Suzuki et al. 1999). Both models show defects in B-cell development and activation, with no effects on T cells. Despite decreased levels and activity of the class 1a catalytic subunits in these mice following the absence of the regulatory subunit, PI3K signaling, as judged by PIP3 production and insulin sensitivity, is actually increased (Fruman et al. 2000) (Terauchi et al.

Fig. 15.2 (continued) **PTEN phosphatase-dependent and phosphatase-independent functions.** (**A**) Phosphatase-dependent effects. PTEN dephosphorylates phosphatidylinositol (3,4,5) trisphosphate (PIP3) to produce phosphatidylinositol (4,5) bisphosphate (PIP2). PIP3 recruits PKB/Akt to the plasma membrane where it is phosphorylated and activated by PDK1 on Thr-308. PKB/Akt is fully activated through the phosphorylation of Ser-473 by mTORC2, comprised of the protein kinase mTOR, and the regulatory subunits Rictor, Gβl, and mSin1. Activated PKB/Akt then phosphorylates a number of substrates that result in increased growth, changes in metabolism, and increased survival. Abbreviations: TSC2 (tuberous sclerosis complex-2), PRAS40 (proline-rich Akt substrate, 40 kDa), AS160 (Akt substrate of 160 kDa), PFK-2 (phosphofructokinase-2), GSK3 (glycogen synthase kinase-3), mdm2 (murine double minute-2), Foxo (Forkhead Box, member O). The left hand panel in the figure shows the effects of PTEN that are thought to be the result of its protein phosphatase activity. Abbreviations: FAK (focal adhesion kinase), TSC2 (tuberous sclerosis protein-2), PRAS40 (proline-rich Akt substrate of 40 kDa), AS160 (Akt substrate of 160 kDa), PFK-2 (phosphofructokinase-2), GSK3 (glycogen synthase kinase-3), mdm2 (mouse double minute-2), BAD (bcl2 antagonist of cell death), Foxo (forkhead box-o), mTOR (mammalian target of rapamycin). (**B**) Phosphatase-independent effects. Non-enzymatic functions of PTEN in the cytoplasm and at the cell membrane regulate cell migration and protein stability, most likely through the C2 domain. Specifically, vinculin is required to maintain β-catenin-MAGI2 (membrane-associated guanylate kinase inverted 2) interactions at adherens junctions and thereby limit ubiquitin-mediated degradation of PTEN (Subauste et al. 2005). Translocation into the nucleus is regulated by the major vault protein (MVP) and RAN, two constituents of nuclear pores (Chung et al. 2005; Gil et al. 2006). Within the nucleus, PTEN regulates transcription activity of p53, enhances Rad51 (radiation sensitivity abnormal-51) expression, promotes chromosome stability by influencing centromere protein C-1 (CENP-C), and can block transformation mediated by MSP-58 (58-kDa microspherule protein)

1999). Similarly, mice lacking regulatory subunit p85β also show hypoinsulinemia, hypoglycemia, and improved insulin sensitivity, suggesting increased PI3K pathway activity. In contrast, mice lacking both p85α and p85β in muscle tissues display a dramatic decrease in PI3K activity, as well as insulin resistance and glucose intolerance. Further studies have suggested that the loss of combinations of p85 subunits can increase PI3K signaling in some tissues, but decrease it in others (Luo et al. 2005). These results, as well as others, suggest that p85 subunits can play an inhibitory role in PI3K activity and signaling, in addition to their stabilizing and scaffolding role to traffic p110 catalytic subunits to activated growth factor receptors.

Similarly, the deletion of class 1 PI3K catalytic subunits has also generated insights into the importance of PI3K signaling during development and disease. Deletion of p110α or p110β results in embryonic lethality (Bi et al. 2002, 1999). Deletion of p110γ results in mice that are viable and healthy, but that show specific defects in neutrophil migration and activation in response to infection (Dekker and Segal 2000). The role of p110δ has also been explored using conventional knockout, as well as kinase-dead knockin approaches. Both of these techniques demonstrated that mice lacking p110δ activity are viable and fertile, but show defects in immune cell functions, including B cells, T cells, and mast cells (Ali et al. 2004; Clayton et al. 2002; Jou et al. 2002; Okkenhaug et al. 2002). More recently, conditional knockout approaches have been used to demonstrate the roles of distinct isoforms of PI3K during tumor progression. This work has demonstrated that p110β, and not p110α, plays a critical role in prostate tumorigenesis induced by tissue-specific loss of the tumor suppressor PTEN. Similar experiments to determine the role of different PI3K isoforms in PTEN-driven glioma models (discussed below) are currently underway and are awaited with anticipation. Clearly the results of such experiments will be critical in understanding the appropriate delivery of PI3K inhibitors as therapy. For example, given the prevalence of PTEN mutations in gliomas, a p110β, or p110α/β, inhibitor might be more efficacious than a p110α-specific inhibitor.

15.6 Pathway Inhibition: PTEN

15.6.1 Loss of Heterozygosity of Chromosome 10 and the Search for Tumor Suppressor Genes

Molecular and cytogenetic analyses of glioblastomas have shown that monosomy of chromosome 10 is frequent, occurring in more than 80% of tumors (Bigner et al. 1990; James et al. 1988), and that allelic losses of chromosome 10 occur in the great majority of glioblastomas, but only occasionally in anaplastic astrocytomas or lower grade gliomas (Fujimoto et al. 1989; Fults et al. 1990; James et al. 1988; Venter and Thomas 1991; von Deimling et al. 1992; Maier et al. 1997). These data suggested the presence of a tumor suppressor gene(s) on chromosome 10 involved in the progression of grade III to grade IV gliomas. Since the entire chromosome is often lost, attempts to map tumor suppressor gene(s) have been challenging. A number of deletion mapping studies have suggested that this chromosome may have as many as three tumor suppressor genes involved in gliomagenesis, mapping near 10q25 (Fults and Pedone 1993; Karlbom et al. 1993; Rasheed et al. 1992; Maier et al. 1998), 10p (Karlbom et al. 1993; von Deimling et al. 1992) and 10q near the centromere (Karlbom et al. 1993).

15.6.2 PTEN *Discovery and Its Link to Genetic Syndromes*

In seminal experiments performed over a decade ago, the relevant 10q25 tumor suppressor gene, involved in glioma as well as several other cancers, was identified by three research groups. Steck et al. fine-mapped homozygous deletions in glioma cell lines and isolated the gene by exon trapping using a bacterial artificial chromosome that spanned the suspect region (Steck et al. 1997). These authors named the identified gene *MMAC1* for *m*utated in *m*ultiple *a*dvanced *c*ancers. Li et al. utilized representational difference analysis in conjunction with mapping of cancer-associated homozygous deletions on 10q23 to identify *PTEN* (Li et al. 1997). Lastly, Li and Sun surveyed Genebank's expressed sequence tag database for sequences containing conserved motifs for tyrosine phosphatase catalytic domains and identified a partial cDNA that was used to clone a gene they termed *TEP1*, for *T*GFβ-regulated and *e*pithelial cell-enriched *p*hosphatase (Li and Sun 1997). This name referred to the high level of gene expression in a keratinocyte cell line, which could be downregulated by TGFβ treatment. Today, *PTEN* has been adopted by the Human Genome Organization Nomenclature Committee, as the official gene name.

Large-scale genetic analysis has shown that *PTEN* is mutated in 24% of glioblastomas (Ohgaki et al. 2004); however, this same study showed that 10q was lost in 69% of glioblastomas, indicating that another critical gene resides in this region or that *PTEN* haploinsufficiency is enough for tumor initiation, the latter theory of which is supported by mouse tumor models and human-inherited genetic syndromes associated with *PTEN* mutation (see below).

In addition to glioblastomas, *PTEN* is frequently mutated in a wide spectrum of late-stage sporadic cancers, including melanoma and carcinomas of the prostate, endometrium, kidney, and lung (Li and Sun 1998; Steck et al. 1997; Dahia 2000). Furthermore, germline mutations have been detected in the autosomal dominant disorders, Cowden syndrome, Bannayan–Zonana syndrome, juvenile polyposis syndromes, Lhermitte–Duclos disease, and Proteus and Proteus-like syndromes (Eng and Peacocke 1998; Liaw et al. 1997), known collectively as PTEN hamartoma tumor syndromes (PHTS), for their shared benign differentiated proliferative lesions within highly disorganized tissue architectures.

In addition to hamartomas, Cowden syndrome individuals have an increased incidence of breast and thyroid cancers, while Bannayan–Zonana syndrome is characterized by macrocephaly, learning disabilities, and freckling, with a reduced cancer risk when compared with Cowden disease. Proteus and Proteus-like syndromes are characterized by tissue and bone overgrowth, with no increased cancer risk, raising the issue of whether different PTEN mutations seen in these syndromes could drive different clinical phenotypes (Zbuk and Eng 2007). This could attest to multiple PTEN functions, or perhaps various genetic modifiers exist in the population that alter PTEN-associated disease presentation.

The human *PTEN* gene maps to chromosomal band 10q23.3 (Li et al. 1997; Steck et al. 1997) and consists of nine exons spanning approximately 100 kb of genomic sequence. The PTEN protein is 403 amino acids of a relative mass of 47 kDa. Its domain structure consists of a 25-amino acid N-terminal motif that binds phosphatidylinositol-4,5-bisphosphate (PtdIns(4,5)P2), a core phosphatase domain (amino acids 25–185) defined by the invariant signature motif, $Cys(X)_5Arg$ (Cantley and Neel 1999) and which also contains homology to tensin and auxilin, a C2 domain that facilitates PTEN's anchoring to negatively charged membranes (Downes et al. 2004; Lee et al. 1999), a C-terminal 50-amino acid region that regulates PTEN activity and stability through multiple phosphorylated residues (discussed later), and the last three amino acids comprise a binding site for membrane-associated PDZ domain-containing proteins (see Figs. 15.2b and 15.4).

15.6.3 Lipid Phosphatase-Specific Functions of PTEN

Sequencing of the *PTEN* gene established that it showed considerable homology to previously identified tyrosine phosphatases, especially dual specificity phosphatases that can dephosphorylate tyrosine, serine, and threonine residues. Indeed, initial experiments showed that it possessed phosphatase activity against these amino acids, but the activity was quite weak and specific to highly acidic substrates (Myers et al. 1997). A seminal paper in 1998 showed that PTEN dephosphorylates PIP3 at the 3′ position of the inositol ring, the same position that PI3K enzymes phosphorylate (Maehama and Dixon 1998). Therefore, PTEN acts as the physiological antagonist of PI3K activity (Fig 15.2A). Confirming this result, deletion of *PTEN* in mice results in massive increases in PI3K-dependent signaling such as PKB/Akt phosphorylation (Stambolic et al. 1998). Abundant genetic evidence in model organisms shows that PTEN acts to antagonize PI3K activity (Stocker et al. 2002). The importance of the lipid phosphatase activity in human tumors is also illustrated by a particular mutant of PTEN found in Cowden's patients and in an endometrial tumor (Risinger et al. 1997; Liaw et al. 1997), G129E, that lies in the conserved phosphatase domain. This mutation greatly attenuates lipid phosphatase activity, by decreasing the size of the substrate-binding pocket to prevent phospholipid binding, but retains phosphotyrosine interaction and phosphotyrosine phosphatase activity (Myers et al. 1998; Lee et al. 1999; Furnari et al. 1998). Revealingly, this mutant form of PTEN is unable to cause cell cycle arrest in glioma cell lines (Furnari et al. 1998) or inhibit cell migration in *PTEN* null mouse fibroblasts (Liliental et al. 2000).

15.6.4 Protein Phosphatase-Specific Functions of PTEN

The view that PTEN acts solely as a lipid phosphatase is probably too simple. While G129E PTEN was unable to cause G1 arrest in U87MG glioblastoma cells, it caused a cell cycle arrest in MCF7 cells (Hlobilkova et al. 2000). Moreover, this mutant also decreased the levels of cyclin D1, an important modulator of the cell cycle machinery in these cells (Weng et al. 2001). Additional protein phosphatase-dependent effects of PTEN have also been observed, such as the inhibition of migration and invasion of *PTEN* null glioma cells (Cai et al. 2005; Raftopoulou et al. 2004; Dey et al. 2008; Maier et al. 1999). Putative protein substrates of PTEN relevant to these effects include focal adhesion kinase (FAK) (Tamura et al. 1998), as well as PTEN itself (Raftopoulou et al. 2004). While wt PTEN required protein phosphatase activity to inhibit glioma cell migration, a T383A mutant does not, suggesting that this site could be the relevant target of PTEN in these experiments. The C2 domain of PTEN was determined to be important in the inhibition of cell migration. Interestingly, the C2 domain has also been implicated in additional, non-phosphatase-dependent functions of PTEN (see below) (Fig 15.2B).

15.6.5 Non-enzymatic Functions of PTEN

In addition to the well-defined enzymatic functions of PTEN as a phosphatase, emerging data indicate that this protein regulates several biological processes in a non-catalytic fashion, chiefly through protein–protein interactions mediated through its C2 domain. Freeman et al. have reported that the PTEN C2 domain binds directly to p53 resulting in stabilization of this tumor suppressor (Tang and Eng 2006) and stimulates its DNA binding and transcriptional activation functions (Freeman et al. 2003) most likely by enhancing p53 acetylation (Li et al. 2006; Mayo et al. 2002) (Fig 15.2b).

In a screen for potential proteins that interact with the C-terminal half of PTEN, Okumura et al. isolated the nuclear proto-oncogene MSP58 (Okumura et al. 2005). Introduction of MSP58 into *Pten* null mouse embryo fibroblasts (MEFs) resulted in transformation, although this outcome was abrogated by co-expression of wt PTEN and, surprisingly, by G129R, a phosphatase inactive PTEN mutant. Interestingly, phosphorylation of PTEN Thr-366 was required for MSP58 interaction and hence suppression of transformation. As this site is phosphorylated by glycogen synthase kinase 3β (GSK3 β) (Al-Khouri et al. 2005), which is itself inactivated by PI3K signaling, this suppressive activity of PTEN could represent a mechanism by which phosphatase-dependent and phosphatase-independent functions act in concert. Furthermore, as the c-Jun transcription factor has been shown to upregulate MSP58 expression (Karagiannidis et al. 2008) as well as downregulate PTEN expression (Hettinger et al. 2007), it will be interesting to determine if glioblastomas with high levels of active c-Jun (Assimakopoulou and Varakis 2001) utilize MSP58 in part to drive their malignant phenotype.

A role for PTEN in the maintenance of chromosomal integrity has been suggested by studies in breast cancer in which loss of *PTEN* is associated with centromere breakage and chromosomal translocations (Puc and Parsons 2005; Shen et al. 2007). In one study, the effect on chromosomal integrity was attributed to AKT-mediated phosphorylation of CHK1, thus causing cytoplasmic sequestration of this important DNA damage checkpoint protein (Puc and Parsons 2005). Subsequently, PTEN was also found to be associated with the centromere in complex with CENP-C (Shen et al. 2007), thus helping to maintain chromosomal stability independent of its phosphatase activity. In a similar non-enzymatic fashion, PTEN has also been shown to control DNA repair through transcriptional regulation of Rad51, a key protein in mediating double-stranded break repair (Shen et al. 2007), and perhaps through modulation of p53 stability and activity (Freeman et al. 2003). The non-enzymatic functions of PTEN are summarized in Fig 15.2B.

15.7 PTEN in Glioma Biology: Primary vs Secondary Glioma

As discussed in Section 15.6.2, *PTEN* is a tumor suppressor on a region of chromosome 10q that is lost in >80% of glioblastomas. Most glioblastomas occur de novo, without any indication of prior disease. However, approximately 5% arise from previously existing lower grade tumors, like grade II astrocytomas and grade III anaplastic astrocytomas, that are treated with surgery, and sometimes radiation and chemotherapy. Although de novo and secondary glioblastomas cannot be distinguished from a pathology standpoint, their molecular signatures allow for their separation. For example, *EGFR* amplification is a common event in de novo glioblastoma, but rare in secondary glioblastoma, whereas p53 mutations occur more frequently in secondary glioblastoma and show a bias toward hot spot mutations at codons 248 and 273 (Ohgaki and Kleihues 2007, 2005). While both de novo and secondary glioblastomas display a high frequency of 10q LOH, only de novo glioblastomas show a high frequency of PTEN mutations (25–40%) (Fig. 15.3). A recent study showed that epigenetic regulation of PTEN in secondary glioblastoma could explain this discrepancy (Wiencke et al. 2007). Nine of 11 (82%)

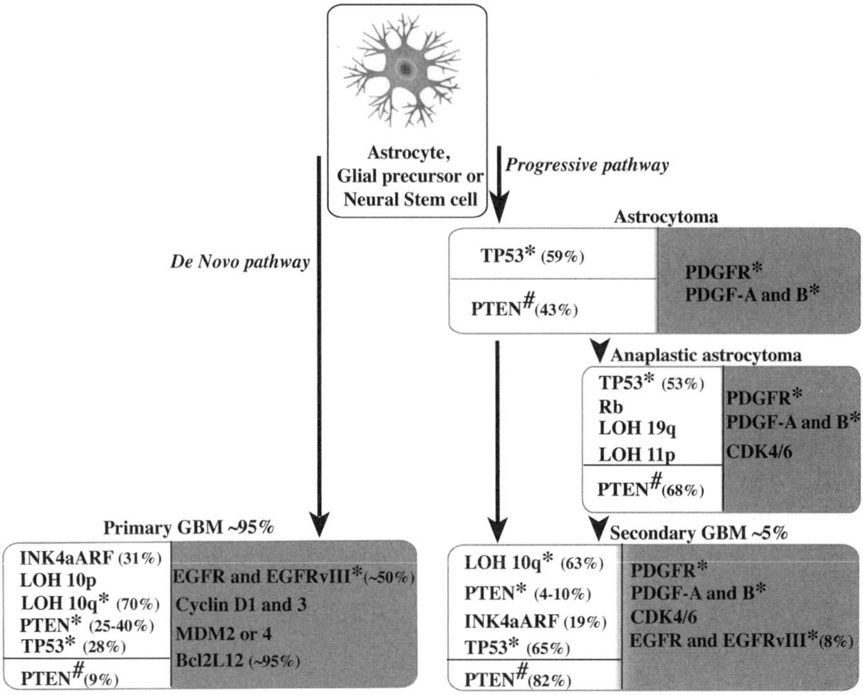

Fig. 15.3 Genetics and epigenetics of PI3K pathway activation in primary and secondary gliomas. Shown are the molecular lesions involved in the genesis of primary glioblastoma (de novo pathway) and secondary glioblastoma (progressive pathway) (for specific details see Furnari et al., 2007). Oncogenes (gray-shaded areas) and tumor suppressors (unshaded areas) are indicated with frequency of their known involvement in parenthesis. Genes involved in the PI3K pathway activation are indicated by an asterisk. In primary glioblastomas, activation of the PI3K pathway is achieved by several cooperative mechanisms, including EGFR amplification and mutation (EGFRvIII), p53 mutation, PTEN mutation, and LOH 10q (encompassing the *PTEN* gene). While in secondary glioblastomas, PDGFR, PDGF-A and B, p53 mutation, *PTEN* promoter methylation (#), and LOH 10q are the major mechanisms of pathway activation, with PTEN mutation and EGFR involvement being rare

secondary glioblastomas examined showed methylation at the *PTEN* promoter, whereas only 2/23 (9%) de novo glioblastomas showed this alteration. Moreover, none of the secondary glioblastomas displayed PTEN mutations, whereas the PTEN mutations present in de novo glioblastoma were mutually exclusive with *PTEN* promoter methylation (Fig 15.3). Therefore, mutations and methylation could be two independent mechanisms to lose function of the remaining *PTEN* allele in glioblastoma tumors. While low-grade gliomas do not show 10q LOH or PTEN mutations, they do display a high incidence of *PTEN* promoter methylation, which is associated with increased PKB/Akt phosphorylation (Wiencke et al. 2007). This appears to correlate with the time and incidence of progression of low-grade tumors (Sean McBryde, DS and Daphne Haas-Kogan, unpublished observations). Therefore, PI3K inhibitor therapy could be suitable for low-grade gliomas prior to the activation of multiple additional pathways that occur in high-grade disease (Stommel et al. 2007).

15.8 PTEN Involvement in Brain Tumor Stem Cells

Data from several studies in which PTEN expressed in the mouse brain had been disrupted have indicated that its function might also play a role in stem cell homeostasis (Backman et al. 2001; Groszer et al. 2001; Kwon et al. 2001) (see Chapters 29, 36, and 44). Macrocephaly and severe brain structure patterning abnormalities in these mice appeared to be the consequence of a combination of decreased cell death, increased proliferation, and an enlargement in neuronal cell size, results which were supported by ex vivo experiments indicating that PTEN loss had a cell autonomous effect. Further experiments (Groszer et al. 2006) illustrated that an enhanced self-renewal capacity and entry into the G1 phase of the cell cycle as well as decreased growth factor dependency of *Pten* null neural/stem progenitor cells was the cause of the brain defects described above. In contrast, *Pten* deficiency in hematopoietic stem cells (HSC) results in exhaustion of normal HSCs and expansion of leukemogenic cells and the eventual development of myeloproliferative disorders and leukemia (Yilmaz et al. 2006; Zhang et al. 2006), both of which were preventable by treating the mice with the mTOR inhibitor, rapamycin (Yilmaz et al. 2006). These organ-specific stem cell phenotypes resulting from *Pten* deletion may be linked to different cellular failsafe responses, where activation of PI3K signaling in the neuronal compartment results in stem cell expansion, while in the hematopoietic lineage *Pten* loss results in stem cell depletion, similar to the p53-dependent senescence response observed in the mouse prostate upon *Pten* deletion (Chen et al. 2005).

In a more recent study, gliomas were generated in a p53 heterozygous mouse upon conditional inactivation in neural cells of the Ras pathway regulator, *Nf1* (Zhu et al. 2005) (see also Chapters 5 and 6). Histopathologic evaluation revealed that the tumors that formed ranged from low- to high-grade astrocytoma, with a majority of the high-grade tumors expressing activated Akt. Introduction of *Pten* heterozygosity to this model resulted in accelerated morbidity, shortened survival, and full penetrance of high-grade astrocytomas. Whereas haploinsufficiency of *Pten* accelerated grade III astrocytoma formation, loss of the remaining *Pten* allele produced grade IV tumors associated with Akt activation (Kwon et al. 2008). This full spectrum of glioma phenotype permitted examination of presymptomatic mice which revealed abnormal proliferation and hyperplasia in the vicinity of the stem/progenitor cell niche, thus supporting the hypothesis of a neural stem/progenitor cell origin for glioma (Hemmati et al. 2003; Singh et al. 2003; Zhu et al. 2005) regulated by PI3K signaling (see also Chapter 29). This hypothesis is further supported by a recent study in which microarray expression profiling defined three prognostic subclasses of high-grade glioma, proneural, proliferative, and mesenchymal (see also Chapter 23). The two molecular subgroups with the poorest prognosis, proliferative and mesenchymal, possessed a signature of low PTEN mRNA, high levels of phosphorylated Akt, and a neural stem cell phenotype, implicating as in the mouse model above that the PI3K pathway may govern processes that regulate cell fate choices during neurogenesis (Phillips et al. 2006).

15.9 Transcriptional Regulation

Due to its robust expression levels and long protein half-life, PTEN was initially thought to be a constitutively expressed gene; however several transcription factors have now been shown to positively and negatively regulate its gene expression (Fig 15.4a). Upon examination of the *PTEN* promoter, two binding sites for EGR1 were found (Virolle et al. 2001) and PTEN was shown to be upregulated in response to EGR1 activators, including radiation treatment (Virolle et al. 2001) and by IGF-II, as part of a negative feedback loop modulating the duration of PI3K pathway activation in the mammary gland (Moorehead et al. 2003). Direct expression correlation between EGR1 and PTEN has been detected in non-small-cell lung cancer (Ferraro et al. 2005) and is associated with poor prognosis. In addition the therapeutic agent, doxorubicin, which has been shown to be toxic to glioblastoma cell lines (Abe et al. 1994; Darling and Thomas 2001; Stan et al. 1999) and has been tested as a treatment for patients with high-grade glioma (Voulgaris et al. 2002), may elicit its antineoplastic action, at least in part, through EGR1-dependent upregulation of PTEN expression (Pan et al. 2007).

PPARγ has also been shown to upregulate *PTEN* transcription (Patel et al. 2001) and use of PPARγ agonists has been shown to have potent anticancer effects in many clinical models, including glioma (Grommes et al. 2006) and liposarcoma (Demetri et al. 1999). However, diminishing the enthusiasm for the use of these agonists in cancer treatment has been data illustrating an increase in colon polyp formation in a preclinical model of intestinal neoplasia (Apc^{Min} mouse) (Saez et al. 1998) and increased cancer incidence in type 2 diabetes patients (Ramos-Nino et al. 2007) when treated with these agonists.

Lastly, Stambolic et al. identified a p53-binding element in the *PTEN* promoter sequence and characterized a p53-mediated apoptosis mechanism that requires the activation of PTEN transcription (Stambolic et al. 2001). This result indicates that such a mechanism is perhaps defective in mutant p53, wild-type PTEN tumors, a genetic signature that describes some glioblastomas (Ohgaki et al. 2004).

In contrast to PTEN activation, much less is known about its negative regulation. The cloning of PTEN by Li et al. was the first study to identify a

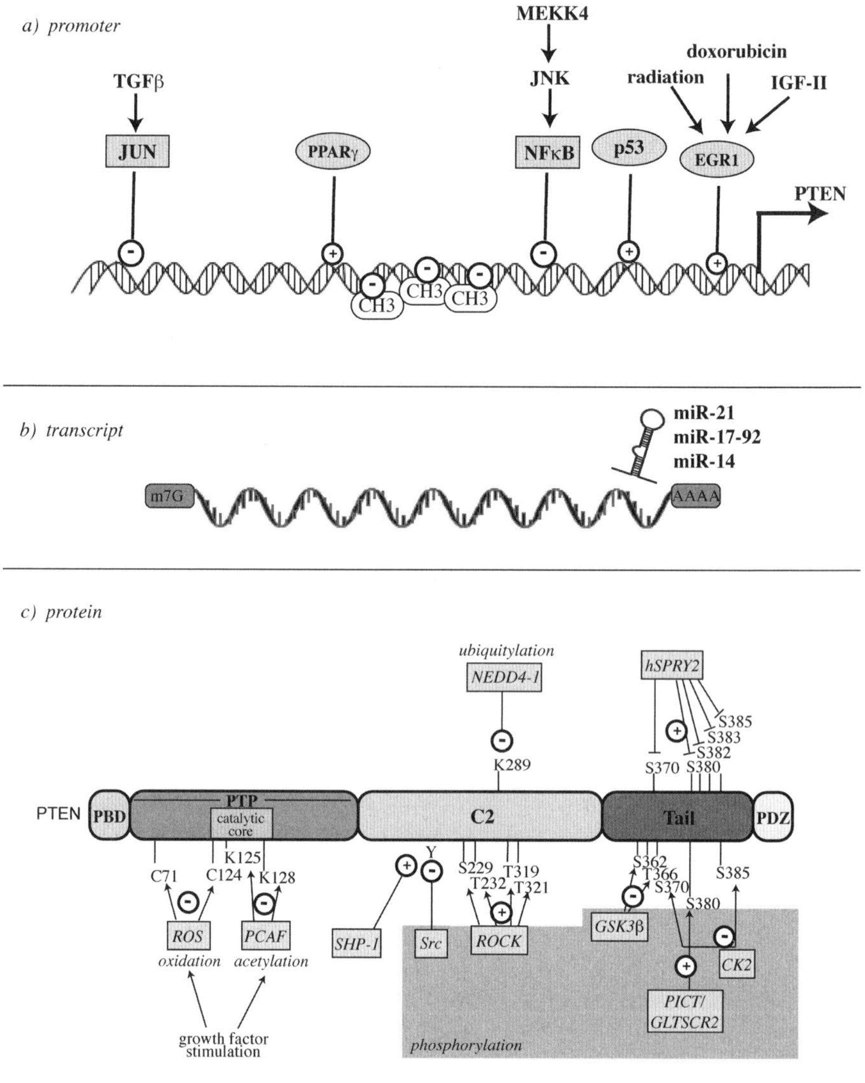

Fig. 15.4 Modes of PTEN regulation. *PTEN* gene expression and protein activity are regulated at the (a) promoter, (b) transcript, and (c) protein modification levels. For simplicity, mechanisms involved or suspected to be involved in glioma are indicated. Transcription factors, pathways, kinases, and phosphatases known to upregulate *PTEN* expression or activity are indicated by (+) and those negatively regulating expression or activity are indicated by (–). Abbreviations: TGFβ (transforming growth factor-β), PPARγ (peroxisome proliferator-activated receptor-γ), MEKK4 (mitogen-activated protein kinase kinase kinase 4), NFκB (nuclear factor-kappa B), EGFR1 (early growth response 1), miR (microRNA), PBD (phosphatidylinositol-4,5-bisphosphate-binding domain), PTP (protein tyrosine phosphatase homology region), PDZ (PDZ domain-binding motif), NEDD4-1 (neural precursor cell expressed, developmentally downregulated 4), hSPRY2 (human sprouty 2), ROS (reactive oxygen species), PCAF (p300/CBP-associated factor), SHP-1 (src homology phosphatase-1), ROCK (Rho-associated kinase), PICT (protein interacting with carboxyl terminus 1), GSK3 β (glycogen synthase kinase 3β), GLTSCR2 (glioma tumor suppressor candidate region 2), CK2 (casein kinase 2)

growth factor, TGFβ, responsible for PTEN downregulation (Li and Sun 1997). Subsequently, RAS-RAF-MEK-ERK signaling (Chow et al. 2007; Vasudevan et al. 2007) leading to c-Jun activation and its binding to a repressor element ~19,600 bp upstream of the *PTEN* transcriptional start site was shown to mediate TGFβ-induced PTEN repression (Hettinger et al. 2007). Moreover, other stress kinase pathways including MEKK4 and JNK promote resistance to apoptosis through PTEN suppression via direct binding of NFκB to the *PTEN* promoter (Xia et al. 2007).

15.10 Inactivation Mechanisms of PTEN

15.10.1 PTEN *Loss and Mutation Spectrum in Glioma*

PTEN is inactivated in 50% of high-grade gliomas by mutations or epigenetic mechanisms (Knobbe and Reifenberger 2003; Ohgaki et al. 2004). Specifically, the bulk of *PTEN* mutations is found in glioblastomas, with reported frequencies ranging from 15% (Duerr et al. 1998) to 40% (Schmidt et al. 1999) and with a strong bias toward primary glioblastomas, giant cell glioblastomas, and gliosarcomas (Peraud et al. 1999; Reis et al. 2000; Tohma et al. 1998; Tortosa et al. 2000). *PTEN* gene alterations in glioblastomas do not correlate with either *EGFR* amplification or *TP53* mutation (Liu et al. 1997; Rasheed et al. 1997; Schmidt et al. 1999; Smith et al. 2001) (Fig. 15.3). Typically the *PTEN* mutations found in gliomas cause premature truncations (~17%), insertions/deletions (26%), or missense mutations (~57%) that alter the PTEN coding sequence and generally reduce phosphatase activity (Sanger Center: Distribution of somatic mutations in PTEN; Sanger Center Catalogue of Somatic Mutations in Cancer (COSMIC); Furnari et al. 1997; Ali, Schriml, and Dean 1999), resulting in loss of its ability to antagonize the signaling output of PI3K. Interestingly, a small proportion of *PTEN* mutations found in glioblastoma do not result in activation of Akt phosphorylation (Downes et al. 2004), supporting data demonstrating non-enzymatic functions of PTEN (see above).

15.10.2 Modulation of PTEN Function by Protein Modifications

Recent investigations have provided great insight into the regulation of PTEN activity by posttranslational modifications (reviewed in Tamguney and Stokoe 2007) (Fig. 15.4c). The best understood of these mechanisms is through casein kinase 2 (CK2)-mediated phosphorylation of Ser-370 and Ser-385 in the C-terminus of PTEN. Phosphorylation of these residues is not required for PTEN enzymatic activity but results in protein stability and cytosolic localization, while dephosphorylated PTEN is more enzymatically active, localized at the plasma membrane and less stable (Vazquez et al. 2000; Torres and Pulido 2001; Vazquez et al. 2001). Additional investigations have illustrated that CK2 phosphorylation of PTEN serves as a priming event for further phosphorylation by GSK3β at Ser-362 and Thr-366, which could serve as part of a negative feedback loop that regulates PTEN and PI3K activity (Al-Khouri et al. 2005) and as a means to promote the association with the oncogene, MSP58 (Okumura et al. 2005) (see above). Moreover, phosphorylation of Ser-385 also likely primes the protein for phosphorylation at Ser-380, Thr-382, and -383 (Odriozola et al. 2007), while glioma tumor suppressor candidate region 2 (GLTSCRs, also known as PICT-1) has also been shown to promote Ser-380 phosphorylation and to cause an increase in PTEN levels (Okahara et al. 2006; Yim et al. 2007). The Rho-associated kinase ROCK has also been shown to phosphorylate PTEN at several serine/threonine residues in the C2 domain causing activation of PTEN and localization to the plasma membrane (Li et al. 2005). In contrast, human sprouty2 (hSPRY2) promotes PTEN dephosphorylation on Ser-370, 380, 382, 383, and 385, resulting in increased PTEN activity (Edwin et al. 2006) and inhibition of cell cycle progression mediated by EGFR signaling (Wong et al. 2002). Recent evidence has suggested that Src-mediated tyrosine phosphorylation of the C-terminus of PTEN may similarly alter the function of PTEN by affecting stability and altering its capacity to bind to the cellular membrane (Lu et al. 2003; Nagata et al. 2004). In a breast cancer cell line, this effect of Src was inhibited by co-expression of SHP-1, an SH2 domain-containing protein tyrosine phosphatase that selectively bound and dephosphorylated PTEN (Lu et al. 2003). Given that the kinase activity of Lyn, a Src family kinase member, has been detected at significantly elevated levels in glioblastoma tumor samples (Stettner et al. 2005), it is interesting to speculate that this could be an additional mechanism attenuating PTEN activity in glioma.

There are several non-phosphorylation modifications that also regulate PTEN activity. Like many lipid and protein phosphatases, PTEN is regulated by oxidation of cysteine-124 in its active catalytic site. Reactive oxygen species (ROS) cause an intramolecular disulfide bond between Cys-124 and Cys-71 (Lee et al. 2002). While initially thought to be by-products of metabolism, ROS are now known to play a significant role in cell signaling mediated by growth factors such as insulin, EGF, PDGF, and lipopolysaccharide and have been shown to contribute to the activation of the PI3K pathway through oxidation and inactivation of PTEN (Kwon et al. 2004; Lee et al. 2002; Leslie et al. 2003). The histone acetyltransferase p300/CBP-associated factor (PCAF) interacts with PTEN and acetylates lysines 125 and 128 in response to growth factor. These residues are located within the catalytic cleft of PTEN and are essential for PIP3 specificity; consequently PCAF acts as a negative regulator of PTEN (Okumura et al. 2006). Ubiquitin-mediated degradation of PTEN due to direct binding and ubiquitination of Lys-13 and -289 by the E3 ligase, NEDD4-1, has also been reported (Trotman et al. 2007; Wang et al. 2007); however, studies have yet to validate a role for NEDD4-1 in human cancer showing the targeting of PTEN to the proteosome (Fouladkou et al. 2008).

15.10.3 MicroRNA Regulation of PTEN Expression

MicroRNAs (miRNAs), endogenous short single-stranded RNAs that repress mRNA translation by base-pairing to sequence located in the 3́UTR of target mRNAs, are emerging as important regulators of cellular processes and have been implicated in the etiology of a variety of human cancers (see also Chapter 27). Recently several studies have profiled miRNAs in gliomas (Ciafre et al. 2005; Silber et al. 2008) and one miRNA in particular, miR-21, has been reported to repress PTEN expression (Meng et al. 2007) and protect glioma (Chan, Krichevsky, and Kosik 2005; Corsten et al. 2007) and breast cancer cells (Si et al. 2007) from cell death. Similarly, miR-17-92 and miR-214 have been shown to suppress PTEN expression in lymphoma (Xiao et al. 2008) and in ovarian cancer (Yang et al. 2008), respectively. These studies suggest that miRNAs can exert oncogenic activity in part through the downregulation of *PTEN* expression and add to the repertoire of posttranslational and epigenetic mechanisms that silence PTEN expression and activity (Fig 15.4b).

15.11 PTEN Localization

The phospholipid substrates for PTEN are localized in cellular membrane compartments, and overexpression of PTEN specifically depletes plasma membrane pools of PIP3 (Lindsay et al. 2006). PTEN also possesses three distinct membrane localization domains: a PI(4,5)P2-binding region at the N-terminus (Walker et al. 2004), a C2 domain that comprises the middle third of the protein (Das et al. 2003), and a C-terminal PDZ domain-binding motif (Bonifant et al. 2007). It is therefore surprising that efforts to confirm an expected membrane localization of PTEN have been generally unsuccessful. In fact, endogenous PTEN appears to be localized to the cytosol and the nucleus (Lachyankar et al. 2000; Gimm et al. 2000). More recent sophisticated approaches have shown that PTEN does interact with the plasma membrane, but for only very short intervals of a few milliseconds (Vazquez et al. 2006). In addition, phosphorylation of the C-terminal tail of PTEN also prevents membrane localization by preventing incorporation into a complex that includes PDZ domain-containing proteins such as MAGI2 (Vazquez et al. 2001) (Fig 15.2b). Although the importance of PDZ domain interactions with PTEN remains to be fully established, there is some circumstantial evidence that it plays a function in the tumor-suppressive role of PTEN in glioblastoma. A critical component of the PDZ domain recognition motif is a free carboxy group on a hydrophobic residue two amino acids after a serine or threonine (Nourry et al. 2003). Therefore, mutations that target the PTEN stop codon would essentially abolish these interactions by extending the carboxy terminal amino acids. Such mutations have indeed been found in three human tumors, and interestingly all occur in glioblastoma specimens (Tohma et al. 1998; Schmidt et al. 1999; Zhou et al. 1999).

Sequences in the C2 domain and phosphatase domain of PTEN are thought to be important for nuclear localization (Chung et al. 2005). There is likely a role for nuclear PTEN in its tumor suppressor function, as nuclear PTEN, but not total PTEN, is lost in thyroid cancers (Gimm et al. 2000). Recently, some of the signals that regulate PTEN localization to the nucleus have been elucidated, such as oxidative stress (Chang et al. 2008), decreased ATP levels (Lobo et al. 2008), and PI3K signaling itself (Liu et al. 2007). Interestingly, there is evidence that the roles and functions of nuclear PTEN could be quite different from those in the cytoplasm and plasma membrane (Denning et al. 2007) (reviewed in Planchon et al. 2008) (Fig 15.2b).

15.12 Other Regulators of Akt Activity

In addition to aberrant PI3K signaling driven by RTK activity, PTEN inactivation, and oncogenic activation of p110α, there are a number of other possible mechanisms by which AKT activation may become dysregulated in glioblastoma. PHLPP (PH domain leucine-rich repeat protein phosphatase), which dephosphorylates Akt S473, is expressed at very low levels in certain glioblastoma cell lines (Gao et al. 2005), as is CTMP (carboxy terminal modulator protein), which binds to AKT and inhibits its phosphorylation (Maira et al. 2001; Knobbe et al. 2004a). Thirdly, PIKE-A, a small GTPase found to be amplified in glioblastomas and glioma cell lines, binds directly to phosphorylated Akt and enhances its anti-apoptotic function (Ahn et al. 2004a; Knobbe et al. 2005; Ahn et al. 2004b). It is unclear whether PIKE-A is targeted for amplification or whether it is a "passenger" in the CDK4 and mdm2 loci-targeted amplifications on chromosome 12.

15.13 Mouse Glioma Models and PTEN Involvement

Given the high frequency with which PTEN is inactivated in brain tumors, many investigators have tried to create mouse models recapitulating human glioma pathology by disrupting *PTEN* expression (see Chapters 2 and 5). As described above, systemic inactivation of *PTEN* results in embryonic lethality, while specific deletion in the neural compartment results in macrocephaly and seizures. These data suggest that inactivation of PTEN is not sufficient for tumor initiation at least in the mouse brain. However, loss of PTEN has been shown to accelerate gliomagenesis, complete with hallmark phenotypes of cell invasion and angiogenesis, when combined with additional genetic alterations such as astrocyte-specific inactivation of the Rb pathway, a close parallel to the progression of high-grade disease in humans coincident with loss of PTEN

(Xiao et al. 2002, 2005) (see Chapter 7). Substantiating these results, studies have shown that key glioma relevant mutations – including those in PTEN and EGFR – may act as an "angiogenic switch" by stabilizing HIF-1α or one of its downstream targets, VEGF (Blum et al. 2005; Phung et al. 2006) (see Chapter 22).

In a different mouse system, PTEN loss was achieved in a subset of astrocytes, via intracranial injection of adenovirus expressing cre recombinase, and when combined with astrocyte-specific expression of oncogenic Ras resulted in high-grade astrocytomas with short latency (Wei et al. 2006) (see Chapter 4).

15.14 Therapeutic Intervention and Conditions for Resistance in Glioma and Breast Cancer: PTEN as a Marker for Drug Response and Resistance

In addition to the effects PTEN loss and mutation have on initiating and sustaining the tumorigenic phenotype, the presence or absence of PTEN function has also been shown to act as a powerful predictive marker of response to therapy. As previously mentioned above, >50% glioblastoma tumors display EGFR amplification, suggesting that this tumor type appears to be ideal for small molecule inhibitors of EGFR such as gefitinib or erlotinib (see also Chapter 20). In a phase 1 trial treating recurrent glioblastoma patients with erlotinib, response rates (as measured by a 50% decrease in radiographically measured tumor volume) were ~20%. Response was correlated with *EGFR* expression and amplification, and it was found that the tumors lacking EGFR protein expression did not respond to treatment as expected under the assumption that these drugs are target specific. However, the presence of increased expression or amplification of *EGFR* in the tumors was not sufficient to predict response. When the activity of the PI3K pathway was also examined, using antibodies specific to phosphorylated PKB/Akt, it became clear that tumors showing strong expression of phosphorylated PKB/Akt failed to respond to treatment. In sum, the most dramatic responses to treatment with erlotinib were found in the tumors expressing high levels of EGFR and low levels of phosphorylated PKB/Akt (Haas-Kogan et al. 2005). A very similar result was also seen in a second study, in which patients whose tumors expressed EGFRvIII and intact PTEN were the most likely to respond to EGFR inhibitors (Mellinghoff et al. 2005). Therefore, low activity of the PI3K pathway in GBM as measured by wild-type *PTEN* gene sequence and low phospho-Akt by immunohistochemistry act as a strong positive predictive markers for response to EGFR therapies.

In contrast, elevated levels of PKB/Akt phosphorylation in tumor tissue were found to be a positive predictive marker of response in a clinical trial with gefitinib in NSCLC (Cappuzzo et al. 2004). However, some NSCLC tumors (unlike glioblastoma) show a reasonable frequency of EGFR mutations. These EGFR mutations result in stronger activation of PI3K signaling compared to wt EGFR, which is a poor activator of PI3K (Sordella et al. 2004). Furthermore, when gefitinib-treated NSCLC patients are stratified by the presence of EGFR mutations, elevated phosphorylated PKB/Akt predicts good response for the mutated EGFR-expressing tumors, but poor response for the wt EGFR-expressing tumors. Therefore, if PI3K activity is driven directly by EGFR, then EGFR inhibitors are likely to be effective therapeutics. However, if PI3K activity is driven by EGFR-independent mechanisms (such as PTEN inactivation), these tumors are likely to be resistant to EGFR monotherapy. Although speculative, this hypothesis is supported by additional experiments in breast cancer cells. In cells expressing wt PTEN, gefitinib inhibited PKB/Akt phosphorylation and caused growth arrest and apoptosis, whereas in cells expressing mutant PTEN, PKB/Akt phosphorylation was not affected and the cells remained viable (Bianco et al. 2003). These results also suggest that EGFR inhibitors and PI3K pathway inhibitors given in combination will be particularly effective in tumors in which PTEN is mutated and EGFR is important in driving tumor cell proliferation and survival. Indeed, initial experiments in glioblastoma preclinical settings have shown that this represents a promising strategy (Wang et al. 2006; Goudar et al. 2005) and is currently being implemented in the clinical setting.

Interestingly, PTEN also appears to act as a predictive marker for responses to other types of therapies. Patients whose tumors show high levels of PTEN expression also show better responses to trastuzumab (an antibody targeted to Her2) (Fujita et al. 2006; Nagata et al. 2004), to tamoxifen (an antagonist of the estrogen receptor) (Shoman et al. 2005) in breast cancer, and progesterone (Milam et al. 2007) in endometrial hyperplasia. PTEN even appears to determine response to some conventional cytotoxic agents, for example cisplatin in ovarian cancer cell lines (Yan et al. 2006). As approaches to monitor the levels of PTEN, and the activity of the PI3K pathway, in tumor samples become more robust and reliable, we anticipate that routine incorporation of these tests into clinical trials will markedly improve response rates to existing and novel therapies.

15.15 Conclusions

Since the discovery of PI3K (Whitman et al. 1988) and its antagonist PTEN (Steck et al. 1997; Li and Sun 1997; Li et al. 1997), the pathway governed by these two enzymes has been determined to be the linchpin in the etiology of a wide number of cancer types, including glioma, as well as to be important in associated biologic features, such as loss of cell cycle control, uncontrolled proliferation, invasion, escape from apoptosis, and aberrant angiogenesis. To date our attempts to target the signaling inputs of this pathway, such as inhibitors directed to amplified or mutated EGFR or the consequential downstream Akt effector, mTOR, have generated relatively poor responses in glioblastoma patients, and the few who do respond eventually progress through therapy (see Furnari et al., 2007, for a summary of therapeutics in clinical trial). As discussed above, we are only beginning to recognize the multitude of mechanisms whereby alterations to PTEN (and PI3K) can lead to such resistance. These include not only mutations but also modulators of function by posttranslational modifications, miRNA targeting of PTEN transcripts, promoter methylation, upstream co-activation of several receptors increasing the input into the pathway, and potential downstream modulation of Akt activity and its effectors. This means that we will have to develop more sophisticated methods to analyze these changes in patient tumors before selecting the most appropriate therapies or identify reliable surrogate markers that will be easy to use in the clinic.

To date, application of this information in the clinical setting has been in the form of immunohistochemistry, genomic DNA sequencing, and Western blotting techniques, all of which have practical drawbacks and interpretation biases. Newer techniques that may circumvent these limitations are assays that analyze the consequence of PI3K/PTEN/Akt pathway alterations such as reliable biomarkers indicative of PTEN mutation (Saal et al. 2007) or PI3K/Akt activation status (Mehrian-Shai et al. 2007), magnetic resonance spectroscopy that detects metabolic changes associated with inhibition in PI3K signaling (Beloueche-Babari et al. 2006), or phospho-flow cytometry that can analyze at the single cell level the activation state of pathway molecules (Krutzik and Nolan 2006; Schulz et al. 2007). Incorporation of some of these technologies into the clinical trials setting could aid in the rapid selection of patients who would best benefit from current therapies and are the best candidates for testing of novel agents.

References

Abe, T., S. Hasegawa, K. Taniguchi, A. Yokomizo, T. Kuwano, M. Ono, T. Mori, S. Hori, K. Kohno, and M. Kuwano. 1994. Possible involvement of multidrug-resistance-associated protein (MRP) gene expression in spontaneous drug resistance to vincristine, etoposide and adriamycin in human glioma cells. *Int J Cancer* 58 (6):860–4.

Ahn, J. Y., Y. Hu, T. G. Kroll, P. Allard, and K. Ye. 2004a. PIKE-A is amplified in human cancers and prevents apoptosis by up-regulating Akt. *Proc Natl Acad Sci USA* 101 (18):6993–8.

Ahn, J. Y., R. Rong, T. G. Kroll, E. G. Van Meir, S. H. Snyder, and K. Ye. 2004b. PIKE (phosphatidylinositol 3-kinase enhancer)-A GTPase stimulates Akt activity and mediates cellular invasion. *J Biol Chem* 279 (16):16441–51.

Al-Khouri, A. M., Y. Ma, S. H. Togo, S. Williams, and T. Mustelin. 2005. Cooperative phosphorylation of the tumor suppressor phosphatase and tensin homologue (PTEN) by casein kinases and glycogen synthase kinase 3beta. *J Biol Chem* 280 (42):35195–202.

Alessi, D. R., M. Andjelkovic, B. Caudwell, P. Cron, N. Morrice, P. Cohen, and B. A. Hemmings. 1996. Mechanism of activation of protein kinase B by insulin and IGF-1. *EMBO J.* 15:6541–51.

Alessi, D. R., S. R. James, C. P. Downes, A. B. Holmes, P. R. J. Gaffney, C. B. Reese, and P. Cohen. 1997. Characterisation of a 3-phosphoinositide-dependent protein kinase which phosphorylates and activates protein kinase Ba. *Current Biology* 7:261–9.

Ali, I. U., L. M. Schriml, and M. Dean. 1999. Mutational spectra of PTEN/MMAC1 gene: a tumor suppressor with lipid phosphatase activity. *J Natl Cancer Inst* 91 (22):1922–32.

Ali, K., A. Bilancio, M. Thomas, W. Pearce, A. M. Gilfillan, C. Tkaczyk, N. Kuehn, A. Gray, J. Giddings, E. Peskett, R. Fox, I. Bruce, C. Walker, C. Sawyer, K. Okkenhaug, P. Finan, and B. Vanhaesebroeck. 2004. Essential role for the p110delta phosphoinositide 3-kinase in the allergic response. *Nature* 431 (7011):1007–11.

Arcaro, A., M. J. Zvelebil, C. Wallasch, A. Ullrich, M. D. Waterfield, and J. Domin. 2000. Class II phosphoinositide 3-kinases are downstream targets of activated polypeptide growth factor receptors. *Mol Cell Biol* 20 (11):3817–30.

Assanah, M., R. Lochhead, A. Ogden, J. Bruce, J. Goldman, and P. Canoll. 2006. Glial progenitors in adult white matter are driven to form malignant gliomas by platelet-derived growth factor-expressing retroviruses. *J Neurosci* 26 (25):6781–90.

Assimakopoulou, M., and J. Varakis. 2001. AP-1 and heat shock protein 27 expression in human astrocytomas. *J Cancer Res Clin Oncol* 127 (12):727–32.

Bachoo, R. M., E. A. Maher, K. L. Ligon, N. E. Sharpless, S. S. Chan, M. J. You, Y. Tang, J. DeFrances, E. Stover, R. Weissleder, D. H. Rowitch, D. N. Louis, and R. A. DePinho. 2002. Epidermal growth factor receptor and Ink4a/Arf: convergent mechanisms governing terminal differentiation and transformation along the neural stem cell to astrocyte axis. *Cancer Cell* 1 (3):269–77.

Backman, S. A., V. Stambolic, A. Suzuki, J. Haight, A. Elia, J. Pretorius, M. S. Tsao, P. Shannon, B. Bolon, G. O. Ivy, and T. W. Mak. 2001. Deletion of Pten in mouse brain causes seizures, ataxia and defects in soma size resembling Lhermitte-Duclos disease. *Nat Genet* 29 (4):396–403.

Barber, M. A., and H. C. Welch. 2006. PI3K and RAC signalling in leukocyte and cancer cell migration. *Bull Cancer* 93 (5):E44–52.

Beloueche-Babari, M., L. E. Jackson, N. M. Al-Saffar, S. A. Eccles, F. I. Raynaud, P. Workman, M. O. Leach, and S. M. Ronen. 2006. Identification of magnetic resonance detectable metabolic changes associated with inhibition of phosphoinositide 3-kinase signaling in human breast cancer cells. *Mol Cancer Ther* 5 (1):187–96.

Bi, L., I. Okabe, D. J. Bernard, and R. L. Nussbaum. 2002. Early embryonic lethality in mice deficient in the p110beta catalytic subunit of PI 3-kinase. *Mamm Genome* 13 (3):169–72.

Bi, L., I. Okabe, D. J. Bernard, A. Wynshaw-Boris, and R. L. Nussbaum. 1999. Proliferative defect and embryonic lethality in mice homozygous for a deletion in the p110alpha subunit of phosphoinositide 3-kinase. *J Biol Chem* 274 (16):10963–8.

Bianco, R., I. Shin, C. A. Ritter, F. M. Yakes, A. Basso, N. Rosen, J. Tsurutani, P. A. Dennis, G. B. Mills, and C. L. Arteaga. 2003. Loss of PTEN/MMAC1/TEP in EGF receptor-expressing tumor cells counteracts the antitumor action of EGFR tyrosine kinase inhibitors. *Oncogene* 22 (18):2812–22.

Bigner, S. H., B. Vogelstein, J. Mark, H. S. Friedman, and D. D. Bigner. 1990. Cytogenetics and molecular genetics: their status and role in understanding the behavior of central nervous system neoplasms. *Monogr Pathol* 32:30–40.

Blum, R., J. Jacob-Hirsch, N. Amariglio, G. Rechavi, and Y. Kloog. 2005. Ras inhibition in glioblastoma down-regulates hypoxia-inducible factor-1alpha, causing glycolysis shutdown and cell death. *Cancer Res* 65 (3):999–1006.

Bonifant, C. L., J. S. Kim, and T. Waldman. 2007. NHERFs, NEP, MAGUKs, and more: Interactions that regulate PTEN. *J Cell Biochem* 102 (4):878–885.

Bozulic, L., B. Surucu, D. Hynx, and B. A. Hemmings. 2008. PKBalpha/Akt1 acts downstream of DNA-PK in the DNA double-strand break response and promotes survival. *Mol Cell* 30 (2):203–13.

Broderick, D. K., C. Di, T. J. Parrett, Y. R. Samuels, J. M. Cummins, R. E. McLendon, D. W. Fults, V. E. Velculescu, D. D. Bigner, and H. Yan. 2004. Mutations of PIK3CA in anaplastic oligodendrogliomas, high-grade astrocytomas, and medulloblastomas. *Cancer Res* 64 (15):5048–50.

Byfield, M. P., J. T. Murray, and J. M. Backer. 2005. hVps34 is a nutrient-regulated lipid kinase required for activation of p70 S6 kinase. *J Biol Chem* 280 (38):33076–82.

Cai, X. M., B. B. Tao, L. Y. Wang, Y. L. Liang, J. W. Jin, Y. Yang, Y. L. Hu, and X. L. Zha. 2005. Protein phosphatase activity of PTEN inhibited the invasion of glioma cells with epidermal growth factor receptor mutation type III expression. *Int J Cancer* 117 (6):905–12.

Calleja, V., D. Alcor, M. Laguerre, J. Park, B. Vojnovic, B. A. Hemmings, J. Downward, P. J. Parker, and B. Larijani. 2007. Intramolecular and Intermolecular Interactions of Protein Kinase B Define Its Activation In Vivo. *PLoS Biol* 5 (4):e95.

Cantley, L. C., and B. G. Neel. 1999. New insights into tumor suppression: PTEN suppresses tumor formation by restraining the phosphoinositide 3-kinase/AKT pathway. *Proc Natl Acad Sci USA* 96 (8):4240–5.

Cappuzzo, F., E. Magrini, G. L. Ceresoli, S. Bartolini, E. Rossi, V. Ludovini, V. Gregorc, C. Ligorio, A. Cancellieri, S. Damiani, A. Spreafico, C. T. Paties, L. Lombardo, C. Calandri, G. Bellezza, M. Tonato, and L. Crino. 2004. Akt phosphorylation and gefitinib efficacy in patients with advanced non-small-cell lung cancer. *J Natl Cancer Inst* 96 (15):1133–41.

Chan, J. A., A. M. Krichevsky, and K. S. Kosik. 2005. MicroRNA-21 is an antiapoptotic factor in human glioblastoma cells. *Cancer Res* 65 (14):6029–33.

Chang, C. J., D. J. Mulholland, B. Valamehr, S. Mosessian, W. R. Sellers, and H. Wu. 2008. PTEN nuclear localization is regulated by oxidative stress and mediates p53-dependent tumor suppression. *Mol Cell Biol* 28 (10):3281–9.

Chen, Z., L. C. Trotman, D. Shaffer, H. K. Lin, Z. A. Dotan, M. Niki, J. A. Koutcher, H. I. Scher, T. Ludwig, W. Gerald, C. Cordon-Cardo, and P. P. Pandolfi. 2005. Crucial role of p53-dependent cellular senescence in suppression of Pten-deficient tumorigenesis. *Nature* 436 (7051):725–30.

Chow, J. Y., K. Quach, B. L. Cabrera, J. Cabral, S. E. Beck, and J. M. Carethers. 2007. RAS/ERK Modulates TGF{beta}-regulated PTEN Expression In Human Pancreatic Adenocarcinoma Cells. *Carcinogenesis* 28 (11):2321–2327.

Chung, J. H., M. E. Ginn-Pease, and C. Eng. 2005. Phosphatase and tensin homologue deleted on chromosome 10 (PTEN) has nuclear localization signal-like sequences for nuclear import mediated by major vault protein. *Cancer Res* 65 (10):4108–16.

Ciafre, S. A., S. Galardi, A. Mangiola, M. Ferracin, C. G. Liu, G. Sabatino, M. Negrini, G. Maira, C. M. Croce, and M. G. Farace. 2005. Extensive modulation of a set of microRNAs in primary glioblastoma. *Biochem Biophys Res Commun* 334 (4):1351–8.

Clarke, I. D., and P. B. Dirks. 2003. A human brain tumor-derived PDGFR-alpha deletion mutant is transforming. *Oncogene* 22 (5):722–33.

Clayton, E., G. Bardi, S. E. Bell, D. Chantry, C. P. Downes, A. Gray, L. A. Humphries, D. Rawlings, H. Reynolds, E. Vigorito, and M. Turner. 2002. A crucial role for the p110delta subunit of phosphatidylinositol 3-kinase in B cell development and activation. *J Exp Med* 196 (6):753–63.

Corsten, M. F., R. Miranda, R. Kasmieh, A. M. Krichevsky, R. Weissleder, and K. Shah. 2007. MicroRNA-21 knockdown disrupts glioma growth in vivo and displays synergistic cytotoxicity with neural precursor cell delivered S-TRAIL in human gliomas. *Cancer Res* 67 (19):8994–9000.

Dahia, P. L. 2000. PTEN, a unique tumor suppressor gene. *Endocr Relat Cancer* 7 (2):115–29.

Dai, C., J. C. Celestino, Y. Okada, D. N. Louis, G. N. Fuller, and E. C. Holland. 2001. PDGF autocrine stimulation dedifferentiates cultured astrocytes and induces oligodendrogliomas and oligoastrocytomas from neural progenitors and astrocytes in vivo. *Genes Dev* 15 (15):1913–25.

Darling, J. L., and D. G. Thomas. 2001. Response of short-term cultures derived from human malignant glioma to aziridinylbenzoquinone, etoposide and doxorubicin: an in vitro phase II trial. *Anticancer Drugs* 12 (9):753–60.

Das, S., J. E. Dixon, and W. Cho. 2003. Membrane-binding and activation mechanism of PTEN. *Proc Natl Acad Sci USA* 100 (13):7491–6.

Dekker, L. V., and A. W. Segal. 2000. Perspectives: signal transduction. Signals to move cells [comment]. *Science* 287 (5455):982–3, 985.

Demetri, G. D., C. D. Fletcher, E. Mueller, P. Sarraf, R. Naujoks, N. Campbell, B. M. Spiegelman, and S. Singer. 1999. Induction of solid tumor differentiation by the peroxisome proliferator-activated receptor-gamma ligand troglitazone in patients with liposarcoma. *Proc Natl Acad Sci USA* 96 (7):3951–6.

Denning, G., B. Jean-Joseph, C. Prince, D. L. Durden, and P. K. Vogt. 2007. A short N-terminal sequence of PTEN controls cytoplasmic localization and is required for suppression of cell growth. *Oncogene* 26 (27):3930–40.

Dey, N., H. E. Crosswell, P. De, R. Parsons, Q. Peng, J. D. Su, and D. L. Durden. 2008. The protein phosphatase activity of PTEN regulates SRC family kinases and controls glioma migration. *Cancer Res* 68 (6):1862–71.

Di Rocco, F., R. S. Carroll, J. Zhang, and P. M. Black. 1998. Platelet-derived growth factor and its receptor expression in human oligodendrogliomas. *Neurosurgery* 42 (2):341–6.

Downes, C. P., S. Walker, G. McConnachie, Y. Lindsay, I. H. Batty, and N. R. Leslie. 2004. Acute regulation of the tumour suppressor phosphatase, PTEN, by anionic lipids and reactive oxygen species. *Biochem Soc Trans* 32 (Pt 2):338–42.

Duerr, E. M., B. Rollbrocker, Y. Hayashi, N. Peters, B. Meyer-Puttlitz, D. N. Louis, J. Schramm, O. D. Wiestler, R. Parsons, C. Eng, and A. von Deimling. 1998. PTEN mutations in gliomas and glioneuronal tumors. *Oncogene* 16 (17):2259–64.

Edwin, F., R. Singh, R. Endersby, S. J. Baker, and T. B. Patel. 2006. The tumor suppressor PTEN is necessary for human Sprouty 2-mediated inhibition of cell proliferation. *J Biol Chem* 281 (8):4816–22.

Eng, C., and M. Peacocke. 1998. PTEN and inherited hamartoma-cancer syndromes. *Nat Genet* 19 (3):223.

Engelman, J. A., J. Luo, and L. C. Cantley. 2006. The evolution of phosphatidylinositol 3-kinases as regulators of growth and metabolism. *Nat Rev Genet* 7 (8):606–19.

Facchinetti, V., W. Ouyang, H. Wei, N. Soto, A. Lazorchak, C. Gould, C. Lowry, A. C. Newton, Y. Mao, R. Q. Miao, W. C. Sessa, J. Qin, P. Zhang, B. Su, and E. Jacinto. 2008. The mammalian target of rapamycin complex 2 controls folding and stability of Akt and protein kinase C. *Embo J* 27 (14):1932–1943.

Falasca, M., W. E. Hughes, V. Dominguez, G. Sala, F. Fostira, M. Q. Fang, R. Cazzolli, P. R. Shepherd, D. E. James, and T. Maffucci. 2007. The role of phosphoinositide 3-kinase C2alpha in insulin signaling. *J Biol Chem* 282 (38):28226–36.

Ferraro, B., G. Bepler, S. Sharma, A. Cantor, and E. B. Haura. 2005. EGR1 predicts PTEN and survival in patients with non-small-cell lung cancer. *J Clin Oncol* 23 (9):1921–6.

Fouladkou, F., T. Landry, H. Kawabe, A. Neeb, C. Lu, N. Brose, V. Stambolic, and D. Rotin. 2008. The ubiquitin ligase Nedd4-1 is dispensable for the regulation of PTEN stability and localization. *Proc Natl Acad Sci USA* 105 (25):8585–90.

Freeman, D. J., A. G. Li, G. Wei, H. H. Li, N. Kertesz, R. Lesche, A. D. Whale, H. Martinez-Diaz, N. Rozengurt, R. D. Cardiff, X. Liu, and H. Wu. 2003. PTEN tumor suppressor regulates p53 protein levels and activity through phosphatase-dependent and -independent mechanisms. *Cancer Cell* 3 (2):117–30.

Fruman, D. A., F. Mauvais-Jarvis, D. A. Pollard, C. M. Yballe, D. Brazil, R. T. Bronson, C. R. Kahn, and L. C. Cantley. 2000. Hypoglycaemia, liver necrosis and perinatal death in mice lacking all isoforms of phosphoinositide 3-kinase p85 alpha. *Nat Genet* 26 (3):379–82.

Fruman, D. A., S. B. Snapper, C. M. Yballe, L. Davidson, J. Y. Yu, F. W. Alt, and L. C. Cantley. 1999. Impaired B cell development and proliferation in absence of phosphoinositide 3-kinase p85alpha. *Science* 283 (5400):393–7.

Fujimoto, M., D. W. Fults, G. A. Thomas, Y. Nakamura, M. P. Heilbrun, R. White, J. L. Story, S. L. Naylor, K. S. Kagan-Hallet, and P. J. Sheridan. 1989. Loss of heterozygosity on chromosome 10 in human glioblastoma multiforme. *Genomics* 4 (2):210–4.

Fujita, T., H. Doihara, K. Kawasaki, D. Takabatake, H. Takahashi, K. Washio, K. Tsukuda, Y. Ogasawara, and N. Shimizu. 2006. PTEN activity could be a predictive marker of trastuzumab efficacy in the treatment of ErbB2-overexpressing breast cancer. *Br J Cancer* 94 (2):247–52.

Fults, D., and C. Pedone. 1993. Deletion mapping of the long arm of chromosome 10 in glioblastoma multiforme. *Genes Chromosomes Cancer* 7 (3):173–7.

Fults, D., C. A. Pedone, G. A. Thomas, and R. White. 1990. Allelotype of human malignant astrocytoma. *Cancer Res* 50 (18):5784–9.

Furnari, F. B., T. Fenton, R. M. Bachoo, A. Mukasa, J. M. Stommel, A. Stegh, W. C. Hahn, K. L. Ligon, D. N. Louis, C. Brennan, L. Chin, R. A. DePinho, and W. K. Cavenee. 2007. Malignant astrocytic glioma: genetics, biology, and paths to treatment. *Genes Dev* 21 (21):2683–710.

Furnari, F. B., H. J. Huang, and W. K. Cavenee. 1998. The phosphoinositol phosphatase activity of PTEN mediates a serum- sensitive G1 growth arrest in glioma cells. *Cancer Res* 58 (22):5002–8.

Furnari, F. B., H. Lin, H. S. Huang, and W. K. Cavenee. 1997. Growth suppression of glioma cells by PTEN requires a functional phosphatase catalytic domain. *Proc Natl Acad Sci USA* 94 (23):12479–84.

Gao, T., F. Furnari, and A. C. Newton. 2005. PHLPP: a phosphatase that directly dephosphorylates Akt, promotes apoptosis, and suppresses tumor growth. *Mol Cell* 18 (1):13–24.

Gil, A., A. Andres-Pons, E. Fernandez, M. Valiente, J. Torres, J. Cervera, and R. Pulido. 2006. Nuclear localization of PTEN by a Ran-dependent mechanism enhances apoptosis: Involvement of an N-terminal nuclear localization domain and multiple nuclear exclusion motifs. *Mol Biol Cell* 17 (9):4002–13.

Gimm, O., A. Perren, L. P. Weng, D. J. Marsh, J. J. Yeh, U. Ziebold, E. Gil, R. Hinze, L. Delbridge, J. A. Lees, G. L. Mutter, B. G. Robinson, P. Komminoth, H. Dralle, and C. Eng. 2000. Differential nuclear and cytoplasmic expression of PTEN in normal thyroid tissue, and benign and malignant epithelial thyroid tumors. *Am J Pathol* 156 (5):1693–700.

Goudar, R. K., Q. Shi, M. D. Hjelmeland, S. T. Keir, R. E. McLendon, C. J. Wikstrand, E. D. Reese, C. A. Conrad, P. Traxler, H. A. Lane, D. A. Reardon, W. K. Cavenee, X. F. Wang, D. D. Bigner, H. S. Friedman, and J. N. Rich. 2005. Combination therapy of inhibitors of epidermal growth factor receptor/vascular endothelial growth factor receptor 2 (AEE788) and the mammalian target of rapamycin (RAD001) offers improved glioblastoma tumor growth inhibition. *Mol Cancer Ther* 4 (1):101–12.

Greenman, C., P. Stephens, R. Smith, G. L. Dalgliesh, C. Hunter, G. Bignell, H. Davies, J. Teague, A. Butler, C. Stevens, S. Edkins, S. O'Meara, I. Vastrik, E. E. Schmidt, T. Avis, S. Barthorpe, G. Bhamra, G. Buck, B. Choudhury, J. Clements, J. Cole, E. Dicks, S. Forbes, K. Gray, K. Halliday, R. Harrison, K. Hills, J. Hinton, A. Jenkinson, D. Jones, A. Menzies, T. Mironenko, J. Perry, K. Raine, D. Richardson, R. Shepherd, A. Small, C. Tofts, J. Varian, T. Webb, S. West, S. Widaa, A. Yates, D. P. Cahill, D. N. Louis, P. Goldstraw, A. G. Nicholson, F. Brasseur, L. Looijenga, B. L. Weber, Y. E. Chiew, A. Defazio, M. F. Greaves, A. R. Green, P. Campbell, E. Birney, D. F. Easton, G. Chenevix-Trench, M. H. Tan, S. K. Khoo, B. T. Teh, S. T. Yuen, S. Y. Leung, R. Wooster, P. A. Futreal, and M. R. Stratton. 2007. Patterns of somatic mutation in human cancer genomes. *Nature* 446 (7132):153–8.

Grommes, C., G. E. Landreth, M. Sastre, M. Beck, D. L. Feinstein, A. H. Jacobs, U. Schlegel, and M. T. Heneka. 2006. Inhibition of in vivo glioma growth and invasion by peroxisome proliferator-activated receptor gamma agonist treatment. *Mol Pharmacol* 70 (5):1524–33.

Groszer, M., R. Erickson, D. D. Scripture-Adams, J. D. Dougherty, J. Le Belle, J. A. Zack, D. H. Geschwind, X. Liu, H. I. Kornblum, and H. Wu. 2006. PTEN negatively regulates neural stem cell self-renewal by modulating G0–G1 cell cycle entry. *Proc Natl Acad Sci USA* 103 (1):111–6.

Groszer, M., R. Erickson, D. D. Scripture-Adams, R. Lesche, A. Trumpp, J. A. Zack, H. I. Kornblum, X. Liu, and H. Wu. 2001. Negative regulation of neural stem/progenitor cell proliferation by the Pten tumor suppressor gene in vivo. *Science* 294 (5549):2186–9.

Guha, A. 1998. Ras activation in astrocytomas and neurofibromas. *Can J Neurol Sci* 25 (4):267–81.

Guillermet-Guibert, J., K. Bjorklof, A. Salpekar, C. Gonella, F. Ramadani, A. Bilancio, S. Meek, A. J. Smith, K. Okkenhaug, and B. Vanhaesebroeck. 2008. The p110beta isoform of phosphoinositide 3-kinase signals downstream of G protein-coupled receptors and is functionally redundant with p110gamma. *Proc Natl Acad Sci USA* 105 (24):8292–7.

Gulati, P., L. D. Gaspers, S. G. Dann, M. Joaquin, T. Nobukuni, F. Natt, S. C. Kozma, A. P. Thomas, and G. Thomas. 2008. Amino acids activate mTOR complex 1 via Ca2+/CaM signaling to hVps34. *Cell Metab* 7 (5):456–65.

Haas-Kogan, D. A., M. D. Prados, T. Tihan, D. A. Eberhard, N. Jelluma, N. D. Arvold, R. Baumber, K. R. Lamborn, A. Kapadia, M. Malec, M. S. Berger, and D. Stokoe. 2005. Epidermal growth factor receptor, protein kinase B/Akt, and glioma response to erlotinib. *J Natl Cancer Inst* 97 (12):880–7.

Hagerstrand, D., G. Hesselager, S. Achterberg, U. Wickenberg Bolin, M. Kowanetz, M. Kastemar, C. H. Heldin, A. Isaksson, M. Nister, and A. Ostman. 2006. Characterization of an imatinib-sensitive subset of high-grade human glioma cultures. *Oncogene* 25 (35):4913–22.

Hartmann, C., L. Devermann, C. Gehlhaar, N. Holtkamp, and A. von Deimling. 2006. PIK3CA mutations in oligodendroglial tumours. *Neuropathol Appl Neurobiol* 32 (2):209–12.

Heldin, C. H. 1996. Protein tyrosine kinase receptors. *Cancer Surv* 27:7–24.

Hemmati, H. D., I. Nakano, J. A. Lazareff, M. Masterman-Smith, D. H. Geschwind, M. Bronner-Fraser, and H. I. Kornblum. 2003. Cancerous stem cells can arise from pediatric brain tumors. *Proc Natl Acad Sci USA* 100 (25):15178–83.

Hermanson, M., K. Funa, M. Hartman, L. Claesson-Welsh, C. H. Heldin, B. Westermark, and M. Nister. 1992. Platelet-derived growth factor and its receptors in human glioma tissue: expression of messenger RNA and protein suggests the presence of autocrine and paracrine loops. *Cancer Res* 52 (11):3213–9.

Hettinger, K., F. Vikhanskaya, M. K. Poh, M. K. Lee, I. de Belle, J. T. Zhang, S. A. Reddy, and K. Sabapathy. 2007. c-Jun promotes cellular survival by suppression of PTEN. *Cell Death Differ* 14 (2):218–29.

Hlobilkova, A., P. Guldberg, M. Thullberg, J. Zeuthen, J. Lukas, and J. Bartek. 2000. Cell cycle arrest by the PTEN tumor suppressor is target cell specific and may require protein phosphatase activity. *Exp Cell Res* 256 (2):571–7.

Holland, E. C., W. P. Hively, R. A. DePinho, and H. E. Varmus. 1998. A constitutively active epidermal growth factor receptor cooperates with disruption of G1 cell-cycle arrest pathways to induce glioma-like lesions in mice. *Genes Dev* 12 (23):3675–85.

Huang, P. H., A. Mukasa, R. Bonavia, R. A. Flynn, Z. E. Brewer, W. K. Cavenee, F. B. Furnari, and F. M. White. 2007. Quantitative analysis of EGFRvIII cellular signaling networks reveals a combinatorial therapeutic strategy for glioblastoma. *Proc Natl Acad Sci USA* 104 (31):12867–72.

Hurtt, M. R., J. Moossy, M. Donovan-Peluso, and J. Locker. 1992. Amplification of epidermal growth factor receptor gene in gliomas: histopathology and prognosis. *J Neuropathol Exp Neurol* 51 (1):84–90.

Ikenoue, T., F. Kanai, Y. Hikiba, T. Obata, Y. Tanaka, J. Imamura, M. Ohta, A. Jazag, B. Guleng, K. Tateishi, Y. Asaoka, M. Matsumura, T. Kawabe, and M. Omata. 2005. Functional analysis of PIK3CA gene mutations in human colorectal cancer. *Cancer Res* 65 (11):4562–7.

Isakoff, S. J., J. A. Engelman, H. Y. Irie, J. Luo, S. M. Brachmann, R. V. Pearline, L. C. Cantley, and J. S. Brugge. 2005. Breast cancer-associated PIK3CA mutations are oncogenic in mammary epithelial cells. *Cancer Res* 65 (23):10992–1000.

James, C. D., E. Carlbom, J. P. Dumanski, M. Hansen, M. Nordenskjold, V. P. Collins, and W. K. Cavenee. 1988. Clonal genomic alterations in glioma malignancy stages. *Cancer Res* 48 (19):5546–51.

Jaros, E., R. H. Perry, L. Adam, P. J. Kelly, P. J. Crawford, R. M. Kalbag, A. D. Mendelow, R. P. Sengupta, and A. D. Pearson. 1992. Prognostic implications of p53 protein, epidermal growth factor receptor, and Ki-67 labelling in brain tumours. *Br J Cancer* 66 (2):373–85.

Jeuken, J., C. van den Broecke, S. Gijsen, S. Boots-Sprenger, and P. Wesseling. 2007. RAS/RAF pathway activation in gliomas: the result of copy number gains rather than activating mutations. *Acta Neuropathol* 114 (2):121–33.

Jou, S. T., N. Carpino, Y. Takahashi, R. Piekorz, J. R. Chao, N. Carpino, D. Wang, and J. N. Ihle. 2002. Essential, nonredundant role for the phosphoinositide 3-kinase p110delta in signaling by the B-cell receptor complex. *Mol Cell Biol* 22 (24):8580–91.

Karagiannidis, A. I., A. G. Bader, M. Hartl, and K. Bister. 2008. TOJ3, a v-jun target with intrinsic oncogenic potential, is directly regulated by Jun via a novel AP-1 binding motif. *Virology* 378 (2):371–376.

Karlbom, A. E., C. D. James, J. Boethius, W. K. Cavenee, V. P. Collins, M. Nordenskjold, and C. Larsson. 1993. Loss of heterozygosity in malignant gliomas involves at least three distinct regions on chromosome 10. *Hum Genet* 92 (2):169–74.

Khan, W. N., F. W. Alt, R. M. Gerstein, B. A. Malynn, I. Larsson, G. Rathbun, L. Davidson, S. Muller, A. B. Kantor, L. A. Herzenberg, and et al. 1995. Defective B cell development and function in Btk-deficient mice. *Immunity* 3 (3):283–99.

Kilic, T., J. A. Alberta, P. R. Zdunek, M. Acar, P. Iannarelli, T. O'Reilly, E. Buchdunger, P. M. Black, and C. D. Stiles. 2000. Intracranial inhibition of platelet-derived growth factor-mediated glioblastoma cell growth by an orally active kinase inhibitor of the 2-phenylaminopyrimidine class. *Cancer Res* 60 (18):5143–50.

Kita, D., Y. Yonekawa, M. Weller, and H. Ohgaki. 2007. PIK3CA alterations in primary (de novo) and secondary glioblastomas. *Acta Neuropathol (Berl)* 113 (3):295–302.

Kleihues, P., D. N. Louis, B. W. Scheithauer, L. B. Rorke, G. Reifenberger, P. C. Burger, and W. K. Cavenee. 2002. The WHO classification of tumors of the nervous system. *J Neuropathol Exp Neurol* 61 (3):215–25; discussion 226–9.

Knobbe, C. B., and G. Reifenberger. 2003. Genetic alterations and aberrant expression of genes related to the phosphatidyl-inositol-3'-kinase/protein kinase B (Akt) signal transduction pathway in glioblastomas. *Brain Pathol* 13 (4):507–18.

Knobbe, C. B., J. Reifenberger, B. Blaschke, and G. Reifenberger. 2004a. Hypermethylation and transcriptional downregulation of the carboxyl-terminal modulator protein gene in glioblastomas. *J Natl Cancer Inst* 96 (6):483–6.

Knobbe, C. B., J. Reifenberger, and G. Reifenberger. 2004b. Mutation analysis of the Ras pathway genes NRAS, HRAS, KRAS and BRAF in glioblastomas. *Acta Neuropathol (Berl)* 108 (6):467–70.

Knobbe, C. B., A. Trampe-Kieslich, and G. Reifenberger. 2005. Genetic alteration and expression of the phosphoinositol-3-kinase/Akt pathway genes PIK3CA and PIKE in human glioblastomas. *Neuropathol Appl Neurobiol* 31 (5):486–90.

Krutzik, P. O., and G. P. Nolan. 2006. Fluorescent cell barcoding in flow cytometry allows high-throughput drug screening and signaling profiling. *Nat Methods* 3 (5):361–8.

Kurosu, H., T. Maehama, T. Okada, T. Yamamoto, S. Hoshino, Y. Fukui, M. Ui, O. Hazeki, and T. Katada. 1997. Heterodimeric phosphoinositide 3-kinase consisting of p85 and p110beta is synergistically activated by the betagamma subunits of G proteins and phosphotyrosyl peptide. *J Biol Chem* 272 (39):24252–6.

Kwon, C. H., D. Zhao, J. Chen, S. Alcantara, Y. Li, D. K. Burns, R. P. Mason, E. Y. Lee, H. Wu, and L. F. Parada. 2008. Pten haploinsufficiency accelerates formation of high-grade astrocytomas. *Cancer Res* 68 (9):3286–94.

Kwon, C. H., X. Zhu, J. Zhang, L. L. Knoop, R. Tharp, R. J. Smeyne, C. G. Eberhart, P. C. Burger, and S. J. Baker. 2001. Pten regulates neuronal soma size: a mouse model of Lhermitte-Duclos disease. *Nat Genet* 29 (4):404–11.

Kwon, J., S. R. Lee, K. S. Yang, Y. Ahn, Y. J. Kim, E. R. Stadtman, and S. G. Rhee. 2004. Reversible oxidation and inactivation of the tumor suppressor PTEN in cells stimulated with peptide growth factors. *Proc Natl Acad Sci U S A* 101 (47):16419–24.

Lachyankar, M. B., N. Sultana, C. M. Schonhoff, P. Mitra, W. Poluha, S. Lambert, P. J. Quesenberry, N. S. Litofsky, L. D. Recht, R. Nabi, S. J. Miller, S. Ohta, B. G. Neel, and A. H. Ross. 2000. A role for nuclear PTEN in neuronal differentiation. *J Neurosci* 20 (4):1404–13.

Lee, J.O., H. Yang, M.-M. Georgescu, A. Di Christofano, T. Maehama, Y. Shi, J. E. Dixon, P. Pandolfi, and N. P. Pavletich. 1999. Crystal Structure of the PTEN Tumor Suppressor: Implications for Its Phosphoinositide Phosphatase Activity and Membrane Association. *Cell* 99:323–34.

Lee, S. R., K. S. Yang, J. Kwon, C. Lee, W. Jeong, and S. G. Rhee. 2002. Reversible inactivation of the tumor suppressor PTEN by H2O2. *J Biol Chem* 277 (23):20336–42.

Leslie, N. R., D. Bennett, Y. E. Lindsay, H. Stewart, A. Gray, and C. P. Downes. 2003. Redox regulation of PI 3-kinase signalling via inactivation of PTEN. *Embo J* 22 (20):5501–10.

Li, A. G., L. G. Piluso, X. Cai, G. Wei, W. R. Sellers, and X. Liu. 2006. Mechanistic insights into maintenance of high p53 acetylation by PTEN. *Mol Cell* 23 (4):575–87.

Li, D. M., and H. Sun. 1997. TEP1, encoded by a candidate tumor suppressor locus, is a novel protein tyrosine phosphatase regulated by transforming growth factor beta. *Cancer Res* 57 (11):2124–9.

Li, D. M., and H. Sun. 1998. PTEN/MMAC1/TEP1 suppresses the tumorigenicity and induces G1 cell cycle arrest in human glioblastoma cells. *Proc Natl Acad Sci USA* 95 (26):15406–11.

Li, J., C. Yen, D. Liaw, K. Podsypanina, S. Bose, S. I. Wang, J. Puc, C. Miliaresis, L. Rodgers, R. McCombie, S. H. Bigner, B. C. Giovanella, M. Ittmann, B. Tycko, H. Hibshoosh, M. H. Wigler, and R. Parsons. 1997. PTEN, a putative protein tyrosine phosphatase gene mutated in human brain, breast, and prostate cancer. *Science* 275 (5308):1943–7.

Li, Z., X. Dong, Z. Wang, W. Liu, N. Deng, Y. Ding, L. Tang, T. Hla, R. Zeng, L. Li, and D. Wu. 2005. Regulation of PTEN by Rho small GTPases. *Nat Cell Biol* 7 (4):399–404.

Liaw, D., D. J. Marsh, J. Li, P. L. Dahia, S. I. Wang, Z. Zheng, S. Bose, K. M. Call, H. C. Tsou, M. Peacocke, C. Eng, and R. Parsons. 1997. Germline mutations of the PTEN gene in Cowden disease, an inherited breast and thyroid cancer syndrome. *Nat Genet* 16 (1):64–7.

Liliental, J., S. Y. Moon, R. Lesche, R. Mamillapalli, D. Li, Y. Zheng, H. Sun, and H. Wu. 2000. Genetic deletion of the Pten tumor suppressor gene promotes cell motility by activation of Rac1 and Cdc42 GTPases. *Curr Biol* 10 (7):401–4.

Lindsay, Y., D. McCoull, L. Davidson, N. R. Leslie, A. Fairservice, A. Gray, J. Lucocq, and C. P. Downes. 2006. Localization of agonist-sensitive PtdIns(3,4,5)P3 reveals a nuclear pool that is insensitive to PTEN expression. *J Cell Sci* 119 (Pt 24):5160–8.

Liu, J. L., Z. Mao, T. A. LaFortune, M. M. Alonso, G. E. Gallick, J. Fueyo, and W. K. Yung. 2007. Cell cycle-dependent nuclear export of phosphatase and tensin homologue tumor suppressor is regulated by the phosphoinositide-3-kinase signaling cascade. *Cancer Res* 67 (22):11054–63.

Liu, W., C. D. James, L. Frederick, B. E. Alderete, and R. B. Jenkins. 1997. PTEN/MMAC1 mutations and EGFR amplification in glioblastomas. *Cancer Res* 57 (23):5254–7.

Lobo, G. P., K. A. Waite, S. M. Planchon, T. Romigh, J. A. Houghton, and C. Eng. 2008. ATP modulates PTEN subcellular localization in multiple cancer cell lines. *Hum Mol Genet* 17 (18):2877–2885.

Lokker, N. A., C. M. Sullivan, S. J. Hollenbach, M. A. Israel, and N. A. Giese. 2002. Platelet-derived growth factor (PDGF) autocrine signaling regulates survival and mitogenic pathways in glioblastoma cells: evidence that the novel PDGF-C and PDGF-D ligands may play a role in the development of brain tumors. *Cancer Res* 62 (13):3729–35.

Lu, Y., Q. Yu, J. H. Liu, J. Zhang, H. Wang, D. Koul, J. S. McMurray, X. Fang, W. K. Yung, K. A. Siminovitch, and G. B. Mills. 2003. Src family protein-tyrosine kinases alter the function of PTEN to regulate phosphatidylinositol 3-kinase/AKT cascades. *J Biol Chem* 278 (41):40057–66.

Luo, J., C. L. Sobkiw, N. M. Logsdon, J. M. Watt, S. Signoretti, F. O'Connell, E. Shin, Y. Shim, L. Pao, B. G. Neel, R. A. Depinho, M. Loda, and L. C. Cantley. 2005. Modulation of epithelial neoplasia and lymphoid hyperplasia in PTEN+/– mice by the p85 regulatory subunits of phosphoinositide 3-kinase. *Proc Natl Acad Sci USA* 102 (29):10238–43.

Maehama, T., and J. E. Dixon. 1998. The tumor suppressor, PTEN/MMAC1, dephosphorylates the lipid second messenger, phosphatidylinositol 3,4,5-trisphosphate. *J Biol Chem* 273 (22):13375–8.

Maier, D., D. Comparone, E. Taylor, Z. Zhang, O. Gratzl, E. G. Van Meir, R. J. Scott, and A. Merlo. 1997. New deletion in low-grade oligodendroglioma at the glioblastoma suppressor locus on chromosome 10q25-26. *Oncogene* 15 (8):997–1000.

Maier, D., G. Jones, X. Li, A. H. Schonthal, O. Gratzl, E. G. Van Meir, and A. Merlo. 1999. The PTEN lipid phosphatase domain is not required to inhibit invasion of glioma cells. *Cancer Res* 59 (21):5479–82.

Maier, D., Z. Zhang, E. Taylor, M. F. Hamou, O. Gratzl, E. G. Van Meir, R. J. Scott, and A. Merlo. 1998. Somatic deletion mapping on chromosome 10 and sequence analysis of PTEN/MMAC1 point to the 10q25-26 region as the primary target in low-grade and high-grade gliomas. *Oncogene* 16 (25):3331–5.

Maira, S. M., I. Galetic, D. P. Brazil, S. Kaech, E. Ingley, M. Thelen, and B. A. Hemmings. 2001. Carboxyl-terminal modulator protein (CTMP), a negative regulator of PKB/Akt and v-Akt at the plasma membrane. *Science* 294 (5541):374–80.

Manning, B. D., and L. C. Cantley. 2007. AKT/PKB signaling: navigating downstream. *Cell* 129 (7):1261–74.

Massion, P. P., W. L. Kuo, D. Stokoe, A. B. Olshen, P. A. Treseler, K. Chin, C. Chen, D. Polikoff, A. N. Jain, D. Pinkel, D. G. Albertson, D. M. Jablons, and J. W. Gray. 2002. Genomic copy number analysis of non-small cell lung cancer using array comparative genomic hybridization: implications of the phosphatidylinositol 3-kinase pathway. *Cancer Res* 62 (13):3636–40.

Mayo, L. D., J. E. Dixon, D. L. Durden, N. K. Tonks, and D. B. Donner. 2002. PTEN protects p53 from Mdm2 and sensitizes cancer cells to chemotherapy. *J Biol Chem* 277 (7):5484–9.

Mehrian-Shai, R., C. D. Chen, T. Shi, S. Horvath, S. F. Nelson, J. K. Reichardt, and C. L. Sawyers. 2007. Insulin growth factor-binding protein 2 is a candidate biomarker for PTEN status and PI3K/Akt pathway activation in glioblastoma and prostate cancer. *Proc Natl Acad Sci USA* 104 (13):5563–8.

Mellinghoff, I. K., M. Y. Wang, I. Vivanco, D. A. Haas-Kogan, S. Zhu, E. Q. Dia, K. V. Lu, K. Yoshimoto, J. H. Huang, D. J. Chute, B. L. Riggs, S. Horvath, L. M. Liau, W. K. Cavenee, P. N. Rao, R. Beroukhim, T. C. Peck, J. C. Lee, W. R. Sellers, D. Stokoe, M. Prados, T. F. Cloughesy, C. L. Sawyers, and P. S. Mischel. 2005. Molecular determinants of the response of glioblastomas to EGFR kinase inhibitors. *N Engl J Med* 353 (19):2012–24.

Meng, F., R. Henson, H. Wehbe-Janek, K. Ghoshal, S. T. Jacob, and T. Patel. 2007. MicroRNA-21 regulates expression of the PTEN tumor suppressor gene in human hepatocellular cancer. *Gastroenterology* 133 (2):647–58.

Milam, M. R., P. T. Soliman, L. H. Chung, K. M. Schmeler, R. L. Bassett, Jr., R. R. Broaddus, and K. H. Lu. 2007. Loss of phosphatase and tensin homologue deleted on chromosome 10 and phosphorylation of mammalian target of rapamycin are associated with progesterone refractory endometrial hyperplasia. *Int J Gynecol Cancer* 18 (1):146–151.

Mizoguchi, M., C. L. Nutt, G. Mohapatra, and D. N. Louis. 2004. Genetic alterations of phosphoinositide 3-kinase subunit genes in human glioblastomas. *Brain Pathol* 14 (4):372–7.

Moorehead, R. A., C. V. Hojilla, I. De Belle, G. A. Wood, J. E. Fata, E. D. Adamson, K. L. Watson, D. R. Edwards, and R. Khokha. 2003. Insulin-like growth factor-II regulates PTEN expression in the mammary gland. *J Biol Chem* 278 (50):50422–7.

Myers, M. P., I. Pass, I. H. Batty, J. Van der Kaay, J. P. Stolarov, B. A. Hemmings, M. H. Wigler, C. P. Downes, and N. K. Tonks. 1998. The lipid phosphatase activity of PTEN is critical for its tumor suppressor function [In Process Citation]. *Proc Natl Acad Sci USA* 95 (23):13513–8.

Myers, M. P., J. P. Stolarov, C. Eno, J. Li, S. I. Wang, M. H. Wigler, R. Parsons, and N. K. Tonks. 1997. P-TEN, the tumor suppressor from human chromosome 10q23, is a dual-specificity phosphatase. *Proc Natl Acad Sci* 94:9052–7.

Nagane, M., A. Levitzki, A. Gazit, W. K. Cavenee, and H. J. Huang. 1998. Drug resistance of human glioblastoma cells conferred by a tumor-specific mutant epidermal growth factor receptor through modulation of Bcl-XL and caspase-3-like proteases. *Proc Natl Acad Sci USA* 95 (10):5724–9.

Nagane, M., H. Lin, W. K. Cavenee, and H. J. Huang. 2001. Aberrant receptor signaling in human malignant gliomas: mechanisms and therapeutic implications. *Cancer Lett* 162 Suppl:S17–S21.

Nagata, Y., K. H. Lan, X. Zhou, M. Tan, F. J. Esteva, A. A. Sahin, K. S. Klos, P. Li, B. P. Monia, N. T. Nguyen, G. N. Hortobagyi, M. C. Hung, and D. Yu. 2004. PTEN activation contributes to tumor inhibition by trastuzumab, and loss of PTEN predicts trastuzumab resistance in patients. *Cancer Cell* 6 (2):117–27.

Narita, Y., M. Nagane, K. Mishima, H. J. Huang, F. B. Furnari, and W. K. Cavenee. 2002. Mutant epidermal growth factor receptor signaling down-regulates p27 through activation of the phosphatidylinositol 3-kinase/Akt pathway in glioblastomas. *Cancer Res* 62 (22):6764–9.

Nobukuni, T., M. Joaquin, M. Roccio, S. G. Dann, S. Y. Kim, P. Gulati, M. P. Byfield, J. M. Backer, F. Natt, J. L. Bos, F. J. Zwartkruis, and G. Thomas. 2005. Amino acids mediate mTOR/raptor signaling through activation of class 3 phosphatidylinositol 3OH-kinase. *Proc Natl Acad Sci USA* 102 (40):14238–43.

Nourry, C., S. G. Grant, and J. P. Borg. 2003. PDZ domain proteins: plug and play! *Sci STKE* 2003 (179):RE7.

Oda, K., D. Stokoe, Y. Taketani, and F. McCormick. 2005. High Frequency of Coexistent Mutations of PIK3CA and PTEN Genes in Endometrial Carcinoma. *Cancer Res* 65 (23):10669–73.

Odriozola, L., G. Singh, T. Hoang, and A. M. Chan. 2007. Regulation of PTEN activity by its carboxyl-terminal autoinhibitory domain. *J Biol Chem* 282 (32):23306–15.

Ohgaki, H., P. Dessen, B. Jourde, S. Horstmann, T. Nishikawa, P. L. Di Patre, C. Burkhard, D. Schuler, N. M. Probst-Hensch, P. C. Maiorka, N. Baeza, P. Pisani, Y. Yonekawa, M. G. Yasargil, U. M. Lutolf, and P. Kleihues. 2004. Genetic pathways to glioblastoma: a population-based study. *Cancer Res* 64 (19):6892–9.

Ohgaki, H., and P. Kleihues. 2005. Population-based studies on incidence, survival rates, and genetic alterations in astrocytic and oligodendroglial gliomas. *J Neuropathol Exp Neurol* 64 (6):479–89.

Ohgaki, H., and P. Kleihues. 2007. Genetic pathways to primary and secondary glioblastoma. *Am J Pathol* 170 (5):1445–53.

Okahara, F., K. Itoh, A. Nakagawara, M. Murakami, Y. Kanaho, and T. Maehama. 2006. Critical role of PICT-1, a tumor suppressor candidate, in phosphatidylinositol 3,4,5-trisphosphate signals and tumorigenic transformation. *Mol Biol Cell* 17 (11):4888–95.

Okkenhaug, K., A. Bilancio, G. Farjot, H. Priddle, S. Sancho, E. Peskett, W. Pearce, S. E. Meek, A. Salpekar, M. D. Waterfield, A. J. Smith, and B. Vanhaesebroeck. 2002. Impaired B and T cell antigen receptor signaling in p110delta PI 3-kinase mutant mice. *Science* 297 (5583):1031–4.

Okumura, K., M. Mendoza, R. M. Bachoo, R. A. DePinho, W. K. Cavenee, and F. B. Furnari. 2006. PCAF modulates PTEN activity. *J Biol Chem* 281 (36):26562–8.

Okumura, K., M. Zhao, R. A. Depinho, F. B. Furnari, and W. K. Cavenee. 2005. Cellular transformation by the MSP58 oncogene is inhibited by its physical interaction with the PTEN tumor suppressor. *Proc Natl Acad Sci USA* 102 (8):2703–6.

Pacold, M. E., S. Suire, O. Perisic, S. Lara-Gonzalez, C. T. Davis, E. H. Walker, P. T. Hawkins, L. Stephens, J. F. Eccleston, and R. L. Williams. 2000. Crystal structure and functional analysis of Ras binding to its effector phosphoinositide 3-kinase gamma. *Cell* 103 (6):931–43.

Pan, L., J. Lu, X. Wang, L. Han, Y. Zhang, S. Han, and B. Huang. 2007. Histone deacetylase inhibitor trichostatin a potentiates doxorubicin-induced apoptosis by up-regulating PTEN expression. *Cancer* 109 (8):1676–88.

Parcellier, A., L. A. Tintignac, E. Zhuravleva, and B. A. Hemmings. 2008. PKB and the mitochondria: AKTing on apoptosis. *Cell Signal* 20 (1):21–30.

Patel, L., I. Pass, P. Coxon, C. P. Downes, S. A. Smith, and C. H. MacPhee. 2001. Tumour suppressor and anti-inflammatory actions of PPARg agonists are mediated via upregulation of PTEN. *Current Biol* 11:764–8.

Peraud, A., K. Watanabe, K. Schwechheimer, Y. Yonekawa, P. Kleihues, and H. Ohgaki. 1999. Genetic profile of the giant cell glioblastoma. *Lab Invest* 79 (2):123–9.

Phillips, H. S., S. Kharbanda, R. Chen, W. F. Forrest, R. H. Soriano, T. D. Wu, A. Misra, J. M. Nigro, H. Colman, L. Soroceanu, P. M. Williams, Z. Modrusan, B. G. Feuerstein, and K. Aldape. 2006. Molecular subclasses of high-grade glioma predict prognosis, delineate a pattern of disease progression, and resemble stages in neurogenesis. *Cancer Cell* 9 (3):157–73.

Phung, T. L., K. Ziv, D. Dabydeen, G. Eyiah-Mensah, M. Riveros, C. Perruzzi, J. Sun, R. A. Monahan-Earley, I. Shiojima, J. A. Nagy, M. I. Lin, K. Walsh, A. M. Dvorak, D. M. Briscoe, M. Neeman, W. C. Sessa, H. F. Dvorak, and L. E. Benjamin. 2006. Pathological angiogenesis is induced by sustained Akt signaling and inhibited by rapamycin. *Cancer Cell* 10 (2):159–70.

Planchon, S. M., K. A. Waite, and C. Eng. 2008. The nuclear affairs of PTEN. *J Cell Sci* 121 (Pt 3):249–53.

Plate, K. H., G. Breier, C. L. Farrell, and W. Risau. 1992. Platelet-derived growth factor receptor-beta is induced during tumor development and upregulated during tumor progression in endothelial cells in human gliomas. *Lab Invest* 67 (4):529–34.

Puc, J., and R. Parsons. 2005. PTEN loss inhibits CHK1 to cause double stranded-DNA breaks in cells. *Cell Cycle* 4 (7):927–9.

Raftopoulou, M., S. Etienne-Manneville, A. Self, S. Nicholls, and A. Hall. 2004. Regulation of cell migration by the C2 domain of the tumor suppressor PTEN. *Science* 303 (5661):1179–81.

Ramos-Nino, M. E., C. D. MacLean, and B. Littenberg. 2007. Association between cancer prevalence and use of thiazolidinediones: results from the Vermont Diabetes Information System. *BMC Med* 5:17.

Rasheed, B. K., G. N. Fuller, A. H. Friedman, D. D. Bigner, and S. H. Bigner. 1992. Loss of heterozygosity for 10q loci in human gliomas. *Gene Chromosome Cancer* 5 (1):75–82.

Rasheed, B. K., T. T. Stenzel, R. E. McLendon, R. Parsons, A. H. Friedman, H. S. Friedman, D. D. Bigner, and S. H. Bigner. 1997. PTEN gene mutations are seen in high-grade but not in low-grade gliomas. *Cancer Res* 57 (19):4187–90.

Reardon, D. A., M. J. Egorin, J. A. Quinn, J. N. Rich, S. Gururangan, J. J. Vredenburgh, A. Desjardins, S. Sathornsumetee, J. M. Provenzale, J. E. Herndon, 2nd, J. M. Dowell, M. A. Badruddoja, R. E. McLendon, T. F. Lagattuta, K. P. Kicielinski, G. Dresemann, J. H. Sampson, A. H. Friedman, A. J. Salvado, and H. S. Friedman. 2005. Phase II study of imatinib mesylate plus hydroxyurea in adults with recurrent glioblastoma multiforme. *J Clin Oncol* 23 (36):9359–68.

Reis, R. M., D. Konu-Lebleblicioglu, J. M. Lopes, P. Kleihues, and H. Ohgaki. 2000. Genetic profile of gliosarcomas. *Am J Pathol* 156 (2):425–32.

Risinger, J. I., A. K. Hayes, A. Berchuck, and J. C. Barrett. 1997. PTEN/MMAC1 mutations in endometrial cancers. *Cancer Res* 57 (21):4736–8.

Rodriguez-Viciana, P., C. Sabatier, and F. McCormick. 2004. Signaling specificity by Ras family GTPases is determined by the full spectrum of effectors they regulate. *Mol Cell Biol* 24 (11):4943–54.

Rodriguez-Viciana, P., P. H. Warne, R. Dhand, B. Vanhaesebroeck, I. Gout, M. J. Fry, M. D. Waterfield, and J. Downward. 1994. Phosphatidylinositol-3-OH kinase as a direct target of Ras. *Nature* 370:527–32.

Rodriguez-Viciana, P., P. H. Warne, B. Vanhaesebroeck, M. D. Waterfield, and J. Downward. 1996. Activation of phosphoinositide 3-kinase by interaction with Ras and by point mutation. *EMBO J.* 15:2442–51.

Saal, L. H., K. Holm, M. Maurer, L. Memeo, T. Su, X. Wang, J. S. Yu, P. O. Malmstrom, M. Mansukhani, J. Enoksson, H. Hibshoosh, A. Borg, and R. Parsons. 2005. PIK3CA mutations correlate with hormone receptors, node metastasis, and ERBB2, and are mutually exclusive with PTEN loss in human breast carcinoma. *Cancer Res* 65 (7):2554–9.

Saal, L. H., P. Johansson, K. Holm, S. K. Gruvberger-Saal, Q. B. She, M. Maurer, S. Koujak, A. A. Ferrando, P. Malmstrom, L. Memeo, J. Isola, P. O. Bendahl, N. Rosen, H. Hibshoosh, M. Ringner, A. Borg, and R. Parsons. 2007. Poor prognosis in carcinoma is associated with a gene expression signature of aberrant PTEN tumor suppressor pathway activity. *Proc Natl Acad Sci USA* 104 (18):7564–9.

Saez, E., P. Tontonoz, M. C. Nelson, J. G. Alvarez, U. T. Ming, S. M. Baird, V. A. Thomazy, and R. M. Evans. 1998. Activators of the nuclear receptor PPARgamma enhance colon polyp formation. *Nat Med* 4 (9):1058–61.

Samuels, Y., Z. Wang, A. Bardelli, N. Silliman, J. Ptak, S. Szabo, H. Yan, A. Gazdar, S. M. Powell, G. J. Riggins, J. K. Willson, S. Markowitz, K. W. Kinzler, B. Vogelstein, and V. E. Velculescu. 2004. High frequency of mutations of the PIK3CA gene in human cancers. *Science* 304 (5670):554.

Sanger Center Catalogue of Somatic Mutations in Cancer (COSMIC).

Sanger Center: Distribution of somatic mutations in PTEN.

Sarbassov dos, D., D. A. Guertin, S. M. Ali, and D. M. Sabatini. 2005. Phosphorylation and regulation of Akt/PKB by the rictor-mTOR complex. *Science* 307 (5712):1098–101.

Schlegel, J., A. Merdes, G. Stumm, F. K. Albert, M. Forsting, N. Hynes, and M. Kiessling. 1994. Amplification of the epidermal-growth-factor-receptor gene correlates with different growth behaviour in human glioblastoma. *Int J Cancer* 56 (1):72–7.

Schmidt, E. E., K. Ichimura, H. M. Goike, A. Moshref, L. Liu, and V. P. Collins. 1999. Mutational profile of the PTEN gene in primary human astrocytic tumors and cultivated xenografts. *J Neuropathol Exp Neurol* 58 (11):1170–83.

Schulz, K. R., E. A. Danna, P. O. Krutzik, and G. P. Nolan. 2007. Single-cell phosphoprotein analysis by flow cytometry. *Curr Protoc Immunol* Chapter 8:Unit 8 17.

Shayesteh, L., Y. Lu, W. L. Kuo, R. Baldocchi, T. Godfrey, C. Collins, D. Pinkel, B. Powell, G. B. Mills, and J. W. Gray. 1999. PIK3CA is implicated as an oncogene in ovarian cancer. *Nat Genet* 21 (1):99–102.

Shen, W. H., A. S. Balajee, J. Wang, H. Wu, C. Eng, P. P. Pandolfi, and Y. Yin. 2007. Essential role for nuclear PTEN in maintaining chromosomal integrity. *Cell* 128 (1):157–70.

Shih, A. H., C. Dai, X. Hu, M. K. Rosenblum, J. A. Koutcher, and E. C. Holland. 2004. Dose-dependent effects of platelet-derived growth factor-B on glial tumorigenesis. *Cancer Res* 64 (14):4783–9.

Shih, A. H., and E. C. Holland. 2006. Platelet-derived growth factor (PDGF) and glial tumorigenesis. *Cancer Lett* 232 (2):139–47.

Shoman, N., S. Klassen, A. McFadden, M. G. Bickis, E. Torlakovic, and R. Chibbar. 2005. Reduced PTEN expression predicts relapse in patients with breast carcinoma treated by tamoxifen. *Mod Pathol* 18 (2):250–9.

Si, M. L., S. Zhu, H. Wu, Z. Lu, F. Wu, and Y. Y. Mo. 2007. miR-21-mediated tumor growth. *Oncogene* 26 (19):2799–803.

Silber, J., D. A. Lim, C. Petritsch, A. I. Persson, A. K. Maunakea, M. Yu, S. R. Vandenberg, D. G. Ginzinger, C. D. James, J. F. Costello, G. Bergers, W. A. Weiss, A. Alvarez-Buylla, and J. G. Hodgson. 2008. miR-124 and miR-137 inhibit proliferation of glioblastoma multiforme cells and induce differentiation of brain tumor stem cells. *BMC Med* 6:14.

Singh, S. K., I. D. Clarke, M. Terasaki, V. E. Bonn, C. Hawkins, J. Squire, and P. B. Dirks. 2003. Identification of a cancer stem cell in human brain tumors. *Cancer Res* 63 (18):5821–8.

Sjolander, A., and E. G. Lapetina. 1992. Agonist-induced association of the p21ras GTPase-activating protein with phosphatidylinositol 3-kinase. *Biochem Biophys Res Commun* 189 (3):1503–8.

Sjolander, A., K. Yamamoto, B. E. Huber, and E. G. Lapetina. 1991. Association of p21ras with phosphatidylinositol 3-kinase. *Proc Natl Acad Sci USA* 88 (18):7908–12.

Smith, J. S., I. Tachibana, S. M. Passe, B. K. Huntley, T. J. Borell, N. Iturria, J. R. O'Fallon, P. L. Schaefer, B. W. Scheithauer, C. D. James, J. C. Buckner, and R. B. Jenkins. 2001. PTEN mutation, EGFR amplification, and outcome in patients with anaplastic astrocytoma and glioblastoma multiforme. *J Natl Cancer Inst* 93 (16):1246–56.

Sordella, R., D. W. Bell, D. A. Haber, and J. Settleman. 2004. Gefitinib-sensitizing EGFR mutations in lung cancer activate anti-apoptotic pathways. *Science* 305 (5687):1163–7.

Stambolic, V., D. MacPherson, D. Sas, Y. Lin, B. Snow, Y. Jang, S. Benchimol, and T. W. Mak. 2001. Regulation of PTEN transcription by p53. *Mol Cell* 8 (2):317–25.

Stambolic, V., A. Suzuki, J. L. de la Pomps, G. M. Brothers, C. Mirtsos, T. Sasaki, J. Ruland, J. M. Penninger, D. P. Siderovski, and T. W. Mak. 1998. Negative Regulation of PKB/Akt-Dependent Cell Survival by the Tumor Suppressor PTEN. *Cell* 95:29–39.

Stan, A. C., S. Casares, D. Radu, G. F. Walter, and T. D. Brumeanu. 1999. Doxorubicin-induced cell death in highly invasive human gliomas. *Anticancer Res* 19 (2A):941–50.

Steck, P. A., M. A. Pershouse, S. A. Jasser, W. K. Yung, H. Lin, A. H. Ligon, L. A. Langford, M. L. Baumgard, T. Hattier, T. Davis, C. Frye, R. Hu, B. Swedlund, D. H. Teng, and S. V. Tavtigian. 1997. Identification of a candidate tumour suppressor gene, MMAC1, at chromosome 10q23.3 that is mutated in multiple advanced cancers. *Nat Genet* 15 (4):356–62.

Stephens, L. R., A. Eguinoa, H. Erdjument-Bromage, M. Lui, F. Cooke, J. Coadwell, A. S. Smrcka, M. Thelen, K. Cadwallader, P. Tempst, and P. T. Hawkins. 1997. The Gbg Sensitivity of a PI3K Is Dependent upon a Tightly Associated Adaptor, p101. *Cell* 89:105–14.
Stettner, M. R., W. Wang, L. B. Nabors, S. Bharara, D. C. Flynn, J. R. Grammer, G. Y. Gillespie, and C. L. Gladson. 2005. Lyn kinase activity is the predominant cellular SRC kinase activity in glioblastoma tumor cells. *Cancer Res* 65 (13):5535–43.
Stocker, H., M. Andjelkovic, S. Oldham, M. Laffargue, M. P. Wymann, B. A. Hemmings, and E. Hafen. 2002. Living with lethal PIP3 levels: viability of flies lacking PTEN restored by a PH domain mutation in Akt/PKB. *Science* 295 (5562):2088–91.
Stokoe, D., L. R. Stephens, T. Copeland, P. R. J. Gaffney, C. B. Reese, G. F. Painter, A. B. Holmes, F. McCormick, and P. T. Hawkins. 1997. Dual Role of Phosphatidylinositol-3,4,5-trisphosphate in the Activation of Protein Kinase B. *Science* 277:567–70.
Stommel, J. M., A. C. Kimmelman, H. Ying, R. Nabioullin, A. H. Ponugoti, R. Wiedemeyer, A. H. Stegh, J. E. Bradner, K. L. Ligon, C. Brennan, L. Chin, and R. A. DePinho. 2007. Coactivation of receptor tyrosine kinases affects the response of tumor cells to targeted therapies. *Science* 318 (5848):287–90.
Stoyanov, B., S. Volinia, T. Hanck, I. Rubio, M. Loubtchenkov, D. Malek, S. Stoyanova, B. Vanhaesebroeck, R. Dhand, B. Nurnberg, and et al. 1995. Cloning and characterization of a G protein-activated human phosphoinositide-3 kinase. *Science* 269 (5224):690–3.
Subauste, M. C., P. Nalbant, E. D. Adamson, and K. M. Hahn. 2005. Vinculin controls PTEN protein level by maintaining the interaction of the adherens junction protein beta-catenin with the scaffolding protein MAGI-2. *J Biol Chem* 280 (7):5676–81.
Suire, S., J. Coadwell, G. J. Ferguson, K. Davidson, P. Hawkins, and L. Stephens. 2005. p84, a new Gbetagamma-activated regulatory subunit of the type IB phosphoinositide 3-kinase p110gamma. *Curr Biol* 15 (6):566–70.
Suire, S., P. Hawkins, and L. Stephens. 2002. Activation of phosphoinositide 3-kinase gamma by Ras. *Curr Biol* 12 (13):1068–75.
Suzuki, H., Y. Terauchi, M. Fujiwara, S. Aizawa, Y. Yazaki, T. Kadowaki, and S. Koyasu. 1999. Xid-like immunodeficiency in mice with disruption of the p85alpha subunit of phosphoinositide 3-kinase. *Science* 283 (5400):390–2.
Tamguney, T., and D. Stokoe. 2007. New insights into PTEN. *J Cell Sci* 120 (Pt 23):4071–9.
Tamura, M., J. Gu, K. Matsumoto, S. Aota, R. Parsons, and K. M. Yamada. 1998. Inhibition of Cell Migration, Spreading, and Focal Adhesions by Tumor Supressor PTEN. *Science* 280:1614–7.
Tang, Y., and C. Eng. 2006. PTEN autoregulates its expression by stabilization of p53 in a phosphatase-independent manner. *Cancer Res* 66 (2):736–42.
Terauchi, Y., Y. Tsuji, S. Satoh, H. Minoura, K. Murakami, A. Okuno, K. Inukai, T. Asano, Y. Kaburagi, K. Ueki, H. Nakajima, T. Hanafusa, Y. Matsuzawa, H. Sekihara, Y. Yin, J. C. Barrett, H. Oda, T. Ishikawa, Y. Akanuma, I. Komuro, M. Suzuki, K. Yamamura, T. Kodama, H. Suzuki, T. Kadowaki, and et al. 1999. Increased insulin sensitivity and hypoglycaemia in mice lacking the p85 alpha subunit of phosphoinositide 3-kinase. *Nat Genet* 21 (2):230–5.
Tohma, Y., C. Gratas, W. Biernat, A. Peraud, M. Fukuda, Y. Yonekawa, P. Kleihues, and H. Ohgaki. 1998. PTEN (MMAC1) mutations are frequent in primary glioblastomas (de novo) but not in secondary glioblastomas. *J Neuropathol Exp Neurol* 57 (7):684–9.
Torres, J., and R. Pulido. 2001. The tumor suppressor PTEN is phosphorylated by the protein kinase CK2 at its C terminus. Implications for PTEN stability to proteasome- mediated degradation. *J Biol Chem* 276 (2):993–8.
Tortosa, A., Y. Ino, N. Odell, S. Swilley, H. Sasaki, D. N. Louis, and J. W. Henson. 2000. Molecular genetics of radiographically defined de novo glioblastoma multiforme. *Neuropathol Appl Neurobiol* 26 (6):544–52.

Trotman, L. C., X. Wang, A. Alimonti, Z. Chen, J. Teruya-Feldstein, H. Yang, N. P. Pavletich, B. S. Carver, C. Cordon-Cardo, H. Erdjument-Bromage, P. Tempst, S. G. Chi, H. J. Kim, T. Misteli, X. Jiang, and P. P. Pandolfi. 2007. Ubiquitination Regulates PTEN Nuclear Import and Tumor Suppression. *Cell* 128 (1):141–56.

Vanhaesebroeck, B., S. J. Leevers, K. Ahmadi, J. Timms, R. Katso, P. C. Driscoll, R. Woscholski, P. J. Parker, and M. D. Waterfield. 2001. Synthesis and function of 3-phosphorylated inositol lipids. *Annu Rev Biochem* 70:535–602.

Vasudevan, K. M., R. Burikhanov, A. Goswami, and V. M. Rangnekar. 2007. Suppression of PTEN expression is essential for antiapoptosis and cellular transformation by oncogenic Ras. *Cancer Res* 67 (21):10343–50.

Vazquez, F., S. R. Grossman, Y. Takahashi, M. V. Rokas, N. Nakamura, and W. R. Sellers. 2001. Phosphorylation of the PTEN tail acts as an inhibitory switch by preventing its recruitment into a protein complex. *J Biol Chem* 276 (52):48627–30.

Vazquez, F., S. Matsuoka, W. R. Sellers, T. Yanagida, M. Ueda, and P. N. Devreotes. 2006. Tumor suppressor PTEN acts through dynamic interaction with the plasma membrane. *Proc Natl Acad Sci USA* 103 (10):3633–8.

Vazquez, F., S. Ramaswamy, N. Nakamura, and W. R. Sellers. 2000. Phosphorylation of the PTEN tail regulates protein stability and function. *Mol Cell Biol* 20 (14):5010–8.

Venter, D. J., and D. G. Thomas. 1991. Multiple sequential molecular abnormalities in the evolution of human gliomas. *Br J Cancer* 63 (5):753–7.

Virolle, T., E. D. Adamson, V. Baron, D. Birle, D. Mercola, T. Mustelin, and I. de Belle. 2001. The Egr-1 transcription factor directly activates PTEN during irradiation-induced signalling. *Nat Cell Biol* 3 (12):1124–8.

von Deimling, A., D. N. Louis, K. von Ammon, I. Petersen, T. Hoell, R. Y. Chung, R. L. Martuza, D. A. Schoenfeld, M. G. Yasargil, O. D. Wiestler, and et al. 1992. Association of epidermal growth factor receptor gene amplification with loss of chromosome 10 in human glioblastoma multiforme. *J Neurosurg* 77 (2):295–301.

Voulgaris, S., M. Partheni, M. Karamouzis, P. Dimopoulos, N. Papadakis, and H. P. Kalofonos. 2002. Intratumoral doxorubicin in patients with malignant brain gliomas. *Am J Clin Oncol* 25 (1):60–4.

Walker, S. M., N. R. Leslie, N. M. Perera, I. H. Batty, and C. P. Downes. 2004. The tumour-suppressor function of PTEN requires an N-terminal lipid-binding motif. *Biochem J* 379 (Pt 2):301–7.

Wang, M. Y., K. V. Lu, S. Zhu, E. Q. Dia, I. Vivanco, G. M. Shackleford, W. K. Cavenee, I. K. Mellinghoff, T. F. Cloughesy, C. L. Sawyers, and P. S. Mischel. 2006. Mammalian Target of Rapamycin Inhibition Promotes Response to Epidermal Growth Factor Receptor Kinase Inhibitors in PTEN-Deficient and PTEN-Intact Glioblastoma Cells. *Cancer Res* 66 (16):7864–9.

Wang, X., L. C. Trotman, T. Koppie, A. Alimonti, Z. Chen, Z. Gao, J. Wang, H. Erdjument-Bromage, P. Tempst, C. Cordon-Cardo, P. P. Pandolfi, and X. Jiang. 2007. NEDD4-1 Is a Proto-Oncogenic Ubiquitin Ligase for PTEN. *Cell* 128 (1):129–39.

Wei, Q., L. Clarke, D. K. Scheidenhelm, B. Qian, A. Tong, N. Sabha, Z. Karim, N. A. Bock, R. Reti, R. Swoboda, E. Purev, J. F. Lavoie, M. L. Bajenaru, P. Shannon, D. Herlyn, D. Kaplan, R. M. Henkelman, D. H. Gutmann, and A. Guha. 2006. High-grade glioma formation results from postnatal pten loss or mutant epidermal growth factor receptor expression in a transgenic mouse glioma model. *Cancer Res* 66 (15):7429–37.

Wen, P. Y., W. K. Yung, K. R. Lamborn, P. L. Dahia, Y. Wang, B. Peng, L. E. Abrey, J. Raizer, T. F. Cloughesy, K. Fink, M. Gilbert, S. Chang, L. Junck, D. Schiff, F. Lieberman, H. A. Fine, M. Mehta, H. I. Robins, L. M. DeAngelis, M. D. Groves, V. K. Puduvalli, V. Levin, C. Conrad, E. A. Maher, K. Aldape, M. Hayes, L. Letvak, M. J. Egorin, R. Capdeville, R. Kaplan, A. J. Murgo, C. Stiles, and M. D. Prados. 2006.

Phase I/II study of imatinib mesylate for recurrent malignant gliomas: North American Brain Tumor Consortium Study 99–08. *Clin Cancer Res* 12 (16):4899–907.

Weng, L. P., J. L. Brown, and C. Eng. 2001. PTEN coordinates G(1) arrest by down-regulating cyclin D1 via its protein phosphatase activity and up-regulating p27 via its lipid phosphatase activity in a breast cancer model. *Hum Mol Genet* 10 (6):599–604.

Westermark, B., C. H. Heldin, and M. Nister. 1995. Platelet-derived growth factor in human glioma. *Glia* 15 (3):257–63.

Whitman, M., C. P. Downes, M. Keeler, T. Keller, and L. Cantley. 1988. Type I phosphatidylinositol kinase makes a novel inositol phospholipid, phosphatidylinositol-3-phosphate. *Nature* 332 (6165):644–6.

Wiencke, J. K., S. Zheng, N. Jelluma, T. Tihan, S. Vandenberg, T. Tamguney, R. Baumber, R. Parsons, K. R. Lamborn, M. S. Berger, M. R. Wrensch, D. A. Haas-Kogan, and D. Stokoe. 2007. Methylation of the PTEN promoter defines low-grade gliomas and secondary glioblastoma. *Neuro Oncol* 9 (3):271–9.

Wong, E. S., C. W. Fong, J. Lim, P. Yusoff, B. C. Low, W. Y. Langdon, and G. R. Guy. 2002. Sprouty2 attenuates epidermal growth factor receptor ubiquitylation and endocytosis, and consequently enhances Ras/ERK signalling. *Embo J* 21 (18):4796–808.

Wood, L. D., D. W. Parsons, S. Jones, J. Lin, T. Sjoblom, R. J. Leary, D. Shen, S. M. Boca, T. Barber, J. Ptak, N. Silliman, S. Szabo, Z. Dezso, V. Ustyanksky, T. Nikolskaya, Y. Nikolsky, R. Karchin, P. A. Wilson, J. S. Kaminker, Z. Zhang, R. Croshaw, J. Willis, D. Dawson, M. Shipitsin, J. K. Willson, S. Sukumar, K. Polyak, B. H. Park, C. L. Pethiyagoda, P. V. Pant, D. G. Ballinger, A. B. Sparks, J. Hartigan, D. R. Smith, E. Suh, N. Papadopoulos, P. Buckhaults, S. D. Markowitz, G. Parmigiani, K. W. Kinzler, V. E. Velculescu, and B. Vogelstein. 2007. The Genomic Landscapes of Human Breast and Colorectal Cancers. *Science* 318 (5853):1108–1113.

Xia, D., H. Srinivas, Y. H. Ahn, G. Sethi, X. Sheng, W. K. Yung, Q. Xia, P. J. Chiao, H. Kim, P. H. Brown, Wistuba, II, B. B. Aggarwal, and J. M. Kurie. 2007. Mitogen-activated protein kinase kinase-4 promotes cell survival by decreasing PTEN expression through an NF kappa B-dependent pathway. *J Biol Chem* 282 (6):3507–19.

Xiao, A., H. Wu, P. P. Pandolfi, D. N. Louis, and T. Van Dyke. 2002. Astrocyte inactivation of the pRb pathway predisposes mice to malignant astrocytoma development that is accelerated by PTEN mutation. *Cancer Cell* 1 (2):157–68.

Xiao, A., C. Yin, C. Yang, A. Di Cristofano, P. P. Pandolfi, and T. Van Dyke. 2005. Somatic induction of Pten loss in a preclinical astrocytoma model reveals major roles in disease progression and avenues for target discovery and validation. *Cancer Res* 65 (12):5172–80.

Xiao, C., L. Srinivasan, D. P. Calado, H. C. Patterson, B. Zhang, J. Wang, J. M. Henderson, J. L. Kutok, and K. Rajewsky. 2008. Lymphoproliferative disease and autoimmunity in mice with increased miR-17-92 expression in lymphocytes. *Nat Immunol* 9 (4):405–14.

Yan, X., M. Fraser, Q. Qiu, and B. K. Tsang. 2006. Over-expression of PTEN sensitizes human ovarian cancer cells to cisplatin-induced apoptosis in a p53-dependent manner. *Gynecol Oncol* 102 (2):348–55.

Yang, H., W. Kong, L. He, J. J. Zhao, J. D. O'Donnell, J. Wang, R. M. Wenham, D. Coppola, P. A. Kruk, S. V. Nicosia, and J. Q. Cheng. 2008. MicroRNA expression profiling in human ovarian cancer: miR-214 induces cell survival and cisplatin resistance by targeting PTEN. *Cancer Res* 68 (2):425–33.

Yang, J., P. Cron, V. M. Good, V. Thompson, B. A. Hemmings, and D. Barford. 2002. Crystal structure of an activated Akt/protein kinase B ternary complex with GSK3-peptide and AMP-PNP. *Nat Struct Biol* 9 (12):940–4.

Yang, J., P. Cron, V. Thompson, V. M. Good, D. Hess, B. A. Hemmings, and D. Barford. 2002. Molecular mechanism for the regulation of protein kinase b/akt by hydrophobic motif phosphorylation. *Mol Cell* 9 (6):1227–40.

Yilmaz, O. H., R. Valdez, B. K. Theisen, W. Guo, D. O. Ferguson, H. Wu, and S. J. Morrison. 2006. Pten dependence distinguishes haematopoietic stem cells from leukaemia-initiating cells. *Nature* 441 (7092):475–82.

Yim, J. H., Y. J. Kim, J. H. Ko, Y. E. Cho, S. M. Kim, J. Y. Kim, S. Lee, and J. H. Park. 2007. The putative tumor suppressor gene GLTSCR2 induces PTEN-modulated cell death. *Cell Death Differ* 14 (11):1872–9.

Zbuk, K. M., and C. Eng. 2007. Cancer phenomics: RET and PTEN as illustrative models. *Nat Rev Cancer* 7 (1):35–45.

Zhang, J., J. C. Grindley, T. Yin, S. Jayasinghe, X. C. He, J. T. Ross, J. S. Haug, D. Rupp, K. S. Porter-Westpfahl, L. M. Wiedemann, H. Wu, and L. Li. 2006. PTEN maintains haematopoietic stem cells and acts in lineage choice and leukaemia prevention. *Nature* 441 (7092):518–22.

Zhou, X. P., Y. J. Li, K. Hoang-Xuan, P. Laurent-Puig, K. Mokhtari, M. Longy, M. Sanson, J. Y. Delattre, G. Thomas, and R. Hamelin. 1999. Mutational analysis of the PTEN gene in gliomas: molecular and pathological correlations. *Int J Cancer* 84 (2):150–4.

Zhu, Y., F. Guignard, D. Zhao, L. Liu, D. K. Burns, R. P. Mason, A. Messing, and L. F. Parada. 2005. Early inactivation of p53 tumor suppressor gene cooperating with NF1 loss induces malignant astrocytoma. *Cancer Cell* 8 (2):119–30.

Chapter 16
Value of 1p/19q and Other LOH Markers for Brain Tumor Diagnosis, Prognosis, and Therapy

Jean-Louis Boulay and Adrian Merlo

Abstract Gliomas frequently show allelic loss of chromosomes 1p and 19q, suggesting the existence of one or more tumor suppressor loci in these genomic segments. Attempts, based mostly on somatic deletion mapping, to identify candidate glioma suppressor genes have focused on the telomeric region of 1p and on chromosome band 19q13. Although telomeric 1p represents a deletion hotspot, it shows no association with patient outcome. In fact, a favorable clinical outcome is linked with centromeric *NOTCH2* loss in both oligodendroglioma (ODG) and glioblastoma (GBM), raising the question of a role of Notch2 in gliomagenesis. While targeting the same gene, 1p deletion patterns are distinct between ODG and GBM in terms of extension, frequency, and association with 19q loss. Centromeric 1p deletion patterns can therefore be used for genetic diagnosis, prognosis, and prediction of response to therapy.

Contents

J.-L. Boulay (✉)
Laboratory of Neuro-Oncology, Department of Biomedicine and Neurosurgery, University Hospital, Basel, CH-4031, Switzerland
e-mail: jean-louis.boulay@unibas.ch

E.G. Van Meir (ed.), *CNS Cancer*, Cancer Drug Discovery and Development, DOI 10.1007/978-1-60327-553-8_16,
© Humana Press, a part of Springer Science+Business Media, LLC 2009

16.1 Introduction

Median survival time of glioma patients varies from less than 12 months in the most aggressive WHO grade IV glioblastoma (GBM) (Ohgaki and Kleihues 2005) to 10 years in WHO grade II oligodendroglioma (ODG) (Reifenberger et al. 1994, Shaw et al. 1992). Even within one histological subtype of glioma, the course of the disease can be highly variable. In fact, the outcome is highly dependent on the genetic background of the tumor (Ohgaki and Kleihues 2005). For these reasons, molecular markers are expected to improve our understanding of the natural course of the disease, to refine diagnosis and prognosis, and to predict response to therapeutic interventions (Merlo 2003, Reifenberger and Louis 2003).

ODG shows frequent (>80%) loss of heterozygosity (LOH) on the entire chromosome 1p, in association with 19q allelic loss (Reifenberger et al. 1994, Bigner et al. 1999). In most, but not all studies, the deletion frequency on chromosome 1p equals the deletion frequency on 19q. This manifest co-deletion results from an unbalanced translocation t(1;19)(q10;p10) in 81% of ODGs (Griffin et al. 2006, Jenkins et al. 2006). 1p/19q allelic loss is associated with a more favorable prognosis for ODG and is considered to be a predictive factor for response to radio- and chemotherapy in ODG WHO grade III (Cairncross et al. 2006, Mirimanoff et al. 2006).

In this manuscript, we review the evidence supporting a role for 1p/19q as a clinical marker, the biology underlying the subgroup of tumors which carry these markers, and the candidate genes that may be involved. Evidence for a role of the *NOTCH2* gene on 1p as a relevant candidate is presented.

16.2 1p/19q Loss Is Associated with Response to Therapy in Grade III Gliomas

The evidence for a role of 1p/19q loss in grade III gliomas derives from several large studies. A large multicenter study on 289 patients compared surgery and radiotherapy with and without early chemotherapy on anaplastic ODG or anaplastic oligoastrocytoma with assessment of 1p and 19q allelic losses. Although highly beneficial in patients with 1p/19q loss, chemotherapy was attenuated by significant toxicity in patients with 1p/19q retention. It was concluded that tumors lacking 1p and 19q alleles are less aggressive, more responsive, or both (Cairncross et al. 2006). On the basis of this study, a singular 1p arm loss, or combined loss of chromosomal arms 1p and 19q, has been considered to represent a good and reliable marker for ODG WHO grade III in two respects. First, because 1p/19q loss appeared to be linked to patient survival, it may serve as a prognostic marker. Secondly, since 1p/19q loss was associated with favorable chemotherapy responsiveness, it may also serve as a predictive marker.

In a retrospective study on 208 glioma WHO grades II and III patients, 1p/19q loss was found in about 80% of ODG, 42% of oligoastrocytomas, and above 20% in astrocytomas. On multivariate analyses, chromosome 1p was found to be a prognostic factor for prolonged progression-free survival in grade II regardless of histologic subtype (Iwamoto et al. 2008).

The value of 1p/19q co-deletion as marker of favorable response to therapy for oligodendroglial tumors is generally accepted in the neuro-oncology field. However, some issues regarding the prognostic value of the 1p/19q deletion remain unresolved, perhaps due to uncertainties on the precise mapping of the regions of loss (Weller et al. 2007). Nevertheless, 1p or 1p/19q allelic loss is being increasingly used to estimate the prognosis in ODG patients. Whether these genetic alterations can reliably be used as predictive factor to guide therapeutic intervention in ODG patients remains open to debate.

16.3 Is There a Common Prognostic Denominator in GBM and ODG on Chromosome 1p?

Bearing in mind the classical Knudson hypothesis where a hemizygous deletion of the wild-type allele unmasks the remaining mutant allele (Knudson 2001), the interpretation that an allelic loss predicts a more favorable outcome is counterintuitive. A genetic loss, which is selected during tumor progression, is not expected to improve survival. However, the genetic alteration may point to an early event in tumorigenesis. This would imply that the 1p/19q genetic alteration represents involvement of genetic pathways that impact on tumor biology in a less aggressive form. It was hypothesized that the consistent deletion on 1p/19q is linked to a distinct pathway of glioma development that is biochemically very different from those oligodendroglial tumors which show a much more aggressive clinical course of the disease. In other words, the 1p/19q deletion is likely to define a subgroup of gliomas possessing a tumor biology entirely different from the smaller subgroup of oligodendroglial tumors that retain both arms on chromosomes 1p and 19q. Since prognosis can also vary considerably in GBM, a genetic link between the more favorable GBM and ODG displaying 1p/19q loss was hypothesized. This hypothesis prompted a large somatic deletion mapping study in which chromosome 1p and also partially 19q were scanned for common deletion patterns and correlated with the clinical course.

The concept that a certain genetic alteration is very tightly linked to prognosis by defining a biochemical pathway is further supported by the observation that within ODG, a predominating 1p loss (81%) was found to mutually exclude a *TP53* mutation (13%) (Reifenberger 1994, Bigner et al. 1999). *TP53* mutations are oncogenic and major effectors of chemo-resistance in tumors of a wide range of cell lineages (Soussi and Lozano 2005). This suggests that 1p loss drives gliomagenesis through a less aggressive pathway than, for example, the p53 pathway. It is significant that ODG with 1p loss shows a genetic profile distinct from other ODG, as assessed by a microarray gene expression study (Mukasa et al. 2002).

16.4 The Search for 1p Glioma Suppressor Genes

The deletions on chromosome 1p span the entire short arm (Bigner et al. 1999, Smith et al. 1999), which covers 120 megabases (Mb) and therefore contains a vast number of potential tumor suppressor genes. Moreover, the structural complexity of chromosome 1, which has only recently been resolved by a very intense sequencing effort (Gregory et al. 2006), had long been a serious obstacle for fine mapping in the search for new disease genes, including tumor suppressor genes.

Telomeric 1p has been found to be a deletion target in malignancies of various lineages, including those of neural, hematopoietic, and epithelial origins. A comprehensive compilation of somatic deletions in this area is provided by Bagchi and Mills (2008). Early somatic deletion mapping on chromosome 1p in ODG revealed two distinct regions of loss, one located on 1p36.3 and another on 1p34–35 (Husemann et al. 1999). However, further refined deletion mapping on 1p34.2-tel only disclosed a few non-overlapping partial deletions (Felsberg et al. 2004).

The 1p36.3 gene *TP73*, encoding a structural homolog of p53 was suggested as a candidate. However, no mutations were detected by sequencing of 20 ODG samples (Mai et al. 1998). Based on the findings of another mapping study, a minimal area of loss located on 1p36.2 was described to contain the transcription factor gene *CAMTA1,* proposed as a candidate ODG suppressor gene (Barbashina et al. 2005). However, sequencing of 10 primary tumor samples did not reveal mutations of the candidate gene *CAMTA1.* Two further candidate genes have been proposed to be involved in oligodendrogliomagenesis. Amongst several genes exposed by the allelic loss at chromosome 1p32, there are the genes coding for the DNA helicase RAD54 and the cyclin-dependent kinase inhibitor $p18^{INK4C}$. However, no mutations were found within the coding sequence of the RAD54 gene in the 25 tumor samples analyzed (Bello et al. 2000), and only a single somatic mutation changing GAA (glutamic acid) into TAA (ochre) at codon 113 of the *CDKN2C* reading frame was detected at a frequency not exceeding the background mutation rate of cancer cells (Husemann et al. 1999). Also, the *ras*-related tumor suppressor gene *DIRAS3*, located at 1p31, was shown to be frequently inactivated by epigenetic silencing in oligodendroglial tumors with 1p loss (Riemenschneider et al. 2008).

Finally, in agreement with a 1p deletion mapping study performed on glioma cell lines (Law et al. 2005), functional mapping of 1p36.22-32 allowed the identification of the gene for the chromodomain helicase DNA binding domain 5 (CHD5) as a positive regulator of p53-mediated pathways (Bagchi et al. 2007). However, since 1p loss was found to mutually exclude a *TP53* mutation, a suppressor gene candidate positively regulating p53 function cannot be considered a good tumor suppressor gene candidate for ODG.

Based on the observation that the telomeric region of chromosome 1p is deleted in about 80% of ODG, the search for glioma tumor suppressor genes has focused on the distal 1p region. However, since the deletion patterns in tumors span the entire short arm of chromosome 1, it is conceivable that the putative tumor suppressor region may have a more centromeric location. All mapping efforts have not yet convincingly identified a gene candidate that is frequently involved in the genesis of ODG.

The finding of large deletions involving the entire 1p arm could mean that several genes need to be lost simultaneously for tumor development. Alternatively, the cause underlying the large deletions observed may be simply structural, as the finding of the translocation t(1;19)(q10;p10) in many ODG suggests. A purely structural argument would preclude the need for an additional telomeric gene as target of recombination.

16.5 The Search for 19q Glioma Suppressor Genes

Chromosome 19 is documented as a specific target for genetic alterations in gliomas (von Deimling et al. 1992) and to a lower extent in ovarian carcinoma (Bicher et al. 1997). The long arm of chromosome 19 is 33-Mb long. Early attempts to delimit the 19q tumor suppressor locus in primary brain tumor biopsies identified a 5-Mb region at 19q13.2-3 (Rubio et al. 1994). This region is still recognized as the major 19q site targeted in gliomas. The region contains several putative suppressor genes, including the DNA repair/DNA metabolism genes *ERCC1, ERCC2, and LIGI* (Rubio et al. 1994). However, these candidates have been excluded by further narrowing down the minimal region of loss to 425 kilobases (kb) (Yong et al. 1995). Within the 5-Mb region, another 900 kb more telomeric interval has been defined (Rosenberg et al. 1996) and from which the *BAX* gene has been excluded as candidate, due to lack of mutations (Chou et al. 1996). Further, another non-overlapping and more distal minimal area of 150 kb has been defined within the 19q13.3 5-Mb segment (Smith et al. 2000).

Using fluorescence in situ hybridization (FISH) probes and supported by microsatellite marker mapping, the breakpoints of primary gliomas with 19q13.3 deletion boundaries were shown to overlap the area delimited by a study performed on cell lines (Law et al. 2005) and the most distal region described above (von Deimling et al. 1992). In addition, silencing of the 19q13.3 gene for the myelin-related epithelial membrane protein 3 (EMP3) by promoter methylation (Alaminos et al. 2005) was found to be associated with 19q loss in oligodendrocytic, but not in astrocytic gliomas, rendering EMP3 a reasonable candidate gene (Kunitz et al. 2007). The issue of glioma suppressor genes on 19q is, however, not yet resolved.

16.6 Fine Mapping of the Deletions in the 1p Arm Reveals that Loss of the Centromeric 1p Region/Area Correlates with Survival in ODG and GBM

In an effort to further refine the location of tumor suppressor(s) located on 1p by comparing deletion profiles between GBM and ODG, a genetic mapping effort involving 3 translational research centers was performed on a total number of 144 tumors (26 ODG and 118 GBM). The chromosome 1p deletion profile was compared between ODG and primary GBM by constructing an extensive 1p somatic deletion map (Fig. 16.1). Three main conclusions emerged from this study. First, in ODG, 1p loss was highly prevalent (81%), was complete and involved the entire 1p arm, and was virtually always combined with 19q loss. Second, in GBM, loss of chromosome 1p was less frequent (32%), usually partial, and was not systematically associated with 19q loss (Fig 16.1), but rather randomly distributed among tumors displaying either retention or deletion on chromosome 1p. Third, four deletion hotspots were detected in GBM: two telomeric (1p36.3 and 1p36.1), one interstitial (1p22), and one centromeric (1p11), with 1p36.3 loss being the most frequent 1p loss in GBM (Fig 16.1).

Analysis of these deletion profiles for impact on survival revealed that chromosome 1p loss in ODG is associated with favorable prognosis. In GBM, interstitial 1p loss is a marker for poor survival with earlier onset of

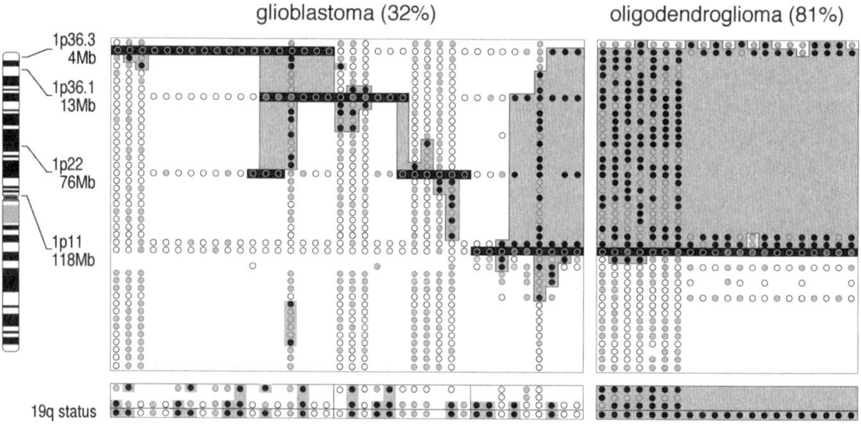

Fig. 16.1 Comparative 1p somatic deletion mapping between GBM and OG. 118 GBM and 26 ODG were analyzed at 43 chromosome 1p and 1q markers (*horizontal lines*). GBM and ODG with 1p LOH are shown. Conclusions on the 19q status are shown below the data from three individual chromosome 19q markers. Vertical columns show results for individual patients. *Open circles*: retention of both parental alleles, *filled circles*: allelic loss, *grey circles*: non-informative data. Deleted areas are shown in grey; deletion hotspots are highlighted in black. Chromosome bands and distances from 1pTel of 1p deletion hotspots are indicated on the left; 1p deletion frequencies are shown at the top

disease, centromeric loss is a marker for better survival, and despite its highest frequency in GBM, telomeric loss has no significant relevance (Boulay et al. 2007). It is noteworthy that loss of the potential telomeric glioma suppressor loci cited above, although all located within the most frequently deleted 1p region in GBM, have no impact on survival. In contrast, centromeric 1p loss appears to be a favorable genetic indicator in a manner analogous to 1p/19q loss in ODG. This suggests a tumor suppressor locus commonly inactivated in both ODG and GBM.

16.7 Gene Mapping Within the Chromosome 1 Pericentric Duplication

The chromosome 1p centromere contains a pericentric duplication, which consists of a 150-kb sequence originating from the 1p11 region duplicated into the 1q21 region, such that chromosome 1 centromere is surrounded by highly similar sequences in opposite orientations (Fig. 16.2, left panel). The duplicated sequence contains the 5' region of the *NOTCH2* gene, forming in 1q21 a new gene called the *NOTCH2 N-terminal (N2N)* gene (Duan et al. 2004). Detailed somatic deletion mapping in the centromeric region of 1p has been complicated by the presence of this duplication. Genomic duplication with a high degree of sequence conservation may render a genetic locus susceptible to rearrangements, such as nonallelic homologous recombination or possibly translocations (Turner et al. 2008). To overcome this problem, a genetic test based on intra-chromosomal dosage between the duplicated areas has been developed. This test, designated "N2/N2N test", evaluates gene copy balance between the duplicated regions by exploiting the sequence polymorphisms between the 1p11 region and its 1q21 duplication (Fig 16.2).

The N2/N2N test reveals a minimally lost area in GBM and homozygous deletions in ODG that both converge to the *NOTCH2* gene (Boulay et al. 2007). Interestingly, *Notch2* hemizygous mice fail to develop a subset of B cells (Saito et al. 2003). Likewise, during *Drosophila* development *Notch* haploidy leads to an expanded population of neuroblasts at the expense of epidermis cells, thereby mimicking loss of Notch function (Heitzler and Simpson 1991). This suggests that haplo-insufficency is a conserved mechanism of *Notch* down-regulation throughout evolution and raises the possibility that *Notch2* haplo-insuffiency may be involved in the disease phenotype, including brain tumorigenesis in mammals.

The N2/N2N test delimits a breakpoint area common to ODG located *between* duplicated segments, while GBM have breakpoints *distal* to the duplicated segments (Fig. 16.2). Thus, the N2/N2N test, besides refining 1p mapping in gliomas, permits the genetic distinction between ODG and GBM with 1p loss and, therefore, has potential utility for diagnostic, prognostic, and predictive purposes. This needs to be further validated in prospective studies.

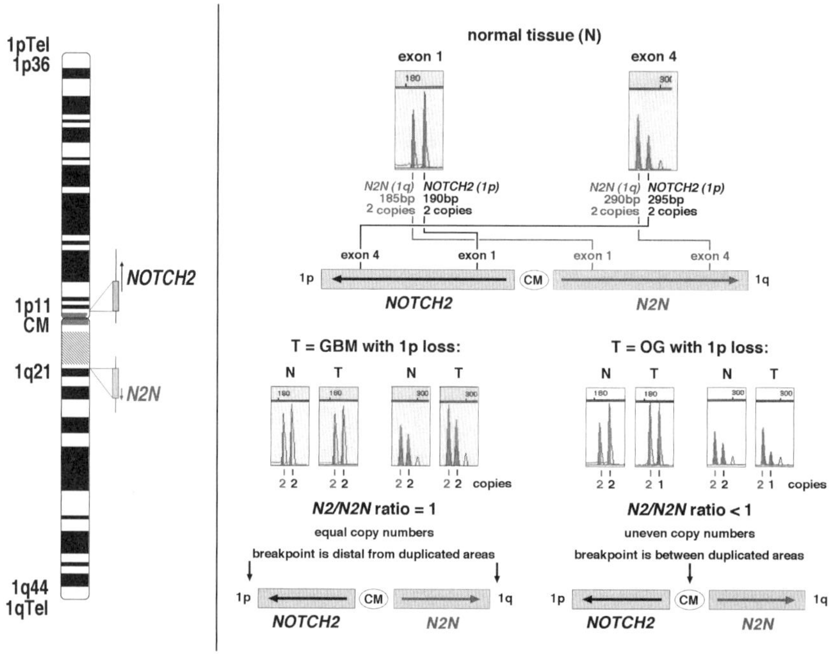

Fig. 16.2 Principle of the N2/N2N assay. *Left panel*. Ideogram of chromosome 1 with enlargement of the N2 and N2N duplicated areas that surround the centromere (CM) and the heterochromatine block on 1q (hatched). The duplicated region is 150-kb long and contains 50 kb of the 5' part of the 150-kb long *NOTCH2* (*N2*) gene on 1p, and basically the whole *Notch2 N-terminal*(*N2N*) gene on 1q. *Right panel*. Comparison between sequences of the *NOTCH2* region (1p11) and *N2N* region (1q21) revealed a few deletion polymorphisms. Primers were designed to amplify such polymorphisms so that *NOTCH2* and *N2N* products can be recognized by size (exon1: 190 bp in *NOTCH2* and 185 bp in *N2N*; exon4: 295 bp in *NOTCH2* and 290 bp in *N2N*). Under semi-quantitative conditions, peak height reflects copy number of the template. Ratio between DNAs extracted from glial tumor (T) and from normal lymphocytes from the same donor (N) allows calculation of local copy number in tumor relative to normal diploidy in germline DNA. When compiled with conventional 1p/1q LOH data, this allows accurate somatic deletion mapping within and between the duplicated areas. Adapted from Boulay et al. 2007 *PLoS ONE* **2**:e576

16.8 ROC Analysis for 1p and Prognosis Shows that N2/N2N Analysis Is Superior to Histology

Compared to conventional telomeric 1p and 19q genetic markers, the use of the N2/N2N markers considerably increases accuracy, expressed as area under the curve (AUC) of receiver operating characteristics (ROC) analysis, with regard to prognosis (Fig 16.3).

The explanation for this marked improvement with an AUC of nearly 95% is that gliomas incidentally having both telomeric 1p loss and 19q loss due to severe genomic instability are retained as false positives with conventional

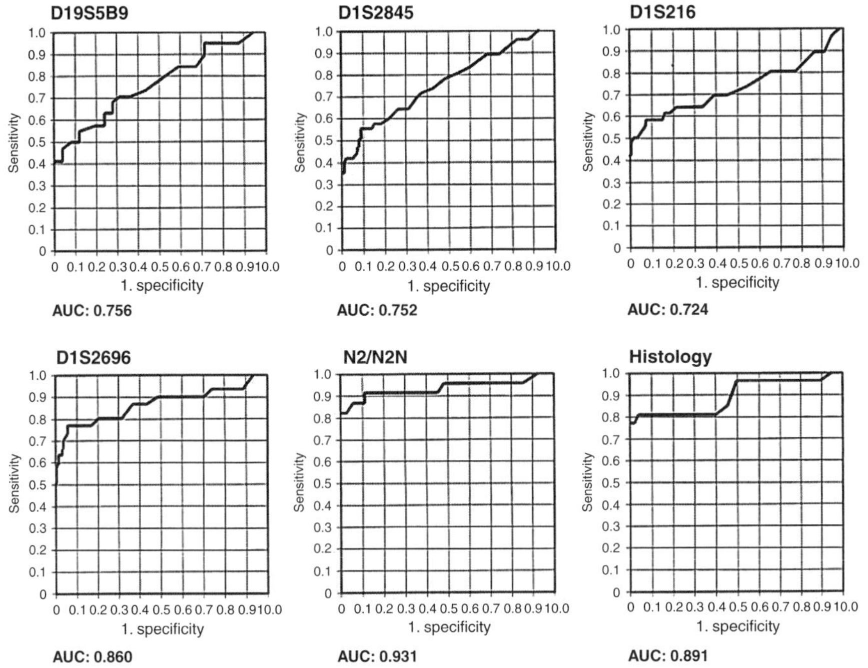

Fig. 16.3 Receiver operating characteristics (ROC) analysis of 1p markers. Prognostic value of D19S589 (19q13), D1S2845 (1p36), D1S216 (1p22), D1S2696 (1p11), N2/N2N (pericentric 1p11-q21) genetic markers, and histology. Compared to more telomeric 1p markers, the 1p centromeric marker D1S2696 selects ODG and GBM with more favorable patient outcome and excludes false positive with more telomeric 1p deletions associated with worse prognosis. D1S2696 shows therefore higher reliability to predict patient outcome, as expressed by an area under the curve (AUC) closer to 1 (0.860), compared to more telomeric 1p markers D1S2845 and D1S216 (0.752 and 0.724, respectively). 19q marker D19S589 identifies GBM with 19q loss together with ODG with 1p/19q loss; its reliability therefore is also lower (0.756) than that of D1S2696 (0.860). This indirectly suggests that 19q loss in absence of association with t(1;19)(q10;p10) may not impact on survival. While D1S2696 selects both ODG with 1p/19q loss and GBM with centromeric 1p loss, the N2/N2N test exclusively selects ODG with 1p/19q, those with the most favorable outcome, resulting in the highest AUC (0.931). Finally, compared to histology, which selects ODG regardless of their genetic background, N2/N2N test only identifies ODG with combined 1p/19q loss which have been found to harbor the translocation t(1;19)(q10;p10) (7,8). This is reflected by a higher AUC for the N2/N2N test (0.931) vs. histology (0.891). From Boulay et al. 2007 *PLoS ONE* **2**:e576

markers, but they are identified as an arbitrary co-deletion and therefore discarded with N2/N2N assay. This supports previous observations that telomeric and interstitial markers on chromosome 1p cannot be linked with more favorable outcome and suggests that 19q per se may not impact on survival loss, irrespective of the 1p status, except in cases with the translocation t(1;19)(q10;p10). Moreover, considering that ODG with 1p/19q loss has by far the longest survival, also compared to ODG with 1p/19q retention (Fig16.4), the prognostic value of the N2/N2N test turns out to be higher

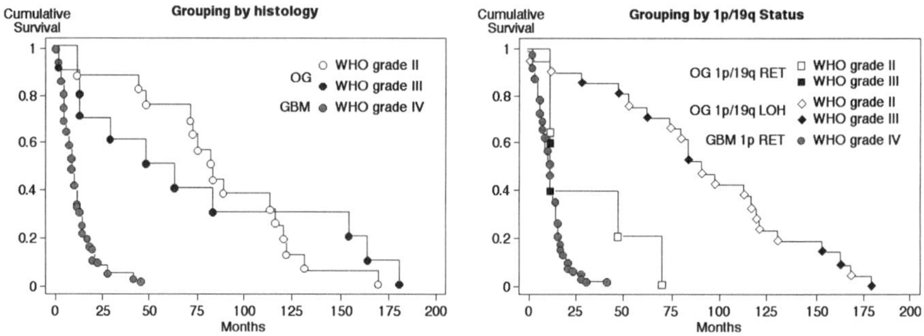

Fig. 16.4 1p/19q status of ODG is superior to tumor grading for evaluation of patient survival. On the left graph, cumulative survival curves do not very well delineate prognosis in ODG if the focus is put on the WHO grading system. However, by focusing on the 1p/19q genetic status, there is a significant difference in survival times. Interestingly, 1p/19q retention in ODG is associated with a tumor behavior, not much different from GBM with 1p retention. From Boulay et al. 2007 *PLoS ONE* **2**:e576

than histological examination, which cannot distinguish between the two molecular subsets of ODG. In sum, the combined status *NOTCH2* and N2/N2N classifies gliomas firstly by identifying those with 1p centromeric loss, regardless of histology, as the ones with better outcome and secondly, among them, by segregating between GBM and ODG.

16.9 An Oncogenic Role of Notch2 in Gliomagenesis?

As shown above, ODG and GBM that have a common loss at the *NOTCH2* locus have a more favorable prognosis relative to tumors with no *NOTCH2* loss. This raises the possibility that gliomas with 1p loss and a positive N2/N2N-assay – targeting either *NOTCH2* or an adjacent gene, or both – may be less aggressive than those gliomas that retain or even have amplified the *NOTCH2* locus and express Notch2 (Sivasankaran et al. 2009).

During normal murine brain development, *Notch2*is expressed in the cerebellar external granule layer and subventricular zones, where it maintains proliferation and prevents differentiation of neuronal precursor cells (Solecki et al. 2001). Notch2 expression in postnatal brain is restricted to ventricular germinal zones and dividing immature glial cells (Tanaka and Marunouchi 2003). These observations suggest that Notch2 may play a role in the maintenance of glial cells in an undifferentiated state. Homozygous Notch2-deficient mutant mice consistently show intense apoptosis in neural tissue normally expressing Notch2 at embryonic day 9.5 (E9.5). This leads to embryonic lethality at E11.5–E12.5 (Hamada et al. 1999), suggesting a role for Notch2 in maintaining the survival of developing cells of the neural lineage. Interestingly, expression of Notch2 protein can frequently be detected in GBM by immunohistochemistry and western blotting. On the other hand, most ODG do not express Notch2 protein (Sivasankaran et al. 2009). Opposition between Notch2 statuses in both glioma types suggests a functional linkage, especially since the prognosis of these 2 tumor types is so fundamentally different. These observations are further supported by the finding that the gene promoters of nestin, a marker for neural precursors and of tenascin-C, an effector of cell migration during development, both expressed in GBM, are both activated by Notch signaling (Shih and Holland 2006; Sivasankaran et al. 2009). The involvement of Notch2, however, is complex, since *HES-1* – a Notch signaling target – drives astrocytic cell fate at the expense of oligodendrocytic differentiation (Wu et al. 2003). It is not clear how long, and to what extent, Notch2 is involved in normal glial cell maturation and differentiation or in gliomagenesis.

Thus, besides Notch2 being a marker for the differentiation status of glioma, it is conceivable that Notch2 also plays a role in the promotion of gliomagenesis. Identification of effectors of gliomagenesis transactivated or indirectly up- or down-regulated by Notch signaling would be of help to support this theory.

16.10 Conclusion

In summary, loss at the *NOTCH2* locus is a predictor of longer survival in subtypes of ODG and GBM and suggests involvement/engagement of less aggressive Notch2-independent pathways. Conversely, gain of Notch2 is associated with less differentiated and more malignant forms of astrocytomas and GBM. In either case the gain or loss of Notch2 expression conveys a tumor phenotype. This invokes dual functions for *NOTCH2* in gliomagenesis, namely as an oncogene or as a tumor suppressor gene, depending on the cellular context as demonstrated for *NOTCH1* (Radtke and Raj 2003).

Abbreviations

AUC	area under the curve
GBM	glioblastoma
kb	kilobase
LOH	loss of heterozygosity
Mb	megabase
N2	Notch2
N2N	Notch2 N-terminal
ODG	oligodendroglioma
ROC	receiver operating characteristics
WHO	World Health Organization

Acknowledgments Supported by Oncosuisse (OCS-01613-12-2004) and Krebsliga beider Basel (Nr. 7 2004). We are grateful to Elisabeth Taylor and Therese Resink for critical reading of the manuscript.

References

Alaminos M, Davalos V, Ropero S, et al. EMP3, a myelin-related gene located in the critical 19q13.3 region, is epigenetically silenced and exhibits features of a candidate tumor suppressor in glioma and neuroblastoma. Cancer Res 2005;65(7):2565–71.

Bagchi A, Mills AA. The quest for the 1p36 tumor suppressor. Cancer Res 2008;68(8):2551–6.

Bagchi A, Papazoglu C, Wu Y, et al. CHD5 is a tumor suppressor at human 1p36. Cell 2007;128(3):459–75.

Barbashina V, Salazar P, Holland EC, Rosenblum MK, Ladanyi M. Allelic losses at 1p36 and 19q13 in gliomas: correlation with histologic classification, definition of a 150 kb minimal deleted region on 1p36, and evaluation of CAMTA1 as a candidate tumor suppressor gene. Clin Cancer Res 2005;11(3):1119–28.

Bello MJ, de Campos JM, Vaquero J, et al. hRAD54 gene and 1p high-resolution deletion-mapping analyses in oligodendrogliomas. Cancer Genet Cytogenet 2000;116(2):142–7.

Bicher A, Ault K, Kimmelman A, Gershenson D, Reed E, Liang B. Loss of heterozygosity in human ovarian cancer on chromosome 19q. Gynecol Oncol 1997;66(1):36–40.

Bigner SH, Matthews MR, Rasheed BK, et al. Molecular genetic aspects of oligodendrogliomas including analysis by comparative genomic hybridization. Am J Pathol 1999;155(2):375–86.

Boulay JL, Miserez AR, Zweifel C, et al. Loss of NOTCH2 positively predicts survival in subgroups of human glial brain tumors. PLoS ONE 2007;2(6):e576.

Cairncross G, Berkey B, Shaw E, et al. Phase III trial of chemotherapy plus radiotherapy compared with radiotherapy alone for pure and mixed anaplastic oligodendroglioma: Intergroup Radiation Therapy Oncology Group Trial 9402. J Clin Oncol 2006;24(18):2707–14.

Chou D, Miyashita T, Mohrenweiser HW, et al. The BAX gene maps to the glioma candidate region at 19q13.3, but is not altered in human gliomas. Cancer Genet Cytogenet 1996;88(2):136–40.

Duan Z, Li FQ, Wechsler J, et al. A novel notch protein, N2N, targeted by neutrophil elastase and implicated in hereditary neutropenia. Mol Cell Biol 2004;24(1):58–70.

Felsberg J, Erkwoh A, Sabel MC, et al. Oligodendroglial tumors: refinement of candidate regions on chromosome arm 1p and correlation of 1p/19q status with survival. Brain Pathol 2004;14(2):121–30.

Gregory SG, Barlow KF, McLay KE, et al. The DNA sequence and biological annotation of human chromosome 1. Nature 2006;441(7091):315–21.

Griffin CA, Burger P, Morsberger L, et al. Identification of der(1;19)(q10;p10) in five oligodendrogliomas suggests mechanism of concurrent 1p and 19q loss. J Neuropathol Exp Neurol 2006;65(10):988–94.

Hamada Y, Kadokawa Y, Okabe M, Ikawa M, Coleman JR, Tsujimoto Y. Mutation in ankyrin repeats of the mouse Notch2 gene induces early embryonic lethality. Development 1999;126(15):3415–24.

Heitzler P, Simpson P. The choice of cell fate in the epidermis of Drosophila. Cell 1991;64(6):1083–92.

Husemann K, Wolter M, Buschges R, Bostrom J, Sabel M, Reifenberger G. Identification of two distinct deleted regions on the short arm of chromosome 1 and rare mutation of the CDKN2C gene from 1p32 in oligodendroglial tumors. J Neuropathol Exp Neurol 1999;58(10):1041–50.

Iwamoto FM, Nicolardi L, Demopoulos A, et al. Clinical relevance of 1p and 19q deletion for patients with WHO grade 2 and 3 gliomas. J Neurooncol 2008;88(3):293–8.

Jenkins RB, Blair H, Ballman KV, et al. A t(1;19)(q10;p10) mediates the combined deletions of 1p and 19q and predicts a better prognosis of patients with oligodendroglioma. Cancer Res 2006;66(20):9852–61.

Knudson AG. Two genetic hits (more or less) to cancer. Nat Rev Cancer 2001;1(2):157–62.

Kunitz A, Wolter M, van den Boom J, et al. DNA hypermethylation and aberrant expression of the EMP3 gene at 19q13.3 in Human Gliomas. Brain Pathol 2007;17(4):363–70.
Law ME, Templeton KL, Kitange G, et al. Molecular cytogenetic analysis of chromosomes 1 and 19 in glioma cell lines. Cancer Genet Cytogenet 2005;160(1):1–14.
Mai M, Huang H, Reed C, et al. Genomic organization and mutation analysis of p73 in oligodendrogliomas with chromosome 1 p-arm deletions. Genomics 1998;51(3):359–63.
Merlo A. Genes and pathways driving glioblastomas in humans and murine disease models. Neurosurg Rev 2003;26(3):145–58.
Mirimanoff RO, Gorlia T, Mason W, et al. Radiotherapy and temozolomide for newly diagnosed glioblastoma: recursive partitioning analysis of the EORTC 26981/22981-NCIC CE3 phase III randomized trial. J Clin Oncol 2006;24(16):2563–9.
Mukasa A, Ueki K, Matsumoto S, et al. Distinction in gene expression profiles of oligodendrogliomas with and without allelic loss of 1p. Oncogene 2002;21(25):3961–8.
Ohgaki H, Kleihues P. Population-based studies on incidence, survival rates, and genetic alterations in astrocytic and oligodendroglial gliomas. J Neuropathol Exp Neurol 2005; 64(6):479–89.
Radtke F, Raj K. The role of Notch in tumorigenesis: oncogene or tumour suppressor? Nat Rev Cancer 2003;3(10):756–67.
Reifenberger G, Louis DN. Oligodendroglioma: toward molecular definitions in diagnostic neuro-oncology. J Neuropathol Exp Neurol 2003;62(2):111–26.
Reifenberger J, Reifenberger G, Liu L, James CD, Wechsler W, Collins VP. Molecular genetic analysis of oligodendroglial tumors shows preferential allelic deletions on 19q and 1p. Am J Pathol 1994;145(5):1175–90.
Riemenschneider MJ, Reifenberger J, Reifenberger G. Frequent biallelic inactivation and transcriptional silencing of the DIRAS3 gene at 1p31 in oligodendroglial tumors with 1p loss. Int J Cancer 2008;122(11):2503–10.
Rosenberg JE, Lisle DK, Burwick JA, et al. Refined deletion mapping of the chromosome 19q glioma tumor suppressor gene to the D19S412-STD interval. Oncogene 1996;13(11): 2483–5.
Rubio MP, Correa KM, Ueki K, et al. The putative glioma tumor suppressor gene on chromosome 19q maps between APOC2 and HRC. Cancer Res 1994;54(17):4760–3.
Saito T, Chiba S, Ichikawa M, et al. Notch2 is preferentially expressed in mature B cells and indispensable for marginal zone B lineage development. Immunity 2003;18(5): 675–85.
Shaw EG, Scheithauer BW, O'Fallon JR, Tazelaar HD, Davis DH. Oligodendrogliomas: the Mayo Clinic experience. J Neurosurg 1992;76(3):428–34.
Shih AH, Holland EC. Notch signaling enhances nestin expression in gliomas. Neoplasia 2006;8(12):1072–82.
Sivasankaran B, Degen M, Ghaffari A, Hegi ME, Hamou MF, Ionescu MCS, Zweifel C, Tolnay M, Wasner M, Mergenthaler S, Miserez AR, Kiss R, Lino MM, Merlo A, Chiquet-Ehrismann R & Boulay JL. Tenascin-C is a novel RBPJk-induced target gene for Notch signaling in gliomas. Cancer Res 2009; 69(2): 458–465.
Smith JS, Alderete B, Minn Y, et al. Localization of common deletion regions on 1p and 19q in human gliomas and their association with histological subtype. Oncogene 1999;18(28): 4144–52.
Smith JS, Tachibana I, Lee HK, et al. Mapping of the chromosome 19 q-arm glioma tumor suppressor gene using fluorescence in situ hybridization and novel microsatellite markers. Genes Chromosomes Cancer 2000;29(1):16–25.
Solecki DJ, Liu XL, Tomoda T, Fang Y, Hatten ME. Activated Notch2 signaling inhibits differentiation of cerebellar granule neuron precursors by maintaining proliferation. Neuron 2001;31(4):557–68.
Soussi T, Lozano G. p53 mutation heterogeneity in cancer. Biochem Biophys Res Commun 2005;331(3):834–42.

Tanaka M, Marunouchi T. Immunohistochemical localization of Notch receptors and their ligands in the postnatally developing rat cerebellum. Neurosci Lett 2003;353(2):87–90.

Turner DJ, Miretti M, Rajan D, et al. Germline rates of de novo meiotic deletions and duplications causing several genomic disorders. Nat Genet 2008;40(1):90–5.

von Deimling A, Louis DN, von Ammon K, Petersen I, Wiestler OD, Seizinger BR. Evidence for a tumor suppressor gene on chromosome 19q associated with human astrocytomas, oligodendrogliomas, and mixed gliomas. Cancer Res 1992;52(15):4277–9.

Weller M, Berger H, Hartmann C, et al. Combined 1p/19q loss in oligodendroglial tumors: predictive or prognostic biomarker? Clin Cancer Res 2007;13(23):6933–7.

Wu Y, Liu Y, Levine EM, Rao MS. Hes1 but not Hes5 regulates an astrocyte versus oligodendrocyte fate choice in glial restricted precursors. Dev Dyn 2003;226(4):675–89.

Yong WH, Chou D, Ueki K, et al. Chromosome 19q deletions in human gliomas overlap telomeric to D19S219 and may target a 425 kb region centromeric to D19S112. J Neuropathol Exp Neurol 1995;54(5):622–6.

Chapter 17
Discovery of Genetic Markers for Brain Tumors by Comparative Genomic Hybridization

Anjan Misra and Burt G. Feuerstein

Abstract The use of DNA microarrays for surveys of cancer genome has grown exponentially in the last few years. So far, array comparative genomic hybridization (aCGH) has been the most powerful tool for studies of DNA copy number. Array CGH, together with other genome-wide profiling techniques such as expression and methylation profiling, along with follow-up biological studies, has yielded important insights ranging from simple DNA copy number information in a tumor to novel oncogene and tumor suppressor gene discoveries. This chapter traces, from a strategic and scientific perspective, aCGH's role in the discovery of genetic markers for brain tumors.

Contents

17.1 Historical Perspective

Comparative Genomic Hybridization (CGH) was conceived at the University of California, San Francisco in the early 1990s (Kallioniemi et al., 1992). Since then, different forms of CGH have been the most popular effective method for

A. Misra (✉)
Barrow Neurological Institute, St. Joseph's Hospital and Medical Center, Phoenix, AZ, USA
e-mail: anjan.misra@chw.edu

E.G. Van Meir (ed.), *CNS Cancer*, Cancer Drug Discovery and Development, DOI 10.1007/978-1-60327-553-8_17,

© Humana Press, a part of Springer Science+Business Media, LLC 2009

detecting genome-wide DNA copy number, especially in cancer research, resulting in more than 3000 publications.

The first generation of CGH used probes made from tumor and sex-matched control DNA, labeled with two different fluorescent colors, and hybridized together to normal human metaphase spreads. The ratios of test and control colors along each chromosome were plotted to represent chromosomal regions with DNA copy number gain or loss for all chromosomes (Kallioniemi et al., 1992). However, limited resolution of CGH, along with required expertise in identifying each chromosome correctly from metaphase spread, posed a significant challenge. Six years later, the same investigators came up with array CGH (aCGH, Pinkel et al., 1998) to address both of these concerns. To hybridize the tumor and normal genome probes, aCGH replaced the human metaphase spread with an array of spotted DNA from individual bacterial artificial chromosomes (BAC) on a glass slide. This process was later mechanized (Snijders et al., 2001), and paved the road for spotting an array of ~32000 BACs, tiling the whole genome (Ishkanian et al., 2004). Each BAC is unique and represents a 50–200 Kb length of human genome. Using one such array for each sample would, in principle, detect most copy number gains and losses in a sample throughout the entire genome; small gains and losses would be undetected. Different aCGH platforms have different resolution. Among commercially available platforms, resolution varies from 50 Kb to ~1 – 1.4 Mb. But custom arrays can be made with overlapping BACs or oligonucleotides to literally cover a region of interest, no matter how big. Since exons are part of cDNA, and mammalian genes have both exons and introns, in theory a cDNA microarray can be used for DNA copy number measurements. However, although the Stanford DNA microarray group used cDNA microarray (Pollack et al., 1999) for aCGH, few others did.

The next advance was oligonucleotide array for DNA copy number analysis, which used arrays that were initially designed to study single nucleotide polymorphisms (Bignell et al., 2004; Huang et al., 2004). Over time, after the human genome sequence was assembled and better algorithms for probe design were available, some oligonucleotide arrays were claimed to work better for detecting DNA copy number than for detecting single nucleotide polymorphisms. Usually, each oligonucleotide is 40–50 bp long and the array resolution can be up to 500 bp.

For any array type, DNA spots are printed in replicates. From a general DNA–DNA hybridization perspective, a sufficiently long stretch of genomic DNA is best suited to be used as a DNA spot on array. Overall, the best performance of a specific platform is subjective based on investigator preference and experience. Many groups use single nucleotide polymorphism arrays to detect DNA copy number, although these arrays tend to result in more noise. With the advent in photolithic and other technologies to synthesize thousands of oligonucleotides on a very small glass surface, better printing heads for printing thousands of DNA spots in neat rows in a small space, and improved surface chemistry, private sector interest in DNA microarray grew.

Commercialization of DNA microarray brought competition, improvement, choices, and, most importantly, more affordability to users. Some companies developed DNA microarrays that covered loci for disease-specific or a biologic process-specific genes (e.g., arrays to study a few pathways heavily involved in cancer, or biological process e.g., apoptosis). Many offered to design, print, and supply custom DNA microarrays, thereby enabling laboratories to study DNA copy number just for genomic regions of interest without exorbitant costs. To keep their competitive edge, universities and research institutes used their DNA microarray cores to offer services to users for a fee. This gave individual laboratories additional choices, without having to invest in their own DNA microarray infrastructure and equipment. As with DNA sequencing, today a laboratory can perform its DNA microarray experiments or get them done for a price at many public and private institutes. The differences in aCGH platforms often necessitate using a set of programs most suitable or custom made for that particular platform. However, one concern is that the data format for one platform is often incompatible with other platforms. Therefore, the choice of a specific platform by a laboratory has long-term consequences.

An essential by-product of DNA microarray technology was the development of different analysis techniques. Since the data generated by DNA microarrays usually have more variables than samples, new statistical methods were developed to aid data analysis. The ability to view an enormous amount of data was also a challenge. Today, many programs for DNA microarray data analysis are in the public domain. These programs are user friendly and free (see resources in Section 17.8). Data analyzed using these programs have been widely published in peer-reviewed journals, and NIH-funded published data are often available for re-analysis by others.

17.2 General Methodology

From the user's perspective, the general methodology for aCGH can be divided into four steps. The first is to make probes by random priming (Sambrook et al., 1989), degenerate oligonucleotide PCR (DOP-PCR) (Telenius et al., 1992), or by other means from test (e.g., tumor) and control (sex-matched leukocyte DNA) samples, each labeled with one fluorochrome (e.g., cy3, cy5), purified from unbound or free fluorochromes in the reaction and used for hybridization (Pinkel et al., 1998; Sinjders et al., 2001; Misra et al., 2005; Nigro et al., 2005). The fluorochrome selection is an important step. For aCGH, two fluorochromes that have an easily distinguishable emission spectrum are used. More than one sample can be hybridized to one DNA microarray (Misra et al., 2006). For this, two test samples are labeled with two different fluorochromes (e.g., Cy3 and FITC), where each fluorochrome has a different excitation and emission spectrum, and the sex-matched control DNA is labeled by a third fluorochrome (e.g., Cy5). This strategy can reduce the cost of using expensive arrays.

The second step is hybridization, where the repeat sequences on the DNA microarray are blocked with DNA from salmon or herring sperm, and the remaining sequences on the array are hybridized to an array, and washed with buffer solution (Misra et al., 2005; Nigro et al., 2005). The stringency of washing is well established (Misra et al., 2005: Nigro et al., 2005). Like other hybridization techniques, e.g., Southern or Northern blotting, stringency can be manipulated to achieve a better signal to noise ratio. The arrays are then counter-stained with 4′,6-diamidino-2-phenylindole (DAPI) to stain DNA spots and mounted with glycerol.

The third step is image acquisition, in which images of the hybridized microarray are acquired using a charged couple device (CCD) camera (Jain et al., 2002) or laser scanner (Graves et al., 2002). The principle for doing either type of imaging is similar. For CCD, a pair of the excitation and emission filters is used for each color channel to minimize background. For each sample, three different images (e.g., DAPI, Cy3, and Cy5 channel) are acquired and used for analysis. The linearity of signal acquisition over a fairly large window of exposure time is the key for good imaging. Though higher exposure time leads to increases in both signal and background, the quantitative increase in signal intensity is more than background and therefore provides a larger range of background subtracted signal intensities. For data from each DNA spot on the array, intensity from a number of pixels covering the DNA spots is considered as 'signal' (detailed in Jain et al., 2002). This consideration is based on how intensity in each pixel vary from their immediate neighbors. The process determines variation within hybridization spots, and also indicates the intensity of local background. This way of measuring local background for each DNA spot is very helpful since, in theory, the whole microarray should have a similar background, but often there are small differences. When more than one sample is used, the image for the second sample hybridized to the same microarray is acquired separately using appropriate filters and analyzed (Misra et al., 2006).

The fourth step is analysis of aCGH data. This entails two steps: converting image data into numerical data and analyzing the data statistically. The basic principle for converting image data into numerical data is the same, no matter what type of imaging equipment and software are used. The whole array is divided into a grid where each cell covers one DNA spot and some of its surrounding area. Within each such cell, the pixels covering the DNA spot are used as signal and the surrounding pixels as background. This is done for every DNA spot in the whole array and is then converted into a numerical table (Jain et al., 2002). Once this table is generated, data from each DNA spot are subtracted from background and normalized either by mean or median intensity for all DNA spots in an array. This is a key step because different segments of genome can have different hybridization properties and kinetics, based on their sequence; normalization such as this helps to scale the intensity data. Normalization also helps standardize batch-to-batch variations in data. Finally, the ratio of test to control probes for each DNA spot (relative ratio or RR) is calculated and then the mean and standard deviation of all replicates for each arrayed DNA spot is tabulated. Once these data are ready, one can plot genome-wide copy number changes as a function of distance along the chromosome or genome. Usually this is done by a 'Macro' written in Excel (Misra et al., 2005).

Generally, aCGH data are $\log_2$ transformed and plotted. Since normal DNA has two copies, $\log_2$ transformation brings the baseline of 2 to 0, and the baseline for normal copy in the plot number for the whole genome becomes 0. The advantage of data transformation is that it stretches the scale of copy number loss so that heterozygous and homozygous deletions are more clearly distinguished. It squeezes the amplification side of the scale, and since amplification of a DNA locus can reach 200–250 copies or more, it can still be plotted for easy viewing. More often than not, a data filtering step is used before data are plotted, to remove those DNA spots that have data from only one replicate or that have an unacceptable standard deviation among replicates. This is an important step to reduce noise in the data. If one repeatedly uses arrays that are printed as a batch, often the same DNA spots show erratic behavior. Therefore, these spots are flagged and not included in analysis. Many laboratories use a smoothing step whereby a running mean of three to five contiguous DNA spots are calculated and then plotted (Willenbrock and Fridlyand, 2005). The primary advantage of this is to reduce the effects of erratic behavior of some individual DNA spots. Despite using replicates of each DNA spot in an array, some spots show far more deviant behavior than their neighbors. Perhaps this can be either attributed to microarray construction or to an inherent property of primary sequence of DNA on that spot.

There are some general principles for statistical analysis of microarray data, but the exact methodology used depends on the specific question. To identify common aberrations such as the frequency of gain or loss or amplification of a DNA spot in a sample set, gain or loss or amplification must first be defined. Many laboratories score a $> 20\%$ deviation from the mean values as loss or gain. This can be an issue if the sensitivities of all the hybridizations are not similar, which usually is the case because sample quality varies and reagents, equipment, and individual handling variations are expected. A more customized approach is to identify a cut-off value for gain and loss scoring for each sample separately (Misra et al., 2005). With this approach, the ratios of test-to-control intensity for each DNA locus (relative ratio or RR) are plotted as a histogram and Gaussian curves are fitted on this histogram. Given that extensive DNA copy number changes occur in less than 50% of the genome in more than 95% of cases, even in the most aggressive brain tumor, glioblastoma multiforme, at least half of the DNA spots will form a population with a bell-shaped distribution of RR (Fig. 17.1). This population becomes the RR distribution of the genome that is normal with respect to copy number, i.e., 2. The other populations with lesser and higher RR values than the middle population become the loci with copy number loss and gain, respectively. This methodology works best with near diploid tumors. If a tumor is an even

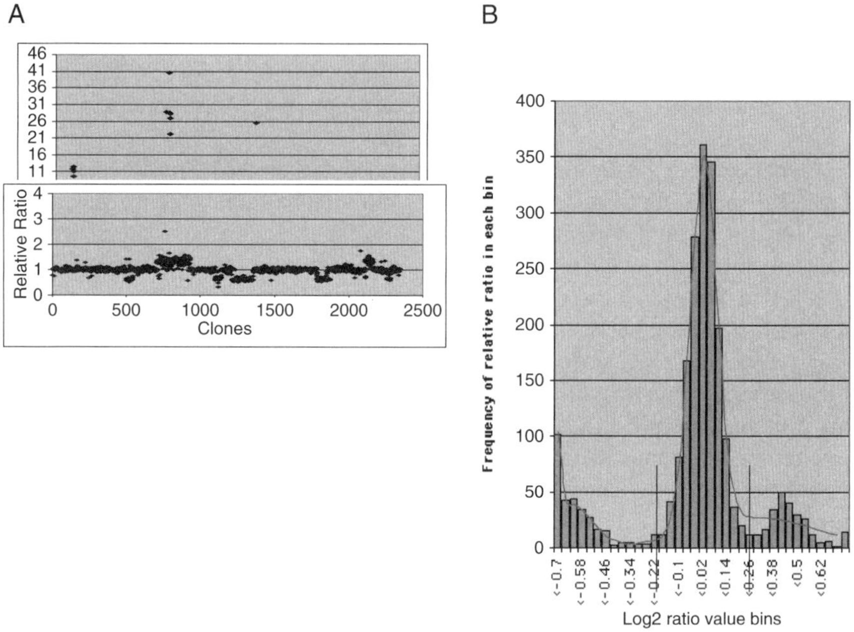

Fig. 17.1 Scoring loss and gain. Relative ratio (RR) values from all the DNA spots (**A**) in an array are plotted as a histogram (**B**). The central population of the histogram (B) forms a Gaussian distribution. The cut-off boundaries are set by the user (here it is 3 standard deviations from the mean on either side) and all the RR values below or above these cut-off values are scored as losses and gains, respectively (Modified from Misra et al., 2005)

mixture of near diploid and near triploid cells, this strategy will not work. However, in a study of over 300 different types of brain tumors, we have seen only few tumors that are not near diploid. Certain tumor types like neuroblastoma have a more near triploid tumors and interpreting the DNA copy number in these cases needs to be done carefully (Tomioka et al., 2007).

The current technical challenge is to combine the power of genetic techniques to make quality cancer DNA probes from a tiny amount of frozen or paraffin-embedded DNA material. Using a small amount of DNA to profile a sample has been tried in many different ways. The key is to get a good representation of the whole genome. Experience with conventional CGH established that proper representation of certain stretches of certain chromosomes (e.g., 1p, 22q) could be a problem, but it turned out that aCGH does not have that kind of representation issue. Using a small amount of DNA forces a user to amplify it while making probe. However, overamplification of probes tends to increase the background. The problem is often the DNA quality and quantity from paraffin-embedded samples. Simple tests such as extracted DNA size or DNAse digestion rate of paraffin-extracted DNA have not been the reliable markers for quality of DNA extracted. In our experience, the data quality of paraffin-extracted DNA has ranged from excellent (indistinguishable from frozen samples) to unusable. Several groups have reported ways to amplify and label probes that work well with aCGH. These include degenerate primer PCR (Daigo et al., 2001; de Vries et al., 2005), two-stage random primer labeling reactions (de Vries et al., 2005), ligation-mediated PCR (Tanabe et al., 2003; Guillaud-Bataille et al., 2004), ligation circularization of degraded DNA (Wang et al., 2004b), balanced PCR (Wang et al., 2004a), and three-stage random priming (Prestagarden et al., 2008). A few studies using paraffin-embedded brain tumor samples have been reported (Maher et al., 2006; Johnson et al., 2006; Mohapatra et al., 2006). The general belief is that formalin, used to fix the tissue before embedding it in paraffin, cross-links DNA. Since pathologist's fixation protocols are not standard, the quality of DNA extracted out of paraffin samples varies. Moreover, as paraffin blocks age, degradation of DNA increases, and this increase is attributed to oxidation over the storage period. All of these problems can compromise DNA quality and therefore lead to varying data quality. When more laboratories are successful in using paraffin-embedded samples to produce quality DNA for profiling genome-wide DNA copy number, we can expect more insights using samples from clinical trials where there are uniform treatments of patients and multiple uses of the tissue samples with longer periods of follow up.

17.3 Interpretation of aCGH Data

Apart from measuring locus by locus DNA copy number, aCGH can inform about a variety of genetic events (Fig. 17.2). It can detect aneuploidy, interstitial deletions, break points, aberration boundaries, amplifications, and non-reciprocal translocations. Identifying amplifications and deletions can lead to recognition of novel candidate oncogenes and tumor suppressor genes (Table 17.1). The improved resolution of aCGH can identify two different regions of deletions in a locus that in the past looked like one large region of loss, and can identify the exact boundary of an amplicon (Fig. 17.3 and Color Plate 18) as well as a break point, or can narrow a region of loss (Fig. 17.4). Genetic classification of tumors has been a hallmark of aCGH data. Many genetically defined groups of tumors can be identified using this technique (Fig. 17.5 and Color Plate 19). The copy number frequency of genetic changes can be generated for a specific tumor type and grade, or a specific genetic group (Fig. 17.6 and Color Plate 20). In addition, a marker for diagnosis and/or prognosis can be identified (Fig. 17.7 and Color Plate 21). Finally, a preexisting marker can be refined on the basis of aCGH data (Fig. 17.8 and Color Plate 22).

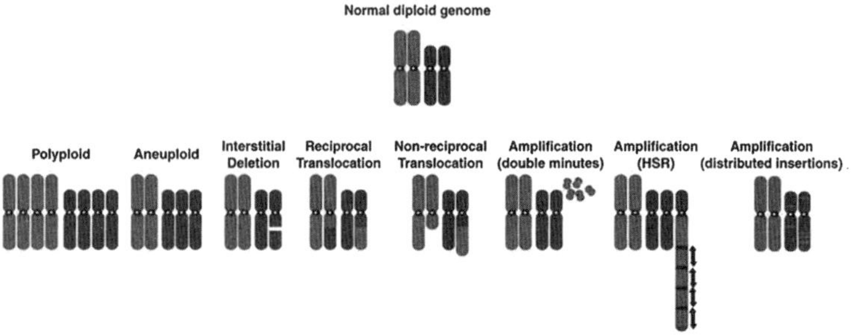

Technique	Detection							
Banding	+	+	+/-	+	+	+	+	-
SKY	+	+	-	+	+	+	+	-
CGH	-	+	+	-	+	+	+	+
LOH	-	+	+	-	+	+	+	+

Fig. 17.2 Comparison of different cytogenetic techniques. CGH can detect aneuploidy, interstitial deletions, non-reciprocal translocation, amplification, and break points (From Pinkel and Albertson, Hum. Mol. Genet. 2003, 12, rev. issue 2)

17.4 Strategy for Identifying Genetic Markers with Clinical Relevance Using Array CGH

Success in identifying genetic markers for brain tumors depends on well-defined sample sets of tumors, like those from a clinical trial. Since it is impossible to use normal adult brain as a control to compare tumor samples, the conventional wisdom has been to use 'non-neoplastic' brain samples (e.g., epileptic foci or accidental death cases); though not equivalent to normal brain, such samples are the best available. However, the need for using 'normal brain' as control is more important for expression arrays than for DNA microarrays. Since all somatic cells are thought to have very similar DNA, a pool of leukocyte DNA from a normal population without blood abnormalities is often used as reference DNA for CGH. This is done separately for male and female DNA.

As a technique, aCGH has its own internal controls. Every DNA sample is hybridized against sex-matched normal DNA; therefore, the DNA copy numbers seen in each sample are relative to copy numbers of normal human genome. If the research question is, 'What are the genetic markers for a tumor type?', then only a group of those tumors are adequate to answer this question. In such cases, these samples are studied for their genetic profiles, the copy number changes are cataloged, and statistical analysis done to identify the changes that are significant in this tumor group. But if the research question is more complex, for example, 'What are the markers for glioblastoma multiforme that result in poor survival?', then the task becomes multistep. Step one must identify the genetic changes that are frequent in glioblastoma multiforme and step two is to analyze their association with a phenotype, e.g., survival, using appropriate statistical methods, such as Cox proportional hazard models. For a

Table 17.1 A list of candidate oncogenes and tumor suppressors in grade 4 astrocytoma, identified by array comperative genomic hybridization

Heterozygous loss				Amplification			
BAC name	Location	Candidate tumor suppressor gene	Reported by	BAC name	Location	Candidate Oncogene	Reported by
RP11-42A17	4p11-4p12	GABRG 1		RP11-100C21	7p14		
CTC-205110				RP11-141P12	7p13	HECW1	
RP11-40D5	4q28			RP11-217010	7P12	ACDY1	
RP11-6L19	4q32-4q33	TLL1		RP11-15L23	7P12	COBL	
RP11-77E2	7q31.1	DLD, LAMB1, LAMB4		CTD-207010	7q21.2-7q21.3		
RP11-26H17	9P23	PELI2		CTB-54J7	7Q31		
RP11-50C21	9P23	PTPRD	Misra et al. (Unpullished)	CTD 2039F11	7q31.3		Misra et al. (Unpublished)
RP11-264011	9p23			CTB-185C18	7q31.2-q31.31		
RP11-3302	10q21.3	CTNNA3		CTD-2041G23	7Q31.2-q31.31		
RP11-1705	10q22.2	KCNMA1		RP11-98J9	7q31.31-7Qq3	CTTNBP2	
RP11-8C15	13Q12.1	EFHA1		RP11-89P14	11P15.2		
					11p14.3-11p	MRGPRX4	
RP11-52N13	17q12	CCDC43, DBF4B, GJC1		GS-561N1	12q13-q14		
CTD-2100E13	18q11.2	RIOK3, NPC1, ANKRD29		CTB-136014	12q14		
RP11-86J21	21q21			RP11-16H12	12q23	SLC17A8	
RP11-4H24	22q13.2						
				HIPK2	7q34		Deshmukh et al. (2008)
RP11157L10 to RP360M22	6q27	WDR27, TGBS2,PHF10, TCTE3	Ichimura et al. (2006)				
Rp11-2J18 toRP180E10	6q27	SYTL3					
				CCND3			Ichimura et al. (2006)
IRF2BP2	1p42.2		Maher et al. (2006)	*SLA/LP, STIM2*	4p15		Ruano et al. (2006)
TMPO/LAP2	12q22			*TNFSF13B, COL4A2*	13q32-34		
				EPS15	1p32		Maher et al. (2006)
				WN17A	3p26.3-24.3		
				RASSF3	12q14.2		
				ERK	8q23-24		
				SKP2	5p13.2		Saiguse et al. (2005)

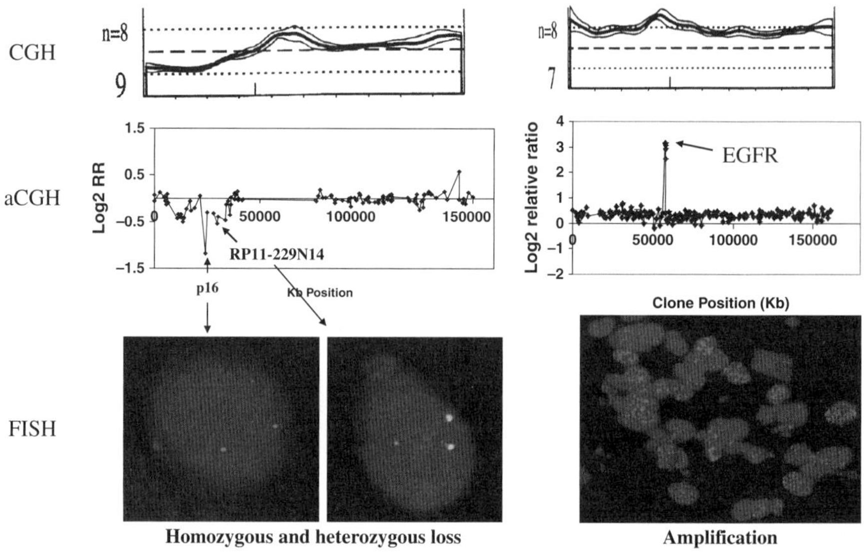

Fig. 17.3 Homozygous and heterozygous losses and amplifications are better defined by aCGH than by conventional CGH. Data from the same tumors analyzed by standard CGH and aCGH show the advantages of aCGH. The left panel shows loss of chromosome 9p in a glioblastoma multiforme (GBM) by conventional CGH. The same region actually has two regions of loss with homozygous deletion of P16 locus. FISH validated the aCGH data. The right panel shows chromosome 7 gain and EGFR amplification. aCGH narrowed the boundary of EGFR amplification much better than conventional CGH did, and FISH validated it (Modified from Misra et al., 2005) (*see* Color Plate 18)

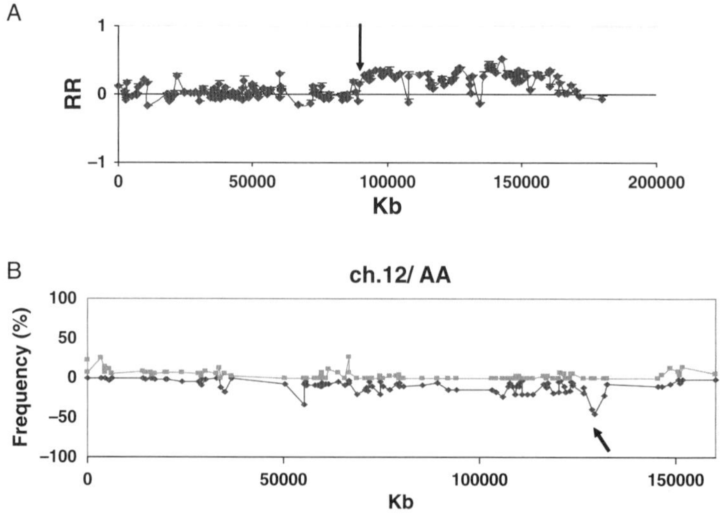

Fig. 17.4 Breakpoint identification and narrowing a region of frequent loss in tumor. (**A**) Profile of chromosome 7 in a GBM showing breakpoint (*arrow*). (**B**) A region of 12q loss frequently seen in grade 3 astrocytoma. 12q loss may be associated with survival in these tumors, and is therefore a potential tumor suppressor locus. The frequency of gain and loss for each BAC clone is plotted as positive and negative values, respectively

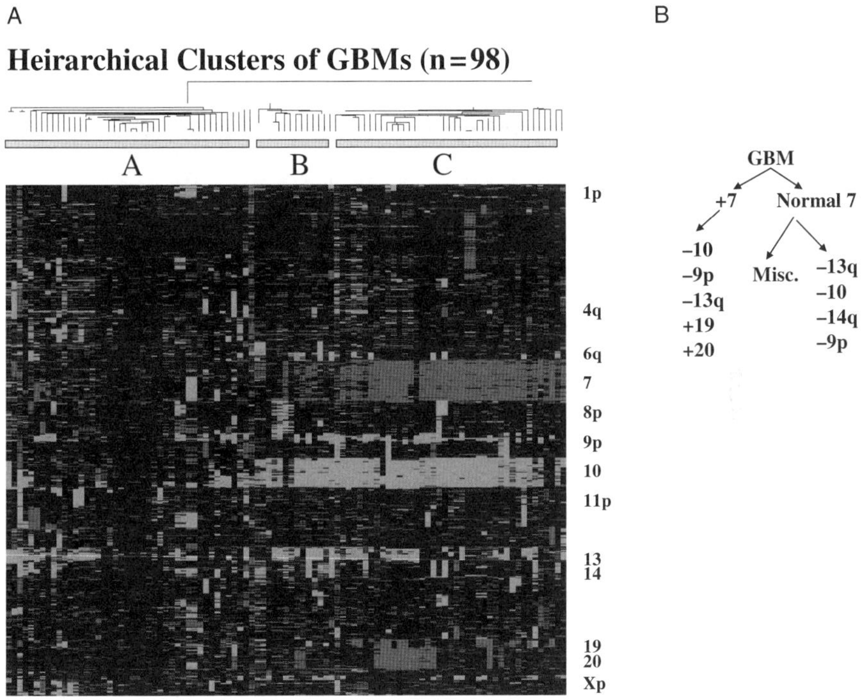

Fig. 17.5 Identification of genetic subgroups in GBM. (**A**) The classification tree shows three sub groups. The genetic signatures defining these groups are shown in the heat map below. In the heat map, each row shows data from one locus and each column shows data from one tumor. DNA copy number gains are shown in red and losses in green. Group C has both chr. 7 gain and 10 loss; group B has predominantly chr. 10 loss without chr. 7 gain; and group A has miscellaneous genetic changes. (**B**) The genetic signatures and how each contributed toward tumor subgroup classification is listed (*see* Color Plate 19)

pilot study, a few samples might be enough to develop a hypothesis, but more definitive studies require power calculations to know precisely how many samples are required to find statistically significant differences or associations, depending on what questions are being asked. When the questions are complex, as is usual for most studies, obtaining numbers of samples necessary for adequate statistical power becomes a challenge.

For even more complex studies, such as an integrated genomic approach using microarray-based data from different platforms, no single statistical approach is usually adequate. Usually more than one statistical approach is used to answer the same question, and similar answers from different approaches are then perceived as having yielded reliable data. Since the number of variables studied exceeds the number of samples by hundreds or even thousands, special statistical analysis software has been designed for this kind of analysis, including Significant Analysis of Microarray (SAM), Prediction Analysis of Microarray (PAM), and cluster analysis. Programs like 'Treeview' can then be used to view the data. All of these are open source programs (see resources in Section 17.8).

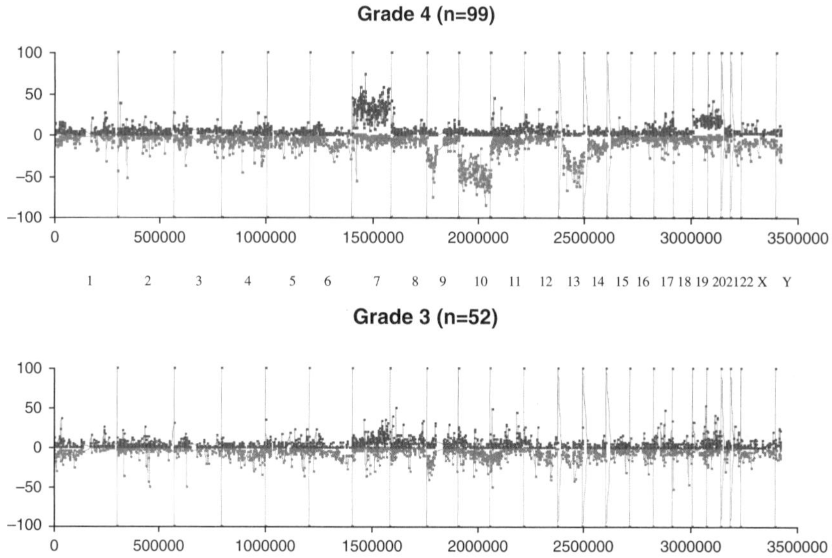

Fig. 17.6 Map showing frequency of copy number aberrations in grade 4 (**A**) and grade 3 (**B**) astrocytoma. The ordinate marks the frequency of gain (positive) and loss (negative). The abscissa shows the genome in 1p to Yq direction (*see* Color Plate 20)

The analysis of microarray data can be 'unsupervised' or 'supervised'. Unsupervised analysis is usually undertaken for questions such as whether there are different genetic groups within a tumor type and grade, where the goal is to determine different possible groups based on similarity of cases to each other. For example, Fig. 17.5 shows the results of an 'unsupervised' hierarchical cluster analysis. In supervised analysis, the user classifies the samples into at least two groups and compares them to identify which aberrations mark each group (Figs. 17.6, 17.9 and Color Plate 23).

17.5 New Insights in Primary Brain Tumors Using Array CGH

The ability to detect different forms of change in DNA copy number has gradually improved our understanding of the relationship between genetics and brain tumors. Cancer in somatic cells is now well established as a disease of the genome. A genetic change detected at any point in a given cancer can be the cause or the effect of development and/or progression. Array CGH can detect genome-wide copy number changes in DNA at a level of resolution limited only by the array. Functionally, any such change can be causal (e.g., oncogene, tumor suppressor gene) or be nonspecifically correlated with behavior (Cairncross et al., IRTOG trial 9402, 2006).

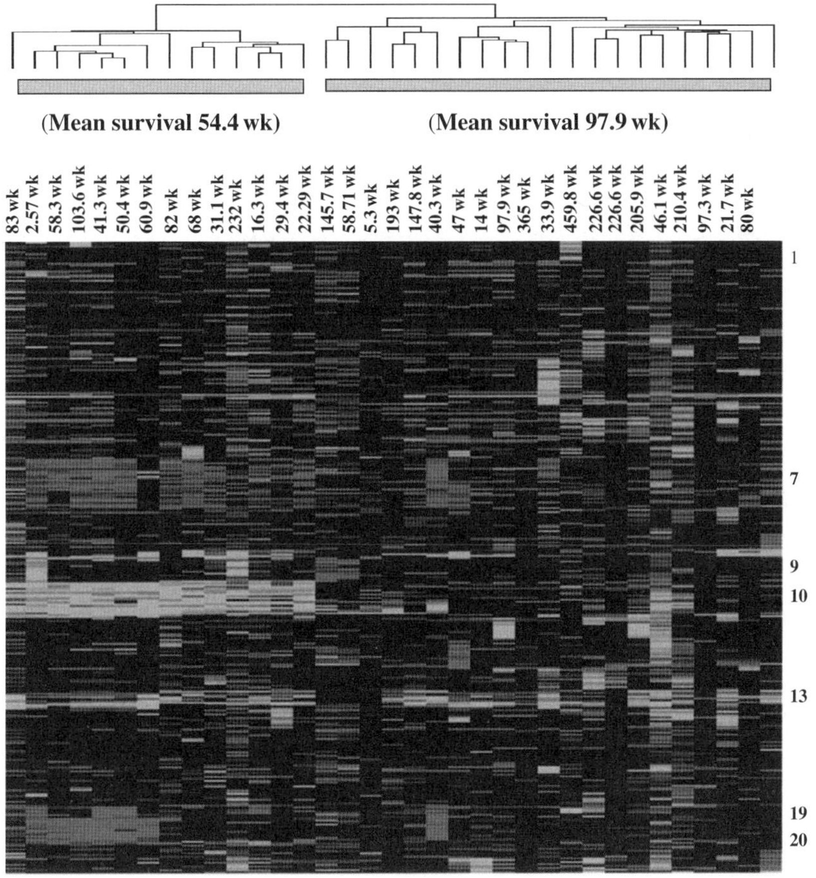

Fig. 17.7 Markers of survival in GBM. In an age-matched comparison of GBM patients with poor (>2 yr) survival and better (<2 yr) survival, frequent 7 gain, 10 loss, and 19 gain were found in those with poor survival. Global gene expression profiles of the same tumors separated the poor and better survivors into almost identical groups (Nigro et al., 2005) (*see* Color Plate 21)

Because copy number change occurs in primarily large segments of chromosomes in brain tumors, using aCGH to identify genome-wide copy number change has not added radical new understanding at the chromosomal level. The most frequent genetic abberations are large and were not missed previously using conventional CGH (Mohapatra et al., 1998). However, aCGH can generate very high resolution maps of the frequency of changes in DNA copy number in different tumor types (Misra et al., 2005; Kitange et al., 2005). In addition, it can successfully identify genetic markers in different types and grades of brain tumors as discussed below.

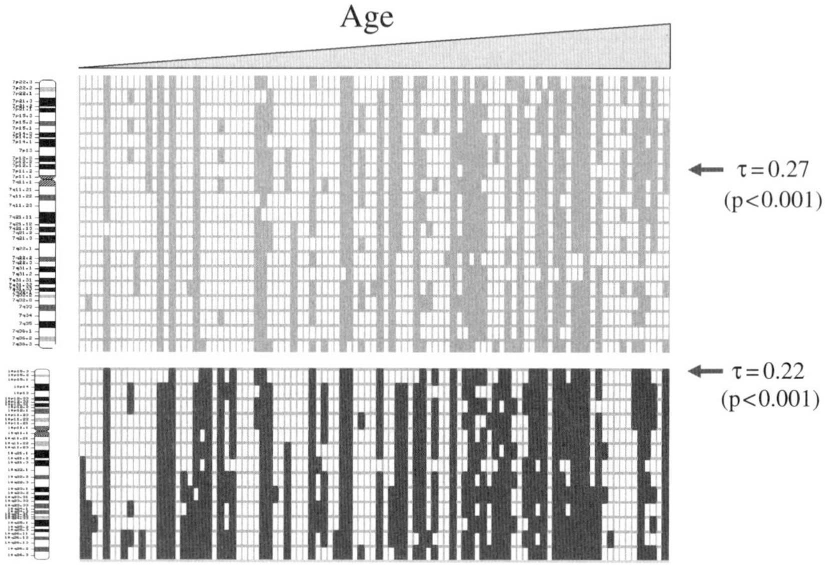

Fig. 17.8 After undergoing surgery followed by radiation and chemotherapy, young patients with GBM do better than older patients. Whether any genetic difference underlies this difference has not been clear. Chromosome 7 gain (*green*) and 10 loss (*red*) are the signature genetic changes seen in patients with poor survival. When each of these chromosomes are divided into roughly 10 Mb blocks and gain and loss of each block were analyzed for associations with survival, a region of 7p gain and a region of 10p loss (marked by *arrows*) were the most statistically significant marker for survival (*see* Color Plate 22)

In grade 4 astrocytoma, the most frequent genetic events are gain of chr. 7, 19, and 20 and loss of 9p, 10, and 13q (Misra et al., 2005; Nigro et al., 2005; Phillips et al., 2006). Two to three percent of cases had loss of 1p and 19q, a signature genetic event for oligodendroglioma. A host of other abberations, e.g., loss of 2p, 8p, 8q, whole 8, 11q, 17p, 22q, and gain of 1p, 1q, 3q, 4q, 5q, 12q, and 16q were observed at a lower frequencies. The implication is that genes located at these regions contribute to initiation and progression of grade 4 astrocytoma. Consequently, many investigators examined these regions to identify candidate tumor suppressors or oncogenes (Table 17.1) and markers.

Most genetic abberations found in grade 4 astrocytomas were present in grade 3 astrocytoma, albeit at a lower frequency. Specifically, grade 4 astrocytoma had more frequent gain of 1p, 4q, 7, 12, and loss of 2p, 8, 10, 11q, 13q than did grade 3 astrocytoma. In both grades, 9p loss and 19 gain occur at a similar frequency. In grade 4 (Nigro et al., 2005; Phillips et al., 2006) and grade 3 (Misra et al., unpublished data), chr. 10 loss and 7 gain were prognostic markers.

Grade 2 astrocytomas show nondescript and/or random genetic events without any signature abberations (Misra et al., unpublished data).

A

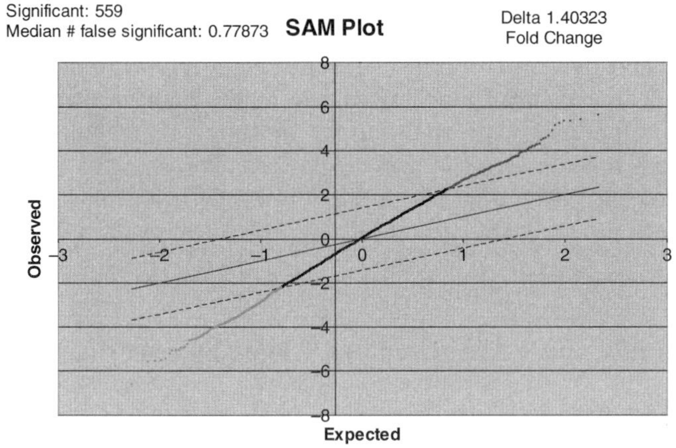

B

	Gain	Loss
1p	15	2
1q	8	6
2p	9	18
3q	8	2
4q	28	2
5q	8	7
7p	53	0
7q	24	0
8p	4	12
8q	1	21
9p	0	9
10p	0	32
10q	0	73
11p	9	1
11q	0	22
12q	20	1
13q	0	20
16q	7	0
17p	0	11
17q	8	6
20p	8	0
22q	0	10

Fig. 17.9 Supervised analysis to identify genetic differences between grade 3 and grade 4 astrocytomas. (**A**) Significance analysis of microarray (SAM) identifies more than 500 BAC clones throughout genome that differ significantly in copy number in anaplastic astrocytoma and GBM. The analysis plots the expected versus the observed frequencies of aberrations. When differences between the two exceed a predetermined value, the change is defined as significant. The losses are shown in green and the gains in red. (**B**) A list of the major aberrations in grade 4 astrocytomas. The number of BAC clones lost and gained for each of these regions shows chr. 7 gain and chr. 10 loss are the most frequent aberrations (see Color Plate 23)

Grade 4 astrocytoma signature aberrations and their frequency were confirmed by other studies (Maher et al., 2006; Beroukhim et al., 2007; The cancer genome atlas network; 2008), but genetic profiling work is rare for grade 3 and grade 2 astrocytomas, presumably because they are infrequent. These grades need further study. From what is currently known, loss of chr. 10 and gain of chr. 7 are robust markers for poor survival among malignant astrocytomas.

In oligodendroglioma, aCGH has shown that the most frequent aberrations are loss of 1p, 19q, and combined loss of 1p/19q. In addition, deletion of 4q, 5p, 9p, 10q, 11p, and 13q, and gain of 7p, 8q, 10p, and 11q were observed. Occasional whole chromosomes 4, 9, and 13 loss; and whole chromosome 7 and 11 gain were also observed (Kitange et al., 2005). In that study, 8q gain was a marker of poor prognosis.

In ependymoma, aCGH has shown that 1q gain is correlated with pediatric patients, intracranial location, and grade 3 (Mendrzyk et al., 2006). Also in that study, 1q21.1–32.1 gain was associated with tumor recurrence, and gain of 1q25 was an independent prognostic marker for recurrence-free and overall survival. EGFR amplification was an independent prognostic marker for intracranial ependymomas. This and another study of ependymomas (Kurian et al., 2008) reported infrequent loss of chr. 6, 8, and 14q.

In meningiomas, aCGH has shown that all three grades (benign, atypical, and malignant) were genetically divided into two molecular groups: 'low-proliferative' and 'high-proliferative' (Carvalho et al., 2007). The atypical meningiomas are genetically a mixture of both benign and proliferative tumors. Loss of 6q, 9p, 13, and 14 were found exclusively in the high-proliferative meningiomas. Additional gene expression studies indicated that higher cell proliferation and transforming growth factor-beta pathway were the major molecular mechanisms that distinguish 'low-proliferative' and 'high-proliferative' groups.

17.6 Array CGH in Cancer Subgroup and Gene Discovery

The power of using aCGH to classify or identify clinically relevant markers comes from the fact that change in DNA copy number is robust when compared to other variables such as expression or methylation. Array CGH has been a powerful tool for discovery when used in conjunction with other assays, such as expression profiling, gene promoter methylation, or miRNA expression. For example, in a small sample of grade 4 astrocytomas, aCGH, and expression array profiling each identified similar subgroups of tumors (Nigro et al., 2005). Genetic signatures in the group that had chr. 10 loss and 7 gain were associated with poor survival. The group that did not have those changes was a mixture of poor and better survivors. These same two groups could also be identified by comparing over expression and under expression of a set of genes. A follow-up larger study confirmed chr. 10 loss and chr. 7 gain as a marker for poor survival (Phillips et al., 2006). This study identified three functional groups: proliferative (Po), mesenchymal (Ms), and proneural (Pn). The Po and Ms groups had chr. 7 gain and 10 loss and poor survival. The Pn group did not have 7 gain and 10 loss and had better survival. This finding has been confirmed by other studies (Maher et al., 2006; Beroukhim et al., 2007; TCGA, 2008).

Another marker and critical gene discovery approach seeks to identify regions of DNA lost by using aCGH first and then identifying which gene located in that region has expression loss of the other copy due to promoter hypermethylation (Zardo et al., 2002; Kim et al., 2006), or degradation mediated by micro RNA, which can bind and degrade mRNA. For this group of tumor suppressors (e.g., CISH1, COE3, RUNX3, TES), typically, the first copy of DNA is lost and the second copy gene is methylated at its promoter. MiRNA copy number loss or gain due to DNA copy number change can lead to up or down regulation of the gene and its associated pathway. Little has been reported about this in astrocytoma. Array CGH chips can also identify the genomic locus targeted by a transcription factor using chip on chip assay.

Array CGH has commonly been used to identify novel candidate tumor suppressor or oncogene loci across tumor types (Table 17.1 and Fig. 17.10). Key roles of a host of oncogenes (e.g., EGFR, PDGFR1A, CDK6) and tumor

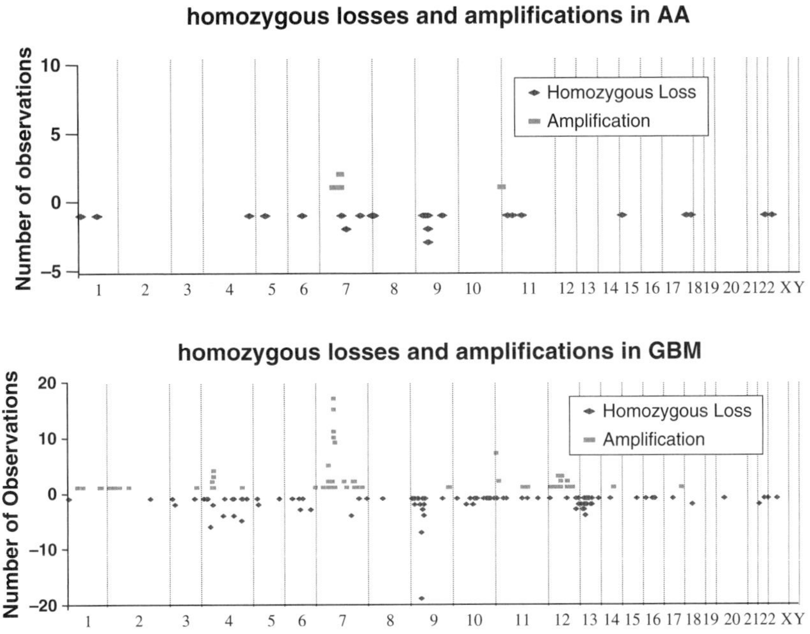

Fig. 17.10 Relative position and frequency of candidate oncogenes and tumor suppressors in grade 3 ($n = 50$) and grade 4 ($n = 50$) astrocytomas. The X-axis shows genome position and chromosome boundaries. The Y-axis shows frequency of events: positive for amplification and negative for homozygous deletions

suppressors (e.g., p16, p53, Rb1, NF1) in the genesis of glioma have been known for a long time. But there are likely many more such genes, and their role in astrocytoma are not yet well established, although functional studies in model cell lines and animals have validated the biological significance of some.

Array CGH data, along with follow-up biological experiments, and expression and mutation analysis, have been successfully used to identify key pathways involved in grade 4 astrocytoma. Several studies have reported that important signaling pathways, e.g., IGF2, RAS/RAF, and MAPK, are driven by DNA copy number in high- and low-grade astrocytoma (Soroceanu et al., 2007, Jeuken et al., 2007, Pfister et al., 2008). These types of pathway profiling studies were further extended by projects that sequenced the human cancer genome. Two such efforts in grade 4 astrocytoma suggest that the RTK/RAS/PI3Kinase, p53 signaling, and p16/INK4 pathways are affected by DNA copy number and/or mutation of their member genes (Fig. 17.11 and Color Plate 24; The Cancer Genome Atlas Network, 2008; Parsons et al., 2008). However, this is just the beginning. It is becoming clear that perhaps 10–15 major signaling pathways act as the ultimate effector routes for all procancerous genes. The future of cancer treatment is to identify the affected

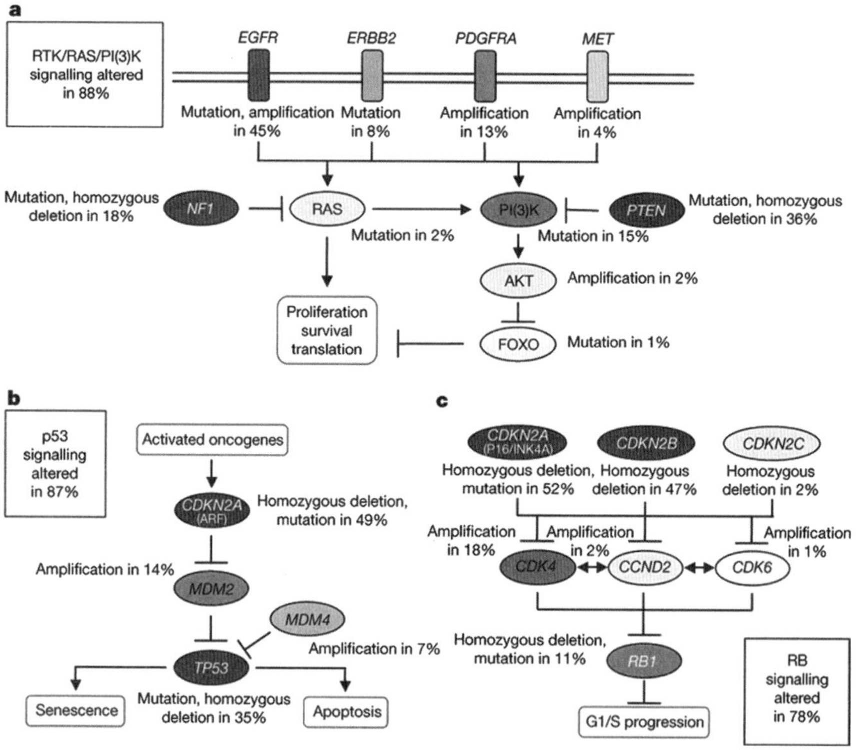

Fig. 17.11 Three major affected pathways (a, b, c) in grade 4 astrocytoma that showed DNA copy number changes, mutation, and amplification of their member genes. More pathways are expected to be added to this list. (TCGA, 2008) (*see* Color Plate 24)

pathways in each case and use personalized intervention. Array CGH will be one of the platforms used for this effort.

In summary, array CGH has been used for a host of purposes, including genome-wide copy number screening, high-resolution analysis of a locus, mapping aberration boundaries or break points, identifying disease-related gene loci (e.g., oncogene and tumor suppressor loci in cancer), classifying tumors, and identifying diagnostic and prognostic markers. Efforts are now underway to use aCGH to predict response to therapy.

17.7 Useful Resources

The following are some of the center and company addresses with accessible useful resources, and freely available programs related to aCGH that are downloadable or available for use over the internet.

UCSF Genome Core: http://cancer.ucsf.edu/array/index.php
The Broad Institute Center for Genotyping and Analysis: http://www.broad.mit.edu/node/306
The Cancer Genome Atlas Project: http://cancergenome.nih.gov/
Affymatrix: http://www.affymetrix.com/products/application/whole_genome.affx
Agilent:http://www.chem.agilent.com/en-US/Products/Instruments/dnamicroarrays/Pages/default.aspx
Nimblegen: http://www.nimblegen.com/products/cgh/
SAM analysis: http://www-stat.stanford.edu/~tibs/SAM/
PAM analysis: http://www-stat.stanford.edu/~tibs/PAM/
Cluster analysis: http://genome-www.stanford.edu/clustering/
Treeview: http://taxonomy.zoology.gla.ac.uk/rod/treeview.html
R for statistical computing: http://www.r-project.org/

Acknowledgments This work was supported by the Arizona Biomedical Research Commission, NIH (NS42927), Diane and Bruce Halle, and the Barrow Neurological Foundations.

References

Beroukhim R, Getz G, Nghiemphu L, Barretina J, Hsueh T, Linhart D, Vivanco I, Lee JC, Huang JH, Alexander S, Du J, Kau T, Thomas RK, Shah K, Soto H, Perner S, Prensner J, Debiasi RM, Demichelis F, Hatton C, Rubin MA, Garraway LA, Nelson SF, Liau L, Mischel PS, Cloughesy TF, Meyerson M, Golub TA, Lander ES, Mellinghoff IK, Sellers WR. Assessing the significance of chromosomal aberrations in cancer: methodology and application to glioma. Proc Natl Acad Sci USA. 2007;104(50):20007–12.

Bignell GR, Huang J, Greshock J, Watt S, Butler A, West S, Grigorova M, Jones KW, Wei W, Stratton MR, Futreal PA, Weber B, Shapero MH, Wooster R. High-resolution analysis of DNA copy number using oligonucleotide microarrays. Genome Res. 2004;14(2):287–95.

Cairncross G, Berkey B, Shaw E, Jenkins R, Scheithauer B, Brachman D, Buckner J, Fink K, Souhami L, Laperierre N, Mehta M, Curran W, Intergroup Radiation Therapy Oncology Group Trial 9402. Phase III trial of chemotherapy plus radiotherapy compared with radiotherapy alone for pure and mixed anaplastic oligodendroglioma: Intergroup Radiation Therapy Oncology Group Trial 9402. J Clin Oncol. 2006;24(18):2707–14.

Carvalho LH, Smirnov I, Baia GS, Modrusan Z, Smith JS, Jun P, Costello JF, McDermott MW, Vandenberg SR, Lal A. Molecular signatures define two main classes of meningiomas. Mol Cancer. 2007; 15;6:64.

Daigo Y, Chin SF, Gorringe KL, Bobrow LG, Ponder BA, et al. Degenerate oligonucleotide primed-polymerase chain reaction-based array comparative genomic hybridization for extensive amplicon profiling of breast cancers: a new approach for the molecular analysis of paraffin-embedded cancer tissue. Am J Pathol. 2001; 158:1623–31.

Deshmukh H, Yeh TH, Yu J, Sharma MK, Perry A, Leonard JR, Watson MA, Gutmann DH, Nagarajan R. High-resolution, dual-platform aCGH analysis reveals frequent HIPK2 amplification and increased expression in pilocytic astrocytomas. Oncogene. 2008;27(34): 4745–51.

DeVries S, Nyante SJ, Korkola JE, Segraves R, Nakao K, et al. Array-based comparative genomic hybridization from formalin-fixed, paraffin-embedded breast tumors. J Mol Diagn. 2005; 7:1–7.

Graves DJ, Su HJ, Addya S, Surrey S, Fortina P. Four-laser scanning confocal system for microarray analysis. Biotechniques. 2002;32(2):346–54.
Guillaud-Bataille M, Valent A, Soularue P, Perot C, Inda MM, Receveur A, Smaïli S, Roest Crollius H, Bénard J, Bernheim A, Gidrol X, Danglot G. Detecting single DNA copy number variations in complex genomes using one nanogram of starting DNA and BAC-array CGH. Nucleic Acids Res. 2004 Jul 29;32(13):e112.
Huang J, Wei W, Zhang J, Liu G, Bignell GR, Stratton MR, Futreal PA, Wooster R, Jones KW, Shapero MH. Whole genome DNA copy number changes identified by high density oligonucleotide arrays. Hum Genomics. 2004;1(4):287–99.
Ichimura K, Mungall AJ, Fiegler H, Pearson DM, Dunham I, Carter NP, Collins VP. Small regions of overlapping deletions on 6q26 in human astrocytic tumours identified using chromosome 6 tile path array-CGH. Oncogene. 2006;25(8):1261–71.
Ishkanian AS, Malloff CA, Watson SK, DeLeeuw RJ, Chi B, Coe BP, Snijders A, Albertson DG, Pinkel D, Marra MA, Ling V, MacAulay C, Lam WL.A tiling resolution DNA microarray with complete coverage of the human genome. Nat Genet. 2004;36(3): 299–303.
Jain AN, Tokuyasu TA, Snijders AM, Segraves R, Albertson DG, Pinkel D. Fully automatic quantification of microarray image data. Genome Res. 2002;12(2):325–32.
Jeuken J, van den Broecke C, Gijsen S, Boots-Sprenger S, Wesseling P. RAS/RAF pathway activation in gliomas: the result of copy number gains rather than activating mutations. Acta Neuropathol. 2007;114(2):121–33.
Johnson NA, Hamoudi RA, Ichimura K, Liu L, Pearson DM, Collins VP, Du MQ. Application of array CGH on archival formalin-fixed paraffin-embedded tissues including small numbers of microdissected cells. Lab Invest. 2006;86(9):968–78.
Kallioniemi A, Kallioniemi OP, Sudar D, Rutovitz D, Gray JW, Waldman F, Pinkel D. Comparative genomic hybridization for molecular cytogenetic analysis of solid tumors. Science. 1992;258(5083):818–21.
Kim B, Kim H, Song BJ, Cha SH, Lee MO, Park SH. Oligonucleotide DNA chips are useful adjuncts in epigenetic studies of glioblastomas. Neuropathology. 2006;26(5):409–16.
Kitange G, Misra A, Law M, Passe S, Kollmeyer TM, Maurer M, Ballman K, Feuerstein BG, Jenkins RB. Chromosomal imbalances detected by array comparative genomic hybridization in human oligodendrogliomas and mixed oligoastrocytomas. Genes Chromosomes Cancer. 2005;42(1):68–77.
Kurian KM, Jones DT, Marsden F, Openshaw SW, Pearson DM, Ichimura K, Collins VP. Genome-wide analysis of subependymomas shows underlying chromosomal copy number changes involving chromosomes 6, 7, 8 and 14 in a proportion of cases. Brain Pathol. 2008;18(4):469–73.
Maher EA, Brennan C, Wen PY, Durso L, Ligon KL, Richardson A, Khatry D, Feng B, Sinha R, Louis DN, Quackenbush J, Black PM, Chin L, DePinho RA. Marked genomic differences characterize primary and secondary glioblastoma subtypes and identify two distinct molecular and clinical secondary glioblastoma entities. Cancer Res. 2006; 66(23): 11502–13.
Mendrzyk F, Korshunov A, Benner A, Toedt G, Pfister S, Radlwimmer B, Lichter P. Identification of gains on 1q and epidermal growth factor receptor overexpression as independent prognostic markers in intracranial ependymoma. Clin Cancer Res. 2006; 12(7 Pt 1):2070–9.
Misra A, Pellarin M, Nigro J, Smirnov I, Moore D, Lamborn KR, Pinkel D, Albertson DG, Feuerstein BG. Array comparative genomic hybridization identifies genetic subgroups in grade 4 human astrocytoma. Clin Cancer Res. 2005;11(8):2907–18.
Misra A, Pellarin M, Hu L, Kunwar S, Perhouse M, Lamborn KR, Deen DF, Feuerstein BG. Chromosome transfer experiments link regions on chromosome 7 to radiation resistance in human glioblastoma multiforme. Genes Chromosomes Cancer. 2006;45(1):20–30.
Misra A, Smirnov I, Yeh R, VandenBerg S, Hong C, Hirose Y, Kharbanda S, Nigro J, Pan E, Prestegarden L, Costello J, Yates A, Pearl D, Scheithauer B, Giannini C, Burger P,

Phillips, H, Aldape K and Feuerstein BG. PTEN Copy number is a better marker for survival than histologic grade in consensus grade 2 and 3 astrocytomas. *Unpublished data.*

Mohapatra G, Bollen AW, Kim DH, Lamborn K, Moore DH, Prados MD, Feuerstein BG. Genetic analysis of glioblastoma multiforme provides evidence for subgroups within the grade. Genes Chromosomes Cancer. 1998;21(3):195–206.

Mohapatra G, Betensky RA, Miller ER, Carey B, Gaumont LD, Engler DA, Louis DN. Glioma test array for use with formalin-fixed, paraffin-embedded tissue: array comparative genomic hybridization correlates with loss of heterozygosity and fluorescence in situ hybridization. J Mol Diagn. 2006;8(2):268–76.

Nigro JM, Misra A, Zhang L, Smirnov I, Colman H, Griffin C, Ozburn N, Chen M, Pan E, Koul D, Yung WK, Feuerstein BG, Aldape KD. Integrated array-comparative genomic hybridization and expression array profiles identify clinically relevant molecular subtypes of glioblastoma. Cancer Res. 2005;65(5):1678–86.

Parsons DW, Jones S, Zhang X, Lin JC, Leary RJ, Angenendt P, Mankoo P, Carter H, Siu IM, Gallia GL, Olivi A, McLendon R, Rasheed BA, Keir S, Nikolskaya T, Nikolsky Y, Busam DA, Tekleab H, Diaz LA Jr, Hartigan J, Smith DR, Strausberg RL, Marie SK, Shinjo SM, Yan H, Riggins GJ, Bigner DD, Karchin R, Papadopoulos N, Parmigiani G, Vogelstein B, Velculescu VE, Kinzler KW. An integrated genomic analysis of human glioblastoma multiforme. Science. 2008;321(5897):1807–12.

Pfister S, Janzarik WG, Remke M, Ernst A, Werft W, Becker N, Toedt G, Wittmann A, Kratz C, Olbrich H, Ahmadi R, Thieme B, Joos S, Radlwimmer B, Kulozik A, Pietsch T, Herold-Mende C, Gnekow A, Reifenberger G, Korshunov A, Scheurlen W, Omran H, Lichter P. BRAF gene duplication constitutes a mechanism of MAPK pathway activation in low-grade astrocytomas. J Clin Invest. 2008;118(5):1739–49.

Phillips HS, Kharbanda S, Chen R, Forrest WF, Soriano RH, Wu TD, Misra A, Nigro JM, Colman H, Soroceanu L, Williams PM, Modrusan Z, Feuerstein BG, Aldape K. Molecular subclasses of high-grade glioma predict prognosis, delineate a pattern of disease progression, and resemble stages in neurogenesis. Cancer Cell. 2006;9 (3):157–73.

Pinkel D, Segraves R, Sudar D, Clark S, Poole I, Kowbel D, Collins C, Kuo WL, Chen C, Zhai Y, Dairkee SH, Ljung BM, Gray JW, Albertson DG. High resolution analysis of DNA copy number variation using comparative genomic hybridization to microarrays. Nat Genet. 1998;20(2):207–11.

Pollack JR, Perou CM, Alizadeh AA, Eisen MB, Pergamenschikov A, Williams CF, Jeffrey SS, Botstein D, Brown PO. Genome-wide analysis of DNA copy-number changes using cDNA microarrays. Nat Genet. 1999;23(1):41–6.

Prestegarden L, Misra A, Ware ML, Yeh RF, Bjerkvig R, Feuerstein BG. Amplifying small amounts of tumor DNA allows detection of DNA copy number abberations with array-CGH. Biotechniques. 2008;44(7):Piii–Pvi.

Ruano Y, Mollejo M, Ribalta T, Fiaño C, Camacho FI, Gómez E, de Lope AR, Hernández-Moneo JL, Martínez P, Meléndez B. Identification of novel candidate target genes in amplicons of Glioblastoma multiforme tumors detected by expression and CGH microarray profiling. Mol Cancer. 2006;5:39–50.

Saigusa K, Hashimoto N, Tsuda H, Yokoi S, Maruno M, Yoshimine T, Aoyagi M, Ohno K, Imoto I, Inazawa J. Overexpressed Skp2 within 5p amplification detected by array-based comparative genomic hybridization is associated with poor prognosis of glioblastomas. Cancer Sci. 2005;96(10):676–83.

Sambrook J, Fritsch EF, MAniatis T. Preparation of radiolabeled DNA and RNA probes, In: Molecularcloning. 2nd ed, Cold Spring Harbor: Cold Spring Harbor laboratory; 1989: p.e3–4; 10.8–10.10; 10.14–15.

Snijders AM, Nowak N, Segraves R, Blackwood S, Brown N, Conroy J, Hamilton G, Hindle AK, Huey B, Kimura K, Law S, Myambo K, Palmer J, Ylstra B, Yue JP, Gray JW, Jain AN, Pinkel D, Albertson DG. Assembly of microarrays for genome-wide measurement of DNA copy number. Nat Genet. 2001;29(3):263–4.

Soroceanu L, Kharbanda S, Chen R, Soriano RH, Aldape K, Misra A, Zha J, Forrest WF, Nigro JM, Modrusan Z, Feuerstein BG, Phillips HS. Identification of IGF2 signaling through phosphoinositide-3-kinase regulatory subunit 3 as a growth-promoting axis in glioblastoma. Proc Natl Acad Sci USA. 2007;104(9):3466–71.

Tanabe C, Aoyagi K, Sakiyama T, Kohno T, Yanagitani N, et al. Evaluation of a whole-genome amplification method based on adaptor-ligation PCR of randomly sheared genomic DNA. Genes Chromosomes Cancer. 2003; 38:168–76.

Telenius H, Pelmear AH, Tunnacliffe A, Carter NP, Behmel A, Ferguson-Smith MA, Nordenskjöld M, Pfragner R, Ponder BA. Cytogenetic analysis by chromosome painting using DOP-PCR amplified flow-sorted chromosomes. Genes Chromosomes Cancer. 1992; 4: 257–63.

The Cancer Genome Atlas Research Network. Comprehensive genomic characterization defines human glioblastoma genes and core pathways. Nature. 2008 Sep 4. [Epub ahead of print]

Tomioka N, Oba S, Ohira M, Misra A, Fridlyand J, Ishii S, Nakamura Y, Isogai E, Hirata T, Yoshida Y, Todo S, Kaneko Y, Albertson DG, Pinkel D, Feuerstein BG, Nakagawara A. Novel risk stratification of patients with neuroblastoma by genomic signature, which is independent of molecular signature. Oncogene. 2007 ;27(4):441–9.

Wang G, Brennan C, Rook M, Wolfe JL, Leo C, et al. Balanced-PCR amplification allows unbiased identification of genomic copy changes in minute cell and tissue samples. Nucleic Acids Res. 2004a; 32:e76

Wang G, Maher E, Brennan C, Chin L, Leo C, et al. DNA amplification method tolerant to sample degradation. Genome Res. 2004b; 14:2357–66.

Willenbrock H, Fridlyand J. A comparison study: applying segmentation to array CGH data for downstream analyses. Bioinformatics. 2005;21(22):4084–91.

Zardo G, Tiirikainen MI, Hong C, Misra A, Feuerstein BG, Volik S, Collins CC, Lamborn KR, Bollen A, Pinkel D, Albertson DG, Costello JF. Integrated genomic and epigenomic analyses pinpoint biallelic gene inactivation in tumors. Nat Genet. 2002;32(3):453–8.

Chapter 18
Genomic Identification of Significant Targets in Brain Cancer

Rameen Beroukhim, Gaddy Getz, and Ingo K. Mellinghoff

Abstract Recent advances in technology have empowered the cancer community to collect an almost unlimited amount of molecular data points from even small, routinely collected primary human tumor samples. It is still unclear, however, how to best extract biologically relevant information from such datasets for subsequent validation studies and biomarker development. The need for robust computational tools is particularly pressing in the systematic analysis of the cancer genome which is hampered by the lack of a statistical framework to distinguish between "driver" mutations and "passenger" mutations. In this chapter, we review a new bioinformatic method, called genomic identification of significant targets in cancer (GISTIC), designed for analyzing chromosomal aberrations in cancer under specific consideration for such random events. This chapter describes the original development of this method on primary glioma tumor samples, its subsequent application to other cancer types, and further modifications of algorithm.

Contents

I.K. Mellinghoff (✉)
Department of Neurology and Human Oncology & Pathogenesis Program, Memorial Sloan-Kettering Cancer Center, 1275 York Avenue, Mailbox 20, New York, NY 10065
e-mail: mellingi@mskcc.org

E.G. Van Meir (ed.), *CNS Cancer*, Cancer Drug Discovery and Development, DOI 10.1007/978-1-60327-553-8_18,
© Humana Press, a part of Springer Science+Business Media, LLC 2009

18.1 Introduction

Recent advances in molecular oncology have generated great optimism that the empiric use of anticancer agents will soon be transformed into a practice of "personalized" cancer medicine where the molecular profile of the patient's tumor, rather than tissue type and population-based trials, will guide the choice of therapeutic interventions (Varmus, 2006). There is compelling evidence that activating mutations in signaling pathways can result in tumor cell "addiction" to this pathway (Weinstein, 2002) and predict clinical responses to pathway inhibition (Sawyers, 2003). This has clearly been shown for chronic myeloid leukemia driven by the protein product of the *BCR-ABL* translocation (Druker et al., 2001), breast cancers harboring *HER2* gene amplifications (Slamon et al., 2001), *EGFR* mutant lung cancers (Paez et al., 2004; Lynch et al., 2004), and selected other human malignancies. The early success and promise of targeted cancer therapy has spurred large-scale efforts to paint a more refined, and perhaps clinically more meaningful, molecular portrait of cancer using new high-resolution tools of mutational profiling (Thomas et al., 2007), gene expression analysis (Chung et al., 2002), and proteomics (Rikova et al., 2007). These advances are slowly making their way into the oncology drug development process as pharmaceutical companies have begun to include gene expression analysis, gene copy-number determinations, and mutational profiling into clinical trial design (Kummar et al., 2007).

While the cancer community is now empowered to collect an almost unlimited amount of molecular data points from even small, routinely collected primary human tumor samples, it is still unclear how to best extract biologically relevant information from such datasets for subsequent validation studies and biomarker development (Sawyers, 2008; Feero et al., 2008). The need for robust computational tools is particularly pressing in the systematic analysis of the cancer genome which is hampered by the lack of a statistical framework to distinguish between "driver" mutations which confer a biological property that allows the tumor to initiate, grow, or persist and "passenger" mutations which represent random somatic events that preceded clonal expansion and are carried along without conferring any fitness advantage (Fig. 18.1 and Color Plate 25).

The distinction between "driver" and "passenger" mutations is critical not only for the interpretation of high-throughput sequencing projects (Wood et al., 2007; Getz et al., 2007; Rubin and Green, 2007; Forrest and Cavet, 2007), but also in the genome-wide analysis of gene copy-number alterations (Pinkel et al., 1998). In the context of chromosomal aberrations such as amplification and deletion, it is common practice to identify and report "regions of interest" as genomic areas that are most frequently affected by gene copy-number alterations within the examined sample set. "Driver" genes are assumed to reside within the chromosomal segment most consistently affected by the gene copy-number alterations, the so-called "minimal common region". It is easily

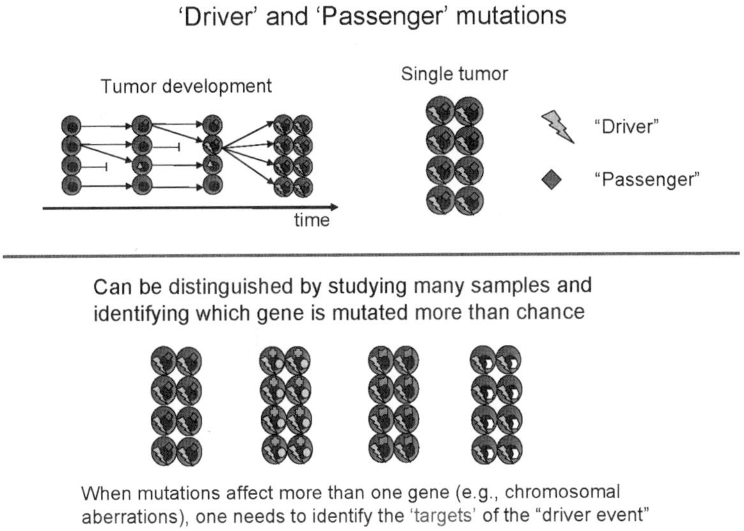

Fig. 18.1 "Driver" and "passenger" mutations in the cancer genome (*see* Color Plate 25)

apparent how the presence of random "passenger" alterations can skew the identification of these minimal common regions in large sample sets (Fig. 18.2), perhaps explaining the poor overlap in "regions of interest" between different studies of copy-number alterations for the same type of tumor. Two recent lung cancer studies of similar sample size and methodology, for example, described a

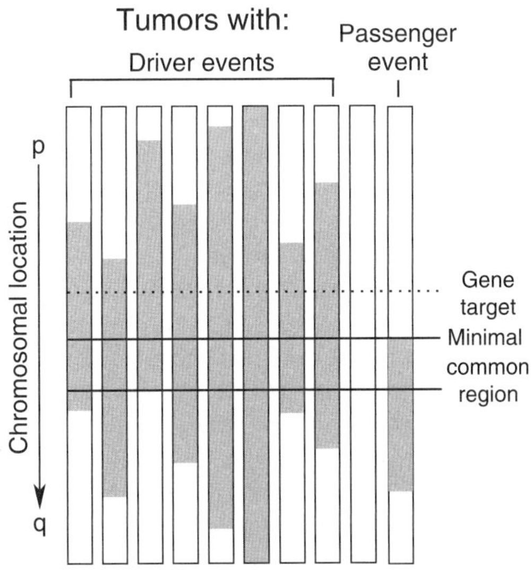

Fig. 18.2 Displacement of minimal common regions by passenger mutations. The cartoon illustrates how passenger mutations in one tumor within a larger dataset can result in the displacement of the minimal common region for the complete group of tumors

large number of regions of interest (48 and 93), but less than 5% of these regions overlapped between the two datasets (Tonon et al., 2005; Zhao et al., 2005). While this discordance might be explained by insufficient size of each study to capture all aberrations for this particular cancer type, it is also possible that many of the regions of interest represented random events which are not explicitly accounted for by current analysis methods.

In this chapter, we review a new bioinformatic method, called Genomic Identification of Significant Targets in Cancer (GISTIC), designed for analyzing chromosomal aberrations in cancer under specific consideration for such random events. This method has been developed on a glioma dataset (Beroukhim et al., 2007) and has subsequently been applied to large genomic datasets for other cancer types (Weir et al., 2007; Takeyama et al., 2008; Lin et al., 2008; Haverty et al., 2008; Chiang et al., 2008).

18.2 Key Features of the GISTIC Algorithm

With data describing chromosomal aberrations in large tumor sets, the aberrations that drive tumorigenesis and the oncogenes and TSGs they most likely target can be identified if the following four issues are addressed. (*i*) The aberrations in each of the tumors must be accurately mapped. (*ii*) Driver aberrations that rise above the background rate of random passenger aberrations must be identified. (*iii*) For each driver aberration, the loci most likely to contain the targeted oncogenes or TSGs must be identified. (*iv*) Tumors must be classified as to whether they are aberrant at the predicted driver loci, so that the effects of those aberrations can be studied. Each of these issues is addressed in a different stage in the GISTIC algorithm (see below).

The core conceptual stage involves the identification of driver events among the total set of aberrations. GISTIC identifies these through a statistical analysis divided into two key steps (Fig. 18.3 and Color Plate 26). First, the method calculates a statistic (*G*-score) that involves both the frequency of occurrence and "amplitude" of the aberration (i.e., the number of gene copies that are gained or lost). Homozygous deletions and high-level gene copy-number gains are given higher scores because they are less likely to occur by chance. Second, it assesses the statistical significance of each aberration by comparing the observed statistic to the results that would be expected by chance, using a permutation test that is based on the overall pattern of aberrations seen across the genome. The method accounts for multiple hypothesis testing using the false-discovery rate (FDR) framework and assigns a q value to each result, reflecting the probability that the event is due to chance fluctuation. For each significant region, the method defines a "peak region" with the greatest frequency and amplitude of aberration. Each peak is tested to determine whether the signal is due primarily to broad events, focal events, or overlapping events of both types.

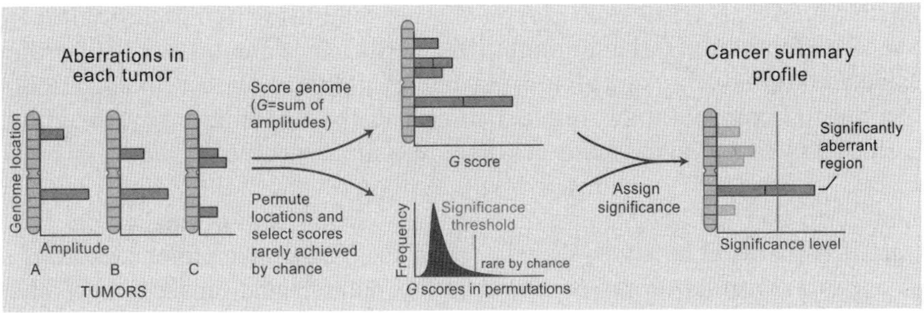

Fig. 18.3 Overview of the GISTIC. After identifying the locations and magnitudes of chromosomal aberrations in multiple tumors (*left*), GISTIC scores each genomic marker with a *G*-score that is proportional to the total magnitude of aberrations at each location. By permuting the locations in each tumor, GISTIC determines the frequency with which a given score would be attained if the events were due to chance and randomly distributed (*center*). A significance threshold (*green line*) is determined such that significant scores are unlikely to occur by chance alone and alterations are considered significant if they occur in regions that surpass this threshold (*right*) (*see* Color Plate 26)

18.3 The Four Stages of the GISTIC: A Detailed View

The goal of stage 1 of the GISTIC algorithm is to determine accurately for each tumor the copy-number changes and, if genotyping data are available, loss-of-heterozygosity events. To accomplish this, the algorithm makes multiple efforts to minimize systematic and random errors and discard poor-quality datasets.

We limit systematic errors in two steps: first, by selecting appropriate controls for each tumor and second, by limiting the effects of the major contributor to systematic error, batch effect. The basis of these steps is the recognition that systematic errors arise when tumor data are generated under slightly different experimental conditions from their normal controls, leading to differences in signal intensities between the tumors and their controls. Examples of such experimental conditions are the day of data generation (batch), day of manufacture of the array, or slight variations in PCR conditions when generating target for the array. Because copy-number changes are called when signal intensities differ between the tumor and its normal controls, such variations in experimental conditions can lead to artifactual copy-number change events. Some array comparative genomic hybridization platforms inherently minimize these types of errors by using two-color systems in which tumor and control DNA are hybridized simultaneously to the same array. Many datasets are produced using single-color systems, however, such as the Affymetrix SNP arrays we used to study chromosomal aberrations in glioma. Rather than using paired normals from the same individual (which might differ in the experimental conditions they have undergone), or using all normal data available, we select for each tumor the normal controls that are most similar in the signal intensity variations induced by noise across the genome. We also specifically address batch effects, in which data generated on different days vary slightly, by identifying and correcting markers that show consistent signal within batches but large variations between batches. We have found that these interventions result in as much as a threefold decrease in noise in our datasets and far fewer artifactual copy-number events.

We limit random error using previously developed methods. Many such methods identify regions of copy-number change and determine the level of change as the average normalized signal intensity for all markers within each region (Lai et al., 2005). Examples include segmentation algorithms such as circular binary segmentation (CBS) (Olshen et al., 2004), gain and loss analysis of DNA (GLAD) (Hupe et al., 2004), hidden Markov model-based approaches (Zhao et al., 2004), and clustering methods (Wang et al., 2005). Each has advantages and disadvantages that may vary with the noise characteristics of the dataset. We used GLAD due to its high sensitivity for identifying copy-number changes (Lai et al., 2005). However, this high level of sensitivity occasionally leads GLAD to report non-existent copy-number changes in very small segments (fewer than four markers), so we filtered those out. In practice, we find that our results are almost identical when we use other algorithms such as CBS.

We also perform a quality control step to remove datasets in which copy-number changes are obscured by noise. We have found that when we generate histograms of signal intensities in each tumor, high-quality datasets exhibit separate peaks, corresponding to different copy-numbers in the tumor. Poor-quality samples, particularly those with extensive contamination with normal DNA, generate insufficient signal to distinguish these separate peaks. We therefore discard them. In the case of SNP array data, we also take advantage of the genotyping information to identify and eliminate duplicate samples from the same individual.

The two core features of GISTIC are contained within stage 2: scoring of the genome and determination of the significance of each score (Fig. 18.3). Each genomic marker is given a *G*-score that reflects the level of evidence that it is in a region affected by driver aberrations. Amplifications, deletions, and LOH events are treated separately to allow for the possibility that a region could be significantly amplified and deleted simultaneously, for instance if an oncogene and TSG neighbor each other. In the cases of amplifications and deletions, we assume that both the prevalence and average amplitude of these events independently indicate the likelihood with which a region is affected by such driver aberrations. Therefore, we use a simple integrated score of the prevalence of the copy-number change times the average ($\log_2$-transformed) amplitude. In the case of LOH, amplitudes do not apply and we therefore score each marker only by the prevalence of events. A separate analysis of LOH reflecting loss of heterozygous genotypes identifies regions of copy-neutral LOH (e.g., "uniparental disomy") in addition to regions of LOH that result from hemizygous deletion.

To determine the significance of each *G*-score, we compare it to the distribution of scores expected if only random aberrations were observed. This distribution can be determined by permuting the marker locations within each sample and then rescoring the genome. To save computing time, we derive a semi-exact estimate of this distribution. We can then compare the scores actually obtained to those generated by our null model of random aberrations to calculate the statistical significance of each *G*-score (represented by false-discovery rate *q*-values), representing the likelihood that the observed data could have been generated by chance alone. We then select regions of the genome that are too frequently or highly aberrant to be explained by chance alone as likely to harbor driver aberrations.

The goal of stage 3 is to identify the regions most likely to harbor the oncogene or TSG targets of the driver aberrations identified in stage 2. Because the genes targeted by an aberration are most likely to lie in the region most frequently aberrant to the highest degree, we select the "peak" regions with maximal *G*-scores and (an equivalent statement) minimal *q*-values as most likely to contain the oncogene or TSG targets.

However, these peak regions may be displaced away from the oncogene or TSG targets of an aberration by occasional random passenger events that happen to occur near, but not overlapping, these oncogenes or TSGs (Fig. 18.2). To account for this possibility, we perform a leave-one-out analysis: we leave each sample out in turn and recalculate the boundaries of the peak region. By taking only the widest boundaries so calculated, we select regions that are robust to the presence of these occasional distractive passenger events.

We also allow for the possibility that a single region may contain two or more independent gene targets by applying a "peel-off" method designed to identify aberrations that overlap but are independently statistically significant. Furthermore, we characterize each event as primarily focal or broad. Primarily broad events may exert their effects through broad-based changes across much of their length, rather than solely through effects on a limited number of genes in the peak region.

The goal of stage 4 is to classify tumors on the basis of the driver aberrations they exhibit. Here, we first classify each tumor according to its copy-number status at the peak regions, since these are most likely to contain the gene targets of each aberration. For broad aberrations, which may be specifically disrupting a large region of the genome, we also classify each tumor as to whether it is aberrant across most of the length of the region. This stage allows the user to identify correlations between events or between events and clinical or other parameters.

18.4 Application of GISTIC to Glioma

We developed the GISTIC algorithm on a newly generated, high-resolution dataset of chromosomal aberrations in 141 gliomas (Beroukhim et al., 2007). We chose glioblastoma as our initial application because we were able to benchmark the results of our GISTIC analysis against the substantial number of previous surveys of the glioblastoma genome (Feuerstein and Mohapatra, 1995; Ichimura et al., 2004) and because the biological significance of the most frequently altered genes in such surveys has already been examined in experimental models (Holland, 2001).

Figure 18.4A and Color Plate 27 shows a color representation (also referred to as "heatmap") of the inferred copy-number values for each of the 100,000 single nucleotide polymorphism (SNP) loci in each tumor sample with red representing copy gain and blue representing copy loss. The overall pattern across the entire sample set (arranged from left to right) is clearly complex with almost every region of the genome being altered in at least one tumor. Figure 18.4B shows the GISTIC output for the 105 primary tumor samples which passed our quality control. The latter group of tumors represents mostly primary glioblastomas (71%), a much smaller fraction of secondary glioblastomas (11%), and lower grade gliomas. Using GISTIC, we identified 32 statistically significant events of genomic amplification or loss. Because of the previously reported differences in gene copy-number alterations between primary and secondary glioblastomas (Maher et al., 2006) and between astrocytic and oligodendroglial tumors (Kraus et al., 1995), we ran a separate GISTIC analysis for our subgroup of primary glioblastomas. This analysis did not uncover any additional statistically significant alterations.

Areas of statistically significant gene copy-number change fell into two major categories: focal events and broad events (near the size of a chromosome arm). In some instances, focal events were superimposed on broad events, including focal events on chromosomes 7, 9, 10, and 13. The 16 broad events in our dataset included six amplifications (chromosomes 7, 8q, 12p, 17q, 19p, and 20), nine deletions (6q, 9p, 10, 11p, 13, 14, 16q, 19q, and 22), and one region of copy-neutral LOH (17p). These events were particularly common (range 10–70%, median 27%). Consistent with previous lower resolution surveys of the glioblastoma genome, copy gain of chr7 and copy loss of chr10 were exceedingly common (>60% of all glioma samples and >80% of our primary GBMs). For broad regions without superimposed focal events, the peak regions were large with a median of 110 genes. Most of the 16 focal events occurred at lower frequencies than the broad aberrations (range 6–49%, median 14%). Among these, amplifications of 4q12 and 7p11.2 and deletions of 1p36.31 and 9p21.3 were the most frequent. Some areas of focal copy gain reached statistical significance based on the high level of copy gain despite their overall rare occurrence (6–7%) across the entire dataset, e.g., regions containing *CDK4*

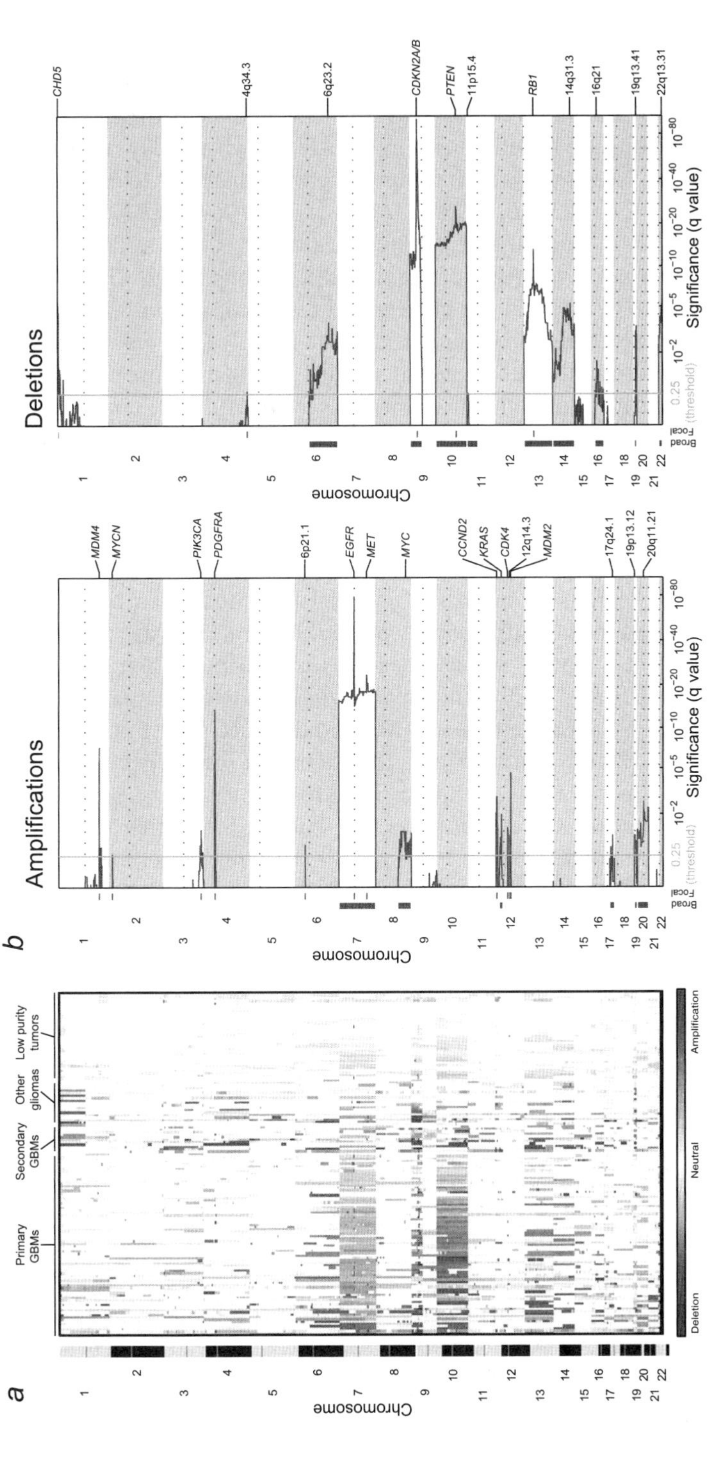

Fig. 18.4 Application of GISTIC to glioma. (**A**) Amplifications (*red*) and deletions (*blue*), determined by segmentation analysis of normalized signal intensities from 100 K SNP arrays are displayed across the genome (chromosome positions indicated along the *y*-axis) for 141 gliomas (*x*-axis, diagnosis

and *MDM2* on chr12. Peak regions for the focal events could generally be localized to small regions of the genome, containing a median of four genes.

One of the most gratifying aspects during the application of GISTIC to our glioma dataset was the frequency with which predicted "driver" mutations in our dataset coincided with genes previously shown to play a role in glioma formation. A recent review of the glioma literature listed 12 such "glioma genes" (*TP53*, *RB1*, *CDKN2A/B*, *PTEN*, *EGFR*, *PDGFRA*, *MET*, *CDK4*, *CDK6*, *MDM2*, *MDM4*, and *MYC*) (Reifenberger and Collins, 2004) and 11/12 genes corresponded with one of the 28 peak regions in our GISTIC analysis. The 12th gene (*CDK6*) did not correspond to a peak region but resided within the broad region of significant amplification on chr7. *TP53* was not identified as a peak of copy-number change, but resided within the single peak region of LOH and thus appears to be primarily inactivated through copy-neutral LOH (and mutation). The finding that *TP53*undergoes LOH (determined by genotyping the tumors) but not deletion (determined by local signal intensities) suggests the possibility that deletion of the region including *TP53* is disadvantageous for the tumor and emphasizes the need to genotype tumors (to identify regions of LOH) in addition to profiling copy-number changes.

Other peak regions in our GISTIC analysis included genes that have not (yet) been implicated in the pathogenesis of glioblastoma, but are believed to play prominent roles in other cancers, such as transcription factor *MYCN*, PI3-kinase subunit *PIK3CA*(also known as *p110α*), cell cycle regulator *CCND2*, ras family member *KRAS*, and chromatin modulator *CHD5* (Futreal et al., 2004; Bagchi et al., 2007; Fujita et al., 2008). Twelve other genomic regions of significant copy-number alteration in GISTIC show no association with known cancer genes and are of particular interest for further study, including amplifications of 6p, 12q, 17q, 19p, and 20q, and deletions of 4q, 6q, 11p, 14q, 16q, 19q, and 22q (Beroukhim et al., 2007).

A critical question in any high-resolution survey of the cancer genome is whether the large number of identified alterations adds up to a representative molecular portrait of the examined cancer type. If our GISTIC results were indeed representative for glioblastoma, we expected to find a very similar pattern of gene copy-number alterations if we ran copy-number data from other glioblastoma sample sets through our GISTIC algorithm. We were particularly interested in this question as two previous studies of copy-number alterations in glioma (178 samples on 100 K SNP arrays; 37 samples on a 16 K CGH arrays) (Maher et al., 2006; Kotliarov et al., 2006) reported many

Fig. 18.4 (continued) is displayed on top). (**B**) GISTIC analysis with statistical significance of the aberrations displayed as FDR *q*-values to account for multiple hypothesis testing. Centromere positions are indicated for each chromosome by a dotted line. The locations of the peak regions and the known cancer-related genes within those peaks are indicated to the right of each panel (*see* Color Plate 27) more regions of interest (208 and 97, respectively), identified fewer of the known "glioma genes", and showed an overall low concordance with one another. When we applied bioinformatic algorithms used in these previous studies to our dataset (i.e., focus on minimal common regions of copy-number change without explicit correction for background noise), we identified a similarly large number of regions (144) and fewer glioma-associated genes. Conversely, we reduced the number of statistically significant copy-number alterations to 24 and 26 regions, respectively, when we applied the raw data from the other two datasets through GISTIC and these regions agreed closely with the regions identified in the initial GISTIC analysis of our dataset. In contrast to the close resemblance of our three glioblastoma datasets, the genome-wide pattern of gene copy-number alterations was distinctly different when we applied GISTIC to a lung cancer dataset (Fig. 18.5 and Color Plate 28).

Collectively, these results demonstrated that GISTIC was able to draw a concordant picture of the glioma genome. After combining both 100K Affymetrix SNP array datasets (total of 319 samples), several regions in our original dataset now exceeded the significance threshold (raising the number of significantly altered regions to a total of 34 regions) and peak regions were further narrowed down from 12 to 5 genes per region (median gene number). Large datasets, as currently being generated in the context of the glioblastoma pilot project of The Cancer Genome Project (TCGA, 2008), may be able to define these regions with even greater precision.

We also examined the question whether overlapping focal and broad events may identify subsets of biologically distinct tumors, using chromosome 7 as an example. Compared with GBMs with broad amplification of chromosome 7 in the absence of focal *EGFR* amplification (7^{gain}), tumors with focal *EGFR* amplification ($7^{gain}EGFR^{amp}$) in our dataset more frequently overexpressed EGFR, were more frequently associated with EGFR mutations, and were less frequently associated with TP53 mutations, as previously reported (Ekstrand et al., 1992; Galanis et al., 1998; Watanabe et al., 1996; Lee et al., 2006). To identify targets genes that might drive a subset of 7^{gain} tumors, we identified genes on the chromosome that show extreme outliers in expression in at least 10% of tumors with 7^{gain} (compared with 7^{normal}), based on the concept that broad events such as 7^{gain} are likely to have heterogeneous effects across various tumors. Two of the top four genes in this "comparative outlier analysis" encoded the receptor MET and its ligand HGF. Approximately one-third of 7^{gain} events were associated with either *MET* or *HGF* overexpression, and tumors that overexpress one were more likely to overexpress both ($P = 0.06$). A combined analysis of gene expression and copy-number data in glioblastoma cell lines demonstrated increased MET receptor activation in the subset of cell lines with 7^{gain} and overexpression of *MET* and *HGF* and these cell lines showed enhanced responsiveness to the MET kinase inhibitor SU11274 (Beroukhim et al., 2007). 7^{gain} with combined overexpression of *MET* and *HGF* may thus provide a mechanism for cell-autonomous activation of the MET signaling pathway in glioma. The finding that HGF does not represent a target of focal

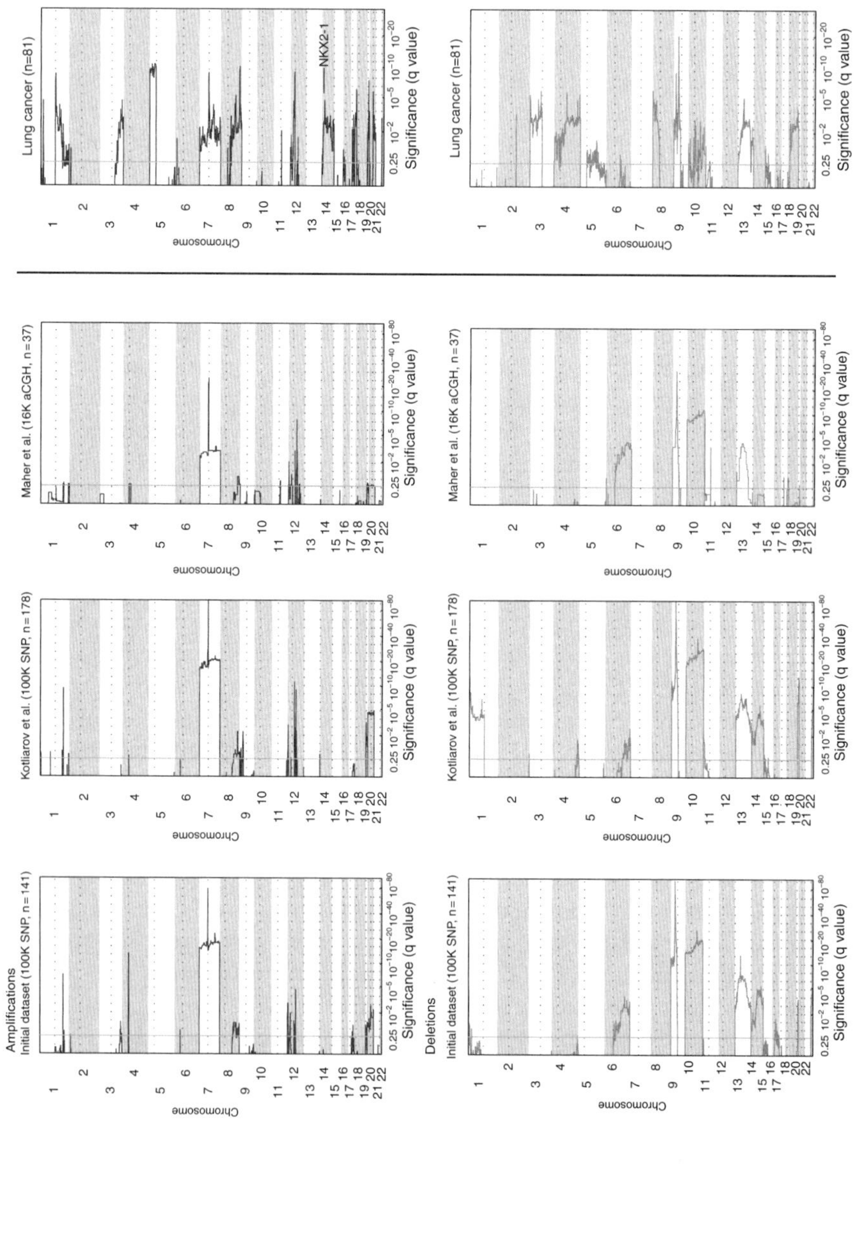

Fig. 18.5 (continued)

gene amplification illustrates the value of adding orthogonal datasets (such as gene expression profiling) to identify target genes within broad genomic events.

18.5 Application of GISTIC to Other Cancers

The ability of GISTIC to provide a concordant picture of the glioma genome has encouraged its further use in the context of systematic cancer genome discovery projects for other cancer types. The largest such study, led by Matthew Meyerson at the Broad Institute, examined gene copy-number alterations in genomic DNA from 371 lung tumors hybridized to Affymetrix 250 k single nucleotide polymorphism arrays and identified a total of 57 significantly recurrent events, including 26 areas of large-scale copy-number gain or loss and 31 recurrent focal events (Weir et al., 2007). The overall pattern of significant copy-number alterations was consistent with the literature on lung cancer and – similar to our experience in glioma – GISTIC identified many disease-relevant genes in this disease as "driver mutations" in areas of focal amplifications (*EGFR*, *KRAS*, and *ERBB2)*and deletions (e.g., CDKN2A/CDKN2B, PTEN, and RB1). Three additional deletion regions each localized to a single gene (AUTS2, PDE4D, and PTPRD) of which one (PTPRD) harbored somatic mutations in 11/188 samples and likely represents a new tumor suppressor phosphatase. GISTIC was also able to narrow down the critical region on the most common focal amplification (chromosome 14q13.3) to a 480-kb interval containing only two known genes, *MBIP* (MAP3K12 binding inhibitory protein 1) and *NKX2-1*(NK2 homeobox 1, also called *TITF1*) which encodes a lineage-specific transcription factor and was functionally validated as a novel candidate proto-oncogene. Of note, when we applied GISTIC to a previously published, lower resolution dataset comprising only 83 lung tumors (Zhao et al., 2005), we found similar peak regions, including the 14q13.3 amplification that contains *NKX2-1*(Fig. 18.5 and Color Plate 28). The use of the smaller dataset resulted in poorer ability to pinpoint target genes. Nevertheless, *NKX2-1* was one of only six genes in its peak region. The finding that GISTIC could pinpoint a novel oncogene in a dataset published 2 years before the discovery of that oncogene suggests the importance of a systematic analytic approach to identifying cancer-related genes.

A second study used GISTIC as part of a systematic genomic analysis of 101 melanoma short-term cultures (Lin et al., 2008) and identified 14 areas of

Fig. 18.5 (continued) GISTIC identifies cancer-specific patterns of gene copy-number alterations. Results of the original GISTIC analysis (displayed as in Fig. 7) are presented alongside similar analyses of 178 tumors on 100 K SNP arrays (Kotliarov et al., 2006) and 37 tumors on 16 K CGH arrays (Maher et al., 2006). A strikingly distinct pattern is seen when the original GISTIC analysis of glioma is compared to a similar analysis of 81 lung cancer samples using 100 K SNP arrays (Zhao et al., 2005) (*see* Color Plate 28) significant copy-number gain and 13 regions of significant copy-number loss. One of the most significant regions of copy gain was located on chromosome 7q34 (65% of samples) and this locus harbors the oncogene *BRAF*, a regulator of the MAP kinase signaling pathway previously shown to be mutated in > 50% of cutaneous melanomas (Davies et al., 2002). Other GISTIC peaks localized exquisitely to the microphthalmia-associated transcription factor *(MITF)* gene, a master transcriptional regulator of melanocyte development, and to the cell cycle regulator cyclin D1. The most prominent region of significant copy loss identified cyclin-dependent kinase inhibitor 2A *(CDKN2A)*, an established tumor suppressor gene in melanoma. To place their findings into the context of gene copy-number alterations identified in other melanoma studies, the authors compared GISTIC plots generated on 250 K SNP arrays from 70 melanoma short-term cultures, 50 K SNP arrays from 31 additional short-term cultures and cell lines, 33 K tiling arrays from 45 independent cell lines, and BAC array CGH data derived from 70 primary cutaneous melanomas. The resulting GISTIC plots were strikingly similar across all datasets, reminiscent of our experience with different genomic platforms and datasets in glioma.

A third study used GISTIC to examine recurrent gene copy-number alterations collected on 238,000 genomic loci in 103 primary tumor samples from early stage hepatitis C-related hepatocellular carcinomas (Chiang et al., 2008). Focal regions of copy gain or loss were rare events in this group of tumors. Only 15% of tumors harbored at least one high-level gain and GISTIC was able to identify the vascular endothelial growth factor A *(VEGFA)* gene as likely target of the high-level copy gain on 6p21. Additional applications of GISTIC include genomic projects in breast cancer (Haverty et al., 2008) and lymphoma (Takeyama et al., 2008).

18.6 Limitations and Future Modifications of the GISTIC Algorithm

Similar to the experience with other computational algorithms aiming to identify the biologically most meaningful alterations in the cancer genome, such as "Significance Testing for Aberrant Copy number" *(STAC)* (Diskin et al., 2006), "Multiple Sample Analysis" *(MSA)* (Guttman et al., 2007), and the "Genome topography scanning" (GTS) (Wiedemeyer et al., 2008), a number of variables limit the identification of "driver events" by GISTIC. The two most obvious confounding factors are germline copy-number polymorphisms, which will score as recurrent events at the same locus, and systematic artifacts during data collection (e.g., batch effects). Special effort has been made in the pre-processing steps of the GISTIC algorithm to correct for both of these variables (Beroukhim et al., 2007).

The relative weighting of copy-number amplitude and frequency in the current GISTIC algorithm represents an estimate that seemed particularly well suited to the glioma dataset on which the algorithm was developed (Beroukhim et al., 2007). In glioma, the frequency with which copy-number changes were seen appeared to correspond to the log of the change in copy-number and we therefore scored copy-number changes by their $\log_2$ ratios rather than the absolute copy-number change. Other tumor types may exhibit a different relationship between amplitude and frequency of key genomic alterations, and a modification of the weighting scheme might generate more accurate estimates of the significance of both rare and common genomic events in such cancers. Also, the overall ploidy of each tumor cannot be determined from array data alone with current copy-number algorithms. Therefore, the amplitude measurements are necessarily relative to the euploid level, rather than measured in absolute number of copies added or deleted. If methods are developed in the future to determine absolute copy-numbers, these data can be easily integrated into the GISTIC algorithm.

The ultimate proof that an event "drives" cancer is functional evidence that it leads to tumor initiation and/or maintenance of the malignant phenotype. By providing a biological advantage to the cancer cell and favoring its clonal expansion, these events should be enriched above the "background" of biologically inert genetic events. An accurate assessment of this background rate of genomic alterations, however, is currently limited by our incomplete understanding of the cancer genome. It is possible and indeed likely, that the frequency and nature of such "background" alterations vary between different cancer types, can be affected by previous exposure to genotoxic agents (e.g., radiation), mutations in the DNA repair machinery which might favor one particular type of genomic change, and/or the genomic context of the mutation itself (i.e., location of the targeted gene relative to the centromere or telomere). All of these factors should ideally be identified and included in determining the *G*-score in the GISTIC algorithm.

Future modifications to GISTIC will address some of the current limitations of this algorithm. For example, the *G*-score in the current GISTIC version does not consider the size of copy-number alterations and it is conceivable that focal events are less likely to occur and by chance than broad events. One approach to separate out focal events is by considering only amplifications and deletions that pass a high-amplitude threshold, as was done in the description of the lung cancer genome (Weir et al., 2007). Future versions of the GISTIC algorithm will include the ability to select copy-number events on the basis of their size.

A major goal in identifying driver events is to determine the genes they target. The peak regions, where the most samples are aberrant to the highest degree, are the most likely to contain these genes, but as noted above (Fig. 18.2), the presence of passenger aberrations near the targeted genes may skew the locations of these peaks. GISTIC currently implements on a leave-one-out approach to identify a wider peak region that is robust to the presence of a single passenger aberration. As datasets get larger, however, the likelihood increases that these peaks will be skewed by more than one nearby passenger event. Future releases of GISTIC will address the more general possibility of any number of nearby passenger events.

GISTIC is publicly available through two sources, namely the website of the Broad Institute (www.broad.mit.edu/cancer/pub/GISTIC) and through GenePattern (http://genepattern.broad.mit.edu/gp/pages/login.jsf).

Acknowledgments We would like to thank Bill Sellers, Charles Sawyers, Matthew Meyerson, and Eric Lander for many helpful discussions during the development of GISTIC. Tim Cloughesy, Paul Mischel, Linda Liau, Howard Fine, Elizabeth Maher, Cameron Brennan, Ron Depinho, and Lynda Chin kindly shared data. Nadav Kupiec and Bang Wong provided help with illustrations. This work was supported by funds from the Broad Institute of Harvard University and Massachusetts Institute of Technology, the Dana-Farber/Harvard Cancer Center Prostate Specialized Program of Research Excellence (RB), Department of Defense Grants (RB and IKM), the Brain Tumor Funders' Collaborative (IKM), the Sontag Foundation (IKM), the Doris Duke Foundation (IKM), and the Sidney Kimmel Foundation (IKM).

References

Bagchi, A., Papazoglu, C., Wu, Y., Capurso, D., Brodt, M., Francis, D., Bredel, M., Vogel, H., and Mills, A.A. (2007). CHD5 is a tumor suppressor at human 1p36. Cell *128*, 459–475.

Beroukhim, R., Getz, G., Nghiemphu, L., Barretina, J., Hsueh, T., Linhart, D., Vivanco, I., Lee, J.C., Huang, J.H., Alexander, S., et al. (2007). Assessing the significance of chromosomal aberrations in cancer: methodology and application to glioma. Proc Natl Acad Sci USA *104*, 20007–20012.

Chiang, D.Y., Villanueva, A., Hoshida, Y., Peix, J., Newell, P., Minguez, B., LeBlanc, A.C., Donovan, D.J., Thung, S.N., Sole, M., et al. (2008). Focal gains of VEGFA and molecular classification of hepatocellular carcinoma. Cancer Res *68*, 6779–6788.

Chung, C.H., Bernard, P.S., and Perou, C.M. (2002). Molecular portraits and the family tree of cancer. Nat Genet *32 Suppl*, 533–540.

Davies, H., Bignell, G.R., Cox, C., Stephens, P., Edkins, S., Clegg, S., Teague, J., Woffendin, H., Garnett, M.J., Bottomley, W., et al. (2002). Mutations of the BRAF gene in human cancer. Nature *417*, 949–954.

Diskin, S.J., Eck, T., Greshock, J., Mosse, Y.P., Naylor, T., Stoeckert, C.J., Jr., Weber, B.L., Maris, J.M., and Grant, G.R. (2006). STAC: A method for testing the significance of DNA copy number aberrations across multiple array-CGH experiments. Genome Res *16*, 1149–1158.

Druker, B.J., Talpaz, M., Resta, D.J., Peng, B., Buchdunger, E., Ford, J.M., Lydon, N.B., Kantarjian, H., Capdeville, R., Ohno-Jones, S., et al. (2001). Efficacy and safety of a specific inhibitor of the BCR-ABL tyrosine kinase in chronic myeloid leukemia. N Engl J Med *344*, 1031–1037.

Ekstrand, A.J., Sugawa, N., James, C.D., and Collins, V.P. (1992). Amplified and rearranged epidermal growth factor receptor genes in human glioblastomas reveal deletions of sequences encoding portions of the N- and/or C-terminal tails. Proc Natl Acad Sci USA *89*, 4309–4313.

Feero, W.G., Guttmacher, A.E., and Collins, F.S. (2008). The genome gets personal – almost. JAMA *299*, 1351–1352.

Feuerstein, B.G., and Mohapatra, G. (1995). Molecular cytogenetic quantitation of gains and losses of genetic material from human gliomas. J Neurooncol *24*, 47–55.

Forrest, W.F., and Cavet, G. (2007). Comment on "The consensus coding sequences of human breast and colorectal cancers". Science *317*, 1500; author reply 1500.

Fujita, T., Igarashi, J., Okawa, E.R., Gotoh, T., Manne, J., Kolla, V., Kim, J., Zhao, H., Pawel, B.R., London, W.B., et al. (2008). CHD 5, a tumor suppressor gene deleted from 1p36.31 in neuroblastomas. J Natl Cancer Inst *100*, 940–949.

Futreal, P.A., Coin, L., Marshall, M., Down, T., Hubbard, T., Wooster, R., Rahman, N., and Stratton, M.R. (2004). A census of human cancer genes. Nat Rev Cancer *4*, 177–183.

Galanis, E., Buckner, J., Kimmel, D., Jenkins, R., Alderete, B., O'Fallon, J., Wang, C.H., Scheithauer, B.W., and James, C.D. (1998). Gene amplification as a prognostic factor in primary and secondary high-grade malignant gliomas. Int J Oncol *13*, 717–724.

Getz, G., Hofling, H., Mesirov, J.P., Golub, T.R., Meyerson, M., Tibshirani, R., and Lander, E.S. (2007). Comment on "The consensus coding sequences of human breast and colorectal cancers". Science *317*, 1500.

Guttman, M., Mies, C., Dudycz-Sulicz, K., Diskin, S.J., Baldwin, D.A., Stoeckert, C.J., Jr., and Grant, G.R. (2007). Assessing the significance of conserved genomic aberrations using high resolution genomic microarrays. PLoS Genet *3*, e143.

Haverty, P.M., Fridlyand, J., Li, L., Getz, G., Beroukhim, R., Lohr, S., Wu, T.D., Cavet, G., Zhang, Z., and Chant, J. (2008). High-resolution genomic and expression analyses of copy number alterations in breast tumors. Genes Chromosomes Cancer *47*, 530–542.

Holland, E.C. (2001). Gliomagenesis: genetic alterations and mouse models. Nat Rev Genet *2*, 120–129.

Hupe, P., Stransky, N., Thiery, J.P., Radvanyi, F., and Barillot, E. (2004). Analysis of array CGH data: from signal ratio to gain and loss of DNA regions. Bioinformatics *20*, 3413–3422.

Ichimura, K., Ohgaki, H., Kleihues, P., and Collins, V.P. (2004). Molecular pathogenesis of astrocytic tumours. J Neurooncol *70*, 137–160.

Kotliarov, Y., Steed, M.E., Christopher, N., Walling, J., Su, Q., Center, A., Heiss, J., Rosenblum, M., Mikkelsen, T., Zenklusen, J.C., et al. (2006). High-resolution global genomic survey of 178 gliomas reveals novel regions of copy number alteration and allelic imbalances. Cancer Res *66*, 9428–9436.

Kraus, J.A., Koopmann, J., Kaskel, P., Maintz, D., Brandner, S., Schramm, J., Louis, D.N., Wiestler, O.D., and von Deimling, A. (1995). Shared allelic losses on chromosomes 1p and 19q suggest a common origin of oligodendroglioma and oligoastrocytoma. J Neuropathol Exp Neurol *54*, 91–95.

Kummar, S., Kinders, R., Rubinstein, L., Parchment, R.E., Murgo, A.J., Collins, J., Pickeral, O., Low, J., Steinberg, S.M., Gutierrez, M., et al. (2007). Compressing drug development timelines in oncology using phase '0' trials. Nat Rev Cancer *7*, 131–139.

Lai, W.R., Johnson, M.D., Kucherlapati, R., and Park, P.J. (2005). Comparative analysis of algorithms for identifying amplifications and deletions in array CGH data. Bioinformatics *21*, 3763–3770.

Lee, J.C., Vivanco, I., Beroukhim, R., Huang, J.H., Feng, W.L., Debiasi, R.M., Yoshimoto, K., King, J.C., Nghiemphu, P., Yuza, Y., et al. (2006). Epidermal growth factor receptor activation in glioblastoma through novel missense mutations in the extracellular domain. PLoS Med *3*, e485.

Lin, W.M., Baker, A.C., Beroukhim, R., Winckler, W., Feng, W., Marmion, J.M., Laine, E., Greulich, H., Tseng, H., Gates, C., et al. (2008). Modeling genomic diversity and tumor dependency in malignant melanoma. Cancer Res *68*, 664–673.

Lynch, T.J., Bell, D.W., Sordella, R., Gurubhagavatula, S., Okimoto, R.A., Brannigan, B.W., Harris, P.L., Haserlat, S.M., Supko, J.G., Haluska, F.G., et al. (2004). Activating mutations in the epidermal growth factor receptor underlying responsiveness of non-small-cell lung cancer to gefitinib. N Engl J Med *350*, 2129–2139.

Maher, E.A., Brennan, C., Wen, P.Y., Durso, L., Ligon, K.L., Richardson, A., Khatry, D., Feng, B., Sinha, R., Louis, D.N., et al. (2006). Marked genomic differences characterize primary and secondary glioblastoma subtypes and identify two distinct molecular and clinical secondary glioblastoma entities. Cancer Res *66*, 11502–11513.

Olshen, A.B., Venkatraman, E.S., Lucito, R., and Wigler, M. (2004). Circular binary segmentation for the analysis of array-based DNA copy number data. Biostatistics *5*, 557–572.

Paez, J.G., Janne, P.A., Lee, J.C., Tracy, S., Greulich, H., Gabriel, S., Herman, P., Kaye, F.J., Lindeman, N., Boggon, T.J., et al. (2004). EGFR mutations in lung cancer: correlation with clinical response to gefitinib therapy. Science *304*, 1497–1500.

Pinkel, D., Segraves, R., Sudar, D., Clark, S., Poole, I., Kowbel, D., Collins, C., Kuo, W.L., Chen, C., Zhai, Y., et al. (1998). High resolution analysis of DNA copy number variation using comparative genomic hybridization to microarrays. Nat Genet *20*, 207–211.

Reifenberger, G., and Collins, V.P. (2004). Pathology and molecular genetics of astrocytic gliomas. J Mol Med *82*, 656–670.

Rikova, K., Guo, A., Zeng, Q., Possemato, A., Yu, J., Haack, H., Nardone, J., Lee, K., Reeves, C., Li, Y., et al. (2007). Global survey of phosphotyrosine signaling identifies oncogenic kinases in lung cancer. Cell *131*, 1190–1203.

Rubin, A.F., and Green, P. (2007). Comment on "The consensus coding sequences of human breast and colorectal cancers". Science *317*, 1500.

Sawyers, C.L. (2003). Opportunities and challenges in the development of kinase inhibitor therapy for cancer. Genes Dev *17*, 2998–3010.

Sawyers, C.L. (2008). The cancer biomarker problem. Nature *452*, 548–552.

Slamon, D.J., Leyland-Jones, B., Shak, S., Fuchs, H., Paton, V., Bajamonde, A., Fleming, T., Eiermann, W., Wolter, J., Pegram, M., et al. (2001). Use of chemotherapy plus a monoclonal antibody against HER2 for metastatic breast cancer that overexpresses HER2. N Engl J Med *344*, 783–792.

Takeyama, K., Monti, S., Manis, J.P., Cin, P.D., Getz, G., Beroukhim, R., Dutt, S., Aster, J.C., Alt, F.W., Golub, T.R., et al. (2008). Integrative analysis reveals 53BP1 copy loss and decreased expression in a subset of human diffuse large B-cell lymphomas. Oncogene *27*, 318–322.

The Cancer Genome Atlas Research Network, McLendon, R., Friedman, A., Bigner, D., Van Meir, E.G., Brat, D.J., Marie Mastrogianakis, G., Olson, J.J., Mikkelsen, T., Lehman, N., Aldape, K., et al. (2008). Comprehensive genomic characterization defines human glioblastoma genes and core pathways. Nature *455*, 1061–1068.

Thomas, R.K., Baker, A.C., Debiasi, R.M., Winckler, W., Laframboise, T., Lin, W.M., Wang, M., Feng, W., Zander, T., Macconnaill, L.E., et al. (2007). High-throughput oncogene mutation profiling in human cancer. Nat Genet *39*, 347–351.

Tonon, G., Wong, K.K., Maulik, G., Brennan, C., Feng, B., Zhang, Y., Khatry, D.B., Protopopov, A., You, M.J., Aguirre, A.J., et al. (2005). High-resolution genomic profiles of human lung cancer. Proc Natl Acad Sci USA *102*, 9625–9630.

Varmus, H. (2006). The new era in cancer research. Science *312*, 1162–1165.

Wang, P., Kim, Y., Pollack, J., Narasimhan, B., and Tibshirani, R. (2005). A method for calling gains and losses in array CGH data. Biostatistics *6*, 45–58.

Watanabe, K., Tachibana, O., Sata, K., Yonekawa, Y., Kleihues, P., and Ohgaki, H. (1996). Overexpression of the EGF receptor and p53 mutations are mutually exclusive in the evolution of primary and secondary glioblastomas. Brain Pathol *6*, 217–223; discussion 223–214.

Weinstein, I.B. (2002). Cancer. Addiction to oncogenes – the Achilles heal of cancer. Science *297*, 63–64.

Weir, B.A., Woo, M.S., Getz, G., Perner, S., Ding, L., Beroukhim, R., Lin, W.M., Province, M.A., Kraja, A., Johnson, L.A., et al. (2007). Characterizing the cancer genome in lung adenocarcinoma. Nature *450*, 893–898.

Wiedemeyer, R., Brennan, C., Heffernan, T.P., Xiao, Y., Mahoney, J., Protopopov, A., Zheng, H., Bignell, G., Furnari, F., Cavenee, W.K., et al. (2008). Feedback circuit among INK4 tumor suppressors constrains human glioblastoma development. Cancer Cell *13*, 355–364.

Wood, L.D., Parsons, D.W., Jones, S., Lin, J., Sjoblom, T., Leary, R.J., Shen, D., Boca, S.M., Barber, T., Ptak, J., et al. (2007). The genomic landscapes of human breast and colorectal cancers. Science *318*, 1108–1113.

Zhao, X., Li, C., Paez, J.G., Chin, K., Janne, P.A., Chen, T.H., Girard, L., Minna, J., Christiani, D., Leo, C., et al. (2004). An integrated view of copy number and allelic alterations in the cancer genome using single nucleotide polymorphism arrays. Cancer Res *64*, 3060–3071.

Zhao, X., Weir, B.A., LaFramboise, T., Lin, M., Beroukhim, R., Garraway, L., Beheshti, J., Lee, J.C., Naoki, K., Richards, W.G., et al. (2005). Homozygous deletions and chromosome amplifications in human lung carcinomas revealed by single nucleotide polymorphism array analysis. Cancer Res *65*, 5561–5570.

Chapter 19
Oncomodulatory Role of the Human Cytomegalovirus in Glioblastoma

Liliana Soroceanu and Charles S. Cobbs

Abstract The most malignant form of primary CNS tumors, *glioblastoma* (GBM), is rapidly fatal in most patients despite current therapies. Recently, it has been shown that a "tumor stem cell-like" population (CD133 positive) exists within GBMs, which can drive tumor initiation and may be responsible for tumor recurrence (Singh et al., 2004). Other studies have shown that a platelet-derived growth factor receptor (PDGFR)-alpha positive *subset of neural precursor cells* (NPCs) in the adult brain may give rise to glioma-like lesions in vivo when PDGFR-alpha (PDGFRα) signaling is activated in these cells and their differentiation is "blocked" (Jackson et al., 2006). These data suggest that a stimulus capable of inducing *chronic activation* of the PDGFR-α in adult NPCs, blocking their differentiation, and promoting oncogenic signaling would be an ideal candidate for a glioma-inducing agent. Our laboratory was the first to show that human cytomegalovirus (HCMV) nucleic acids and proteins are present in over 90% of human malignant gliomas (Cobbs et al., 2002), and these data were recently confirmed by others (Mitchell et al., 2008). HCMV, a neurotropic beta-herpesvirus, persistently infects over 70% of the adult population worldwide, is the most common cause of congenital CNS disease in humans and can establish a lifelong persistent CNS infection (Britt and Alford, 1996). Mouse models of CMV infection show that the virus can be reactivated from latency specifically in the NPCs of the subventricular zone (SVZ) (Tsutsui et al., 2002). In human embryonic neural precursor stem cells, HCMV gene expression is activated at the onset of differentiation (Odeberg et al., 2006) and can arrest the progression from the NPC state toward terminal neuronal/glial phenotypes. In addition, HCMV gene products (such as the immediate-early-1, IE1, gene) can cause DNA mutations and deregulation of myriad pathways involved in maintaining cell homeostasis (Castillo and Kowalik, 2002). Our unpublished data demonstrate that the HCMV IE1 gene product is

C.S. Cobbs (✉)
Department of Neuroscience, California Pacific Medical Center Research Institute, 475 Brannan Street, Suite 220, San Francisco, CA, 94107, USA
e-mail: Charles.Cobbs@gmail.com

E.G. Van Meir (ed.), *CNS Cancer*, Cancer Drug Discovery and Development, DOI 10.1007/978-1-60327-553-8_19,
© Humana Press, a part of Springer Science+Business Media, LLC 2009

preferentially expressed in the CD133+, stem-like subpopulation of glioblastoma-derived primary neurospheres, suggesting that the virus may be selectively reactivated in and modulate the biology of this tumor cell pool (Fig. 19.1). In addition, we recently discovered that HCMV infection potently and selectively activates the PDGFRα tyrosine kinase signaling pathway in human glioma and fibroblast cells (Fig. 19.2) and that the HCMV IE1 and PDGFRα proteins co-localize in human primary GBM in situ (Fig. 19.3). We showed that HCMV infection causes activation of signaling pathways downstream of PDGFRα that promote glioma cell survival, proliferation, and invasion, such as PI3K-Akt, PLC-gamma, and FAK (Cobbs et al., 2007). Using genetic approaches to knock down the receptor, we determined that PDGFRα is *required* for cellular infection by HCMV (Soroceanu et al., 2008). We also found that sustained expression of the essential IE1 viral gene augments the proliferation rate and cell cycle progression of glioblastoma cells by sustained activation of Akt, down-regulation of p53, and inactivation of the Rb tumor suppressor protein (Cobbs et al., 2008). Taken together, our data suggest that HCMV infection and gene expression in human NPCs, particularly in the PDGFRα positive subpopulation of NPC, could potentially cause oncogenic transformation by blockade of differentiation, by increased proliferation, and by causing increased self-renewal capacity of neural stem cells and accumulation of genetic alterations. Therefore, HCMV is an important marker of brain tumors and a potential target for novel therapies.

Contents

19.1 Human Cytomegalovirus Background

19.1.1 HCMV Is Widely Prevalent and Persistently Infects Adult Human Stem Cells

HCMV, a beta-herpesvirus, persistently infects over 70% of the world's adult population and is the most common cause of congenital central nervous system (CNS) infection in humans (Britt and Alford, 1996). Most HCMV infections are thought to remain asymptomatic throughout the individual's life, although recurrent reactivations of virus are known to occur with stress, inflammation, and immunosuppression. Stem cell populations in various organ systems harbor persistent latent HCMV infection (Goodrum et al., 2002). In fetuses or immunosuppressed patients, such as transplant or AIDS patients, HCMV can cause life-threatening infections of multiple organ systems.

19.1.2 HCMV and Human Malignant Gliomas

Association of HCMV with several human malignancies has been reported, including brain, prostate, and colon cancers (Cobbs et al., 2002; Harkins et al., 2002; Samanta et al., 2003; Scheurer et al., 2007). A recent study by Duke University investigators (Mitchell et al., 2008) confirmed our findings (Cobbs et al., 2002) that HCMV nucleic acids and proteins are detectable in over 90% of malignant gliomas, while not present in the surrounding normal brain tissue. In this study, the majority of GBM patients had detectable HCMV in the peripheral blood, indicating the presence of an active viral infection. Recently, a report has addressed the discrepancies that exist among results reported by different groups in identification of HCMV in human GBMs (Poltermann et al., 2006). The authors conclude that seemingly minor but *critical technical deficiencies* are the most likely reason for which some studies (Lau et al., 2005; Sabatier et al., 2005) could not confirm the presence of HCMV in human glioma tissues. Most recently, evidence was found that the level of HCMV infection in human GBMs has predictive value for patient survival (Rahbar et al., 2007). These latest studies (conducted at the Karolinska Institute) have prompted initiation of a clinical trial in GBM patients using antiviral drugs, entitled: *Efficacy and Safety of Valcyte® as an Add-On Therapy in Patients with Malignant Glioblastoma and CMV Infection.* In addition, Duke University researchers have developed a new anti-CMV^{pp65} autologous dendritic cell vaccine therapy, and a clinical trial using this vaccine has been initiated for patients with malignant gliomas (Mitchell, 2007). Preliminary evidence from this phase II trial indicates that immunotherapy against HCMV is safe and may increase time to progression and survival (Mitchell, 2007). Below, we discuss published and unpublished experimental data that describe how the biological properties of this virus could contribute to glioma pathogenesis.

19.2 Oncomodulatory Properties of HCMV and Their Contribution to Glioma Pathogenesis

19.2.1 The Role of Inflammatory Chemokines and Chemokine Receptors

HCMV infection in the fetus or immunocompromised adult can cause severe and even fatal encephalitis (Britt and Alford, 1996). In vitro, fetal and malignant human astrocytes provide an excellent environment for HCMV replication, and human glioma tumor cells are among the rare cell types that can support persistent and productive HCMV infection without cytopathic effect (Cheeran et al., 2005; Cobbs et al., 2008). HCMV induces an inflammatory response in infected cells, as evidenced by increased production of NO, superoxide, and COX-2 (Suzuki et al., 1998). HCMV encodes four G protein-coupled receptors (GPCR), US27, US28, UL33, and UL78 with high homology to human chemokine receptors (Chee et al., 1990). The viral US28 GPCR is a homolog for the cellular CCR1, binding a variety of chemokines, including CCL2/MCP-1, CCL5/RANTES, and CX3CL1/Fraktalkine, and exhibits constitutive activity (Casarosa et al., 2001), which has been linked to induction of an angiogenic phenotype in glioma cell lines (Maussang et al., 2006). US28 activation in glioma cells results in the induced expression of the chemokines monocyte chemoattractant protein-1 (MCP-1), IL-8, TNF-α, and IFN-gamma-inducible protein-10 (Bezzi et al., 2001; Oh et al., 2001; Pleskoff et al., 1997). The COX-2 pathway is induced strongly at both the transcriptional and post-translational levels after HCMV infection, and this leads to a marked increase in the production of inflammatory prostaglandins, especially prostaglandin E2 (PGE-2). PGE-2 and other inflammatory cytokines, such as IL-1β and TNFα, in turn directly activate the HCMV immediate-early promoter region, which further promotes viral replication (Kline et al., 1998). PGE-2 also increases the production of glutamate in glioma cells (Takano et al., 2001), which further promotes inflammation and tumor growth (Bezzi et al., 2001).

In transgenic mice, the CMV immediate-early (IE) gene promoter activity is upregulated specifically in astrocytes, and especially in response to inflammation (Aiba-Masago et al., 1999; Fritschy et al., 1996). In summary, CMV promotes chronic inflammatory pathways that could support a pro-oncogenic environment.

19.2.2 HCMV Immediate-Early (IE) Gene Products Dysregulate Cell Cycle Controls, Are Mutagenic, Are Anti-Apoptotic, and Promote Oncogenic Transformation

Once activated, the HCMV IE gene products (IE1 and IE2) can dysregulate cell cycle checkpoint controls by interacting with the p53 and Rb tumor suppressor proteins. In some cell types, IE1 and IE2 can mediate a growth arrest in G1 in infected cells to allow viral DNA replication at the expense of host replication. In other cell types, IE1 and IE2 can alter the cell cycle distribution toward S- and G2/M-phases to generate an environment conducive to proliferation (Castillo et al., 2005; Castillo and Kowalik, 2002). IE2, but not IE1, can induce quiescent cells into S-phase and delay cell cycle exit, and in the presence of non-functioning p53 tumor suppressor protein, IE1 induces S-phase and delays cell cycle exit. When combined with other viral oncogenic proteins that disinhibit cell cycle checkpoint controls such as adenovirus E1A protein, the IE1 and IE2 gene products are able to induce oncogenic transformation of cells (Shen et al., 1997).

In addition to dysregulating the cell cycle, IE1-72 and IE2-86 gene products block TNF-α-mediated apoptosis and are mutagenic (Shen et al., 1997; Zhu et al., 1995). We have shown that the HCMV IE1 gene product has the potential to promote glioblastoma cell proliferation by dysregulating key tumor pathways. We determined that sustained IE1 expression can suppress p53 and Rb tumor suppressor activity, while simultaneously driving the PI3K/Akt oncogenic signaling pathway in U87MG and U118MG glioblastoma cells. We also found that this effect may depend on the cellular state of differentiation and/or immortalization, such that viral gene expression may play a paradoxical role, promoting growth in tumor cells while blocking growth in non-transformed astrocytes or fibroblasts (Cobbs et al., 2007, 2008).

Another HCMV protein, UL69, is required for the HCMV-mediated G1 arrest seen in HCMV-infected cells (Hayashi et al., 2000). HCMV deletion mutants lacking UL69 are unable to efficiently induce G1 arrest in infected cells (Hayashi et al., 2000). Thus, it is conceivable that a mutant HCMV virus that expresses IE proteins in the absence of UL69 could promote unabated cell cycle progression and mutagenesis. In addition, HCMV expresses two proteins, pp71 and UL97, that can phosphorylate and inactivate the Rb family of tumor suppressor proteins (Hume et al., 2008; Kalejta et al., 2003). The UL97 protein causes constitutive phosphorylation of Rb, which is not able to be suppressed by normal cellular cyclin-dependent kinase inhibitor proteins such as p21/Waf1. Finally, recent evidence indicates that the HCMV IE1 gene product can cause sustained hTERT telomerase activity in glioblastoma cells and that hTERT expression co-localizes with IE1 detection in human tumors in vivo (C. Soderberg-Naucler, personal communication).

19.2.3 HCMV Infection Modulates Cell Proliferation and Cell Survival Signaling Pathways

HCMV infection activates cellular proto-oncogenes, cyclins, and kinases involved in cell mitogenic and cell survival pathways including *c-myc, c-fos, c-jun,* cyclin-B, cyclin-E, MAPK, ERK 1/2, and PI3-kinase (Chen et al., 2001; Hagemeier et al., 1992; Jault et al., 1995; Johnson et al., 2000, 2001). HCMV can also induce transcription factors such as NF-κB that activate cell survival pathways (Yurochko et al., 1995) (see also Chapter 42) and provide positive feedback for further HCMV immediate-early gene transcription. In persistently infected neuroblastoma cells, HCMV induces the anti-apoptotic protein Bcl-2 resulting in acquired resistance to cytotoxic drugs such as cisplatin and etoposide, which can be reversed after treating the cells with the antiviral drug ganciclovir (GCV) (Cinatl et al., 1998).

19.2.4 HCMV Infection Modulates Cellular Pathways that Promote Cell Migration and Invasion

Expression of the HCMV homolog (US28) to the human CC chemokine receptor CCR1 promotes cell migration toward chemokines RANTES and MCP-1 (Streblow et al., 1999). In HCMV-infected neuroblastoma cells, cell invasiveness is increased via activation of $\alpha5\beta1$ integrin and increased activity of extracellular matrix proteases (Scholz et al., 2000). As stated, HCMV infection activates the COX-2 and prostaglandin synthesis pathway. The downstream products of this pathway are known to promote migration and invasion in glioma cells. Our published results demonstrate that HCMV infection promotes glioma cell invasion and induces activation of the PIK3-AKT and FAK pathways (Cobbs et al., 2007).

19.2.5 HCMV Promotes Angiogenesis

Human brain capillary endothelial cells are permissive for infection by HCMV, and infection of endothelial cells by HCMV results in cytoplasmic p53 sequestration and escape from apoptosis (Kovacs et al., 1996). The HCMV IE1-72 and IE2-86 proteins increase vascular smooth muscle cell migration, proliferation, and expression of PDGF-β-receptor (Reinhardt et al., 2005) and IE2-86 can promote endothelial proliferation by binding and inactivating p53 in endothelial cells (Kovacs et al., 1996) . Expression of thrombospondin-1 (TSP-1), a potent inhibitor of angiogenesis in gliomas, is suppressed after HCMV infection of human fibroblasts and glioma cells. Inhibition of TSP-1 expression in glioma cells promotes glioma angiogenesis in vivo and is associated with a more malignant glioma phenotype (Cinatl et al., 2000, 1999; Kawataki et al., 2000; Margraf et al., 2001; Tenan et al., 2000). HCMV-mediated activation of COX-2 may also promote angiogenesis in tumor cells since COX-2 induces the expression of VEGF, bFGF, PDGF, iNOS, and TGF-α in tumor cells and promotes capillary endothelial cell migration and tube formation (Liu et al., 1998; Zhu et al., 2002). Furthermore, as stated, HCMV US28 constitutive activity induces an angiogenic phenotype in human glioma cell lines (Maussang et al., 2006).

19.2.6 HCMV Strain Variability and Gene Expression Patterns Influence Viral Neurotropism

HCMV strain-to-strain variability affects the tissue tropism and survival of HCMV-infected cells. Some HCMV strains are more tropic for certain cell types than others (e.g., for endothelial cells and monocytes) (Fish et al., 1995). The viral genes responsible for this phenotype have not been identified. Productive HCMV infection typically causes a cytopathic effect, yet some cell types in vivo, including macrophages and endothelial cells, appear to tolerate persistent HCMV infection without obvious cytopathology (Fish et al., 1995). In vitro, neural crest-derived tumor cells (GBM and neuroblastoma cells) are unique in their ability to be persistently infected by HCMV over long periods of time. In the case of GBM cells, prolonged infection with HCMV was associated with mutations in the viral genotype, which was thought to account for the non-cytopathic persistent infection. In neuroblastoma cells, long-term HCMV infection results in induction of Bcl-2, and an anti-apoptotic phenotype, suggesting that alterations in viral gene expression patterns in certain cell types may allow HCMV to persist in tumor cells and perhaps inhibit cell death (Cinatl et al., 1998, 1996).

Due to the vast heterogeneity found in HCMV clinical isolates, it has been postulated that viral strains with a particular tropism for proliferating astrocytic cells may infect these cells and contribute to the malignant phenotype. Defective virus particles arising spontaneously in an infected individual could express a subset of the viral genes including IE1 and IE2 and contribute to the malignant phenotype without full expression of the viral genome (Bresnahan and Shenk, 2000). Alternatively, the wild-type virus might express only subsets of its genes in certain cell types, as has been suggested for the interaction of HCMV with peripheral blood mononuclear cells (Grefte et al., 1994; Maciejewski et al., 1993). Nonproductive infections could induce the accumulation of mutations in cellular growth regulatory genes, ultimately leading to cell transformation.

19.3 HCMV Reactivation in Patients with Malignant Gliomas: The Role of the Immune System and Lessons from Animal Models

19.3.1 The Impact of the Immunosuppressed Status of GBM Patients on HCMV Reactivation

A significant body of evidence indicates that HCMV is reactivated in the host by inflammation or immunosuppression (Soderberg-Naucler, 2006). This would be potentially very important in the setting of malignant glioma since most patients with the diagnosis of GBM are profoundly immunosuppressed (Gomez and Kruse, 2006). Markers for cell-mediated immunity in glioma patients suggest that these patients have helper and cytotoxic T cell anergy. This fact, in combination with a high percentage of immunosuppressive regulatory T cells and inflammatory microglial cells, would support an environment conducive to HCMV reactivation and persistent infection. Indeed, a recent report suggests that patients with glioblastomas may harbor HCMV infection in their tumors, although their immunological response to HCMV is compromised (Prins et al., 2008). Nevertheless, it appears that the potential exists for artificially reactivating the immune response against HCMV, and this may be associated with a dramatic reactivation of specific T cell effector response to HCMV antigen. Such a response was demonstrated by Prins et al. in a patient with an aggressive glioblastoma, who had a potent anti-HCMV immune response after his tumor lysate was pulsed into autologous dendritic cells and then re-administered as an immunotherapy. This patient has had a complete response without evidence of tumor recurrence in over 5 years (Prins et al., 2008). Below, we are discussing experimental evidence from mouse models of CMV reactivation within the stem cell pool of the CNS, which may suggest potential mechanisms for virus reactivation during gliomagenesis.

19.3.2 Reactivation of CMV During Neural Precursor Differentiation: Evidence from Mouse Models

Studies of both human and murine CMV (MCMV) indicate that although embryonic stem cells (ES cells) are not permissive to viral infection, *at the onset of differentiation* of these stem cells into neural precursor stem cells (NPCs) and immature glial cells, an induction of the viral immediate-early (IE) genes occurs and subsequent viral gene expression is activated (Odeberg et al. , 2006). In studies of adult mice infected in utero with MCMV, IE gene expression could be detected in nestin + /GFAP + cells in the SVZ later in life, suggesting that viral gene products are expressed in these neuro-glial stem cells throughout adult life (Tsutsui et al., 2002). These studies in mouse models may, in fact, reflect the course of human CNS disease. *These data therefore suggest that HCMV is likely to persistently infect the neural precursor stem cell population in the adult human brain.*

19.3.3 HCMV Infection Can Arrest Differentiation of Stem Cells

Experiments using human *embryonic* neural stem cells (NSCs) indicate that these cells are permissive for HCMV infection at the onset of differentiation along neuronal and glial lineages, and that HCMV infection causes a dramatic decrease in the number of differentiated neurons (Odeberg et al., 2006) . Subsequent studies demonstrated that HCMV late-gene products inhibit embryonic NPC differentiation into astrocytes (Odeberg et al., 2007).

19.4 The Glioma Cell of Origin: The Role of Glioma Stem-Like Cells

19.4.1 Glioma Stem Cells

In the past decade, self-renewing NSCs have been identified in the adult mammalian brain, supporting the hypothesis that neurogenesis can occur throughout adult life (Hemmati et al., 2003; Holland, 2001b). The cell surface protein CD133 (Prominin 1) has been proven useful in the enrichment of NSC (Pfenninger et al., 2007). The concept of glioma stem cells is based on the striking similarities observed between the self-renewal capacity of stem cells and that of a CD133 positive subpopulation of cancer cells, freshly isolated from GBM patient tissue (see also Chapters 29 and 44). The ability of CD133 positive glioma-derived cells to form tumors in nude mice (Singh et al., 2003) further supports the hypothesis that this cell subpopulation may indeed comprise the "tumor-propagating cells." Recent studies show that the CD133 positive fraction of tumor cells contribute to glioma radio-resistance through preferential activation of the DNA damage checkpoint response and an increase in DNA repair capacity (Bao et al., 2006). Our unpublished data (Fig. 19.1 and Color Plate 29) demonstrate that HCMV IE1 and CD133 co-localize in human GBM in situ.

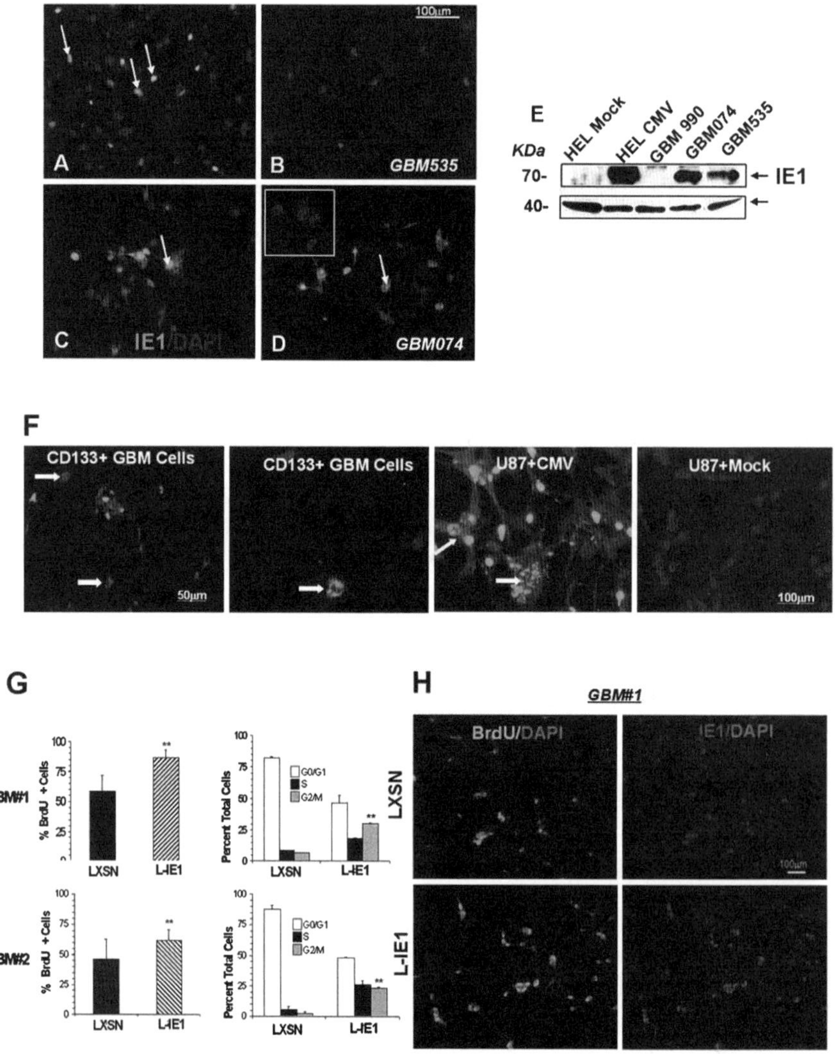

Fig. 19.1 Primary GBM cells endogenously expressed HCMV IE1. Primary glioma-derived cultures were processed for IE1 immunofluorescence using MAB810 (Chemicon) and Alexa 488-labeled secondary antibody. Nuclei were counterstained using DAPI. Panel **A** shows nuclear localization of endogenous IE1 in one GBM culture; panels **C** and **D** illustrate IE1 perinuclear staining in a different GBM primary culture. Panel **B** and the inset in panel **D**

19.4.2 Evidence for a Role of HCMV IE1 Expression in Glioma Stem-Like Cells

We have performed studies to characterize HCMV protein IE1 expression in primary GBM cells. We screened ten acutely dissociated primary GBM cultures maintained in neurosphere growth media within 48 h from initial culturing, using immunofluorescence and western blotting. Figure 19.1 shows an example of such analyses. Two of three cultures shown below are IE1 positive by western blot (panel E). Immunofluorescence detection of IE1 in two of the same samples is shown in panels A–D. In one case, we have found nuclear localization of IE1 (GBM 535, panel A). Most samples displayed a perinuclear, cytoplasmic IE1 localization (panels C,D GBM 074), as it has been recently described for HCMV "microinfections" associated with human malignancies, including gliomas (Soderberg-Naucler, 2008). These data unequivocally demonstrate the presence of endogenous IE1 in human GBM primary cultures grown in conditions that prevent differentiation and promote stem cell maintenance.

Since HCMV latently resides in stem cells of the bone marrow (Goodrum et al., 2002), we investigated whether HCMV gene products are present within the "stem-like," CD133+, glioma-derived cultures. Primary GBM tissue obtained from patients undergoing surgical resection was subjected to enzymatic digest, and cells were further sorted for CD133 using the Myltenyi CD133-coated magnetic beads in conjunction with the Automacs sorter, according to the manufacturer's instructions. CD133+ GBM primary cells and control U87MG/Mock and U87MG/HCMV cells were cultured in chamber slides for 48 h, fixed with cold methanol and processed for IE1 immunocytochemistry (Fig. 19.1F).These data demonstrate that the HCMV IE1 gene product is preferentially expressed in the stem-like cell pool within human

Fig 19.1 (continued) illustrate isotype control IgG staining. Cell lysates obtained from the same cultures demonstrate the presence of IE1 by western blotting in 2 out of 3 cases analyzed (panel **E**). Actin blots are shown to illustrate equivalent loading. Lysates from mock- and HCMV-treated HEL (panel **E**) cells are shown as negative and positive controls, respectively. **F** The presence of IE1 in sorted CD133 positive primary (passage 0) human GBM cells (*left two panels, arrows*) is detected in the perinuclear and cytoplasmic space. As positive control, U87 human glioma cells infected with HCMV display IE1 staining (72 hpi) not only, mostly, in the nuclei but also in the perinuclear space which is comparable to the IE1 expression detected in primary GBM cells (*third panel from the left, arrows*). Mock-infected U87 cells do not stain positive for IE1 (*right panel*). **G–H DNA synthesis and cell cycle distribution in primary GBM cells over-expressing IE1.** Retrovirally mediated HCMV IE1 over-expression in primary human GBM cultures increased the number of cells in S and G2M in both GBMs (**G** – *left panels*). **H** Representative fields of L-IE1 and control GBM cells "pulsed" with BrdU are shown in the right panels. Double immunofluorescence for BrdU and IE1 demonstrates that IE1-transduced primary glioma cells actively incorporate BrdU as a measure of increased DNA synthesis (*see* Color Plate 29)

GBMs, suggesting that HCMV may be selectively reactivated in, and may modulate the oncogenic phenotype of this tumor cell subpopulation.

In situ double immunofluorescence detection of CD133 and IE1 in GBM frozen tissue sections showed that CD133+ glioma cells express HCMV IE1 in a majority of the gliomas we have sampled to date, with HCMV (IE1) expression occurring in about 40–60% of the CD133 positive cells (not shown). Identification of the essential HCMV gene product IE1 in glioma "stem-like" cells in situ constitutes evidence that CD133+ positive cells may be *persistently* infected with HCMV in glioma patients.

Our published data show that over-expression of HCMV IE1 in primary GBM-derived cells promotes cell cycle progression and BrdU incorporation (Fig. 19.1G, H), indicating that upon reactivation, HCMV IE1 could modulate critical oncogenic features of glioma cells, including cell proliferation and survival. We have previously shown that sustained IE1 expression in glioma cell lines can profoundly alter their cell cycle progression and growth rates by inducing Akt phosphorylation, inhibition of p53, and Rb phosphorylation. Figure 19.1G and H illustrates examples of two primary GBM cultures transduced with IE1 (L-IE1) which incorporate BrdU and progress through the cell cycle at significantly higher rates as compared to the control cultures (L-XSN).

In addition to *acute* HCMV treatment, we wished to determine whether *chronic* expression of a critical HCMV gene (such as IE1) could modulate key signaling pathways controlling glioma progression. Therefore, we expressed the IE1 gene (and the control vector) using a retroviral construct, in three different cell types, including the glioblastoma U87 cell line. We found that IE1 stable expression led to increased cell proliferation in the U87 GBM cell line (40% increase over control transfected cells (Cobbs et al., 2008)). We subsequently investigated the pathways controlling cell proliferation, survival, and cell cycle progression. We found that IE1 stable expression in the U87 glioma cells induces p-Akt, inhibits Rb by promoting phosphorylation of Rb, and decreases the expression levels of p53 family proteins (Cobbs et al., 2008). Taken together, these data indicate that HCMV IE1 gene product can act as a viral oncogene and modulate proliferation, survival, and cell cycle progression of human glioblastoma.

19.5 The Role of PDGF/PDGFRα Signaling in Gliomagenesis

19.5.1 The PDGF/PDGFR System Is Genetically Altered in GBMs

The PDGFα-receptor gene is amplified in a subset (13%) of human glioblastoma (2008) suggesting that activation of PDGF receptor signaling confers a selective growth advantage in tumor growth. Evidence from mouse models of gliomas suggests that genetic alterations such as loss of *Ink4Arf* locus in cooperation with exacerbated growth factor/growth factor receptor signaling in neural precursor cells can drive gliomagenesis (Holland, 2001a) (see also Chapter 2). In vivo gene transfer of PDGF to neural precursor cells and astrocytes induces the formation of high-grade gliomas in a dose-dependent manner (Shih and Holland, 2006), suggesting that *chronic activation* of the PDGF receptors can promote proliferation of glial precursors and furthermore activate downstream signaling pathways (such as the PI3K-Akt) sufficient to drive tumorigenesis. Recent experimental evidence revealed that *adult neural precursors driven to express high levels of PDGF had the capacity to give rise to gliomas* and recruit resident progenitor cells in the mitogenic environment of the tumor (Assanah et al., 2006). Recently, a subpopulation of the neural progenitor cells located in the subventricular zone and positive for PDGFRα has been shown to have neural stem cell characteristics and respond to increased PDGF signaling by generating "glioma-like" lesions in the adult brain (Erlandsson et al., 2006) (see also Chapter 1). Chronic activation of the receptor in the SVZ B cells resulted in *blocked differentiation*, increased proliferation, and generation of hyperplastic lesions, thus supporting the notion that this subpopulation of cells may serve the role of tumor-initiating stem cell (Jackson et al., 2006).

19.5.2 PDGFRα Is a Required *Cellular Receptor for HCMV*

To directly examine the possibility that HCMV can initiate oncogenic signaling, we conducted experiments to determine whether HCMV infection and gene expression could modulate key signaling pathways in human cells, including immortalized astrocytes and glioblastoma cells. Using whole virus, we found that short-term stimulation with HCMV activates Akt, PLCγ, and FAK signaling in human glioma cells (Cobbs et al., 2007). Since we detected phosphorylation of a likely receptor tyrosine kinase (RTK), distinct from EGFR (Cobbs et al., 2007) and engaging Akt, PLCγ, and FAK, we explored the possibility that another RTK might be activated by HCMV. We utilized a human phospho-RTK array as a screening tool to detect the relative phosphorylation of 42 different human RTKs. We discovered that *PDGFRα phosphorylation is significantly induced* in response to short-term HCMV infection (Fig. 19.2A (Soroceanu et al., 2008)). This finding was confirmed by western blot analysis, indicating that only PDGFRα is activated by HCMV, while the related PDGFRβ receptor is not phosphorylated (Soroceanu et al., 2008) (Fig. 19.2). These data suggest that HCMV may initiate oncogenic signaling in these tumors by engaging this tyrosine kinase receptor. To identify whether HCMV-infected cells also harbor active PDGFRα, we performed immunocytochemical analyses of short-term-stimulated U87MG glioma cells. Double immunofluorescence labeling of U87MG human GBM cells (Fig. 19.2D) demonstrated that HCMV short-term treatment induces phosphorylation of PDGFRα in infected cells, similar

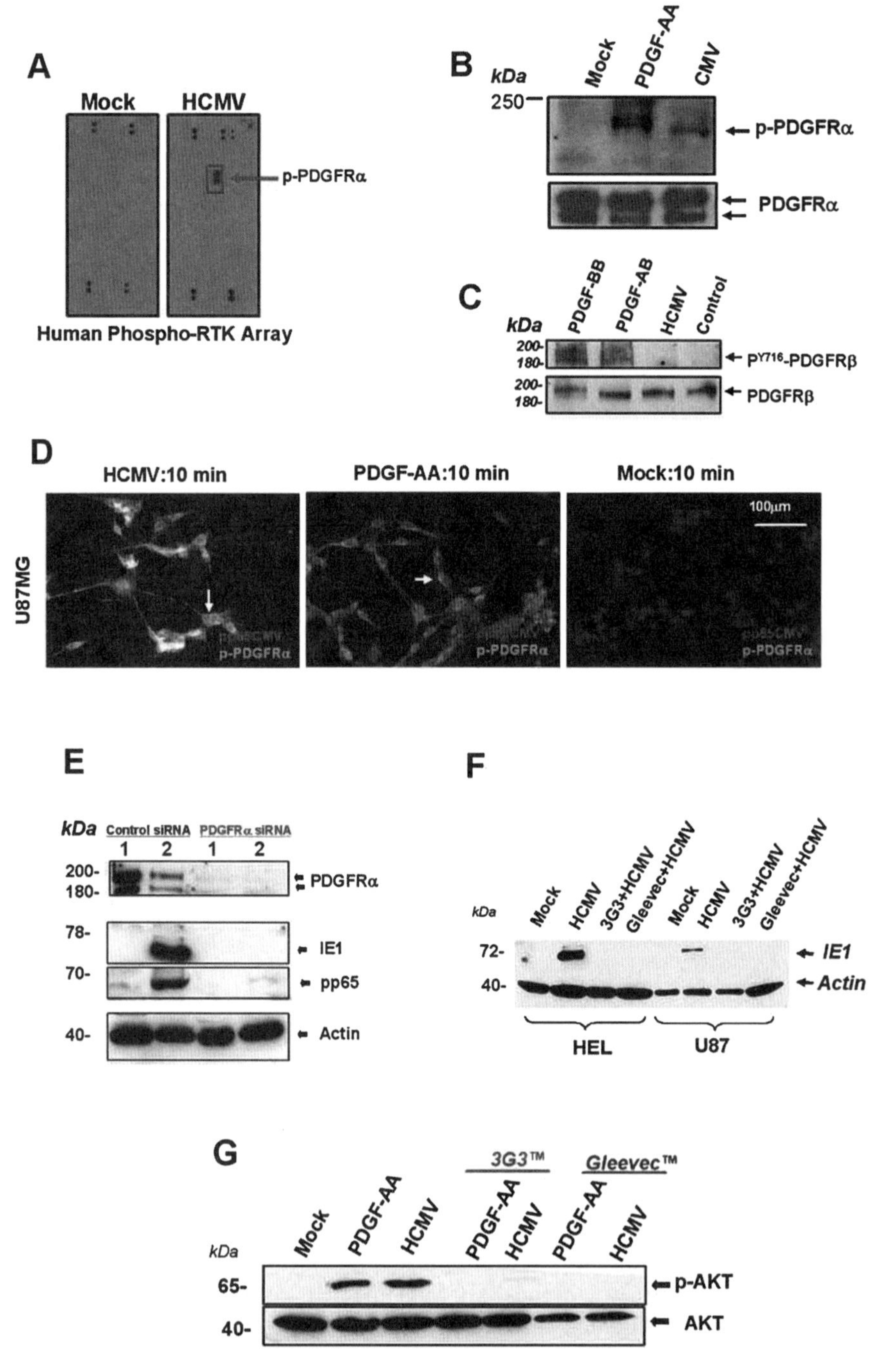

19.2 HCMV induces selective PDGFRα phosphorylation. A–C Short-term stimulation with HCMV induces tyrosine phosphorylation of the human PDGFRα. Lysates of HEL cells, mock to the stimulation using the genuine ligand, PDGF-AA. To ascertain specificity of the HCMV-induced PDGFRα phosphorylation, we used siRNA technology to knock down the PDGFRα in human fibroblast cells and tested whether they are susceptible to HCMV infection. We determined that in the absence of a functional PDGFRα, we could not detect IE1 immediate-early gene product 12 h following HCMV infection of PDGFR KD cells, while the control siRNA treated cells were readily infected (Fig. 19.2E). This suggests that PDFGRα is a necessary cellular receptor for HCMV infection and IE1 gene expression. We next tested the ability of currently available PDGFRα blocking reagents to inhibit HCMV entry, gene expression, and virus production. Our data show that using either the IMC-3G3 PDGFRα blocking antibody (a gift from Nick Loizos, Imclone, Inc.) or the small molecule Gleevec (STI-571, which inhibits receptor tyrosine kinase function) could inhibit HCMV gene expression (Fig. 19.2F) and downstream HCMV-induced oncogenic signaling, such as the PI3K-Akt pathway (Fig. 19.2G).

Fig 19.2 (continued) infected or treated with HCMV for 10 min, were hybridized to a human phosphor-RTK array which contains 42 different human RTKs (R&D systems). The membranes were further incubated with HRP-linked secondary antibody and visualized using chemiluminescence reagents (Pierce). HCMV-treated HEL cells (but not mock infected) clearly display tyrosine phosphorylation of the PDGFRα (**A**, *right panel*). To validate these findings, we stimulated HEL cells with PDGF (5 ng/ml, 10 min), mock, or HCMV (~ 1 MOI, 10 min) and subjected the cell lysates to western blot analysis. Panel **B** shows that PDGFRα becomes phosphorylated in response to both growth factor and HCMV treatment (*upper panel*), while the levels of total PDGFRα are similar across all samples (*lower panel*). **C** By contrast, hPDGFRβ is not tyrosine phosphorylated by HCMV, as shown by western blot analysis using a PDGFRβ phospho-specific antibody. **D U87MG human GBM cells infected with HCMV show phosphorylation of PDGFRα.** HCMV pp65 and p-PDGFRα are detected in the same cells infected by HCMV (*left panel, arrows*); p-PDGFRα pattern induced by HCMV infection is comparable to that induced by PDGF-AA treatment (**D**, *middle panel*). Mock-treated cells were negative for both pp65CMV and p-PDGFRα, as shown in panel **5C.E–G PDGFRα is *required* for cellular infection by HCMV. E** 1 – Mock, 2 – HCMV. HEL cells were transfected with siRNA targeting the human PDGFRα and control siRNA, following manufacturer's (Dharmacon) protocol. Sixty hours following transfection, cells were either mock infected or HCMV infected and cultured for an additional 12 h. Western blot analysis showed that IE1 and pp65 viral gene products are only detected in the control siRNA/HCMV treated cells (*middle panels*, lane 2 in the siRNA-treated cells); knocking down PDGFRα renders the cells complete resistant to HCMV infection (lane 2 in PDGFRα siRNA-treated samples). The extent of PDGFRα knockdown was significant (upper panel). The actin blots demonstrate equivalent loading of the samples. **F** IE1 expression is not detectable in U87 and HEL cells in the presence of PDGFRα–blocking antibodies (lane 3, IMC-3G3) or kinase inhibitors (lane 4, Gleevec). **G.** Pre-treatment with IMC-3G3 or Gleevec inhibits HCMV-induced phosphorylation of Akt, as shown by the upper panel which is a western blot for phosphor-Akt. PDGF-induced Akt phosphorylation is also inhibited by IMC-3G3 and Gleevec, as previously reported. Total Akt levels are not affected, as shown in the lower panel. IMC-3G3 was used at 10 μg/ml, 6 h pre-treatment. Gleevec was used at 40 μM, 30 min pre-treatment

19.6 Evidence in Support of a Role for HCMV-Induced Oncogenesis by Activation of Human PDGFRα

19.6.1 PDGFRα and HMCV IE1 Co-localize in Primary Human GBM Tissues and Cells

Given our hypothesis that HCMV reactivation in a PDGFRα positive neural stem cell subpopulation may lead to sustained PDGFRα activation, we investigated the degree of co-localization between HCMV IE1 product and

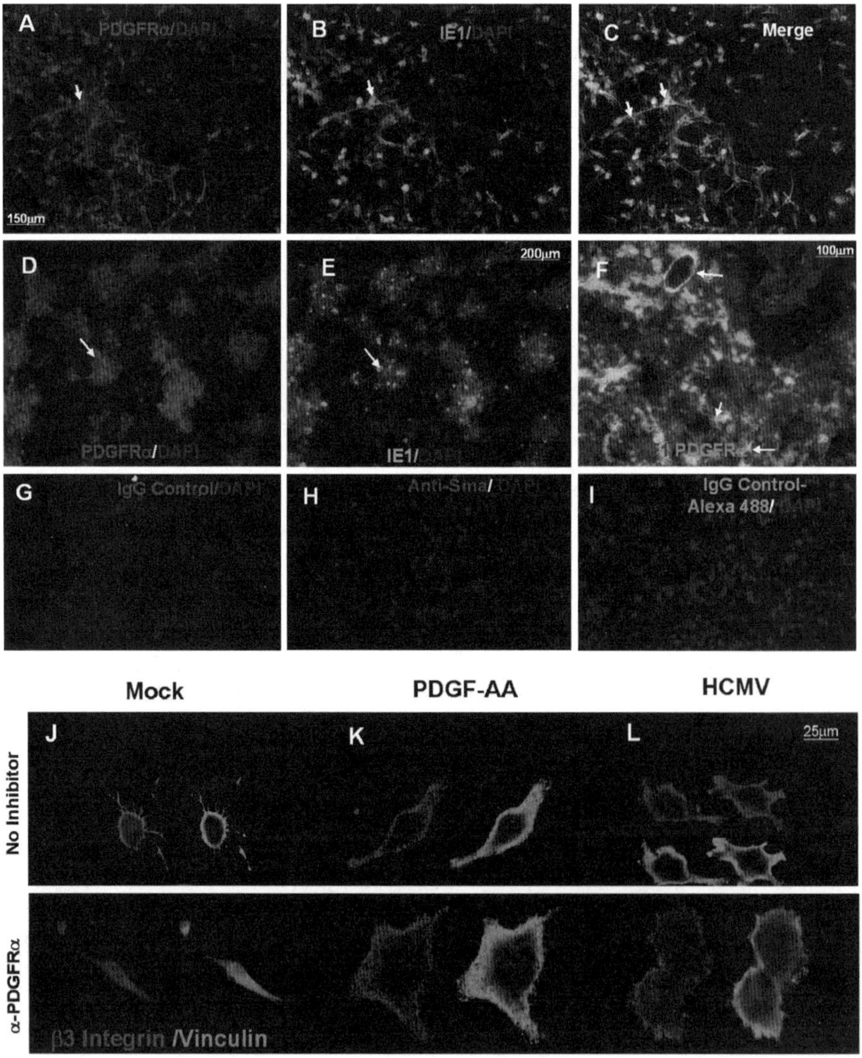

Fig. 19.3 Co-localization of PDGFRα and IE1 in primary human GBM samples. GBM primary cultures and tissues were examined for the presence of IE1 and PDGFRα using

PDGFRα in GBM-primary-derived cultures and GBM tissues using double immunofluorescence. Figure 19.3A, B, C, D, E, F, G, H, I and Color Plate 30 illustrates representative cases of IE1 and PDGFRα co-localization in GBM tissues and cells.

19.6.2 HCMV Promotes Glioma Cell Invasiveness by Engaging PDGFRα and the αvβ3 Integrin

We have previously demonstrated that HCMV can promote glioma cell invasiveness (Cobbs et al., 2007). Given the documented role of integrins and the PDGFRs in mediating glioma cell motility (Ding et al., 2003), we have performed experiments to investigate the role of integrins and PDGFRα in HCMV-induced cell motility. Scrape-wound assays showed that both αvβ3 and PDGFRα blocking antibodies inhibited HCMV-induced cell migration (not shown). Double immunofluorescence analyses showed that HCMV can induce αvβ3 recruitment to the focal adhesions to the same extent as PDGF-AA, and that PDGFRα blocking antibodies can reverse this effect (Fig. 19.3 J, K, L), suggesting that HCMV may act through αvβ3 integrin/PDGFRα to promote glioma cell invasiveness.

19.6.3 Mechanisms of HCMV-Induced Oncogenesis in Human Adult Neural Precursor Cells

We next investigated possible mechanisms of HCMV-induced oncogenesis using adult human neural precursor cells (NPC) obtained by culturing surgically removed tissue from a patient with intractable epilepsy. Figure 19.4A, B, C, D, E, F, G, H and Color Plate 31) illustrates the growth of NPC as

Fig 19.3 (continued) double immunofluorescence. Panels **A and D** represent immunofluorescence detection of PDGFRα in primary cultures, panels **B** and **E** show IE1 detection in the same cells. Panels **C** and **F** show examples of cells double positive for HCMV IE1 and PDGFRα.(superimposed single-staining photographs). Control stained sections were negative for both antigens (**G, H, I**). **J, K, L**. HMCV treatment induces recruitment of the αvβ3 integrin to focal adhesions in a PDGFRα-dependent manner. U87 glioma cells were serum starved for 24 h, and pre-treated with a PDGFRα blocking antibody (10 μg/ml, R&D systems, lower panels) or mock (upper panels) for 2 h, followed by Mock (**J**) PDGF-AA (**K**, 5 ng/ml) or HCMV (**L**, MOI = 1) stimulation for 10 min. Confocal images of cells processed for immunofluorescence show cellular localization of the β3 integrin (Rhodamine) and Vinculin (FITC) – a marker of focal adhesions. PDGF-AA and HCMV-induced recruitment of αvβ3 to focal adhesions shown by co-localization with vinculin at the cell cortex (**K**, **L**, *upper panels*) is inhibited by pre-treatment with receptor blocking antibodies (note diffuse cytoplasmic staining in **K**, **L** *lower panels*) (*see* Color Plate 30)

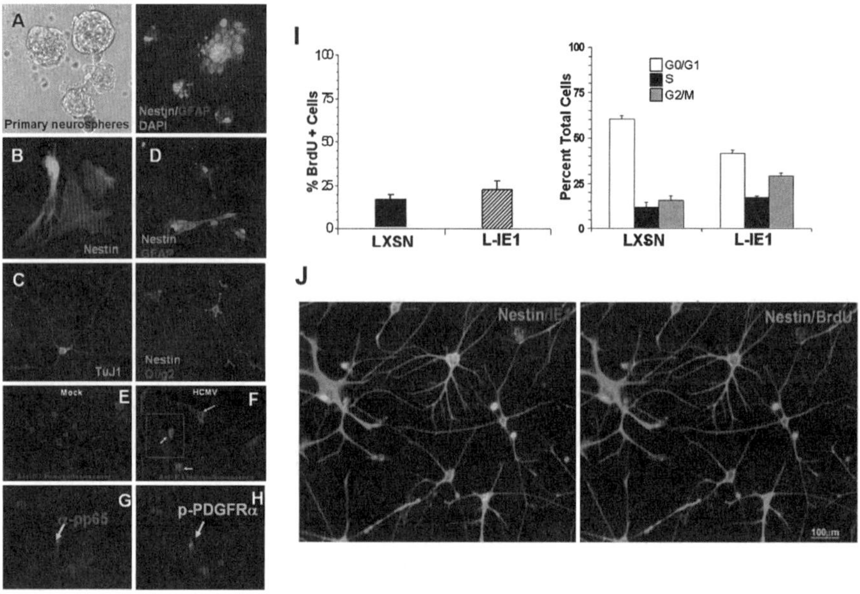

Fig. 19.4 Adult human normal NPCs can be grown as neurospheres and are permissive to HCMV infection. **A, B, C, D.** Neural precursor cells (NPCs) isolated from these adult brain specimens were grown in neurosphere conditions and re-seeded in adherent conditions for an additional 48 h. Nestin antibody was used to identify undifferentiated neuro-glial precursors, GFAP staining indicates the presence of astrocytes; Tuj1 staining identifies neurons, while Olig2 is used as a marker for oligodendrocytes. **E, F.** NPCs obtained from acutely dissociated adult SVZ brain tissue were grown as neurospheres and mock treated or infected with HCMV 3 days following culturing on adhesive substrate. Six hours following infection, cells were stained for HMCV IE1. Immunofluorescence demonstrates the characteristic nuclear and perinuclear IE1 localization in infected NPC (red- IE1, blue-DAPI). **G, H.** Short-term stimulation with HCMV induces PDGFRα phosphorylation in NPC – pp65 HCMV **(G)** gene product is co-localized with p-PDGFRα **(H). I, J. IE1 expression induces NPC proliferation. I.** NPCs retrovirally transduced with L-IE1 or LXSN control vector were subjected to BrdU incorporation and cell cycle analysis using FACS. IE1-NPC cells accumulate in S and G2/M, indicating increased DNA synthesis. **J.** BrdU is actively incorporated by nestin positive NPCs transduced with IE1. Overall, these data suggest that HCMV gene expression could increase cell proliferation of adult neural precursor cells and potentially contribute to tumor initiation (*see* Color Plate 31)

neurospheres, which can be induced to differentiate along neuronal, astrocytic, and oligodendrocytic lineages upon stimulation with specific growth factors or serum.

NPCs obtained from acutely dissociated adult SVZ brain tissue were grown as neurospheres and mock treated or infected with HCMV 3 days following culturing on an adhesive substrate. Twelve hours following infection, cells were stained for HMCV IE1. Immunofluorescence was used to visualize detection of IE1 which displays characteristic nuclear and perinuclear localization in infected

NPC (right panel, arrows; red-IE1, blue-DAPI). Furthermore, immunofluorescence analyses demonstrate that HCMV induces PDGFRα phosphorylation in adult human NPCs, as shown in Fig. 19.4. Our published data demonstrate that HCMV glycoprotein B (gB) directly binds to and activates human PDGFRα (Soroceanu et al., 2008). Furthermore, gB-neutralizing antibodies could prevent HCMV-induced PDGFRα phosphorylation (Soroceanu et al., 2008), suggesting that gB may be the viral moiety that initiates oncogenic signaling in the PDGFRα positive subpopulation of neural stem-like cells. On-going experiments in our laboratory are testing this hypothesis.

We have also performed preliminary experiments in which we retrovirally expressed IE1 in human NPC. Three to five days following IE1 retroviral transduction, pooled NPC clones were subjected to cell cycle analysis. As shown in Fig. 19.4, IE1 expression induced cell cycle progression in NPC (Fig. 19.4I compares L-IE1 with LXSN controls). BrdU incorporation was also enhanced by 10–20% in the IE1 compared to control-transduced cultures (Fig. 19.4I, J).

19.7 HCMV Association with Glioblastoma: Implications for Cancer Prevention, Detection, and Therapy

19.7.1 HCMV Association with Glioblastoma: Cause or Consequence?

The fact that HCMV infection is highly associated with malignant glioma might either represent a "passenger" phenomenon or conversely, this virus may play a causal role in the etiology and pathogenesis of this cancer. While more than 70% of adults carry persistent HCMV infection, it is known that malignant glioma patients have profound defects in their cell-mediated immunity, putting them at high risk for reactivation of an opportunistic pathogen such as HCMV. Indeed, it appears that glioma patients may develop a "specific HCMV immunocompromise" (John Sampson, personal communication). In such circumstances, it would be conceivable that reactivation of HCMV could occur in persistently infected neuronal precursor stem cells within the brain, as has been reported in the mouse model of CMV brain infection (Li et al., 2001; Tsutsui et al., 2002). Alternatively, glioma precursor lesions in the brain may become infiltrated with bone marrow-derived stem cells, which are known to both harbor persistent HCMV infection and have a strong affinity for infiltration of gliomas (Nakamizo et al., 2005). During differentiation of bone marrow-derived monocytic cells, HCMV would likely become reactivated (Smith, 2004). Once activated, this glioma-tropic virus could easily establish a low level of non-cytopathic infection with expression of only a subset of viral genes that allow the virus to coexist with the infected tumor cells, and perhaps mutate into defective viral strains that have altered growth-promoting properties as has been described (Luo and Fortunato, 2007) (Ogura et al., 1986). Persistent expression of HCMV genes such as IE1, UL97, and US28 could promote growth and invasion of the infected tumor. Thus, while HCMV may be a mere passenger of malignant glioma, the well-established biological properties of this pathogen suggests that it could play a profound role in oncogenesis and tumor promotion.

19.7.2 Clinical Impact of HCMV Association with Glioblastoma: Implications for Cancer Prevention, Detection, Screening, and Treatment

Should additional investigations reveal that HCMV is involved in the oncogenesis and pathogenesis of malignant glioma, this could open the door to several novel avenues of screening, prevention, and treatment. As in the case of *Helicobacter pylori* and human papillomavirus (HPV) infections, which are causally implicated in human gastric carcinoma and cervical cancer respectively, a causal association of HCMV and glioma could lead to early detection, early intervention, and potentially even tumor prevention. Ongoing clinical trials are aimed at determining whether the antiviral drug valganciclovir (Valcyte^{TM}) can inhibit glioblastoma progression after surgical removal of the primary tumor and recurrence (Rahbar et al., 2007). If these clinical trials document an antitumor effect of valganciclovir, it would immediately raise the possibility that antiviral therapy of HCMV-infected grade II and grade III astrocytomas may prevent progression to glioblastoma. Unpublished findings by investigators at Karolinska Institute have already suggested that the degree of HCMV viral expression found in tumors is inversely correlated with survival in these patients (Cecilia Soderberg-Naucler, personal communication). Hence, detection of HCMV could serve as a biomarker for tumor aggressiveness and a target for tumor therapy. Furthermore, given our data showing that HCMV engages the PDGFRα tyrosine kinase and activates downstream oncogenic signaling in glioma cells, receptor blocking reagents (i.e., IMC-3G3 or Gleevec) may prove useful in combination with antiviral therapies to target both HCMV and HCMV-induced oncogenic signaling.

19.8 Summary

In summary, HCMV is a ubiquitous human herpesvirus that demonstrates a specific tropism to brain and is the most common cause of fetal brain infection in humans. Substantial evidence exists to suggest that HCMV might persistently infect the human brain and that persistent infection in neural precursor stem cells in the subventricular zone may occur. In the setting of inflammation

Table 19.1 HCMV expresses several gene products that are known to modulate key oncogenic and apoptotic signaling pathways (Castillo and Kowalik, 2004)

HCMV gene product	Mechanism of action
pp71	Promotes early S-phase, binds all three Rb family members, transactivates major immediate-early promoter (MIEP)
UL97	Constitutively phosphorylates Rb
IE1	Promotes S-phase entry, binds Rb family members, induces E2F activity, can decrease p53 family member expression, can activate PI3-K/Akt, can inhibit apoptosis by activating NF-κB
IE2	Essential for HCMV infection; induces cells to enter S-phase; specifically interacts with Rb; induces c-myc, cyclin E, cdk-2, E2F1; can inhibit apoptosis by activating NF-κB
pUL69	Inhibits cell cycle progression to early S-phase-like state
US28	Viral chemokine receptor promotes angiogenesis and migration
pUL36, pUL37	Block caspase-8 apoptotic pathways
gB	Viral glycoprotein, phosphorylates PDGFRα

or immunocompromised host, reactivation of virus is likely to occur. Should a persistent viral expression occur in a SVZ NPC, this could lead to further downstream oncogenic features since HCMV encodes for multiple gene products that can dysregulate the cell cycle and promote important tumor signaling pathways. Our data indicate that the PDGFRα receptor may be a target of HCMV-mediated signal transduction, which could potentially promote gliomagenesis. In addition we have shown that persistent expression of the HCMV IE1 gene could lead to sustained expression of Akt and inactivation of Rb and P53 tumor suppressor pathway. We have demonstrated that HCMV IE1 expression occurs in the CD133+ stem-like pool of glioblastoma cells in vivo, and it is possible that viral expression in these tumor stem cells may enhance the malignant features of these cells. Recent clinical trials by our colleagues suggest that therapeutic strategies for glioblastoma patients with a HCMV vaccine/immunotherapy approach or antiviral drug approach may hold promise for treating this malignancy. A better understanding of the involvement of HCMV in glioma biology will no doubt lead to an improvement in our understanding of these tumors and potential novel therapeutics.

Acknowledgments We are grateful to Dr. William Britt (UAB) for reagents and useful discussions. We thank Dr. Cecilia Soderberg Naucler (Karolinska Institute) and Dr. Duane Mitchell (Duke University) for sharing with us unpublished results of ongoing clinical trials using anti-CMV therapies in glioma patients. We thank Dr. Nick Loizos (Imclone, Inc.) for the IMC-3G3 antibody and Loui Harkins for technical help with immunohistochemical analyses. We thank Alex Zider for help with the immunofluorescence and confocal microscopy and Roxanne Martinez for help with editing this chapter.

References

Aiba-Masago, S., Baba, S., Li, R.Y., Shinmura, Y., Kosugi, I., Arai, Y., Nishimura, M., and Tsutsui, Y. (1999). Murine cytomegalovirus immediate-early promoter directs astrocyte-specific expression in transgenic mice. Am J Pathol *154*, 735–743.

Assanah, M., Lochhead, R., Ogden, A., Bruce, J., Goldman, J., and Canoll, P. (2006). Glial progenitors in adult white matter are driven to form malignant gliomas by platelet-derived growth factor-expressing retroviruses. J Neurosci *26*, 6781–6790.

Bao, S., Wu, Q., McLendon, R., Hao, Y., Shi, Q., Hjelmeland, A., Dewhirst, M., Bigner, D.D., and Rich, J.N. (2006). Glioma stem cells promote radioresistance by preferential activation of the DNA damage response. Nature *444*, 756–760.

Bezzi, P., Domercq, M., Brambilla, L., Galli, R., Schols, D., De Clercq, E., Vescovi, A., Bagetta, G., Kollias, G., Meldolesi, J., et al. (2001). CXCR4-activated astrocyte glutamate release via TNFalpha: amplification by microglia triggers neurotoxicity. Nat Neurosci *4*, 702–710.

Bresnahan, W.A., and Shenk, T. (2000). A subset of viral transcripts packaged within human cytomegalovirus particles. Science *288*, 2373–2376.

Britt, W.J., and Alford, C.A. (1996). Cytomegalovirus. In Fields Virology, Third Edition, B.N. Fields, D.M. Knipe, and P.M. Howley, eds. (New York, Raven Press), pp. 2493–2523.

Cancer Genome Atlas Research Network (2008). Comprehensive genomic characterization defines human glioblastoma genes and core pathways. Nature *455*, 1061–1068.

Casarosa, P., Bakker, R.A., Verzijl, D., Navis, M., Timmerman, H., Leurs, R., and Smit, M.J. (2001). Constitutive signaling of the human cytomegalovirus-encoded chemokine receptor US28. J Biol Chem *276*, 1133–1137.

Castillo, J.P., Frame, F.M., Rogoff, H.A., Pickering, M.T., Yurochko, A.D., and Kowalik, T.F. (2005). Human cytomegalovirus IE1-72 activates ataxia telangiectasia mutated kinase and a p53/p21-mediated growth arrest response. J Virol *79*, 11467–11475.

Castillo, J.P., and Kowalik, T.F. (2002). Human cytomegalovirus immediate early proteins and cell growth control. Gene *290*, 19–34.

Castillo, J.P., and Kowalik, T.F. (2004). HCMV infection: modulating the cell cycle and cell death. Int Rev Immunol *23*, 113–139.

Chee, M.S., Satchwell, S.C., Preddie, E., Weston, K.M., and Barrell, B.G. (1990). Human cytomegalovirus encodes three G protein-coupled receptor homologues. Nature *344*, 774–777.

Cheeran, M.C., Hu, S., Ni, H.T., Sheng, W., Palmquist, J.M., Peterson, P.K., and Lokensgard, J.R. (2005). Neural precursor cell susceptibility to human cytomegalovirus diverges along glial or neuronal differentiation pathways. J Neurosci Res *82*, 839–850.

Chen, Z., Knutson, E., Kurosky, A., and Albrecht, T. (2001). Degradation of p21cip1 in cells productively infected with human cytomegalovirus. J Virol *75*, 3613–3625.

Cinatl, J., Jr., Bittoova, M., Margraf, S., Vogel, J.U., Cinatl, J., Preiser, W., and Doerr, H.W. (2000). Cytomegalovirus infection decreases expression of thrombospondin-1 and - 2 in cultured human retinal glial cells: effects of antiviral agents. J Infect Dis *182*, 643–651.

Cinatl, J., Jr., Cinatl, J., Vogel, J.U., Kotchetkov, R., Driever, P.H., Kabickova, H., Kornhuber, B., Schwabe, D., and Doerr, H.W. (1998). Persistent human cytomegalovirus infection induces drug resistance and alteration of programmed cell death in human neuroblastoma cells. Cancer Res *58*, 367–372.

Cinatl, J., Jr., Cinatl, J., Vogel, J.U., Rabenau, H., Kornhuber, B., and Doerr, H.W. (1996). Modulatory effects of human cytomegalovirus infection on malignant properties of cancer cells. Intervirology *39*, 259–269.

Cinatl, J., Jr., Kotchetkov, R., Scholz, M., Cinatl, J., Vogel, J.U., Driever, P.H., and Doerr, H.W. (1999). Human cytomegalovirus infection decreases expression of thrombospondin- 1 independent of the tumor suppressor protein p53. Am J Pathol *155*, 285–292.

Cobbs, C.S., Harkins, L., Samanta, M., Gillespie, G.Y., Bharara, S., King, P.H., Nabors, L.B., Cobbs, C.G., and Britt, W.J. (2002). Human cytomegalovirus infection and expression in human malignant glioma. Cancer Res *62*, 3347–3350.

Cobbs, C.S., Soroceanu, L., Denham, S., Zhang, W., Britt, W.J., Pieper, R., and Kraus, M.H. (2007). Human cytomegalovirus induces cellular tyrosine kinase signaling and promotes glioma cell invasiveness. J Neurooncol *85*, 271–280.

Cobbs, C.S., Soroceanu, L., Denham, S., Zhang, W., and Kraus, M.H. (2008). Modulation of oncogenic phenotype in human glioma cells by cytomegalovirus IE1-mediated mitogenicity. Cancer Res *68*, 724–730.

Ding, Q., Stewart, J., Jr., Olman, M.A., Klobe, M.R., and Gladson, C.L. (2003). The pattern of enhancement of Src kinase activity on platelet-derived growth factor stimulation of glioblastoma cells is affected by the integrin engaged. J Biol Chem *278*, 39882–39891.

Erlandsson, A., Brannvall, K., Gustafsdottir, S., Westermark, B., and Forsberg-Nilsson, K. (2006). Autocrine/Paracrine platelet-derived growth factor regulates proliferation of neural progenitor cells. Cancer Res *66*, 8042–8048.

Fish, K.N., Stenglein, S.G., Ibanez, C., and Nelson, J.A. (1995). Cytomegalovirus persistence in macrophages and endothelial cells. Scand J Infect Dis Suppl *99*, 34–40.

Fritschy, J.M., Brandner, S., Aguzzi, A., Koedood, M., Luscher, B., and Mitchell, P.J. (1996). Brain cell type specificity and gliosis-induced activation of the human cytomegalovirus immediate-early promoter in transgenic mice. J Neurosci *16*, 2275–2282.

Gomez, G.G., and Kruse, C.A. (2006). Mechanisms of malignant glioma immune resistance and sources of immunosuppression. Gene Ther Mol Biol *10*, 133–146.

Goodrum, F.D., Jordan, C.T., High, K., and Shenk, T. (2002). Human cytomegalovirus gene expression during infection of primary hematopoietic progenitor cells: a model for latency. Proc Natl Acad Sci USA *99*, 16255–16260.

Grefte, A., Harmsen, M.C., van der Giessen, M., Knollema, S., van Son, W.J., and The, T.H. (1994). Presence of human cytomegalovirus (HCMV) immediate early mRNA but not ppUL83 (lower matrix protein pp65) mRNA in polymorphonuclear and mononuclear leukocytes during active HCMV infection. J Gen Virol *75*, 1989–1998.

Hagemeier, C., Walker, S.M., Sissons, P.J., and Sinclair, J.H. (1992). The 72 K IE1 and 80 K IE2 proteins of human cytomegalovirus independently trans-activate the c-fos, c-myc and hsp70 promoters via basal promoter elements. J Gen Virol *73*, 2385–2393.

Harkins, L., Volk, A.L., Samanta, M., Mikolaenko, I., Britt, W.J., Bland, K.I., and Cobbs, C.S. (2002). Specific localisation of human cytomegalovirus nucleic acids and proteins in human colorectal cancer. Lancet *360*, 1557–1563.

Hayashi, M.L., Blankenship, C., and Shenk, T. (2000). Human cytomegalovirus UL69 protein is required for efficient accumulation of infected cells in the G1 phase of the cell cycle. Proc Natl Acad Sci USA *97*, 2692–2696.

Hemmati, H.D., Nakano, I., Lazareff, J.A., Masterman-Smith, M., Geschwind, D.H., Bronner-Fraser, M., and Kornblum, H.I. (2003). Cancerous stem cells can arise from pediatric brain tumors. Proc Natl Acad Sci USA *100*, 15178–15183.

Holland, E.C. (2001a). Gliomagenesis: genetic alterations and mouse models. Nat Rev Genet *2*, 120–129.

Holland, E.C. (2001b). Progenitor cells and glioma formation. Curr Opin Neurol *14*, 683–688.

Hume, A.J., Finkel, J.S., Kamil, J.P., Coen, D.M., Culbertson, M.R., and Kalejta, R.F. (2008). Phosphorylation of retinoblastoma protein by viral protein with cyclin-dependent kinase function. Science *320*, 797–799.

Jackson, E.L., Garcia-Verdugo, J.M., Gil-Perotin, S., Roy, M., Quinones-Hinojosa, A., VandenBerg, S., and Alvarez-Buylla, A. (2006). PDGFR alpha-positive B cells are neural stem cells in the adult SVZ that form glioma-like growths in response to increased PDGF signaling. Neuron *51*, 187–199.

Jault, F.M., Jault, J.M., Ruchti, F., Fortunato, E.A., Clark, C., Corbeil, J., Richman, D.D., and Spector, D.H. (1995). Cytomegalovirus infection induces high levels of cyclins, phosphorylated Rb, and p53, leading to cell cycle arrest. J Virol *69*, 6697–6704.

Johnson, R.A., Huong, S.M., and Huang, E.S. (2000). Activation of the mitogen-activated protein kinase p38 by human cytomegalovirus infection through two distinct pathways: a novel mechanism for activation of p38. J Virol *74*, 1158–1167.

Johnson, R.A., Wang, X., Ma, X.L., Huong, S.M., and Huang, E.S. (2001). Human cytomegalovirus up-regulates the phosphatidylinositol 3-kinase (PI3-K) pathway: inhibition of PI3-K activity inhibits viral replication and virus-induced signaling. J Virol *75*, 6022–6032.

Kalejta, R.F., Bechtel, J.T., and Shenk, T. (2003). Human cytomegalovirus pp71 stimulates cell cycle progression by inducing the proteasome-dependent degradation of the retinoblastoma family of tumor suppressors. Mol Cell Biol *23*, 1885–1895.

Kawataki, T., Naganuma, H., Sasaki, A., Yoshikawa, H., Tasaka, K., and Nukui, H. (2000). Correlation of thrombospondin-1 and transforming growth factor-beta expression with malignancy of glioma. Neuropathology *20*, 161–169.

Kline, J.N., Hunninghake, G.M., He, B., Monick, M.M., and Hunninghake, G.W. (1998). Synergistic activation of the human cytomegalovirus major immediate early promoter by prostaglandin E2 and cytokines. Exp Lung Res *24*, 3–14.

Kovacs, A., Weber, M.L., Burns, L.J., Jacob, H.S., and Vercellotti, G.M. (1996). Cytoplasmic sequestration of p53 in cytomegalovirus-infected human endothelial cells. Am J Pathol *149*, 1531–1539.

Lau, S.K., Chen, Y.Y., Chen, W.G., Diamond, D.J., Mamelak, A.N., Zaia, J.A., and Weiss, L.M. (2005). Lack of association of cytomegalovirus with human brain tumors. Mod Pathol *18*, 838–843.

Li, R.Y., Baba, S., Kosugi, I., Arai, Y., Kawasaki, H., Shinmura, Y., Sakakibara, S.I., Okano, H., and Tsutsui, Y. (2001). Activation of murine cytomegalovirus immediate-early promoter in cerebral ventricular zone and glial progenitor cells in transgenic mice. Glia *35*, 41–52.

Liu, Y., Tonna-DeMasi, M., Park, E., Schuller-Levis, G., and Quinn, M.R. (1998). Taurine chloramine inhibits production of nitric oxide and prostaglandin E2 in activated C6 glioma cells by suppressing inducible nitric oxide synthase and cyclooxygenase-2 expression. Brain Res Mol Brain Res *59*, 189–195.

Luo, M.H., and Fortunato, E.A. (2007). Long-term infection and shedding of human cytomegalovirus in T98G glioblastoma cells. J Virol *81*, 10424–10436.

Maciejewski, J.P., Bruening, E.E., Donahue, R.E., Sellers, S.E., Carter, C., Young, N.S., and St Jeor, S. (1993). Infection of mononucleated phagocytes with human cytomegalovirus. Virology *195*, 327–336.

Margraf, S., Bittoova, M., Vogel, J.U., Kotchekov, R., Doerr, H.W., and Cinatl, J., Jr. (2001). Antisense oligonucleotide ISIS 2922 targets IE-expression and prevents HCMV-IE-induced suppression of TSP-1 and TSP-2 expression. Nucleosides Nucleotides Nucleic Acids *20*, 1425–1428.

Maussang, D., Verzijl, D., van Walsum, M., Leurs, R., Holl, J., Pleskoff, O., Michel, D., van Dongen, G.A., and Smit, M.J. (2006). Human cytomegalovirus-encoded chemokine receptor US28 promotes tumorigenesis. Proc Natl Acad Sci USA *103*, 13068–13073.

Mitchell, D., Archer G, Bigner D, Friedman A, Friedman H, Reardon D, Vredenburgh J, Herndon J, McLendon R, Sampson JH (2007). RNA loaded dendritic cells targeting cytomegalovirus in patients with malignant gliomas. Neuro-Oncology *9*, 509.

Mitchell, D., Xie, W, Schmittling, R, Learn C, Friedman, A, McLendon RE, Sampson JH (2008). Sensitive detection of human cytomegalovirus in tumors and peripheral blood of patients diagnosed with glioblastoma. Neuro-Oncology *10*, 10–18.

Color Plates

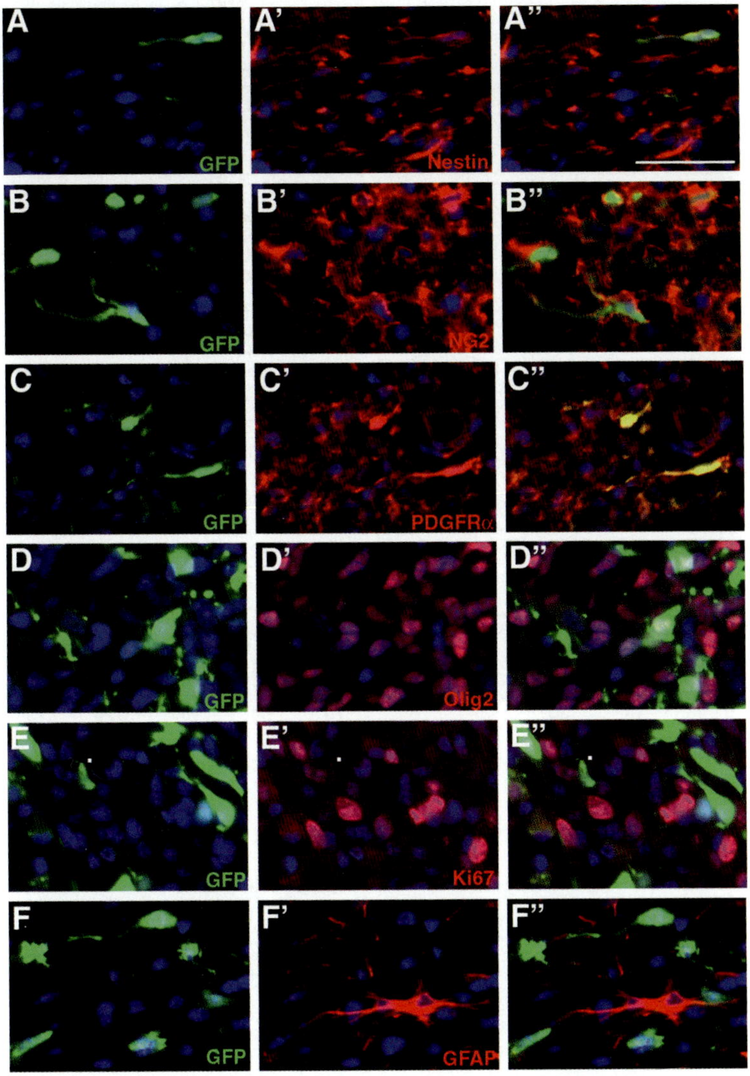

Adapted from Assanah M et al. (2006) J Neurosci 26(25):6781-6790

Color Plate 1. GFP + and GFP– tumor cells express markers of proliferative glial progenitor cells. Double-immunofluorescence analysis of tumors at 17 dpi with the PDGF-IRES-GFP retrovirus shows that GFP (*green*) is expressed in only a subset of tumor cells. However, nestin (A′, A″), NG2 (B′, B″), PDGFR-α (C′, C″), and olig2 (D′, D″), each stained red, are expressed in the vast majority of GFP + and GFP– tumor cells. Ki67 proliferation marker is expressed in a significant number of both GFP + and GFP– cells (E′, E″). GFAP + /GFP– reactive astrocytes (*red*) are seen scattered throughout the tumor (F′, F″). Rare GFAP + /GFP + cells were seen (<3%) (Chapter 1, Fig. 2; *see* discussion on p.12).

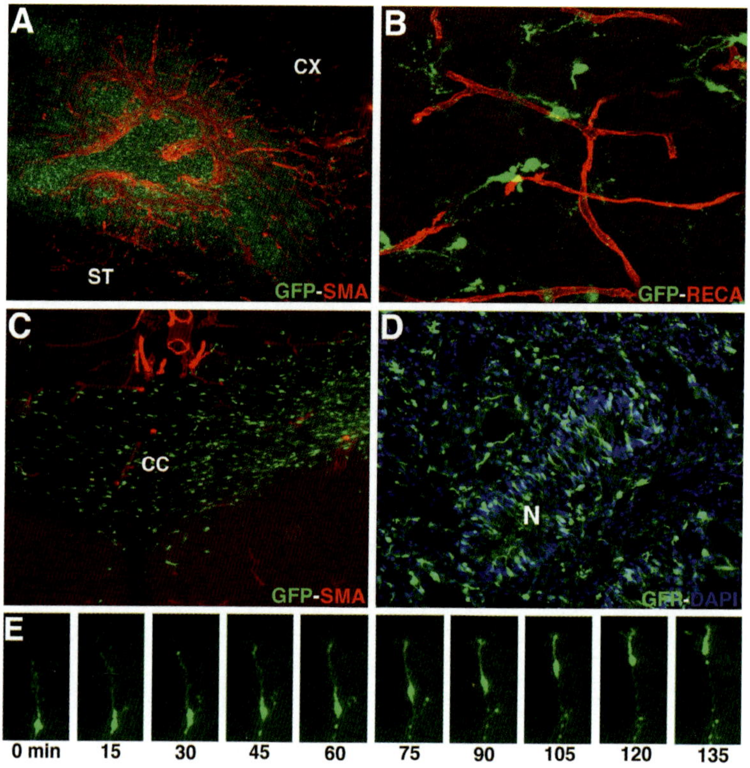

Color Plate 2. GFP expression reveals the distribution of retrovirally infected cells (Chapter 1, Fig. 3; *see* complete caption on p. 15 and discussion on p. 16).

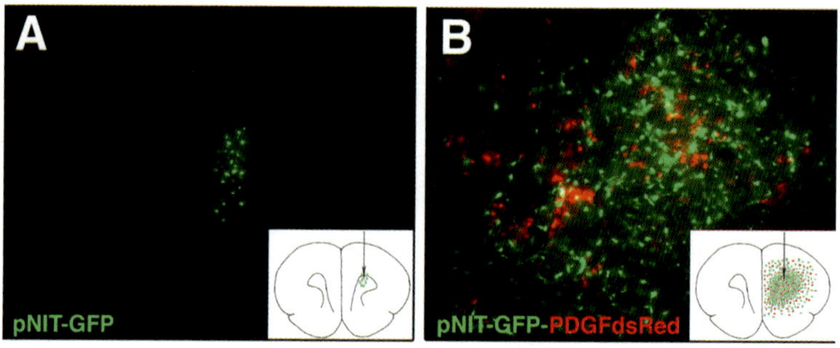

Adapted from Assanah M et al. (2006). J Neurosci 26(25):6781-6790

Color Plate 3. A. Adult rat glial progenitors infected in vitro with a pNIT-GFP retrovirus (*green*) do not proliferate, migrate, or form tumors when reinjected into subcortical white matter (diagram inset) (Chapter 1, Fig. 4; *see* complete caption and discussion on p. 18).

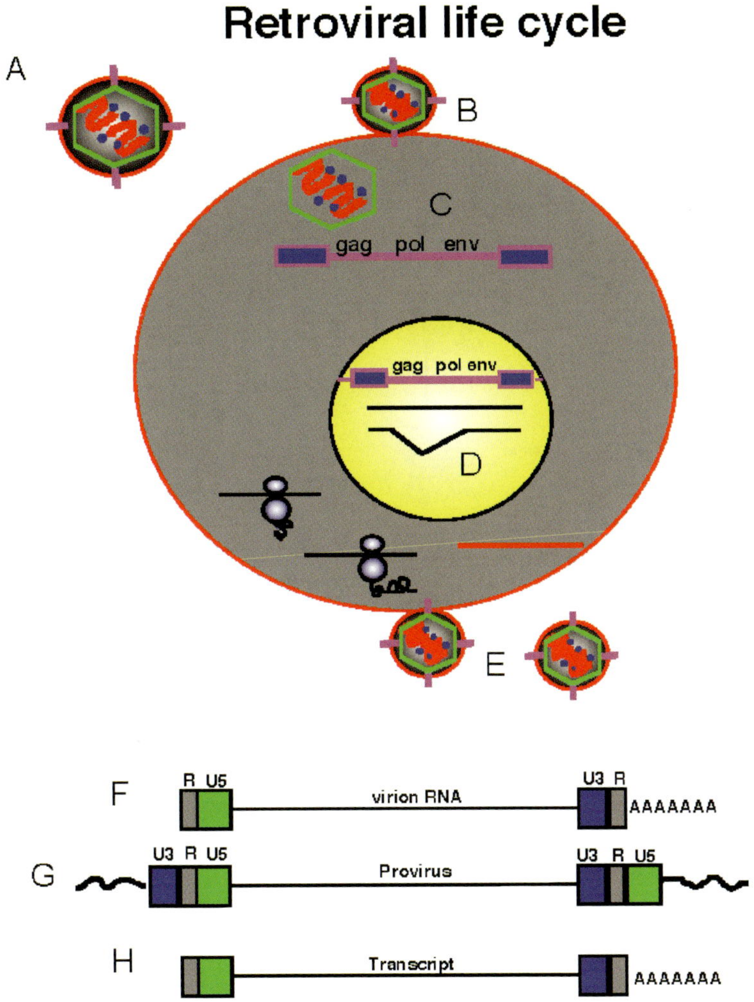

Color Plate 4. Retroviral virion (**A**) binds to the target cell via interaction of envelope protein with its receptor (**B**). The nucleocapsid enters the cytoplasm and RNA genome (**F**) is converted to double-stranded DNA (**C**), which is integrated into the genome as a provirus (**G**) and transcribed (**D, H**). The proviral transcripts are translated into viral proteins and full-length transcripts serve as the viral genome of the next generation of virus (**E**) (Chapter 2, Fig. 1; *see* discussion on p. 32).

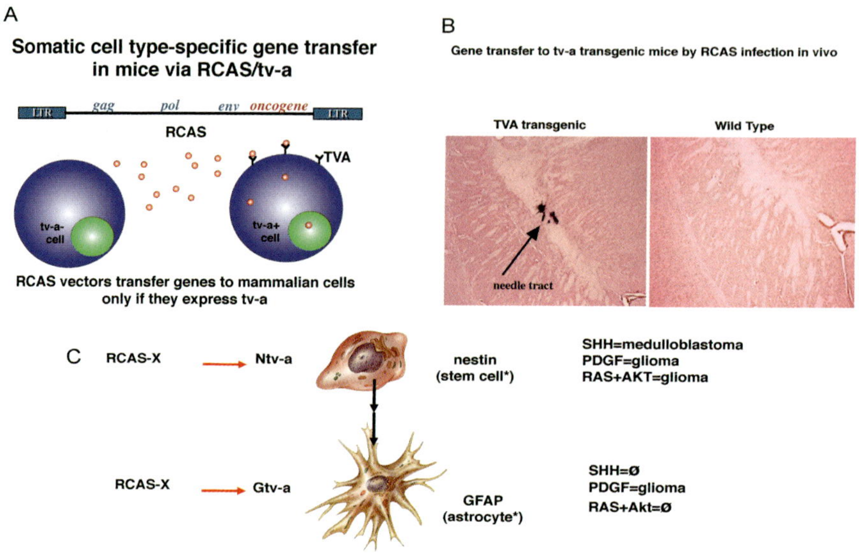

Color Plate 5. RCAS/tv-a-based somatic cell gene transfer. RCAS vectors are engineered to encode a gene downstream of the *env* gene and will only infect mammalian cells if they express the RCAS receptor TVA (**A**) (Chapter 2, Fig. 2; *see* complete caption on p. 35 and discussion on p. 34).

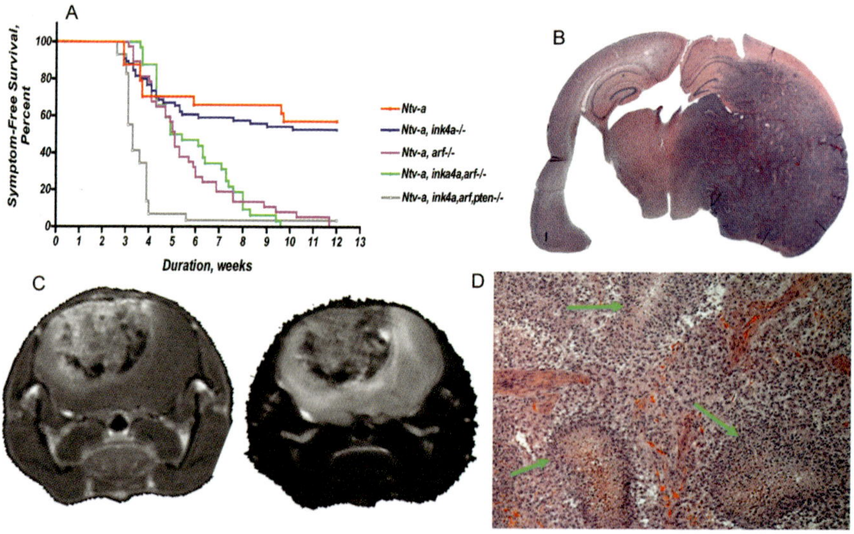

Color Plate 6. Glioma formation with the RCAS/tv-a system. (**A**) Survival curves for mice of different genetic backgrounds infected with RCAS-PDGF demonstrating cooperativity between gain of function oncogenes and loss of tumor suppressors (Chapter 2, Fig. 3; *see* complete caption on p. 37 and discussion on p. 36).

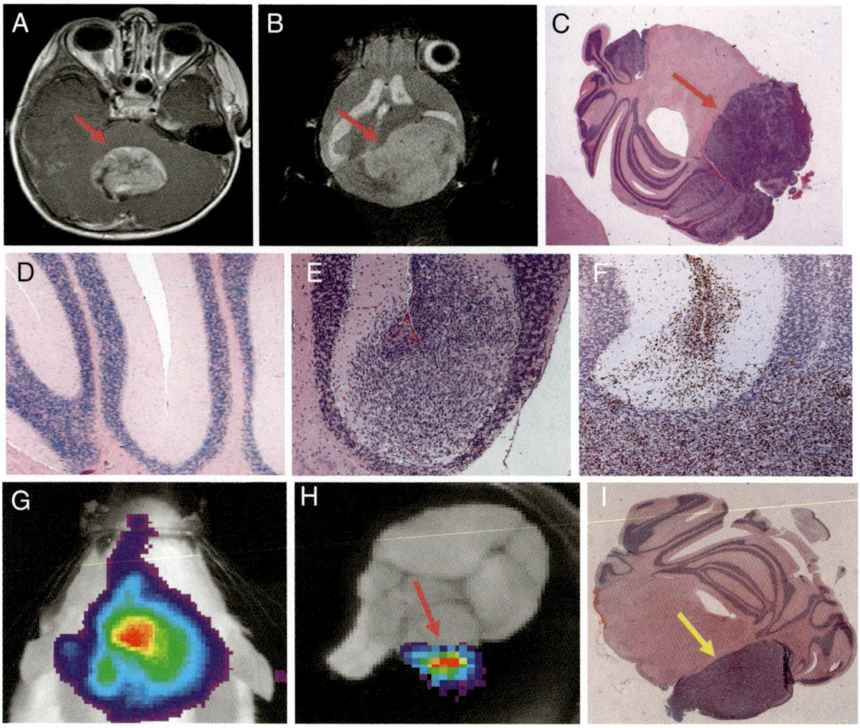

Color Plate 7. RCAS/tv-a-mediated medulloblastoma and bioluminescence imaging. (**A**) MRI scan of human medulloblastoma. (**B**) MRI scan of RCAS–SHH-induced medulloblastoma (courtesy of Jason Koutcher MSKCC) with (**C**) H&E-stained whole mount. (**D**) Normal adult cerebellum. (**E**) Cluster of cells trapped in the region of the external granule cell layer by SHH autocrine signaling showing proliferation by Ki67 staining (**F**). Medulloblastoma bearing mouse in a gli-luciferase reporter background (**G**). Brain removed from mouse showing light production arising from the medulloblastoma (**H**) shown on whole mount (**I**) (Chapter 2, Fig. 4; *see* discussion on p. 39).

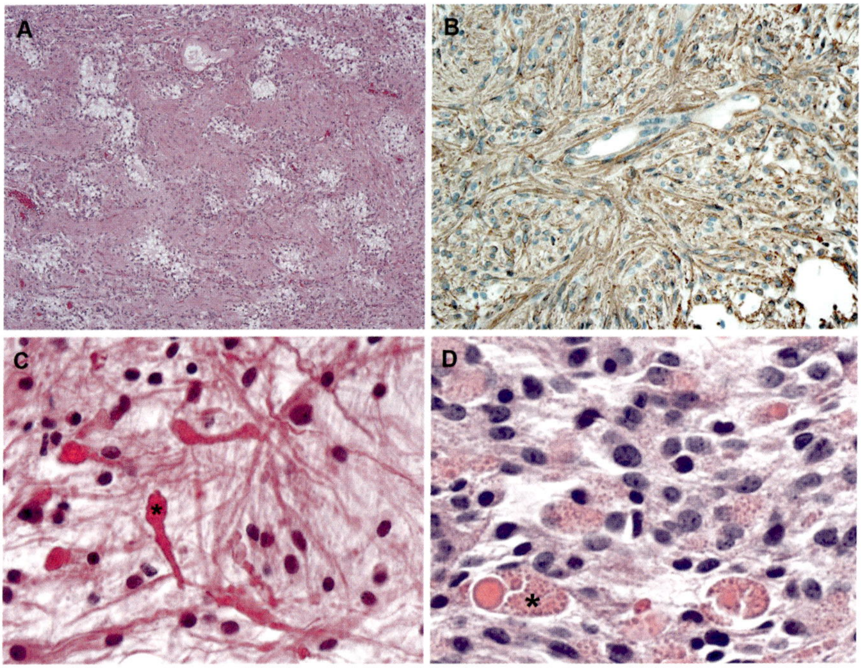

Color Plate 8. Histologic features of human pilocytic astrocytomas. (**A**) Biphasic pattern of regions with more compact cellularity alternating with regions with more loosely structured architecture (Chapter 3, Fig. 1; *see* complete caption and discussion on p. 46).

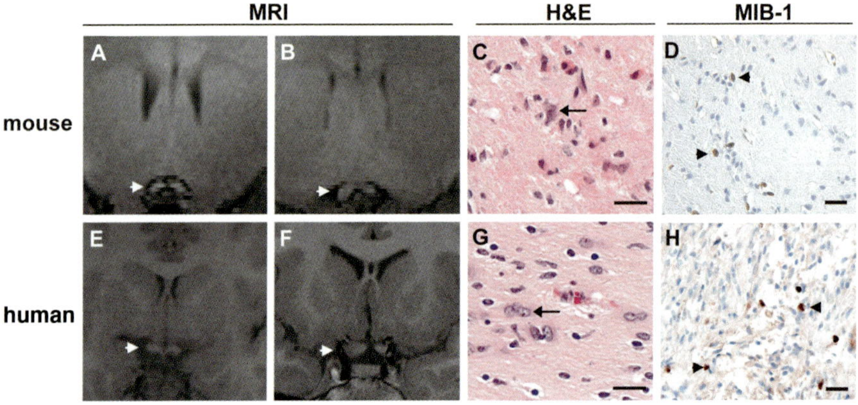

Color Plate 9. *Nf1*+/−^{GFAP}CKO mice develop optic gliomas similar to those observed in children with neurofibromatosis-1 (Chapter 3, Fig. 3; *see* complete caption and discussion on p. 51).

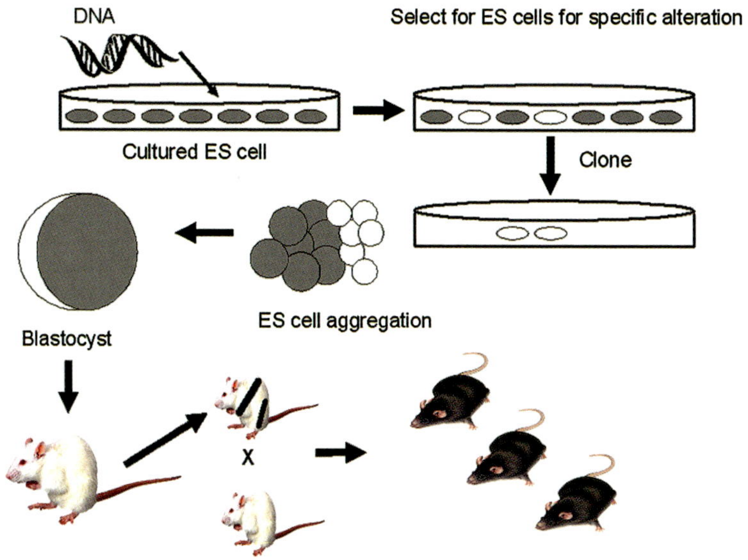

Color Plate 10. General principle of classical ES transgenesis. DNA Vector carrying gene of interest is transfected into cultured mouse ES cells. In our case we used a retrovirus carrying the ^{V12}Ha-Ras gene under the control of the astrocyte-specific human GFAP promoter and a neomycin selection marker expression cassette. Selection of ES cells with the transgene of interest is first accomplished by selecting for neomycin-resistant clones. Thereafter NeoR ES clones are tested for their ability to express the transgene by in vitro differentiation to astrocytes. This process confirms activation of the GFAP promoter expression and specificity. Positive ES cells undergo aggregations and are transferred to a pseudo-pregnant female mouse to create chimeric embryos (striped mouse in picture). The chimeric mice are bred to normal mice and those mice having incorporated the transgene in their germ-line will generate transgenic offspring (Chapter 4, Fig. 1; *see* discussion on p. 63).

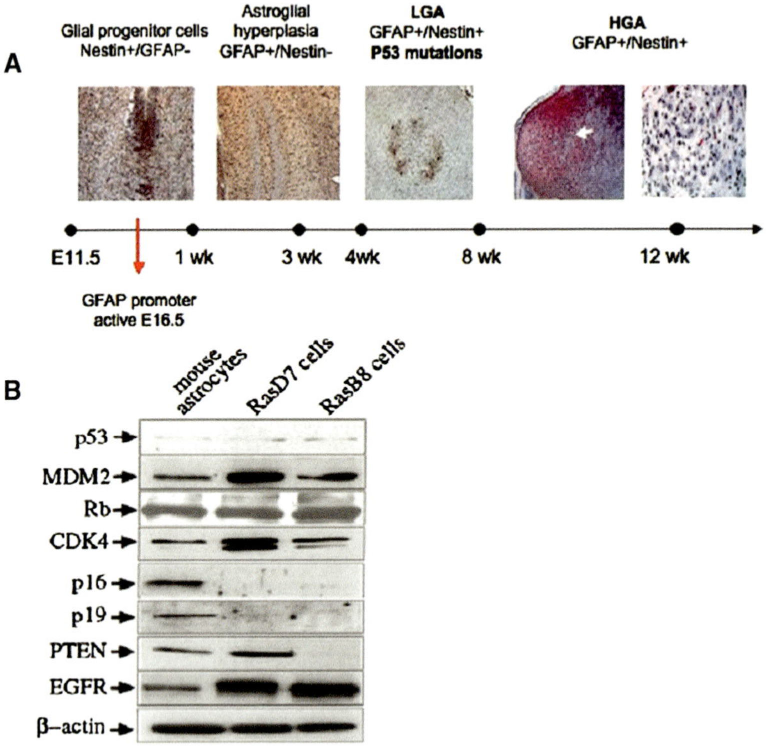

Color Plate 11. RasB8-pathologocal/molecular progression. **A.** *RasB8 GEM-Pathological progression.* The hGFAP-regulated transgene is expressed as early as E13.5 where the mice are similar to normal littermates. For the first few weeks there are no astrocytomas, but diffuse astroglial hyperplasia. At 3–4 weeks LGA appear with p53 mutations, as demonstrated by microdissection. At 12 weeks and beyond one sees HGA with infiltrative and necrotic tumors. **B.** *RasB8-Molecular progression.* Astrocytes isolated at 1 week are not transformed, in contrast, astrocytoma cells from the HGA after 12 weeks show genetic alterations which are known to be associated with human GBMs: loss of p16, p19, PTEN, and overexpression of EGFR (Chapter 4, Fig. 3; *see* discussion on p. 66).

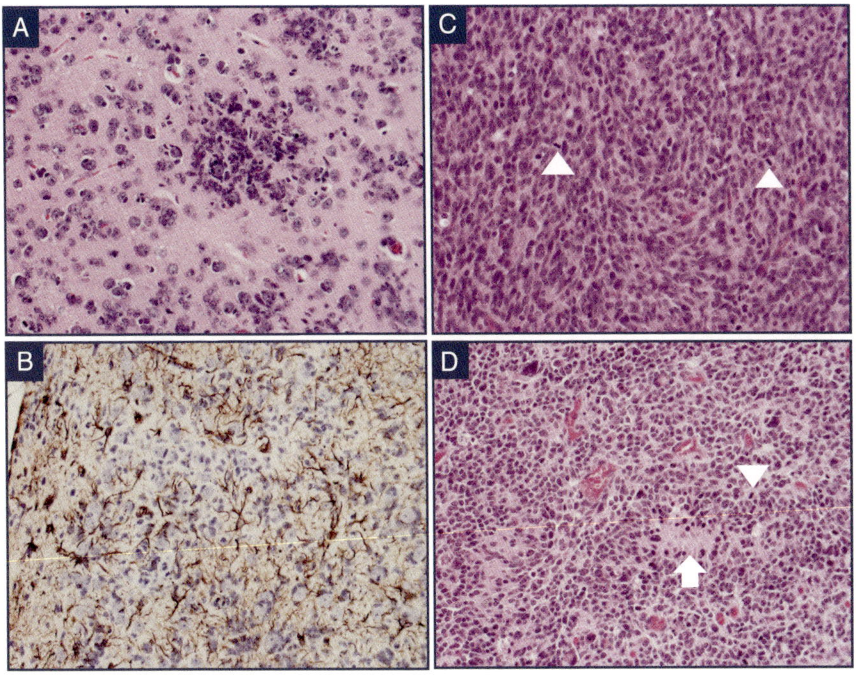

Color Plate 12. Inducible GEM astrocytomas. T mice developed diffuse astrocytomas, WHO grade II (**A**). Tumors were immunoreactive for GFAP (**B**). TR mice developed anaplastic astrocytomas, WHO grade III (**C**), characterized by numerous mitoses (*arrowheads*). $TRP^{+/-}$ (not shown) and $TRP^{-/-}$ mice (D) developed glioblastomas, WHO grade IV, characterized by numerous mitoses (*arrowhead*) and areas of pseudopalisading necrosis (*arrow*) (Chapter 7, Fig. 5; *see* discussion on p. 129).

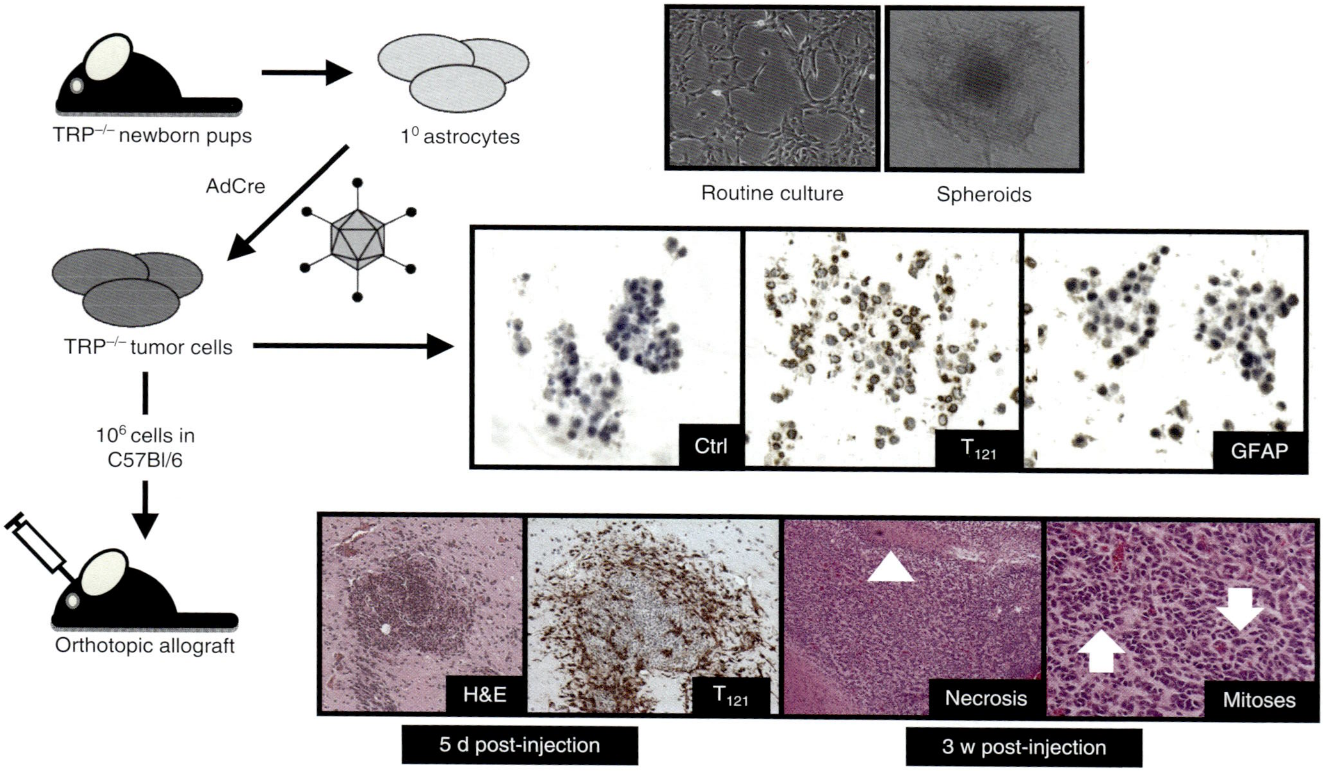

Color Plate 13. Generation and characterization of cell lines derived from conditional GEM models of astrocytomas (Chapter 7, Fig. 10; *see* complete caption on p. 139 and discussion on p. 137).

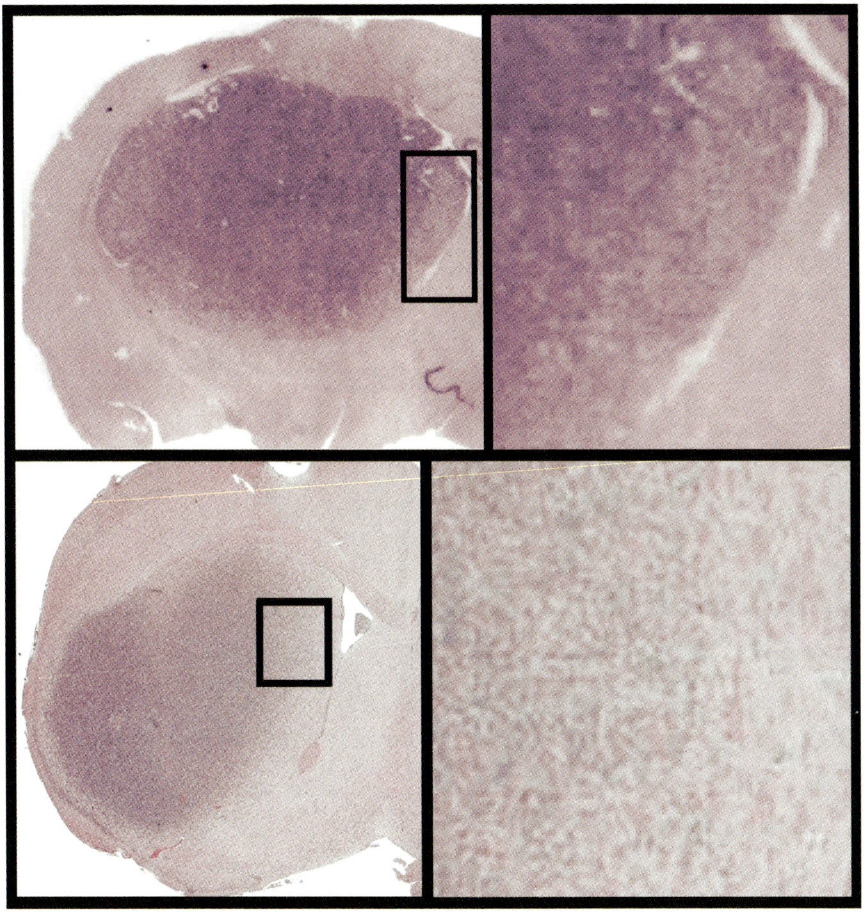

Color Plate 14. Comparing the intracranial invasiveness of GBM cell lines propagated as monolayer cultures in serum-supplemented media (*upper panels*) vs. propagation as neurospheres in EGF + FGF supplemented media (*lower panels*). Upper panels show a well-circumscribed intracranial tumor established from U-87 MG monolayer culture (image shown to the right is an enlargement of the area indicated by the black rectangle in *left panel*). Note the well-delineated plane of separation between U-87 MG tumor and surrounding normal brain (*upper right panel*). In contrast, intracranial tumors established from GS2 cells propagated as a neurosphere culture (*bottom panels*) show diffuse infiltration, as highlighted by the enlargement image shown in the lower right section of the figure (Chapter 8, Fig. 1; *see* discussion on p. 151).

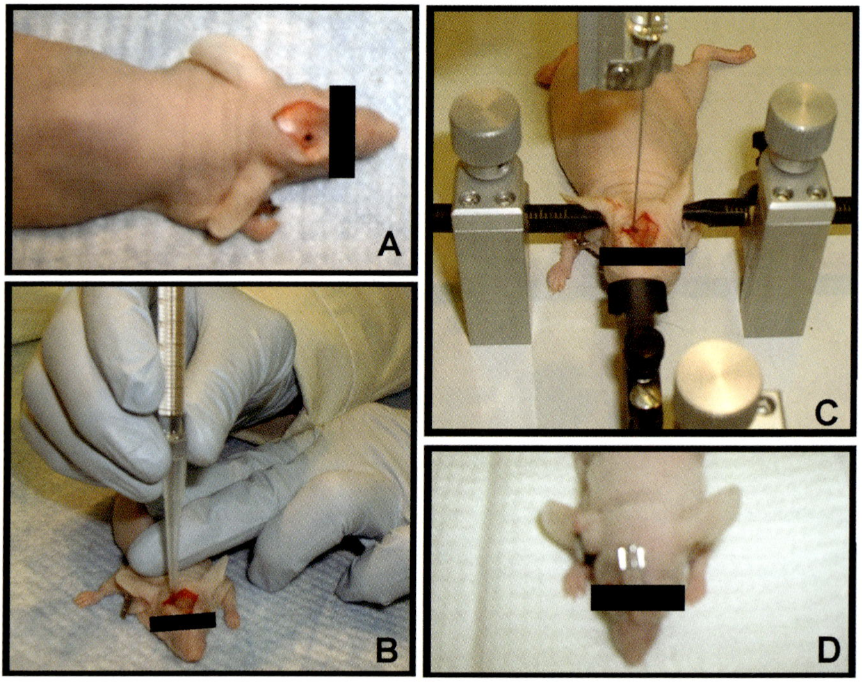

Color Plate 15. Approaches to establishing orthotopic brain tumor xenografts. Following the midline incision and separation of the skin covering the skull (panel **A**: *pen mark* shows location for injection of cells, approximately 2.5–3 mm right from the bregma and just behind the coronal suture), tumor cells can either be injected "freehand" (panel **B**), or by use of a small animal stereotactic frame (panel **C**), which provides increased stability and control of injection depth. The opening in the skull for injection can be created either with a small drill or by simply pricking the skull with a 25 gauge needle. For the freehand method, injection depth is limited by a pipette tip (shown) or rubber sleeve covering all but the exposed end of the needle. Once the hole has been created, tumor cells are injected 3 mm below the outer table of the skull for routine supratentorial tumor establishment. Following injection, the separated skin is closed by use of clip (panel **D**) that eventually dislodges as the skin closes (heals). Especially when injecting large series of mice (>50), we recommend the freehand method as it increases throughput 3–4× relative to use of the stereotactic frame. For example, as many as 50 mice can be injected in an hour when two investigators are working in tandem (i.e., one investigator exposing the skull and the other performing the injection), whereas 12–16 mice per hour is an achievable rate when using a stereotactic frame (Chapter 8, Fig. 3; *see* discussion on p. 153).

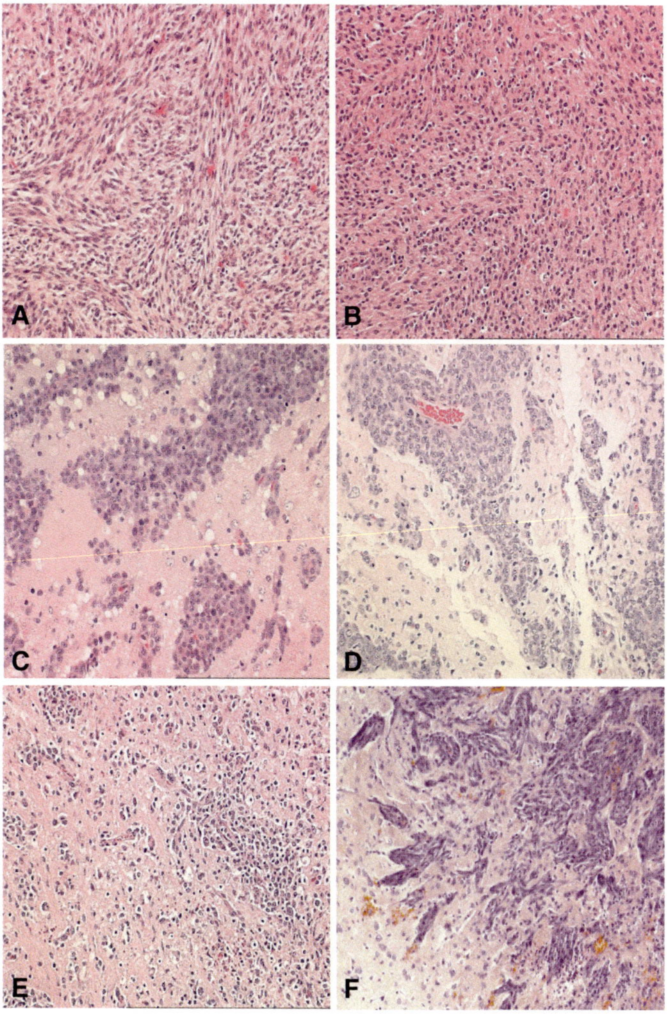

Color Plate 16. Histopathologic features of the C6, 9L, RG2, F98, CNS-1, and BT4C brain tumors. **A** (Chapter 10, Fig. 1; *see* complete caption on p. 187 and discussion on p. 186).

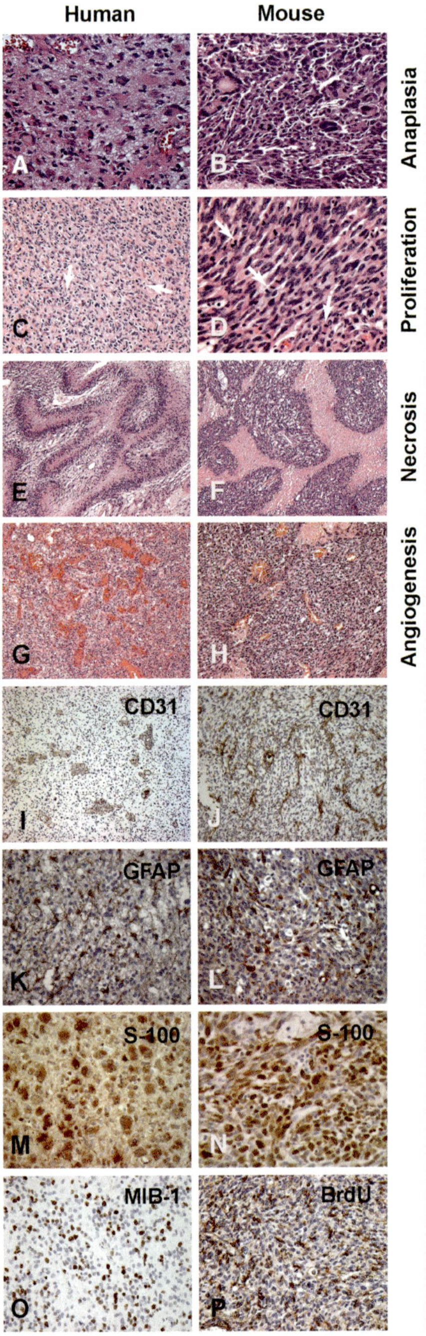

Color Plate 17. Histopathology: Comparison between high-grade human gliomas and the murine GL261 glioma (Chapter 12, Fig. 2; *see* complete caption on p. 233 and discussion on p. 231).

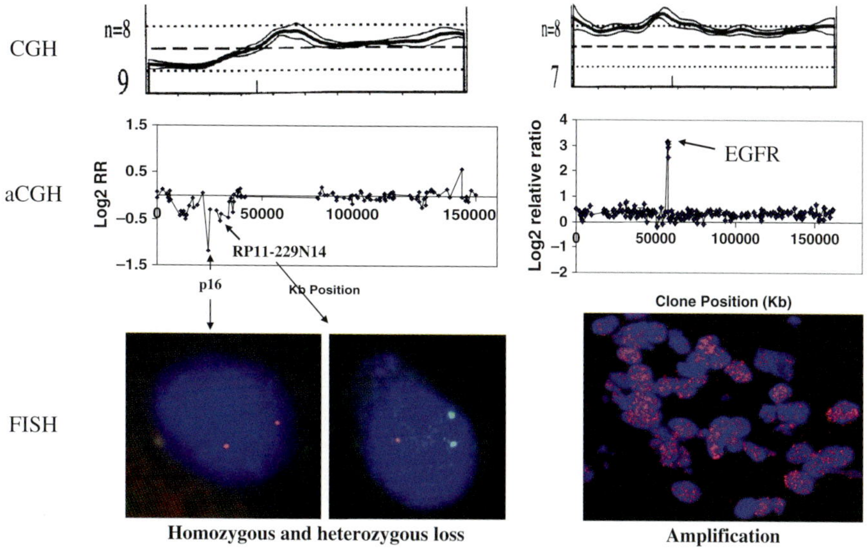

Color Plate 18. Homozygous and heterozygous losses and amplifications are better defined by aCGH than by conventional CGH (Chapter 17, Fig. 3; *see* complete caption on p. 382 and discussion on p. 379).

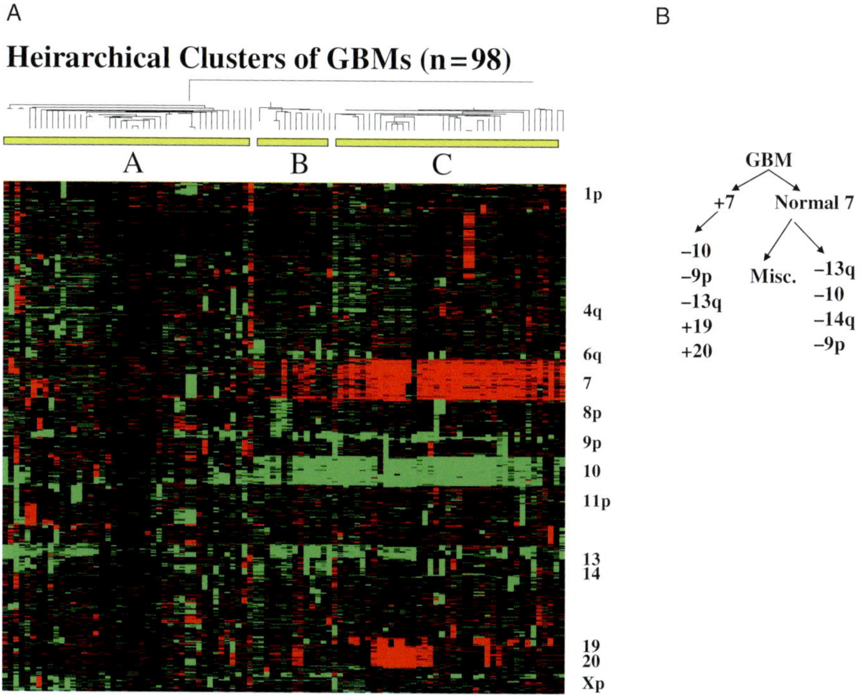

Color Plate 19. Identification of genetic subgroups in GBM. (**A**) The classification tree shows three sub groups (Chapter 17, Fig. 5; *see* complete caption on p. 383 and discussion on p. 379).

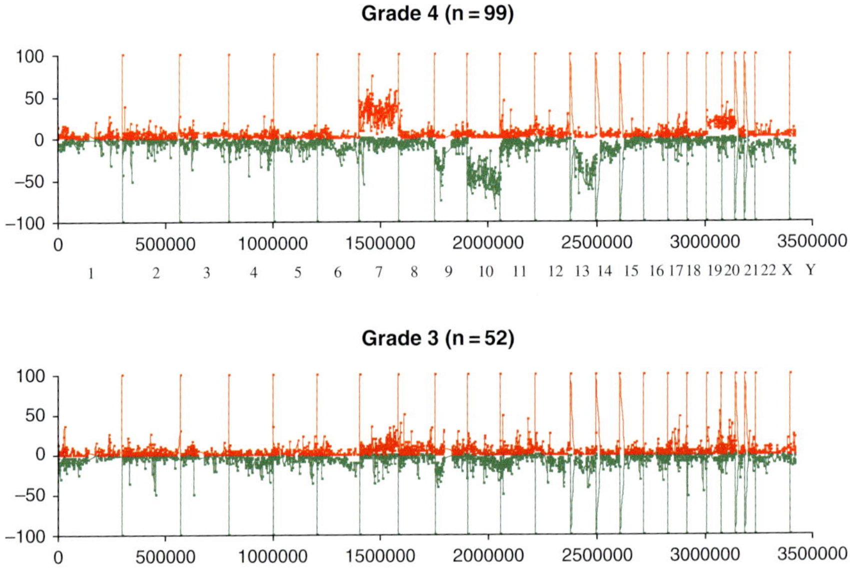

Color Plate 20. Map showing frequency of copy number aberrations in grade 4 (**A**) and grade 3 (**B**) astrocytoma. The ordinate marks the frequency of gain (positive) and loss (negative). The abscissa shows the genome in 1p to Yq direction (Chapter 17, Fig. 6; *see* discussion on p. 379).

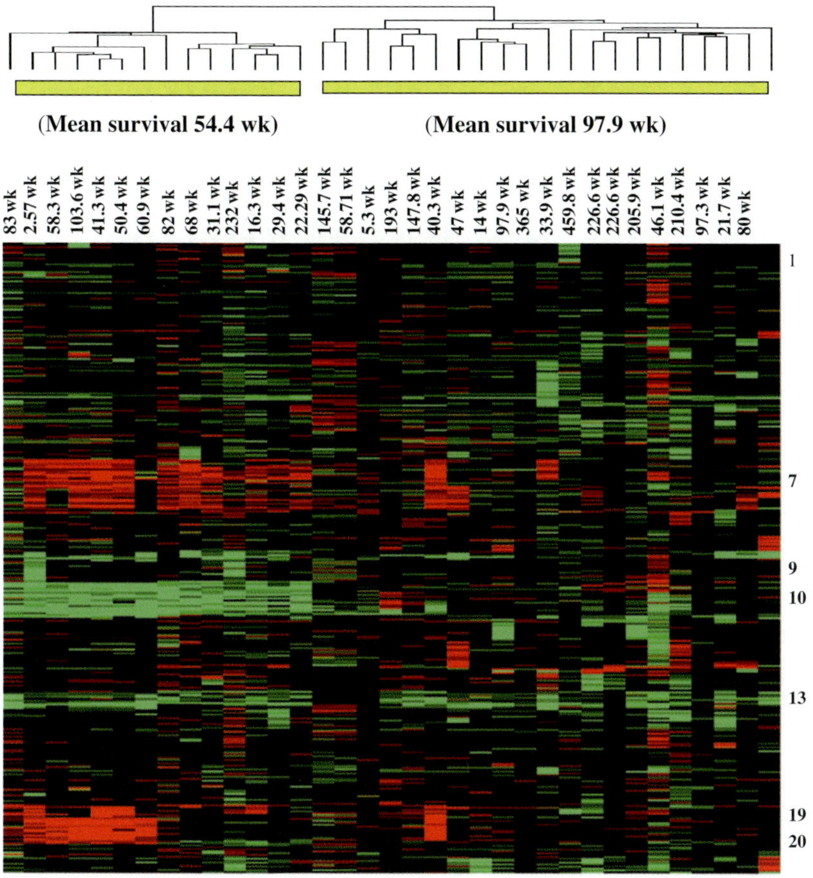

Color Plate 21. Markers of survival in GBM. In an age-matched comparison of GBM patients with poor (>2 yr) survival and better (<2 yr) survival, frequent 7 gain, 10 loss, and 19 gain were found in those with poor survival. Global gene expression profiles of the same tumors separated the poor and better survivors into almost identical groups (Nigro et al., 2005) (Chapter 17, Fig. 7; *see* discussion on p. 379).

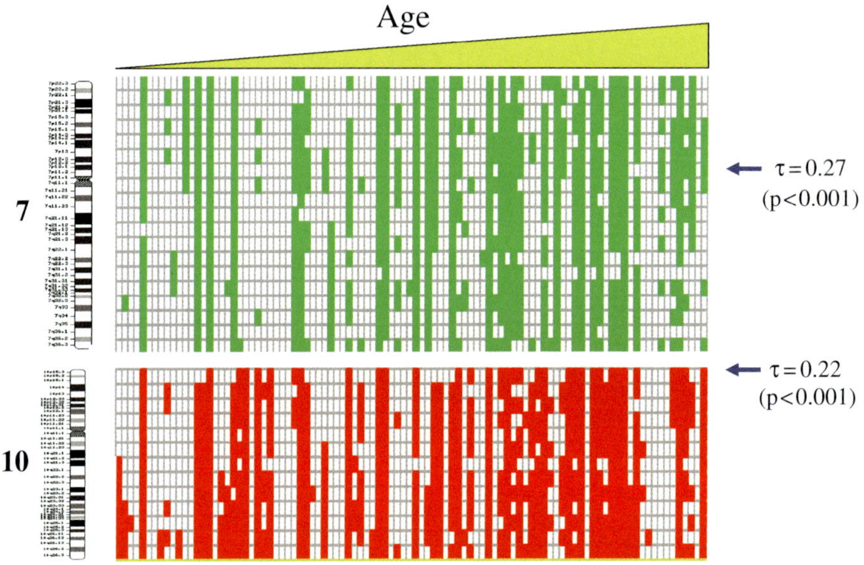

Color Plate 22. After undergoing surgery followed by radiation and chemotherapy, young patients with GBM do better than older patients (Chapter 17, Fig. 8; *see* complete caption on p. 386 and discussion on p. 379)

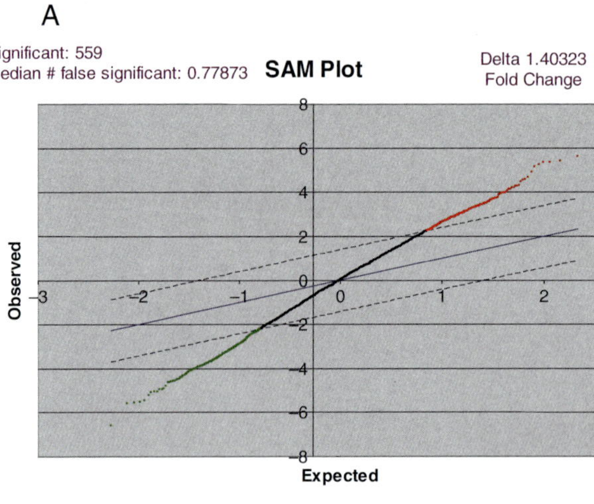

B

	Gain	Loss
1p	15	2
1q	8	6
2p	9	18
3q	8	2
4q	28	2
5q	8	7
7p	53	0
7q	24	0
8p	4	12
8q	1	21
9p	0	9
10p	0	32
10q	0	73
11p	9	1
11q	0	22
12q	20	1
13q	0	20
16q	7	0
17p	0	11
17q	8	6
20p	8	0
22q	0	10

Color Plate 23. Supervised analysis to identify genetic differences between grade 3 and grade 4 astrocytomas (Chapter 17, Fig. 9; *see* complete caption on p. 387 and discussion on p. 384).

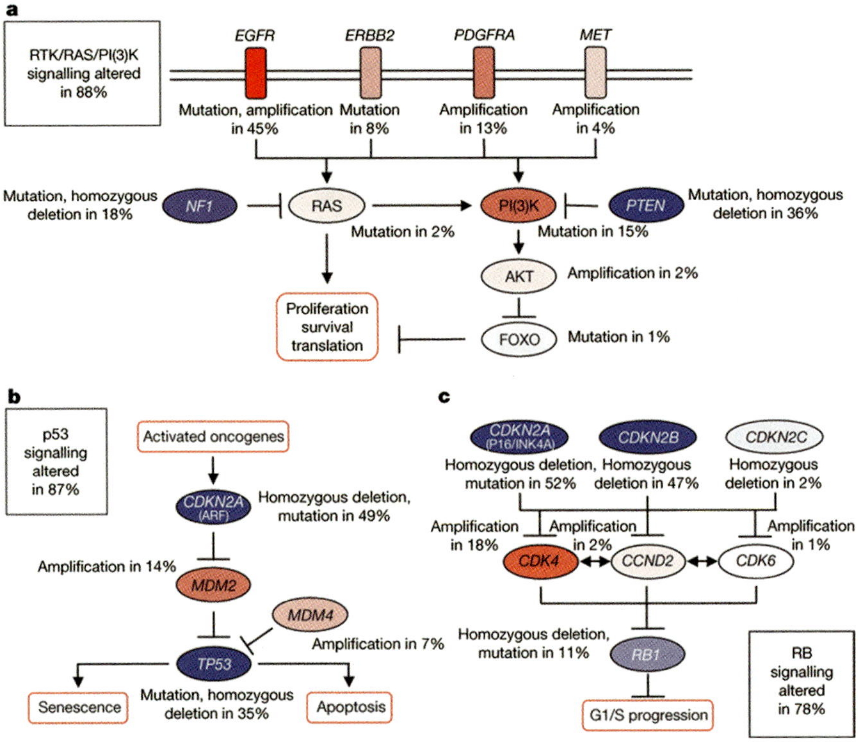

Color Plate 24. Three major affected pathways (a, b, c) in grade 4 astrocytoma that showed DNA copy number changes, mutation, and amplification of their member genes. More pathways are expected to be added to this list. (TCGA, 2008) (Chapter 17, Fig. 11; *see* discussion on p. 389).

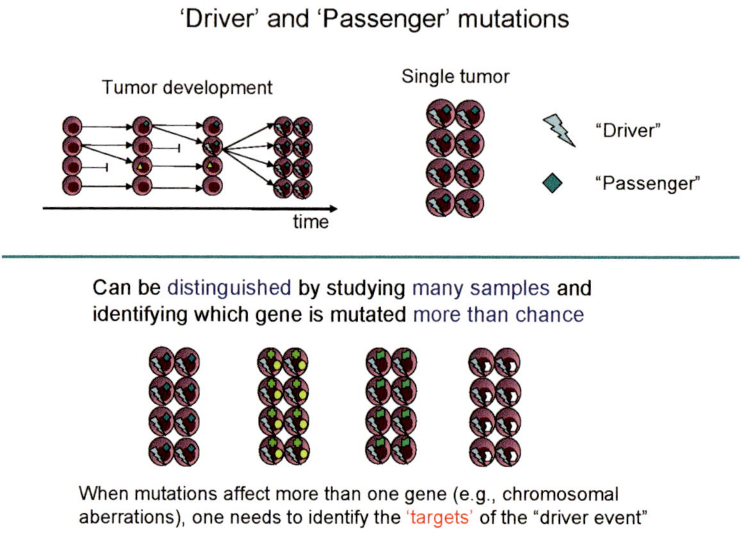

Color Plate 25. "Driver" and "passenger" mutations in the cancer genome (Chapter 18, Fig. 1; *see* discussion on p. 396).

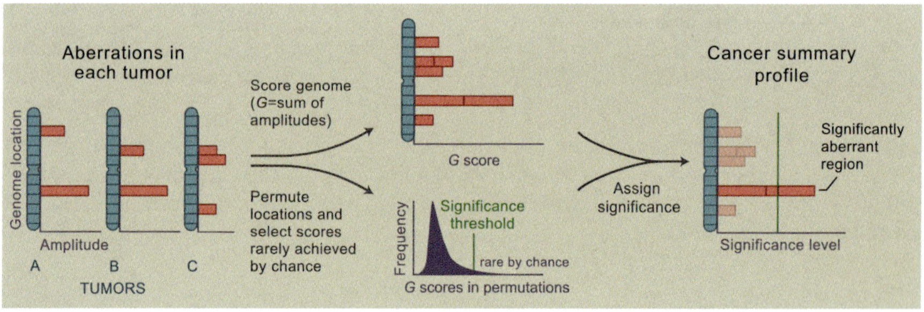

Color Plate 26. Overview of the GISTIC. After identifying the locations and magnitudes of chromosomal aberrations in multiple tumors (*left*), GISTIC scores each genomic marker with a *G*-score that is proportional to the total magnitude of aberrations at each location. By permuting the locations in each tumor, GISTIC determines the frequency with which a given score would be attained if the events were due to chance and randomly distributed (*center*). A significance threshold (*green line*) is determined such that significant scores are unlikely to occur by chance alone and alterations are considered significant if they occur in regions that surpass this threshold (*right*) (Chapter 18, Fig. 3; *see* discussion on p. 398).

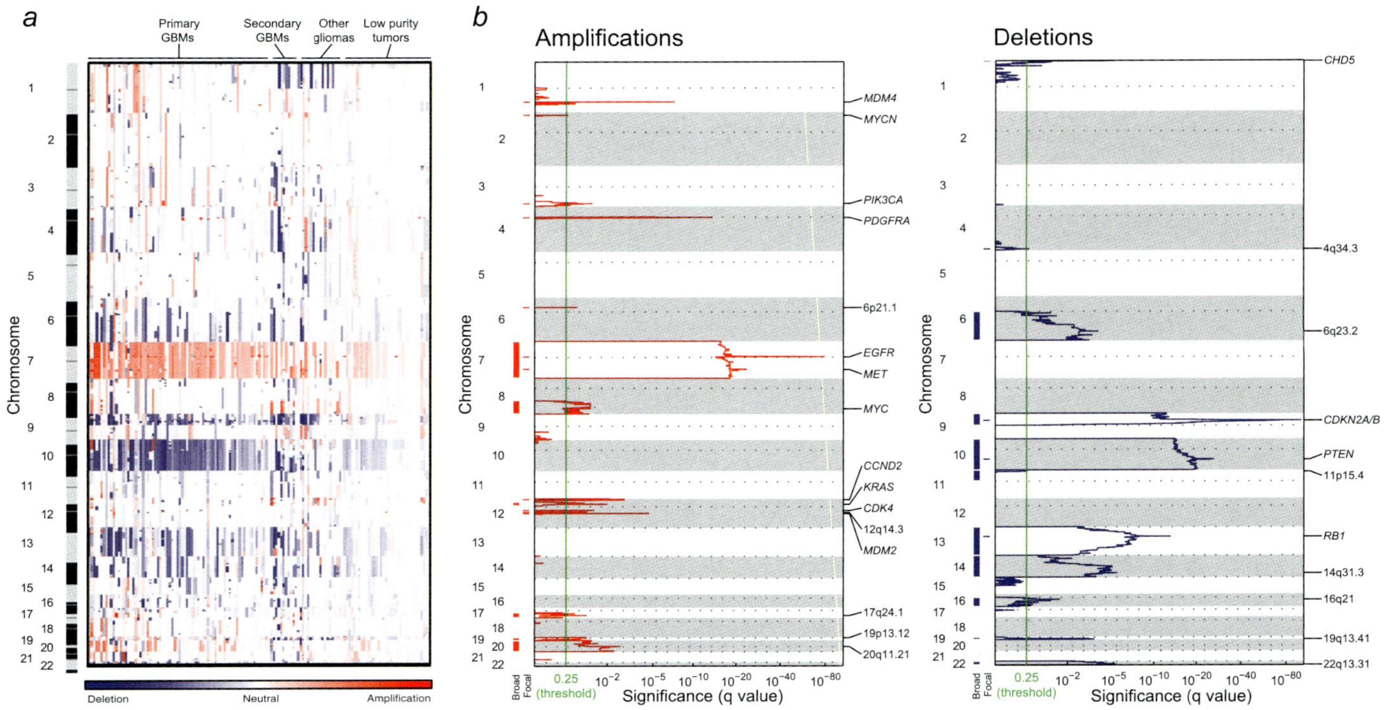

Color Plate 27. Application of GISTIC to glioma. (**A**) Amplifications (*red*) and deletions (*blue*), determined by segmentation analysis of normalized signal intensities from 100 K SNP arrays are displayed across the genome (chromosome positions indicated along the *y*-axis) for 141 gliomas (*x*-axis, diagnosis is displayed on top). (**B**) GISTIC analysis with statistical significance of the aberrations displayed as FDR *q*-values to account for multiple hypothesis testing. Centromere positions are indicated for each chromosome by a dotted line. The locations of the peak regions and the known cancer-related genes within those peaks are indicated to the right of each panel (Chapter 18, Fig. 4; *see* discussion on p. 402).

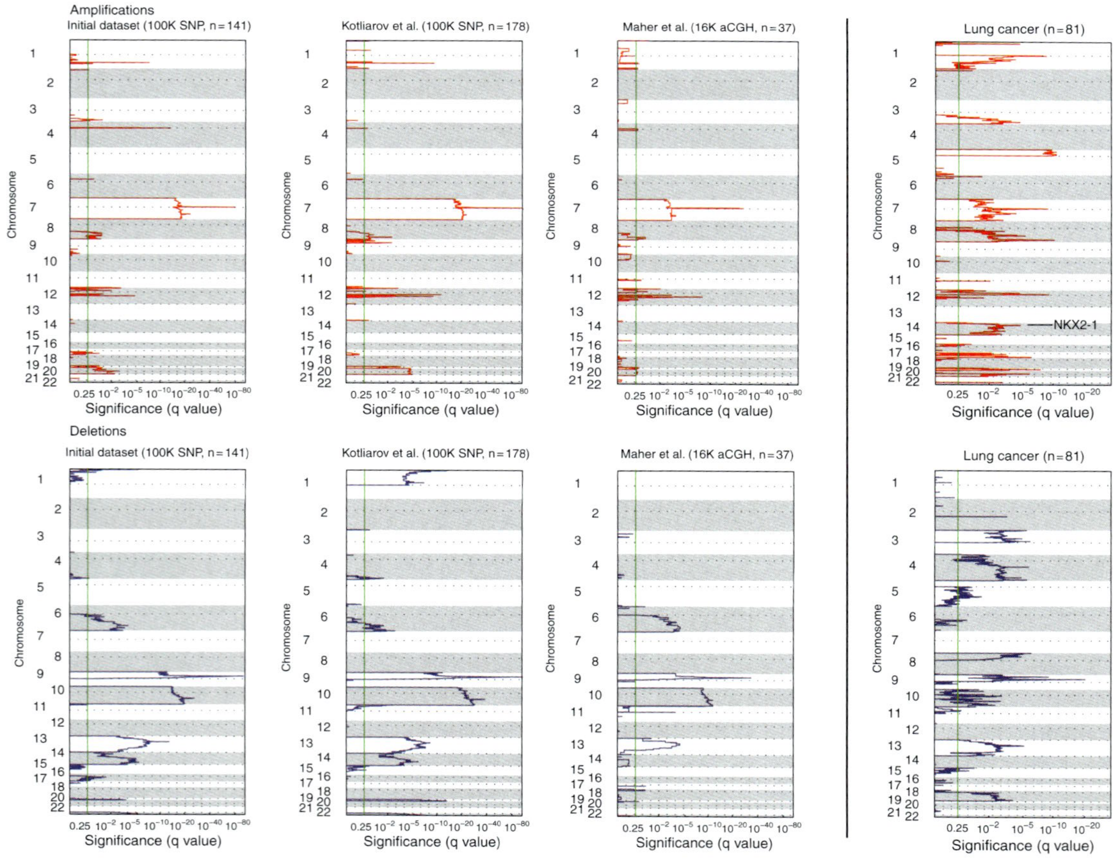

Color Plate 28. GISTIC identifies cancer-specific patterns of gene copy-number alterations. (Chapter 18, Fig. 5; *see* complete caption on p. 407 and discussion on p. 405).

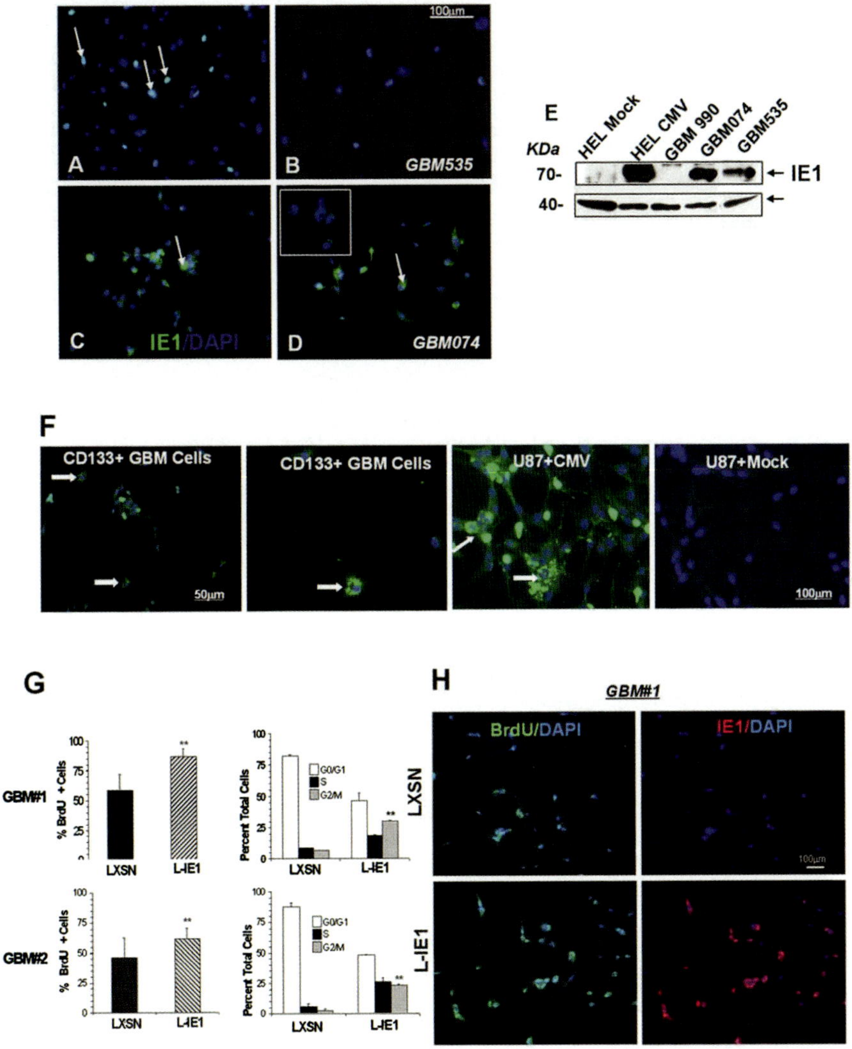

Color Plate 29. Primary GBM cells endogenously expressed HCMV IE1. Primary glioma-derived cultures were processed for IE1 immunofluorescence using MAB810 (Chemicon) and Alexa 488-labeled secondary antibody. Nuclei were counterstained using DAPI. Panel **A** shows nuclear localization of endogenous IE1 in one GBM culture; panels **C** and **D** illustrate IE1 perinuclear staining in a different GBM primary culture (Chapter 19, Fig. 1; *see* complete caption and discussion on p. 424).

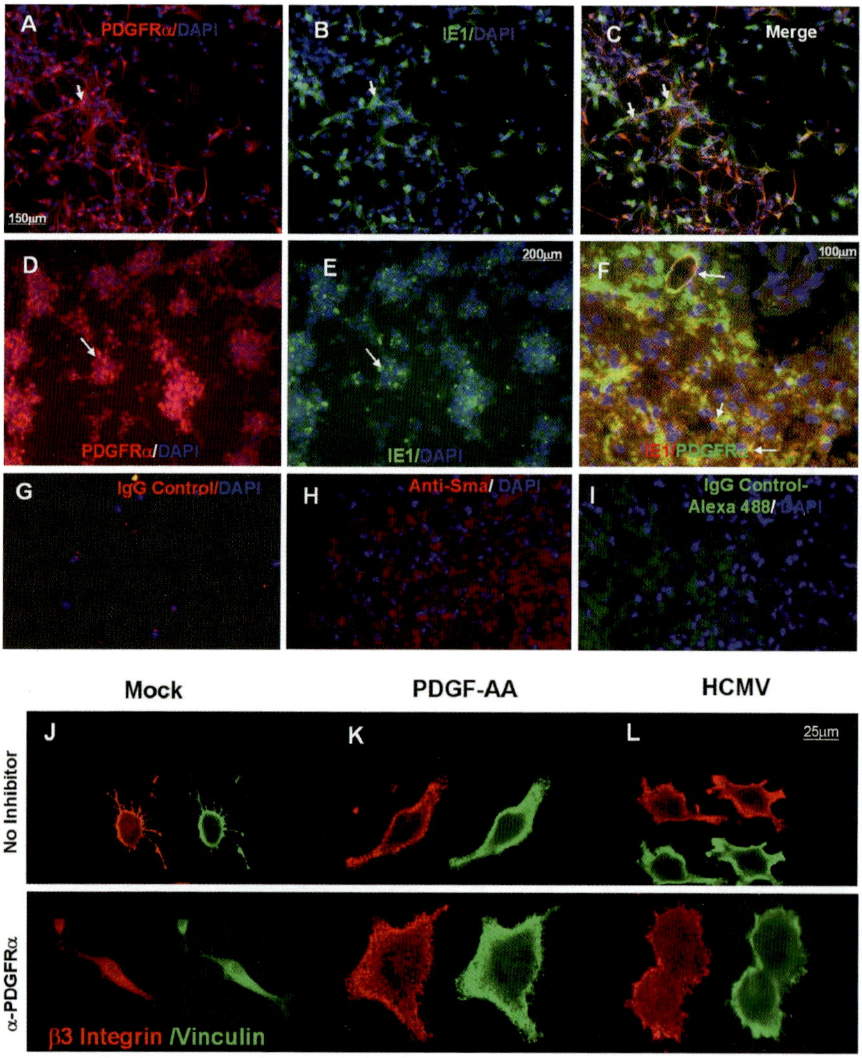

Color Plate 30. Co-localization of PDGFRα and IE1 in primary human GBM samples. GBM primary cultures and tissues were examined for the presence of IE1 and PDGFRα using double immunofluorescence. Panels **A and D** represent immunofluorescence detection of PDGFRα in primary cultures, panels **B** and **E** show IE1 detection in the same cells. Panels **C** and **F** show examples of cells double positive for HCMV IE1 and PDGFRα.(superimposed single-staining photographs). Control stained sections were negative for both antigens (**G, H, I**). **J, K, L**. HMCV treatment induces recruitment of the $\alpha v\beta 3$ integrin to focal adhesions in a PDGFRα-dependent manner (Chapter 19, Fig. 3; *see* complete caption and discussion on p. 431).

Nakamizo, A., Marini, F., Amano, T., Khan, A., Studeny, M., Gumin, J., et al. (2005). Human bone marrow-derived mesenchymal stem cells in the treatment of gliomas. Cancer Res *65*, 3307–3318.

Odeberg, J., Wolmer, N., Falci, S., Westrgren, M., Seiger, A., Soderberg-Naucler, C. (2006). Human cytomegalovirus inhibits neuronal differentiation and induces apoptosis in human neural precursor cells. J Virol *80*, 8929–8939.

Odeberg, J., Wolmer, N., Falci, S., Westgren, M., Sundtrom, E., Seiger, A., Soderberg-Naucler, C. (2007). Late human cytomegalovirus (HCMV) proteins inhibit differentiation of human neural precursor cells into astrocytes. J Nerosci Res *85*, 583–593.

Ogura, T., Tanaka, J., Kamiya, S., Sato, H., Ogura, H., and Hatano, M. (1986). Human cytomegalovirus persistent infection in a human central nervous system cell line: production of a variant virus with different growth characteristics. J Gen Virol *67*, 2605–2616.

Oh, J.W., Drabik, K., Kutsch, O., Choi, C., Tousson, A., and Benveniste, E.N. (2001). CXC chemokine receptor 4 expression and function in human astroglioma cells. J Immunol *166*, 2695–2704.

Pfenninger, C.V., Roschupkina, T., Hertwig, F., Kottwitz, D., Englund, E., Bengzon, J., Jacobsen, S.E., and Nuber, U.A. (2007). CD133 is not present on neurogenic astrocytes in the adult subventricular zone, but on embryonic neural stem cells, ependymal cells, and glioblastoma cells. Cancer Res *67*, 5727–5736.

Pleskoff, O., Treboute, C., Brelot, A., Heveker, N., Seman, M., and Alizon, M. (1997). Identification of a chemokine receptor encoded by human cytomegalovirus as a cofactor for HIV-1 entry. Science *276*, 1874–1878.

Poltermann, S., Schlehofer, B., Steindorf, K., Schnitzler, P., Geletneky, K., and Schlehofer, J.R. (2006). Lack of association of herpesviruses with brain tumors. J Neurovirol *12*, 90–99.

Prins, R.M., Cloughesy, T.F., and Liau, L.M. (2008). Cytomegalovirus immunity after vaccination with autologous glioblastoma lysate. N Engl J Med *359*, 539–541.

Rahbar A, P.I., Orrego A, Straat K, Wolmer N, Tammik L, Soderberg-Naucler C (2007). The level of HCMV infection in human malignant glioblastoma is of predictive value for patient survival. In 11-th International CMV Workshop Abstract Book, pp. 158.

Reinhardt, B., Mertens, T., Mayr-Beyrle, U., Frank, H., Luske, A., Schierling, K., and Waltenberger, J. (2005). HCMV infection of human vascular smooth muscle cells leads to enhanced expression of functionally intact PDGF beta-receptor. Cardiovasc Res *67*, 151–160.

Sabatier J, U.-C.E., Pommepuy I, Labrousse F, Allart S, (2005). Detection of human cytomegalovirus genome and gene products in central nervous system tumours. Br J Cancer *92*, 747–750.

Samanta, M., Harkins, L., Klemm, K., Britt, W.J., and Cobbs, C.S. (2003). High prevalence of human cytomegalovirus in prostatic intraepithelial neoplasia and prostatic carcinoma. J Urol *170*, 998–1002.

Scheurer, M.E., El-Zein, R., Bondy, M.L., Harkins, L., and Cobbs, C.S. (2007). RE: "Lack of association of herpesviruses with brain tumors". J Neurovirol *13*, 85; author reply 86–87.

Scholz, M., Blaheta, R.A., Wittig, B., Cinatl, J., Vogel, J.U., Doerr, H.W., and Cinatl, J., Jr. (2000). Cytomegalovirus-infected neuroblastoma cells exhibit augmented invasiveness mediated by beta1alpha5 integrin (VLA-5). Tissue Antigens *55*, 412–421.

Shen, Y., Zhu, H., and Shenk, T. (1997). Human cytomagalovirus IE1 and IE2 proteins are mutagenic and mediate "hit-and-run" oncogenic transformation in cooperation with the adenovirus E1A proteins. Proc Natl Acad Sci USA *94*, 3341–3345.

Shih, A.H., and Holland, E.C. (2006). Platelet-derived growth factor (PDGF) and glial tumorigenesis. Cancer Lett *232*, 139–147.

Singh, S.K., Clarke, I.D., Terasaki, M., Bonn, V.E., Hawkins, C., Squire, J., and Dirks, P.B. (2003). Identification of a cancer stem cell in human brain tumors. Cancer Res *63*, 5821–5828.

Singh, S.K., Hawkins, C., Clarke, I.D., Squire, J.A., Bayani, J., Hide, T., Henkelman, R.M., Cusimano, M.D., and Dirks, P.B. (2004). Identification of human brain tumour initiating cells. Nature *432*, 396–401.

Smith, S., Bentz GL, Alexander S, Yuorochko AD (2004). Human cytomegalovirus induces monocyte differentiation and migration as a strategy for dissemination and persistence. J Virol *78*, 4444–4453.

Soderberg-Naucler, C. (2006). Does cytomegalovirus play a causative role in the development of various inflammatory diseases and cancer? J Intern Med *259*, 219–246.

Soderberg-Naucler, C. (2008). HCMV microinfections in inflammatory diseases and cancer. J Clin Virol *41*, 218–223.

Soroceanu, L., Akhavan, A., and Cobbs, C.S. (2008). Platelet-derived growth factor-alpha receptor activation is required for human cytomegalovirus infection. Nature *455*, 391–395.

Streblow, D.N., Soderberg-Naucler, C., Vieira, J., Smith, P., Wakabayashi, E., Ruchti, F., Mattison, K., Altschuler, Y., and Nelson, J.A. (1999). The human cytomegalovirus chemokine receptor US28 mediates vascular smooth muscle cell migration. Cell *99*, 511–520.

Suzuki, S., Kimura, T., and Ikuta, K. (1998). [Superoxide generation and human cytomegalovirus infection]. Nippon Rinsho *56*, 75–78.

Takano, T., Lin, J.H., Arcuino, G., Gao, Q., Yang, J., and Nedergaard, M. (2001). Glutamate release promotes growth of malignant gliomas. Nat Med *7*, 1010–1015.

Tenan, M., Fulci, G., Albertoni, M., Diserens, A.C., Hamou, M.F., El Atifi-Borel, M., Feige, J.J., Pepper, M.S., and Van Meir, E.G. (2000). Thrombospondin-1 is downregulated by anoxia and suppresses tumorigenicity of human glioblastoma cells. J Exp Med *191*, 1789–1798.

Tsutsui, Y., Kawasaki, H., and Kosugi, I. (2002). Reactivation of latent cytomegalovirus infection in mouse brain cells detected after transfer to brain slice cultures. J Virol *76*, 7247–7254.

Yurochko, A.D., Kowalik, T.F., Huong, S.M., and Huang, E.S. (1995). Human cytomegalovirus upregulates NF-kappa B activity by transactivating the NF-kappa B p105/p50 and p65 promoters. J Virol *69*, 5391–5400.

Zhu, H., Cong, J.P., Yu, D., Bresnahan, W.A., and Shenk, T.E. (2002). From the Cover: Inhibition of cyclooxygenase 2 blocks human cytomegalovirus replication. Proc Natl Acad Sci USA *99*, 3932–3937.

Zhu, H., Shen, Y., and Shenk, T. (1995). Human cytomegalovirus IE1 and IE2 proteins block apoptosis. J Virol *69*, 7960–7970.

Chapter 20
Aberrant EGFR Signaling in Glioma

YeoHyeon Hwang, Khatri Latha, Anupama Gururaj, Marta Rojas, and Oliver Bogler

Abstract Dysregulation of receptor tyrosine kinase (RTK) signaling is a major contributor to cancer, including glioma (Pawson and Hunter 1994). In glioma, epidermal growth factor receptor (EGFR) is frequently amplified at the genomic level and mutated, and this is associated with poorer survival (Libermann et al., 1985; Wong et al., 1987; Ekstrand et al., 1992; Hurtt et al., 1992; Jaros et al., 1992; Schlegel et al., 1994). Here we review what is known about abnormal EGFR signaling in glioma, focusing on recent advances made with proteomics approaches, and discuss two new areas just being investigated: localization of EGFR in new cellular compartments and point mutations in its extracellular domain.

Contents

20.1 ΔEGFR

The most common of the rearrangements of the EGFR gene in glioma leads to the deletion of exons 2–7, causing an in-frame deletion of 801 bp in the extracellular domain (Sugawa et al., 1990; Ekstrand et al., 1992; Wong et al., 1992; Frederick et al., 2000a) (Fig. 20.1). The resulting protein, deleted-(2–7) EGFR

O. Bogler (✉)
Department of Neurosurgery and Neuro-Oncology, Brain Tumor Center, University of Texas M.D. Anderson Cancer Center, Unit BSRB 1004, Room S5.8136, 1515 Holcombe Blvd. Houston TX 77030, USA
e-mail: obogler@mdanderson.org

E.G. Van Meir (ed.), *CNS Cancer*, Cancer Drug Discovery and Development, DOI 10.1007/978-1-60327-553-8_20,
© Humana Press, a part of Springer Science+Business Media, LLC 2009

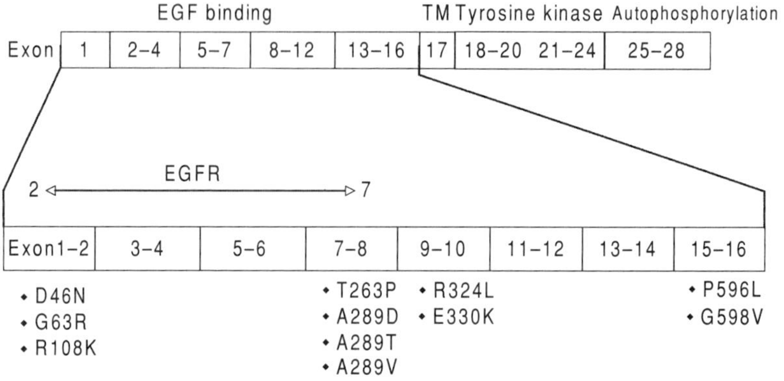

Fig. 20.1 Cartoon of point mutations and EGFR localization. Point mutations in the ectodomain are cartooned in relation to the deletion found in ΔEGFR/EGFRvIII. Mutations are from Lee et al. (2006) and data from The Cancer Genome Atlas

(also known as EGFRvIII, EGFR* and ΔEGFR – referred to as ΔEGFR here), can be detected on the basis of a neo-epitope created by the in-frame fusion of exons 1 and 8 (LEEKKGNYVVTDHC where G is a new amino acid not found in wild-type EGFR). ΔEGFR can also be detected by antibodies that recognize an activation state common to ΔEGFR and EGFR when expressed at high levels (Humphrey et al., 1990; Johns et al., 2002). There is consensus that ΔEGFR is expressed in high-grade gliomas, and higher in glioblastoma/astrocytoma grade IV (Humphrey et al., 1990; Johns et al., 2002). ΔEGFR is only rarely found in pediatric high-grade astrocytomas (Liang et al., 2008).

Detection of ΔEGFR in other cancers has also been reported, but the evidence is not always incontrovertible. In breast cancer the existence of ΔEGFR alongside EGFR is supported by several studies. In a small series of infiltrating ductal breast carcinomas close to 80% were suspected of expressing ΔEGFR by western blot, and in two instances this was supported by RT-PCR data across the deletion junction (Moscatello et al., 1995). A more recent analysis found a similar frequency of around 70% in another small series of invasive breast carcinoma, again using RT-PCR and western blot, this time based on laser capture microdissected material (Ge et al., 2002). The altered subcellular location of ΔEGFR in breast cancer found in these studies suggests that its trafficking may somehow differ from wild type, and that this may lead to sustained tyrosine kinase activity, and a more potent, aggressive and oncogenic effect. Interestingly, ΔEGFR mRNA could also be detected in the blood of breast cancer patients, and the prevalence correlated with the aggressiveness of the disease, suggesting that it could be used as a biomarker (Silva et al., 2006).

Analyses of non-small cell lung cancer by RT-PCR suggest a low incidence of 2–8% for ΔEGFR, which is almost entirely restricted to squamous cell carcinoma; when present, levels of the transcript appear comparable to those found in glioblastoma and increased copy number of the EGFR gene was also observed more commonly in tumors with the ΔEGFR mutation (Ji et al., 2006; Sasaki et al., 2007). Higher rates of ΔEGFR expression have been found in lung cancer by immunohistochemistry only (Okamoto et al., 2003; Sonnweber et al., 2006), but this may reflect non-specific cross-reaction with amplified EGFR or other antigens.

A similar series of observations were made in bladder cancer, where an initially positive result on the basis of staining of tissue arrays suggested that about half of tumors had a signal, but when this was followed up by RT-PCR no positive tumors could be identified (Blehm et al., 2006). The authors conclude that the immunohistochemistry signal may not be reliable. Studies in several other tumor types rely either exclusively on staining of sections, such as reports on ovarian (Moscatello et al., 1995), prostate (Olopade et al., 1992) or colorectal cancer (Cunningham et al., 2005), or use RT-PCR only on a few samples for confirmation, such as in head and neck cancer (Sok et al., 2006). The findings in these studies, at least of a high level of prevalence of the ΔEGFR mutation, have to be treated with skepticism until broad confirmation at the RT-PCR level (Yoshimoto et al., 2008) is reported.

The oncogenic impact of ΔEGFR on cells is significant, as has been established in a variety of models. ΔEGFR can transform NIH3T3 cells like wild-type EGFR (Batra et al., 1995; Moscatello et al., 1996). More significantly, it confers enhanced tumorigenicity on human glioma cells in vivo, lending greater take and growth rates (Nishikawa et al., 1994), and does so by reducing apoptosis and increasing proliferation (Nagane et al., 1996; Narita et al., 2002). When glioma cells expressing ΔEGFR are mixed with parental cells, the enhanced growth rate conferred by the mutant receptor drives clonal selection in implanted tumor models, and glioma cells expressing ΔEGFR rapidly outgrow their parental cells (Nagane et al., 1996). In the RCAS/tv-a mouse model ΔEGFR can co-operate with loss of cell cycle control, either by the co-expression of cdk4 or by use of mice bearing a disrupted INK4A-ARF locus, to cause gliomas (Holland et al., 1998). Similarly, glial or neural stem cells from INK4A knockout mice can be transformed by ΔEGFR and form high-grade gliomas when implanted (Bachoo et al., 2002). Therefore, ΔEGFR is a potent glioma oncogene, and understanding its signal in order to target it therapeutically is an important goal.

ΔEGFR is phosphorylated in a ligand-independent fashion and signals constitutively in the absence of significant internalization and downregulation (Nishikawa et al., 1994; Chu et al., 1997; Huang et al., 1997). ΔEGFR autophosphorylation occurs primarily at tyrosines 1068, 1148 and 1173, with 1173 alone accounting for about half (Huang et al., 1997). This is also the preferred phosphorylation site of wild-type EGFR (Downward et al., 1984), suggesting that the pattern of modification of the active ΔEGFR and wild-type EGFR C-terminus may not be qualitatively very different. However, ΔEGFR shows almost 10-fold lower levels of autophosphorylation than ligand-stimulated EGFR (Huang et al., 1997), implying that persistence rather than intensity of signal may be a major contributor to ΔEGFR tumorigenicity. One consequence of this low level of signaling is that mutation of even a single tyrosine autophosphorylation site in ΔEGFR is sufficient to ablate its promotion of glioma growth (Huang et al., 1997), in contrast to the wild-type receptor where multiple tyrosines need to be eliminated to significantly reduce signaling (Helin et al., 1991).

The lack of interaction with ligand and low level of signaling suggest that ΔEGFR may not dimerize efficiently, and the balance of published evidence supports this interpretation. Therefore, although a band of approximately twice the molecular weight of the ΔEGFR monomer had been observed in ΔEGFR-transfected NIH3T3 fibroblasts, following cross-linking and immunoprecipitation (Moscatello et al., 1996) subsequent analysis failed to confirm this, using the same cell lines and a more specific antibody against ΔEGFR (Chu et al., 1997). In a third study, very low levels of dimerization were detected for ΔEGFR in glioma cells (Huang et al., 1997).

Similarly, the cellular localization of ΔEGFR has been reported variously as predominantly at the surface or approximately evenly split between the outside and inside of the cell. For example, transfection of ΔEGFR into CHO (Ekstrand et al., 1995) or NIH3T3 (Moscatello et al., 1996) cells results in a significant portion localizing intracellularly in the endoplasmic reticulum or the Golgi. In contrast, in glioma cells ΔEGFR localized predominantly and consistently to the cell surface; indeed this is an important prerequisite for efforts to use immunological approaches against ΔEGFR (Huang et al., 1997; Wikstrand et al., 1997; Heimberger et al., 2003). It is likely that the reported variation in distribution of ΔEGFR represents differences in cell type, and perhaps reagents. The consistent observation that antibodies can cause internalization of ΔEGFR (Humphrey et al., 1990; Johns et al., 2002) demonstrates that a significant amount is exposed on the cell surface.

Direct analysis of whether ΔEGFR interacts with the molecular complexes that regulate the internalization of the activated wild-type EGFR suggested that such interactions do not occur. Members of the Cbl E3 ubiquitin ligases are thought to mediate ubiquitination of active receptor tyrosine kinases, and are essential for receptor degradation and cessation of receptor-induced signal transduction (Thien and Langdon, 2001). The Cbls work together with other adaptor proteins, including CIN85/SETA (Cbl-interacting protein of 85 K/SH3 containing expressed in tumorigenic astrocytes) and endophilins to form a complex with activated EGF receptors, thus controlling receptor internalization (Soubeyran et al., 2002). Analysis of ΔEGFR complexes failed to show Cbls, CIN85/SETA, or endophilins, and no ubiquitination of the ΔEGFR could be observed (Schmidt et al., 2003). This lack of interaction appears to be because of the lower level of activity of ΔEGFR (Schmidt et al., 2003) and may be specifically related to hypophosphorylation on Y1045 (Han et al., 2006). Interestingly, ΔEGFR is not immune to other modes of negative regulation, such as that mediated extracellularly by LR1G1 (Stutz et al., 2008).

Whether the differences in the behavior of the ΔEGFR outlined above result in a qualitatively different signal from that of the wild-type receptor has been a long-standing question. As already noted the pattern of tyrosine phosphorylation of ΔEGFR does not differ markedly from EGFR (Huang et al., 1997). Analysis of downstream targets has suggested that certain elements in the EGFR pathway are activated to a greater degree, or in a more sustained fashion by ΔEGFR. Starting proximally to the receptor, ΔEGFR binds to the adaptor proteins Grb2 and Shc constitutively, while overall reducing their levels, and also induces higher levels of Shc phosphorylation (Moscatello et al., 1996; Chu et al., 1997). An approximately two-fold elevation of activated ras is induced by ΔEGFR in glioma cells and microinjection of anti-Ras antibodies inhibits the ΔEGFR signal to the MAPK pathway (Prigent et al., 1996). In turn a two-fold increase in the phosphorylation of p42/p44 MAPK1/3 (also known as Erk2 and Erk1, respectively) is observed (Montgomery et al., 1995), and inhibition of Erk2 suppresses proliferation of glioma cells expressing ΔEGFR (Klingler-Hoffmann et al., 2001). Interestingly, the level of JNK is significantly upregulated by ΔEGFR, and this is mediated by PI3K (Antonyak et al., 2002) and so does not occur via the more commonly encountered ras pathway. Furthermore, the induction of apoptosis that often accompanies the elevation of JNK is not engendered by ΔEGFR, suggesting that the nature of this JNK activation is different from that normally encountered in stress responses, and so is able to promote cellular transformation (Antonyak et al., 2002). The PI3K dependence is in agreement with reports that the activity of PI3K is elevated in cells expressing ΔEGFR, and furthermore that this elevation is necessary for the transformation of fibroblasts (Moscatello et al., 1998) and for the enhanced proliferation of U87MG glioma cells (Klingler-Hoffmann et al., 2003) induced by ΔEGFR. ΔEGFR interacts with PI3K directly, but also via the docking protein Gab1, to induce a sustained elevation in its activity (Holgado-Madruga et al., 1996; Antonyak et al., 1998; Moscatello et al., 1998). ΔEGFR-induced elevated PI3K activity results in sustained activation of Akt, reduction of levels of the cyclin-dependent kinase inhibitor p27 and elevation of CDK2-CyclinA activity in U87MG glioma cells (Narita et al., 2002). It is possible that this occurs via Akt-mediated inhibition of the Forkhead transcription factors that stimulate p27 expression. These reduced levels of p27 may be directly responsible for the elevated CDK2-CyclinA activity, which in turn hyperphosphorylates Rb, promotes cell division, and helps to overcome the G1 cell cycle arrest that normally occurs when serum is withdrawn from cultured cells (Nagane et al., 1996; Narita et al., 2002).

The first open-ended analysis of ΔEGFR signaling, using shotgun phosphoproteomics delineated quantitative differences between downstream signaling in cells expressing different levels of ΔEGFR (Huang et al., 2007). The overall finding was that ΔEGFR signaled predominantly via the PI3Kinase pathway and demonstrated that the c-Met receptor could be activated by and was responsive to ΔEGFR in glioma cells, and this suggested that c-Met inhibitors could be used to circumvent resistance to therapy (Huang et al., 2007).

20.2 Other Glioma-Associated Mutations of the EGFR

In addition to ΔEGFR, other EGFR mutants are found in glioma. Two other deletion mutants that have been described are ΔjmEGFR and C-958EGFR, which have an in-frame deletion extracellularly at the juxtamembrane region and a truncation in the C-terminus, respectively (Frederick et al., 2000b). ΔjmEGFR results in an in-frame deletion of 83 amino acids in domain IV of the extracellular domain of the EGFR, and while it shows intrinsic kinase activity, retains the ability to bind ligand at high affinity and is activated by this (Humphrey et al., 1991). C-958EGFR, in contrast to ΔjmEGFR or ΔEGFR, has an intact ligand-binding domain, but lacks both the internalization domain and the tyrosine residues which interact with the Cbl proteins when they become phosphorylated (Chen et al., 1989; Lipkowitz, 2002), suggesting that a lack of ubiquitin-mediated endosomal attenuation contributes to its tumorigenic signal (Peschard and Park, 2003).

More recently point mutations in the extracellular, ligand-binding domain of EGFR have been identified in glioma (Fig. 20.1). One publication reported missense mutations in around 15% of tumors from a cohort of more than 100 glioblastoma, and these mutants were demonstrated to be constitutively active and to promote tumorigenic behavior in cells (Lee et al., 2006). This study suggests that these missense mutations could be a novel mechanism of oncogenic EGFR signaling in glioblastoma, and interestingly while these mutants were capable of ligand-independent signaling, they could still be further activated by ligand (Lee et al., 2006). Additional mutations in that class are now being identified in gliomas by The Cancer Genome Atlas (TCGA), a pilot project of the National Cancer Institute and the National Human Genome Research Institute that allows the integration of clinical genomic characterization, large-scale genome sequencing data from different cancer types (http://cancergeome.nih.gov). The role of these novel EGFR mutants in this disease remains to be explored more thoroughly.

20.3 Clinical Significance of EGFR Abnormalities: Biomarker and Target

The utility of ΔEGFR expression for identifying or confirming the identity of malignant astrocytomas whose clinical behavior is consistent with that of glioblastoma was demonstrated in a series of astrocytic tumors analyzed by immunohistochemistry, after confirmation of agreement between staining and RT-PCR in a smaller series of glioblastoma (Aldape et al., 2004). Among the glioblastomas, ΔEGFR expression was found in 19 of 46 cases (41.3%) with EGFR amplification, and in only 3 of 59 tumors lacking amplified EGFR (5.1%) but had no prognostic significance. Among the grade III astrocytomas, ΔEGFR expression was observed in 3 of 14 cases with amplified EGFR (21.4%) and in 6 of 49 cases without EGFR amplification (12.2%), but was highly associated with reduced survival (Aldape et al., 2004). A similar study found the ΔEGFR rearrangement in 54% of glioblastomas and 75% of grade III astrocytomas with amplification, as well as in 8% of glioblastomas and 5% of grade III astrocytomas without amplification (Liu et al., 2005). Again no significant association between EGFR amplification or rearrangement, and age or survival was found in the glioblastoma patients, while there was a tendency toward decreased survival with any EGFR abnormality in the 41 patients with grade III astrocytoma (Liu et al.,

2005). Hence neither EGFR amplification nor the presence of the ΔEGFR transcript can predict patient outcome in conventionally treated glioblastoma. However, in grade III astrocytoma, although uncommon, EGFR aberrations appear to be associated with shorter survival. Interestingly, the newly described ectodomain mutants of EGFR may be indicative of sensitivity to erlotinib treatment (Lee et al., 2006).

EGFR abnormalities do not exist in isolation but in the context of other mutations, and the elevated signal they generate at the membrane is dependent on internal signaling molecules for propagation. In this context the function of the PTEN tumor suppressor, which is an enzyme that removes the third phosphate from the key downstream second messenger, phosphatidylinositol-3 (PIP3) and so antagonizes PI3K, is particularly important (see Chapter 15). If PTEN is non-functional, then PIP3 levels can more easily accumulate and stimulate downstream processes such as cell division and survival. This suggests that the PTEN status could well be a key determinant of whether blockade of

Table 20.1 Clinical trials with EGFR inhibitors in glioma

Study focus	Analyses included	Findings	Reference
Response to erlotinib	EGFR expression IHC ΔEGFR IHC phospho Akt IHC EGFR gene amplification FISH PTEN mutation PCR SEQ EGFR mutation PCR SEQ	8/42 patients responded overall Response assoc. w/EGFR ampl. No association with ΔEGFR found 8/18 with low pAkt responded 0/22 with high pAkt responded	Haas-Kogan et al. (2005)
Response to erlotinib and gefitinib	ΔEGFR RT-PCR EGFR gene amplification FISH PTEN mutation PCR SEQ EGFR mutation PCR SEQ	9/49 patients responded overall 13/15 responders ΔEGFR+ 17/44 non-responders ΔEGFR+ 12/15 responders PTEN+ 10/44 non-responders PTEN+ 11/15 responders ΔEGFR/PTEN+ 3/44 non-responders ΔEGFR/PTEN+	Mellinghoff et al. (2005)
Response to erlotinib and gefitinib	EGFR mutation PCR SEQ EGFR gene amplification aCGH pEGFR, pERK, pAkt WB	No correlation between EGFR amplification and response No consistent impact on pEGFR of either agent	Lassman et al. (2005)

IHC: immunohistochemistry; PCR: polymerase chain reaction; SEQ: sequencing; FISH: fluorescence in situ hybridization; aCGH: array-based comparative genome hybridization; WB: western blot; pEGFR: phosphorylated EGFR; pERK: phosphorylated ERK; pAkt: phosphorylated Akt.

the EGFR signal is therapeutically effective, if its inactivation allows sufficient signaling regardless of the upstream status of EGFR. This hypothesis is supported by preclinical data from mouse xenografts showing that the co-expression of ΔEGFR and wild-type PTEN is significantly associated with response to EGFR tyrosine kinase inhibitors, such as erlotinib or gefinitib (Mellinghoff et al., 2005). In a similar study using serially propagated glioblastoma xenografts, which have been shown to maintain corresponding patient morphologic and molecular characteristics including EGFR amplification, sensitivity to erlotinib was also restricted to tumors with EGFR abnormalities and intact PTEN (Sarkaria et al., 2007). Consistent with these laboratory studies are retrospective analyses of GBM patients that investigated EGFR and PTEN status and response to EGFR inhibitors. Patients with co-expression of ΔEGFR and wild-type PTEN had the highest rate of response (Mellinghoff et al., 2005) and in another study lower levels of phospho-Akt pre-treatment were associated with response (Haas-Kogan et al., 2005); for details see Table 20.1. However, analysis of the phosphorylation status of EGFR in post-treatment glioma samples showed that neither erlotinib or gefitinib were able to reduce the activity of their target, suggesting a more complicated biological mechanism at play (Lassman et al., 2005). Therefore, the possibility remains that the "beautiful hypothesis" that an oncogene addiction to EGFR,

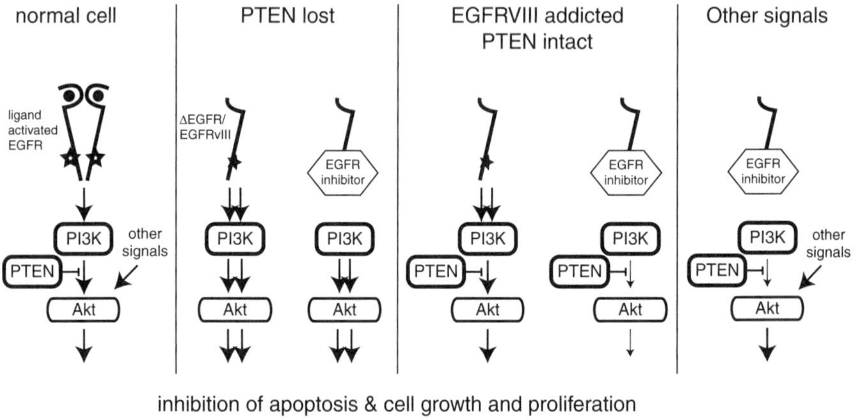

Fig. 20.2 A model of EGFRvIII and PTEN interaction. The interaction of EGFR activation and PTEN loss determine the activity of Akt in glioblastoma cells. In normal cells activation of EGFR leads to a controlled signal due to the negative regulation by PTEN; Akt receives signals from other pathways as well. In glioma cells that have an activated EGFR signal, e.g., downstream of ΔEGFR, and have lost PTEN the Akt signal is elevated, and inhibition of EGFR is ineffective because PI3K remains overactive; whether Akt receives signals from other pathways does not matter. In the third panel, glioma cells are both addicted to abnormal EGFR signaling, as Akt does not receive other signals, and PTEN remains intact. In such cells inhibition of EGFR can effectively reduce the Akt signal. However, as the fourth panel shows, it is possible that other signals exist that can activate Akt when EGFR is shut down; such cells would not be considered to be addicted to abnormal EGFR signals

due to EGFR amplification or mutation, combined with a PI3K pathway that can be switched off at the receptor tyrosine kinase level, due to intact PTEN, is necessary and sufficient for response to EGFR inhibitors "will be slain" by the accumulation of additional observations (Lassman et al., 2006) (see Fig. 20.2 for a possible model). What seems clear is that EGFR inhibitors alone are not going to provide the clinical breakthrough in glioblastoma, and this will hopefully usher in combination therapies targeting other nodes in connected pathways, for example, mTOR (Doherty et al., 2006; Wang et al., 2006a) or PI3K (Ihle et al., 2005).

20.4 EGFR Localization Beyond the Plasma Membrane

EGFR signaling is traditionally viewed as being primarily at the level of the plasma membrane, where the receptor encounters ligand, dimerizes and causes the formation of signaling complex on the inner surface. From there, the receptor is typically internalized and its signal attenuated, by the endosomal pathway, where additional signaling has been recognized to take place (Stasyk et al., 2007). More recently, new aspects of EGFR biology, involving the regulation of nuclear and mitochondrial functions through translocation to these organelles, are being demonstrated (summarized in Fig. 20.3).

Mitochondrial translocation of EGFR was observed in breast cancer cells, following EGF stimulation, and this was dependent on interaction of the

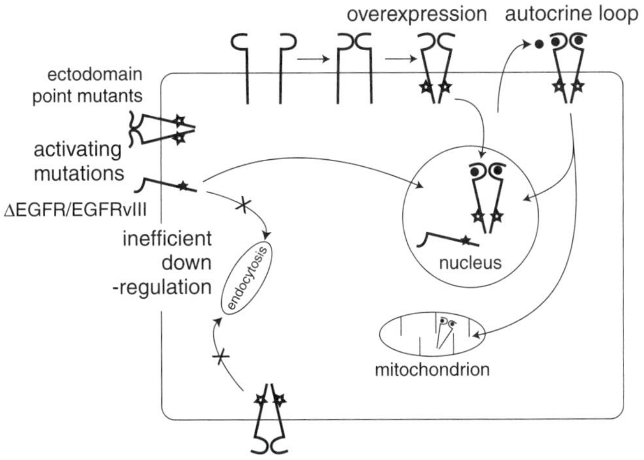

Fig. 20.3 Cartoon of different mechanisms of EGFR aberrant signaling. Abnormal EGFR signals can arise from a variety of mechanisms, illustrated here. These include, clockwise from top, overexpression due to genomic amplification, autocrine stimulation, inefficient downregulation, deletion and point mutations. More recently the importance of signaling by EGFR in the nucleus and mitochondria has been demonstrated, and these may represent new venues for abnormal EGFR signals

receptor with cytochrome c oxidase subunit II (CoxII), and protected the cells from serum deprivation- and adriamycin-induced apoptosis (Boerner et al., 2004). A recent report also demonstrated that EGFR translocates to the mitochondrion during autophagy where it again promoted cell survival (Yue et al., 2008), implying that mitochondrial localization of EGFR could potentially be an important survival strategy for cells.

Nuclear EGFR has been more broadly detected than mitochondrial, particularly in rapidly proliferating tissues such as regenerating liver (Marti et al., 1991), sweat glands (Saga and Jimbow 2001), placenta (Cao et al., 1995), and in tumors of the thyroid (Marti et al., 2001), breast (Lo et al., 2005b), esophagus (Hoshino et al., 2007), head and neck (Psyrri et al., 2008), bladder (Lipponen and Eskelinen, 1994) and adrenal gland (Kamio et al., 1990). These studies suggest that nuclear localization of EGFR is a context-specific physiological event that is amplified in pathological situations such as cancer. Interestingly, in addition to cancers, nuclear EGFR has also been implicated in glaucoma and neuropathy of the optic nerve (Liu and Neufeld, 2003). This allows that a similar role for nuclear EGFR may be found in gliomas.

The presence of nuclear EGFR in tumors has been associated with tumor stage, metastasis, patient survival and response to therapy, including radiation (for a summary, see Table 20.2). In breast carcinoma the presence of EGFR in the nucleus correlated with proliferation markers such as cyclin D1 and Ki-67,

Table 20. 2 Correlations of nuclear EGFR in clinical samples

Cancer type	% Nuclear EGFR	Sample size	Positive correlates	Negative correlates	Reference
Thyroid	100	10	Proliferation	–	Marti et al. (2001)
Breast	38	130	Cyclin D1, Ki-67	Survival	Lo et al. (2005b)
Esophagus	37 (pEGFR)	52	Stage, lymph node metastasis	Survival	Hoshino et al. (2007)
Head and neck	24	37	–	Survival	Lo et al. (2005b)
	58	72	Cytoplasmic EGFR, nuclear ERK2, nuclear PCNA	–	Psyrri et al. (2008)
Bladder	31	234	–	–	Lipponen and Eskelinen (1994)
Adrenal gland	80	94	–	–	Kamio et al. (1990)

The prevalence of nuclear EGFR has been found to correlate with other histological characteristics and survival, in several cancers.

and inversely correlated with survival (Lo et al., 2005b). A study in esophageal squamous cell carcinoma using antibodies specific for phosphorylated EGFR showed that pEGFR not only localized to the nucleus but also correlated with disease stage, lymph node positivity and poor outcome (Hoshino et al., 2007). The presence of nuclear EGFR and its association with increased local recurrence rate and inferior overall survival was shown in oropharyngeal cancer, using an automated quantitative protein analysis with subcellular localization on a tissue microarray (Psyrri et al., 2005). Tumors bearing high nuclear EGFR levels had a significantly decreased likelihood of attaining a complete response to treatment. In a more comprehensive follow-up analysis this group found that nuclear EGFR correlated with non-nuclear EGFR, nuclear ERK2 and very strongly with PCNA (Psyrri et al., 2008) corroborating the previous finding that PCNA is a substrate for EGFR in the nucleus.

Translocation of EGFR to the nucleus occurs in response to ligand stimulation (both EGF and TGF-alpha), and nuclear EGFR is highly tyrosine phosphorylated (Holt et al., 1994; Lin et al., 2001). Although an EGFR mutant which lacked the transmembrane domain could also translocate to the nucleus, this movement required active ligand signaling (Marti and Wells, 2000). Both the intracellular and extracellular domains of EGFR appear to move to the nucleus in a ligand-bound form. While the mechanism of nuclear translocation of the full-length protein is intricate and incompletely understood, recent studies have shed light on some aspects of the process. It has been shown that the juxtamembrane region of EGFR harbors a tripartite nuclear localization sequence that mediates the nuclear translocation (Hsu and Hung, 2007). EGFR has also been demonstrated to interact with importins $\alpha 1/\beta 1$ for which the NLS appears to be indispensable (Lo et al., 2006). The same study also showed that the endosomal machinery and CRM1 exportin were involved in nuclear–cytoplasmic shuttling of EGFR. In human bladder cells, HB-EGF and urothelial cell growth factor stimulated nuclear translocation of EGFR. For this nuclear trafficking, PIKfyve, a phosphoinositide kinase was an essential component (Kim et al., 2007). Stimuli other than ligand can also promote nuclear EGFR, by allowing it to escape receptor internalization and degradation and translocate to the nucleus, including ionizing radiation, heat shock, H_2O_2, and cisplatin (Khan et al., 2006). Radiation-induced nuclear translocation of EGFR seems to require the binding of importins, α and β, which interact with the EGFR nuclear localization signal and mediate its nuclear import (Dittmann et al., 2005; Lo et al., 2006) through the EGFR-dependent activation of the PI3K/AKT signaling pathway (Toulany et al., 2005).

The functions of nuclear EGFR are also beginning to be defined (see Fig. 20.4 for a summary). EGFR lacks a DNA-binding domain; however, nuclear EGFR can physically interact with transcription factors containing DNA-binding domains such as STAT3 and E2F1 (Lo et al., 2005a); it can thereby upregulate the expression of target genes, including cyclin D1, iNOS, and B-myb (Lin et al., 2001). Interestingly, iNOS was also induced by EGFR in reactive astrocytes of human glaucomatous optic nerve (Liu and Neufeld,

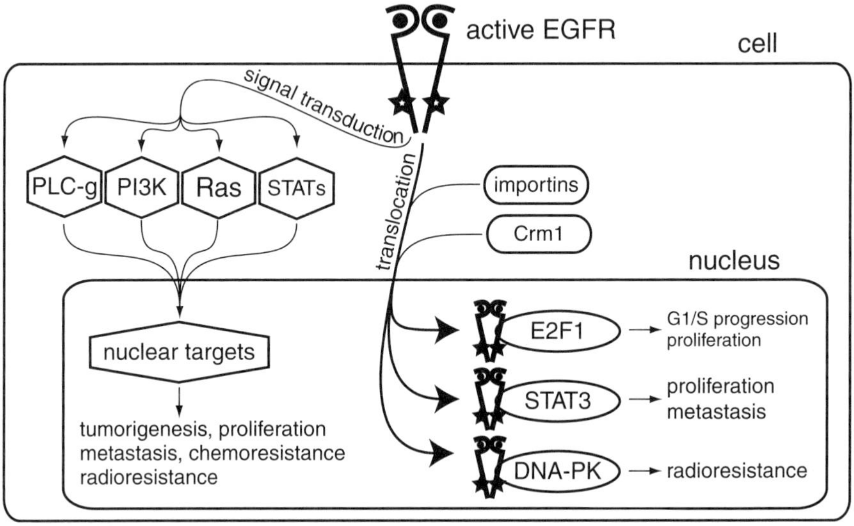

Fig. 20.4 Nuclear functions of EGFR. A summary of EGFR signals reaching the nucleus, divided into indirect signal transduction that occurs via intermediates and more direct effects following translocation of EGFR to the nucleus. After Lo and Hung (2006)

2003). In addition, nuclear EGFR phosphorylates and stabilizes proliferating cell nuclear antigen (PCNA) in its chromatin-bound form and phosphorylates it on Tyr211, and this phosphorylation is required for maintaining PCNA function on chromatin, and was associated with a pronounced increase in cell proliferation and reduced survival of breast cancer patients (Wang et al., 2006b). How EGFR affects gene transcription is not entirely clear yet, but a strong proline-rich nuclear transactivation domain, similar to those found in transcription factors, has been identified in its carboxy terminus, and this is capable of mediating nuclear transactivation functions (Lin et al., 2001). EGFR also influences DNA repair, which was first suggested by the physical interaction between EGFR and the DNA-PKs (Bandyopadhyay et al., 1998). More recent studies show that EGFR is normally present in the perinuclear space of unirradiated cells and that radiation induces the ligand-independent translocation of the EGFR into the nucleoplasm in a process that involves free radicals (Harari and Huang, 2000; Huang and Harari, 2000; Dittmann et al., 2005). Moreover, nuclear EGFR binds to the catalytic subunit DNA-PKs, and the regulatory subunit Ku70 of DNA-PK.

Whether mutants of the EGFR go to the nucleus in the same manner as the wild type is under active investigation. A recent study has identified ΔEGFR as an interacting partner with STAT3 in the nucleus of gliomas (de la Iglesia et al., 2008), and demonstrated a critical role for STAT3 in ΔEGFR-induced tumorigenesis. Further, they also showed a physical interaction between STAT3 and ΔEGFR in primary tumors, suggesting a potentially important role for this interaction in the human disease.

In summary, while it is clear that abnormalities in EGFR status, including expression level and mutations, make an important contribution to malignancy of glioblastoma, the question of whether there are distinguishing characteristics to the signals emanating from abnormal EGFRs remains unanswered. With new mutations and new arenas of signaling in the nucleus and mitochondria being discovered, this question has increased in scope, and hopefully also in translational potential. Whether the interruption of the EGFR signal can be clinically exploited ultimately awaits the results from a new generation of combination therapy trials.

References

Aldape, K. D., Ballman, K., Furth, A., Buckner, J. C., Giannini, C., Burger, P. C., Scheithauer, B. W., Jenkins, R. B. and James, C. D. 2004. Immunohistochemical detection of EGFRvIII in high malignancy grade astrocytomas and evaluation of prognostic significance. J Neuropathol Exp Neurol 63: 700–707.

Antonyak, M. A., Kenyon, L. C., Godwin, A. K., James, D. C., Emlet, D. R., Okamoto, I., Tnani, M., Holgado-Madruga, M., Moscatello, D. K. and Wong, A. J. 2002. Elevated JNK activation contributes to the pathogenesis of human brain tumors. Oncogene 21: 5038–5046.

Antonyak, M. A., Moscatello, D. K. and Wong, A. J. 1998. Constitutive activation of c-Jun N-terminal kinase by a mutant epidermal growth factor receptor. J Biol Chem 273: 2817–2822.

Bachoo, R. M., Maher, E. A., Ligon, K. L., Sharpless, N. E., Chan, S. S., You, M. J., Tang, Y., DeFrances, J., Stover, E., Weissleder, R., Rowitch, D. H., Louis, D. N. and DePinho, R. A. 2002. Epidermal growth factor receptor and Ink4a/Arf: convergent mechanisms governing terminal differentiation and transformation along the neural stem cell to astrocyte axis. Cancer Cell 1: 269–277.

Bandyopadhyay, D., Mandal, M., Adam, L., Mendelsohn, J. and Kumar, R. 1998. Physical interaction between epidermal growth factor receptor and DNA-dependent protein kinase in mammalian cells. J Biol Chem 273: 1568–1573.

Batra, S. K., Castelino-Prabhu, S., Wikstrand, C. J., Zhu, X., Humphrey, P. A., Friedman, H. S. and Bigner, D. D. 1995. Epidermal growth factor ligand-independent, unregulated, cell-transforming potential of a naturally occurring human mutant EGFRvIII gene. Cell Growth Differ 6: 51251–1259.

Blehm, K. N., Spiess, P. E., Bondaruk, J. E., Dujka, M. E., Villares, G. J., Zhao, Y. J., Bogler, O., Aldape, K. D., Grossman, H. B., Adam, L., McConkey, D. J., Czerniak, B. A., Dinney, C. P. and Bar-Eli, M. 2006. Mutations within the kinase domain and truncations of the epidermal growth factor receptor are rare events in bladder cancer: implications for therapy. Clin Cancer Res 12: 4671–4677.

Boerner, J. L., Demory, M. L., Silva, C. and Parsons, S. J. 2004. Phosphorylation of Y845 on the epidermal growth factor receptor mediates binding to the mitochondrial protein cytochrome c oxidase subunit II. Mol Cell Biol 24: 7059–7071.

Cao, H., Lei, Z. M., Bian, L. and Rao, C. V. 1995. Functional nuclear epidermal growth factor receptors in human choriocarcinoma JEG-3 cells and normal human placenta. Endocrinology 136: 3163–3172.

Chen, W. S., Lazar, C. S., Lund, K. A., Welsh, J. B., Chang, C. P., Walton, G. M., Der, C. J., Wiley, H. S., Gill, G. N. and Rosenfeld, M. G. 1989. Functional independence of the epidermal growth factor receptor from a domain required for ligand-induced internalization and calcium regulation. Cell 59: 33–43.

Chu, C. T., Everiss, K. D., Wikstrand, C. J., Batra, S. K., Kung, H. J. and Bigner, D. D. 1997. Receptor dimerization is not a factor in the signalling activity of a transforming variant epidermal growth factor receptor (EGFRvIII). Biochem J 324 (Pt 3): 855–861.

Cunningham, M. P., Essapen, S., Thomas, H., Green, M., Lovell, D. P., Topham, C., Marks, C. and Modjtahedi, H. 2005. Coexpression, prognostic significance and predictive value of EGFR, EGFRvIII and phosphorylated EGFR in colorectal cancer. Int J Oncol 27: 317–325.

de la Iglesia, N., Konopka, G., Puram, S. V., Chan, J. A., Bachoo, R. M., You, M. J., Levy, D. E., Depinho, R. A. and Bonni, A. 2008. Identification of a PTEN-regulated STAT3 brain tumor suppressor pathway. Genes Dev 22: 449–462.

Dittmann, K., Mayer, C., Fehrenbacher, B., Schaller, M., Raju, U., Milas, L., Chen, D. J., Kehlbach, R. and Rodemann, H. P. 2005. Radiation-induced epidermal growth factor receptor nuclear import is linked to activation of DNA-dependent protein kinase. J Biol Chem 280: 31182–31189.

Doherty, L., Gigas, D. C., Kesari, S., Drappatz, J., Kim, R., Zimmerman, J., Ostrowsky, L. and Wen, P. Y. 2006. Pilot study of the combination of EGFR and mTOR inhibitors in recurrent malignant gliomas. Neurology 67: 156–158.

Downward, J., Parker, P. and Waterfield, M. D. 1984. Autophosphorylation sites on the epidermal growth factor receptor. Nature 311: 483–485.

Ekstrand, A. J., Liu, L., He, J., Hamid, M. L., Longo, N., Collins, V. P. and James, C. D. 1995. Altered subcellular location of an activated and tumour-associated epidermal growth factor receptor. Oncogene 10: 1455–1460.

Ekstrand, A. J., Sugawa, N., James, C. D. and Collins, V. P. 1992. Amplified and rearranged epidermal growth factor receptor genes in human glioblastomas reveal deletions of sequences encoding portions of the N- and/or C-terminal tails. Proc Natl Acad Sci USA 89: 4309–4313.

Frederick, L., Eley, G., Wang, X. Y. and James, C. D. 2000a. Analysis of genomic rearrangements associated with EGRFvIII expression suggests involvement of Alu repeat elements. Neuro Oncol 2: 159–163.

Frederick, L., Wang, X. Y., Eley, G. and James, C. D. 2000b. Diversity and frequency of epidermal Growth Factor Receptor Mutations in Human Glioblastomas. Cancer Res 60: 1383.

Ge, H., Gong, X. and Tang, C. K. 2002. Evidence of high incidence of EGFRvIII expression and coexpression with EGFR in human invasive breast cancer by laser capture microdissection and immunohistochemical analysis. Int J Cancer 98: 357–361.

Haas-Kogan, D. A., Prados, M. D., Tihan, T., Eberhard, D. A., Jelluma, N., Arvold, N. D., Baumber, R., Lamborn, K. R., Kapadia, A., Malec, M., Berger, M. S. and Stokoe, D. 2005. Epidermal growth factor receptor, protein kinase B/Akt, and glioma response to erlotinib. J Natl Cancer Inst 97: 880–887.

Han, W., Zhang, T., Yu, H., Foulke, J. and Tang, C. 2006. Hypophosphorylation of residue Y1045 leads to defective downregulation of EGFRvIII. Cancer Biol Ther 5: 1361–1368.

Harari, P. M. and Huang, S. M. 2000. Modulation of molecular targets to enhance radiation. Clin Cancer Res 6: 323–325.

Heimberger, A. B., Crotty, L. E., Archer, G. E., Hess, K. R., Wikstrand, C. J., Friedman, A. H., Friedman, H. S., Bigner, D. D. and Sampson, J. H. 2003. Epidermal growth factor receptor VIII peptide vaccination is efficacious against established intracerebral tumors. Clin Cancer Res 9: 4247–4254.

Helin, K., Velu, T., Martin, P., Vass, W. C., Allevato, G., Lowy, D. R. and Beguinot, L. 1991. The biological activity of the human epidermal growth factor receptor is positively regulated by its C-terminal tyrosines. Oncogene 6: 825–832.

Holgado-Madruga, M., Emlet, D. R., Moscatello, D. K., Godwin, A. K. and Wong, A. J. 1996. A Grb2-associated docking protein in EGF- and insulin-receptor signalling. Nature 379: 560–564.

Holland, E. C., Hively, W. P., DePinho, R. A. and Varmus, H. E. 1998. A constitutively active epidermal growth factor receptor cooperates with disruption of G1 cell-cycle arrest pathways to induce glioma-like lesions in mice. Genes Dev 12: 3675–3685.
Holt, S. J., Alexander, P., Inman, C. B. and Davies, D. E. 1994. Epidermal growth factor induced tyrosine phosphorylation of nuclear proteins associated with translocation of epidermal growth factor receptor into the nucleus. Biochem Pharmacol 47: 117–126.
Hoshino, M., Fukui, H., Ono, Y., Sekikawa, A., Ichikawa, K., Tomita, S., Imai, Y., Imura, J., Hiraishi, H. and Fujimori, T. 2007. Nuclear expression of phosphorylated EGFR is associated with poor prognosis of patients with esophageal squamous cell carcinoma. Pathobiology 74: 15–21.
Hsu, S. C. and Hung, M. C. 2007. Characterization of a novel tripartite nuclear localization sequence in the EGFR family. J Biol Chem 282: 10432–10440.
Huang, H. S., Nagane, M., Klingbeil, C. K., Lin, H., Nishikawa, R., Ji, X. D., Huang, C. M., Gill, G. N., Wiley, H. S. and Cavenee, W. K. 1997. The enhanced tumorigenic activity of a mutant epidermal growth factor receptor common in human cancers is mediated by threshold levels of constitutive tyrosine phosphorylation and unattenuated signaling. J Biol Chem 272: 2927–2935.
Huang, P. H., Mukasa, A., Bonavia, R., Flynn, R. A., Brewer, Z. E., Cavenee, W. K., Furnari, F. B. and White, F. M. 2007. Quantitative analysis of EGFRvIII cellular signaling networks reveals a combinatorial therapeutic strategy for glioblastoma. Proc Natl Acad Sci USA 104: 12867–12872.
Huang, S. M. and Harari, P. M. 2000. Modulation of radiation response after epidermal growth factor receptor blockade in squamous cell carcinomas: inhibition of damage repair, cell cycle kinetics, and tumor angiogenesis. Clin Cancer Res 6: 2166–2174.
Humphrey, P. A., Gangarosa, L. M., Wong, A. J., Archer, G. E., Lund-Johansen, M., Bjerkvig, R., Laerum, O. D., Friedman, H. S. and Bigner, D. D. 1991. Deletion-mutant epidermal growth factor receptor in human gliomas: effects of type II mutation on receptor function. Biochem Biophys Res Commun 178: 1413–1420.
Humphrey, P. A., Wong, A. J., Vogelstein, B., Zalutsky, M. R., Fuller, G. N., Archer, G. E., Friedman, H. S., Kwatra, M. M., Bigner, S. H. and Bigner, D. D. 1990. Anti-synthetic peptide antibody reacting at the fusion junction of deletion-mutant epidermal growth factor receptors in human glioblastoma. Proc Natl Acad Sci USA 87: 4207–4211.
Hurtt, M. R., Moossy, J., Donovan-Peluso, M. and Locker, J. 1992. Amplification of epidermal growth factor receptor gene in gliomas: histopathology and prognosis. J Neuropathol Exp Neurol 51: 84–90.
Ihle, N. T., Paine-Murrieta, G., Berggren, M. I., Baker, A., Tate, W. R., Wipf, P., Abraham, R. T., Kirkpatrick, D. L. and Powis, G. 2005. The phosphatidylinositol-3-kinase inhibitor PX-866 overcomes resistance to the epidermal growth factor receptor inhibitor gefitinib in A-549 human non-small cell lung cancer xenografts. Mol Cancer Ther 4: 1349–1357.
Jaros, E., Perry, R. H., Adam, L., Kelly, P. J., Crawford, P. J., Kalbag, R. M., Mendelow, A. D., Sengupta, R. P. and Pearson, A. D. 1992. Prognostic implications of p53 protein, epidermal growth factor receptor, and Ki-67 labelling in brain tumours. Br J Cancer 66: 373–385.
Ji, H., Zhao, X., Yuza, Y., Shimamura, T., Li, D., Protopopov, A., Jung, B. L., McNamara, K., Xia, H., Glatt, K. A., Thomas, R. K., Sasaki, H., Horner, J. W., Eck, M., Mitchell, A., Sun, Y., Al-Hashem, R., Bronson, R. T., Rabindran, S. K., Discafani, C. M., Maher, E., Shapiro, G. I., Meyerson, M. and Wong, K. K. 2006. Epidermal growth factor receptor variant III mutations in lung tumorigenesis and sensitivity to tyrosine kinase inhibitors. Proc Natl Acad Sci USA 103: 7817–7822.
Johns, T. G., Stockert, E., Ritter, G., Jungbluth, A. A., Huang, H. J., Cavenee, W. K., Smyth, F. E., Hall, C. M., Watson, N., Nice, E. C., Gullick, W. J., Old, L. J., Burgess, A. W. and Scott, A. M. 2002. Novel monoclonal antibody specific for the de2-7 epidermal growth factor receptor (EGFR) that also recognizes the EGFR expressed in cells containing amplification of the EGFR gene. Int J Cancer 98: 398–408.

Kamio, T., Shigematsu, K., Sou, H., Kawai, K. and Tsuchiyama, H. 1990. Immunohistochemical expression of epidermal growth factor receptors in human adrenocortical carcinoma. Hum Pathol 21: 277–282.

Khan, E. M., Heidinger, J. M., Levy, M., Lisanti, M. P., Ravid, T. and Goldkorn, T. 2006. Epidermal growth factor receptor exposed to oxidative stress undergoes Src- and caveolin-1-dependent perinuclear trafficking. J Biol Chem 281: 14486–14493.

Kim, J., Jahng, W. J., Di Vizio, D., Lee, J. S., Jhaveri, R., Rubin, M. A., Shisheva, A. and Freeman, M. R. 2007. The phosphoinositide kinase PIKfyve mediates epidermal growth factor receptor trafficking to the nucleus. Cancer Res 67: 9229–9237.

Klingler-Hoffmann, M., Bukczynska, P. and Tiganis, T. 2003. Inhibition of phosphatidylinositol 3-kinase signaling negates the growth advantage imparted by a mutant epidermal growth factor receptor on human glioblastoma cells. Int J Cancer 105: 331–339.

Klingler-Hoffmann, M., Fodero-Tavoletti, M. T., Mishima, K., Narita, Y., Cavenee, W. K., Furnari, F. B., Huang, H. J. and Tiganis, T. 2001. The protein tyrosine phosphatase TCPTP suppresses the tumorigenicity of glioblastoma cells expressing a mutant epidermal growth factor receptor. J Biol Chem 276: 46313–46318.

Lassman, A. B., Abrey, L. E. and Gilbert, M. R. 2006. Response of glioblastomas to EGFR kinase inhibitors. N Engl J Med 354: 525–526; author reply 525–526.

Lassman, A. B., Rossi, M. R., Raizer, J. J., Razier, J. R., Abrey, L. E., Lieberman, F. S., Grefe, C. N., Lamborn, K., Pao, W., Shih, A. H., Kuhn, J. G., Wilson, R., Nowak, N. J., Cowell, J. K., DeAngelis, L. M., Wen, P., Gilbert, M. R., Chang, S., Yung, W. A., Prados, M. and Holland, E. C. 2005. Molecular study of malignant gliomas treated with epidermal growth factor receptor inhibitors: tissue analysis from North American Brain Tumor Consortium Trials 01-03 and 00-01. Clin Cancer Res 11: 7841–7850.

Lee, J. C., Vivanco, I., Beroukhim, R., Huang, J. H., Feng, W. L., DeBiasi, R. M., Yoshimoto, K., King, J. C., Nghiemphu, P., Yuza, Y., Xu, Q., Greulich, H., Thomas, R. K., Paez, J. G., Peck, T. C., Linhart, D. J., Glatt, K. A., Getz, G., Onofrio, R., Ziaugra, L., Levine, R. L., Gabriel, S., Kawaguchi, T., O'Neill, K., Khan, H., Liau, L. M., Nelson, S. F., Rao, P. N., Mischel, P., Pieper, R. O., Cloughesy, T., Leahy, D. J., Sellers, W. R., Sawyers, C. L., Meyerson, M. and Mellinghoff, I. K. 2006. Epidermal growth factor receptor activation in glioblastoma through novel missense mutations in the extracellular domain. PLoS Med 3: e485.

Liang, M. L., Ma, J., Ho, M., Solomon, L., Bouffet, E., Rutka, J. T. and Hawkins, C. 2008. Tyrosine kinase expression in pediatric high grade astrocytoma. J Neurooncol 87: 247–253.

Libermann, T. A., Nusbaum, H. R., Razon, N., Kris, R., Lax, I., Soreq, H., Whittle, N., Waterfield, M. D., Ullrich, A. and Schlessinger, J. 1985. Amplification, enhanced expression and possible rearrangement of EGF receptor gene in primary human brain tumours of glial origin. Nature 313: 144–147.

Lin, S. Y., Makino, K., Xia, W., Matin, A., Wen, Y., Kwong, K. Y., Bourguignon, L. and Hung, M. C. 2001. Nuclear localization of EGF receptor and its potential new role as a transcription factor. Nat Cell Biol 3: 802–808.

Lipkowitz, S. 2002. The role of the ubiquitination-proteasome pathway in breast cancer: ubiquitin mediated degradation of growth factor receptors in the pathogenesis and treatment of cancer. Breast Cancer Res 5: 8–15.

Lipponen, P. and Eskelinen, M. 1994. Expression of epidermal growth factor receptor in bladder cancer as related to established prognostic factors, oncoprotein (c-erbB-2, p53) expression and long-term prognosis. Br J Cancer 69: 1120–1125.

Liu, B. and Neufeld, A. H. 2003. Activation of epidermal growth factor receptor signals induction of nitric oxide synthase-2 in human optic nerve head astrocytes in glaucomatous optic neuropathy. Neurobiol Dis 13: 109–123.

Liu, L., Backlund, L. M., Nilsson, B. R., Grander, D., Ichimura, K., Goike, H. M. and Collins, V. P. 2005. Clinical significance of EGFR amplification and the aberrant EGFRvIII transcript in conventionally treated astrocytic gliomas. J Mol Med 83: 917–926.

Lo, H. W., Ali-Seyed, M., Wu, Y., Bartholomeusz, G., Hsu, S. C. and Hung, M. C. 2006. Nuclear-cytoplasmic transport of EGFR involves receptor endocytosis, importin beta1 and CRM1. J Cell Biochem 98: 1570–1583.

Lo, H. W., Hsu, S. C., Ali-Seyed, M., Gunduz, M., Xia, W., Wei, Y., Bartholomeusz, G., Shih, J. Y. and Hung, M. C. 2005a. Nuclear interaction of EGFR and STAT3 in the activation of the iNOS/NO pathway. Cancer Cell 7: 575–589.

Lo, H. W. and Hung, M. C. 2006. Nuclear EGFR signalling network in cancers: linking EGFR pathway to cell cycle progression, nitric oxide pathway and patient survival. Br J Cancer 94: 184–188.

Lo, H. W., Xia, W., Wei, Y., Ali-Seyed, M., Huang, S. F. and Hung, M. C. 2005b. Novel prognostic value of nuclear epidermal growth factor receptor in breast cancer. Cancer Res 65: 338–348.

Marti, U., Burwen, S. J., Wells, A., Barker, M. E., Huling, S., Feren, A. M. and Jones, A. L. 1991. Localization of epidermal growth factor receptor in hepatocyte nuclei. Hepatology 13: 15–20.

Marti, U., Ruchti, C., Kampf, J., Thomas, G. A., Williams, E. D., Peter, H. J., Gerber, H. and Burgi, U. 2001. Nuclear localization of epidermal growth factor and epidermal growth factor receptors in human thyroid tissues. Thyroid 11: 137–145.

Marti, U. and Wells, A. 2000. The nuclear accumulation of a variant epidermal growth factor receptor (EGFR) lacking the transmembrane domain requires coexpression of a full-length EGFR. Mol Cell Biol Res Commun 3: 8–14.

Mellinghoff, I. K., Wang, M. Y., Vivanco, I., Haas-Kogan, D. A., Zhu, S., Dia, E. Q., Lu, K. V., Yoshimoto, K., Huang, J. H., Chute, D. J., Riggs, B. L., Horvath, S., Liau, L. M., Cavenee, W. K., Rao, P. N., Beroukhim, R., Peck, T. C., Lee, J. C., Sellers, W. R., Stokoe, D., Prados, M., Cloughesy, T. F., Sawyers, C. L. and Mischel, P. S. 2005. Molecular determinants of the response of glioblastomas to EGFR kinase inhibitors. N Engl J Med 353: 2012–2024.

Montgomery, R. B., Moscatello, D. K., Wong, A. J., Cooper, J. A. and Stahl, W. L. 1995. Differential modulation of mitogen-activated protein (MAP) kinase/extracellular signal-related kinase kinase and MAP kinase activities by a mutant epidermal growth factor receptor. J Biol Chem 270: 30562.

Moscatello, D. K., Holgado-Madruga, M., Emlet, D. R., Montgomery, R. B. and Wong, A. J. 1998. Constitutive activation of phosphatidylinositol 3-kinase by a naturally occurring mutant epidermal growth factor receptor. J Biol Chem 273: 200–206.

Moscatello, D. K., Holgado-Madruga, M., Godwin, A. K., Ramirez, G., Gunn, G., Zoltick, P. W., Biegel, J. A., Hayes, R. L. and Wong, A. J. 1995. Frequent expression of a mutant epidermal growth factor receptor in multiple human tumors. Cancer Res. 55: 5536–5539.

Moscatello, D. K., Montgomery, R. B., Sundareshan, P., McDanel, H., Wong, M. Y. and Wong, A. J. 1996. Transformational and altered signal transduction by a naturally occurring mutant EGF receptor. Oncogene 13: 85–96.

Nagane, M., Coufal, F., Lin, H., Bögler, O., Cavenee, W. K. and Huang, H. J. 1996. A common mutant epidermal growth factor receptor confers enhanced tumorigenicity on human glioblastoma cells by increasing proliferation and reducing apoptosis. Cancer Res 56: 5079–5086.

Narita, Y., Nagane, M., Mishima, K., Huang, H. J., Furnari, F. B. and Cavenee, W. K. 2002. Mutant epidermal growth factor receptor signaling down-regulates p27 through activation of the phosphatidylinositol 3-kinase/Akt pathway in glioblastomas. Cancer Res 62: 6764–6769.

Nishikawa, R., Ji, X. D., Harmon, R. C., Lazar, C. S., Gill, G. N., Cavenee, W. K. and Huang, H. J. 1994. A mutant epidermal growth factor receptor common in human glioma confers enhanced tumorigenicity. Proc Natl Acad Sci USA 91: 7727–7731.

Okamoto, I., Kenyon, L. C., Emlet, D. R., Mori, T., Sasaki, J., Hirosako, S., Ichikawa, Y., Kishi, H., Godwin, A. K., Yoshioka, M., Suga, M., Matsumoto, M. and Wong, A. J. 2003.

Expression of constitutively activated EGFRvIII in non-small cell lung cancer. Cancer Sci 94: 50–56.
Olopade, O. I., Jenkins, R. B., Ransom, D. T., Malik, K., Pomykala, H., Nobori, T., Cowan, J. M., Rowley, J. D. and Diaz, M. O. 1992. Molecular analysis of deletions of the short arm of chromosome 9 in human gliomas. Cancer Res 52: 2523–2529.
Pawson, T. and Hunter, T. 1994. Signal transduction and growth control in normal and cancer cells. Curr Opin Genet Dev 4: 1–4.
Peschard, P. and Park, M. 2003. Escape from Cbl-mediated downregulation. A recurrent theme for oncogenic deregulation of receptor tyrosine kinases. Cancer Cell 3: 519–523.
Prigent, S. A., Nagane, M., Lin, H., Huvar, I., Boss, G. R., Feramisco, J. R., Cavenee, W. K. and Huang, H. S. 1996. Enhanced tumorigenic behavior of glioblastoma cells expressing a truncated epidermal growth factor receptor is mediated through the Ras-Shc-Grb2 pathway. J Biol Chem 271: 25639–25645.
Psyrri, A., Egleston, B., Weinberger, P., Yu, Z., Kowalski, D., Sasaki, C., Haffty, B., Rimm, D. and Burtness, B. 2008. Correlates and determinants of nuclear epidermal growth factor receptor content in an oropharyngeal cancer tissue microarray. Cancer Epidemiol Biomarkers Prev 17: 1486–1492.
Psyrri, A., Yu, Z., Weinberger, P. M., Sasaki, C., Haffty, B., Camp, R., Rimm, D. and Burtness, B. A. 2005. Quantitative determination of nuclear and cytoplasmic epidermal growth factor receptor expression in oropharyngeal squamous cell cancer by using automated quantitative analysis. Clin Cancer Res 11: 5856–5862.
Saga, K. and Jimbow, K. 2001. Immunohistochemical localization of activated EGF receptor in human eccrine and apocrine sweat glands. J Histochem Cytochem 49: 597–602.
Sarkaria, J. N., Yang, L., Grogan, P. T., Kitange, G. J., Carlson, B. L., Schroeder, M. A., Galanis, E., Giannini, C., Wu, W., Dinca, E. B. and James, C. D. 2007. Identification of molecular characteristics correlated with glioblastoma sensitivity to EGFR kinase inhibition through use of an intracranial xenograft test panel. Mol Cancer Ther 6: 1167–1174.
Sasaki, H., Kawano, O., Endo, K., Yukiue, H., Yano, M. and Fujii, Y. 2007. EGFRvIII mutation in lung cancer correlates with increased EGFR copy number. Oncol Rep 17: 319–323.
Schlegel, J., Merdes, A., Stumm, G., Albert, F. K., Forsting, M., Hynes, N. and Kiessling, M. 1994. Amplification of the epidermal-growth-factor-receptor gene correlates with different growth behaviour in human glioblastoma. Int J Cancer 56: 72–77.
Schmidt, M. H. H., Furnari, F. B., Cavenee, W. K. and Bogler, O. 2003. Epidermal growth factor receptor signaling intensity determines intracellular protein interactions, ubiquitination, and internalization. Proc Natl Acad Sci USA 100: 6505.
Silva, H. A., Abraul, E., Raimundo, D., Dias, M. F., Marques, C., Guerra, C., de Oliveira, C. F. and Regateiro, F. J. 2006. Molecular detection of EGFRvIII-positive cells in the peripheral blood of breast cancer patients. Eur J Cancer 42: 2617–2622.
Sok, J. C., Coppelli, F. M., Thomas, S. M., Lango, M. N., Xi, S., Hunt, J. L., Freilino, M. L., Graner, M. W., Wikstrand, C. J., Bigner, D. D., Gooding, W. E., Furnari, F. B. and Grandis, J. R. 2006. Mutant epidermal growth factor receptor (EGFRvIII) contributes to head and neck cancer growth and resistance to EGFR targeting. Clin Cancer Res 12: 5064–5073.
Sonnweber, B., Dlaska, M., Skvortsov, S., Dirnhofer, S., Schmid, T. and Hilbe, W. 2006. High predictive value of epidermal growth factor receptor phosphorylation but not of EGFRvIII mutation in resected stage I non-small cell lung cancer (NSCLC). J Clin Pathol 59: 255–259.
Soubeyran, P., Kowanetz, K., Szymkiewicz, I., Langdon, W. Y. and Dikic, I. 2002. Cbl-CIN85-endophilin complex mediates ligand-induced downregulation of EGF receptors. Nature 416: 183–187.
Stasyk, T., Schiefermeier, N., Skvortsov, S., Zwierzina, H., Peranen, J., Bonn, G. K. and Huber, L. A. 2007. Identification of endosomal epidermal growth factor receptor signaling targets by functional organelle proteomics. Mol Cell Proteomics 6: 908–922.

Stutz, M., Shattuck, D., Laederich, M., Carraway, K. and Sweeney, C. 2008. LRIG1 negatively regulates the oncogenic EGF receptor mutant EGFRvIII. Oncogene 27: 5741–5752.

Sugawa, N., Ekstrand, A. J., James, C. D. and Collins, V. P. 1990. Identical splicing of aberrant epidermal growth factor receptor transcripts from amplified rearranged genes in human glioblastomas. Proc Natl Acad Sci USA 87: 8602–8606.

Thien, C. B. and Langdon, W. Y. 2001. Cbl: many adaptations to regulate protein tyrosine kinases. Nat.Rev.Mol Cell Biol 2: 294–307.

Toulany, M., Dittmann, K., Kruger, M., Baumann, M. and Rodemann, H. P. 2005. Radioresistance of K-Ras mutated human tumor cells is mediated through EGFR-dependent activation of PI3K-AKT pathway. Radiother Oncol 76: 143–150.

Wang, M. Y., Lu, K. V., Zhu, S., Dia, E. Q., Vivanco, I., Shackleford, G. M., Cavenee, W. K., Mellinghoff, I. K., Cloughesy, T. F., Sawyers, C. L. and Mischel, P. S. 2006a. Mammalian target of rapamycin inhibition promotes response to epidermal growth factor receptor kinase inhibitors in PTEN-deficient and PTEN-intact glioblastoma cells. Cancer Res 66: 7864–7869.

Wang, S. C., Nakajima, Y., Yu, Y. L., Xia, W., Chen, C. T., Yang, C. C., McIntush, E. W., Li, L. Y., Hawke, D. H., Kobayashi, R. and Hung, M. C. 2006b. Tyrosine phosphorylation controls PCNA function through protein stability. Nat Cell Biol 8: 1359–1368.

Wikstrand, C. J., McLendon, R. E., Friedman, A. H. and Bigner, D. D. 1997. Cell surface localization and density of the tumor-associated variant of the epidermal growth factor receptor, EGFRvIII. Cancer Res 57: 4130–4140.

Wong, A. J., Bigner, S. H., Bigner, D. D., Kinzler, K. W., Hamilton, S. R. and Vogelstein, B. 1987. Increased expression of the epidermal growth factor receptor gene in malignant gliomas is invariably associated with gene amplification. Proc Natl Acad Sci USA 84: 6899–6903.

Wong, A. J., Ruppert, J. M., Bigner, S. H., Grzeschik, C. H., Humphrey, P. A., Bigner, D. S. and Vogelstein, B. 1992. Structural alterations of the epidermal growth factor receptor gene in human gliomas. Proc Natl Acad Sci USA 89: 2965–2969.

Yoshimoto, K., Dang, J., Zhu, S., Nathanson, D., Huang, T., Dumont, R., Seligson, D. B., Yong, W. H., Xiong, Z., Rao, N., Winther, H., Chakravarti, A., Bigner, D. D., Mellinghoff, I. K., Horvath, S., Cavenee, W. K., Cloughesy, T. F. and Mischel, P. S. 2008. Development of a real-time RT-PCR assay for detecting EGFRvIII in glioblastoma samples. Clin Cancer Res 14: 488–493.

Yue, X., Song, W., Zhang, W., Chen, L., Xi, Z., Xin, Z. and Jiang, X. 2008. Mitochondrially localized EGFR is subjected to autophagic regulation and implicated in cell survival. Autophagy 4: 641–649.

Chapter 21
Mechanisms of Brain Tumor Angiogenesis

Bo Hu and Shi-Yuan Cheng

Abstract The growth of brain tumors is dependent on the development of new vessels, a process called angiogenesis. In the clinic, neovascularization has been used as an independent prognostic marker, and is also a promising therapeutic target for treatments of patients with brain tumors. A large body of evidence demonstrates that brain tumor angiogenesis is an orchestrated process modulated by an array of factors, both pro-angiogenic and anti-angiogenic, in tumors and their microenvironment. Of great interest, vascular endothelial growth factors (VEGF), angiopoietins (Ang), platelet-derived growth factors (PDGF) and their respective receptors as well as hypoxia (low oxygen tensions) and hypoxia-inducible factor-1 (HIF-1) are considered the most critical molecules and agents in modulation of brain tumor angiogenesis. Additional factors such as hepatocyte growth factor (HGF) and its receptor, c-Met, transforming growth factor β (TGF-β), interleukin-8 (IL-8), integrins, and nitric oxide (NO) are also important in brain tumor angiogenesis. This chapter summarizes data from glioma angiogenesis studies, as malignant gliomas count for nearly 40% incidence of brain tumors in humans, and results of these studies should apply to angiogenesis occurring in other types of brain tumors. A better understanding of the complex process of brain tumor angiogenesis will lead to further advances in development of new and more effective drugs and treatment for patients with malignant brain tumors.

Keywords Brain tumor · Glioma · Angiogenesis · VEGF · PDGF · Angiopoietin · Integrins · Hypoxia · HIF-1 · NO · p53

S.-Y. Cheng (✉)
Cancer Institute and Department of Pathology, University of Pittsburgh, Pittsburgh, PA 15213, USA
e-mail: chengs@upmc.edu

E.G. Van Meir (ed.), *CNS Cancer*, Cancer Drug Discovery and Development, DOI 10.1007/978-1-60327-553-8_21,
© Humana Press, a part of Springer Science+Business Media, LLC 2009

Contents

21.1 Angiogenesis in Brain Tumors

Angiogenesis generally refers to a process of the growth of vessel sprouts from capillary blood vessels, including endothelial cell (EC) migration toward the stimuli in microenvironment, EC proliferation, tube formation, and intussusceptions followed by recruitment of peri-EC and synthesis of extracellular matrix (ECM) (Carmeliet and Jain, 2000). It has been established that the growth and progression of human solid tumors including brain tumors is dependent on pathological growth of new blood vessels (neovascularization) (Carmeliet and Jain, 2000; Jain et al., 2007). This chapter will primarily focus on findings in glioma angiogenesis that may be generally applied to neovascularization in other types of tumors in the central nervous system (CNS), as gliomas account for approximately 40% of cancerous malignancies in the CNS (Kleihues and Cavenee, 2000), and most of the available data of the mechanisms of brain tumor angiogenesis are derived from studies using glioma as a model system.

21.1.1 Neovascularization as an Independent Prognostic Marker for Brain Tumors

Glioma angiogenesis is characterized by endothelial hyperplasia, microvascular proliferation, high blood vessel density, and glomeruloid formation (Fig. 21.1, thin arrow). In low-grade gliomas (WHO grade II), although glioma cells are actively proliferating, expression of angiogenic factors such as vascular endothelial growth factor (VEGF) and hepatocyte growth factor (HGF) is not upregulated and density of neo-vessels is low. When low-grade gliomas progress to WHO grade III tumors, significant upregulation of angiogenic factors such as VEGF is observed, resulting in marked increases in blood vessel growth in these tumors (Fig. 21.1). In WHO grade IV gliomas (glioblastoma

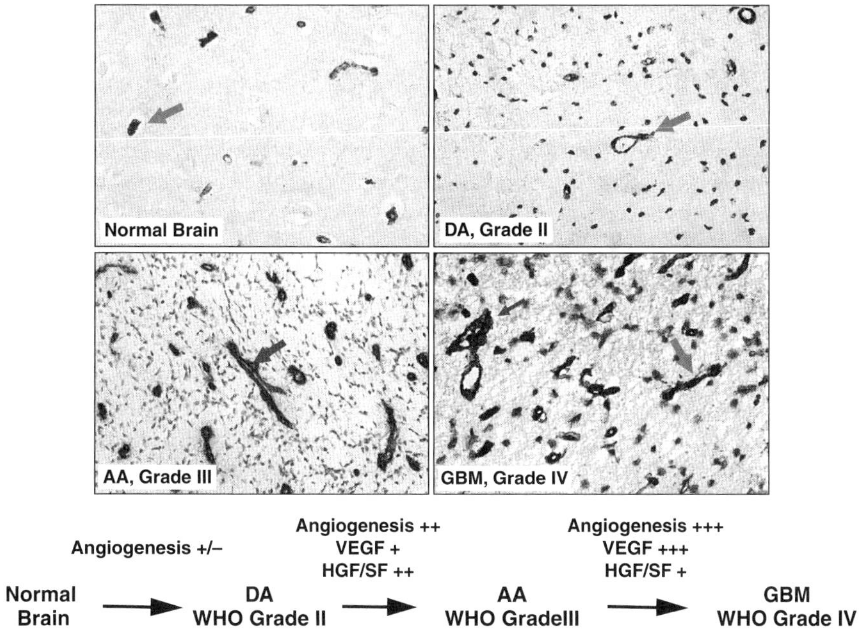

Fig. 21.1 Tumor angiogenesis and expression of angiogenic factors (VEGF and HGF) are upregulated in high-grade gliomas. Photographs show immuohistochemical analyses (IHC) of clinical glioma specimens and a normal brain. Paraffin-embedded tissue sections in 5-μm thickness were stained using an anti-von Williebrand factor antibody. A total of 92 primary glioma specimens including WHO grade II–IV tumors and 4 normal brain tissues that had no pathological alterations were analyzed. Thick arrows indicate stained tumor vessels. A thin arrow indicates stained glomeruloid. DA, a diffuse astrocytoma; AA, an anaplastic astrocytoma; GBM, glioblastoma multiforme. Angiogenesis, using microvessel density (MVD) as an indicator, was evaluated as previously reported (Cheng et al., 1997). Symbols +/–, basal level of angiogenesis (MVD); +, 1.5- to 2-fold increase in protein expression; ++, 2- to 3-fold increase in MVD or protein expression; +++, 3- to 5-fold increase in protein expression or MVD. Original magnification: 400×. IHC analyses were performed two independent times on the same set of clinical specimens and similar results were obtained

multiforme, GBM), high expression of VEGF is detected with a further increase in neovascularization compared to WHO grade III gliomas. Based on the studies of glioma angiogenesis using different cohorts of primary human glioma specimens (Abdulrauf et al., 1998; Burger et al., 1985; Daumas-Duport et al., 1997; Jain et al., 2007; Nishikawa et al., 1998; Straume et al., 2002), the WHO classification distinguishes low-grade diffuse astrocytomas (WHO grade II tumors) from high-grade gliomas (WHO grade III tumors and grade IV GBM) by the presence of hyperproliferation of EC and peri-EC as a diagnostic criterion and an independent prognostic marker (Kleihues and Cavenee, 2000). It is established that increased neovascularization in gliomas directly associates with aggressive pathological phenotype, degrees of malignancy, and frequency of tumor reoccurrence and directly correlates with high morbidity of patients with gliomas (Fischer et al., 2005).

21.1.2 How Angiogenesis Occurs in Brain Tumors

The process of angiogenesis is orchestrated by an array of angiogenic stimulators and inhibitors (Carmeliet and Jain, 2000). Within the tumor microenvironment, tumor cells and tumor-associated stromal cells such as macrophages and other immune cells produce angiogenic factors such as VEGF, HGF, and fibroblast growth factor (FGF) as well as endogenous inhibitors such as angiostatin and thrombospondin-1. A balance between expressions of angiogenic factors and inhibitors determines whether angiogenesis proceeds or halts during progression of malignant gliomas. Currently, there are two accepted hypotheses supported with experimental evidence that describe how angiogenesis occurs during glioma progression (Bergers and Benjamin, 2003; Bergers and Hanahan, 2008). One is a classical view of neovascularization. During active glioma growth, tumor cells activate cellular programs resulting in increased expression of angiogenic factors such as VEGF. One mechanism by which this occurs results from the hypoxic regions generated in the center of gliomas or the far distance of single infiltrating glioma cells from blood vessels. A second theory describes a co-option between tumor cells and host blood vessels. According to this model, glioma cells actively proliferate around existing viable blood vessels or single invading glioma cells migrate along the white matter tracks and the vasculature in the brain. The host vascular EC becomes apoptotic, resulting in degradation of host blood vessels. Disappearance of viable capillaries causes necrosis and hypoxia within the tumors and near single infiltrating glioma cells. Hypoxia induces angiogenic factors through the activation of hypoxia-induced factor-1 (HIF-1) (Semenza, 2004). Upregulated angiogenic factors in glioma cells stimulate EC migration and proliferation in nearby capillaries, leading to an increase in vessel sprouting toward the hypoxic region of gliomas or hypoxic individual invading glioma cells. Additionally, in both models, de novo growth of tumor vessels (vasculogenesis) and active recruitment of circulating endothelial progenitor cells (EPS) originating from the bone marrow, stromal cells including glial cells, astrocytes, and various immune cells also occur in the fast-growing gliomas, thus contributing to the exuberant angiogenesis in gliomas (please see Chapter 31 for more detailed information). In general, both modes of tumor angiogenesis can occur in the same glioma, either in different regions of the tumor or during different stages of tumor progression (Bergers and Benjamin, 2003; Bergers and Hanahan, 2008; Carmeliet and Jain, 2000).

21.1.3 Morphology of Neo-Vessels and Blood–Brain Barrier (BBB) in Gliomas

Neovasculatures in gliomas are abnormal in their structure and functions. Studies in patients with gliomas, clinical glioma specimens, and preclinical glioma xenografts in animals have revealed that rapid grown neovasculatures in gliomas lack typical morphologies in normal brain vessels. Neo-vessels are tortuous, disorganized, highly permeable, and characterized by abnormalities and holes in their endothelial wall covered with few pericytes and astrocytes. These abnormal vessels have larger diameters and thicker basement membranes than those in the normal brain vasculature. A common feature of aberrant neovasculature in gliomas is the formation of glomeruloids in the tumor mass, consisting of multilayered, mitotically active EC and peri-EC (Fig. 21.1, indicated by a thin arrow) (Kleihues and Cavenee, 2000).

In contrast, normal blood vessels in the brain are well organized with distinct functions. EC and peri-EC, including pericytes and astrocytes, form and maintain the blood–brain barrier (BBB) that restricts the exchange of molecules between the intracerebral and extracerebral circulatory systems and also functions as a major barrier for drug delivery (Neuwelt, 2004). During glioma growth, when tumors expand beyond 2.0 mm^3 in volume, the BBB is destroyed, losing control of the traffic of molecules between the intracerebral and extracerebral blood vessel systems. Loss of BBB and aberrant morphologies in glioma blood vessels results in a significant increase in permeability in tumor vasculature. Abnormal blood flow and uneven distribution of oxygen caused by the leakiness in these vessels leads to lower red blood cell velocity than that in normal brain vessels. Additionally, upregulation of VEGF in glioma tissues further increases the permeability of these vessels (Batchelor et al., 2007; Fukumura et al., 2001; Wolf et al., 2005; Yuan et al., 1994), leading to increases in interstitial fluid pressure and edema within the brain parenchyma which are major causes of patient symptoms.

21.2 Regulation in Brain Tumor Angiogenesis

Figure 21.2 depicts functions of several most of the important growth factors and their receptors that modulate glioma angiogenesis. These factors are vascular endothelial growth factor (VEGF), angiopoietins (Ang), platelet-derived

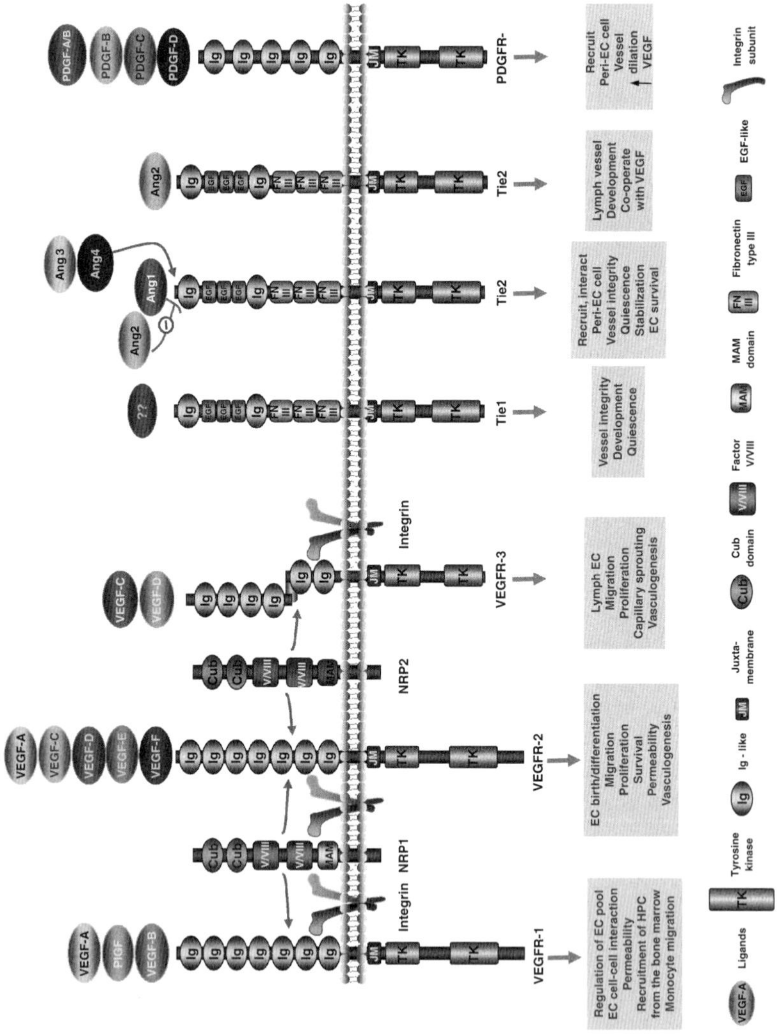

Fig. 21.2 (continued)

growth factors (PDGF), hepatocyte growth factor (HGF), transforming growth factor beta (TGF-β), and interleukin-8 (IL-8). Among them, VEGF, Ang, and PDGF are considered to be the most critical factors in glioma angiogenesis. Additionally, hypoxic conditions (hypoxia) and nitric oxide (NO) are also crucial in glioma angiogenesis.

21.2.1 *VEGF-A and Its Isoforms*

The VEGF (referred to as VEGF-A thereafter) gene was cloned in 1989 from a pituitary tumor cell line and two other tumor cell lines (Connolly et al., 1989; Keck et al., 1989; Leung et al., 1989; Senger et al., 1990). In vivo and in vitro, VEGF-A functions as a stimulus and pro-survival factor for EC. Remarkably, deletion of a single VEGF allele in mice resulted in embryonic lethality between days 11 and 12. VEGF-A$^{+/-}$ embryos die from widespread defects in their developmental abnormalities in organ formation and in the vasculature (Carmeliet et al., 1996; Ferrara et al., 1996). Modulation of VEGF-A by various genetic approaches in early postnatal mice resulted in increased mortality, impaired development and growth of multiple organs in these animals (Carmeliet and Storkebaum, 2002; Compernolle et al., 2002; Dor et al., 2001, 2002; Eremina et al., 2003; Gerber et al., 1999a; Haigh et al., 2000; Kitamoto et al., 1997; Ryan et al., 1999; Stalmans et al., 2003). These studies support a notion that there is a threshold level of VEGF-A expression critical for angiogenesis during development. In gliomas, VEGF-A mRNA and proteins were highly expressed in clinical glioma specimens (Fischer et al., 2005; Jain et al., 2007; Plate et al., 1992). Inhibition of VEGF-A expression by an antisense DNA construct in a highly tumorigenic human glioma cell line led to significant suppression of tumor growth and angiogenesis in the brain of mice (Cheng et al., 1996).

Fig. 21.2 (continued) **Roles of angiogenic growth factors and their receptors in angiogenesis.** Ligands are shown at the top of their cognate receptors. The receptors are transmembrane tyrosine kinases. Integrins and neuropilins (NRP-1 and NRP-2) function as co-receptors by interacting with VEGFRs enhancing their functions. Angiogenic factors, various isoforms of vascular endothelial growth factor (VEGF), placenta growth factor (PlGF), angiopoietins (Ang), and platelet-derived growth factor (PDGF) bind to their receptors, leading to receptor dimerization and activation of receptor tyrosine kinase phosphorylation. This leads to activation of various downstream signal cascades, resulting in various biological effects on endothelial cells and lymphatic endothelial cells and their precursors in vitro and in vivo. Biological functions of angiogenesis receptor signaling during development and in cellular functions are described below each receptor. Functional or structural domains are indicated as symbols at the bottom of the figure

Human VEGF-A has four major protein isoforms generated by alternative splicing having 121, 165, 189, and 206 amino acids ($VEGF_{121}$, $VEGF_{165}$, $VEGF_{189}$, and $VEGF_{206}$), respectively. Less frequent splicing variants have also been reported such as $VEGF_{145}$ and $VEGF_{183}$. Due to the lack of its heparin-binding domains, $VEGF_{121}$ is a freely diffused protein, while $VEGF_{189}$ and $VEGF_{206}$ are almost completely associated with ECM in cells. $VEGF_{165}$ has an intermediate capacity of heparin binding and can be secreted out and associated with glioma cells (Cheng et al., 1997; Ferrara et al., 2003). In the brain of mice, expression of $VEGF_{121}$ and $VEGF_{165}$ in U87MG intracranial gliomas induced formation of dilated and leaky blood vessels, leading to tumor-associated intracerebral hemorrhages, whereas expression of $VEGF_{189}$ promoted glioma angiogenesis similar to that by $VEGF_{121}$ and $VEGF_{165}$ without causing vessel disruption (Cheng et al., 1997). At subcutaneous sites of mice with inoculation of the same set of U87MG glioma cell lines that separately overexpressed VEGF-A isoforms, expression of $VEGF_{165}$ and $VEGF_{189}$ significantly promoted tumor growth while $VEGF_{121}$ had minimal impact on tumor formation in mice (Guo et al., 2001). However, overexpression of $VEGF_{121}$ and $VEGF_{165}$ in U251MG, but not NG-1 glioma cells, promoted tumor angiogenesis and growth in the brain and $VEGF_{165}$ appears to be more potent than $VEGF_{121}$ in stimulating tumor angiogenesis (Ke et al., 2002). These results suggest that different isoforms of VEGF-A have different functions in angiogenesis in different biological contexts.

This hypothesis was soon corroborated by studies in transgenic mice demonstrating that $VEGF_{188}$ (VEGF-A variants in mice are one amino acid less than in humans) decreases luminal diameter, whereas $VEGF_{120}$ and $VEGF_{164}$ increase lumen formation as well as vessel length (Carmeliet and Collen, 1999; Carmeliet and Storkebaum, 2002; Dor et al., 2002; Mattot et al., 2002; Stalmans et al., 2002). Mice that expressed exclusively $VEGF_{120}$ displayed deficiencies in the distribution of EC and impaired filopodia extension, leading to impaired myocardial angiogenesis and ischemic cardiomyopathy (Carmeliet and Collen, 1999; Carmeliet et al., 1999). Mice with $VEGF_{188}$ expression only had impaired arterial development (Stalmans et al., 2002), whereas mice with $VEGF_{164}$ expression showed no abnormality or deficiency in development and angiogenesis (Carmeliet and Collen, 1999; Stalmans et al., 2002). Nonetheless, the molecular mechanisms by which different VEGF-A isoforms exert distinct functions remain to be elucidated.

21.2.2 Other VEGF Family Members

The VEGF superfamily comprises seven members encoded by separate genes: VEGF-A, -B, -C, -D, -E, -F, and placenta growth factor (PlGF). VEGFs and PlGF separately bind to VEGFR-1, -2, and -3 with different affinities

(Fig. 21.2). VEGF-B has two splicing variants, VEGF-B_{167} and VEGF-B_{186}, that differ in the sequence and length of the *C*-terminal portion of the molecule (Grimmond et al., 1996). VEGF-B binds to VEGFR-1 but not to VEGFR-2 or -3, causing weak signaling in promoting EC proliferation (Nash et al., 2006). Mice deficient in VEGF-B had smaller hearts and impaired recovery after experimentally induced myocardial infarctions, suggesting a role of VEGF-B in arteriogenesis during heart development (Bellomo et al., 2000).

VEGF-C is produced as a precursor protein and processed by proteolysis into mature forms (Joukov et al., 1997; Siegfried et al., 2003). VEGF-C and VEGFR-3 are co-expressed in developing lymph vessels during development (Karkkainen et al., 2004; Kukk et al., 1996). VEGF-C binds to VEGFR-2 and -3 with high affinities, inducing mitogenesis, migration, and survival of lymph EC and EC (Saharinen et al., 2004). VEGF-C activation of VEGFR-3 induces selective lymphangiogenesis in animals. Transgenic mice overexpressing VEGF-C had increases in lymph vessels (Alitalo and Carmeliet, 2002; Enholm et al., 2001; Jeltsch et al., 1997). VEGF-C null mice failed to develop lymphatic vessels and died due to edema (Karkkainen et al., 2004). VEGF-C also stimulates the migration of macrophages, and its receptor, VEGFR-3, is found in a fraction of peripheral blood monocytes and macrophages in activated tissues (Schoppmann et al., 2002; Skobe et al., 2001).

VEGF-D is processed by proteolyses at its *N*-terminal and *C*-terminal. VEGF-D stimulates growth of vascular EC and lymphatic EC through VEGFR-2- and -3-mediated signal pathways (Fig. 21.2) (Akahane et al., 2006; Saharinen et al., 2004). Overexpression of VEGF-D in tumor cells promoted lymphangiogenesis and lymphatic metastasis in mice (Stacker et al., 2001). VEGF-E is encoded by the Orf virus genome and specifically activates VEGFR-2, promoting angiogenesis (Lyttle et al., 1994; Meyer et al., 1999; Ogawa et al., 1998). VEGF-E has three isoforms: VEGF-E_{NZ-7}, VEGF-E_{NZ-2}, and VEGF-E_{D1701} (Meyer et al., 1999; Wise et al., 1999). VEGF-F was identified from viper venom with two related proteins, vammin (110 amino acid residues) and VR-1 (109 residues). It has 50% homology with VEGF-A_{165} and activates VEGFR-2-mediated signaling (Suto et al., 2005).

PlGF was originally identified in the placenta and has four isoforms, PlGF-1, -2, -3, and -4, which are different in size and affinities for receptor bindings (Nagy et al., 2003). PlGF binds to VEGFR-1 and NRP-1, but not to VEGFR-2 and -3, inducing VEGFR-1-mediated gene expression (Fig. 21.2) (Autiero et al., 2003; Nagy et al., 2003; Park et al., 1994). Mice deficient in PlGF had impaired angiogenesis, collateral growth during ischemia, wound healing, inflammation, and cancer (Carmeliet et al., 2001). PlGF gene transduction in the skin of mice induced dermal vessel growth with enlarged sizes and increased vascular permeability (Odorisio et al., 2002; Oura et al., 2003). PlGF null mice were deficient in the inflammatory response, and had reduced angiogenesis and developed edema (Oura et al., 2003).

Studies of the roles of these VEGF family members in brain tumor angiogenesis so far are descriptive, mainly reporting levels of their mRNA or proteins in primary brain tumor specimens (Donnini et al., 1999; Gollmer et al., 2000; Grau et al., 2007; Jenny et al., 2006; Moffat et al., 2006; Takeuchi et al., 2007). The precise roles of these VEGF family members in modulation of brain tumor angiogenesis are still to be elucidated.

21.2.3 VEGF Receptors (VEGFR)

As shown in Fig. 21.2, there are two tyrosine kinase receptors for VEGF-A: VEGFR-1 (fms like tyrosine-1, Flt-1); VEGFR-2 (fetal liver kinase-1/kinase insert domain-containing receptor, flk-1/KDR); and two VEGF co-receptors, neuropilin (NRP)-1 and -2 that are non-tyrosine kinase receptors. VEGFR-1 and -2 are expressed primarily in vascular EC, whereas NRP-1 and -2 are found in various types of cells including endothelial, glial, neuronal, and brain tumor cells (Klagsbrun et al., 2002; Soker, 2001). VEGFR-2 appears to be the principal signal receptor that mediates the pro-angiogenic activity of VEGF in differentiated EC and endothelial precursor cells (Ferrara et al., 2003; Olsson et al., 2006). Mice deficient in VEGFR-2 die in utero between embryonic days 8.5 and 9.5, due to the lack of vasculogenesis and failure to develop blood islands and organized blood vessels (Shalaby et al., 1995).

VEGFR-1 was the first-identified VEGFR and has higher affinity with VEGF-A compared to that with VEGFR-2 (Barleon et al., 1997; de Vries et al., 1992). Mice deficient in VEGFR-1 die in utero between days 8.5 and 9.5 not due to the lack of differentiation of EC but to excess proliferation of angioblasts, resulting in failure to organize vascular channels (Fong et al., 1995, 1999). Transgenic mice that expressed a mutant VEGFR-1 lacking its signaling module, the intracellular tyrosine kinase domain developed normally, suggesting that VEGFR-1 is a negative regulator of VEGF-A action (Hiratsuka et al., 1998). It is generally agreed that VEGFR-1 may function as a "decoy" receptor that sequestrates VEGF-A and prevents its binding to VEGFR-2, thus negatively regulating angiogenesis (Ferrara et al., 2003; Gille et al., 2000). Moreover, since PlGF specifically binds to VEGFR-1 (Fig. 21.2) and $PlGF^{-/-}$ mice displayed impaired tumorigenicity and vascular leakage, VEGFR-1 could modulate a synergism between VEGF-A and PlGF in vivo, especially during tumorigenesis (Carmeliet et al., 2001).

NRP-1 was identified as a VEGF-A co-receptor in breast cancer cells (Soker et al., 1998). Moreover, NRP-1 was initially studied as a repelling receptor to semaphorins during neuronal development (Kolodkin et al., 1997; Takahashi et al., 1999). Mice deficient in NRP-1 or overexpressing NRP-1 not only had abnormalities in the nervous system but also in their vasculature accompanied with hemorrhages in several organs (Kitsukawa et al., 1995; Takahashi et al., 1999). Neuropilin-1 is required for development of the yolk sac in embryonic vessel formation and endothelial tip cell guidance in the developing central nervous system (Gerhardt et al., 2004; Kawasaki et al., 1999; Takashima et al., 2002; Yamada et al., 2001). Interaction of NRP-1 with $VEGF_{165}$ and $VEGF_{189}$, but not $VEGF_{121}$, did not stimulate EC proliferation and migration but potentiated angiogenic activities when co-expressed with VEGFR-2 in EC (Soker et al., 1998). Since NRP-1 does not possess a signal domain in its cytoplasmic segment, it has been proposed that NRP-1 presents $VEGF_{165}$ to VEGFR-2 to enhance the binding of $VEGF_{165}$ to VEGFR-2 and VEGFR-2-mediated signaling in EC (Klagsbrun et al., 2002; Soker, 2001). NRP-2 is expressed in venous and lymphatic vessel, and mice deficient in NRP-2 had abnormal lymphatic vessels (Herzog et al., 2001; Yuan et al., 2002). NRP-2 binds to $VEGF_{145}$ and $VEGF_{164}$ and interacts with VEGFR-2 and -3, promoting EC survival and migration (Favier et al., 2006; Gluzman-Poltorak et al., 2000; Shraga-Heled et al., 2007).

Multiple lines of evidence indicate the critical roles of VEGFRs in glioma angiogenesis. Early work in human glioma tissue demonstrated that VEGFR-1 and -2 were expressed at high levels in neovasculature in primary glioma specimens (Plate et al., 1994, 1992). Gene transfer of a truncated (soluble) flk-1 lacking its signaling domain into intracranial gliomas inhibited glioma growth and angiogenesis in the brain of mice (Millauer et al., 1994). Soluble VEGFR-1 comprising the first 1–3 or 1–5 extracellular EGF-like segments was also capable of sequestrating VEGF-A from angiogenesis, inhibiting angiogenesis in animal models (Barleon et al., 1997; Gerber et al., 1999b). VEGFR-1 is expressed in macrophages that infiltrate into malignant gliomas. Recruitment of macrophages into rapidly growing tumors is mediated in part by VEGF–VEGFR-1 paracrine signaling between glioma cells and macrophages (Barleon et al., 1996; Murdoch et al., 2008). High levels of expression of NRP-1 were also found in clinical glioma specimens (Ding et al., 2000). Overexpression of NRP-1 in glioma cells led to a significant increase in tumor vasculatures in gliomas in the brain (Hu et al., 2007). Additionally, therapeutic blockage of NRP-2 inhibited VEGF-C-induced lymphatic EC migration, tumor growth, and metastasis in animals (Caunt et al., 2008; Gray et al., 2008).

21.2.4 VEGFR-Mediated Signaling

VEGFR-2 is the principal receptor that mediates signal transduction stimulated by VEGF-A and other family members (Ferrara et al., 2003; Olsson et al., 2006). The VEGF–VEGFR-2-signal cascades in angiogenesis depicted in Fig. 21.3 are well documented by a large number of investigations and have recently been summarized in two excellent reviews (Ferrara et al., 2003; Olsson et al., 2006). Briefly, upon the binding of VEGF to VEGFR-2, VEGFR-2 dimerizes and becomes phosphorylated at tyrosine residues in its cytoplasmic domain. Src homology 2 (SH2) domain-containing proteins such as PLC-γ, Shb, Shc, Grb2, SHP-1, and -2 bind to phosphorylated tyrosine residues, activating downstream pathways. VEGF-stimulated EC proliferation and survival involve activation of

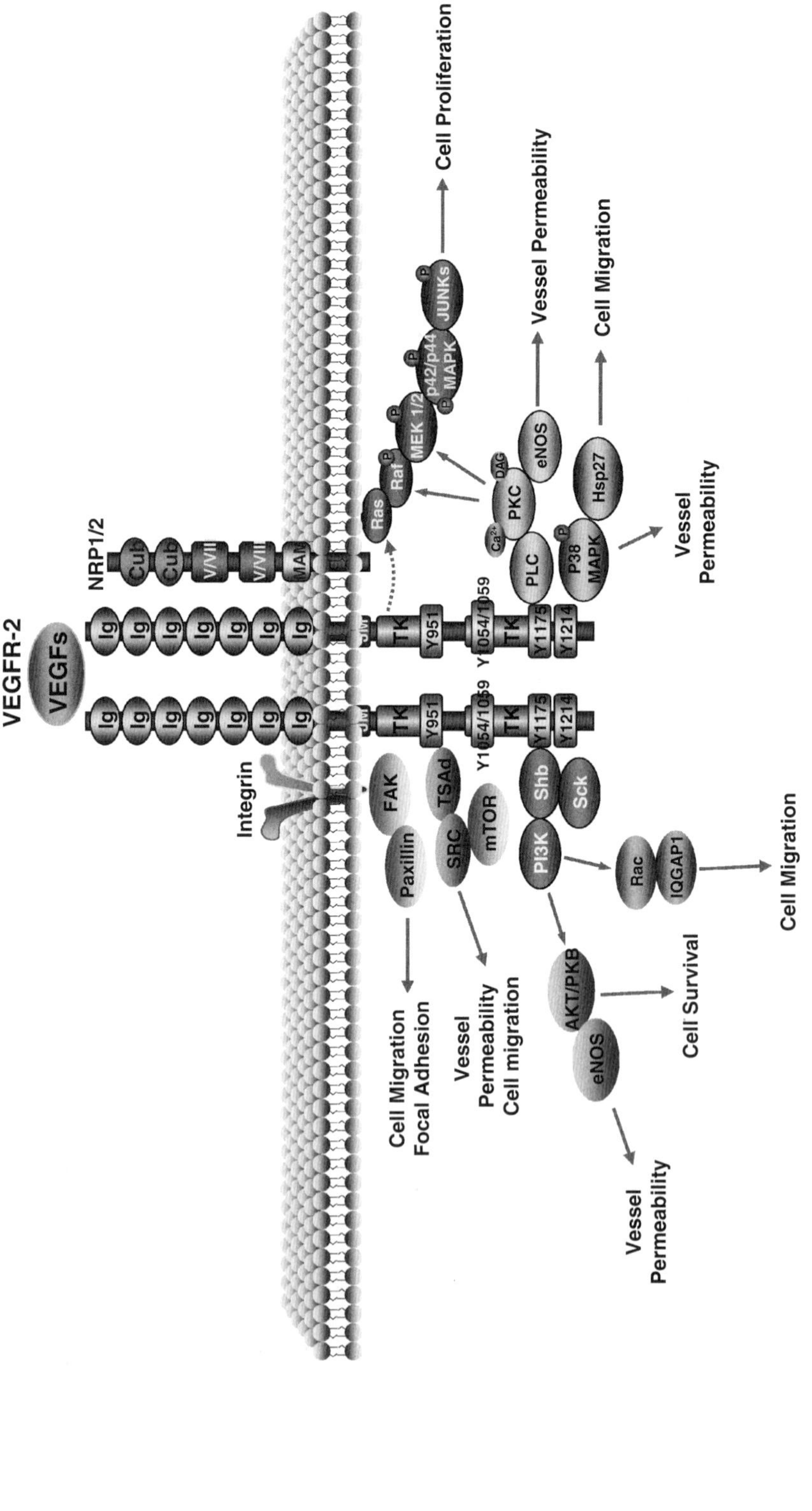

Fig. 21.3 (continued)

the Ras-Raf-MEK-MAPK-JUNKs, the PLC-γ-PKC-MEK-MAPK, and the Shb-Sck-PI3K-Akt/PKB pathways. VEGF-induced EC migration activates the TSAd-Src, the Shb-Sck-PI3K-Rac-IQGAP1, the p38/MAPK-HSP27, and the FAK-paxillin pathways. VEGF-induced vascular permeability is mediated by the TSAd-Src, the PLC-γ-PKC-eNOS, the p38/MAPK-HSP27, and the Shb-Sck-PI3K-Akt/PKB-eNOS pathways.

In contrast, VEGFR-1-mediated signal cascades remain unclear (Fig. 21.4). The "decoy" role of VEGFR-1 was initially supported by identification of an inhibitory segment for VEGF-A stimulation at the cytoplasmic region near the transmembrane domain (Gille et al., 2000). Subsequently, PlGF was shown to stimulate angiogenesis through VEGFR-1 in vivo and EC migration and proliferation in vitro (Ziche et al., 1997a). VEGFR-1 was also found to mediate the response of cell migration and tissue factor expression in monocytes and EC (Barleon et al., 1996; Clauss et al., 1996), and modulate MMP expression and production in smooth muscle cells (Wang and Keiser, 1998). Stimulation of VEGFR-1 by VEGF-A and PlGF induced tyrosine phosphorylation at its *C*-terminal that recruits SH3-domain-containing proteins such as PLC-γ and Grb2, leading to the enhancement of vessel permeability, monocyte migration, recruitment of EC progenitors from bone marrow, and regulation of EC pool during development (Fig. 21.4). It is still unclear how signal transduction is mediated by VEGF-A activation of VEGFR-1 in primary cells such as EC and monocytes (Ferrara et al., 2003; Olsson et al., 2006).

VEGF-C and -D activate VEGFR-3 (Flt-4) inducing phosphorylation at tyrosine residues at the *C*-terminal of VEGFR-3 (Fig. 21.4). Phosphorylated VEGFR-3 binds to Shc-Grb2 and activates the PI3K-Akt and the PKC-ERK1/2 pathways as well as PLC-γ, SHIP2, and Stat3, stimulating lymphatic EC migration, survival, and capillary sprouting (Fournier et al., 1995; Makinen

Fig. 21.3 (continued) **VEGFR-2-signal cascades and their biological functions in angiogenesis.** The schematic illustrates the VEGFR-2-signal pathways in angiogenesis. Integrins and neuropilins (NRP-1 and NRP-2) function as co-receptors by interacting with VEGFR-2 enhancing its functions.Various signal molecules are depicted as ovals. Circle R indicates the use of phosphorylation sites at various signal molecules that is activated by VEGF binding to VEGFR-2. Upon VEGF (see Fig. 21.2) binding, VEGFR-2 are dimerized and autophosphorylated at various tyrosine residues (indicated as Y951, etc.) at its tyrosine kinase-insertion domain (TK), resulting in recruitment of various signal molecules that contain Src homologous domains (SH) or other protein–protein interaction modules and activating downstream signal cascades. These lead to specific biological responses and functions described after the arrows. FAK, focal adhesion kinase; TSAd, T-cell-specific adaptor; mTOR, mammalian target of rapamycin; PI3K, phosphatidylinositol 3-kinase; Hsp27, heat-shock protein-27; MAPK, mitogen-activated protein kinase; MEK, MAPK and ERK kinase; PKC, protein kinase C; PLCγ, phospholipase C gamma; Shb, SH2 and β-cells; eNOS, endothelial nitric oxide synthase; JUNK, c-Jun *N*-terminal kinase; DAG, diacylglycerol; Shb, src homology 2 domain-containing transforming protein B; Sck, src-family tyrosine kinase; IQGAP1, IQ-domain GTPase-activating protein 1

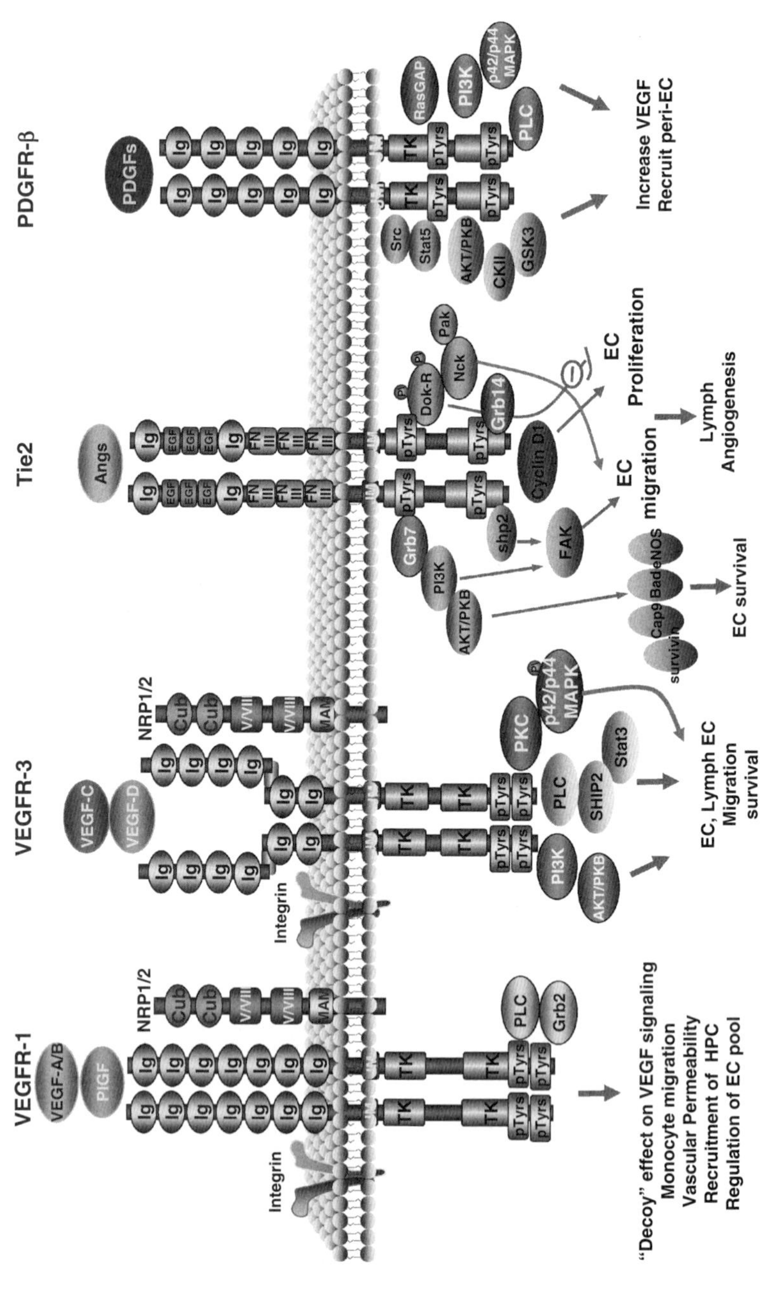

Fig. 21.4 (continued)

et al., 2001; Saharinen et al., 2004; Wang et al., 2004). Additionally, VEGFR-3 forms heterodimers with VEGFR-2 in both EC and lymphatic EC in response to mature VEGF-C activation (Saharinen et al., 2004).

21.2.5 Angiopoietins

The angiopoietin (Ang) family has four members: Ang1, Ang2, Ang3, and Ang4; and two related tyrosine kinase receptors, Tie2 and Tie1 (Shim et al., 2007). Ang3 and Ang4 have not been well studied and thus will not be discussed. In vivo, Ang1 and Ang2 have complementary functions in maintaining vascular functions and integrity. Ang1 maintains the integrity of vasculature through recruiting peri-EC into blood vessels (Carmeliet and Jain, 2000). Transgenic mice deficient in Ang1 or overexpressing Ang2 have disrupted interactions between EC and peri-EC cells that severely impaired vascular function, leading to embryonic death of mice (Davis et al., 1996; Maisonpierre et al., 1997). Transgenic mice overexpressing VEGF-A in the skin induced hyperpermeable vessels. Moreover, vessels in Ang1-overexpressing mice were not leaky and resistant to leaks caused by inflammatory agents (Suri et al., 1998). Co-expression of Ang1 and VEGF-A had an additive effect on angiogenesis and resulted in leakage-resistant vessels typical of Ang1-expressing vessels (Thurston et al., 1999). Ang2 was initially thought of as an antagonist of Ang1 in vascular development and angiogenesis (Davis et al., 1996; Maisonpierre et al., 1997). Unexpectedly, mice lacking Ang2 exhibit major lymphatic vessel defects without affecting vascular development. At birth, vasculature in newborn Ang2 null pulps was indistinguishable from wild-type pulps. However, postnatal Ang2–/– mice had dramatic defects in subsequent vascular remodeling. In the eye,

Fig. 21.4 (continued) **Signal cascades and their biological functions of VEGF-1 and -3, Tie1 and 2, and PDGFR-β in angiogenesis.** The schematic illustrates the various angiogenic receptor signal pathways in angiogenesis. Integrins and neuropilins (NRP-1 and NRP-2) function as co-receptors by interacting with VEGFR-1 and -3 enhancing their functions. Various signal molecules are depicted as ovals. Circle R indicates the use of phosphorylation sites at various signal molecules that are activated by ligand binding to its cognate receptor. Upon ligand (see Fig. 21.2) binding, the receptors are dimerized and auto-phosphorylated at various tyrosine residues (indicated as pTyrs) at its tyrosine kinase-insertion domain (TK), resulting in recruitment of various signal molecules that contain Src homologous domains (SH) or other protein–protein interaction modules and activating downstream signal cascades. These lead to specific biological responses and functions described after the arrows. FAK, focal adhesion kinase; PI3K, phosphatidylinositol 3-kinase; MAPK, mitogen-activated protein kinase; MEK, MAPK and ERK kinase; PKC, protein kinase C; PLCγ, phospholipase C gamma; eNOS, endothelial nitric oxide synthase; JUNK, c-Jun *N*-terminal kinase; CKII, casein kinase II; GSK3β, glucose synthase 3 beta; Dok-R, docking protein; Pak, p21-activated kinase; HPC, hematopoietic progenitor cell; EC, endothelial cell; Cap 9, caspase-9; Stat1/3, signal transducers and activators of transcriptions 1 and 3; CrkII, v-crk sarcoma virus CT10 oncogene homolog (avian) II; Grb, growth factor receptor-bound protein; shp2, shatterproof 2; Bad, Bcl2 antagonist of cell death the hyaloid vasculature normally had largely regressed in wild-type and heterozygous mice by postnatal day 10. In contrast, the hyaloid vasculature was aberrantly maintained in Ang2-deficient mice at this age. This and other postnatal defects in vasculatures of Ang2 null mice revealed that Ang2 is absolutely required for the coupled vascular regression and sprouting events that comprise normal angiogenic remodeling of the ocular vasculature. Genetic rescue with Ang1 corrected the lymphatic, but not the postnatal angiogenesis defects, suggesting that Ang2 acts as a Tie2 agonist in the former setting, but as an antagonist in the latter setting (Gale et al., 2002).

The role of Ang1 in tumor angiogenesis and growth has been controversial (Shim et al., 2007). Clinical studies in primary glioma specimens as well as samples of other types of human cancers showed a strong association of upregulated Ang1 expression with tumor malignancy (Ding et al., 2001; Martoglio et al., 2000; Nakayama et al., 2004a; Shirakawa et al., 2001; Stratmann et al., 1998; Takahama et al., 1999; Tangkeangsirisin et al., 2004; Wang et al., 2005). Overexpression of Ang1 in several glioma cell lines increased tumor angiogenesis and growth in mice (Machein et al., 2004; Zadeh et al., 2004). Ang1 dose-dependently induced the proliferation and increased the labeling index of a murine brain capillary EC, IBE, and human umbilical vein EC (HUVEC) (Kanda et al., 2005). A potent Ang1 variant, COMP-Ang1 long-term administered by an adenoviral vector induced long-lasting vascular enlargement and increased tracheal blood flow. In contrast, short-term administration of COMP-Ang1 induced transient vascular enlargement that spontaneously reversed within a month. In both cases, the vascular enlargement observed in COMP-Ang1-treated animals resulted from endothelial proliferation in the pre-existing blood vessels (Cho et al., 2005). Additionally, Ang1 enhanced brain tumor angiogenesis through mobilization of bone marrow-derived endothelial progenitor cells in animals (Udani et al., 2005). Moreover, in cell lines of colon cancer, breast cancer, squamous cell carcinomas, and Lewis lung carcinomas, overexpression of Ang1 inhibited tumor angiogenesis and growth due to its capacity of recruiting peri-EC that prevented further growth of neo-vessels (Ahmad et al., 2001; Hawighorst et al., 2002; Hayes et al., 2000; Yu and Stamenkovic, 2001).

The role of Ang2 in tumor angiogenesis has also been similarly arguable (Shim et al., 2007). Upregulation of Ang2 correlates with tumor malignancy in gliomas and other types of human cancers (Caine et al., 2003; Ding et al., 2001; Hatanaka et al., 2001; Nakayama et al., 2004b; Osada et al., 2001; Tanaka et al., 2002; Torimura et al., 2004). Overexpression of Ang2 in glioma cells and other cancer cell lines augmented tumor angiogenesis and growth in mice (Ahmad et al., 2001; Etoh et al., 2001; Tanaka et al., 1999). However, other reports demonstrated that specific induction of Ang2 in gliomas, mammary carcinomas, and lung carcinomas inhibits tumor growth and metastasis (Machein et al., 2004; Yu and Stamenkovic, 2001). Systemic overexpression of Ang2 leads to unexpected massive tumor vessel regression within 24 h, even without concomitant inhibition of VEGF. By impairing pericyte coverage of the tumor vasculature, Ang2 induced massive tumor vascular regression while improving perfusion in surviving tumor vessels and transiently exacerbates tumor hypoxia without affecting ATP levels. This significantly inhibits tumor angiogenesis, promotes tumor apoptosis, and suppresses tumor growth (Cao et al., 2007).

In addition to its role in tumor angiogenesis, expression of Ang2 by tumor cells has been linked with invasive and metastatic phenotypes of gliomas, gastric, colon, brain, prostate, and breast cancers (Etoh et al., 2001; Koga et al., 2001; Lind et al., 2005; Ochiumi et al., 2004; Ogawa et al., 2004; Sfiligoi et al., 2003; Tanaka et al., 2002). We recently reported that Ang2 is co-upregulated with matrix metalloprotease (MMP)-2, mèmbrane type-1 (MT1)-MMP, and laminin γ2 in invasive areas, but not in the central regions of clinical primary glioma specimens. Statistical analyses revealed a significant link between the preferential expression of these molecules and invasiveness (Guo et al., 2005). Consonant with these features, intracranial xenografts of U87MG glioma cells engineered to express Ang2 were highly invasive into adjacent brain parenchyma compared to isogenic control tumors. In regions of the Ang2-expressing tumors that were actively invading the brain, high levels of expression of MMP-2 and increased angiogenesis were also evident. A link between these two features was apparent as stable expression of Ang2 by U87MG cells or treatment of several glioma cell lines with recombinant Ang2 in vitro caused activation of MMP-2 and acquisition of increased invasiveness. Conversely, MMP inhibitors suppressed Ang2-stimulated activation of MMP-2 and Ang2-induced cell invasion (Hu et al., 2003). Our observations of Ang2 promotion of glioma cell invasion were supported by other studies in gliomas, gastric cancers, and our own results in breast cancers using various tumor xenograft models in animals (Etoh et al., 2001; Imanishi et al., 2007; Koga et al., 2001; Machein et al., 2004).

21.2.6 Tie2-Mediated Signaling

As shown in Fig. 21.4, Ang1 and Ang2 interact with their cognate receptor Tie2 that is most frequently expressed in EC. Upon binding to Angs, the Tie2 receptor dimerizes and becomes phosphorylated in tyrosine residues at its *C*-terminal (Eklund and Olsen, 2006). Activated Tie2 stimulates PI3K-dependent activation of Akt that leads to increase in cell survival, suppression of caspases-3, -7, and -9 activities as well as attenuation of mitochondrial-derived activator of caspase (smac) release (Dimmeler and Zeiher, 2000; Harfouche et al., 2002; Papapetropoulos et al., 1999). Ang1 also stimulates Tie2 activating the Dok-R-Pak, Nck, and Grb14 pathways, inhibiting EC proliferation, displaying an anti-angiogenic property (Huang et al., 1995; Jones and Dumont, 1999; Jones et al., 2001; Jones et al., 1999). On the contrary, Ang1 was shown to upregulate the expression of cyclin D1 and activate MAPK and phosphatidylinositol 3-kinase (PI3K) in murine IBE cells and HUVECs (Kanda et al., 2005). In addition, the COMP-Ang1-induced vascular enlargement and blood flow are mediated mainly through Tie2 activation, and sustained overexpression of Tie2 could participate in the maintenance of vascular changes (Cho et al., 2005). The protective role of EC from apoptosis by Ang1 or in synergy with VEGF-A has been widely observed in vitro and in vivo (Baffert et al., 2004; Hayes et al., 1999; Kwak et al., 1999; Papapetropoulos et al., 1999; Peirce et al., 2004) and under various stress conditions (Kim et al., 2001; Kwak et al., 1999; Lund et al., 2000).

Ang2 was initially found as an antagonist for Ang1 by inhibiting Ang1 activation of Tie2 activities (Maisonpierre et al., 1997; Suri et al., 1996). However, it has been reported that Ang2 is also an agonist for Tie2-mediated signaling enhancing EC survival and angiogenesis (Kim et al., 2000; Teichert-Kuliszewska et al., 2001; Witzenbichler et al., 1998). Moreover, it has been proposed that the major role of Ang2 in angiogenesis is in cooperation with VEGF-A function. In the presence of VEGF-A, Ang2 promotes vascular sprouting and destabilizes blood vessels through disruption of interactions between EC and peri-EC, thus enhancing VEGF-A stimulation. In the absence of VEGF-A, however, Ang2 acts as a suppressor that accelerates vessel regression (Benjamin et al., 1998; Grosskreutz et al., 1999; Holash et al., 1999; Zagzag et al., 2000a). This hypothesis has been validated by studies of neovascularization in rat cornea (Lobov et al., 2002). Additionally, in a panel of glioma cell lines, Ang2 inhibited VEGF-A expression at both mRNA and protein levels in Tie2-expressing glioma cells, but not in Tie2-negative tumor cells. Ang2 regulated VEGF expression at the transcriptional level in relation to a decrease in HIF-1α expression and HIF-DNA-binding activity. Tie2 silencing by siRNA rescued the Ang2-mediated downmodulation of VEGF, suggesting an essential role for Tie2 in this regulatory loop (Lee et al., 2008).

21.2.7 Interaction Between Angiopoietins and Integrins

Although Ang2 modulates angiogenesis through interaction with the Tie2 receptor (Yancopoulos et al., 2000), it contains a highly conserved *C*-terminal fibrinogen-like receptor-binding domain which may form a functional association with certain integrin receptors (Davis et al., 2003; Weber et al., 2005). Ang1 and Ang2 were shown to stimulate Tie2-independent cell adhesion of endothelial cells and fibroblasts to Ang1- or Ang2-coated surfaces through $\alpha_5\beta_1$ and $\alpha_v\beta_5$ integrin-mediated activation of ERK and focal adhesion kinase (FAK) signaling (Carlson et al., 2001). Skeletal myocytes lacking Tie2 adhere to Ang1- and Ang2-coated surfaces in a similar manner as to laminin, fibronectin, and vitronectin. The Ang-stimulated skeletal myocyte adhesion is mediated by integrin receptors such as $\alpha_5\beta_1$, activating ERK, FAK signaling, and promoting cell survival (Dallabrida et al., 2005). It has been postulated that the interaction of Ang with integrins is likely through the fibrinogen-like receptor-binding domain present in the Ang protein structure (Davis et al., 2003). This theory has been recently examined showing that a monomeric Ang1 variant (△Ang), comprised only of the fibrinogen-like receptor-binding domain, ligates Tie2 without activating the receptor. Moreover, △Ang binds to $\alpha_5\beta_1$ integrin with similar affinity compared to Tie2. When EC were plated on △Ang-coated surfaces, △Ang displays similar biological effects as the full-length Ang1 stimulating cell adhesion, ERK signaling, and vascular maturation (Weber et al., 2005).

Modulation of EC function and angiogenesis by Ang1 through direct interaction with integrins was also demonstrated in EC that expresses the Tie2 receptor. Immobilized Ang1 was shown to selectively mediate $\alpha_5\beta_1$ integrin outside-in signaling leading to a cross talk between Tie2 and $\alpha_5\beta_1$ and promotion of angiogenesis (Cascone et al., 2005). In tumor cells that lack Tie2 expression, we showed that Ang2 induces glioma cell invasion by stimulating MMP-2 expression through the $\alpha_v\beta_1$ integrin and FAK pathways (Hu et al., 2006). We also reported that Ang2 associates with $\alpha_5\beta_1$ integrin in Tie2-deficient breast cancer cells. Ang2 activates an integrin-mediated signaling pathway leading to breast cancer cell invasion and metastasis. Inhibition of β_1 or α_5, but not other integrins, attenuates Ang2 modulation of integrin-linked kinase (ILK), Akt, glucose synthase kinase (GSK)-3β, Snail, E-cadherin and vimentin, and Ang2-stimulated breast cancer cell motility (Imanishi et al., 2007). Furthermore, similar to the association of Ang2 with integrins in skeletal myocytes (Dallabrida et al., 2005) and PG-MV/vesican with integrin in glioma cells (Wu et al., 2002), the association of Ang2 with integrins was highly calcium and manganese-dependent in our system. These studies establish a critical role of Ang2 in promoting tumor cell invasion and metastasis through stimulation of cell motility and invasion mediated by the $\alpha_v\beta_1$ integrin/FAK pathway in glioma cells and the $\alpha_5\beta_1$ integrin/ILK pathway in breast cancer cells independent of Tie2.

21.2.8 PDGF and Their Receptors

Platelet-derived growth factors (PDGF) belong to a superfamily including VEGF family members. There are four PDGF isoforms, PDGF-A, -B, -C, and -D encoded by different genes. PDGF-A and -B form homodimers and heterodimers, while -C and -D only form homodimers (Heldin et al., 2002; Shih and Holland, 2006; Tallquist and Kazlauskas, 2004). There are two protein tyrosine kinase PDGF receptors, PDGFR-α and -β. PGDF-AA, -AB, -BB, and -CC bind to the -α receptor, -AB and -BB bind to the -αβ dimer, and -BB and -DD interact with the -β receptor (Fig. 21.2) (Fredriksson et al., 2004; Heldin and Westermark, 1999). Mice deficient in PDGF-B or the -β receptor have dilated aorta, heart and capillaries, frequent microaneurysms and hemorrhages due to marked reduction of peri-EC (vascular smooth muscle cells and pericytes) in the vessels, resulting in death at birth (Lindahl et al., 1998, 1997a). In contrast, PDGF-A null mice displayed defective myelination and lung emphysema (Betsholtz et al., 2001; Heldin et al., 2002; Lindahl et al., 1997b). During glioma progression, PDGF-A, -B and PDGFR-α, -β are overexpressed in early stages of glioma formation (Furnari et al., 2007; Wiedemeyer et al., 2008). Upregulation of PDGFR-α is localized in tumor cells, whereas high levels of expression of PDGFR-β were found in the endothelial compartment (Hermanson et al., 1992, 1995). In vitro, PDGF-B induces angiogenesis in chick chorioallantonic membrane assays and rat aorta ring assays (Battegay et al., 1994; Nicosia et al., 1994; Risau et al., 1992). We reported that overexpression of PDGF-B in U87MG glioma cells markedly promoted glioma angiogenesis and growth in the brain of mice while co-expression of PDGF-B with VEGF-A in gliomas inhibited VEGF-A-induced intratumoral hemorrhage through recruitment of peri-EC (Guo et al., 2003). Expression of PDGF-C and -D are very low or absent in normal adult and fetal brains. However, both PDGF-C and -D were found in brain tumor cells and clinical brain tumors such as meduloblastomas and activating PDGFR-α through autocrine pathways (Andrae et al., 2002; Lokker et al., 2002).

PDGFR-mediated signaling has been investigated in fibroblasts, smooth muscle cells, and EC in detail (Heldin and Westermark, 1999; Tallquist and Kazlauskas, 2004). As shown in Figs. 21.2 and 21.4, PDGF-B and other PDGF isoforms bind to PDGFR-β activating Stat1 and Stat3, the PI3K-CrK-Grbs pathway, PLCγ, and the Akt-CKII-GSK3β pathway, resulting in recruitment of peri-EC into growing vessels (Heldin and Westermark, 1999; Tallquist and Kazlauskas, 2004). Additionally, PDGF-B was shown to stimulate VEGF expression in endothelial cells through the PDGFR-β-PI3K-mediated pathway (Wang et al., 1999).

21.2.9 Other Growth Factors and Their Receptors: HGF/c-Met

HGF/c-Met are expressed at high levels in primary glioma specimens (Furnari et al., 2007; Wiedemeyer et al., 2008). In vitro, HGF stimulates EC proliferation, migration, invasion and tube-like structure formation and VEGF-A expression in a hindlimb ischemia model (Rosen et al., 1991; Van Belle et al., 1998). In glioma cells, overexpression of HGF promoted tumor growth and angiogenesis, while inhibition of the HGF decreased vascular density and tumor growth in mice (Abounader et al., 2002, 1999; Laterra et al., 1997). The roles and molecular signaling of HGF/c-Met pathway in angiogenesis, tumor growth, and progression of brain tumors including gliomas are discussed in detail in Chapter 39.

21.2.10 FGF/FGFR

Fibroblast growth factor (FGF) and its receptor (FGFR) are a family that has 23 FGF and 4 FGFR members. FGF-1 and FGF-2 have been shown to be potent angiogenic factors (Powers et al., 2000). FGF-2 was the first proangiogenic molecule identified and is a strong promoter for angiogenesis in vitro and in vivo. In gliomas, several studies provide evidence for an involvement in glioma angiogenesis (Auguste et al., 2001; Stan et al., 1995). Moreover, due to the fact that FGFs are secreted out of cells through an unclear mechanism and targeting a wide range of cells including EC, peri-EC, and tumor cells, studies of the role of FGF–FGFR signaling in glioma angiogenesis have not been very active in the past decade.

21.2.11 TGF-β

The role of TGF-β in angiogenesis is debatable since TGF-β has been described as both an angiogenic and anti-angiogenic factor toward EC depending on the assay systems used. In gliomas, TGF-β and its receptors were found in tumor cells and their expressions correlate with tumor malignancy and neovascularization (Horst et al., 1992; Stiles et al., 1997; Yamada et al., 1995). TGF-β1 and TGF-β2 stimulate VEGF-A production in glioma cells (Koochekpour et al., 1996) and induce expression of PDGF-A, -B, and PDGFR-β in EC (Kavanaugh et al., 1988). Although overexpression of TGF-β1 was shown to promote tumor growth of subcutaneous tumors, no enhanced angiogenesis was found, suggesting that TGF-β1-stimulated tumor growth was independent of the status of neovascularization (Ashley et al., 1998).

21.2.12 Integrins

Integrins belong to a family of heterodimeric transmembrane receptors comprised of at least 16 α and 8 β subunits. They are the primary receptors that mediate cell adhesion to the ECM and play an important role in angiogenesis. Involvement of integrin receptors in angiogenesis is mostly attributed to EC-expressed integrins that activate an array of signal pathways regulating EC functions and angiogenesis. In particular, endothelial integrins $\alpha_1\beta_1$, $\alpha_2\beta_1$, $\alpha_4\beta_1$, $\alpha_5\beta_1$, $\alpha_9\beta_1$, and $\alpha_6\beta_4$ as well as α_v integrins have been shown to be important in angiogenesis. Recently, the involvement of $\alpha_9\beta_1$, $\alpha_1\beta_1$, $\alpha_2\beta_1$, and $\alpha_4\beta_1$ integrins in lymphangiogenesis has also been reported (Avraamides et al., 2008). In addition to interactions with molecules in the ECM and the tumor microenvironment, integrins also interact with growth factors and VEGFRs to modulate angiogenesis. For example, angiogenesis induced by FGF or TNF-α was shown to be dependent on $\alpha_v\beta_3$ integrin-mediated signaling whereas in vivo vessel growth stimulated by VEGF was found to be dependent on $\alpha_v\beta_5$-mediated signaling (Friedlander et al., 1995). Integrin $\alpha_v\beta_3$ was also shown to interact with FGF-2 promoting angiogenesis (Eliceiri, 2001) and mediate VEGF-enhanced EC adhesion and migration (Byzova et al., 2000). In the latter study, involvement of $\alpha_v\beta_3$ as well as $\alpha_v\beta_5$, $\alpha_5\beta_1$, $\alpha_2\beta_1$ integrins in VEGF-stimulated angiogenesis was shown via interactions with the VEGFR-2 receptor, which activates the PI3K-Akt-PTEN signaling axis (Byzova et al., 2000). Based on the critical roles of integrins in tumor angiogenesis, cyclic RGD-containing peptides and their derivates such as cilengitide or EMD 121974 that inhibit binding of the substrate to integrins in tumor-associated EC, have been developed as therapeutic drugs and used in clinical trials for glioma treatment (MacDonald et al., 2008; Nabors et al., 2007). An excellent review by Avraamides et al. (2008) discussed the roles of integrins in angiogenesis and lymphatic angiogenesis in detail.

21.2.13 Interleukin-8 (IL-8)

IL-8 is a known angiogenic factor, and expression of IL-8 correlates with glioma progression and angiogenesis. High levels of IL-8 were found in pseudopalisading around areas of necrosis (Desbaillets et al., 1999, 1997; Van Meir et al., 1992). Stimulation of IL-8 expression in gliomas was attributed to hypoxia, Fas ligation, death receptor activation, cytosolic Ca^{2+}, TNF-α, IL-1, and other cytokines and various cellular stresses (Brat et al., 2005). A potential tumor suppressor ING4 was identified in glioma cells as a mediator for NF-κB-stimulated IL-8 transcription. Knockdown of ING4 accelerated angiogenesis compared with control in gliomas, suggesting an indirect role of IL-8 in promoting NF-κB-mediated angiogenesis (Garkavtsev et al., 2004). IL-8 was also shown to induce CXCR1 and CXCR2 expression, promoting angiogenesis and tumor growth. However, the specific mechanisms by which IL-8 exerts its pro-angiogenic functions are not well studied (Brat et al., 2005).

21.2.14 Nitric Oxide (NO)

NO is an important signaling molecule that regulates a variety of physiological and pathological processes (Moncada and Higgs, 1993). NO is produced by three NO synthases (NOS): neuronal NOS (nNOS), endothelial NO (eNOS), and inducible NOS (iNOS) (Kerwin et al., 1995). In vitro and in vivo administrations of NO donors to EC led to increased mitogenesis of vascular EC and potentiation of neovascularization (Ziche et al., 1994, 1993). NO is involved in VEGF-stimulated angiogenesis through cGMP-MAPK signaling. Thus inhibition of NO signaling attenuates the response to VEGF in endothelium (Ziche et al., 1997b). NO has been shown to play an important role in tumor angiogenesis. Increased levels of NO and NOS are found in brain tumors and other types of human cancers (Cobbs et al., 1995; Feng et al., 2002; Kashiwagi et al., 2008; Klotz et al., 1998; Kong et al., 2001a, b; Thomsen et al., 1994; Yin et al., 2008; Zheng et al., 2007). nNOS, eNOS, and iNOS are upregulated in brain tumor tissues and cell lines (Bakshi et al., 1998; Broholm et al., 2001; Cobbs et al.,

1995; Ellie et al., 1995; Fujisawa et al., 1995; Hara et al., 1996). NO production modulates aspects of tumor angiogenesis such as tonic vasodilatation of tumor vessels, vessel permeability, edema formation, and neovascularization (Bian et al., 2001; Garbossa et al., 2001). Modulation of NO production through NOS expression in glioma cells affects tumor growth, angiogenesis, tumor blood flow, and delivery of anti-cancer drugs to tumor tissue (Fukumura et al., 1997; Shinoda and Whittle, 2001; Tozer et al., 1997). Moreover, whether NO enhances or attenuates chemotherapeutic efficacy in malignant gliomas has not been determined (Lam-Himlin et al., 2006).

21.2.15 Hypoxia in Brain Tumor Angiogenesis

Like normal eukaryotic cells, glioma cells need oxygen for their metabolism and survival. However, due to the fast growth of gliomas, supplies of nutrients and oxygen are often insufficient, resulting in low oxygen tension (hypoxia) in regions throughout the tumor mass. To adapt to hypoxic conditions, glioma cells respond by activating an array of gene expression. These hypoxia-inducible genes have functions in cell proliferation, survival, apoptosis, angiogenesis, gene transcription, metabolism of energy and iron, pH regulation, and ECM molecules. As a result, malignant gliomas maintain their fast growth with increases in cell proliferation, invasion, and neovascularization (Fischer et al., 2005; Kaur et al., 2005b). Importantly, recent studies suggest that hypoxia induces appearance of necrosis associated with the pseudopalisading seen in malignant glioblastoma multiforme (Brat et al., 2004; Brat and Van Meir, 2004).

21.2.16 Hypoxia-Inducible Factor-1 (HIF-1)

Among the large group of hypoxia-inducible genes, hypoxia-inducible factor-1 (HIF-1) has been considered as a master regulator of hypoxic responses in cells (Semenza, 2004). HIF-1 is transcription factor with two basic helix loop helix (bHLH)-PAS subunits, HIF-1α and HIF-1β (also called aryl hydrocarbon nuclear translocator, ARNT). HIF-2α and HIF-3α are two other HIF proteins with several splice variants of HIF-3α (Kaur et al., 2005b). Mice deficient in HIF-1α, HIF-1β, and HIF-2α displayed different defects in vascular development as well as in different organs, suggesting distinct functions of specific HIF proteins in vasculogenesis and angiogenesis (Semenza, 2004). In cells, HIF-1β is constitutively expressed while HIF-1α and -2α are hypoxia stabilized. Under normoxic conditions, HIF-1α is hydroxylated at its prolyl residues by prolyl hydrolase (PHD) enzymes, resulting in rapid ubiquitination of HIF-1α and subsequent proteasomal degradation (Semenza, 2002).

Under hypoxic conditions, lack of oxygen leads to inactivation of PHD enzymes, and HIF-1α accumulates and translocates into the nucleus where it dimerizes with HIF-1β and binds to hypoxia response elements (HRE) in its target (hypoxia-inducible) genes, thus promoting cell growth and survival (Semenza, 2004). HIF-1α is also regulated by hydroxylation at its asparagine residues, acetylation, phosphorylation, and SUMOylation (Brahimi-Horn et al., 2005; Jeong et al., 2002; Semenza, 2004; Shao et al., 2004). In addition, a number of growth factors such as EGF, TGF-α, PDGF-A, IGF-1, and -2, insulin, angiotensin, and thrombin also modulate expression of HIF-1α at the transcriptional level via the PI3K and MAPK pathways (Acker and Plate, 2002; Hu et al., 1992; Richard et al., 2000; Zelzer et al., 1998). In glioma cells, expression of EGFRvIII, a common mutation of EGFR in gliomas, induces expression of HIF-1α. PTEN loss further potentiated the stimulation of HIF-1α through the EGFRvIII-activated PI3K/Akt/FRAP/mTOR pathway (Clarke et al., 2001; Haas-Kogan and Stokoe, 2008).

HIF-1α is considered as an activator for glioma angiogenesis, primarily through control of the most important angiogenic factors, VEGF-A. In response to hypoxia, HIF-1α binds to the HRE element in the VEGF-A gene promoter to increase VEGF expression. HIF-1α can also stabilize mRNA of VEGF-A by directly interacting with the 3'-untranslated region of the VEGF-A transcript (Claffey et al., 1992; Shih and Claffey, 1999). Additionally, HIF-1α stimulates expression of other angiogenic factors aforementioned such as PlGF, PDGF-B, Ang1, and Ang2 as well as molecules that are implicated in angiogenesis and EC functions such as cathepsin D, MMP-2, urokinase plasminogen activator receptor (uPRA), endothelin-1, iNOS, adrenomedullin, erythropoietin, fibronectin, TGF-α, and TGF-β (Kaur et al., 2005b; Semenza, 2004). Expression of HIF-1α in glioma cells induced expressions of SDF receptor CXCR4 and VEGF-A. Since VEGF-A stimulates CXCR4 in EC, VEGF-mediated CXCR4 expression in EC contributed to an increase in glioma angiogenesis (Zagzag et al., 2006). A recent study showed that in an intracranial glioma model, HIF-1α induced recruitment of bone marrow-derived CD45+ myeloid cells containing Tie2+, VEGFR-1+, CD11b+, and F4/80+ subpopulations as well as endothelial and pericyte progenitor cells to promote neovascularization in gliomas (Du et al., 2008). In primary gliomas, HIF-1α is expressed in psuedopalisading cells around necrotic foci, co-localizing with upregulated VEGF-A in clinical tumor specimens (Plate et al., 1992; Shweiki et al., 1992; Zagzag et al., 2000b). This unique expression pattern has been utilized for developing anti-brain tumor therapies to deliver an oncolytic virus into the hypoxic regions of fast-growing gliomas, thus inhibiting glioma growth and angiogenesis in vivo (Post et al., 2007; Post and Van Meir, 2001, 2003).

21.2.17 Induction of Angiogenic Inhibitors by Tumor Suppressor Genes

During glioma progression, three tumor suppressor genes are commonly lost or mutated: p53, PTEN, and RB (Furnari et al., 2007; Wen and Kesari, 2008). These tumor suppressor genes were shown to modulate tumor angiogenesis by upregulation of angiogenic inhibitors and downregulation of angiogenic promoters. p53 controls glioma angiogenesis by upregulating thrombospondin-1 (TSP-1) (Dameron et al., 1994; Good et al., 1990; Lawler et al., 2001) which inhibits angiogenesis through multiple mechanisms (Ren et al., 2006). p53 was also shown to induce a brain-specific angiogenesis inhibitor 1 (BAI-1) (Nishimori et al., 1997) which is processed by proteolytic degradation to generate an anti-angiogenic peptide called vasculostatin, inhibiting glioma angiogenesis in mice (Kaur et al., 2005a). Additionally, p53 was also shown to induce a not yet identified anti-angiogenic peptide named glioma-derived angiogenesis inhibitory factor (GD-AIF) that inhibits EC migration in vitro and angiogenesis in vivo (Van Meir et al., 1994). In contrast to p53, tumor suppressors PTEN and RB negatively regulate glioma angiogenesis indirectly. PTEN inhibits angiogenesis primarily through inhibiting VEGF expression by downregulating PI3K-Akt-HIF-1 activities (Gomez-Manzano et al., 2003; Zhong et al., 2000), while loss of PTEN results in upregulation of HIF-1-mediated expression of VEGF and other angiogenic factors, thus facilitating angiogenesis (Zundel et al., 2000). RB and its family members, pRb2/p130, were shown to downregulate angiogenic factors VEGF, FGFR-1, and IL-8 directly or indirectly, thereby attenuating glioma angiogenesis (Claudio et al., 2001; Lasorella et al., 2005; Tashiro et al., 2003; Wegiel et al., 2005; Zhang et al., 1999).

21.2.18 Contribution of Tumor Angiogenesis by Stem Cell-Like Glioma Cells

Stem cell-like glioma cells (SCLGC) are a subpopulation of tumor cells within gliomas that share characteristics with neural stem cells. SCLGC isolated from human glioblastoma biopsy specimens and xenografts potently generated tumors with widespread tumor angiogenesis, necrosis, and hemorrhage (Bao et al., 2006a; Galli et al., 2004; Singh et al., 2003, 2004). In comparison with matched non-SCLGC populations, SCLGC consistently secret markedly elevated levels of VEGF-A, which were further induced by hypoxia. The pro-angiogenic effects of SCLGC on EC were specifically abolished by an anti-VEGF neutralizing antibody, bevacizumab. Furthermore, bevacizumab displayed potent anti-angiogenic efficacy in vivo and suppressed growth of xenografts derived from SCLGC. This data indicates that stem cell-like tumor cells can be a crucial source of key angiogenic factors in gliomas and that targeting pro-angiogenic factors from stem cell-like tumor populations may be critical for patient therapy (Bao et al., 2006b). The roles of SCLGC in glioma tumorigenesis, progression, and angiogenesis as well as their use as diagnostic markers and therapeutic targets for brain tumors are discussed in detail in Chapters 29 and 44.

21.2.19 Anti-angiogenic Therapy of Brain Tumors: Clinical Applications and Challenges

The balance of orchestrated angiogenesis constitutes an attractive target for anti-angiogenic therapy of brain tumors. Extensive studies in orthotopic brain tumors in animals and increasing numbers of clinical trials for various types of human cancer therapies using angiogenic inhibitors have been well documented (Jain et al., 2007). Most, if not all, anti-angiogenic inhibitors are designed to target the signal pathways depicted in Figs. 21.3 and 21.4, with a focus on inhibiting the VEGF–VEGFR-2-signal pathway. In addition to slowing glioma growth, anti-angiogenic therapies normalize tumor vasculature to create a therapeutic window for other means of anti-cancer treatment, such as radiation or chemotherapy, has emerged as a promising approach. In a preclinical study, VEGFR-2 blockade by a neutralizing anti-VEGFR-2 antibody, DC101, creates a "normalization window," a period during which combined radiation therapy gives the best outcome. This window is characterized by an increase in tumor oxygenation, which is known to enhance radiation response. During the normalization window, but not before or after it, the VEGFR-2 blockade increases pericyte coverage of brain tumor vessels via upregulation of Ang1 and degrades their pathologically thick basement membrane via MMP activation (Winkler et al., 2004).

A follow-up study using contrast-enhanced magnetic resonance imaging (MRI) further supports this theory. Cediranib (AZD2171, an oral, pan anti-VEGFR tyrosine kinase inhibitor with activity toward PDGFR-α and -β, and c-Kit) temporarily induced a "normalization time window" in tumor vessels in recurrent glioblastoma patients by daily administration. Such a window is prolonged but reversible, and has the significant clinical benefit of reduced tumor-associated vasogenic edema. Basic FGF, SDF1-α, and viable circulating endothelial cells (CECs) increased when tumors escaped treatment, and circulating progenitor cells (CPCs) increased when tumors progressed after drug interruption (Batchelor et al., 2007).

Anti-angiogenic therapies in combination with other regimens have been developed to treat patients with malignant gliomas (Jain et al., 2007). Several recent Phase II trials using bevacizumab and irinotecan (a telomerase inhibitor) also showed initial effects on reducing tumor volume and enhanced contrast areas in MRI imaging (Bokstein et al., 2008; Pope et al., 2006; Sathornsumetee et al., 2008; Vredenburgh et al., 2007a, b). Simultaneous targeting of tumor vessels and cancer cells provides an excellent opportunity to obtain a better outcome in therapy of brain tumors. In this book, Chapters 31, 32, and 33 have been devoted to "targeting tumor vasculature" and describe in further detail the current status and progress of anti-angiogenic therapy for brain tumors.

21.3 Summary

In conclusion, a large number of studies on angiogenesis from animal development, cell culture models, and tumor xenografts in animals as well as clinical investigations have considerably advanced our knowledge of the mechanisms of brain tumor angiogenesis. However, the challenge of studying brain tumor angiogenesis is to understand the underlying mechanisms of the angiogenic process within a proper biological context. As described in this chapter, the complexity of brain tumor angiogenesis and its regulation involve orchestrated interactions among various growth factors, their receptors, molecules, and stress from the tumor microenvironment and tumor stromal compartment, areas that will be further discussed in Chapter 31. Although multiple clinical trials have shown promise for brain tumor treatment by targeting angiogenesis or tumor vasculature, the reality of limited effectiveness for prolonging the survival of patients with gliomas in the clinic presents an urgent need to further understand the mechanisms of brain tumor angiogenesis and the interplays by each of the critical molecules and their signaling. As discussed in Chapters 30, 31, 32, and 33 as well as in several recent reviews (Ellis and Hicklin, 2008; Folkman, 2007; Kiselyov et al., 2007), a better understanding of the biology of brain tumors will lead to future advances in developing effective anti-angiogenic and anti-brain tumor therapies.

Acknowledgments We would like to thank Ryo Nishikawa and Takanori Hirose for providing clinical glioma specimens for data showed in Fig. 21.1, Ping Guo, Hou-Quan Tao, and Christopher Schafer for performing IHC staining of tumor vessels and statistical analyses. We would also like to thank Mrs. Sarah Cork for her excellent help in editing this chapter. This work was supported in part by grants from the National Institutes of Health (CA102011 and CA130966), American Cancer Society (RSG CSM-107144), and the Hillman Fellows Program for Innovative Cancer Research to Shi-Yuan Cheng and Bo Hu.

References

Abdulrauf, S. I., Edvardsen, K., Ho, K. L., Yang, X. Y., Rock, J. P., and Rosenblum, M. L. 1998. Vascular endothelial growth factor expression and vascular density as prognostic markers of survival in patients with low-grade astrocytoma. J Neurosurg 88:513–520.

Abounader, R., Lal, B., Luddy, C., Koe, G., Davidson, B., Rosen, E. M., and Laterra, J. 2002. In vivo targeting of SF/HGF and c-met expression via U1snRNA/ribozymes inhibits glioma growth and angiogenesis and promotes apoptosis. Faseb J 16:108–110.

Abounader, R., Ranganathan, S., Lal, B., Fielding, K., Book, A., Dietz, H., Burger, P., and Laterra, J. 1999. Reversion of human glioblastoma malignancy by U1 small nuclear RNA/ribozyme targeting of scatter factor/hepatocyte growth factor and c-met expression. J Natl Cancer Inst 91:1548–1556.
Acker, T., and Plate, K. H. 2002. A role for hypoxia and hypoxia-inducible transcription factors in tumor physiology. J Mol Med 80:562–575.
Ahmad, S. A., Liu, W., Jung, Y. D., Fan, F., Wilson, M., Reinmuth, N., Shaheen, R. M., Bucana, C. D., and Ellis, L. M. 2001. The effects of angiopoietin-1 and -2 on tumor growth and angiogenesis in human colon cancer. Cancer Res 61:1255–1259.
Akahane, M., Akahane, T., Matheny, S. L., Shah, A., Okajima, E., and Thorgeirsson, U. P. 2006. Vascular endothelial growth factor-D is a survival factor for human breast carcinoma cells. Int J Cancer 118:841–849.
Alitalo, K., and Carmeliet, P. 2002. Molecular mechanisms of lymphangiogenesis in health and disease. Cancer Cell 1:219–227.
Andrae, J., Molander, C., Smits, A., Funa, K., and Nister, M. 2002. Platelet-derived growth factor-B and -C and active alpha-receptors in medulloblastoma cells. Biochem Biophys Res Commun 296:604–611.
Ashley, D. M., Kong, F. M., Bigner, D. D., and Hale, L. P. 1998. Endogenous expression of transforming growth factor beta1 inhibits growth and tumorigenicity and enhances Fas-mediated apoptosis in a murine high-grade glioma model. Cancer Res 58:302–309.
Auguste, P., Gursel, D. B., Lemiere, S., Reimers, D., Cuevas, P., Carceller, F., Di Santo, J. P., and Bikfalvi, A. 2001. Inhibition of fibroblast growth factor/fibroblast growth factor receptor activity in glioma cells impedes tumor growth by both angiogenesis-dependent and -independent mechanisms. Cancer Res 61:1717–1726.
Autiero, M., Waltenberger, J., Communi, D., Kranz, A., Moons, L., Lambrechts, D., Kroll, J., Plaisance, S., De Mol, M., Bono, F., Kliche, S., Fellbrich, G., Ballmer-Hofer, K., Maglione, D., Mayr-Beyrle, U., Dewerchin, M., Dombrowski, S., Stanimirovic, D., Van Hummelen, P., Dehio, C., Hicklin, D. J., Persico, G., Herbert, J. M., Communi, D., Shibuya, M., Collen, D., Conway, E. M., and Carmeliet, P. 2003. Role of PlGF in the intra- and intermolecular cross talk between the VEGF receptors Flt1 and Flk1. Nat Med 9:936–943.
Avraamides, C. J., Garmy-Susini, B., and Varner, J. A. 2008. Integrins in angiogenesis and lymphangiogenesis. Nat Rev Cancer 8:604–617.
Baffert, F., Thurston, G., Rochon-Duck, M., Le, T., Brekken, R., and McDonald, D. M. 2004. Age-related changes in vascular endothelial growth factor dependency and angiopoietin-1-induced plasticity of adult blood vessels. Circ Res 94:984–992.
Bakshi, A., Nag, T. C., Wadhwa, S., Mahapatra, A. K., and Sarkar, C. 1998. The expression of nitric oxide synthases in human brain tumours and peritumoral areas. J Neurol Sci 155:196–203.
Bao, S., Wu, Q., McLendon, R. E., Hao, Y., Shi, Q., Hjelmeland, A. B., Dewhirst, M. W., Bigner, D. D., and Rich, J. N. 2006a. Glioma stem cells promote radioresistance by preferential activation of the DNA damage response. Nature 444:756–760.
Bao, S., Wu, Q., Sathornsumetee, S., Hao, Y., Li, Z., Hjelmeland, A. B., Shi, Q., McLendon, R. E., Bigner, D. D., and Rich, J. N. 2006b. Stem cell-like glioma cells promote tumor angiogenesis through vascular endothelial growth factor. Cancer Res 66:7843–7848.
Barleon, B., Sozzani, S., Zhou, D., Weich, H. A., Mantovani, A., and Marme, D. 1996. Migration of human monocytes in response to vascular endothelial growth factor (VEGF) is mediated via the VEGF receptor flt-1. Blood 87:3336–3343.
Barleon, B., Totzke, F., Herzog, C., Blanke, S., Kremmer, E., Siemeister, G., Marme, D., and Martiny-Baron, G. 1997. Mapping of the sites for ligand binding and receptor dimerization at the extracellular domain of the vascular endothelial growth factor receptor FLT-1. J Biol Chem 272:10382–10388.
Batchelor, T. T., Sorensen, A. G., di Tomaso, E., Zhang, W. T., Duda, D. G., Cohen, K. S., Kozak, K. R., Cahill, D. P., Chen, P. J., Zhu, M., Ancukiewicz, M., Mrugala, M. M.,

Plotkin, S., Drappatz, J., Louis, D. N., Ivy, P., Scadden, D. T., Benner, T., Loeffler, J. S., Wen, P. Y., and Jain, R. K. 2007. AZD2171, a pan-VEGF receptor tyrosine kinase inhibitor, normalizes tumor vasculature and alleviates edema in glioblastoma patients. Cancer Cell 11:83–95.

Battegay, E. J., Rupp, J., Iruela-Arispe, L., Sage, E. H., and Pech, M. 1994. PDGF-BB modulates endothelial proliferation and angiogenesis in vitro via PDGF beta-receptors. J Cell Biol 125:917–928.

Bellomo, D., Headrick, J. P., Silins, G. U., Paterson, C. A., Thomas, P. S., Gartside, M., Mould, A., Cahill, M. M., Tonks, I. D., Grimmond, S. M., Townson, S., Wells, C., Little, M., Cummings, M. C., Hayward, N. K., and Kay, G. F. 2000. Mice lacking the vascular endothelial growth factor-B gene (Vegfb) have smaller hearts, dysfunctional coronary vasculature, and impaired recovery from cardiac ischemia. Circ Res 86:E29–35.

Benjamin, L. E., Hemo, I., and Keshet, E. 1998. A plasticity window for blood vessel remodelling is defined by pericyte coverage of the preformed endothelial network and is regulated by PDGF- B and VEGF. Development 125:1591–1598.

Bergers, G., and Benjamin, L. E. 2003. Tumorigenesis and the angiogenic switch. Nat Rev Cancer 3:401–410.

Bergers, G., and Hanahan, D. 2008. Modes of resistance to anti-angiogenic therapy. Nat Rev Cancer 8:592–603.

Betsholtz, C., Karlsson, L., and Lindahl, P. 2001. Developmental roles of platelet-derived growth factors. Bioessays 23:494–507.

Bian, X., Du, L., Chen, Z., Shi, J., and Liu, F. 2001. [A quantitative pathological study on angiogenesis, vascular endothelial growth factor and inducible nitric oxide synthase in astrocytomas]. Zhonghua Bing Li Xue Za Zhi 30:23–26.

Bokstein, F., Shpigel, S., and Blumenthal, D. T. 2008. Treatment with bevacizumab and irinotecan for recurrent high-grade glial tumors. Cancer 112:2267–2273.

Brahimi-Horn, C., Mazure, N., and Pouyssegur, J. 2005. Signalling via the hypoxia-inducible factor-1alpha requires multiple posttranslational modifications. Cell Signal 17:1–9.

Brat, D. J., Bellail, A. C., and Van Meir, E. G. 2005. The role of interleukin-8 and its receptors in gliomagenesis and tumoral angiogenesis. Neuro Oncol 7:122–133.

Brat, D. J., Castellano-Sanchez, A. A., Hunter, S. B., Pecot, M., Cohen, C., Hammond, E. H., Devi, S. N., Kaur, B., and Van Meir, E. G. 2004. Pseudopalisades in glioblastoma are hypoxic, express extracellular matrix proteases, and are formed by an actively migrating cell population. Cancer Res 64:920–927.

Brat, D. J., and Van Meir, E. G. 2004. Vaso-occlusive and prothrombotic mechanisms associated with tumor hypoxia, necrosis, and accelerated growth in glioblastoma. Lab Invest 84:397–405.

Broholm, H., Braendstrup, O., and Lauritzen, M. 2001. Nitric oxide synthase expression of oligodendrogliomas. Clin Neuropathol 20:233–238.

Burger, P. C., Vogel, F. S., Green, S. B., and Strike, T. A. 1985. Glioblastoma multiforme and anaplastic astrocytoma. Pathologic criteria and prognostic implications. Cancer 56:1106–1111.

Byzova, T. V., Goldman, C. K., Pampori, N., Thomas, K. A., Bett, A., Shattil, S. J., and Plow, E. F. 2000. A mechanism for modulation of cellular responses to VEGF: activation of the integrins. Mol Cell 6:851–860.

Caine, G. J., Blann, A. D., Stonelake, P. S., Ryan, P., and Lip, G. Y. 2003. Plasma angiopoietin-1, angiopoietin-2 and Tie-2 in breast and prostate cancer: a comparison with VEGF and Flt-1. Eur J Clin Invest 33:883–890.

Cao, Y., Sonveaux, P., Liu, S., Zhao, Y., Mi, J., Clary, B. M., Li, C. Y., Kontos, C. D., and Dewhirst, M. W. 2007. Systemic overexpression of angiopoietin-2 promotes tumor microvessel regression and inhibits angiogenesis and tumor growth. Cancer Res 67:3835–3844.

Carlson, T. R., Feng, Y., Maisonpierre, P. C., Mrksich, M., and Morla, A. O. 2001. Direct cell adhesion to the angiopoietins mediated by integrins. J Biol Chem 276:26516–26525.

Carmeliet, P., and Collen, D. 1999. Role of vascular endothelial growth factor and vascular endothelial growth factor receptors in vascular development. Curr Top Microbiol Immunol 237:133–158.

Carmeliet, P., Ferreira, V., Breier, G., Pollefeyt, S., Kieckens, L., Gertsenstein, M., Fahrig, M., Vandenhoeck, A., Harpal, K., Eberhardt, C., Declercq, C., Pawling, J., Moons, L., Collen, D., Risau, W., and Nagy, A. 1996. Abnormal blood vessel development and lethality in embryos lacking a single VEGF allele. Nature 380:435–439.

Carmeliet, P., and Jain, R. K. 2000. Angiogenesis in cancer and other diseases. Nature 407:249–257.

Carmeliet, P., Moons, L., Luttun, A., Vincenti, V., Compernolle, V., De Mol, M., Wu, Y., Bono, F., Devy, L., Beck, H., Scholz, D., Acker, T., DiPalma, T., Dewerchin, M., Noel, A. Stalmans, I., Barra, A., Blacher, S., Vandendriessche, T., Ponten, A., Eriksson, U., Plate, K. H., Foidart, J. M., Schaper, W., Charnock-Jones, D. S., Hicklin, D. J., Herbert, J. M., Collen, D., and Persico, M. G. 2001. Synergism between vascular endothelial growth factor and placental growth factor contributes to angiogenesis and plasma extravasation in pathological conditions. Nat Med 7:575–583.

Carmeliet, P., Ng, Y. S., Nuyens, D., Theilmeier, G., Brusselmans, K., Cornelissen, I., Ehler, E., Kakkar, V. V., Stalmans, I., Mattot, V., Perriard, J. C., Dewerchin, M., Flameng, W., Nagy, A., Lupu, F., Moons, L., Collen, D., D'Amore, P. A., and Shima, D. T. 1999. Impaired myocardial angiogenesis and ischemic cardiomyopathy in mice lacking the vascular endothelial growth factor isoforms VEGF164 and VEGF188. Nat Med 5:495–502.

Carmeliet, P., and Storkebaum, E. 2002. Vascular and neuronal effects of VEGF in the nervous system: implications for neurological disorders. Semin Cell Dev Biol 13:39–53.

Cascone, I., Napione, L., Maniero, F., Serini, G., and Bussolino, F. 2005. Stable interaction between alpha5beta1 integrin and Tie2 tyrosine kinase receptor regulates endothelial cell response to Ang-1. J Cell Biol 170:993–1004.

Caunt, M., Mak, J., Liang, W. C., Stawicki, S., Pan, Q., Tong, R. K., Kowalski, J., Ho, C., Reslan, H. B., Ross, J., Berry, L., Kasman, I., Zlot, C., Cheng, Z., Le Couter, J., Filvaroff, E. H., Plowman, G., Peale, F., French, D., Carano, R., Koch, A. W., Wu, Y., Watts, R. J., Tessier-Lavigne, M., and Bagri, A. 2008. Blocking neuropilin-2 function inhibits tumor cell metastasis. Cancer Cell 13:331–342.

Cheng, S. Y., Huang, H. J., Nagane, M., Ji, X. D., Wang, D., Shih, C. C., Arap, W., Huang, C. M., and Cavenee, W. K. 1996. Suppression of glioblastoma angiogenicity and tumorigenicity by inhibition of endogenous expression of vascular endothelial growth factor. Proc Natl Acad Sci USA 93:8502–8507.

Cheng, S.-Y., Nagane, M., Su Huang, H.-J., and Cavenee, W. K. 1997. Intracerebral Tumor-Associated Hemorrhage Caused By Overexpression of Vascular Endothelial Growth Factor (VEGF) Isoforms, $VEGF_{121}$ and VEGF $_{165}$ But Not $VEGF_{189}$. Proc Natl Acad Sci USA 94:12081–12087.

Cho, C. H., Kim, K. E., Byun, J., Jang, H. S., Kim, D. K., Baluk, P., Baffert, F., Lee, G. M., Mochizuki, N., Kim, J., Jeon, B. H., McDonald, D. M., and Koh, G. Y. 2005. Long-term and sustained COMP-Ang1 induces long-lasting vascular enlargement and enhanced blood flow. Circ Res 97:86–94.

Claffey, K. P., Wilkison, W. O., and Spiegelman, B. M. 1992. Vascular endothelial growth factor. Regulation by cell differentiation and activated second messenger pathways. J Biol Chem 267:16317–16322.

Clarke, K., Smith, K., Gullick, W. J., and Harris, A. L. 2001. Mutant epidermal growth factor receptor enhances induction of vascular endothelial growth factor by hypoxia and insulin-like growth factor-1 via a PI3 kinase dependent pathway. Br J Cancer 84:1322–1329.

Claudio, P. P., Stiegler, P., Howard, C. M., Bellan, C., Minimo, C., Tosi, G. M., Rak, J., Kovatich, A., De Fazio, P., Micheli, P., Caputi, M., Leoncini, L., Kerbel, R., Giordano, G. G., and Giordano, A. 2001. RB2/p130 gene-enhanced expression down-regulates vascular endothelial growth factor expression and inhibits angiogenesis in vivo. Cancer Res 61:462–468.

Clauss, M., Weich, H., Breier, G., Knies, U., Rockl, W., Waltenberger, J., and Risau, W. 1996. The vascular endothelial growth factor receptor Flt-1 mediates biological activities. Implications for a functional role of placenta growth factor in monocyte activation and chemotaxis. J Biol Chem 271:17629–17634.

Cobbs, C. S., Brenman, J. E., Aldape, K. D., Bredt, D. S., and Israel, M. A. 1995. Expression of nitric oxide synthase in human central nervous system tumors. Cancer Res 55:727–730.

Compernolle, V., Brusselmans, K., Acker, T., Hoet, P., Tjwa, M., Beck, H., Plaisance, S., Dor, Y., Keshet, E., Lupu, F., Nemery, B., Dewerchin, M., Van Veldhoven, P., Plate, K., Moons, L., Collen, D., and Carmeliet, P. 2002. Loss of HIF-2alpha and inhibition of VEGF impair fetal lung maturation, whereas treatment with VEGF prevents fatal respiratory distress in premature mice. Nat Med 8:702–710.

Connolly, D. T., Olander, J. V., Heuvelman, D., Nelson, R., Monsell, R., Siegel, N., Haymore, B. L., Leimgruber, R., and Feder, J. 1989. Human vascular permeability factor. Isolation from U937 cells. J Biol Chem 264:20017–20024.

Dallabrida, S. M., Ismail, N., Oberle, J. R., Himes, B. E., and Rupnick, M. A. 2005. Angiopoietin-1 promotes cardiac and skeletal myocyte survival through integrins. Circ Res 96:e8–24.

Dameron, K. M., Volpert, O. V., Tainsky, M. A., and Bouck, N. 1994. Control of angiogenesis in fibroblasts by p53 regulation of thrombospondin-1. Science 265:1582–1584.

Daumas-Duport, C., Tucker, M. L., Kolles, H., Cervera, P., Beuvon, F., Varlet, P., Udo, N., Koziak, M., and Chodkiewicz, J. P. 1997. Oligodendrogliomas. Part II: A new grading system based on morphological and imaging criteria. J Neurooncol 34:61–78.

Davis, S., Aldrich, T. H., Jones, P. F., Acheson, A., Compton, D. L., Jain, V., Ryan, T. E., Bruno, J., Radziejewski, C., Maisonpierre, P. C., and Yancopoulos, G. D. 1996. Isolation of angiopoietin-1, a ligand for the TIE2 receptor, by secretion-trap expression cloning [see comments]. Cell 87:1161–1169.

Davis, S., Papadopoulos, N., Aldrich, T. H., Maisonpierre, P. C., Huang, T., Kovac, L., Xu, A., Leidich, R., Radziejewska, E., Rafique, A., Goldberg, J., Jain, V., Bailey, K., Karow, M., Fandl, J., Samuelsson, S. J., Ioffe, E., Rudge, J. S., Daly, T. J., Radziejewski, C., and Yancopoulos, G. D. 2003. Angiopoietins have distinct modular domains essential for receptor binding, dimerization and superclustering. Nat Struct Biol 10:38–44.

de Vries, C., Escobedo, J. A., Ueno, H., Houck, K., Ferrara, N., and Williams, L. T. 1992. The fms-like tyrosine kinase, a receptor for vascular endothelial growth factor. Science 255:989–991.

Desbaillets, I., Diserens, A. C., de Tribolet, N., Hamou, M. F., and Van Meir, E. G. 1999. Regulation of interleukin-8 expression by reduced oxygen pressure in human glioblastoma. Oncogene 18:1447–1456.

Desbaillets, I., Diserens, A. C., Tribolet, N., Hamou, M. F., and Van Meir, E. G. 1997. Upregulation of interleukin 8 by oxygen-deprived cells in glioblastoma suggests a role in leukocyte activation, chemotaxis, and angiogenesis. J Exp Med 186:1201–1212.

Dimmeler, S., and Zeiher, A. M. 2000. Akt takes center stage in angiogenesis signaling. Circ Res 86:4–5.

Ding, H., Roncari, L., Wu, X., Lau, N., Shannon, P., Nagy, A., and Guha, A. 2001. Expression and hypoxic regulation of angiopoietins in human astrocytomas. Neuro Oncol 3:1–10.

Ding, H., Wu, X., Roncari, L., Lau, N., Shannon, P., Nagy, A., and Guha, A. 2000. Expression and regulation of neuropilin-1 in human astrocytomas. Int J Cancer 88:584–592.

Donnini, S., Machein, M. R., Plate, K. H., and Weich, H. A. 1999. Expression and localization of placenta growth factor and PlGF receptors in human meningiomas. J Pathol 189:66–71.

Dor, Y., Camenisch, T. D., Itin, A., Fishman, G. I., McDonald, J. A., Carmeliet, P., and Keshet, E. 2001. A novel role for VEGF in endocardial cushion formation and its potential contribution to congenital heart defects. Development 128:1531–1538.

Dor, Y., Djonov, V., Abramovitch, R., Itin, A., Fishman, G. I., Carmeliet, P., Goelman, G., and Keshet, E. 2002. Conditional switching of VEGF provides new insights into adult neovascularization and pro-angiogenic therapy. Embo J 21:1939–1947.

Du, R., Lu, K. V., Petritsch, C., Liu, P., Ganss, R., Passegue, E., Song, H., Vandenberg, S., Johnson, R. S., Werb, Z., and Bergers, G. 2008. HIF1alpha induces the recruitment of bone marrow-derived vascular modulatory cells to regulate tumor angiogenesis and invasion. Cancer Cell 13:206–220.

Eklund, L., and Olsen, B. R. 2006. Tie receptors and their angiopoietin ligands are context-dependent regulators of vascular remodeling. Exp Cell Res 312:630–641.

Eliceiri, B. P. 2001. Integrin and growth factor receptor crosstalk. Circ Res 89:1104–1110.

Ellie, E., Loiseau, H., Lafond, F., Arsaut, J., and Demotes-Mainard, J. 1995. Differential expression of inducible nitric oxide synthase mRNA in human brain tumours. Neuroreport 7:294–296.

Ellis, L. M., and Hicklin, D. J. 2008. VEGF-targeted therapy: mechanisms of anti-tumour activity. Nat Rev Cancer 8:579–591.

Enholm, B., Karpanen, T., Jeltsch, M., Kubo, H., Stenback, F., Prevo, R., Jackson, D. G., Yla-Herttuala, S., and Alitalo, K. 2001. Adenoviral expression of vascular endothelial growth factor-C induces lymphangiogenesis in the skin. Circ Res 88:623–629.

Eremina, V., Sood, M., Haigh, J., Nagy, A., Lajoie, G., Ferrara, N., Gerber, H. P., Kikkawa, Y., Miner, J. H., and Quaggin, S. E. 2003. Glomerular-specific alterations of VEGF-A expression lead to distinct congenital and acquired renal diseases. J Clin Invest 111:707–716.

Etoh, T., Inoue, H., Tanaka, S., Barnard, G. F., Kitano, S., and Mori, M. 2001. Angiopoietin-2 is related to tumor angiogenesis in gastric carcinoma: possible in vivo regulation via induction of proteases. Cancer Res 61:2145–2153.

Favier, B., Alam, A., Barron, P., Bonnin, J., Laboudie, P., Fons, P., Mandron, M., Herault, J. P., Neufeld, G., Savi, P., Herbert, J. M., and Bono, F. 2006. Neuropilin-2 interacts with VEGFR-2 and VEGFR-3 and promotes human endothelial cell survival and migration. Blood 108:1243–1250.

Feng, C. W., Wang, L. D., Jiao, L. H., Liu, B., Zheng, S., and Xie, X. J. 2002. Expression of p53, inducible nitric oxide synthase and vascular endothelial growth factor in gastric precancerous and cancerous lesions: correlation with clinical features. BMC Cancer 2:8.

Ferrara, N., Carver-Moore, K., Chen, H., Dowd, M., Lu, L., O'Shea, K. S., Powell-Braxton, L., Hillan, K. J., and Moore, M. W. 1996. Heterozygous embryonic lethality induced by targeted inactivation of the VEGF gene. Nature 380:439–442.

Ferrara, N., Gerber, H. P., and LeCouter, J. 2003. The biology of VEGF and its receptors. Nat Med 9:669–676.

Fischer, I., Gagner, J. P., Law, M., Newcomb, E. W., and Zagzag, D. 2005. Angiogenesis in gliomas: biology and molecular pathophysiology. Brain Pathol 15:297–310.

Folkman, J. 2007. Angiogenesis: an organizing principle for drug discovery? Nat Rev Drug Discov 6:273–286.

Fong, G. H., Rossant, J., Gertsenstein, M., and Breitman, M. L. 1995. Role of the Flt-1 receptor tyrosine kinase in regulating the assembly of vascular endothelium. Nature 376:66–70.

Fong, G. H., Zhang, L., Bryce, D. M., and Peng, J. 1999. Increased hemangioblast commitment, not vascular disorganization, is the primary defect in flt-1 knock-out mice. Development 126:3015–3025.

Fournier, E., Dubreuil, P., Birnbaum, D., and Borg, J. P. 1995. Mutation at tyrosine residue 1337 abrogates ligand-dependent transforming capacity of the FLT4 receptor. Oncogene 11:921–931.

Fredriksson, L., Li, H., and Eriksson, U. 2004. The PDGF family: four gene products form five dimeric isoforms. Cytokine Growth Factor Rev 15:197–204.
Friedlander, M., Brooks, P. C., Shaffer, R. W., Kincaid, C. M., Varner, J. A., and Cheresh, D. A. 1995. Definition of two angiogenic pathways by distinct alpha v integrins. Science 270:1500–1502.
Fujisawa, H., Ogura, T., Hokari, A., Weisz, A., Yamashita, J., and Esumi, H. 1995. Inducible nitric oxide synthase in a human glioblastoma cell line. J Neurochem 64:85–91.
Fukumura, D., Xu, L., Chen, Y., Gohongi, T., Seed, B., and Jain, R. K. 2001. Hypoxia and acidosis independently up-regulate vascular endothelial growth factor transcription in brain tumors in vivo. Cancer Res 61:6020–6024.
Fukumura, D., Yuan, F., Endo, M., and Jain, R. K. 1997. Role of nitric oxide in tumor microcirculation. Blood flow, vascular permeability, and leukocyte-endothelial interactions. Am J Pathol 150:713–725.
Furnari, F. B., Fenton, T., Bachoo, R. M., Mukasa, A., Stommel, J. M., Stegh, A., Hahn, W. C., Ligon, K. L., Louis, D. N., Brennan, C., Chin, L., DePinho, R. A., and Cavenee, W. K. 2007. Malignant astrocytic glioma: genetics, biology, and paths to treatment. Genes Dev 21:2683–2710.
Gale, N. W., Thurston, G., Hackett, S. F., Renard, R., Wang, Q., McClain, J., Martin, C., Witte, C., Witte, M. H., Jackson, D., Suri, C., Campochiaro, P. A., Wiegand, S. J., and Yancopoulos, G. D. 2002. Angiopoietin-2 is required for postnatal angiogenesis and lymphatic patterning, and only the latter role is rescued by Angiopoietin-1. Dev Cell 3:411–423.
Galli, R., Binda, E., Orfanelli, U., Cipelletti, B., Gritti, A., De Vitis, S., Fiocco, R., Foroni, C., Dimeco, F., and Vescovi, A. 2004. Isolation and characterization of tumorigenic, stem-like neural precursors from human glioblastoma. Cancer Res 64:7011–7021.
Garbossa, D., Fontanella, M., Pagni, C. A., and Vercelli, A. 2001. Nitric oxide synthase and cytochrome c oxidase changes in the tumoural and peritumoural cerebral cortex. Acta Neurochir (Wien) 143:897–908.
Garkavtsev, I., Kozin, S. V., Chernova, O., Xu, L., Winkler, F., Brown, E., Barnett, G. H., and Jain, R. K. 2004. The candidate tumour suppressor protein ING4 regulates brain tumour growth and angiogenesis. Nature 428:328–332.
Gerber, H. P., Hillan, K. J., Ryan, A. M., Kowalski, J., Keller, G. A., Rangell, L., Wright, B. D., Radtke, F., Aguet, M., and Ferrara, N. 1999a. VEGF is required for growth and survival in neonatal mice. Development 126:1149–1159.
Gerber, H. P., Vu, T. H., Ryan, A. M., Kowalski, J., Werb, Z., and Ferrara, N. 1999b. VEGF couples hypertrophic cartilage remodeling, ossification and angiogenesis during endochondrial bone formation. Nat Med 5:623–628.
Gerhardt, H., Ruhrberg, C., Abramsson, A., Fujisawa, H., Shima, D., and Betsholtz, C. 2004. Neuropilin-1 is required for endothelial tip cell guidance in the developing central nervous system. Dev Dyn 231:503–509.
Gille, H., Kowalski, J., Yu, L., Chen, H., Pisabarro, M. T., Davis-Smyth, T., and Ferrara, N. 2000. A repressor sequence in the juxtamembrane domain of Flt-1 (VEGFR-1) constitutively inhibits vascular endothelial growth factor-dependent phosphatidylinositol 3'-kinase activation and endothelial cell migration. Embo J 19:4064–4073.
Gluzman-Poltorak, Z., Cohen, T., Herzog, Y., and Neufeld, G. 2000. Neuropilin-2 is a receptor for the vascular endothelial growth factor (VEGF) forms VEGF-145 and VEGF-165 [corrected]. J Biol Chem 275:18040–18045.
Gollmer, J. C., Ladoux, A., Gioanni, J., Paquis, P., Dubreuil, A., Chatel, M., and Frelin, C. 2000. Expression of vascular endothelial growth factor-b in human astrocytoma. Neuro Oncol 2:80–86.
Gomez-Manzano, C., Fueyo, J., Jiang, H., Glass, T. L., Lee, H. Y., Hu, M., Liu, J. L., Jasti, S. L., Liu, T. J., Conrad, C. A., and Yung, W. K. 2003. Mechanisms underlying PTEN regulation of vascular endothelial growth factor and angiogenesis. Ann Neurol 53:109–117.

Good, D. J., Polverini, P. J., Rastinejad, F., Le Beau, M. M., Lemons, R. S., Frazier, W. A., and Bouck, N. P. 1990. A tumor suppressor-dependent inhibitor of angiogenesis is immunologically and functionally indistinguishable from a fragment of thrombospondin. Proc Natl Acad Sci USA 87:6624–6628.

Grau, S. J., Trillsch, F., Herms, J., Thon, N., Nelson, P. J., Tonn, J. C., and Goldbrunner, R. 2007. Expression of VEGFR3 in glioma endothelium correlates with tumor grade. J Neurooncol 82:141–150.

Gray, M. J., Van Buren, G., Dallas, N. A., Xia, L., Wang, X., Yang, A. D., Somcio, R. J., Lin, Y. G., Lim, S., Fan, F., Mangala, L. S., Arumugam, T., Logsdon, C. D., Lopez-Berestein, G., Sood, A. K., and Ellis, L. M. 2008. Therapeutic targeting of neuropilin-2 on colorectal carcinoma cells implanted in the murine liver. J Natl Cancer Inst 100:109–120.

Grimmond, S., Lagercrantz, J., Drinkwater, C., Silins, G., Townson, S., Pollock, P., Gotley, D., Carson, E., Rakar, S., Nordenskjold, M., Ward, L., Hayward, N., and Weber, G. 1996. Cloning and characterization of a novel human gene related to vascular endothelial growth factor. Genome Res 6:124–131.

Grosskreutz, C. L., Anand-Apte, B., Duplaa, C., Quinn, T. P., Terman, B. I., Zetter, B., and D'Amore, P. A. 1999. Vascular endothelial growth factor-induced migration of vascular smooth muscle cells in vitro. Microvasc Res 58:128–136.

Guo, P., Hu, B., Gu, W., Xu, L., Wang, D., Huang, H. J., Cavenee, W. K., and Cheng, S. Y. 2003. Platelet-derived growth factor-B enhances glioma angiogenesis by stimulating vascular endothelial growth factor expression in tumor endothelia and by promoting pericyte recruitment. Am J Pathol 162:1083–1093.

Guo, P., Imanishi, Y., Cackowski, F. C., Jarzynka, M. J., Tao, H. Q., Nishikawa, R., Hirose, T., Hu, B., and Cheng, S. Y. 2005. Up-regulation of angiopoietin-2, matrix metalloprotease-2, membrane type 1 metalloprotease, and laminin 5 gamma 2 correlates with the invasiveness of human glioma. Am J Pathol 166:877–890.

Guo, P., Xu, L., Pan, S., Brekken, R. A., Yang, S. T., Whitaker, G. B., Nagane, M., Thorpe, P. E., Rosenbaum, J. S., Su Huang, H. J., Cavenee, W. K., and Cheng, S. Y. 2001. Vascular endothelial growth factor isoforms display distinct activities in promoting tumor angiogenesis at different anatomic sites. Cancer Res 61:8569–8577.

Haas-Kogan, D., and Stokoe, D. 2008. PTEN in brain tumors. Expert Rev Neurother 8:599–610.

Haigh, J. J., Gerber, H. P., Ferrara, N., and Wagner, E. F. 2000. Conditional inactivation of VEGF-A in areas of collagen2a1 expression results in embryonic lethality in the heterozygous state. Development 127:1445–1453.

Hara, E., Takahashi, K., Tominaga, T., Kumabe, T., Kayama, T., Suzuki, H., Fujita, H., Yoshimoto, T., Shirato, K., and Shibahara, S. 1996. Expression of heme oxygenase and inducible nitric oxide synthase mRNA in human brain tumors. Biochem Biophys Res Commun 224:153–158.

Harfouche, R., Hassessian, H. M., Guo, Y., Faivre, V., Srikant, C. B., Yancopoulos, G. D., and Hussain, S. N. 2002. Mechanisms which mediate the antiapoptotic effects of angiopoietin-1 on endothelial cells. Microvasc Res 64:135–147.

Hatanaka, H., Abe, Y., Naruke, M., Tokunaga, T., Oshika, Y., Kawakami, T., Osada, H., Nagata, J., Kamochi, J., Tsuchida, T., Kijima, H., Yamazaki, H., Inoue, H., Ueyama, Y., and Nakamura, M. 2001. Significant correlation between interleukin 10 expression and vascularization through angiopoietin/TIE2 networks in non-small cell lung cancer. Clin Cancer Res 7:1287–1292.

Hawighorst, T., Skobe, M., Streit, M., Hong, Y. K., Velasco, P., Brown, L. F., Riccardi, L., Lange-Asschenfeldt, B., and Detmar, M. 2002. Activation of the tie2 receptor by angiopoietin-1 enhances tumor vessel maturation and impairs squamous cell carcinoma growth. Am J Pathol 160:1381–1392.

Hayes, A. J., Huang, W. Q., Mallah, J., Yang, D., Lippman, M. E., and Li, L. Y. 1999. Angiopoietin-1 and its receptor Tie-2 participate in the regulation of capillary-like tubule formation and survival of endothelial cells. Microvasc Res 58:224–237.

Hayes, A. J., Huang, W. Q., Yu, J., Maisonpierre, P. C., Liu, A., Kern, F. G., Lippman, M. E., McLeskey, S. W., and Li, L. Y. 2000. Expression and function of angiopoietin-1 in breast cancer. Br J Cancer 83:1154–1160.

Heldin, C. H., Eriksson, U., and Ostman, A. 2002. New members of the platelet-derived growth factor family of mitogens. Arch Biochem Biophys 398:284–290.

Heldin, C. H., and Westermark, B. 1999. Mechanism of action and in vivo role of platelet-derived growth factor. Physiol Rev 79:1283–1316.

Hermanson, M., Funa, K., Hartman, M., Claesson-Welsh, L., Heldin, C. H., Westermark, B., and Nister, M. 1992. Platelet-derived growth factor and its receptors in human glioma tissue: expression of messenger RNA and protein suggests the presence of autocrine and paracrine loops. Cancer Res 52:3213–3219.

Hermanson, M., Olsson, T., Westermark, B., and Funa, K. 1995. PDGF and its receptors following facial nerve axotomy in rats: expression in neurons and surrounding glia. Exp Brain Res 102:415–422.

Herzog, Y., Kalcheim, C., Kahane, N., Reshef, R., and Neufeld, G. 2001. Differential expression of neuropilin-1 and neuropilin-2 in arteries and veins. Mech Dev 109:115–119.

Hiratsuka, S., Minowa, O., Kuno, J., Noda, T., and Shibuya, M. 1998. Flt-1 lacking the tyrosine kinase domain is sufficient for normal development and angiogenesis in mice. Proc Natl Acad Sci USA 95:9349–9354.

Holash, J., Maisonpierre, P. C., Compton, D., Boland, P., Alexander, C. R., Zagzag, D., Yancopoulos, G. D., and Wiegand, S. J. 1999. Vessel cooption, regression, and growth in tumors mediated by angiopoietins and VEGF. Science 284:1994–1998.

Horst, H. A., Scheithauer, B. W., Kelly, P. J., and Kovach, J. S. 1992. Distribution of transforming growth factor-beta 1 in human astrocytomas. Hum Pathol 23:1284–1288.

Hu, B., Guo, P., Bar-Joseph, I., Imanishi, Y., Jarzynka, M. J., Bogler, O., Mikkelsen, T., Hirose, T., Nishikawa, R., and Cheng, S. Y. 2007. Neuropilin-1 promotes human glioma progression through potentiating the activity of the HGF/SF autocrine pathway. Oncogene 26:5577–5586.

Hu, B., Guo, P., Fang, Q., Tao, H. Q., Wang, D., Nagane, M., Huang, H. J., Gunji, Y., Nishikawa, R., Alitalo, K., Cavenee, W. K., and Cheng, S. Y. 2003. Angiopoietin-2 induces human glioma invasion through the activation of matrix metalloprotease-2. Proc Natl Acad Sci USA 100:8904–8909.

Hu, B., Jarzynka, M. J., Guo, P., Imanishi, Y., Schlaepfer, D. D., and Cheng, S. Y. 2006. Angiopoietin 2 Induces Glioma Cell Invasion by Stimulating Matrix Metalloprotease 2 Expression through the {alpha}v{beta}1 Integrin and Focal Adhesion Kinase Signaling Pathway. Cancer Res 66:775–783.

Hu, P., Margolis, B., Skolnik, E. Y., Lammers, R., Ullrich, A., and Schlessinger, J. 1992. Interaction of phosphatidylinositol 3-kinase-associated p85 with epidermal growth factor and platelet-derived growth factor receptors. Mol Cell Biol 12:981–990.

Huang, L., Turck, C. W., Rao, P., and Peters, K. G. 1995. GRB2 and SH-PTP2: potentially important endothelial signaling molecules downstream of the TEK/TIE2 receptor tyrosine kinase. Oncogene 11:2097–2103.

Imanishi, Y., Hu, B., Jarzynka, M. J., Guo, P., Elishaev, E., Bar-Joseph, I., and Cheng, S. Y. 2007. Angiopoietin-2 stimulates breast cancer metastasis through the {alpha}5{beta}1 integrin-mediated pathway. Cancer Res 67:4254–4263.

Jain, R. K., di Tomaso, E., Duda, D. G., Loeffler, J. S., Sorensen, A. G., and Batchelor, T. T. 2007. Angiogenesis in brain tumours. Nat Rev Neurosci 8:610–622.

Jeltsch, M., Kaipainen, A., Joukov, V., Meng, X., Lakso, M., Rauvala, H., Swartz, M., Fukumura, D., Jain, R. K., and Alitalo, K. 1997. Hyperplasia of lymphatic vessels in VEGF-C transgenic mice. Science 276:1423–1425.

Jenny, B., Harrison, J. A., Baetens, D., Tille, J. C., Burkhardt, K., Mottaz, H., Kiss, J. Z., Dietrich, P. Y., De Tribolet, N., Pizzolato, G. P., and Pepper, M. S. 2006. Expression and localization of VEGF-C and VEGFR-3 in glioblastomas and haemangioblastomas. J Pathol 209:34–43.

Jeong, J. W., Bae, M. K., Ahn, M. Y., Kim, S. H., Sohn, T. K., Bae, M. H., Yoo, M. A., Song, E. J., Lee, K. J., and Kim, K. W. 2002. Regulation and destabilization of HIF-1alpha by ARD1-mediated acetylation. Cell 111:709–720.

Jones, N., and Dumont, D. J. 1999. Recruitment of Dok-R to the EGF receptor through its PTB domain is required for attenuation of Erk MAP kinase activation. Curr Biol 9:1057–1060.

Jones, N., Iljin, K., Dumont, D. J., and Alitalo, K. 2001. Tie receptors: new modulators of angiogenic and lymphangiogenic responses. Nat Rev Mol Cell Biol 2:257–267.

Jones, N., Master, Z., Jones, J., Bouchard, D., Gunji, Y., Sasaki, H., Daly, R., Alitalo, K., and Dumont, D. J. 1999. Identification of Tek/Tie2 binding partners. Binding to a multifunctional docking site mediates cell survival and migration. J Biol Chem 274:30896–30905.

Joukov, V., Sorsa, T., Kumar, V., Jeltsch, M., Claesson-Welsh, L., Cao, Y., Saksela, O., Kalkkinen, N., and Alitalo, K. 1997. Proteolytic processing regulates receptor specificity and activity of VEGF-C. Embo J 16:3898–3911.

Kanda, S., Miyata, Y., Mochizuki, Y., Matsuyama, T., and Kanetake, H. 2005. Angiopoietin 1 is mitogenic for cultured endothelial cells. Cancer Res 65:6820–6827.

Karkkainen, M. J., Haiko, P., Sainio, K., Partanen, J., Taipale, J., Petrova, T. V., Jeltsch, M., Jackson, D. G., Talikka, M., Rauvala, H., Betsholtz, C., and Alitalo, K. 2004. Vascular endothelial growth factor C is required for sprouting of the first lymphatic vessels from embryonic veins. Nat Immunol 5:74–80.

Kashiwagi, S., Tsukada, K., Xu, L., Miyazaki, J., Kozin, S. V., Tyrrell, J. A., Sessa, W. C., Gerweck, L. E., Jain, R. K., and Fukumura, D. 2008. Perivascular nitric oxide gradients normalize tumor vasculature. Nat Med 14:255–257.

Kaur, B., Brat, D. J., Devi, N. S., and Van Meir, E. G. 2005a. Vasculostatin, a proteolytic fragment of brain angiogenesis inhibitor 1, is an antiangiogenic and antitumorigenic factor. Oncogene 24:3632–3642.

Kaur, B., Khwaja, F. W., Severson, E. A., Matheny, S. L., Brat, D. J., and Van Meir, E. G. 2005b. Hypoxia and the hypoxia-inducible-factor pathway in glioma growth and angiogenesis. Neuro Oncol 7:134–153.

Kavanaugh, W. M., Harsh, G. R. t., Starksen, N. F., Rocco, C. M., and Williams, L. T. 1988. Transcriptional regulation of the A and B chain genes of platelet-derived growth factor in microvascular endothelial cells. J Biol Chem 263:8470–8472.

Kawasaki, T., Kitsukawa, T., Bekku, Y., Matsuda, Y., Sanbo, M., Yagi, T., and Fujisawa, H. 1999. A requirement for neuropilin-1 in embryonic vessel formation. Development 126:4895–4902.

Ke, L. D., Shi, Y. X., and Yung, W. K. 2002. VEGF(121), VEGF(165) overexpression enhances tumorigenicity in U251 MG but not in NG-1 glioma cells. Cancer Res 62:1854–1861.

Keck, P. J., Hauser, S. D., Krivi, G., Sanzo, K., Warren, T., Feder, J., and Connolly, D. T. 1989. Vascular permeability factor, an endothelial cell mitogen related to PDGF. Science 246:1309–1312.

Kerwin, J. F., Jr., Lancaster, J. R., Jr., and Feldman, P. L. 1995. Nitric oxide: a new paradigm for second messengers. J Med Chem 38:4343–4362.

Kim, I., Kim, J. H., Moon, S. O., Kwak, H. J., Kim, N. G., and Koh, G. Y. 2000. Angiopoietin-2 at high concentration can enhance endothelial cell survival through the phosphatidylinositol 3'-kinase/Akt signal transduction pathway. Oncogene 19: 4549–4552.

Kim, I., Moon, S. O., Han, C. Y., Pak, Y. K., Moon, S. K., Kim, J. J., and Koh, G. Y. 2001. The angiopoietin-tie2 system in coronary artery endothelium prevents oxidized low-density lipoprotein-induced apoptosis. Cardiovasc Res 49:872–881.

Kiselyov, A., Balakin, K. V., and Tkachenko, S. E. 2007. VEGF/VEGFR signalling as a target for inhibiting angiogenesis. Expert Opin Investig Drugs 16:83–107.

Kitamoto, Y., Tokunaga, H., and Tomita, K. 1997. Vascular endothelial growth factor is an essential molecule for mouse kidney development: glomerulogenesis and nephrogenesis. J Clin Invest 99:2351–2357.

Kitsukawa, T., Shimono, A., Kawakami, A., Kondoh, H., and Fujisawa, H. 1995. Over-expression of a membrane protein, neuropilin, in chimeric mice causes anomalies in the cardiovascular system, nervous system and limbs. Development 121:4309–4318.

Klagsbrun, M., Takashima, S., and Mamluk, R. 2002. The role of neuropilin in vascular and tumor biology. Adv Exp Med Biol 515:33–48.

Kleihues, P., and Cavenee, W. K., eds. (2000). Pathology & Genetics: Tumours of the Nervous System (Lyon: IARC Press).

Klotz, T., Bloch, W., Volberg, C., Engelmann, U., and Addicks, K. 1998. Selective expression of inducible nitric oxide synthase in human prostate carcinoma. Cancer 82:1897–1903.

Koga, K., Todaka, T., Morioka, M., Hamada, J., Kai, Y., Yano, S., Okamura, A., Takakura, N., Suda, T., and Ushio, Y. 2001. Expression of angiopoietin-2 in human glioma cells and its role for angiogenesis. Cancer Res 61:6248–6254.

Kolodkin, A. L., Levengood, D. V., Rowe, E. G., Tai, Y. T., Giger, R. J., and Ginty, D. D. 1997. Neuropilin is a semaphorin III receptor. Cell 90:753–762.

Kong, G., Kim, E., Kim, W., Lee, Y., Lee, J., Paik, S., Rhee, J., Choi, K., and Lee, K. 2001a. Inducible nitric oxide synthase (iNOS) Immunoreactivity and its relationship to cell proliferation, apoptosis, angiogenesis, clinicopathologic characteristics, and patient survival in pancreatic cancer. Int J Gastrointest Cancer 29:133–140.

Kong, G., Kim, E. K., Kim, W. S., Lee, Y. W., Lee, J. K., Paik, S. W., Rhee, J. C., Choi, K. W., and Lee, K. T. 2001b. Inducible nitric oxide synthase (iNOS) immunoreactivity and its relationship to cell proliferation, apoptosis, angiogenesis, clinicopathologic characteristics, and patient survival in pancreatic cancer. Int J Pancreatol 29:133–140.

Koochekpour, S., Merzak, A., and Pilkington, G. J. 1996. Vascular endothelial growth factor production is stimulated by gangliosides and TGF-beta isoforms in human glioma cells in vitro. Cancer Lett 102:209–215.

Kukk, E., Lymboussaki, A., Taira, S., Kaipainen, A., Jeltsch, M., Joukov, V., and Alitalo, K. 1996. VEGF-C receptor binding and pattern of expression with VEGFR-3 suggests a role in lymphatic vascular development. Development 122:3829–3837.

Kwak, H. J., So, J. N., Lee, S. J., Kim, I., and Koh, G. Y. 1999. Angiopoietin-1 is an apoptosis survival factor for endothelial cells. FEBS Lett 448:249–253.

Lam-Himlin, D., Espey, M. G., Perry, G., Smith, M. A., and Castellani, R. J. 2006. Malignant glioma progression and nitric oxide. Neurochem Int 49:764–768.

Lasorella, A., Rothschild, G., Yokota, Y., Russell, R. G., and Iavarone, A. 2005. Id2 mediates tumor initiation, proliferation, and angiogenesis in Rb mutant mice. Mol Cell Biol 25:3563–3574.

Laterra, J., Nam, M., Rosen, E., Rao, J. S., Lamszus, K., Goldberg, I. D., and Johnston, P. 1997. Scatter factor/hepatocyte growth factor gene transfer enhances glioma growth and angiogenesis in vivo. Lab Invest 76:565–577.

Lawler, J., Miao, W. M., Duquette, M., Bouck, N., Bronson, R. T., and Hynes, R. O. 2001. Thrombospondin-1 gene expression affects survival and tumor spectrum of p53-deficient mice. Am J Pathol 159:1949–1956.

Lee, O. H., Xu, J., Fueyo, J., Alonso, M. M., Liu, D., Martin, V., Jiang, H., Piao, Y., Liu, T. J., and Gomez-Manzano, C. 2008. Angiopoietin-2 decreases vascular endothelial growth factor expression by modulating HIF-1 alpha levels in gliomas. Oncogene 27:1310–1314.

Leung, D. W., Cachianes, G., Kuang, W. J., Goeddel, D. V., and Ferrara, N. 1989. Vascular endothelial growth factor is a secreted angiogenic mitogen. Science 246:1306–1309.

Lind, A. J., Wikstrom, P., Granfors, T., Egevad, L., Stattin, P., and Bergh, A. 2005. Angiopoietin 2 expression is related to histological grade, vascular density, metastases, and outcome in prostate cancer. Prostate 62:394–399.

Lindahl, P., Hellstrom, M., Kalen, M., Karlsson, L., Pekny, M., Pekna, M., Soriano, P., and Betsholtz, C. 1998. Paracrine PDGF-B/PDGF-Rbeta signaling controls mesangial cell development in kidney glomeruli. Development 125:3313–3322.

Lindahl, P., Johansson, B. R., Leveen, P., and Betsholtz, C. 1997a. Pericyte loss and microaneurysm formation in PDGF-B-deficient mice. Science 277:242–245.

Lindahl, P., Karlsson, L., Hellstrom, M., Gebre-Medhin, S., Willetts, K., Heath, J. K., and Betsholtz, C. 1997b. Alveogenesis failure in PDGF-A-deficient mice is coupled to lack of distal spreading of alveolar smooth muscle cell progenitors during lung development. Development 124:3943–3953.

Lobov, I. B., Brooks, P. C., and Lang, R. A. 2002. Angiopoietin-2 displays VEGF-dependent modulation of capillary structure and endothelial cell survival in vivo. Proc Natl Acad Sci USA 99:11205–11210.

Lokker, N. A., Sullivan, C. M., Hollenbach, S. J., Israel, M. A., and Giese, N. A. 2002. Platelet-derived growth factor (PDGF) autocrine signaling regulates survival and mitogenic pathways in glioblastoma cells: evidence that the novel PDGF-C and PDGF-D ligands may play a role in the development of brain tumors. Cancer Res 62:3729–3735.

Lund, E. L., Bastholm, L., and Kristjansen, P. E. 2000. Therapeutic synergy of TNP-470 and ionizing radiation: effects on tumor growth, vessel morphology, and angiogenesis in human glioblastoma multiforme xenografts. Clin Cancer Res 6:971–978.

Lyttle, D. J., Fraser, K. M., Fleming, S. B., Mercer, A. A., and Robinson, A. J. 1994. Homologs of vascular endothelial growth factor are encoded by the poxvirus orf virus. J Virol 68:84–92.

MacDonald, T. J., Stewart, C. F., Kocak, M., Goldman, S., Ellenbogen, R. G., Phillips, P., Lafond, D., Poussaint, T. Y., Kieran, M. W., Boyett, J. M., and Kun, L. E. 2008. Phase I clinical trial of cilengitide in children with refractory brain tumors: pediatric brain tumor consortium study PBTC-012. J Clin Oncol 26:919–924.

Machein, M. R., Knedla, A., Knoth, R., Wagner, S., Neuschl, E., and Plate, K. H. 2004. Angiopoietin-1 promotes tumor angiogenesis in a rat glioma model. Am J Pathol 165:1557–1570.

Maisonpierre, P. C., Suri, C., Jones, P. F., Bartunkova, S., Wiegand, S. J., Radziejewski, C., Compton, D., McClain, J., Aldrich, T. H., Papadopoulos, N., Daly, T. J., Davis, S., Sato, T. N., and Yancopoulos, G. D. 1997. Angiopoietin-2, a natural antagonist for Tie2 that disrupts in vivo angiogenesis [see comments]. Science 277:55–60.

Makinen, T., Veikkola, T., Mustjoki, S., Karpanen, T., Catimel, B., Nice, E. C., Wise, L., Mercer, A., Kowalski, H., Kerjaschki, D., Stacker, S. A., Achen, M. G., and Alitalo, K. 2001. Isolated lymphatic endothelial cells transduce growth, survival and migratory signals via the VEGF-C/D receptor VEGFR-3. Embo J 20:4762–4773.

Martoglio, A. M., Tom, B. D., Starkey, M., Corps, A. N., Charnock-Jones, D. S., and Smith, S. K. 2000. Changes in tumorigenesis- and angiogenesis-related gene transcript abundance profiles in ovarian cancer detected by tailored high density cDNA arrays. Mol Med 6:750–765.

Mattot, V., Moons, L., Lupu, F., Chernavvsky, D., Gomez, R. A., Collen, D., and Carmeliet, P. 2002. Loss of the VEGF(164) and VEGF(188) isoforms impairs postnatal glomerular angiogenesis and renal arteriogenesis in mice. J Am Soc Nephrol 13:1548–1560.

Meyer, M., Clauss, M., Lepple-Wienhues, A., Waltenberger, J., Augustin, H. G., Ziche, M., Lanz, C., Buttner, M., Rziha, H. J., and Dehio, C. 1999. A novel vascular endothelial growth factor encoded by Orf virus, VEGF-E, mediates angiogenesis via signalling through VEGFR-2 (KDR) but not VEGFR-1 (Flt-1) receptor tyrosine kinases. Embo J 18:363–374.

Millauer, B., Shawver, L. K., Plate, K. H., Risau, W., and Ullrich, A. 1994. Glioblastoma growth inhibited in vivo by a dominant-negative Flk-1 mutant. Nature 367:576–579.

Moffat, B. A., Chen, M., Kariaapper, M. S., Hamstra, D. A., Hall, D. E., Stojanovska, J., Johnson, T. D., Blaivas, M., Kumar, M., Chenevert, T. L., Rehemtulla, A., and Ross, B. D. 2006. Inhibition of vascular endothelial growth factor (VEGF)-A causes a paradoxical increase in tumor blood flow and up-regulation of VEGF-D. Clin Cancer Res 12:1525–1532.

Moncada, S., and Higgs, A. 1993. The L-arginine-nitric oxide pathway. N Engl J Med 329:2002–2012.

Murdoch, C., Muthana, M., Coffelt, S. B., and Lewis, C. E. 2008. The role of myeloid cells in the promotion of tumour angiogenesis. Nat Rev Cancer 8:618–631.

Nabors, L. B., Mikkelsen, T., Rosenfeld, S. S., Hochberg, F., Akella, N. S., Fisher, J. D., Cloud, G. A., Zhang, Y., Carson, K., Wittemer, S. M., Colevas, A. D., and Grossman, S. A. 2007. Phase I and correlative biology study of cilengitide in patients with recurrent malignant glioma. J Clin Oncol 25:1651–1657.

Nagy, J. A., Dvorak, A. M., and Dvorak, H. F. 2003. VEGF-A(164/165) and PlGF: roles in angiogenesis and arteriogenesis. Trends Cardiovasc Med 13:169–175.

Nakayama, T., Yao, L., and Tosato, G. 2004a. Mast cell-derived angiopoietin-1 plays a critical role in the growth of plasma cell tumors. J Clin Invest 114:1317–1325.

Nakayama, T., Yoshizaki, A., Kawahara, N., Ohtsuru, A., Wen, C. Y., Fukuda, E., Nakashima, M., and Sekine, I. 2004b. Expression of Tie-1 and 2 receptors, and angiopoietin-1, 2 and 4 in gastric carcinoma; immunohistochemical analyses and correlation with clinicopathological factors. Histopathology 44:232–239.

Nash, A. D., Baca, M., Wright, C., and Scotney, P. D. 2006. The biology of vascular endothelial growth factor-B (VEGF-B). Pulm Pharmacol Ther 19:61–69.

Neuwelt, E. A. 2004. Mechanisms of disease: the blood-brain barrier. Neurosurgery 54:131–140; discussion 141–132.

Nicosia, R. F., Nicosia, S. V., and Smith, M. 1994. Vascular endothelial growth factor, platelet-derived growth factor, and insulin-like growth factor-1 promote rat aortic angiogenesis in vitro. Am J Pathol 145:1023–1029.

Nishikawa, R., Cheng, S. Y., Nagashima, R., Huang, H. J., Cavenee, W. K., and Matsutani, M. 1998. Expression of vascular endothelial growth factor in human brain tumors. Acta Neuropathol 96:453–462.

Nishimori, H., Shiratsuchi, T., Urano, T., Kimura, Y., Kiyono, K., Tatsumi, K., Yoshida, S., Ono, M., Kuwano, M., Nakamura, Y., and Tokino, T. 1997. A novel brain-specific p53-target gene, BAI1, containing thrombospondin type 1 repeats inhibits experimental angiogenesis. Oncogene 15:2145–2150.

Ochiumi, T., Tanaka, S., Oka, S., Hiyama, T., Ito, M., Kitadai, Y., Haruma, K., and Chayama, K. 2004. Clinical significance of angiopoietin-2 expression at the deepest invasive tumor site of advanced colorectal carcinoma. Int J Oncol 24:539–547.

Odorisio, T., Schietroma, C., Zaccaria, M. L., Cianfarani, F., Tiveron, C., Tatangelo, L., Failla, C. M., and Zambruno, G. 2002. Mice overexpressing placenta growth factor exhibit increased vascularization and vessel permeability. J Cell Sci 115:2559–2567.

Ogawa, M., Yamamoto, H., Nagano, H., Miyake, Y., Sugita, Y., Hata, T., Kim, B. N., Ngan, C. Y., Damdinsuren, B., Ikenaga, M., Ikeda, M., Ohue, M., Nakamori, S., Sekimoto, M., Sakon, M., Matsuura, N., and Monden, M. 2004. Hepatic expression of ANG2 RNA in metastatic colorectal cancer. Hepatology 39:528–539.

Ogawa, S., Oku, A., Sawano, A., Yamaguchi, S., Yazaki, Y., and Shibuya, M. 1998. A novel type of vascular endothelial growth factor, VEGF-E (NZ-7 VEGF), preferentially utilizes KDR/Flk-1 receptor and carries a potent mitotic activity without heparin-binding domain. J Biol Chem 273:31273–31282.

Olsson, A. K., Dimberg, A., Kreuger, J., and Claesson-Welsh, L. 2006. VEGF receptor signalling – in control of vascular function. Nat Rev Mol Cell Biol 7:359–371.
Osada, H., Tokunaga, T., Hatanaka, H., Kawakami, T., Tsuchida, T., Abe, Y., Tsugu, A., Kijima, H., Yamazaki, H., Shima, K., Osamura, Y., Ueyama, Y., and Nakamura, M. 2001. Gene expression of angiogenesis related factors in glioma. Int J Oncol 18:305–309.
Oura, H., Bertoncini, J., Velasco, P., Brown, L. F., Carmeliet, P., and Detmar, M. 2003. A critical role of placental growth factor in the induction of inflammation and edema formation. Blood 101:560–567.
Papapetropoulos, A., Garcia-Cardena, G., Dengler, T. J., Maisonpierre, P. C., Yancopoulos, G. D., and Sessa, W. C. 1999. Direct actions of angiopoietin-1 on human endothelium: evidence for network stabilization, cell survival, and interaction with other angiogenic growth factors. Lab Invest 79:213–223.
Park, J. E., Chen, H. H., Winer, J., Houck, K. A., and Ferrara, N. 1994. Placenta growth factor. Potentiation of vascular endothelial growth factor bioactivity, in vitro and in vivo, and high affinity binding to Flt-1 but not to Flk-1/KDR. J Biol Chem 269:25646–25654.
Peirce, S. M., Price, R. J., and Skalak, T. C. 2004. Spatial and temporal control of angiogenesis and arterialization using focal applications of VEGF164 and Ang-1. Am J Physiol Heart Circ Physiol 286:H918–925.
Plate, K. H., Breier, G., Weich, H. A., Mennel, H. D., and Risau, W. 1994. Vascular endothelial growth factor and glioma angiogenesis: coordinate induction of VEGF receptors, distribution of VEGF protein and possible in vivo regulatory mechanisms. Int J Cancer 59:520–529.
Plate, K. H., Breier, G., Weich, H. A., and Risau, W. 1992. Vascular endothelial growth factor is a potential tumour angiogenesis factor in human gliomas in vivo. Nature 359:845–848.
Pope, W. B., Lai, A., Nghiemphu, P., Mischel, P., and Cloughesy, T. F. 2006. MRI in patients with high-grade gliomas treated with bevacizumab and chemotherapy. Neurology 66:1258–1260.
Post, D. E., Sandberg, E. M., Kyle, M. M., Devi, N. S., Brat, D. J., Xu, Z., Tighiouart, M., and Van Meir, E. G. 2007. Targeted cancer gene therapy using a hypoxia inducible factor dependent oncolytic adenovirus armed with interleukin-4. Cancer Res 67:6872–6881.
Post, D. E., and Van Meir, E. G. 2001. Generation of bidirectional hypoxia/HIF-responsive expression vectors to target gene expression to hypoxic cells. Gene Ther 8:1801–1807.
Post, D. E., and Van Meir, E. G. 2003. A novel hypoxia-inducible factor (HIF) activated oncolytic adenovirus for cancer therapy. Oncogene 22:2065–2072.
Powers, C. J., McLeskey, S. W., and Wellstein, A. 2000. Fibroblast growth factors, their receptors and signaling. Endocr Relat Cancer 7:165–197.
Ren, B., Yee, K. O., Lawler, J., and Khosravi-Far, R. 2006. Regulation of tumor angiogenesis by thrombospondin-1. Biochim Biophys Acta 1765:178–188.
Richard, D. E., Berra, E., and Pouyssegur, J. 2000. Nonhypoxic pathway mediates the induction of hypoxia-inducible factor 1alpha in vascular smooth muscle cells. J Biol Chem 275:26765–26771.
Risau, W., Drexler, H., Mironov, V., Smits, A., Siegbahn, A., Funa, K., and Heldin, C. H. 1992. Platelet-derived growth factor is angiogenic in vivo. Growth Factors 7:261–266.
Rosen, E. M., Grant, D., Kleinman, H., Jaken, S., Donovan, M. A., Setter, E., Luckett, P. M., and Carley, W. (1991). Scatter Factor Stimulates Migration of Accused Endothelium and Capillary-like Tube Formation, In Cell Motility Factors, I. D. Golberg, and E. M. Rosen, eds. (Basel: Birkhauser-Verlag), pp. 76–88.
Ryan, A. M., Eppler, D. B., Hagler, K. E., Bruner, R. H., Thomford, P. J., Hall, R. L., Shopp, G. M., and O'Neill, C. A. 1999. Preclinical safety evaluation of rhuMAbVEGF, an antiangiogenic humanized monoclonal antibody. Toxicol Pathol 27:78–86.
Saharinen, P., Tammela, T., Karkkainen, M. J., and Alitalo, K. 2004. Lymphatic vasculature: development, molecular regulation and role in tumor metastasis and inflammation. Trends Immunol 25:387–395.

Sathornsumetee, S., Cao, Y., Marcello, J. E., Herndon, J. E., 2nd, McLendon, R. E., Desjardins, A., Friedman, H. S., Dewhirst, M. W., Vredenburgh, J. J., and Rich, J. N. 2008. Tumor angiogenic and hypoxic profiles predict radiographic response and survival in malignant astrocytoma patients treated with bevacizumab and irinotecan. J Clin Oncol 26:271–278.

Schoppmann, S. F., Birner, P., Stockl, J., Kalt, R., Ullrich, R., Caucig, C., Kriehuber, E., Nagy, K., Alitalo, K., and Kerjaschki, D. 2002. Tumor-associated macrophages express lymphatic endothelial growth factors and are related to peritumoral lymphangiogenesis. Am J Pathol 161:947–956.

Semenza, G. 2002. Signal transduction to hypoxia-inducible factor 1. Biochem Pharmacol 64:993–998.

Semenza, G. L. 2004. O2-regulated gene expression: transcriptional control of cardiorespiratory physiology by HIF-1. J Appl Physiol 96:1173–1177; discussion 1170–1172.

Senger, D. R., Connolly, D. T., Van de Water, L., Feder, J., and Dvorak, H. F. 1990. Purification and NH2-terminal amino acid sequence of guinea pig tumor-secreted vascular permeability factor. Cancer Res 50:1774–1778.

Sfiligoi, C., de Luca, A., Cascone, I., Sorbello, V., Fuso, L., Ponzone, R., Biglia, N., Audero, E., Arisio, R., Bussolino, F., Sismondi, P., and De Bortoli, M. 2003. Angiopoietin-2 expression in breast cancer correlates with lymph node invasion and short survival. Int J Cancer 103:466–474.

Shalaby, F., Rossant, J., Yamaguchi, T. P., Gertsenstein, M., Wu, X. F., Breitman, M. L., and Schuh, A. C. 1995. Failure of blood-island formation and vasculogenesis in Flk-1-deficient mice. Nature 376:62–66.

Shao, R., Zhang, F. P., Tian, F., Anders Friberg, P., Wang, X., Sjoland, H., and Billig, H. 2004. Increase of SUMO-1 expression in response to hypoxia: direct interaction with HIF-1alpha in adult mouse brain and heart in vivo. FEBS Lett 569:293–300.

Shih, A. H., and Holland, E. C. 2006. Platelet-derived growth factor (PDGF) and glial tumorigenesis. Cancer Lett 232:139–147.

Shih, S. C., and Claffey, K. P. 1999. Regulation of human vascular endothelial growth factor mRNA stability in hypoxia by heterogeneous nuclear ribonucleoprotein L. J Biol Chem 274:1359–1365.

Shim, W. S., Ho, I. A., and Wong, P. E. 2007. Angiopoietin: a TIE(d) balance in tumor angiogenesis. Mol Cancer Res 5:655–665.

Shinoda, J., and Whittle, I. R. 2001. Nitric oxide and glioma: a target for novel therapy? Br J Neurosurg 15:213–220.

Shirakawa, K., Tsuda, H., Heike, Y., Kato, K., Asada, R., Inomata, M., Sasaki, H., Kasumi, F., Yoshimoto, M., Iwanaga, T., Konishi, F., Terada, M., and Wakasugi, H. 2001. Absence of endothelial cells, central necrosis, and fibrosis are associated with aggressive inflammatory breast cancer. Cancer Res 61:445–451.

Shraga-Heled, N., Kessler, O., Prahst, C., Kroll, J., Augustin, H., and Neufeld, G. 2007. Neuropilin-1 and neuropilin-2 enhance VEGF121 stimulated signal transduction by the VEGFR-2 receptor. Faseb J 21:915–926.

Shweiki, D., Itin, A., Soffer, D., and Keshet, E. 1992. Vascular endothelial growth factor induced by hypoxia may mediate hypoxia-initiated angiogenesis. Nature 359:843–845.

Siegfried, G., Basak, A., Cromlish, J. A., Benjannet, S., Marcinkiewicz, J., Chretien, M., Seidah, N. G., and Khatib, A. M. 2003. The secretory proprotein convertases furin, PC5, and PC7 activate VEGF-C to induce tumorigenesis. J Clin Invest 111:1723–1732.

Singh, S. K., Clarke, I. D., Terasaki, M., Bonn, V. E., Hawkins, C., Squire, J., and Dirks, P. B. 2003. Identification of a cancer stem cell in human brain tumors. Cancer Res 63:5821–5828.

Singh, S. K., Hawkins, C., Clarke, I. D., Squire, J. A., Bayani, J., Hide, T., Henkelman, R. M., Cusimano, M. D., and Dirks, P. B. 2004. Identification of human brain tumour initiating cells. Nature 432:396–401.

Skobe, M., Hamberg, L. M., Hawighorst, T., Schirner, M., Wolf, G. L., Alitalo, K., and Detmar, M. 2001. Concurrent induction of lymphangiogenesis, angiogenesis, and macrophage recruitment by vascular endothelial growth factor-C in melanoma. Am J Pathol 159:893–903.

Soker, S. 2001. Neuropilin in the midst of cell migration and retraction. Int J Biochem Cell Biol 33:433–437.

Soker, S., Takashima, S., Miao, H. Q., Neufeld, G., and Klagsbrun, M. 1998. Neuropilin-1 is expressed by endothelial and tumor cells as an isoform- specific receptor for vascular endothelial growth factor. Cell 92:735–745.

Stacker, S. A., Caesar, C., Baldwin, M. E., Thornton, G. E., Williams, R. A., Prevo, R., Jackson, D. G., Nishikawa, S., Kubo, H., and Achen, M. G. 2001. VEGF-D promotes the metastatic spread of tumor cells via the lymphatics. Nat Med 7:186–191.

Stalmans, I., Lambrechts, D., De Smet, F., Jansen, S., Wang, J., Maity, S., Kneer, P., von der Ohe, M., Swillen, A., Maes, C., Gewillig, M., Molin, D. G., Hellings, P., Boetel, T., Haardt, M., Compernolle, V., Dewerchin, M., Plaisance, S., Vlietinck, R., Emanuel, B., Gittenberger-de Groot, A. C., Scambler, P., Morrow, B., Driscol, D. A., Moons, L., Esguerra, C. V., Carmeliet, G., Behn-Krappa, A., Devriendt, K., Collen, D., Conway, S. J., and Carmeliet, P. 2003. VEGF: a modifier of the del22q11 (DiGeorge) syndrome? Nat Med 9:173–182.

Stalmans, I., Ng, Y. S., Rohan, R., Fruttiger, M., Bouche, A., Yuce, A., Fujisawa, H., Hermans, B., Shani, M., Jansen, S., Hicklin, D., Anderson, D. J., Gardiner, T., Hammes, H. P., Moons, L., Dewerchin, M., Collen, D., Carmeliet, P., and D'Amore, P. A. 2002. Arteriolar and venular patterning in retinas of mice selectively expressing VEGF isoforms. J Clin Invest 109:327–336.

Stan, A. C., Nemati, M. N., Pietsch, T., Walter, G. F., and Dietz, H. 1995. In vivo inhibition of angiogenesis and growth of the human U-87 malignant glial tumor by treatment with an antibody against basic fibroblast growth factor. J Neurosurg 82:1044–1052.

Stiles, J. D., Ostrow, P. T., Balos, L. L., Greenberg, S. J., Plunkett, R., Grand, W., and Heffner, R. R., Jr. 1997. Correlation of endothelin-1 and transforming growth factor beta 1 with malignancy and vascularity in human gliomas. J Neuropathol Exp Neurol 56:435–439.

Stratmann, A., Risau, W., and Plate, K. H. 1998. Cell type-specific expression of angiopoietin-1 and angiopoietin-2 suggests a role in glioblastoma angiogenesis [see comments]. Am J Pathol 153:1459–1466.

Straume, O., Chappuis, P. O., Salvesen, H. B., Halvorsen, O. J., Haukaas, S. A., Goffin, J. R., Begin, L. R., Foulkes, W. D., and Akslen, L. A. 2002. Prognostic importance of glomeruloid microvascular proliferation indicates an aggressive angiogenic phenotype in human cancers. Cancer Res 62:6808–6811.

Suri, C., Jones, P. F., Patan, S., Bartunkova, S., Maisonpierre, P. C., Davis, S., Sato, T. N., and Yancopoulos, G. D. 1996. Requisite role of angiopoietin-1, a ligand for the TIE2 receptor, during embryonic angiogenesis [see comments]. Cell 87:1171–1180.

Suri, C., McClain, J., Thurston, G., McDonald, D. M., Zhou, H., Oldmixon, E. H., Sato, T. N., and Yancopoulos, G. D. 1998. Increased vascularization in mice overexpressing angiopoietin-1. Science 282:468–471.

Suto, K., Yamazaki, Y., Morita, T., and Mizuno, H. 2005. Crystal structures of novel vascular endothelial growth factors (VEGF) from snake venoms: insight into selective VEGF binding to kinase insert domain-containing receptor but not to fms-like tyrosine kinase-1. J Biol Chem 280:2126–2131.

Takahama, M., Tsutsumi, M., Tsujiuchi, T., Nezu, K., Kushibe, K., Taniguchi, S., Kotake, Y., and Konishi, Y. 1999. Enhanced expression of Tie2, its ligand angiopoietin-1, vascular endothelial growth factor, and CD31 in human non-small cell lung carcinomas. Clin Cancer Res 5:2506–2510.

Takahashi, T., Fournier, A., Nakamura, F., Wang, L. H., Murakami, Y., Kalb, R. G., Fujisawa, H., and Strittmatter, S. M. 1999. Plexin-neuropilin-1 complexes form functional semaphorin-3A receptors. Cell 99:59–69.

Takashima, S., Kitakaze, M., Asakura, M., Asanuma, H., Sanada, S., Tashiro, F., Niwa, H., Miyazaki Ji, J., Hirota, S., Kitamura, Y., Kitsukawa, T., Fujisawa, H., Klagsbrun, M., and Hori, M. 2002. Targeting of both mouse neuropilin-1 and neuropilin-2 genes severely impairs developmental yolk sac and embryonic angiogenesis. Proc Natl Acad Sci USA 99:3657–3662.

Takeuchi, H., Matsuda, K., Kitai, R., Sato, K., and Kubota, T. 2007. Angiogenesis in primary central nervous system lymphoma (PCNSL). J Neurooncol 84:141–145.

Tallquist, M., and Kazlauskas, A. 2004. PDGF signaling in cells and mice. Cytokine Growth Factor Rev 15:205–213.

Tanaka, F., Ishikawa, S., Yanagihara, K., Miyahara, R., Kawano, Y., Li, M., Otake, Y., and Wada, H. 2002. Expression of angiopoietins and its clinical significance in non-small cell lung cancer. Cancer Res 62:7124–7129.

Tanaka, S., Mori, M., Sakamoto, Y., Makuuchi, M., Sugimachi, K., and Wands, J. R. 1999. Biologic significance of angiopoietin-2 expression in human hepatocellular carcinoma. J Clin Invest 103:341–345.

Tangkeangsirisin, W., Hayashi, J., and Serrero, G. 2004. PC cell-derived growth factor mediates tamoxifen resistance and promotes tumor growth of human breast cancer cells. Cancer Res 64:1737–1743.

Tashiro, E., Maruki, H., Minato, Y., Doki, Y., Weinstein, I. B., and Imoto, M. 2003. Overexpression of cyclin D1 contributes to malignancy by up-regulation of fibroblast growth factor receptor 1 via the pRB/E2F pathway. Cancer Res 63:424–431.

Teichert-Kuliszewska, K., Maisonpierre, P. C., Jones, N., Campbell, A. I., Master, Z., Bendeck, M. P., Alitalo, K., Dumont, D. J., Yancopoulos, G. D., and Stewart, D. J. 2001. Biological action of angiopoietin-2 in a fibrin matrix model of angiogenesis is associated with activation of Tie2. Cardiovasc Res 49:659–670.

Thomsen, L. L., Lawton, F. G., Knowles, R. G., Beesley, J. E., Riveros-Moreno, V., and Moncada, S. 1994. Nitric oxide synthase activity in human gynecological cancer. Cancer Res 54:1352–1354.

Thurston, G., Suri, C., Smith, K., McClain, J., Sato, T. N., Yancopoulos, G. D., and McDonald, D. M. 1999. Leakage-resistant blood vessels in mice transgenically overexpressing angiopoietin-1. Science 286:2511–2514.

Torimura, T., Ueno, T., Kin, M., Harada, R., Taniguchi, E., Nakamura, T., Sakata, R., Hashimoto, O., Sakamoto, M., Kumashiro, R., Sata, M., Nakashima, O., Yano, H., and Kojiro, M. 2004. Overexpression of angiopoietin-1 and angiopoietin-2 in hepatocellular carcinoma. J Hepatol 40:799–807.

Tozer, G. M., Prise, V. E., and Chaplin, D. J. 1997. Inhibition of nitric oxide synthase induces a selective reduction in tumor blood flow that is reversible with L-arginine. Cancer Res 57:948–955.

Udani, V., Santarelli, J., Yung, Y., Cheshier, S., Andrews, A., Kasad, Z., and Tse, V. 2005. Differential expression of angiopoietin-1 and angiopoietin-2 may enhance recruitment of bone-marrow-derived endothelial precursor cells into brain tumors. Neurol Res 27:801–806.

Van Belle, E., Witzenbichler, B., Chen, D., Silver, M., Chang, L., Schwall, R., and Isner, J. M. 1998. Potentiated angiogenic effect of scatter factor/hepatocyte growth factor via induction of vascular endothelial growth factor: the case for paracrine amplification of angiogenesis. Circulation 97:381–390.

Van Meir, E., Ceska, M., Effenberger, F., Walz, A., Grouzmann, E., Desbaillets, I., Frei, K., Fontana, A., and de Tribolet, N. 1992. Interleukin-8 is produced in neoplastic and infectious diseases of the human central nervous system. Cancer Res 52:4297–4305.

Van Meir, E. G., Polverini, P. J., Chazin, V. R., Su Huang, H. J., de Tribolet, N., and Cavenee, W. K. 1994. Release of an inhibitor of angiogenesis upon induction of wild type p53 expression in glioblastoma cells. Nat Genet 8:171–176.

Vredenburgh, J. J., Desjardins, A., Herndon, J. E., 2nd, Dowell, J. M., Reardon, D. A., Quinn, J. A., Rich, J. N., Sathornsumetee, S., Gururangan, S., Wagner, M., Bigner, D. D.,

Friedman, A. H., and Friedman, H. S. 2007a. Phase II trial of bevacizumab and irinotecan in recurrent malignant glioma. Clin Cancer Res 13:1253–1259.
Vredenburgh, J. J., Desjardins, A., Herndon, J. E., 2nd, Marcello, J., Reardon, D. A., Quinn, J. A., Rich, J. N., Sathornsumetee, S., Gururangan, S., Sampson, J., Wagner, M., Bailey, L., Bigner, D. D., Friedman, A. H., and Friedman, H. S. 2007b. Bevacizumab plus irinotecan in recurrent glioblastoma multiforme. J Clin Oncol 25:4722–4729.
Wang, D., Huang, H. J., Kazlauskas, A., and Cavenee, W. K. 1999. Induction of vascular endothelial growth factor expression in endothelial cells by platelet-derived growth factor through the activation of phosphatidylinositol 3-kinase. Cancer Res 59: 1464–1472.
Wang, H., and Keiser, J. A. 1998. Vascular endothelial growth factor upregulates the expression of matrix metalloproteinases in vascular smooth muscle cells: role of flt-1. Circ Res 83:832–840.
Wang, J., Wu, K., Zhang, D., Tang, H., Xie, H., Hong, L., Pan, Y., Lan, M., Hu, S., Ning, X., and Fan, D. 2005. Expressions and clinical significances of angiopoietin-1, -2 and Tie2 in human gastric cancer. Biochem Biophys Res Commun 337:386–393.
Wang, J. F., Zhang, X., and Groopman, J. E. 2004. Activation of vascular endothelial growth factor receptor-3 and its downstream signaling promote cell survival under oxidative stress. J Biol Chem 279:27088–27097.
Weber, C. C., Cai, H., Ehrbar, M., Kubota, H., Martiny-Baron, G., Weber, W., Djonov, V., Weber, E., Mallik, A. S., Fussenegger, M., Frei, K., Hubbell, J. A., and Zisch, A. H. 2005. Effects of protein and gene transfer of the angiopoietin-1 fibrinogen-like receptor-binding domain on endothelial and vessel organization. J Biol Chem 280:22445–22453.
Wegiel, B., Bjartell, A., Ekberg, J., Gadaleanu, V., Brunhoff, C., and Persson, J. L. 2005. A role for cyclin A1 in mediating the autocrine expression of vascular endothelial growth factor in prostate cancer. Oncogene 24:6385–6393.
Wen, P. Y., and Kesari, S. 2008. Malignant gliomas in adults. N Engl J Med 359:492–507.
Wiedemeyer, R., Brennan, C., Heffernan, T. P., Xiao, Y., Mahoney, J., Protopopov, A., Zheng, H., Bignell, G., Furnari, F., Cavenee, W. K., Hahn, W. C., Ichimura, K., Collins, V. P., Chu, G. C., Stratton, M. R., Ligon, K. L., Futreal, P. A., and Chin, L. 2008. Feedback circuit among INK4 tumor suppressors constrains human glioblastoma development. Cancer Cell 13:355–364.
Winkler, F., Kozin, S. V., Tong, R. T., Chae, S. S., Booth, M. F., Garkavtsev, I., Xu, L., Hicklin, D. J., Fukumura, D., di Tomaso, E., Munn, L. L., and Jain, R. K. 2004. Kinetics of vascular normalization by VEGFR2 blockade governs brain tumor response to radiation: role of oxygenation, angiopoietin-1, and matrix metalloproteinases. Cancer Cell 6:553–563.
Wise, L. M., Veikkola, T., Mercer, A. A., Savory, L. J., Fleming, S. B., Caesar, C., Vitali, A., Makinen, T., Alitalo, K., and Stacker, S. A. 1999. Vascular endothelial growth factor (VEGF)-like protein from orf virus NZ2 binds to VEGFR2 and neuropilin-1. Proc Natl Acad Sci USA 96:3071–3076.
Witzenbichler, B., Maisonpierre, P. C., Jones, P., Yancopoulos, G. D., and Isner, J. M. 1998. Chemotactic properties of angiopoietin-1 and -2, ligands for the endothelial-specific receptor tyrosine kinase Tie2. J Biol Chem 273:18514–18521.
Wolf, R. L., Wang, J., Wang, S., Melhem, E. R., O'Rourke, D. M., Judy, K. D., and Detre, J. A. 2005. Grading of CNS neoplasms using continuous arterial spin labeled perfusion MR imaging at 3 Tesla. J Magn Reson Imaging 22:475–482.
Wu, Y., Chen, L., Zheng, P. S., and Yang, B. B. 2002. beta 1-Integrin-mediated glioma cell adhesion and free radical-induced apoptosis are regulated by binding to a C-terminal domain of PG-M/versican. J Biol Chem 277:12294–12301.
Yamada, N., Kato, M., Yamashita, H., Nister, M., Miyazono, K., Heldin, C. H., and Funa, K. 1995. Enhanced expression of transforming growth factor-beta and its type-I and type-II receptors in human glioblastoma. Int J Cancer 62:386–392.

Yamada, Y., Takakura, N., Yasue, H., Ogawa, H., Fujisawa, H., and Suda, T. 2001. Exogenous clustered neuropilin 1 enhances vasculogenesis and angiogenesis. Blood 97:1671–1678.
Yancopoulos, G. D., Davis, S., Gale, N. W., Rudge, J. S., Wiegand, S. J., and Holash, J. 2000. Vascular-specific growth factors and blood vessel formation. Nature 407:242–248.
Yin, D., Wang, X., Konda, B. M., Ong, J. M., Hu, J., Sacapano, M. R., Ko, M. K., Espinoza, A. J., Irvin, D. K., Shu, Y., and Black, K. L. 2008. Increase in brain tumor permeability in glioma-bearing rats with nitric oxide donors. Clin Cancer Res 14:4002–4009.
Yu, Q., and Stamenkovic, I. 2001. Angiopoietin-2 is implicated in the regulation of tumor angiogenesis. Am J Pathol 158:563–570.
Yuan, F., Salehi, H. A., Boucher, Y., Vasthare, U. S., Tuma, R. F., and Jain, R. K. 1994. Vascular permeability and microcirculation of gliomas and mammary carcinomas transplanted in rat and mouse cranial windows. Cancer Res 54:4564–4568.
Yuan, L., Moyon, D., Pardanaud, L., Breant, C., Karkkainen, M. J., Alitalo, K., and Eichmann, A. 2002. Abnormal lymphatic vessel development in neuropilin 2 mutant mice. Development 129:4797–4806.
Zadeh, G., Koushan, K., Pillo, L., Shannon, P., and Guha, A. 2004. Role of Ang1 and its interaction with VEGF-A in astrocytomas. J Neuropathol Exp Neurol 63:978–989.
Zagzag, D., Amirnovin, R., Greco, M. A., Yee, H., Holash, J., Wiegand, S. J., Zabski, S., Yancopoulos, G. D., and Grumet, M. 2000a. Vascular apoptosis and involution in gliomas precede neovascularization: a novel concept for glioma growth and angiogenesis. Lab Invest 80:837–849.
Zagzag, D., Lukyanov, Y., Lan, L., Ali, M. A., Esencay, M., Mendez, O., Yee, H., Voura, E. B., and Newcomb, E. W. 2006. Hypoxia-inducible factor 1 and VEGF upregulate CXCR4 in glioblastoma: implications for angiogenesis and glioma cell invasion. Lab Invest 86:1221–1232.
Zagzag, D., Zhong, H., Scalzitti, J. M., Laughner, E., Simons, J. W., and Semenza, G. L. 2000b. Expression of hypoxia-inducible factor 1alpha in brain tumors: association with angiogenesis, invasion, and progression. Cancer 88:2606–2618.
Zelzer, E., Levy, Y., Kahana, C., Shilo, B. Z., Rubinstein, M., and Cohen, B. 1998. Insulin induces transcription of target genes through the hypoxia-inducible factor HIF-1alpha/ARNT. Embo J 17:5085–5094.
Zhang, H., Shepherd, A. T., Eason, D. D., Wei, S., Diaz, J. I., Djeu, J. Y., Wu, G. D., and Blanck, G. 1999. Retinoblastoma protein expression leads to reduced Oct-1 DNA binding activity and enhances interleukin-8 expression. Cell Growth Differ 10:457–465.
Zheng, P. P., Hop, W. C., Luider, T. M., Sillevis Smitt, P. A., and Kros, J. M. 2007. Increased levels of circulating endothelial progenitor cells and circulating endothelial nitric oxide synthase in patients with gliomas. Ann Neurol 62:40–48.
Zhong, H., Chiles, K., Feldser, D., Laughner, E., Hanrahan, C., Georgescu, M. M., Simons, J. W., and Semenza, G. L. 2000. Modulation of hypoxia-inducible factor 1alpha expression by the epidermal growth factor/phosphatidylinositol 3-kinase/PTEN/AKT/FRAP pathway in human prostate cancer cells: implications for tumor angiogenesis and therapeutics. Cancer Res 60:1541–1545.
Ziche, M., Maglione, D., Ribatti, D., Morbidelli, L., Lago, C. T., Battisti, M., Paoletti, I., Barra, A., Tucci, M., Parise, G., Vincenti, V., Granger, H. J., Viglietto, G., and Persico, M. G. 1997a. Placenta growth factor-1 is chemotactic, mitogenic, and angiogenic. Lab Invest 76:517–531.
Ziche, M., Morbidelli, L., Choudhuri, R., Zhang, H. T., Donnini, S., Granger, H. J., and Bicknell, R. 1997b. Nitric oxide synthase lies downstream from vascular endothelial growth factor-induced but not basic fibroblast growth factor-induced angiogenesis. J Clin Invest 99:2625–2634.
Ziche, M., Morbidelli, L., Masini, E., Amerini, S., Granger, H. J., Maggi, C. A., Geppetti, P., and Ledda, F. 1994. Nitric oxide mediates angiogenesis in vivo and endothelial cell growth and migration in vitro promoted by substance P. J Clin Invest 94:2036–2044.

Ziche, M., Morbidelli, L., Parenti, A., Amerini, S., Granger, H. J., and Maggi, C. A. 1993. Substance P increases cyclic GMP levels on coronary postcapillary venular endothelial cells. Life Sci 53:PL229–234.

Zundel, W., Schindler, C., Haas-Kogan, D., Koong, A., Kaper, F., Chen, E., Gottschalk, A. R., Ryan, H. E., Johnson, R. S., Jefferson, A. B., Stokoe, D., and Giaccia, A. J. 2000. Loss of PTEN facilitates HIF-1-mediated gene expression. Genes Dev 14:391–396.

Chapter 22
Vaso-occlusive Mechanisms that Intiate Hypoxia and Necrosis in Glioblastoma: The Role of Thrombosis and Tissue Factor

Yuan Rong and Daniel J. Brat

Abstract Glioblastoma (GBM) is a highly malignant, rapidly progressive astrocytoma that is distinguished from lower grade tumors by necrosis, severe hypoxia and microvascular hyperplasia. While the development of hypoxia and necrosis are known to be ominous prognostic features, precise mechanisms that underlie their development have not been elucidated. Pathologic observations and experimental evidence now suggest that vaso-occlusion and intravascular thrombosis may initiate or propagate hypoxia and necrosis. This emerging model suggests that thrombosis arises within the vasculature of high grade gliomas secondary to the overexpression of the highly pro-thrombotic protein tissue factor. This protein is dramatically upregulated in response to EGFR activation, *PTEN* loss and hypoxia, which occur at the transition from grade III to grade IV astrocytoma. A pro-thrombotic enviroment also activates the family of protease-activated receptors (PARs) on tumor cells, which are G-protein coupled and enhance invasive and pro-angiogenic properties. Vaso-occlusive and pro-thrombotic mechanisms in GBM could readily explain the rapid peripheral expansion seen on neuroimaging and the dramatic shift to an acceleration in clinical progression due to hypoxia-induced angiogenesis.

Contents

D.J. Brat (✉)
Department of Pathology and Laboratory Medicine, Emory University Hospital, H-176, 1364 Clifton Rd. NE, Atlanta, GA 30322, USA
e-mail: dbrat@emory.edu

E.G. Van Meir (ed.), *CNS Cancer*, Cancer Drug Discovery and Development, DOI 10.1007/978-1-60327-553-8_22,
© Humana Press, a part of Springer Science+Business Media, LLC 2009

22.1 Introduction

Most clinicians and investigators in neuro-oncology are well aware of the features of glioblastoma (GBM), as it remains the most predictably devastating disease in the field. This tumor is the highest grade astrocytoma (WHO grade IV), characterized by widespread infiltration, necrosis, angiogenesis, rapid growth, and a dismal prognosis (CBTRUS 2002, Kleihues et al. 2000, Ohgaki and Kleihues 2005). Following the most advanced treatment, including neurosurgery, radiotherapy, and chemotherapy, mean survival of patients with GBM is only 60 weeks (Stupp et al. 2005). When patients receive only surgical resection but are not treated with adjuvant therapy, mean survival is a mere 14 weeks, underscoring the tremendous natural growth properties of these tumors (Shapiro and Young 1976). Lower grade infiltrative astrocytomas (i.e., WHO grade II and III astrocytomas) are also fatal tumors but are characterized by much slower growth rates and longer survivals (3–8 years) (Brat et al. 2002, Gupta et al. 2005). Only once these lower grade tumors have progressed to GBM do they demonstrate accelerated growth and rapid progression to death. This review explores potential mechanisms that might account for the rapid clinical progression associated with the GBM histology, emphasizing mechanisms that initiate the hypoxia and necrosis that are the hallmarks of this tumor.

22.2 Distinctive Features of Glioblastoma

GBMs (grade IV) are sufficiently distinct from the lower grade astrocytomas (grade II and III) in their clincial behavior and biologic potential that they can be thought of as a quantum leap in malignancy rather than a small step along a disease spectrum. The unique neuroimaging and pathologic features that emerge during the transition to GBM provide the best insight into the mechanisms that might account for these enhanced growth properties. Grade II and III astrocytomas show hyperintense T2-weighted (or FLAIR) signal abnormalities on magnetic resonance imaging (MRI), reflecting vasogenic edema generated in response to diffuse infiltration by individual tumor cells. These lower grade tumors expand the involved brain and distort its architecture to the point of producing clinical symptoms, but tissue destruction and necrosis are not observed. There is only mild or no contrast-enhancement, suggesting a relatively intact blood–brain barrier (Henson et al. 2005, Zhu et al. 2000). Radial growth rates of these tumors are modest, with annual increases in diameter of 2–4 mm/yr (Mandonnet et al. 2003, Swanson et al. 2003). Histologic sections of grade II–III tumors reflect the imaging properties: neoplastic cells are seen diffusely infiltrating between neuronal and glial processes, leading to architectural disruption and edema (Bellail et al. 2004, Gupta et al. 2005). As astrocytomas advance through the pathologic spectrum from the lower end of grade II to the upper end of grade III, the degree of nuclear anaplasia increases and the proliferative capacity edges upward, resulting in a more densely cellular tumor with greater malignant potential (Brat et al. 2002). Thus, grade II–III astrocytomas can be conceptualized as a continuum of gradually increasing tumor grade and growth, with clinical properties generally correlating with the density and malignancy of tumor cells.

Tumor imaging, histology, and dynamics change dramatically during the transition to GBM, suggesting that a fundamentally altered neoplasm has emerged. Radial growth rates can accelerate to values nearly 10 times greater than those in grade II astrocytomas (Mandonnet et al. 2003, Swanson et al. 2003). MRI typically reveals a central, contrast-enhancing component ("ring-enhancing mass") that arises from within the infiltrative astrocytoma and rapidly expands outward, causing a much larger T2-weighted signal abnormality in the tumor's periphery (Fig. 22.1) (Henson et al. 2005, Zhu et al. 2000). The histopathologic features that disinguish GBM from lower grade astrocytomas are found near this contrast-enhancing rim and include (1) foci of necrosis, usually with evidence of surrounding cellular pseudopalisades ("pseudopalisading necrosis") and (2) microvascular hyperplasia, a form of angiogenesis morphologically recognized as endothelial proliferation within newly sprouted vessels (Fig. 22.2 and Color Plate 32) (Brat et al. 2002, Brat and Van Meir 2001, Burger and Green 1987, Kleihues et al. 2000). These two diagnostic findings of GBM are independent of tumor

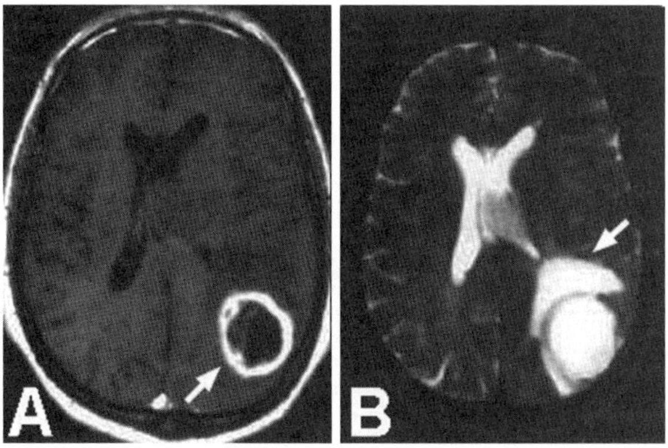

Fig. 22.1 Glioblastoma (WHO grade IV) has a distinct growth pattern on magnetic resonance imaging (MRI). (**A**) Axial post-contrast MRI of GBM shows a ring-like pattern of contrast-enhancement (*arrow*) surrounding a central zone of necrosis. (**B**) Axial T2-weighted MRI demonstrates a hyperintense region (*arrow*) peripheral to the central necrotic zone, which represents diffusely infiltrating tumor cells and the accompanying vasogenenic edema

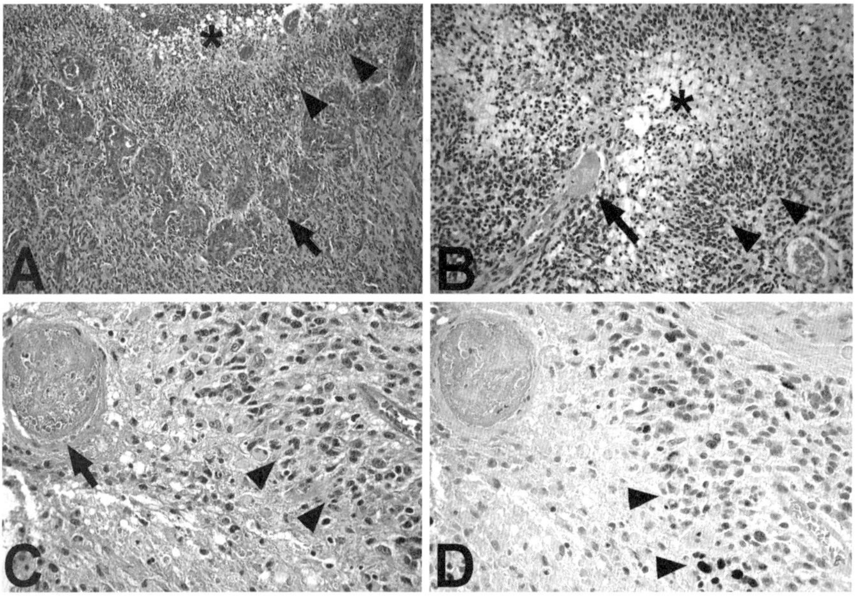

Fig. 22.2 Pathologic features of glioblastoma. (**A**) Pseudopalisades (*arrowheads*) are characterized by an accumulation of tumor cells around a central necrotic zone (*asterisk*). Microvascular hyperplasia (*arrow*) is a form of angiogenesis that is induced by hypoxic pseudopalisading cells and can be noted in regions adjacent to necrosis. (**B**) A central vessel within a GBM is occluded by an intravascular thrombus (*arrow*) in close proximity to an emerging region of necrosis (*asterisk*) with surrounding pseudopalisading cells (*arrowheads*). (**C**) H&E staining of a GBM demonstrates intravascular thrombosis occluding and distending a vessel (*arrow*) within the center of a pseudopalisade (*arrowheads*). (**D**) Immunohistochemistry for HIF-1α on a serial tissue section shows increased nuclear staining in pseudopalisades, indicating an adaptive response to hypoxia (*arrowheads*) (*see* Color Plate 32)

cell characteristics, yet carry an inordinant degree of prognostic power (Nelson et al. 1983, Raza et al. 2002). Given their remarkable prognostic significance, it is almost certain that these structures are mechanistically linked to the accelerated growth properties that characterize the grade III–IV transition.

An emerging model of tumor progression may explain the development of necrosis, the relationship between necrosis and angiogenesis, and the strong association between necrosis and aggressive clinical behavior (Figs. 22.2, 22.3 and Color Plate 33) (Brat et al. 2002, Brat and Van Meir 2001, Holash et al. 1999, Zagzag et al. 2000). This model hypothesizes a sequence that begins with an infiltrating astocytoma of moderate to high cellularity (i.e., grade III astrocytoma) and continues with (see Fig. 22.3): (1) vascular occlusion within the tumor that is often associated with intravascular thrombosis; (2) hypoxia in regions surrounding vascular pathology; (3) outward migration

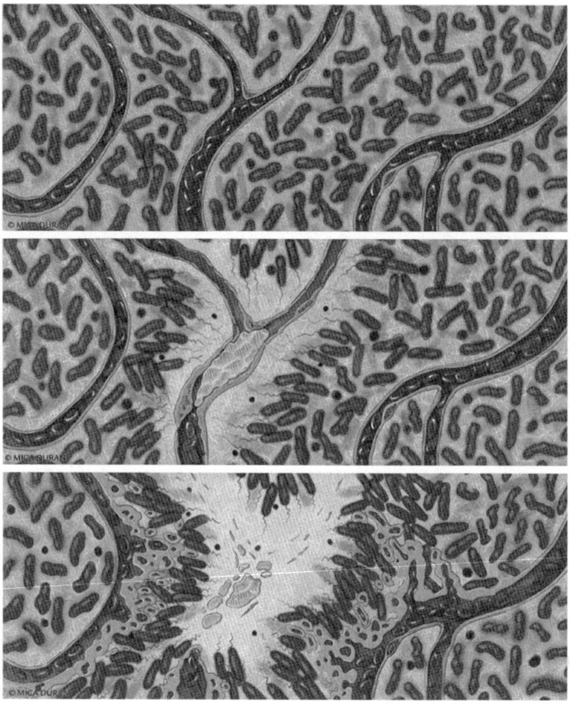

Fig. 22.3 Potential mechanism of pseudopalisade formation. (*Upper panel*) In grade III astrocytoma, tumor cells with moderate to high-density infiltrate through the CNS and receive oxygen and nutrient supplies through intact native blood vessels. (*Middle panel*) A vascular insult occurs as a result of tumor growth and causes endothelial injury, expression of procoagulant factors and intravascular thrombosis, leading to hypoxia in regions surrounding vascular pathology. Tumor cells begin to migrate away from hypoxia, creating a peripherally moving wave that is seen microscopically as pseudopalisading cells. (*Lower panel*) The zone of hypoxia and central necrosis expands, while the hypoxic tumor cells of pseudopalisades secrete pro-angiogenic factors (VEGF, IL-8) leading to microvascular proliferation in regions adjacent to central hypoxia causing an accelerated outward expansion of tumor cells toward a new vasculature. Illustration by Mica Duran. Reproduced with permission from Blackwell Press from Tehrani M et al. (2008) *Brain Pathology* **18**:164–171 (*see* Color Plate 33)

of tumor cells away from hypoxia, creating a peripherally moving wave (pseudopalisade) and central necrosis; (4) secretion of hypoxia-inducible, pro-angiogenic factors (VEGF, IL-8) by pseudopalisading cells; (5) an exuberant angiogenic response creating microvascular proliferation in regions adjacent to central hypoxia; (6) accelerated outward expansion of tumor cells toward a new vasculature. The global growth properties of GBM within the brain reflect a coalescence of these microscopic processes and result in a peripherally expanding tumor with a large degree of central necrosis.

22.3 The Significance of Pseudopalisades, Necrosis, and Hypoxia

It is widely agreed that pseudopalisades represent hypercellular zones that surround necrotic foci in GBM (Fig. 22.2) (Burger and Green 1987, Kleihues et al. 2000). Pseudopalisading of cells around central degeneration has been recognized for nearly a century as both a defining feature of GBM and a morphologic finding that predicts aggressive behavior (Bailey and Cushing 1926). In light of this, it is curious that there is only scattered data on their nature or their role in tumor progression. Analysis of the shapes and sizes of pseudopalisades suggests that these structures evolve and enlarge over time, giving rise to wider and wider expanses of coagulative necrosis (Brat et al. 2004). A commonly held belief has been that pseudopalisades represent a rim of residual tumor cells around a centrally degenerating clone of highly proliferative cells. The term "pseudopalisade" itself implies that cells have not truly aggregated around necrosis, but only give this impression due to the absence of a cental hypercellular zone.

Recent studies have attempted to more precisely define underlying mechanisms of necrosis and pseudopalisading in GBM (Brat et al. 2004). These began by considering that this hypercellular population around central necrosis could represent (1) a clone of rapid proliferating neoplastic cells that "outgrew its blood supply" and underwent central necrosis (clonal expansion theory); (2) a population of neoplastic cells that was resistant to apoptosis and accumulated due to increased cell survival; (3) a mixed population of neoplastic and inflammatory cells adjacent to necrosis; or (4) a population of rapidly moving tumor cells that superimposed themselves on a more stationary population, causing increased cell density. Perhaps surprisingly, these investigations determined that pseudopalisading cells were *less* proliferative than adjacent tumor, indicating they do not likely accumulate due to clonal expansion (Brat et al. 2004, Schiffer et al. 1995). Second, pseudopalisades are composed almost entirely of tumor cells and do not include a significant population of non-neoplastic cells (e.g., inflammatory cells). Third, pseudopalisades show *increased* levels of apoptosis compared to adjacent tumor, indicating they do not accumulate due to a survival advantage (Brat et al. 2004, Tachibana et al. 1996).

These investigations instead supported a model in which pseudopalisades represent a wave of actively migrating tumor cells that are moving away from an area of central hypoxia. Pseudopalisading cells are known to be hypoxic, as demonstrated by their dramatic upregulation of hypoxia-inducible factor-1 (HIF-1), a nuclear transcription factor that orchestrates the cell's adaptive response to low oxygen (Fig. 22.2) (Brat et al. 2004, Brat and Mapstone 2003, Semenza 2001, Zagzag et al. 2000). Gene expression studies performed on microdissected pseudopalisading cells from human GBMs have also supported that pseudopalisading cells have a hypoxic gene signature (Dong et al. 2005). In one study, a total of 314 up- and 385 downregulated genes were identified in pseudopalisading cells as compared to adjacent brain tumor cells. Pathway analysis of specific gene families revealed a pattern indicating a hypoxic environment, high levels of glycolosis, and cell cycle regulation. Aldolase A, pyruvate kinase, phosphoglycerate kinase and glyceraldehyde-3-phosphate dehydrogenase,and GLUT1, a glucose transporter, were glycolytic genes that were all upregulated in pseudopalisades.

Also supporting the contention that pseudopalisades represent a highly migratory population is the demonstration that hypoxic GBM cells in culture are more motile and that HIF-1 itself can regulate critical pro-migratory mechanisms (Brat et al. 2004, Graham et al. 1999, Krishnamachary et al. 2003, Pennacchietti et al. 2003). Hypoxic upregulation of c-Met, a tyrosine kinase receptor, as well as the potentiation of hepatocyte growth factor (HGF) signaling through c-Met, could account for at least some of the promigratory effects of HIF-1 activation (Abounader and Laterra 2005, Pennacchietti et al. 2003). Moreover, hypoxic pseudopalisades express increased levels of extracellular matrix proteases associated with invasion, including MMP-2 and uPAR (Bellail et al. 2004, Brat et al. 2004, Graham et al. 1999, Mori et al. 2000, Pennacchietti et al. 2003, Yamamoto et al. 1996). Thus, the combined evidence suggests that the pseudopalisades in GBM are formed by a population of hypoxic, actively migrating neoplastic cells that create a hypercellular zone around an evolving area of central necrosis.

22.4 Vascular Pathology Underlies Hypoxia, Necrosis, and Pseudopalisades

The hypoxia that leads to increased tumor cell migration to form pseudopalisades could result from limitations in vascular perfusion within the tumor (i.e., disruption of the blood supply) or from reduced oxygen diffusion within the growing neoplasm, in part due to increased metabolic demands (Brat and Van Meir 2001). A growing body of experimental and observational evidence favors the hypothesis that pseudopalisades represent tumor cells migrating away from a dysfunctional vasculature (Brat et al. 2004, Holash et al. 1999, Zagzag et al. 2000). The majority of pseudopalisades are ring-like or ovoid, but others have a long, narrow and winding (i.e., serpiginous) pattern when viewed in longitudinal tissue sections – a pattern that suggests an underlying vascular substrate (Kleihues et al. 2000). Perhaps less appreciated, abnormal vessels can often be noted within the lumina of at least a subset of pseudopalisades. A comprehensive survey of human GBM specimens found that over 50% of pseudopalisades had evidence of a central vascular lumen that was either degenerating or thrombosed (Fig. 22.2) (Brat et al. 2004). Twenty percent contained a vessel with complete luminal occlusion caused by intravascular thrombosis (Fig. 22.2). Analysis of pseudopalisade sizes and shapes led to the conclusion that tissue sampling and tangential sections result in an underestimation of the true frequency of vascular pathology and intravascular thrombosis within pseudopalisades, which has led to an under-appreciation of their relevance to necrosis in GBM. Moreover, it is worth considering that the vasculature upstream and downstream of intravascular thrombosis will not adequately perfuse the tumor in its distribution, which will ultimately lead to hypoxia and necrosis without histologic evidence of thrombus.

22.5 Initiators of Vascular Pathology

Experimental evidence indicates that vaso-occlusion within gliomas occurs before the development of hypoxia-induced angiogenesis. Inifiltrating tumor cells of low-grade tumors, such as those in grade II astrocytoma, gain access to oxygen and nutrients through a vascular supply by "co-opting" the host's blood vessels (Holash et al. 1999, Zagzag et al. 2000). In response, vascular endothelial cells eventually undergo a number of changes that include hypertrophy, discohesion, and even apoptosis. One suggestion is that endothelial damage is first initiated by the effects of Angiopoietin-2 (Ang-2) on endothelial cell. Ang-2 is thought to act in an autocrine fashion on tumoral blood vessels as a Tie-2 receptor antagonist. In the absence of VEGF, Tie-2 blockage leads to vascular destabilization, endothelial cell apoptosis, and vascular regression (Holash et al. 1999, Maisonpierre et al. 1997). In human specimens, Ang-2 is expressed by endothelial cells of high-grade gliomas but not low-grade gliomas or normal brain, and its upregulation precedes endothelial apoptosis, suggesting that it could cause vascular injury (Stratmann et al. 1998, Zagzag et al. 2000, 1999). Other arguments hold that Ang-2 causes structural changes of vessels that are required for angiogenesis but does not induce apoptosis (Vajkoczy et al. 2002, Zhang et al. 2003). Factors released from glioma cells following genetic alteration (*EGFR* amplication or *PTEN* loss), such as VEGF and TNF-α, could also precipitate vascular injury and thrombosis (Shen et al. 2001). VEGF induces changes in vascular permeability, while both VEGF and TNF-α have been demonstrated to induce endothelial tissue factor expression through activation of the transcription factor Egr-1 (Mechtcheriakova et al. 2001).

22.6 Intravascular Thrombosis Accentuates and Propagates Tumor Hypoxia

While precise initiators of vascular pathology in GBM continue to be studied, it is becoming clear that intravascular thrombosis within these neoplasms can accentuate and propagate tumoral hypoxia and necrosis. A strong relationship between abnormal blood clotting and human malignancy is well established in gliomas and other forms of cancer (Rickles and Falanga 2001). Patients with GBM are at high risk for developing systemic disorders of coagulation, with nearly 30% suffering from deep vein thrombosis or pulmonary thrombo-embolism (Walsh and Kakkar 2001). Intravascular thrombosis within the tumoral tissue of GBM is a frequent finding at the time of operation. Even more impressively, thrombosed vessels within resected GBM specimens can almost always be identified under the microscope (Brat et al. 2004). Both the frequencies of associated systemic coagulopathy and the finding of intravascular thrombosis within neoplastic tissue are much higher in GBMs (grade IV) than AAs (grade III), indicating that critical pro-thrombotic events must occur in this transition (Brat et al. 2004, Sawaya et al. 1995, Walsh and Kakkar 2001).

In order to determine whether intravascular thrombosis was a specific finding associated with the GBM histology, Tehrani et al. investigated the histologic presence of thrombosis in a representative cross section of 297 adult CNS malignancies, including 103 GBMs (Tehrani et al. 2008). Among newly diagnosed (i.e., untreated) tumors, thrombosis was present in 92% of GBM resections, significantly greater than any of the other types of CNS neoplasm. The sensitivity of thrombosis for the diagnosis of GBM in this set of tumors was 92% and the specificity was 91%. Thus, intravascular thrombosis seemed to be a near constant feature of GBM, but not other tumor types. Interestingly, intravascular thrombosis was an uncommon finding in AAs and was only noted in a small number of stereotactic biopsies. This subset of AA patients had significantly shorter survivals than those AAs without thrombosis. This could imply that stereotactic biopsies were actually undersampled GBMs or that these AAs with thrombosis represented an aggressive subset whose progression to the GBM phenotype was imminent. The development of intravascular thrombosis within GBM and the emergence of hypoxia and necrosis are too interrelated, both spatially and temporally, to be coincidental. It is highly probable that intravascular thrombosis initiates or propagates hypoxia and necrosis in GBM (Brat and Van Meir 2004).

22.7 Tissue Factor, a Potent Pro-Coagulant, Is Upregulated in GBM

Multiple factors likely contribute to intravascular thrombosis in GBM, including abnormal blood flow within a distorted vasculature, increased interstitial edema and pressure resulting in vascular collapse, dysregulation of pro- and anti-coagulant factors, and access of plasma clotting factors to tumoral tissue. Normal CNS blood vessels allow only limited diffusion through their walls due to a highly restrictive blood–brain barrier, which is formed primarily by endothelial tight junctions, but also has contributions from astrocytic foot plates, extracellular matrix, and endothelial-pericytic interactions (Dinda et al. 1993). This barrier becomes breached in GBM and can be visualized radiologically by the presence of contrast-enhancement due to increased vascular permeability to contrast agents (e.g., Gadolinium) and to proteins that bind them, such as albumin (Fig. 22.1) (Henson et al. 2005, Zhu et al. 2000).

Damaged vessels appear fenestrated, show detachment of pericytes, and exhibit extracellular matrix alterations (Dinda et al. 1993). All the factors that contribute to increased permeability have not been defined, but VEGF secretion by neoplastic cells is known to cause vascular leakage (Fischer et al. 1999, Senger et al. 1983). One result is the leakage of plasma coagulation factors such as Factor VII into the tissue spaces where they are activated and result in thrombosis.

A large number of plasma clotting factors are dysregulated in GBM and favor thrombosis. For example, the pro-coagulant plasminogen activator inhibitor 1 (PAI-1) is markedly elevated in GBMs, while the expression of anti-coagulants, such as the fibrinolytic tissue type plasminogen activator (tPA), is decreased (Sawaya et al. 1991, 1995). One of the most highly upregulated pro-thrombotic factors in GBM is tissue factor (TF), a 47 kDa transmembrane glycoprotein receptor that is a critical regulator of tissue hemostasis and one of the body's most potent stimulants of thrombosis (Versteeg et al. 2003). In normal tissue, TF is expressed almost exclusively by stromal cells and a disruption of vascular integrity is required to bring TF into contact with its activating ligand from the plasma, Factor VII/VIIa (Morrissey 2001). In turn, TF/Factor VIIa activation promotes the generation of thrombin from prothrombin, ultimately leading to platelet aggregation, fibrin deposition, and local hemostasis. The normally tight regulation of TF is lost in a variety of pathologic conditions including neoplasia and numerous cancers show increased expression by tumor cells, stroma, and endothelium (Rickles et al. 2003). A direct correlation between TF levels and tumor grade has been noted for multiple tumor types (Contrino et al. 1996, Seto et al. 2000), including gliomas (Guan et al. 2002, Hamada et al. 1996). Indeed, TF is highly expressed by over 90% of malignant astrocytomas, but only 10% of grade I and II astrocytomas (Guan et al. 2002). The pro-thrombotic effects of TF at the cell surface are largely mediated through downstream activation of coagulation proteases Factor VII (VIIa), Factor X (Xa), and thrombin.

22.8 PTEN, EGFR, and Hypoxia Regulate Tissue Factor Expression in GBM

Recent investigations have attempted to define the genetic and physiologic triggers that might cause increased TF expression and thrombosis in human malignancy (Boccaccio et al. 2005, Rak et al. 2006, Rong et al. 2005, Yu et al. 2005). Genetic events that arise during astrocytoma progression have been well characterized and include *PTEN* and *TP53* mutations, *p16(CDKN2A)* and $p14^{ARF}$ deletions, *EGFR* and *MDM2* amplifications (Hunter et al. 2003). Among these, *EGFR* amplification and *PTEN* mutations are prime candidates to explore for regulation of pro-thrombotic factors since they occur precisely during the transition from AA to GBM, when thrombosis and pseudopalisades emerge (Rak et al. 2006, Yu et al. 2004). *PTEN* is a tumor suppressor located at 10q23.3 (Li et al. 1997). Inactivating mutations of *PTEN* occur in 30–40% of GBMs and gene inactivation through promoter methylation leads to lost expression of PTEN in over 70% (Duerr et al. 1998, Rasheed et al. 1997, Wang et al. 1997). The effects of PTEN on TF expression and pro-coagulant properties by malignant gliomas were recently studied by introducing a wild-type *PTEN* gene into a *PTEN* null glioma cell line (U87MG). The expression TF protein at the cell surface of glioma cells was dramatically suppressed by PTEN, which in turn led to prolonged plasma clotting times using in vitro measures of coagulation. Although many of PTEN's biologic effects depend on its lipid phosphatase activity and ability to antagonize PI-3 kinase, these studies indicated that regulation of TF depended at least in part on PTEN's protein phosphatase activity. Potential downstream signaling mechanisms relevant to the control of TF by PTEN were investigated using a series of human astrocytes that were sequentially transformed with E6/E7/hTERT, Ras, and Akt expression vectors, which have been used to recapitulate astrocytoma progression both in vitro and in vivo (Sonoda et al. 2001a, b). Cells transfected with either Akt or Ras showed upregulation of TF, while those transformed with combined Ras and Akt showed the highest TF expression, suggesting that both signaling pathways may participate as downstream regulators of PTEN (Rong et al. 2005, Yu et al. 2005). Other investigations have emphasized that activated forms of Ras are critical for the expression of TF and its tumorigenic effects (Yu et al. 2005). Thus, PTEN loss during astrocytoma progression likely leads to increased TF expression and plasma coagulation, both through Akt/Ras-dependent and protein phosphatase-dependent mechansism.

EGFR amplification is a second genetic alteration present in a subset of GBMs (40–50%) that could be responsible for TF upregulation. The most frequent *EGFR* mutation in GBM involves deletion of exon 2–7 resulting in the constitutively active form EGFRvIII. It has recently been shown that overexpression of either EGFR or EGFRvIII in human glioma cells in vitro consistently leads to increased basal expression of TF. When EGFR overexpressing gliomas are stimulated with EGF, there is a striking upregulation of TF that occurs within 6 hours (Fig. 22.4). In all cases, increased TF expression by GBM leads to accelerated plasma coagulation in vitro. The EGFR-mediated increases in TF expression depended most strongly on AP-1 transcriptional activity and were associated with c-Jun N-terminal kinase (JNK) and JunD activation. Interestingly, the restoration of PTEN expression in *PTEN*-deficient GBM cells diminished EGFR-induced TF expression by inhibiting this same JunD/AP-1 transcriptional activity. PTEN mediated this effect by antagonizing PI-3 K activity, which in turn attenuated both Akt and JNK activities. It was also suggested that these mechanisms are likely at work in vivo, since amplification of *EGFR* and expression of EGFR protein were associated with the expression of TF and the presence of thrombosis in human high-grade astrocytoma specimens (Fig. 22.5 and Color Plate 34).

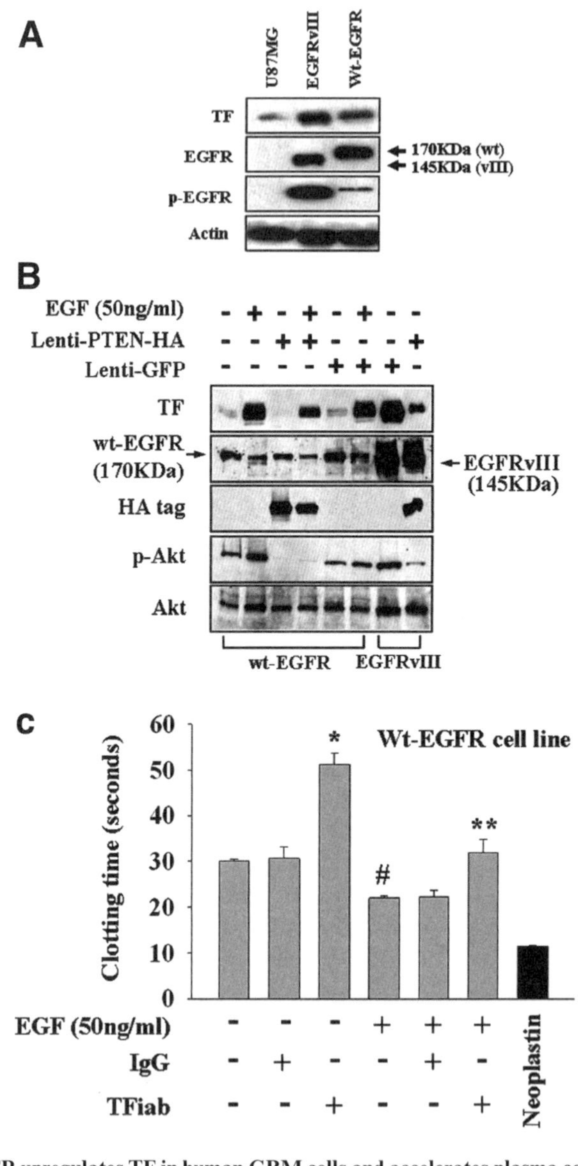

Fig. 22.4 EGFR upregulates TF in human GBM cells and accelerates plasma coagulation, while PTEN suppresses TF expression (A) Western blot of cell lysates from U87MG, U87MG-EGFRvIII, and U87MG-wt-EGFR cells demonstrates higher basal TF expression by U87MG-EGFRvIII cells (lane 2) and U87MG-EGFRwt (lane 3). U87MG-EGFRvIII has a high level of constitutively active tyrosine kinase activity as demonstrated by the phosphorylated form of EGFR. (**B**) Western blot of cell lysates from U87MG-wt-EGFR cells following Lentiviral infection of PTEN-HA or GFP shows reduced TF expression under both basal and EGF-stimulated (50 ng/ml, 24 h) conditions. Western blot of U87MG-EGFRvIII cell lysates following Lentiviral infection of PTEN-HA or GFP shows reduced expression of TF in PTEN-HA infected cells. (**C**) The addition of 10^6 U87MG-EGFRwt

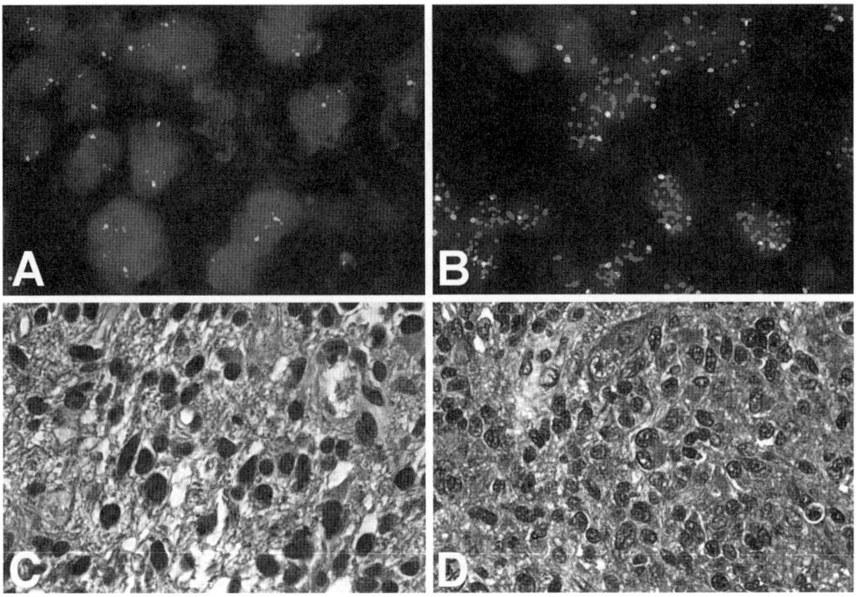

Fig. 22.5 Fluorescence in situ hybridization (FISH) analysis of *EGFR* gene status and IHC analysis of EGFR and TF protein in human GBM and AA specimens. (**A, B**) Representative fluorescence images showing the *EGFR* (*orange*) and chromosome 7 centromeric (*green*) signals in interphase GBM cells. (**A**) A GBM specimen that is non-amplified for *EGFR* shows roughly equal numbers of *EGFR* and centromeric signals per nuclei (typically 2 *EGFR* signals per nucleus). (**B**) GBM with *EGFR* gene amplification shows greatly increased signals for *EGFR* compared to centromeric signal (>10 *EGFR* signals per nucleus). (**C, D**) IHC for TF protein expression in AA and GBM specimens using DAB (*brown*) for detection. (**C**) Representative image of AA showing weak TF expression (1+, *brown color*) in the cytoplasm on scattered tumor cells. (**D**) GBM specimen showing strong TF staining (3+ *brown color*) within the cytoplasm of nearly all tumor cells (*see* Color Plate 34)

Thus, both EGFR activation and PTEN loss, which both occur in the transition to GBM, favor the upregulation of TF.

In addition to genetic regulation, TF is also strongly upregulated by hypoxia in GBM (Rong et al. 2005). Hypoxic GBM cells placed directly into human plasma cause a marked acceleration of plasma clotting times compared to

Fig. 22.4 (continued) glioma cells to human plasma causes plasma clotting in 30 sec (control, neoplastin causes plasma clotting in 12 sec). Stimulation of these cells with EGF (50 ng/ml) causes a significant shortening of the clotting time to 23 sec (#p < 0.001). An inhibitory antibody directed at TF (TFiab) causes a dramatic prolongation of plasma clotting time in both the unstimulated and the EGF-stimulated conditions (*, ** p < 0.001), while nonspecific IgG has no effect on plasma clotting normoxic cells. This effect can be prevented by both the pre-incubation of cells with inhibitory antibodies to TF (Fig. 22.4C) and by using plasma that lacks Factor VII (not shown), strongly implicating TF-dependent mechanisms. Similar hypoxic conditions also cause a rapid increase in TF mRNA and protein expression by GBM cells in vitro, which are modestly suppressed by PTEN expression (Rong et al. 2005). Within human GBM specimens, the severely hypoxic pseudopalisading cells around necrosis show the highest level of TF expression, corroborating in vitro studies (Rong et al. 2005). Mechanisms responsible for the hypoxic upregulation of TF are challenging to investigate since the TF promoter contains binding sites for a variety of transcriptional regulators that can be induced by hypoxia, including Egr-1, Sp1, NF-κB, and AP-1 (Mackman 1997). The accumulated evidence in animal models and in vitro indicates that Egr-1 is the transcription factor that is most important to the hypoxic upregulation of TF and that these mechanisms do not depend on the increased expression of HIF-1 (Rong et al. 2006, Yan et al. 1999a, b). Thus, both *PTEN* loss and hypoxia upregulate TF expression and promote plasma clotting by GBM cells in vitro, which might suggest that these mechanisms promote intravascular thrombosis and pseudopalisading necrosis in the transition from AA to GBM.

22.9 TF Intitiates Signaling Through Its Cytoplasmic Tail and Through PARs

As a transmembrane receptor, TF is activated by binding to Factor VII/VIIa and transduces independent intracellular signals through its cytoplasmic tail and through interactions with the G-protein-coupled protease-activated receptors (PARs) that promote tumorigenesis. Activation of pro-coagulant function of TF is accompanied by the formation of stabilizing disulfide bonds between two cystein residues within its extracellular domain (Rehemtulla et al. 1991). A cell surface protein-disulfide isomerase (PDI) targets the disulfide bond and inactivates pro-coagulant activity but maintains intracellular signaling throughout the cytoplasmic tail (Ahamed et al. 2006). Activation of TF following Factor VIIa binding leads to the downstream activation of the mitogen-activated protein (MAP) kinase members p38 MAP kinase, p42/p44 MAP kinase, and c-Jun N-terminal kinase (JNK) (Versteeg and Ruf 2006). Other downstream pathways activated include Src-like kinases, PI3-kinase, and c-Akt/PKB Rac and Cdc42. Many of these signaling cascades cause interactions with cytoskeletal elements including actin to induce a pro-migratory phenotype (Ott et al. 1998, 2005, Versteeg et al. 2000). Intracellular signaling mechanisms induced by TF strongly promote tumorigenesis through pro-angiogenic and pro-metastatic mechanisms (Belting et al. 2004, Versteeg et al. 2003, Versteeg and Ruf 2006, Versteeg et al. 2008, 2004).

The activation of TF by Factor VIIa also has biologic significance beyond specific pro-coagulant function and signaling through its cytoplasmic tail. For example, thrombin, Factor VIIa, and Factor Xa are proteases that act as potent physiologic activators of protease-activated receptors (PARs), a family of G-protein-coupled, transmembrane receptors (Versteeg and Ruf 2006). PAR1, the family's prototype, is activated most strongly by thrombin, which cleaves the amino-terminal extracellular domain of PAR1 and unmasks a new N-terminus, which then serves as the receptor's ligand (Coughlin 2000). Both PAR1 and PAR2 can also be activated by Factors VIIa and Factor Xa. Activated PARs tranduce intracellular signals by coupling through G-proteins, predominantly Gαi, Gαq, and Gα12/13. Secondary signals are generated through Rho, phopholipase C (IP3 and diacylglycerol), and inhibition of adenyl cyclase. Although PARs are expressed at low levels in most normal epithelia, they are aberrantly overexpressed by a variety of carcinomas including those of breast, colon, lung, and stomach (Darmoul et al. 2003, Even-Ram et al. 1998, 2001). PAR1 activation can transform cells and is able to enhance tumorigenicity, in large part by signaling through Gαq and Gα13 (Marinissen et al. 2003, Wang et al. 2002). It is also clear that PAR1 and PAR2 activation by coagulation factors promotes invasive and metastatic properties of malignant cells (Even-Ram et al. 1998, Hjortoe et al. 2004, Morris et al. 2006, Nguyen et al. 2005, Versteeg et al. 2008). Mechanisms of increased invasion include its ability to direct cytoskeletal actin rearrangements, phosphorylation of focal adhesion kinases, and recruitment of αvβ5 integrin to contact sites (Even-Ram et al. 2001).

PAR1 protein is present in both the human and the mouse central nervous system, mostly in astrocytes, where it can be activated by thrombin (Junge et al. 2004, 2003). Investigations of human GBM cell lines and short-term cultures of resected human GBM specimens have demonstrated that PAR1 is present on the surface of tumor cells where it can be activated by both thrombin and PAR1 agonists. Such activation leads to increased phospho-inositol (PI) hydrolysis and calcium mobilization, presumably coupling through Gαq (Junge et al. 2004). Although more evidence is required to determine the biologic relevance of TF activation of thrombin and consequent PAR1 signaling in gliomas, it is highly probable that the activation of PAR1 by pro-coagulant proteases directs the migration of tumor cells in a manner similar to other malignancies. In the context of human GBM, activation would be expected to direct migration away from vaso-occlusion and hypoxia to form pseudopalisades.

22.10 Angiogenesis Supports Peripheral Tumor Growth

The emerging models of GBM progression indicate that vascular pathology may underlie the development of hypoxia and necrosis in GBM. While necrosis has long been recognized as a marker of aggressive behavior in diffuse gliomas, it does not explain rapid tumor progression per se (Burger and Green 1987, Raza et al. 2002). Instead, pseudopalisades that surround necrosis in GBM are intimately related to microvascular hyperplasia, a defining morphologic feature of GBM that is most often noted in regions directly adjacent to pseudopalisades (Figs. 22.2, 22.3) (Brat et al. 2002, Brat and Mapstone 2003, Brat and Van Meir 2001). This angiogenic response attempts to lay down a new vasculature for rapid neoplastic expansion, yet the proper function of these distorted vessels has not been established.

One of the most critical pro-angiogenic factors produced by hypoxic pseudopalisades that is responsible for directing nearby angiogenesis in GBM is vascular endothelial growth factor (VEGF). The *VEGF* gene contains an hypoxia responsive element (HRE) within its promoter that binds HIF-1, thereby activating transcription (Plate 1999, Plate et al. 1992, Semenza 2001, Shweiki et al. 1992). VEGF concentrations in the cystic fluid of human GBMs can reach levels that are 200- to 300-fold higher than in serum (Takano et al. 1996). Inhibition of the HIF/VEGF pathway suppresses tumor growth experimentally (Kung et al. 2000). Once expressed and secreted, extracellular VEGF binds to its high-affinity receptors, VEGFR-1 and VEGFR-2, which are upregulated on endothelial cells of high-grade gliomas but not present in normal brain (Plate 1999). Receptor activation then leads to angiogenesis in regions adjacent to pseudopalisades, eventually leading to a vascular density in GBMs that is among the highest of all human neoplasms (Figs. 22.2, 22.3).

A second pro-angiogenic factor that is highly upregulated in GBMs is interleukin-8 (IL-8, CXCL8) (Brat et al. 2005). Much like VEGF, hypoxia/anoxia strongly stimulates IL-8 expression and its expression is also found at highest levels within the pseudopalisades of GBM (Desbaillets et al. 1999, 1997). Unlike VEGF, IL-8 has a more punctate distribution within pseudopalisades and it remains unclear if tumor cells or scattered infiltrating macrophages are responsible for the majority of its expression. Hypoxic upregulation of the *IL-8* gene is not directly due to HIF activation, since there is no HRE within its promoter. Rather, the IL-8 promoter contains binding sites for other transcription factors, including NF-κB, AP-1, and C-EBP/NF-IL-6. AP-1 appears to mediate much of IL-8's upregulation by hypoxia/anoxia (Desbaillets et al. 1999, 1997, Garkavtsev et al. 2004). IL-8 is also strongly upregulated by tumor cells in response to activation of Factor VIIa by TF. Such overexpression of IL-8 by neoplastic cells may have autocrine effects on the malignant behavior of tumor cells (i.e., invasion or metastasis) in addition to inducing angiogenesis (Hjortoe et al. 2004). The IL-8 receptors that could potentially contribute to IL-8-mediated tumorigenic and angiogenic responses in GBM include CXCR1 and CXCR2, both of which are G-protein coupled.

The precise type of angiogenesis that is most evident in GBM, microvascular hyperplasia, is characterized by numerous enlarged, rapidly dividing endothelial cells, pericytes, and smooth muscle cells that form tufted micro-aggregates at the leading edge of sprouting vessels (Fig. 22.2A) (Brat and Van Meir 2001). In its most florid form, angiogenesis takes the shape of "glomeruloid bodies" – a feature that is most characteristic of GBM but is also an independent marker of poor prognosis in other forms of cancer (Straume et al. 2002). Since necrosis and hypoxia are located in the GBM's core and near the contrast-enhancing rim, hypoxia-induced angiogenesis occurs further peripherally, favoring neoplastic growth outward. The permissive nature of the CNS parenchymal matrix to diffuse infiltration by individual glioma cells allows for this burst of peripheral expansion (Bellail et al. 2004).

22.11 Conclusion

The development of hypoxia and necrosis within a diffuse glioma has critical biologic implications and results in a highly aggressvie tumor, GBM. The pseudopalisades around necrosis and the ensuing microvascular hyperplasia may suggest an underlying mechanism responsible for this accelerated growth. We have proposed that a sequence of events that includes vaso-occlusion and intravascular thrombosis leads to the development of the biologically aggressive hypoxic growth phase in GBM. These mechanisms could readily explain the dramatic change in behavior as tumors transition to the GBM histology. Since both necrosis and vascular proliferation are also markers of poor prognosis in other types of cancer, the identification of their underlying mechanisms may have more general implications for tumor angiogenesis and malignant progression. Once identified, the pathophysiologic triggers underlying vaso-occlusion will become attractive, novel targets for anti-tumor therapy.

References

Abounader R, Laterra J (2005) Scatter factor/hepatocyte growth factor in brain tumor growth and angiogenesis. Neuro Oncol 7:436–451

Ahamed J, Versteeg HH, Kerver M, et al. (2006) Disulfide isomerization switches tissue factor from coagulation to cell signaling. Proc Natl Acad Sci USA 103:13932–13937

Bailey P, Cushing H (1926) Tumors of the glioma group. Lippincott Philadelphia

Bellail AC, Hunter SB, Brat DJ, et al. (2004) Microregional extracellular matrix heterogeneity in brain modulates glioma cell invasion. Int J Biochem Cell Biol 36:1046–1069

Belting M, Dorrell MI, Sandgren S, et al. (2004) Regulation of angiogenesis by tissue factor cytoplasmic domain signaling. Nat Med 10:502–509

Boccaccio C, Sabatino G, Medico E, et al. (2005) The MET oncogene drives a genetic programme linking cancer to haemostasis. Nature 434:396–400

Brat DJ, Bellail AC, Van Meir EG (2005) The role of interleukin-8 and its receptors in gliomagenesis and tumoral angiogenesis. Neuro Oncol 7:122–133

Brat DJ, Castellano-Sanchez A, Kaur B, et al. (2002) Genetic and biologic progression in astrocytomas and their relation to angiogenic dysregulation. Adv Anat Pathol 9:24–36

Brat DJ, Castellano-Sanchez AA, Hunter SB, et al. (2004) Pseudopalisades in glioblastoma are hypoxic, express extracellular matrix proteases, and are formed by an actively migrating cell population. Cancer Res 64:920–927

Brat DJ, Mapstone TB (2003) Malignant glioma physiology: cellular response to hypoxia and its role in tumor progression. Ann Intern Med 138:659–668

Brat DJ, Van Meir EG (2001) Glomeruloid microvascular proliferation orchestrated by VPF/ VEGF: a new world of angiogenesis research. Am J Pathol 158:789–796
Brat DJ, Van Meir EG (2004) Vaso-occlusive and prothrombotic mechanisms associated with tumor hypoxia, necrosis, and accelerated growth in glioblastoma. Lab Invest 84:397–405
Burger PC, Green SB (1987) Patient age, histologic features, and length of survival in patients with glioblastoma multiforme. Cancer 59:1617–1625
Central Brain Tumor Registry of the United States (CBTRUS) (2002) Statistical report: primary brain tumors in the United States 1995–1999. Central Brain Tumor Registry of the United States (CBTRUS), Chicago, IL
Contrino J, Hair G, Kreutzer DL, et al. (1996) In situ detection of tissue factor in vascular endothelial cells: correlation with the malignant phenotype of human breast disease. Nat Med 2:209–215
Coughlin SR (2000) Thrombin signalling and protease-activated receptors. Nature 407:258–264
Darmoul D, Gratio V, Devaud H, et al. (2003) Aberrant expression and activation of the thrombin receptor protease-activated receptor-1 induces cell proliferation and motility in human colon cancer cells. Am J Pathol 162:1503–1513
Desbaillets I, Diserens AC, de Tribolet N, et al. (1999) Regulation of interleukin-8 expression by reduced oxygen pressure in human glioblastoma. Oncogene 18:1447–1456
Desbaillets I, Diserens AC, Tribolet N, et al. (1997) Upregulation of interleukin 8 by oxygen-deprived cells in glioblastoma suggests a role in leukocyte activation, chemotaxis, and angiogenesis. J Exp Med 186:1201–1212
Dinda AK, Sarkar C, Roy S, et al. (1993) A transmission and scanning electron microscopic study of tumoral and peritumoral microblood vessels in human gliomas. J Neurooncol 16:149–158
Dong S, Nutt CL, Betensky RA, et al. (2005) Histology-based expression profiling yields novel prognostic markers in human glioblastoma. J Neuropathol Exp Neurol 64:948–955
Duerr EM, Rollbrocker B, Hayashi Y, et al. (1998) PTEN mutations in gliomas and glioneuronal tumors. Oncogene 16:2259–2264
Even-Ram S, Uziely B, Cohen P, et al. (1998) Thrombin receptor overexpression in malignant and physiological invasion processes. Nat Med 4:909–914
Even-Ram SC, Maoz M, Pokroy E, et al. (2001) Tumor cell invasion is promoted by activation of protease activated receptor-1 in cooperation with the alpha vbeta 5 integrin. J Biol Chem 276:10952–10962
Fischer S, Clauss M, Wiesnet M, et al. (1999) Hypoxia induces permeability in brain microvessel endothelial cells via VEGF and NO. Am J Physiol 276:C812–820
Garkavtsev I, Kozin SV, Chernova O, et al. (2004) The candidate tumour suppressor protein ING4 regulates brain tumour growth and angiogenesis. Nature 428:328–332
Graham CH, Forsdike J, Fitzgerald CJ, et al. (1999) Hypoxia-mediated stimulation of carcinoma cell invasiveness via upregulation of urokinase receptor expression. Int J Cancer 80:617–623
Guan M, Jin J, Su B, et al. (2002) Tissue factor expression and angiogenesis in human glioma. Clin Biochem 35:321–325
Gupta M, Djalilvand A, Brat DJ (2005) Clarifying the diffuse gliomas: an update on the morphologic features and markers that discriminate oligodendroglioma from astrocytoma. Am J Clin Pathol 124:755–768
Hamada K, Kuratsu J, Saitoh Y, et al. (1996) Expression of tissue factor correlates with grade of malignancy in human glioma. Cancer 77:1877–1883
Henson JW, Gaviani P, Gonzalez RG (2005) MRI in treatment of adult gliomas. Lancet Oncol 6:167–175
Hjortoe GM, Petersen LC, Albrektsen T, et al. (2004) Tissue factor-factor VIIa-specific up-regulation of IL-8 expression in MDA-MB-231 cells is mediated by PAR-2 and results in increased cell migration. Blood 103:3029–3037

Holash J, Maisonpierre PC, Compton D, et al. (1999) Vessel cooption, regression, and growth in tumors mediated by angiopoietins and VEGF. Science 284:1994–1998
Hunter SB, Brat DJ, Olson JJ, et al. (2003) Alterations in molecular pathways of diffusely infiltrating glial neoplasms: application to tumor classification and anti-tumor therapy (Review). Int J Oncol 23:857–869
Junge CE, Lee CJ, Hubbard KB, et al. (2004) Protease-activated receptor-1 in human brain: localization and functional expression in astrocytes. Exp Neurol 188:94–103
Junge CE, Sugawara T, Mannaioni G, et al. (2003) The contribution of protease-activated receptor 1 to neuronal damage caused by transient focal cerebral ischemia. Proc Natl Acad Sci USA 100:13019–13024
Kleihues P, Burger PC, Collins VP, et al. (2000) Pathology and genetics of tumours of the nervous systems. International Agency for Research on Cancer Lyon
Krishnamachary B, Berg-Dixon S, Kelly B, et al. (2003) Regulation of colon carcinoma cell invasion by hypoxia-inducible factor 1. Cancer Res 63:1138–1143
Kung AL, Wang S, Klco JM, et al. (2000) Suppression of tumor growth through disruption of hypoxia-inducible transcription. Nat Med 6:1335–1340
Li J, Yen C, Liaw D, et al. (1997) PTEN, a putative protein tyrosine phosphatase gene mutated in human brain, breast, and prostate cancer. Science 275:1943–1947
Mackman N (1997) Regulation of the tissue factor gene. Thromb Haemost 78:747–754
Maisonpierre PC, Suri C, Jones PF, et al. (1997) Angiopoietin-2, a natural antagonist for Tie2 that disrupts in vivo angiogenesis. Science 277:55–60
Mandonnet E, Delattre JY, Tanguy ML, et al. (2003) Continuous growth of mean tumor diameter in a subset of grade II gliomas. Ann Neurol 53:524–528
Marinissen MJ, Servitja JM, Offermanns S, et al. (2003) Thrombin protease-activated receptor-1 signals through Gq- and G13-initiated MAPK cascades regulating c-Jun expression to induce cell transformation. J Biol Chem 278:46814–46825
Mechtcheriakova D, Schabbauer G, Lucerna M, et al. (2001) Specificity, diversity, and convergence in VEGF and TNF-alpha signaling events leading to tissue factor up-regulation via EGR-1 in endothelial cells. Faseb J 15:230–242
Mori T, Abe T, Wakabayashi Y, et al. (2000) Up-regulation of urokinase-type plasminogen activator and its receptor correlates with enhanced invasion activity of human glioma cells mediated by transforming growth factor-alpha or basic fibroblast growth factor. J Neurooncol 46:115–123
Morris DR, Ding Y, Ricks TK, et al. (2006) Protease-activated receptor-2 is essential for factor VIIa and Xa-induced signaling, migration, and invasion of breast cancer cells. Cancer Res 66:307–314
Morrissey JH (2001) Tissue factor: an enzyme cofactor and a true receptor. Thromb Haemost 86:66–74
Nelson JS, Tsukada Y, Schoenfeld D, et al. (1983) Necrosis as a prognostic criterion in malignant supratentorial, astrocytic gliomas. Cancer 52:550–554
Nguyen QD, De Wever O, Bruyneel E, et al. (2005) Commutators of PAR-1 signaling in cancer cell invasion reveal an essential role of the Rho-Rho kinase axis and tumor microenvironment. Oncogene 24:8240–8251
Ohgaki H, Kleihues P (2005) Epidemiology and etiology of gliomas. Acta Neuropathol (Berl) 109:93–108
Ott I, Fischer EG, Miyagi Y, et al. (1998) A role for tissue factor in cell adhesion and migration mediated by interaction with actin-binding protein 280. J Cell Biol 140:1241–1253
Ott I, Weigand B, Michl R, et al. (2005) Tissue factor cytoplasmic domain stimulates migration by activation of the GTPase Rac1 and the mitogen-activated protein kinase p38. Circulation 111:349–355
Pennacchietti S, Michieli P, Galluzzo M, et al. (2003) Hypoxia promotes invasive growth by transcriptional activation of the met protooncogene. Cancer Cell 3:347–361
Plate KH (1999) Mechanisms of angiogenesis in the brain. J Neuropathol Exp Neurol 58:313–320

Plate KH, Breier G, Weich HA, et al. (1992) Vascular endothelial growth factor is a potential tumour angiogenesis factor in human gliomas in vivo. Nature 359:845–848
Rak J, Milsom C, May L, et al. (2006) Tissue factor in cancer and angiogenesis: the molecular link between genetic tumor progression, tumor neovascularization, and cancer coagulopathy. Semin Thromb Hemost 32:54–70
Rasheed BK, Stenzel TT, McLendon RE, et al. (1997) PTEN gene mutations are seen in high-grade but not in low-grade gliomas. Cancer Res 57:4187–4190
Raza SM, Lang FF, Aggarwal BB, et al. (2002) Necrosis and glioblastoma: a friend or a foe? A review and a hypothesis. Neurosurgery 51:2–12; discussion 12–13
Rehemtulla A, Ruf W, Edgington TS (1991) The integrity of the cysteine 186-cysteine 209 bond of the second disulfide loop of tissue factor is required for binding of factor VII. J Biol Chem 266:10294–10299
Rickles FR, Falanga A (2001) Molecular basis for the relationship between thrombosis and cancer. Thromb Res 102:V215–224
Rickles FR, Patierno S, Fernandez PM (2003) Tissue factor, thrombin, and cancer. Chest 124:58S–68S
Rong Y, Hu F, Huang R, et al. (2006) Early growth response gene-1 regulates hypoxia-induced expression of tissue factor in glioblastoma multiforme through hypoxia-inducible factor-1-independent mechanisms. Cancer Res 66:7067–7074
Rong Y, Post DE, Pieper RO, et al. (2005) PTEN and hypoxia regulate tissue factor expression and plasma coagulation by glioblastoma. Cancer Res 65:1406–1413
Sawaya R, Ramo OJ, Shi ML, et al. (1991) Biological significance of tissue plasminogen activator content in brain tumors. J Neurosurg 74:480–486
Sawaya R, Yamamoto M, Ramo OJ, et al. (1995) Plasminogen activator inhibitor-1 in brain tumors: relation to malignancy and necrosis. Neurosurgery 36:375–380; discussion 380–371
Schiffer D, Cavalla P, Migheli A, et al. (1995) Apoptosis and cell proliferation in human neuroepithelial tumors. Neurosci Lett 195:81–84
Semenza GL (2001) Hypoxia-inducible factor 1: oxygen homeostasis and disease pathophysiology. Trends Mol Med 7:345–350
Senger DR, Galli SJ, Dvorak AM, et al. (1983) Tumor cells secrete a vascular permeability factor that promotes accumulation of ascites fluid. Science 219:983–985
Seto S, Onodera H, Kaido T, et al. (2000) Tissue factor expression in human colorectal carcinoma: correlation with hepatic metastasis and impact on prognosis. Cancer 88:295–301
Shapiro WR, Young DF (1976) Treatment of malignant glioma. A controlled study of chemotherapy and irradiation. Arch Neurol 33:494–450
Shen BQ, Lee DY, Cortopassi KM, et al. (2001) Vascular endothelial growth factor KDR receptor signaling potentiates tumor necrosis factor-induced tissue factor expression in endothelial cells. J Biol Chem 276:5281–5286
Shweiki D, Itin A, Soffer D, et al. (1992) Vascular endothelial growth factor induced by hypoxia may mediate hypoxia-initiated angiogenesis. Nature 359:843–845
Sonoda Y, Ozawa T, Aldape KD, et al. (2001a) Akt pathway activation converts anaplastic astrocytoma to glioblastoma multiforme in a human astrocyte model of glioma. Cancer Res 61:6674–6678
Sonoda Y, Ozawa T, Hirose Y, et al. (2001b) Formation of intracranial tumors by genetically modified human astrocytes defines four pathways critical in the development of human anaplastic astrocytoma. Cancer Res 61:4956–4960
Stratmann A, Risau W, Plate KH (1998) Cell type-specific expression of angiopoietin-1 and angiopoietin-2 suggests a role in glioblastoma angiogenesis. Am J Pathol 153:1459–1466
Straume O, Chappuis PO, Salvesen HB, et al. (2002) Prognostic importance of glomeruloid microvascular proliferation indicates an aggressive angiogenic phenotype in human cancers. Cancer Res 62:6808–6811
Stupp R, Mason WP, van den Bent MJ, et al. (2005) Radiotherapy plus concomitant and adjuvant temozolomide for glioblastoma. N Engl J Med 352:987–996

Swanson KR, Bridge C, Murray JD, et al. (2003) Virtual and real brain tumors: using mathematical modeling to quantify glioma growth and invasion. J Neurol Sci 216:1–10
Tachibana O, Lampe J, Kleihues P, et al. (1996) Preferential expression of Fas/APO1 (CD95) and apoptotic cell death in perinecrotic cells of glioblastoma multiforme. Acta Neuropathol (Berl) 92:431–434
Takano S, Yoshii Y, Kondo S, et al. (1996) Concentration of vascular endothelial growth factor in the serum and tumor tissue of brain tumor patients. Cancer Res 56:2185–2190
Tehrani M, Friedman, T, Olson, JJ, Brat, DJ. (2008) Intravascular thrombosis in central nervous system malignancies: a potential role in astrocytoma progression. Brain Pathol 18:164–171
Vajkoczy P, Farhadi M, Gaumann A, et al. (2002) Microtumor growth initiates angiogenic sprouting with simultaneous expression of VEGF, VEGF receptor-2, and angiopoietin-2. J Clin Invest 109:777–785
Versteeg HH, Hoedemaeker I, Diks SH, et al. (2000) Factor VIIa/tissue factor-induced signaling via activation of Src-like kinases, phosphatidylinositol 3-kinase, and Rac. J Biol Chem 275:28750–28756
Versteeg HH, Peppelenbosch MP, Spek CA (2003) Tissue factor signal transduction in angiogenesis. Carcinogenesis 24:1009–1013
Versteeg HH, Ruf W (2006) Emerging insights in tissue factor-dependent signaling events. Semin Thromb Hemost 32:24–32
Versteeg HH, Schaffner F, Kerver M, et al. (2008) Inhibition of tissue factor signaling suppresses tumor growth. Blood 111:190–199
Versteeg HH, Spek CA, Peppelenbosch MP, et al. (2004) Tissue factor and cancer metastasis: the role of intracellular and extracellular signaling pathways. Mol Med 10:6–11
Walsh DC, Kakkar AK (2001) Thromboembolism in brain tumors. Curr Opin Pulm Med 7:326–331
Wang H, Ubl JJ, Stricker R, et al. (2002) Thrombin (PAR-1)-induced proliferation in astrocytes via MAPK involves multiple signaling pathways. Am J Physiol Cell Physiol 283:C1351–1364
Wang SI, Puc J, Li J, et al. (1997) Somatic mutations of PTEN in glioblastoma multiforme. Cancer Res 57:4183–4186
Yamamoto M, Mohanam S, Sawaya R, et al. (1996) Differential expression of membrane-type matrix metalloproteinase and its correlation with gelatinase A activation in human malignant brain tumors in vivo and in vitro. Cancer Res 56:384–392
Yan SF, Lu J, Zou YS, et al. (1999a) Hypoxia-associated induction of early growth response-1 gene expression. J Biol Chem 274:15030–15040
Yan SF, Mackman N, Kisiel W, et al. (1999b) Hypoxia/Hypoxemia-Induced activation of the procoagulant pathways and the pathogenesis of ischemia-associated thrombosis. Arterioscler Thromb Vasc Biol 19:2029–2035
Yu JL, May L, Klement P, et al. (2004) Oncogenes as regulators of tissue factor expression in cancer: implications for tumor angiogenesis and anti-cancer therapy. Semin Thromb Hemost 30:21–30
Yu JL, May L, Lhotak V, et al. (2005) Oncogenic events regulate tissue factor expression in colorectal cancer cells: implications for tumor progression and angiogenesis. Blood 105:1734–1741
Zagzag D, Amirnovin R, Greco MA, et al. (2000) Vascular apoptosis and involution in gliomas precede neovascularization: a novel concept for glioma growth and angiogenesis. Lab Invest 80:837–849
Zagzag D, Hooper A, Friedlander DR, et al. (1999) In situ expression of angiopoietins in astrocytomas identifies angiopoietin-2 as an early marker of tumor angiogenesis. Exp Neurol 159:391–400
Zagzag D, Zhong H, Scalzitti JM, et al. (2000) Expression of hypoxia-inducible factor 1alpha in brain tumors: association with angiogenesis, invasion, and progression. Cancer 88:2606–2618

Zhang L, Yang N, Park JW, et al. (2003) Tumor-derived vascular endothelial growth factor up-regulates angiopoietin-2 in host endothelium and destabilizes host vasculature, supporting angiogenesis in ovarian cancer. Cancer Res 63:3403–3412

Zhu XP, Li KL, Kamaly-Asl ID, et al. (2000) Quantification of endothelial permeability, leakage space, and blood volume in brain tumors using combined T1 and T2* contrast-enhanced dynamic MR imaging. J Magn Reson Imaging 11:575–585

Chapter 23
Transcription Profiling of Brain Tumors: Tumor Biology and Treatment Stratification

Erik P. Sulman, Marisol Guerrero, and Ken Aldape

Abstract The spectrum and diversity of primary brain tumors has made prognostic determinations based purely on clinicopathologic variables inexact. For the most frequently occurring and lethal tumors, the malignant astrocytomas, the use of large-scale gene expression profiling experiments has led to a better understanding of the biology of these tumors, giving insights into their origin and development, as well as more powerful outcome prediction. It has also paved the way for the possibility of personalized medicine, where a patient's tumor expression profile can be used to design treatment specific to that individual with the greatest possibility of response. This chapter will focus on the use and development of transcriptional profiles as biomarkers of outcome and treatment response in patients with brain tumors. The discussion will be limited to array-based profiling, as other techniques, such as serial analysis of gene expression (SAGE), have had less widespread use (Ljubimova et al. 2001a; Boon et al. 2003; Boon and Riggins 2003; Beaty et al. 2007; Kavsan et al. 2007). While mRNA-based profiles have been described for a variety of tumors that affect the central nervous system, this chapter will focus particularly on malignant gliomas, to which the majority of large-scale efforts have been focused to date, both due to the larger tumor populations available for analyses and due to the poorer outcome of patients with these devastating tumors (Kleihues et al. 2000; Behin et al. 2003).

Contents

K. Aldape (✉)
Department of Pathology and Radiation Oncology, M. D. Anderson Cancer Center, Houston, TX, USA
e-mail: kaldape@mdanderson.org

E.G. Van Meir (ed.), *CNS Cancer*, Cancer Drug Discovery and Development, DOI 10.1007/978-1-60327-553-8_23,
© Humana Press, a part of Springer Science+Business Media, LLC 2009

23.1 Microarray Profiling

Prior to the development of microarray technologies, assessment of expression was accomplished on a gene-by-gene basis, typically by Northern blotting. While arrays of cDNA probes were developed using membrane substrates similar to that used in blotting techniques (Kulesh et al. 1987), the first miniaturized microarrays were developed in the mid-1990s and used initially to measure gene expression in model organisms, such as yeast or plants (Schena et al. 1995; Lashkari et al. 1997). Rapid advances in the technology with the use of oligonucleotide probes, high-density arrays, and precision manufacturing, such as the Affymetrix GeneChips, have allowed for comparison of expression among large numbers of tumors with little concern for technical, chip-to-chip variation (Pease et al. 1994; Bammler et al. 2005).

Microarray profiling assesses the relative quantity of messenger RNA (mRNA) in a biologic specimen (target) for each cDNA or oligonucleotide on the array (probe) (Fig. 23.1 and Color Plate 35). In practice, target mRNA is usually converted to a fluorescently tagged-form of either complementary DNA (cDNA) or RNA (cRNA) which is hybridized to either a glass slide- or a silicon chip-based array. The relative amount of mRNA in the target is determined by the amount of fluorescence signal at that particular probe. Fluorescence intensities are normalized to that of a reference mRNA source labeled with a different fluorophore with non-overlapping fluorescence spectra (two-color arrays) or by more complex control gene and/or whole array-based normalization (one-color arrays). The end result is a set of relative expression values for all probes on the array for that target which can be compared to other targets processed on the same array platform in a similar manner. Currently available commercial microarrays contain probes, and typically multiple probes, for every known gene and for most predicted genes as determined by human genome sequence analysis. Thus, it is possible to assess the entire mRNA signature, the "transcriptome", for a given biologic specimen.

Gene signatures have been reported that are capable of distinguishing molecular subtypes of tumors that appear histologically indistinguishable, but often have very different effects on clinical outcome, such as the groundbreaking study profiling diffuse large B-cell lymphoma (DLBCL) (Alizadeh et al. 2000). In that report, two molecular subtypes of DLBCL were identified with vastly different patient survivals. Extensive work of this type has also been reported for breast cancer, where gene expression profiling has identified five subtypes of tumors not observed previously, each with a different level of tumor aggressiveness (Perou et al. 2000; Sorlie et al. 2001, 2003). Recently, these signatures have been incorporated into clinical diagnostic tools (Glas et al. 2006; Baker 2007).

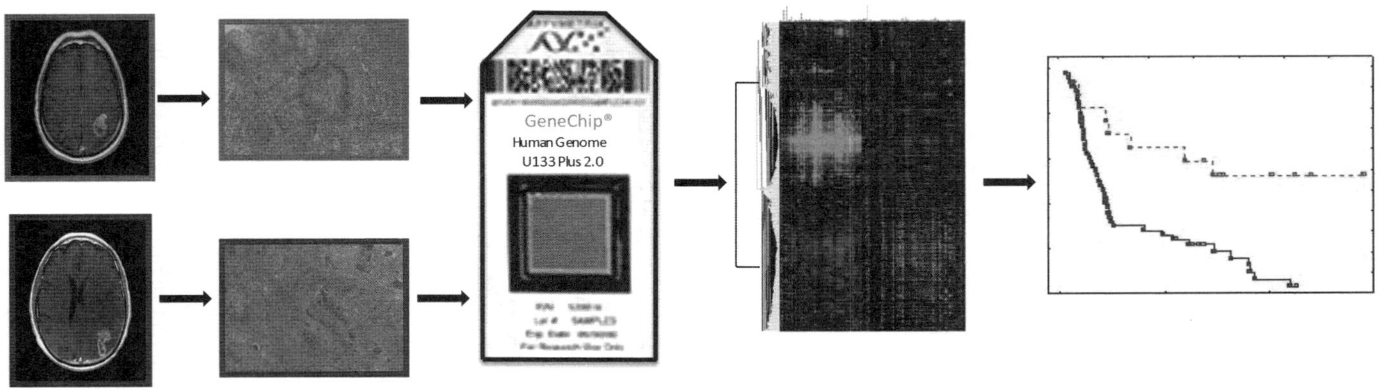

Fig. 23.1 Gene expression profiling in brain tumors. Tumor-specific, such as tumor imaging and histopathology, as well as patient-specific information, such as age and sex, is used to provide prognostic information. Tissue obtained at diagnosis, either from biopsy or from surgical resection, is utilized to develop a complex profile of gene expression in the tumor. Labeled (typically fluorescently) target samples are made from total RNA that is enzymatically processed into complementary DNA (or RNA) and represent relative messenger RNA (mRNA) abundance within the tumor for all expressed genes. This is hybridized to filter-, glass slide-, or silicon chip-based arrays of cDNA or oligonucleotide probes and the signals are measured and normalized. Clustering provides a means to identify sets of genes with similar expression and group tumors based on these clusters (unsupervised), thus identifying unique molecular signatures or group genes based on known characteristics of the tumors (supervised). Gene signatures identified may have prognostic significance. Tumors that appear similar on imaging and histologic examination may be shown to exhibit differing molecular profiles and therefore different clinical outcomes using microarray technologies (*see* Color Plate 35)

A particular limitation of the microarray approach rests in the need for fresh or frozen biologic samples (Auer et al. 2003; Bustin and Nolan 2004; Farragher et al. 2008), as opposed to the paraffin-embedded archival tissue most readily available in clinical pathology laboratories. While analytes derived from frozen tissue are nearly always preferable, the existence of many archival paraffin tissues in repositories has spawned efforts to identify methods for extracting high-throughput data from this source. In this regard, methods for profiling the fragmented mRNA obtained from archival tissue have recently become available that should allow for even larger collections of data (Bibikova et al. 2004; Scicchitano et al. 2006; Haque et al. 2007; Penland et al. 2007; Farragher et al. 2008; Furusato et al. 2008; Srivastava et al. 2008).

To analyze microarray data, some general approaches have been employed. Unsupervised clustering is a statistical method which utilizes correlation of expression among probes to group samples (Eisen et al. 1998; Eisen and Brown 1999; Tavazoie et al. 1999). These groups share molecular signatures and, presumably, an underlying biology. Supervised clustering can be used to determine gene signatures specific for known classes of samples (Allison et al. 2006; Michiels et al. 2007). For example, tumors can be grouped based on patient outcome (for example, survivors vs. deaths) or by known molecular changes (for example, retention vs. loss of human chromosomes 1p/19q in oligodendrogliomas) and particular signatures for each type identified. In attempting to identify particular genes that might play a role in tumorigenesis or malignant progression, a correction must be employed for the large number of statistical comparisons needed, and an expected false-discover rate threshold set. Validation, either by the use of independent datasets, in the case of gene signatures, or by the use of independent platforms, such as real-time quantitative PCR (qRT-PCR), is required to guard against false-positive results (Allison et al. 2006). Validation can be “technical” where the subset of genes examined in the array analysis is tested in the same tumor samples using a different analytic method to ensure concordance. While important in the early days, this may be less important currently, as experience with robust microarray platforms (such as Affymetrix) indicates reliable performance with most genes, especially those which are expressed at moderate to high levels.

In contrast, to technical validation, testing to ensure reproducibility of results in independent sample sets remains a critical but sometimes overlooked requirement. The high-throughput nature of expression microarrays leads to an issue familiar to statisticians termed “the multiple comparisons problem”. The reader is referred to the bioinformatic literature for a more thorough description, but this problem, in essence, results from the fact that false-positive results are inevitable when testing a large number of variables (gene expression measurements) using a limited number of samples. Efforts to reduce false positives, including validation of results using a large independent sample, are therefore required to ensure generalizability of results. Failure to do this may in part explain a previous lack of reproducibility among optimal gene lists for a single tumor type.

A powerful use for gene signatures is as biomarkers of tumor prognosis and response to therapy. Microarray profiles have been used as prognostic (i.e., predictive of outcome) markers and, more recently, have been proposed as predictive (i.e., predictive of response to a treatment) markers. An important consideration in any new biomarker, and gene expression profiles are no exception, is that it augment the existing clinical and pathological prognostic markers commonly used to predict outcome in brain tumors. The complex and comprehensive nature of gene expression profiles allows for the potential determination of response to a wide range of therapies and the personalization of care. However, as stated above, caution is warranted when moving from microarray data to clinically useful biomarkers. Biomarker studies are optimal when the number of samples far exceeds the number of markers tested, which is impossible for microarray experiments. Several rounds of validation are therefore needed to address this problem and find biomarkers that are reproducible among independent datasets.

23.2 Expression Profiling in Human Brain Tumors

Early studies of cDNA array-based profiling in brain tumors were reported within just a few years of the development of the technology. Initial studies relied on the use of large, filter-based arrays (Fuller et al. 1999; Caskey et al. 2000; Huang et al. 2000; Sallinen et al. 2000; Chakravarti et al. 2001; Raza et al. 2004; Somasundaram et al. 2005). In one such report using glioma specimens, expression of 20 tumors [5 glioblastoma (GBM), 5 anaplastic astrocytoma (AA), 5 anaplastic oligodendroglioma (AO), and 5 oligodendroglioma] was compared to two normal brain specimens using commercial filters of 597 genes. The insulin-like growth factor-binding protein 2 (*IGFBP2*) gene was found to be specifically upregulated in GBM and has subsequently been proposed to have a biological function in these tumors. Nevertheless, such early profiling studies underscore the need for high-resolution arrays to identify more than just a single upregulated gene and for the use of microarrays that allow for much larger sample sizes.

With the exception of gliomas, expression profiling of brain tumors has relied on relatively small cohorts of tumors. For example, limited studies have been performed using meningioma- or schwannoma-derived specimens (Watson et al. 2002; Sasaki et al. 2003; Cuevas et al. 2005; Wrobel et al. 2005; Sayagues et al. 2006; Aarhus et al. 2008; Keller et al. 2008; Martinez-Glez et al. 2008) and novel biomarkers from these studies have yet to emerge. Nevertheless, a number of important studies have been undertaken with medulloblastoma. Using 23 tumors from metastatic and non-metastatic tumors, a subset of 85 genes was sufficient to accurately classify the tumors (MacDonald et al. 2001). The results suggested that the platelet-derived growth factor receptor (*PDGFR*)- signaling pathway was important in medulloblastoma metastasis, a finding validated by immunohistochemical and in vitro studies. A larger study of 60 tumors identified an eight-gene signature capable of predicting survival independent of the existing clinical stratification scheme used for medulloblastoma (Pomeroy et al. 2002). Importantly, this study demonstrated that medulloblastoma represented a molecularly distinct group of pediatric tumors compared to other embryonal tumors, and provided evidence that activation of the sonic hedgehog (SHH) pathway was important for medulloblastoma tumorigenesis. In a third study, comparison of six medulloblastomas to normal cerebellum identified a number upregulated genes, including ezrin, cyclin D2, high mobility group protein 2, microtubule-associated protein Rb/EB family member 1, histone deacetylase 2, and ornithine decarboxylase 1; however, the small size of the study requires further validation (Park et al. 2003). The aurora kinase A gene (*AURA*, *STK15*), whose protein product plays a role in mitosis, was identified as a marker of overall survival among 35 medulloblastomas using both cDNA microarrays and immunohistochemical validation (Neben et al. 2004). In another report, 46 medulloblastomas were partitioned into five molecular subtypes, each with associated molecular abnormalities previously associated with medulloblastoma tumorigenesis, such as mutation of the wingless gene (*WNT*), deletion of chromosome 6, or mutations in the sonic hedgehog pathway (SHH) (Thompson et al. 2006). Profiling of 31 additional tumors showed that the expression signatures accurately predicted the genetic alteration associated with each subtype. To summarize, profiling data of medulloblastoma are still underdeveloped but indicate that analysis of additional samples will likely elucidate molecular signatures of clinical relevance.

Similar to medulloblastoma, small cohort studies have been performed using ependymoma tumors (Korshunov et al. 2003; Lau 2005; Suarez-Merino et al. 2005; Taylor et al. 2005; Gilbertson 2006; Modena et al. 2006; Sowar et al. 2006; Lukashova-v Zangen et al. 2007; de Bont et al. 2008). In one example, a microarray of >4700 cDNA probes representing >2600 genes was used to profile 39 tumors from adult and pediatric patients by 2-color hybridization (Korshunov et al. 2003). Gene expression signatures clustered based on tumor location (brain vs. spinal cord), patient age, and grade (for supratentorial tumors). The data suggested that activation of proliferation-associated genes and downregulation of the phosphate and tensin homolog gene (*PTEN*) tumor suppressor gene may lead to progression from World Health Organization (WHO) grade II to III. Generalization of these findings will require analysis of larger sample sets. In another study, 19 pediatric ependymomas were profiled against >12,000 genes and expression compared to normal brain. Additional information including loss of heterozygosity (LOH) analysis was also included. A panel of 112 genes emerged as candidate genes for tumorigenesis based on their relative expression and position within regions of allelic imbalance (e.g., the long-arm of chromosome 22), but the prognostic role of this signature was not investigated (Suarez-Merino et al. 2005). In a landmark analysis of 29 ependymomas profiled on Affymetrix GeneChips, supervised clustering based on tumor location (supratentorial, posterior fossa, or spinal) identified gene signatures that recapitulated the expression of the neural precursors from each of those sites (Taylor et al. 2005; Gilbertson 2006). For example, expression of *EPHB-EPHRIN* and *NOTCH*-signaling pathway genes that are found in the developing cells of the brain subventricular zone (SVZ) were also found in supratentorial tumors. Similarly, the developmentally regulated homeobox (*HOX*) genes were seen in spinal tumors, where they play a role in anteroposterior tissue patterning around the cord and where their dysregulation may lead to tumor formation. Microarray results were validated by immunohistochemical staining of corresponding protein products. Based on the observation that ependymoma gene signatures recapitulate expression seen in developing glia, the authors then proposed that ependymal tumors are derived from a stem-like, radial glial cell-like precursor and that identification of these cells in tumors will have prognostic and therapeutic implications (Taylor et al. 2005; Gilbertson 2006). In another report, profiling of ependymomas was undertaken in order to develop a biomarker of tumor recurrence (Sowar et al. 2006). Thirteen specimens, seven from patients who experienced recurrent tumor and six from those that did not, were analyzed on Affymetrix GeneChips. A minimal gene subset including pleckstrin (*PLEK*), nuclear factor kappa β2 (*NFKB2*), and a pseudogene homologous to transmembrane phosphatase with tensin homology (*TPTE*) and *PTEN* were sufficient to accurately distinguish recurrent from non-recurrent tumors. Further validation with larger sample sizes will be needed for these findings. In an analysis of 47 ependymomas, unique gene signatures were identified to distinguish long (>10 year) vs. typical-duration survivors (Lukashova-v Zangen et al. 2007). A poor-outcome signature was also identified and associated with proliferation-related genes. Additional profiles were identified based on tumor location. However, minimal overlap exists between these profiles and the other profiles reported for ependymomas using similarly small tumor sample numbers. Finally, differential expression of sex-determining region on Y box (*SOX*) genes has been identified by comparison of expression profiles between medulloblastomas and ependymo(de Bont et al. 2008). Medulloblastoma and ependymoma-specific expression signatures were identified by comparison of each tumor type with normal cerebellum. A total of 27 medulloblastoma, 13 ependymoma, and 5 normal cerebellum specimens were used and expression of specific *SOX* genes appeared to have prognostic significance. Nevertheless, the small sample size again precludes generalization of these results, and robust conclusions await the generation of additional data.

23.3 Expression Profiling of Human Gliomas

Of all the brain tumor types, by far the largest numbers of profiled tumors have been gliomas (mainly astrocytic and oligodendroglial tumors), largely due to the greater availability of specimens as well as the research interest in discovery because of the poor outcome of high-grade gliomas (Table 23.1). Using first

Table 23.1 Expression profiling studies in gliomas*

First author name	Tumor type	Samples	Array	References
Aronica	Ganglioglioma	4	U133Plus2.0	Aronica et al. (2008)
Beetz	Astrocytoma	25	U95Av2	Beetz et al. (2006)
Bozinov	Astrocytoma	16	Research genetics (gf201)	Bozinov et al. (2008)
Bredel	Glioma	50	Custom array	Bredel et al. (2005)
Bruna	Astrocytoma	52	U133A	Bruna et al. (2007)
Carlson	Glioma	71	U133A	Carlson et al. (2007)
Czernicki	Glioma	28	Clontech	Czernicki et al. (2007)
Diehn	Glioblastoma	22	Custom array	Diehn et al. (2008)
Dong	Glioblastoma	28	U133A	Dong et al. (2005)
Ducray	Glioma	13	U133Plus2.0	Ducray et al. (2008)
Faury	Glioblastoma	25	Custom array	Faury et al. (2007)
Freije	Astrocytoma	74	U133A and U133B	Freije et al. (2004)
French	Glioma	48	Affymetrix human exon 1.0	French et al. (2007)
French	Oligodendroglioma	38	U133Plus2.0	French et al. (2005)
Fuller	Glioma	24	Clontech	Fuller et al. (1999)
Godard	Astrocytoma	53	Clontech	Godard et al. (2003)
Hagerstrand	Glioma	23	Custom array	Hagerstrand et al. (2008)
Haque	Glioblastoma	16	Custom array	Haque et al. (2007)
Horvath	Glioblastoma	120	U133A	Horvath et al. (2006)
Huang	Astrocytoma Gr II	11	Clontech	Huang et al. (2000)
Huang	Glioma	32	Clontech	Huang et al. (2004)
Khatua	Astrocytoma	13	U95Av2	Khatua et al. (2003)
Kim	Gliomas	25	Clontech	Kim et al. (2002)
Korshunov	Ependymoma	39	Clontech	Korshunov et al. (2003)
Liang	Glioma	105	Custom array	Liang et al. (2005)
Liu	Glioblastoma	21	U133A	Liu et al. (2006a)
Ljubimova	Glioma	22	Incyte genomics	Ljubimova et al. (2001a)
Ljubimova	Astrocytoma	7	Incyte genomics	Ljubimova et al. (2001b)
Lukashova-v Zangen	Ependymoma	47	Custom array	Lukashova-v Zangen et al. (2007)
MacDonald	Medulloblastoma	23	Affymetrix G110 array	MacDonald et al. (2001)
Markert	Glioblastoma	7	Affymetrix HU6800	Markert et al. (2001)
Marko	Glioblastoma	20	U133Plus2.0	Marko et al. (2008)
McDonald	Glioma	143	Custom array	McDonald et al. (2007)
Mischel	Glioblastoma	13	U95Av2	Mischel et al. (2003)
Mukasa	Glioma	22	U95A	Mukasa et al. (2002)
Mukasa	Oligodendroglioma	13	U95A	Mukasa et al. (2004)
Neben	Medulloblastoma	35	Custom array	Neben et al. (2004)
Nigro	Glioblastoma	34	U95Av2	Nigro et al. (2005)
Nutt	Gliomas	50	U95Av2	Nutt et al. (2003)
Park	Medulloblastoma	6	Clontech	Park et al. (2003)

Table 23.1 (continued)

First author name	Tumor type	Samples	Array	References
Persson	Glioma	36	Custom array	Persson et al. (2007)
Petalidis	Astrocytoma	65	U133A	Petalidis et al. (2008)
Phillips	Astrocytoma	76	U133A and U133B	Phillips et al. (2006)
Pomeroy	Glioma	99	Affymetrix HU6800	Pomeroy et al. (2002)
Pope	Glioblastoma	52	U133A and U133B	Pope et al. (2008)
Qi	Glioma	3	BioDoor gene technology	Qi et al. (2005)
Raza	Astrocytoma	20	Clontech	Raza et al. (2004)
Reddy	Astrocytoma	25	Custom array	Reddy et al. (2008)
Rich	Glioma	41	U133A	Rich et al. (2005)
Rickman	Astrocytoma	45	Affymetrix HU6800	Rickman et al. (2001)
Riemenschneider	Glioblastoma	30	GE healthcare	Riemenschneider et al. (2005)
Ruano	Glioblastoma	20	Custom array	Ruano et al. (2008)
Sallinen	Astrocytoma	9	Clontech	Sallinen et al. (2000)
Scrideli	Glioblastoma	6	GE healthcare	Scrideli et al. (2008)
Shai	Glioma	35	U95Av2	Shai et al. (2003)
Sharma	Astrocytoma (PA)	8	U95A	Sharma et al. (2006)
Somasundaram	Astrocytoma	7	Genomic solutions	Somasundaram et al. (2005)
Sowar	Ependymoma	13	U133Plus2.0	Sowar et al. (2006)
Suarez-Merino	Ependymoma	6	U95Av2	Suarez-Merino et al. (2005)
Tanwar	Astrocytoma	19	Incyte genomics	Tanwar et al. (2002)
Tews	Glioma	35	Custom array	Tews et al. (2006)
Thompson	Medulloblastoma	46	U133A	Thompson et al. (2006)
van den boom	Glioma	43	Affymetrix HU6800	van den Boom et al. (2003)
Van meter	Glioblastoma	6	U133A	Van Meter et al. (2006)
Watson	Oligodendroglioma	7	Affymetrix HU6800	Watson et al. (2001)
Wong	Astrocytoma (PA)	21	U133A	Wong et al. (2005)

(PA) Pilocytic Astrocytoma.
* We apologize for exclusion of reports not available for review.

generation Affymetrix chips (HU6800), 45 astrocytic tumors (19 grade I, 5 grade II, and 21 grade IV), and 6 normal brain specimens were profiled on approximately 6800 probes (Rickman et al. 2001). A unique profile of 360 genes was identified that distinguishes pilocytic (grade I) tumors from GBM (grade IV). Five genes upregulated in GBM, but not previously known to play a role in the tumor, were validated by qRT-PCR and immunohistochemical staining of clinical tissue specimens. Some of these genes, such as *FOXM1*, have been subsequently reported by others to play functional roles in glioma tumorigenesis and progression (Teh et al. 2002; van den Boom et al. 2003; Liu et al. 2006b; Dai et al. 2007). The complexity and robustness of the microarray data obtained has improved based on improving technology, such that not only is nearly every known and predicted gene represented on a single, current-generation microarray, but gene splice variants can also be profiled using arrays containing oligonucleotides from potentially spiced exons. Such "exon" arrays have been utilized for glioma profiling (French et al. 2007; Cheung et al. 2008). Interesting, glioma-specific alternative splicing was a rare event in one study, with only 14 genes identified with tumor-specific splice variants (Cheung et al. 2008).

A number of investigations have attempted to identify individual genes or signaling pathways from microarray data that are prognostic in malignant gliomas (Tanwar et al. 2002; Khatua et al. 2003; Liang et al. 2005; Nigro et al. 2005; Liu et al. 2006a; Faury et al. 2007; McDonald et al. 2007; Reddy et al. 2008; Ruano et al. 2008; Scrideli et al. 2008). Using a group of only 19 gliomas, the chitinase-3-like-1 gene (*CHI3L1)*, which encodes for the glycoprotein YKL-40, was found to be upregulated compared to normal brain and its expression correlated to tumor grade (Tanwar et al. 2002). Using a larger set of 34 GBMs, *CHI3L1* again emerged as a significant gene and its expression correlated with decreased overall survival and in vitro radioresistance (Nigro et al. 2005). Subsequent studies have validated the role of *CHI3L1* as a biomarker and suggested a functional role for YKL-40 in tumor progression (Nutt et al. 2005; Pelloski et al. 2005, 2006). The epidermal growth factor receptor (EGFR) and hypoxia-inducible factor-2α (HIF-2α) pathway have been implicated in high-grade pediatric astrocytomas based on microarray analysis (Khatua et al. 2003). An examination of genes overexpressed in GBMs identified a 70-gene signature that differentiated long term from typical-survivors (Liang et al. 2005). One of the genes in the signature, fatty acid-binding protein 7 (*FABP7*), was prognostic in an independent set of 105 patients. The ephrin receptor *EPHA2* gene was found to be a prognostic marker based on a novel integrative analysis of comparative genomic hybridization (CGH) and mRNA microarray data (Liu et al. 2006a). Other studies have attempted to combine genomic structural information with expression profiling data to best identify prognostic genes and this type integrative approach represents the future of biomarker discovery (Nigro et al. 2005; Liu et al. 2006a; Persson et al. 2007).

Similar to the earliest studies mentioned previously (Rickman et al. 2001), a number of groups have taken the approach of attempting to predict tumor classification (e.g., pathologic grade) based on expression profiling (Kim et al. 2002; Pomeroy et al. 2002; Godard et al. 2003; Nutt et al. 2003; Shai et al. 2003; van den Boom et al. 2003; Czernicki et al. 2007; Margareto et al. 2007; Bozinov et al. 2008). For example, analysis of 35 gliomas using Affymetrix U95A GeneChips identified a 170-gene signature that accurately classified tumors based on grade. Another group attempted to develop a molecular classifier based on microarray data which could be used to help classify gliomas with "non-classic" histologies (Nutt et al. 2003). Twenty-one tumors were used to build a gene classifier that was then applied to an additional 29 tumors with ambiguous histology (GBM vs. AO). Survival prediction based on the classifier was superior to that based on histologic diagnosis.

Specific studies have focused on oligodendroglioma array analysis (Watson et al. 2001; Mukasa et al. 2002; Huang et al. 2004; Mukasa et al. 2004; French et al. 2005; Tews et al. 2006; Ducray et al. 2008; Hagerstrand et al. 2008). In one report, a gene signature of approximately 1100 probes was capable of classifying based on grade (WHO grade II vs. III) (Watson et al. 2001). As response to treatment in these tumors is related to deletion of human chromosome 1p/19q (Cairncross et al. 1998), several of the studies have attempted to identify unique expression profiles based on the 1p/19q status (Mukasa et al. 2002; French et al. 2005; Tews et al. 2006; Ducray et al. 2008). Expression of unique genes or gene signatures has been identified to correlate with 1p/19q deletion, such a neuron-related genes (Mukasa et al. 2004; Ducray et al. 2008) or candidate tumor suppressor genes (Tews et al. 2006). The concept of functional gene signatures that may be independent of histologic grade, but that reflect the underlying tumor biology, has been developed by a number of groups.

23.4 Molecular Subtypes of Infiltrating Gliomas

Expression profiling followed by clustering of infiltrating gliomas (using both k-means and hierarchical methods) has led to the concept of molecular subtypes defined by genes overexpressed within each group. A group from the University of California, Los Angeles (UCLA) identified several subtypes, in a set of 84 tumors, which they termed extracellular matrix, mitosis, neurogenesis, and synaptic transmission (Freije et al. 2004). An independent study (see Figure 23.2 and Color Plate 36) then found subtypes with some similarities found by the UCLA group, specifically a "mesenchymal" group (corresponding to the extracellular matrix) proneural (corresponding to neural development) and "proliferative" (corresponding to mitosis) (Phillips et al. 2006). The subtype termed by the UCLA group as "synaptic transmission" was not found, and it is possible that this group represents cases with a high degree of normal/non-neoplastic brain within the sample. Subsequently, a group from the United Kingdom in an independent study highlighted the mesenchymal/angiogenic subtype (called "angio" by the authors) as clinically aggressive and characteristic of grade IV tumors (Petalidis et al. 2008). This picture is still evolving, and the specific genes that describe each subtype are not identical among the various studies. However, a preliminary conclusion that can be reached is that a subset of gliomas exist that overexpress genes associated with mesenchyme and angiogenesis. This subgroup is composed almost solely of GBMs and is particularly aggressive and generally resistant to therapy. A second group exists that may correspond to the "proneural" subtype. This group is overrepresented with lower grade gliomas. Some GBMs also are included in this group, and these tend to be more responsive to therapy. This concept has also been extended to oligodendroglioma, which has been reported as having a proneural phenotype (Mukasa et al. 2004; Ducray et al. 2008). While future work will clarify the robustness of these molecular subtypes, the concept of mesenchymal vs. proneural gliomas does seems to be supported by

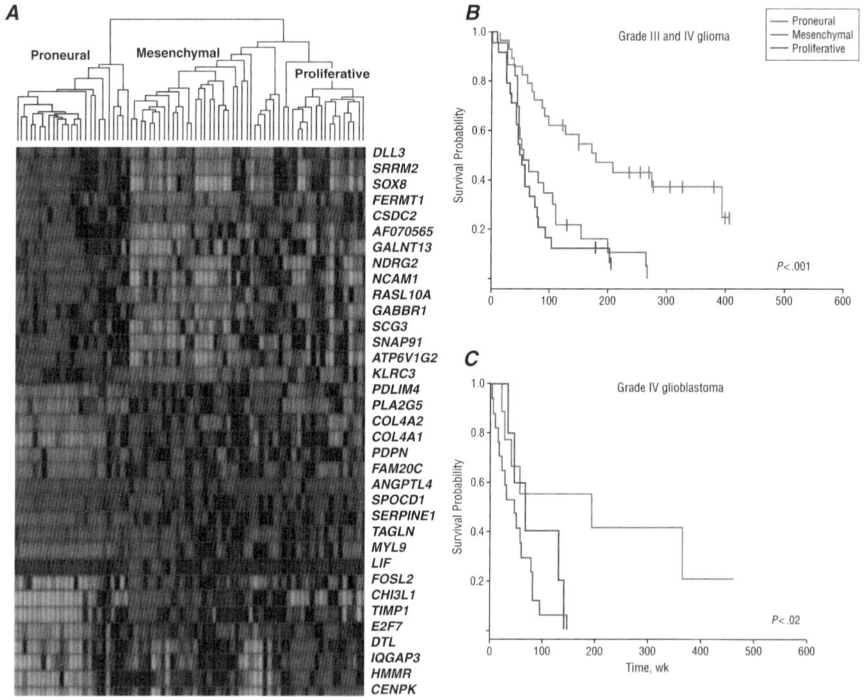

Fig. 23.2 A mesenchymal molecular signature in GBM is prognostic for poor survival. (**A**) Identification of distinct molecular subtypes of malignant gliomas from gene expression profiling consisting of proneural, mesenchymal, and proliferative phenotypes (Phillips et al. 2006). Genes with high expression are shown in *red*, while those with low expression are shown in *green*. The proneural, mesenchymal, and proliferative subtypes demonstrate statistically significant associations with patient outcome in both grade III and IV glioma (**B**) and in an independent data set consisting only of grade IV GBM with necrosis (**C**). Adapted with permission from Elsevier Limited (*see* Color Plate 36)

several independent studies and represents a paradigm for future biologic investigations. Whether or not specific therapies are more or less effective within each molecular subgroup will no doubt be examined in future clinical trials.

23.5 Stem-Cell Biomarkers

As noted previously for ependymoma, microarray analysis has been used to gain insight into the stem cell of origin for brain tumors (Taylor et al. 2005; Gilbertson 2006; Lee et al. 2006). A wealth of data has begun to accumulate on glioma cancer stem cells, a small population of cells within the tumor hypothesized to be the initiators of tumorigenesis, to be resistant to conventional treatment, and to regrow the tumor following therapy (Reya et al. 2001; Hemmati et al. 2003; Singh et al. 2003, 2004; Yuan et al. 2004; Bao et al.

2006). Primary culture of human gliomas under stem-cell promoting conditions (i.e., as neurospheres) identified unique gene signatures which closely matched those of the primary tumor but which were lost once the cells were allowed to differentiate in vitro (Lee et al. 2006). These data pave the way for identifying novel stem-cell-specific biomarkers and therapeutic targets in gliomas.

23.6 The Future of Profiling: Multiplatform Integration

As demonstrated by those studies that incorporated both genomic information (copy number alterations, chromosomal loss of heterozygosity, etc.) and mRNA expression data from microarrays (Mukasa et al. 2002, 2004; Nigro et al. 2005; Liu et al. 2006a; Tews et al. 2006; Persson et al. 2007; Ducray et al. 2008), more robust analyses are often possible by combining profiling platforms. It is possible to envision situations in which the combined profile from several methodologies is used to generate the most robust classifier. Such an approach is already underway. The Cancer Genome Atlas (TCGA) project, sponsored by the National Cancer Institute, aims to profile a large cohort of GBMs (approximately 500) at the DNA, mRNA, microRNA, and epigenetic (DNA methylation) levels (TCGA, 2008). Preliminary analysis of the first 206 GBMs to be studied has already provided validation of known genes and pathways previously implicated in GBM and new targets not otherwise known. The vastness of this data collection will require complex bioinformatics integration and robust statistical analysis but should lead to powerful prognostic tools.

The importance of developing biomarkers is not limited to determining the natural history of the tumor in a specific patient. Prognostic markers in themselves do not necessarily impact patient care unless they alter treatment choice. In the case of GBM, for example, newly diagnosed patients are currently treated uniformly with temozolomide chemoradiation, despite knowledge of the molecular heterogeneity of these tumors. Recent experience in breast cancer (van de Vijver et al. 2002; Paik et al. 2004) suggests that a multimarker panel may be more robust predictor of outcomes in patients with cancer. While gene expression data have begun to help define molecular subgroups of GBM, no such clinical gene expression predictor for GBM currently exists. Development of a multigene/multiplatform predictor in response to standard therapy could serve to identify the subset of patients with GBM who will experience durable tumor response and survival to this therapy alone. Patients identified prospectively based on this predictor as having a poor likelihood of response to standard therapy could be offered participation in more aggressive clinical trials with the knowledge that accepting the possibility of higher toxicity has a favorable risk-benefit ratio owing to the low likelihood of significant benefit from standard therapy alone. Future trials could incorporate both molecular inclusion criteria (identifying sensitive and refractory tumors) and hypothesis-based targeted therapies for resistant tumors based on molecular phenotype. Such an approach would allow for personalization of treatment for brain tumors.

23.7 Conclusions

Transcriptional profiling of brain tumors has provided a wealth of candidate biomarkers and biologic data. Unique molecular signatures have been identified which are prognostic markers, independent of existing clinical and pathologic criteria. In the future, it is expected that these signatures and genes will be included as part of the diagnostic workup of brain tumors and utilized in treatment stratification in clinical trials. Ultimately, combining expression profiling data with data from other high-throughput genomic platforms will allow for the most robust prognostic determination and for customization of therapy to fit an individual patients molecular makeup.

References

Aarhus, M., Bruland, O., Bredholt, G., Lybaek, H., Husebye, E.S., Krossnes, B.K., Vedeler, C., Wester, K., Lund-Johansen, M., and Knappskog, P.M. 2008. Microarray analysis reveals down-regulation of the tumour suppressor gene WWOX and up-regulation of the oncogene TYMS in intracranial sporadic meningiomas. *J Neurooncol* **88**(3): 251–259.

Alizadeh, A.A., Eisen, M.B., Davis, R.E., Ma, C., Lossos, I.S., Rosenwald, A., Boldrick, J.C., Sabet, H., Tran, T., Yu, X., Powell, J.I., Yang, L., Marti, G.E., Moore, T., Hudson, J., Jr., Lu, L., Lewis, D.B., Tibshirani, R., Sherlock, G., Chan, W.C., Greiner, T.C., Weisenburger, D.D., Armitage, J.O., Warnke, R., Levy, R., Wilson, W., Grever, M.R., Byrd, J.C., Botstein, D., Brown, P.O., and Staudt, L.M. 2000. Distinct types of diffuse large B-cell lymphoma identified by gene expression profiling. *Nature* **403**(6769): 503–511.

Allison, D.B., Cui, X., Page, G.P., and Sabripour, M. 2006. Microarray data analysis: From disarray to consolidation and consensus. *Nat Rev Genet* **7**(1): 55–65.

Aronica, E., Boer, K., Becker, A., Redeker, S., Spliet, W.G., van Rijen, P.C., Wittink, F., Breit, T., Wadman, W.J., Lopes da Silva, F.H., Troost, D., and Gorter, J.A. 2008. Gene expression profile analysis of epilepsy-associated gangliogliomas. *Neuroscience* **151**(1): 272–292.

Auer, H., Lyianarachchi, S., Newsom, D., Klisovic, M.I., Marcucci, U., and Kornacker, K. 2003. Chipping away at the chip bias: RNA degradation in microarray analysis [2]. *Nat Genet* **35**(4): 292–293.

Baker, J. 2007. Genomic Health, Inc. *Pharmacogenomics* **8**(4): 397–399.

Bammler, T., Beyer, R.P., Bhattacharya, S., Boorman, G.A., Boyles, A., Bradford, B.U., Bumgarner, R.E., Bushel, P.R., Chaturvedi, K., Choi, D., Cunningham, M.L., Deng, S., Dressman, H.K., Fannin, R.D., Farin, F.M., Freedman, J.H., Fry, R.C., Harper, A., Humble, M.C., Hurban, P., Kavanagh, T.J., Kaufmann, W.K., Kerr, K.F., Jing, L., Lapidus, J.A., Lasarev, M.R., Li, J., Li, Y.J., Lobenhofer, E.K., Lu, X., Malek, R.L., Milton, S., Nagalla, S.R., O'Malley J, P., Palmer, V.S., Pattee, P., Paules, R.S., Perou, C. M., Phillips, K., Qin, L.X., Qiu, Y., Quigley, S.D., Rodland, M., Rusyn, I., Samson, L.D., Schwartz, D.A., Shi, Y., Shin, J.L., Sieber, S.O., Slifer, S., Speer, M.C., Spencer, P.S., Sproles, D.I., Swenberg, J.A., Suk, W.A., Sullivan, R.C., Tian, R., Tennant, R.W., Todd, S.A., Tucker, C.J., Van Houten, B., Weis, B.K., Xuan, S., and Zarbl, H. 2005. Standardizing global gene expression analysis between laboratories and across platforms. *Nat Methods* **2**(5): 351–356.

Bao, S., Wu, Q., McLendon, R.E., Hao, Y., Shi, Q., Hjelmeland, A.B., Dewhirst, M.W., Bigner, D.D., and Rich, J.N. 2006. Glioma stem cells promote radioresistance by preferential activation of the DNA damage response. *Nature* **444** (7120): 756–760.

Beaty, R.M., Edwards, J.B., Boon, K., Siu, I.M., Conway, J.E., and Riggins, G.J. 2007. PLXDC1 (TEM7) is identified in a genome-wide expression screen of glioblastoma endothelium. *J Neurooncol* **81**(3): 241–248.

Beetz, C., Bergner, S., Brodoehl, S., Brodhun, M., Ewald, C., Kalff, R., Kruger, J., Patt, S., Kiehntopf, M., and Deufel, T. 2006. Outcome-based profiling of astrocytic tumours identifies prognostic gene expression signatures which link molecular and morphology-based pathology. *Int J Oncol* **29**(5): 1183–1191.

Behin, A., Hoang-Xuan, K., Carpentier, A.F., and Delattre, J.Y. 2003. Primary brain tumours in adults. *Lancet* **361** (9354): 323–331.

Bibikova, M., Yeakley, J.M., Chudin, E., Chen, J., Wickham, E., Wang-Rodriguez, J., and Fan, J.B. 2004. Gene expression profiles in formalin-fixed, paraffin-embedded tissues obtained with a novel assay for microarray analysis. *Clin Chem* **50**(12): 2384–2386.

Boon, K., Edwards, J.B., Siu, I.M., Olschner, D., Eberhart, C.G., Marra, M.A., Strausberg, R.L., and Riggins, G.J. 2003. Comparison of medulloblastoma and normal neural transcriptomes identifies a restricted set of activated genes. *Oncogene* **22**(48): 7687–7694.

Boon, K. and Riggins, G.J. 2003. SAGE as a strategy to isolate cancer-related genes. *Methods Mol Biol* **222**: 463–479.

Bozinov, O., Kohler, S., Samans, B., Benes, L., Miller, D., Ritter, M., Sure, U., and Bertalanffy, H. 2008. Candidate genes for the progression of malignant gliomas identified by microarray analysis. *Neurosurg Rev* **31**(1): 83–89; discussion 89–90.

Bredel, M., Bredel, C., Juric, D., Harsh, G.R., Vogel, H., Recht, L.D., and Sikic, B.I. 2005. Functional network analysis reveals extended gliomagenesis pathway maps and three novel MYC-interacting genes in human gliomas. *Cancer Res* **65**(19): 8679–8689.

Bruna, A., Darken, R.S., Rojo, F., Ocana, A., Penuelas, S., Arias, A., Paris, R., Tortosa, A., Mora, J., Baselga, J., and Seoane, J. 2007. High TGFbeta-Smad activity confers poor prognosis in glioma patients and promotes cell proliferation depending on the methylation of the PDGF-B gene. *Cancer Cell* **11**(2): 147–160.

Bustin, S.A. and Nolan, T. 2004. Pitfalls of quantitative real-time reverse-transcription polymerase chain reaction. *J Biomol Tech JBT* **15**(3): 155–166.

Cairncross, J.G., Ueki, K., Zlatescu, M.C., Lisle, D.K., Finkelstein, D.M., Hammond, R.R., Silver, J.S., Stark, P.C., Macdonald, D.R., Ino, Y., Ramsay, D.A., and Louis, D.N. 1998. Specific genetic predictors of chemotherapeutic response and survival in patients with anaplastic oligodendrogliomas. *J Natl Cancer Inst* **90**(19): 1473–1479.

Carlson, M.R., Pope, W.B., Horvath, S., Braunstein, J.G., Nghiemphu, P., Tso, C.L., Mellinghoff, I., Lai, A., Liau, L.M., Mischel, P.S., Dong, J., Nelson, S.F., and Cloughesy, T.F. 2007. Relationship between survival and edema in malignant gliomas: role of vascular endothelial growth factor and neuronal pentraxin 2. *Clin Cancer Res* **13**(9): 2592–2598.

Caskey, L.S., Fuller, G.N., Bruner, J.M., Yung, W.K., Sawaya, R.E., Holland, E.C., and Zhang, W. 2000. Toward a molecular classification of the gliomas: histopathology, molecular genetics, and gene expression profiling. *Histol Histopathol* **15**(3): 971–981.

Chakravarti, A., Delaney, M.A., Noll, E., Black, P.M., Loeffler, J.S., Muzikansky, A., and Dyson, N.J. 2001. Prognostic and pathologic significance of quantitative protein expression profiling in human gliomas. *Clin Cancer Res* **7**(8): 2387–2395.

Cheung, H.C., Baggerly, K.A., Tsavachidis, S., Bachinski, L.L., Neubauer, V.L., Nixon, T.J., Aldape, K.D., Cote, G.J., and Krahe, R. 2008. Global analysis of aberrant pre-mRNA splicing in glioblastoma using exon expression arrays. *BMC Genomics* **9**: 216.

Cuevas, I.C., Slocum, A.L., Jun, P., Costello, J.F., Bollen, A.W., Riggins, G.J., McDermott, M.W., and Lal, A. 2005. Meningioma transcript profiles reveal deregulated Notch signaling pathway. *Cancer Res* **65**(12): 5070–5075.

Czernicki, T., Zegarska, J., Paczek, L., Cukrowska, B., Grajkowska, W., Zajaczkowska, A., Brudzewski, K., Ulaczyk, J., and Marchel, A. 2007. Gene expression profile as a prognostic factor in high-grade gliomas. *Int J Oncol* **30**(1): 55–64.

Dai, B., Kang, S.H., Gong, W., Liu, M., Aldape, K.D., Sawaya, R., and Huang, S. 2007. Aberrant FoxM1B expression increases matrix metalloproteinase-2 transcription and enhances the invasion of glioma cells. *Oncogene* **26**(42): 6212–6219.

de Bont, J.M., Kros, J.M., Passier, M.M., Reddingius, R.E., Sillevis Smitt, P.A., Luider, T.M., den Boer, M.L., and Pieters, R. 2008. Differential expression and prognostic significance of SOX genes in pediatric medulloblastoma and ependymoma identified by microarray analysis. *Neuro Oncol* **10**(5): 648–660.

Diehn, M., Nardini, C., Wang, D.S., McGovern, S., Jayaraman, M., Liang, Y., Aldape, K., Cha, S., and Kuo, M.D. 2008. Identification of noninvasive imaging surrogates for brain tumor gene-expression modules. *Proc Natl Acad Sci USA* **105**(13): 5213–5218.

Dong, S., Nutt, C.L., Betensky, R.A., Stemmer-Rachamimov, A.O., Denko, N.C., Ligon, K.L., Rowitch, D.H., and Louis, D.N. 2005. Histology-based expression profiling yields novel prognostic markers in human glioblastoma. *J Neuropathol Exp Neurol* **64**(11): 948–955.

Ducray, F., Idbaih, A., de Reynies, A., Bieche, I., Thillet, J., Mokhtari, K., Lair, S., Marie, Y., Paris, S., Vidaud, M., Hoang-Xuan, K., Delattre, O., Delattre, J.Y., and Sanson, M. 2008. Anaplastic oligodendrogliomas with 1p19q codeletion have a proneural gene expression profile. *Mol Cancer* **7**: 41.

Eisen, M.B. and Brown, P.O. 1999. DNA arrays for analysis of gene expression. *Methods Enzymol* **303**: 179–205.

Eisen, M.B., Spellman, P.T., Brown, P.O., and Botstein, D. 1998. Cluster analysis and display of genome-wide expression patterns. *Proc Natl Acad Sci USA* **95**(25): 14863–14868.

Farragher, S.M., Tanney, A., Kennedy, R.D., and Paul Harkin, D. 2008. RNA expression analysis from formalin fixed paraffin embedded tissues. *Histochem Cell Biol* **130**(3): 435–445.

Faury, D., Nantel, A., Dunn, S.E., Guiot, M.C., Haque, T., Hauser, P., Garami, M., Bognar, L., Hanzely, Z., Liberski, P.P., Lopez-Aguilar, E., Valera, E.T., Tone, L.G., Carret, A.S., Del Maestro, R.F., Gleave, M., Montes, J.L., Pietsch, T., Albrecht, S., and Jabado, N. 2007. Molecular profiling identifies prognostic subgroups of pediatric glioblastoma and shows increased YB-1 expression in tumors. *J Clin Oncol* **25**(10): 1196–1208.

Freije, W.A., Castro-Vargas, F.E., Fang, Z., Horvath, S., Cloughesy, T., Liau, L.M., Mischel, P.S., and Nelson, S.F. 2004. Gene expression profiling of gliomas strongly predicts survival. *Cancer Res* **64**(18): 6503–6510.

French, P.J., Peeters, J., Horsman, S., Duijm, E., Siccama, I., van den Bent, M.J., Luider, T.M., Kros, J.M., van der Spek, P., and Sillevis Smitt, P.A. 2007. Identification of differentially regulated splice variants and novel exons in glial brain tumors using exon expression arrays. *Cancer Res* **67**(12): 5635–5642.

French, P.J., Swagemakers, S.M., Nagel, J.H., Kouwenhoven, M.C., Brouwer, E., van der Spek, P., Luider, T.M., Kros, J.M., van den Bent, M.J., and Sillevis Smitt, P.A. 2005. Gene expression profiles associated with treatment response in oligodendrogliomas. *Cancer Res* **65**(24): 11335–11344.

Fuller, G.N., Rhee, C.H., Hess, K.R., Caskey, L.S., Wang, R., Bruner, J.M., Yung, W.K., and Zhang, W. 1999. Reactivation of insulin-like growth factor binding protein 2 expression in glioblastoma multiforme: a revelation by parallel gene expression profiling. *Cancer Res* **59**(17): 4228–4232.

Furusato, B., Shaheduzzaman, S., Petrovics, G., Dobi, A., Seifert, M., Ravindranath, L., Nau, M.E., Werner, T., Vahey, M., McLeod, D.G., Srivastava, S., and Sesterhenn, I.A. 2008. Transcriptome analyses of benign and malignant prostate epithelial cells in formalin-fixed paraffin-embedded whole-mounted radical prostatectomy specimens. *Prostate Cancer Prostatic Dis* **11**(2): 194–197.

Gilbertson, R.J. 2006. Brain tumors provide new clues to the source of cancer stem cells: does oncology recapitulate ontogeny? *Cell Cycle* **5**(2): 135–137.

Glas, A.M., Floore, A., Delahaye, L.J., Witteveen, A.T., Pover, R.C., Bakx, N., Lahti-Domenici, J.S., Bruinsma, T.J., Warmoes, M.O., Bernards, R., Wessels, L.F., and Van't Veer, L.J. 2006. Converting a breast cancer microarray signature into a high-throughput diagnostic test. *BMC Genomics* **7**: 278.

Godard, S., Getz, G., Delorenzi, M., Farmer, P., Kobayashi, H., Desbaillets, I., Nozaki, M., Diserens, A.C., Hamou, M.F., Dietrich, P.Y., Regli, L., Janzer, R.C., Bucher, P., Stupp, R., de Tribolet, N., Domany, E., and Hegi, M.E. 2003. Classification of human astrocytic gliomas on the basis of gene expression: a correlated group of genes with angiogenic activity emerges as a strong predictor of subtypes. *Cancer Res* **63**(20): 6613–6625.

Hagerstrand, D., Smits, A., Eriksson, A., Sigurdardottir, S., Olofsson, T., Hartman, M., Nister, M., Kalimo, H., and Ostman, A. 2008. Gene expression analyses of grade II gliomas and identification of rPTPbeta/zeta as a candidate oligodendroglioma marker. *Neuro Oncol* **10**(1): 2–9.

Haque, T., Faury, D., Albrecht, S., Lopez-Aguilar, E., Hauser, P., Garami, M., Hanzely, Z., Bognar, L., Del Maestro, R.F., Atkinson, J., Nantel, A., and Jabado, N. 2007. Gene expression profiling from formalin-fixed paraffin-embedded tumors of pediatric glioblastoma. *Clin Cancer Res* **13**(21): 6284–6292.

Hemmati, H.D., Nakano, I., Lazareff, J.A., Masterman-Smith, M., Geschwind, D.H., Bronner-Fraser, M., and Kornblum, H.I. 2003. Cancerous stem cells can arise from pediatric brain tumors. *Proc Natl Acad Sci USA* **100**(25): 15178–15183.

Horvath, S., Zhang, B., Carlson, M., Lu, K.V., Zhu, S., Felciano, R.M., Laurance, M.F., Zhao, W., Qi, S., Chen, Z., Lee, Y., Scheck, A.C., Liau, L.M., Wu, H., Geschwind, D.H., Febbo, P.G., Kornblum, H.I., Cloughesy, T.F., Nelson, S.F., and Mischel, P.S. 2006. Analysis of oncogenic signaling networks in glioblastoma identifies ASPM as a molecular target. *Proc Natl Acad Sci USA* **103**(46): 17402–17407.

Huang, H., Colella, S., Kurrer, M., Yonekawa, Y., Kleihues, P., and Ohgaki, H. 2000. Gene expression profiling of low-grade diffuse astrocytomas by cDNA arrays. *Cancer Res* **60**(24): 6868–6874.

Huang, H., Okamoto, Y., Yokoo, H., Heppner, F.L., Vital, A., Fevre-Montange, M., Jouvet, A., Yonekawa, Y., Lazaridis, E.N., Kleihues, P., and Ohgaki, H. 2004. Gene expression profiling and subgroup identification of oligodendrogliomas. *Oncogene* **23**(35): 6012–6022.

Kavsan, V.M., Dmitrenko, V.V., Shostak, K.O., Bukreieva, T.V., Vitak, N.Y., Simirenko, O.E., Malisheva, T.A., Shamayev, M.I., Rozumenko, V.D., and Zozulya, Y.A. 2007. Comparison of microarray and sage techniques in gene expression analysis of human glioblastoma. *Tsitol Genet* **41**(1): 36–55.

Keller, A., Ludwig, N., Comtesse, N., Henn, W., Steudel, W.I., Lenhof, H.P., and Meese, E. 2008. Combining gene expression signatures and autoantibody profiles in human meningioma. *Gene Ther* **16**(2): 184–189.

Khatua, S., Peterson, K.M., Brown, K.M., Lawlor, C., Santi, M.R., LaFleur, B., Dressman, D., Stephan, D.A., and MacDonald, T.J. 2003. Overexpression of the EGFR/FKBP12/HIF-2alpha pathway identified in childhood astrocytomas by angiogenesis gene profiling. *Cancer Res* **63**(8): 1865–1870.

Kim, S., Dougherty, E.R., Shmulevich, I., Hess, K.R., Hamilton, S.R., Trent, J.M., Fuller, G.N., and Zhang, W. 2002. Identification of combination gene sets for glioma classification. *Mol Cancer Ther* **1**(13): 1229–1236.

Kleihues P, B.P., Collins VP, Newcomb EW, Ohgaki H, Cavenee WK. 2000. Glioblastoma. in *Pathology and Genetics of Tumours of the Nervous System* (ed. C.W. Kleihues P), pp. 29–39. International Agency for Research on Cancer (IARC) *Press*, Lyon, France.

Korshunov, A., Neben, K., Wrobel, G., Tews, B., Benner, A., Hahn, M., Golanov, A., and Lichter, P. 2003. Gene expression patterns in ependymomas correlate with tumor location, grade, and patient age. *Am J Pathol* **163**(5): 1721–1727.

Kulesh, D.A., Clive, D.R., Zarlenga, D.S., and Greene, J.J. 1987. Identification of interferon-modulated proliferation-related cDNA sequences. *Proc Natl Acad Sci USA* **84**(23): 8453–8457.

Lashkari, D.A., DeRisi, J.L., McCusker, J.H., Namath, A.F., Gentile, C., Hwang, S.Y., Brown, P.O., and Davis, R.W. 1997. Yeast microarrays for genome wide parallel genetic and gene expression analysis. *Proc Natl Acad Sci USA* **94**(24): 13057–13062.

Lau, C.C. 2005. Genomic profiling in pediatric brain tumors. *Cancer J* **11**(4): 283–293.

Lee, J., Kotliarova, S., Kotliarov, Y., Li, A., Su, Q., Donin, N.M., Pastorino, S., Purow, B.W., Christopher, N., Zhang, W., Park, J.K., and Fine, H.A. 2006. Tumor stem cells derived from glioblastomas cultured in bFGF and EGF more closely mirror the phenotype and genotype of primary tumors than do serum-cultured cell lines. *Cancer Cell* **9**(5): 391–403.

Liang, Y., Diehn, M., Watson, N., Bollen, A.W., Aldape, K.D., Nicholas, M.K., Lamborn, K.R., Berger, M.S., Botstein, D., Brown, P.O., and Israel, M.A. 2005. Gene expression profiling reveals molecularly and clinically distinct subtypes of glioblastoma multiforme. *Proc Natl Acad Sci USA* **102**(16): 5814–5819.

Liu, F., Park, P.J., Lai, W., Maher, E., Chakravarti, A., Durso, L., Jiang, X., Yu, Y., Brosius, A., Thomas, M., Chin, L., Brennan, C., DePinho, R.A., Kohane, I., Carroll, R.S., Black, P.M., and Johnson, M.D. 2006a. A genome-wide screen reveals functional gene clusters in the cancer genome and identifies EphA2 as a mitogen in glioblastoma. *Cancer Res* **66**(22): 10815–10823.

Liu, M., Dai, B., Kang, S.H., Ban, K., Huang, F.J., Lang, F.F., Aldape, K.D., Xie, T.X., Pelloski, C.E., Xie, K., Sawaya, R., and Huang, S. 2006b. FoxM1B is overexpressed in human glioblastomas and critically regulates the tumorigenicity of glioma cells. *Cancer Res* **66**(7): 3593–3602.

Ljubimova, J.Y., Khazenzon, N.M., Chen, Z., Neyman, Y.I., Turner, L., Riedinger, M.S., and Black, K.L. 2001a. Gene expression abnormalities in human glial tumors identified by gene array. *Int J Oncol* **18**(2): 287–295.

Ljubimova, J.Y., Lakhter, A.J., Loksh, A., Yong, W.H., Riedinger, M.S., Miner, J.H., Sorokin, L.M., Ljubimov, A.V., and Black, K.L. 2001b. Overexpression of alpha4 chain-containing laminins in human glial tumors identified by gene microarray analysis. *Cancer Res* **61**(14): 5601–5610.

Lukashova-v Zangen, I., Kneitz, S., Monoranu, C.M., Rutkowski, S., Hinkes, B., Vince, G.H., Huang, B., and Roggendorf, W. 2007. Ependymoma gene expression profiles associated with histological subtype, proliferation, and patient survival. *Acta Neuropathol* **113**(3): 325–337.

MacDonald, T.J., Brown, K.M., LaFleur, B., Peterson, K., Lawlor, C., Chen, Y., Packer, R.J., Cogen, P., and Stephan, D.A. 2001. Expression profiling of medulloblastoma: PDGFRA and the RAS/MAPK pathway as therapeutic targets for metastatic disease. *Nat Genet* **29**(2): 143–152.

Margareto, J., Leis, O., Larrarte, E., Idoate, M.A., Carrasco, A., and Lafuente, J.V. 2007. Gene expression profiling of human gliomas reveals differences between GBM and LGA related to energy metabolism and notch signaling pathways. *J Mol Neurosci* **32**(1): 53–63.

Markert, J.M., Fuller, C.M., Gillespie, G.Y., Bubien, J.K., McLean, L.A., Hong, R.L., Lee, K., Gullans, S.R., Mapstone, T.B., and Benos, D.J. 2001. Differential gene expression profiling in human brain tumors. *Physiol Genomics* **5**(1): 21–33.

Marko, N.F., Toms, S.A., Barnett, G.H., and Weil, R. 2008. Genomic expression patterns distinguish long-term from short-term glioblastoma survivors: a preliminary feasibility study. *Genomics* **91**(5): 395–406.

Martinez-Glez, V., Franco-Hernandez, C., and Rey, J.A. 2008. Microarray gene expression profiling in meningiomas and schwannomas. *Curr Med Chem* **15**(8): 826–833.

McDonald, K.L., O'Sullivan, M.G., Parkinson, J.F., Shaw, J.M., Payne, C.A., Brewer, J.M., Young, L., Reader, D.J., Wheeler, H.T., Cook, R.J., Biggs, M.T., Little, N.S., Teo, C., Stone, G., and Robinson, B.G. 2007. IQGAP1 and IGFBP2: valuable biomarkers for determining prognosis in glioma patients. *J Neuropathol Exp Neurol* **66**(5): 405–417.

Michiels, S., Koscielny, S., and Hill, C. 2007. Interpretation of microarray data in cancer. *Brit J Cancer* **96**(8): 1155–1158.

Mischel, P.S., Shai, R., Shi, T., Horvath, S., Lu, K.V., Choe, G., Seligson, D., Kremen, T.J., Palotie, A., Liau, L.M., Cloughesy, T.F., and Nelson, S.F. 2003. Identification of molecular subtypes of glioblastoma by gene expression profiling. *Oncogene* **22**(15): 2361–2373.

Modena, P., Lualdi, E., Facchinetti, F., Veltman, J., Reid, J.F., Minardi, S., Janssen, I., Giangaspero, F., Forni, M., Finocchiaro, G., Genitori, L., Giordano, F., Riccardi, R., Schoenmakers, E.F., Massimino, M., and Sozzi, G. 2006. Identification of tumor-specific molecular signatures in intracranial ependymoma and association with clinical characteristics. *J Clin Oncol* **24**(33): 5223–5233.

Mukasa, A., Ueki, K., Ge, X., Ishikawa, S., Ide, T., Fujimaki, T., Nishikawa, R., Asai, A., Kirino, T., and Aburatani, H. 2004. Selective expression of a subset of neuronal genes in oligodendroglioma with chromosome 1p loss. *Brain Pathol* **14**(1): 34–42.

Mukasa, A., Ueki, K., Matsumoto, S., Tsutsumi, S., Nishikawa, R., Fujimaki, T., Asai, A., Kirino, T., and Aburatani, H. 2002. Distinction in gene expression profiles of oligodendrogliomas with and without allelic loss of 1p. *Oncogene* **21**(25): 3961–3968.

Neben, K., Korshunov, A., Benner, A., Wrobel, G., Hahn, M., Kokocinski, F., Golanov, A., Joos, S., and Lichter, P. 2004. Microarray-based screening for molecular markers in medulloblastoma revealed STK15 as independent predictor for survival. *Cancer Res* **64**(9): 3103–3111.

Nigro, J.M., Misra, A., Zhang, L., Smirnov, I., Colman, H., Griffin, C., Ozburn, N., Chen, M., Pan, E., Koul, D., Yung, W.K., Feuerstein, B.G., and Aldape, K.D. 2005. Integrated array-comparative genomic hybridization and expression array profiles identify clinically relevant molecular subtypes of glioblastoma. *Cancer Res* **65**(5): 1678–1686.

Nutt, C.L., Betensky, R.A., Brower, M.A., Batchelor, T.T., Louis, D.N., and Stemmer-Rachamimov, A.O. 2005. YKL-40 is a differential diagnostic marker for histologic subtypes of high-grade gliomas. *Clin Cancer Res* **11**(6): 2258–2264.

Nutt, C.L., Mani, D.R., Betensky, R.A., Tamayo, P., Cairncross, J.G., Ladd, C., Pohl, U., Hartmann, C., McLaughlin, M.E., Batchelor, T.T., Black, P.M., von Deimling, A., Pomeroy, S.L., Golub, T.R., and Louis, D.N. 2003. Gene expression-based classification of malignant gliomas correlates better with survival than histological classification. *Cancer Res* **63**(7): 1602–1607.

Paik, S., Shak, S., Tang, G., Kim, C., Baker, J., Cronin, M., Baehner, F.L., Walker, M.G., Watson, D., Park, T., Hiller, W., Fisher, E.R., Wickerham, D.L., Bryant, J., and Wolmark, N. 2004. A multigene assay to predict recurrence of tamoxifen-treated, node-negative breast cancer. *N Engl J Med* **351**(27): 2817–2826.

Park, P.C., Taylor, M.D., Mainprize, T.G., Becker, L.E., Ho, M., Dura, W.T., Squire, J., and Rutka, J.T. 2003. Transcriptional profiling of medulloblastoma in children. *J Neurosurg* **99**(3): 534–541.

Pease, A.C., Solas, D., Sullivan, E.J., Cronin, M.T., Holmes, C.P., and Fodor, S.P. 1994. Light-generated oligonucleotide arrays for rapid DNA sequence analysis. *Proc Natl Acad Sci USA* **91**(11): 5022–5026.

Pelloski, C.E., Lin, E., Zhang, L., Yung, W.K., Colman, H., Liu, J.L., Woo, S.Y., Heimberger, A.B., Suki, D., Prados, M., Chang, S., Barker, F.G., 3rd, Fuller, G.N., and Aldape, K.D. 2006. Prognostic associations of activated mitogen-activated protein kinase and Akt pathways in glioblastoma. *Clin Cancer Res* **12**(13): 3935–3941.

Pelloski, C.E., Mahajan, A., Maor, M., Chang, E.L., Woo, S., Gilbert, M., Colman, H., Yang, H., Ledoux, A., Blair, H., Passe, S., Jenkins, R.B., and Aldape, K.D. 2005. YKL-40 expression is associated with poorer response to radiation and shorter overall survival in glioblastoma. *Clin Cancer Res* **11**(9): 3326–3334.

Penland, S.K., Keku, T.O., Torrice, C., He, X., Krishnamurthy, J., Hoadley, K.A., Woosley, J.T., Thomas, N.E., Perou, C.M., Sandler, R.S., and Sharpless, N.E. 2007. RNA expression analysis of formalin-fixed paraffin-embedded tumors. *Lab Invest* **87**(4): 383–391.

Perou, C.M., Sorlie, T., Eisen, M.B., van de Rijn, M., Jeffrey, S.S., Rees, C.A., Pollack, J.R., Ross, D.T., Johnsen, H., Akslen, L.A., Fluge, O., Pergamenschikov, A., Williams, C., Zhu, S.X., Lonning, P.E., Borresen-Dale, A.L., Brown, P.O., and Botstein, D. 2000. Molecular portraits of human breast tumours. *Nature* **406** (6797): 747–752.

Persson, O., Krogh, M., Saal, L.H., Englund, E., Liu, J., Parsons, R., Mandahl, N., Borg, A., Widegren, B., and Salford, L.G. 2007. Microarray analysis of gliomas reveals chromosomal position-associated gene expression patterns and identifies potential immunotherapy targets. *J Neurooncol* **85**(1): 11–24.

Petalidis, L.P., Oulas, A., Backlund, M., Wayland, M.T., Liu, L., Plant, K., Happerfield, L., Freeman, T.C., Poirazi, P., and Collins, V.P. 2008. Improved grading and survival prediction of human astrocytic brain tumors by artificial neural network analysis of gene expression microarray data. *Mol Cancer Ther* **7**(5): 1013–1024.

Phillips, H.S., Kharbanda, S., Chen, R., Forrest, W.F., Soriano, R.H., Wu, T.D., Misra, A., Nigro, J.M., Colman, H., Soroceanu, L., Williams, P.M., Modrusan, Z., Feuerstein, B.G., and Aldape, K. 2006. Molecular subclasses of high-grade glioma predict prognosis, delineate a pattern of disease progression, and resemble stages in neurogenesis. *Cancer Cell* **9**(3): 157–173.

Pomeroy, S.L., Tamayo, P., Gaasenbeek, M., Sturla, L.M., Angelo, M., McLaughlin, M.E., Kim, J.Y., Goumnerova, L.C., Black, P.M., Lau, C., Allen, J.C., Zagzag, D., Olson, J.M., Curran, T., Wetmore, C., Biegel, J.A., Poggio, T., Mukherjee, S., Rifkin, R., Califano, A., Stolovitzky, G., Louis, D.N., Mesirov, J.P., Lander, E.S., and Golub, T.R. 2002. Prediction of central nervous system embryonal tumour outcome based on gene expression. *Nature* **415** (6870): 436–442.

Pope, W.B., Chen, J.H., Dong, J., Carlson, M.R., Perlina, A., Cloughesy, T.F., Liau, L.M., Mischel, P.S., Nghiemphu, P., Lai, A., and Nelson, S.F. 2008. Relationship between gene expression and enhancement in glioblastoma multiforme: exploratory DNA microarray analysis. *Radiology* **249**(1): 268–277.

Qi, Z.Y., Hui, G.Z., Li, Y., Zhou, Z.X., Gu, S.H., Ying, K., and Xie, Y. 2005. cDNA microarray in isolation of novel differentially expressed genes related to human glioma and clone of a novel full-length gene. *Chin Med J (Engl)* **118**(10): 799–805.

Raza, S.M., Fuller, G.N., Rhee, C.H., Huang, S., Hess, K., Zhang, W., and Sawaya, R. 2004. Identification of necrosis-associated genes in glioblastoma by cDNA microarray analysis. *Clin Cancer Res* **10** (1 Pt 1): 212–221.

Reddy, S.P., Britto, R., Vinnakota, K., Aparna, H., Sreepathi, H.K., Thota, B., Kumari, A., Shilpa, B.M., Vrinda, M., Umesh, S., Samuel, C., Shetty, M., Tandon, A., Pandey, P., Hegde, S., Hegde, A.S., Balasubramaniam, A., Chandramouli, B.A., Santosh, V., Kondaiah, P., Somasundaram, K., and Rao, M.R. 2008. Novel glioblastoma markers with diagnostic and prognostic value identified through transcriptome analysis. *Clin Cancer Res* **14**(10): 2978–2987.

Reya, T., Morrison, S.J., Clarke, M.F., and Weissman, I.L. 2001. Stem cells, cancer, and cancer stem cells. *Nature* **414** (6859): 105–111.

Rich, J.N., Hans, C., Jones, B., Iversen, E.S., McLendon, R.E., Rasheed, B.K., Dobra, A., Dressman, H.K., Bigner, D.D., Nevins, J.R., and West, M. 2005. Gene expression profiling and genetic markers in glioblastoma survival. *Cancer Res* **65**(10): 4051–4058.

Rickman, D.S., Bobek, M.P., Misek, D.E., Kuick, R., Blaivas, M., Kurnit, D.M., Taylor, J., and Hanash, S.M. 2001. Distinctive molecular profiles of high-grade and low-grade gliomas based on oligonucleotide microarray analysis. *Cancer Res* **61**(18): 6885–6891.

Riemenschneider, M.J., Mueller, W., Betensky, R.A., Mohapatra, G., and Louis, D.N. 2005. In situ analysis of integrin and growth factor receptor signaling pathways in human glioblastomas suggests overlapping relationships with focal adhesion kinase activation. *Am J Pathol* **167**(5): 1379–1387.

Ruano, Y., Mollejo, M., Camacho, F.I., Rodriguez de Lope, A., Fiano, C., Ribalta, T., Martinez, P., Hernandez-Moneo, J.L., and Melendez, B. 2008. Identification of survival-related genes of the phosphatidylinositol 3'-kinase signaling pathway in glioblastoma multiforme. *Cancer* **112**(7): 1575–1584.

Sallinen, S.L., Sallinen, P.K., Haapasalo, H.K., Helin, H.J., Helen, P.T., Schraml, P., Kallioniemi, O.P., and Kononen, J. 2000. Identification of differentially expressed genes in human gliomas by DNA microarray and tissue chip techniques. *Cancer Res* **60**(23): 6617–6622.

Sasaki, T., Hankins, G.R., and Helm, G.A. 2003. Comparison of gene expression profiles between frozen original meningiomas and primary cultures of the meningiomas by GeneChip. *Neurosurgery* **52**(4): 892–898; discussion 898–899.

Sayagues, J.M., Tabernero, M.D., Maillo, A., Trelles, O., Espinosa, A.B., Sarasquete, M.E., Merino, M., Rasillo, A., Vera, J.F., Santos-Briz, A., de Alava, E., Garcia-Macias, M.C., and Orfao, A. 2006. Microarray-based analysis of spinal versus intracranial meningiomas: different clinical, biological, and genetic characteristics associated with distinct patterns of gene expression. *J Neuropathol Exp Neurol* **65**(5): 445–454.

Schena, M., Shalon, D., Davis, R.W., and Brown, P.O. 1995. Quantitative monitoring of gene expression patterns with a complementary DNA microarray. *Science* **270** (5235): 467–470.

Scicchitano, M.S., Dalmas, D.A., Bertiaux, M.A., Anderson, S.M., Turner, L.R., Thomas, R.A., Mirable, R., and Boyce, R.W. 2006. Preliminary comparison of quantity, quality, and microarray performance of RNA extracted from formalin-fixed, paraffin-embedded, and unfixed frozen tissue samples. *J Histochem Cytochem* **54**(11): 1229–1237.

Scrideli, C.A., Carlotti, C.G., Jr., Okamoto, O.K., Andrade, V.S., Cortez, M.A., Motta, F.J., Lucio-Eterovic, A.K., Neder, L., Rosemberg, S., Oba-Shinjo, S.M., Marie, S.K., and Tone, L.G. 2008. Gene expression profile analysis of primary glioblastomas and non-neoplastic brain tissue: identification of potential target genes by oligonucleotide microarray and real-time quantitative PCR. *J Neurooncol* **88**(3): 281–291.

Shai, R., Shi, T., Kremen, T.J., Horvath, S., Liau, L.M., Cloughesy, T.F., Mischel, P.S., and Nelson, S.F. 2003. Gene expression profiling identifies molecular subtypes of gliomas. *Oncogene* **22**(31): 4918–4923.

Sharma, M.K., Watson, M.A., Lyman, M., Perry, A., Aldape, K.D., Deak, F., and Gutmann, D.H. 2006. Matrilin-2 expression distinguishes clinically relevant subsets of pilocytic astrocytoma. *Neurology* **66**(1): 127–130.

Singh, S.K., Clarke, I.D., Terasaki, M., Bonn, V.E., Hawkins, C., Squire, J., and Dirks, P.B. 2003. Identification of a cancer stem cell in human brain tumors. *Cancer Res* **63**(18): 5821–5828.

Singh, S.K., Hawkins, C., Clarke, I.D., Squire, J.A., Bayani, J., Hide, T., Henkelman, R.M., Cusimano, M.D., and Dirks, P.B. 2004. Identification of human brain tumour initiating cells. *Nature* **432** (7015): 396–401.

Somasundaram, K., Reddy, S.P., Vinnakota, K., Britto, R., Subbarayan, M., Nambiar, S., Hebbar, A., Samuel, C., Shetty, M., Sreepathi, H.K., Santosh, V., Hegde, A.S., Hegde, S., Kondaiah, P., and Rao, M.R. 2005. Upregulation of ASCL1 and inhibition of Notch signaling pathway characterize progressive astrocytoma. *Oncogene* **24**(47): 7073–7083.

Sorlie, T., Perou, C.M., Tibshirani, R., Aas, T., Geisler, S., Johnsen, H., Hastie, T., Eisen, M.B., van de Rijn, M., Jeffrey, S.S., Thorsen, T., Quist, H., Matese, J.C., Brown, P.O., Botstein, D., Eystein Lonning, P., and Borresen-Dale, A.L. 2001. Gene expression patterns of breast carcinomas distinguish tumor subclasses with clinical implications. *Proc Natl Acad Sci USA* **98**(19): 10869–10874.

Sorlie, T., Tibshirani, R., Parker, J., Hastie, T., Marron, J.S., Nobel, A., Deng, S., Johnsen, H., Pesich, R., Geisler, S., Demeter, J., Perou, C.M., Lonning, P.E., Brown, P.O., Borresen-Dale, A.L., and Botstein, D. 2003. Repeated observation of breast tumor subtypes in independent gene expression data sets. *Proc Natl Acad Sci USA* **100**(14): 8418–8423.

Sowar, K., Straessle, J., Donson, A.M., Handler, M., and Foreman, N.K. 2006. Predicting which children are at risk for ependymoma relapse. *J Neurooncol* **78**(1): 41–46.

Srivastava, P.K., Kuffer, S., Brors, B., Shahi, P., Li, L., Kenzelmann, M., Gretz, N., and Grone, H.J. 2008. A cut-off based approach for gene expression analysis of formalin-fixed and paraffin-embedded tissue samples. *Genomics* **91**(6): 522–529.

Suarez-Merino, B., Hubank, M., Revesz, T., Harkness, W., Hayward, R., Thompson, D., Darling, J.L., Thomas, D.G., and Warr, T.J. 2005. Microarray analysis of pediatric ependymoma identifies a cluster of 112 candidate genes including four transcripts at 22q12.1–q13.3. *Neuro Oncol* **7**(1): 20–31.

Tanwar, M.K., Gilbert, M.R., and Holland, E.C. 2002. Gene expression microarray analysis reveals YKL-40 to be a potential serum marker for malignant character in human glioma. *Cancer Res* **62**(15): 4364–4368.

Tavazoie, S., Hughes, J.D., Campbell, M.J., Cho, R.J., and Church, G.M. 1999. Systematic determination of genetic network architecture. *Nat Genet* **22**(3): 281–285.

Taylor, M.D., Poppleton, H., Fuller, C., Su, X., Liu, Y., Jensen, P., Magdaleno, S., Dalton, J., Calabrese, C., Board, J., Macdonald, T., Rutka, J., Guha, A., Gajjar, A., Curran, T., and Gilbertson, R.J. 2005. Radial glia cells are candidate stem cells of ependymoma. *Cancer Cell* **8**(4): 323–335.

Teh, M.T., Wong, S.T., Neill, G.W., Ghali, L.R., Philpott, M.P., and Quinn, A.G. 2002. FOXM1 is a downstream target of Gli1 in basal cell carcinomas. *Cancer Res* **62**(16): 4773–4780.

Tews, B., Felsberg, J., Hartmann, C., Kunitz, A., Hahn, M., Toedt, G., Neben, K., Hummerich, L., von Deimling, A., Reifenberger, G., and Lichter, P. 2006. Identification of novel oligodendroglioma-associated candidate tumor suppressor genes in 1p36 and 19q13 using microarray-based expression profiling. *Int J Cancer* **119**(4): 792–800.

The Cancer Genome Atlas Research Network, McLendon, R. Friedman, A. Bigner, D. Van Meir, E.G. Brat, D.J. Mastrogianakis, M. Olson, J.J. Mikkelsen, T. Lehman, N. Aldape, K. Alfred Yung, W.K. Bogler, O. Vandenberg, S. Berger, M. Prados, M. Muzny, D. Morgan, M. Scherer, S. Sabo, A. Nazareth, L. Lewis, L. Hall, O. Zhu, Y. Ren, Y. Alvi, O. Yao, J. Hawes, A. Jhangiani, S. Fowler, G. San Lucas, A. Kovar, C. Cree, A. Dinh, H. Santibanez, J. Joshi, V. Gonzalez-Garay, M.L. Miller, C.A. Milosavljevic, A. Donehower, L. Wheeler, D.A. Gibbs, R.A. Cibulskis, K. Sougnez, C. Fennell, T. Mahan, S. Wilkinson, J. Ziaugra, L. Onofrio, R. Bloom, T. Nicol, R. Ardlie, K. Baldwin, J. Gabriel, S. Lander, E.S. Ding, L. Fulton, R.S. McLellan, M.D. Wallis, J. Larson, D.E. Shi, X. Abbott, R. Fulton, L. Chen, K. Koboldt, D.C. Wendl, M.C. Meyer, R. Tang, Y. Lin, L. Osborne, J.R. Dunford-Shore, B.H. Miner, T.L. Delehaunty, K. Markovic, C. Swift, G. Courtney, W. Pohl, C. Abbott, S. Hawkins, A. Leong, S. Haipek, C. Schmidt, H. Wiechert, M. Vickery, T. Scott, S. Dooling, D.J. Chinwalla, A. Weinstock, G.M. Mardis, E.R. Wilson, R.K. Getz, G. Winckler, W. Verhaak, R.G. Lawrence, M.S. O'Kelly, M. Robinson, J. Alexe, G. Beroukhim, R. Carter, S. Chiang, D. Gould, J. Gupta, S. Korn, J. Mermel, C. Mesirov, J. Monti, S. Nguyen, H. Parkin, M. Reich, M. Stransky, N. Weir, B.A. Garraway, L. Golub, T. Meyerson, M. Chin, L. Protopopov, A. Zhang, J. Perna, I. Aronson, S. Sathiamoorthy, N. Ren, G. Wiedemeyer, W.R. Kim, H. Won Kong, S. Xiao, Y. Kohane, I.S. Seidman, J. Park, P.J. Kucherlapati, R. Laird, P.W. Cope, L. Herman, J.G. Weisenberger, D.J. Pan, F. Van Den Berg, D. Van Neste, L. Mi Yi, J. Schuebel, K.E. Baylin, S.B. Absher, D.M. Li, J.Z. Southwick, A. Brady, S. Aggarwal, A. Chung, T. Sherlock, G. Brooks, J.D. Myers, R. M. Spellman, P.T. Purdom, E. Jakkula, L.R. Lapuk, A.V. Marr, H. Dorton, S. Gi Choi, Y. Han, J. Ray, A. Wang, V. Durinck, S. Robinson, M. Wang, N.J. Vranizan, K. Peng, V.

Van Name, E. Fontenay, G.V. Ngai, J. Conboy, J.G. Parvin, B. Feiler, H.S. Speed, T.P. Gray, J.W. Brennan, C. Socci, N.D. Olshen, A. Taylor, B.S. Lash, A. Schultz, N. Reva, B. Antipin, Y. Stukalov, A. Gross, B. Cerami, E. Qing Wang, W. Qin, L.X. Seshan, V.E. Villafania, L. Cavatore, M. Borsu, L. Viale, A. Gerald, W. Sander, C. Ladanyi, M. Perou, C.M. Neil Hayes, D. Topal, M.D. Hoadley, K.A. Qi, Y. Balu, S. Shi, Y. Wu, J. Penny, R. Bittner, M. Shelton, T. Lenkiewicz, E. Morris, S. Beasley, D. Sanders, S. Kahn, A. Sfeir, R. Chen, J. Nassau, D. Feng, L. Hickey, E. Weinstein, J.N. Barker, A. Gerhard, D.S. Vockley, J. Compton, C. Vaught, J. Fielding, P. Ferguson, M.L. Schaefer, C. Madhavan, S. Buetow, K.H. Collins, F. Good, P. Guyer, M. Ozenberger, B. Peterson, J. and Thomson, E. 2008. Comprehensive genomic characterization defines human glioblastoma genes and core pathways. *Nature* **455**(7216): 1061–1068.

Thompson, M.C., Fuller, C., Hogg, T.L., Dalton, J., Finkelstein, D., Lau, C.C., Chintagumpala, M., Adesina, A., Ashley, D.M., Kellie, S.J., Taylor, M.D., Curran, T., Gajjar, A., and Gilbertson, R.J. 2006. Genomics identifies medulloblastoma subgroups that are enriched for specific genetic alterations. *J Clin Oncol* **24**(12): 1924–1931.

van de Vijver, M.J., He, Y.D., van't Veer, L.J., Dai, H., Hart, A.A., Voskuil, D.W., Schreiber, G.J., Peterse, J.L., Roberts, C., Marton, M.J., Parrish, M., Atsma, D., Witteveen, A., Glas, A., Delahaye, L., van der Velde, T., Bartelink, H., Rodenhuis, S., Rutgers, E.T., Friend, S.H., and Bernards, R. 2002. A gene-expression signature as a predictor of survival in breast cancer. *N Engl J Med* **347**(25): 1999–2009.

van den Boom, J., Wolter, M., Kuick, R., Misek, D.E., Youkilis, A.S., Wechsler, D.S., Sommer, C., Reifenberger, G., and Hanash, S.M. 2003. Characterization of gene expression profiles associated with glioma progression using oligonucleotide-based microarray analysis and real-time reverse transcription-polymerase chain reaction. *Am J Pathol* **163**(3): 1033–1043.

Van Meter, T., Dumur, C., Hafez, N., Garrett, C., Fillmore, H., and Broaddus, W.C. 2006. Microarray analysis of MRI-defined tissue samples in glioblastoma reveals differences in regional expression of therapeutic targets. *Diagn Mol Pathol* **15**(4): 195–205.

Watson, M.A., Gutmann, D.H., Peterson, K., Chicoine, M.R., Kleinschmidt-DeMasters, B.K., Brown, H.G., and Perry, A. 2002. Molecular characterization of human meningiomas by gene expression profiling using high-density oligonucleotide microarrays. *Am J Pathol* **161**(2): 665–672.

Watson, M.A., Perry, A., Budhraja, V., Hicks, C., Shannon, W.D., and Rich, K.M. 2001. Gene expression profiling with oligonucleotide microarrays distinguishes World Health Organization grade of oligodendrogliomas. *Cancer Res* **61**(5): 1825–1829.

Wong, K.K., Chang, Y.M., Tsang, Y.T., Perlaky, L., Su, J., Adesina, A., Armstrong, D.L., Bhattacharjee, M., Dauser, R., Blaney, S.M., Chintagumpala, M., and Lau, C.C. 2005. Expression analysis of juvenile pilocytic astrocytomas by oligonucleotide microarray reveals two potential subgroups. *Cancer Res* **65**(1): 76–84.

Wrobel, G., Roerig, P., Kokocinski, F., Neben, K., Hahn, M., Reifenberger, G., and Lichter, P. 2005. Microarray-based gene expression profiling of benign, atypical and anaplastic meningiomas identifies novel genes associated with meningioma progression. *Int J Cancer* **114**(2): 249–256.

Yuan, X., Curtin, J., Xiong, Y., Liu, G., Waschsmann-Hogiu, S., Farkas, D.L., Black, K.L., and Yu, J.S. 2004. Isolation of cancer stem cells from adult glioblastoma multiforme. *Oncogene* **23**(58): 9392–9400.

Chapter 24
Proteomic Profiling of Human Brain Tumors

Rongcai Jiang, Jian Yi Li, Gregory N. Fuller, and Wei Zhang

Abstract Although challenging, proteomic profiling has recently become a hot area in cancer research, and a majority of the currently available methodologies, such as two-dimensional polyacrylamide gel electrophoresis, two-dimensional difference gel electrophoresis, liquid chromatography, matrix-assisted laser desorption/ionization time-of-flight mass spectrometry, surface-enhanced laser desorption/ionization time-of-flight MS, tissue microarrays, and protein and antibody arrays, have been used in human brain tumor research. These studies have generated an enormous amount of data, and, in the postproteomics era, more powerful bioinformatics tools are needed to effectively mine proteomics data efficiently and accurately. The design, execution, and interpretation of in vitro and in vivo biological confirmatory experiments constitute major tasks for scientists who seek to identify clinically meaningful diagnostic and prognostic makers.

Contents

W. Zhang (✉)
Department of Pathology, University of Texas M. D. Anderson Cancer Center, Houston, TX, USA
e-mail: wzhang@mdanderson.org

E.G. Van Meir (ed.), *CNS Cancer*, Cancer Drug Discovery and Development, DOI 10.1007/978-1-60327-553-8_24,

© Humana Press, a part of Springer Science+Business Media, LLC 2009

24.1 Background

Technological advances have constituted a major force in the drive to increase our understanding of human brain tumors. Conventional molecular biologic approaches, such as Southern blotting, northern hybridization, western blot analysis, genotyping, polymerase chain reaction (PCR), and nucleotide sequencing, have led to the identification of many genetic and molecular events associated with human brain tumor initiation and progression. Among the signature events associated with the development of human diffuse gliomas, some of the most exciting include the amplification of the epidermal growth factor receptor (EGFR) gene and the deletion or mutation of tumor suppressor genes *TP53, PTEN,* and *p16INK4A* (Caskey et al., 2000).

The development and advancement of high-throughput genomic technologies, such as DNA microarrays, have led to an exponential growth in the knowledge of the molecular and genetic characteristics of gliomas. In the first reported studies of gene expression profiling of diffuse gliomas, we profiled 25 gliomas of different histologic subtypes and grades using the first commercially available microarray product, which permitted the evaluation of approximately 600 genes. These studies led to the discovery of the overexpression of insulin-like growth factor binding protein 2 (IGFBP2) in high-grade gliomas, and to the identification of combination gene sets that could be used for accurately classifying four major subtypes of diffuse glioma (oligodendroglioma, anaplastic oligodendroglioma, anaplastic astrocytoma, and glioblastoma) (Fuller et al., 1999; Kim et al., 2002). Even more studies identifying diagnostic and prognostic markers using much higher density DNA microarrays have been reported since then, many of which have independently confirmed the earlier discoveries of us and further established IGFBP2 as an oncogene for glioma development and progression through Akt pathway (Sallinen et al., 2000; Dunlap et al., 2007; Fukushima et al., 2007; Mehrian-Shai et al., 2007).

A major limitation of RNA-based assays is that relative mRNA expression level neither corresponds with the level of protein expression nor reveals post-translational protein modifications, which are critical for the function of many regulatory proteins. Moreno et al. performed genomic profiling by cDNA array and, concurrently, proteomic profiling by two-dimensional polyacrylamide gel electrophoresis (2D PAGE)-matrix-assisted laser desorption/ionization time-of-flight mass spectrometry (MALDI-TOF-MS) on a series of pituitary adenomas. A comparison of the results revealed that only 40% of the proteins identified by proteomic assay had the corresponding genes identified by the gene chip analysis, and the overall agreement of the proteomic and mRNA expression data was only 43%. It was also found that some genes, such as *thioredoxin domain containing 9*, exhibited an increased mRNA expression level with a paradoxically decreased corresponding protein expression level (Moreno et al., 2005). An additional recent report found a negative correlation between mRNA and protein levels during mouse embryonic stem cell differentiation (Baharvand et al., 2008).

Genomic profiling is one side of the equation; the other side, proteomic profiling, has also been a focus of intensive investigation in cancer research. Although a much more challenging endeavor, proteomic study has several advantages. First, protein identification and profiling by immunohistochemical techniques have been critical for accurate diagnosis of many types of tumors for many years. Secondly, body fluids, which are relatively easy to obtain through non-invasive methods, are quite amenable to proteomic analysis. Finally, a survey of protein activation status provides insight into the signaling pathways that operate in a given tumor, thereby delineating the tumor's pathobiology and also potentially identifying relevant pathways for therapeutic intervention.

Protein profiling based on 2D PAGE has been conducted since the early 1980s. However, the concept has been expanded to broadly encompass 2D PAGE-based and 2D PAGE-free protein profiling, protein arrays, tissue micro-arrays (TMAs), and protein identification through mass spectrometry (MS)-based technologies. Excluding protein and tissue arrays, proteomics analyses always include four steps: (1) sample collection and protein isolation, (2) protein separation, (3) protein identification and data extraction, and (4) protein function confirmation.

For sample collection and protein isolation, protein prefractionation technologies, such as laser microdissection, can be utilized to isolate a relatively "pure" tumor cell population from the mixed cell population that the native tissue specimen comprises, thus enhancing protein profiling precision. For protein separation, gel-free technologies, such as liquid chromatography (LC) and MS, have been developed that are based on direct protein identification from body fluids, and are used in addition to classical 2D PAGE. Also, significant advances have appeared in peptide measurement and data extraction in conjunction with the rapid development of MS and bioinformatics procedures. For protein functional confirmation, traditional molecular biological technologies, such as western blotting, immunohistochemical staining, and cell proliferation assays, are advantageously coupled with modern molecular biologic technologies for the assessment of overexpression or downregulation of particular genes of interest. One current trend is to combine several different proteomic-related technologies with multiple bioinformatic approaches to facilitate protein profiling and subsequent data analysis. Herein, we review the proteomics approach to brain tumor investigation according to key technologies in current use.

24.2 Protein Separation

24.2.1 Two-Dimensional Polyacrylamide Gel Electrophoresis (2D PAGE)

Protein separation is the key step in proteome analysis in both gel-based and gel-free procedures. Gel-based protein separation is synonymous with 2D

PAGE, which was developed as a method to separate proteins based on charge and size (O'Farrell, 1975; Narayan et al., 1986). 2D PAGE remains the dominant methodology for protein separation and can be used to analyze hundreds of different proteins in a single experiment, despite inherent limitations, such as limited throughput, relatively large sample volume requirements, gel-to-gel variability, and the inability to accurately detect and measure low-abundance proteins.

The utility of 2D PAGE coupled with MS is illustrated by the studies of Dasgupta et al., in which levels of the eIF2α-binding protein MetAP2 were significantly higher in the cerebrospinal fluid of NF1-deficient mice with optic pathway gliomas compared to tumor-free NF1 mice. Highly expressed MetAP2 was confirmed in the optic pathway glioma tissues and the optic nerves from the genetically engineered NF1-deficient mice. Furthermore, MetAP2 was determined to be higher only in the pilocytic astrocytomas of NF1-deficient mice, but not in sporadic astrocytomas (Dasgupta et al., 2005b).

To uncover the intracellular signaling pathways in NF1-deficient astrocytes, 2D PAGE coupled with MS was used to analyze protein lysates derived from primary NF1+/+ and NF1–/– murine neocortical astrocyte cultures. The results revealed that a series of ribosome biogenesis-promoting proteins, as well as mTOR pathway signaling, was upregulated in the NF1–/– astrocytes. The inhibition of mTOR resulted in the growth abrogation of the NF1–/– astrocytes and restoration of normal proliferation rates (Dasgupta et al., 2005a).

Khwaja et al. collected 60 cerebrospinal fluid and cyst fluid specimens from 32 astrocytomas, 7 primary brain tumors, 8 metastatic brain tumors, 3 infectious disease samples, and 10 normal controls (Khwaja et al., 2007). Based on the combined results from 2D PAGE, MALDI-TOF and TOF-MS, high-performance liquid chromatography (HPLC), and cleavable isotope-coded affinity tag analyses, attractin was found to be specially secreted by astrocytoma cells. Western blotting analysis and immunohistochemical staining both confirmed that the expression level of attractin was high in high-grade astrocytomas and slightly increased in metastatic brain tumors and low-grade astrocytomas. However, within the various cellular constituents of normal brain tissue, attractin expression was confined to the neuronal population. No attractin expression was detected in schwannoma cells. Furthermore, scratch-wound assays and Boyden chamber migration assays both demonstrated a key role of attractin in glioma invasiveness (Khwaja et al., 2006a).

Using 2D PAGE, Li et al. identified nine proteins that were exclusively expressed in astrocytomas of different histologic grades but not in normal astrocytes, four proteins that presented in high-grade astrocytomas (WHO grades III and IV) but not in low-grade astrocytomas (WHO grade II), and four proteins that were expressed only in glioblastoma. The expression of three of these proteins, Ki-67, N-CoR, and IRS-2, was validated by immunohistochemical staining. Low-grade diffuse astrocytomas exhibited a low MIB-1 (Ki-67) proliferation index. Anaplastic astrocytomas expressed increased

N-CoR and had a moderate MIB-1 (Ki-67) proliferation index. Glioblastomas strongly expressed N-CoR and IRS-2 and had very high MIB-1 (Ki-67) proliferation indices.

Using the combination of 2D PAGE and cICAT (cleavable isotope-coded affinity tags) in a LN-Z308 (p53-null) human glioblastoma cell line in the presence or absence of reconstituted wild-type p53 expression, Khwaja et al. found that of the 111 proteins identified as secreted by the cells, 39 were enhanced and 21 were inhibited in response to wild-type p53 expression. None of these were direct transcriptional targets of wild-type p53 transcription factor activity, indicating that wild-type p53 indirectly affects the stability or secretion of these proteins (Khwaja et al., 2006c).

24.2.2 Two-Dimensional Difference Gel Electrophoresis (2D DIGE)

2D DIGE was developed to overcome the irreproducibility issue associated with gels, which constitutes the most troubling shortcoming of 2D PAGE. In 2D DIGE, two proteins, from an experimental and a control sample, are labeled with different cyanine-based fluorescent dyes, Cy3-NHS and Cy5-NHS being the most popular (Gong et al., 2004), and then run on the same gel. Thus, the pattern of the protein of interest in the experimental sample is superimposed on that of its counterpart in the control sample. 2D DIGE is very sensitive and is capable of detecting as little as 0.5 fmol of protein without electrophoretic mobility shift arising between the differentially labeled samples (Gong et al., 2004). Because of 2D DIGE's high sensitivity, sample variation, such as that introduced by contamination from neighboring tissues or that resulting from sample clean up and fractionation, can result in significant errors. Fortunately, several groups have shown that the use of laser capture microdissection can significantly mitigate error attributable to sample variation (Kondo et al., 2003; Mustafa et al., 2008).

Beckner et al. reported using 2D DIGE with Cy3 and Cy5 to investigate the invasiveness of U87MG glioma cells by comparing the protein composition of cell pseudopodia with that of whole cells. MALDI-TOF-MS revealed that levels of HGF, Met, actin, total AnxI, and four other proteins were increased in pseudopodia compared to their levels in whole cells. AnxI and AnxII had been previously found to be associated with glioma progression (Beckner et al., 2005); however, actin is a "housekeeping" protein, and its elevation indicated a 2D DIGE error.

It is well known that oligodendrogliomas that exhibit the favorable genetic signature of co-deletion of chromosomal arms 1p and 19q are sensitive to a number of treatment modalities, including chemotherapy with PCV (procarbazine, 1-(2-chloroethyl)-3-cyclohexyl-l-nitrosourea (CCNU), and vincristine) or temozolomide, and radiation therapy. However, the mechanism underlying this response is not clear. Therefore, Ngo et al., using a proteomics approach consisting of 2D DIGE and MS coupled with classical protein-induction, cytotoxicity testing, cytogenetic analysis, and western blotting, analyzed two malignant glioma cell lines with 1p+/+ and 1p+/–. A biomarker protein, stathmin, was identified and determined to be highly associated with 1p status. Downregulated stathmin was associated with 1p+/– and with better chemotherapeutic response, thus providing a hypothesis for the relationship between 1p deletion and chemoresponsiveness (Ngo et al., 2007).

24.2.3 Liquid Chromatography (LC)

LC is another advanced technology that separates proteins in a gel-free environment and is currently applied broadly with MS to profile proteins in biofluid samples. Adkins et al. published the first proteomics study using LC–MS/MS for human biofluid protein profiling in 2002 (Adkins et al., 2002). Since then, the number of LC–MS-based applications for human biofluid analysis has increased exponentially. In LC–MS or LC–MS/MS, the protein mixtures from cellular lysates or biofluids are digested into polypeptides by proteases, such as trypsin, separated by capillary LC, and analyzed by MS online via an electrospray ionization interface. Using strong cation exchange chromatography, thousands of proteins from complex mammalian tissues and cells can be identified by LC–MS/MS. Many peptides can be identified by high-throughput LC–MS through the established accurate mass and time tag reference library (Qian et al., 2006). Furthermore, when suitable depletion, fractionation, and/or enrichment techniques have been applied, the proteome coverage offered by current LC–MS or LC–MS/MS extends to 100–300, and the dynamic range is enhanced to 10^3–10^7 (Lee et al., 2006; Qian et al., 2006). The peak capacities and dynamic range can be further enhanced by using higher pressure, smaller particles, nanoelectrospray interfaces, long gradients for separations, and columns that are longer or have smaller inner diameters (Tolley et al., 2001; Shen et al., 2002, 2005).

Despite the advantages of LC–MS and LC–MS/MS, both have a number of limitations in global protein profiling, including a high requirement for protein purification when the buffers and/or detergents used interfere with analysis. For example, in one study, Okamoto et al. used 2D PAGE and LC/MS to analyze oligodendrogliomas with or without 1p loss of heterozygosity (LOH). They found seven candidate proteins were overexpressed in oligodendrogliomas without 1p LOH, including Glyoxalase I and Rho GDP dissociation inhibitor, which enhance chemoresistance in other tumors (Okamoto et al., 2007). Twelve overexpressed proteins in tumors with 1p LOH have previously been reported to induce chemosensitivity in other forms of human tumors (Okamoto et al.,

2007). In one protein profiling study using the malignant glioma cell line D54MG, Westman-Brinkmalm et al. reported that prefractionation with microsolution isoelectric focusing strengthened the protein identification power of LC–MS/MS compared to that of 2D PAGE coupled with MALDI-MS. As an additional benefit, the prefractionation procedure depleted detergents before the samples were applied to LC–MS/MS. Moreover, the authors speculated that a delipidization process might facilitate the detection of intracellular proteins by opening membranes (Westman-Brinkmalm et al., 2005). With the development of LC–MS technologies and the advance of fractionation approaches, the range of proteins detectable in human biofluids and tissues by global profiling has been greatly expanded. However, no single technology can currently be considered to be the best method of protein profiling, and more effort is required to improve and optimize protein separation and identification.

Vogel et al. used nanospray LC, a recently developed LC technology, to profile four glioblastoma cell lines and eight surgically resected glioblastoma tissue samples (Vogel et al., 2005). The authors found that more than 60 proteins were lost and more than 160 proteins were gained during cell culture. Among these 220 proteins, six that were found to be expressed in all of the surgically resected human glioblastomas were sequenced, and all were associated in one way or another with cell growth by virtue of a role in enhancing cell signaling, transcription, or cell division. Vogel et al. also identified other proteins exclusively expressed in the glioblastoma cell lines that were related to cytoskeleton movement or scaffolding. Other investigators have observed similar findings in cultured fibroblasts (Chang et al., 2004, 2002).

24.3 MS-Based Protein Identification

MS determines structural information from the analysis of ionized peptides based on the mass-to-charge (m/z) principle. MS technologies have evolved rapidly over the past decade, with matrix-assisted laser desorption/ionization MS (MALDI-MS) and electrospray ionization MS (ESI-MS) among the most commonly used methods.

In MALDI-MS, a protein and peptide sample is mixed with a small energy-absorbing matrix to form a crystal lattice, which is then irradiated by a laser. The matrix absorbs the energy from the laser and subsequently passes it to the sample peptides to induce ionization. The peptide ions in their gas phase are subsequently ejected into a mass analyzer, and the peptide ion intensity versus m/z is measured to facilitate identification.

Although the protein identification procedure in ESI-MS is also based on the mass-to-charge principle, in ESI-MS the liquid proteins and peptides are sprayed out through a microcapillary tube in a very fine mist, during which they are ionized using high voltage. The sample particles are further ionized by being passed through a heated capillary or a curtain of nitrogen, after which they enter the MS analyzer, which detects and calculates ion intensity versus m/z.

24.3.1 Matrix-Assisted Laser Desorption/Ionization Time-of-Flight Mass Spectrometry (MALDI-TOF-MS)

Currently, one of the most popular MS procedures is MALDI-TOF-MS, which takes advantage of the physical property of time-of-flight (TOF). In MALDI-TOF-MS, the gas ions of the MALDI-generated protein and peptide sample are directed through a flight tube and strike a detector. The time required for the ions to travel the length of the flight tube correlates with the m/z value; ion intensity versus m/z is then determined. MALDI-TOF-MS has gained popularity because of several inherent advantages, including its simplicity, sensitivity, and fully automatic data analysis and database search capabilities (Smith et al., 2006).

Using MALDI-MS, Schwartz et al. accurately separated glioma from non-tumor cells, stratified individual tumor grades, and distinguished patients who survived long term (>90 months) from those who survived short term (<15 months). In patients with short-term survival, protein profiles were found to be an independent biomarker of patient survival. Furthermore, six expressed proteins were identified as glioma specific. Among these, calcyclin was predominantly expressed in patients with short-term survival, dynein light chain 2 was overexpressed in patients with long-term survival, and PEA-15 expression was higher in low-grade gliomas than in glioblastoma (Schwartz et al., 2005).

Drug response experiments have also been performed using LC coupled with MALDI-TOF-MS. For example, Billecke et al. treated the LNZ308 glioma cell line with platinum chemotherapeutic agents, profiled protein peak changes using 2D chromatography, and analyzed the resultant data using MetaComparison Tool and ProteomeLab PF2D software (Beckman Coulter). The authors found that the response protein peaks were either unique to the treatment with trinuclear platinum, BBR3464, BBR3610, or cisplatin, or common to the combination of two of these agents. They also identified two interesting protein peaks in the cisplatin- and BBR3610-treated cells, which were subsequently determined by MALDI-TOF-MS and MALDI-TOF/TOF-MS to represent triosephosphate isomerase 1. These experiments demonstrated that a proteomic approach based on LC and MALDI-TOF-MS could be effectively applied to drug design and selection (Beckner et al., 2005).

MALDI-Fourier transform ion cyclotron resonance MS (MALDI-FTICR-MS) and MALDI-Fourier transform MS (MALDI-FTMS) have been utilized to study the proteomics of glioma microvasculature. Using these methods, fibronectin, colligin2, non-muscular myosin-9, calcium-binding protein 22, and Cdc42 effector protein 3 were shown to be overexpressed in glioma vessels (Mustafa et al., 2007; Titulaer et al., 2008).

24.3.2 Surface-Enhanced Laser Desorption/Ionization Time-of-Flight Mass Spectrometry (SELDI-TOF-MS)

SELDI-TOF-MS, which is being increasingly utilized, takes advantage of the fact that chemical or biological surfaces can serve as the platforms for protein retention, which, in turn, can serve as a prefractionation step that permits detection of less-abundant proteins. In brief, SELDI-TOF-MS produces differential mass spectra between two experimental proteins. For example, in one recent study of cerebrospinal fluid samples from 32 pediatric brain tumor patients and 70 pediatric control patients, the combined application of SELDI-MS, ProteinChip array technology, and statistical analysis revealed that of 247 identified protein peaks, 123 were differentially expressed in the brain tumor patient cohort, which permitted differentiation of the control and brain tumor cohorts with 88% accuracy and 88% specificity. Of the 123 peaks, one that was highly overexpressed in brain tumor patients was selected for further evaluation and, using SDS-PAGE, was identified as apolipoprotein A-II. Expression of this protein, which was confirmed by western blotting and immunohistochemistry, correlated significantly with the cerebrospinal fluid albumin concentration, suggesting an association with blood–brain barrier disruption (de Bont et al., 2006).

Apolipoprotein A-II was also sequenced using a SELDI-based analysis by the application of protein tryptic digestion and MS/MS in a secondary processing (Smith et al., 2006). Khwaja et al. used SELDI-TOF-MS to analyze cerebrospinal fluid from 10 patients with central nervous system malignancies (six glioblastomas, one diffuse astrocytoma, one ependymoma, two melanomas, and one metastatic carcinoma), 12 with inflammatory or reactive conditions, and 10 with unknown central nervous system diseases. The authors found that carbonic anhydrase was overexpressed in many central nervous system malignancies, including glioblastoma. Non-neoplastic cerebrospinal fluid, especially in inflammatory conditions, exhibited prominent levels of cystatin C. The study thus demonstrated that cerebrospinal fluid proteomics can be used to detect, diagnose, and monitor central nervous system disease (Khwaja et al., 2006b).

Recently, a MALDI-MS-based technique called imaging MS, or direct-tissue proteomics, has been developed that can produce an MS image, or molecular weight-specific map, of a given tissue sample (Stoeckli et al., 2001). Direct-tissue proteomics can be combined with molecular enrichment using different surfaces. In one study, a gold surface was used to differentiate healthy brain from glioma tissue, and an achromatographic surface helped determine tumor type and also revealed three tumor biomarkers of molecular weight 4535 Da, 9896 Da, and 20246 Da. The 4533-Da protein was found to be a potential diagnostic marker for glioblastoma (Bouamrani et al., 2006).

A summary of the above technologies and their application is shown in Fig. 24.1 and Color Plate 37.

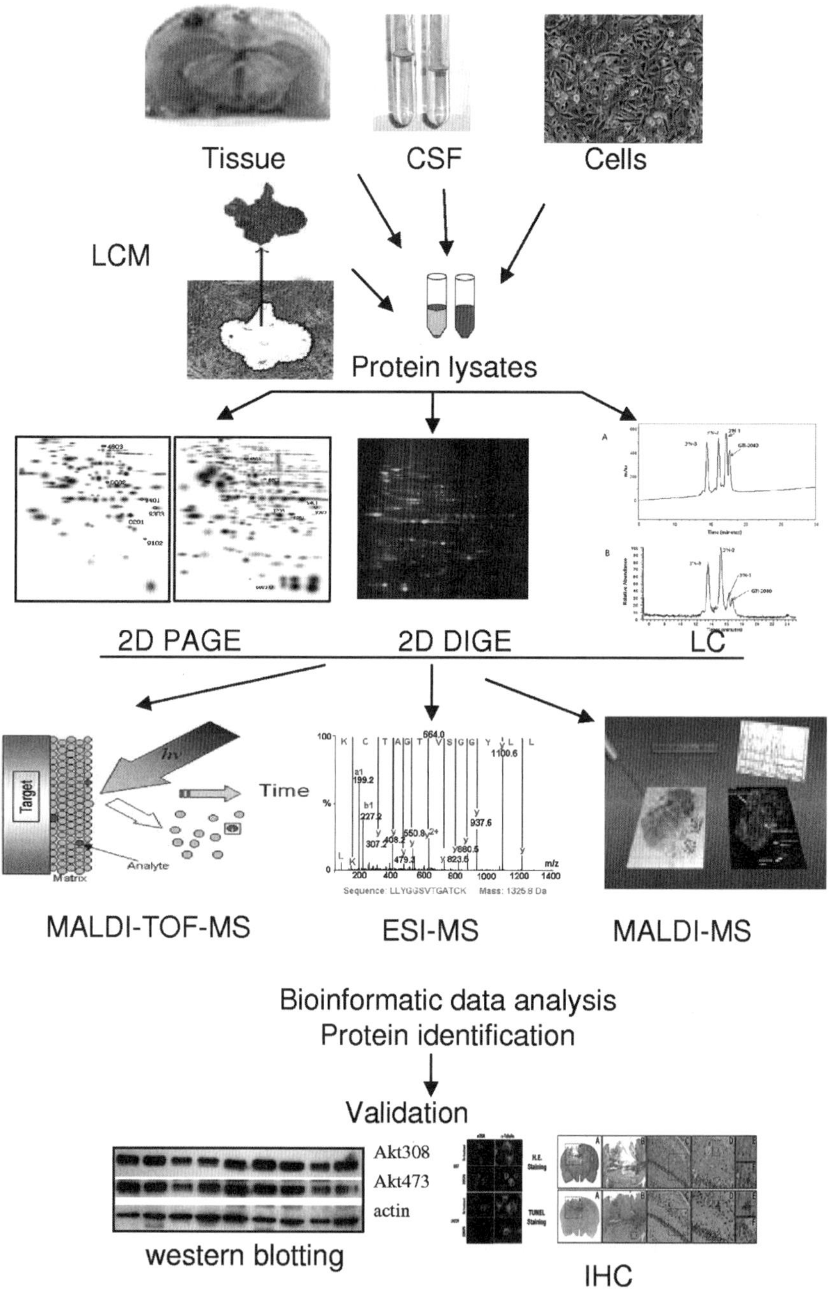

Fig. 24.1 Summary of the protein separation and the MS-based protein identification. The cellular lysates come from tissue, cerebral spinal fluid, or cell line cultured in vitro. Laser capture microdissection can be applied to purify the tumor cells from the tumor tissue block. 2D PAGE, 2D DIGE, or liquid chromatography is often used to separate the proteins. With

24.4 Tissue Microarray (TMA)

As an alternative proteomic technology, TMA plays a key role in accelerating the translation of basic research findings into clinical applications. TMA permits in situ histopathological analysis to occur simultaneously with in situ hybridization and/or immunohistochemical analysis of hundreds of different archival tissue samples on a single glass slide array. TMA has become a widely utilized tool for all types of tissue-based research (Bubendorf et al., 2001, Wang et al., 2002). Figure 24.2 and Color Plate 38 provides an example of a high-density TMA.

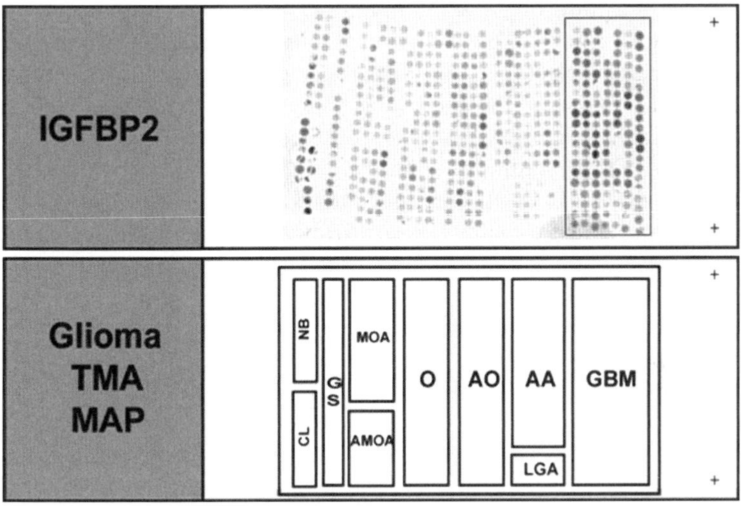

Fig. 24.2 Detection of IGFBP2 expression in a glioma TMA. GBM, glioblastoma; AA, anaplastic astrocytoma; LGA, low grade astrocytoma; AO, anaplastic oligodendroglioma; O, oligodendroglioma; MOA, mixed oligoastrocytoma; AMOA, anaplastic mixed oligoastrocytoma; GS, gliosarcoma; NB, normal brain; CL, cell lines (see Color Plate 38)

In cancer, specifically, TMAs permit the detection of tumor-associated protein expression through the rapid screening of a large number of tumors. In one study by Brat et al., 189 surgical formalin-fixed, paraffin-embedded tissue samples of human gliomas of WHO grades I–IV and 23 normal human brain tissues were collected and incorporated into a TMA (Brat et al., 2004). Using immunohistochemical staining, the investigators observed that aquaporin 4 (AQP4) expression and distribution were greater in high-grade

---

Fig. 24.1 (continued) the bioinformatics support, the proteins from the lysate can be identified by the mass spectrometry-based technologies, such as MALDI-TOF-MS, ESI-MS, and MALDI-MS. Finally, the interesting proteins are selectively further confirmed by western blotting or immunohistochemical analysis (*see* Color Plate 37) astrocytomas (WHO grades III and IV) than in low-grade astrocytomas (WHO grade II). In contrast, pilocytic astrocytomas (WHO grade I) had a higher expression score than low-grade diffuse astrocytomas. Also, the group found that the central region of glioblastomas had a significantly higher AQP4 score than the peripheral infiltration zone. No significant differential AQP4 expression was found between primary and secondary glioblastomas. In another study, Warth et al. also found that a higher AQP4 score was associated with more prominent brain edema and blood–brain barrier disturbance but not with patient survival (Warth et al., 2007).

The combination of TMA with other techniques, such as genome-wide screening and fluorescence in situ hybridization (FISH), constitutes a powerful tool for the detection of differential gene expression and abnormal chromosomes in tumors. For example, Neben et al. profiled gene expression in 35 newly diagnosed medulloblastomas to detect genes associated with unfavorable clinical course. Nine of the most promising candidate genes were selected for further analysis using a TMA of 189 medulloblastoma tissue cores. The expression of STK15, stathmin 1, and cyclin D1 was found to be associated with unfavorable survival. Of these three genes, STK15 was identified as an independent prognostic factor for survival regardless of clinical parameters such as patient gender or age; the metastatic stage, grade, or extent of tumor resection; and whether chemotherapy had been used. Moreover, the FISH analysis revealed that additional gene copy numbers of MYC and STK15 predicted poor survival. These results show that genes associated with proliferation, transcription, and mitosis, including cyclin D1, MYC, and STK15, play a key role in medulloblastoma pathogenesis (Neben et al., 2004).

The expression of AKT, NFκB, and PTEN in gliomas is well known. However, the correlation of expression of these proteins in human gliomas is not well described. Huang et al. constructed a TMA using 259 glioma samples and used it with other technologies, including western blotting, to determine the expression and correlation of AKT, NFκB, and PTEN. A strong positive correlation was found between the expression of AKT and NFκB and histological tumor grade. The expression of AKT was inhibited by stable PTEN expression in U251 cells. These results suggest that the regulation of AKT, NFκB, and PTEN expression may constitute a target for therapeutic intervention (Wang et al., 2004).

Another study by Wang et al. demonstrated that the expression of IGFBP5, but not IGFBP3, increased with anaplastic progression of gliomas. The results suggest that IGFBP5, like IGFBP2, may also play a role in glioma progression (Wang et al., 2006).

24.5 Protein and Antibody Array Analysis

Driven by the fact that many targets in cancer therapy are related to signaling pathway, investigators have recently developed a new method of profiling based on the activation status of cellular signal pathways. The method, parallel analysis of protein function, uses a biochip to provide high-throughput characterization of protein expression (Haab et al., 2001; Knezevic et al., 2001; Templin et al., 2003). This approach informs the clinician about the activated signaling pathways operative in a given tumor and thus enables the rational selection of specific targeted therapy as well as permitting the monitoring of total and phosphorylated proteins before and after treatment and between disease and non-disease states (Sheehan et al., 2005).

The antibody array (forward-phase protein array) and the reverse-phase protein array, which was developed later, are the two basic protein array formats (see Fig. 24.3 and Color Plate 39) (Haab, 2005). In the antibody array, hundreds of antibodies are immobilized on a substratum and act as bait molecules that capture the solution phase analyte molecules

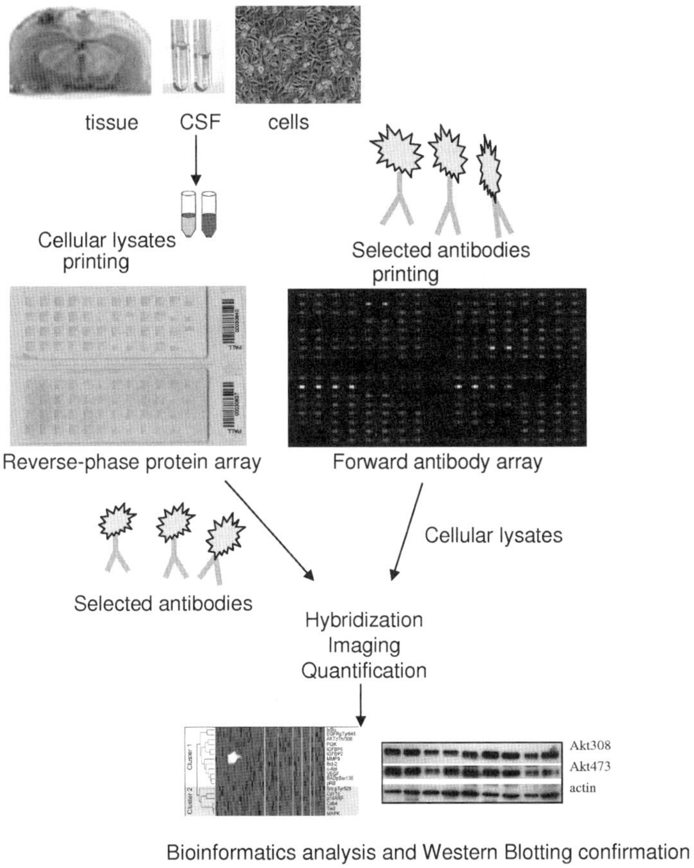

Fig. 24.3 Protein arrays. Antibody array (forward-phase protein array) is formatted by printing the selective antibodies on a slide, while the reverse-phase protein array is printed with the cellular lysate extracted from tissue, cerebral spinal fluid, or cell lines (see Color Plate 39)

(from serum or tissue protein lysates). Antibody arrays have been successfully used in breast cancer research to identify a linkage between the ErbB2 receptor, AP-2 transcription factors, and differential G1 cyclin expression (Yeretssian et al., 2005). Leukemia researchers have also used antibody arrays to concurrently evaluate 50 or more CD antigens on leukocytes or leukemia cells in a single analysis. Using this approach, the expression of 48 CD antigens as determined by microarray correlated well with flow cytometry results (Belov et al., 2001) (*see* Color Plate 39).

In the reverse-phase protein array, hundreds of test samples (protein lysates from serum or tissues) are immobilized on a suitable surface, permitting the antigen responses of multiple samples to be compared directly when incubated with an antibody. Generally, the reverse-phase methodology assesses only one protein per slide, which allows multiple samples to be compared side by side. Efforts are under way to develop dual-color infrared dye-labeled antibodies and quantum dots to permit the measurement of protein expression levels from multiple patient samples on the same spot in the same array (Geho et al., 2005). Reverse-phase protein arrays have two additional advantages: (1) only a very limited quantity of protein lysate is required for each spot, which allows the analysis of signaling pathways in a small number of cultured cells or cells isolated by laser capture microdissection; and (2) both denatured lysates and non-denatured lysates can be used, thus avoiding the problem of antigen retrieval; and, in addition, protein–protein, protein–DNA, and/or protein–RNA complexes can be detected and characterized (Sheehan et al., 2005).

Paweletz et al. analyzed prostate cancer samples with reverse-phase protein arrays and confirmed that prostate cancer progression was associated with the increased phosphorylation of Akt, the suppression of apoptosis pathways, and the decreased phosphorylation of ERK. The protocol Paweletz et al. described was designed to accomplish several aims: to retain proteins in a largely unfolded state, to avoid the boiling of proteins, to allow the microtiter plates used in robotic spotting to be frozen and thawed between uses, to keep a high relative humidity during spotting to prevent the evaporation of liquid, and to include staining for total protein after the normalization of the negative control (Paweletz et al., 2001). In another study, reverse-phase protein array analysis revealed that protein kinase C was downregulated in prostate cancer progression (Grubb et al., 2003). These findings demonstrate that reverse-phase protein arrays show promise for monitoring disease-related protein expression and for investigating the cellular effects of pharmaceutical agents (Nishizuka et al., 2003; Espina et al., 2003; Grubb et al., 2003; Wulfkuhle et al., 2003).

In our laboratory, a glioma protein lysate array was constructed from 82 primary glioma tissue samples and used to survey the expression and phosphorylation of 46 proteins involved in the signaling pathways of cell proliferation, cell survival, apoptosis, angiogenesis, and cell invasion. We then employed an analysis algorithm to robustly estimate the protein expression in these samples. When ranked by their discriminating power to separate 37 glioblastomas from

45 lower-grade gliomas, the following 12 proteins were identified as the most powerful discriminators: IBα, EGFRpTyr845, AKTpThr308, PI3K, BadpSer136, IGFBP2, IGFBP5, MMP9, VEGF, pRB, Bcl-2, and c-Abl. Clustering analysis showed a close link between PI3K and AKTpThr308, IGFBP5 and IGFBP2, and EGFRpTyr845 and IBα. Another cluster consisted of MMP9, Bcl-2, VEGF, and pRB. These patterns suggest functional relationships that warrant further investigation. The association of phosphorylation of AKT at Thr308, but not at Ser473, with glioblastoma suggests that a specific PI3K pathway event activates glioma progression (Jiang et al., 2006). Figure 24.4 and Color Plate 40 provides an example of a glioma protein lysate array.

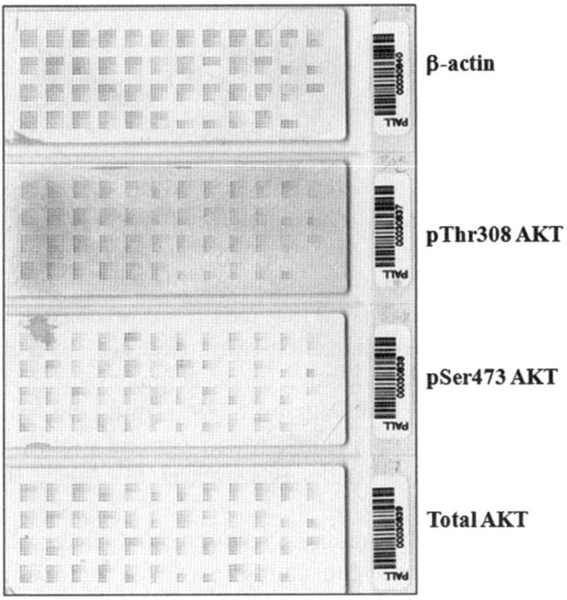

Fig. 24.4 Glioma protein lysate array. Protein was isolated from frozen glioma tissues and adjusted to 20 mg/mL with lysis buffer tissue. The serially diluted protein lysates were printed on PVDF-coated glass slides in triplicate using a robotic spotter (G3, Genomics Solutions). Detection was conducted with a DakoCytomation-catalyzed signal amplification system kit. Individual glass slide can be hybridized with antibodies against β-actin, pThr308 AKT, pSer473 AKT, total AKT, or other proteins; β-actin served as a positive control. The hybridized slides were scanned at an optical resolution of 1200 dpi and saved as uncompressed TIFF files (*see* Color Plate 40)

Despite its strengths, protein array technology still has some defects, including issues with cross-reactivity between sample proteins, suboptimal signal detection systems, poor detection of low-abundance proteins, posttranslational modifications and protein–protein interactions of individual proteins, difficulty in attaining high quality specific antibodies or suitable protein-binding ligands, and inability to detect unknown antigens with predictable affinity and specificity (Templin et al., 2002; Molloy et al., 1999). For example, Aoki et al. used a reverse-phase protein array in an attempt to validate the observation that DNA oligonucleotides homologous to the telomere 3' overhang (T-oligos) induce autophagy in malignant glioma cells through the inhibition of mTOR and STAT3. The results, however, from western blotting performed to confirm the protein array data were only partially consistent with the initial findings. The authors hypothesized that the discrepancy between the protein array and western blotting data might have resulted from a lack of antibody monospecificity and from non-specific labeling. As the authors noted, the data reinforce the critical importance of cross-correlating protein array and western blotting results (Aoki et al., 2007).

24.6 Conclusion

The proteomic approach is increasingly employed in many medical fields and the technology continues to advance. Developments include procedures for the subcellular fractionation and separation of compartment proteins, such as the membrane fraction from whole tissues, and the development of direct proteomics, which obviates the need for time-consuming and labor-intensive laser capture microdissection (Molloy et al., 1999; Encheva et al., 2006). Additional advances include the development of gel-free 2D chromatography (Davidsson and Nilsson, 1999) and the combination of SELDI-TOF-MS with ProteinChips, which can be rapidly analyzed and provide extremely sensitive results (Cazares et al., 2002; Bast Jr., 2003; Mannes et al., 2003).

Nevertheless, existing proteomics techniques, such as 2D PAGE/MS and protein arrays, are time-consuming, expensive, and often technically challenging, which greatly hinders their use in the clinical setting. In addition, a majority of the published literature purporting to identify protein biomarkers using proteomics describe only a few proteins that are differentially expressed among tumor subsets and do not explore the clinical implications or potential applications of the findings in any depth. In fact, of the literally hundreds of brain tumor biomarkers identified through the use of proteomics techniques (summarized in Table 24.1), none have attained broad application for use in clinical prognosis, therapeutic target selection, or molecular classification. In this regard, it is likely that accurate diagnosis and prediction of disease behavior will require a panel of protein markers rather than single protein (Hale et al., 2003; Khwaja et al., 2007). Finally, bioinformatics and confirmatory in vitro and in vivo biological experiments are expected to play an ever increasing and critical role in the postproteomics era.

Table 24.1 New brain tumor markers identified from proteomics studies

Markers	Observed function	Samples	Identification techniques	Confirmation techniques	References
IGFBP2	Glioma oncogene, cell migration and invasion	Glioma tissues	cDNA microarray, tissue micorarray	Immunohistochemical staining, tissue-specific transgenic mouse model	Fuller et al. Cancer Res (1999) Wang et al. Brain Pathology (2002) Dunlap SM, et al. Proc Natl Acad Sci USA (2007)
AMPM2 (MetAp2)	Regulating NF1 pathway	CSF	2D PAGE and MS	Immunohistochemistry, western blotting, cell proliferation assay	Dasgupta et al. Cancer Res (2005b)
ATRN (attractin)	Glioma cells migration	CSF	2D PAGE and MALDI-TOF-MS, HPLC, cleavable isotope-coded affinity tag analysis	Immunohistochemical staining, western blotting, scratch-wound assay, Boyden chamber migration assay	Khwaja et al. J Proteome Res (2007)
N-COR IRS-2	Associated with the malignancy of gliomas	Glioma tissues	LCM, 2D PAGE, protein sequence	Immunohistochemical staining	Li J, et al. Neurology (2006)
STATHMIN	Strongly associated with the sensitivity to nitrosourea and overall survival of anaplastic oligodendrogliomas	Anaplastic oligodendrogliomas cell lines	2D DIGE, MALDI-TOF-MS	Protein induction, cell cytotoxicity testing, cytogenetic analysis and western blotting, immunohisto-chemistry, survival analysis	Ngo et al. J Natl Cancer Inst (2007)
CALCYLIN (calcyclin), DC1L2 (dynein light chain2), PEA-15	Discriminating the different grade gliomas and indicate the overall survival	Glioma tissues	MALDI-TOF-MS	Immunohistochemical staining	Schwartz et al. Cancer Res (2005)
APOA-II (apolipoprotein-II)	Correlated with blood–brain barrier disruption	Glioma tissues	SELDI-TOF-MS, 2D PAGE, MS-MS	western blotting, immunohistochemistry	De Bont et al. Clin Chem (2006)
CAH (carbonic anhydrase)	Correlated with the malignancy of the brain tumors	CSF	SELDI-TOF-MS, MALDI-TOF-MS		Khwaja et al. Proteomics (2006b)

Table 24.1 (continued)

Markers	Observed function	Samples	Identification techniques	Confirmation techniques	References
AURKA (STK15), STMN1 (stathmin 1), CCND1 (cyclin D1)	Predicting unfavorable overall survival of medulloblastomas	Medulloblastoma tissues	cDNA array, TMA, FISH		Neben et al. Cancer Res (2004)
IGFBP5	Correlated with the histological grade of the gliomas	Gliomas tissue	TMA	Immunohistochemistry	Wang et al. Technol Cancer Res Treat (2006)
FINC (fibronectin), CBP2 (colligin 2)	Activating angiogenesis in gliomas	Glioma tissues	Nano-LC, MALDI-TOF-MS, MALDI-FTMS	Immunohistochemistry	Mustafa et al. Mol Cell Proteomics (2007)
Stathmin, ANXA1 (annexin A1), CAPS calcyphonsine	Tumor specific proteins in pediatric PNET and ependymomas	Tumor tissues	2D DIGE, MALDI-TOF-MS	Immunohistochemistry	De Bont, et al. J Neurolpath Exp Neurol (2007)

Abbreviations

2D PAGE	two-dimensional polyacrylamide gel electrophoresis
2D DIGE	two-dimensional difference gel electrophoresis
AQP4	aquaporin 4
EGFR	epidermal growth factor receptor
ESI-MS	electrospray ionization mass spectrometry
FISH	fluorescence in situ hybridization
HPLC	high-performance liquid chromatography
IGFBP2	insulin-like growth factor binding protein 2
LC	liquid chromatography
LOH	loss of heterozygosity
MALDI-FTICR-MS	MALDI-Fourier transform ion cyclotron resonance mass spectrometry
MALDI-FTMS	MALDI-Fourier transform mass spectrometry
MALDI-TOF-MS	matrix-assisted laser desorption/ionization time-of-flight mass spectrometry
MS	mass spectrometry
PCR	polymerase chain reaction
SELDI-TOF-MS	surface-enhanced laser desorption/ionization time-of-flight mass spectrometry
TMA	tissue microarray

Acknowledgments We thank Angelique Geehan of the Department of Scientific Publications for her editing of this chapter.

References

Adkins JN, Varnum SM, Auberry KJ et al. (2002) Toward a human blood serum proteome: analysis by multidimensional separation coupled with mass spectrometry. Mol Cell Proteomics 1:947–955

Aoki H, Iwado E, Eller MS et al. (2007) Telomere 3′ overhang-specific DNA oligonucleotides induce autophagy in malignant glioma cells. FASEB J 21:2918–2930

Baharvand H, Fathi A, Gourabi H et al. (2008) Identification of mouse embryonic stem cell-associated proteins. J Proteome Res 7:412–423

Bast RC, Jr. (2003) Status of tumor markers in ovarian cancer screening. J Clin Oncol 21:200s–205s

Beckner ME, Chen X, An J et al. (2005) Proteomic characterization of harvested pseudopodia with differential gel electrophoresis and specific antibodies. Lab Invest 85:316–327

Belov L, de l, V, dos Remedios CG et al. (2001) Immunophenotyping of leukemias using a cluster of differentiation antibody microarray. Cancer Res 61:4483–4489

Bouamrani A, Ternier J, Ratel D et al. (2006) Direct-tissue SELDI-TOF mass spectrometry analysis: a new application for clinical proteomics. Clin Chem 52:2103–2106

Brat DJ, Seiferheld WF, Perry A et al. (2004) Analysis of 1p, 19q, 9p, and 10q as prognostic markers for high-grade astrocytomas using fluorescence in situ hybridization on tissue microarrays from Radiation Therapy Oncology Group trials. Neuro Oncol 6:96–103

Bubendorf L, Nocito A, Moch H et al. (2001) Tissue microarray (TMA) technology: miniaturized pathology archives for high-throughput in situ studies. J Pathol 195:72–79

Caskey LS, Fuller GN, Bruner JM et al. (2000) Toward a molecular classification of the gliomas: histopathology, molecular genetics, and gene expression profiling. Histol Histopathol 15:971–981

Cazares LH, Adam BL, Ward MD et al. (2002) Normal, benign, preneoplastic, and malignant prostate cells have distinct protein expression profiles resolved by surface enhanced laser desorption/ionization mass spectrometry. Clin Cancer Res 8: 2541–2552

Chang HY, Chi JT, Dudoit S et al. (2002) Diversity, topographic differentiation, and positional memory in human fibroblasts. Proc Natl Acad Sci USA 99:12877–12882

Chang HY, Sneddon JB, Alizadeh AA et al. (2004) Gene expression signature of fibroblast serum response predicts human cancer progression: similarities between tumors and wounds. PLoS Biol 2:E7

Dasgupta B, Yi Y, Chen DY et al. (2005a) Proteomic analysis reveals hyperactivation of the mammalian target of rapamycin pathway in neurofibromatosis 1-associated human and mouse brain tumors. Cancer Res 65:2755–2760

Dasgupta B, Yi Y, Hegedus B et al. (2005b) Cerebrospinal fluid proteomic analysis reveals dysregulation of methionine aminopeptidase-2 expression in human and mouse neurofibromatosis 1-associated glioma. Cancer Res 65:9843–9850

Davidsson P, Nilsson CL (1999) Peptide mapping of proteins in cerebrospinal fluid utilizing a rapid preparative two-dimensional electrophoretic procedure and matrix-assisted laser desorption/ionization mass spectrometry. Biochim Biophys Acta 1473:391–399

de Bont JM, den Boer ML, Reddingius RE et al. (2006) Identification of apolipoprotein A-II in cerebrospinal fluid of pediatric brain tumor patients by protein expression profiling. Clin Chem 52:1501–1509

Dunlap SM, Celestino J, Wang H et al. (2007) Insulin-like growth factor binding protein 2 promotes glioma development and progression. Proc Natl Acad Sci USA 104: 11736–11741

Encheva V, Gharbia SE, Wait R et al. (2006) Comparison of extraction procedures for proteome analysis of Streptococcus pneumoniae and a basic reference map. Proteomics 6:3306–3317

Espina V, Mehta AI, Winters ME et al. (2003) Protein microarrays: molecular profiling technologies for clinical specimens. Proteomics 3:2091–2100

Fukushima T, Tezuka T, Shimomura T et al. (2007) Silencing of insulin-like growth factor-binding protein-2 in human glioblastoma cells reduces both invasiveness and expression of progression-associated gene CD24. J Biol Chem 282:18634–18644

Fuller GN, Rhee CH, Hess KR et al. (1999) Reactivation of insulin-like growth factor binding protein 2 expression in glioblastoma multiforme: a revelation by parallel gene expression profiling. Cancer Res 59:4228–4232

Geho D, Lahar N, Gurnani P et al. (2005) Pegylated, steptavidin-conjugated quantum dots are effective detection elements for reverse-phase protein microarrays. Bioconjug Chem 16:559–566

Gong L, Puri M, Unlu M et al. (2004) Drosophila ventral furrow morphogenesis: a proteomic analysis. Development 131:643–656

Grubb RL, Calvert VS, Wulkuhle JD et al. (2003) Signal pathway profiling of prostate cancer using reverse phase protein arrays. Proteomics 3:2142–2146

Haab BB (2005). Antibody arrays in cancer research. Mol Cell Proteomics 4:377–383

Haab BB, Dunham MJ, Brown PO (2001). Protein microarrays for highly parallel detection and quantitation of specific proteins and antibodies in complex solutions. Genome Biol 2: Research0004.1-Research0004.13

Hale JE, Gelfanova V, Ludwig JR et al. (2003) Application of proteomics for discovery of protein biomarkers. Brief Funct Genomic Proteomic 2:185–193

Jiang R, Mircean C, Shmulevich I et al. (2006) Pathway alterations during glioma progression revealed by reverse phase protein lysate arrays. Proteomics 6:2964–2971

Khwaja FW, Duke-Cohan JS, Brat DJ, et al. (2006a) Attractin is elevated in the cerebrospinal fluid of patients with malignant astrocytoma and mediates glioma cell migration. Clin Cancer Res 12:6331–6336

Khwaja FW, Nolen JD, Mendrinos SE et al. (2006b) Proteomic analysis of cerebrospinal fluid discriminates malignant and nonmalignant disease of the central nervous system and identifies specific protein markers. Proteomics 6:6277–6287

Khwaja FW, Svoboda P, Reed M et al. (2006c) Proteomic identification of the wt-p53-regulated tumor cell secretome. Oncogene 25:7650–7661

Khwaja FW, Reed MS, Olson JJ, Schmotzer BJ, Gillespie GY, Guha A, Groves MD, Kesari S, Pohl J and Van Meir EG (2007) Proteomic identification of biomarkers in the cerebrospinal fluid (CSF) of astrocytoma patients. J Proteome Res 6:559–570

Kim S, Dougherty ER, Shmulevich I et al. (2002) Identification of combination gene sets for glioma classification. Mol Cancer Ther 1:1229–1236

Knezevic V, Leethanakul C, Bichsel VE et al. (2001) Proteomic profiling of the cancer microenvironment by antibody arrays. Proteomics 1:1271–1278

Kondo T, Seike M, Mori Y et al. (2003) Application of sensitive fluorescent dyes in linkage of laser microdissection and two-dimensional gel electrophoresis as a cancer proteomic study tool. Proteomics 3:1758–1766

Lee HJ, Lee EY, Kwon MS et al. (2006) Biomarker discovery from the plasma proteome using multidimensional fractionation proteomics. Curr Opin Chem Biol 10:42–49

Li J, Zhuang Z, Okamoto H et al. (2006) Proteomic profiling distinguishes astrocytomas and identifies differential tumor markers. Neurology 66:733–736

Mannes AJ, Martin BM, Yang HY et al. (2003) Cystatin C as a cerebrospinal fluid biomarker for pain in humans. Pain 102:251–256

Mehrian-Shai R, Chen CD, Shi T et al. (2007) Insulin growth factor-binding protein 2 is a candidate biomarker for PTEN status and PI3K/Akt pathway activation in glioblastoma and prostate cancer. Proc Natl Acad Sci USA 104:5563–5568

Molloy MP, Herbert BR, Williams KL et al. (1999) Extraction of Escherichia coli proteins with organic solvents prior to two-dimensional electrophoresis. Electrophoresis 20:701–704

Moreno CS, Evans CO, Zhan X et al. (2005) Novel molecular signaling and classification of human clinically nonfunctional pituitary adenomas identified by gene expression profiling and proteomic analyses. Cancer Res 65:10214–10222

Mustafa DA, Burgers PC, Dekker LJ et al. (2007) Identification of glioma neovascularization-related proteins by using MALDI-FTMS and nano-LC fractionation to microdissected tumor vessels. Mol Cell Proteomics 6:1147–1157

Mustafa D, Kros JM, Luider T (2008). Combining laser capture microdissection and proteomics techniques. Methods Mol Biol 428:159–178

Narayan RK, Heydorn WE, Creed GJ et al. (1986) Protein patterns in various malignant human brain tumors by two-dimensional gel electrophoresis. Cancer Res 46: 4685–4694

Neben K, Korshunov A, Benner A et al. (2004) Microarray-based screening for molecular markers in medulloblastoma revealed STK15 as independent predictor for survival. Cancer Res 64:3103–3111

Ngo TT, Peng T, Liang XJ et al. (2007) The 1p-encoded protein stathmin and resistance of malignant gliomas to nitrosoureas. J Natl Cancer Inst 99:639–652

Nishizuka S, Charboneau L, Young L et al. (2003) Proteomic profiling of the NCI-60 cancer cell lines using new high-density reverse-phase lysate microarrays. Proc Natl Acad Sci USA 100:14229–14234

O'Farrell PH (1975). High resolution two-dimensional electrophoresis of proteins. J Biol Chem 250:4007–4021
Okamoto H, Li J, Glasker S et al. (2007) Proteomic comparison of oligodendrogliomas with and without 1pLOH. Cancer Biol Ther 6:391–396
Paweletz CP, Charboneau L, Bichsel VE et al. (2001) Reverse phase protein microarrays which capture disease progression show activation of pro-survival pathways at the cancer invasion front. Oncogene 20:1981–1989
Qian WJ, Jacobs JM, Liu T et al. (2006) Advances and challenges in liquid chromatography-mass spectrometry-based proteomics profiling for clinical applications. Mol Cell Proteomics 5:1727–1744
Sallinen SL, Sallinen PK, Haapasalo HK et al. (2000) Identification of differentially expressed genes in human gliomas by DNA microarray and tissue chip techniques. Cancer Res 60:6617–6622
Schwartz SA, Weil RJ, Thompson RC et al. (2005) Proteomic-based prognosis of brain tumor patients using direct-tissue matrix-assisted laser desorption ionization mass spectrometry. Cancer Res 65:7674–7681
Sheehan KM, Calvert VS, Kay EW et al. (2005). Use of reverse phase protein microarrays and reference standard development for molecular network analysis of metastatic ovarian carcinoma. Mol Cell Proteomics 4:346–355
Shen Y, Zhao R, Berger SJ et al. (2002) High-efficiency nanoscale liquid chromatography coupled on-line with mass spectrometry using nanoelectrospray ionization for proteomics. Anal Chem 74:4235–4249
Shen Y, Zhang R, Moore RJ et al. (2005) Automated 20 kpsi RPLC-MS and MS/MS with chromatographic peak capacities of 1000–1500 and capabilities in proteomics and metabolomics. Anal Chem 77:3090–3100
Smith L, Lind MJ, Welham KJ et al. (2006) Cancer proteomics and its application to discovery of therapy response markers in human cancer. Cancer 107:232–241
Stoeckli M, Chaurand P, Hallahan DE et al. (2001) Imaging mass spectrometry: a new technology for the analysis of protein expression in mammalian tissues. Nat Med 7:493–496
Templin MF, Stoll D, Schrenk M et al. (2002) Protein microarray technology. Trends Biotechnol 20:160–166
Templin MF, Stoll D, Schwenk JM et al. (2003) Protein microarrays: promising tools for proteomic research. Proteomics 3:2155–2166
Titulaer MK, Mustafa DA, Siccama I et al. (2008) A software application for comparing large numbers of high resolution MALDI-FTICR MS spectra demonstrated by searching candidate biomarkers for glioma blood vessel formation. BMC Bioinformatics 9:133
Tolley L, Jorgenson JW, Moseley MA (2001) Very high pressure gradient LC/MS/MS. Anal Chem 73:2985–2991
Vogel TW, Zhuang Z, Li J et al. (2005) Proteins and protein pattern differences between glioma cell lines and glioblastoma multiforme. Clin Cancer Res 11:3624–3632
Wang, H, Wang H, Zhang W, Fuller GN. (2002) Tissue microarrays: applications in neuropathology research, diagnosis and education. Brain Pathol 12: 95–107
Wang H, Wang H, Zhang W et al. (2004) Analysis of the activation status of Akt, NFkappaB, and Stat3 in human diffuse gliomas. Lab Invest 84:941–951
Wang H, Wang H, Zhang W et al. (2006) Overexpression of IGFBP5, but not IGFBP3, correlates with the histologic grade of human diffuse glioma: a tissue microarray and immunohistochemical study. Technol Cancer Res Treat 5:195–199
Warth A, Simon P, Capper D et al. (2007) Expression pattern of the water channel aquaporin-4 in human gliomas is associated with blood-brain barrier disturbance but not with patient survival. J Neurosci Res 85:1336–1346
Westman-Brinkmalm A, Karlsson G, Brive LM et al. (2005) Analysis of proteins from a glioma cell line by using micro-scale solution isoelectric focusing in combination with

liquid chromatography/tandem mass spectrometry. Rapid Commun Mass Spectrom 19:3651–3658

Wulfkuhle JD, Aquino JA, Calvert VS et al. (2003) Signal pathway profiling of ovarian cancer from human tissue specimens using reverse-phase protein microarrays. Proteomics 3:2085–2090

Yeretssian G, Lecocq M, Lebon G et al. (2005) Competition on nitrocellulose-immobilized antibody arrays: from bacterial protein binding assay to protein profiling in breast cancer cells. Mol Cell Proteomics 4:605–617

Chapter 25
Proteomic Discovery of Biomarkers in the Cerebrospinal Fluid of Brain Tumor Patients

Fatima W. Khwaja and Erwin G. Van Meir

Abstract Central nervous system (CNS) diseases often induce changes in the protein composition of the cerebrospinal fluid (CSF) as this liquid bathes the brain and collects its secreted products. The detection and monitoring of such pathology-related changes can be exploited for their relation to tumor growth in the brain. The potential of using differential proteomic profiling in CNS malignancies to identify diagnostic, prognostic, and therapeutic response markers as well as therapeutic targets is currently being actively investigated. Furthermore, elucidation of the CSF oncoproteome may yield important biological insights into the pathogenesis of CNS neoplasms. New proteomic technology forecasts rapid screening, low sample consumption, and accurate protein identification in the CSF. These technological improvements will permit the gathering of reliable data on CSF protein composition in a clinically relevant microchip format in the foreseeable future. Here we review the current status of proteomic technology and its application to CNS cancers, with a focus on translational studies.

Contents

E.G. Van Meir (✉)
Laboratory of Molecular Neuro-Oncology, Departments of Neurosurgery, Hematology and Medical Oncology, and Winship Cancer Institute, Emory University School of Medicine, Atlanta, GA 30322, USA
e-mail: evanmei@emory.edu

E.G. Van Meir (ed.), *CNS Cancer*, Cancer Drug Discovery and Development, DOI 10.1007/978-1-60327-553-8_25,
© Humana Press, a part of Springer Science+Business Media, LLC 2009

25.1 Introduction

Body fluids are a valuable source of disease markers as they represent drainage products from involved tissues, including proteins secreted by normal, diseased, and dying cells, including inflammatory markers, immunoglobulins or cytokines, vasoactive compounds, and mediators of cell signaling and/or growth pathways. The detection and measurement of these leakage products and secreted proteins can potentially be used to diagnose a specific pathological process and to monitor its evolution (Kennedy 2001; D'Aguanno et al. 2007). For all these reasons, there is heightened interest in developing reliable methods for the quantitative detection of biomarkers associated with disease. This is a particular challenge but also a unique opportunity for neoplastic disease in the central nervous system (CNS).

25.2 Why Proteomics?

The proteome has been described as all of the proteins that are produced at a given time in a cell, tissue, or fluid. Proteomics offers a comprehensive, bird's-eye view to analyze, at a systems level, all of the proteins that might result from, or contribute to, each different CNS disorder. The CSF proteome could provide unique biomarkers for the early stage diagnosis or the staging of a CNS malignancy, offer potential insights into the biochemical characterization of the affected cell populations, and clarify the principal molecular basis of brain tumor pathologies (Jin et al. 2007).

Proteomics has led to a greater understanding of genomic data generated from genome-wide expression and sequencing projects. However, for several reasons, correlating proteomic with genomic information is not an easy task. The expression level of a given protein varies widely within a cell and its relationship with mRNA levels is rather poor. Furthermore, post-translational modifications and differential splicing, especially in higher organisms, can significantly blur the information gained at the DNA or RNA levels. Moreover, while many putatively expressed proteins have been found through complete genomic sequencing; their functional relevance still remains to be established (Kennedy 2001). Computational methods are currently being developed for rapidly assigning predicted functions to proteins based on genomic information. In contrast, proteomic studies allow us to identify proteins that are most useful in a particular cell or system based on their expression.

25.3 Cerebrospinal Fluid as a Biomarker Repository

Until recently, serum has been the most common sample source for human biomarker research. Serum is a complex medium containing proteins with concentrations that span 12 orders of magnitude. Identification of disease biomarkers within such intricate protein samples is challenging, especially since these markers are expected to be present in far lower concentrations than proteins that constitute the bulk of the mixture. Furthermore, due to the large volume of blood in circulation (5 l) any disease marker gets diluted many fold versus its concentration at the production site. Limitations of serum biomarkers studies are even greater when dealing with diseases of the brain and the nervous system, as they are relatively isolated from the remaining body due to the blood–brain barrier (BBB) and blood–CSF barrier (Abbott 2005; Righetti et al. 2005). To bypass these shortcomings, an increasing number of studies are using the cerebrospinal fluid (CSF) as a source of biomarker for CNS diseases.

25.3.1 Composition of the CSF

The CSF is a clear, colorless, and mostly cell-free liquid that circulates within the ventricles, in the spinal column, and around the brain in a cavity called the subarachnoid space (Fig. 25.1 and Color Plate 41). The CSF is not a simple filtrate of serum but is rather actively secreted from the ventricular choroid plexus epithelium and is reabsorbed at the arachnoid granulations into the venous circulation. The total volume of the CSF in the human ventricular system is estimated at 150 ml, about 20% resides in the ventricles and 80% in the subarachnoid space. Remarkably, 500 ml of new CSF is produced each day allowing it to have a high turnover rate (7–8 h) (Fountoulakis and Kossida 2006). About 70% of CSF is produced by the choroid plexus and another 30% from metabolic water production, including complete oxidation of glucose. The CSF serves multiple functions, it isolates the brain from the general blood circulation, provides buoyancy to the brain (reduces weight from 1,500 g in air to 50 g in CSF), and cushions it against impact damage.

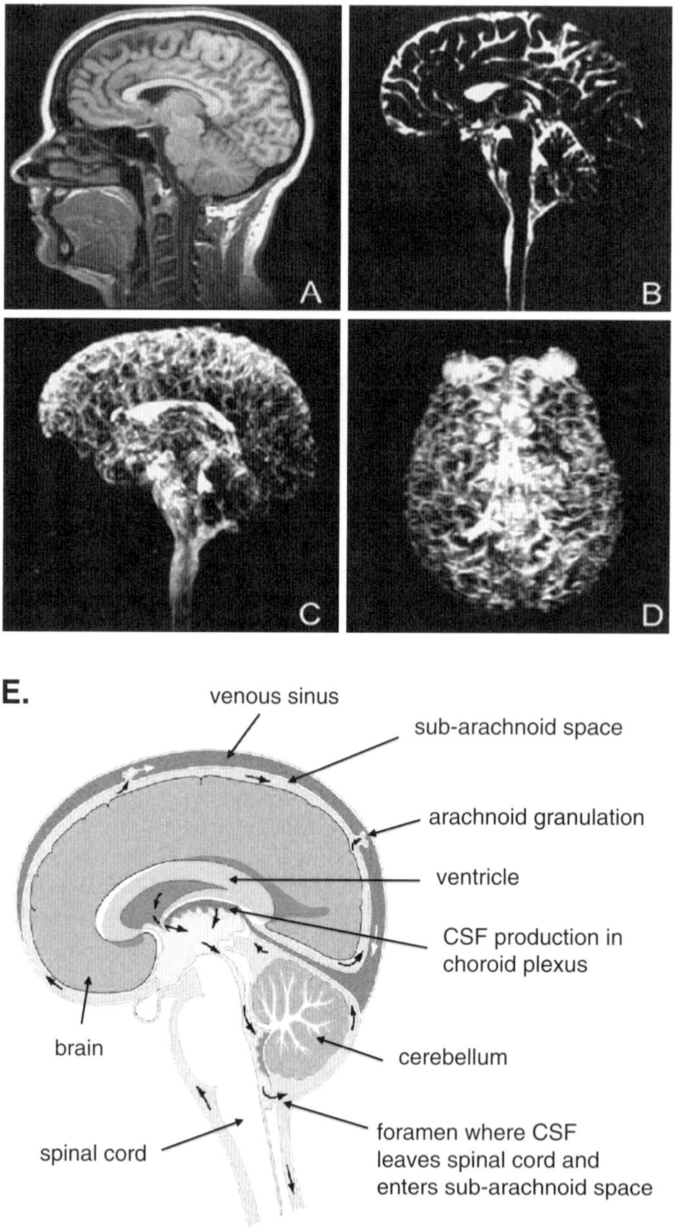

Fig. 25.1 Magnetic resonance imaging enables to noninvasively visualize whole brain structures and CSF at high resolution and sharp contrast. **A.** A sagittal section of T1-weighted spin echo imaging gives dark CSF (e.g., in ventricle) in contrast to the gray and white matter tissue. **B.** A sagittal section of T2-weighted fast spin echo imaging with gray and white matter signal suppressed shows bright CSF. **C, D.** Maximum intensity projection of a whole brain T2-weighted imaging with suppression of brain tissues provides 3-D rendering views of CSF distribution in the whole brain. (Images and image reconstructions are contributed by

CSF is composed of water, glucose, salts (potassium, calcium, magnesium and relatively large amounts of sodium chloride), small molecules, nucleic acids, peptides, proteins, and enzymes that all play critical roles in many physiological processes (Table 25.1). Thus, any change in concentration and/or modification of these constituents, including proteins and peptides, could reflect pathological processes in the CNS. In the case of CNS malignancies, CSF can be thought of as a reservoir of proteins secreted during brain tumor development. As each type of neoplasm has its own characteristics, one would expect that each histologic type of brain tumor might have its own unique proteomic profile (Romeo et al. 2005; Huhmer et al. 2006).

Table 25.1 Comparison between contents of human CSF and serum

	CSF	Serum
Volume	100–160 ml	5,000 ml
Electrolytes		
Sodium (Na)	137–145 mM	136–145 mM
Potassium (K)	2.7–3.9 mM	3.5–5 mM
Calcium (Ca)	1–1.15 mM	2.2–2.6 mM
Chloride (Cl)	116–122 mM	98–106 mM
pH	7.31–7.34	7.38–7.44
Protein		
Total protein	0.2–0.5 g/l	55–80 g/l
Albumin	56–75%	50–60%
IgG	0.01–0.014 g/l	8–15 g/l

CSF shares many properties with serum (Table 25.1). Like serum, the concentration of proteins present in CSF spans several orders of magnitude. Furthermore, over 75% of CSF protein composition is accounted for by albumin and immunoglobulins very similar to serum constitution. Finally, CSF contains high levels of salt and ions and maintains a pH very close to that of the serum. An important difference, however, is that CSF is at least an order of magnitude less complex than serum. The protein concentration in CSF and plasma is 25 and 6,500 mg/100 g, respectively. The overall protein content of the CSF is estimated to be less than 0.5% that of serum with less than 1,000 proteins and peptide products as compared to nearly 40,000 in the serum (Zougman et al. 2008). Lastly, the CSF protein content largely originates

Fig. 25.1 (continued) Dr. Hui Mao, Department of Radiology, Emory University.) **E.** Visualization of CSF circulation in a sagittal section of the human brain. CSF is produced mainly in the choroid plexus (*purple*), then it circulates in the ventricles (*dark tan*) and around the spinal cord from which it enters into the subarachnoid space (*light blue*). The CSF is reabsorbed in the venous circulation at the granuloid villi which herniated into the venous sinus (*see* Color Plate 41) from the CNS due to the absence of a barrier at the CSF–brain interface and the presence of the blood–brain barrier (BBB), which excludes serum proteins from the brain and CSF. In contrast, serum contains proteins produced throughout the body, including those that are reabsorbed from the CSF circulation at the arachnoid villi (Huhmer et al. 2006).

25.3.2 Significance of CNS Barriers

The CNS is a largely closed system that is protected from systemic effects through two separate barriers: the BBB and the blood to cerebrospinal fluid barrier (B-CSF) (Fig. 25.2 and Color Plate 42) (Abbott 2005). The

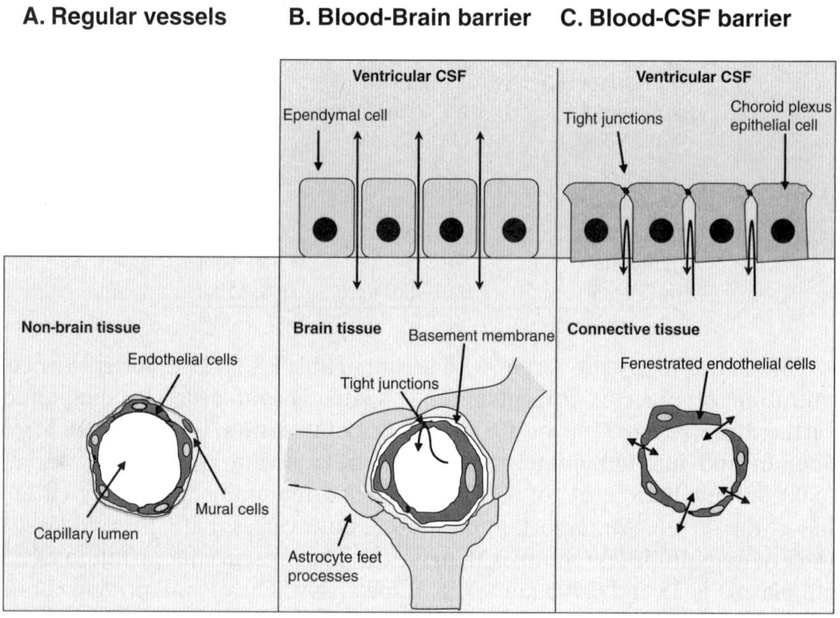

Fig. 25.2 Blood–brain barrier and blood–CSF barrier. **A.** Simplified structure of normal blood vessel not present in the brain. In normal blood vessels, the endothelial cells (shown in *pink*) are surrounded by mural cells such as pericytes and smooth muscle cells. **B.** Blood–brain barrier: In normal brain, the endothelial cells of the capillaries contain tight junctions creating a strong barrier that prevents diffusion of hydrophilic substances from CNS capillaries into the surrounding tissues and vice versa. However, necessary nutrients and metabolites such as glucose are transported with the aid of specific transport mechanisms. **C.** Blood–CSF barrier: In the choroid plexus, the blood–brain barrier is absent as the capillary endothelial cells here are fenestrated. This allows substances to pass freely from the bloodstream into the brain tissue and also in the opposite direction. However, here, tight junctions are present in the overlying ependyma (choroid plexus epithelium), thus creating a two-way barrier between brain tissue and ventricular CSF (*see* Color Plate 42)

discovery of these barriers and their impact on brain tumor imaging and therapy are described in Chapter 33. Disruption or dysfunction of these barriers is a complication of neurodegenerative diseases and brain injuries including those associated with CNS malignancies (Hawkins and Egleton 2008).

The BBB is a structure in the CNS vasculature that blocks the passage of microscopic organisms and most immune cells, as well as selectively restricts movement of chemical substances between the arterial and the venous bloodstream that irrigates the brain and the nervous system. The passage of molecules necessary for proper metabolic functions such as oxygen is unimpeded or facilitated by carrier-mediated transport (D-glucose). The "barrier" is created through tight junctions connecting the endothelial cells constituting the CNS vasculature and is reinforced by associated astrocytes that further restrict the movement of solutes (Marchi et al. 2003). Therefore, very limited amounts of proteins cross from the blood to the brain tissue.

In contrast to the BBB, the B-CSF is a barrier system established through epithelial cell layers connected by tight junctions in different locations in the brain. The first is the choroid plexus, a cauliflower-shaped organ that has many narrow tissue protrusions where blood capillaries are enveloped by a layer of choroid plexus epithelial cells (Fig. 25.2). The majority of the CSF is produced by the choroid plexus, where the blood capillaries provide the incoming flow of liquid to the choroid plexus epithelial cells that actively secrete CSF. The blood capillaries in this area have no tight junctions (Fig. 25.1C) and are fenestrated so as to allow movement of small molecules freely between blood and the epithelial cells that line the external surface of the choroid plexus (Fig. 25.2B). The B-CSF at the choroid plexus is physically formed by the tight junctions that link the choroid plexus epithelial cells. The second part of this barrier, the neurothelium (a layer of meningiothelial cells) covering the arachnoid membrane, envelopes the brain and the surrounding arachnoid space filled with CSF. The meningiothelial cells are also linked by tight junctions, which prevent passage of substances from the blood through this membrane (Marchi et al. 2003; Abbott 2005). The arachnoid membrane is a thin layer of connective tissue resembling a cobweb with numerous threadlike strands attached to the innermost layer of the meninges. The space under the arachnoid membrane, the subarachnoid space, is filled with CSF. The CSF circulation ends when it is reabsorbed by arachnoid granulations, which are tufted prolongations that protrude through the dura into the draining venous sinuses (Fig. 25.2).

While the movement of substances from the blood to the brain tissue or to the CSF is tightly controlled by these two barriers, there is no such restriction at the brain–CSF interface. Ependymal cells lining the ventricles and the pia-glial membrane cells on the surface of the brain are not connected by tight junctions and permit macromolecular exchanges. Consequently, products secreted by normal or tumoral brain tissue in the extracellular space can freely diffuse into the CSF, a process possibly enhanced by the increased interstitial pressure found in tumors. In the case of CNS disease, the concentration of brain-derived protein products can increase in the CSF itself due to the inability to cross the

BBB and the B-CSF. The selective protein permeability at the arachnoid granulations where CSF is reabsorbed to the venous blood is incompletely understood. Overall, the lack of barrier between CSF and brain tissue makes it a valuable source in biomarker research for CNS disease and malignancies (Abbott 2005).

25.4 CSF Proteomics for the Identification of CNS Neoplasia

The CSF can be thought of as a window to study CNS disease and its access is less invasive than neurosurgical procedures (Maurer et al. 2003). The limitations of traditional CSF cytology have spurred the investigation of new techniques for the rapid screening and accurate identification of proteins secreted into the CSF by tumor and stromal cells. Proteomic technologies are particularly suited for investigating biological fluids like CSF in order to identify disease-related alterations and to develop individualized molecular signatures for disease processes, thus realizing personalized proteomic medicine.

25.4.1 The Promise of CSF Proteomics: The Identification of Markers of CNS Neoplasia for Patient Diagnosis, Prognosis, and Follow-Up After Therapy

At present, brain tumors are mainly diagnosed through imaging studies such as CT/MRI scans followed by the difficult task of histologic examination of tissue obtained through stereotactic biopsy or tumor resection. In addition to tumor classification and grading, other prognostic factors include patient age and performance status. To improve prognostication, research is underway to develop molecular approaches for classification of CNS malignancies. These include identification, characterization, and expansion of molecular (genetic and proteomic) factors with diagnostic, prognostic, and therapeutic potential.

Due to recent technological advances in proteomics, the identification of comprehensive "fingerprints" of protein and peptide profiles within biological fluids like CSF has become possible (Hanash et al. 2002; Huhmer et al. 2006; Glasker et al. 2007; Jain 2007). Molecular biology has contributed numerous tools for manipulating proteins and for elucidating their interactions and their occurrence as part of complexes. Biochemical strategies have been used to sort proteins into classes and to identify post-translation modifications. Decades of biochemical research also provide insight into functional aspects of proteins. At the same time, genomics has provided a sequence-based framework for mining this protein data as well through homology search of new sequences against those with known structures and properties. With the availability of these tools, researchers have shown a tremendous interest in the potential ability of proteomics to address many unfulfilled needs in clinical research (Kennedy 2001; Jain 2007; Micallef et al. 2008).

Consider the hypothetical patient presenting to clinic with neurological symptoms, such as a seizure, compatible with a CNS neoplasm. Currently, the presence of a brain lesion will be identified through neurological examination followed by CT scan/MRI imaging studies. A stereotactic biopsy for histologic analysis allows for a tissue-based diagnosis (for example, anaplastic astrocytoma, WHO grade III). The patient would then undergo chemo-/radiation therapy sometimes followed by partial or complete tumor resection through surgery. However, despite these treatments, astrocytoma patients carry a dismal prognosis with most dying within 5 years of initial diagnosis due to tumor recurrence and malignant progression. At present there are no clear prognostic markers available to predict recurrence or to follow the patient's status when no visible tumor is present by neuroimaging. Most recurrences are identified when the tumor becomes visible on imaging studies, and it is usually difficult to distinguish tumor recurrence from radiation necrosis by these methods. Although not currently available, the detection of molecular marker(s) easily accessible through CSF could be immediately informative on the status of the recurrence without an invasive surgical procedure. It is imperative to select appropriate monitoring of tumor growth, response to therapy and recurrence, in a manner similar to how plasma levels of CA-125 protein can be used to follow ovarian cancer and predict recurrent disease before it becomes visible on imaging analyses.

25.4.2 Proteomic Methods for CSF Profiling

Methods for CSF processing and preparation, as this will result in higher levels of resolution, facilitate subsequent image analyses and improve confidence for accurately determining differential protein expression profiles. CSF proteomics itself employs two basic technologies: (1) some form of gel-based or liquid 2-D separation followed by (2) identification of individual proteins using mass spectrometry.

The first 2-DE map of the CSF was published in 1985 (Gallo et al. 1985; Wiederkehr and Vonderschmitt 1985). Since that time, protein spot detection and identification technologies have improved and updated CSF maps have been published. In the latest studies, over 700 specific peptide and protein products were identified as compared to only 70 presented in the first map (Zougman et al. 2008). Recent improvements in protein detection have increased sensitivity of these methods along with increased compatibility with subsequent MS and bioinformatics analyses. Here we briefly discuss the basic techniques for CSF protein mapping. An overview of some basic workflow plans for proteomic analyses of CSF can be seen in Fig. 25.3 and Color Plate 43.

A

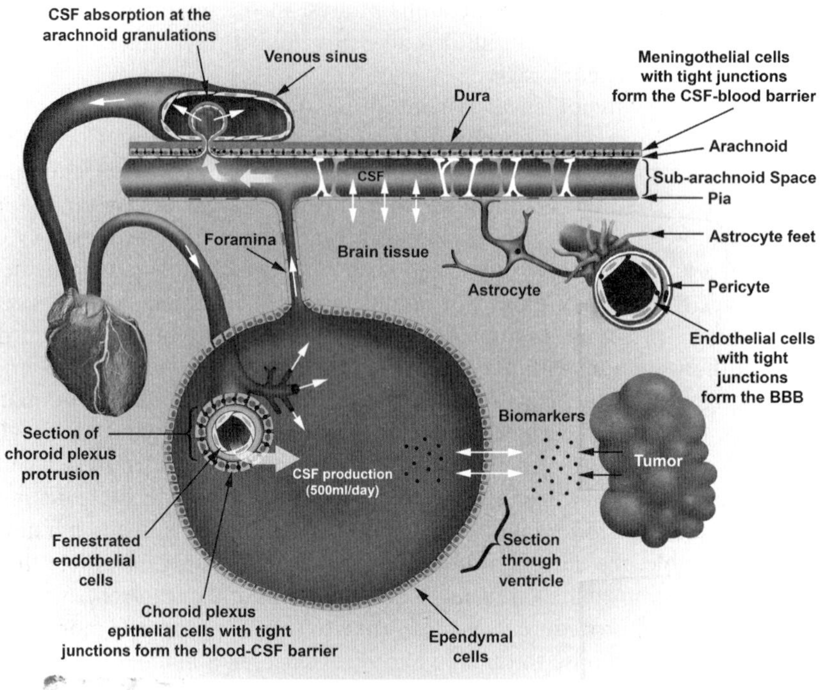

B

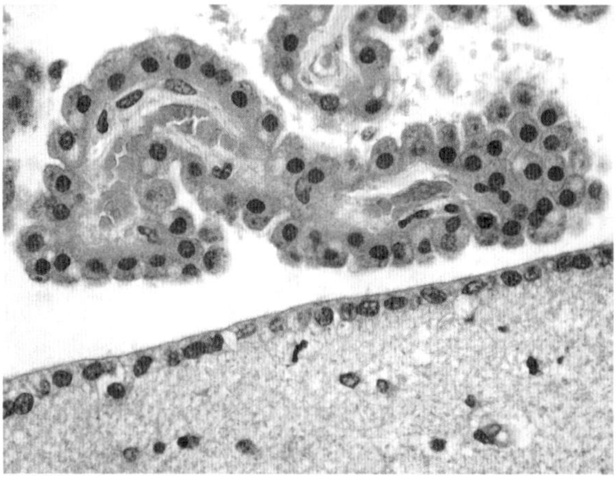

Fig. 25.3 **A.** Schematic illustration of the flow of CSF in the brain and the different cellular structures that create the blood–CSF barrier. This representation is not intended to be entirely anatomically correct and does not show many ultrastructural details. Incoming arterial blood flow from the heart connects to the choroid plexus, a cauliflower-shaped organ where blood is "filtered" through a double cellular layer, endothelial cells lining the arterial capillary and the choroid plexus epithelial cells that are connected through tight junctions. This constitutes the first component of the blood–CSF barrier. Note that the endothelial cells in the choroid plexus are not connected by tight junctions. The CSF is released from the choroid plexus into the ventricles, which are lined by ependymal cells where exchanges between the normal and

25.4.2.1 1-D and 2-D Gel Electrophoresis

Protein separation in a gel medium using electrokinetic methods (most typically electrophoresis) is the simplest and most classical of proteomic techniques. Proteins are either separated in one dimension through isoelectric focusing [to segregate proteins by their isoelectric point (pI)] on immobilized, gel-based pH gradients or, alternatively, using sodium dodecyl sulfate-polyacrylamide electrophoresis (SDS-PAGE) where all proteins get uniformly negatively charged and get separated solely by their relative molecular weight (MW). Neither technique alone is capable of isolating individual proteins with enough purity for downstream identification. However, the combination of the two in 2-DE format provides a powerful tool to theoretically obtain a unique “fingerprint” of all proteins present in a particular sample (Fig. 25.4) (Carrette et al. 2006; D’Aguanno et al. 2007). However, typically only major proteins will be visualized in complex samples and minor proteins will go undetected. The application of commercially available immobilized pH gradient (IPG) strips has improved 2-DE reproducibility immensely. Similarly, the accessibility of IPG strips in various lengths and pH ranges has increased the electrophoretic resolution of proteins by allowing increased sample load. Some new 2-DE systems can simultaneously analyze up to 12 gels, further minimizing any difference between gels that would be caused by varying running conditions. Once run, the proteins are visualized with coomassie brilliant blue, silver, or the newer fluorescent (Sypro-Ruby) stains. Until recently, silver staining was considered the most sensitive as it could allow for visualization of proteins at nanogram levels. However, many silver staining methods are incompatible with downstream protein identification procedures employing mass

Fig. 25.3 (continued) tumor brain tissue extracellular content and the CSF can occur. The hydrostatic pressure of incoming CSF creates CSF flow through foramens like the median aperture at the skull base and the CSF enters a second larger compartment called the subarachnoid space, which surrounds the brain. In this space the CSF–blood barrier is established by the neurothelium, a layer of meningothelial cells that cover the arachnoid and are connected by tight junctions, constituting the second component of the CSF–blood barrier. The CSF is reabsorbed into the venous circulation through multiple arachnoid granulations, which are small tufted protrusions that herniate through the dura mater and serve as one-way pressure-dependent valves. Positive hydrostatic pressure of the CSF moves fluid into the large superior sagittal sinus back into the venous circulation along with limited number of proteins and other markers of the CNS environment. In addition, for comparison, a blood vessel irrigating the brain is shown on the right. The permeation of blood components into the brain parenchyma is restricted by the blood–brain barrier (BBB), which is constituted by endothelial cells with tight junctions, surrounded by pericytes and astrocyte feet (Drawing by Eric Jablonowski, Department of Radiology, Emory University.) **B.** Cross-section of a human ventricle showing the choroid plexus cellular structure (*upper part*) and the ependymal cell layer (*lower part*) separating the ventricular space (clear) from the brain tissue. The section was formalin-fixed and stained with hematoxylin and eosin. (Photography by Daniel J Brat, Department of Pathology, Emory University) (*see* Color Plate 43)

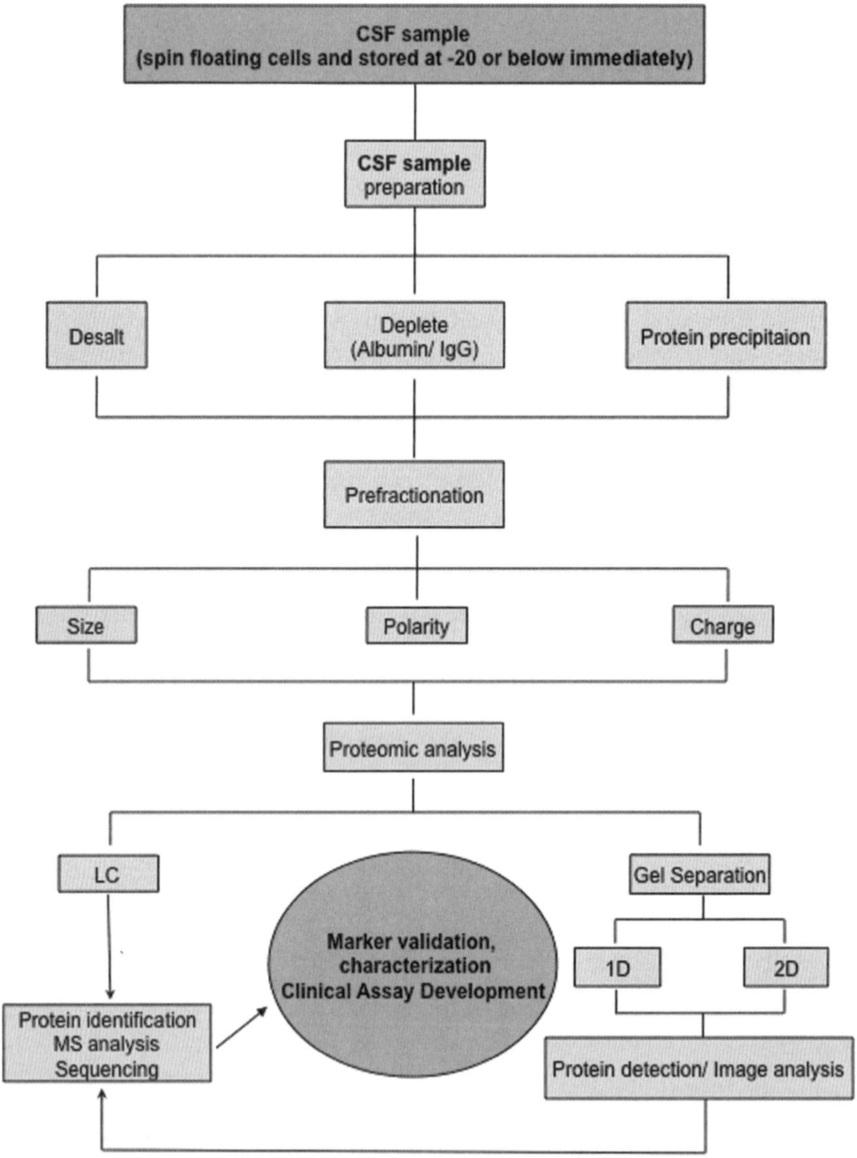

Fig. 25.4 Flowchart for proteomic analysis of CSF using available techniques. CSF samples require processing prior to their use in a proteomic platform. These include depletion of albumin/IgG as well as removal of salt and concentration of remaining protein. Once precipitated the protein should then be prefractionated using either of its properties, such as size, charge, or polarity. This allows for simpler mixtures that can be visualized at a much higher resolution during the downstream studies. Finally, the samples are subjected to proteomic analyses using either a gel-based or a liquid chromatography-based approach. The resulting fingerprint is visualized and interesting proteins are sequenced to gain information about their identity. Potential biomarkers of disease processes can then be validated on independent data sets and characterized for their functional significance

spectrometry. Even recently developed non-glutaraldehyde-based silver staining protocols still reduce the protein coverage during identification. Further MS-compatible staining methods are being developed in the market and will greatly improve the resolution of future studies.

25.4.2.2 Preparative 2-D Liquid-Phase Electrophoresis

To enhance the quality of proteomic analyses, a preparative 2-D liquid-phase electrophoresis system for the preseparation of CSF proteins has been recently promoted (Davidsson et al. 2001). This method is similar to 2-DE except that the first dimension of IEF is performed in the liquid phase. This allows further separation of CSF proteins into multiple (up to 20) fractions that are then individually resolved on SDS-PAGE. This allows for increased sample loading and less discrimination of membrane proteins, which normally have lower transfer efficiency from the first to the second dimension in 2-DE. Also, it results in higher resolution of each pI range and identification of additional proteins that might otherwise be lost due to inefficient focusing. The downside of using this technique is the requirement of larger initial sample as much sample is lost during the liquid-phase step.

25.4.2.3 MS Identification of 2-DE-Separated Proteins

Once the individual proteins in a given sample are well separated, the next step is to find their identity. The recent developments in mass spectrometry have improved the research capabilities in proteomic studies immensely. These methods include surface-enhanced laser desorption/ionization (SELDI), matrix-assisted laser desorption/ionization (MALDI) time-of-flight (TOF) MS, and electrospray ionization (ESI). MALDI-TOF-MS is a relatively straightforward, fast, and sensitive method to identify 2-DE-separated proteins. MALDI-TOF-MS is used to obtain peptide mass fingerprint (PMF) followed by MALDI-post-source decay-MS, which provides product ion (MS/MS) spectra that can be correlated with the amino acid sequence data of the corresponding precursor ions using sophisticated algorithms. This method is generally used for fractionated mixtures of peptides obtained from tryptic digests of single proteins or very simple protein mixtures. Using this approach, nearly 1,000 protein spots from 2-D gels of a single CSF sample have been analyzed with MS (Chaurand et al. 2005). SELDI-TOF-MS analysis on the other hand can be performed on intact protein samples and has been used successfully to find potential peaks of interest in both tissue and CSF samples from brain tumor patients (Bouamrani et al. 2006; Khwaja et al. 2006b). These two techniques are usually coupled to get the most accurate data. In a recent study, a protein from 30.0 to 32.0 kDa peak range was found specifically in neoplastic CSF when compared to non-neoplastic and inflammatory patients. This protein was identified by MALDI-TOF analysis as carbonic anhydrase, a protein overexpressed in many malignancies including high-grade gliomas (Khwaja et al. 2006b). However, this method is best suited for "profiling" small proteins of usually <20 kDa and/or peptides and protein fragments (Bouamrani et al. 2006; Guerreiro et al. 2006). Furthermore, unlike MALDI-TOF or nanoLC-ESI MS/MS it cannot by itself provide for unambiguous positive identification of the proteins in the peaks of interest.

Another analytical tool for rapid screening of complex biological fluid samples is Fourier transform ion cyclotron resonance (FTICR) mass spectrometry (MS). In this method, tryptically digested body fluids (plasma, urine, CSF, and saliva) are directly analyzed without any prior separation, purification, or selection. The information gained from this method is comparable to traditional 2-DE data, consumes only a few microliters of sample, and the data are acquired in only a few minutes. However, it is important to separate the proteins and/or peptides prior to analysis in order to detect low-abundance proteins and other proteins of biological relevance (Bergquist et al. 2002).

25.4.3 Quantitative Proteomics

Quantitative or comparative proteomics is essential for characterizing a disease proteome in relation to its normal counterpart. In traditional 2-DE–MS analyses, the staining intensity of protein spots is compared between gels to determine relative protein concentrations and positive identification is accomplished by mass spectrometry following in-gel digestion. A more recent method, however, can visualize multiple protein samples on a single gel using a differential fluorescent-labeling technique [called 2-D difference gel electrophoresis (2DIGE)], thus improving reproducibility by avoiding gel-to-gel variation. In contrast to "gel-based" quantifications, nongel-based approaches rely on the analysis of the surrogate peptides obtained from digests of unfractionated or partially fractionated protein mixtures. In its simplest form, label-free nanobore LC-MS has been shown to detect differentially expressed proteins with confidence even without prior depletion of abundant proteins (Huang et al. 2007). When using a nanobore LC-MS/MS approach for quantification purposes, an approach based on stable isotope dilution, mass spectrometry adds additional advantages for enumeration. In this approach, the samples being compared are chemically or metabolically labeled with structurally identical yet isotopically distinct (i.e., different mass) tags as done in the case of its prototypic variety, the isotope-coded affinity tag (ICAT) technology (Gygi et al. 1999). This allows comparison of the relative abundance of each labeled peptide in two or more samples by analysis of peptides identical in sequence but differing in mass. This method still remains a technical challenge, however, because protein coverage could be compromised by inefficient chemical labeling, limited representation of peptides in a protein because of amino acid-specific labeling chemistry, sample loss due to additional purification steps, and chemical side reactions. To overcome these limitations, other nanobore LC-MS/MS approaches that do not involve differential isotopic labeling are also being developed. For instance, recent studies indicate that the number of unique peptides identified for a single protein can serve as a measure of protein abundance. In a study examining CSF samples from astrocytoma patients, we employed both 2-DE and ICAT analyses to find differentially expressed proteins between each grade of astrocytoma. Our data suggest that while there is some overlap, still, 2-DE and ICAT work more as complementary techniques rather than validating one another. Using ICAT alone, we were able to identify and provide relative quantitation for several potential biomarkers for each grade of astrocytoma compared to nontumoral control CSF (Khwaja et al. 2007). Another recent study examined individual CSF proteins in patients with CNS lymphoma against those with benign focal brain lesions using a similar liquid chromatography/mass spectrometry-based method. Several hundred CSF proteins in CNS lymphoma were identified and differentially quantified, and further characterized for their expression pattern and quantification within tumor tissue, compared to control patients. Their results were confirmed using ELISA for one of these potential markers, antithrombin III (ATIII), on an independent validation set of 101 patients (Roy et al. 2008).

Although this method is semiquantitative and tends to be biased against low-abundance proteins, it can detect 2.5- to 5-fold changes in protein abundance with high confidence and is suitable for high-throughput proteome profiling using many samples. Improvements in MS instrumentation are also making it possible to quantify differentially expressed proteins on the basis of the ion volume calculated for individual samples by integrating the extracted ion chromatogram for a peptide of interest. In this application, the high-throughput, high-protein coverage, and automation capability of LC-MS/MS remain intact, facilitating its use for large-scale differential expression analysis and biomarker detection as recently accomplished with a large group of human serum samples.

25.4.4 Initial Results and First Biomarker Panel for Brain Tumor CSF

To date, only two studies have been performed to analyze the CSF from brain tumor patients using proteomic approaches. The first one found two candidate tumor-related proteins, the N-myc oncoprotein and the low-molecular-weight caldesmon (l-CaD) in CSF samples of patients with primary brain tumors using 2-DE followed by MALDI-TOF-MS analysis. However, this study was performed on only 10 patient samples that spanned a range of neoplastic histologies, limiting the conclusions that can be drawn (Zheng et al. 2003). A more recent study examined 60 samples of patients with CNS neoplasia and compared them with 11 nontumoral controls. The samples were derived from astrocytomas WHO grade II (6), III (7), and IV (19), schwannomas (5), metastatic brain tumors (10), inflammatory samples (3), and non-neoplastic controls (11). Using two proteomic techniques, 2-D gel electrophoresis (2-DE) and cleavable isotope-coded affinity tag (cICAT), the CSF proteomes were compared and over 200 proteins identified (Khwaja et al. 2007). The number of protein spots in each group correlated directly with malignancy grade where an average of 86 proteins in nontumor controls (range 76–90), 101 in AII (85–104), 136 in AIII (123–148), and 175 in CSF or cyst fluids from AIV patients (168–198) were observed. Both ventricular and lumbar punctures were used to access the CSF with very similar results. Additionally, the 19 AIV samples included 11 cyst fluids from tumor space, thus adding another variable to the analyses. To address the reliability of the assay, biomarkers discovered in the 11 AIV samples derived from fluid-filled tumor cysts were compared with those resulting from the 8 CSF samples from the same group. The distribution and levels of biomarkers identified in CSF and tumor cyst fluid were similar, providing a strong internal control of reliability. This finding also suggested that the proteins in CSF likely originated mostly from the tumor and would be present in the immediate tumor microenvironment. Among the identified proteins, there were 103 tumor and 20 astrocytoma-specific candidate protein biomarkers.

On close observation, one can see that there is variability in the demographic character, disease type, and treatments used within each study group. This is unavoidable as brain tumors are rare and CSF availability sparse, thus it is impossible to collect large groups of CSF that are homogeneous for many clinical parameters. As an example, the underlying diagnosis in the control group included headache, CSF leak, hydrocephalus, and arteriovenous malformation (AVM). Similarly in the high-grade study group, some individuals were early in their therapy and had undergone only diagnostic surgery, while others had advanced disease, were receiving radiation therapy, chemotherapy, and possibly had more than one prior surgery. Another variable was the relationship of the tumor to the CSF containing spaces. In some individuals, the lesions were adjacent to or communicated with ventricles, while others were away from ventricular or subarachnoid spaces. All these variables further complicate the proteomic studies and pose many challenges to data analyses (Khwaja et al. 2007).

The results from this first comprehensive proteomic screen of the CSF from brain tumor patients allowed us to develop tentative biomarker panels that could be used as a starting point to generate a diagnostic and/or prognostic tool for the clinic. Initial results suggest that these panels could potentially differentiate between all types of primary CNS tumors. Two panels were designed: the first contained 31 proteins that differentiated between tumor versus astrocytoma-specific proteins (Fig. 25.5), while the second panel contained the minimal number of proteins ($n = 13$) necessary for the pattern of expression to correlate most strongly with diagnostic grade. These proteins were chosen as they were most consistently seen differentially expressed within the grade they represent. Both potential protein panels were cross-validated using k-nearest neighbors (kNN) to determine how well they could correctly classify astrocytoma grade based on the 2-DE data. Using the kNN algorithm ($k = 1$), all subjects in the original training set of data were correctly classified with a misclassification rate of zero. Additionally, the panel was further validated using an independent prospective set of 11 patients (4 C, 1 AII, and 6 AIV) collected over a period of

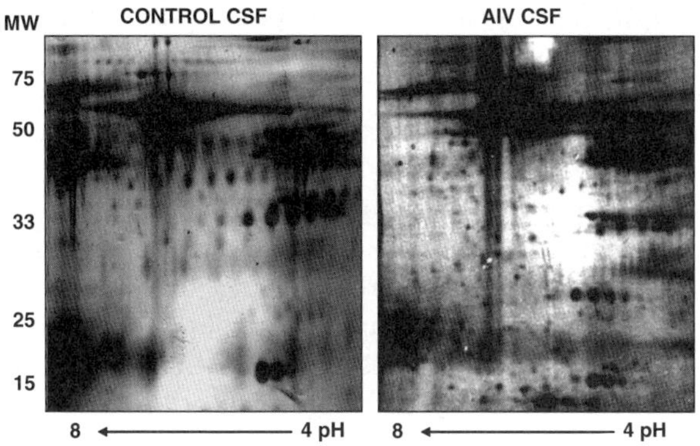

Fig. 25.5 Representative 2-DE gels of CSF. Albumin and IgG-depleted and TCA-precipitated CSF samples from patients with nontumoral control astrocytoma WHO grade IV were analyzed by 2-DE analysis using IEF strips (pH 4–7) and 12.5% SDS-PAGE. Spots were visualized by silver staining and spot patterns were analyzed using ImageMaster software (Reproduced from Khwaja et al. Journal of Proteome Research 2007.)

6 months. This test set also yielded a misclassification rate of zero, thus providing proof-of-principle evidence for the use of biomarker panels in the clinical assessment of brain tumors in the future (Khwaja et al. 2007). Clearly, these studies are still preliminary, and a validation with larger sets of patients is necessary before a biomarker panel with clinical applicability is developed.

The above study identified several known markers of neoplastic disease, including secreted protein with acidic-rich cysteines (SPARC), vascular endothelial growth factor (VEGF), and fibroblast growth factor (FGF), which were differentially expressed in the CSF from glioma patients compared to nontumoral controls (Khwaja et al. 2007). Some of these proteins had already been shown to be involved in enhancing tumor development, growth, and migration of brain tumors (Shi et al. 2004; Tang et al. 2005). Gene expression for many of these secreted proteins has also been found upregulated in microarray expression-profiling studies of brain tumors, indicating that tumor, and not the surrounding normal stroma, is the source for secretion of these proteins into the CSF (Godard et al. 2003; Liang et al. 2005; Rich et al. 2005). Previously unreported proteins like attractin, pro-angiotensinogen, beta-defensins, FGF-14 and others were found to be differentially secreted in glioma CSF for the first time.

Among these, FGF-14 was especially interesting as it was produced in all samples at about similar levels. However, there was a difference in the size of the protein product. While the wild-type form described in the literature has a molecular weight of 34 kDa, we identified a new shorter form of 27 kDa. Specifically, there appeared to be a switch from the larger isoform to the smaller one with transition to higher grade (AIII and AIV) in CSF from astrocytoma patients. The precise identity of the smaller form has not yet been established, but it may represent an alternatively spliced or cleaved form of the protein

(Khwaja et al. 2007). This apparent reduced protein size could also result from a lack of post-translational modifications. This specific finding is an example of how a unique tumor-specific protein product can be identified by proteomics but would not likely have been detected through genomic profiling or expression analyses.

Another of these proteins is the attractin which was found to be a novel marker for malignant astrocytoma (WHO grade III and IV) in the CSF (Khwaja et al. 2007). To verify these results, attractin expression was examined in an independent set of 100 brain tumor samples and was found elevated in 97% of malignant astrocytomas. This secreted attractin was found to act as a promotility factor for glioma cells in vitro, an important finding as invasiveness is a critical feature of glioma malignancy (Khwaja et al. 2006a). This discovery demonstrates that CSF contains proteins that may be biomarkers as well as active players in the pathobiology of the disease.

The production site of these new proteins found in the CSF remains unknown but could arise from either the tumor cells or the normal cells present in its surrounding microenvironment. For example, attractin was demonstrated to be produced and secreted by the tumor cells using immunohistochemical analyses (Khwaja et al. 2006a). Other proteins however could be the result of BBB breakdown during the process of tumorigenesis or they could be present in the CSF due to glioma-induced neuronal damage or tumor factor-induced stimulation of nontransformed glial and stromal cells.

25.4.5 Lessons Learned from Initial CSF Proteomic Studies

The above studies were based on 2-D gel electrophoresis coupled with protein identification through mass spectrometry, as well as ICAT. These are commonly used techniques to identify protein products that are differentially expressed between samples or groups of samples and are only semiquantitative. However, even with the combination of the "gold standard" proteomic technique, 2-DE, and the latest quantitative proteomic technology of cICAT, only 200 different proteins were identified in the CSF. This number represents only 20% of the total 1,000 protein products thought to be present in the CSF (Khwaja et al. 2007). Additionally, despite their semiquantitative nature, the potential biomarkers identified by 2-DE and cICAT analyses were largely confirmed either through each other or via western blot analysis. In some cases, 2-DE and cICAT failed to detect low levels of protein, likely representing the higher sensitivity of the western technique. Cleavable ICAT also proved less reliable than 2-DE for semiquantitative assessment, as quantification in cICAT is disrupted by overlapping MS spectrum peaks, a problem that might be overcome by new technology (Abdi et al. 2006; Ogata et al. 2007). Additionally, the identification and quantification can be improved immensely if the CSF samples are prefractionated post-depletion of albumin and IgG. These individual fractions should then be run separately to enhance the quality of the data and allow for increased number of identified proteins.

25.5 Importance of Experimental Design in CSF Proteomics

While even simplistic studies may reveal proteins that are differentially expressed, these are often not significant when subjected to rigorous statistical analyses. This problem can be addressed through appropriate well-developed experimental design (Hunt et al. 2005).

25.5.1 Accounting for Individual Variation Through Appropriate Biostatistical Design

Prior to comparing CSF samples between individuals to identify patterns of disease-associated proteins, it is essential to examine variation within individuals. This would allow better interpretation of potentially important changes in CSF within and between individuals due to disease processes. As an illustration, one study of six individuals with Alzheimer's disease evaluated two samples of CSF from each individual at 2 weeks interval (Hu et al. 2005). These two samples were processed using multiaffinity depletion for high-abundance proteins. Afterward, the pairs of samples were run on the same gel using 2D-DIGE analysis. The intraindividual variations, hierarchical clustering, and other statistical analyses of the proteomic profiles revealed that two CSF samples from the same individual clustered closer together than samples from different individuals. However, a number of proteins with varied expression between the two time points from the same patient were identified by tandem mass spectrometry (Hu et al. 2005). These results have important implications for the design of CSF biomarker studies for CNS disorders as they show how even CSF samples from the same individual can differ over time without any disease manifestation. On the other hand, another study examined differential expression in pooled male versus female samples using a new proteomic technique employing isobaric tags after depletion of six highly abundant proteins using a multiple affinity removal system. They found only 12 out of nearly 300 proteins with altered expression, indicating marked similarity between male and female CSF and suggesting little variation in CSF composition of healthy individuals (Ogata et al. 2007). These seemingly contradictory conclusions from the two studies could simply be due to the fact that in the first study each sample was analyzed individually, while the second group used pooled samples from all subjects within each group. These results further stress the importance of study design and sample selection for obtaining meaningful results from proteomic studies.

It is also imperative to consider the impact of the sources of variation (both analytical and biological) on the statistical strength of the results. The design should address the number of samples that must be analyzed to achieve statistical significance for the desired question and the number of replicates per sample, in the context of a particular minimum difference that one is seeking to demonstrate. Sample size calculation is important in any study design but is even more relevant in microarray or proteomic experiments since only a few repetitions are usually feasible. As a result of these experiments information is generated about a large number of proteins. This results in problems during statistical analyses, termed multiple testing problem, as it requires multiple tests to be performed simultaneously. Several approaches have been designed to compensate for this drawback. The two most commonly used methods are to calculate the false discovery rate (FDR) or the family-wise error rate (FWER) to identify the most significant results. FDR reflects the expected percent of false predictions in a given data set, while FWER calculates only the probability of making one or more false discoveries among all the various hypotheses when analyzing multiple pairwise tests (Liu and Hwang 2007). Therefore, in these experiments, it is more powerful and more reasonable to control false discovery rate (FDR) or positive FDR (pFDR) instead of type I error, e.g., family-wise error rate (FWER).

25.5.2 Sample Selection and Processing

After appropriate design, choosing the right CSF sample is probably the single most important step in any proteomic study. Additionally, this sample must also be processed properly for optimal results. First, it is essential to make sure that the CSF obtained from the patients is as clean as possible, free of contaminating blood, immune cells, and/or infectious particles that could mask real results during downstream analyses. Once this sample is acquired, it is equally important to store all samples under uniform conditions, preferably at –20°C or below to ensure minimum loss of proteins due to degradation and proteolysis (Hale et al. 2008). The CSF sample should then be further processed prior to experimentation to maximize the results. CSF normally contains a high salt concentration (>150 mmol/l) and a low protein content (200–700 μg/ml). The excessive level of salt interferes with the electrophoretic mobility of proteins in many gel-based proteomic methods due to high electrical current carried by the salt load. Additionally, similar to plasma, the majority of CSF proteins are isoforms of serum albumin, transferrin, and immunoglobulins, which represent more than 70% of the total protein amount. Furthermore, proteins found in the CSF can span a wide range of concentrations, making the detection of scarce proteins, which are likely to be significant, extremely challenging with the current analytical methods. To bypass these problems, CSF samples have to be prefractionated, desalted, and depleted of the higher abundance proteins in order to observe potential biomarkers (Hale et al. 2008) (Fig. 25.6 and Color Plate 44, Fig. 25.7 and Color Plate 45).

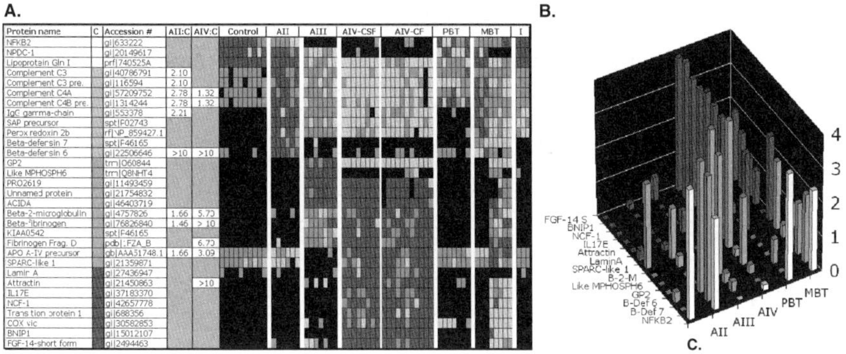

Fig. 25.6 Potential biomarker panels differentiate between astrocytoma grades using CSF. **A.** Panel of 32 proteins that can be used to differentiate between AII–IV patients, nontumoral controls, and other forms of brain tumors. *Black* = no expression, *yellow* = low expression, *orange* = moderate expression, and *red* = high expression level as determined from Image-Master analysis of 2-DE gels. C = Biomarker class; *white* = control specific, *light blue* = AII, *green* = AIII, and *pink* = AIV biomarker. **B.** Restricted panel containing top 13 proteins from panel **A**. *White* = control, *light blue* = AII, *green* = AIII, and *purple* = AIV biomarkers. Vertical axis represents relative level (0–4) of each protein as estimated from 2-DE (Reproduced from Khwaja et al. Journal of Proteome Research 2007.) (*see* Color Plate 44)

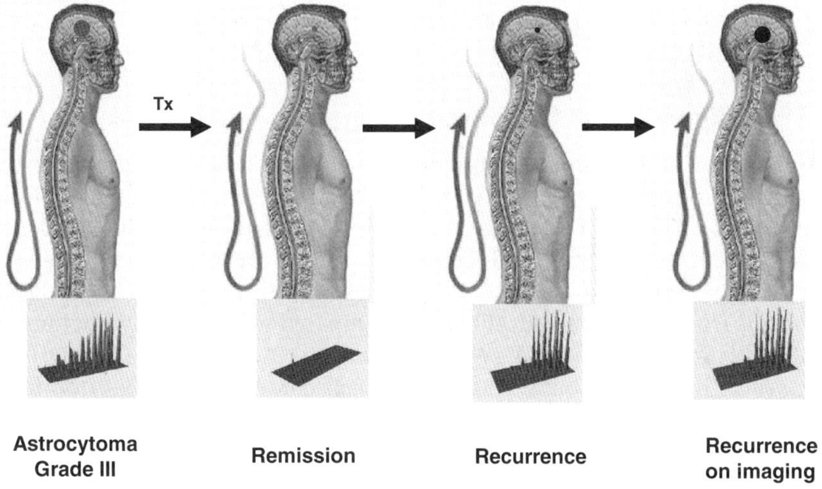

Fig. 25.7 Possible future applications of CSF biomarkers. Protein markers found in the CSF through a spinal tap could be used individually or in combination in a biomarker panel to diagnose CNS malignancies. A protein or an antibody array developed using identified biomarkers would allow for personalized medicine based on the unique limited protein profile. These markers could also allow for early detection of original, residual, or recurrent disease in a minimally invasive procedure compared to biopsy or surgery. Furthermore, the specific protein profile before and after therapeutic treatment (Tx) or upon tumor recurrence will provide information about the biological status of the tumor and on whether the treatment has an impact. Precautions need to be taken when drawing spinal CSF in patients with a cerebral mass due to elevated intraventricular pressure (*see* Color Plate 45)

25.5.2.1 Prefractionation and Depletion of CSF

Since the high-abundance proteins frequently precipitate during proteomic analyses leading to increased background while the sparse proteins are not detected either due to their minuscule levels or due to the interference on the gel from neighboring high-abundance proteins, prefractionation of CSF is crucial to preferentially enrich low-abundance proteins. This can be achieved through several methods prior to protein precipitation (Kennedy 2001).

The first successful method to deplete CSF of high-abundance albumin and immunoglobulins took advantage of the affinity interactions between albumin and Cibacron Blue F3G-A (Blue Sepharose 6 Fast Flow) and between immunoglobulins and protein G (Prosep-G) to deplete the high-abundance CSF protein–albumin and immunoglobulins (Hammack et al. 2003; Ramstrom et al. 2005). Similar methods have been used in many commercial affinity albumin-removal kits. However, these methods have been designed specifically for use with serum. Since the protein concentration is much higher in serum than that in CSF, these kits are usually not found to be compatible for use with CSF. To bypass this limitation, alternate methods have recently been developed specifically for depletion of CSF (Ramstrom et al. 2008). These include prefractionation with liquid-phase isoelectric focusing (IEF) (Davidsson et al. 2001) and solid-phase extraction that uses variable hydrophobic properties of CSF proteins (Yuan and Desiderio 2005a).

25.5.2.2 Preparation of CSF Samples

In complement with simple prefractionation, there are several different ways to optimize CSF samples for proteomic analyses. These include the use of ultrafiltration (Yuan and Desiderio 2005b), dialysis or Biospin columns to desalt and concentrate the proteins followed by protein precipitation using acetone, TCA, or a combination of the two. Studies have found improved recovery of proteins from CSF using ultrafiltration compared to dialysis for desalting. The recovery of protein is less (40–60%) (Hammack et al. 2003) with dialysis than that of ultrafiltration but contains lower salt content and would thus lead to better resolution in downstream analyses. Biospin columns employ a new method of protein precipitation that has been reported to provide greater than 99% protein recovery, yet their quality remains to be assessed (Yuan et al and Terry and Desiderio).

Overall, these preparations result in variable purity and protein recovery (20–90%) depending on the method used. For example, even though protein recovery is highest using an acetone–protein precipitation method (90%) (Yuan and Desiderio 2005b), horizontal and vertical streaks on the gel caused by the high salt concentration lead to excessive level of background (Chen et al. 2006), reducing the number of proteins that can be easily distinguished by image analysis software. For proteomic analyses, precipitation of CSF proteins with TCA in water followed by acetone wash appears to give the cleanest results.

25.6 Data Analysis and Validation

Proteomic studies have generated numerous data sets of potential diagnostic, prognostic, and therapeutic significance in human cancer. Before characterizing biomarkers unique to each disease, it is necessary to categorize CSF proteins systematically and extensively. However, the enormous complexity, great dynamic range of protein concentrations, and tremendous protein heterogeneity due to post-translational modification of CSF create significant challenges to the existing proteomic technologies for an in-depth, unbiased profiling of the human CSF proteome.

In the last few years, several separation methodologies and mass spectrometric platforms that greatly enhance the identification coverage and the depth of protein profiling of CSF to characterize CSF proteome have been utilized. For example, in recent studies, a total of 2,594 proteins were identified in well-characterized pooled human CSF samples using stringent proteomics criteria (Pan et al. 2007). However, this data means little if not analyzed properly. The proteomic techniques vary largely and often show little overlap between studies conducted with even the same approach. Therefore, confirmation of these advanced technologies remains a priority. This problem is further exacerbated by lack of uniform patient inclusion and exclusion criteria, low patient numbers, poor supporting clinical data, absence of standardized sample preparation, and limited analytical reproducibility (in particular of 2-DE).

Despite these difficulties, there is little doubt that the proteomic approach has the potential to identify novel diagnostic biomarkers in cancer. Many programs and strategies have been developed to examine and analyze the large data sets produced through proteomic studies for biomarker discovery, statistical analyses, and/ or validation purposes. These include commercial as well as free web-based programs utilizing the wealth of information found in public DNA and protein sequence databases. Images from techniques like 2-DE can now be examined using softwares like Image Master (GE-Amersham Biosciences) and PDQuest (BioRad). In addition, some websites provide their own softwares for analysis free of charge, e.g., ExPASY proteomic tools and Mascot search engine. To use these programs, users first upload images to the software followed by automatic detection of the spots for each image according to parameters set by the user. After detection, automated matching of spots between gels is performed. This matching should be confirmed manually by the user. Once all spots are matched, users can perform data analysis using the analysis manager (i.e., t-test, fold change, and multivariate analyses). Users can also export data for more advanced statistical analysis using Excel or other software packages. These programs when used in combination provide quite advanced capabilities for data set analyses. In 2002, the human proteome organization (HUPO) developed the HUPO proteomics standard initiative (PSI) that defines community standards for data representation in proteomics to facilitate data comparison, exchange, and verification (Hamacher et al. 2006). The standards being developed by this community will vastly improve the quality of proteomics data and allow for it to be more useful in the future.

25.7 Future Directions

Until recently, the focus of most proteomic experiments was qualitative identification of proteins in simple and complex mixtures. However, protein quantification using multiplexed samples is rapidly becoming necessary. New technologies such as 2D-DIGE and ICAT allow for at least semiquantitative comparison of two or more samples at once. These techniques allow for not only identification of peptides but also relative quantification of these peptide levels. A recent variation on ICAT is isobaric tagging for relative and absolute quantification (iTRAQ), where the comparative abundances of peptides in up to eight samples can be compared through the labeling of each with eight different reporter ions. This technique has already been employed to identify potential markers of various neurodegenerative disorders including Alzheimer's, Parkinson's, and dementia (Abdi et al. 2006; Dayon et al. 2008). Newer techniques like MRM MS/MS for quantitation and profiling of selected proteins, both relative and absolute, can go down to high nanograms per milliliter in serum samples (Anderson 2006 #421).

However, even with such quantification, the proteomic analyses are still in their infancy as this provides only the basic information about the proteins present in the samples. Proteomic analyses are much more complex than genomic studies as proteins can be modified in multiple ways. These include glycosylation, phosphorylation, acetylation, ubiquitination, and others. These post-translational modifications are essential for the proper functions of proteins and are often altered in disease states. Therefore, future work is needed to increase the sensitivity of proteomic techniques to identify and analyze these post-translational changes.

25.7.1 Glyco-/Phospho Proteomics

Glycoproteins are enriched in bodily fluids such as human CSF and consequently can serve as diagnostic and/or therapeutic markers for CNS diseases. In a recent study, researchers reported an in-depth identification of glycoproteins in human CSF using a complementary proteomic approach, which integrated hydrazide chemistry and lectin affinity column for glycoprotein enrichment followed by multidimensional chromatography separation and tandem mass spectrometric analysis (Pan et al. 2006). Using stringent criteria, a total of 216 glycoproteins, including many low-abundance proteins, were identified with high confidence.

Approximately one-third of these proteins were already known to be relevant to the CNS structurally or functionally. This investigation, for the first time, not only categorized many glycoproteins in human CSF but also expanded the existing overall CSF protein database (Ogata et al. 2005; Pan et al. 2006).

25.7.2 Protein and Peptide Arrays

Layered peptide array (LPA) is a new methodology for simultaneous measurements of proteins, peptides, and/ or antibodies in a variety of patient specimens. A recent study described an indirect layered peptide array (iLPA) that is capable of measuring proteins on a solid surface, such as target antigens on a tissue section. This group developed an iLPA system and subsequently examined it for reproducibility and specificity when compared with standard immunohistochemistry. Semiquantitative, multiplex proteomic analysis of histological sections was achieved with up to 20 membranes with about 18% variability. Overall, the data suggest that iLPA technology will be a relatively simple and inexpensive method for molecular measurements from tissue sections (Gannot et al. 2007). Similar technique can also be used to create reverse-phase CSF protein arrays with the CSF of multiple patients on one slide that can then be analyzed simultaneously for different markers. This technology can be easily translated into the clinic once appropriate biomarkers are identified.

25.7.3 Antibody Arrays

Antibody arrays represent one of the high-throughput techniques enabling detection of multiple proteins concurrently. One of the main advantages of the technology over other proteomic approaches is that the identities of the measured proteins are known at the time of experimental design or can be readily characterized, facilitating a biological interpretation of the obtained results. Clinical applications of antibody arrays vary from biomarker discovery for diagnosis, prognosis, and drug response to characterization of protein pathways and modification changes associated with disease development and progression, especially when using biological fluids like CSF. As a high-throughput tool addressing protein levels and post-translational modifications, it improves the functional characterization of molecular bases for cancer. Furthermore, the identification and validation of protein expression patterns characteristic of cancer progression and tumor subtypes may enable tailored therapeutic intervention and improvement in the clinical management of cancer patients (Sanchez-Carbayo 2008). Technical requirements such as lower sample volume, antibody concentration, format versatility, and high reproducibility support their increasing impact in cancer research. Commercial arrays are already available for research and are offered by many companies for specific processes and pathways such as apoptosis and cytokines. Such antibody arrays would allow for potential biomarker panels to be translated into clinical applications in an affordable and convenient manner.

25.7.4 Biomarker Panel

The understanding of gliomagenesis could be tremendously accelerated with the ability to perform expression-profiling studies on proteins present in gliomas as well as those in the tumor microenvironment. Such studies could provide mechanistic insights on how tumor cells interact with surrounding tissues to evade programmed cell death (apoptosis), induce new blood vessel formation (angiogenesis), and escape host immune response. The results from published CSF studies confirm that proteomic technologies can indeed be used to find potential biomarkers of brain tumor formation and progression (Zhang et al. 2005; Khwaja et al. 2006a, b; Khalil 2007; Khwaja et al. 2007). Eventually, one important outcome of such studies might be fine-tuning of the glioma grading system, which is presently determined purely on histological criteria. There will be a need to expand the search for biomarker panels to include all types of primary and metastatic brain tumors and not just astrocytomas. Any such proposed panels would need to be tested in a multicenter study for validation of individual proteins. To this effect, while 2-DE and cICAT are excellent screening methods, they are not feasible for such large-scale studies. Therefore, to achieve optimal results, high-throughput, more quantitative and reproducible methods need to be developed. This could include employing tissue microarrays, protein chips, dot blots, or ELISA for specific protein markers for verification process. Once verified, the specific proteins could be used as markers of progression, therapeutic response, and/or survival (Fig. 25.6).

25.8 Conclusion

The introduction of lumbar puncture into clinical medicine over a century ago by German physician Heinrich Quincke marks the beginning of the study of CNS diseases using human CSF (Huhmer et al. 2006). Ever since, CSF has been analyzed in great detail to examine the physiological and biochemical basis of neurological diseases. The proximity of CSF to brain makes it a good target for studying the pathophysiology of brain functions but the BBB and B-CSF functions of the CSF also impede its diagnostic value. Up until recently, CSF analyses were confined to routine measurements to determine alterations in the composition of CSF in response to disease states, particularly CSF cytology. More recently, detailed analyses have been undertaken to examine detailed protein composition of CSF. Such comprehensive analysis of lower abundance CSF protein has the potential to uncover new disease markers. With novel proteomic techniques, CSF biomarkers will likely become invaluable for diagnosis, prognosis, and predicting response to therapy. However, CSF proteomic analysis is not trivial, as this fluid combines many of the difficulties of serum analysis (complexity, dynamic range, etc.) with specific issues of CSF collection and physiological variations. So far, few studies have resulted in significant clinical application, but the use of prefractionation methods and new high-end proteomic technologies on CSF and serum collected in controlled preanalytical conditions could lead to future relevant biomarkers.

Abbreviations

CSF	cerebrospinal fluid
BBB	blood–brain barrier
B-CSF	blood to cerebrospinal fluid barrier
2-DE	two-dimensional polyacrylamide gel electrophoresis
2-D DIGE	two-dimensional difference gel electrophoresis
ESI-MS	electrospray ionization mass spectrometry
LC	liquid chromatography
MALDI-FTICR-MS	matrix-assisted laser desorption/ionization Fourier transform ion cyclotron resonance mass spectrometry
MALDI-TOF-MS	matrix-assisted laser desorption/ionization time-of-flight mass spectrometry
MS	mass spectrometry
SELDI-TOF-MS	surface-enhanced laser desorption/ionization time-of-flight mass spectrometry

Acknowledgments We thank Drs Daniel J Brat and Jan Pohl for reading and commenting on the manuscript.

Glossary

2-DE-(two-dimensional gel electrophoresis) A type of gel electrophoresis-based separation technique in which proteins are first separated based on differences in their net charges [mostly based on differences in isoelectric point (p*I*)] followed by separations based on their relative molecular weight (M*r*). This powerful combination enables the analysis of complex protein mixtures in the form of a unique fingerprint (p*I*-M*r* space) for the given sample; up to several thousands of proteins, isoforms, and variants can be separated and visualized on a single 2-DE gel.

Ampholytes These are molecules that contain both acidic and basic groups and will exist mostly as zwitterions in a certain range of pH. The pH at which the average charge is zero is defined as the molecule's isoelectric point (p*I*).

Angiogenesis The formation of new blood vessels.

Arachnoid membrane A delicate fibrous membrane forming the middle of the three coverings of the brain and spinal cord, closely attached to the dura mater, from which it is separated only by the subdural cleft, but separated from the pia mater by the subarachnoid space.

Apoptosis Disintegration of cells into membrane-bound particles that are then eliminated by phagocytosis or by shedding.

Astrocyte A specific cell type of the brain that is star-shaped and expresses unique differentiation markers such as intermediate filament protein GFAP (glial fibrillary astrocytic protein).

Astrocytoma Tumors of the central nervous system that have morphological characteristics and express markers of the astrocytic lineage. This tumor type comes in different grades of malignancy: diffusely infiltrating astrocytoma (WHO grade II), anaplastic astrocytoma (grade III), and glioblastoma (grade IV). They are believed to originate from the transformation of normal astrocytes or a type of stem cell or neural progenitor cell in the brain.

ATIII Antithrombin III, a natural α-globulin coagulation inhibitor.

BBB (blood–brain barrier) A physical barrier that alters the permeability of brain capillaries, so that some substances, such as certain drugs, are prevented from entering brain tissue, while other substances are allowed to enter freely. The barrier is constituted by endothelial cells lining the capillaries and connected by tight junctions. It is reinforced by extensions from astrocytes called astrocytic feet.

B-CSF (blood–CSF barrier) A physical barrier that separates the CSF compartments (ventricles and subarachnoid space) from the blood and serves as a filtering device to allow water and selected substances to circulate between the blood and the CSF. The barrier is generated by the tight junctions that connect the epithelial cells on the surface of the choroid plexus and the neurothelium covering the arachnoid ceiling.

cICAT (cleavable isotope-coded affinity tag) Method developed and commercialized by Applied Biosystems to compare two different sample states based on cysteine-specific protein labeling strategy. This allows both identification and relative quantitation of proteins present in the two samples during protein expression analysis studies. The cleavable ICAT reagent is composed of four main segments: (1) a protein reactive group composed of iodoacetamide, (2) an affinity tag made of biotin used to purify labeled peptides out of the protein mixture, (3) an acid cleavage site to allow simplification of molecule following labeling and purification, and (4) an isotopically labeled linker ($C_{10}H_{17}N_3O_3$) that contains up to nine ^{12}C (light reagent) or ^{13}C (heavy reagent) atoms. Chemically, the light and heavy molecules are identical except for the differing mass as the heavy version of the reagent with nine ^{13}C atoms is 9 Da heavier than the light version of the reagent. During mass spectrometric analysis, the light and heavy versions of the surrogate, ICAT-labeled peptides are mass-resolved allowing comparison of the parent proteins labeled with heavy and light reagent providing a ratio of the concentration of the proteins in the original sample.

CNS (central nervous system) The portion of the vertebrate nervous system consisting of the brain and spinal cord.

CSF (cerebrospinal fluid) The serum-like fluid that circulates through the ventricles of the brain, the cavity of the spinal cord, and the subarachnoid space.

CT scan An image produced by a CAT scanner. Computed tomography (also known as CT, CT scan, CAT, or computerized axial tomography) scans use X-rays to produce precise cross-sectional images of anatomical structures.

2-D-DIGE (Two-Dimensional Differential Gel Electrophoresis) 2-D-DIGE is a gel-based proteomic profiling technique that enables the detection and quantitation of differences in protein abundance between two differentially labeled proteomes. In principle, differences between two protein samples are detected by fluorescently tagging the samples with different dyes having identical mass and charge yet distinguishable by their fluorescence emission maxima allowing coseparation and visualization in a single conventional 2-D gel. Differences between the samples are analyzed by overlaying the two false color marker fluorescent channels. Irregularities associated with pattern comparison between individual gels are significantly minimized or eliminated due to comigration of differentially labeled protein species.

Electrophoresis An electrokinetic separation method of separating charged substances, such as proteins, which is based on differential mobilities of each component while under the influence of an electric field.

ESI (Electrospray ionization) It is a mass spectrometry technique used to produce ions and introduce them into mass analyzers. It is often termed "soft ionization technique" as it is especially useful in producing ions from macromolecules such as proteins and nucleic acids because it overcomes or diminishes their propensity to fragment when ionized.

FDR (False discovery rate) It is a statistical method used in multiple hypothesis testing requiring simultaneous multiple comparisons.

FGF (Fibroblast growth factor) A family of proteins important in the development of the nervous and skeletal systems.

FTICR (Fourier transform ion cyclotron resonance mass spectrometry) Also known as Fourier transform mass spectrometry, is a type of mass analyzer (or mass spectrometer) for determining the mass-to-charge (m/z) ratio of ions based on the cyclotron frequency of the ions in a fixed magnetic field. Generally externally formed ions are trapped in a FTICR analyzer cell, which is at the center of a strong magnetic field. A cyclotron motion results when ions spiral rapidly around the magnetic field lines. The cyclotron frequencies are dependent upon the mass-to-charge ratios of the different ions in a uniform magnetic field strength. Detection of the ions is performed by recording transient image current signals, which are induced by the ions passing a pair of receiver plates. Frequencies recorded are more precise than any other parameter and lead to mass spectra with very high resolution and mass accuracy. For simultaneous measurement of ions with different mass-to-charge ratios, Fourier transform analysis is used to convert the complex transient from a time-dependent to a frequency-dependent function, which is converted to generate the mass spectra.

FWER (Family-wise error rate) In statistics, when a series of significance tests (such as multiple pairwise comparisons) is conducted, the family-wise error rate is the probability that one or more of the significance tests results in a type 1 (or false-positive) error.

HUPO (Human Proteome Organization) The Human Proteome Organization is an international scientific organization representing and promoting proteomics through international cooperation and collaborations by fostering the development of new technologies, techniques, and training. http://www.hupo.org/

IEF (Isoelectric focusing, also known as electrofocusing) Electrokinetic separation technique in which a mixture of polyelectrolytes such as protein is resolved into its components by subjecting the mixture to an electric field in a supporting gel or free liquid medium having a previously established or transiently formed pH gradient. The proteins will cease to migrate once their net charge becomes zero, specified as their isoelectric point (p*I*).

iLPA (indirect layered peptide array) Recent technology for multiplex molecular measurement of clinical samples capable of measuring proteins on a solid surface, such as target antigens on a tissue section as in the form of tissue microarray. iLPA is used to measure antigens bound to a surface (histological tissue sections, immunoblots) using antibodies as a reporter system. In an analysis of a tissue section, for example, a cocktail of exogenous antibodies is added to the histologic section using standard incubation and washing conditions, and then the membrane set is placed adjacent to the slide. The reporter antibodies subsequently detach from the tissue section, traverse through the membranes, and are captured by their respective peptide-coated layer. The 2-D architecture of the sample is maintained during the process; thus all of the cellular subcomponents within the tissue section can be individually analyzed.

IPG (Immobilized pH gradient) IPG gels are the acrylamide matrix copolymerized with immobilized synthetic polyelectrolytes (ampholytes) of predetermined range of acidities that are used to form transient pH gradient within the gel in an electric field, practically achievable in the pH range of 3–12. The immobilized pH gradient is obtained through covalent incorporation of a mixture of acidic and basic buffering groups into the polyacrylamide gel at the time it is cast. The buffers called acrylamido buffers are a set of well-characterized molecules, each with a single acidic or basic buffering group linked to an acrylamide monomer. This alternative IPG method of gradient formation eliminated the problems of gradient instability and poor sample-loading capacity associated with "free" ampholytes (molecules that contain both acidic and basic groups) pH gradient that were originally developed for use in IEF.

iTRAQ (Isobaric tags for relative and absolute quantification) Recently developed technology to simultaneously analyze and compare up to eight different protein samples. The technique is based on using differential labeling with a set of multiplexed, amine-specific, stable isotope reagents that can label all peptides having amino or imino groups as compared to only those containing specific amino acid residues, e.g., cysteinyl residues as in the case of classical ICAT reagents. This enables simultaneous identification and quantitation, both relative and absolute, while retaining important post-translational modifications.

LC (Liquid chromatography) It is a separation technique in which a sample mixture (analytes) solubilized in a suitable solvent (liquid phase) is passed through a column packed with solid particles (solid phase) to achieve phase distribution. With the proper solvents, packing phase and elution conditions, some components in the sample will travel the column more slowly than others resulting in the desired separation. Liquid chromatography can be carried out either in a column or in a plane (thin layer chromatography). Present day liquid chromatography generally utilizes very small packing particles (typically 1.5–20 μm particle size) for increased resolution and requires relatively high pressures to achieve optimal linear flow rates and is therefore referred to as high-pressure liquid chromatography (HPLC) or ultra-high-pressure liquid chromatography (UPLC).

LC–MS (Liquid chromatography–mass spectrometry) It is an analytical chemistry technique that combines the physical separation capabilities of liquid chromatography with the mass analysis capabilities of mass spectrometry.

LPA (Layered Peptide Array) It is a new methodology for multiplex molecular measurements from 2-D life science platforms. It permits multiple proteins to be identified in tumors and other tissues while maintaining the shape and morphology of the starting material. In this method, different peptides are coated onto individual capture membranes. The membrane stack is then exposed to a sample that is allowed to permeate for a given period of time. Next, the membrane stack is removed and the capture membrane to which the biomolecule adheres is identified.

kNN (k-Nearest Neighbor) In pattern recognition, the *k*NN is a biostatistical method for classifying objects based on closest training examples in the feature space. *k*NN is a type of instance-based learning or lazy learning where the function is only approximated locally and all computations are deferred until classification. It can also be used for regression.

MALDI (Matrix-assisted laser desorption/ionization) It is a "soft ionization technique" used in conjunction with mass spectrometry, allowing the intact mass analysis of biomolecules and other large organic molecules that tend to be fragile and fragment when ionized by other more conventional ionization methods. In this method, the sample is dispersed in a large excess of matrix material which will strongly absorb the incident light. The matrix contains chromophore for the laser light and since the matrix is in a large molar excess, it will absorb essentially all of the laser radiation. The matrix isolates sample molecules in a chemical environment which enhances the probability of ionization without fragmentation. Short pulses of laser light are focused onto the sample "spot" (cocrystallized matrix with the analytes) and cause the analyte and the matrix to volatilize. In the most typical arrangement, the ions thus formed in the MALDI process are accelerated by an applied high voltage and are then allowed to drift down a flight tube of the time-of-flight (TOF) analyzer where they separate according to their mass-to-charge ratio (m/z). Arrival of these ions at the end of the flight tube is detected, the ions are counted and recorded by a high-speed recording device, and the signal is converted to the mass spectrum.

TOF-MS- (Time-of-flight mass spectrometry) It is a mass spectrometry method of ion separation and detection in which proteins or peptides ionized typically via the ESI or the MALDI process are accelerated by an electric field of known strength. TOF mass spectrometers operate on the principle that when a temporally and spatially well-defined group of ions of differing mass-to-charge (m/z) ratios are subjected to the same applied electric field [$K.E. = (mv^2)/2 = zeEs$ where K.E. = kinetic energy; m = the mass of the ion; v = velocity of the ion; z = number of charges; e = the charge on an electron in coulombs; E = electric field gradient; and s = the distance of the ion source region] and allowed to drift in a region of constant electric field, they will traverse this region in a time which depends upon their m/z ratios.

MRI imaging Magnetic resonance imaging (MRI) is the versatile, medical imaging technology by which doctors can get highly refined images of the body's interior without surgery. The basis of MRI is the directional magnetic field, or moment, associated with charged particles in motion. Nuclei containing an odd number of protons and/or neutrons have a characteristic motion or *precession*. Because nuclei are charged particles, this precession produces a small magnetic moment. When a human body is placed in a large magnetic field, many of the free hydrogen nuclei align themselves with the direction of the magnetic field. The nuclei move about the magnetic field direction like gyroscopes. The MR images are obtained either using the proton density (PD) or the transverse relaxation time of these protons (T2). The two images are said to be proton density-weighted (PD-weighted) and T2-weighted, respectively.

mRNA The form of ribonucleic acid (RNA) known as messenger RNA that mediates the transfer of genetic information from the cell nucleus to ribosomes in the cytoplasm, where it serves as a template for protein synthesis. It is synthesized from a DNA template during the process of transcription.

MS/MS (Tandem mass spectrometry) It involves multiple steps of mass spectrometry analyses, with some form of fragmentation occurring in between each round.

MW (molecular weight) The sum of the atomic weights of all atoms making up a molecule.

pI (isoelectric point) The pH of the solution at which a protein or an ampholyte has a net neutral charge and therefore does not move in an electric field.

PMF (probability mass function) It is a biostatistical function that gives the probability that a discrete random variable is exactly equal to some actual value.

Proteomics Proteomics is a term that refers to all the proteins expressed by a given genome. Proteomics involves the identification of proteins in the body and the determination of their role in physiological and pathophysiological conditions. Proteomic techniques refer to defined methods that allow to analyze simultaneously multiple proteins present in a biological samples and evaluate their relative abundance (expression level profiling) as well as other physicochemical characteristics such as post-translational modifications (phosphorylation, glycosylation, ubiquitination, etc.) as compared to a control sample.

Prosep-G A reagent developed by Millipore based on IgG binding properties of Protein-G by which antibody purification is performed to concentrate and enrich antigen-specific antibodies and to lower background by removing any nonspecific immunoglobulins.

PTM (Post-translational modification) It is the chemical modification of a protein after its translation; however, the term is broadly used to also include cotranslational and xenobiotic protein modifications. As one of the later steps in proteosynthesis of many proteins, PTMs are the major factor contributing to structural complexity, diversity, and dynamic nature of the proteomes. This is due to the chemical variability, temporary or permanent nature, and varied stoichiometry of PTMs. These may include multitopic (site-specific) additions or subtractions of carbohydrate residues (glycosylation), lipids (lipoylation), phosphate groups (phosphorylation), conjugation to other proteins such as ubiquitin (ubiquitinylation), acylations (e.g., acetylation, myristoylation), and proteolytic processing, among many other modifications, of which many are of (patho)physiological significance.

SDS-PAGE Sodium dodecyl sulfate-polyacrylamide (SDS) gel electrophoresis is an electrophoretic technique in which proteins complexed with SDS separate according to their molecular size (M*r*) in a gel medium (typically polyacrylamide). The monodirectional electrophoretic mobility of the proteins is achieved by uniformly labeling them negatively through addition of negatively charged SDS molecules. Sodium dodecyl sulfate is an anionic detergent that denatures proteins by "wrapping around" the polypeptide backbone. In doing so, SDS confers a negative charge to the polypeptide in proportion to its length – i.e., the denatured polypeptides become "rods" of negative charge cloud with equal charge densities per polypeptide unit length.

SELDI (Surface-enhanced laser desorption/ionization) is a MALDI-TOF type mass spectrometric ionization method that is typically used for the analysis of protein mixtures. Proteins are captured by adsorption, partition, electrostatic interaction, or affinity chromatography on a solid-phase protein surface ("chip"). Next, a laser ionization of the analytes cocrystallized with the matrix on a target surface and their mass analysis are achieved via the MALDI-TOF process. The protein chip chromatographic surfaces in SELDI are uniquely designed to retain proteins from complex mixtures according to their specific properties.

SPARC (secreted protein acidic and rich in cysteine) A protein that regulates endothelial cell shape and barrier function amongst other functions.

TOF (time of flight) It describes the mass spectrometry method used in proteomics research to measure the molecular masses of molecular ions such as proteins and peptides.

VEGF (vascular endothelial growth factor or vascular permeability factor) A secreted protein that acts through specific cell-surface receptors on endothelial cells to critically regulate vasculogenesis.

References

Abbott, N. J. (2005). "Dynamics of CNS barriers: evolution, differentiation, and modulation." *Cell Mol Neurobiol* **25**(1): 5–23.

Abdi, F., J. F. Quinn, J. Jankovic, M. McIntosh, J. B. Leverenz, E. Peskind, R. Nixon, J. Nutt, K. Chung, C. Zabetian, A. Samii, M. Lin, S. Hattan, C. Pan, Y. Wang, J. Jin, D. Zhu, G. J. Li, Y. Liu, D. Waichunas, T. J. Montine and J. Zhang (2006). "Detection of biomarkers with a multiplex quantitative proteomic platform in cerebrospinal fluid of patients with neurodegenerative disorders." *J Alzheimers Dis* **9**(3): 293–348.

Bergquist, J., M. Palmblad, M. Wetterhall, P. Hakansson and K. E. Markides (2002). "Peptide mapping of proteins in human body fluids using electrospray ionization Fourier transform ion cyclotron resonance mass spectrometry." *Mass Spectrom Rev* **21**(1): 2–15.

Bouamrani, A., J. Ternier, D. Ratel, A. L. Benabid, J. P. Issartel, E. Brambilla and F. Berger (2006). "Direct-tissue SELDI-TOF mass spectrometry analysis: a new application for clinical proteomics." *Clin Chem* **52**(11): 2103–6.

Carrette, O., P. R. Burkhard, J. C. Sanchez and D. F. Hochstrasser (2006). "State-of-the-art two-dimensional gel electrophoresis: a key tool of proteomics research." *Nat Protoc* **1**(2): 812–23.

Chaurand, P., S. A. Schwartz, M. L. Reyzer and R. M. Caprioli (2005). "Imaging mass spectrometry: principles and potentials." *Toxicol Pathol* **33**(1): 92–101.

Chen, R. L., E. A. Sage, M. J. Dunn, R. Wait and J. E. Preston (2006). "Optimising ovine cerebrospinal fluid preparation for two-dimensional gel electrophoresis." *Proteomics* **6**(10): 3170–5.
D'Aguanno, S., P. Del Boccio, S. Bernardini, E. Ballone, C. Di Ilio, G. Federici and A. Urbani (2007). "Electrophoretic separations of cerebrospinal fluid proteins in clinical investigations." *Clin Chem Lab Med* **45**(4): 437–49.
Davidsson, P., L. Paulson, C. Hesse, K. Blennow and C. L. Nilsson (2001). "Proteome studies of human cerebrospinal fluid and brain tissue using a preparative two-dimensional electrophoresis approach prior to mass spectrometry." *Proteomics* **1**(3): 444–52.
Dayon, L., A. Hainard, V. Licker, N. Turck, K. Kuhn, D. F. Hochstrasser, P. R. Burkhard and J. C. Sanchez (2008). "Relative quantification of proteins in human cerebrospinal fluids by MS/MS using 6-plex isobaric tags." *Anal Chem* **80**(8): 2921–31.
Fountoulakis, M. and S. Kossida (2006). "Proteomics-driven progress in neurodegeneration research." *Electrophoresis* **27**(8): 1556–73.
Gallo, P., F. Bracco, S. Morara, L. Battistin and B. Tavolato (1985). "The cerebrospinal fluid transferrin/tau proteins. A study by two-dimensional polyacrylamide gel electrophoresis (2D) and agarose isoelectrofocusing (IEF) followed by double-antibody peroxidase labeling and avidin–biotin amplification." *J Neurol Sci* **70**(1): 81–92.
Gannot, G., M. A. Tangrea, H. S. Erickson, P. A. Pinto, S. M. Hewitt, R. F. Chuaqui, J. W. Gillespie and M. R. Emmert-Buck (2007). "Layered peptide array for multiplex immunohistochemistry." *J Mol Diagn* **9**(3): 297–304.
Glasker, S., R. R. Lonser, H. Okamoto, J. Li, H. Jaffee, E. H. Oldfield, Z. Zhuang and A. O. Vortmeyer (2007). "Proteomic profiling: a novel method for differential diagnosis?" *Cancer Biol Ther* **6**(3): 343–5.
Godard, S., G. Getz, M. Delorenzi, P. Farmer, H. Kobayashi, I. Desbaillets, M. Nozaki, A. C. Diserens, M. F. Hamou, P. Y. Dietrich, L. Regli, R. C. Janzer, P. Bucher, R. Stupp, N. de Tribolet, E. Domany and M. E. Hegi (2003). "Classification of human astrocytic gliomas on the basis of gene expression: a correlated group of genes with angiogenic activity emerges as a strong predictor of subtypes." *Cancer Res* **63**(20): 6613–25.
Guerreiro, N., B. Gomez-Mancilla and S. Charmont (2006). "Optimization and evaluation of surface-enhanced laser-desorption/ionization time-of-flight mass spectrometry for protein profiling of cerebrospinal fluid." *Proteome Sci* **4**: 7.
Gygi, S. P., B. Rist, et al. (1999). "Quantitative analysis of complex protein mixtures using isotope-coded affinity tags." *Nat Biotechnol* **17**(10): 994–9.
Hale, J. E., V. Gelfanova, J. S. You, M. D. Knierman and R. A. Dean (2008). "Proteomics of cerebrospinal fluid: methods for sample processing." *Methods Mol Biol* **425**: 53–66.
Hamacher, M., C. Stephan, M. Bluggel, D. Chamrad, G. Korting, L. Martens, M. Muller, H. Hermjakob, D. Parkinson, A. Dowsey, K. A. Reidegeld, K. Marcus, M. J. Dunn, H. E. Meyer and R. Apweiler (2006). "The HUPO Brain Proteome Project jamboree: centralised summary of the pilot studies." *Proteomics* **6**(6): 1719–21.
Hammack, B. N., G. P. Owens, M. P. Burgoon and D. H. Gilden (2003). "Improved resolution of human cerebrospinal fluid proteins on two-dimensional gels." *Mult Scler* **9**(5): 472–5.
Hanash, S. M., M. P. Bobek, D. S. Rickman, T. Williams, J. M. Rouillard, R. Kuick and E. Puravs (2002). "Integrating cancer genomics and proteomics in the post-genome era." *Proteomics* **2**(1): 69–75.
Hawkins, B. T. and R. D. Egleton (2008). "Pathophysiology of the blood–brain barrier: animal models and methods." *Curr Top Dev Biol* **80**: 277–309.
Hu, Y., J. P. Malone, A. M. Fagan, R. R. Townsend and D. M. Holtzman (2005). "Comparative proteomic analysis of intra- and interindividual variation in human cerebrospinal fluid." *Mol Cell Proteomics* **4**(12): 2000–9.
Huang, J. T., T. McKenna, C. Hughes, F. M. Leweke, E. Schwarz and S. Bahn (2007). "CSF biomarker discovery using label-free nano-LC-MS based proteomic profiling: technical aspects." *J Sep Sci* **30**(2): 214–25.

Huhmer, A. F., R. G. Biringer, H. Amato, A. N. Fonteh and M. G. Harrington (2006). "Protein analysis in human cerebrospinal fluid: Physiological aspects, current progress and future challenges." *Dis Markers* **22**(1–2): 3–26.

Hunt, S. M., M. R. Thomas, L. T. Sebastian, S. K. Pedersen, R. L. Harcourt, A. J. Sloane and M. R. Wilkins (2005). "Optimal replication and the importance of experimental design for gel-based quantitative proteomics." *J Proteome Res* **4**(3): 809–19.

Jain, K. K. (2007). "Recent advances in clinical oncoproteomics." *J Buon***12 Suppl 1**: S31–8.

Jin, T., L. S. Hu, M. Chang, J. Wu, B. Winblad and J. Zhu (2007). "Proteomic identification of potential protein markers in cerebrospinal fluid of GBS patients." *Eur J Neurol* **14**(5): 563–8.

Kennedy, S. (2001). "Proteomic profiling from human samples: the body fluid alternative." *Toxicol Lett* **120**(1–3): 379–84.

Khalil, A. A. (2007). "Biomarker discovery: a proteomic approach for brain cancer profiling." *Cancer Sci* **98**(2): 201–13.

Khwaja, F. W., J. S. Duke-Cohan, D. J. Brat and E. G. Van Meir (2006a). "Attractin is elevated in the cerebrospinal fluid of patients with malignant astrocytoma and mediates glioma cell migration." *Clin Cancer Res* **12**(21): 6331–6.

Khwaja, F. W., J. D. Nolen, S. E. Mendrinos, M. M. Lewis, J. J. Olson, J. Pohl, E. G. Van Meir, J. C. Ritchie and D. J. Brat (2006b). "Proteomic analysis of cerebrospinal fluid discriminates malignant and nonmalignant disease of the central nervous system and identifies specific protein markers." *Proteomics* **6**(23): 6277–87.

Khwaja, F. W., M. S. Reed, J. J. Olson, B. J. Schmotzer, G. Y. Gillespie, A. Guha, M. D. Groves, S. Kesari, J. Pohl and E. G. Meir (2007). "Proteomic identification of biomarkers in the cerebrospinal fluid (CSF) of astrocytoma patients." *J Proteome Res* **6**(2): 559–70.

Liang, Y., M. Diehn, N. Watson, A. W. Bollen, K. D. Aldape, M. K. Nicholas, K. R. Lamborn, M. S. Berger, D. Botstein, P. O. Brown and M. A. Israel (2005). "Gene expression profiling reveals molecularly and clinically distinct subtypes of glioblastoma multiforme." *Proc Natl Acad Sci USA* **102**(16): 5814–9.

Liu, P. and J. T. Hwang (2007). "Quick calculation for sample size while controlling false discovery rate with application to microarray analysis." *Bioinformatics* **23**(6): 739–46.

Marchi, N., V. Fazio, L. Cucullo, K. Kight, T. Masaryk, G. Barnett, M. Vogelbaum, M. Kinter, P. Rasmussen, M. R. Mayberg and D. Janigro (2003). "Serum transthyretin monomer as a possible marker of blood-to-CSF barrier disruption." *J Neurosci* **23**(5): 1949–55.

Maurer, M. H., C. Berger, M. Wolf, C. D. Futterer, R. E. Feldmann, Jr., S. Schwab and W. Kuschinsky (2003). "The proteome of human brain microdialysate." *Proteome Sci* **1**(1): 7.

Micallef, J., A. Gajadhar, J. Wiley, L. V. DeSouza, K. W. Michael Siu and A. Guha (2008). "Proteomics: present and future implications in neuro-oncology." *Neurosurgery* **62**(3): 539–55; discussion 539–55.

Ogata, Y., M. C. Charlesworth, L. Higgins, B. M. Keegan, S. Vernino and D. C. Muddiman (2007). "Differential protein expression in male and female human lumbar cerebrospinal fluid using iTRAQ reagents after abundant protein depletion." *Proteomics* **7**(20): 3726–34.

Ogata, Y., M. C. Charlesworth and D. C. Muddiman (2005). "Evaluation of protein depletion methods for the analysis of total-, phospho- and glycoproteins in lumbar cerebrospinal fluid." *J Proteome Res* **4**(3): 837–45.

Pan, S., Y. Wang, J. F. Quinn, E. R. Peskind, D. Waichunas, J. T. Wimberger, J. Jin, J. G. Li, D. Zhu, C. Pan and J. Zhang (2006). "Identification of glycoproteins in human cerebrospinal fluid with a complementary proteomic approach." *J Proteome Res* **5**(10): 2769–79.

Pan, S., D. Zhu, J. F. Quinn, E. R. Peskind, T. J. Montine, B. Lin, D. R. Goodlett, G. Taylor, J. Eng and J. Zhang (2007). "A combined dataset of human cerebrospinal fluid proteins identified by multi-dimensional chromatography and tandem mass spectrometry." *Proteomics* **7**(3): 469–73.

Ramstrom, M., C. Hagman, J. K. Mitchell, P. J. Derrick, P. Hakansson and J. Bergquist (2005). "Depletion of high-abundant proteins in body fluids prior to liquid chromatography Fourier transform ion cyclotron resonance mass spectrometry." *J Proteome Res* **4**(2): 410–6.

Ramstrom, M., A. Zuberovic, C. Gronwall, J. Hanrieder, J. Bergquist and S. Hober (2008). "Development of affinity columns for the removal of high-abundant proteins in cerebrospinal fluid." *Biotechnol Appl Biochem* **52**(2): 159–166.

Rich, J. N., C. Hans, B. Jones, E. S. Iversen, R. E. McLendon, B. K. Rasheed, A. Dobra, H. K. Dressman, D. D. Bigner, J. R. Nevins and M. West (2005). "Gene expression profiling and genetic markers in glioblastoma survival." *Cancer Res* **65**(10): 4051–8.

Righetti, P. G., A. Castagna, F. Antonucci, C. Piubelli, D. Cecconi, N. Campostrini, C. Rustichelli, P. Antonioli, G. Zanusso, S. Monaco, L. Lomas and E. Boschetti (2005). "Proteome analysis in the clinical chemistry laboratory: myth or reality?" *Clin Chim Acta* **357**(2): 123–39.

Romeo, M. J., V. Espina, M. Lowenthal, B. H. Espina, E. F. Petricoin, 3rd and L. A. Liotta (2005). "CSF proteome: a protein repository for potential biomarker identification." *Expert Rev Proteomics* **2**(1): 57–70.

Roy, S., S. A. Josephson, et al. (2008). "Protein biomarker identification in the CSF of patients with CNS lymphoma." *J Clin Oncol* **26**(1): 96–105.

Sanchez-Carbayo, M. (2008). "Dissecting cancer serum protein profiles using antibody arrays." *Methods Mol Biol* **428**: 263–87.

Shi, Q., S. Bao, J. A. Maxwell, E. D. Reese, H. S. Friedman, D. D. Bigner, X. F. Wang and J. N. Rich (2004). "Secreted protein acidic, rich in cysteine (SPARC), mediates cellular survival of gliomas through AKT activation." *J Biol Chem* **279**(50): 52200–9.

Tang, Y., M. T. Nakada, P. Kesavan, F. McCabe, H. Millar, P. Rafferty, P. Bugelski and L. Yan (2005). "Extracellular matrix metalloproteinase inducer stimulates tumor angiogenesis by elevating vascular endothelial cell growth factor and matrix metalloproteinases. " *Cancer Res* **65**(8): 3193–9.

Wiederkehr, F. and D. J. Vonderschmitt (1985). "[2-dimensional electrophoresis of cerebrospinal fluid in various neurological patients]." *Schweiz Med Wochenschr* **115**(11): 368–73.

Yuan, X. and D. M. Desiderio (2005a). "Human cerebrospinal fluid peptidomics." *J Mass Spectrom* **40**(2): 176–81.

Yuan, X. and D. M. Desiderio (2005b). "Proteomics analysis of prefractionated human lumbar cerebrospinal fluid." *Proteomics* **5**(2): 541–50.

Zhang, J., D. R. Goodlett and T. J. Montine (2005). "Proteomic biomarker discovery in cerebrospinal fluid for neurodegenerative diseases." *J Alzheimers Dis* **8**(4): 377–86.

Zheng, P. P., T. M. Luider, R. Pieters, C. J. Avezaat, M. J. van den Bent, P. A. Sillevis Smitt and J. M. Kros (2003). "Identification of tumor-related proteins by proteomic analysis of cerebrospinal fluid from patients with primary brain tumors." *J Neuropathol Exp Neurol* **62**(8): 855–62.

Zougman, A., B. Pilch, A. Podtelejnikov, M. Kiehntopf, C. Schnabel, C. Kumar and M. Mann (2008). "Integrated analysis of the cerebrospinal fluid peptidome and proteome." *J Proteome Res* **7**(1): 386–99.

Chapter 26
Epigenetic Profiling of Gliomas

Raman P. Nagarajan and Joseph F. Costello

Abstract Glioma is understood as a genetic disease in that it is caused and exacerbated by genetic lesions in specific genes that control cell growth, apoptosis, angiogenesis, and invasion. Epigenetics, mitotically heritable changes in gene expression not due to changes in the primary DNA sequence, provides additional mechanisms by which cancer genes can be dysregulated. Gliomas are affected by genetic and epigenetic lesions that can be independent of each other or interacting. The relative contribution of genetic and epigenetic mechanisms in gliomagenesis is currently unknown but under active investigation. Epigenetic analyses in gliomas, to date mostly involving DNA methylation, have identified new tumor suppressor genes; pinpointed mechanisms for inactivation of pathways controlling genome integrity, cell-cycle regulation, proliferation, and invasion; uncovered epigenetic mechanisms regulating drug and radiation resistance that influence prognosis; provided a rationale for epigenetic-based therapies; and provided clinically useful biomarkers of drug response. Newer technologies such as next-generation sequencing will undoubtedly bring more rapid advancements in glioma epigenome profiling, and allow direct integration of DNA methylation and histone modification profiles. Considering that epigenetic enzymes are critical targets for drugs that are already in clinical trials for gliomas, the paucity of information on the glioma epigenome is surprising.

Contents

J.F. Costello (✉)
Department of Neurosurgery, Brain Tumor Research Center, University of California San Francisco, San Francisco, CA, 94143, USA
e-mail: jcostello@cc.ucsf.edu

E.G. Van Meir (ed.), *CNS Cancer*, Cancer Drug Discovery and Development, DOI 10.1007/978-1-60327-553-8_26,

© Humana Press, a part of Springer Science+Business Media, LLC 2009

26.1 A Central Role for Epigenetics in Biology

Epigenetic mechanisms of gene regulation involve enzymatic modifications of DNA and associated histone proteins. Other potential mechanisms such as non-coding RNAs (e.g., microRNAs), nucleosome positioning, chromatin remodeling and higher nuclear organization may also be considered epigenetic, although this is debatable given the lack of knowledge of the potential mitotic heritability of these molecular events and given that epigenetics is defined as a mitotically heritable mechanism.

26.1.1 DNA Methylation and DNA Methyltransferases

DNA methylation is an enzymatic mechanism found in animals, plants, bacteria, and some fungi that adds a methyl group to cytosine to create 5-methylcytosine. In mammals, this occurs almost always in the context of a 5′-CpG-3′ dinucleotide, where the "p" refers to the intervening phosphate. DNA methylation is controlled by DNA methyltransferases (DNMT) that create (DNMT3A, DNMT3B) or maintain (DNMT1) patterns of methylation (Bestor 1988, Okano et al. 1998). DNMT1 acts on hemimethylated DNA generated after replication, methylating the CpG in the newly synthesized strand opposite a methylated CpG on the parental strand, thereby maintaining methylation patterns through cell division. *Dnmt1–/–* knockout mice die during prenatal development and display apoptosis in multiple tissues including brain (Li et al. 1992). DNMT3A and DNMT3B add methyl groups de novo to unmethylated DNA, and thereby help establish methylation patterns. *Dnmt3a–/–* mice develop to term and are apparently normal at birth, but die approximately 4 weeks after birth (Okano et al. 1999). Homozygous deletion of *Dnmt3b* in mice is embryonic lethal and causes multiple severe developmental defects, including growth impairment and neural tube defects. Mice heterozygous null for any one of the three DNA methyltransferases appear normal and are fertile (Li et al. 1992, Okano et al. 1999). Two other DNMTs, DNMT2, and DNMT3L, possess sequence similarity to the other DNMTs, but do not act as methyltransferases on DNA. DNMT2 methylates aspartic acid transfer RNA (Goll et al. 2006), whereas DNMT3L, which also lacks DNA methyltransferase activity, promotes de novo DNA methylation by association with histone H3 unmethylated at lysine 4 and recruitment or activation of DNMT3A2. These and other studies demonstrate that DNA methylation can be directed by histone modifications (Ooi et al. 2007).

26.1.2 Histone Modifications

A second major epigenetic mechanism is the post-translational modification of N-terminal tails of histone proteins by acetylation, methylation, phosphorylation, ubiquitylation, sumoylation, ADP ribosylation, biotinylation and potentially other modifications (Turner 2005). Combinatorial histone modifications create a putative "histone code" that determines chromatin states and thus regulates gene expression. In general, chromatin (defined as DNA, histones, and associated non-histone proteins) can be subdivided into categories by structure and potential for gene expression. Heterochromatin is a relatively compacted chromatin structure and is associated with gene silencing. It is characterized by certain histone modifications, for example, histone H3 lysine 9 trimethylation. Euchromatin is decondensed chromatin that has the potential for gene expression, although it may be transcriptionally active or inactive. Active euchromatin is associated with acetylation of lysines on histone H3, whereas inactive euchromatin is found with H3K27 trimethylation.

Several families of enzymes catalyze post-translational modifications of histones and include acetyltransferases and deacetylases, methyltransferases and demethylases, and others. Multiple types of modifications can be present on a single histone molecule, increasing combinatorial complexity. In addition, histone methylation can be mono-, di-, or trimethylation on a single, specific lysine (e.g., H3K4). Histone variant proteins can substitute for some of the canonical histones (H2A and H3) and, like histone modifications, carry epigenetic information that regulates gene expression and can define chromatin boundaries. Finally, different types of epigenetic modifications do not act alone but interact to create specific chromatin structures and transcriptional states. For example, histone modifications and DNA methylation often work in concert to set up the epigenetic landscape at a particular locus or genomic region (Jia et al. 2007, Meissner et al. 2008, Ooi et al. 2007).

26.1.3 Other Potential Epigenetic Factors

In addition to DNA methylation and histone modifications, there are other interrelated, potentially epigenetic mechanisms including non-coding RNAs, chromatin remodeling and nucleosome positioning, and higher nuclear organization. Together these add additional layers of regulation on gene expression in both normal and disease states. Non-coding RNAs are transcribed from the genome yet unlike mRNAs do not code for proteins. Examples include microRNAs (miRNAs), antisense RNAs, piwi-interacting RNAs (piRNAs), and small nucleolar RNA (snoRNA) [for review see (Kawaji and Hayashizaki 2008)]. miRNAs are 19–25 nt and are cleaved from 60–110 nt hairpin precursors (pre-miRNAs) derived from larger primary transcripts (pri-miRNAs). They regulate gene expression through interactions with mRNA by regions of sequence complementary, and can exert their control through multiple mechanisms, including stimulating the degradation of specific mRNAs or blocking of their translation, the latter being the main mechanism known in mammals (Stefani and Slack 2008).

Nucleosomes are the main functional unit of chromatin. Each nucleosome is composed of a core octamer of histone proteins wrapped around 147 bp of DNA. As described above, the modification of histone tails affects the properties of the chromatin in which a particular nucleosome resides. The spacing of nucleosomes is also an important determinant of transcriptional activity. Nucleosome position can be affected by protein complexes such as the ATP-dependent chromatin remodeling factor SWI/SNF, which utilize energy to cause nucleosome sliding and noncovalent changes in conformation. This regulation of nucleosome position is important for transcriptional activation (Narlikar et al. 2002). Furthermore, nucleosomes can be irregularly packed and folded into higher order structures. This contributes to epigenetic phenomena such as nuclear organization, homologous chromosome pairing, chromosome territories, transcription factories, etc., that are beyond the scope of this review but have the potential for involvement in human disease.

An example of the importance of epigenetic mechanisms and nuclear organization in human disease comes from the study of immunodeficiency, centromere instability, and facial anomalies (ICF) syndrome. ICF syndrome is caused by mutations in the DNA methyltransferase *DNMT3B*, leading to DNA hypomethylation at particular sites, including CpG islands on the inactive X chromosome in females (Hansen et al. 1999, Xu et al. 1999). Matarazzo et al. examined chromosome territories, which are non-random areas of the cell nucleus that are occupied by a particular chromosome, corresponding to the inactive X and Y chromosomes in cells from ICF patients (Matarazzo et al. 2007). They observed that the human pseudoautosomal region (PAR)2 was relocalized toward the outside of the Y and inactive X chromosome territories in cells from ICF patients. On the inactive X, this relocalization can occur for genes distant from the actual site of DNA hypomethylation. Studies like this are still in the early stages but are likely to provide fascinating mechanistic insights into the complex interplay between different forms of epigenetic regulation of chromosomes.

26.1.4 Epigenetic Regulation of Promoter CpG Islands

CpG nucleotides are five times more abundant compared to the rest of the genome in genomic regions of ~ 500 bp – 1 kb called CpG islands (CGIs), which often overlap with gene promoters (McClelland and Ivarie 1982). CGIs in promoters of actively expressed genes are not DNA methylated and are in an open chromatin conformation, characterized by high levels of histone H3 lysine 9 (H3K9) acetylation (Fig. 26.1A and Color Plate 46). CGI promoters of transcriptionally silent genes are also generally not DNA methylated but are in a more closed chromatin conformation, characterized by a lack of H3K9 acetylation and the presence of H3K27 methylation (Fig. 26.1B). The addition of H3K27 methylation is catalyzed by enhancer of zeste 2 (EZH2), a member of the polycomb repressor complex 2 (PRC2) (Cao et al. 2002). These silent promoters are often also bound by polycomb repressor complex 1 (PRC1), preventing transcription initiation by RNA polymerase II (Boyer

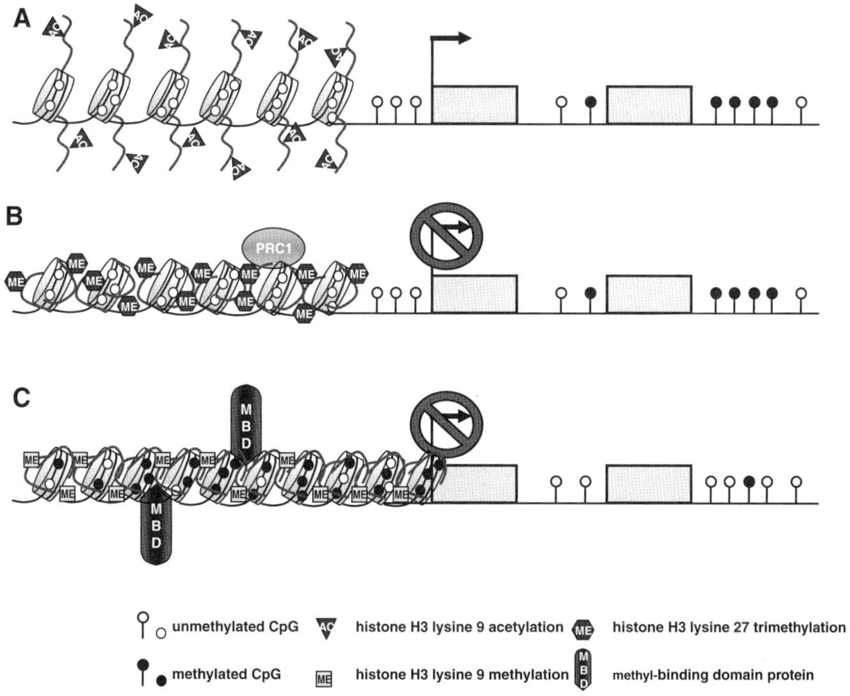

Fig. 26.1 (continued)

et al. 2006, Cao et al. 2002, Dellino et al. 2004). Thus, in normal cells, DNA methylation may play only a minor role in regulating CpG island promoters and associated genes. In cancer cells, many CGI promoters have hypermethylated DNA in addition to having a closed chromatin configuration, marked by addition of histone H3 lysine 9 methylation, loss of H3K9 acetylation, nucleosome occupancy, and the recruitment of methyl-binding domain proteins (MBDs) (Fig. 26.1C).

26.1.5 Functions of DNA Methylation

Epigenetic regulation is involved in diverse biological phenomena including mating-type locus silencing in yeast, position effect variegation in Drosophila, and transgene silencing in both animals and plants. DNA methylation has several specific biological roles. In X chromosome inactivation in mammals, in which one of the two X chromosomes in females is randomly silenced, DNA methylation is required for silencing of genes on the inactive X (Hansen and Gartler 1990, Mohandas et al. 1981, Wolf et al. 1984). However, recent data show that gene bodies (genomic regions corresponding to the exons and introns of a gene) exhibit a methylation pattern opposite to promoter methylation on the X chromosomes, i.e., gene bodies are methylated on the active X and undermethylated on the inactive X, suggesting that gene body methylation might influence gene expression differently than promoter methylation (Hellman and Chess 2007). Indeed, the role of gene body methylation in gene expression has been controversial, but at some loci is conserved evolutionarily, suggesting it has functional importance. DNA methylation also controls allele-specific gene expression of some imprinted loci (Li et al. 1993), is required

◀

Fig. 26.1 (continued) Role of DNA methylation and histone modifications at promoter CpG islands in normal cells and cancer. In normal cells, most promoter CpG islands do not exhibit DNA methylation. Thus the expression status of CpG island-containing genes is primarily determined by the presence or absence of transcription factors and by histone modifications around the promoters of such genes. **(A)** In general, transcriptionally active CpG island loci exhibit unmethylated DNA and high levels of histone H3 lysine 9 acetylation, which are accompanied by an open chromatin configuration. **(B)** Transcriptionally silent genes, however, are marked by histone H3 lysine 27 trimethylation, a modification catalyzed by EZH2 (enhancer of zeste 2), a member of the Polycomb repressor complex 2 (PRC2). Following H3 lysine 27 trimethylation, these promoters can be bound by members of the Polycomb repressor complex 1 (PRC1), which blocks transcription initiation by RNA polymerase II. This is also a mechanism of abnormal gene silencing in cancer, in the absence of aberrant DNA methylation. **(C)** In cancer, a large number of CpG islands are hypermethylated at their DNA, which generally correlates with transcriptional repression of the associated genes. These CpG islands generally exhibit a closed chromatin configuration, marked by histone H3 lysine 9 methylation, loss of acetylation, nucleosome occupancy around the transcription start site and various types of methyl-binding domain proteins. Altogether, these modifications render the chromatin non-permissive for transcription initiation (*see* Color Plate 46) for silencing transposable elements and maintaining genome stability (Eden et al. 2003, Walsh et al. 1998), and is a critical regulator of pluripotency genes (Fouse et al. 2008, Mikkelsen et al. 2008, Takahashi and Yamanaka 2006).

26.1.6 Environment and Epigenetics

An important, newly invigorated paradigm in epigenetics is that the environment can directly impact epigenetic modifications resulting in gene expression changes and phenotypic variation. There is evidence for this in both epidemiological studies and model organisms. In humans, deficiency for dietary folate, a methyl donor, causes global hypomethylation in peripheral white blood cells which can be reversed by folate repletion (Jacob et al. 1998).

In mice, a striking example of the epigenetic effects of an environmental factor, the amount of dietary methyl donors, has been observed. Methyl donors are essential for DNA methylation by supplying one carbon units and cofactors into a biochemical pathway that provides DNMTs with methyl groups for transfer to DNA. Wild-type mice of the C3H/HeJ-*A*/A strain are brown. A spontaneous mutation created the viable yellow allele of the gene *agouti* (*Avy*), resulting in variable coat color depending on the epigenetic status of this allele. The allele is the result of mutational insertion of an intracisternal A-particle (IAP) retrotransposon ~100 kb upstream from *agouti*. A cryptic promoter embedded in this transposon is normally active in *Avy* mice and usurps transcriptional control of *agouti* and drives ectopic expression of its gene product (Duhl et al. 1994, Waterland and Jirtle 2003). The resulting phenotypes include yellow fur, obesity, type II diabetes, and predisposition to tumors. However, the phenotypes display variability on an isogenic background, hinting at epigenetic regulation (Wolff et al. 1999).

Increased dietary methyl donors fed to pregnant *Avy* mothers can cause DNA hypermethylation of the *Avy* cryptic promoter, leading to normal *agouti* gene expression and mottled or brown coat color in offspring (Waterland and Jirtle 2003). Dietary modulation of methyl donors in *Avy* mice also has an effect on susceptibility to diabetes, obesity, and cancer, although the molecular mechanisms for this are unclear (Waterland and Jirtle 2003). The diet-induced epigenetic silencing of the agouti genetic insertion mutation can be transmitted through at least two generations of mice as a result of incomplete erasure of the DNA methylation in the germ line (Cropley et al. 2006, Morgan et al. 2008).

In humans, inter-individual variability and familial clustering of DNA methylation has been observed at specific Alu repeat elements and at the differentially methylated regions (DMRs) of two imprinted loci, *IGF2/H19* and *IGF2R* (Sandovici et al. 2005). Furthermore, intra-individual changes in global methylation occur over time and the magnitude of change appears to have a familial component (Bjornsson et al. 2008). Thus the extent and consequences of epigenetic variability and potential transgenerational inheritance are just beginning to be explored and this may become an entirely new field of inquiry within epigenetics. These studies have important implications for understanding how epigenetic mechanisms might arise in and contribute to clonal selection during tumor initiation and progression.

26.1.7 Epigenetic Regulation in the CNS

Proper epigenetic regulation is critical to development and function of the mammalian CNS. Human and mouse brain exhibit high levels of methylcytosine compared to other tissues (Ehrlich et al. 1982, Tawa et al. 1990). DNA methylation levels are dynamic during brain development (Tawa et al. 1990), and different brain regions also show variable DNA methylation patterns at certain loci (Ladd-Acosta et al. 2007). The relationship between brain-region-specific gene expression (Lein et al. 2007) and brain-region-specific DNA methylation has not been fully explored. Even within specific brain regions, distinct cell types may be differentially marked by DNA methylation. In murine astrogliogenesis, DNA demethylation of the *Gfap* promoter and subsequent unblocking of a DNA sequence containing a binding site for transcription factor STAT3 is associated with *Gfap* transcription, a marker of astroglial lineage (Takizawa et al. 2001). A single CpG site within the *Gfap* promoter is methylated in neural precursors and postmitotic neurons and becomes unmethylated in astrocytes (Condorelli et al. 1997, 1994, Takizawa et al. 2001).

26.1.8 Role of DNA Methyltransferases in the CNS

DNA methyltransferases are important in CNS development and function. The maintenance methyltransferase DNMT1 is expressed highly in the mammalian brain (Goto et al. 1994, Inano et al. 2000, Trasler et al. 1996) including in postmitotic neurons, despite its proposed primary role in copying methylation during DNA replication. Conditional *Dnmt1* deletion in murine postmitotic neurons did not affect DNA methylation levels or cell survival (Fan et al. 2001). On the other hand, conditional *Dnmt1* deletion in embryonic day 12 neuroblasts resulted in DNA hypomethylation and lethality immediately after birth due to respiratory failure, indicating a requirement for DNA methylation in neural precursor cells. Mosaic mice with ~30% *Dnmt1–/–* cells survived into adulthood, but mutant cells were rapidly eliminated from the brain within 3 weeks of birth (Fan et al. 2001). Dnmt3b is expressed in the murine CNS for a short time during neurogenesis, whereas Dnmt3a is expressed in both the prenatal and postnatal CNS (Feng et al. 2005). *Dnmt3b–/–* mice exhibit prenatal lethality and neural tube defects, demonstrating a critical role for DNMT3b in neurodevelopment (Okano et al. 1999). Mice with conditional deletion of *Dnmt3a* in the nervous system are born apparently healthy but die prematurely, displaying hypoactivity, abnormal walking, and poor performance on tests of neuromuscular function and motor coordination (Nguyen et al. 2007). The specific effects of Dnmt deficiency on neurons vs. glia are not well established and warrant further investigation.

Epigenetic-modifying enzymes are also critical in the development and function of the CNS in humans. Several neurodevelopmental disorders are caused by mutations in genes encoding proteins involved in epigenetic mechanisms. Rett syndrome, for example, is a severe neurodevelopmental disorder caused by mutations in *MECP2* which encodes a protein that can bind to methylated DNA and regulate gene expression (Amir et al. 1999). Human ICF syndrome, which includes mental retardation, is caused by mutations in the de novo DNA methyltransferase *DNMT3B* (Hansen et al. 1999, Tuck-Muller et al. 2000, Xu et al. 1999). Furthermore, the dependence of the CNS on epigenetic regulation extends beyond DNA methylation and DNA methyltransferases: mutations in genes encoding other epigenetic regulatory proteins can cause neurodevelopmental disorders. One example is *JARID1/SMCX*, encoding a JmjC-domain-containing histone demethylase which, when mutated, causes a form of X-linked mental retardation (Jensen et al. 2005, Tahiliani et al. 2007).

These studies illustrate the importance of epigenetic control of gene expression in the development and function of the CNS. This knowledge of the critical role of epigenetic mechanisms and marks in the CNS provides a foundation for understanding the role of epigenetic regulation in tumors arising from CNS cells. Brain tumor research will continue to gain insights from basic neuroepigenetics.

26.2 Epigenetic Dysregulation in Cancer

26.2.1 DNA Hypomethylation in Cancer

Epigenetics alterations were first reported in human cancer in the early 1980s. These initial studies focused on a pronounced decrease in the total 5-methylcytosine content in the genome, referred to as global DNA hypomethylation, occurring in both benign and malignant tumors, including glioblastomas (Diala et al. 1983, Feinberg et al. 1988, Feinberg and Vogelstein 1983a, Gama-Sosa et al. 1983, Goelz et al. 1985, Hoffman 1982). DNA hypomethylation also was observed in particular genes, such as the oncogene *HRAS*, indicating that individual loci relevant to cancer might be targets of epigenetic dysregulation (Feinberg and Vogelstein 1983b). However, these changes were not specifically in the *HRAS* gene promoter and have not been shown to directly increase HRAS expression. Since these initial discoveries, aberrant DNA hypomethylation has been found in many cancer types, affecting single-copy genes and often repetitive genomic sequences, and its molecular consequences are beginning to be unraveled. Repetitive elements, which comprise approximately half of the human genome, account for the majority of global hypomethylation in cancer (Ehrlich 2002). In addition, gene-specific hypomethylation is associated with the degree of global hypomethylation. For example, the demethylation of the promoter of the melanoma antigen family A, 1 (*MAGEA1*) gene and its transcriptional activation are linked to global hypomethylation and tumor progression in multiple cancers (Cadieux et al. 2006, De Smet et al. 1996).

There are multiple consequences of aberrant DNA hypomethylation in cancer cells. One consequence is an increased genetic mutation rate. Murine embryonic stem cells nullizygous for *Dnmt1*, resulting in genomic hypomethylation, displayed elevated mutation rates at both the endogenous hypoxanthine phosphoribosyltransferase (*Hprt*) gene and an integrated viral thymidine kinase transgene, with deletions being the predominant mutations at both loci (Chen et al. 1998). The mechanism for this is unknown but could be related to aberrant genetic recombination. In human ICF syndrome, lymphocytes from patients show hypomethylation of particular repetitive sequences such as pericentromeric satellite 2 and 3 repeats leading to chromosomal instability and subsequent chromosomal breakage (Ehrlich et al. 2008).

In addition to demonstrating an increased mutation rate, experiments in mice have shown that DNA hypomethylation can contribute to and sometimes be sufficient for tumorigenesis. Hypomethylation induced by a hypomorphic allele of DNA methyltransferase 1 (*Dnmt1Chip/–)* (that reduces Dnmt1 expression to 10% of wild-type levels and causes genome-wide hypomethylation in all tissues) is sufficient to initiate tumorigenesis in mice (aggressive T-cell lymphomas) (Gaudet et al. 2003). DNA hypomethylation can also increase genomic instability and tumor incidence in a murine *Nf1*$^{+/-}$ *p53*$^{+/-}$ genetic model of sarcoma (Eden et al. 2003). Mouse lymphomas induced by DNA hypomethylation can activate endogenous retroviral elements resulting in increased retrotransposition. In mice, hypomethylation causes relatively frequent IAP somatic insertion into the *Notch1* genomic locus, generating an oncogenic form of Notch1 (Howard et al. 2008). In human cancers, however, the disruption of cancer genes by retrotransposition appears to be rare relative to other mutational mechanisms. Finally, murine models of defective imprinting provide evidence for a causal role in tumorigenesis. Imprinting refers to the parental-specific allelic expression of some mammalian genes which is often mediated by differential allele-specific DNA methylation. Hypomethylation- induced loss of imprinting (LOI), caused by transient experimentally induced demethylation of imprints in embryonic stem cells, leads to widespread solid tumors in chimeric adult mice (Holm et al. 2005).

26.2.2 DNA Hypermethylation in Cancer

Following the initial discovery of global and gene-specific hypomethylation in cancer, aberrant DNA hypermethylation of CpG island promoters was also reported, and the extensive list of hypermethylated genes in cancer now rivals the list of genetically altered genes. Promoter CpG hypermethylation usually involves high levels of methylation affecting a large portion of CpG sites in a promoter. The first observation of hypermethylation was at the calcitonin gene promoter, and the first observation at a known tumor suppressor was at the retinoblastoma (*RB*) gene promoter, which was shown to be associated with transcriptional silencing in cultured tumor cells (Baylin et al. 1986, Greger et al. 1994, 1989, Ohtani-Fujita et al. 1993, Sakai et al. 1991). Since the mid-1990s, promoter hypermethylation has been found in many tumor suppressor genes, such as *INK4/p16*, *MLH1*, and *VHL*. Dense promoter methylation is thought to contribute to transcriptional silencing through several potential mechanisms, including (1) direct blocking of transcription factor binding and (2) binding of methyl-DNA binding proteins that recruit transcriptional repressors such as histone deacetylase, creating a more compact chromatin structure that precludes transcription. Nevertheless, the causal nature of the relationship between aberrant promoter methylation and gene silencing, and their temporal order, is still debated (Baylin and Bestor 2002).

Alterations in DNA methylation at specific loci in cancer can occur in conjunction with or independent from genetic mutations. Consistent with the Knudson two-hit hypothesis, DNA hypermethylation can (1) inactivate both alleles of tumor suppressor genes in sporadic cancer; (2) provide a second "hit" resulting in loss of heterozygosity in familial cancer (Grady et al. 2000, Yanagisawa et al. 2000); or (3) can be a first hit in some familial cancers (Chan et al. 2006, Suter et al. 2004). In addition, the late age of onset of many cancers is consistent with a contributing epigenetic etiology, since both genetic and epigenetic alterations increase with aging (Bjornsson et al. 2008).

Loss of imprinting (LOI) can be caused by DNA hypermethylation in human cancers. The imprinting disorder Beckwith-Weidemann syndrome (BWS), which is caused by maternal deficiency at the 11p15 locus, results in increased tumors including Wilms tumors. LOI was found in Wilms tumors in 1993–1994, caused by gain of methylation and silencing of the gene *H19*, whereas the co-regulated and reciprocally imprinted gene *IGF2* is upregulated (Moulton et al. 1994, Ogawa et al. 1993a, b, Rainier et al. 1993, Steenman et al. 1994). Notably, this epimutation (an epigenetic alteration not affecting the primary DNA sequence) was found in local surrounding non-tumor tissue and was the earliest molecular change observed, suggesting a gatekeeper role for epigenetic alterations in some cancers. Although the number of known imprinted genes in the mammalian genome is small (100–200) (Morison et al. 2001) they appear to have a disproportional role in cancer, likely due to their propensity to encode for proteins that regulate cell growth.

26.2.3 Histone Code Modifications and Cancer

Neither genes encoding DNMTs nor histone-modifying enzymes are frequently mutated in human cancers, except for some acute leukemias which have common translocations involving the mixed lineage leukemia (*MLL*) gene, which encodes an H3K4 methyltransferase that promotes gene expression. These translocations result in MLL fusion proteins that have lost H3K4 methyltransferase activity. Despite the lack of common mutations in epigenetic-modifying enzymes in cancer, epigenetically silenced loci, in addition to being DNA hypermethylated, are characterized by aberrant patterns of histone modifications. Silenced CpG island promoters are characterized by increased histone H3K9 methylation and loss of H3K9 acetylation (Fig. 26.1C). Some silenced genes in cancer cells may result from a chromatin structure similar to that found in developmentally regulated genes in embryonic stem (ES) cells. This pattern is characterized by the dual presence of H3K27 methylation and H3K4 methylation (bivalent domains) and is thought to create a "poised" chromatin state for developmentally regulated genes, allowing silencing in ES cells and subsequent transcriptional activation or repression in differentiated cells (Bernstein et al. 2006). In cancer cells, promoter DNA hypermethylation is sometimes associated with enhancer of zeste 2 (EZH2)-mediated H3K27 methylation (Schlesinger et al. 2007, Widschwendter et al. 2007, Vire et al. 2006). Furthermore, histone modification patterns similar to bivalent domains are found in at promoters of genes silenced by DNA hypermethylation in cancer. These histone modifications are hypothesized to predispose tumor suppressor genes to DNA hypermethylation and heritable silencing (McGarvey et al. 2008, Ohm et al. 2007).

For silencing of some genes in cancer, DNA hypermethylation might not be causal or required. The EZH2 histone methyltransferase silences approximately 5% of gene promoters in prostate cancer cells by histone H3K27 trimethylation independent of DNA methylation (Kondo et al. 2008). The order and hierarchy of epigenetic modifications in the process of gene silencing is an area of extensive investigation and will likely yield clues about potential primary causes of epigenetic alterations in cancer.

26.2.4 Nucleosome Positioning Alterations in Cancer

Nucleosome positioning in promoters might also be a critical regulator of epigenetic gene silencing in cancer. *MLH1* promoter hypermethylation is correlated with nucleosome occupancy and gene silencing in cancer cell lines (Lin et al. 2007), whereas unmethylated CpG islands have nucleosome-free zones. Furthermore, single molecule analysis of demethylation induced by 5-aza-2′-deoxycytidine (5-aza) showed long-term loss of promoter nucleosomes. However, many demethylated promoters contained nucleosomes 72 hours after treatment, suggesting that DNA demethylation might indirectly cause promoter nucleosome depletion as a result of destabilization of nucleosomes, resulting in eventual gene reactivation.

26.2.5 Causes of Epigenetic Modifications in Cancer

The causes and consequences of these different types of epigenetic dysregulation in cancer remain an area of intense investigation, with significant progress being made in understanding the consequences. The causes, however, remain mostly obscure. For aberrant DNA methylation in cancer cells, multiple causes have been proposed. Alterations in DNA methyltransferase enzymes are one obvious possibility, and although mutations in *DNMT* genes have not been reported in cancer, there is evidence for their aberrant expression. In particular, expression of DNMT3B splice variants and aberrant transcripts are associated with several cancers, including GBM (Kanai et al. 2004, Ostler et al. 2007, Saito et al. 2002). In the $Apc^{min/+}$ mouse model of intestinal cancer, induced overexpression of Dnmt3b1 caused increased tumor number accompanied by gene-specific de novo methylation (Linhart et al. 2007). In GBM cell lines, increased DNMT1 and decreased DNMT3A mRNA and protein have been reported (Fanelli et al. 2008).

Alterations in epigenetic regulatory proteins other than DNMTs also might cause changes in DNA methylation, albeit indirectly. For example, in ATRX disorder (α-thalassemia, myelodysplasia) mutations in *ATRX*, encoding a DNA helicase, lead to hypomethylation of repetitive sequences including ribosomal DNA (Gibbons et al. 2000). This example illustrates that an epigenetic regulatory protein other than a DNMT can indirectly affect DNA methylation levels at specific subsets of genomic loci, though it is not known if this indirect mechanism is relevant in cancer.

In theory, either an initial genetic or an epigenetic abnormality could result in tumorigenesis and cause further downstream genetic and epigenetic changes. In glioma, epigenetic silencing of the tumor suppressor gene WNK lysine deficient protein kinase 2 (*WNK2)* was significantly associated with combined deletion of chromosomes 1p and 19q (Hong et al. 2007). WNK2 in directly inhibits MEK1, enhancing growth-promoting signals through EGFR (Moniz et al. 2008, 2007). Thus, it is possible that the epigenetic silencing of *WNK2* interacts on a pathway level with genetic alteration of EGFR signaling, a common abnormality in glioblastomas. In contrast to gliomas, more commonly occurring cancers exhibit genetic point mutations in all four *WNK* genes.

26.2.6 Environmental Factors Affecting Epigenetic Modifications in Cancer

There is also evidence that environmental factors can directly promote tumorigenesis through epigenetic dysregulation. For example, arsenic induces genome-wide and *Ras*-specific hypomethylation in mice (Okoji et al. 2002) and low-dose benzene exposure in humans causes DNA methylation defects at multiple loci, including *MAGEA1* hypomethylation and *p15* hypermethylation (Bollati et al. 2007). More research into this area is needed and should help to determine which environmental risk factors can cause epigenetic dysregulation contributing to cancer.

26.3 Epigenetic Dysregulation in Gliomas

26.3.1 Overview of Epigenetic Alterations in Gliomas

Similar to other tumor types, gliomas exhibit extensive epigenetic abnormalities, including gene-specific hypermethylation, gene-specific and global hypomethylation, and LOI. An important early discovery was global decrease in 5-methylcytosine in a subset of GBM and astrocytoma samples (Gama-Sosa et al. 1983). Recent follow-up studies show that global hypomethylation occurs at a high frequency (~80%) in primary glioblastomas (Cadieux et al. 2006). As in other cancer types, the causes and consequences of global DNA hypomethylation in gliomas have not been fully elucidated.

The best example of locus-specific hypomethylation in gliomas is at the cancer-testis antigen gene *MAGEA1*, which has been observed in astrocytoma and GBM (Cadieux et al. 2006, Yu et al. 2004). *MAGEA1*, a member of the MAGE family of genes, is one of a group of germline-specific genes that become transcriptionally activated in multiple tumors, and this activation is correlated with genome-wide hypomethylation and increased cellular proliferation (Cadieux et al. 2006, De Smet et al. 1996). The expression of the protein products of these "cancer-testis antigen" genes in tumors results in the recognition of tumor-specific antigens on the cell surface by cytolytic T lymphocytes and also inhibits p53 function and response to chemotherapy (Liu et al. 2004, Van Der Bruggen et al. 2002).

Locus-specific hypermethylation, mostly at CpG island promoters, is a frequent observation in gliomas, including low-grade astrocytomas and oligodendrogliomas. These silencing events occur at genes with diverse functions related to tumorigenesis and tumor progression, including cell-cycle regulation, DNA repair, apoptosis, angiogenesis, invasion, and drug resistance. The RB and PI3K pathways are examples of pathways affected by epigenetic silencing (including *CDKN2/p16, RB,* and *PTEN*) (Baeza et al. 2003, Costello et al. 1996, Nakamura et al. 2001). Promoter methylation is also frequent in genes within the p53 pathway, including *TP53* and $p14^{ARF}$ (Amatya et al. 2005, Bello and Rey 2006, Watanabe et al. 2001).

Genome-scale epigenetic analyses have identified new tumor suppressor candidates as well as *bona fide* tumor suppressors in gliomas. One example is at chromosome 19q. Deletions in this region in gliomas and neuroblastomas have suggested the presence of an unknown tumor suppressor. Expression array analysis of glioma cells treated with a DNA demethylating agent discovered a candidate tumor suppressor, epithelial membrane protein 3 (*EMP3),* a myelin-related gene involved in cell proliferation and cell–cell interactions (Alaminos et al. 2005).

EMP3 is silenced by hypermethylation in primary gliomas and reintroduction of *EMP3* in neuroblastoma cell lines with *EMP3* silencing resulted in reduced colony formation in vitro and decreased xenograft growth in mice, suggesting tumor suppressor function (Alaminos et al. 2005).

The oncogenic, pro-proliferative transforming growth factor (TGF)-beta signaling pathway in aggressive, highly proliferative gliomas is affected by an interesting type of epigenetic dysregulation. High levels of TGF-beta signaling are normally associated with poor prognosis in glioma. TGF-beta signaling promotes proliferation through the induction of platelet-derived growth factor *(PDGF)-B*. However, epigenetic silencing of *PDGF-B* can override the pro-proliferative effects of TGF-beta signaling. Specifically, *PDGF-B* promoter hypermethylation prevents *PDGF-B* transcriptional activation by TGF-beta-induced Smad proteins (Bruna et al. 2007). The oncogenic affect of the TGF-beta pathway is therefore blocked by epigenetic alteration of one of its targets.

Genes involved in invasion and metastasis can also be affected by hypermethylation in gliomas. A high frequency of astrocytomas (88%), GBMs (87%), and glioma cell lines (100%) tested exhibit CpG island hypermethylation of the protocadherin-gamma subfamily A11 (*PCDH-gamma-A11*) gene, which is thought to be important in invasion of cancer cells into normal brain parenchyma (Waha et al. 2005). However, the use of the sensitive MSP method for detecting methylation may overestimate the percentage of tumors in which methylation reaches a biologically meaningful level.

26.3.2 Epigenetic Silencing of MGMT *and Drug Resistance to Alkylating Agents*

One particularly important example of epigenetic silencing of a drug resistance gene is promoter hypermethylation of O6-methylguanine-DNA methyltransferase (*MGMT*) in glioma. *MGMT* encodes a DNA repair protein, O6-methylguanine-DNA methyltransferase, that removes alkyl adducts at the O6 position of guanine and (less frequently) at the O4 position of thymine (Gerson 2004). Expression of *MGMT* protects normal cells from carcinogens; however, it can also protect cancer cells from chemotherapeutic alkylating agents. *MGMT* promoter methylation is negatively correlated with expression and is associated with decreased transcription factor binding in glioma cell lines (Costello et al. 1994a, b). An initial report suggested a paradoxical positive correlation between *MGMT* methylation and expression in cancer cell lines (Pieper et al. 1991). However, updates in the genomic structure of the *MGMT* gene showed that the paradoxically higher level of methylation in MGMT-expressing cells was located 60–240 kb downstream of the *MGMT* promoter. Hypermethylation of the *MGMT* promoter, leading to transcriptional silencing, occurs in multiple primary human tumors, including glioma, lymphoma, breast cancer, prostate cancer, and retinoblastoma (Esteller et al. 1999a). In human colorectal cancer, *MGMT* promoter methylation is associated with increased G to A transition mutations in *TP53* and *K-RAS* (Esteller et al. 2001, 2000).

MGMT hypermethylation is associated with significantly longer survival in glioblastomas and low-grade gliomas treated with radiation and alkylating agents, including temozolomide (Everhard et al. 2006, Hegi et al. 2005), although it is unclear if this is directly due to reduced MGMT expression (see also Chapter 28). Furthermore, *MGMT* hypermethylation is a predictor of the incidence and outcome of pseudoprogression (progressive and enhancing lesions observed by MRI immediately after the end of treatment that are not actual tumor progression, but rather are an effect of the radiotherapy and temozolomide treatment) (Brandes et al. 2008). *MGMT* hypermethylation is a late event in progressive oligodendrogliomas, leading to the hypothesis that *MGMT* methylation may have a different prognostic value for oligodendrogliomas compared to GBMs and low-grade gliomas (Lavon et al. 2007). The predictive value of *MGMT* methylation may be increased when used in conjunction with gene expression data (Murat et al. 2008). However, further technical refinement is needed for the commonly used *MGMT* methylation assay: particularly when applied to fixed tissue, the methylation-specific PCR (MSP) method is prone to false positives (Rand et al. 2002).

26.3.3 Patterns of Epigenetic Alterations in Gliomas

CpG island hypermethylation can occur on both alleles of a tumor suppressor or on one allele while the other allele is altered by a genetic mechanism. However, most aberrant methylation events in glioma are focal and independent of deletions, suggesting a widespread and independent role for epigenetic dysregulation (Zardo et al. 2002). Glioma hypermethylation events can occur concurrently, suggestive of a hypermethylator phenotype, such as the observation that the *ER* and *N33* genes display concordant methylation in GBM (Li et al. 1998). As in other cancers, imprinted genes can also be affected by hypermethylation in glioma. LOI of *IGF2* has been reported in primary glioma (Uyeno et al. 1996) and *PEG3* is epigenetically silenced resulting in LOI in some glioma cell lines (Maegawa et al. 2001).

Different glioma subtypes and tumor grades display distinct aberrant DNA methylation profiles (Uhlmann et al. 2003). Secondary GBMs have a higher overall frequency of promoter methylation compared to primary GBMs, at least for the promoters of $p14^{ARF}$, $p16^{INK4a}$, *RB1*, *MGMT*, and *TIMP-3* (Ohgaki and Kleihues 2007). Low-grade gliomas and secondary GBMs show *PTEN* promoter methylation and activation of the PI3K pathway as measured by protein kinase B (PKB/AKT) phosphorylation, whereas *PTEN* promoter methylation is a rare occurrence in primary GBMs (Wiencke et al. 2007). On the other hand, the same epigenetic alterations can be shared by different types of brain tumors, even in different species. For example, *SLC5A8* is inactivated in human oligodendrogliomas and astrocytomas and in mouse models of oligodendroglial tumors by an epigenetic mechanism, suggesting that aberrant epigenetic silencing of this locus is common in mammalian gliomas (Hong et al. 2005). CNS cancers other than gliomas also display distinct methylation profiles: for example, *hMLH1*, *TIMP3*, *MGMT*, *p73*, and *THBS1* are frequently hypermethylated in schwannomas (Bello et al. 2007), and *NF2* is genetically and epigenetically altered in meningioma (Lomas et al. 2005).

The progression of glioma over time is associated with distinct epigenetic patterns. Malignant progression and shorter survival in astrocytoma are associated with $p14^{ARF}$ but not *MGMT* hypermethylation, suggesting that these are two distinct pathways in astrocytoma with different clinical consequences (Watanabe et al. 2007). Recurrence is also characterized by specific epigenetic marks: hypermethylation of the pro-apoptotic gene caspase-8 is frequently associated with relapsed GBM (Martinez et al. 2007). Increased recurrence-free survival is associated with *CITED4* hypermethylation at 1p43.2 and 1p and 19q losses (Tews et al. 2007). Murine glioma models also provide evidence of a role for epigenetic mechanisms in modifying tumor progression. In a mouse model of astrocytoma with mutant *Trp53* and *Nf1*, a genetic modifier controlling susceptibility to progression is itself epigenetically modified (Reilly et al. 2004).

Epigenetic alterations affecting gene expression may modulate sensitivity to drugs (i.e., *MGMT* methylation) and radiotherapy. Re-expression of suppressors of cytokine signaling 1 (*SOCS1*) in GBMs with *SOCS1* hypermethylation and transcriptional silencing caused sensitization to ionizing radiation and decreased activation of MAPKs associated with the ERK pathway (Zardo et al. 2002, Zhou et al. 2007). Thus, epigenetic profiling might be one way to molecularly categorize gliomas and to apply rationally designed therapy in a patient-specific manner.

26.3.4 Epigenetics of Glioma Tumor Initiating Cells

Epigenetic mechanisms appear to be important in regulating putative cancer stem cells, also called tumor initiating cells (TICs). Recent data show that DNA hypermethylation can alter the differentiation properties of the fraction of glioma cells thought to be TICs. Normal astroglial differentiation is regulated by the bone morphogenetic protein (BMP) – and ciliary neurotrophic factor (CNTF) – mediated Jak/STAT pathway. In a subset of glioblastoma TICs, this differentiation pathway is inhibited by epigenetic silencing of the BMP receptor 1B (*BMPR1B*) gene (Lee et al. 2008). This silencing is dependent on the histone methyltransferase enhancer of zeste 2 (EZH2) and DNA methylation and could be reversed by treatment with a DNA demethylating agent. These data demonstrate that a subset of human GBM cells are blocked from differentiation though a defect in the BMP signaling pathway. Furthermore, forced expression of *BMPR1B* could restore the differentiation potential of these cells and can decrease tumorigenicity. These findings reinforce the idea that future epigenetic therapies might be applied rationally, guided by patient-specific epigenetic profiling.

The gene encoding the CD133 cell surface marker used to identify and enrich glioma TICs is itself subject to epigenetic regulation. In glioma cell lines, *CD133* promoter CGI DNA methylation was negatively correlated with CD133 expression (Yi et al. 2008). In pure CD133+ cell lines, this methylation was absent. Furthermore, *CD133* methylation was not observed in normal brain but only in cultured and primary tumors, suggesting that it could be an epigenetic tumor-specific marker.

26.3.5 Identification of Genome-Wide Methylation Patterns in Brain Tumors

There are multiple strategies for discovering epigenetic alterations in brain tumors. One approach is to examine candidate loci that are affected by deletion or mutation on one allele, based on the idea that DNA hypermethylation might inactivate the other allele, leading to complete silencing. This strategy, by design, is more likely to discover hypermethylation of tumor suppressors rather than hypomethylation events. A more unbiased approach is to scan the entire genome for both hyper- and hypomethylation events. For gliomas, this was achieved first through the use of methyl-sensitive restriction enzymes (MREs) using a method called restriction landmark genomic scanning (RLGS) (Costello et al. 2000, 1997, Nakamura et al. 1998, 1997a, b, c). Newer, more advanced methods include reduced representation bisulfite sequencing (Meissner et al. 2005) and methylated DNA immunoprecipitation (MeDIP) combined with DNA microarrays (Weber et al. 2005) or massively parallel sequencing (Down et al. 2008), which will surely advance our understanding of epigenetic dysregulation in brain tumors.

One additional approach to uncovering epigenetically altered genes is to use chemical treatment with DNMT1 and histone deacetylase inhibitors such as 5-aza-2′-deoxycytidine (5-aza) and trichostatin A (TSA), respectively, combined with expression microarrays (Karpf et al. 1999). This strategy led to the identification of brain expressed, X-linked 1 (*BEX1)* and 2 (*BEX2)* as candidate tumor suppressors in glioma (Foltz et al. 2006). Another study identified >160 genes upregulated by combined 5-aza and TSA treatment in glioma cell lines and in separate experiments provided evidence that some epigenetically silenced loci are aberrantly methylated by the combined action of DNMT1 and DNMT3B, whereas others are regulated only by a single DNMT (Kim et al. 2006). 5-aza treatment of short-term cultured primary GBMs identified two genes, runt-related transcription factor 3 (*RUNX3)* and testin (*TES*), with aberrant methylation (Mueller et al. 2007). In this chemical approach, numerous genes may be activated indirectly. Thus, follow-up analyses of the epigenetic marks at the activated genes in primary tumors are essential.

26.3.6 Aberrant Expression of MicroRNAs in Gliomas

MicroRNAs are important in normal development and dysregulation of their expression has been observed in multiple cancers. In gliomas, multiple miRNAs can be aberrantly expressed in both primary tumors and cell lines [(Nicoloso and Calin 2008); Chapter 27]. Primary GBMs and cell lines overexpress miR-221, whereas a set of brain-enriched miRNAs (miR-128, miR-181a, miR-181b, and miR-181c) show decreased expression (Ciafre et al. 2005). Another study showed that miR-124 and miR-137 are underexpressed in primary GBM and anaplastic astrocytoma (Silber et al. 2008). MiR-137 expression was increased in GBM cell lines U87 and U251 following treatment with 5-aza-2′-deoxycytidine, suggesting regulation of this microRNA by DNA methylation. Functionally, miR-124 and -137 inhibit proliferation in GBM and can induce differentiation of normal brain tumor stem cells. Additional publications have demonstrated that miR-124 is underexpressed in primary oligodendrogliomas, astroblastomas, and GBM cell lines (Gaur et al. 2007, Landgraf et al. 2007, Nelson et al. 2006) indicating a potentially central role for this non-coding RNA in brain tumors. Overall, microRNAs appear to play multiple roles in cancer biology; for example in GBM miR-21 has both anti-apoptotic and pro-invasion functions (Chan et al. 2005, Gabriely et al. 2008).

26.4 Targeting Epigenetic Events for Therapy in Gliomas

26.4.1 Overview of Epigenetic Therapy for Gliomas

Epigenetic-based therapy is currently being tested in multiple cancers including gliomas. In contrast to genetic mutations which are "hard-wired' and difficult to change once mutated, epimutations such as promoter hypermethylation are theoretically reversible by drug treatment or possibly diet. The main epigenetic-based drugs being tested are DNMT inhibitors and HDAC inhibitors (HDACi) that are proposed to reactivate epigenetically silenced genes such as tumor suppressors, and to open chromatin to expose the DNA to chemotherapeutic agents. For HDACi a proposed mechanism involves inhibition of histone lysine acetylation at promoters of silenced genes leading to increased histone acetylation, more open, accessible chromatin, and transcriptional activation. The activation of these genes would lead to tumor suppression through multiple pathways, such as cell-cycle inhibition and induction of apoptosis.

A major unresolved issue for epigenetic therapy of cancer is target specificity. First, some genes that require DNA methylation or histone deacetylation for silencing in normal cells could be aberrantly activated by agents that inhibit DNMTs or HDACs. The effects of this, if any, are unknown. Second, cancer genomes are characterized by both DNA hyper- and hypomethylation.

Therefore, using drugs that reactivate silenced tumor suppressors may have the undesired effect of further activating oncogenes. These problems should be addressed to gain a more complete understanding of the molecular events resulting from epigenetic-based therapy.

26.4.2 Histone Deacetylase (HDAC) Inhibitors for Glioma Treatment

DNMT inhibitors, such as decitabine (5-aza-2′-deoxycytidine; Dacogen, MGI Pharma, Bloomington, MN) and HDACi such as suberoylanilide hydroxamic acid (SAHA; Vorinostat; Aton Pharma, Lawrenceville, NJ) are in clinical trials for treatment of multiple cancers. Currently only HDACi are in trials for gliomas; at the moment, there are no clinical trials using agents blocking DNA methylation in gliomas.

HDACs catalyze the deacetylation of lysine residues within the N-terminal tails of core histones and also within non-histone proteins. As a result, their effects are complex and involve many protein substrates, and the mechanism of specificity for each HDAC is not well understood. There are 18 known HDACs in humans, divided into five main classes, with different target specificities (Dokmanovic et al. 2007). HDACs of Class I (HDACs 1, 2, 3, and 8), Class IIA (HDACs 4, 5, 7, and 9), Class IIB (HDACs 6 and 10), and Class IV (HDAC 11) all contain zinc in their active sites and are inhibited by TSA and SAHA. Class III HDACs (sirtuins) do not contain zinc and are not inhibited by TSA or SAHA.

HDACi are comprised of several classes of compounds, including hydroxymates (SAHA, TSA), cyclic peptides (depsipeptide), aliphatic acids (valproic acid, butyrate), and benzamides. None of the HDACi are effective against all HDACs, and the mechanism(s) by which cancer cells are affected by HDACi is only partially understood. HDACi can cause increased acetylation of histone and non-histone proteins and reactivate *p21*, which contributes to cell-cycle arrest (Gui et al. 2004, Yin et al. 2007). SAHA treatment increased *p21* promoter histone H3 acetylation in the U87 glioma cell line and inhibited the proliferation of GL26 glioma cells implanted in mice (Yin et al. 2007). Non-cancerous cells are more resistant to the effects of HDACi, but the reasons for this selective sensitivity are unclear (Qiu et al. 1999). HDACi alter the expression levels of only a subset of genes in transformed cells (~2–10%), and both increases and decreases in transcript levels are observed (Gray et al. 2004, Lee et al. 2006b, Mitsiades et al. 2004, Peart et al. 2005).

Three HDACi are in phase I and II clinical trials for gliomas (Table 26.1). SAHA was found to sensitize glioma cells in vitro, ex vivo, and in vivo to chemotherapy and radiation in preclinical studies (Chinnaiyan et al. 2005, Eyupoglu et al. 2005, Kumagai et al. 2007, Ugur et al. 2007) and is now being used as both monotherapy and combination therapy in 5 phase I or I–II clinical trials. Two of these trials use SAHA in combination with temozolomide, and

Table 26.1 Clinical trials of agents targeting HDACs in gliomas

	Disease(s)	HDAC classes targeted	Phase	Sponsor(s)	Status	Clinicaltrials.gov ID
SAHA, Isotretinoin, Carboplatin	GBM	I,II	I,II	M.D. Anderson Cancer Center/Merck	Active	NCT00555399
SAHA, Temozolomide, radiation	GBM	I,II	I,II	NCI/North Central Cancer Treatment Group	Approved, not yet active	NCT00731731
SAHA	GBM	I,II	II	NCI/North Central Cancer Treatment Group	Active	NCT00238303
SAHA, Bortezomib	GBM	I,II	II	NCI/North Central Cancer Treatment Group	Active	NCT00641706
SAHA, Temozolomide	malignant gliomas	I,II	I	NCI/North American Brain Tumor Consortium	Active	NCT00268385
Valproic acid, Temozolomide, radiation	GBM	I,IIA	II	NCI	Active	NCT00313664
Valproate, Etoposide	neuronal tumors and brain metastases	I,IIA	I	M.D. Anderson Cancer Center	Active	NCT00513162
Depsipeptide	High-grade gliomas	I	I,II	NCI/North American Brain Tumor Consortium	Closed	NCT00085540

one of these also includes radiotherapy. A third trial is SAHA plus Isotretinoin and Carboplatin, a fourth uses SAHA plus Bortezomib, and a fifth trial is testing SAHA as a monotherapy. SAHA targets class I and II HDACs at micromolar concentrations.

Trials are also currently underway for two additional HDACi, valproic acid (Depakene, Abbott Labs, Abbott Park, IL) and depsipeptide (Romedepsin; FK-228; Gloucester Pharmaceuticals, Cambridge, MA). Valproic acid is being tested against GBM in combination with temozolomide plus radiation, and in a broader second trial against neuronal tumors and brain metastases in combination with etoposide. Depsipeptide monotherapy was tested against recurrent high-grade gliomas; this study is now closed. Valproic acid is active against Class I and IIA HDACs at millimolar concentrations; depsipeptide is active against Class I HDACs at nanomolar concentrations.

There are additional promising HDACi that might be effective in clinical trials. Butyrate is an aliphatic acid HDACi effective against Class I and IIA HDACs at millimolar concentrations. A derivative of butyrate, pivaloyloxymethyl butyrate (AN-9; Titan Pharmaceuticals, South San Francisco, CA) shows efficacy in GBM cell culture and animal models (Entin-Meer et al. 2005, 2007). AN-9 sensitized GBM mouse xenografts to radiation and showed decreased tumor growth and increased survival. There are several HDACi that have shown efficacy against cancer cells but not yet specifically for gliomas. For example, Panobinostat (LBH589, Novartis) is in clinical trials for the treatment of both solid tumors and hematologic malignancies. It is well tolerated and induces clinical responses in cutaneous T-cell lymphoma (CTCL) patients (Ellis et al. 2008) Another HDAC that is in clinical trials for both multiple cancer types and that could be considered for glioma treatment is Belinostat (PXD101, TopoTarget A/S) (Gimsing et al. 2008). The discovery and development of new epigenetic enzyme-targeting compounds is an area of active research in the pharmaceutical industry.

26.4.3 Epigenetic Marks as Biomarkers for Clinical Evaluation

Blood plasma in cancer patients contains DNA derived from tumor cells due to necrotic or apoptotic cancer cells releasing genomic DNA. This potentially provides a less invasive method for biomarker detection. Aberrantly hypermethylated cancer genes found in plasma could be one such type of biomarker. This type of analysis may provide clinically useful information such as diagnosis, prognosis, and follow-up post-therapy. Methylated tumor-specific biomarkers have in fact been found in plasma and serum for several types of cancer (Esteller et al. 1999b, Wong et al. 1999). There is a measureable amount of tumor DNA in the plasma of high-grade glioma patients, and in 60% of patients the same methylated promoters (*p16INK4a*, *MGMT*, *p73*, and *RARbeta* were tested) could be detected in both tumor and plasma DNA (Weaver et al. 2006).

The frequency of detection of methylated promoters in plasma of GBM patients was similar to that in other cancers, suggesting that the blood–brain barrier does not completely block the transfer of tumor DNA to plasma. This method is theoretically highly sensitive, since small amounts of methylated DNA can be detected in a sample by methylation-specific PCR.

26.5 Future Directions for Epigenetics of Gliomas

Epigenetic research into gliomas is poised to make substantial contributions to understanding glioma biology, adding predictive biomarkers and identifying new targets for therapy. New glioma models, such as patient GBM-derived tumor stem cells grown as neurospheres, may be a valuable addition to epigenetic research into GBM, particularly if the epigenetic profiles of the corresponding primary tumor are retained, as has been shown for gene expression patterns and invasive growth patterns of these cells (Lee et al. 2006a, Li et al. 2008). Epigenomic profiling of DNA methylation, histone modifications and non-coding RNAs (such as microRNAs) in primary tumors, orthotopic xenografts, and tumor neurospheres are strategies that will likely uncover many additional epigenetic alterations in gliomas, and therefore targets for therapy.

There are still many questions remaining about the role of epigenetics in gliomas and in all cancers. The causes and consequences of epigenetic alterations are still mostly unknown, and the relative contributions of genetic and environmental factors in causing epigenetic alterations have not been quantified. Why are some genes or pathways more affected by epigenetic rather than genetic alterations or vice versa? It is clear that approaches simultaneously examining both genetic and epigenetic defects, complemented with functional studies, will be essential. It will also be prudent to further study the effects of HDACi on the cancer genome as a whole to understand the molecular consequences of this treatment strategy.

Combination therapy with both DNMT and HDAC inhibitors might be one strategy against gliomas. This dual treatment approach may have a synergistic effect and allow lower doses of each drug to be used. An area that is mostly unexplored in glioma is the development and testing of drugs directed against histone modifications other than acetylation. H3K27 methylation at silenced tumor suppressor promoters could be targeted to reactivate these genes, for example using the S-adenosylhomocysteine hydrolase inhibitor 3-Deazaneplanocin A (DZNep), although the specificity of DZNep for H3K27 methylation remains to be determined (Tan et al. 2007).

Reflecting the increased interest in epigenetics in cancer, The Cancer Genome Atlas (TCGA; http://cancergenome.nih.gov/about/mission.asp) is examining genomic changes and DNA methylation in three cancers: GBM, lung, and ovarian cancer. DNA methylation is being profiled in candidate genes by the Illumina GoldenGate® BeadArray. Currently available data are from the Illumina Cancer Panel I, which includes 1,505 CpG loci selected from 807 genes.

A recent TCGA publication demonstrated that *MGMT* promoter hypermethylation was found to be associated with a hypermutator phenotype due to deficient mismatch repair in temozolomide-treated GBMs (TCGA, 2008). A complementary, project sequenced the exons of 20,661 protein coding genes in GBM (Parsons et al. 2008). The International Cancer Genome Consortium (ICGC) is an additional effort, currently in the planning stages, which will include epigenomic profiling of DNA methylation. Considering there are 30,000 CpG islands in the human genome, next-generation sequencing methods may be required to fully investigate aberrant DNA methylation in CNS tumors. A truly genome-scale map of DNA methylation and histone modifications in GBM will be one key to accelerating understanding of epigenetic mechanisms underlying this deadly disease.

Abbreviations

5-aza	5-aza-2′-deoxycytidine
CGI	CpG island
DNMT	DNA methyltransferase
GBM	glioblastoma multiforme
HDAC	histone deacetylase
HDACi	histone deacetylase inhibitor
ICF	immunodeficiency, centromere instability and facial anomalies
LOI	loss of imprinting
MGMT	O6-methylguanine-DNA methyltransferase
SAHA	suberoylanilide hydroxamic acid
TIC	tumor initiating cell
TSA	trichostatin A

Acknowledgments The authors thank Dan Zhu for providing critical comments on the manuscript and Martin Brena for contributing to the generation of figures and figure legends.

References

Alaminos M, Davalos V, Ropero S, Setien F, Paz MF, Herranz M, Fraga MF, Mora J, Cheung NK, Gerald WL, Esteller M (2005) EMP3, a myelin-related gene located in the critical 19q13.3 region, is epigenetically silenced and exhibits features of a candidate tumor suppressor in glioma and neuroblastoma. Cancer Res 65:2565–2571

Amatya VJ, Naumann U, Weller M, Ohgaki H (2005) TP53 promoter methylation in human gliomas. Acta Neuropathol 110:178–184

Amir RE, Van den Veyver IB, Wan M, Tran CQ, Francke U, Zoghbi HY (1999) Rett syndrome is caused by mutations in X-linked MECP2, encoding methyl-CpG-binding protein 2. Nat Genet 23:185–188

Baeza N, Weller M, Yonekawa Y, Kleihues P, Ohgaki H (2003) PTEN methylation and expression in glioblastomas. Acta Neuropathol 106:479–485

Baylin S, Bestor TH (2002) Altered methylation patterns in cancer cell genomes: cause or consequence? Cancer Cell 1:299–305

Baylin SB, Hoppener JW, de Bustros A, Steenbergh PH, Lips CJ, Nelkin BD (1986) DNA methylation patterns of the calcitonin gene in human lung cancers and lymphomas. Cancer Res 46:2917–2922

Bello MJ, Martinez-Glez V, Franco-Hernandez C, Pefla-Granero C, de Campos JM, Isla A, Lassaletta L, Vaquero J, Rey JA (2007) DNA methylation pattern in 16 tumor-related genes in schwannomas. Cancer Genet Cytogenet 172:84–86

Bello MJ, Rey JA (2006) The p53/Mdm2/p14ARF cell cycle control pathway genes may be inactivated by genetic and epigenetic mechanisms in gliomas. Cancer Genet Cytogenet 164:172–173

Bernstein BE, Mikkelsen TS, Xie X, Kamal M, Huebert DJ, Cuff J, Fry B, Meissner A, Wernig M, Plath K, Jaenisch R, Wagschal A, Feil R, Schreiber SL, Lander ES (2006) A bivalent chromatin structure marks key developmental genes in embryonic stem cells. Cell 125:315–326

Bestor TH (1988) Cloning of a mammalian DNA methyltransferase. Gene 74:9–12

Bjornsson HT, Sigurdsson MI, Fallin MD, Irizarry RA, Aspelund T, Cui H, Yu W, Rongione MA, Ekstrom TJ, Harris TB, Launer LJ, Eiriksdottir G, Leppert MF, Sapienza C, Gudnason V, Feinberg AP (2008) Intra-individual change over time in DNA methylation with familial clustering. JAMA 299:2877–2883

Bollati V, Baccarelli A, Hou L, Bonzini M, Fustinoni S, Cavallo D, Byun HM, Jiang J, Marinelli B, Pesatori AC, Bertazzi PA, Yang AS (2007) Changes in DNA methylation patterns in subjects exposed to low-dose benzene. Cancer Res 67:876–880

Boyer LA, Plath K, Zeitlinger J, Brambrink T, Medeiros LA, Lee TI, Levine SS, Wernig M, Tajonar A, Ray MK, Bell GW, Otte AP, Vidal M, Gifford DK, Young RA, Jaenisch R (2006) Polycomb complexes repress developmental regulators in murine embryonic stem cells. Nature 441:349–353

Brandes AA, Franceschi E, Tosoni A, Blatt V, Pession A, Tallini G, Bertorelle R, Bartolini S, Calbucci F, Andreoli A, Frezza G, Leonardi M, Spagnolli F, Ermani M (2008) MGMT promoter methylation status can predict the incidence and outcome of pseudoprogression after concomitant radiochemotherapy in newly diagnosed glioblastoma patients. J Clin Oncol 26:2192–2197

Bruna A, Darken RS, Rojo F, Ocana A, Penuelas S, Arias A, Paris R, Tortosa A, Mora J, Baselga J, Seoane J (2007) High TGFbeta-Smad activity confers poor prognosis in glioma patients and promotes cell proliferation depending on the methylation of the PDGF-B gene. Cancer Cell 11:147–160

Cadieux B, Ching TT, VandenBerg SR, Costello JF (2006) Genome-wide hypomethylation in human glioblastomas associated with specific copy number alteration, methylenetetrahydrofolate reductase allele status, and increased proliferation. Cancer Res 66:8469–8476

Cao R, Wang L, Wang H, Xia L, Erdjument-Bromage H, Tempst P, Jones RS, Zhang Y (2002) Role of histone H3 lysine 27 methylation in Polycomb-group silencing. Science New York, NY 298:1039–1043

Chan JA, Krichevsky AM, Kosik KS (2005) MicroRNA-21 is an antiapoptotic factor in human glioblastoma cells. Cancer Res 65:6029–6033

Chan TL, Yuen ST, Kong CK, Chan YW, Chan AS, Ng WF, Tsui WY, Lo MW, Tam WY, Li VS, Leung SY (2006) Heritable germline epimutation of MSH2 in a family with hereditary nonpolyposis colorectal cancer. Nat Genet 38:1178–1183

Chen RZ, Pettersson U, Beard C, Jackson-Grusby L, Jaenisch R (1998) DNA hypomethylation leads to elevated mutation rates. Nature 395:89–93

Chinnaiyan P, Vallabhaneni G, Armstrong E, Huang SM, Harari PM (2005) Modulation of radiation response by histone deacetylase inhibition. Int J Radiat Oncol Biol Phys 62:223–229

Ciafre SA, Galardi S, Mangiola A, Ferracin M, Liu CG, Sabatino G, Negrini M, Maira G, Croce CM, Farace MG (2005) Extensive modulation of a set of microRNAs in primary glioblastoma. Biochem Biophys Res Commun 334:1351–1358

Condorelli DF, Dell'Albani P, Conticello SG, Barresi V, Nicoletti VG, Caruso A, Kahn M, Vacanti M, Albanese V, de Vellis J, Giuffrida AM (1997) A neural-specific hypomethylated domain in the 5′ flanking region of the glial fibrillary acidic protein gene. Dev Neurosci 19:446–456

Condorelli DF, Nicoletti VG, Barresi V, Caruso A, Conticello S, de Vellis J, Giuffrida Stella AM (1994) Tissue-specific DNA methylation patterns of the rat glial fibrillary acidic protein gene. J Neurosci Res 39:694–707

Costello JF, Berger MS, Huang HS, Cavenee WK (1996) Silencing of p16/CDKN2 expression in human gliomas by methylation and chromatin condensation. Cancer Res 56:2405–2410

Costello JF, Fruhwald MC, Smiraglia DJ, Rush LJ, Robertson GP, Gao X, Wright FA, Feramisco JD, Peltomaki P, Lang JC, Schuller DE, Yu L, Bloomfield CD, Caligiuri MA, Yates A, Nishikawa R, Su Huang H, Petrelli NJ, Zhang X, O'Dorisio MS, Held WA, Cavenee WK, Plass C (2000) Aberrant CpG-island methylation has non-random and tumour-type-specific patterns. Nat Genet 24:132–138

Costello JF, Futscher BW, Kroes RA, Pieper RO (1994a) Methylation-related chromatin structure is associated with exclusion of transcription factors from and suppressed expression of the O-6-methylguanine DNA methyltransferase gene in human glioma cell lines. Mol Cell Biol 14:6515–6521

Costello JF, Futscher BW, Tano K, Graunke DM, Pieper RO (1994b) Graded methylation in the promoter and body of the O6-methylguanine DNA methyltransferase (MGMT) gene correlates with MGMT expression in human glioma cells. J Biol Chem 269:17228–17237

Costello JF, Plass C, Arap W, Chapman VM, Held WA, Berger MS, Su Huang HJ, Cavenee WK (1997) Cyclin-dependent kinase 6 (CDK6) amplification in human gliomas identified using two-dimensional separation of genomic DNA. Cancer Res 57:1250–1254

Costello JF, Plass C, Cavenee WK (2000) Aberrant methylation of genes in low-grade astrocytomas. Brain Tumor Pathol 17:49–56

Cropley JE, Suter CM, Beckman KB, Martin DI (2006) Germ-line epigenetic modification of the murine A vy allele by nutritional supplementation. Proc Nat Acad of Sci U S A 103:17308–17312

De Smet C, De Backer O, Faraoni I, Lurquin C, Brasseur F, Boon T (1996) The activation of human gene MAGE-1 in tumor cells is correlated with genome-wide demethylation. Proc Nat Acad Sci USA 93:7149–7153

Dellino GI, Schwartz YB, Farkas G, McCabe D, Elgin SC, Pirrotta V (2004) Polycomb silencing blocks transcription initiation. Mol Cell 13:887–893

Diala ES, Cheah MS, Rowitch D, Hoffman RM (1983) Extent of DNA methylation in human tumor cells. J Natl Cancer Inst 71:755–764

Dokmanovic M, Clarke C, Marks PA (2007) Histone deacetylase inhibitors: overview and perspectives. Mol Cancer Res 5:981–989

Down TA, Rakyan VK, Turner DJ, Flicek P, Li H, Kulesha E, Graf S, Johnson N, Herrero J, Tomazou EM, Thorne NP, Backdahl L, Herberth M, Howe KL, Jackson DK, Miretti MM, Marioni JC, Birney E, Hubbard TJ, Durbin R, Tavare S, Beck S (2008) A Bayesian deconvolution strategy for immunoprecipitation-based DNA methylome analysis. Nat Biotechnol 26:779–785

Duhl DM, Vrieling H, Miller KA, Wolff GL, Barsh GS (1994) Neomorphic agouti mutations in obese yellow mice. Nat Genet 8:59–65

Eden A, Gaudet F, Waghmare A, Jaenisch R (2003) Chromosomal instability and tumors promoted by DNA hypomethylation. Science, New York, NY 300:455

Ehrlich M (2002) DNA methylation in cancer: too much, but also too little. Oncogene 21:5400–5413

Ehrlich M, Gama-Sosa MA, Huang LH, Midgett RM, Kuo KC, McCune RA, Gehrke C (1982) Amount and distribution of 5-methylcytosine in human DNA from different types of tissues of cells. Nucleic Acids Res 10:2709–2721

Ehrlich M, Sanchez C, Shao C, Nishiyama R, Kehrl J, Kuick R, Kubota T, Hanash SM (2008) ICF, an immunodeficiency syndrome: DNA methyltransferase 3B involvement, chromosome anomalies, and gene dysregulation. Autoimmunity 41:253–271

Ellis L, Pan Y, Smyth GK, George DJ, McCormack C, Williams-Truax R, Mita M, Beck J, Burris H, Ryan G, Atadja P, Butterfoss D, Dugan M, Culver K, Johnstone RW, Prince HM (2008) Histone deacetylase inhibitor panobinostat induces clinical responses with associated alterations in gene expression profiles in cutaneous T-cell lymphoma. Clin Cancer Res 14:4500–4510

Entin-Meer M, Rephaeli A, Yang X, Nudelman A, VandenBerg SR, Haas-Kogan DA (2005) Butyric acid prodrugs are histone deacetylase inhibitors that show antineoplastic activity and radiosensitizing capacity in the treatment of malignant gliomas. Mol Cancer Ther 4:1952–1961

Entin-Meer M, Yang X, VandenBerg SR, Lamborn KR, Nudelman A, Rephaeli A, Haas-Kogan DA (2007) In vivo efficacy of a novel histone deacetylase inhibitor in combination with radiation for the treatment of gliomas. Neuro-oncology 9:82–88

Esteller M, Hamilton SR, Burger PC, Baylin SB, Herman JG (1999a) Inactivation of the DNA repair gene O6-methylguanine-DNA methyltransferase by promoter hypermethylation is a common event in primary human neoplasia. Cancer Res 59:793–797

Esteller M, Risques RA, Toyota M, Capella G, Moreno V, Peinado MA, Baylin SB, Herman JG (2001) Promoter hypermethylation of the DNA repair gene O(6)-methylguanine-DNA methyltransferase is associated with the presence of G:C to A:T transition mutations in p53 in human colorectal tumorigenesis. Cancer Res 61:4689–4692

Esteller M, Sanchez-Cespedes M, Rosell R, Sidransky D, Baylin SB, Herman JG (1999b) Detection of aberrant promoter hypermethylation of tumor suppressor genes in serum DNA from non-small cell lung cancer patients. Cancer Res 59:67–70

Esteller M, Toyota M, Sanchez-Cespedes M, Capella G, Peinado MA, Watkins DN, Issa JP, Sidransky D, Baylin SB, Herman JG (2000) Inactivation of the DNA repair gene O6-methylguanine-DNA methyltransferase by promoter hypermethylation is associated with G to A mutations in K-ras in colorectal tumorigenesis. Cancer Res 60:2368–2371

Everhard S, Kaloshi G, Criniere E, Benouaich-Amiel A, Lejeune J, Marie Y, Sanson M, Kujas M, Mokhtari K, Hoang-Xuan K, Delattre JY, Thillet J (2006) MGMT methylation: a marker of response to temozolomide in low-grade gliomas. Ann Neurol 60:740–743

Eyupoglu IY, Hahnen E, Buslei R, Siebzehnrubl FA, Savaskan NE, Luders M, Trankle C, Wick W, Weller M, Fahlbusch R, Blumcke I (2005) Suberoylanilide hydroxamic acid (SAHA) has potent anti-glioma properties in vitro, ex vivo and in vivo. J Neurochem 93:992–999

Fan G, Beard C, Chen RZ, Csankovszki G, Sun Y, Siniaia M, Biniszkiewicz D, Bates B, Lee PP, Kuhn R, Trumpp A, Poon C, Wilson CB, Jaenisch R (2001) DNA hypomethylation perturbs the function and survival of CNS neurons in postnatal animals. J Neurosci 21:788–797

Fanelli M, Caprodossi S, Ricci-Vitiani L, Porcellini A, Tomassoni-Ardori F, Amatori S, Andreoni F, Magnani M, De Maria R, Santoni A, Minucci S, Pelicci PG (2008) Loss of pericentromeric DNA methylation pattern in human glioblastoma is associated with altered DNA methyltransferases expression and involves the stem cell compartment. Oncogene 27:358–365

Feinberg AP, Gehrke CW, Kuo KC, Ehrlich M (1988) Reduced genomic 5-methylcytosine content in human colonic neoplasia. Cancer Res 48:1159–1161

Feinberg AP, Vogelstein B (1983a) Hypomethylation distinguishes genes of some human cancers from their normal counterparts. Nature 301:89–92

Feinberg AP, Vogelstein B (1983b) Hypomethylation of ras oncogenes in primary human cancers. Biochem Biophys Res Communicat 111:47–54
Feng J, Chang H, Li E, Fan G (2005) Dynamic expression of de novo DNA methyltransferases Dnmt3a and Dnmt3b in the central nervous system. J Neurosci Res 79:734–746
Foltz G, Ryu GY, Yoon JG, Nelson T, Fahey J, Frakes A, Lee H, Field L, Zander K, Sibenaller Z, Ryken TC, Vibhakar R, Hood L, Madan A (2006) Genome-wide analysis of epigenetic silencing identifies BEX1 and BEX2 as candidate tumor suppressor genes in malignant glioma. Cancer Res 66:6665–6674
Fouse SD, Shen Y, Pellegrini M, Cole S, Meissner A, Van Neste L, Jaenisch R, Fan G (2008) Promoter CpG methylation contributes to ES cell gene regulation in parallel with Oct4/Nanog, PcG complex, and histone H3 K4/K27 trimethylation. Cell Stem Cell 2:160–169
Gabriely G, Wurdinger T, Kesari S, Esau CC, Burchard J, Linsley PS, Krichevsky AM (2008) MiR-21 promotes glioma invasion by targeting MMP regulators. Mol Cell Biol 28:5369–5380
Gama-Sosa MA, Slagel VA, Trewyn RW, Oxenhandler R, Kuo KC, Gehrke CW, Ehrlich M (1983) The 5-methylcytosine content of DNA from human tumors. Nucleic Acids Res 11:6883–6894
Gaudet F, Hodgson JG, Eden A, Jackson-Grusby L, Dausman J, Gray JW, Leonhardt H, Jaenisch R (2003) Induction of tumors in mice by genomic hypomethylation. Science New York, NY 300:489–492
Gaur A, Jewell DA, Liang Y, Ridzon D, Moore JH, Chen C, Ambros VR, Israel MA (2007) Characterization of microRNA expression levels and their biological correlates in human cancer cell lines. Cancer Res 67:2456–2468
Gerson SL (2004) MGMT: its role in cancer aetiology and cancer therapeutics. Nat Rev Cancer 4:296–307
Gibbons RJ, McDowell TL, Raman S, O'Rourke DM, Garrick D, Ayyub H, Higgs DR (2000) Mutations in ATRX, encoding a SWI/SNF-like protein, cause diverse changes in the pattern of DNA methylation. Nat Genet 24:368–371
Gimsing P, Hansen M, Knudsen LM, Knoblauch P, Christensen IJ, Ooi CE, Buhl-Jensen P (2008) A phase I clinical trial of the histone deacetylase inhibitor belinostat in patients with advanced hematological neoplasia. Eur J Haematol 81:170–176
Goelz SE, Vogelstein B, Hamilton SR, Feinberg AP (1985) Hypomethylation of DNA from benign and malignant human colon neoplasms. Science, New York, NY 228:187–190
Goll MG, Kirpekar F, Maggert KA, Yoder JA, Hsieh CL, Zhang X, Golic KG, Jacobsen SE, Bestor TH (2006) Methylation of tRNAAsp by the DNA methyltransferase homolog Dnmt2. Science New York, NY 311:395–398
Goto K, Numata M, Komura JI, Ono T, Bestor TH, Kondo H (1994) Expression of DNA methyltransferase gene in mature and immature neurons as well as proliferating cells in mice. Differentiation 56:39–44
Grady WM, Willis J, Guilford PJ, Dunbier AK, Toro TT, Lynch H, Wiesner G, Ferguson K, Eng C, Park JG, Kim SJ, Markowitz S (2000) Methylation of the CDH1 promoter as the second genetic hit in hereditary diffuse gastric cancer. Nature genetics 26:16–17
Gray SG, Qian CN, Furge K, Guo X, Teh BT (2004) Microarray profiling of the effects of histone deacetylase inhibitors on gene expression in cancer cell lines. Int J Oncol 24:773–795
Greger V, Debus N, Lohmann D, Hopping W, Passarge E, Horsthemke B (1994) Frequency and parental origin of hypermethylated RB1 alleles in retinoblastoma. Hum Genet 94:491–496
Greger V, Passarge E, Hopping W, Messmer E, Horsthemke B (1989) Epigenetic changes may contribute to the formation and spontaneous regression of retinoblastoma. Hum Genet 83:155–158
Gui CY, Ngo L, Xu WS, Richon VM, Marks PA (2004) Histone deacetylase (HDAC) inhibitor activation of p21WAF1 involves changes in promoter-associated proteins, including HDAC1. Proc Natl Acad Sci USA 101:1241–1246

Hansen RS, Gartler SM (1990) 5-Azacytidine-induced reactivation of the human X chromosome-linked PGK1 gene is associated with a large region of cytosine demethylation in the 5′ CpG island. Proc Natl Acad Sci USA 87:4174–4178

Hansen RS, Wijmenga C, Luo P, Stanek AM, Canfield TK, Weemaes CM, Gartler SM (1999) The DNMT3B DNA methyltransferase gene is mutated in the ICF immunodeficiency syndrome. Proc Natl Acad Sci USA 96:14412–14417

Hegi ME, Diserens AC, Gorlia T, Hamou MF, de Tribolet N, Weller M, Kros JM, Hainfellner JA, Mason W, Mariani L, Bromberg JE, Hau P, Mirimanoff RO, Cairncross JG, Janzer RC, Stupp R (2005) MGMT gene silencing and benefit from temozolomide in glioblastoma. N Engl J Med 352:997–1003

Hellman A, Chess A (2007) Gene body-specific methylation on the active X chromosome. Science, New York, NY 315:1141–1143

Hoffman RM (1982) Methionine dependence in cancer cells – a review. In Vitro 18:421–428

Holm TM, Jackson-Grusby L, Brambrink T, Yamada Y, Rideout WM, 3rd, Jaenisch R (2005) Global loss of imprinting leads to widespread tumorigenesis in adult mice. Cancer Cell 8:275–285

Hong C, Maunakea A, Jun P, Bollen AW, Hodgson JG, Goldenberg DD, Weiss WA, Costello JF (2005) Shared epigenetic mechanisms in human and mouse gliomas inactivate expression of the growth suppressor SLC5A8. Cancer Res 65:3617–3623

Hong C, Moorefield KS, Jun P, Aldape KD, Kharbanda S, Phillips HS, Costello JF (2007) Epigenome scans and cancer genome sequencing converge on WNK2, a kinase-independent suppressor of cell growth. Proc Natl Acad Sci USA 104:10974–10979

Howard G, Eiges R, Gaudet F, Jaenisch R, Eden A (2008) Activation and transposition of endogenous retroviral elements in hypomethylation induced tumors in mice. Oncogene 27:404–408

Inano K, Suetake I, Ueda T, Miyake Y, Nakamura M, Okada M, Tajima S (2000) Maintenance-type DNA methyltransferase is highly expressed in post-mitotic neurons and localized in the cytoplasmic compartment. J Biochem 128:315–321

Jacob RA, Gretz DM, Taylor PC, James SJ, Pogribny IP, Miller BJ, Henning SM, Swendseid ME (1998) Moderate folate depletion increases plasma homocysteine and decreases lymphocyte DNA methylation in postmenopausal women. J Nutr 128:1204–1212

Jensen LR, Amende M, Gurok U, Moser B, Gimmel V, Tzschach A, Janecke AR, Tariverdian G, Chelly J, Fryns JP, Van Esch H, Kleefstra T, Hamel B, Moraine C, Gecz J, Turner G, Reinhardt R, Kalscheuer VM, Ropers HH, Lenzner S (2005) Mutations in the JARID1C gene, which is involved in transcriptional regulation and chromatin remodeling, cause X-linked mental retardation. Am J Human Genet 76:227–236

Jia D, Jurkowska RZ, Zhang X, Jeltsch A, Cheng X (2007) Structure of Dnmt3a bound to Dnmt3L suggests a model for de novo DNA methylation. Nature 449:248–251

Kanai Y, Saito Y, Ushijima S, Hirohashi S (2004) Alterations in gene expression associated with the overexpression of a splice variant of DNA methyltransferase 3b, DNMT3b4, during human hepatocarcinogenesis. J Cancer Res Clin Oncol 130:636–644

Karpf AR, Peterson PW, Rawlins JT, Dalley BK, Yang Q, Albertsen H, Jones DA (1999) Inhibition of DNA methyltransferase stimulates the expression of signal transducer and activator of transcription 1, 2, and 3 genes in colon tumor cells. Proc Natl Acad Sci USA 96:14007–14012

Kawaji H, Hayashizaki Y (2008) Exploration of small RNAs. PLoS Genet 4:e22

Kim TY, Zhong S, Fields CR, Kim JH, Robertson KD (2006) Epigenomic profiling reveals novel and frequent targets of aberrant DNA methylation-mediated silencing in malignant glioma. Cancer Res 66:7490–7501

Kondo Y, Shen L, Cheng AS, Ahmed S, Boumber Y, Charo C, Yamochi T, Urano T, Furukawa K, Kwabi-Addo B, Gold DL, Sekido Y, Huang TH, Issa JP (2008) Gene silencing in cancer by histone H3 lysine 27 trimethylation independent of promoter DNA methylation. Nature Genet 40:741–750

Kumagai T, Wakimoto N, Yin D, Gery S, Kawamata N, Takai N, Komatsu N, Chumakov A, Imai Y, Koeffler HP (2007) Histone deacetylase inhibitor, suberoylanilide hydroxamic acid (Vorinostat, SAHA) profoundly inhibits the growth of human pancreatic cancer cells. Int J Cancer 121:656–665

Ladd-Acosta C, Pevsner J, Sabunciyan S, Yolken RH, Webster MJ, Dinkins T, Callinan PA, Fan JB, Potash JB, Feinberg AP (2007) DNA methylation signatures within the human brain. Am J Human Genet 81:1304–1315

Landgraf P, Rusu M, Sheridan R, Sewer A, Iovino N, Aravin A, Pfeffer S, Rice A, Kamphorst AO, Landthaler M, Lin C, Socci ND, Hermida L, Fulci V, Chiaretti S, Foa R, Schliwka J, Fuchs U, Novosel A, Muller RU, Schermer B, Bissels U, Inman J, Phan Q, Chien M, Weir DB, Choksi R, De Vita G, Frezzetti D, Trompeter HI, Hornung V, Teng G, Hartmann G, Palkovits M, Di Lauro R, Wernet P, Macino G, Rogler CE, Nagle JW, Ju J, Papavasiliou FN, Benzing T, Lichter P, Tam W, Brownstein MJ, Bosio A, Borkhardt A, Russo JJ, Sander C, Zavolan M, Tuschl T (2007) A mammalian microRNA expression atlas based on small RNA library sequencing. Cell 129:1401–1414

Lavon I, Zrihan D, Zelikovitch B, Fellig Y, Fuchs D, Soffer D, Siegal T (2007) Longitudinal assessment of genetic and epigenetic markers in oligodendrogliomas. Clin Cancer Res 13:1429–1437

Lee J, Kotliarova S, Kotliarov Y, Li A, Su Q, Donin NM, Pastorino S, Purow BW, Christopher N, Zhang W, Park JK, Fine HA (2006a) Tumor stem cells derived from glioblastomas cultured in bFGF and EGF more closely mirror the phenotype and genotype of primary tumors than do serum-cultured cell lines. Cancer Cell 9:391–403

Lee J, Son MJ, Woolard K, Donin NM, Li A, Cheng CH, Kotliarova S, Kotliarov Y, Walling J, Ahn S, Kim M, Totonchy M, Cusack T, Ene C, Ma H, Su Q, Zenklusen JC, Zhang W, Maric D, Fine HA (2008) Epigenetic-mediated dysfunction of the bone morphogenetic protein pathway inhibits differentiation of glioblastoma-initiating cells. Cancer Cell 13:69–80

Lee JH, Park JH, Jung Y, Kim JH, Jong HS, Kim TY, Bang YJ (2006b) Histone deacetylase inhibitor enhances 5-fluorouracil cytotoxicity by down-regulating thymidylate synthase in human cancer cells. Mol Cancer Ther 5:3085–3095

Lein ES, Hawrylycz MJ, Ao N, Ayres M, Bensinger A, Bernard A, Boe AF, Boguski MS, Brockway KS, Byrnes EJ, Chen L, Chen TM, Chin MC, Chong J, Crook BE, Czaplinska A, Dang CN, Datta S, Dee NR, Desaki AL, Desta T, Diep E, Dolbeare TA, Donelan MJ, Dong HW, Dougherty JG, Duncan BJ, Ebbert AJ, Eichele G, Estin LK, Faber C, Facer BA, Fields R, Fischer SR, Fliss TP, Frensley C, Gates SN, Glattfelder KJ, Halverson KR, Hart MR, Hohmann JG, Howell MP, Jeung DP, Johnson RA, Karr PT, Kawal R, Kidney JM, Knapik RH, Kuan CL, Lake JH, Laramee AR, Larsen KD, Lau C, Lemon TA, Liang AJ, Liu Y, Luong LT, Michaels J, Morgan JJ, Morgan RJ, Mortrud MT, Mosqueda NF, Ng LL, Ng R, Orta GJ, Overly CC, Pak TH, Parry SE, Pathak SD, Pearson OC, Puchalski RB, Riley ZL, Rockett HR, Rowland SA, Royall JJ, Ruiz MJ, Sarno NR, Schaffnit K, Shapovalova NV, Sivisay T, Slaughterbeck CR, Smith SC, Smith KA, Smith BI, Sodt AJ, Stewart NN, Stumpf KR, Sunkin SM, Sutram M, Tam A, Teemer CD, Thaller C, Thompson CL, Varnam LR, Visel A, Whitlock RM, Wohnoutka PE, Wolkey CK, Wong VY, Wood M, Yaylaoglu MB, Young RC, Youngstrom BL, Yuan XF, Zhang B, Zwingman TA, Jones AR (2007) Genome-wide atlas of gene expression in the adult mouse brain. Nature 445:168–176

Li A, Walling J, Kotliarov Y, Center A, Steed ME, Ahn SJ, Rosenblum M, Mikkelsen T, Zenklusen JC, Fine HA (2008) Genomic changes and gene expression profiles reveal that established glioma cell lines are poorly representative of primary human gliomas. Mol Cancer Res 6:21–30

Li E, Beard C, Jaenisch R (1993) Role for DNA methylation in genomic imprinting. Nature 366:362–365

Li E, Bestor TH, Jaenisch R (1992) Targeted mutation of the DNA methyltransferase gene results in embryonic lethality. Cell 69:915–926

Li Q, Jedlicka A, Ahuja N, Gibbons MC, Baylin SB, Burger PC, Issa JP (1998) Concordant methylation of the ER and N33 genes in glioblastoma multiforme. Oncogene 16:3197–3202

Lin JC, Jeong S, Liang G, Takai D, Fatemi M, Tsai YC, Egger G, Gal-Yam EN, Jones PA (2007) Role of nucleosomal occupancy in the epigenetic silencing of the MLH1 CpG island. Cancer Cell 12:432–444

Linhart HG, Lin H, Yamada Y, Moran E, Steine EJ, Gokhale S, Lo G, Cantu E, Ehrich M, He T, Meissner A, Jaenisch R (2007) Dnmt3b promotes tumorigenesis in vivo by gene-specific de novo methylation and transcriptional silencing. Gene Dev 21: 3110–3122

Liu G, Ying H, Zeng G, Wheeler CJ, Black KL, Yu JS (2004) HER-2, gp100, and MAGE-1 are expressed in human glioblastoma and recognized by cytotoxic T cells. Cancer Res 64:4980–4986

Lomas J, Bello MJ, Arjona D, Alonso ME, Martinez-Glez V, Lopez-Marin I, Aminoso C, de Campos JM, Isla A, Vaquero J, Rey JA (2005) Genetic and epigenetic alteration of the NF2 gene in sporadic meningiomas. Gene Chromosomes Cancer 42:314–319

Maegawa S, Yoshioka H, Itaba N, Kubota N, Nishihara S, Shirayoshi Y, Nanba E, Oshimura M (2001) Epigenetic silencing of PEG3 gene expression in human glioma cell lines. Mol Carcinog 31:1–9

Martinez R, Setien F, Voelter C, Casado S, Quesada MP, Schackert G, Esteller M (2007) CpG island promoter hypermethylation of the pro-apoptotic gene caspase-8 is a common hallmark of relapsed glioblastoma multiforme. Carcinogenesis 28:1264–1268

Matarazzo MR, Boyle S, D'Esposito M, Bickmore WA (2007) Chromosome territory reorganization in a human disease with altered DNA methylation. Proc Natl Acad Sci USA 104:16546–16551

McClelland M, Ivarie R (1982) Asymmetrical distribution of CpG in an 'average' mammalian gene. Nucleic Acids Res 10:7865–7877

McGarvey KM, Van Neste L, Cope L, Ohm JE, Herman JG, Van Criekinge W, Schuebel KE, Baylin SB (2008) Defining a chromatin pattern that characterizes DNA-hypermethylated genes in colon cancer cells. Cancer research 68:5753–5759

Meissner A, Gnirke A, Bell GW, Ramsahoye B, Lander ES, Jaenisch R (2005) Reduced representation bisulfite sequencing for comparative high-resolution DNA methylation analysis. Nucleic Acids Res 33:5868–5877

Meissner A, Mikkelsen TS, Gu H, Wernig M, Hanna J, Sivachenko A, Zhang X, Bernstein BE, Nusbaum C, Jaffe DB, Gnirke A, Jaenisch R, Lander ES (2008) Genome-scale DNA methylation maps of pluripotent and differentiated cells. Nature

Mikkelsen TS, Hanna J, Zhang X, Ku M, Wernig M, Schorderet P, Bernstein BE, Jaenisch R, Lander ES, Meissner A (2008) Dissecting direct reprogramming through integrative genomic analysis. Nature 454:49–55

Mitsiades CS, Mitsiades NS, McMullan CJ, Poulaki V, Shringarpure R, Hideshima T, Akiyama M, Chauhan D, Munshi N, Gu X, Bailey C, Joseph M, Libermann TA, Richon VM, Marks PA, Anderson KC (2004) Transcriptional signature of histone deacetylase inhibition in multiple myeloma: biological and clinical implications. Proc Natl Acad Sci USA 101:540–545

Mohandas T, Sparkes RS, Shapiro LJ (1981) Reactivation of an inactive human X chromosome: evidence for X inactivation by DNA methylation. Science, New York, NY 211:393–396

Moniz S, Matos P, Jordan P (2008) WNK2 modulates MEK1 activity through the Rho GTPase pathway. Cell Signal 20:1762–1768

Moniz S, Verissimo F, Matos P, Brazao R, Silva E, Kotelevets L, Chastre E, Gespach C, Jordan P (2007) Protein kinase WNK2 inhibits cell proliferation by negatively modulating the activation of MEK1/ERK1/2. Oncogene 26:6071–6081

Morison IM, Paton CJ, Cleverley SD (2001) The imprinted gene and parent-of-origin effect database. Nucleic Acids Res 29:275–276

Moulton T, Crenshaw T, Hao Y, Moosikasuwan J, Lin N, Dembitzer F, Hensle T, Weiss L, McMorrow L, Loew T et al. (1994) Epigenetic lesions at the H19 locus in Wilms' tumour patients. Nat Genet 7:440–447
Mueller W, Nutt CL, Ehrich M, Riemenschneider MJ, von Deimling A, van den Boom D, Louis DN (2007) Downregulation of RUNX3 and TES by hypermethylation in glioblastoma. Oncogene 26:583–593
Murat A, Migliavacca E, Gorlia T, Lambiv WL, Shay T, Hamou MF, de Tribolet N, Regli L, Wick W, Kouwenhoven MC, Hainfellner JA, Heppner FL, Dietrich PY, Zimmer Y, Cairncross JG, Janzer RC, Domany E, Delorenzi M, Stupp R, Hegi ME (2008) Stem cell-related "self-renewal" signature and high epidermal growth factor receptor expression associated with resistance to concomitant chemoradiotherapy in glioblastoma. J Clin Oncol 26:3015–3024
Nakamura M, Konishi N, Inui T, Hiasa Y, Nagai H, Tsunoda S, Nakase H, Tsuzuki T, Aoki H, Sakitani H, Aoyama N, Sakaki T (1998) Genetic variations in recurrent astrocytic tumors detected by restriction landmark genomic scanning. Brain Tumor Pathol 15:1–6
Nakamura M, Konishi N, Tsunoda S, Hiasa Y, Takemura K, Tsuzuki T, Kobitsu K, Sakaki T (1997a) Genomic alterations of human gliomas detected by restriction landmark genomic scanning. Brain Tumor Pathol 14:13–17
Nakamura M, Konishi N, Tsunoda S, Hiasa Y, Tsuzuki T, Aoki H, Kobitsu K, Nagai H, Sakaki T (1997b) Analyses of human gliomas by restriction landmark genomic scanning. J Neurooncol 35:113–120
Nakamura M, Konishi N, Tsunoda S, Hiasa Y, Tsuzuki T, Takemura K, Kobitsu K, Sakaki T (1997c) Genomic alterations in human glioma cell lines detected by restriction landmark genomic scanning. J Neurooncol 34:203–209
Nakamura M, Yonekawa Y, Kleihues P, Ohgaki H (2001) Promoter hypermethylation of the RB1 gene in glioblastomas. Lab Invest 81:77–82
Narlikar GJ, Fan HY, Kingston RE (2002) Cooperation between complexes that regulate chromatin structure and transcription. Cell 108:475–487
Nelson PT, Baldwin DA, Kloosterman WP, Kauppinen S, Plasterk RH, Mourelatos Z (2006) RAKE and LNA-ISH reveal microRNA expression and localization in archival human brain. RNA 12:187–191
Nguyen S, Meletis K, Fu D, Jhaveri S, Jaenisch R (2007) Ablation of de novo DNA methyltransferase Dnmt3a in the nervous system leads to neuromuscular defects and shortened lifespan. Dev Dyn 236:1663–1676
Nicoloso MS, Calin GA (2008) MicroRNA involvement in brain tumors: from bench to bedside. Brain Pathol 18:122–129
Ogawa O, Becroft DM, Morison IM, Eccles MR, Skeen JE, Mauger DC, Reeve AE (1993a) Constitutional relaxation of insulin-like growth factor II gene imprinting associated with Wilms' tumour and gigantism. Nat Genet 5:408–412
Ogawa O, Eccles MR, Szeto J, McNoe LA, Yun K, Maw MA, Smith PJ, Reeve AE (1993b) Relaxation of insulin-like growth factor II gene imprinting implicated in Wilms' tumour. Nature 362:749–751
Ohgaki H, Kleihues P (2007) Genetic pathways to primary and secondary glioblastoma. Am J Pathol 170:1445–1453
Ohm JE, McGarvey KM, Yu X, Cheng L, Schuebel KE, Cope L, Mohammad HP, Chen W, Daniel VC, Yu W, Berman DM, Jenuwein T, Pruitt K, Sharkis SJ, Watkins DN, Herman JG, Baylin SB (2007) A stem cell-like chromatin pattern may predispose tumor suppressor genes to DNA hypermethylation and heritable silencing. Nat Genet 39:237–242
Ohtani-Fujita N, Fujita T, Aoike A, Osifchin NE, Robbins PD, Sakai T (1993) CpG methylation inactivates the promoter activity of the human retinoblastoma tumor-suppressor gene. Oncogene 8:1063–1067
Okano M, Bell DW, Haber DA, Li E (1999) DNA methyltransferases Dnmt3a and Dnmt3b are essential for de novo methylation and mammalian development. Cell 99:247–257

Okano M, Xie S, Li E (1998) Cloning and characterization of a family of novel mammalian DNA (cytosine-5) methyltransferases. Nature genetics 19:219–220

Okoji RS, Yu RC, Maronpot RR, Froines JR (2002) Sodium arsenite administration via drinking water increases genome-wide and Ha-ras DNA hypomethylation in methyl-deficient C57BL/6 J mice. Carcinogenesis 23:777–785

Ooi SK, Qiu C, Bernstein E, Li K, Jia D, Yang Z, Erdjument-Bromage H, Tempst P, Lin SP, Allis CD, Cheng X, Bestor TH (2007) DNMT3L connects unmethylated lysine 4 of histone H3 to de novo methylation of DNA. Nature 448:714–717

Ostler KR, Davis EM, Payne SL, Gosalia BB, Exposito-Cespedes J, Le Beau MM, Godley LA (2007) Cancer cells express aberrant DNMT3B transcripts encoding truncated proteins. Oncogene 26:5553–5563

Parsons DW, Jones S, Zhang X, Lin JC, Leary RJ, Angenendt P, Mankoo P, Carter H, Siu IM, Gallia GL, Olivi A, McLendon R, Rasheed BA, Keir S, Nikolskaya T, Nikolsky Y, Busam DA, Tekleab H, Diaz LA, Jr., Hartigan J, Smith DR, Strausberg RL, Marie SK, Shinjo SM, Yan H, Riggins GJ, Bigner DD, Karchin R, Papadopoulos N, Parmigiani G, Vogelstein B, Velculescu VE, Kinzler KW (2008) An Integrated Genomic Analysis of Human Glioblastoma Multiforme. Science, New York, NY

Peart MJ, Smyth GK, van Laar RK, Bowtell DD, Richon VM, Marks PA, Holloway AJ, Johnstone RW (2005) Identification and functional significance of genes regulated by structurally different histone deacetylase inhibitors. Proc Natl Acad Sci USA 102:3697–3702

Pieper RO, Costello JF, Kroes RA, Futscher BW, Marathi U, Erickson LC (1991) Direct correlation between methylation status and expression of the human O-6-methylguanine DNA methyltransferase gene. Cancer Commun 3:241–253

Qiu L, Kelso MJ, Hansen C, West ML, Fairlie DP, Parsons PG (1999) Anti-tumour activity in vitro and in vivo of selective differentiating agents containing hydroxamate. Br J Cancer 80:1252–1258

Rainier S, Johnson LA, Dobry CJ, Ping AJ, Grundy PE, Feinberg AP (1993) Relaxation of imprinted genes in human cancer. Nature 362:747–749

Rand K, Qu W, Ho T, Clark SJ, Molloy P (2002) Conversion-specific detection of DNA methylation using real-time polymerase chain reaction (ConLight-MSP) to avoid false positives. Methods 27:114–120

Reilly KM, Tuskan RG, Christy E, Loisel DA, Ledger J, Bronson RT, Smith CD, Tsang S, Munroe DJ, Jacks T (2004) Susceptibility to astrocytoma in mice mutant for Nf1 and Trp53 is linked to chromosome 11 and subject to epigenetic effects. Proc Natl Acad Sci USA 101:13008–13013

Saito Y, Kanai Y, Sakamoto M, Saito H, Ishii H, Hirohashi S (2002) Overexpression of a splice variant of DNA methyltransferase 3b, DNMT3b4, associated with DNA hypomethylation on pericentromeric satellite regions during human hepatocarcinogenesis. Proc Natl Acad Sci USA 99:10060–10065

Sakai T, Toguchida J, Ohtani N, Yandell DW, Rapaport JM, Dryja TP (1991) Allele-specific hypermethylation of the retinoblastoma tumor-suppressor gene. Am J Human Genet 48:880–888

Sandovici I, Kassovska-Bratinova S, Loredo-Osti JC, Leppert M, Suarez A, Stewart R, Bautista FD, Schiraldi M, Sapienza C (2005) Interindividual variability and parent of origin DNA methylation differences at specific human Alu elements. Human Molecular Genetics 14:2135–2143

Schlesinger Y, Straussman R, Keshet I, Farkash S, Hecht M, Zimmerman J, Eden E, Yakhini Z, Ben-Shushan E, Reubinoff BE, Bergman Y, Simon I, Cedar H (2007) Polycomb-mediated methylation on Lys27 of histone H3 pre-marks genes for de novo methylation in cancer. Nat Genet 39:232–236

Silber J, Lim DA, Petritsch C, Persson AI, Maunakea AK, Yu M, Vandenberg SR, Ginzinger DG, James CD, Costello JF, Bergers G, Weiss WA, Alvarez-Buylla A, Hodgson JG (2008)

miR-124 and miR-137 inhibit proliferation of glioblastoma multiforme cells and induce differentiation of brain tumor stem cells. BMC Med 6:14

Steenman MJ, Rainier S, Dobry CJ, Grundy P, Horon IL, Feinberg AP (1994) Loss of imprinting of IGF2 is linked to reduced expression and abnormal methylation of H19 in Wilms' tumour. Nat Genet 7:433–439

Stefani G, Slack FJ (2008) Small non-coding RNAs in animal development. Nat Rev Mol Cell Biol 9:219–230

Suter CM, Martin DI, Ward RL (2004) Germline epimutation of MLH1 in individuals with multiple cancers. Nat Genet 36:497–501

Tahiliani M, Mei P, Fang R, Leonor T, Rutenberg M, Shimizu F, Li J, Rao A, Shi Y (2007) The histone H3K4 demethylase SMCX links REST target genes to X-linked mental retardation. Nature 447:601–605

Takahashi K, Yamanaka S (2006) Induction of pluripotent stem cells from mouse embryonic and adult fibroblast cultures by defined factors. Cell 126:663–676

Takizawa T, Nakashima K, Namihira M, Ochiai W, Uemura A, Yanagisawa M, Fujita N, Nakao M, Taga T (2001) DNA methylation is a critical cell-intrinsic determinant of astrocyte differentiation in the fetal brain. Dev Cell 1:749–758

Tan J, Yang X, Zhuang L, Jiang X, Chen W, Lee PL, Karuturi RK, Tan PB, Liu ET, Yu Q (2007) Pharmacologic disruption of Polycomb-repressive complex 2-mediated gene repression selectively induces apoptosis in cancer cells. Gene Dev 21:1050–1063

Tawa R, Ono T, Kurishita A, Okada S, Hirose S (1990) Changes of DNA methylation level during pre- and postnatal periods in mice. Differentiation 45:44–48

Tews B, Roerig P, Hartmann C, Hahn M, Felsberg J, Blaschke B, Sabel M, Kunitz A, Toedt G, Neben K, Benner A, Deimling A, Reifenberger G, Lichter P (2007) Hypermethylation and transcriptional downregulation of the CITED4 gene at 1p34.2 in oligodendroglial tumours with allelic losses on 1p and 19q. Oncogene 26:5010–5016

The Cancer Genome Atlas Research Network, McLendon R, Friedman A, Bigner D, Van Meir EG, Brat DJ, Mastrogianakis M, Olson JJ, Mikkelsen T, Lehman N, Aldape K, Alfred Yung WK, Bogler O, Vandenberg S, Berger M, Prados M, Muzny D, Morgan M, Scherer S, Sabo A, Nazareth L, Lewis L, Hall O, Zhu Y, Ren Y, Alvi O, Yao J, Hawes A, Jhangiani S, Fowler G, San Lucas A, Kovar C, Cree A, Dinh H, Santibanez J, Joshi V, Gonzalez-Garay ML, Miller CA, Milosavljevic A, Donehower L, Wheeler DA, Gibbs RA, Cibulskis K, Sougnez C, Fennell T, Mahan S, Wilkinson J, Ziaugra L, Onofrio R, Bloom T, Nicol R, Ardlie K, Baldwin J, Gabriel S, Lander ES, Ding L, Fulton RS, McLellan MD, Wallis J, Larson DE, Shi X, Abbott R, Fulton L, Chen K, Koboldt DC, Wendl MC, Meyer R, Tang Y, Lin L, Osborne JR, Dunford-Shore BH, Miner TL, Delehaunty K, Markovic C, Swift G, Courtney W, Pohl C, Abbott S, Hawkins A, Leong S, Haipek C, Schmidt H, Wiechert M, Vickery T, Scott S, Dooling DJ, Chinwalla A, Weinstock GM, Mardis ER, Wilson RK, Getz G, Winckler W, Verhaak RG, Lawrence MS, O'Kelly M, Robinson J, Alexe G, Beroukhim R, Carter S, Chiang D, Gould J, Gupta S, Korn J, Mermel C, Mesirov J, Monti S, Nguyen H, Parkin M, Reich M, Stransky N, Weir BA, Garraway L, Golub T, Meyerson M, Chin L, Protopopov A, Zhang J, Perna I, Aronson S, Sathiamoorthy N, Ren G, Wiedemeyer WR, Kim H, Won Kong S, Xiao Y, Kohane IS, Seidman J, Park PJ, Kucherlapati R, Laird PW, Cope L, Herman JG, Weisenberger DJ, Pan F, Van Den Berg D, Van Neste L, Mi Yi J, Schuebel KE, Baylin SB, Absher DM, Li JZ, Southwick A, Brady S, Aggarwal A, Chung T, Sherlock G, Brooks JD, Myers RM, Spellman PT, Purdom E, Jakkula LR, Lapuk AV, Marr H, Dorton S, Gi Choi Y, Han J, Ray A, Wang V, Durinck S, Robinson M, Wang NJ, Vranizan K, Peng V, Van Name E, Fontenay GV, Ngai J, Conboy JG, Parvin B, Feiler HS, Speed TP, Gray JW, Brennan C, Socci ND, Olshen A, Taylor BS, Lash A, Schultz N, Reva B, Antipin Y, Stukalov A, Gross B, Cerami E, Qing Wang W, Qin LX, Seshan VE, Villafania L, Cavatore M, Borsu L, Viale A, Gerald W, Sander C, Ladanyi M, Perou CM, Neil Hayes D, Topal MD, Hoadley KA, Qi Y, Balu S, Shi Y, Wu J, Penny R, Bittner M, Shelton T, Lenkiewicz E,

Morris S, Beasley D, Sanders S, Kahn A, Sfeir R, Chen J, Nassau D, Feng L, Hickey E, Weinstein JN, Barker A, Gerhard DS, Vockley J, Compton C, Vaught J, Fielding P, Ferguson ML, Schaefer C, Madhavan S, Buetow KH, Collins F, Good P, Guyer M, Ozenberger B, Peterson J, Thomson E (2008) Comprehensive genomic characterization defines human glioblastoma genes and core pathways. Nature 321:1807–1812

Trasler JM, Trasler DG, Bestor TH, Li E, Ghibu F (1996) DNA methyltransferase in normal and Dnmtn/Dnmtn mouse embryos. Dev Dyn 206:239–247

Tuck-Muller CM, Narayan A, Tsien F, Smeets DF, Sawyer J, Fiala ES, Sohn OS, Ehrlich M (2000) DNA hypomethylation and unusual chromosome instability in cell lines from ICF syndrome patients. Cytogenet Cell Genet 89:121–128

Turner BM (2005) Reading signals on the nucleosome with a new nomenclature for modified histones. Nat Struct Mol Biol 12:110–112

Ugur HC, Ramakrishna N, Bello L, Menon LG, Kim SK, Black PM, Carroll RS (2007) Continuous intracranial administration of suberoylanilide hydroxamic acid (SAHA) inhibits tumor growth in an orthotopic glioma model. J Neurooncol 83:267–275

Uhlmann K, Rohde K, Zeller C, Szymas J, Vogel S, Marczinek K, Thiel G, Nurnberg P, Laird PW (2003) Distinct methylation profiles of glioma subtypes. Int J Cancer 106:52–59

Uyeno S, Aoki Y, Nata M, Sagisaka K, Kayama T, Yoshimoto T, Ono T (1996) IGF2 but not H19 shows loss of imprinting in human glioma. Cancer Res 56:5356–5359

Van Der Bruggen P, Zhang Y, Chaux P, Stroobant V, Panichelli C, Schultz ES, Chapiro J, Van Den Eynde BJ, Brasseur F, Boon T (2002) Tumor-specific shared antigenic peptides recognized by human T cells. Immunol Rev 188:51–64

Vire E, Brenner C, Deplus R, Blanchon L, Fraga M, Didelot C, Morey L, Van Eynde A, Bernard D, Vanderwinden JM, Bollen M, Esteller M, Di Croce L, de Launoit Y, Fuks F (2006) The Polycomb group protein EZH2 directly controls DNA methylation. Nature 439:871–874

Waha A, Guntner S, Huang TH, Yan PS, Arslan B, Pietsch T, Wiestler OD (2005) Epigenetic silencing of the protocadherin family member PCDH-gamma-A11 in astrocytomas. Neoplasia 7:193–199

Walsh CP, Chaillet JR, Bestor TH (1998) Transcription of IAP endogenous retroviruses is constrained by cytosine methylation. Nature genetics 20:116–117

Watanabe T, Katayama Y, Yoshino A, Yachi K, Ohta T, Ogino A, Komine C, Fukushima T (2007) Aberrant hypermethylation of p14ARF and O6-methylguanine-DNA methyltransferase genes in astrocytoma progression. Brain Pathol 17:5–10

Watanabe T, Yokoo H, Yokoo M, Yonekawa Y, Kleihues P, Ohgaki H (2001) Concurrent inactivation of RB1 and TP53 pathways in anaplastic oligodendrogliomas. J Neuropathol Exp Neurol 60:1181–1189

Waterland RA, Jirtle RL (2003) Transposable elements: targets for early nutritional effects on epigenetic gene regulation. Mol Cell Biol 23:5293–5300

Weaver KD, Grossman SA, Herman JG (2006) Methylated tumor-specific DNA as a plasma biomarker in patients with glioma. Cancer Invest 24:35–40

Weber M, Davies JJ, Wittig D, Oakeley EJ, Haase M, Lam WL, Schubeler D (2005) Chromosome-wide and promoter-specific analyses identify sites of differential DNA methylation in normal and transformed human cells. Nat Genet 37:853–862

Widschwendter M, Fiegl H, Egle D, Mueller-Holzner E, Spizzo G, Marth C, Weisenberger DJ, Campan M, Young J, Jacobs I, Laird PW (2007) Epigenetic stem cell signature in cancer. Nature genetics 39:157–158

Wiencke JK, Zheng S, Jelluma N, Tihan T, Vandenberg S, Tamguney T, Baumber R, Parsons R, Lamborn KR, Berger MS, Wrensch MR, Haas-Kogan DA, Stokoe D (2007) Methylation of the PTEN promoter defines low-grade gliomas and secondary glioblastoma. Neuro-oncology 9:271–279

Wolf SF, Jolly DJ, Lunnen KD, Friedmann T, Migeon BR (1984) Methylation of the hypoxanthine phosphoribosyltransferase locus on the human X chromosome: implications for X-chromosome inactivation. Proc Nat Acad Sci USA 81:2806–2810

Wolff GL, Roberts DW, Mountjoy KG (1999) Physiological consequences of ectopic agouti gene expression: the yellow obese mouse syndrome. Physiol Genomics 1:151–163
Wong IH, Lo YM, Zhang J, Liew CT, Ng MH, Wong N, Lai PB, Lau WY, Hjelm NM, Johnson PJ (1999) Detection of aberrant p16 methylation in the plasma and serum of liver cancer patients. Cancer Res 59:71–73
Xu GL, Bestor TH, Bourc'his D, Hsieh CL, Tommerup N, Bugge M, Hulten M, Qu X, Russo JJ, Viegas-Pequignot E (1999) Chromosome instability and immunodeficiency syndrome caused by mutations in a DNA methyltransferase gene. Nature 402:187–191
Yanagisawa Y, Akiyama Y, Iida S, Ito E, Nomizu T, Sugihara K, Yuasa Y, Maruyama K (2000) Methylation of the hMLH1 promoter in familial gastric cancer with microsatellite instability. Int J Cancer 85:50–53
Yi JM, Tsai HC, Glockner SC, Lin S, Ohm JE, Easwaran H, James CD, Costello JF, Riggins G, Eberhart CG, Laterra J, Vescovi AL, Ahuja N, Herman JG, Schuebel KE, Baylin SB (2008) Abnormal DNA methylation of CD133 in colorectal and glioblastoma tumors. Cancer Res 68:8094–8103
Yin D, Ong JM, Hu J, Desmond JC, Kawamata N, Konda BM, Black KL, Koeffler HP (2007) Suberoylanilide hydroxamic acid, a histone deacetylase inhibitor: effects on gene expression and growth of glioma cells in vitro and in vivo. Clin Cancer Res 13:1045–1052
Yu J, Zhang H, Gu J, Lin S, Li J, Lu W, Wang Y, Zhu J (2004) Methylation profiles of thirty four promoter-CpG islands and concordant methylation behaviours of sixteen genes that may contribute to carcinogenesis of astrocytoma. BMC Cancer 4:65
Zardo G, Tiirikainen MI, Hong C, Misra A, Feuerstein BG, Volik S, Collins CC, Lamborn KR, Bollen A, Pinkel D, Albertson DG, Costello JF (2002) Integrated genomic and epigenomic analyses pinpoint biallelic gene inactivation in tumors. Nat Genet 32:453–458
Zhou H, Miki R, Eeva M, Fike FM, Seligson D, Yang L, Yoshimura A, Teitell MA, Jamieson CA, Cacalano NA (2007) Reciprocal regulation of SOCS 1 and SOCS3 enhances resistance to ionizing radiation in glioblastoma multiforme. Clin Cancer Res 13:2344–2353

Chapter 27
MicroRNAs in the Central Nervous System and Potential Roles of RNA Interference in Brain Tumors

Benjamin Purow

Abstract The study of RNA interference, in the form of endogenous microRNAs (miRNAs) or exogenous small interfering RNAs (siRNAs), is revealing powerful regulatory mechanisms throughout biology. Though small, these short RNA duplexes can lead to potent suppression of their targets. Numerous miRNAs are dysregulated in cancers, and several have been shown to play oncogenic or tumor suppressor roles. miRNAs are also pivotal in the development and function of the central nervous system. Brain tumors, positioned at the intersection of both, are strongly influenced by miRNAs. Early studies have shown upregulated miRNAs such as miR-21 and miR-221/222 to act in an oncogenic fashion, while the underexpressed miR-124 and miR-7 appear to suppress brain tumor formation. miRNAs and siRNAs also offer novel targeted approaches to the treatment of brain tumors. In this chapter we will discuss miRNAs in the central nervous system, their roles in brain tumors, and potential miRNA- and siRNA-based therapeutic strategies in neuro-oncology.

Contents

B. Purow (✉)
Neuro-Oncology Division, Neurology Department, University of Virginia, One Hospital Drive, Old Medical School, Room 4814, Charlottesville, VA 22908, USA
e-mail: bwp5g@virginia.edu

E.G. Van Meir (ed.), *CNS Cancer*, Cancer Drug Discovery and Development, DOI 10.1007/978-1-60327-553-8_27,

© Humana Press, a part of Springer Science+Business Media, LLC 2009

27.1 Introduction

RNA interference refers generally to short double-stranded RNA oligonucleotides which are complementary to target mRNAs and lead to their silencing. This silencing occurs via an ancient and evolutionarily conserved pathway that may be accessed in two ways – either through synthetic small interfering RNAs (siRNAs) or through their endogenous analog, the microRNAs (miRNAs). siRNAs, designed to target a single gene product, have been a powerful research tool over the last 10 years and are now beginning to reach the clinic. The more recently recognized miRNAs are quite different. Found throughout plant and animal cells, these 21–22 base RNA oligonucleotides play critical roles in biology and form complex regulatory webs with their numerous targets. The central nervous system (CNS) is no exception and may represent the richest site for miRNA activity. miRNAs have been demonstrated to be vitally important not only in normal development and cellular function, but also in cancer cells. Given their potent effects in neurobiology and in oncology, it is perhaps not surprising that a growing number of reports have shown that they regulate brain tumors as well. In this chapter we will review miRNA and siRNA processing and mechanisms, miRNA roles in CNS development and function, and potential therapeutic applications of miRNAs and siRNAs in neuro-oncology.

27.2 miRNA and siRNA Background

RNA interference was initially recognized in *Caenorhabditis elegans* as a phenomenon of specific gene silencing when a matching double-stranded RNA was introduced (Fire et al. 1998). This biological phenomenon was also found to be present in Drosophila (Hammond et al. 2000), but was not demonstrated in vertebrates until short RNA duplexes were delivered instead of longer ones. It was discovered that long double-stranded RNAs were processed to short 20–22 nucleotide RNA duplexes in the cytoplasm by the RNA-cleaving enzyme Dicer, and that these short RNA duplexes were the active element (Hamilton and Baulcombe 1999; Hammond et al. 2000; Bernstein et al. 2001; Grishok et al. 2001). Long double-stranded RNAs >30 bases triggered a non-specific interferon response in vertebrate cells that globally degraded mRNAs (Brown et al. 1976), but synthetic small interfering RNAs did not and were noted to induce specific gene suppression. Later, miRNAs were recognized as an endogenous form of RNA interference utilizing the same or similar mechanisms. miRNAs were actually discovered much earlier in *C. elegans* as short double-stranded loops of RNA encoded within the genome (Ambros 1989; Wightman et al. 1993), though their ubiquity initially went unnoticed. Later, they were also found to be present in plants and animals, including humans (Lagos-Quintana et al. 2001; Reinhart et al. 2002). miRNAs are located in areas of the genome previously thought to be "junk DNA," either in introns or in transcriptional units within intergenic areas (Lee and Ambros 2001; Lagos-Quintana et al. 2003). It is now recognized that these areas are far from silent, often producing powerful regulatory non-coding RNAs, and miRNAs may be the most vital of these. It is estimated that the human genome may hold approximately one thousand of these short hairpins, with up to one-third of human genes potently regulated by them. Many of the miRNAs identified in mammals have been found in brain samples and are more highly expressed in the CNS than elsewhere. Numerous reports have shown very striking effects from some of these miRNAs in differentiation and function of neurons and glia, supporting their importance in the CNS.

miRNAs are originally transcribed from the genome as part of large primary transcripts, called pri-microRNAs (pri-miRNAs or pri-miRs) (Fig. 27.1). Sometimes these pri-miRs include more than one miRNA hairpin. These large transcripts are processed in the nucleus by the Drosha protein complex to form roughly 70-base pre-microRNA hairpins (pre-miRNAs or pre-miRs) (Lee et al. 2003). Other RNA-binding proteins may regulate processing of particular miRNAs, but this has not yet been well explored. One recently reported example, lin28 regulation of the processing of let-7 miRNAs, suggests that this may be an important phenomenon (Newman et al. 2008; Viswanathan et al. 2008). Following processing to the pre-miR form, the miRNAs are transported from the nucleus to the cytoplasm by the exportin-5 protein (Lund et al. 2004). Once in the cytoplasm, pre-miRs are processed further by the Dicer complex to create mature double-stranded miRNAs of 20–23 base pairs (Hutvagner and Zamore 2002). These mature miRNAs are then bound by the RISC complex (RNA-induced silencing complex) of the RNA interference pathway. The miRNA/RISC complex then targets mRNAs with sites in their 3′-untranslated regions (3′-UTR) complementary to the miRNA (Ha et al. 1996). This usually results in suppression of translation by an unknown mechanism, though it may involve routing of target mRNAs to the P-body organelle in the cytoplasm (Liu et al. 2005; Sen and Blau 2005). miRNA target inhibition can also cause degradation of target mRNAs, particularly if there is a very high degree of complementarity between the miRNA and the target region in the 3′-UTR. Degradation of target mRNAs was originally thought to be quite rare in humans, but more recent work suggests that it may be more common than was previously thought (Yu et al. 2007; Baek et al. 2008; Selbach et al. 2008). In general, it appears important that the region of complementarity includes the "seed region," bases 2-8 or 1–7 of the miRNA (Lai et al. 2005). Generally, the more seed matches for a given miRNA present in a gene's 3′-UTR, the stronger the inhibition. Two recent proteomics studies have

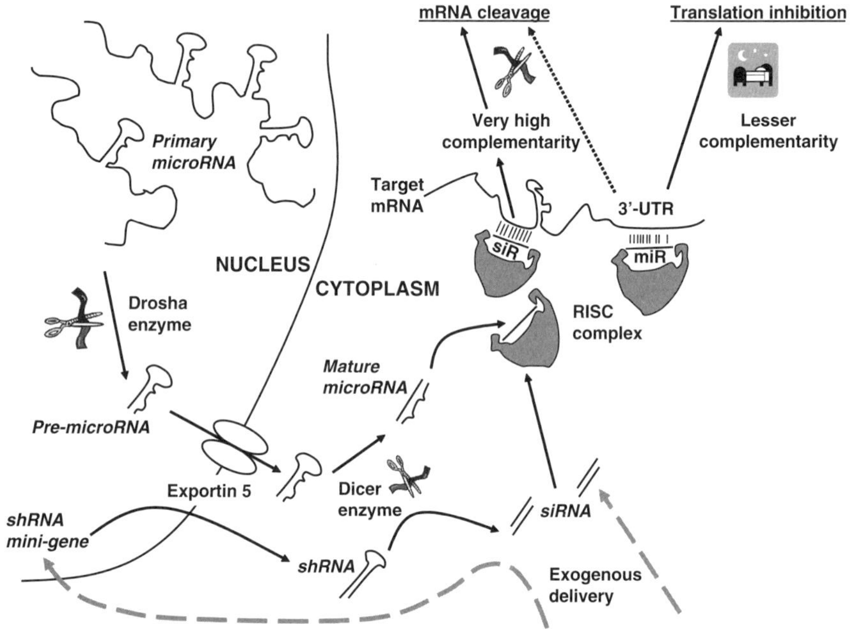

Fig. 27.1 Overview of RNA interference in the cell. MicroRNAs are initially small microRNA hairpins within larger transcripts from introns or intergenic regions. These are then processed within the nucleus by the Drosha enzyme to generate small pre-microRNA hairpins, which are then exported from the nucleus by exportin-5. Within the cytoplasm, the pre-microRNAs are then processed by the Dicer enzyme to form mature double-stranded microRNAs 19–21 bases long. These mature microRNAs are picked up by the RISC complex and one strand discarded. The single strand held by the RISC complex is then used to find partly complementary sites in the 3′-untranslated regions (3′-UTRs) of target genes. "Seed matches" with bases 2–8 or 1–7 at the 5′-end of the microRNA are particularly important. High levels of complementarity of the microRNA to the target sequence can lead to cleavage of the target mRNA, but more commonly there is less complementarity and instead there is suppression of translation by an unknown mechanism. Small interfering RNAs (siRNAs) are introduced exogenously into the cytoplasm already as short double-stranded RNAs, already able to be picked up by the RISC complex. They are designed to be perfectly complementary to the target mRNA at any point and lead to its cleavage. Minigenes also may be introduced to cells with a short hairpin RNA (shRNA) encoding an siRNA; the shRNA is cleaved by Dicer to produce the desired siRNA

confirmed that individual miRNAs can weakly affect the expression of hundreds of genes, but strongly affect expression in quite few (Baek et al. 2008; Selbach et al. 2008). Notably, one report indicates that miRNA binding to the 5′-untranslated region of target mRNAs is just as effective as binding to 3′-UTRs (Lytle et al. 2007), but this may be far less significant given the relatively smaller size of 5′-UTRs versus 3′-UTRs and findings from extensive proteomics analysis (Selbach et al. 2008). miRNA and siRNA processing is summarized in Fig. 27.1.

Since the recognition that delivery of 20–22 base RNA duplexes perfectly complementary to a target mRNA led to its degradation, siRNAs rapidly became the method of choice for inhibiting expression of a target gene – supplanting antisense and ribozymes. While the success of these synthetic siRNAs was initially quite hit-or-miss, the criteria for their design have been continuously refined and now the likelihood of efficient target suppression with a given siRNA is much higher. Small interfering RNAs appear to utilize part of the RNA interference pathway described above, but enter at a late point at which one strand can be bound to the RISC complex. siRNAs are designed to be perfectly complementary to a single mRNA, so cleavage of the target results. Importantly, siRNAs may be complementary to the target mRNA at any point, not just in the UTRs. In some cell types, their use is limited by the ability to deliver them efficiently to the cytoplasm. Additionally, siRNAs can only suppress a target for a short period measured in days. To get around this, the siRNA can be delivered in an expression vector in the form of a short hairpin RNA, or shRNA, analogous to a pre-miRNA. Such shRNAs may be stably expressed in cells through delivery modalities such as viruses. Following shRNA expression, the hairpin loop is cleaved off by Dicer to leave the 20–22 base double-stranded siRNA. Use of siRNAs to silence a target gene is also complicated by off-target silencing of other genes, reducing the specificity of suppression and potentially affecting the resulting phenotype (Scacheri et al. 2004). It may be possible to reduce this by avoiding complementarity in the siRNA's 5′-area to non-targeted genes – the equivalent of "seed matches" if the siRNA were a miRNA.

27.3 MicroRNAs in CNS Development and Function

Several studies over the past 5 years have performed global profiling of miRNA expression in various animal and human tissues, including the CNS (Dostie et al. 2003; Krichevsky et al. 2003; Ambros and Lee 2004; Babak et al. 2004; Barad et al. 2004; Kim et al. 2004; Liu et al. 2004; Sun et al. 2004; Thomson et al. 2004). Usually this has been done with microRNA microarrays, typically custom made but now available commercially or as a contract service. These studies have shown numerous miRNAs to be preferentially or exclusively expressed in the nervous system, with many fewer organ-specific miRNAs found for other organ systems. Other profiling studies have shown that expression of this large group of nervous system miRNAs varies widely across both space and time; miRNA expression changes dramatically from one area of the brain to the next and as the nervous system develops (Krichevsky et al. 2003; Kapsimali et al. 2007; Bak et al. 2008). The nervous system-specific expression of many of these miRNAs is evolutionarily conserved, supporting their importance. Additionally, many new central nervous system-specific miRNAs were identified in one study comparing miRNAs in the central nervous system of primates versus lower organisms (Berezikov et al. 2006). It is tempting to speculate from an evolutionary perspective that miRNAs may be a major factor in the expansion of brain size and function, given that miRNAs differ far more than the genome as a whole in the evolution of recent species such as primates. Additionally, miRNAs may also be a major determinant of intraspecies variability in brain function among humans; one interesting recent report showed that variability in gene expression in human brain cortex across different individuals correlated with the number of miRNA seed matches in the genes' 3′-UTRs (Zhang and Su 2008).

The critical role of miRNAs in the CNS is indicated by studies in which the expression of the Dicer processing protein is knocked out in specific brain areas. Elimination of Dicer in the mouse forebrain led to microcephaly and dendritic spine abnormalities (Davis et al. 2008). In a second study by the same groups, Dicer knockout in striatal neurons was found to cause severe neuromotor phenotypes but did not lead to neuronal death (Cuellar et al. 2008). Many other studies have probed the role of individual miRNAs expressed highly in the central nervous system.

27.4 Individual MicroRNAs in the CNS

While miRNAs as a whole are clearly essential for the development of the nervous system, the power of individual miRNAs is quite striking. The earliest and perhaps most notable example of this came in zebrafish. Giraldez and colleagues created Dicer knockout mice in which the brain defects could be rescued by adding back processed miR-430 – suggesting that the brain deficits were due almost exclusively to a deficiency of miR-430 (Giraldez et al. 2005). A similar central role for miR-430 in the mammalian central nervous system has not yet been shown. However, single miRNAs may be pivotal in the human nervous system as well, with miRNA-124 standing out as the best studied and most prominent. miR-124a and b are highly and specifically expressed in neurons (Sempere et al. 2004; Bak et al. 2008) and play a key role in the differentiation of precursors to mature neurons. One potential mechanism for this (Makeyev et al. 2007) is miR-124 targeting of PTBP1, a potent regulator of alternative mRNA splicing found in non-nervous system cells. This downregulation leads to upregulation of functional PTBP2, another mRNA splicing regulator in nervous system cells. The expression of PTBP2 and not PTBP1 leads to proper splicing patterns in nervous system cells, a far-reaching consequence for a single miRNA target. Another mechanism for the proneural importance of miR-124 stems from the demonstration that miR-124a inhibits expression of both the RE1 silencing transcription factor (REST) and its partner small C-terminal phosphatase 1 (SCP1), and neuronal fate is opposed by REST/SCP1 (Conaco et al. 2006; Visvanathan et al. 2007). Interestingly, REST/SCP1 also inhibits expression of miR-124, suggesting that there is a miR-124/REST-SCP1 axis determining neuronal fate. In addition to the importance of miR-124 in neuronal differentiation, recent evidence indicates that its downregulation may be important in certain brain tumors, and this will be addressed later in this chapter.

miRNAs may have especially prominent roles in the dendritic spines involved in synapses. Several pre- and mature miRNAs have been found to be localized in post-synaptic densities, suggesting they are processed there and act at that location within the cell (Lugli et al. 2008). An individual miRNA, miR-134, has been shown to drive the formation of dendritic spines (Schratt et al. 2006). A different miRNA, miR-132, has been demonstrated to increase synaptic plasticity, and interestingly the expression of this miRNA is increased by the CREB transcription factor dependent on neuronal activity (Wayman et al. 2008).

Other work has suggested roles for individual miRNAs in specific parts of the brain. For example, Choi and colleagues have shown in zebrafish and mice that terminal differentiation of olfactory neurons requires the miR-200 family, though mature olfactory neurons do not require it (Choi et al. 2008). miR-9, one of the highest-expressed miRNAs in the central nervous system, also plays a role in brain development through the determination of midbrain/hindbrain separation (Leucht et al. 2008). miR-7 may be important in the pituitary and hypothalamus, where its expression is high. Its expression is particularly high in the human pituitary, presumably due to the fact that one of its three isoforms lies within an intron of a highly expressed pituitary-specific gene (Farh et al. 2005; Bak et al. 2008). Lee and colleagues demonstrated one role for miR-7b in the mouse hypothalamus, where it is upregulated in response to hyperosmolar stress and downregulates Fos expression (Lee et al. 2006). As with miR-124, downregulation of miR-7 appears significant in brain tumors and will be discussed later in the chapter.

27.5 MicroRNAs in Cancer

Prior to considering potential roles for miRNAs in brain tumors, their impact on oncology as a whole should be discussed. The study of miRNAs is generating increasing enthusiasm among cancer researchers, yielding new insights into cancer biology as well as potential tools for diagnosis and treatment. miRNA profiling can be used to identify cancer types or subtypes, and may in fact be better at this than standard expression profiling with oligonucleotide microarrays (Lu et al. 2005). Expression of numerous miRNAs is dysregulated in cancer, and miRNAs are disproportionately located in areas of amplification or deletion in cancer (Calin et al. 2004). For a few such loci, the genes targeted by these genetic alterations had been unsuccessfully hunted for many years before it was realized that the relevant local feature was a miRNA and not a gene (Calin et al. 2002). miRNAs can have oncogenic properties through their targeting of major tumor suppressor genes, while others act as tumor suppressors through their inhibition of oncogenes (prominent oncogenic and tumor suppressor miRNAs are listed in Table 27.1 and also described in more detail below).

The miR-17-92 miRNA cluster was the first to be formally demonstrated as an oncogenic microRNA or oncomiR. This region is amplified in B-cell lymphomas, and driving its expression in mouse B cells accelerated cancer

Table 27.1 Selected prominent microRNAs in cancer. Oncogenic microRNAs upregulated in multiple cancers are shown at the top of the chart, with potential mechanisms and key targets tabulated on the right. This set includes potential oncomiRs in brain tumors. At the bottom of the table are microRNAs commonly downregulated in various cancers, with potential tumor suppressor functions

Oncogenic microRNAs	Dysregulated in cancers	Potential functions/relevant targets
miR-17-92 cluster	B-cell CLL (He et al. 2005b)	Cooperates with myc (He et al. 2005b)
miR-21	Glioblastoma (Chan et al. 2005; Silber et al. 2008); breast, colon, lung, pancreas, prostate, stomach (Iorio et al. 2005; Volinia et al. 2006; Lee et al. 2007); HNSCC (Tran et al. 2007)	Promotes cell survival – targets PDCD4 (Frankel et al. 2008), PTEN (Meng et al. 2007), TPM1 (Zhu et al. 2007); promotes invasion – targets RECK, TIMP3 (Gabriely et al. 2008)
miR-221	Glioblastoma (Ciafre et al. 2005); melanoma (Felicetti et al. 2008); prostate (Galardi et al. 2007); pancreatic (Lee et al. 2007); thyroid (Nikiforova et al. 2008); kidney/bladder (Gottardo et al. 2007); thyroid (He et al. 2005a); ovarian (Dahiya et al. 2008)	Targets tumor suppressors p27 and p57 (Gillies and Lorimer 2007; Fornari et al. 2008)
miR-155	Glioblastoma (Silber et al. 2008); breast, colon, lung (Iorio et al. 2005; Volinia et al. 2006); tongue SCC (Wong et al. 2008); lung (Yanaihara et al. 2006); lymphoma (Kluiver et al. 2005)	Targets hematopoietic development genes (O'Connell et al. 2008); targets TP53INP1 (Gironella et al. 2007)
miR-10b	Glioblastoma (Ciafre et al. 2005; Silber et al. 2008); breast (Ma et al. 2007)	Promotes metastasis – Inhibits HOXD10 (Ma et al. 2007)
Tumor suppressor microRNA		
miR-15/16	B-cell CLL (Calin et al. 2002); pituitary (Bottoni et al. 2005)	Inhibits survival by targeting Bcl-2 (Cimmino et al. 2005)
let-7 family	Lung, colon (Takamizawa et al. 2004; Akao et al. 2006), likely most others	Target ras, myc (Johnson et al. 2005; Sampson et al. 2007)
miR-34 a,b,c	Neuroblastoma (Welch et al. 2007); colon (Tazawa et al. 2007)	A mediator of p53; targets CDK6, c-met, CCND1 (He et al. 2007; Sun et al. 2008) and N-myc (Wei et al. 2008a)

formation in conjunction with overexpression of the myc oncogene (He et al. 2005b). The miRNAs within the cluster appeared to protect the B cells from the apoptosis triggered by myc overexpression alone. Other potential oncogenic miRNAs have been identified in various cancers through profiling studies (Volinia et al. 2006). miRNA-21 stands out as perhaps the most universally overexpressed in different cancer types, including brain tumors, and will be discussed in more detail later (Chan et al. 2005; Iorio et al. 2005; Volinia et al. 2006; Lee et al. 2007; Tran et al. 2007). miRNA-221 is dysregulated in a wide variety of tumors, including brain tumors, and will also be addressed in more detail in a subsequent section (Ciafre et al. 2005; He et al. 2005a; Gottardo et al. 2007; Lee et al. 2007; Nikiforova et al. 2008). miRNA-155 is overexpressed in a number of cancers, particularly hematopoietic, and is also a major regulator of normal lymphocytes (Iorio et al. 2005; Kluiver et al. 2005; Ramkissoon et al. 2006; Tam and Dahlberg 2006; Volinia et al. 2006; Yanaihara et al. 2006; Vigorito et al. 2007; Wong et al. 2008).

miRNAs have also been reported to drive specific malignant behaviors, such as invasiveness and chemoresistance. miR-10b is upregulated in metastatic breast cancer cells and increases breast cancer invasion and metastasis, possibly via inhibition of the HOXD10 gene that normally represses the pro-metastatic RHOC gene (Ma et al. 2007). Another group screened a miRNA library in a non-invasive breast cancer line and noted that miRs -373 and -520c strongly promoted invasiveness (Huang et al. 2008). Endogenous miR-373 was important for cell migration in a number of cancer lines, and this was associated with inhibition of CD44. Other miRNAs, including miR-21 and miR-7, have also been shown to promote or inhibit invasiveness (Gabriely et al. 2008; Kefas et al. 2008; Zhu et al. 2008). Resistance to chemotherapy has also been linked to miRNAs. One report associated expression of miR-21, let-7i, and other miRNAs to chemoresistance (Blower et al. 2008), while others demonstrated that miRs -15b and -16 played this role in gastric cancer (Xia et al. 2008).

Some miRNAs have been discovered which normally act as inhibitors of oncogenes and which are downregulated in cancers. A case in point is the 13q14 genomic region deleted in a majority of cases of chronic lymphocytic leukemia (CLL), a region found to hold miR-15a and miR-16-1 (Calin et al. 2002). These miRNAs target the survival protein Bcl-2, providing a rationale for their downregulation in CLL (Cimmino et al. 2005). The most widely downregulated miRNAs in cancer are the let-7 family, which includes numerous variants. Nearly all are highly expressed in normal tissues and minimally expressed in cancers (Sempere et al. 2004; Takamizawa et al. 2004; Akao et al. 2006). The let-7 family targets key oncogenes such as myc and ras, so downregulation of this miRNA family provides cancers with a single means to upregulate both pathways (Johnson et al. 2005; Sampson et al. 2007). Recent exciting reports suggest that the key stem cell protein lin-28 suppresses processing of the let-7 miRNAs, and that upregulation of lin-28 is one mechanism by which cancers downregulate let-7 (Newman et al. 2008; Viswanathan et al. 2008). The miRNA-34 family is another group downregulated in some cancers and with important biological roles. Several groups showed recently that the tumor suppressor p53 drives expression of miR-34 a, b, and c, and that miR-34 is an important mediator of the pro-apoptotic effects of p53 (Chang et al. 2007; Corney et al. 2007; He et al. 2007; Raver-Shapira et al. 2007). Key targets of miR-34 include the oncogenes CDK6, c-met, and cyclin D1 (CCND1) (He et al. 2007; Sun et al. 2008).

27.6 MicroRNAs in Brain Tumors

The study of miRNAs in brain tumors is one in which the number of review articles may exceed the actual reports, to paraphrase a colleague. Given the apparent centrality of miRNAs in the human nervous system and their increasingly recognized roles in cancer, it has almost been assumed that they would be important in brain tumors. However, there have been relatively few reports to date specifically addressing miRNAs in brain tumors. Despite this slow start, the number of published reports in this area has been increasing and promises to offer vital new understanding and therapeutic approaches for brain tumors. These early reports indicate that some of the oncogenic or tumor suppressor miRNAs important in other cancer types are significant in brain tumors as well, but there also appear to be miRNAs uniquely relevant in neuro-oncology.

Beginning a few years ago, reports of global miRNA profiling in brain tumors began to appear. This has generally been performed with microarrays similar to typical oligonucleotide microarrays, though there are now commercially available formats that allow quantitative real-time PCR of 400–500 miRNAs simultaneously in multiple plates. Both cell lines and tissues have been studied. One report assessed miRNA expression in the NCI-60 panel of cell lines, identifying trends among cell lines of a few tumor types (Gaur et al. 2007). Numerous miRNAs were downregulated among brain tumor lines, particularly miR-124 and miR-7 – both of which shall be revisited later in this chapter. The first study with brain tumor tissues compared miRNA expression in a small number of glioblastomas (GBMs) to normal brain samples (Ciafre et al. 2005). Several miRNAs were found to be upregulated in some of the GBMs, including miRNAs mentioned earlier that play roles in several cancers: miR-21, miR-221, and miR-10b. miR-125b also had increased expression in GBMs, and this miRNA has previously been shown to play a role in proliferation in cancer cell lines (Lee et al. 2005). Among the downregulated miRNAs were miR-128 and the miR-181 family. miR-128 has been found to be upregulated in neurons (Smirnova et al. 2005), so its downregulation in glioblastomas may reflect their greater similarity to astrocytes than to neurons. miR-181 has been shown to correlate with differentiation and to inhibit the pro-survival oncogene TCL1 (Naguibneva et al. 2006; Pekarsky et al. 2006), possibly explaining pressure to downregulate its expression in tumors.

Brain tumors other than GBM have also undergone preliminary profiling studies. One early report compared expression of a few miRNAs in oligodendroglioma, brain with astrocytosis, fetal brain, and adult brain (Nelson et al. 2006). mir-9 had increased expression in oligodendrogliomas versus adult cortex and astrocytosis, miR-124a was decreased in oligodendrogliomas versus adult and fetal cortex, and miR-125b showed negligible change. miR-9 was also highlighted in a recent profiling study of primary brain tumors versus metastases to brain; the authors found that expression of miR-9/miR-9* (miR-9* is the opposite strand in the miR-9 duplex) and miR-92b could be used to accurately distinguish the two groups (Nass et al. 2008). miRNA profiling has been performed for pituitary tumors as well, comparing miRNA expression in 32 pituitary adenomas versus that in 6 normal samples (Bottoni et al. 2007). Numerous miRNAs were up- or downregulated, and the downregulated miRNAs included miR-128a, miR-7-1 and miR-7-3, three let-7 family members, and miR-9-3. The same group also showed earlier that miR-15 and miR-16 are downregulated in pituitary tumors, potentially elevating their expression of the prosurvival factor Bcl-2 (Bottoni et al. 2005).

Further results on miRNA profiling in glioblastomas is expected from The Cancer Genome Atlas (TCGA), a U.S. government-sponsored project spanning multiple centers for the purpose of profiling three different cancers on numerous fronts. Glioblastoma is among the TCGA's three cancers, which were chosen for the large amounts of high-quality stored tissue and for their poor prognoses. Initial miRNA profiling results of glioblastomas are publicly available online, though registration and approval are required for higher level access to any patient information associated with the samples. Some early analyses of TCGA data on miRNA and gene expression in GBMs were presented at the 2008 American Association for Cancer Research (AACR) meeting (Qi et al. 2008). Three subtypes were identified by gene expression and by miRNA expression analyses, with agreement between both groups and also with a previous report on classification of high-grade gliomas (Phillips et al. 2006). While the TCGA data on miRNA expression in GBMs will no doubt continue to bear fruit, it will be helpful in the future to have such high-throughput efforts also include non-neoplastic brain samples for comparison. Additionally, miRNA profiling across different grades of brain tumors, or between primary and secondary GBMs, would be useful as well. Such global miRNA profiling will not only enhance subsequent efforts to classify brain tumors but also enable new insights into their biology and suggests individual miRNAs for further study.

27.6.1 Oncogenic miRNAs in Brain Tumors

Early profiling work in this young field indicated that miR-21 was upregulated in GBMs versus fetal and adult brain and non-neoplastic tissues (Krichevsky et al. 2003). The inhibition of this miRNA with short antisense 2′-O-methyl oligonucleotides or LNA (locked nucleic acid) oligonucleotides triggered apoptosis in glioblastoma cells, suggesting that miR-21 played an important role in GBM cell survival. Furthermore, the combination of LNA oligonucleotide inhibition of miR-21 with neural precursor cell delivery of a soluble form of tumor necrosis factor-related apoptosis inducing ligand (S-TRAIL) showed synergistic anti-tumor effects in vitro and in vivo. These studies established miR-21 as an oncogenic miRNA in glioblastoma that can be targeted for therapy (Corsten et al. 2007). This appears to match its role in many other tumor types as well. In other cancers miR-21 expression has been shown to be a prognostic factor, but this has not yet been reported in brain tumors (Roldo et al. 2006; Schetter et al. 2008). The mechanism for miR-21 upregulation in GBMs has not been elucidated but may involve the activity of the transcription factors Stat3 (Loffler et al. 2007) or AP-1 (Fujita et al. 2008) which are both upregulated in GBM (de la Iglesia et al. 2008) (Desbaillets et al. 1999).

The mechanism(s) for the oncogenic effects of miR-21 has not yet been identified precisely and indeed may vary across different tumor types. A few targets of miR-21 have been documented and proposed as the most relevant, but its effects may stem from combined inhibition of these and other targets. Four groups have proposed that miR-21 targeting of the PDCD4 gene (programmed cell death 4) is central to its effects (Asangani et al. 2008; Frankel et al. 2008; Lu et al. 2008; Zhu et al. 2008). PDCD4 has not been specifically linked to brain tumors to date, but it plays a role in apoptosis and suppression of invasion and metastasis. Notably, one group described a successful "rescue" experiment in which siRNA to PDCD4 could largely spare a breast cancer line from the effects of a miR-21 inhibitor on cell viability (Frankel et al. 2008). Such rescue experiments are critical in miRNA studies to demonstrate the importance of a particular target. However, they are rarely reported, likely due to the relevance of multiple targets in the effects of most miRNAs. Other groups have not described rescue experiments with miR-21 inhibitors but have shown targeting of important cancer genes. PTEN, a critical tumor suppressor gene in glioblastoma and other advanced cancers, is a target of miR-21 (Meng et al. 2007). The tumor suppressor gene tropomyosin 1 (TPM1) has also been reported as a key miR-21 target (Zhu et al. 2007). Sprouty 2, a negative regulator of receptor tyrosine kinase signaling, is inhibited by miR-21 as well (Sayed et al. 2008). miR-21 downregulation of invasion and metastasis may be partially mediated by its inhibition of the RECK and TIMP-3 genes, which are matrix metalloprotease (MMP) inhibitors (Gabriely et al. 2008).

miR-221 is overexpressed in GBMs, as noted earlier, and appears to be another key oncomiR across multiple cancers (Ciafre et al. 2005). It has been noted to be elevated in melanoma, pancreatic cancer, prostate cancer, bladder cancer, ovarian cancer, hepatocellular carcinoma, and papillary thyroid carcinoma (He et al. 2005a; Galardi et al. 2007; Gottardo et al. 2007; Lee et al. 2007; Dahiya et al. 2008; Felicetti et al. 2008; Nikiforova et al. 2008). The mechanisms behind its tumor-promoting effects have not been investigated as extensively as those for miR-21, but Lorimer and colleagues have shown in GBM that miR-221/miR-222 inhibits p27 (Gillies and Lorimer 2007). Fornari and colleagues have also demonstrated in hepatocellular carcinoma that miR-221 targets the tumor suppressors p27 and p57 (Fornari et al. 2008). How miR-221 is upregulated in GBMs is unknown, but in other cancers the oncogenes driving its overexpression include mycN and PLZF (Felicetti et al. 2008; Schulte et al. 2008).

27.6.2 miRNAs with Tumor Suppressor Properties in Brain Tumors

No miRNAs have yet been conclusively demonstrated as classic tumor suppressor genes in brain tumors, with evidence that their downregulation promotes tumorigenesis in the nervous system. However, three groups to date have shown tumor suppressor properties of a few miRNAs in brain tumors (tabulated in Table 27.2).

Expression profiling of 192 miRNAs with quantitative real-time PCR in anaplastic astrocytomas, GBMs, and non-neoplastic brain tissue (Silber et al. 2008) disclosed numerous up- and downregulated miRNAs, with the upregulated miRNAs in GBMs comprised of known oncomiRs such as miR-10b, miR-21, and miR-155. miR-210 also demonstrated increased expression, and this miRNA has been shown in breast cancer to be hypoxia-regulated and a negative prognostic indicator (Camps et al. 2008). The authors then focused on the miRNAs with decreased expression in high-grade gliomas, in particular miR-124 and miR-137. miR-124 is a well-known pro-neuronal miRNA described earlier in this chapter, and miR-137 is also highly expressed in neurons. Transfection of either of these miRNAs into glioblastoma tumor stem cells increased neuronal differentiation upon serum exposure, as indicated

Table 27.2 Tumor-suppressive microRNAs in brain tumors. This chart summarizes the microRNAs with potential tumor suppressor functions reported to date in brain tumors. Unlike the situation for oncogenic microRNAs, these may often be specific to brain tumors and include microRNAs with important functions in normal brain

MicroRNA	Expression in brain tumors	Potential functions/relevant targets
miR-124 miR-137	Downregulated in glioblastomas (Silber et al. 2008) Downregulated in medulloblastomas (mir-124) (Pierson et al. 2008)	Cause cell cycle arrest, promote neuronal differentiation in GBM tumor stem cells (Silber et al. 2008)
miR-7	Downregulated in glioblastomas (Kefas et al. 2008; Silber et al. 2008)	Inhibits proliferation, survival and migration; targets the EGF receptor and Akt pathway (Kefas et al. 2008)
miR-15/16	Downregulated in pituitary adenomas (Bottoni et al. 2005)	Targets the p43 gene, which regulates angiogenesis and inflammation and is anti-neoplastic (Bottoni et al. 2005); also known to target the pro-survival gene Bcl-2 (Cimmino et al. 2005)

by both morphology and marker profile. miR-124 and miR-137 also triggered G1-cell cycle arrest in glioblastoma cells, and the authors suggest that this may have been due to the potent inhibition of cdk6 they demonstrated for both miRNAs. The mechanism for miR-137 downregulation appeared to involve methylation, as the de-methylating agent 5-aza-2′-deoxycytidine (5-aza-dC) markedly increased its expression in glioma cells. Thus both of these neuronal miRNAs act as potential tumor suppressors in gliomas, and their delivery may have therapeutic potential. They may also have relevance in other brain tumors; miR-124 downregulation, inhibition of cell proliferation, and targeting of cdk6 have been described in medulloblastomas as well (Pierson et al. 2008).

miRNA-7 was shown in another report to be downregulated in GBMs relative to non-neoplastic brain (Kefas et al. 2008), and this was subsequently confirmed in the work described above. Kefas and colleagues demonstrated potent targeting by miR-7 of the epidermal growth factor receptor (EGFR) and of the Akt pathway, both of which appear to play prominent roles in the genesis of GBMs (Libermann et al. 1985; Haas-Kogan et al. 1998; Holland et al. 2000) (see also Chapters 15, 20, 38). Insulin receptor substrate-1 and -2 (IRS-1 and -2), upstream regulators of Akt activation, were both downregulated by transfection with pre-miR-7. The mechanism for miR-7 downregulation in GBMs appeared to be at the level of pri-miR to pre-miR processing, possibly involving unidentified RNA-binding regulatory proteins. Transfection with miR-7 slowed glioma cell growth, increased apoptosis, and decreased invasion in multiple glioma cell types, raising the prospect of miR-7 delivery as a potential therapy for glioma.

27.7 Potential miRNA- and siRNA-Based Therapies for Brain Tumors

27.7.1 Delivery of siRNAs or miRNAs as Therapy

miRNA- and siRNA-based approaches offer a number of novel therapeutic strategies against brain tumors. While the hope is that these strategies can be targeted in an elegant fashion against tumor cells while sparing normal cells, achieving this is not straightforward. At the simplest level, siRNAs to some essential tumor gene, perhaps an oncogene, will be efficiently delivered to brain tumor cells. Targeting could result from selective toxicity of the siRNA to the tumor cells, selective delivery, or a combination of both. Numerous groups have shown the in vitro effectiveness of knockdown of a given gene against brain tumor cells (e.g., Purow et al. 2005; Amos et al. 2007; Pyrko et al. 2007; Li et al. 2008; Saito et al. 2008; Wei et al. 2008b, to cite a few), and recent work in animal models has indicated its feasibility against brain tumors in vivo (Arwert et al. 2007; Zhao et al. 2007; Chen et al. 2008; Kargiotis et al. 2008). Significant challenges remain in optimizing the use of short RNAs as cancer therapy. If the

RNAs are delivered in an unmodified form, they are rapidly degraded. Several approaches are being pursued to modify or conjugate short RNAs to protect them in an in vivo milieu and to help them reach the cytoplasm of target cells. Perhaps an even more daunting challenge lies in identifying an efficient method for delivering short RNAs to tumor cells, though progress continues to be made with viral delivery of shRNAs and liposomal delivery of siRNAs. The state-of-the-art has recently been reviewed elsewhere (Pirollo and Chang 2008). Delivery of RNAs seems especially challenging for brain tumors, which are frequently disseminated through normal and essential brain tissue. However, we may ultimately have more success with brain tumors than other cancer types, given the potential of convection-enhanced delivery (CED) to saturate a brain region (Nguyen et al. 2003; Chen et al. 2005) and the inability of most brain tumors to metastasize outside the brain.

27.7.2 Oncogenic miRNA-Based Therapies

Oncogenic miRNAs are a new class of targets for brain tumor therapy. Inhibition of miR-21, miR-221, and miR-10b may all represent promising approaches, with miR-21 inhibition already showing efficacy in glioma models. These miRNAs can be inhibited through delivery of short modified oligonucleotides (oligos) complementary to their sequence. Such oligonucleotides may take various forms, such as locked nucleic acid (LNA) oligos or antagomiRs previously shown to act as efficient and specific blockers of microRNAs (Krutzfeldt et al. 2005; Orom et al. 2006). Alternatively, it may be possible to diminish activity of an oncogenic miRNA through delivery of a "decoy" transgene with an artificial 3′-UTR containing multiple target sites for that miRNA, monopolizing available copies (Ebert et al. 2007). This decoy approach may also permit the design of transgenic mice with the activity of a given miRNA diminished. Other approaches to inhibiting oncomiRs could involve downregulation of their transcription or processing.

27.7.3 Tumor-Suppressive miRNA-Based Therapies

Downregulated miRNAs with tumor suppressor properties could also be the basis of new brain tumor therapies. In this case, therapy could consist of simple delivery of the miRNA itself. Candidate miRNAs to date include miR-124, miR-137, and miR-7. One potential advantage of such treatments is that the miRNAs are found in normal brain, so spillover of delivery to surrounding normal cells would hopefully be non-toxic. Combinations of such miRNAs may be even more effective, but this has not yet been evaluated. As an alternative to endogenous tumor-suppressive miRNAs, it is possible to design artificial miRNAs that may offer theoretical advantages (Zeng et al. 2002;

Schwab et al. 2006). An artificial miRNA can be engineered to inhibit multiple desired targets, as opposed to the single target offered by an siRNA (Schwab et al. 2006; Ossowski et al. 2008). They can also be designed to avoid undesirable targets such as tumor suppressor genes, offering a potential advantage versus endogenous miRNAs as therapy; it seems likely that endogenous tumor-suppressive miRNAs lose efficacy against cancer cells because of tumor suppressor genes among their numerous targets.

27.7.4 Indirect miRNA-Based Strategies for Brain Tumor Therapy

While delivery of siRNAs, shRNAs, miRNAs, or miRNA inhibitors offers the potential for targeted therapies against brain tumors, there are at least two major risks that have been identified to date. Delivery of double-stranded RNAs longer than 30 bases triggers an interferon response mediated by Toll-like receptor 3 (Sledz et al. 2003; Kariko et al. 2004), but the same response may be triggered by too high a concentration of short RNA duplexes (Bridge et al. 2003). This could require modulation of the quantity of short RNAs delivered in vivo. It has also been found that overexpression of shRNA in vivo may be toxic through another mechanism. Grimm and colleagues noted in mice that viral delivery of high amounts of shRNAs to the liver often led to potentially lethal hepatotoxicity, apparently due to competition with endogenous miRNAs for factors such as exportin 5 (Grimm et al. 2006). However, it did appear that this could be bypassed by modulating the amount and fashion of shRNA delivery.

One exciting strategy that avoids such side effects is the use of miRNA-regulated transgenes or viruses to attack tumors through their miRNA expression profile. A number of studies in recent years have investigated the use of selective viruses against brain tumors, and these have proven the viability of such viral strategies (see Chapters 46 and 47). If a miRNA is identified that is expressed in normal brain but lacking in brain tumor cells, then a therapeutic/toxic transgene can be virally delivered with an artificial 3′-UTR containing complementary sites for that miRNA (Fig. 27.2). Transgene expression will be inhibited in normal cells containing the miRNA but not in cancer cells lacking it. This strategy of using miRNA expression profiles to selectively target transgenes has been demonstrated in hematopoietic and stem cells in three intriguing recent reports (Brown et al. 2006, 2007a, b). A subsequent study used underexpression of the let-7 miRNA family to develop a tumor-selective virus, given the low expression of let-7 miRNAs in most cancer types and their high expression in normal tissues (Edge et al. 2008). The authors cloned let-7 target sites behind the vesicular stomatitis virus (VSV) M gene necessary for VSV propagation, yielding an engineered VSV that selectively propagated in cancer cells. It may also be possible to design similar strategies targeting transgenes or viruses to cells overexpressing a miRNA such as miR-21, but this will require more intricate approaches.

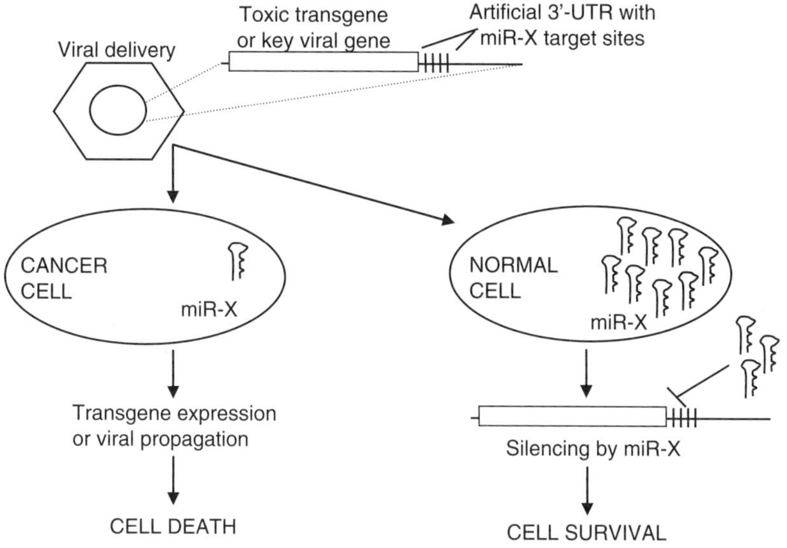

Fig. 27.2 Schematic of an anti-cancer strategy utilizing microRNA-regulated transgenes or viruses. Given a microRNA-X that is highly underexpressed in cancer cells versus normal cells, a virus may be utilized to deliver a transgene or modified viral gene with an artificial 3′-UTR with multiple complementary target sites for miR-X. Since miR-X is expressed minimally in a cancer cell, the transgene or viral gene will be expressed fully, leading to cell death or lethal viral replication. In a normal cell, miR-X will block expression of the transgene/viral gene, preserving the cell

There is no doubt that other miRNA-related strategies will be developed to combat brain tumors and other cancers in the coming years. One area that may bear fruit is the modulation of miRNA expression or processing. Recent reports by two groups describe the ability of the lin28 protein to bind pri-let-7 miRNAs, inhibiting their processing to pre-let-7 (Newman et al. 2008; Viswanathan et al. 2008). It seems certain that such regulatory RNA-binding proteins exist for other important miRNAs as well, and conceivably small-molecule inhibitors of these interactions could be developed.

27.8 Conclusion

The impact of the young field of RNA interference has been felt nowhere more keenly than in oncology, with the possible exception of neuroscience. With brain tumors at the intersection of both disciplines, it makes sense that powerful roles for miRNAs are being discovered in brain tumors. Early studies of miRNA expression in brain tumors have already provided important leads. In general, oncogenic miRNAs overexpressed in many cancers are also overexpressed in brain tumors, including miR-21, miR-10b, and miR-221.

Underexpressed miRNAs with tumor-suppressive function in brain tumors, such as miR-124 and miR-7, have also been identified and may be more selectively relevant to neuro-oncology. Key oncogene and tumor suppressor targets of these miRNAs have been identified, yielding new mechanistic insights into the regulation of genes such as EGFR and PTEN. Investigation of miRNAs and siRNAs in neuro-oncology offers the hope of novel targeted therapies to these resistant tumors. Initial strategies will involve delivery of siRNAs or shRNAs, tumor-suppressive miRNAs, or inhibitors of oncogenic miRNAs, but ultimately may also include more creative approaches such as miRNA-regulated viruses or modulators of miRNA processing.

References

Akao Y, Nakagawa Y Naoe T (2006) let-7 microRNA functions as a potential growth suppressor in human colon cancer cells. Biol Pharm Bull 29(5): 903–6

Ambros V (1989) A hierarchy of regulatory genes controls a larva-to-adult developmental switch in C. elegans. Cell 57(1): 49–57

Ambros V Lee RC (2004) Identification of microRNAs and other tiny noncoding RNAs by cDNA cloning. Methods Mol Biol 265: 131–58

Amos S, Mut M, diPierro CG, Carpenter JE, Xiao A, Kohutek ZA, Redpath GT, Zhao Y, Wang J, Shaffrey ME Hussaini IM (2007) Protein kinase C-alpha-mediated regulation of low-density lipoprotein receptor related protein and urokinase increases astrocytoma invasion. Cancer Res 67(21): 10241–51

Arwert E, Hingtgen S, Figueiredo JL, Bergquist H, Mahmood U, Weissleder R Shah K (2007) Visualizing the dynamics of EGFR activity and antiglioma therapies in vivo. Cancer Res 67(15): 7335–42

Asangani IA, Rasheed SA, Nikolova DA, Leupold JH, Colburn NH, Post S Allgayer H (2008) MicroRNA-21 (miR-21) post-transcriptionally downregulates tumor suppressor Pdcd4 and stimulates invasion, intravasation and metastasis in colorectal cancer. Oncogene 27(15): 2128–36

Babak T, Zhang W, Morris Q, Blencowe BJ Hughes TR (2004) Probing microRNAs with microarrays: tissue specificity and functional inference. Rna 10(11): 1813–9

Baek B, Villen J, Shin C, Camargo FD, Gygi SP Bartel B (2008) The impact of microRNAs on protein output. Nature: Epub ahead of print

Bak M, Silahtaroglu A, Moller M, Christensen M, Rath MF, Skryabin B, Tommerup N Kauppinen S (2008) MicroRNA expression in the adult mouse central nervous system. Rna 14(3): 432–44

Barad O, Meiri E, Avniel A, Aharonov R, Barzilai A, Bentwich I, Einav U, Gilad S, Hurban P, Karov Y, Lobenhofer EK, Sharon E, Shiboleth YM, Shtutman M, Bentwich Z Einat P (2004) MicroRNA expression detected by oligonucleotide microarrays: system establishment and expression profiling in human tissues. Genome Res 14(12): 2486–94

Berezikov E, Thuemmler F, van Laake LW, Kondova I, Bontrop R, Cuppen E Plasterk RH (2006) Diversity of microRNAs in human and chimpanzee brain. Nat Genet 38(12): 1375–7

Bernstein E, Caudy AA, Hammond SM Hannon GJ (2001) Role for a bidentate ribonuclease in the initiation step of RNA interference. Nature 409(6818): 363–6

Blower PE, Chung JH, Verducci JS, Lin S, Park JK, Dai Z, Liu CG, Schmittgen TD, Reinhold WC, Croce CM, Weinstein JN Sadee W (2008) MicroRNAs modulate the chemosensitivity of tumor cells. Mol Cancer Ther 7(1): 1–9

Bottoni A, Piccin D, Tagliati F, Luchin A, Zatelli MC degli Uberti EC (2005) miR-15a and miR-16-1 down-regulation in pituitary adenomas. J Cell Physiol 204(1): 280–5

Bottoni A, Zatelli MC, Ferracin M, Tagliati F, Piccin D, Vignali C, Calin GA, Negrini M, Croce CM Degli Uberti EC (2007) Identification of differentially expressed microRNAs by microarray: a possible role for microRNA genes in pituitary adenomas. J Cell Physiol 210(2): 370–7

Bridge AJ, Pebernard S, Ducraux A, Nicoulaz AL Iggo R (2003) Induction of an interferon response by RNAi vectors in mammalian cells. Nat Genet 34(3): 263–4

Brown BD, Cantore A, Annoni A, Sergi LS, Lombardo A, Della Valle P, D'Angelo A Naldini L (2007a) A microRNA-regulated lentiviral vector mediates stable correction of hemophilia B mice. Blood 110(13): 4144–52

Brown BD, Gentner B, Cantore A, Colleoni S, Amendola M, Zingale A, Baccarini A, Lazzari G, Galli C Naldini L (2007b) Endogenous microRNA can be broadly exploited to regulate transgene expression according to tissue, lineage and differentiation state. Nat Biotechnol 25(12): 1457–67

Brown BD, Venneri MA, Zingale A, Sergi Sergi L Naldini L (2006) Endogenous microRNA regulation suppresses transgene expression in hematopoietic lineages and enables stable gene transfer. Nat Med 12(5): 585–91

Brown GE, Lebleu B, Kawakita M, Shaila S, Sen GC Lengyel P (1976) Increased endonuclease activity in an extract from mouse Ehrlich ascites tumor cells which had been treated with a partially purified interferon preparation: dependence of double-stranded RNA. Biochem Biophys Res Commun 69(1): 114–22

Calin GA, Dumitru CD, Shimizu M, Bichi R, Zupo S, Noch E, Aldler H, Rattan S, Keating M, Rai K, Rassenti L, Kipps T, Negrini M, Bullrich F Croce CM (2002) Frequent deletions and down-regulation of micro- RNA genes miR15 and miR16 at 13q14 in chronic lymphocytic leukemia. Proc Natl Acad Sci USA 99(24): 15524–9

Calin GA, Sevignani C, Dumitru CD, Hyslop T, Noch E, Yendamuri S, Shimizu M, Rattan S, Bullrich F, Negrini M Croce CM (2004) Human microRNA genes are frequently located at fragile sites and genomic regions involved in cancers. Proc Natl Acad Sci USA 101(9): 2999–3004

Camps C, Buffa FM, Colella S, Moore J, Sotiriou C, Sheldon H, Harris AL, Gleadle JM Ragoussis J (2008) hsa-miR-210 Is induced by hypoxia and is an independent prognostic factor in breast cancer. Clin Cancer Res 14(5): 1340–8

Chan JA, Krichevsky AM Kosik KS (2005) MicroRNA-21 is an antiapoptotic factor in human glioblastoma cells. Cancer Res 65(14): 6029–33

Chang TC, Wentzel EA, Kent OA, Ramachandran K, Mullendore M, Lee KH, Feldmann G, Yamakuchi M, Ferlito M, Lowenstein CJ, Arking DE, Beer MA, Maitra A Mendell JT (2007) Transactivation of miR-34a by p53 broadly influences gene expression and promotes apoptosis. Mol Cell 26(5): 745–52

Chen H, Huang Q, Dong J, Zhai DZ, Wang AD Lan Q (2008) Overexpression of CDC2/CyclinB1 in gliomas, and CDC2 depletion inhibits proliferation of human glioma cells in vitro and in vivo. BMC Cancer 8: 29

Chen MY, Hoffer A, Morrison PF, Hamilton JF, Hughes J, Schlageter KS, Lee J, Kelly BR Oldfield EH (2005) Surface properties, more than size, limiting convective distribution of virus-sized particles and viruses in the central nervous system. J Neurosurg 103(2): 311–9

Choi PS, Zakhary L, Choi WY, Caron S, Alvarez-Saavedra E, Miska EA, McManus M, Harfe B, Giraldez AJ, Horvitz RH, Schier AF Dulac C (2008) Members of the miRNA-200 family regulate olfactory neurogenesis. Neuron 57(1): 41–55

Ciafre SA, Galardi S, Mangiola A, Ferracin M, Liu CG, Sabatino G, Negrini M, Maira G, Croce CM Farace MG (2005) Extensive modulation of a set of microRNAs in primary glioblastoma. Biochem Biophys Res Commun 334(4): 1351–8

Cimmino A, Calin GA, Fabbri M, Iorio MV, Ferracin M, Shimizu M, Wojcik SE, Aqeilan RI, Zupo S, Dono M, Rassenti L, Alder H, Volinia S, Liu CG, Kipps TJ, Negrini M Croce CM (2005) miR-15 and miR-16 induce apoptosis by targeting BCL2. Proc Natl Acad Sci USA 102(39): 13944–9

Conaco C, Otto S, Han JJ Mandel G (2006) Reciprocal actions of REST and a microRNA promote neuronal identity. Proc Natl Acad Sci USA 103(7): 2422–7

Corney DC, Flesken-Nikitin A, Godwin AK, Wang W Nikitin AY (2007) MicroRNA-34b and MicroRNA-34c are targets of p53 and cooperate in control of cell proliferation and adhesion-independent growth. Cancer Res 67(18): 8433–8

Corsten MF, Miranda R, Kasmieh R, Krichevsky AM, Weissleder R Shah K (2007) MicroRNA-21 knockdown disrupts glioma growth in vivo and displays synergistic cytotoxicity with neural precursor cell delivered S-TRAIL in human gliomas. Cancer Res 67(19): 8994–9000

Cuellar TL, Davis TH, Nelson PT, Loeb GB, Harfe BD, Ullian E McManus MT (2008) Dicer loss in striatal neurons produces behavioral and neuroanatomical phenotypes in the absence of neurodegeneration. Proc Natl Acad Sci USA 105(14): 5614–9

Dahiya N, Sherman-Baust CA, Wang TL, Davidson B, Shih Ie M, Zhang Y, Wood W, 3rd, Becker KG Morin PJ (2008) MicroRNA expression and identification of putative miRNA targets in ovarian cancer. PLoS ONE 3(6): e2436

Davis TH, Cuellar TL, Koch SM, Barker AJ, Harfe BD, McManus MT Ullian EM (2008) Conditional loss of Dicer disrupts cellular and tissue morphogenesis in the cortex and hippocampus. J Neurosci 28(17): 4322–30

de la Iglesia N, Konopka G, Lim KL, Nutt CL, Bromberg JF, Frank DA, Mischel PS, Louis DN Bonni A (2008) Deregulation of a STAT3-interleukin 8 signaling pathway promotes human glioblastoma cell proliferation and invasiveness. J Neurosci 28(23): 5870–8

Desbaillets I, Diserens AC, de Tribolet N, Hamou MF Van Meir EG (1999) Regulation of interleukin-8 expression by reduced oxygen pressure in human glioblastoma. Oncogene 18(7): 1447–56

Dostie J, Mourelatos Z, Yang M, Sharma A Dreyfuss G (2003) Numerous microRNPs in neuronal cells containing novel microRNAs. Rna 9(2): 180–6

Ebert MS, Neilson JR Sharp PA (2007) MicroRNA sponges: competitive inhibitors of small RNAs in mammalian cells. Nat Methods 4(9): 721–6

Edge RE, Falls TJ, Brown CW, Lichty BD, Atkins H Bell JC (2008) A let-7 MicroRNA-sensitive vesicular stomatitis virus demonstrates tumor-specific replication. Mol Ther: Epub ahead of print

Farh KK, Grimson A, Jan C, Lewis BP, Johnston WK, Lim LP, Burge CB Bartel DP (2005) The widespread impact of mammalian MicroRNAs on mRNA repression and evolution. Science 310(5755): 1817–21

Felicetti F, Errico MC, Bottero L, Segnalini P, Stoppacciaro A, Biffoni M, Felli N, Mattia G, Petrini M, Colombo MP, Peschle C Care A (2008) The promyelocytic leukemia zinc finger-microRNA-221/-222 pathway controls melanoma progression through multiple oncogenic mechanisms. Cancer Res 68(8): 2745–54

Fire A, Xu S, Montgomery MK, Kostas SA, Driver SE Mello CC (1998) Potent and specific genetic interference by double-stranded RNA in Caenorhabditis elegans. Nature 391(6669): 806–11

Fornari F, Gramantieri L, Ferracin M, Veronese A, Sabbioni S, Calin GA, Grazi GL, Giovannini C, Croce CM, Bolondi L Negrini M (2008) MiR-221 controls CDKN1C/p57 and CDKN1B/p27 expression in human hepatocellular carcinoma. Oncogene: Epub ahead of print

Frankel LB, Christoffersen NR, Jacobsen A, Lindow M, Krogh A Lund AH (2008) Programmed cell death 4 (PDCD4) is an important functional target of the microRNA miR-21 in breast cancer cells. J Biol Chem 283(2): 1026–33

Fujita S, Ito T, Mizutani T, Minoguchi S, Yamamichi N, Sakurai K Iba H (2008) miR-21 Gene expression triggered by AP-1 is sustained through a double-negative feedback mechanism. J Mol Biol 378(3): 492–504
Gabriely G, Wurdinger T, Kesari S, Esau CC, Burchard J, Linsley PS Krichevsky AM (2008) MiR-21 Promotes Glioma Invasion by Targeting MMP Regulators. Mol Cell Biol: Epub ahead of print
Galardi S, Mercatelli N, Giorda E, Massalini S, Frajese GV, Ciafre SA Farace MG (2007) miR-221 and miR-222 expression affects the proliferation potential of human prostate carcinoma cell lines by targeting p27Kip1. J Biol Chem 282(32): 23716–24
Gaur A, Jewell DA, Liang Y, Ridzon D, Moore JH, Chen C, Ambros VR Israel MA (2007) Characterization of microRNA expression levels and their biological correlates in human cancer cell lines. Cancer Res 67(6): 2456–68
Gillies JK Lorimer IA (2007) Regulation of p27Kip1 by miRNA 221/222 in glioblastoma. Cell Cycle 6(16): 2005–9
Giraldez AJ, Cinalli RM, Glasner ME, Enright AJ, Thomson JM, Baskerville S, Hammond SM, Bartel DP Schier AF (2005) MicroRNAs regulate brain morphogenesis in zebrafish. Science 308(5723): 833–8
Gironella M, Seux M, Xie MJ, Cano C, Tomasini R, Gommeaux J, Garcia S, Nowak J, Yeung ML, Jeang KT, Chaix A, Fazli L, Motoo Y, Wang Q, Rocchi P, Russo A, Gleave M, Dagorn JC, Iovanna JL, Carrier A, Pebusque MJ Dusetti NJ (2007) Tumor protein 53-induced nuclear protein 1 expression is repressed by miR-155, and its restoration inhibits pancreatic tumor development. Proc Natl Acad Sci USA 104(41): 16170–5
Gottardo F, Liu CG, Ferracin M, Calin GA, Fassan M, Bassi P, Sevignani C, Byrne D, Negrini M, Pagano F, Gomella LG, Croce CM Baffa R (2007) Micro-RNA profiling in kidney and bladder cancers. Urol Oncol 25(5): 387–92
Grimm D, Streetz KL, Jopling CL, Storm TA, Pandey K, Davis CR, Marion P, Salazar F Kay MA (2006) Fatality in mice due to oversaturation of cellular microRNA/short hairpin RNA pathways. Nature 441(7092): 537–41
Grishok A, Pasquinelli AE, Conte D, Li N, Parrish S, Ha I, Baillie DL, Fire A, Ruvkun G Mello CC (2001) Genes and mechanisms related to RNA interference regulate expression of the small temporal RNAs that control C. elegans developmental timing. Cell 106(1): 23–34
Ha I, Wightman B Ruvkun G (1996) A bulged lin-4/lin-14 RNA duplex is sufficient for Caenorhabditis elegans lin-14 temporal gradient formation. Genes Dev 10(23): 3041–50
Haas-Kogan D, Shalev N, Wong M, Mills G, Yount G Stokoe D (1998) Protein kinase B (PKB/Akt) activity is elevated in glioblastoma cells due to mutation of the tumor suppressor PTEN/MMAC. Curr Biol 8(21): 1195–8
Hamilton AJ Baulcombe DC (1999) A species of small antisense RNA in posttranscriptional gene silencing in plants. Science 286(5441): 950–2
Hammond SM, Bernstein E, Beach D Hannon GJ (2000) An RNA-directed nuclease mediates post-transcriptional gene silencing in Drosophila cells. Nature 404(6775): 293–6
He H, Jazdzewski K, Li W, Liyanarachchi S, Nagy R, Volinia S, Calin GA, Liu CG, Franssila K, Suster S, Kloos RT, Croce CM de la Chapelle A (2005a) The role of microRNA genes in papillary thyroid carcinoma. Proc Natl Acad Sci USA 102(52): 19075–80
He L, He X, Lim LP, de Stanchina E, Xuan Z, Liang Y, Xue W, Zender L, Magnus J, Ridzon D, Jackson AL, Linsley PS, Chen C, Lowe SW, Cleary MA Hannon GJ (2007) A microRNA component of the p53 tumour suppressor network. Nature 447(7148): 1130–4
He L, Thomson JM, Hemann MT, Hernando-Monge E, Mu D, Goodson S, Powers S, Cordon-Cardo C, Lowe SW, Hannon GJ Hammond SM (2005b) A microRNA polycistron as a potential human oncogene. Nature 435(7043): 828–33
Holland EC, Li Y, Celestino J, Dai C, Schaefer L, Sawaya RA Fuller GN (2000) Astrocytes give rise to oligodendrogliomas and astrocytomas after gene transfer of polyoma virus middle T antigen in vivo. Am J Pathol 157(3): 1031–7

Huang Q, Gumireddy K, Schrier M, le Sage C, Nagel R, Nair S, Egan DA, Li A, Huang G, Klein-Szanto AJ, Gimotty PA, Katsaros D, Coukos G, Zhang L, Pure E Agami R (2008) The microRNAs miR-373 and miR-520c promote tumour invasion and metastasis. Nat Cell Biol 10(2): 202–10

Hutvagner G Zamore PD (2002) A microRNA in a multiple-turnover RNAi enzyme complex. Science 297(5589): 2056–60

Iorio MV, Ferracin M, Liu CG, Veronese A, Spizzo R, Sabbioni S, Magri E, Pedriali M, Fabbri M, Campiglio M, Menard S, Palazzo JP, Rosenberg A, Musiani P, Volinia S, Nenci I, Calin GA, Querzoli P, Negrini M Croce CM (2005) MicroRNA gene expression deregulation in human breast cancer. Cancer Res 65(16): 7065–70

Johnson SM, Grosshans H, Shingara J, Byrom M, Jarvis R, Cheng A, Labourier E, Reinert KL, Brown D Slack FJ (2005) RAS is regulated by the let-7 microRNA family. Cell 120(5): 635–47

Kapsimali M, Kloosterman WP, de Bruijn E, Rosa F, Plasterk RH Wilson SW (2007) MicroRNAs show a wide diversity of expression profiles in the developing and mature central nervous system. Genome Biol 8(8): R173

Kargiotis O, Chetty C, Gondi CS, Tsung AJ, Dinh DH, Gujrati M, Lakka SS, Kyritsis AP Rao JS (2008) Adenovirus-mediated transfer of siRNA against MMP-2 mRNA results in impaired invasion and tumor-induced angiogenesis, induces apoptosis in vitro and inhibits tumor growth in vivo in glioblastoma. Oncogene: Epub ahead of print

Kariko K, Bhuyan P, Capodici J Weissman D (2004) Small interfering RNAs mediate sequence-independent gene suppression and induce immune activation by signaling through toll-like receptor 3. J Immunol 172(11): 6545–9

Kefas B, Godlewski J, Comeau L, Li Y, Abounader R, Hawkinson M, Lee J, Fine H, Chiocca EA, Lawler S Purow B (2008) microRNA-7 inhibits the epidermal growth factor receptor and the Akt pathway and is down-regulated in glioblastoma. Cancer Res 68(10): 3566–72

Kim J, Krichevsky A, Grad Y, Hayes GD, Kosik KS, Church GM Ruvkun G (2004) Identification of many microRNAs that copurify with polyribosomes in mammalian neurons. Proc Natl Acad Sci USA 101(1): 360–5

Kluiver J, Poppema S, de Jong D, Blokzijl T, Harms G, Jacobs S, Kroesen BJ van den Berg A (2005) BIC and miR-155 are highly expressed in Hodgkin, primary mediastinal and diffuse large B cell lymphomas. J Pathol 207(2): 243–9

Krichevsky AM, King KS, Donahue CP, Khrapko K Kosik KS (2003) A microRNA array reveals extensive regulation of microRNAs during brain development. Rna 9(10): 1274–81

Krutzfeldt J, Rajewsky N, Braich R, Rajeev KG, Tuschl T, Manoharan M Stoffel M (2005) Silencing of microRNAs in vivo with 'antagomirs'. Nature 438(7068): 685–9

Lagos-Quintana M, Rauhut R, Lendeckel W Tuschl T (2001) Identification of novel genes coding for small expressed RNAs. Science 294(5543): 853–8

Lagos-Quintana M, Rauhut R, Meyer J, Borkhardt A Tuschl T (2003) New microRNAs from mouse and human. Rna 9(2): 175–9

Lai EC, Tam B Rubin GM (2005) Pervasive regulation of Drosophila Notch target genes by GY-box-, Brd-box-, and K-box-class microRNAs. Genes Dev 19(9): 1067–80

Lee EJ, Gusev Y, Jiang J, Nuovo GJ, Lerner MR, Frankel WL, Morgan DL, Postier RG, Brackett DJ Schmittgen TD (2007) Expression profiling identifies microRNA signature in pancreatic cancer. Int J Cancer 120(5): 1046–54

Lee HJ, Palkovits M Young WS, 3rd (2006) miR-7b, a microRNA up-regulated in the hypothalamus after chronic hyperosmolar stimulation, inhibits Fos translation. Proc Natl Acad Sci USA 103(42): 15669–74

Lee RC Ambros V (2001) An extensive class of small RNAs in Caenorhabditis elegans. Science 294 (5543): 862–4

Lee Y, Ahn C, Han J, Choi H, Kim J, Yim J, Lee J, Provost P, Radmark O, Kim S Kim VN (2003) The nuclear RNase III Drosha initiates microRNA processing. Nature 425 (6956): 415–9

Lee YS, Kim HK, Chung S, Kim KS Dutta A (2005) Depletion of human micro-RNA miR-125b reveals that it is critical for the proliferation of differentiated cells but not for the down-regulation of putative targets during differentiation. J Biol Chem 280(17): 16635–41

Leucht C, Stigloher C, Wizenmann A, Klafke R, Folchert A Bally-Cuif L (2008) MicroRNA-9 directs late organizer activity of the midbrain-hindbrain boundary. Nat Neurosci 11(6): 641–8

Li Y, Guessous F, Kwon S, Kumar M, Ibidapo O, Fuller L, Johnson E, Lal B, Hussaini I, Bao Y, Laterra J, Schiff D Abounader R (2008) PTEN has tumor-promoting properties in the setting of gain-of-function p53 mutations. Cancer Res 68(6): 1723–31

Libermann TA, Nusbaum HR, Razon N, Kris R, Lax I, Soreq H, Whittle N, Waterfield MD, Ullrich A Schlessinger J (1985) Amplification, enhanced expression and possible rearrangement of EGF receptor gene in primary human brain tumours of glial origin. Nature 313 (5998): 144–7

Liu CG, Calin GA, Meloon B, Gamliel N, Sevignani C, Ferracin M, Dumitru CD, Shimizu M, Zupo S, Dono M, Alder H, Bullrich F, Negrini M Croce CM (2004) An oligonucleotide microchip for genome-wide microRNA profiling in human and mouse tissues. Proc Natl Acad Sci USA 101(26): 9740–4

Liu J, Valencia-Sanchez MA, Hannon GJ Parker R (2005) MicroRNA-dependent localization of targeted mRNAs to mammalian P-bodies. Nat Cell Biol 7(7): 719–23

Loffler D, Brocke-Heidrich K, Pfeifer G, Stocsits C, Hackermuller J, Kretzschmar AK, Burger R, Gramatzki M, Blumert C, Bauer K, Cvijic H, Ullmann AK, Stadler PF Horn F (2007) Interleukin-6 dependent survival of multiple myeloma cells involves the Stat3-mediated induction of microRNA-21 through a highly conserved enhancer. Blood 110(4): 1330–3

Lu J, Getz G, Miska EA, Alvarez-Saavedra E, Lamb J, Peck D, Sweet-Cordero A, Ebert BL, Mak RH, Ferrando AA, Downing JR, Jacks T, Horvitz HR Golub TR (2005) MicroRNA expression profiles classify human cancers. Nature 435 (7043): 834–8

Lu Z, Liu M, Stribinskis V, Klinge CM, Ramos KS, Colburn NH Li Y (2008) MicroRNA-21 promotes cell transformation by targeting the programmed cell death 4 gene. Oncogene 27(31): 4373–9

Lugli G, Torvik VI, Larson J Smalheiser NR (2008) Expression of microRNAs and their precursors in synaptic fractions of adult mouse forebrain. J Neurochem: Epub ahead of print

Lund E, Guttinger S, Calado A, Dahlberg JE Kutay U (2004) Nuclear export of microRNA precursors. Science 303 (5654): 95–8

Lytle JR, Yario TA Steitz JA (2007) Target mRNAs are repressed as efficiently by microRNA-binding sites in the 5' UTR as in the 3' UTR. Proc Natl Acad Sci USA 104(23): 9667–72

Ma L, Teruya-Feldstein J Weinberg RA (2007) Tumour invasion and metastasis initiated by microRNA-10b in breast cancer. Nature 449 (7163): 682–8

Makeyev EV, Zhang J, Carrasco MA Maniatis T (2007) The MicroRNA miR-124 promotes neuronal differentiation by triggering brain-specific alternative pre-mRNA splicing. Mol Cell 27(3): 435–48

Meng F, Henson R, Wehbe-Janek H, Ghoshal K, Jacob ST Patel T (2007) MicroRNA-21 regulates expression of the PTEN tumor suppressor gene in human hepatocellular cancer. Gastroenterology 133(2): 647–58

Naguibneva I, Ameyar-Zazoua M, Polesskaya A, Ait-Si-Ali S, Groisman R, Souidi M, Cuvellier S Harel-Bellan A (2006) The microRNA miR-181 targets the homeobox protein Hox-A11 during mammalian myoblast differentiation. Nat Cell Biol 8(3): 278–84

Nass D, Rosenwald S, Meiri E, Gilad S, Tabibian-Keissar H, Schlosberg A, Kuker H, Sion-Vardy N, Tobar A, Kharenko O, Sitbon E, Yanai G, Elyakim E, Cholakh H, Gibori H, Spector Y, Bentwich Z, Barshack I Rosenfeld N (2008) MiR-92b and miR-9/9* Are Specifically Expressed in Brain Primary Tumors and Can Be Used to Differentiate Primary from Metastatic Brain Tumors. Brain Pathol: Epub ahead of print

Nelson PT, Baldwin DA, Kloosterman WP, Kauppinen S, Plasterk RH Mourelatos Z (2006) RAKE and LNA-ISH reveal microRNA expression and localization in archival human brain. Rna 12(2): 187–91

Newman MA, Thomson JM Hammond SM (2008) Lin-28 interaction with the Let-7 precursor loop mediates regulated microRNA processing. Rna: Epub ahead of print

Nguyen TT, Pannu YS, Sung C, Dedrick RL, Walbridge S, Brechbiel MW, Garmestani K, Beitzel M, Yordanov AT Oldfield EH (2003) Convective distribution of macromolecules in the primate brain demonstrated using computerized tomography and magnetic resonance imaging. J Neurosurg 98(3): 584–90

Nikiforova MN, Tseng GC, Steward D, Diorio D Nikiforov YE (2008) MicroRNA expression profiling of thyroid tumors: biological significance and diagnostic utility. J Clin Endocrinol Metab 93(5): 1600–8

O'Connell RM, Rao DS, Chaudhuri AA, Boldin MP, Taganov KD, Nicoll J, Paquette RL Baltimore D (2008) Sustained expression of microRNA-155 in hematopoietic stem cells causes a myeloproliferative disorder. J Exp Med 205(3): 585–94

Orom UA, Kauppinen S Lund AH (2006) LNA-modified oligonucleotides mediate specific inhibition of microRNA function. Gene 372: 137–41

Ossowski S, Schwab R Weigel D (2008) Gene silencing in plants using artificial microRNAs and other small RNAs. Plant J 53(4): 674–90

Pekarsky Y, Santanam U, Cimmino A, Palamarchuk A, Efanov A, Maximov V, Volinia S, Alder H, Liu CG, Rassenti L, Calin GA, Hagan JP, Kipps T Croce CM (2006) Tcl1 expression in chronic lymphocytic leukemia is regulated by miR-29 and miR-181. Cancer Res 66(24): 11590–3

Phillips HS, Kharbanda S, Chen R, Forrest WF, Soriano RH, Wu TD, Misra A, Nigro JM, Colman H, Soroceanu L, Williams PM, Modrusan Z, Feuerstein BG Aldape K (2006) Molecular subclasses of high-grade glioma predict prognosis, delineate a pattern of disease progression, and resemble stages in neurogenesis. Cancer Cell 9(3): 157–73

Pierson J, Hostager B, Fan R Vibhakar R (2008) Regulation of cyclin dependent kinase 6 by microRNA 124 in medulloblastoma. J Neurooncol: Epub ahead of print

Pirollo KF Chang EH (2008) Targeted delivery of small interfering RNA: approaching effective cancer therapies. Cancer Res 68(5): 1247–50

Purow BW, Haque RM, Noel MW, Su Q, Burdick MJ, Lee J, Sundaresan T, Pastorino S, Park JK, Mikolaenko I, Maric D, Eberhart CG Fine HA (2005) Expression of Notch-1 and its ligands, Delta-like-1 and Jagged-1, is critical for glioma cell survival and proliferation. Cancer Res 65(6): 2353–63

Pyrko P, Schonthal AH, Hofman FM, Chen TC Lee AS (2007) The unfolded protein response regulator GRP78/BiP as a novel target for increasing chemosensitivity in malignant gliomas. Cancer Res 67(20): 9809–16

Qi Y, Hoadley K, Topal M, Perou CM Hayes DN (2008) Parallel microRNA and gene expression strategies of human glioblastomas. abstract/presentation, 2008 Annual Meeting: 4965

Ramkissoon SH, Mainwaring LA, Ogasawara Y, Keyvanfar K, McCoy JP, Jr., Sloand EM, Kajigaya S Young NS (2006) Hematopoietic-specific microRNA expression in human cells. Leuk Res 30(5): 643–7

Raver-Shapira N, Marciano E, Meiri E, Spector Y, Rosenfeld N, Moskovits N, Bentwich Z Oren M (2007) Transcriptional activation of miR-34a contributes to p53-mediated apoptosis. Mol Cell 26(5): 731–43

Reinhart BJ, Weinstein EG, Rhoades MW, Bartel B Bartel DP (2002) MicroRNAs in plants. Genes Dev 16(13): 1616–26

Roldo C, Missiaglia E, Hagan JP, Falconi M, Capelli P, Bersani S, Calin GA, Volinia S, Liu CG, Scarpa A Croce CM (2006) MicroRNA expression abnormalities in pancreatic endocrine and acinar tumors are associated with distinctive pathologic features and clinical behavior. J Clin Oncol 24(29): 4677–84

Saito T, Hama S, Izumi H, Yamasaki F, Kajiwara Y, Matsuura S, Morishima K, Hidaka T, Shrestha P, Sugiyama K Kurisu K (2008) Centrosome amplification induced by survivin suppression enhances both chromosome instability and radiosensitivity in glioma cells. Br J Cancer 98(2): 345–55

Sampson VB, Rong NH, Han J, Yang Q, Aris V, Soteropoulos P, Petrelli NJ, Dunn SP Krueger LJ (2007) MicroRNA let-7a down-regulates MYC and reverts MYC-induced growth in Burkitt lymphoma cells. Cancer Res 67(20): 9762–70

Sayed D, Rane S, Lypowy J, He M, Chen IY, Vashistha H, Yan L, Malhotra A, Vatner D Abdellatif M (2008) MicroRNA-21 Targets Sprouty2 and Promotes Cellular Outgrowths. Mol Biol Cell: Epub ahead of print

Scacheri PC, Rozenblatt-Rosen O, Caplen NJ, Wolfsberg TG, Umayam L, Lee JC, Hughes CM, Shanmugam KS, Bhattacharjee A, Meyerson M Collins FS (2004) Short interfering RNAs can induce unexpected and divergent changes in the levels of untargeted proteins in mammalian cells. Proc Natl Acad Sci USA 101(7): 1892–7

Schetter AJ, Leung SY, Sohn JJ, Zanetti KA, Bowman ED, Yanaihara N, Yuen ST, Chan TL, Kwong DL, Au GK, Liu CG, Calin GA, Croce CM Harris CC (2008) MicroRNA expression profiles associated with prognosis and therapeutic outcome in colon adenocarcinoma. Jama 299(4): 425–36

Schratt GM, Tuebing F, Nigh EA, Kane CG, Sabatini ME, Kiebler M Greenberg ME (2006) A brain-specific microRNA regulates dendritic spine development. Nature 439 (7074): 283–9

Schulte JH, Horn S, Otto T, Samans B, Heukamp LC, Eilers UC, Krause M, Astrahantseff K, Klein-Hitpass L, Buettner R, Schramm A, Christiansen H, Eilers M, Eggert A Berwanger B (2008) MYCN regulates oncogenic MicroRNAs in neuroblastoma. Int J Cancer 122(3): 699–704

Schwab R, Ossowski S, Riester M, Warthmann N Weigel D (2006) Highly specific gene silencing by artificial microRNAs in Arabidopsis. Plant Cell 18(5): 1121–33

Selbach M, Schwanhausser B, Thierfelder N, Fang Z, Khanin R Rajewsky N (2008) Widespread changes in protein synthesis induced by microRNAs. Nature: Epub ahead of print

Sempere LF, Freemantle S, Pitha-Rowe I, Moss E, Dmitrovsky E Ambros V (2004) Expression profiling of mammalian microRNAs uncovers a subset of brain-expressed microRNAs with possible roles in murine and human neuronal differentiation. Genome Biol 5(3): R13

Sen GL Blau HM (2005) Argonaute 2/RISC resides in sites of mammalian mRNA decay known as cytoplasmic bodies. Nat Cell Biol 7(6): 633–6

Silber J, Lim DA, Petritsch C, Persson AI, Maunakea AK, Yu M, Vandenberg SR, Ginzinger DG, James CD, Costello JF, Bergers G, Weiss WA, Alvarez-Buylla A Hodgson JG (2008) miR-124 and miR-137 inhibit proliferation of glioblastoma multiforme cells and induce differentiation of brain tumor stem cells. BMC Med 6: 14

Sledz CA, Holko M, de Veer MJ, Silverman RH Williams BR (2003) Activation of the interferon system by short-interfering RNAs. Nat Cell Biol 5(9): 834–9

Smirnova L, Grafe A, Seiler A, Schumacher S, Nitsch R Wulczyn FG (2005) Regulation of miRNA expression during neural cell specification. Eur J Neurosci 21(6): 1469–77

Sun F, Fu H, Liu Q, Tie Y, Zhu J, Xing R, Sun Z Zheng X (2008) Downregulation of CCND1 and CDK6 by miR-34a induces cell cycle arrest. FEBS Lett 582(10): 1564–8

Sun Y, Koo S, White N, Peralta E, Esau C, Dean NM Perera RJ (2004) Development of a micro-array to detect human and mouse microRNAs and characterization of expression in human organs. Nucleic Acids Res 32(22): e188

Takamizawa J, Konishi H, Yanagisawa K, Tomida S, Osada H, Endoh H, Harano T, Yatabe Y, Nagino M, Nimura Y, Mitsudomi T Takahashi T (2004) Reduced expression of the let-7 microRNAs in human lung cancers in association with shortened postoperative survival. Cancer Res 64(11): 3753–6

Tam W Dahlberg JE (2006) miR-155/BIC as an oncogenic microRNA. Gene Chromosome Cancer 45(2): 211–2

Tazawa H, Tsuchiya N, Izumiya M Nakagama H (2007) Tumor-suppressive miR-34a induces senescence-like growth arrest through modulation of the E2F pathway in human colon cancer cells. Proc Natl Acad Sci USA 104(39): 15472–7

Thomson JM, Parker J, Perou CM Hammond SM (2004) A custom microarray platform for analysis of microRNA gene expression. Nat Methods 1(1): 47–53

Tran N, McLean T, Zhang X, Zhao CJ, Thomson JM, O'Brien C Rose B (2007) MicroRNA expression profiles in head and neck cancer cell lines. Biochem Biophys Res Commun 358(1): 12–7

Vigorito E, Perks KL, Abreu-Goodger C, Bunting S, Xiang Z, Kohlhaas S, Das PP, Miska EA, Rodriguez A, Bradley A, Smith KG, Rada C, Enright AJ, Toellner KM, Maclennan IC Turner M (2007) microRNA-155 regulates the generation of immunoglobulin class-switched plasma cells. Immunity 27(6): 847–59

Visvanathan J, Lee S, Lee B, Lee JW Lee SK (2007) The microRNA miR-124 antagonizes the anti-neural REST/SCP1 pathway during embryonic CNS development. Genes Dev 21(7): 744–9

Viswanathan SR, Daley GQ Gregory RI (2008) Selective blockade of microRNA processing by Lin28. Science 320 (5872): 97–100

Volinia S, Calin GA, Liu CG, Ambs S, Cimmino A, Petrocca F, Visone R, Iorio M, Roldo C, Ferracin M, Prueitt RL, Yanaihara N, Lanza G, Scarpa A, Vecchione A, Negrini M, Harris CC Croce CM (2006) A microRNA expression signature of human solid tumors defines cancer gene targets. Proc Natl Acad Sci USA 103(7): 2257–61

Wayman GA, Davare M, Ando H, Fortin D, Varlamova O, Cheng HY, Marks D, Obrietan K, Soderling TR, Goodman RH Impey S (2008) An activity-regulated microRNA controls dendritic plasticity by down-regulating p250GAP. Proc Natl Acad Sci USA 105(26): 9093–8

Wei JS, Song YK, Durinck S, Chen QR, Cheuk AT, Tsang P, Zhang Q, Thiele CJ, Slack A, Shohet J Khan J (2008a) The MYCN oncogene is a direct target of miR-34a. Oncogene: Epub ahead of print

Wei LC, Shi M, Cao R, Chen LW Chan YS (2008b) Nestin small interfering RNA (siRNA) reduces cell growth in cultured astrocytoma cells. Brain Res 1196: 103–12

Welch C, Chen Y Stallings RL (2007) MicroRNA-34a functions as a potential tumor suppressor by inducing apoptosis in neuroblastoma cells. Oncogene 26(34): 5017–22

Wightman B, Ha I Ruvkun G (1993) Posttranscriptional regulation of the heterochronic gene lin-14 by lin-4 mediates temporal pattern formation in C. elegans. Cell 75(5): 855–62

Wong TS, Liu XB, Wong BY, Ng RW, Yuen AP Wei WI (2008) Mature miR-184 as Potential Oncogenic microRNA of Squamous Cell Carcinoma of Tongue. Clin Cancer Res 14(9): 2588–92

Xia L, Zhang D, Du R, Pan Y, Zhao L, Sun S, Hong L, Liu J Fan D (2008) miR-15b and miR-16 modulate multidrug resistance by targeting BCL2 in human gastric cancer cells. Int J Cancer 123(2): 372–9

Yanaihara N, Caplen N, Bowman E, Seike M, Kumamoto K, Yi M, Stephens RM, Okamoto A, Yokota J, Tanaka T, Calin GA, Liu CG, Croce CM Harris CC (2006) Unique microRNA molecular profiles in lung cancer diagnosis and prognosis. Cancer Cell 9(3): 189–98

Yu Z, Jian Z, Shen SH, Purisima E Wang E (2007) Global analysis of microRNA target gene expression reveals that miRNA targets are lower expressed in mature mouse and Drosophila tissues than in the embryos. Nucleic Acids Res 35(1): 152–64

Zeng Y, Wagner EJ Cullen BR (2002) Both natural and designed micro RNAs can inhibit the expression of cognate mRNAs when expressed in human cells. Mol Cell 9(6): 1327–33

Zhang R Su B (2008) MicroRNA regulation and the variability of human cortical gene expression. Nucleic Acids Res: Epub ahead of print
Zhao P, Wang C, Fu Z, You Y, Cheng Y, Lu X, Lu A, Liu N, Pu P, Kang C, Salford LG Fan X (2007) Lentiviral vector mediated siRNA knock-down of hTERT results in diminished capacity in invasiveness and in vivo growth of human glioma cells in a telomere length-independent manner. Int J Oncol 31(2): 361–8
Zhu S, Si ML, Wu H Mo YY (2007) MicroRNA-21 targets the tumor suppressor gene tropomyosin 1 (TPM1). J Biol Chem 282(19): 14328–36
Zhu S, Wu H, Wu F, Nie D, Sheng S Mo YY (2008) MicroRNA-21 targets tumor suppressor genes in invasion and metastasis. Cell Res 18(3): 350–9

Chapter 28
Of *Escherichia coli* and Man: Understanding Glioma Resistance to Temozolomide Therapy

Clark C. Chen, Kristopher T. Kahle, Kimberly Ng, Masayuki Nitta, and Alan D'Andrea

Abstract Our understanding of the human cellular response to DNA alkylating agents has its origin in a rich history of genetic experimentation in prokaryotic model systems, including the bacterium *Escherichia coli*. The recent clinical finding that chemotherapy with the DNA alkylating agent, temozolomide, improved survival in patients afflicted with malignant gliomas has heightened interests in translating this understanding into therapeutic strategies. Because the molecular responses to temozolomide and other DNA alkylating agents are similar between humans and many prokaryotes, insights garnered from bacterial genetics may facilitate such translation. Studies in both prokaryotic and human systems reveal that the cellular response to temozolomide involves a dynamic network of interacting pathways. Given this complexity, it is perhaps not surprising that any single genetic alteration may confer either sensitivity or resistance to temozolomide depending on the context of other interacting pathways. Thus, models of the cellular resistance to temozolomide should account for the network of interacting pathways rather than focusing on any single canonical pathway.

Contents

C.C. Chen (✉)
Division of Neurosurgery, Beth Israel Deaconess Medical Center, Harvard Medical School, Boston, MA, USA; Division of Genomic Stability and DNA Repair, Department of Radiation Oncology, Dana-Farber Cancer Institute, Jimmy Fund 518, 44 Binney Street, Boston, MA 02115–6084, USA
e-mail: cchen1@partners.org

E.G. Van Meir (ed.), *CNS Cancer*, Cancer Drug Discovery and Development, DOI 10.1007/978-1-60327-553-8_28,
© Humana Press, a part of Springer Science+Business Media, LLC 2009

28.1 Introduction

Despite therapeutic advances, malignant glioma remains a devastating disease, causing death in nearly all patients within 5 years of diagnosis. Historically, the cornerstones of therapy for malignant gliomas involve surgery and radiotherapy; however, these treatment modalities provide only marginal survival benefits (Reardon et al., 2006). Given the inherent radiation resistance of malignant gliomas and their infiltrative nature (Burger et al., 2002), it is anticipated that chemotherapeutic agents would be required for meaningful improvement in clinical prognosis. The first chemotherapeutic agent to demonstrate efficacy for malignant glioma is the DNA damaging agent temozolomide (TMZ). In the landmark-randomized trial by Stupp et al., incorporation of TMZ was shown to confer significant survival benefit. The 2-year survival of patients treated with surgery and radiation alone was 10.4%. In contrast, patients treated with the same regimen and TMZ was 26.5% (Stupp et al., 2005).

The therapeutic benefit of TMZ, however, was modest due to either intrinsic or acquired chemoresistance (Giese et al., 2004; Reardon et al., 2006; Sarkaria et al., 2008). Understanding the cellular mechanisms underlying resistance to TMZ remains a critical aspect of therapeutic development.

Our understanding of the cellular response to DNA alkylating agents (see Glossary) is largely derived from genetic and biochemical studies performed in prokaryotic systems (Wei et al., 1996). Since both prokaryotic and eukaryotic genomes are subject to similar chemical reactions, they are liable to the formation of similar damaged substrates. As such, it is not surprising that human cells employ many of the same repair mechanisms as those observed in bacteria (Friedberg et al., 1995). Further, the repair proteins between humans and bacteria share a high degree of amino acid sequence conservation. In most instances, human repair proteins are identified by virtue of their sequence or functional homology to their prokaryotic counterparts (Friedberg et al., 1995; Friedberg et al., 2004; Tano et al., 1990). Experimental interrogations of these proteins in mammalian systems are often interpreted in light of the paradigms developed in prokaryotic systems. Thus, a discussion of human repair processes in the context of the prokaryotic models should be helpful in sparking insights in terms of therapeutic strategies.

Of the prokaryotic systems, our knowledge of DNA repair is most comprehensive in the bacteria *Escherichia coli* (Friedberg et al., 1995). As such, this chapter will discuss the mechanisms of resistance to TMZ in glioma cells in light of the paradigms previously established in *E. coli*. We will begin by giving a brief overview of the chemical properties of TMZ and the various types of lesions in DNA that it causes. Subsequently, we will discuss the clinically relevant effects of each lesion type and the repair mechanisms involved in their correction.

28.2 Temozolomide (TMZ): Chemical Properties

Temozolomide (8-carbamoyl-3-methylimidazo[5,1-*d*]-1,2,3,5-tetrazin-4(3*H*)-one) is a bicyclic heterocyclic compound (Fig. 28.1a) derived from imidazotetrazine (Stevens et al., 1984). In a neutral or basic environment (pH>7), the electrophilic C4 of the tetrazinone ring is susceptible to nucleophilic attack by water molecules, leading to the formation of the active drug 5-(3-methyltriazen-1-yl)imidazole-4-carboxamide (MTIC) (Denny et al., 1994). MTIC rapidly degrades into an inactive carboxylic acid derivative and a highly reactive methyldiazonium cation. The half-life of MTIC in an aqueous environment is approximately 2 hours (Kim et al., 1997).

The reactive methyldiazonium ion reacts with electron donors within DNA, yielding transfer of a methyl group from the ion to the DNA. This reaction can occur at all O- and N-atoms of nucleobases (see Glossary) as well as on O-atoms in the phosphodiester backbone. The most common nucleophilic centers within duplex DNA that are accessible to methylation by TMZ are the following (Fig. 28.1b): N7 position of guanine (70% of adducts), N3 position of adenine and cytosine (25% of adducts), and O6 position of guanine (5%) of adducts (Darkes et al., 2002; Denny et al., 1994; Friedberg et al., 1995). The biologic effects of these modifications differ, as do their repair mechanisms.

28.3 Repair of Temozolomide-Induced DNA Damage in *E. coli*

The biologic effects of the various nucleotide modifications listed above are, for the most part, elucidated in *E. coli* and subsequently extrapolated to human cells (Friedberg et al., 1995). To better understand the effects of TMZ in humans, we will first review the biologic effect of these lesions in the *E. coli* model.

28.3.1 N7-Methyl Guanine

In *E. coli*, the N7-methyl guanine, which accounts for ~70% of TMZ-induced adducts, predominantly undergoes rapid spontaneous depurination (see

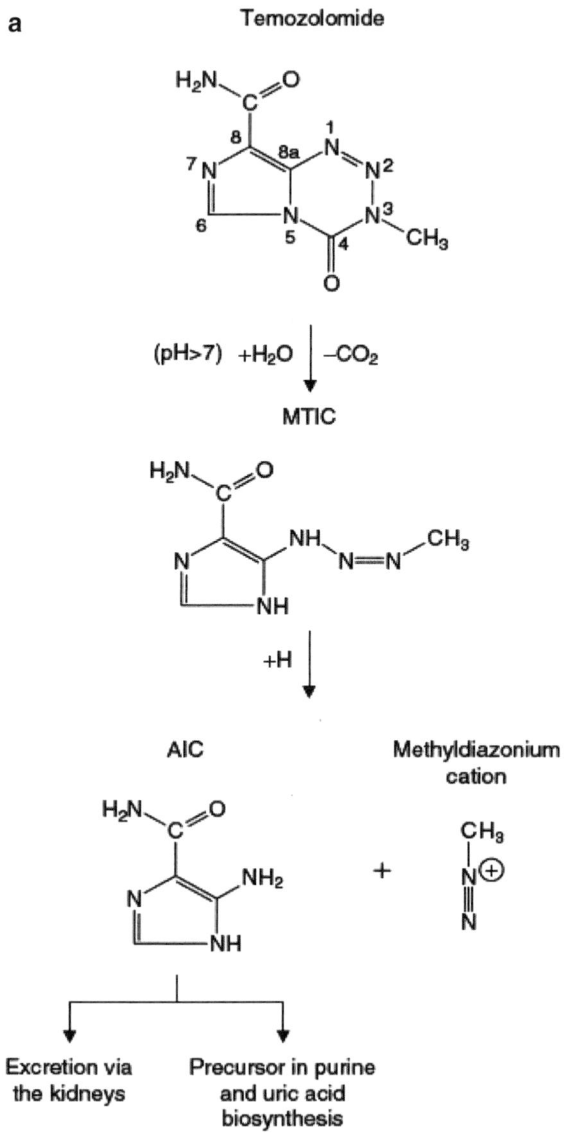

Fig. 28.1 **(a) Formation of reactive ion from temozolomide.** In a neutral or basic environment, the electrophilic C4 of the tetrazinone ring is susceptible to nucleophilic attack by water molecules, leading to the formation of the active drug MTIC. MTIC rapidly degrades into an inactive carboxylic acid derivative and a highly reactive methyldiazonium ion (adapted from Darkes et al., 2002). **(b) Sites of methylation by temozolomide.** The most common nucleophilic centers within duplex DNA that are accessible to methylation by TMZ are N7 position of guanine (70% of adducts), N3 position of adenine and cytosine (25% of adducts), and O6 position of guanine (5% of adducts) (Darkes et al., 2002; Denny et al., 1994; Friedberg et al., 1995)

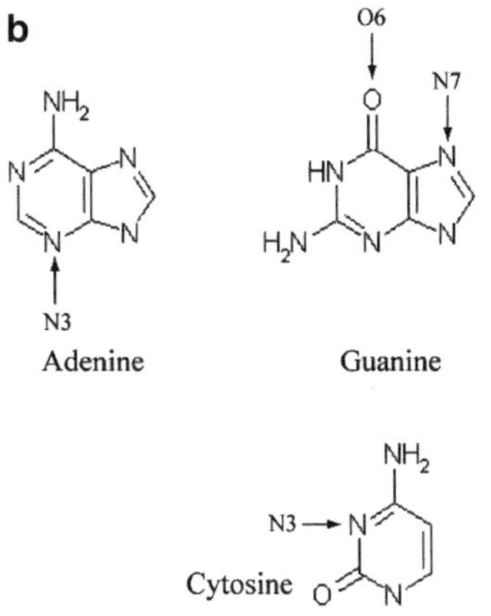

Fig. 28.1 (continued)

Glossary) resulting in the formation of abasic sites (see Glossary). These abasic sites are prohibitive to DNA replication and are ultimately converted into cytotoxic double-stranded breaks (Drablos et al., 2004). A small portion of the N7-methyl guanine are recognized by AlkA, a broad specificity glycosylase (see Glossary and below). This enzyme removes the N7-methyl guanine nucleobase, leaving behind an abasic site (Krokan et al., 1997; Seeberg et al., 1995; Wyatt et al., 1999). AlkA is a 30 kDa glycosylase that recognizes a wide variety of damaged bases, including alkylation products N7-methyl guanine and N3-methyl adenine, deamination products, ring-opened purines, oxidation products, and others (Krokan et al., 1997; Seeberg et al., 1995; Wyatt et al., 1999). *alkA* gene expression is strongly induced by treatment with DNA alkylating agents.

Following the removal of the damaged nucleobase, the abasic sites are repaired via a process referred to as base excision repair (BER, see Glossary). In this process (Fig. 28.2a for *E. coli* BER, Fig. 28.2b for mammalian BER), an enzyme known as apurinic and apyrimidinic endonuclease (also known as AP endonuclease) hydrolyzes the phosphodiester backbone 5′ to the lesion and a DNA deoxyribophosphodiesterase (dRpase) excises the residual 2-deoxyribose-5-phosphate, generating a gap of one nucleotide. The gap is filled by DNA polymerase β, and the continuity of the DNA is restored by DNA ligase. As the BER process is extremely efficient in wild-type *E. coli*, the cytotoxic effect of N7 methylated guanine is detectable only in mutants defective in the process (Krokan et al., 1997; Seeberg et al., 1995; Wyatt et al., 1999).

28.3.2 N3-Methyl Adenine

N3-methyl adenine is a major cytotoxic adduct in *E coli* and accounts for approximately 12% of TMZ-induced DNA lesions (Darkes et al., 2002;

a

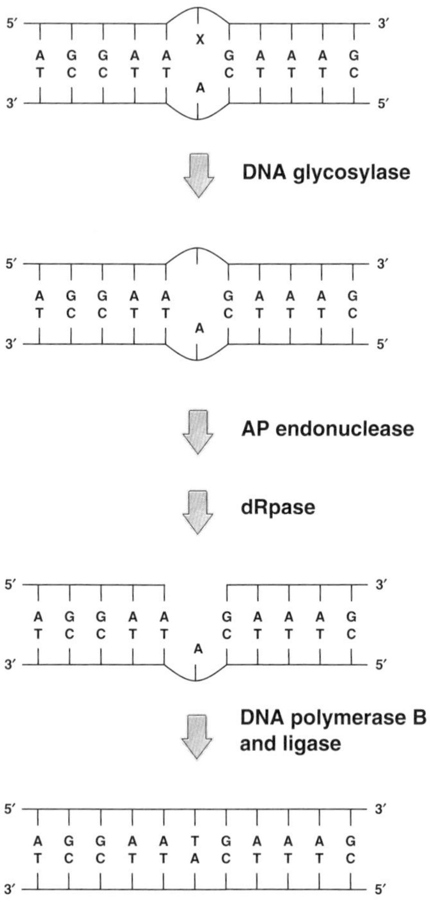

Fig. 28.2 (a) Mechanism of base excision repair (BER) in *E. coli*. During base excision repair, AP endonucleases hydrolyze the phosphodiester backbone 5′ to the lesion and a dRpase excises the residual 2-deoxyribose-5-phosphate, generating a gap of one nucleotide. The gap is filled by DNA polymerase β, and the continuity of the DNA is restored by DNA ligase. X denotes a damaged nucleobase that triggered BER. **(b) Mechanism of base excision repair in mammalian cells.** Similar to bacteria, abasic sites resulting from spontaneous depurination of N7-methyl guanine or from glycosylase processing of N3-methyl adenine in mammals are processed by the mechanism of base excision repair. The abasic sites are processed by the AP endonuclease to produce a single base gap. The strand is detected by PARP1, which catalyzes the synthesis of a polymer of ADP-ribose on various nuclear proteins including histone H1. These modifications alter chromatin structure and facilitate the access of other DNA repair proteins to the site of strand break. PARP2 is also activated in response to DNA strand breaks and facilitates ADP ribosylation of histone H2. Following chromatin modification, PARP1 stimulates the activity of polymerase β to hydrolyze the 5′dRP moiety and fills the single nucleotide gap. The continuity of the phosphodiesterase backbone is then restored by the ligase activity of the XRCC1/LIG3 complex

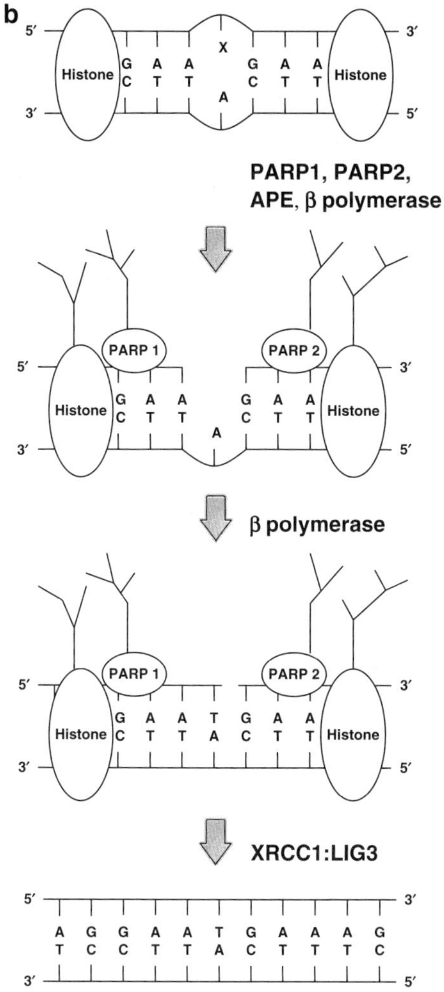

Fig. 28.2 (continued)

Denny et al., 1994; Friedberg et al., 1995). N3-methyl adenine does not undergo spontaneous depurination. However, if not removed from the DNA, 3-methyl adenine causes the formation of double-stranded DNA breaks and, to a lesser extent, single-stranded DNA breaks (for detailed mechanisms, see Friedberg et al., 1995). N3-methyl adenine is excised from DNA by two distinct glycosylases named TagA and AlkA. TagA specifically recognizes N3 methyl-modified purines, while AlkA recognizes a wide variety of damaged bases as mentioned above. The abasic site is subsequently repaired via BER as shown in Fig. 28.2a.

tagA encodes a 21-kDa protein that is expressed constitutively and is not induced upon treatment with DNA alkylating agents (Steium and Seeberg, 1986). The encoded protein recognizes only N3-methyl adenine and N3-methyl guanine. Mutants defective in the *tagA* gene function specifically accumulate N3-methyl adenine and are moderately hypersensitive to DNA alkylation (Sancar and Sancar, 1998). Moreover, overexpression of *E. coli tagA* in mammalian cells conferred resistance to DNA alkylating agents (Klungland et al., 1992).

Like *alkA* mutants, *tagA* mutants are only moderately sensitive to DNA alkylating agents. The *alkA tagA* double mutant, however, exhibits extreme sensitivity to alkylation exposure, suggesting the functional redundancy between these two glycosylases (Sancar and Sancar, 1998).

28.3.3 N3-Methyl Cytosine

N3-methyl cytosine accounts for approximately 13% of TMZ-induced lesions and is typically generated when the MTIC-derived methyldiazonium ions interact with the single-stranded regions of the genome (Darkes et al., 2002; Denny et al., 1994; Friedberg et al., 1995). This alkylated nucleotide blocks DNA replication in *E. coli* and is, therefore, cytotoxic (Sedgwick et al., 2007). In *E. coli*, the major mechanism of repair for N3-methyl cytosine is by direct restoration through the protein AlkB (Dinglay et al., 2000). Unlike AlkA, which recognizes a broad range of substrates, AlkB specifically recognizes N3-methyl cytosine. *alkB* encodes a 24-kDa protein that belongs to a large class of enzymes known as the 2-oxoglutarate and Fe(II)-dependent oxygenase superfamily (Drablo 1397). This enzyme utilizes Fe^{2+} and 2-oxoglutarate as cofactors to oxidize the N3-methyl group of the damaged cytosine. The oxidized methyl moiety is spontaneously released as formaldehyde, thereby restoring the native cytosine (Sedgwick and Lindahl, 2002). *E. coli alkB* mutants are extremely sensitive to alkylation exposure (Kataoka et al., 1983). Interestingly, overexpression of the *E. coli alkB* gene in human cells confers resistance to DNA alkylating agents (Chen et al., 1994).

28.3.4 O6-Methyl Guanine

For N3-methyl cytosine, the methyl group protrudes into the minor grove of the DNA duplex (which is normally free of methyl groups) in a conformation that inhibits DNA polymerase function. O6-methyl guanine (O6MeG for short), on the other hand, can mispair with thymine to allow polymerase bypass. While the O6-methyl guanine moiety is not inherently cytotoxic, the mispair with thymine (O6MeG:T) is processed by DNA mismatch repair (MMR for short, see Glossary) to yield cytotoxic intermediates. DNA mismatch repair is a ubiquitous repair process that normally serves to correct non-Watson–Crick paired duplexes (see Glossary) that arise either

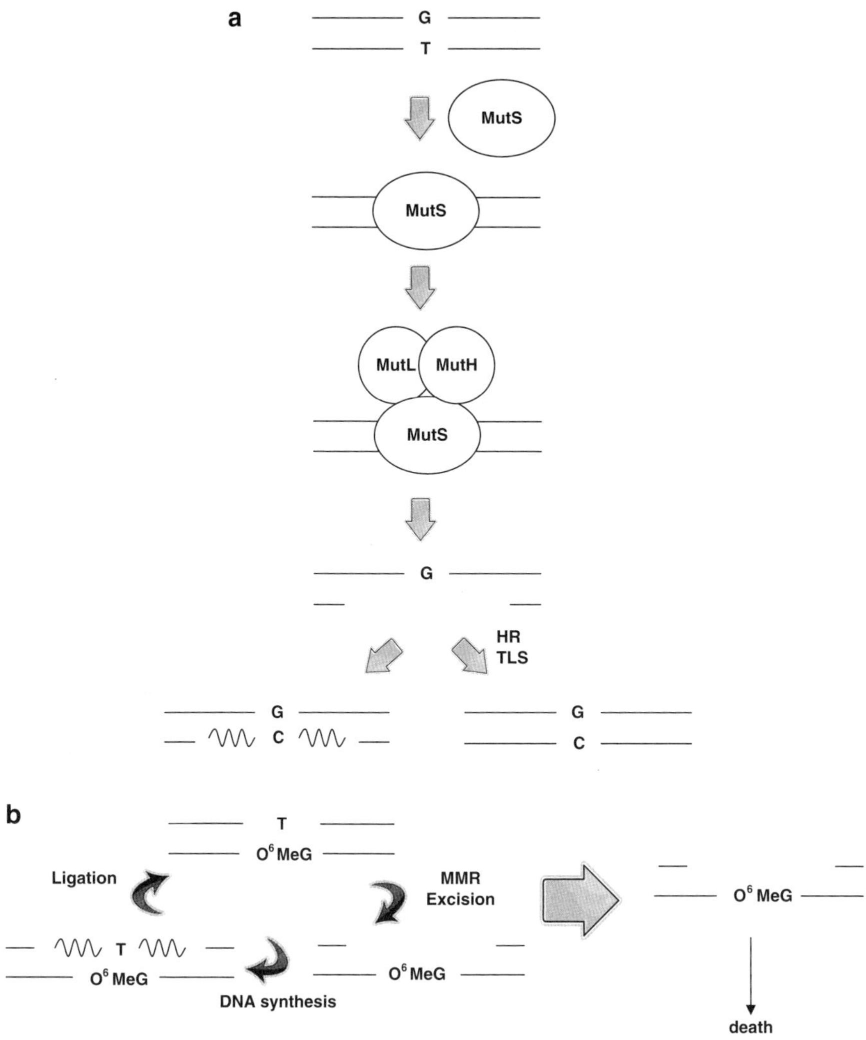

Fig. 28.3 (a) Normal mechanism of mismatch repair (MMR) in *E. coli*. *E. coli* mismatch repair begins with MutS, a protein that binds specifically to mismatched DNA. This binding in turn recruits MutL and MutH, activating the latent endonuclease activity of MutH. MutH cleaves the newly synthesized strand, generating a nick. The nick is used by Helicase II to unwind the DNA into a single-stranded region that is digested by either 3′ or 5′ exonucleases. The gapped DNA is subsequently resynthesized by DNA polymerase III and the continuity of DNA restored by DNA ligase. Here, resynthesized DNA is indicated by the zigzag line. The DNA gap can alternatively be restored by homologous recombination (HR) with or without DNA translesion synthesis (TLS). **(b) Mechanism of mismatch repair in *E. coli* in the presence of O6-methyl guanine**. During DNA replication, the O6MeG mispairs with thymine. This mispair triggers the activation of mismatch repair, which excises the thymine-containing strand. However, during gap filling DNA synthesis, another thymine is inserted across from O6MeG. The second mispair triggers another round of DNA mismatch repair. Multiple cycles of "futile" repair are subsequently triggered, culminating in the generation of

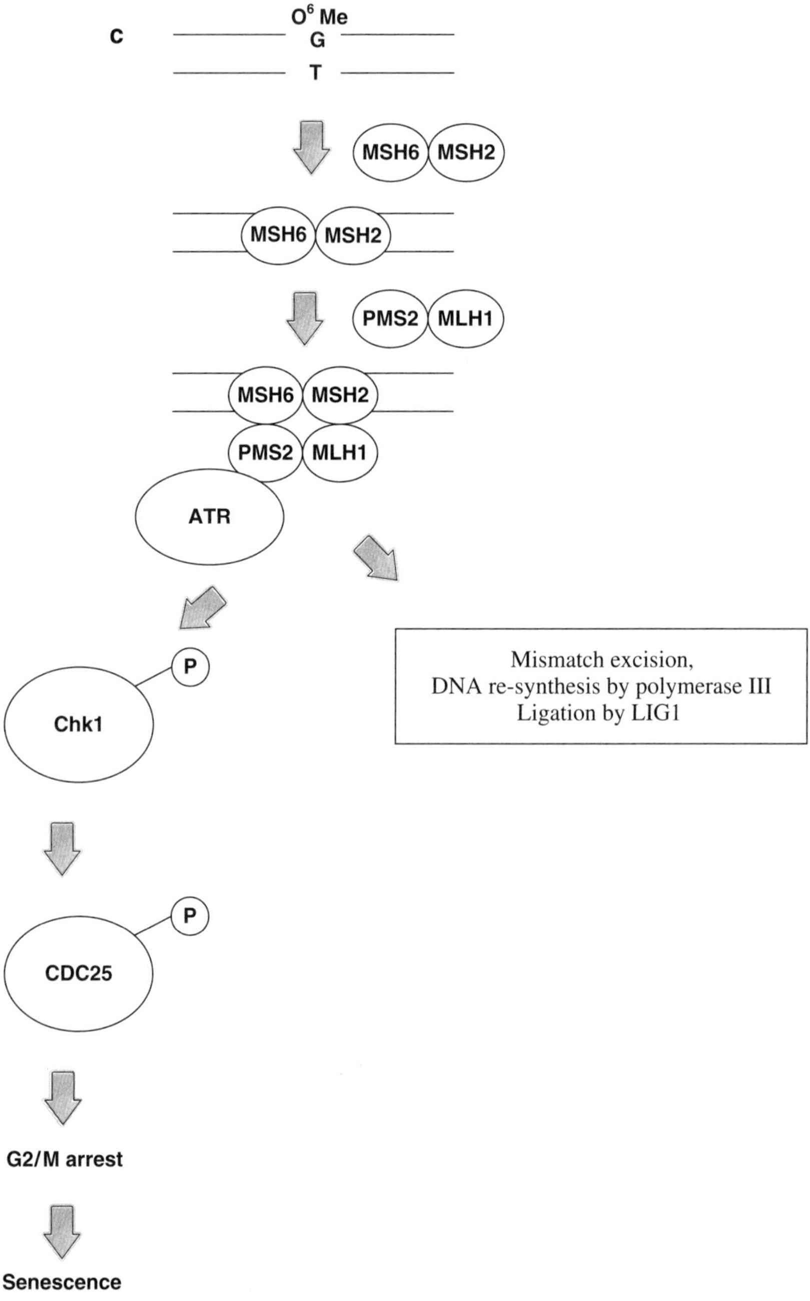

Fig. 28.3 (continued)

spontaneously or in response to DNA damage. The mechanistic details of this process are complex and remain the subject of intense investigation (Kunkel and Erie, 2005). In *E. coli*, this process begins with MutS, a protein that binds specifically to mismatched DNA (Fig. 28.3a). This binding in turn recruits MutL and MutH, activating the latent endonuclease activity of MutH. MutH cleaves the newly synthesized strand, generating a nick. The nick is used by Helicase II to unwind the DNA into a single-stranded region. The unwound single-stranded DNA is digested by either 3′ or 5′ exonucleases, yielding a gap. This gap is subsequently resynthesized by DNA polymerase III using the parental strand as template, and the continuity of DNA restored by DNA ligase (Kunkel and Erie, 2005). Unfortunately, this repair process does not remove the mutated O6MeG since it is typically located on the parental strand. Therefore, during gap filling DNA synthesis, another thymine is inserted across from O6MeG restoring the DNA to the pre-repair state. This second mispair triggers another round of DNA mismatch repair. Ultimately, repeated cycles of "futile" repair are triggered, culminating in the generation of single-stranded DNA gaps (Fig. 28.3b). The mechanistic details underlying this process remain an area of active investigation.

These gaps are ultimately repaired by two different repair processes, either by homologous recombination (HR, see Glossary) or translesion synthesis (TLS, see Glossary). However, when the number of gaps exceeds cellular capacity for repair, cell death ensues (Friedman et al., 1997; Lage and Dietel, 1999; Liu et al., 1996; Stojic et al., 2004).

Since DNA damaged by alkylation requires MMR processing for its cytotoxic effect, MMR-deficient *E. coli* is highly resistant to DNA alkylating agents (Jones and Wagner, 1981; Karran and Marinus, 1982). Because HR and TLS facilitate the repair of DNA gaps resulting from MMR processing of alkylated DNA, mutants defective in homologous recombination or translesion synthesis exhibit heightened sensitivity to alkylation exposure (Bjedov et al., 2007; Nowosielska et al., 2006).

Fig. 28.3 (continued) single-stranded DNA gaps. When the number of gaps exceeds cellular capacity for repair, cell death occurs. **(c) Mechanism of mismatch repair in human cells in the presence of O6-methyl guanine**. Eukaryotic mismatch repair shares many features of the *E. coli* system, but the proteins involved differ depending on the nature of the mismatch. Repair of the O6-methyl guanine– thymine mismatch is initiated when heterodimers of MutS homologs (MSH2–MSH6) bind to a mispair. This binding recruits the MLH1–PMS2 complex (the human homologue of MutL). This complex harbors an endonuclease activity that nicks the strand bearing the thymine. This nick is ultimately processed into a gap catalyzing the futile cycles described in Fig. 28.3b. Ultimately, the gap triggers G2 arrest. This arrest requires an intact ATR/CHK1 axis. The activated CHK1 phosphorylates CDC25C, causing its degradation and G2 arrest

The O6MeG:T mispairs that escape MMR repair ultimately result in mutagenesis. Because the strand bearing thymine base pairs with an adenine in the subsequent round of replication, the outcome is a G->A transition (Horsfall et al., 1990).

Besides MMR activation, *E. coli* harbors two repair pathways that remove O6MeGs. The pathways involve the enzymatic activity of two methyltransferases: Ada and Ogt. These enzymes directly remove the O6 methyl moiety and restore the chemical integrity of guanine (Potter et al., 1987). *ada* encodes a 38-kDa protein that consists of two functional domains linked by a hinge region. The two domains can function independently. The C-terminal domain directly transfers the O6 methyl moiety onto its Cys-321 residue (Sedgwick et al., 1988). The N-terminal domain contains a zinc finger motif that is required for transcriptional modulation of itself (*ada*), *alkA*, and *alkB* in response to alkylation exposure (Myers et al., 1992). Ogt has biochemical properties similar to those exhibited by Ada in that they shared a high affinity for O6MeG. Not surprisingly, the region containing the methyl acceptor cysteine in Ogt exhibits extensive amino acid homology to Ada (Rebeck et al., 1989). Unlike Ada, however, Ogt levels are not induced upon alkylation exposure (Potter et al., 1989). Both *ada* and *ogt E. coli* mutants, are highly sensitive to alkylation exposure (Drablos et al., 2004). Overexpression of both *E. coli* proteins in mammalian cells confers resistance against DNA alkylating agents (Drablos et al., 2004).

28.4 Evolutionarily Conserved Temozolomide Resistance Mechanisms

As discussed, the molecular mechanisms underlying DNA repair were first elucidated in prokaryotic models such as *E. coli.* With the recent cloning and characterization of the homologous genes in higher organisms, there has been an explosion of information about eukaryotic DNA repair. With regard to the process of DNA repair, the proteins and mechanisms involved appear highly similar despite the significant evolutionary distance between humans and *E. coli.* However, as human cells have evolved complexities in subcellular organization (e.g., chromatin structures) and cell growth regulation (e.g., cell cycle progression and cell death), human repair proteins have developed additional functionalities to accommodate these complexities. In many instances, proteins unique to the eukaryotes are recruited to the site of damage (Ame et al., 2004; Schreiber et al., 2002). In other situations, a single ancestral DNA repair gene evolves into multiple homologues, each with specialized functions (Aas et al., 2003; Dinglay et al., 2000; Duncan et al., 2002; Wei et al., 1996). The human homologues of the various DNA alkylation repair pathways discussed above will be reviewed here.

28.4.1 N7-Methyl Guanine

Analogous to the bacterial repair system, human cells accumulate abasic sites as a result of spontaneous depurination of N7-methyl guanine. These basic sites are then repaired by the human BER machinery (Fig. 28.2b). Analogous to the bacteria system, the abasic sites in human cells are subsequently processed by the AP endonuclease, APE, to generate a single base gap (Demple et al., 1991; Hansen and Kelley, 2000).

In contrast to the *E. coli* DNA repair system where higher order chromatin structures are absent, the human repair proteins face the challenge of negotiating these structures during repair. In BER, the chromatin structure is, in part, modulated by a group of proteins called poly(ADP-ribose) polymerase (PARP). The strand discontinuity produced during BER is detected by PARP1, the founding member of a superfamily of 18 proteins (Ame et al., 2004; Haince et al., 2005). In response to the DNA strand break, PARP1 synthesizes polymers of ADP-ribose onto the various nuclear proteins including histone H1 (Poirier et al., 1982). These modifications alter chromatin structure (Poirier et al., 1982; Tulin et al., 2006) and facilitate the access of DNA repair proteins to the site of strand break. Another member of the PARP family, PARP2, is also involved in this process. PARP2 catalyzes ADP ribosylation of a host of nuclear proteins including histone H2 (Ame et al., 2004; Schreiber et al., 2002). Mice deficient in *Parp1* or *Parp2* exhibit sensitivity to DNA alkylating agents as well as delay in the processing of DNA strand breaks (Ménissier de Murcia et al., 2003; Shall and De Murcia, 2000). Of note, PARP1 inhibitors have been shown to sensitize glioma to TMZ in both in vivo and in vitro models (Curtin et al., 2004; Sarkaria et al., 2008).

Following chromatin modification, PARP1 stimulates the activity of polymerase β to hydrolyze the 5′-deoxyribose phosphate (5′dRP) moiety and fills the single nucleotide gap (Wood et al., 2005). The continuity of the phosphodiesterase backbone is subsequently restored by the ligase activity of the XRCC1/LIG3 complex (see Glossary) (Caldecott et al., 1994, 1995). XRCC1, in turn, specifically associates with and inactivates PARP1 (Masson et al., 1998). As would be expected, genetic silencing or inactivation of APE, polymerase β, XRCC1, or LIG3 individually confers sensitivity to DNA alkylating agents (Elleberger and Tomkinson, 2008; Fritz et al., 2003; Trivedi et al., 2005). However, the interplay between these proteins is complex. For instance, overexpression of APE is frequently seen in certain tumor types (Morgan et al., 1999; Xu et al., 1997). Overexpression of APE in an XRCC1-proficient cell is protective against alkylation exposure (Grosch et al., 1998; Ramana et al., 1998). However, the same overexpression in an XRCC1-deficient tumor sensitizes cells to DNA alkylation. Mechanistically, by virtue of its endonuclease activity, APE overexpression increases DNA strand break accumulation in response to alkylation exposure. The repair of these strand breaks normally requires an intact XRCC1/LIG3 complex. XRCC1 mutants suffer diminutive capacity in strand break repair and are, therefore, hypersensitive to APE1 overexpression (Sossou et al., 2005). This example illustrates how a genetic alteration can confer either sensitivity or resistance to TMZ depending on the cellular context.

28.4.2 N3-Methyl Adenine

The human protein alkyl-adenine glycosylase (AAG; also known as methylpurine DNA glycosylase or MPG) is the primary glycosylase responsible for the repair of N3-methyl adenine. In contrast to other human DNA repair proteins that are identified by virtue of their sequence homology to bacterial repair proteins, AAG is not related to the *E. coli* AlkA or TagA at the sequence level. However, its glycosylase specificity is broad and similar to that described for AlkA (Krokan et al., 1997; Seeberg et al., 1995; Wyatt et al., 1999). Moreover, overexpression of human *AAG* restores alkylation resistance in *E. coli alkA* mutants, suggesting functional conservation between these genes (Bonanno et al., 2002). As such, the human AAG protein is considered an orthologue of the *E. coli* AlkA.

The human AAG exists in two isoforms, resulting from differential splicing of either exon 1a (hAAG1) or exon 1b (hAAG2) (O'Connor, 1993; Vickers et al., 1993). Both isoforms appear expressed in all tissues examined. No functional differences between these isoforms have been found to date (O'Connor, 1993; Pendlebury et al., 1994).

In terms of sensitivity to DNA alkylating agents, the effects of inactivating human AAG appear variable and dependent on the cellular context. *Aag* null mouse embryonic stem cells are hypersensitive to DNA alkylating agents (Allan et al., 1998; Engelward et al., 1996). However, the bone marrow cells derived from the same mice are hyper-resistant to alkylation exposure (Roth and Samson, 2002). To add to this complexity, overexpression of human AAG in human cells conferred sensitivity to TMZ, while the same overexpression in an *E. coli alkA* mutant conferred resistance (Bonanno et al., 2002; Trivedi et al., 2005). While the mechanisms underlying these observations remain elusive, it is clear that the physiologic effects of AAG on TMZ resistance differ pending on cellular context.

To date, no human homologue or orthologue of the *E. coli* TagA protein has been identified.

28.4.3 N3-Methyl Cytosine

The *E. coli* AlkB protein is critical in repairing TMZ-induced N3-methyl cytosine (Dinglay et al., 2000). The first human homologue of the *E. coli* AlkB (ABH1) was found in 1996 (Wei et al., 1996). Two others, ABH2 and ABH3, were subsequently identified by sequence analysis and functional complementation (Aas et al., 2003; Duncan et al., 2002). Using domains conserved in these three homologues, ABH4-8 were identified (Kurowski et al., 2003).

Of these homologues, only two (ABH2 and ABH3) have been shown to act on N3-methyl cytosine to directly reverse the alkylation damage (Aas et al., 2003). ABH2 preferentially repairs double-stranded DNA substrates, while ABH3 preferentially repairs single-stranded RNA substrates. When expressed in *E. coli alkB* mutants, ABH2 best restores alkylation resistance (Ringvoll et al., 2008). These results combine to suggest that ABH2 is the key homologue of the *E coli* AlkB in terms of DNA damage repair. Indeed, mice deficient in *Abh2*, but not *Abh3*, are hypersensitive to DNA alkylating agents (Ringvoll et al., 2006). These studies suggest that ABH2 is a potential determinant of cellular sensitivity to TMZ. This hypothesis awaits experimental validation.

28.4.4 O6-Methyl Guanine

In human cells, the primary mechanism of repair for O6-methyl guanine involves the protein O6-methyl guanine methyltransferase (MGMT). The human *MGMT* was initially cloned from a cDNA library by virtue of its ability to correct DNA alkylation sensitivity of *E. coli ogt* mutants (see Section 7.3.4) (Tano et al., 1990). At the amino acid level, it is 28% identical to the *E coli* Ogt. In the C-terminal region where the catalytic site is located, the two proteins share 60–65% homology (Tano et al., 1990). The human *MGMT* encodes a 22-kDa protein that repairs O6-alkylation adducts in a one-step reaction that transfers the adduct from the O6 position of guanine to a cysteine residue in the catalytic pocket (Kaina et al., 2007). The alkylated MGMT subsequently undergoes poly-ubiquitination followed by proteolysis (Srivenugopal et al., 1996). As one MGMT molecule can repair only one alkyl adduct, the cellular repair capacity depends on the rate at which the cell can resynthesize MGMT. Indeed, *MGMT* is one of the handful of DNA repair genes that are transcriptionally upregulated in response to alkylation exposure (Christmann et al., 2003; Fritz et al., 1991; Grombacher and Kaina, 1995).

As with other eukaryotic DNA repair processes, MGMT activity is regulated by post-translational modification and subcellular localization. MGMT is localized in the cytoplasm and translocates into the nucleus upon DNA damage (Lim and Li, 1996). Its activity is inhibited by phosphorylation (Mullapudi et al., 2000; Srivenugopal et al., 2000) and facilitated by open chromatin structures (Ryan et al., 1986).

As the O6-methyl adduct is one of the major products of TMZ treatment, constituting approximately 5% of the TMZ-induced lesion (Darkes et al., 2002; Denny et al., 1994; Friedberg et al., 1995), cells deficient in MGMT are more sensitive to TMZ (Futscher et al., 1989; Glassner et al., 1999; Smith and Brent, 1989). MGMT expression levels have been inversely correlated to favorable response to DNA alkylating agents in both experimental models and malignant glioma specimens (Anda et al., 2003; Belanich et al., 1996; Jaeckle et al., 1998; Wang et al., 1996).

The human *MGMT* gene possesses a CpG island (Gardiner-Garden and Frommer, 1987), which spans approximately 1,000 bases around the transcriptional start site. Direct sequencing after bisulfite treatment yielded 108 CpG sites (Mikeska et al., 2007) that are methylated. Methylation of a subset of these CpGs has been associated with transcriptional silencing in tissue culture models (Herfarth et al., 1999; Watts et al., 1997).

If the observations made in the tissue culture models can be extended to tumor specimens, one would anticipate that the extent of *MGMT* promoter methylation would correlate with MGMT protein level and, therefore, therapeutic response. This hypothesis was examined in 206 GBM patients who were randomized to radiation or radiation plus TMZ in a phase III clinical trial. Tumor specimens were collected and examined for *MGMT* promoter methylation using methylation-specific PCR. For patients with tumors containing a methylated *MGMT* promoter, a survival benefit was observed with TMZ and radiation treatment as compared to those receiving only radiation (21 months versus 15 months). Such benefit was not observed in patients with tumors containing unmethylated *MGMT* promoters (Hegi et al., 2005). Similar observations have been made by others though none of these previous studies were done with specimens collected from a randomized trial (Balana et al., 2003; Esteller, 2000; Hegi et al., 2004; Kamiryo et al., 2004; Komine et al., 2003; Watanabe et al., 2005). These findings demonstrate that the methylation status of the *MGMT* gene promoter is a marker of therapeutic response to TMZ in patients with glioblastoma.

While none of the above cited studies rigorously tested the correlation between *MGMT* promoter methylation and gene expression, it was widely assumed that in the methylated group of patients low to no MGMT expression would be found. Similarly, it was expected that all the patients in the other group would show strong MGMT expression. Therefore, it came as a surprise when poor to no correlations were found between *MGMT* promoter methylation status and MGMT protein in tumor specimens (Brell et al., 2005; Maxwell et al., 2006; Preusser et al., 2008; Rodriguez et al., 2008; Sasai et al., 2008). In these studies, a significant portion of the tumor harboring methylated *MGMT* promoter still expressed high levels of MGMT protein. Likewise, a significant portion of tumor harboring unmethylated *MGMT* promoter showed low level of MGMT protein.

In the nonmethylated patient group, the discrepancy between *MGMT* promoter methylation and MGMT protein levels can be explained by poor specimen processing. For instance, *MGMT* mRNA and protein degrade if there is significant delay between specimen procurement and processing. Another issue relates to the semiquantitative nature of immunohistochemistry and the notorious difficulties with such technique in avoiding artifacts due to antibody quality and antigen retrieval procedures. Further, the presence of stromal elements in tumor can bias methylation-specific PCR.

In the methylated group, however, the inconsistency between *MGMT* promoter methylation and protein levels cannot be as easily explained. This discrepancy suggests the possibility that *MGMT* promoter methylation and MGMT protein level may capture distinct, though likely overlapping, aspects of malignant glioma biology. This hypothesis postulates that *MGMT* promoter methylation might simply be a surrogate marker of the overall methylation status of the genome (Herfarth et al., 1999; Jacinto and Esteller, 2007; Paz et al., 2003; Turker, 2002; Watts et al., 1997). This raises the interesting possibility that *MGMT*-independent gene functions may determine or contribute to the cellular response to TMZ. Such hypothesis would explain the limited efficacy of MGMT inhibitors in the clinical setting (Mrugala and Chamberlain, 2008). In sum, the hypothesis proposed here awaits further experimental validation. Global profiling of promoter methylation status with correlation to *MGMT* promoter methylation and clinical outcome may be a helpful first step in testing this hypothesis.

28.4.5 MMR and DNA Damage Checkpoint Activation

The increased resistance of DNA mismatch repair-deficient cells to DNA alkylating agents has been the subject of multiple rounds of rediscoveries. The observation was initially made in *E. coli* over 20 years ago (Shanabruch et al., 1983). With the discovery of eukaryotic mismatch repair systems, the observation was remade in yeast, plant, mouse, and ultimately human tumor cells (Friedberg et al., 1995).

Eukaryotic mismatch repair shares many features of the *E. coli* system, but the proteins involved differ, depending on the nature of the mismatch (Fig. 28.3c). Repair is initiated when heterodimers of MutS homologues [either MSH2–MSH6 (MutSα) or MSH2–MSH3 (mutSβ)] bind to a DNA mismatch. MutSα (MSH2–MSH6) is primarily responsible for the repair of single base mispairs, whereas the MutSβ (MSH2-MSH3) is critical in the repair of insertion deletion loops. This binding recruits the MLH1–PMS2 complex (the human homologue of MutL). The MLH1–PMS2 complex harbors an endonuclease activity that nicks the mismatch-bearing strand. This nick is processed into a gap by a combination of exonucleases. The gapped DNA is ultimately repaired by DNA polymerase III and ligase I (Kunkel and Erie, 2005).

Similar to observations made in *E. coli*, alkylation exposure in human cells causes accumulation of single-stranded DNA gaps in a mismatch repair-dependent manner (Mojas et al., 2007). For reasons that are not clear, these gaps are tolerated during the first cell cycle after alkylation exposure but trigger G2/M checkpoint activation during the second cell cycle (Stojic et al., 2004). It has been proposed that the gaps generated during the first S phase are converted into double-stranded breaks during the second S phase. These breaks, in turn, trigger G2/M checkpoint activation (Plant and Roberts, 1971).

The G2/M checkpoint activation following gap generation requires an intact ATR/CHK1 axis but not ATM (see Glossary) (Stojic et al., 2004). ATM and ATR are critical kinases that are activated in response to DNA damage. ATM is rapidly activated by clastogenic damages such as ionizing radiation (Bakkenist and Kastan, 2003). On the other hand, ATR is known to be preferentially activated by replication fork arrest (Abraham, 2001). Upon TMZ treatment, ATR phosphorylates the CHK1 kinase that in turn phosphorylates CDC25C. This phosphorylation facilitates the degradation of CDC25C, resulting in G2 arrest (see Glossary). Inactivation of ATR function by expression of a dominant negative mutant or pharmacologic CHK1 inhibition abolishes the TMZ-induced G2 arrest (Stojic et al., 2004) and sensitizes the U87 glioblastoma cell line to TMZ toxicity (Hirose et al., 2001a). Evidence suggests that the activation of ATR in this context may involve direct physical interaction between MSH2 and ATR (Wang and Qin, 2003) or via a p38 kinase cascade (Hirose et al., 2003).

In contrast to hematopoietic neoplasms that undergo extensive apoptosis after TMZ treatment, only a small portion (approximately 10–20%) of glioblastoma cells treated with TMZ undergo apoptosis (Chakravarti et al., 2006; Gunther et al., 2003). The remaining cells undergo prolonged G2/M arrest (8–10 days) followed by cellular senescence (Hirose et al., 2001b). Loss of G2/M arrest is associated with the accumulation of micronuclei, a feature consistent with mitotic catastrophe (Hirose et al., 2001a; Hirose et al., 2005, 2003).

Over the past 20 years, MMR deficiency has been shown to confer resistance to DNA alkylating agents in a number of experimental models. However, the pertinence of these observations in the clinical setting remains controversial (Friedberg et al., 1995). Clinical interests in DNA mismatch repair were recently ignited by the identification of a *MSH6* inactivating mutation in a high-grade glioma specimen that recurred after TMZ therapy (Hunter et al., 2006). This mutation was associated with loss of protein expression as assessed by immunohistochemistry (IHC). Subsequent analyses of MSH6 expression in a panel of matched pretreatment and recurrent tumors revealed that MSH6 expression was present in all pretreatment samples but lost in 41% of post-treatment cases. The authors concluded that mismatch repair inactivation by *MSH6* mutation contributes to TMZ resistance and tumor recurrence (Cahill et al., 2007). However, a follow-up study examining this hypothesis reports that *MSH6* mutation or loss of MSH6 protein expression in clinical specimens did not correlate with TMZ resistance (Maxwell et al., 2008).

The importance of MMR in TMZ resistance was also examined in the first report put forth by The Cancer Genome Atlas project (TCGA). In this study, 601 selected genes were exhaustively sequenced in a total of 91 GBM specimens. Of the 91 specimens, seven were derived from recurrent tumor after treatment with DNA alkylating agents. Six of the seven tumors harbored mutations in MMR genes including *MLH1*, *MSH2*, *MSH6*, and *PMS2*

(TCGA Research Network et. al., 2008). However, the study did not test whether these mutations inactivated the encoded protein. Moreover, it was unclear whether these mutations were the result of TMZ therapy or the cause of resistance. Since that mutations in the MMR genes were exceedingly rare in GBM specimens prior to TMZ therapy (TCGA, 2008), it is conceivable that DNA alkylating agents induced mutations in "hot spots" located within MMR genes.

In sum, the notion that MMR plays a critical role in TMZ resistance is an attractive one, especially given findings in the various experimental systems. There are some data supporting this notion in the clinical setting though caveats of these data sets need to be taken into consideration. In this context, molecular profiling of MMR as a determinant for whether TMZ therapy should be administered remains premature at the present time.

28.4.6 Fanconi Anemia (FA) DNA Repair Pathway

In *E. coli*, mutants defective in homologous recombination and DNA translesion synthesis are sensitive to alkylation exposure. Since these processes are highly conserved evolutionarily, it is likely that these processes participate in glioma response to TMZ (Friedberg et al., 1995).

In higher eukaryotes, HR and TLS are modulated by the Fanconi anemia (FA) pathway. The regulation of the FA pathway is highly complex, involving at least 12 proteins (FANCA, B, C, D1, D2, E, F, G, I, J, L, M) (Medhurst et al., 2001; Pace et al., 2002; Taniguchi and D'Andrea, 2002). In response to DNA damage, coordinated regulation of these proteins leads to mono-ubiquitination of the downstream FANCD2 protein. This modification, in turn, causes the FANCD2 and the FANCI protein to cluster at sites of DNA damage, leading to nuclear foci formation (Garcia-Higuera et al., 2001). Interactions between FANCD2/FANCI complex and the proteins involved in homologous recombination and DNA translesion synthesis at these sites facilitate the process of DNA repair (Garcia-Higuera et al., 2001; Howlett et al., 2002; Taniguchi et al., 2002).

Extrapolating from the *E. coli* paradigm where HR and TLS play critical roles in alkylation response, the coordination of HR and TLS by the FA repair pathway may affect cellular resistance to alkylation exposure. Indeed, TMZ treatment of FA-proficient cell lines led to a dose- and time-dependent increase in FANCD2 mono-ubiquitination as well as FANCD2 nuclear foci formation, both hallmarks of FA pathway activation. Importantly, glioblastoma cell lines deficient in the FA repair pathway exhibited increased sensitivity to TMZ relative to the FA-proficient glioma cell lines. Moreover, inhibition of FA pathway activation caused hypersensitivity to TMZ in the U87MG glioma cell line. The TMZ sensitizing effect of FA inhibition was additive to that of

MGMT inhibition. These results suggest the importance of eukaryotic homologous recombination and DNA translesion synthesis in alkylation resistance (Chen et al., 2007).

In summary, cellular resistance to TMZ is determined by a complex network of DNA repair pathways that are highly analogous to models developed in *E. coli*. A diagrammatic summary of these pathways is shown in Fig. 28.4.

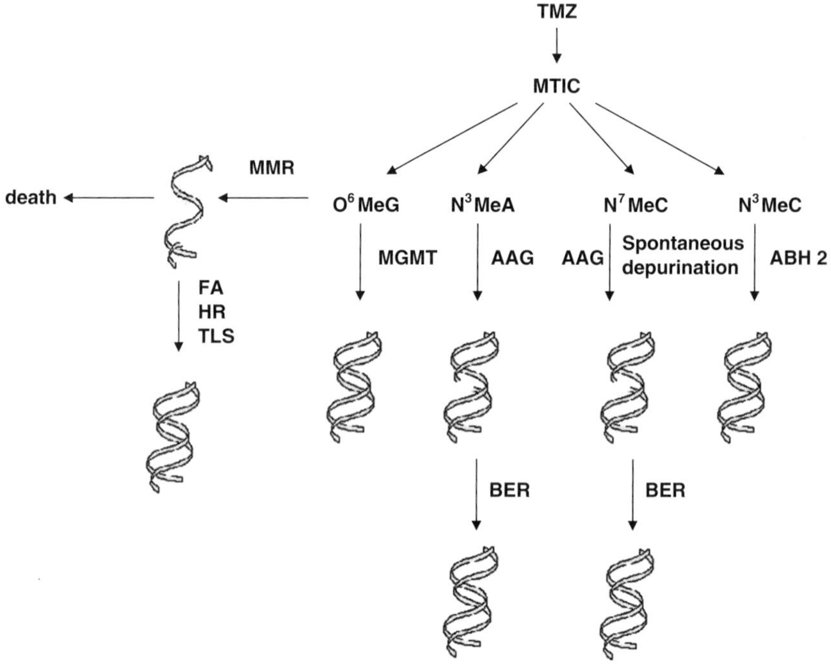

Fig. 28.4 Mechanisms of cellular resistance to temozolomide. Toxicity of temozolomide is derived from methylation of the various nucleotides. The most common damages produced by temozolomide are N7 position of guanine (70% of adducts), N3 position of adenine and cytosine (25% of adducts), and O6 position of guanine (5% of adducts). The O6-methyl guanines are primarily repaired by MGMT in a single-step reaction that transfers the methyl moiety from the damaged nucleoside to the MGMT protein. The O6-methyl guanines that escape MGMT repair are processed by mismatch repair into secondary cytotoxic lesions. These lesions are repaired by various DNA repair pathways, including Fanconi anemia (FA) repair pathway. N3-methyl adenine is excised from DNA by AAG, and the abasic site is subsequently repaired by base excision repair. N7-methyl guanine undergoes rapid spontaneous depurination, resulting in the formation of cytotoxic abasic sites. A small portion of the N7-methyl guanine is also recognized by AAG to yield abasic sites. These abasic sites are repaired via base excision repair. N3-methyl cytosines are directly restored to cytosine by ABH2

28.5 Temozolomide Resistance Mechanism Unique to Higher Eukaryotes

With the development of subcellular organization and the need for cell growth regulation, eukaryotic cells evolved unique cellular processes that are not present in prokaryotic cells. Some of these processes affect cellular resistance to TMZ and will be discussed here.

28.5.1 p53

The p53 tumor-suppressor gene encodes critical functions that modulate cell division and death in higher eukaryotes. These functions appear unique to higher eukaryotes, as no homologue has been identified in lower eukaryotes or prokaryotes (Levine, 1997). Because mutations in the *p53* gene are found in more than 50% of human glioblastomas (Hayashi et al., 1997; Newcomb et al., 1997) (see also Chapter 14), a large number of investigations have been devoted to understanding the mechanism of p53 activity. These studies revealed that p53 acts primarily as a transcription factor that is activated in response to genotoxic stress, including DNA damage. This activation results in either cell cycle arrest or apoptosis (Levine, 1997).

Studies of p53 effect on TMZ resistance suggest a complex picture, with contradictory results from independent groups. There are reports that glioblastoma cell lines with functional p53 responses exhibit increased sensitivity to DNA alkylation relative to those with dysfunctional p53 (Bocangel et al., 2002). However, in another study where TMZ sensitivity was compared between isogenic cell lines differing only in p53 status, the opposite was found. In this study, inactivation of the p53 response in the U87MG cell line (normally wild type for p53) by expression of the HPV E6 protein resulted in increased TMZ sensitivity. Further investigation revealed that E6 expression in U87MG cells facilitated escape from the G2/M arrest. These cells ultimately die from mitotic catastrophe (Hirose et al., 2001b). Consistent with this second study, a small molecule inhibitor of p53 enhanced TMZ sensitivity in a GBM xenograft model (Dinca et al., 2008). The discrepancy between these studies raises the possibility that the effect of p53 on TMZ response may be modulated by other genetic determinants.

Given the wide spectrum of genes transcriptionally regulated by p53, it is conceivable that any of the p53-regulated genes involved in apoptosis, cell cycle regulation, mitogen response, cell survival, or DNA repair may modulate TMZ response (Levine, 1997). Any predictive model of cellular response to TMZ will require a comprehensive integration of all aspects of p53 biology. For instance, the expression of MGMT requires a wild-type p53 protein (Blough et al., 2007). The loss of MGMT expression in a p53-deficient tumor would predict that the cells should become hypersensitive to TMZ. However, it is equally conceivable that this loss of *MGMT* expression may be overshadowed by the loss of pro-apoptosis or pro-senescence genes that are similarly dependent on a wild-type p53 (Levine, 1997).

28.5.2 Autophagy

Autophagy is one of the two major protein degradation systems that are found in eukaryotes (Fig. 28.5). The other is the ubiquitin–proteasome system. In autophagy, a small volume of cytoplasm is enclosed by membranes to form the autophagosome. The autophagosome, in turn, fuses with the lysosome, where the cytoplasm-derived materials are degraded (Mizushima, 2004). Autophagy is thought to be required for normal turnover of cellular components. It is also induced in cancer cells in response to a variety of anticancer agents to either promote cell survival or programmed cell death (Kondo et al., 2005; Levine and Yuan, 2005).

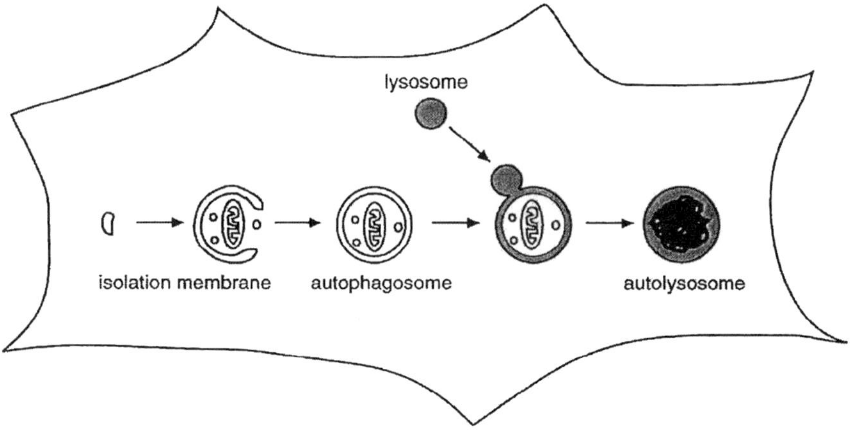

Fig. 28.5 The process of autophagy. Autophagy is one of the two major protein degradation systems found in eukaryotes. The other is the ubiquitin–proteasome system. In autophagy, a small volume of cytoplasm is enclosed by membranes to form the autophagosome. The autophagosome, in turn, fuses with the lysosome, where the cytoplasm-derived materials are degraded (adapted from Mizushima, 2004)

In multiple glioblastoma cell lines, treatment with TMZ is associated with the induction of autophagy (Kanzawa et al., 2004). Moreover, pharmacologic inhibition of this process results in sensitization to TMZ (Kanzawa et al., 2004).TMZ-induced autophagy is associated with elevated steady-state levels of cellular ATP. Together, these results suggest that cellular response to TMZ include increased autophagy and associated catabolic processes that provide the energy necessary to ensure cell survival (Katayama et al., 2007). It is important to note that these observations have yet been validated using clinically derived specimens.

28.6 Conclusion

To date, the alkylating agent TMZ remains one of the few chemotherapeutic agents that has demonstrated definitive efficacy in the treatment of malignant gliomas. It is currently the standard of treatment for glioblastoma in the clinic in conjunction with radiation therapy. Understanding the molecular mechanisms underlying glioma resistance to this agent is a prerequisite in devising future therapeutic strategies. Many of the mechanisms of alkylation resistance were previously defined in *E. coli* and subsequently extrapolated to human cells. Other resistance mechanisms appear unique to human cells. Irrespective of evolutionary conservation, cellular mechanisms of alkylation response appear highly complex, since the same genetic alteration may confer drug resistance in one setting while producing sensitivity in another. As such, new paradigms of cellular resistance should include assessments of the dynamic interplay among many critical pathways rather than a narrow focus on any particular genetic alteration. An understanding of this dynamic interplay would allow for customized treatment regimens individually tailored to the genetic landscape of each tumor and optimization of clinical efficacy.

Abbreviations

Temozolomide	TMZ
N7-methyl guanine	N7MeG
N3-methyl adenine	N3MeA
N3-methyl cytosine	N3MeC
O6-methyl guanine	O6MeG
Base excision repair	BER
DNA mismatch repair	MMR

Acknowledgments We are grateful to Dr. Paul Doetsch (Emory University) and Dr. Erwin Van Meir (Emory University) for their comments and careful reading of this manuscript.

Glossary

DNA alkylating agents Agents that transfer alkyl group from one molecule to another. Alkyl groups refer to groups of carbon and hydrogen atoms arranged in a chain. Common alkyl groups include methyl (CH3) or ethyl (CH2–CH3) moieties.

Nucleotides The structural units of DNA. These molecules consist of three joined structures (Fig. 28.1b): a base moiety (adenine, guanine, cytosine, or thymine), a sugar, and a phosphate group

Nucleobases Another name for the base moiety of the nucleotide.

Abasic sites Sites within DNA where the nucleobases have been removed.

Depurination A DNA alteration involving hydrolysis of the bond between a purine base (i.e., adenine or guanine) and the sugar moiety of the DNA.

Glycosylase Enzymes that remove the nucleobase while leaving the sugar–phosphate backbone intact.

Base excision repair (BER) A cellular process that repairs damaged nucleobases by direct excision of the nucleobase. This process is followed by the removal of the remaining nucleotide. The single nucleotide gap is then resynthesized by a specific DNA polymerase (Fig. 28.2a).

Mismatch repair (MMR) A cellular process that recognizes and repairs non-Watson–Crick base-paired nucleotides. The same system is also involved in the repair of damaged nucleotides (Fig. 28.3a).

Non-Watson–Crick pairing Base pairing that deviate from A:T and G:C.

Homologous recombination (HR) A cellular process that results in physical exchange between two strands of DNA. The process involves the alignment of similar sequences followed by breaking and rejoining of the phosphate backbone. It is a major mechanism for repairing gapped or fragmented DNA.

Translesion synthesis (TLS) A cellular process that allows DNA replication machinery to replicate past damaged DNA. It involves the switching of replicative polymerases for specialized translesion polymerases that carry out the insertion of bases opposite the damaged nucleotides. By allowing for bypass of these DNA damages, TLS allows for completion of DNA synthesis/repair and thereby confers resistance to the various DNA damaging agents.

XRCC1/LIG3 complex The human ligase 3 (LIG3) is the ligase responsible for restoring continuity of DNA during BER. All human DNA ligases function as a complex with a "partner" protein. For instance, LIG1 associates with replication factor proliferating cell nuclear antigen (PCNA) and LIG4 associates with XRCC4. These partners modulate the activity of the associated ligase as well as the respective repair process. The partner for LIG3 is XRCC1. These two proteins form a tight complex, and both proteins are required for BER. XRCC1 is short for *X*-ray *R*epair *C*omplementing defective repair in *C*hinese hamster cells. As the name implies, the gene is cloned by virtue of its ability to restore radiation resistance in a Chinese hamster cell line that is otherwise highly sensitive to ionizing radiation. Please see Friedberg et al. (1995) for additional details.

ATM *A*taxia *T*elangiectasia *M*utated. The gene that is mutated in the disease that bears the same name. ATM is a member of the phosphoinositide 3-kinase-like kinase (PIKK) family, which includes several proteins that are required for DNA repair. The ATM kinase is activated by damaged or broken DNA strands. This process initiates a phosphorylation cascade that ultimately triggers DNA damage checkpoint activation and facilitates DNA repair.

ATR *AT*M and *R*ad3-Related. As the name implies, the ATR kinase is closely related to ATM and is a member of the PIKK family. In contrast to ATM, ATR primarily responds to stalled replication forks. In response to these structures, ATR phosphorylates several downstream target proteins, eventually leading to DNA damage checkpoint activation.

CHK1 *CH*eckpoint *K*inase 1. CHK1 is a critical downstream effector ATR. In response to stalled replication fork, ATR is activated to phosphorylate CHK1. This phosphorylation activates the kinase activity of CHK1. Activated CHK1, in turn, phosphorylates downstream effectors, including CDC25.

CDC25 Short for *C*ell *D*ivision *C*ycle 25. The yeast gene was cloned by virtue of its ability to complement a mutant defective in cell cycle progression. Historically, this yeast mutant was the 25th mutant that exhibited this phenotype (hence CDC25). The gene product was found to harbor a phosphatase activity. The human homologue was subsequently cloned and found to play roles in cell cycle progression highly analogous to that observed in yeast. Both the yeast and human CDC25 remove an inhibitory phosphate residue in critical downstream proteins to allow progression through the cell cycle.

References

Aas, P. A., Otterlei, M., Falnes, P. O., Vagbo, C. B., Skorpen, F., Akbari, M., Sundheim, O., Bjoras, M., Slupphaug, G., Seeberg, E., and Krokan, H. E. (2003) Human and bacterial oxidative demethylases repair alkylation damage in both RNA and DNA.[see comment]. Nature 421: 859–863.

Abraham, R. T. (2001) Cell cycle checkpoint signaling through the ATM and ATR kinases. Genes Dev 15: 2177–2196.

Allan, J. M., Engelward, B. P., Dreslin, A. J., Wyatt, M. D., Tomasz, M., and Samson, L. D. (1998) Mammalian 3-methyladenine DNA glycosylase protects against the toxicity and clastogenicity of certain chemotherapeutic DNA cross-linking agents. Cancer Res 58: 3965–3973.

Ame, J. C., Spenlehauer, C., and de Murcia, G. (2004) The PARP superfamily. Bioessays 26: 882–893.

Anda, T., Shabani, H. K., Tsunoda, K., Tokunaga, Y., Kaminogo, M., Shibata, S., Hayashi, T., and Iseki, M. (2003) Relationship between expression of O6-methylguanine-DNA methyltransferase, glutathione-S-transferase pi in glioblastoma and the survival of the patients treated with nimustine hydrochloride: an immunohistochemical analysis. Neurol Res 25: 241–248.

Bakkenist, C. J., and Kastan, M. B. (2003) DNA damage activates ATM through intermolecular autophosphorylation and dimer dissociation.[see comment]. Nature 421: 499–506.

Balana, C., Ramirez, J. L., Taron, M., Roussos, Y., Ariza, A., Ballester, R., Sarries, C., Mendez, P., Sanchez, J. J., and Rosell, R. (2003) O6-methyl-guanine-DNA methyltransferase methylation in serum and tumor DNA predicts response to 1,3-bis(2-chloroethyl)-1-nitrosourea but not to temozolamide plus cisplatin in glioblastoma multiforme. Clin Cancer Res 9: 1461–1468.

Belanich, M., Pastor, M., Randall, T., Guerra, D., Kibitel, J., Alas, L., Li, B., Citron, M., Wasserman, P., White, A., Eyre, H., Jaeckle, K., Schulman, S., Rector, D., Prados, M., Coons, S., Shapiro, W., and Yarosh, D. (1996) Retrospective study of the correlation between the DNA repair protein alkyltransferase and survival of brain tumor patients treated with carmustine. Cancer Res 56: 783–788.

Bjedov, I., Dasgupta, C. N., Slade, D., Le Blastier, S., Selva, M., and Matic, I. (2007) Involvement of Escherichia coli DNA polymerase IV in tolerance of cytotoxic alkylating DNA lesions in vivo. Genetics 176: 1431–1440.

Blough, M. D., Zlatescu, M. C., and Cairncross, J. G. (2007) O6-methylguanine-DNA methyltransferase regulation by p53 in astrocytic cells. Cancer Res 67: 580–584.

Bocangel, D. B., Finkelstein, S., Schold, S. C., Bhakat, K. K., Mitra, S., and Kokkinakis, D. M. (2002) Multifaceted resistance of gliomas to temozolomide. Clinical Cancer Res 8: 2725–2734.

Bonanno, K., Wyrzykowski, J., Chong, W., Matijasevic, Z., and Volkert, M. R. (2002) Alkylation resistance of E. coli cells expressing different isoforms of human alkyladenine DNA glycosylase (hAAG). DNA Repair 1: 507–516.

Brell, M., Tortosa, A., Verger, E., Gil, J. M., Vinolas, N., Villa, S., Acebes, J. J., Caral, L., Pujol, T., Ferrer, I., Ribalta, T., and Graus, F. (2005) Prognostic significance of O6-methylguanine-DNA methyltransferase determined by promoter hypermethylation and immunohistochemical expression in anaplastic gliomas. Clin Cancer Res 11: 5167–5174.

Burger, P., Scheithauer, B., and Vogel, F. (2002) Surgical Pathology of the Nervous System and Its Coverings Elsevier Science, Philadelphia.

Cahill, D. P., Levine, K. K., Betensky, R. A., Codd, P. J., Romany, C. A., Reavie, L. B., Batchelor, T. T., Futreal, P. A., Stratton, M. R., Curry, W. T., Iafrate, A. J., and Louis, D. N. (2007) Loss of the mismatch repair protein MSH6 in human glioblastomas is associated with tumor progression during temozolomide treatment. Clinical Cancer Res 13: 2038–2045.

Caldecott, K. W., McKeown, C. K., Tucker, J. D., Ljungquist, S., and Thompson, L. H. (1994) An interaction between the mammalian DNA repair protein XRCC1 and DNA ligase III. Mol Cell Biol 14: 68–76.

Caldecott, K. W., Tucker, J. D., Stanker, L. H., and Thompson, L. H. (1995) Characterization of the XRCC1-DNA ligase III complex in vitro and its absence from mutant hamster cells. Nucleic Acids Res 23: 4836–4843.

Chakravarti, A., Erkkinen, M. G., Nestler, U., Stupp, R., Mehta, M., Aldape, K., Gilbert, M. R., Black, P. M., and Loeffler, J. S. (2006) Temozolomide-mediated radiation enhancement in glioblastoma: a report on underlying mechanisms. Clinical Cancer Res 12: 4738–4746.

Chen, B. J., Carroll, P., and Samson, L. (1994) The *Escherichia coli* AlkB protein protects human cells against alkylation-induced toxicity. J Bact 176: 6255–6261.

Chen, C. C., Taniguchi, T., and D'Andrea, A. (2007) The Fanconi anemia (FA) pathway confers glioma resistance to DNA alkylating agents. J Mol Med 85: 497–509. Epub 2007 Jan 2013.

Christmann, M., Tomicic, M. T., Roos, W. P., and Kaina, B. (2003) Mechanisms of human DNA repair: an update. Toxicology 193: 3–34.

Curtin, N. J., Wang, L. Z., Yiakouvaki, A., Kyle, S., Arris, C. A., Canan-Koch, S., Webber, S. E., Durkacz, B. W., Calvert, H. A., Hostomsky, Z., and Newell, D. R. (2004) Novel poly (ADP-ribose) polymerase-1 inhibitor, AG14361, restores sensitivity to temozolomide in mismatch repair-deficient cells. Clinical Cancer Res 10: 881–889.

Darkes, M. J. M., Plosker, G. L., and Jarvis, B. (2002) Temozolomide: A review of its use in the treatment of malignant gliomas, malignant melanoma, and other advanced cancers. Am J Cancer 1: 55–80.

Demple, B., Herman, T., and Chen, D. S. (1991) Cloning and expression of APE, the cDNA encoding the major human apurinic endonuclease: definition of a family of DNA repair enzymes. Proc Natl Acad Sci USA 88: 11450–11454.

Denny, B. J., Wheelhouse, R. T., Stevens, M. F., Tsang, L. L., and Slack, J. A. (1994) NMR and molecular modeling investigation of the mechanism of activation of the antitumor drug temozolomide and its interaction with DNA. Biochemistry 33: 9045–9051.

Dinca, E. B., Lu, K. V., Sarkaria, J. N., Pieper, R. O., Prados, M. D., Haas-Kogan, D. A., Vandenberg, S. R., Berger, M. S., and James, C. D. (2008) p53 small molecule inhibitor enhances temozolomide cytotoxic activity against intracranial glioblastoma xenografts. Cancer Res 68(24): 10034–10038.

Dinglay, S., Trewick, S. C., Lindahl, T., and Sedgwick, B. (2000) Defective processing of methylated single-stranded DNA by E. coli AlkB mutants. Genes Dev 14: 2097–2105.

Drablos, F., Feyzi, E., Aas, P. A., Vaagbo, C. B., Kavli, B., Bratlie, M. S., Pena-Diaz, J., Otterlei, M., Slupphaug, G., and Krokan, H. E. (2004) Alkylation damage in DNA and RNA – repair mechanisms and medical significance. DNA Repair (Amst) 3: 1389–1407.

Duncan, T., Trewick, S. C., Koivisto, P., Bates, P. A., Lindahl, T., and Sedgwick, B. (2002) Reversal of DNA alkylation damage by two human dioxygenases. Proc Natl Acad Sci USA 99: 16660–16665.

Elleberger, T., and Tomkinson, A. E. (2008) Eukaryotic DNA ligases: structural and functional insights. Annu Rev Biochem 77: 313–338.

Engelward, B. P., Dreslin, A., Christensen, J., Huszar, D., Kurahara, C., and Samson, L. (1996) Repair-deficient 3-methyladenine DNA glycosylase homozygous mutant mouse cells have increased sensitivity to alkylation-induced chromosome damage and cell killing. EMBO J 15: 945–952.

Esteller, M. (2000) Epigenetic lesions causing genetic lesions in human cancer: promoter hypermethylation of DNA repair genes. Eur J Cancer 36: 2294–2300.

Friedberg, E. C., Graham, W. C., and Siede, W., eds. (1995). DNA Repair and Mutagenesis (Washington D. C.: American Society for Microbiology).

Friedberg, E. C., McDaniel, L. D., and Schultz, R. A. (2004) The role of endogenous and exogenous DNA damage and mutagenesis. Curr Opin Genet Dev 14: 5–10.

Friedman, H. S., Johnson, S. P., Dong, Q., Schold, S. C., Rasheed, B. K., Bigner, S. H., Ali-Osman, F., Dolan, E., Colvin, O. M., Houghton, P., Germain, G., Drummond, J. T., Keir, S., Marcelli, S., Bigner, D. D., and Modrich, P. (1997) Methylator resistance mediated by mismatch repair deficiency in a glioblastoma multiforme xenograft. Cancer Res 57: 2933–2936.

Fritz, G., Grosch, S., Tomicic, M., and Kaina, B. (2003) APE/Ref-1 and the mammalian response to genotoxic stress. Toxicology 193: 67–78.

Fritz, G., Tano, K., Mitra, S., and Kaina, B. (1991) Inducibility of the DNA repair gene encoding O6-methylguanine-DNA methyltransferase in mammalian cells by DNA-damaging treatments. Mol Cell Biol 11: 4660–4668.

Futscher, B. W., Micetich, K. C., Barnes, D. M., Fisher, R. I., and Erickson, L. C. (1989) Inhibition of a specific DNA repair system and nitrosourea cytotoxicity in resistant human cancer cells. Cancer Commun 1: 65–73.

Garcia-Higuera, I., Taniguchi, T., Ganesan, S., Meyn, M. S., Timmers, C., Hejna, J., Grompe, M., and D'Andrea, A. D. (2001) Interaction of the Fanconi anemia proteins and BRCA1 in a common pathway. Mol Cell 7: 249–262.

Gardiner-Garden, M., and Frommer, M. (1987) CpG islands in vertebrate genomes. J Mol Biol 196: 261–282.

Giese, A., Kucinski, T., Knopp, U., Goldbrunner, R., Hamel, W., Mehdorn, H. M., Tonn, J. C., Hilt, D., and Westphal, M. (2004) Pattern of recurrence following local chemotherapy with biodegradable carmustine (BCNU) implants in patients with glioblastoma. J Neurooncol 66: 351–360.

Glassner, B. J., Weeda, G., Allan, J. M., Broekhof, J. L., Carls, N. H., Donker, I., Engelward, B. P., Hampson, R. J., Hersmus, R., Hickman, M. J., Roth, R. B., Warren, H. B., Wu, M. M., Hoeijmakers, J. H., and Samson, L. D. (1999) DNA repair methyltransferase (Mgmt) knockout mice are sensitive to the lethal effects of chemotherapeutic alkylating agents. Mutagenesis 14: 339–347.

Grombacher, T., and Kaina, B. (1995) Constitutive expression and inducibility of O6-methylguanine-DNA methyltransferase and N-methylpurine-DNA glycosylase in rat liver cells exhibiting different status of differentiation. Biochimica et Biophysica Acta 1270: 63–72.

Grosch, S., Fritz, G., and Kaina, B. (1998) Apurinic endonuclease (Ref-1) is induced in mammalian cells by oxidative stress and involved in clastogenic adaptation. Cancer Res 58: 4410–4416.

Gunther, W., Pawlak, E., Damasceno, R., Arnold, H., and Terzis, A. J. (2003) Temozolomide induces apoptosis and senescence in glioma cells cultured as multicellular spheroids. Brit J Cancer 88: 463–469.

Haince, J. F., Rouleau, M., Hendzel, M. J., Masson, J. Y., and Poirier, G. G. (2005) Targeting poly(ADP-ribosyl)ation: a promising approach in cancer therapy. Trends Mol Med 11: 456–463.

Hansen, W. K., and Kelley, M. R. (2000) Review of mammalian DNA repair and translational implications. J Pharmacol Exp Ther 295: 1–9.

Hayashi, Y., Ueki, K., Waha, A., Wiestler, O. D., Louis, D. N., and von Deimling, A. (1997) Association of EGFR gene amplification and CDKN2 (p16/MTS1) gene deletion in glioblastoma multiforme. Brain Pathol 7: 871–875.

Hegi, M. E., Diserens, A. C., Godard, S., Dietrich, P. Y., Regli, L., Ostermann, S., Otten, P., Van Melle, G., de Tribolet, N., and Stupp, R. (2004) Clinical trial substantiates the predictive value of O-6-methylguanine-DNA methyltransferase promoter methylation in glioblastoma patients treated with temozolomide. Clin Cancer Res 10: 1871–1874.

Hegi, M. E., Diserens, A. C., Gorlia, T., Hamou, M. F., de Tribolet, N., Weller, M., Kros, J. M., Hainfellner, J. A., Mason, W., Mariani, L., Bromberg, J. E., Hau, P., Mirimanoff, R. O., Cairncross, J. G., Janzer, R. C., and Stupp, R. (2005) MGMT gene silencing and benefit from temozolomide in glioblastoma. N Engl J Med 352: 997–1003.

Herfarth, K. K., Brent, T. P., Danam, R. P., Remack, J. S., Kodner, I. J., Wells, S. A., Jr., and Goodfellow, P. J. (1999) A specific CpG methylation pattern of the MGMT promoter region associated with reduced MGMT expression in primary colorectal cancers. Mol Carcinog 24: 90–98.

Hirose, Y., Berger, M. S., and Pieper, R. O. (2001a) Abrogation of the Chk1-mediated G(2) checkpoint pathway potentiates temozolomide-induced toxicity in a p53-independent manner in human glioblastoma cells. Cancer Res 61: 5843–5849.

Hirose, Y., Berger, M. S., and Pieper, R. O. (2001b) p53 effects both the duration of G2/M arrest and the fate of temozolomide-treated human glioblastoma cells. Cancer Res 61: 1957–1963.

Hirose, Y., Katayama, M., Mirzoeva, O. K., Berger, M. S., and Pieper, R. O. (2005) Akt activation suppresses Chk2-mediated, methylating agent-induced G2 arrest and protects from temozolomide-induced mitotic catastrophe and cellular senescence. Cancer Res 65: 4861–4869.

Hirose, Y., Katayama, M., Stokoe, D., Haas-Kogan, D. A., Berger, M. S., and Pieper, R. O. (2003) The p38 mitogen-activated protein kinase pathway links the DNA mismatch repair system to the G2 checkpoint and to resistance to chemotherapeutic DNA-methylating agents. Mol Cell Biol 23: 8306–8315.

Horsfall, M. J., Gordon, A. J., Burns, P. A., Zielenska, M., van der Vliet, G. M., and Glickman, B. W. (1990) Mutational specificity of alkylating agents and the influence of DNA repair. Environ Mol Mutagen 15: 107–122.

Howlett, N. G., Taniguchi, T., Olson, S., Cox, B., Waisfisz, Q., De Die-Smulders, C., Persky, N., Grompe, M., Joenje, H., Pals, G., Ikeda, H., Fox, E. A., and D'Andrea, A. D. (2002) Biallelic inactivation of BRCA2 in Fanconi anemia. Science 297: 606–609.

Hunter, C., Smith, R., Cahill, D. P., Stephens, P., Stevens, C., Teague, J., Greenman, C., Edkins, S., Bignell, G., Davies, H., O'Meara, S., Parker, A., Avis, T., Barthorpe, S., Brackenbury, L., Buck, G., Butler, A., Clements, J., Cole, J., Dicks, E., Forbes, S., Gorton, M., Gray, K., Halliday, K., Harrison, R., Hills, K., Hinton, J., Jenkinson, A., Jones, D., Kosmidou, V., Laman, R., Lugg, R., Menzies, A., Perry, J., Petty, R., Raine, K., Richardson, D., Shepherd, R., Small, A., Solomon, H., Tofts, C., Varian, J., West, S., Widaa, S., Yates, A., Easton, D. F., Riggins, G., Roy, J. E., Levine, K. K., Mueller, W., Batchelor, T. T., Louis, D. N., Stratton, M. R., Futreal, P. A., and Wooster, R. (2006) A hypermutation phenotype and somatic MSH6 mutations in recurrent human malignant gliomas after alkylator chemotherapy. Cancer Res 66: 3987–3991.

Jacinto, F. V., and Esteller, M. (2007) Mutator pathways unleashed by epigenetic silencing in human cancer. Mutagenesis 22: 247–253. Epub 2007 Apr 2004.

Jaeckle, K. A., Eyre, H. J., Townsend, J. J., Schulman, S., Knudson, H. M., Belanich, M., Yarosh, D. B., Bearman, S. I., Giroux, D. J., and Schold, S. C. (1998) Correlation of tumor O6 methylguanine-DNA methyltransferase levels with survival of malignant astrocytoma patients treated with bis-chloroethylnitrosourea: a southwest oncology group study. J Clin Oncol 16: 3310–3315.

Jones, M., and Wagner, R. (1981) N-Methyl-N'-nitro-N-nitrosoguanidine sensitivity of E. coli mutants deficient in DNA methylation and mismatch repair. Mol Gen Genet 184: 562–563.

Kaina, B., Christmann, M., Naumann, S., and Roos, W. P. (2007) MGMT: key node in the battle against genotoxicity, carcinogenicity and apoptosis induced by alkylating agents. DNA Repair 6: 1079–1099.

Kamiryo, T., Tada, K., Shiraishi, S., Shinojima, N., Kochi, M., and Ushio, Y. (2004) Correlation between promoter hypermethylation of the O6-methylguanine-deoxyribonucleic acid methyltransferase gene and prognosis in patients with high-grade astrocytic tumors treated with surgery, radiotherapy, and 1-(4-amino-2-methyl-5-pyrimidinyl)methyl-3-(2-chloroethyl)-3-nitrosourea-based chemotherapy. Neurosurgery 54: 349–357; discussion 357.

Kanzawa, T., Germano, I. M., Komata, T., Ito, H., Kondo, Y., and Kondo, S. (2004) Role of autophagy in temozolomide-induced cytotoxicity for malignant glioma cells. Cell Death Differ 11: 448–457.

Karran, P., and Marinus, M. G. (1982) Mismatch correction at O6-methylguanine residues in E. coli DNA. Nature 296: 868–869.

Kataoka, H., Yamamoto, Y., and Sekiguchi, M. (1983) A new gene (alkb) of *Escherichia coli* that controls sensitivity to methyl methanesulfonate. J Bacteriol 153: 1301–1307.

Katayama, M., Kawaguchi, T., Berger, M. S., and Pieper, R. O. (2007) DNA damaging agent-induced autophagy produces a cytoprotective adenosine triphosphate surge in malignant glioma cells. Cell Death Differ 14: 548–558.

Kim, H. K., Lin, C. C., Parker, D., Veals, J., Lim, J., Likhari, P., Statkevich, P., Marco, A., and Nomeir, A. A. (1997) High-performance liquid chromatographic determination and stability of 5-(3-methyltriazen-1-yl)-imidazo-4-carboximide), the biologically active product of antitumor agent temozolomide, in human plasma. J Chromatogr B Biomed Sci Appl 703: 225–233.

Klungland, A., Fairbairn, L., Watson, A. J., Margison, G. P., and Seeberg, E. (1992) Expression of the *E.coli* 3-methyladenine DNA glycosylase I gene in mammalian cells reduces the toxic and mutagenic effects of methylating agents. EMBO J 11: 4439–4444.

Komine, C., Watanabe, T., Katayama, Y., Yoshino, A., Yokoyama, T., and Fukushima, T. (2003) Promoter hypermethylation of the DNA repair gene O6-methylguanine-DNA methyltransferase is an independent predictor of shortened progression free survival in patients with low-grade diffuse astrocytomas. Brain Pathol 13: 176–184.

Kondo, Y., Kanzawa, T., Sawaya, R., and Kondo, S. (2005) The role of autophagy in cancer development and response to therapy. Nat Rev Cancer 5: 726–734.

Krokan, H. E., Standal, R., and Slupphaug, G. (1997) DNA glycosylases in the base excision repair of DNA. Biochem J 325: 1–16.

Kunkel, T. A., and Erie, D. A. (2005) DNA mismatch repair. Annu Rev Biochem 74: 681–710.

Kurowski, M. A., Bhagwat, A. S., Papaj, G., and Bujnicki, J. M. (2003) Phylogenomic identification of five new human homologs of the DNA repair enzyme AlkB. BMC Genomics 4: 48.

Lage, H., and Dietel, M. (1999) Involvement of the DNA mismatch repair system in antineoplastic drug resistance. J Cancer Res Clin Oncol 125: 156–165.

Levine, A. J. (1997) p53, the cellular gatekeeper for growth and division. Cell 88: 323–331.

Levine, B., and Yuan, J. (2005) Autophagy in cell death: an innocent convict?[erratum appears in J Clin Invest. 2006 Dec;116(12):3293]. J Clin Invest 115: 2679–2688.

Lim, A., and Li, B. F. (1996) The nuclear targeting and nuclear retention properties of a human DNA repair protein O6-methylguanine-DNA methyltransferase are both required for its nuclear localization: the possible implications. EMBO J 15: 4050–4060.

Liu, L., Markowitz, S., and Gerson, S. L. (1996) Mismatch repair mutations override alkyltransferase in conferring resistance to temozolomide but not to 1,3-bis(2-chloroethyl)nitrosourea. Cancer Res 56: 5375–5379.

Masson, M., Niedergang, C., Schreiber, V., Muller, S., Menissier-de Murcia, J., and de Murcia, G. (1998) XRCC1 is specifically associated with poly(ADP-ribose) polymerase and negatively regulates its activity following DNA damage. Mol Cell Biol 18: 3563–3571.

Maxwell, J. A., Johnson, S. P., McLendon, R. E., Lister, D. W., Horne, K. S., Rasheed, A., Quinn, J. A., Ali-Osman, F., Friedman, A. H., Modrich, P. L., Bigner, D. D., and Friedman, H. S. (2008) Mismatch repair deficiency does not mediate clinical resistance to temozolomide in malignant glioma. Clin Cancer Res 1: 4859–4868.

Maxwell, J. A., Johnson, S. P., Quinn, J. A., McLendon, R. E., Ali-Osman, F., Friedman, A. H., Herndon, J. E., 2nd, Bierau, K., Bigley, J., Bigner, D. D., and Friedman, H. S. (2006) Quantitative analysis of O6-alkylguanine-DNA alkyltransferase in malignant glioma. Mol Cancer Ther 5: 2531–2539.

Medhurst, A. L., Huber, P. A., Waisfisz, Q., de Winter, J. P., and Mathew, C. G. (2001) Direct interactions of the five known Fanconi anaemia proteins suggest a common functional pathway. Hum Mol Genet 10: 423–429.

Ménissier de Murcia, J., Ricoul, M., Tartier, L., Niedergang, C., Huber, A., Dantzer, F., Schreiber, V., Amé, J. C., Dierich, A., LeMeur, M., Sabatier, L., Chambon, P., and de Murcia, G. (2003) Functional interaction between PARP-1 and PARP-2 in chromosome stability and embryonic development in mouse. EMBO J 22: 2255–2263.

Mikeska, T., Bock, C., El-Maarri, O., Hubner, A., Ehrentraut, D., Schramm, J., Felsberg, J., Kahl, P., Buttner, R., Pietsch, T., and Waha, A. (2007) Optimization of quantitative MGMT promoter methylation analysis using pyrosequencing and combined bisulfite restriction analysis. J Mol Diagn 9: 368–381.

Mizushima, N. (2004) Methods for monitoring autophagy. Int J Biochem Cell Biol 36: 2491–2502.

Mojas, N., Lopes, M., and Jiricny, J. (2007) Mismatch repair-dependent processing of methylation damage gives rise to persistent single-stranded gaps in newly replicated DNA. Gene Dev 21: 3342–3355.

Morgan, M. A., Chu, C. S., Benjamin, I., Randall, T. C., Boyd, J., and Rubin, S. C. (1999) Alterations in the expression of the DNA repair/redox enzyme APE/Ref-1 in epithelial ovarian cancers. Gyn Oncol 72: 520.

Mrugala, M. M., and Chamberlain, M. C. (2008) Mechanisms of disease: temozolomide and glioblastoma – look to the future. Nat Clin Pract Oncol 5: 476–486.

Mullapudi, S. R., Ali-Osman, F., Shou, J., and Srivenugopal, K. S. (2000) DNA repair protein O6-alkylguanine-DNA alkyltransferase is phosphorylated by two distinct and novel protein kinases in human brain tumour cells. Biochem J 351 Pt 2: 393–402.

Myers, L. C., Terranova, M. P., Nash, H. M., Markus, M. A., and Verdine, G. L. (1992) Zinc binding by the methylation signaling domain of the Escherichia coli Ada protein. Biochemistry 31: 4541–4547.

Newcomb, E. W., Bhalla, S. K., Parrish, C. L., Hayes, R. L., Cohen, H., and Miller, D. C. (1997) bcl-2 protein expression in astrocytomas in relation to patient survival and p53 gene status. Acta Neuropathol 94: 369–375.

Nowosielska, A., Smith, S. A., Engelward, B. P., and Marinus, M. G. (2006) Homologous recombination prevents methylation-induced toxicity in Escherichia coli. Nucleic Acids Res 34: 2258–2268.

O'Connor, T. R. (1993) Purification and characterization of human 3-methyladenine-DNA glycosylase. Nucleic Acids Res 21: 5561–5569.

Pace, P., Johnson, M., Tan, W. M., Mosedale, G., Sng, C., Hoatlin, M., de Winter, J., Joenje, H., Gergely, F., and Patel, K. J. (2002) FANCE: the link between Fanconi anaemia complex assembly and activity. EMBO J 21: 3414–3423.

Paz, M. F., Fraga, M. F., Avila, S., Guo, M., Pollan, M., Herman, J. G., and Esteller, M. (2003) A systematic profile of DNA methylation in human cancer cell lines. Cancer Res 63: 1114–1121.

Pendlebury, A., Frayling, I. M., Santibanez Koref, M. F., Margison, G. P., and Rafferty, J. A. (1994) Evidence for the simultaneous expression of alternatively spliced alkylpurine N-glycosylase transcripts in human tissues and cells. Carcinogenesis 15: 2957–2960.

Plant, J. E., and Roberts, J. J. (1971) A novel mechanism for the inhibition of DNA synthesis following methylation: the effect of N-methyl-N-nitrosourea on HeLa cells. Chem Biol Interact 3: 337–342.

Poirier, G. G., de Murcia, G., Jongstra-Bilen, J., Niedergang, C., and Mandel, P. (1982) Poly(ADP-ribosyl)ation of polynucleosomes causes relaxation of chromatin structure. Proc Natl Acad Sci USA 79: 3423–3427.

Potter, P. M., Kleibl, K., Cawkwell, L., and Margison, G. P. (1989) Expression of the ogt gene in wild-type and ada mutants of E. coli. Nucleic Acids Res 17: 8047–8060.

Potter, P. M., Wilkinson, M. C., Fitton, J., Carr, F. J., Brennand, J., Cooper, D. P., and Margison, G. P. (1987) Characterization and nucleotide sequence of ogt. Nucleic Acids Res 15: 9177–9193.

Preusser, M., Janzer, R. C., Felsberg, J., Reifenberger, G., Hamou, M. F., Diserens, A. C., Stupp, R., Gorlia, T., Marosi, C., Heinzl, H., Hainfellner, J. A., and Hegi, M. (2008) Anti-O6-Methylguanine-Methyltransferase (MGMT) Immunohistochemistry in glioblastoma multiforme: observer variability and lack of association with patient survival impede its use as clinical biomarker. Brain Pathol 8: 8.

Ramana, C. V., Boldogh, I., Izumi, T., and Mitra, S. (1998) Activation of apurinic/apyrimidinic endonuclease in human cells by reactive oxygen species and its correlation with their adaptive response to genotoxicity of free radicals. Proc Natl Acad Sci USA 95: 5061–5066.

Reardon, D. A., Rich, J. N., Friedman, H. S., and Bigner, D. D. (2006) Recent advances in the treatment of malignant astrocytoma. J Clin Oncol 24: 1253–1265.

Rebeck, G. W., Smith, C. M., Goad, D. L., and Samson, L. (1989) Characterization of the major DNA repair methyltransferase activity in unadapted Escherichia coli and identification of a similar activity in Salmonella typhimurium. J Bacteriol 171: 4563–4568.

Ringvoll, J., Moen, M. N., Nordstrand, L. M., Meira, L. B., Pang, B., Bekkelund, A., Dedon, P. C., Bjelland, S., Samson, L. D., Falnes, P. Ø., and Klungland, A. (2008) AlkB homologue 2-mediated repair of ethenoadenine lesions in mammalian DNA. Cancer Res 68: 4142–4149.

Ringvoll, J., Nordstrand, L. M., Vagbo, C. B., Talstad, V., Reite, K., Aas, P. A., Lauritzen, K. H., Liabakk, N. B., Bjork, A., Doughty, R. W., Falnes, P. O., Krokan, H. E., and Klungland, A. (2006) Repair deficient mice reveal mABH2 as the primary oxidative demethylase for repairing 1meA and 3meC lesions in DNA. EMBO J 25: 2189–2198.

Rodriguez, F. J., Thibodeau, S. N., Jenkins, R. B., Schowalter, K. V., Caron, B. L., O'Neill B, P., David James, C., Passe, S., Slezak, J., and Giannini, C. (2008) MGMT immunohistochemical expression and promoter methylation in human glioblastoma. Appl Immunohistochem Mol Morphol 16: 59–65.

Roth, R. B., and Samson, L. D. (2002) 3-Methyladenine DNA glycosylase-deficient Aag null mice display unexpected bone marrow alkylation resistance. Cancer Res 62: 656–660.

Ryan, A. J., Billett, M. A., and O'Connor, P. J. (1986) Selective repair of methylated purines in regions of chromatin DNA. Carcinogenesis 7: 1497–1503.

Sancar, A., and Sancar, G. B. (1998) DNA repair enzymes. Ann Rev Biochem 57: 29–62.

Sarkaria, J. N., Kitange, G. J., James, C. D., Plummer, R., Calvert, H., Weller, M., and Wick, W. (2008) Mechanisms of chemoresistance to alkylating agents in malignant glioma. Clinical Cancer Res 14: 2900–2908.

Sasai, K., Nodagashira, M., Nishihara, H., Aoyanagi, E., Wang, L., Katoh, M., Murata, J., Ozaki, Y., Ito, T., Fujimoto, S., Kaneko, S., Nagashima, K., and Tanaka, S. (2008) Careful exclusion of non-neoplastic brain components is required for an appropriate evaluation of O6-methylguanine-DNA methyltransferase status in glioma: relationship between immunohistochemistry and methylation analysis. Am J Surg Pathol 19: 19.

Schreiber, V., Ame, J. C., Dolle, P., Schultz, I., Rinaldi, B., Fraulob, V., De Murcia, J., and De Murcia, G. (2002) PARP-2 is required for efficient base excision DNA repair in association with PARP-1 and XRCC-1. J Biol Chem 277: 23028–23036.

Sedgwick, B., Bates, P. A., Paik, J., Jacobs, S. C., and Lindahl, T. (2007) Repair of alkylated DNA: recent advances. DNA Repair 6: 429–442.

Sedgwick, B., and Lindahl, T. (2002) Recent progress on the Ada response for inducible repair of DNA alkylation damage. Oncogene 21: 8886–8894.

Sedgwick, B., Robins, P., Totty, N., and Lindahl, T. (1988) Functional domains and methyl acceptor sites of the Escherichia coli ada protein. J Biol Chem 263: 4430–4433.

Seeberg, E., Eide, L., and Bjoras, M. (1995) The base excision repair pathway. Trends Biochem Sci 20: 391–397.

Shall, S., and De Murcia, G. (2000) Poly(ADP-ribose) polymerase-1: what have we learned from the deficient mouse model? Mutat Res 460: 1–15.

Shanabruch, W. G., Rein, R. P., Behlau, I., and Walker, G. C. (1983) Mutagenesis, by methylating and ethylating agents, in mutH, mutL, mutS, and uvrD mutants of Salmonella typhimurium LT2. J Bacteriol 153: 33–44.

Smith, D. G., and Brent, T. P. (1989) Response of cultured human cell lines from rhabdomyosarcoma xenografts to treatment with chloroethylnitrosoureas. Cancer Res 49: 883–886.

Sossou, M., Flohr-Beckhaus, C., Schulz, I., Daboussi, F., Epe, B., and Radicella, J. P. (2005) APE1 overexpression in XRCC1-deficient cells complements the defective repair of oxidative single strand breaks but increases genomic instability. Nucleic Acids Res 33: 298–306.

Srivenugopal, K. S., Mullapudi, S. R., Shou, J., Hazra, T. K., and Ali-Osman, F. (2000) Protein phosphorylation is a regulatory mechanism for O6-alkylguanine-DNA alkyltransferase in human brain tumor cells. Cancer Res 60: 282–287.

Srivenugopal, K. S., Yuan, X. H., Friedman, H. S., and Ali-Osman, F. (1996) Ubiquitination-dependent proteolysis of O6-methylguanine-DNA methyltransferase in human and murine tumor cells following inactivation with O6-benzylguanine or 1,3-bis(2-chloroethyl)-1-nitrosourea. Biochemistry 35: 1328–1334.

Steium, A., and Seeberg, E. (1986) Nucleotide sequence of the *tag* gene from *Escherichia coli.* Nucleic Acid Res 14: 3763–3772.

Stevens, M. F., Hickman, J. A., Stone, R., Gibson, N. W., Baig, G. U., Lunt, E., and Newton, C. G. (1984) Antitumor imidazotetrazines. 1. Synthesis and chemistry of 8-carbamoyl-3-(2-chloroethyl)imidazo[5,1-d]-1,2,3,5-tetrazin-4(3 H)-one , a novel broad-spectrum antitumor agent. J Med Chem 27: 196–201.

Stojic, L., Mojas, N., Cejka, P., Di Pietro, M., Ferrari, S., Marra, G., and Jiricny, J. (2004) Mismatch repair-dependent G2 checkpoint induced by low doses of SN1 type methylating agents requires the ATR kinase. Gene Dev 18: 1331–1344.

Stupp, R., Mason, W. P., van den Bent, M. J., Weller, M., Fisher, B., Taphoorn, M. J., Belanger, K., Brandes, A. A., Marosi, C., Bogdahn, U., Curschmann, J., Janzer, R. C.,

Ludwin, S. K., Gorlia, T., Allgeier, A., Lacombe, D., Cairncross, J. G., Eisenhauer, E., and Mirimanoff, R. O. (2005) Radiotherapy plus concomitant and adjuvant temozolomide for glioblastoma. N Engl J Med 352: 987–996.

Taniguchi, T., and D'Andrea, A. D. (2002) The Fanconi Anemia Protein, FANCE, Promotes the Nuclear Accumulation of FANCC. Blood prepublished online June 7.

Taniguchi, T., Garcia-Higuera, I., Xu, B., Andreassen, P. R., Gregory, R. C., Kim, S. T., Lane, W. S., Kastan, M. B., and D'Andrea, A. D. (2002) Convergence of the Fanconi anemia and ataxia telangiectasia signaling pathways. Cell 109: 459–472.

Tano, K., Shiota, S., Collier, J., Foote, R. S., and Mitra, S. (1990) Isolation and structural characterization of a cDNA clone encoding the human DNA repair protein for O6-alkylguanine.[erratum appears in Proc Natl Acad Sci USA 1990 Apr;87(8):3253]. Proc Natl Acad Sci USA 87: 686–690.

The Cancer Genome Atlas Research Network et al., (2008) Comprehensive genomic characterization defines human glioblastoma genes and core pathways. Nature [Epub ahead of print].

Trivedi, R. N., Almeida, K. H., Fornsaglio, J. L., Schamus, S., and Sobol, R. W. (2005) The role of base excision repair in the sensitivity and resistance to temozolomide-mediated cell death. Cancer Res 65: 6394–6400.

Tulin, A., Naumova, N. M., Menon, A. K., and Spradling, A. C. (2006) Drosophila poly (ADP-ribose) glycohydrolase mediates chromatin structure and SIR2-dependent silencing. Genetics 172: 363–371.

Turker, M. S. (2002) Gene silencing in mammalian cells and the spread of DNA methylation. Oncogene 21: 5388–5393.

Vickers, M. A., Vyas, P., Harris, P. C., Simmons, D. L., and Higgs, D. R. (1993) Structure of the human 3-methyladenine DNA glycosylase gene and localization close to the 16p telomere. Proc Natl Acad Sci USA 90: 3437–3441.

Wang, G., Weiss, C., Sheng, P., and Bresnick, E. (1996) Retrovirus-mediated transfer of the human O6-methylguanine-DNA methyltransferase gene into a murine hematopoietic stem cell line and resistance to the toxic effects of certain alkylating agents. Biochem Pharmacol 51: 1221–1228.

Wang, Y., and Qin, J. (2003) MSH2 and ATR form a signaling module and regulate two branches of the damage response to DNA methylation. Proc Natl Acad Sci USA 100: 15387–15392.

Watanabe, T., Katayama, Y., Komine, C., Yoshino, A., Ogino, A., Ohta, T., and Fukushima, T. (2005) O6-methylguanine-DNA methyltransferase methylation and TP53 mutation in malignant astrocytomas and their relationships with clinical course. Int J Cancer 113: 581–587.

Watts, G. S., Pieper, R. O., Costello, J. F., Peng, Y. M., Dalton, W. S., and Futscher, B. W. (1997) Methylation of discrete regions of the O6-methylguanine DNA methyltransferase (MGMT) CpG island is associated with heterochromatinization of the MGMT transcription start site and silencing of the gene. Mol Cell Biol 17: 5612–5619.

Wei, Y. F., Carter, K. C., Wang, R. P., and Shell, B. K. (1996) Molecular cloning and functional analysis of a human cDNA encoding an Escherichia coli AlkB homolog, a protein involved in DNA alkylation damage repair. Nucleic Acids Res 24: 931–937.

Wood, R. D., Mitchell, M., and Lindahl, T. (2005) Human DNA repair genes, 2005. Mutation Res 577: 275–283.

Wyatt, M. D., Allan, J. M., Lau, A. Y., Ellenberger, T. E., and Samson, L. D. (1999) 3-Methyladnine DNA glycosylases: structure, function, and biological importance. Bioassay 21: 668–676.

Xu, Y., Moore, D. H., Broshears, J., Liu, L., Wilson, T. M., and Kelley, M. R. (1997) The apurinic/apyrimidinic endonuclease (APE/Ref-1) DNA repair enzyme is elevated in pre-malignant and malignant cervical cancer. Anticancer Res 17: 3713–3719.

Chapter 29
Brain Tumor Stem Cell Markers

Jeremy N. Rich

Abstract Brain tumors display striking heterogeneity of cellular morphology and differentiation status. Recent studies have identified tumor subpopulations in several brain tumor types that self-renew and can propagate tumor formation in mice models. These cells, called tumor stem cells, are defined functionally but several markers are under investigation to identify brain tumor stem cells. Although no marker has proven absolutely informative for the identification of brain tumor stem cells, several markers show promise for either prospective enrichment of some populations of brain tumor stem cells or for their identification in immunohistologic studies. The use of stem cell markers must be approached with caution as the method of detection and context are essential in interpretation. Several studies have investigated the relationship between expression of stem cell markers and patient prognosis with variable findings. The information provided by tumor stem cell markers may depend on the subtypes of tumors generated from different tumor cells of origin or oncogenic stimuli. Future studies may refine the utility of stem cell markers to the study of cancer stem cells through the identification of improved or additional markers and/or new methodologies. It is imperative to realize that brain tumor stem cells remain defined through functional assays (self-renewal, multilineage differentiation, and tumor propagation) and the expression of any marker is not definitive for a tumor stem cell phenotype.

Contents

J.N. Rich (✉)
Department of Stem Cell Biology and Regenerative Medicine, Cleveland Clinic,
9500 Euclid Avenue, Mailstop NE30, Cleveland, OH 44195, USA
e-mail: richj@ccf.org

E.G. Van Meir (ed.), *CNS Cancer*, Cancer Drug Discovery and Development, DOI 10.1007/978-1-60327-553-8_29,
© Humana Press, a part of Springer Science+Business Media, LLC 2009

29.1 Introduction

Cancers are complex organ systems that are aberrantly regulated and are formed from neoplastic cells and associated vasculature, inflammatory cells, and recruited nonneoplastic cells (Reya et al. 2001). Within the neoplastic compartment, brain tumors exhibit cellular heterogeneity with differences in morphology and marker expression, suggesting a potential hierarchy in differentiation status. This cellular diversity is reflected in clinical observations in neuro-oncology. For example, noninvasive imaging of the tumor bulk poorly predicts overall survival. Brain tumors commonly do not globally recur but rather show nodular enhancement, suggesting growth from a small tumor cell population. The outgrowth of a selected set of tumor cells has been explained through two model systems: the classic stochastic model in which all tumor cells are equally likely to acquire further genetic changes creating an advantage in growth and a hierarchical model in which some tumor populations are less differentiated and are capable of generating the differentiated bulk of tumor cells. These models are likely nonexclusive and improved models may be created with elements of both systems. The hierarchical model of tumor growth supports the presence of tumor cells that reproduce characteristics of normal adult stem cells, which are long-lived and are functionally defined by their ability to self-renew (create at least one daughter cell, that is, an exact replica of the parental cell), sustain proliferation, and differentiate into relevant cellular identities. Tumor stem cells are tumor populations that share the ability to self-renew and propagate tumors. Radiation oncologists have appreciated the fact that not all neoplastic cells are equally sensitive to irradiation, so have defined tumor stem cells as cells capable of regenerating tumors after irradiation. More recently, seminal studies have demonstrated that rare cells within leukemias were capable of propagating tumors (Lapidot et al. 1994; Bonnet and Dick 1997). These approaches have been extended to several solid cancers, including several primary brain tumors, suggesting that cellular heterogeneity may be present in many (but not necessarily all) cancers with a hierarchy in tumor propagation potential and the presence of tumor stem cells (Al-Hajj et al. 2003; Ignatova et al. 2002; Hemmati et al. 2003; Singh et al. 2003; Galli et al. 2004; Singh et al. 2004; Yuan et al. 2004; Hope et al. 2004; Taylor et al. 2005; Li et al. 2007; O'Brien et al. 2007; Ricci-Vitiani et al. 2007; Dalerba et al. 2007). However, the tumor stem cell hypothesis is poorly understood and highly controversial. Not all tumors need to be driven by tumor stem cells and tumor stem cells need not be rare. In addition, a tumor stem cell does not imply a stem cell of origin but may have acquired similar capabilities as a stem or progenitor cell due to genetic and epigenetic alterations. Among the solid cancers, brain tumors have been witness to a large number of tumor stem cell studies that have delineated roles of tumor stem cells in therapeutic resistance, angiogenesis, and invasion/metastasis. Therefore, understanding tumor stem cells may hold benefit for brain tumor therapy.

29.2 Tumor Stem Cell Markers

Defining a tumor stem cell remains a central challenge in the field. As noted above, tumor stem cells are defined through functional assays of self-renewal and tumor propagation. The use of functional assays necessitates a retrospective identification of tumor stem cells. Unfortunately, this prevents direct comparison of tumor stem cells to the tumor bulk or nonstem tumor cells. To identify tumor stem cells, many groups have applied techniques pioneered in normal stem cell biology. Normal neural stem cells can grow as three-dimensional nonadherent multicellular structures (neurospheres) in growth factor-defined media. The repeated generation of neurospheres has been taken as evidence for self-renewal but caution must be exercised as the neurosphere assay is subject to significant artifact due to clumping of small cellular structures (Singec et al. 2006). Ultimately, in vivo tumor generation remains the gold standard and must be part of any tumor stem cell study. The use of functional assays presents difficulties in comparative analyses of tumor stem and nonstem cells necessitating the development of tumor stem cell markers that would permit to prospectively enrich for populations that fulfill the criteria for tumor stem cells. Preliminary studies have demonstrated modest success supporting the utility of markers that inform the selection of brain tumor cells that self-renew and propagate tumors. Broadly, two classes of markers are under development (Fig. 29.1). Cell surface markers can segregate viable tumor populations by flow cytometry or magnetic bead sorting that are enriched or depleted for tumor stem cells for further study. Intracellular markers have been identified that may also be informative of a tumor stem cell identity but are more challenging to use for viable cell studies, yet may be useful in genetic models, immunohistochemical studies, or in some enzymatic/function studies [e.g., aldehyde dehydrogenase 1 (ALDH1) or side population (SP)]. To date, no tumor stem cell marker has been absolutely informative. Not all marker-positive cells are tumor stem cells and not all tumor stem cells express tested stem cell markers. Therefore, the expression of a marker cannot be interpreted as proof of tumor stem cell identity.

Stem cell markers must be interpreted within specific contexts. The methodology employed to assay a marker must be approached with caution. The mRNA of a marker often does not correlate with the protein levels of the same

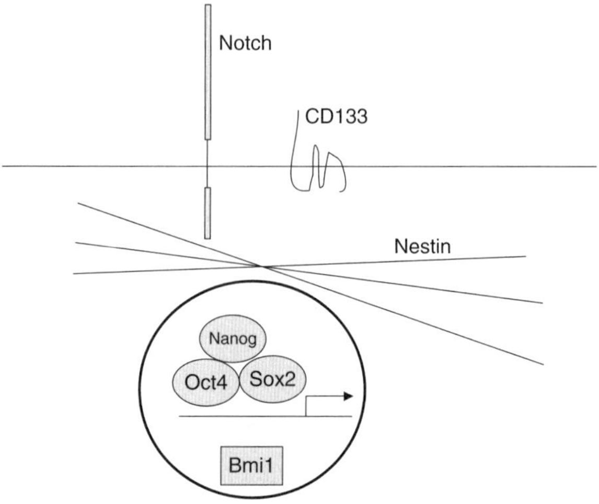

Fig. 29.1 Brain tumor stem cell markers. Notch receptors are cell surface proteins that may hold promise as brain tumor stem cell markers. CD133/Prominin-1 is a pentaspan transmembrane glycoprotein in most common use to prospectively segregate brain tumor stem cells. Nestin is an intermediate filament expressed by brain tumor stem cells. Sox2 is a transcription factor that binds with Octamer 4 (Oct4) and Nanog in a complex to regulate stem cell-related genes. Bmi1 is a chromatin regulator that may function as an oncogene. Not pictured: Musashi 1 (Mash1), an RNA-binding protein, and A2B5, a ganglioside antigen

gene product and the presentation of an antigen in flow cytometry requires additional post-translational modification and localization that may differ from denatured proteins on immunoblotting. The expression of a marker may also be highly variable within the same tumor type and may be altered upon changes in tumor grade or stage. Many stem cell markers are associated with polarized cells. Cells exhibit highly altered morphology when cultured outside of the native microenvironment, particularly when cultured on plastic. Therefore, a marker may be informative when used on uncultured cells from a tumor but may be uninformative with long-term cultured cells. To date, few standardized protocols are available, so marker-positive cells from one lab may be very different from those derived from other investigators. The application of tumor stem cell markers to clinical studies faces many of the same challenges of other biomarkers requiring analysis with carefully selected methods in appropriate patient and control cohorts. Some of the criticisms leveled against the cancer stem cell hypothesis are directed against weaknesses in tumor stem cell markers. Although great strides have been made in brain tumor stem cell biology, the currently available markers require additional study and new markers are required but early indications suggest that stem cell markers may have some utility in prognosis.

There are few validated markers and each may have strengths and weaknesses. We cannot separate a stem cell stage of differentiation from a more restricted progenitor stage at this time in the CNS, so it is likely that the current markers that are largely based on neural stem/progenitor markers may identify a mixed population of cells. The current diagnoses of brain tumors may contain subgroups represented by a diversity of tumor stem cells that may require the development of multiple tumor stem cell markers. Due to the limited state of our understanding, the discussion of brain tumor stem cell markers is by necessity brief.

29.3 Prominin-1/CD133

Prominin-1 [cluster of differentiation 133 (CD133)] is the most developed brain tumor stem cell marker. Prominin-1 is a pentaspan transmembrane glycoprotein located on cellular protrusions that was originally identified separately through the development of antibodies against the mouse neuroepithelium (Weigmann et al. 1997) and CD34^{bright} hematopoietic stem and progenitor cells derived from human fetal liver and bone marrow and blood (Yin et al. 1997; Miraglia et al. 1997). The function of prominin-1 is unknown but mutations in prominin-1 are detected in patients with familiar macular degeneration and disrupt photoreceptor disk morphogenesis in a genetic mouse model (Yang et al. 2008). These studies further showed that prominin-1 binds to protocadherin 21, a photoreceptor-specific cadherin, and actin filaments. A frameshift prominin-1 mutation that impairs proper photoreceptor localization was found in a pedigree with autosomal-recessive retinal degeneration (Maw et al. 2000). Prominin-1 is localized within the cell surface membrane in cholesterol-based lipid microdomains (lipid rafts) and may function in membrane topology (Röper et al. 2000). The expression of prominin-1 is controversial and may be dependent on the assay method. CD133 is expressed by embryonic neural stem cells (Uchida et al. 2000) but similar populations are not detected in the adult brain, although ependymal cells are CD133+ in the adult (Pfenninger et al. 2007). Clearly, CD133 is a useful marker for functional endothelial precursors (Peichev et al. 2000) in addition to the aforementioned stem/progenitor populations. Most studies have employed the AC133 antibodies that are directed against the glycosylated protein (Weigmann et al. 1997; Yin et al. 1997). However, another research group developed a different antiserum directed against recombinant prominin-1 (Florek et al. 2005). This antibody (αhE2) bound to a much broader spectrum of cells in normal tissues. A genetically engineered murine model in which the lacZ reporter was placed under the control of the CD133 promoter demonstrated that prominin-1/CD133 is expressed in non-stem cells as well as stem cells (Shmelkov et al. 2008). Other models under development may provide a more complex understanding of CD133 expression and, by extension, function in normal physiology. Another recent genetic model demonstrates CD133 expression in intestinal stem cells that are potential cells of origin for cancers (Zhu et al. 2009).

CD133 was found to be useful in enriching tumor-repopulating cells initially in leukemia (Horn et al. 1999; Bühring et al. 1999) and contains prognostic information (Lee et al. 2001). Based on its expression on neural stem/progenitor cells, CD133 was investigated in its utility as a brain tumor stem cell marker. In elegant studies first performed in vitro and then in vivo, brain tumor stem cells were exclusively detected in CD133+ cells from gliomas and medulloblastomas (Singh et al. 2003; Singh et al. 2004). In other studies, tumor-derived neurospheres from pediatric brain tumors also expressed CD133 in addition to other stem cell markers (Sox2, musashi-1, bmi-1, maternal embryonic leucine zipper kinase, and phosphoserine phosphatase) (Hemmati et al. 2003). Even in these earliest reports, investigators recognized variation between tumors in marker expression. CD133 is also informative in ependymomas in conjunction with other markers (nestin and BLBP) (Taylor et al. 2005). Many reports have confirmed the utility of CD133 in prospective isolation of brain tumor stem cells (Bao et al. 2006a; Bao et al. 2006b; Piccirillo et al. 2006; Calabrese et al. 2007; Bao et al. 2008) and CD133 has proven useful in a number of other solid cancers, including colorectal cancers (O'Brien et al. 2007; Ricci-Vitiani et al. 2007). However, challenges to the universal expression of CD133 have been raised and some tumors have tumor-propagating potential without significant numbers of CD133+ cells (Beier et al. 2007). Interestingly, in these studies primary glioblastomas had much higher levels of CD133+ cells than recurrent tumors. The difficulties posed by CD133 as a marker likely have multiple explanations. First, the AC133 reagents are challenging to use (Bidlingmaier et al. 2008). In flow cytometry assays, CD133+ peaks are not fully separated from isotype antibody control peaks in most tumor preparations. Without a clear separation, the delineation between CD133– and CD133+ populations poses challenges. In addition, the precise methodologies used to disaggregate tissues and purify cellular populations can have profound effects on CD133 fractions (Panchision et al. 2007). The culture conditions are critical to maintain appropriate tumor stem cell populations (Lee et al. 2006) but direct transfer to an in vivo environment may be optimal to preservation of a CD133+ tumor cell fraction (Shu et al. 2008). CD133 is a target of promoter methylation alterations in cancers (Tabu et al. 2008; Yi et al. 2008) and may be regulated during the cell cycle (Jaksch et al. 2008). It is almost certainly the case, however, that morphologically identical brain tumors have underlying complex cellular differences due to different cell of origin or oncogenic changes that are represented with different brain tumor stem cells that may express different marker immunophenotypes.

CD133 analysis has also been applied to immunohistochemical studies of brain tumor specimens. Not surprisingly, variability in these studies has also been noted, likely due to the combination of tumor heterogeneity and reagent specificity. Within tumors, CD133+ cells reside in a perivascular niche (Bao et al. 2006a; Calabrese et al. 2007; Christensen et al. 2008). Variability in the costaining for CD133 and proliferation markers has been noted (Christensen et al. 2008; Ma et al. 2008). Several studies have shown that CD133 informs prognosis (Zeppernick et al. 2008; Beier et al. 2008; Thon et al. 2008; Howard and Boockvar 2008) but some investigators have found that CD133 expression is not informative (Christensen et al. 2008). It is premature to consider CD133 as a validated prognostic indicator.

In conclusion, CD133 is undergoing an evolution in its use and limitations as a brain tumor stem cell marker but appears to be informative and useful when present in a tumor.

29.4 Nestin

Nestin is an intermediate filament protein expressed by neural stem cells (Lendahl et al. 1990; Reynolds and Weiss 1992). Shortly after nestin was recognized as a neural stem cell marker, studies demonstrated its expression in brain tumor cells (Valtz et al. 1991; Tohyama et al. 1992; Fults et al. 1992; Dahlstrand et al. 1992). Genetically engineered models have demonstrated that the expression of oncogenes under the control of the *Nestin* gene promoter can drive brain tumor formation (Holland et al. 1998; Holland et al. 2000). Activating Notch signaling that is active in brain tumor stem cells (Fan et al. 2006) increases nestin expression (Shih and Holland 2006). However, nestin is widely expressed in brain tumors including the proliferative endothelium of these cancers (Sugawara et al. 2002). The expression of nestin is highly variable but may correlate with tumor grade and sometimes survival (Dahlstrand et al. 1992; Almqvist et al. 2002; Ikota et al. 2006; Rani et al. 2006; Mao et al. 2007; Strojnik et al. 2007; Ma et al. 2008; Yang et al. 2008). Nestin + cells are also expressed at sites of glioma infiltration (Kong et al. 2008). As nestin is an intracellular protein, it is less useful in the prospective sorting of viable tumor cells outside of genetic models. Thus, nestin is an important marker but is not necessarily specific for brain tumor stem cells.

29.5 Bmi1

Bmi1 is a polycomb ring finger oncogene that regulates chromatin remodeling. Bmi1 was initially identified as target of viral integration in the E mu-myc transgenic mouse model (van Lohuizen et al. 1991). Bmi1 is recognized as a core stem cell regulator but its role in brain tumors is less clear. Bmi1 regulates normal cerebellar development and is overexpressed in human medulloblastoma biopsy specimens (Leung et al. 2004). Bmi1 is also expressed in astrocytomas (Tirabosco et al. 2008; Häyry et al. 2008b). Copy number alterations of the *BMI1* locus, located on the short arm of chromosome 10 (10p13) (Alkema et al. 1993), are frequently detected in gliomas (Nakahara et al. 2004; Häyry et al. 2008a, b). Bmi1 is expressed in brain tumor stem cells (Hemmati et al. 2003) and is required for tumor initiation in brain tumor models (Bruggeman et al. 2007). Although no studies have directly linked Bmi1 to prognosis in brain cancer patients, the Bmi1 gene signature is informative for survival in gliomas and medulloblastomas (Glinsky et al. 2005).

29.6 Musashi1

Musashi1 is a highly conserved RNA-binding protein expressed in neural stem/progenitors (Nakamura et al. 1994; Sakakibara et al. 1996; Kaneko et al. 2000). Musashi1 regulates mammary progenitor cell proliferation through regulation of the Wnt and Notch pathways through increased secretion of the PLF1 growth factor and inhibition of the secreted Wnt inhibitor, DKK3 (Wang et al. 2008). Musashi1 is expressed by brain tumor stem cells (Hemmati et al. 2003; Bao et al. 2006b; Thon et al. 2008). Musashi1 is expressed by gliomas (Strojnik et al. 2007; Ma et al. 2008; Kong et al. 2008) and medulloblastomas (Yokota et al. 2004). RNA interference against Musashi1 in the medulloblastoma cell line Daoy restricted proliferation and downregulated proliferation-related genes (Sanchez-Diaz et al. 2008).

29.7 Notch

The Notch signaling pathway is a highly conserved cell–cell communication pathway originally discovered due to the presence of notched wings in *Drosophila* mutants. There are four Notch proteins that are single pass receptors for the Delta and Serrate ligands. Upon binding of Notch with the appropriate ligands, two sequential cleavage events of the Notch protein are required for the intracellular domain of Notch to become liberated and regulate transcription. The second Notch cleavage event is catalyzed by gamma secretase. Notch signaling regulates neural stem cells (Androutsellis-Theotokis et al. 2006) and is expressed by gliomas (Purow et al. 2005; Phillips et al. 2006; Boulay et al. 2007), medulloblastomas (Yokota et al. 2004), and ependymomas (Modena et al. 2006). Notch is frequently expressed by brain tumor stem cells (Ignatova et al. 2002; Fan et al. 2006). Notch1 and Notch2 may play differential roles in tumor biology but the importance of each protein remains unclear. Gamma secretase inhibitors have been used to inhibit Notch activity and decrease brain tumor stem cell function both in culture and in vivo (Fan et al. 2006).

29.8 Sox2

SRY (sex determining region Y)-box 2 (Sox2) is a transcription factor that is essential in self-renewal of stem cells. Sox2 forms a transcription complex in stem cells with Oct4 and Nanog to regulate pluripotency (Wang et al. 2006). Sox2 has been recently recognized as a critical regulator of an induced pluripotent stem (iPS) cell state (Takahashi and Yamanaka 2006). Interestingly, neural stem cells express high levels of Sox2 at baseline and can undergo induced pluripotency without the addition of exogenous Sox2 (Kim et al. 2008). Sox2 is expressed by brain tumor stem cells (Hemmati et al. 2003; Bao et al. 2006b). Targeting Sox2 attenuates glioma stem cell proliferation (Gangemi et al. 2008).

29.9 A2B5

A2B5 is a ganglioside antigen presented on neural cell membranes (Eisenbarth et al. 1979). A2B5 binds to some central nervous system tumors (Coakham et al. 1985; Bodey et al. 1990). A2B5 appears to mark progenitor cells rather than neural stem cells (Abney et al. 1983; Raff et al. 1983). A recent report demonstrated that subsets of tumors display tumor propagation in a CD133-A2B5+ population, suggesting potentially a progenitor cell rather than stem cell origin (Ogden et al. 2008).

29.10 Other Potential Brain Tumor Stem Cell Markers

Self-renewal and embryonic stem cell gene expression signatures may be informative for brain tumors (Murat et al. 2008; Ben-Porath et al. 2008), suggesting that many new brain tumor stem cell markers may await discovery. Many other gene products are in early stages of investigation as brain tumor stem/transit amplifying cell markers, including MELK (Hemmati et al. 2003; Nakano et al. 2008), L1CAM (Bao et al. 2008), inhibitor of differentiation 4 (ID4) (Jeon et al. 2008), and IQGAP1 (Balenci et al. 2006). CD44 has been demonstrated to be useful as a tumor stem cell marker in other cancers (Al-Hajj et al. 2003) and is expressed in brain tumors (Kuppner et al. 1992; Li et al. 1993; Baltuch et al. 1995; Bouvier-Labit et al. 2002), so may be useful in brain tumor stem cell studies as well. Other neural stem cell markers, particularly CD15/stage-specific embryonic antigen-1 (SSEA-1)/Lewis x structure (Le^x), may be useful (Read et al. 2009). These markers await validation in larger studies.

29.11 Perspectives

The tumor stem cell field has largely advanced due to improved functional assays and identification of stem cell markers. Improved stem cell markers may permit a more reliable isolation and characterization of tumor stem cell populations. Cell surface markers have the advantage of utility in viable cell assays to segregate populations for more focused studies. The functional ALDH1 enzyme may permit additional assays but validation is required. Brain tumor stem cell markers will also need improvement to better determine in patients whether tumor stem cells are functionally important.

29.12 Conclusions

Several brain tumor stem cell markers are under investigation. The most prominent is CD133 but others may confer additional information. No single marker is likely to be definitive and all marker assays require validation with functional tumor stem cell assays. To date, the value of stem cell markers in brain tumor prognosis is unresolved but holds promise for the near future.

References

Abney ER, Williams BP, Raff MC (1983) Tracing the development of oligodendrocytes from precursor cells using monoclonal antibodies, fluorescence-activated cell sorting, and cell culture. Dev Biol 100:166–171

Al-Hajj M, Wicha MS, Benito-Hernandez A, Morrison SJ, Clarke MF (2003) Prospective identification of tumorigenic breast cancer cells. Proc Natl Acad Sci U S A 100:3983–3988

Alkema MJ, Wiegant J, Raap AK, Berns A, van Lohuizen M (1993) Characterization and chromosomal localization of the human proto-oncogene BMI-1. Hum Mol Genet 2:1597–1603

Almqvist PM, Mah R, Lendahl U, Jacobsson B, Hendson G (2002) Immunohistochemical detection of nestin in pediatric brain tumors. J Histochem Cytochem 50:147–158

Androutsellis-Theotokis A, Leker RR, Soldner F, Hoeppner DJ, Ravin R, Poser SW, Rueger MA, Bae SK, Kittappa R, McKay RD (2006) Notch signalling regulates stem cell numbers in vitro and in vivo. Nature 442:823–826

Balenci L, Clarke ID, Dirks PB, Assard N, Ducray F, Jouvet A, Belin MF, Honnorat J, Baudier J (2006) IQGAP1 protein specifies amplifying cancer cells in glioblastoma multiforme. Cancer Res 66:9074–9082

Baltuch G, de Tribolet N, Van Meir EG (1995) Expression of the CD44 adhesion molecule in tumours of the central and peripheral nervous system. J Neuro-Oncol 26:191–198

Bao S, Wu Q, Sathornsumetee S, Hao Y, Li Z, Hjelmeland AB, Shi Q, McLendon RE, Bigner DD, Rich JN (2006a) Stem cell-like glioma cells promote tumor angiogenesis through vascular endothelial growth factor. Cancer Res 66:7843–7848

Bao S, Wu Q, McLendon RE, Hao Y, Shi Q, Hjelmeland AB, Dewhirst MW, Bigner DD, Rich JN (2006b) Glioma stem cells promote radioresistance by preferential activation of the DNA damage response. Nature 444:756–760

Bao S, Wu Q, Li Z, Sathornsumetee S, Wang H, McLendon RE, Hjelmeland AB, Rich JN (2008) Targeting cancer stem cells through L1CAM suppresses glioma growth. Cancer Res 68:6043–6048

Beier D, Hau P, Proescholdt M, Lohmeier A, Wischhusen J, Oefner PJ, Aigner L, Brawanski A, Bogdahn U, Beier CP (2007) CD133(+) and CD133(-) glioblastoma-derived cancer stem cells show differential growth characteristics and molecular profiles. Cancer Res 67:4010–4015

Beier D, Wischhusen J, Dietmaier W, Hau P, Proescholdt M, Brawanski A, Bogdahn U, Beier CP (2008) CD133 expression and cancer stem cells predict prognosis in high-grade oligodendroglial tumors. Brain Pathol 18:370–377

Ben-Porath I, Thomson MW, Carey VJ, Ge R, Bell GW, Regev A, Weinberg RA (2008) An embryonic stem cell-like gene expression signature in poorly differentiated aggressive human tumors. Nat Genet 40:499–507

Bidlingmaier S, Zhu X, Liu B (2008) The utility and limitations of glycosylated human CD133 epitopes in defining cancer stem cells. J Mol Med 86:1025–1032

Bodey B, Zeltzer PM, Saldivar V, Kemshead J (1990) Immunophenotyping of childhood astrocytomas with a library of monoclonal antibodies. Int J Cancer 45:1079–1087

Bonnet D, Dick JE (1997) Human acute myeloid leukemia is organized as a hierarchy that originates from a primitive hematopoietic cell. Nature Med 3:730–737

Boulay JL, Miserez AR, Zweifel C, Sivasakaran B, Kana V, Ghaffari A, Luyken C, Sabel M, Zerrouqi A, Wasner M, Van Meir EG, Tolnay M, Reifenberger G Merlo A (2007) Loss of Notch2 positively predicts survival in distinct subgroups of human oligodendroglioma and glioblastoma PloS ONE 2:e576

Bouvier-Labit C, Liprandi A, Monti G, Pellissier JF, Figarella-Branger D (2002) CD44H is expressed by cells of the oligodendrocyte lineage and by oligodendrogliomas in humans. J Neurooncol 60:127–134

Bruggeman SW, Hulsman D, Tanger E, Buckle T, Blom M, Zevenhoven J, van Tellingen O, van Lohuizen M. (2007) Bmi1 controls tumor development in an Ink4a/Arf-independent manner in a mouse model for glioma. Cancer Cell 12:328–341

Bühring HJ, Seiffert M, Marxer A, Weiss B, Faul C, Kanz L, Brugger W (1999) AC133 antigen expression is not restricted to acute myeloid leukemia blasts but is also found on acute lymphoid leukemia blasts and on a subset of CD34+ B-cell precursors. Blood 94:832–833

Calabrese C, Poppleton H, Kocak M, Hogg TL, Fuller C, Hamner B, Oh EY, Gaber MW, Finklestein D, Allen M, Frank A, Bayazitov IT, Zakharenko SS, Gajjar A, Davidoff A, Gilbertson RJ (2007) A perivascular niche for brain tumor stem cells. Cancer Cell 11:69–82

Christensen K, Schrøder HD, Kristensen BW (2008) CD133 identifies perivascular niches in grade II-IV astrocytomas. J Neurooncol 90:157–170

Coakham HB, Garson JA, Allan PM, Harper EI, Brownell B, Kemshead JT, Lane EB (1985) Immunohistological diagnosis of central nervous system tumours using a monoclonal antibody panel. J Clin Pathol 38:165–173

Dahlstrand J, Collins VP, Lendahl U (1992) Expression of the class VI intermediate filament nestin in human central nervous system tumors. Cancer Res 52:5334–5341

Dalerba P, Dylla SJ, Park IK, Liu R, Wang X, Cho RW, Hoey T, Gurney A, Huang EH, Simeone DM, Shelton AA, Parmiani G, Castelli C, Clarke MF (2007) Phenotypic characterization of human colorectal cancer stem cells. Proc Natl Acad Sci U S A 104:10158–10163

Eisenbarth GS, Walsh FS, Nirenberg M (1979) Monoclonal antibody to a plasma membrane antigen of neurons. Proc Natl Acad Sci U S A 76:4913–4917

Fan X, Matsui W, Khaki L, Stearns D, Chun J, Li YM, Eberhart CG (2006) Notch pathway inhibition depletes stem-like cells and blocks engraftment in embryonal brain tumors. Cancer Res 66:7445–7452

Florek M, Haase M, Marzesco AM, Freund D, Ehninger G, Huttner WB, Corbeil D (2005) Prominin-1/CD133, a neural and hematopoietic stem cell marker, is expressed in adult human differentiated cells and certain types of kidney cancer. Cell Tissue Res 319:15–26

Fults D, Pedone CA, Morse HG, Rose JW, McKay RD (1992) Establishment and characterization of a human primitive neuroectodermal tumor cell line from the cerebral hemisphere. J Neuropathol Exp Neurol 51:272–280

Galli R, Binda E, Orfanelli U, Cipelletti B, Gritti A, De Vitis S, Fiocco R, Foroni C, Dimeco F, Vescovi A (2004) Isolation and characterization of tumorigenic, stem-like neural precursors from human glioblastoma. Cancer Res 64:7011–7021

Gangemi RM, Griffero F, Marubbi D, Perera M, Capra MC, Malatesta P, Ravetti GL, Zona GL, Daga A, Corte G (2008) SOX2 silencing in glioblastoma tumor initiating cells causes stop of proliferation and loss of tumorigenicity. Stem Cells [Epub ahead of print]

Glinsky GV, Berezovska O, Glinskii AB (2005) Microarray analysis identifies a death-from-cancer signature predicting therapy failure in patients with multiple types of cancer. J Clin Invest 115:1503–1521

Häyry V, Tanner M, Blom T, Tynninen O, Roselli A, Ollikainen M, Sariola H, Wartiovaara K, Nupponen NN (2008a) Copy number alterations of the polycomb gene BMI1 in gliomas. Acta Neuropathol 116:97–102

Häyry V, Tynninen O, Haapasalo HK, Wölfer J, Paulus W, Hasselblatt M, Sariola H, Paetau A, Sarna S, Niemelä M, Wartiovaara K, Nupponen NN (2008b) Stem cell protein BMI-1 is an independent marker for poor prognosis in oligodendroglial tumours. Neuropathol Appl Neurobiol 34:555–563

Hemmati HD, Nakano I, Lazareff JA, Masterman-Smith M, Geschwind DH, Bronner-Fraser M, Kornblum HI (2003) Cancerous stem cells can arise from pediatric brain tumors. Proc Natl Acad Sci U S A 100:15178–15183

Holland EC, Hively WP, DePinho RA, Varmus HE (1998) A constitutively active epidermal growth factor receptor cooperates with disruption of G1 cell-cycle arrest pathways to induce glioma-like lesions in mice. Genes Dev 12:3675–3685

Holland EC, Celestino J, Dai C, Schaefer L, Sawaya RE, Fuller GN (2000) Combined activation of Ras and Akt in neural progenitors induces glioblastoma formation in mice. Nat Genet 25:55–57

Hope KJ, Jin L, Dick JE (2004) Acute myeloid leukemia originates from a hierarchy of leukemic stem cell classes that differ in self-renewal capacity. Nat Immunol 5:738–743

Horn PA, Tesch H, Staib P, Kube D, Diehl V, Voliotis D (1999) Expression of AC133, a novel hematopoietic precursor antigen, on acute myeloid leukemia cells. Blood 93:1435–1437

Howard BM, Boockvar JA (2008) Stem Cell Marker CD133 Expression Predicts Outcome in Glioma Patients. Neurosurgery 62:N8

Ignatova TN, Kukekov VG, Laywell ED, Suslov ON, Vrionis FD, Steindler DA (2002) Human cortical glial tumors contain neural stem-like cells expressing astroglial and neuronal markers in vitro. Glia 39:193–206

Ikota H, Kinjo S, Yokoo H, Nakazato Y (2006) Systematic immunohistochemical profiling of 378 brain tumors with 37 antibodies using tissue microarray technology. Acta Neuropathol 111:475–482

Jaksch M, Múnera J, Bajpai R, Terskikh A, Oshima RG (2008) Cell cycle-dependent variation of a CD133 epitope in human embryonic stem cell, colon cancer, and melanoma cell lines. Cancer Res 68:7882–7886

Jeon HM, Jin X, Lee JS, Oh SY, Sohn YW, Park HJ, Joo KM, Park WY, Nam DH, DePinho RA, Chin L, Kim H (2008) Inhibitor of differentiation 4 drives brain tumor-initiating cell genesis through cyclin E and notch signaling. Genes Dev 22:2028–2033

Kaneko Y, Sakakibara S, Imai T, Suzuki A, Nakamura Y, Sawamoto K, Ogawa Y, Toyama Y, Miyata T, Okano H (2000) Musashi1: an evolutionally conserved marker for CNS progenitor cells including neural stem cells. Dev Neurosci 22:139–153

Kim JB, Zaehres H, Wu G, Gentile L, Ko K, Sebastiano V, Araúzo-Bravo MJ, Ruau D, Han DW, Zenke M, Schöler HR (2008) Pluripotent stem cells induced from adult neural stem cells by reprogramming with two factors. Nature 454:646–650

Kong DS, Kim MH, Park WY, Suh YL, Lee JI, Park K, Kim JH, Nam DH (2008) The progression of gliomas is associated with cancer stem cell phenotype. Oncol Rep 19:639–643

Kuppner MC, Van Meir EG, Gauthier T, Hamou MF, de Tribolet N (1992) Differential expression of the CD44 molecule in human brain tumors. Int J Cancer 50: 572–577

Lapidot T, Sirard C, Vormoor J, Murdoch B, Hoang T, Caceres-Cortes J, Minden M, Paterson B, Caligiuri MA, Dick JE (1994) A cell initiating human acute myeloid leukaemia after transplantation into SCID mice. Nature 367:645–648

Lee J, Kotliarova S, Kotliarov Y, Li A, Su Q, Donin NM, Pastorino S, Purow BW, Christopher N, Zhang W, Park JK, Fine HA (2006) Tumor stem cells derived from glioblastomas cultured in bFGF and EGF more closely mirror the phenotype and genotype of primary tumors than do serum-cultured cell lines. Cancer Cell 9:391–403

Lee ST, Jang JH, Min YH, Hahn JS, Ko YW (2001) AC133 antigen as a prognostic factor in acute leukemia. Leuk Res 25:757–767

Lendahl U, Zimmerman LB, McKay RD (1990) CNS stem cells express a new class of intermediate filament protein. Cell 60:585–595

Leung C, Lingbeek M, Shakhova O, Liu J, Tanger E, Saremaslani P, Van Lohuizen M, Marino S (2004) Bmi1 is essential for cerebellar development and is overexpressed in human medulloblastomas. Nature 428:337–341

Li C, Heidt DG, Dalerba P, Burant CF, Zhang L, Adsay V, Wicha M, Clarke MF, Simeone DM (2007) Identification of pancreatic cancer stem cells. Cancer Res 67:1030–1037

Li H, Hamou M-F, de Tribolet N, Jaufeerally R, Hofmann M, Diserens A-C, Van Meir EG (1993) Variant CD44 adhesion molecules are expressed in human brain metastases but not in glioblastomas. Cancer Res 53:5345–5349

Ma YH, Mentlein R, Knerlich F, Kruse ML, Mehdorn HM, Held-Feindt J (2008) Expression of stem cell markers in human astrocytomas of different WHO grades. J Neurooncol 86:31–45

Mao Y, Zhou L, Zhu W, Wang X, Yang G, Xie L, Mao X, Jin K (2007) Proliferative status of tumor stem cells may be correlated with malignancy grade of human astrocytomas. Front Biosci 12:2252–2259

Maw MA, Corbeil D, Koch J, Hellwig A, Wilson-Wheeler JC, Bridges RJ, Kumaramanickavel G, John S, Nancarrow D, Röper K, Weigmann A, Huttner WB, Denton MJ (2000) A frameshift mutation in prominin (mouse)-like 1 causes human retinal degeneration. Hum Mol Genet 9:27–34

Miraglia S, Godfrey W, Yin AH, Atkins K, Warnke R, Holden JT, Bray RA, Waller EK, Buck DW (1997) A novel five-transmembrane hematopoietic stem cell antigen: isolation, characterization, and molecular cloning. Blood 90:5013–5021

Modena P, Lualdi E, Facchinetti F, Veltman J, Reid JF, Minardi S, Janssen I, Giangaspero F, Forni M, Finocchiaro G, Genitori L, Giordano F, Riccardi R, Schoenmakers EF, Massimino M, Sozzi G (2006) Identification of tumor-specific molecular signatures in intracranial ependymoma and association with clinical characteristics. J Clin Oncol 24:5223–5233

Murat A, Migliavacca E, Gorlia T, Lambiv WL, Shay T, Hamou MF, de Tribolet N, Regli L, Wick W, Kouwenhoven MC, Hainfellner JA, Heppner FL, Dietrich PY, Zimmer Y, Cairncross JG, Janzer RC, Domany E, Delorenzi M, Stupp R, Hegi ME (2008) Stem cell-related "self-renewal" signature and high epidermal growth factor receptor expression associated with resistance to concomitant chemoradiotherapy in glioblastoma. J Clin Oncol 26:3015–3024

Nakahara Y, Shiraishi T, Okamoto H, Mineta T, Oishi T, Sasaki K, Tabuchi K (2004) Detrended fluctuation analysis of genome-wide copy number profiles of glioblastomas using array-based comparative genomic hybridization. Neuro Oncol 6:281–289

Nakamura M, Okano H, Blendy JA, Montell C (1994) Musashi, a neural RNA-binding protein required for Drosophila adult external sensory organ development. Neuron 13:67–81

Nakano I, Masterman-Smith M, Saigusa K, Paucar AA, Horvath S, Shoemaker L, Watanabe M, Negro A, Bajpai R, Howes A, Lelievre V, Waschek JA, Lazareff JA, Freije WA, Liau LM, Gilbertson RJ, Cloughesy TF, Geschwind DH, Nelson SF, Mischel PS, Terskikh AV, Kornblum HI (2008) Maternal embryonic leucine zipper kinase is a key regulator of the proliferation of malignant brain tumors, including brain tumor stem cells. J Neurosci Res 86:48–60

O'Brien CA, Pollett A, Gallinger S, Dick JE (2007) A human colon cancer cell capable of initiating tumour growth in immunodeficient mice. Nature 445:106–110

Ogden AT, Waziri AE, Lochhead RA, Fusco D, Lopez K, Ellis JA, Kang J, Assanah M, McKhann GM, Sisti MB, McCormick PC, Canoll P, Bruce JN (2008) Identification of A2B5 + CD133- tumor-initiating cells in adult human gliomas. Neurosurgery 62:505–514

Panchision DM, Chen HL, Pistollato F, Papini D, Ni HT, Hawley TS (2007) Optimized flow cytometric analysis of central nervous system tissue reveals novel functional relationships among cells expressing CD133, CD15, and CD24. Stem Cells 25:1560–1570

Peichev M, Naiyer AJ, Pereira D, Zhu Z, Lane WJ, Williams M, Oz MC, Hicklin DJ, Witte L, Moore MA, Rafii S (2000) Expression of VEGFR-2 and AC133 by circulating human

CD34(+) cells identifies a population of functional endothelial precursors. Blood 95:952–958
Pfenninger CV, Roschupkina T, Hertwig F, Kottwitz D, Englund E, Bengzon J, Jacobsen SE, Nuber UA (2007) CD133 is not present on neurogenic astrocytes in the adult subventricular zone, but on embryonic neural stem cells, ependymal cells, and glioblastoma cells. Cancer Res 67:5727–5736
Phillips HS, Kharbanda S, Chen R, Forrest WF, Soriano RH, Wu TD, Misra A, Nigro JM, Colman H, Soroceanu L, Williams PM, Modrusan Z, Feuerstein BG, Aldape K (2006) Molecular subclasses of high-grade glioma predict prognosis, delineate a pattern of disease progression, and resemble stages in neurogenesis. Cancer Cell 9:157–173
Piccirillo SG, Reynolds BA, Zanetti N, Lamorte G, Binda E, Broggi G, Brem H, Olivi A, Dimeco F, Vescovi AL (2006) Bone morphogenetic proteins inhibit the tumorigenic potential of human brain tumour-initiating cells. Nature 444:761–765
Purow BW, Haque RM, Noel MW, Su Q, Burdick MJ, Lee J, Sundaresan T, Pastorino S, Park JK, Mikolaenko I, Maric D, Eberhart CG, Fine HA (2005) Expression of Notch-1 and its ligands, Delta-like-1 and Jagged-1, is critical for glioma cell survival and proliferation. Cancer Res 65:2353–2363
Raff MC, Abney ER, Cohen J, Lindsay R, Noble M (1983) Two types of astrocytes in cultures of developing rat white matter: differences in morphology, surface gangliosides, and growth characteristics. J Neurosci 3:1289–1300
Rani SB, Mahadevan A, Anilkumar SR, Raju TR, Shankar SK. (2006) Expression of nestin – a stem cell associated intermediate filament in human CNS tumours. Indian J Med Res 124:269–280
Read TA, Fogarty MP, Markant SL, McLendon RE, Wei Z, Ellison DW, Febbo PG, Wechsler-Reya RJ (2009) Identification of CD15 as a marker for tumor-propagating cells in a mouse model of medulloblastoma. Cancer Cell 15:135–147
Reya T, Morrison SJ, Clarke MF, Weissman IL (2001) Stem cells, cancer, and cancer stem cells. Nature 414:105–111
Reynolds BA, Weiss S (1992) Generation of neurons and astrocytes from isolated cells of the adult mammalian central nervous system. Science 255:1707–1710
Ricci-Vitiani L, Lombardi DG, Pilozzi E, Biffoni M, Todaro M, Peschle C, De Maria R (2007) Identification and expansion of human colon-cancer initiating cells. Nature 445:111–115
Röper K, Corbeil D, Huttner WB (2000) Retention of prominin in microvilli reveals distinct cholesterol-based lipid micro-domains in the apical plasma membrane. Nat Cell Biol 2:582–592
Sakakibara S, Imai T, Hamaguchi K, Okabe M, Aruga J, Nakajima K, Yasutomi D, Nagata T, Kurihara Y, Uesugi S, Miyata T, Ogawa M, Mikoshiba K, Okano H (1996) Mouse-Musashi-1, a neural RNA-binding protein highly enriched in the mammalian CNS stem cell. Dev Biol 176:230–242
Sanchez-Diaz PC, Burton TL, Burns SC, Hung JY, Penalva LO (2008) Musashi1 modulates cell proliferation genes in the medulloblastoma cell line Daoy. BMC Cancer 8:280
Shih AH, Holland EC (2006) Notch signaling enhances nestin expression in gliomas. Neoplasia 8:1072–1082
Shmelkov SV, Butler JM, Hooper AT, Hormigo A, Kushner J, Milde T, St Clair R, Baljevic M, White I, Jin DK, Chadburn A, Murphy AJ, Valenzuela DM, Gale NW, Thurston G, Yancopoulos GD, D'Angelica M, Kemeny N, Lyden D, Rafii S (2008) CD133 expression is not restricted to stem cells, and both CD133+ and CD133- metastic colon cancer cells initiate tumours. J Clin Invest 118:2111–2120
Shu Q, Wong KK, Su JM, Adesina AM, Yu LT, Tsang YT, Antalffy BC, Baxter P, Perlaky L, Yang J, Dauser RC, Chintagumpala M, Blaney SM, Lau CC, Li XN (2008) Direct orthotopic transplantation of fresh surgical specimen preserves CD133+ tumor cells in

clinically relevant mouse models of medulloblastoma and glioma. Stem Cells 26:1414–1424

Singec I, Knoth R, Meyer RP , Maciaczyk J, Volk B, Nikkhah G, Frotscher M, Synder EY (2006) Defining the actual sensitivity and specificity of the neurosphere assay in stem cell biology. Nat Methods 3:801–806

Singh SK, Clarke ID, Terasaki M, Bonn VE, Hawkins C, Squire J, Dirks PB (2003) Identification of a cancer stem cell in human brain tumors. Cancer Res 63:5821–5828

Singh SK, Hawkins C, Clarke ID, Squire JA, Bayani J, Hide T, Henkelman RM, Cusimano MD, Dirks PB (2004) Identification of human brain tumour initiating cells. Nature 432:396–401

Strojnik T, Røsland GV, Sakariassen PO, Kavalar R, Lah T (2007) Neural stem cell markers, nestin and musashi proteins, in the progression of human glioma: correlation of nestin with prognosis of patient survival. Surg Neurol 68:133–143

Sugawara K, Kurihara H, Negishi M, Saito N, Nakazato Y, Sasaki T, Takeuchi T (2002) Nestin as a marker for proliferative endothelium in gliomas. Lab Invest 82:345–351

Tabu K, Sasai K, Kimura T, Wang L, Aoyanagi E, Kohsaka S, Tanino M, Nishihara H, Tanaka S (2008) Promoter hypomethylation regulates CD133 expression in human gliomas. Cell Res 18:1037–1046

Takahashi K, Yamanaka S (2006) Induction of pluripotent stem cells from mouse embryonic and adult fibroblast cultures by defined factors. Cell 126:663–676

Taylor MD, Poppleton H, Fuller C, Su X, Liu Y, Jensen P, Magdaleno S, Dalton J, Calabrese C, Board J, Macdonald T, Rutka J, Guha A, Gajjar A, Curran T, Gilbertson RJ (2005) Radial glia cells are candidate stem cells of ependymoma. Cancer Cell 8:323–335

Thon N, Damianoff K, Hegermann J, Grau S, Krebs B, Schnell O, Tonn JC, Goldbrunner R (2008) Presence of pluripotent CD133(+) cells correlates with malignancy of gliomas. Mol Cell Neurosci [Epub ahead of print]

Tirabosco R, De Maglio G, Skrap M, Falconieri G, Pizzolitto S (2008) Expression of the Polycomb-Group protein BMI1 and correlation with p16 in astrocytomas an immunohistochemical study on 80 cases. Pathol Res Pract 204:625–631

Tohyama T, Lee VM, Rorke LB, Marvin M, McKay RD, Trojanowski JQ (1992) Nestin expression in embryonic human neuroepithelium and in human neuroepithelial tumor cells. Lab Invest 66:303–313

Uchida N, Buck DW, He D, Reitsma MJ, Masek M, Phan TV, Tsukamoto AS, Gage FH, Weissman IL (2000) Direct isolation of human central nervous system stem cells. Proc Natl Acad Sci U S A 97:14720–14725

Valtz NL, Hayes TE, Norregaard T, Liu SM, McKay RD (1991) An embryonic origin for medulloblastoma. New Biol. 3:364–371.

van Lohuizen M, Verbeek S, Scheijen B, Wientjens E, van der Gulden H, Berns A (1991) Identification of cooperating oncogenes in E mu-myc transgenic mice by provirus tagging. Cell 65:737–752

Wang J, Rao S, Chu J, Shen X, Levasseur DN, Theunissen TW, Orkin SH (2006) A protein interaction network for pluripotency of embryonic stem cells. Nature 444:364–368

Wang XY, Yin Y, Yuan H, Sakamaki T, Okano H, Glazer RI (2008) Musashi1 modulates mammary progenitor cell expansion through proliferin-mediated activation of the Wnt and Notch pathways. Mol Cell Biol 28:3589–3599

Weigmann A, Corbeil D, Hellwig A, Huttner WB (1997) Prominin, a novel microvilli-specific polytopic membrane protein of the apical surface of epithelial cells, is targeted to plasmalemmal protrusions of non-epithelial cells. Proc Natl Acad Sci U S A 94:12425–12430

Yang XH, Wu QL, Yu XB, Xu CX, Ma BF, Zhang XM, Li SN, Lahn BT, Xiang AP (2008) Nestin expression in different tumours and its relevance to malignant grade. J Clin Pathol 61:467–473

Yang Z, Chen Y, Lillo C, Chien J, Yu Z, Michaelides M, Klein M, Howes KA, Li Y, Kaminoh Y, Chen H, Zhao C, Chen Y, Al-Sheikh YT, Karan G, Corbeil D, Escher P, Kamaya S, Li C,

Johnson S, Frederick JM, Zhao Y, Wang C, Cameron DJ, Huttner WB, Schorderet DF, Munier FL, Moore AT, Birch DG, Baehr W, Hunt DM, Williams DS, Zhang K (2008) Mutant prominin 1 found in patients with macular degeneration disrupts photoreceptor disk morphogenesis in mice. J Clin Invest 118:2908–2916

Yi JM, Tsai HC, Glöckner SC, Lin S, Ohm JE, Easwaran H, James CD, Costello JF, Riggins G, Eberhart CG, Laterra J, Vescovi AL, Ahuja N, Herman JG, Schuebel KE, Baylin SB (2008) Abnormal DNA methylation of CD133 in colorectal and glioblastoma tumors. Cancer Res 68:8094–8103

Yin AH, Miraglia S, Zanjani ED, Almeida-Porada G, Ogawa M, Leary AG, Olweus J, Kearney J, Buck DW (1997) AC133, a novel marker for human hematopoietic stem and progenitor cells. Blood 90:5002–5012

Yokota N, Mainprize TG, Taylor MD, Kohata T, Loreto M, Ueda S, Dura W, Grajkowska W, Kuo JS, Rutka JT (2004) Identification of differentially expressed and developmentally regulated genes in medulloblastoma using suppression subtraction hybridization. Oncogene 23:3444–3453

Yuan X, Curtin J, Xiong Y, Liu G, Waschsmann-Hogiu S, Farkas DL, Black KL, Yu JS (2004) Isolation of cancer stem cells from adult glioblastoma multiforme. Oncogene 23:9392–9400

Zeppernick F, Ahmadi R, Campos B, Dictus C, Helmke BM, Becker N, Lichter P, Unterberg A, Radlwimmer B, Herold-Mende CC (2008) Stem cell marker CD133 affects clinical outcome in glioma patients. Clin Cancer Res 14:123–129

Zhu L, Gibson P, Currle DS, Tong Y, Richardson RJ, Bayazitov IT, Poppleton H, Zakharenko S, Ellison DW, Gilbertson RJ (2009) Prominin 1 marks intestinal stem cells that are susceptible to neoplastic transformation. Nature 457:603–607

Part III
Therapeutic Targets and Targeting Approaches

Chapter 30
Clinical Agents for the Targeting of Brain Tumor Vasculature

Elizabeth R. Gerstner and Tracy T. Batchelor

Abstract Glioblastomas are characterized by a robust, abnormal vascular network that leads to heterogeneous blood flow. Some tumor areas receive adequate flow, while others become hypoxic from poor flow. Radiation and chemotherapy require sufficient oxygenation to be maximally effective, so hypoxia decreases tumor response to therapy. Vascular endothelial growth factor (VEGF), predominately through its receptor VEGFR-2, interacts with a variety of intracellular signaling pathways to promote this abnormal tumor angiogenesis and permits glioblastoma growth. Consequently, a variety of drugs that target the VEGF pathway are being tested in clinical trials with promising results. The precise role of these agents in glioblastoma treatment needs to be optimized but likely will entail combating peritumoral edema, inducing vascular normalization, and destroying the cancer stem cell niche. Unfortunately, most patients treated with anti-VEGF agents eventually relapse and potential mechanisms of tumor escape such as upregulation of alternate angiogenesis pathways are actively being studied. Anti-VEGF agents have clearly prolonged progression-free survival in recurrent glioblastoma patients and have been a significant addition to our drug armamentarium for many patients while at the same time providing important clues into underlying tumor physiology.

Contents

T. Batchelor (✉)
Executive Director, Stephen E. and Catherine Pappas Center for Neuro-Oncology, Yawkey 9E, Massachusetts General Hospital Cancer Center, 55 Fruit Street, Boston, MA 02114, USA
e-mail: tbatchelor@partners.org

E.G. Van Meir (ed.), *CNS Cancer*, Cancer Drug Discovery and Development, DOI 10.1007/978-1-60327-553-8_30,
© Humana Press, a part of Springer Science+Business Media, LLC 2009

30.1 Introduction

Glioblastoma (GBM) is the most common type of malignant primary brain tumor. There are approximately 10,000 GBMs diagnosed each year in the United States and the 5-year survival rate is under 10%. Current treatment for patients with GBM entails maximal safe resection, focal, fractionated radiation with concurrent temozolomide, an oral alkylating chemotherapeutic agent, followed by 6–12 monthly cycles of post-radiation temozolomide. Despite this treatment, the median survival is only 15 months (Stupp et al. 2005, 2009). Because of this poor prognosis, new therapeutic options are desperately needed. Current research efforts have begun to exploit the fact that GBMs are highly vascularized tumors. Consequently, agents that target the tumor vascular network are increasingly being explored in clinical trials with encouraging results.

30.2 Angiogenesis in Gliomas

Angiogenesis in GBM involves complicated interactions between glioma cells, stromal cells, and endothelial cells. A detailed review of glioma angiogenesis is beyond the scope of this chapter, so we will focus on the VEGF signaling pathway which appears to promote the majority of new blood vessel formation in GBMs (see Chapter 21) (Jain et al. 2007).

Growing tumors eventually reach a point at which the existing blood supply is no longer adequate and areas within the tumor become hypoxic leading to cell death and necrosis (see Chapter 22). In response to hypoxia, GBMs undergo an "angiogenic switch" and increase secretion of various growth factors to promote new blood vessel formation. VEGF appears to play a critical role in this process and GBMs have a 50-fold greater expression of VEGF than lower grade astrocytomas which are not characterized by robust angiogenesis (Plate et al. 1992). Low oxygen levels increase the stability of hypoxia-inducible factor-1 (HIF-1) which binds to the *VEGF* gene promoter to increase VEGF mRNA transcription (Forsythe et al. 1996, Jensen et al. 2006). Elevated HIF-1 and VEGF correlate with advanced tumor grade and HIF-1 inhibition leads to inhibition of VEGF secretion (Jensen et al. 2006).

Signaling of VEGF through its tyrosine kinase receptors VEGFR-1 and R-2 on endothelial cells is mediated by a variety of intracellular pathways including PTEN/pI3-kinase/Akt (Gomez-Manzano et al. 2003), MAPK/ERK (Yoshino et al. 2006), and nitric oxide (Saino et al. 2004). VEGFR-2 is considered the critical receptor associated with cancer-related angiogenesis. In addition, VEGF upregulates Notch-Deltalike ligand 4 (DLL4) expression in tumor vasculature (Kerbel 2008). The DLL4 pathway has been recognized as an important mediator of tumor-related angiogenesis although the precise role of DLL4 in angiogenesis is unclear. Both VEGFR-1 and R-2 and the downstream molecules in the VEGF signaling pathway represent possible points of therapeutic intervention (Table 30.1

Table 30.1 Anti-VEGF agents

Drug	Mechanism	Most advanced phase	Results
Antibodies			
Bevacizumab	VEGF antibody	Phase II*	*Bevacizumab alone*: 35.1 % APF6 *Bevacizumab + irinotecan*: 50.2% APF6 (Cloughesy et al. 2008)
Aflibercept	VEGF-A & -B, PlGF "receptor body"	Phase II	30% response rate (De Groot et al. 2008)
Small-molecule inhibitors			
Cediranib	VEGFR-1/-2/-3, c-kit, PDGFR-α/β inhibitor, weak FGFR-1, EGFR inhibitor	Phase II*	25.8% APF6 (Batchelor et al. 2007)
Vatalanib	VEGFR-1/-2/-3, PDGFR-β, c-kit inhibitor	Phase II	33/47 patients with PR/SD (Conrad et al. 2004)
Sunitinib	VEGFR-2, PDGFR, c-kit inhibitor	Phase II	Ongoing
XL184	VEGFR-2, c-met, Tie-2, c-kit inhibitor	Phase II	Ongoing
Pazopanib	VEGFR-1/-2/-3, PDGFR-α/β, c-kit inhibitor	Phase I/II	Ongoing
AEE788	VEGFR-1/-2, EGFR inhibitor	Phase I/II	Results pending
Sorafenib	VEGFR-2/-3, PDGFR-β, Flt-3, Raf inhibitor	Phase I/II	Ongoing
Vandetanib	VEGFR-1/-2, EGFR, Ret kinases inhibitor	Phase I/II	Ongoing
SU6668	VEGFR-2, FGFR, PDGFR, c-kit inhibitor	Phase I	Ongoing
AAL881	VEGFR-2, Raf inhibitor	Preclinical	

VEGF, vascular endothelial growth factor; VEGFR, vascular endothelial growth factor receptor; PlGF, placental growth factor; EGFR, epidermal growth factor receptor; PDGFR, platelet-derived growth factor receptor; FGFR, fibroblast growth factor receptor. *Phase III to open soon (2008–2009).

and Fig. 30.1). In principle, inhibiting VEGF-induced angiogenesis should selectively target actively dividing tumor endothelial cells because normal brain endothelial cells rarely participate in active angiogenesis, making this pathway an attractive target.

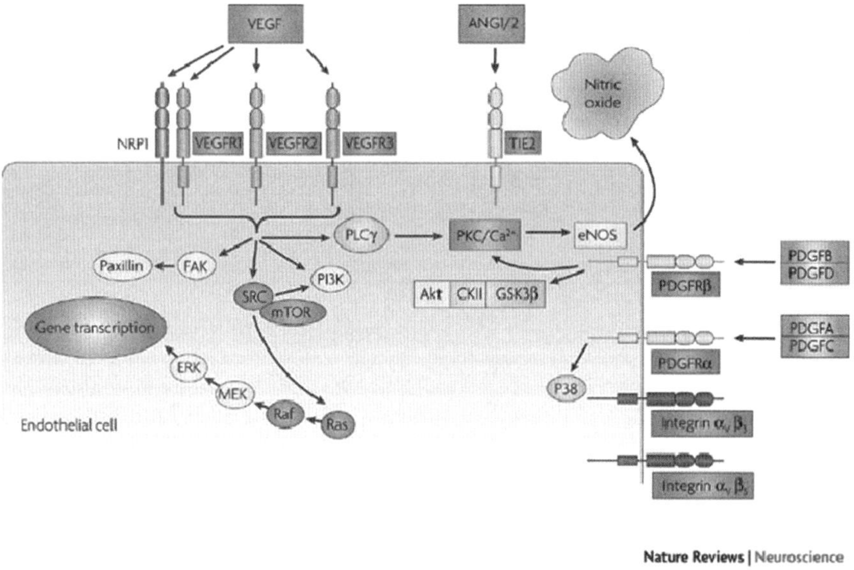

Fig. 30.1 Simplified brain tumor angiogenesis pathway and potential points of intervention. VEGF is targeted by bevacizumab, whereas tyrosine kinase inhibitors such as cediranib target mainly VEGF receptors 1–3 (VEGFR-1–3), TIE2 (as well as TIE1, which interacts with TIE2), and platelet-derived growth factor receptors α and β (PDGFR-α and PDGFR-). Agents targeting other pathways, such as inhibitors of mammalian target of rapamycin (mTOR) (e.g., temsirolimus), Src, or integrins (such as αvβ3 and αvβ5), are also in clinical development for brain tumors. ANG1/2, angiopoietin 1/2; CKII, casein kinase II; eNOS, endothelial nitric oxide synthase; ERK, extracellular signal-regulated kinase; FAK, focal adhesion kinase 1; GSK3β, glycogen synthase kinase-3β; MEK, mitogen-activated protein kinase ERK kinase; NRP1, neuropilin 1; PI3K, phosphatidylinositol-3 kinase; PKC, protein kinase C; PLCγ, phospholipase-Cγ. Reprinted with permission from *Angiogenesis in brain tumors*. NRN 2007;8:610–22

Several other growth factors interact with the VEGF pathway to promote the growth and survival of tumor and endothelial cells through stimulation of alternate tyrosine kinase receptors (TKR). Platelet-derived growth factor-B (PDGF-B) (Brockmann et al. 2003, Tsai et al. 1995), epidermal growth factor (EGF) (Goldman et al. 1993, Mellinghoff et al. 2005), tumor necrosis factor-α (TNF-α) (Ryuto et al. 1996), and basic fibroblast growth factor (bFGF) (Morrison et al. 1990, Tsai et al. 1995) can all upregulate expression of VEGF in gliomas. The angiopoietins, Ang-1 and Ang-2, have a complicated interaction with VEGF through their TKRs, Tie1 and Tie2. In the presence of VEGF, Ang-2 promotes vessel sprouting but in the absence of VEGF, Ang-2 causes vessel regression (Reiss et al. 2005). In addition, other proangiogenic peptides independent of VEGF are upregulated in gliomas. For example, IL-8 is strongly expressed in areas of GBM hypoxia (e.g., around pseudopallisading necrosis) and may contribute to glioma angiogenesis through modulation of NFκB (Brat et al. 2005, Desbaillets et al. 1997, Garkavtsev et al. 2004). Consequently, effective tumor control will ultimately require targeting more than just VEGF and its receptor.

Preventing angiogenesis is hypothesized to arrest tumor growth through several mechanisms. The traditional notion is that antiangiogenic agents prevent new blood vessel formation and prune the existing tumor vessels leading to tumor deprivation of oxygen and nutrients (Folkman 2007). Vascular normalization is another potential mechanism by which antiangiogenic agents may achieve an antitumor effect when combined with other cytotoxic therapies. Glioblastoma vessels are highly abnormal and are characterized by enlarged vessel diameter, increased permeability, lack of adequate pericyte coverage, and abnormally thickened basement membranes. Often, lumen diameter is decreased and there is evidence for vascular degeneration and thrombosis (see Chapter 22). A number of antiangiogenic agents have been shown to normalize this abnormal vascular network associated with GBMs (see Chapter 21) (Jain et al. 2006, Kragh et al. 2002, Tenan et al. 2000, Winkler et al. 2004). The vessel abnormalities enumerated above may prevent effective delivery of chemotherapeutic agents to tumor cells and also contribute to the abnormal hypoxic tumor microenvironment that accounts for some of the intrinsic resistance of these tumors to cytotoxic therapies (Brat et al. 2004, Jain et al. 2005). As opposed to pruning or destroying blood vessels, vascular normalization induces structural and functional changes in the abnormal tumor vasculature that transforms these vessels to a more “normal” morphological state. Through normalization, anti-VEGF agents may improve the efficacy of chemotherapy by facilitating the delivery of cytotoxic drugs to the tumor and by diminishing tumor hypoxia (Jain et al. 2005). Finally, another possible mechanism of action of antiangiogenic drugs is disruption of the perivascular niche of cancer stem cells. GBM stem cells, the self-renewable cells thought to give rise to gliomas, exist in a stem cell–vascular niche that allows these cells to remain in a self-renewing state (Calabrese et al. 2007). Antiangiogenic agents may disrupt the critical interaction between these GBM stem cells and endothelial cells, thus contributing to their death.

30.3 Antibodies to Growth Factors/Receptors

Antibodies have the advantage of being highly specific for their target so that there is little cross reactivity and fewer “off-target” side effects. The half-life of an antibody is generally long allowing for less frequent dosing. Conversely, antibodies are costly to produce and must be administered by intravenous infusion. Moreover, antibodies are large molecular weight protein molecules with limited penetration of the normal blood–brain barrier (BBB). However, when targeting endothelial cells that line tumor blood vessels or in the setting of a disrupted BBB, this may be less of an impediment.

30.3.1 Bevacizumab (Avastin)

Bevacizumab, a recombinant, humanized monoclonal antibody to VEGF with a half-life of approximately 20 days, is being studied in patients with GBM with encouraging preliminary results. Bevacizumab inhibits VEGFR-mediated cell signaling by sequestration of its ligand VEGF-A (commonly referred to as VEGF). VEGF-A is the best characterized VEGF isoform and likely the most important for brain tumor angiogenesis. The role of the other isoforms, VEGF-B, -C, and -D, has not been fully characterized. A phase II study of 35 patients with recurrent GBM treated with bevacizumab and irinotecan, a cytotoxic chemotherapeutic that inhibits topoisomerase I, demonstrated promising results. Forty-six percent of patients were alive and progression-free at 6 months (APF6), a commonly used metric in recurrent malignant glioma studies, and median progression-free survival was 24 weeks (Vredenburgh et al. 2007a, b). Median overall survival was 42 weeks. This compares favorably to a historical database of various phase II studies in recurrent GBM in which the median APF6 was 15% (Wong et al. 1999). High VEGF expression in the original tumor tissue correlated with radiographic response, while high expression of carbonic anhydrase 9 (CA9), a marker of hypoxia and acidosis, was correlated with reduced survival (Sathornsumetee et al. 2008a, b).

A subsequent randomized phase II trial of patients with recurrent GBM confirmed the impact on APF6. One hundred and sixty-seven patients were randomized to bevacizumab alone (85 patients) or bevacizumab concomitantly with irinotecan (82 patients) (Cloughesy et al. 2008). Because of the possible normalizing effects on tumor vasculature, bevacizumab in combination with irinotecan (a cytotoxic agent) was postulated to be more effective than bevacizumab alone (Friedman et al. 1999). The APF6 was 35.1% in the bevacizumab alone arm and 50.2% in the combination therapy arm but there was significant overlap in the confidence intervals. Median overall survival was 9.7 months in the bevacizumab arm and 8.9 months in the combination arm with more frequent Grade 3 toxicity in the bevacizumab and irinotecan arm (67% versus 48%). Consequently, it is unclear whether or not there is a significant advantage to combining bevacizumab with irinotecan over bevacizumab alone considering the increased rate of toxicity observed in the combination arm and the similar median overall survival between the two arms of the study. Alternate drug combinations with bevacizumab such as erlotinib, an EGFR tyrosine kinase inhibitor, and etoposide are being explored in patients with recurrent GBM (Rich et al. 2008). In addition, bevacizumab is being studied in combination with temozolomide and radiation in newly diagnosed GBM patients and this regimen was determined to be relatively safe in a small pilot study (Lai et al. 2008).

30.3.2 Aflibercept (VEGF-Trap)

Aflibercept is a recombinant human chimeric fusion protein that contains segments of the extracellular domain of human VEGFR-1 and R-2 fused with the constant region (Fc) of human IgG1. The protein blocks two VEGF subtypes, VEGF-A and VEGF-B, as well as placental growth factor (PlGF), another ligand for VEGFR-Z. It has a higher affinity for VEGF than bevacizumab, a half-life of approximately 25 days, and works by sequestering extracellular VEGF and preventing its interaction with VEGFRs (Holash et al. 2002). Preliminary data from a phase II trial of aflibercept in recurrent malignant glioma patients demonstrated a 30% radiographic response rate in the GBM subset (14 patients with stable disease, 8 patients with a partial response) (De Groot et al. 2008). Twelve patients (25%) had to terminate treatment due to toxicity; one patient had CNS ischemia and one patient had a systemic hemorrhage. In a mouse xenograft model, aflibercept combined with radiation was shown to be more effective than radiation alone, suggesting that it might be beneficial in combination with radiation and temozolomide in newly diagnosed GBM patients, so a trial is planned in this patient population (Wachsberger et al. 2007).

30.4 Tyrosine Kinase Inhibitors

Small molecule tyrosine kinase inhibitors (TKIs) interfere with tyrosine or serine/threonine kinase growth factor receptor signaling by attaching to the intracellular ATP-binding pocket of the receptor. These agents have the advantage of being orally active. Most of the agents in this class lack specificity for one TKR, thus allowing for broad inhibition of a variety of growth factor pathways, albeit at the risk of increasing potential side effects.

30.4.1 Cediranib (Recentin)

Cediranib is a TKI that blocks all VEGFRs (-1/-2/-3), c-kit, and PDGFR-α/β. It is administered orally and has a half-life of 12.5–35.4 hours, so it can be administered once daily. In a phase II study of 30 patients with recurrent GBM treated with cediranib alone, the radiographic response proportion was 56%, median PFS was 117 days, and the overall survival was 231 days (Batchelor et al. 2007). In this study, the APF6 was 25.8% which compares favorably to historical controls. Application of a number of MRI techniques in this study led to the observation that cediranib transiently normalizes the glioblastoma vascular network as measured by significant reduction in tumor vessel diameter and permeability. This was the first study to identify a "normalization window" secondary to anti-VEGF therapy in human cancer patients. A consequence of reduced vascular permeability in these patients was reduction of vasogenic cerebral edema, a cause of major morbidity in this patient population. The antiedema effect of cediranib also resulted in a steroid-sparing effect in this population with most subjects able to reduce or discontinue corticosteroids that had been previously prescribed for vasogenic cerebral edema. A randomized phase III trial of cediranib versus cediranib with lomustine, an oral alkylating agent that has been a standard therapeutic in the GBM population, is ongoing. In addition, a phase Ib/II trial of cediranib in patients with newly diagnosed GBM in combination with radiation and temozolomide is underway.

30.4.2 Vatalanib

Vatalanib (PTK787) is a pan-VEGFR, PDGFR, and c-kit inhibitor with a short half-life that requires twice a day dosing (Wood et al. 2000). Preclinical studies using C6 glioma cell lines that expressed VEGF demonstrated that vatalanib treatment leads to smaller tumor volumes and increased necrosis (Goldbrunner et al. 2004). In a phase I/II trial of 47 patients with recurrent GBM treated with vatalanib alone, 2 patients had a partial response and 31 patients had stable disease as measured by MRI (Conrad et al. 2004). The drug was well tolerated with dose limiting toxicities observed only in patients taking $\geq$1000 mg daily. Vatalanib has also been studied in combination with other drugs. In a phase I/II trial of 51 recurrent GBM patients treated with vatalanib and lomustine or temozolomide, 4 subjects had a partial response (3 with vatalanib + temozolomide, 1 with vatalanib + lomustine) and 27 had stable disease (19 with vatalanib + temozolomide, 8 with vatalanib + lomustine) (Reardon et al. 2004). The median time to progression was 15.7 weeks for these patients. In another study, 8 of 37 patients with recurrent GBM had a partial response when treated with imatanib, hydroxyurea, and vatalanib (Kirkpatrick et al. 2008). Imatinib is a PDGFR inhibitor and hydroxyurea induces double-strand DNA breaks, so the combination was thought to affect multiple tumor targets. Since temozolomide has now become standard of care for newly diagnosed GBM, vatalanib is being studied in combination with this alkylating drug as well. However, Novartis, the manufacturer of this drug, has halted further develop of vatalanib.

30.4.3 Other TKIs

There are several broader spectrum TKIs that target VEGFRs currently under study in the GBM patient population (Table 30.1). Sorafenib has a wide spectrum of targets in tumor cells including VEGFR-1/-2, PDGFR-β, c-kit, bRAF, and RAF1 kinases. It was determined to be safe in a phase I trial of patients with recurrent malignant glioma (Nabors et al. 2007). A phase I/II study exploring sorafenib in combination with temsirolimus (an mTOR inhibitor) or erlotinib (an EGFR inhibitor) is ongoing.

Vandetanib (ZD6474) inhibits VEGFR-1/-2, EGFR, and Ret kinases. In preclinical glioma mouse models, vandetanib prolonged survival, decreased tumor growth, decreased VEGF secretion, and disrupted tumor vascularity (Rich et al. 2005, Sandstrom et al. 2004). Clinical studies of vandetanib in the GBM patient population are ongoing.

AEE788 is a combined inhibitor of EGFR and VEGFR-1/-2 which inhibited VEGFR-driven angiogenesis in preclinical models (Traxler et al. 2004). In one such mouse model of glioma, AEE788 was shown to decrease tumor growth and to increase median survival when used in combination with an mTOR inhibitor (RAD001) (Goudar et al. 2005). A phase I/II trial in recurrent GBM patients has been completed with acceptable toxicity but the final results have not been published (Reardon et al. 2005).

30.5 Resistance to Anti-VEGF Therapy

Although anti-VEGF therapies have been associated with prolonged progression-free and overall survival in several clinical trials in glioma patients, the tumors eventually relapse in most cases. In addition, there appears to be a subset of patients who do not respond at all to anti-VEGF therapy. It is possible that these latter patients have a tumor that is not dependent on VEGF for angiogenesis or growth. The former patients who initially respond but then relapse have likely developed escape mechanisms to bypass VEGF inhibition. Hypothesized escape mechanisms include upregulation of alternate proangiogenic pathways, improved protection of tumor neovasculature by increasing pericyte coverage, increased invasiveness of tumor cells that co-opt native brain blood vessels, and increased metastatic seeding at distant sites (more typical with systemic cancer) (Bergers and Hanahan 2008). Support for these mechanisms has predominately come from preclinical models. In one clinical study, patients with recurrent GBM who relapsed after treatment with cediranib had elevated stromal-derived growth factor 1 (SDF1α), bFGF, and tie-2, all of which have been implicated in alternate angiogenesis pathways (Batchelor et al. 2007).

30.6 Toxicities of Anti-VEGF Agents

Agents that target the VEGF pathway have several uncommon but serious complications (Table 30.2) (Verheul and Pinedo 2007). Hypertension has been a notable side effect because VEGF blocks nitric oxide and prostacyclin synthesis, impairs baroreceptor response, and perturbs endothelial cell function. Many patients, particularly those with borderline hypertension, require

Table 30.2 Anti-VEGF agent toxicities

Toxicity	Possible mechanism
Bleeding	Platelet dysfunction
Impaired wound healing	
Thrombotic events	EC apoptosis, platelet activation
Hypertension	Blockade of NO and prostacyclins, decreased capillary density, impaired baroreceptor response
Proteinuria	Podocyte dysfunction in kidney glomeruli
Rash	Epidermal cell apoptosis, EC dysfunction
Hand–foot syndrome	
GI perforation	Mucosal cell apoptosis, EC dysfunction
Hypothyroidism	Decreased thyroid vascularity
Fatigue	Hypothyroidism

EC, endothelial cell; NO, nitric oxide; GI, gastrointestinal.

treatment with antihypertensive agents. Both arterial and venous thrombosis as well as hemorrhage have been reported a concern in the GBM patient population which is already at risk for intratumoral hemorrhage and deep vein thrombosis. Reassuringly, though, intracerebral hemorrhage has been reported in only a small percentage of GBM patients treated with anti-VEGF therapy in studies to date. Poor wound healing because of angiogenic blockade has been observed and is a particular worry in patients who have recently undergone craniotomy for resection of their tumor. Bowel perforation has also been rarely reported.

30.7 VEGF-Inhibitors as Anti-edema Therapies

Malignant gliomas are often associated with a significant amount of vasogenic edema requiring chronic corticosteroid use. Unfortunately, this often leads to steroid-related toxicity such as osteoporosis, weight gain, insomnia, and psychiatric effects, all of which decrease quality of life in these patients. Vasogenic edema is the result of over secretion of VEGF leading to disruption of the BBB and increased vascular permeability. Vascular permeability permits the influx of macromolecules and fluid into brain tissue, resulting in vasogenic edema and elevated interstitial fluid pressure (Korfman et al. 1957). By blocking VEGF, anti-VEGF agents restore the integrity of the BBB and decrease vasogenic edema. Vatalanib, cediranib, and bevacizumab have all been shown to decrease vasogenic edema as measured by serial MRI scans (Batchelor et al. 2007, Conrad et al. 2004, Drevs et al. 2002, Gonzalez et al. 2007, Pope et al. 2006).

The antipermeability effect of anti-VEGF therapies may be beneficial in a related condition associated with elevated vessel permeability – cerebral radiation necrosis. Radiation necrosis occurs several months to years after therapeutic doses of radiation and is thought to be caused by endothelial cell damage and the release of VEGF. Patients with cerebral radiation necrosis develop progressive vasogenic brain edema and typically require long-term corticosteroid use to control swelling. Bevacizumab was shown to ameliorate radiation necrosis in eight patients based on the improvement in MRI scans (decreased T2 signal and contrast enhancement) and decreased requirement for corticosteroids (Gonzalez et al. 2007).

30.8 Assessing Glioblastoma Response and Progression with Anti-VEGF Therapies

By convention, glioma response to therapy is determined by a reduction in contrast enhancement on post-contrast images. GBMs enhance after the intravenous administration of contrast agent (typically gadolinium) because the tumor vasculature has a permeable BBB that allows the leakage of contrast from the intravascular space into the brain parenchyma where the tumor is located. Therefore, a decrease in enhancement after therapy with standard cytotoxic chemotherapy agents is interpreted as a decrease in tumor burden. However, in the setting of antiangiogenic agents, the association between reduction in contrast enhancement and decreased tumor burden is less clear. Anti-VEGF agents restore the integrity of the BBB which results in a reduction in permeability and contrast leakage on post-contrast MRI scans (Fig. 30.2). Because of reduced vessel permeability subsequent tumor growth may not be visible on standard post-contrast MRI sequences.

Preclinical models have suggested that blocking VEGF and thus angiogenesis may lead to the tumor co-opting native brain blood vessels as an alternate way of maintaining an adequate blood supply (Kunkel et al. 2001, Rubenstein et al. 2000). Histological sections from gliomas in rats treated with a VEGF antibody have demonstrated tumor cells infiltrating into normal surrounding brain and tracking along native brain blood vessels (Kunkel et al. 2001). These blood vessels maintain an intact BBB, so tumor surrounding them will not be visible on contrast-enhanced MRI. While yet to be demonstrated in humans with histological confirmation, there is a concern that observed changes on fluid attenuation inversion recovery (FLAIR) images, which are sensitive to changes in white matter (e.g., edema or infiltrating tumor), or diffusion imaging, which is sensitive to changes in cell density, may represent tumor growth without an associated increase in contrast enhancement (Gerstner et al. 2008). Therefore, new neuroimaging criteria or biomarkers may be needed to assess glioma response in the setting of anti-VEGF therapy.

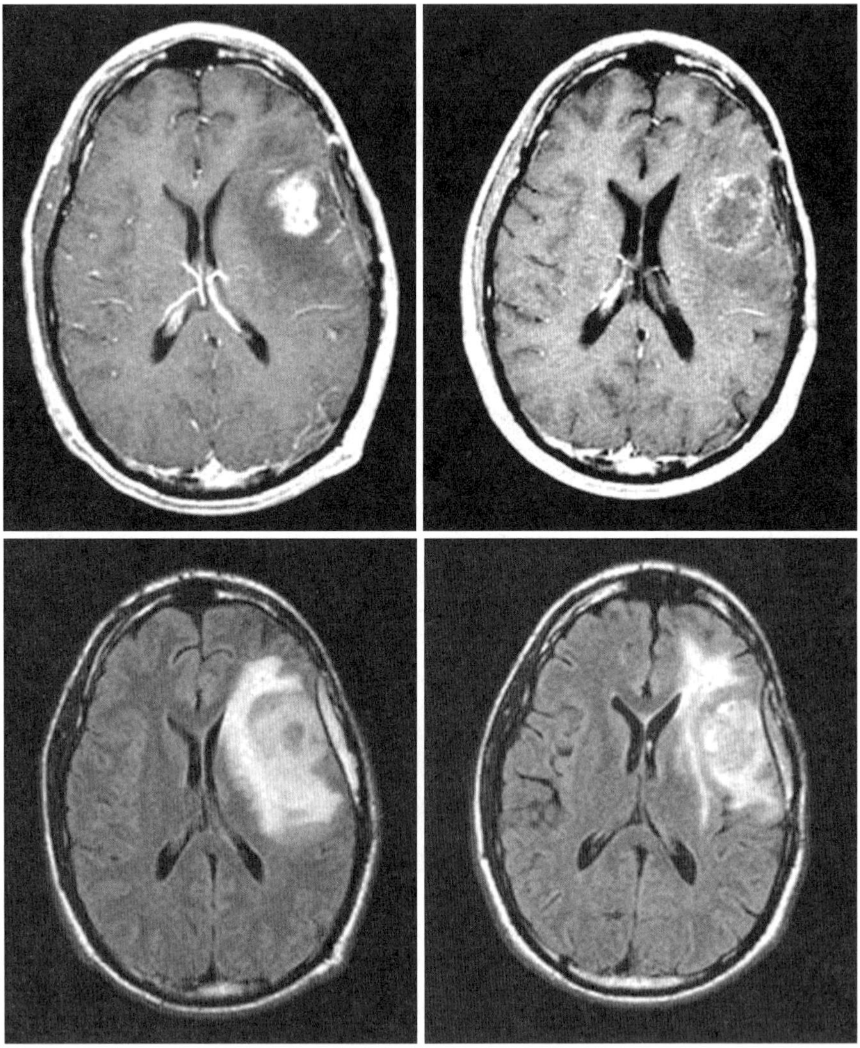

Fig. 30.2 MRI scan of a patient with a recurrent left frontal GBM. *Top row*: Contrast-enhanced MRI prior to anti-VEGF therapy (*left*) and 1 month later (*right*). *Second row*: Fluid attenuation inversion recovery (FLAIR) prior to anti-VEGF therapy (*left*) and 1 month later (*right*). Note the remarkable decrease in contrast enhancement and reduction in FLAIR hyperintensity with decreased mass effect on the lateral ventricle

30.9 Future Role of Anti-VEGF Agents in the Therapy of Glioblastoma

Results to date of anti-VEGF therapies for GBM have been encouraging. These results are preliminary and await validation in prospective phase III trials but there appears to be some positive impact on progression-free survival and overall survival in glioblastoma patients. Unfortunately, all therapies eventually fail, so additional approaches will be required. Tumor angiogenesis is a pathophysiological process characterized by redundant pathways and multiple potential escape mechanisms. Agents that target other components of the angiogenesis pathway (FGF, PDGF, angiopoietins, etc.) will be necessary for a sustained antiangiogenic effect. The long-term effects of prolonged inhibition of angiogenesis on normal organs have not been adequately studied and may ultimately limit application of this type of therapy. Improved identification of the normalization window in GBM by noninvasive serial imaging may allow exploitation of this anti-VEGF effect by identification of the optimal time intervals in which to combine anti-VEGF and cytotoxic therapies. In addition, anti-VEGF therapies may prove effective in the treatment of conditions associated with increased permeability including vasogenic edema in the brain or spinal cord or malignant effusions.

References

Batchelor, T. T., Sorensen, A. G., di Tomaso, E., Zhang, W. T., Duda, D. G., Cohen, K. S., Kozak, K. R., Cahill, D. P., Chen, P. J., Zhu, M., Ancukiewicz, M., Mrugala, M. M., Plotkin, S., Drappatz, J., Louis, D. N., Ivy, P., Scadden, D. T., Benner, T., Loeffler, J. S., Wen, P. Y. and Jain, R. K. AZD2171, a pan-VEGF receptor tyrosine kinase inhibitor, normalizes tumor vasculature and alleviates edema in glioblastoma patients. Cancer Cell. 2007; 11: 83–95.

Bergers, G. and Hanahan, D. Modes of resistance to anti-angiogenic therapy. Nat Rev Cancer. 2008; 8: 592–603.

Brat, D. J., Bellail, A. C. and Van Meir, E. G. The role of interleukin-8 and its receptors in gliomagenesis and tumoral angiogenesis. Neuro Oncol. 2005; 7: 122–33.

Brat, D. J. and Van Meir, E. G. Vaso-occlusive and prothrombotic mechanisms associated with tumor hypoxia, necrosis, and accelerated growth in glioblastoma. Lab Invest. 2004; 84: 397–405.

Brockmann, M., Ulbricht, U., Gruner, K., Fillbrandt, R., Westphal, M. and Lamszus, K. Glioblastoma and cerebral microvascular endothelial cell migration in response to tumor-associated growth factors. Neurosurg. 2003; 52: 1391–9.

Calabrese, C., Poppleton, H., Kocak, M., Hogg, T. L., Fuller, C., Hamner, B., Oh, E. Y., Gaber, M. W., Finklestein, D., Allen, M., Frank, A., Bayazitov, I. T., Zakharenko, S. S., Gajjar, A., Davidoff, A. and Gilbertson, R. J. A perivascular niche of brain tumor stem cells. Cancer Cell. 2007; 11: 69–82.

Cloughesy, T. F., Prados, M. D., Wen, P. Y., Mikkelsen, T., Abrey, L. E., Schiff, D., Yung, W. K. A., Maoxia, Z., Dimery, I. and Friedman, H. S. A phase II, randomized, non-comparative clinical trial of the effect of bevacizumab (BV) alone or in combination with irinotecan (CPT) on 6-month progression free survival (PFS6) in recurrent, treatment-refractory glioblastoma (GBM). J Clin Oncol 26: 2008 (May 20 suppl; abstr 2010b).

Conrad, C., Friedman, H., Reardon, D., Provenzale, J., Jackson, E., Serajuddin, H., Laurent, D., Chen, B. and Yung, W. K. A. A phase I/II trial of single-agent PTK 787/ZK 222584 (PTK/ZK), a novel, oral angiogenesis inhibitor, in patients with recurrent glioblastoma multiforme (GBM). ASCO Annual Meeting Proceedings: Abstr 1512. 2004;

De Groot, J. F., Wen, P. Y., Lamborn, K., Chang, S., Cloughesy, T. F., Chen, A. P., DeAngelis, L. M., Mehta, M. P., Gilbert, M. R., Yung, W. K. A. and Prados, M. D.

Phase II single arm trial of aflibercept in patients with recurrent temozolomide-resistant glioblastoma: NABTC 0601. J Clin Oncol 26: 2008 (May 20 suppl; abstr 2020).
Desbaillets, I., Diserens, A. C., Tribolet, N., Hamou, M. F. and Van Meir, E. G. Upregulation of interleukin 8 by oxygen-deprived cells in glioblastoma suggests a role in leukocyte activation, chemotaxis, and angiogenesis. J Exp Med. 1997; 186: 1201–12.
Drevs, J., Muller-Driver, R., Wittig, C., Fuxius, S., Esser, N., Hugenschmidt, H., Konerding, M., Allegrini, P., Wood, J., Hennig, J., Unger, C. and Marme, D. PTK787/ZK 222584, a specific vascular endothelial growth factor-receptor tyrosine kinase inhibitor, affects the anatomy of the tumor vascular bed and the functional vascular properties as detected by dynamic enhanced magnetic resonance imaging. Cancer Res. 2002; 62: 4015–22.
Folkman, J. Angiogenesis: an organizing principle for drug discovery? Nature Rev Drug Discovery. 2007; 6: 273–286.
Forsythe, J., Jiang, B., Iyer, N., Agani, F., Leung, S., Koos, R. and Semenza , G. Activation of vascular endothelial growth factor gene transcription by hypoxia-inducible factor 1. Mol Cell Biol. 1996; 16: 4604–13.
Friedman, H. S., Petros, W. P., Friedman, A. H., Schaaf, L. J., Kerby, T., Lawyer, J., Parry, M., Houghton, P. J., Lovell, S., Rasheed, K., Cloughsey, T., Stewart, E. S., Colvin, O. M., Provenzale, J. M., McLendon, R. E., Bigner, D. D., Cokgor, I., Haglund, M., Rich, J., Ashley, D., Malczyn, J., Elfring, G. L. and Miller, L. L. Irinotecan therapy in adults with recurrent or progressive malignant glioma. J Clin Oncol. 1999; 17: 1516–25.
Garkavtsev, I., Kozin, S. V., Chernova, O., Xu, L., Winkler, F., Brown, E., Barnett, G. H. and Jain, R. K. The candidate tumour suppressor protein ING4 regulates brain tumour growth and angiogenesis. Nature. 2004; 428: 328–32.
Gerstner, E., Chen, P., Batchelor, T. and Gregory Sorensen, A. Role of diffusion MRI in detecting infiltrative tumor in the setting of cediranib therapy. Society for Neuro-Oncology Meeting, Abstract 0481. 2008;
Goldbrunner, R., Bendszus, M., Wood, J., Kiderlen, M., Sasaki, M. and Tonn, J. PTK787/ZK222584, an inhibitor of vascular endothelial growth factor receptor tyrosine kinases, decreases glioma growth and vascularization. Neurosurgery. 2004; 55: 426–32.
Goldman, C., Kim, J., Wong, W., King, V., Brock, T. and Gillespie, G. Epidermal growth factor stimulates vascular endothelial growth factor production by human malignant glioma cells: a model of glioblastoma multiforme pathophysiology. Mol Biol Cell. 1993; 4: 121–33.
Gomez-Manzano, C., Fueyo, J., Jiang, H., Glass, T. L., Lee, H.-Y., Hu, M., Liu, J.-L., Jasti, S. L., Liu, T.-J., Conrad, C. A. and Yung, W. K. A. Mechanisms underlying PTEN regulation of vascular endothelial growth factor and angiogenesis. Ann Neurol. 2003; 53: 109–17.
Gonzalez, J., Kumar, A., Conrad, C. and Levin, V. Effect of bevacizumab on radiation necrosis of the brain. Int J Radiat Oncol Biol Phys. 2007; 67: 323–6.
Goudar, R. K., Shi, Q., Hjelmeland, M. D., Keir, S. T., McLendon, R. E., Wikstrand, C. J., Reese, E. D., Conrad, C. A., Traxler, P., Lane, H. A., Reardon, D. A., Cavenee, W. K., Wang, X.-F., Bigner, D. D., Friedman, H. S. and Rich, J. N. Combination therapy of inhibitors of epidermal growth factor receptor/vascular endothelial growth factor receptor 2 (AEE788) and the mammalian target of rapamycin (RAD001) offers improved glioblastoma tumor growth inhibition. Mol Cancer Therapeut. 2005; 4: 101–12.
Holash, J., Davis, S., Papadopoulos, N., Croll, S., Ho, L., Russell, M., Boland, P., Leidich, R., Hylton, D., Burova, E., Ioffe, E., Huang, T., Radziejewski, C., Bailey, K., Fandl, J., Daly, T., Wiegand, S., Yancopoulos, G. and Rudge, J. VEGF-Trap: a VEGF blocker with potent antitumor effects. Proc Natl Acad Sci USA. 2002; 99: 11393–8.
Jain, R. K. Normalization of tumor vasculature: an emerging concept in antiangiogenic therapy. Science. 2005; 307: 58–62.
Jain, R. K., di Tomaso, E., Duda, D. G., Loeffler, J. S., Sorensen, A. G. and Batchelor, T. T. Angiogenesis in brain tumours. Nat Rev Neurosci. 2007; 8: 610–22.

Jain, R. K., Duda, D. G., Clark, J. W. and Loeffler, J. S. Lessons from phase III clinical trials on anti-VEGF therapy for cancer. Nature Clin Pract Oncol. 2006; 3: 24–40.

Jensen, R. L., Ragel, B. T., Whang, K. and Gillespie, D. Inhibition of hypoxia inducible factor-1alpha (HIF-1alpha) decreases vascular endothelial growth factor (VEGF) secretion and tumor growth in malignant gliomas. J Neuro Oncol. 2006; 78: 233–47.

Kerbel, R. S. Tumor angiogenesis. N Engl J Med. 2008; 358: 2039–2049.

Kirkpatrick, J. P., Rich, J. N., Vredenburgh, J. J., Desjardins, A., Quinn, J. A., Gururangan, S., Sathornsumetee, S., Egorin, M. J., Friedman, H. S. and Reardon, D. A. Final report: Phase I trial of imatinib mesylate, hydroxyurea, and vatalanib for patients with recurrent malignant glioma (MG). J Clin Oncol 26: 2008 (May 20 suppl; abstr 2057).

Korfman, S., Garvin, J., Nagamani, D. and Taylor, S. Treatment of cerebral metastases from breast carcinoma with prednisolone. JAMA. 1957; 163: 1473–1476.

Kragh, M., Quistorff, B., Tenan, M., Van Meir, E. G. and Kristjansen, P. E. Overexpression of thrombospondin-1 reduces growth and vascular index but not perfusion in glioblastoma. Cancer Res. 2002; 62: 1191–5.

Kunkel, P., Ulbricht, U., Bohlen, P., Brockmann, M. A., Fillbrandt, R., Stavrou, D., Westphal, M. and Lamszus, K. Inhibition of glioma angiogenesis and growth in vivo by systemic treatment with a monoclonal antibody against vascular endothelial growth factor receptor-2. Cancer Res. 2001; 61: 6624–8.

Lai, A., Filka, E., McGibbon, B., Nghiemphu, P. L., Graham, C., Yong, W. H., Mischel, P., Liau, L. M., Bergsneider, M., Pope, W., Selch, M. and Cloughesy, T. Phase II Pilot Study of Bevacizumab in Combination With Temozolomide and Regional Radiation Therapy for Up-Front Treatment of Patients With Newly Diagnosed Glioblastoma Multiforme: Interim Analysis of Safety and Tolerability. Int J Radiat Oncol Biol Phys. 2008; 71; 1372–80.

Mellinghoff, I. K., Wang, M. Y., Vivanco, I., Haas-Kogan, D. A., Zhu, S., Dia, E. Q., Lu, K. V., Yoshimoto, K., Huang, J. H., Chute, D. J., Riggs, B. L., Horvath, S., Liau, L. M., Cavenee, W. K., Rao, P. N., Beroukhim, R., Peck, T. C., Lee, J. C., Sellers, W. R., Stokoe, D., Prados, M., Cloughesy, T. F., Sawyers, C. L., Mischel, P. S., Molecular determinants of the response of glioblastomas to EGFR kinase inhibitors. NE J Med. 2005; 353: 2012–24.

Morrison, R. S., Gross, J. L., Herblin, W. F., Reilly, T. M., LaSala, P. A., Alterman, R. L., Moskal, J. R., Kornblith, P. L., Dexter, D. L., Morrison, R. S., Gross, J. L., Herblin, W. F., Reilly, T. M., LaSala, P. A., Alterman, R. L., Moskal, J. R., Kornblith, P. L. and Dexter, D. L. Basic fibroblast growth factor-like activity and receptors are expressed in a human glioma cell line. Cancer Res. 1990; 50: 2524–9.

Nabors, L. B., Rosenfeld, M., Chamberlain, M., Phuphanich, S., Batchelor, T., Supko, J., Desideri, S., Xiaobu, Y., Wright, J. and Grossman, S. A. A phase I trial of sorafenib (BAY 43-9006) for patients with recurrent or progressive malignant glioma (NABTT 0401). ASCO Annual Meeting Proceedings Part I. Vol 25, No. 18S (June 20 Supplement), 2007: 2058.

Plate, K. H., Breier, G., Weich, H. A. and Risau, W. Vascular endothelial growth factor is a potential tumour angiogenesis factor in human gliomas in vivo. Nature. 1992; 359: 845–848.

Pope, W. B., Lai, A., Nghiemphu, P., Mischel, P. and Cloughesy, T. F. MRI in patients with high-grade gliomas treated with bevacizumab and chemotherapy. Neurology. 2006; 66: 1258–60.

Reardon, D., Cloughesy, T., Conrad, C., Prados, M., Xia, J., Mietlowski, W., Dugan, M., Mischel, P., Friedman, H. and Yung, A. A phase I study of AEE788, a novel multitargeted inhibitor of ErbB and VEGF receptor family tyrosine kinases, in recurrent GBM patients. ASCO Annual Meeting Proceedings: Abst 3063. 2005;

Reardon, D., Friedman, H., Yung, W. K. A., Brada, M., Conrad, C., Provenzale, J., Jackson, E., Serajuddin, H., Chen, B. and Laurent, D. A phase I/II trial of PTK787/ZK 222584 (PTK/ZK), a novel, oral angiogenesis inhibitor, in combination with either temozolomide or lomustine for patients with recurrent glioblastoma multiforme (GBM). ASCO Annual Meeting Proceedings: Abstr 1513. 2004;

Reiss, Y., Machein, M. R. and Plate, K. H. The role of angiopoietins during angiogenesis in gliomas. Brain Pathol. 2005; 15: 311–7.

Rich, J. N., Desjardins, A., Sathornsumetee, S., Vredenburgh, J. J., Quinn, J. A., Gururangan, S., Friedman, A. H., Friedman, H. S. and Reardon, D. A. Phase II study of bevacizumab and etoposide in patients with recurrent malignant glioma. J Clin Oncol 26: 2008 (May 20 suppl; abstr 2022).

Rich, J. N., Sathornsumetee, S., Keir, S. T., Kieran, M. W., Laforme, A., Kaipainen, A., McLendon, R. E., Graner, M. W., Rasheed, B. K. A., Wang, L., Reardon, D. A., Ryan, A. J., Wheeler, C., Dimery, I., Bigner, D. D. and Friedman, H. ZD6474, a novel tyrosine kinase inhibitor of vascular endothelial growth factor receptor and epidermal growth factor receptor, inhibits tumor growth of multiple nervous system tumors. Clin Cancer Res. 2005; 11: 8145–57.

Rubenstein, J. L., Kim, J., Ozawa, T., Zhang, M., Westphal, M., Deen, D. F. and Shuman, M. A. Anti-VEGF antibody treatment of glioblastoma prolongs survival but results in increased vascular cooption. Neoplasia. 2000; 2: 306–14.

Ryuto, M., Ono, M., Izumi, H., Yoshida, S., Weich, H. A., Kohno, K., Kuwano, M., Ryuto, M., Ono, M., Izumi, H., Yoshida, S., Weich, H. A., Kohno, K. and Kuwano, M. Induction of vascular endothelial growth factor by tumor necrosis factor alpha in human glioma cells. Possible roles of SP-1. J Biol Chem. 1996; 271: 28220–8.

Saino, M., Maruyama, T., Sekiya, T., Kayama, T., Murakami, Y., Saino, M., Maruyama, T., Sekiya, T., Kayama, T. and Murakami, Y. Inhibition of angiogenesis in human glioma cell lines by antisense RNA from the soluble guanylate cyclase genes, GUCY1A3 and GUCY1B3. Oncol Rep. 2004; 12: 47–52.

Sandstrom, M., Johansson, M., Andersson, U., Bergh, A., Bergenheim, A. T. and Henriksson, R. The tyrosine kinase inhibitor ZD6474 inhibits tumour growth in an intracerebral rat glioma model. Br J Cancer. 2004; 91: 1174–80.

Sathornsumetee, S., Cao, Y., Marcello, J. E., Herndon, J. E., 2nd, McLendon, R. E., Desjardins, A., Friedman, H. S., Dewhirst, M. W., Vredenburgh, J. J. and Rich, J. N. Tumor angiogenic and hypoxic profiles predict radiographic response and survival in malignant astrocytoma patients treated with bevacizumab and irinotecan. J Clin Oncol. 2008a; 26: 271–8.

Sathornsumetee, S., Vredenburgh, J. J., Rich, J. N., Desjardins, A., Quinn, J. A., Mathe, A. E., Gururangan, S., Friedman, A. H., Friedman, H. S. and Reardon, D. A. Phase II study of bevacizumab and erlotinib in patients with recurrent glioblastoma multiforme. J Clin Oncol 26: 2008b (May 20 suppl; abstr 13008).

Stupp, R., Hegi, M. E., Mason, W. P., van den Bent, M. J., Taphoorn, M. J., Janzer, R. C., Ludwin, S. K., Allgeier, A., Fisher, B., Belanger, K., Hau, P., Brandes, A. A., Gijtenbeek, J., Marosi, C., Vecht, C. J., Mokhtari, K., Wesseling, P., Villa, S., Eisenhauer, E., Gorlia, T., Weller, M., Lacombe, D., Cairncross, J. G. and Mirimanoff, R. O. Effects of radiotherapy with concomitant and adjuvant temozolomide versus radiotherapy alone on survival in glioblastoma in a randomised phase III study: 5-year analysis of the EORTC-NCIC trial. Lancet Oncol. EPub date 2009/03/10.

Stupp, R., Mason, W. P., van den Bent, M. J., Weller, M., Fisher, B., Taphoorn, M. J., Belanger, K., Brandes, A. A., Marosi, C., Bogdahn, U., Curschmann, J., Janzer, R. C., Ludwin, S. K., Gorlia, T., Allgeier, A., Lacombe, D., Cairncross, J. G., Eisenhauer, E. and Mirimanoff, R. O. Radiotherapy plus concomitant and adjuvant temozolomide for glioblastoma. NE J Med. 2005; 352: 987–96.

Tenan, M., Fulci, G., Albertoni, M., Diserens, A. C., Hamou, M. F., El Atifi-Borel, M., Feige, J. J., Pepper, M. S. and Van Meir, E. G. Thrombospondin-1 is downregulated by anoxia and suppresses tumorigenicity of human glioblastoma cells. J Exp Med. 2000; 191: 1789–98.

Traxler, P., Allegrini, P. R., Brandt, R., Brueggen, J., Cozens, R., Fabbro, D., Grosios, K., Lane, H. A., McSheehy, P., Mestan, J., Meyer, T., Tang, C., Wartmann, M., Wood, J. and Caravatti, G. AEE788: a dual family epidermal growth factor receptor/ErbB2 and vascular endothelial growth factor receptor tyrosine kinase inhibitor with antitumor and antiangiogenic activity. Cancer Res. 2004; 64: 4931–41.

Tsai, J. C., Goldman, C. K., Gillespie, G. Y., Vascular endothelial growth factor in human glioma cell lines: induced secretion by EGF, PDGF-BB, and bFGF. J Neurosurg. 1995; 82: 864–73.

Verheul, H. M. and Pinedo, H. M. Possible molecular mechanisms involved in the toxicity of angiogenesis inhibition. Nat Rev Cancer. 2007; 7: 475–485.

Vredenburgh, J. J., Desjardins, A., Herndon, J. E., 2nd, Marcello, J., Reardon, D. A., Quinn, J. A., Rich, J. N., Sathornsumetee, S., Gururangan, S., Sampson, J., Wagner, M., Bailey, L., Bigner, D. D., Friedman, A. H. and Friedman, H. S. Bevacizumab plus irinotecan in recurrent glioblastoma multiforme. J Clin Oncol. 2007a; 25: 4722–9.

Vredenburgh, J. J., Desjardins, A., Herndon, J. E., Dowell, J. M., Reardon, D., Quinn, J. A., Rich, J. N., Sathornsumetee, S., Grurangan, S., Wagner, M., Bigner, D. D., Friedman, A. H. and Friedman, H. Phase II trial of bevacizumab and irinotecan in recurrent malignant glioma. Clin Cancer Res. 2007b; 13: 1253–59.

Wachsberger, P., Burd, R., Cardi, C., Thakur, M., Daskalakis, C., Holash, J., Yancopoulos, G. and Dicker, A. VEGF trap in combination with radiotherapy improves tumor control in u87 glioblastoma. Int J Radiat Oncol Biol Phys. 2007; 67: 1526–37.

Winkler, F., Kozin, S. V., Tong, R. T., Chae, S. S., Booth, M. F., Garkavtsev, I., Xu, L., Hicklin, D. J., Fukumura, D., di Tomaso, E., Munn, L. L., Jain, R. K., Winkler, F., Kozin, S. V., Tong, R. T., Chae, S.-S., Booth, M. F., Garkavtsev, I., Xu, L., Hicklin, D. J., Fukumura, D., di Tomaso, E., Munn, L. L. and Jain, R. K. Kinetics of vascular normalization by VEGFR-2 blockade governs brain tumor response to radiation: role of oxygenation, angiopoietin-1, and matrix metalloproteinases. Cancer Cell. 2004; 6: 553–63.

Wong, E. T., Hess, K. R., Gleason, M. J., Jaeckle, K. A., Kyritsis, A. P., Prados, M. D., Levin, V. A., Yung, W. K., Wong, E. T., Hess, K. R., Gleason, M. J., Jaeckle, K. A., Kyritsis, A. P., Prados, M. D., Levin, V. A. and Yung, W. K. Outcomes and prognostic factors in recurrent glioma patients enrolled onto phase II clinical trials. J Clin Oncol. 1999; 17: 2572–8.

Wood, J., Bold, G., Buchdunger, E., Cozens, R., Ferrari, S., Frei, J., Hofmann, F., Mestan, J., Mett, H., O'Reilly, T., Persohn, E., Rosel, J., Schnell, C., Stover, D., Theuer, A., Towbin, H., Wenger, F., Woods-Cook, K., Menrad, A., Siemeister, G., Schirner, M., Thierauch, K., Schneider, M., Drevs, J., Martiny-Baron, G. and Totzke, F. PTK787/ZK 222584, a novel and potent inhibitor of vascular endothelial growth factor receptor tyrosine kinases, impairs vascular endothelial growth factor-induced responses and tumor growth after oral administration. Cancer Res. 2000; 60: 2178–89.

Yoshino, Y., Aoyagi, M., Tamaki, M., Duan, L., Morimoto, T., Ohno, K., Yoshino, Y., Aoyagi, M., Tamaki, M., Duan, L., Morimoto, T. and Ohno, K. Activation of p38 MAPK and/or JNK contributes to increased levels of VEGF secretion in human malignant glioma cells. Int J Oncol. 2006; 29: 981–7.

Chapter 31
Bone Marrow-Derived Cells in GBM Neovascularization

Gabriele Bergers

Abstract Historically, the formation of new blood vessels was thought to depend upon the activation of existing endothelial cells within the injured tissue or tumor. Based on a wealth of studies from different laboratories over the last 10 years, there has now been increasing appreciation that angiogenesis in the adult is also supported by the mobilization and recruitment of bone marrow-derived circulating vascular progenitor cells and proangiogenic myeloid support cells to generate a new tumor vasculature. Although the functional significance of endothelial progenitor cells (EPC) and pericyte progenitors (PPC) as major contributors to tumor vessel formation is controversial due to their extremely variable and in general rather low frequencies of incorporation into tumor vessels, there is more evidence that innate bone marrow-derived cells (BMDC) contribute to the formation and maintenance of tumor vessels. Influx of BMDC appears to be dependent on the degree of hypoxia and can make up to more than 20% of the cellular content in tumors such as glioblastoma (GBM). Congruent with observations in various tumor types, incorporation of EPC and PPC into the growing brain tumor vasculature is nevertheless observed at a modest rate but can vary significantly between different GBM mouse models, while myeloid proangiogenic support cells display the majority of BMDC and even have been shown to be sufficient to initiate neovascularization in GBM. Importantly, intratumoral hypoxia appears to be a driving force in GBM neovascularization. It induces various proangiogenic growth factors including VEGF, PlGF, and SDF-1α that besides activating residing endothelial cells can also regulate BMDC influx into sites of vascular remodeling in the tumor. These results prompt an agenda to assess the prevalence and functional significance of BMDC in GBM propagation and vascularization.

G. Bergers (✉)
Department of Neurological Surgery, Brain Tumor Research Center and UCSF Helen Diller Family Comprehensive Cancer Center, University of California San Francisco, 513 Parnassus Avenue, San Francisco, CA-94143-0520, USA
e-mail: gabriele.bergers@ucsf.edu

E.G. Van Meir (ed.), *CNS Cancer*, Cancer Drug Discovery and Development, DOI 10.1007/978-1-60327-553-8_31,

© Humana Press, a part of Springer Science+Business Media, LLC 2009

Contents

31.1 Introduction

31.1.1 Neovascularization Is a Prerequisite for Tumor Progression

In the early 1970s, Dr. Judah Folkman proposed that tumor growth and progression is dependent on the tumor's ability to form new blood vessels, a concept that has been validated in nearly all tumor types (Folkman, 1971). Based on the restriction of oxygen diffusion in tissues, most tumors can grow to a limited size of about 1–2 mm in diameter where they can stay dormant for long time periods by reaching a steady state between proliferation and apoptosis. Such dormant lesions have been identified not only in mouse models of tumorigenesis but also during autopsies of individuals who died of causes other than cancer, supporting the notion that only a small percentage of dormant lesions will progress to become full-blown cancers (Black and Welch, 1993). Indeed, tumors require an additional discrete step to further expand and progress, coined the "angiogenic switch," to fuel the growing and progressing tumor with new blood vessels (Folkman et al., 1989; Hanahan and Folkman, 1996; Hanahan and Weinberg, 2000). Given that the ability of blood vessels to stay in either a quiescent or an activated stage depends on the levels of pro- and antiangiogenic factors, induction of the angiogenic switch depends on how heavily the balance tips in favor of proangiogenesis (Bergers and Benjamin, 2003; Folkman, 2006). Depending on the tumor type, the angiogenic switch can occur at different stages of tumor progression or in premalignant lesions as demonstrated in mouse models of multistep tumorigenesis and can be correlated with the onset of tumor growth in advanced premalignant stages in various human cancers such as mammary, cervical, and prostate carcinomas (Hanahan and Folkman, 1996).

There are, however, exceptions in which tumors can grow in the absence of neovascularization. Low-grade and anaplastic astrocytomas (grade II and III astrocytomas, respectively) are unable to promote angiogenesis but are still capable of propagating by co-opting the dense normal brain vasculature (Berger and Wilson, 1999; Kleihues et al., 2007b). When, however, astrocytomas progress to their most aggressive form referred to as glioblastoma multiforme (GBM or

WHO grade IV astrocytoma), then neovascularization needs to be initiated, making GBM one of the most vascularized and angiogenic tumors (Brat et al., 2002; Eberhard et al., 2000; Holash et al., 1999; Kleihues et al., 2007a; Zagzag et al., 2000). These data support the notion that although neovascularization can occur at distinct and different stages of tumorigenesis, it is usually a rate-limiting step and a prerequisite for tumor progression.

31.1.2 Tumor Neovascularization Is Driven by Angiogenic and Vasculogenic Mechanisms

New blood vessels in tumors are predominantly derived from the existing vasculature by a process referred to as angiogenesis. Upon activation of the quiescent vasculature by angiogenic factors, specifically by vascular endothelial growth factor (VEGF), blood vessels (mother vessels) loosen their pericyte coat and exhibit vasodilation and increased vascular permeability (Dvorak, 2000). The vascular basement membrane and extracellular matrix are then locally degraded by various proteases. All these morphological changes enable plasma proteins to extravasate into the perivascular space to lay down a provisional matrix on which endothelial cells migrate into the perivascular space toward angiogenic stimuli. During this process, endothelial cells multiply and form a migration column that is directed by a migratory endothelial tip cell and followed by proliferating endothelial stalk cells. Finally, the latter adhere to each other and form a lumen at which pericytes are recruited concomitant with the formation of a new vascular membrane to support vessel maturation and stability (Bergers and Benjamin, 2003; Gerhardt et al., 2003). While in physiological angiogenesis, this process is tightly regulated by a balance of pro- and antiangiogenic molecules, tumor angiogenesis has lost the appropriate control mechanisms and, therefore, blood vessels fail to become quiescent, enabling the constant growth of new tumor vessels. Partly due to the imbalanced vascular activity, tumor blood vessels are architecturally quite different from normal blood vessels (Baluk et al., 2005). For example, normal brain vessels are slim and smoothly shaped, while the vasculature of GBM is hyperdilated, tortuous, and hemorrhagic with glomeruloid bodies containing clusters of endothelial cells and pericytes, a phenotype that is partly attributed to the abnormally high levels of VEGF in these tumors (Blouw et al., 2003; Dvorak, 2000; Jain et al., 2007). Factors that stimulate angiogenesis like VEGF, fibroblast growth factor (FGF), and placental growth factor (PIGF) (see Chapter 21) are produced by either tumor cells and/or the host cell compartment, which includes bone marrow-derived proangiogenic myeloid cells. In addition, neovascularization can be further supported by the recruitment of vascular progenitor cells, which upon incorporation into growing blood vessels differentiate into endothelial cells or pericytes (Aghi and Chiocca, 2005; Bababeygy et al., 2008; Du et al., 2008a; Kopp et al., 2006; Lyden et al., 2001; Nolan et al., 2007; Peters et al., 2005; Rajantie et al., 2004; Schmid and Varner, 2007; Song et al., 2005). Since this situation mimics the vasculogenic process used by the early embryo in which blood vessels coalesce with vascular progenitor cells, it is commonly described as adult vasculogenesis (Carmeliet, 2005).

31.2 Bone Marrow-Derived Cells Contribute to Neovascularization in GBM

There is an increasing appreciation that tumors recruit heterogeneous populations of bone marrow-derived cells that not only are directly incorporated into tumor vessels and facilitate vasculogenesis but also indirectly regulate and support blood vessel growth by providing crucial proangiogenic factors (De Palma et al., 2005; Du et al., 2008a; Grunewald et al., 2006; Lin et al., 2006; Murdoch et al., 2008; Pollard, 2004; Schmid and Varner, 2007; Shojaei et al., 2008b). At least two major pathways have been described for the attraction of bone marrow-derived cells to the tumor, of which both can be initiated by intratumoral hypoxia. In the first pathway, growth factors such as VEGF and PlGF (placental growth factor), which are released by the tumor, induce and activate matrix metalloproteinase MMP-9 in hematopoietic and stromal cells in the bone marrow to release soluble Kit-ligand (sKitL, stem cell factor, steel factor), which in turn permits the transfer of endothelial and hematopoietic stem cells from a quiescent to a proliferative niche and promotes their mobilization into the bloodstream (Hattori et al., 2002; Heissig et al., 2002). In the second pathway, stromal-derived factor-1α (SDF-1α/CXCL12), the ligand for CXCR4, which can be induced by hypoxia and VEGF, and is expressed in perivascular, endothelial, or tumor cells, is involved in the recruitment of CXCR4$^+$ hematopoietic progenitors to tumors (Ceradini et al., 2004; Hattori et al., 2003; Petit et al., 2007). In the adult, SDF-1α/CXCL12 plays a pivotal role in the retention and homing of hematopoietic stem cells into the bone marrow environment. When SDF-1α is elevated in tumors, it retains infiltrating CXCR4$^+$ bone marrow-derived cells in close proximity to angiogenic blood vessels (Aghi and Chiocca, 2005; Du et al., 2008a; Grunewald et al., 2006; Petit et al., 2007).

A very common technique to detect BMDC in xenograft tumors is based on reconstituting lethally irradiated donor mice with GFP-labeled bone marrow cells from transgenic mice expressing a *GFP* gene under the β-actin promoter. After successful bone marrow transplantation, tumor cells are then inoculated and the recruitment of BMDC to the tumor visualized by their green color (GFP) (Fig. 31.1 and Color Plate 47). Several laboratories have utilized this technique to analyze BMDC influx into various xenograft tumor mouse models, both subcutaneously and orthotopically, as well as in endogenous mouse models of cancer (Aghi and Chiocca, 2005; De Palma and Naldini, 2006; Ganss, 2006; Song et al., 2005). This review will give a general overview about the distinct BMDC populations involved in tumor

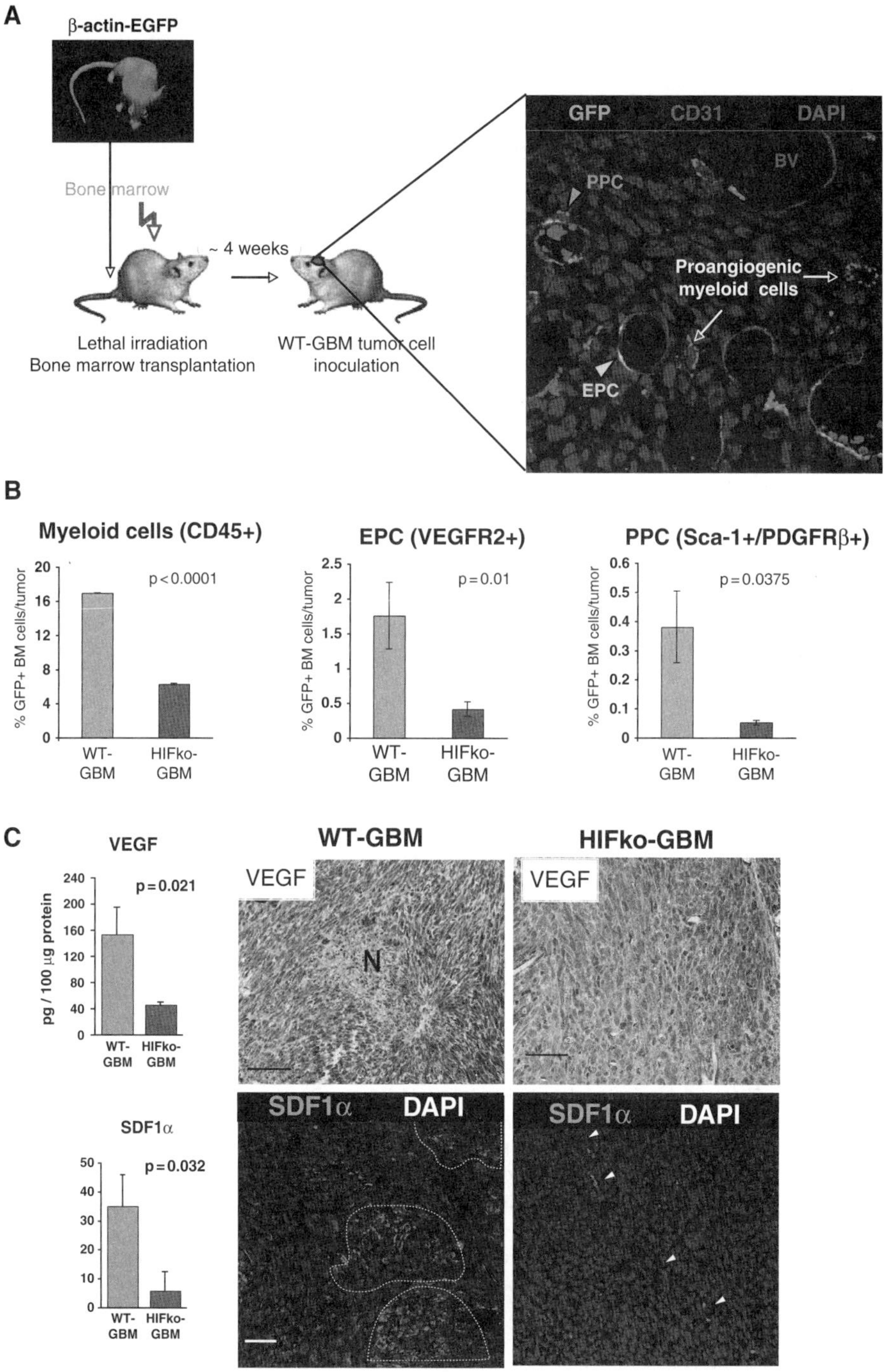

Fig. 31.1 (continued)

neovascularization and highlight the observations of BMD constituents and their function in GBM.

31.2.1 Vascular Progenitor Cells

Vascular progenitor cells have been described to mainly stem from the bone marrow where they are mobilized into the bloodstream upon specific angiogenic stimuli. While endothelial progenitor cells (EPC) incorporate into the

Fig. 31.1 (continued) HIF1 recruits bone marrow-derived cells (BMDC) to orthotopic glioblastomas (GBM). (**A**) Adult bone marrow constitutes a reservoir of various stem and progenitor cells capable of contributing to neovascularization and progression in tumors. Methods whereby genetically marked bone marrow is transplanted into tumor-bearing recipient mice have allowed for the positive identification and visualization of bone marrow-derived cells (BMDC) within tumors. Not only do such approaches permit the tracking and quantification of BMDC recruitment in various tumor systems, they further allow for the isolation and functional characterization of the various BMDC populations in promoting tumor vessel growth. One example of this approach is to transplant GFP-expressing bone marrow cells from β-actin-eGFP donor mice into lethally irradiated, nonfluorescent recipient animals (e.g. FvBN Ragko mice) to fluorescently mark BMDC. About 4 weeks after transplantation, successful bone marrow reconstitution can be verified in peripheral blood, and then tumor cells (e.g., murine SV40 Tag + Hras + astrocytes aka WT-GBM) are inoculated. This approach provides several advantages: (1) it allows for the analysis of bone marrow reconstitution at any time by simply taking a peripheral blood sample and analyzing it by flow-activated cell sorting (FACS) for GFP + cells; (2) BMDC in tumor sections can be easily detected by their green color without additional immunohistochemical analysis; and (3) it permits the detection, fractionation, quantification, and marker characterization of tissue-incorporated BMDC by FACS. In this example, tumor sections are stained with an antibody against CD31 in red to visualize blood vessels. Recruitment of BMDC was detected by the presence of GFP-positive cells in tumor sections. EPC are detected as green cells that have been incorporated into red tumor vessels and therefore appear yellow (*yellow arrow*). PPC are wrapped around tumor vessels (*green arrow*) and CD45 + myeloid cells are located between blood vessels (*white arrow*). The exact identities of BMDC in tumor sections can be determined by further immunohistochemical or immunofluorescent staining procedures of lineage-specific markers. (**B**) A more efficient and versatile way to quantify and characterize BMDC from single tumor cell suspension by FACS. For example, EPC can be detected as GFP + /VEGFR2 + or VE-cadherin + cells, PPC can be determined as GFP + Sca-1 + /PDGFR-β + cells, and myeloid cells can be identified with the marker CD45. In order to determine the various subtypes of CD45 + myeloid cells, additional markers like Tie-2, VEGFR1, GR1, CD11b, and F4/80 can be utilized. Modified from (Du et al., 2008). (**C**) Hypoxia in GBM induces at least two factors involved in recruitment of BMDC, i.e., VEGF as well as SDF-1α in an HIF-1-dependent manner. An ELISA assay revealed that intratumoral VEGF and SDF-1α levels were about four times higher in WT-GBM than in GBM that were genetically deficient in HIF-1α (HIFko-GBM). Congruently, VEGF expression was elevated in WT-GBM tumor sections, specifically around necrotic areas (N), whereas HIFko-GBM exhibited a severe reduction in VEGF expression. Similarly, WT-GBM contained clusters of SDF-1α + cells (*green*; encircled), whereas SDF-1α expression in HIFko-GBM was limited to a few single cells (*white arrows*). Modified from Du et al. (2008) and Blouw et al. (2003) (*see* Color Plate 47) vasculature and differentiate into endothelial cells, pericyte progenitor cells (PPC) envelop blood vessels and mature into pericytes and vascular smooth muscle cells (Carmeliet, 2005; Carmeliet and Tessier-Lavigne, 2005; Ergun et al., 2008; Kopp et al., 2006; Lamagna and Bergers, 2006).

31.2.1.1 Endothelial Progenitor Cells (EPC)

EPC were first isolated from peripheral blood as CD34+ VEGFR2+ mononuclear cells that upon culture in endothelial growth medium expressed the endothelial lineage markers CD31, Tie-2, and VEGFR2/flk-1 and incorporated into blood vessels of ischemic tissues (Asahara et al., 1997). Interestingly, CD133 (AC133), an orphan surface glycoprotein receptor, now also known to be expressed in neural stem cells and a variety of tumor stem cells, was the first marker that helped to differentiate between EPC and mature endothelial cells. CD133 is expressed in endothelial progenitors but downregulated during endothelial cell differentiation (Gehling et al., 2000; Peichev et al., 2000). Other studies have demonstrated that EPC can also be derived from monocytic CD14+ or CD11b+ cells from blood or CD34+/CD11b+ cell populations from bone marrow or spleen or even dendritic precursor cells (CD11c+ CD8+), since they display phenotypical aspects of endothelial cells in vitro such as expression of endothelial markers and the ability to form vascular tubes (Rehman et al., 2003; Rohde et al., 2006; Schmeisser et al., 2001; Yang et al., 2004). These data suggest that differentiated endothelial cells originate from bone marrow-derived cells, either primitive hematopoietic progenitor populations or more differentiated myeloid cell populations that acquire an endothelial cell-like phenotype. In addition, one cannot exclude that EPC and monocytes develop from a common precursor (Murdoch et al., 2008; Schmid and Varner, 2007).

Over the past 10 years, various laboratories have studied the presence and integration of endothelial progenitors into neovessels in tumors of mouse models with varying results (Aghi and Chiocca, 2005; De Palma and Naldini, 2006; Ganss, 2006). In general, EPC incorporation has been found to be a rather rare event in most tumor mouse models with the exception of murine lymphomas in which more than 50% of blood vessels contain EPC. One of the first demonstrations that EPC are functionally incorporated into growing tumor vessels came from studies on the early phases of tumor growth in lymphoma and Lewis lung carcinoma using xenograft mouse models (Lyden et al., 2001). The first evidence confirming the existence of EPC in human tumors was described in a more recent study demonstrating 0.5–12% incorporation of donor-derived endothelial cells into human patients who had undergone hematopoietic stem cell transplantation and developed secondary tumors (Peters et al., 2005). Like in mouse tumor models, EPC incorporation into vessels of various human tumors except for lymphomas was found to be a rather rare event in this study.

How is EPC influx regulated and why are there such differences in EPC recruitment? It is known that the angiogenic factors VEGF and PlGF induce matrix metalloproteinase-9 (MMP-9) expression in the bone marrow (Heissig et al., 2002). In turn, MMP-9 cleaves and activates KitL (steel factor, stem cell factor), thereby permitting mobilization of vascular progenitor cells and hematopoietic stem cells from the bone marrow to the blood circulation (Heissig et al., 2002). Congruently, circulating EPC were detected at increased frequency in the circulation of cancer patients including glioma patients, and tumor volume and tumor VEGF production correlated with EPC mobilization from bone marrow into circulation (Bertolini et al., 2006; Mancuso et al., 2001). Recent findings in mouse xenograft models, however, pointed to the direction that VEGF alone might not be sufficient to induce EPC influx into GBM but that rather elevated levels of SDF-1α appeared to be instrumental for EPC incorporation into glioma vessels (Aghi et al., 2006; Machein et al., 2003). Interestingly, combined overexpression of VEGF and SDF-1α in GBM xenografts revealed synergistic effects in EPC tumor influx (Aghi et al., 2006). These data suggest that although VEGF is a mobilizing factor of EPC into the bloodstream, additional factors such as SDF-1α might be necessary to actually retain EPC in the tumor and enable incorporation into tumor vessels. How is then BMDC recruitment orchestrated? Several studies revealed that intratumoral HIF-1 is the critical main regulator of EPC influx, partly due to inducing expression of both intratumoral VEGF and SDF-1α. It is notable in this context that EPC incorporation was found to be an early and critical event in tumor propagation and metastasis formation (Nolan et al., 2007). In contrast, others identified EPC in late-stage bulky tumors but not in early lesions in transgenic mouse models of pancreatic islet and liver tumors (Spring et al., 2005). Although these results appear to be contradictory, it is likely that it is the degree of low-oxygen tension and subsequent HIF-1 induction in either small avascular lesions or large hypoxic and necrotic lesions that leads to increased influx of EPC. Further support for hypoxia as the main regulator of BMDC recruitment stems from the observation that upon ablation of tumor vessels by vascular disrupting agents in xenograft tumor models, the resulting acute hypoxia and necrosis were accompanied by transient recruitment of EPC to the tumor margins, thus facilitating revascularization (Shaked et al., 2006). These results collectively suggest that EPC influx may be dependent on a threshold of hypoxia or on the degree of low-oxygen tension (Dewhirst et al., 2008).

While GBM are considered as highly hypoxic and very angiogenic tumors, the incorporation of bone marrow-derived EPC into various xenograft mouse GBM models was found to be modest and with highly variable frequencies ranging from 0.2 to 26% of vessels (Table 31.1). Besides variations in the sensitivity of the techniques used to visualize EPC in tumors, the varying numbers of EPC observed might also relate to variability in the degree of low-oxygen tension observed in tumors derived from different glioma cell lines. Indeed, the frequency of EPC incorporation correlated with the inherent hypoxic status of the respective GBM models used (Aghi et al., 2006). Further substantiation stems from a GBM mouse model in which HIF-1 activity was absent by genetic ablation (Blouw et al., 2003). In the absence of HIF-1, the

Table 31.1 Frequency of vascular progenitor cells (EPC, PPC) and CD45+ myeloid support cells in orthotopic and subcutaneous glioma mouse models

Glioma model	EPC (% of vessel)	PPC (% of vessel)	CD45 + BMDC (% of GFP + cells)	Detection	References
GL261 s.c. + i.c.	0.3%	n.d.	n.d.	IHC	Machein et al. (2003)
GL261-VEGF s.c. + i.c.	0.6%	n.d.	n.d.	IHC	
GL261 i.c.	0–0.5%	0%	n.d.	IHC	Aghi et al. (2006)
GL261 s.c.	0%	1.2%	n.d.		
GL261-pSDF-1α i.c.	20.5%	Yes	n.d.	IHC	
GL261-pSDF-1α s.c.	19.9%	11.9 (22.3% FACS)	n.d.	IHC/FACS	
KR158/ΔEGFR s.c.	19.7%	12–22%	n.d.	IHC/FACS	
KR158//ΔEGFR i.c.	25–26%	n.d.	n.d.	IHC	
RT-2/RAG glioma	0.49%	n.d.	n.d.	IHC	Yung et al. (2004)
RT-2/RAG glioma i.c.	8%	n.d.	n.d.	IHC	Udani et al. (2005)
RT-2/RAG glioma i.c.	4%	n.d.	n.d.	IHC	Santarelli et al. (2006)
RT-2/RAG glioma	n.d.	9.1% (NG2+) 24.1% (PDGFR-β+) 12.0% (α-SMA+)	n.d.	IHC	Bababeygy et al. (2008)
U87 s.c.	10–25%	n.d.	n.d.	IHC	Ferrari et al. (2003)
U87 i.c.	0%	0%	100%	IHC/FACS	De Palma et al. (2005)
0627-NSC-GBM	0%	<2%	100% (85% F4/80+)	IHC/FACS	De Palma et al. (2005)
Tag/Hras GBM i.c.	10.3%	2.2%	98% (of GFP+ cells) 11.5% TEM 1.8% Hemangiocytes, 45% F4/80+30% CD11b+ monocytes	IHC/FACS	Du et al. (2008)
	1.8%	0.4%	16% (of all cells within tumor)		

Table 31.1 (continued)

Glioma model	EPC (% of vessel)	PPC (% of vessel)	CD45 + BMDC (% of GFP + cells)	Detection	References
HIFko Tag/Hras i.c.	0.4%	0.05%	5% (of cells within tumor)	IHC/FACS	Du et al. (2008)
	6.39%	0.8%	97% (of all GFP+ cells)		
			8.6% TEM		
			2.2% Hemangiocytes, 45% F4/80+31% CD11b+ monocytes		

Frequency of EPC incorporation is calculated as the percentage of tumor vessels with GFP+ or galactosidase+ cells, or as the percentage of VEGFR2+ cells in the GFP+ cell population that resides within a tumor, or as the percentage of GFP+/VEGFR2+ cells within a tumor. PPC incorporation is calculated as the percentage of NG2+ or CD11b+ cells (Aghi et al., 2006), or as Sca-1+/PDGFR-β+ cells within the GFP population (Du et al., 2008), or as GFP+ Sca-1, PDGFR-β+ cells within the tumor (Du et al., 2008), or as GFP populations either expressing PDGFR-β, α-SMA, or NG2 (Bababeygy et al., 2008). CD45+ myeloid BMDCs are quantified as percentage of the GFP population (De Palma et al., 2005; Du et al., 2008) or as percentage of the tumor (Du et al., 2008). Abbreviations: IHC, immunohistochemistry on tissue sections; FACS, fluorescence-activated cell sorting of tumors; n.d., not determined.

hypoxic response was impaired, leading to decreased levels of SDF-1α and VEGF and subsequent reduction of EPC incorporation into the tumor vessels (Fig. 31.1) (Du et al., 2008a). Collectively, these data reveal that gliomas recruit EPC, albeit at a modest rate, to their growing blood vessels when they undergo rapid growth and become highly hypoxic.

31.2.1.2 Pericyte Progenitor Cells (PPC)

Pericytes (mural cells; vascular smooth muscle cells) are perivascular cells with long cytoplasmic processes and contractile abilities, which envelop microvessels (capillaries and postcapillary venules) (Bergers and Song, 2005). They are implicated in hemostatic regulation of blood vessels and support stabilization and maturation of growing blood vessels. In contrast to endothelial cells, there exist no specific markers for pericytes, but they commonly express myofilaments such as α-smooth muscle actin (α-SMA) or desmin and also PDGFR-β (platelet-derived growth factor receptor-β), NG2 (HMW-MMA), a proteoglycan, and RGS5, a regulator of G-protein signaling, which has recently been implicated in blood vessel normalization (Andrae et al., 2008; Bergers and Song, 2005; Hamzah et al., 2008). A growing number of studies have demonstrated the presence of bone marrow-derived pericyte progenitor cells (PPC) that give rise to pericytes. One of the early studies revealed bone marrow-derived CD11b+ and CD45+ hematopoietic cells, expressing the pericyte marker NG2, in close proximity to blood vessels in a subcutaneous Bl6-F1 melanoma model (Rajantie et al., 2004). The existence of bone marrow-derived PPC was further corroborated by the identification of PDGFR-β^+ Sca-1+ pericyte progenitors (PPP) in a transgenic mouse model of neuroendocrine pancreatic tumorigenesis. PPC were able to differentiate into pericytes and regulate vessel stability and vascular survival in these tumors. The majority of pericytic cells were found to be PDGFR-β-positive but negative for the mature pericyte markers NG2, α-SMA, and desmin (~46%). More than 50% of these cells expressed the hematopoietic marker Sca-1 and elicited the pericyte progenitor pool as they were able to differentiate into mature pericytes in vitro. About 15–26% were double-positive for PDGFR-β and NG2, α-SMA, or desmin, and surprisingly about 28% expressed only mature pericyte markers but not PDGFR-β (Song et al., 2005). Thus, in these murine pancreatic tumors exist a heterogeneous population of pericytes that are composed of distinct maturation stages. So far only three studies have provided evidence for the existence of bone marrow-derived pericyte progenitors in mouse models for GBM (Table 31.1). The first study used mature pericyte markers in combination with GFP and found distinct populations of immature and mature bone marrow-derived pericytes (Bababeygy et al., 2008), nicely confirming the observations about pericyte progenitors and their differentiation capability in the pancreatic endocrine tumor model (Song et al., 2005). The second study focused on the pericyte progenitor population in GBM (PDGFR-β+/Sca-1+) but did not investigate bone marrow-derived pericytes that already had undergone differentiation (Du et al., 2008a). The third study detected pericytes from the bone marrow in different GBM xenograft models by using the markers NG2 or CD11b (Aghi et al., 2006). The higher incidence of bone marrow-derived pericytes in the latter study might be attributed to the marker CD11b, which albeit expressed by some PPC is not considered a pericyte marker and is found in a variety of different myeloid cells (Rajantie et al., 2004). In all three studies, PPC incorporated into GBM vessels at differing but still modest rates depending on the xenograft tumor model, the use of markers, and the detection method. In general, like for EPC, recruitment of bone marrow-derived PPC was regulated by hypoxia in GBM that depended on active MMP-9 in the bone marrow to facilitate mobilization into the bloodstream (Aghi et al., 2006; Du et al., 2008a). Given the early stage of these studies that are also limited to xenograft tumor models, it remains to be elucidated how significant PPC are for human GBM and other tumors to promote neovascularization.

31.2.2 Proangiogenic Myeloid Support Cells

CD45+ myeloid cells constitute the largest and most heterogeneous group of tumor-infiltrating BMDC that have important roles in regulating formation and maintenance of blood vessels in tumors. In contrast to vascular progenitors, these cells reside in close proximity to tumor vessels but are physically not part of the vasculature. They function as proangiogenic support cells because they produce a variety of proangiogenic factors, cytokines, and proteases (Murdoch et al., 2008; Schmid and Varner, 2007). The most prominent subpopulations include tumor-associated macrophages (TAM) (Pollard, 2004) and immature monocytic cells including Tie2+ monocytes (TEM) (De Palma et al., 2005), VEGFR1+ CXCR4+ hemangiocytes (Rafii et al., 2002b), and CD11b+ Gr1+ myeloid-derived suppressive cells (MDSC) (Yang et al., 2004). In addition, neutrophils, mast cells, and dendritic cells have also been described to be able to support neovascularization (Murdoch et al., 2008). While there is now a wealth of data emphasizing the functional significance of CD45 myeloid cells in a variety of different tumor types, so far only few publications have emerged that besides describing the presence of myeloid cells also highlight their importance in GBM biology (Table 31.1). Like EPC and PPC, CD45+ BMDC infiltration is regulated by hypoxia since ablation of HIF-1 in a GBM model dramatically reduced infiltration of CD45+ cells, rendering these tumors unable to induce neovascularization (Fig. 31.1) (Du et al., 2008a). One of the critical hypoxia-regulated factors involved in the recruitment and retention of CD45+ myeloid cells appears to be again SDF-1α (Aghi et al., 2006; Du et al., 2008a). In the aforementioned GBM model, the VEGF-MMP-9 pathway did not substantially affect the influx of CD45+ monocytes. Tumors of SV40Tag/Hras-transformed astrocytes that were genetically deficient in MMP-9 and grown in MMP-9 knockout mice, exhibited low

VEGF activity and a defect in progenitor mobilization due to lack of MMP-9 in the bone marrow but harbored the same amount of CD45+ cells as tumors propagating in wild-type animals (Du et al., 2008a; Rafii et al., 2003). The reason why these tumors did not show differences in CD45 recruitment was based on the comparably high levels of SDF-1α between wild-type GBM and tumors devoid of MMP-9. Further, treatment of wild-type tumor-bearing mice with the CXCR4 inhibitor AMD3100 resulted in reduction of intratumoral CD45+ myeloid cells (Du et al., 2008a). These data support the results from other laboratories that VEGF, albeit a strong mobilization factor, is not critical for the retention of BMDC in GBM xenografts, which relies on intratumoral SDF-1α (Aghi et al., 2006; Machein et al., 2003).

Nevertheless, one of the major mechanisms that CD45+ cells utilize to promote angiogenesis still lies in MMP-9, which these infiltrating cells express in the tumors where it acts as an angiogenesis-modulating factor to facilitate VEGF activity (Du et al., 2008a). This mechanism has also been observed in an endogenous mouse model of multistep pancreatic endocrine tumorigenesis in which infiltrating neutrophils secrete MMP-9 into premalignant lesions to enable VEGF activation and subsequently the onset of angiogenesis (Bergers et al., 2000; Nozawa et al., 2006). As mentioned before, many of the CD45+ cells also express CXCR4, the receptor for SDF-1α (CXCL12). The first indication that this subpopulation of myeloid cells is critical for promoting tumor angiogenesis came from studies where CXCR4 was inhibited with AMD3100 in different mouse tumor models including GBM (Du et al., 2008a; Grunewald et al., 2006) (see also Chapter 34). Upon treatment, tumor vessels looked more normalized, were reduced in numbers, and this was accompanied by a reduction in tumor-infiltrating CXCR4+ BMDC, supporting the notion that SDF-1α (CXCL12) is a pivotal factor for CD45+ BMDC influx (Du et al., 2008a; Grunewald et al., 2006). It is important to note, however, that AMD3100 also targets CXCR4+ endothelial progenitor cells that, albeit rare, still might have supplemental effects in neovascularization. In addition, glioma cells and tumor stem cells were found to express CXCR4+, which when targeted very likely contribute to the benefits of AMD3100 therapy (Hermann et al., 2007; Kucia et al., 2005; Ratajczak et al., 2006; Zagzag et al., 2008). Clearly, myeloid cell populations share various proangiogenic factors but little is known so far what distinct roles the heterogeneous CD45+ myeloid cell populations play in tumor neovascularization. The functions of some of the proangiogenic myeloid subpopulations that have been found in GBMs are described in more detail below.

31.2.2.1 Tumor-Associated Macrophages (TAM)

Historically, macrophages were merely thought to engulf invading microbes or cell debris from injured sites and kill tumor cells. Many human tumors are infiltrated with tumor-associated macrophages (TAM) but clinical reports have highlighted a correlation between the macrophage infiltration in tumors and a poor clinical prognosis obscuring their function in tumors (de Palma and Coussens, 2008). Macrophage infiltration is also correlated with astrocytoma progression; low levels are found in WHO grade II and III, while their levels are highly increased in GBM (Nishie et al., 1999). These results are congruent with the observation that macrophage infiltration is induced under low-oxygen conditions, which are apparent in GBM but not in lower grade astrocytomas, leading to preferential cell accumulation at necrotic and hypoxic areas in various murine and human tumors including GBM where they scavenge cellular debris and may cooperate with tumor cells to promote angiogenesis (Du et al., 2008a; Komohara et al., 2008; Lewis and Murdoch, 2005; Lin et al., 2006; Strik et al., 2004). Once in hypoxic areas of tumors, TAM are known to endorse proangiogenic activities by producing various proangiogenic and angiogenesis-modulating factors including VEGF, basic fibroblast growth factor (bFGF, FGF2), platelet-derived growth factor (PDGF), interleukin-8 (IL-8, CXCL8), and several matrix metalloproteinases like MMP7, MMP9, and MMP12 and urokinase-type plasminogen activator (uPA) (Murdoch et al., 2008; Pollard, 2004). It is also notable that TAM release nitric oxide (NO), which provokes vasodilation and increases vascular flow, through the activity of inducible NO synthase (iNOS) (de Palma and Coussens, 2008).

Among various chemoattractants like CSF-1 (colony-stimulating factor-1) and CCL-5 (RANTES), MCP-1 (CCL-2) induces macrophage recruitment, and its expression increases during astrocytoma progression and is highly elevated in GBM (Desbaillets et al., 1994; Leung et al., 1997; Murdoch et al., 2004). TAM can be derived from locally recruited tissue macrophages or from circulating monocytes. In general, there are two pathways to produce activated macrophages in vivo (Mantovani et al., 2006). M1 macrophage activation in human and mice occurs in response to lipopolysaccharide and interferon-γ (IFN-γ) and is characterized by high production of IL-12 and IL-23 (Verreck et al., 2004). This activates a type I response and is characterized by high capacity to present antigen and to produce factors that promote T-cell proliferation and activity, criteria that allow M1 macrophages to kill microorganisms and tumor cells. In contrast, exposure to glucocortoid hormones, IL-10, and IL-13 induces polarized type II or M2 macrophages that have poor antigen-presenting capability and an immunosuppressive phenotype. These cells are better adapted to scavenging debris, promoting angiogenesis, and repairing and remodeling wounded tissues (Allavena et al., 2008; Guruvayoorappan, 2008; Mantovani et al., 2006). Interestingly, various documentations exist from murine and human tumors describing that when monocytes infiltrate into the tumor, they often differentiate into activated, tumor-associated macrophages that reflect a M2 macrophage phenotype. Thus, the tumor produces a cytokine profile that is able to polarize macrophages in a way that they exhibit protumoral functions. A recent study revealed that tumor macrophages in human GBM tissues were also prevalent as M2 polarized macrophages, supporting their implications in GBM progression as they are capable of producing factors that facilitate tumor progression, angiogenesis, and extracellular matrix degradation and suppressing antitumor immune activities (Komohara et al., 2008).

31.2.2.2 TIE2-Expressing Monocytes (TEM)

A subpopulation of circulating blood monocytes was recently discovered that can be distinguished from other circulating monocytes by its expression of the angiopoietin receptor TIE2 (TEK) (De Palma et al., 2005). TEM have been identified in the peripheral blood of both humans and mice and are distinct from the previously described circulating endothelial cells or endothelial progenitors cells that also express TIE2 (Murdoch et al., 2007, De Palma, 2005 #518). TEM are found in close proximity to the vasculature in various human tumors and have also been identified in spontaneous and orthotopically implanted tumors, including GBM, in mice (Table 31.1) (De Palma et al., 2005; Du et al., 2008a). Unlike peripheral blood monocytes, TEM do not express chemokine (C–C motif) receptor 2 (CCR2) and are unlikely to respond to MCP-1 (CCL2). This suggests that TEM are recruited to tumors by a mechanism different from that of monocytes that are destined to differentiate into TAM (Murdoch et al., 2008). Recent studies have indicated that TEM could be recruited by the TIE2 ligand, angiopoietin-2 (Murdoch et al., 2007; Venneri et al., 2007), a cytokine abundantly expressed by both hypoxic tumor cells and endothelial cells in tumor blood vessels (Stratmann et al., 1998)(see also Chapter 21). Indeed, upregulation of angiopoietin-2 was found to be an early event in vascular remodeling in GBM (Holash et al., 1999). These results support the notion that early infiltration of monocytes and macrophages triggered by hypoxia and angiopoietin-2 could initiate the angiogenic switch in GBM. The functional significance of TEM in neovascularization was demonstrated by generating a system in which Tie2+ monocytes could be specifically ablated by the administration of ganciclovir using a gene-directed enzyme–prodrug therapy (De Palma et al., 2005). Ganciclovir treatment completely ablated TEM in intracerebral U87MG xenografts, resulting in a marked reduction in angiogenesis and tumor growth. Importantly, ablation of TEM did not affect the recruitment of TAM or neutrophils to these tumors, suggesting that, rather than being precursors of TAM, TEM comprise a distinct monocyte subpopulation with potent proangiogenic activity. What these studies also demonstrate is that TEM contributed to only about 5% of the monocytic tumor infiltrate population, yet were the most potent source of proangiogenic signals in these experimental models, suggesting that TEM significantly contribute to tumor angiogenesis. These results are in accordance with other findings demonstrating that in contrast to TAM and CD11b+ monocytes, nearly all TEM expressed high levels of the protease MMP-9, sufficient to initiate the angiogenic switch in experimental GBM (Du et al., 2008a). Besides basic fibroblast growth factor (bFGF), which was expressed by TEM in a glioma xenograft model, little is known about other TEM-produced factors in angiogenesis, an area that is under current investigation (De Palma et al., 2005).

31.2.2.3 VEGFR1+ CXCR4+ Hemangiocytes

Recently, a VEGFR1+/CXCR4+ hematopoietic cell population (HPC) was first described in mice that has potent pro-angiogenic properties in vivo in non-malignant tissues, where they appear to restore tissue perfusion and counteract ischemia. These cells have now also been shown to promote angiogenesis in various murine and human tumors and metastatic lesions (Hattori et al., 2001b; Kaplan et al., 2005; Lyden et al., 2001; Rafii et al., 2002b). As with TEM, VEGR1+ HPC reside mainly in perivascular regions where they are thought to help stabilize blood vessels through the release of angiogenic factors (Hattori et al., 2001a; Rafii et al., 2002a). Mobilization of these cells from the bone marrow and their recruitment to ischemic tissues was first shown to be regulated by CXCL12/SDF-1α and VEGF (Hattori et al., 2003). Based on the observations that hypoxic tumor cells upregulate SDF-1α and VEGF, and HIF-1-deficient GBM exhibit a reduced number of VEGFR1+ hemangiocytes, increased levels of these cytokines also appear to be instrumental in recruiting hemangiocytes to hypoxic areas of tumors including GBM to promote tumor angiogenesis (Table 31.1) (Du et al., 2008b; Grunewald et al., 2006; Rafii et al., 2002a). Accordingly, a recent study demonstrated that loss of VEGFR-1 (Flt-1) signaling in bone marrow-derived myeloid cells led to a significant decrease in tumor volume and vascularization in gliomas (Kerber et al., 2008).

31.2.2.4 Myeloid-Derived Suppressor Cells (MDSC)

Myeloid-derived suppressor cells (MDSC) are a heterogeneous population of cells comprising precursors of monocytes and neutrophils that display immunosuppressive features. These cells express both myeloid differentiation antigen Gr1 and α_M integrin CD11b. In contrast to mature neutrophils, MDSC potently suppress dendritic cell (DC) maturation and the antitumor functions of T and natural killer (NK) cells, a phenotype that currently provides the most effective way of identifying MDSC (Gabrilovich et al., 2007) (see also Chapter 48). While MDSC are primarily located in the bone marrow in the adult, elevated levels of these cells have been found in the spleen and tumors in tumor-bearing mice as well as in blood and tumors of human patients. In humans, MDSC are generally defined as CD14– CD11b+ cells or as cells that express the common myeloid marker CD33 but lack mature myeloid and lymphoid cells (Nagaraj and Gabrilovich, 2008). First, indirect indication that monocytes with immunosuppressive functions might also be prevalent in human GBM came from early studies in which supernatants from human GBM cultures were shown to suppress T-cell responses and alter the cytokine profile of monocytic cells. This result suggested that monocytes can develop immunosuppressive functions in GBM (Zou et al., 1999). A recent study described infiltration of CD11b+ myeloid cells in a subcutaneous GL261 GBM xenograft model of which more than 90% were positive for the macrophage marker F4/80. Some of these cells were also defined as MDSC as they suppressed the proliferation of activated spleenic CD8+ T cells and had a CD11b+ CD11c+Gr1^{low}IL-4Rα+ phenotype (Umemura et al., 2008). MDSC, however, do promote tumor propagation not only by their immunosuppressive activity but also by their ability to endorse neovascularization in various tumor types including GBM (Table 31.1) (Shojaei et al., 2008a; Yang et al., 2004). Like the other proangiogenic monocytic populations, MDSC express high levels of MMP-9 that trigger VEGF release from the ECM, which then activates VEGF receptors on endothelial cells (Du et al., 2008a; Yang et al., 2004). Tumor-bearing animals have been shown to elicit increased levels of MDSC in the blood and spleen, which are mediated, in part, by the cytokines Bv8 and endocrine gland-derived VEGF (EG-VEGF) produced in the tumor (Ferrara et al., 2004; LeCouter et al., 2004; Shojaei et al., 2008a; Yang et al., 2004). Both Bv8 and EG-VEGF bind to G-protein-coupled receptors EG-VEGFR1 and EG-VEGFR2, thereby partly stimulating migration of CD11b+ Gr1+ MDSC in vitro (Ferrara et al., 2004; Yang et al., 2008). Recruitment of MDSC to the tumor site is then governed by chemotactic factors like CXCL12/SDF-1α, MCP-1 (CCL2), and CXCL5 and KIT ligand [stem cell factor (SCF; KITL)] that bind to and activate their respective receptors CXCR4, CCR2, CXCR2, and KIT (CD117) on MDSC (Murdoch et al., 2008).

So far the prevalence and function of MDSC in GBM have not been thoroughly studied, but given their importance in immune suppression and angiogenesis, these studies are highly warranted. Interestingly, a recent preclinical study revealed that infiltrating CD11b+ Gr1+ cells were responsible for the nonresponsiveness of murine transplant tumors to anti-VEGF therapy, likely because they express alternative factors that overcome angiogenic inhibition. Pharmacological impairment of myeloid cell recruitment rendered the otherwise resistant tumors responsive to the VEGF blockade (Shojaei et al., 2007). This raises the important question as to whether hypoxia-induced influx of this and other myeloid populations provoked by tumor vessel reduction can potentially endorse adaptive resistance to antiangiogenic agents in GBM and other tumors, given that in both preclinical and clinical settings, the benefits of antiangiogenic therapy are transitory and are followed by a restoration of tumor growth and progression (Bergers and Hanahan, 2008).

31.3 Conclusions

The angiogenic switch in GBM is predominantly triggered by hypoxia and necrosis, which activate the production of proangiogenic factors by the tumor and host cells. Neovascularization occurs by activating residing endothelial cells and pericytes and by the recruitment of vascular progenitors and myeloid angiogenic support cells from the bone marrow (Fig. 31.2). The threshold of or the degree of low-oxygen tension in gliomas and other tumors appears to be pivotal for BMDC infiltration. Such influx is predominantly governed by the hypoxia-inducible factors VEGF, PlGF, SDF-1α, and angiopoietin-2, which

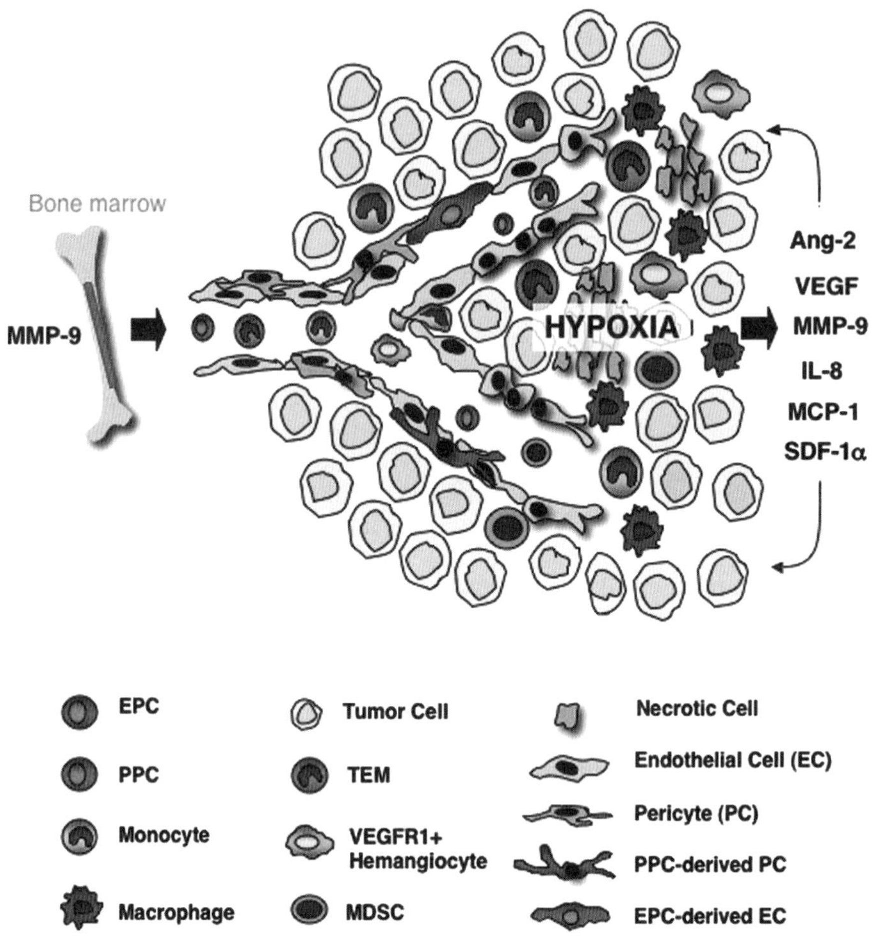

Fig. 31.2 Hypoxia-induced factors promote vasculogenesis and angiogenesis by recruiting vascular progenitors and proangiogenic myeloid cells. Hypoxia in GBM increases HIF1, which in part, by inducing VEGF and SDF-1α in tumor cells, recruits BMDC including EPC, PPC, and distinct CD45+ myeloid proangiogenic cell populations to endorse vascular remodeling in GBM. While VEGF acts as a mobilization factor for vascular progenitor cells and VEGFR1+ myeloid cells, SDF-1α predominantly serves as a retention factor of CXCR4+ vascular progenitor and monocytic BMDC. Similarly, hypoxia-induced angiopoietin-2 has been suggested to retain Tie-2+ monocytes (TEM). Tumor-produced MCP-1 (CCL-2), CSF-1, and IL-8 (CXCL8) serve as chemoattractants for macrophages and granulocytes, respectively. Besides the incorporation of EPC and PPC into growing vessels, the influx of myeloid cells into the tumor provides additional proangiogenic factors such as MMP-9, VEGF, PDGF, and very likely also FGF that foster GBM tumor neovascularization and progression

mobilize BMDC from the bone marrow into the bloodstream or retain them to the tumor. While endothelial and pericyte progenitors are incorporated at rather modest levels into growing GBM vessels, the majority of BDMC consist of a heterogeneous group of CD45+ myeloid cells that all facilitate neovascularization by expressing proangiogenic and angiogenesis-modulating factors pivotal to the formation and maintenance of GBM and other tumor vessels. In GBM xenograft models, BMDC can make up to 20% of the total tumor population underscoring their potential impact on tumor propagation and progression. While macrophages have been repeatedly observed in GBM, yet hardly anything is known about the other BMDC populations in murine and human GBM.

Investigations into BMDC appear to not only be instrumental for nascent tumors but may also be very important in the context of antiangiogenic therapy. Notably, there are reports suggesting that antiangiogenesis-induced hypoxia can elicit BMDC recruitment and thereby foster an adaptive mechanism that enables tumors, including GBM, to overcome hypoxia and induce reneovascularization. Indeed, there is indirect but intriguing evidence from clinical investigations that this evasion mechanism operates in patients with GBM who are undergoing anti-VEGF therapy. One study suggests that hypoxia determines survival outcome in bevacizumab-treated GBM patients and a second study reported that GBM patients treated with a pan-VEGFR kinase inhibitor exhibited elevated levels of SDF-1α (as well as of bFGF) in the blood at the time of tumor progression and relapse (Batchelor et al., 2007; Sathornsumetee et al., 2008). Inferentially, SDF-1α could be a potential effector of and bioresponse marker of response for relapsing GBM, raising the possibility that this form of evasive resistance could be operative in glioblastoma.

Taken together, all these data support the notion that BMDC are pivotal contributors in tumor progression and angiogenesis. The significant variation in recruitment and utilization of vascular progenitor cells and the predominant influx of myeloid proangiogenic support cells in GBM and other tumor models underscore the need to further delineate the mechanisms by which they are activated and recruited, as well as their contributions to tumor neovascularization in these contexts. In particular, it will be critical to dissect in more detail the specific BMDC populations recruited to various tumors and better characterize their functional roles in promoting angiogenesis. More data are just emerging that highlight their prevalence in GBM, further motivating an agenda to assess the functional significance and contribution of the distinct myeloid BMDC populations in neovascularization and progression in GBM.

Abbreviations

BMDC	bone marrow-derived cells
EPC	endothelial progenitor cells
PPC	pericyte progenitor cells
TAM	Tumor-associated macrophages
TEM	Tie2+ monocytes
MDSC	myeloid-derived suppressive cells

References

Aghi, M. and Chiocca, E. A. (2005). Contribution of bone marrow-derived cells to blood vessels in ischemic tissues and tumors. Mol Ther *12*, 994–1005.

Aghi, M., Cohen, K. S., Klein, R. J., Scadden, D. T., and Chiocca, E. A. (2006). Tumor stromal-derived factor-1 recruits vascular progenitors to mitotic neovasculature, where microenvironment influences their differentiated phenotypes. Cancer Res *66*, 9054–9064.

Allavena, P., Garlanda, C., Borrello, M. G., Sica, A., and Mantovani, A. (2008). Pathways connecting inflammation and cancer. Curr Opin Genet Dev *18*, 3–10.

Andrae, J., Gallini, R., and Betsholtz, C. (2008). Role of platelet-derived growth factors in physiology and medicine. Genes Dev *22*, 1276–1312.

Asahara, T., Murohara, T., Sullivan, A., Silver, M., van der Zee, R., Li, T., Witzenbichler, B., Schatteman, G., and Isner, J. M. (1997). Isolation of putative progenitor endothelial cells for angiogenesis. Science *275*, 964–967.

Bababeygy, S. R., Cheshier, S. H., Hou, L. C., Higgins, D. M., Weissman, I. L., and Tse, V. C. (2008). Hematopoietic stem cell-derived pericytic cells in brain tumor angio-architecture. Stem Cells Dev *17*, 11–18.

Baluk, P., Hashizume, H. and McDonald, D. M. (2005). Cellular abnormalities of blood vessels as targets in cancer. Curr Opin Genet Dev *15*, 102–111.

Batchelor, T. T., Sorensen, A. G., di Tomaso, E., Zhang, W. T., Duda, D. G., Cohen, K. S., Kozak, K. R., Cahill, D. P., Chen, P. J., Zhu, M., et al. (2007). AZD2171, a pan-VEGF receptor tyrosine kinase inhibitor, normalizes tumor vasculature and alleviates edema in glioblastoma patients. Cancer Cell *11*, 83–95.

Berger, M. S. and Wilson, C. B. (1999). The Gliomas. WB Saunders, Philadelphia.

Bergers, G. and Benjamin, L. E. (2003). Tumorigenesis and the angiogenic switch. Nat Rev Cancer *3*, 401–410.

Bergers, G., Brekken, R., McMahon, J., Vu, T., Itoh, T., Tamakki, k., Tanzawa, K., Thorpe, P., Itohara, S., Werb, Z., and Hanahan, D. (2000). Matrix Metalloproteinase-9 triggers the angiogenic switch during carcinogenesis. Nat Cell Biol *2*, 737.

Bergers, G. and Hanahan, D. (2008). Modes of resistance to anti-angiogenic therapy. Nat Rev Cancer *8*, 592–603.

Bergers, G. and Song, S. (2005). The role of pericytes in blood-vessel formation and maintenance. Neuro-oncol *7*, 452–464.

Bertolini, F., Shaked, Y., Mancuso, P., and Kerbel, R. S. (2006). The multifaceted circulating endothelial cell in cancer: towards marker and target identification. Nat Rev Cancer *6*, 835–845.

Black, W. C. and Welch, H. G. (1993). Advances in diagnostic imaging and overestimations of disease prevalence and the benefits of therapy. N Engl J Med *328*, 1237–1243.

Blouw, B., Song, H., Tihan, T., Bosze, J., Ferrara, N., Gerber, H. P., Johnson, R. S., and Bergers, G. (2003). The hypoxic response of tumors is dependent on their microenvironment. Cancer Cell *4*, 133–146.

Brat, D. J., Castellano-Sanchez, A., Kaur, B., and Van Meir, E. G. (2002). Genetic and biologic progression in astrocytomas and their relation to angiogenic dysregulation. Adv Anat Pathol *9*, 24–36.

Carmeliet, P. (2005). Angiogenesis in life, disease and medicine. Nature *438*, 932–936.

Carmeliet, P. and Tessier-Lavigne, M. (2005). Common mechanisms of nerve and blood vessel wiring. Nature *436*, 193–200.

Ceradini, D. J., Kulkarni, A. R., Callaghan, M. J., Tepper, O. M., Bastidas, N., Kleinman, M. E., Capla, J. M., Galiano, R. D., Levine, J. P., and Gurtner, G. C. (2004). Progenitor cell trafficking is regulated by hypoxic gradients through HIF-1 induction of SDF-1. Nat Med *10*, 858–864.

de Palma, M. and Coussens, L. M. (2008). Immune Cells and Inflammatory Mediators as Regulators of Tumor Angiogenesis. In Angiogenesis: An Integrative Approach from Science to Medicine, W.D. Figg, and J. Folkman, eds. (New York: Springer Science+ Business Media, LLC).

De Palma, M. and Naldini, L. (2006). Role of haematopoietic cells and endothelial progenitors in tumour angiogenesis. Biochim Biophys Acta *1766*, 159–166.

De Palma, M., Venneri, M. A., Galli, R., Sergi, L. S., Politi, L. S., Sampaolesi, M., and Naldini, L. (2005). Tie2 identifies a hematopoietic lineage of proangiogenic monocytes required for tumor vessel formation and a mesenchymal population of pericyte progenitors. Cancer Cell *8*, 211–226.

Desbaillets, I., Tada, M., de Tribolet, N., Diserens, A. C., Hamou, M. F., and Van Meir, E. G. (1994). Human astrocytomas and glioblastomas express monocyte chemoattractant protein-1 (MCP-1) in vivo and in vitro. Int J Cancer *58*, 240–247.

Dewhirst, M. W., Cao, Y., and Moeller, B. (2008). Cycling hypoxia and free radicals regulate angiogenesis and radiotherapy response. Nat Rev Cancer *8*, 425–437.

Du, R., Lu, K. V., Petritsch, C., Liu, P., Ganss, R., Passegue, E., Song, H., Vandenberg, S., Johnson, R. S., Werb, Z., and Bergers, G. (2008a). HIF1alpha Induces the Recruitment of Bone Marrow-Derived Vascular Modulatory Cells to Regulate Tumor Angiogenesis and Invasion. Cancer Cell *13*, 206–220.

Du, R., Petritsch, C., Lu, K., Liu, P., Haller, A., Ganss, R., Song, H., Vandenberg, S., and Bergers, G. (2008b). Matrix metalloproteinase-2 regulates vascular patterning and growth affecting tumor cell survival and invasion in GBM. Neuro Oncol *10*, 254–264.

Dvorak, H. F. (2000). VPF/VEGF and the angiogenic response. Semin Perinatol *24*, 75–78.

Eberhard, A., Kahlert, S., Goede, V., Hemmerlein, B., Plate, K. H., and Augustin, H. G. (2000). Heterogeneity of angiogenesis and blood vessel maturation in human tumors: implications for antiangiogenic tumor therapies. Cancer Res *60*, 1388–1393.

Ergun, S., Hohn, H. P., Kilic, N., Singer, B. B., and Tilki, D. (2008). Endothelial and hematopoietic progenitor cells (EPCs and HPCs): hand in hand fate determining partners for cancer cells. Stem Cell Rev *4*, 169–177.

Ferrara, N., LeCouter, J., Lin, R., and Peale, F. (2004). EG-VEGF and Bv8: a novel family of tissue-restricted angiogenic factors. Biochim Biophys Acta *1654*, 69–78.

Folkman, J. (1971). Tumor angiogenesis: therapeutic implications. N Engl J Med *285*, 1182–1186.

Folkman, J. (2006). Angiogenesis. Annu Rev Med *57*, 1–18.

Folkman, J., Watson, K., Ingber, D., and Hanahan, D. (1989). Induction of angiogenesis during the transition from hyperplasia to neoplasia. Nature *339*, 58–61.

Gabrilovich, D. I., Bronte, V., Chen, S. H., Colombo, M. P., Ochoa, A., Ostrand-Rosenberg, S., and Schreiber, H. (2007). The terminology issue for myeloid-derived suppressor cells. Cancer Res *67*, 425; author reply 426.

Ganss, R. (2006). Tumor stroma fosters neovascularization by recruitment of progenitor cells into the tumor bed. J Cell Mol Med *10*, 857–865.

Gehling, U. M., Ergun, S., Schumacher, U., Wagener, C., Pantel, K., Otte, M., Schuch, G., Schafhausen, P., Mende, T., Kilic, N., et al. (2000). In vitro differentiation of endothelial cells from AC133-positive progenitor cells. Blood *95*, 3106–3112.

Gerhardt, H., Golding, M., Fruttiger, M., Ruhrberg, C., Lundkvist, A., Abramsson, A., Jeltsch, M., Mitchell, C., Alitalo, K., Shima, D., and Betsholtz, C. (2003). VEGF guides angiogenic sprouting utilizing endothelial tip cell filopodia. J Cell Biol *161*, 1163–1177.

Grunewald, M., Avraham, I., Dor, Y., Bachar-Lustig, E., Itin, A., Jung, S., Chimenti, S., Landsman, L., Abramovitch, R., and Keshet, E. (2006). VEGF-induced adult neovascularization: recruitment, retention, and role of accessory cells. Cell *124*, 175–189.

Guruvayoorappan, C. (2008). Tumor versus tumor-associated macrophages: how hot is the link? Integr Cancer Ther *7*, 90–95.

Hamzah, J., Jugold, M., Kiessling, F., Rigby, P., Manzur, M., Marti, H. H., Rabie, T., Kaden, S., Grone, H. J., Hammerling, G. J., et al. (2008). Vascular normalization in Rgs5-deficient tumours promotes immune destruction. Nature *453*, 410–414.

Hanahan, D. and Folkman, J. (1996). Patterns and emerging mechanisms of the angiogenic switch during tumorigenesis. Cell *86*, 353.

Hanahan, D., and Weinberg, R. A. (2000). The hallmarks of cancer. Cell *100*, 57–70.

Hattori, K., Dias, S., Heissig, B., Hackett, N. R., Lyden, D., Tateno, M., Hicklin, D. J., Zhu, Z., Witte, L., Crystal, R. G., et al. (2001a). Vascular endothelial growth factor and angiopoietin-1 stimulate postnatal hematopoiesis by recruitment of vasculogenic and hematopoietic stem cells. J Exp Med *193*, 1005–1014.

Hattori, K., Heissig, B., and Rafii, S. (2003). The regulation of hematopoietic stem cell and progenitor mobilization by chemokine SDF-1. Leuk Lymphoma *44*, 575–582.

Hattori, K., Heissig, B., Tashiro, K., Honjo, T., Tateno, M., Shieh, J. H., Hackett, N. R., Quitoriano, M. S., Crystal, R. G., Rafii, S., and Moore, M. A. (2001b). Plasma elevation of stromal cell-derived factor-1 induces mobilization of mature and immature hematopoietic progenitor and stem cells. Blood *97*, 3354–3360.

Hattori, K., Heissig, B., Wu, Y., Dias, S., Tejada, R., Ferris, B., Hicklin, D. J., Zhu, Z., Bohlen, P., Witte, L., et al. (2002). Placental growth factor reconstitutes hematopoiesis by recruiting VEGFR1(+) stem cells from bone-marrow microenvironment. Nat Med *8*, 841–849.

Heissig, B., Hattori, K., Dias, S., Friedrich, M., Ferris, B., Hackett, N. R., Crystal, R. G., Besmer, P., Lyden, D., Moore, M. A., et al. (2002). Recruitment of stem and progenitor cells from the bone marrow niche requires MMP-9 mediated release of kit-ligand. Cell *109*, 625–637.

Hermann, P. C., Huber, S. L., Herrler, T., Aicher, A., Ellwart, J. W., Guba, M., Bruns, C. J., and Heeschen, C. (2007). Distinct populations of cancer stem cells determine tumor growth and metastatic activity in human pancreatic cancer. Cell Stem Cell *1*, 313–323.

Holash, J., Maisonpierre, P. C., Compton, D., Boland, P., Alexander, C. R., Zagzag, D., Yancopoulos, G. D., and Wiegand, S. J. (1999). Vessel cooption, regression, and growth in tumors mediated by angiopoietins and VEGF. Science *284*, 1994–1998.

Jain, R. K., di Tomaso, E., Duda, D. G., Loeffler, J. S., Sorensen, A. G., and Batchelor, T. T. (2007). Angiogenesis in brain tumours. Nat Rev Neurosci *8*, 610–622.

Kaplan, R. N., Riba, R. D., Zacharoulis, S., Bramley, A. H., Vincent, L., Costa, C., MacDonald, D. D., Jin, D. K., Shido, K., Kerns, S. A., et al. (2005). VEGFR1-positive haematopoietic bone marrow progenitors initiate the pre-metastatic niche. Nature *438*, 820–827.

Kerber, M., Reiss, Y., Wickersheim, A., Jugold, M., Kiessling, F., Heil, M., Tchaikovski, V., Waltenberger, J., Shibuya, M., Plate, K. H., and Machein, M. R. (2008). Flt-1 signaling in macrophages promotes glioma growth in vivo. Cancer Res *68*, 7342–7351.

Kleihues, P., Burger, P. C., Adalpe, K. D., Brat, D. J., Biernat, W., Bigner, D. D., Nakazato, Y., Plate, K. H., Giangaspero, F., von Deimling, A., and Cavanee, W. K. (2007a). Glioblastoma. In WHO Classification of Tumours of the Central Nervous System, D.N. Louis, H. Ohgaki, O.D. Wiestler, and W.K. Cavenee, eds. (Lyon, France: International Agency for Research on Cancer (IARC)), pp. 33–52.

Kleihues, P., Burger, P. C., Rosenblum, M. K., Paulus, W., and Scheithauser, B. W. (2007b). Anaplastic Astrocytoma. In WHO Classification of Tumours of the Central Nervous System, D.N. Louis, H. Ohgaki, O.D. Wiestler, and W.K. Cavenee, eds. (Lyon, France: International Agency for Research on Cancer (IARC)), pp. 30–32.

Komohara, Y., Ohnishi, K., Kuratsu, J., and Takeya, M. (2008). Possible involvement of the M2 anti-inflammatory macrophage phenotype in growth of human gliomas. J Pathol *216*, 15–24.

Kopp, H. G., Ramos, C. A., and Rafii, S. (2006). Contribution of endothelial progenitors and proangiogenic hematopoietic cells to vascularization of tumor and ischemic tissue. Curr Opin Hematol *13*, 175–181.

Kucia, M., Reca, R., Miekus, K., Wanzeck, J., Wojakowski, W., Janowska-Wieczorek, A., Ratajczak, J., and Ratajczak, M. Z. (2005). Trafficking of normal stem cells and metastasis of cancer stem cells involve similar mechanisms: pivotal role of the SDF-1-CXCR4 axis. Stem Cells *23*, 879–894.

Lamagna, C. and Bergers, G. (2006). The bone marrow constitutes a reservoir of pericyte progenitors. J Leukoc Biol *80*, 677–681.

LeCouter, J., Zlot, C., Tejada, M., Peale, F., and Ferrara, N. (2004). Bv8 and endocrine gland-derived vascular endothelial growth factor stimulate hematopoiesis and hematopoietic cell mobilization. Proc Natl Acad Sci U S A *101*, 16813–16818.

Leung, S. Y., Wong, M. P., Chung, L. P., Chan, A. S., and Yuen, S. T. (1997). Monocyte chemoattractant protein-1 expression and macrophage infiltration in gliomas. Acta Neuropathol *93*, 518–527.

Lewis, C. and Murdoch, C. (2005). Macrophage responses to hypoxia: implications for tumor progression and anti-cancer therapies. Am J Pathol *167*, 627–635.

Lin, E. Y., Li, J. F., Gnatovskiy, L., Deng, Y., Zhu, L., Grzesik, D. A., Qian, H., Xue, X. N., and Pollard, J. W. (2006). Macrophages regulate the angiogenic switch in a mouse model of breast cancer. Cancer Res *66*, 11238–11246.

Lyden, D., Hattori, K., Dias, S., Costa, C., Blaikie, P., Butros, L., Chadburn, A., Heissig, B., Marks, W., Witte, L., et al. (2001). Impaired recruitment of bone-marrow-derived endothelial and hematopoietic precursor cells blocks tumor angiogenesis and growth. Nat Med *7*, 1194–1201.

Machein, M. R., Renninger, S., de Lima-Hahn, E., and Plate, K. H. (2003). Minor contribution of bone marrow-derived endothelial progenitors to the vascularization of murine gliomas. Brain Pathol *13*, 582–597.

Mancuso, P., Burlini, A., Pruneri, G., Goldhirsch, A., Martinelli, G., and Bertolini, F. (2001). Resting and activated endothelial cells are increased in the peripheral blood of cancer patients. Blood *97*, 3658–3661.

Mantovani, A., Schioppa, T., Porta, C., Allavena, P., and Sica, A. (2006). Role of tumor-associated macrophages in tumor progression and invasion. Cancer Metastasis Rev *25*, 315–322.

Murdoch, C., Giannoudis, A., and Lewis, C. E. (2004). Mechanisms regulating the recruitment of macrophages into hypoxic areas of tumors and other ischemic tissues. Blood *104*, 2224–2234.

Murdoch, C., Muthana, M., Coffelt, S. B., and Lewis, C. E. (2008). The role of myeloid cells in the promotion of tumour angiogenesis. Nat Rev Cancer *8*, 618–631.

Murdoch, C., Tazzyman, S., Webster, S., and Lewis, C. E. (2007). Expression of Tie-2 by human monocytes and their responses to angiopoietin-2. J Immunol *178*, 7405–7411.

Nagaraj, S., and Gabrilovich, D. I. (2008). Tumor escape mechanism governed by myeloid-derived suppressor cells. Cancer Res *68*, 2561–2563.

Nishie, A., Ono, M., Shono, T., Fukushi, J., Otsubo, M., Onoue, H., Ito, Y., Inamura, T., Ikezaki, K., Fukui, M., et al. (1999). Macrophage infiltration and heme oxygenase-1 expression correlate with angiogenesis in human gliomas. Clin Cancer Res *5*, 1107–1113.

Nolan, D. J., Ciarrocchi, A., Mellick, A. S., Jaggi, J. S., Bambino, K., Gupta, S., Heikamp, E., McDevitt, M. R., Scheinberg, D. A., Benezra, R., and Mittal, V. (2007). Bone marrow-derived endothelial progenitor cells are a major determinant of nascent tumor neovascularization. Genes Dev *21*, 1546–1558.

Nozawa, H., Chiu, C., and Hanahan, D. (2006). Infiltrating neutrophils mediate the initial angiogenic switch in a mouse model of multistage carcinogenesis. Proc Natl Acad Sci USA *103*, 12493–12498.

Peichev, M., Naiyer, A. J., Pereira, D., Zhu, Z., Lane, W. J., Williams, M., Oz, M. C., Hicklin, D. J., Witte, L., Moore, M. A., and Rafii, S. (2000). Expression of VEGFR-2 and AC133 by circulating human CD34(+) cells identifies a population of functional endothelial precursors. Blood *95*, 952–958.

Peters, B. A., Diaz, L. A., Polyak, K., Meszler, L., Romans, K., Guinan, E. C., Antin, J. H., Myerson, D., Hamilton, S. R., Vogelstein, B., et al. (2005). Contribution of bone marrow-derived endothelial cells to human tumor vasculature. Nat Med *11*, 261–262.

Petit, I., Jin, D., and Rafii, S. (2007). The SDF-1-CXCR4 signaling pathway: a molecular hub modulating neo-angiogenesis. Trends Immunol *28*, 299–307.

Pollard, J. W. (2004). Tumour-educated macrophages promote tumour progression and metastasis. Nat Rev Cancer *4*, 71–78.

Rafii, S., Avecilla, S., Shmelkov, S., Shido, K., Tejada, R., Moore, M. A., Heissig, B., and Hattori, K. (2003). Angiogenic factors reconstitute hematopoiesis by recruiting stem cells from bone marrow microenvironment. Ann N Y Acad Sci *996*, 49–60.

Rafii, S., Lyden, D., Benezra, R., Hattori, K., and Heissig, B. (2002a). Vascular and haematopoietic stem cells: novel targets for anti-angiogenesis therapy? Nat Rev Cancer *2*, 826–835.

Rafii, S., Meeus, S., Dias, S., Hattori, K., Heissig, B., Shmelkov, S., Rafii, D., and Lyden, D. (2002b). Contribution of marrow-derived progenitors to vascular and cardiac regeneration. Semin Cell Dev Biol *13*, 61–67.

Rajantie, I., Ilmonen, M., Alminaite, A., Ozerdem, U., Alitalo, K., and Salven, P. (2004). Adult bone marrow-derived cells recruited during angiogenesis comprise precursors for periendothelial vascular mural cells. Blood *104*, 2084–2086.

Ratajczak, M. Z., Zuba-Surma, E., Kucia, M., Reca, R., Wojakowski, W., and Ratajczak, J. (2006). The pleiotropic effects of the SDF-1-CXCR4 axis in organogenesis, regeneration and tumorigenesis. Leukemia *20*, 1915–1924.

Rehman, J., Li, J., Orschell, C. M., and March, K. L. (2003). Peripheral blood "endothelial progenitor cells" are derived from monocyte/macrophages and secrete angiogenic growth factors. Circulation *107*, 1164–1169.

Rohde, E., Malischnik, C., Thaler, D., Maierhofer, T., Linkesch, W., Lanzer, G., Guelly, C., and Strunk, D. (2006). Blood monocytes mimic endothelial progenitor cells. Stem Cells *24*, 357–367.

Sathornsumetee, S., Cao, Y., Marcello, J. E., Herndon, J. E., 2nd, McLendon, R. E., Desjardins, A., Friedman, H. S., Dewhirst, M. W., Vredenburgh, J. J., and Rich, J. N. (2008). Tumor angiogenic and hypoxic profiles predict radiographic response and survival in malignant astrocytoma patients treated with bevacizumab and irinotecan. J Clin Oncol *26*, 271–278.

Schmeisser, A., Garlichs, C. D., Zhang, H., Eskafi, S., Graffy, C., Ludwig, J., Strasser, R. H., and Daniel, W. G. (2001). Monocytes coexpress endothelial and macrophagocytic lineage markers and form cord-like structures in Matrigel under angiogenic conditions. Cardiovasc Res *49*, 671–680.

Schmid, M. C. and Varner, J. A. (2007). Myeloid cell trafficking and tumor angiogenesis. Cancer Lett *250*, 1–8.

Shaked, Y., Ciarrocchi, A., Franco, M., Lee, C. R., Man, S., Cheung, A. M., Hicklin, D. J., Chaplin, D., Foster, F. S., Benezra, R., and Kerbel, R. S. (2006). Therapy-induced acute recruitment of circulating endothelial progenitor cells to tumors. Science *313*, 1785–1787.

Shojaei, F., Singh, M., Thompson, J. D., and Ferrara, N. (2008a). Role of Bv8 in neutrophil-dependent angiogenesis in a transgenic model of cancer progression. Proc Natl Acad Sci USA *105*, 2640–2645.

Shojaei, F., Wu, X., Malik, A. K., Zhong, C., Baldwin, M. E., Schanz, S., Fuh, G., Gerber, H. P., and Ferrara, N. (2007). Tumor refractoriness to anti-VEGF treatment is mediated by CD11b+Gr1+ myeloid cells. Nat Biotechnol *25*, 911–920.

Shojaei, F., Zhong, C., Wu, X., Yu, L., and Ferrara, N. (2008b). Role of myeloid cells in tumor angiogenesis and growth. Trends Cell Biol *18*, 372–378.

Song, S., Ewald, A. J., Stallcup, W., Werb, Z., and Bergers, G. (2005). PDGFR-β+ perivascular progenitor cells in tumours regulate pericyte differentiation and vascular survival. Nat Cell Biol *7*, 870–879.

Spring, H., Schuler, T., Arnold, B., Hammerling, G. J., and Ganss, R. (2005). Chemokines direct endothelial progenitors into tumor neovessels. Proc Natl Acad Sci U S A *102*, 18111–18116.

Stratmann, A., Risau, W., and Plate, K. H. (1998). Cell type-specific expression of angiopoietin-1 and angiopoietin-2 suggests a role in glioblastoma angiogenesis. Am J Pathol *153*, 1459–1466.

Strik, H. M., Stoll, M., and Meyermann, R. (2004). Immune cell infiltration of intrinsic and metastatic intracranial tumours. Anticancer Res *24*, 37–42.

Umemura, N., Saio, M., Suwa, T., Kitoh, Y., Bai, J., Nonaka, K., Ouyang, G. F., Okada, M., Balazs, M., Adany, R., et al. (2008). Tumor-infiltrating myeloid-derived suppressor cells are pleiotropic-inflamed monocytes/macrophages that bear M1- and M2-type characteristics. J Leukoc Biol *83*, 1136–1144.

Venneri, M. A., De Palma, M., Ponzoni, M., Pucci, F., Scielzo, C., Zonari, E., Mazzieri, R., Doglioni, C., and Naldini, L. (2007). Identification of proangiogenic TIE2-expressing monocytes (TEMs) in human peripheral blood and cancer. Blood *109*, 5276–5285.

Verreck, F. A., de Boer, T., Langenberg, D. M., Hoeve, M. A., Kramer, M., Vaisberg, E., Kastelein, R., Kolk, A., de Waal-Malefyt, R., and Ottenhoff, T. H. (2004). Human IL-23-producing type 1 macrophages promote but IL-10-producing type 2 macrophages subvert immunity to (myco)bacteria. Proc Natl Acad Sci U S A *101*, 4560–4565.

Yang, L., DeBusk, L. M., Fukuda, K., Fingleton, B., Green-Jarvis, B., Shyr, Y., Matrisian, L. M., Carbone, D. P., and Lin, P. C. (2004). Expansion of myeloid immune suppressor Gr+CD11b+ cells in tumor-bearing host directly promotes tumor angiogenesis. Cancer Cell *6*, 409–421.

Yang, L., Huang, J., Ren, X., Gorska, A. E., Chytil, A., Aakre, M., Carbone, D. P., Matrisian, L. M., Richmond, A., Lin, P. C., and Moses, H. L. (2008). Abrogation of TGF beta signaling in mammary carcinomas recruits Gr-1+CD11b+ myeloid cells that promote metastasis. Cancer Cell *13*, 23–35.

Zagzag, D., Amirnovin, R., Greco, M. A., Yee, H., Holash, J., Wiegand, S. J., Zabski, S., Yancopoulos, G. D., and Grumet, M. (2000). Vascular apoptosis and involution in gliomas precede neovascularization: a novel concept for glioma growth and angiogenesis. Lab Invest *80*, 837–849.

Zagzag, D., Esencay, M., Mendez, O., Yee, H., Smirnova, I., Huang, Y., Chiriboga, L., Lukyanov, E., Liu, M., and Newcomb, E. W. (2008). Hypoxia- and vascular endothelial growth factor-induced stromal cell-derived factor-1alpha/CXCR4 expression in glioblastomas: one plausible explanation of Scherer's structures. Am J Pathol *173*, 545–560.

Zou, J. P., Morford, L. A., Chougnet, C., Dix, A. R., Brooks, A. G., Torres, N., Shuman, J. D., Coligan, J. E., Brooks, W. H., Roszman, T. L., and Shearer, G. M. (1999). Human glioma-induced immunosuppression involves soluble factor(s) that alters monocyte cytokine profile and surface markers. J Immunol *162*, 4882–4892.

Chapter 32
Vascular Targeting of Brain Tumors – Bridging the Gap with Phage Display

Michael G. Ozawa, Fernanda I. Staquicini, Richard L. Sidman, Renata Pasqualini, and Wadih Arap

Abstract The development of targeted therapies for cancer remains an enormous challenge. Despite advances in the understanding of molecular pathways involved in tumor growth and rational design of new agents, a gap exists between drug development and patient survival. Ligand-directed delivery of drugs to the tumor is one approach to improve therapeutic indices and help close this gap. Tumor blood vessels are an attractive systemic target for site-directed delivery, as the endothelial lining is uniquely altered by the tumor microenvironment at early stages of disease progression. In the case of brain tumors, the normally restrictive blood–brain barrier becomes molecularly and structurally abnormal permitting specific systemic targeting. Phage display is ideally suited as a method to identify accessible ligand–receptor pairs in an unbiased, functional assay. Discovery of such specific directive systems for brain tumors would have wide-reaching applications for therapeutics and diagnostics.

Contents

R. Pasqualini (✉)
David H. Koch Center, The University of Texas M. D. Anderson Cancer Center, Houston, TX 77030, USA
e-mail: rpasqual@mdanderson.org

E.G. Van Meir (ed.), *CNS Cancer*, Cancer Drug Discovery and Development, DOI 10.1007/978-1-60327-553-8_32,
© Humana Press, a part of Springer Science+Business Media, LLC 2009

32.1 Introduction

Targeted medicine holds the promise to improve therapeutic efficacy while decreasing systemic toxicity. In oncology, early targeted agents have relied on differential functional attributes or gene/protein activities between normal and diseased cells for a therapeutic effect. The classic example is chemotherapies directed against mitotic cells. However, the lack of sufficient specificity for disease sites leads to unwanted effects in normal tissues undergoing rapid division, such as the intestine and bone marrow.

Improvements in the understanding of genetic alterations, protein modifications, and signal transduction pathways in cancer have brought newer and more selective molecularly targeted agents into development. In malignant gliomas, amplification of the epidermal growth factor receptor (EGFR) is seen in nearly 50% of all tumors, with nearly half of those abnormalities being a constitutively active form lacking a ligand-binding domain for EGF (Furnari et al. 2007). The prevalence of this mutation makes selective inhibition of EGFR signaling an attractive therapeutic strategy, either via small molecule inhibitors, blocking antibodies, or by other approaches. (Milano et al. 2008). Despite this targeted approach, overall, molecular agents have a less than 15% response rate with no improvement in 6 month progression-free survival (reviewed in Sathornsumetee et al. 2007). Moreover, growth factor inhibition can still affect other sites, as many growth factors have metabolic functions or promote downstream cascades not solely focused on cell proliferation or survival. This leads to undesired side effects and/or requires dose escalation for efficacy. Thus, alternative strategies are being explored intensively to improve therapeutic indices for patients.

One such approach is the site-specific delivery of agents by targeting ligands. This method relies on the identification of receptors that are distributed with sufficient differences between normal and diseased tissues to permit selective delivery. To become a reality, unique markers on pathological cells need to be identified and targeting molecules need to be developed. Tumor cells often have mutated proteins, overexpressed or differentially expressed proteins, or molecules present in abnormal subcellular locations (Hanahan and Weinberg 2000; Kinzler and Vogelstein 1997). These molecules would, in principle, be exclusive to the tumor microenvironment permitting targeted delivery of drugs. Yet, a fundamental requirement of tumor cell-directed agents is the need for systemic therapies to have access to the target cells. Complicated by changes in blood flow and interstitial pressures, among other physiological barriers, tumor cell targeting agents can have limited and unpredictable therapeutic profiles (Neri and Bicknell 2005).

The evidence has been building in recent years that vital structures associated with tumors, such as the tumor blood vessels, are valid components to target as a therapeutic strategy (Sessa et al. 2008). Tumor blood vessels possess markers that distinguish them from vessels in comparable normal organs, and thus they present a potentially powerful system for targeted therapeutics (Hajitou et al. 2006a). In this chapter, we will discuss the basic concepts of vascular targeting and in that context will describe bacteriophage (phage) display as a means to identify and develop ligand-directed therapeutics. While these concepts are applicable to numerous tumor subtypes, we will highlight the utility and pitfalls of vascular targeting for brain tumors as a new paradigm for disease monitoring and treatment.

32.2 The Principles of Phage Display

Phage display was initially used as a method to probe and identify the binding sites of antibodies in vitro (Smith 1985). The first report demonstrated that fragments of an *Eco*RI endonuclease could be fused to the amino-terminal portion of the pIII minor coat protein from filamentous phage creating chimeric proteins (Smith 1985) (Fig. 32.1). These phage particles retained

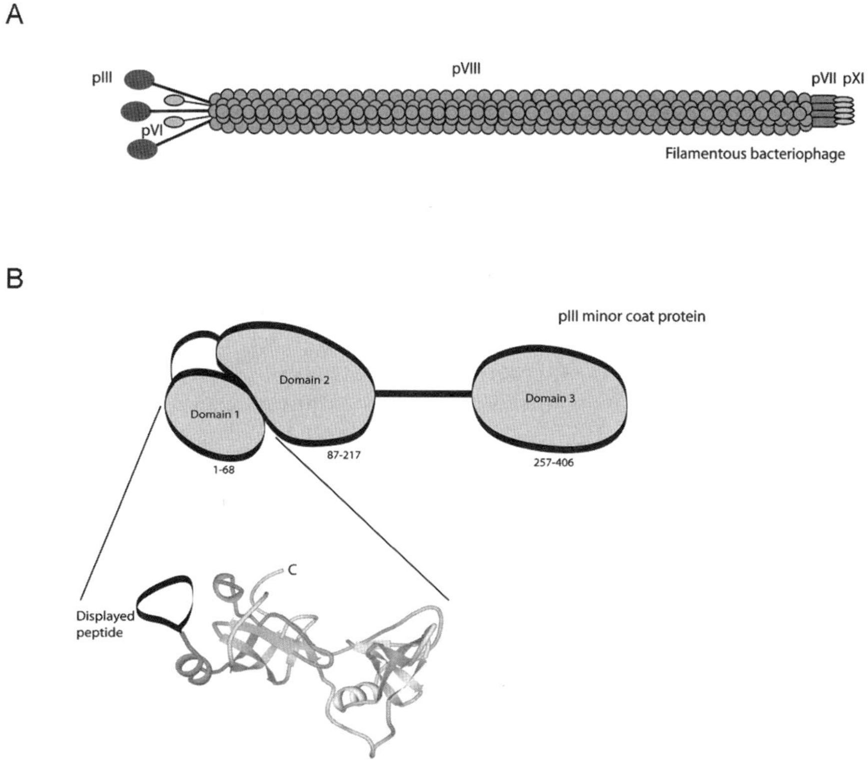

Fig. 32.1 (**A**) Schematic representation of filamentous phage depicting the organization of major (pVIII) and minor (pIII, pVI, pVII, pXI) coat proteins. (**B**) Illustration of the domain structure of pIII, with a detailed ribbon diagram of pIII domain 1 showing the location of phage-displayed peptides (black ribbon)

bacterial infectivity and were able to mediate specific binding to cognate antibodies of the *Eco*RI antibody. Further, following several rounds of affinity selection on the *Eco*RI antibody, phage displaying the *Eco*RI fragment was enriched compared to wild-type phage.

Subsequently, it was demonstrated that large peptide libraries of phage could be constructed as a method to identify specific epitopes binding to the variable region of antibodies (Parmley and Smith 1988; Scott and Smith 1990). The process, termed panning, uses a combinatorial peptide library created through DNA cloning techniques combining purified degenerate oligonucleotide primers with the phage DNA plasmid. The vectors are then transfected into host *Escherichia coli* bacteria for propagation and purification. This approach typically generates a library of up to 10^9 different permutations of peptides with sufficient diversity to probe protein–protein interactions in numerous experimental settings. Sequential rounds of phage binding, elution, and amplification on antibodies enrich for selective phage that can be analyzed by DNA sequencing to determine the peptides mediating binding. Lastly, through biochemical and bioinformatics-based analyses, the cognate proteins that the peptides mimic would then allow for further characterization and validation.

Since then, numerous groups have expanded this general screening approach to identify the antigenic repertoire of circulating antibodies in serum and ascitic fluid and the binding site of isolated molecules. For instance, screening of the humoral response in a prostate cancer patient identified an intracellular chaperone, glucose regulated protein-78 (GRP78) as an antigen eliciting an antibody response (Mintz et al. 2003). Further, the approach has been applied to cells in culture, isolating peptides that bind to cell surface molecules such as urokinase plasminogen activator, thrombin receptor, melanocortin receptor MC-1, integrins, and vascular endothelial growth factor receptors (VEGFR)-1 and -2 (Goodson et al. 1994; Doorbar and Winter 1994; Szardenings et al. 1997; Koivunen et al. 1993; Koivunen et al. 1994; Giordano et al. 2001).

Phage display has also been applied to the NCI-60 cancer cell panel as a high-throughput approach to profile cellular surface and evaluate tumor subtype similarities (Kolonin et al. 2006). First, the BRASIL method, a separation technique based on centrifugation through a non-miscible organic gradient, was used to identify distinct peptides specific to each cell line (Giordano et al. 2001). Next, 96 phage clones recovered from three sequential rounds of panning on each cell line were collected and sequenced. The amino acid sequences were analyzed with the aid of a computer-assisted survey that revealed a total of 26,031 tripeptide motifs (or three amino acid signatures). Bioinformatics-based analyses revealed that the peptide distribution within the NCI-60 set was nonrandom, yielding similarities among and across tumor subtypes, resulting in a collection of potential targets for validation.

With the early success of the phage display approach, the method was eagerly applied in vivo to explore the diversity of endothelial surfaces in normal and pathological conditions. Similar to the in vitro phage display approach, in vivo phage display involves intravenous injection of a random library of phage, removal of the tissue of interest, and recovery of bound phage by growth and amplification in host bacteria (Pasqualini et al. 2001). The first pioneering study systemically injected a combinatorial library in normal mice and demonstrated nonrandom distribution of peptides to the brain and kidney (Pasqualini and Ruoslahti 1996). The same approach was later applied to tumor xenografts and resulted in the characterization of tripeptide motifs (RGD and NGR, single-letter amino acid code) that would preferentially target tumor vasculature (also known as "vascular addresses") (Arap et al. 1998). The target for the RGD sequence was identified as integrin $\alpha v\beta 3$ and that of NGR, aminopeptidase A/CD13. It was shown that these motifs could be coupled to chemotherapeutics and upon systemic delivery to tumor-bearing models could generate a striking reduction in tumor burden at lower doses compared to standard systemic therapy (Arap et al. 1998). In this manner, the concept of vascular targeting was established, and subsequently, targeting peptides have been identified that can specifically recognize vasculature in normal organs such as the brain, kidney, lung, skin, pancreas, intestine, uterus, adrenal gland, and retina, as well as in sub-organ vascular beds such as the pancreatic islets, and in angiogenic blood vessels (Pasqualini and Ruoslahti 1996; Rajotte et al. 1998; Yao et al. 2005).

From a more translational perspective, phage display libraries have recently been used in a terminal wean cancer patient (Arap et al. 2002; Pentz et al. 2003). One of the selected peptides from the prostate demonstrated similarity to human interleukin-11 (IL-11). Further study of the native cytokine, as well as the corresponding peptide, identified a previously unrecognized binding site of IL-11 to its receptor IL-11Rα as well as provided insights into the biology of the IL-11/IL-11Rα in the context of human tumors and metastases (Cardó-Vila et al. 2008; Zurita et al. 2004). Moreover, phage display libraries have been approved for use in living cancer patients, demonstrating the safety and potential utility of phage as screening tools (Krag et al. 2006).

32.3 The Blood–Brain Barrier

Maintenance of normal brain function is highly dependent on a delicate relationship between the vasculature supplying oxygen and nutrients and the neuronal network. Critical to this balance is the highly specialized blood–brain barrier (BBB), which serves to limit entry of components of plasma into the brain parenchyma. The functional unit of the BBB, also known as the neurovascular unit, is composed of endothelial cells joined by tight junctions, neurons, astrocyte "foot processes," and other non-neuronal cells (Pardridge 2008; Neuwelt et al. 2008; Pardridge 2002). The combined effect of the neurovascular unit is the restriction of large and polar molecules present in the circulation from entering the central nervous system unless they transferred by one of the five main classes of specific transport pathways: carrier-mediated transport, receptor-mediated transport, ion transport, active transport, and caveolae-mediated transport (reviewed in Zlokovic 2008).

The selectivity and specificity of BBB transport makes design and use of drugs targeting the CNS, a formidable task. Indeed, nearly 100% of high-molecular weight drugs and greater than 98% of low-molecular weight drugs do not cross the BBB (Abbott et al. 2006; Friden et al. 1991; Spencer and Verma 2007) (see also Chapters 25 and 33). To circumvent this problem, many neurotherapeutic agents have been designed to be lipid soluble, allowing passive diffusion across membranes (Pardridge 1998). Yet, due to the propensity for lipid-soluble drugs to accumulate non-specifically and the difficulties associated with their formulation in the blood, there is a clear advantage and need to identify more specific therapies for delivery to the brain.

32.4 Glioblastoma and Angiogenesis

Malignant gliomas remain the most common primary brain tumor (Jemal et al. 2008). Glioblastomas account for the majority of malignant gliomas and have a median survival of 15 months with standard therapies (Stupp et al. 2005; Omuro et al. 2007; Wen and Kesari 2008). Its biological features have been well reviewed (Furnari et al. 2007; Wen and Kesari 2008). The pathogenesis of glioblastomas have been intimately linked to angiogenesis, as increases in microvascular density are prevalent histologically and the proangiogenic factor VEGF is expressed in all high-grade gliomas (Furnari et al. 2007; Jain et al. 2007). Moreover, high levels of proangiogenic factors such as VEGF, fibroblast growth factor (FGF), and hypoxia inducible factor-1α (HIF-1α) have been found to correlate with poor patient prognosis (Kaur et al. 2004; Samoto et al. 1995; Kaur et al. 2005; Stefanik et al. 1991) (see also Chapter 21).

Angiogenic blood vessels demonstrate organizational, structural, and functional abnormalities compared to the vasculature in normal organs (reviewed in Pasqualini et al. 2002). Vascular hierarchy is typically absent, demonstrated by irregularities in wall and luminal diameters throughout the length of the vascular network (McDonald and Foss 2000). The endothelial lining develops intercellular gaps and cellular sprouting, permitting the overlapping of cellular surfaces. The culmination of these changes results in a vasculature with reduced and unpredictable blood flow as well as disruptions in barrier function permitting non-specific leakage of macromolecules from the circulation into the tumor parenchyma (Jain 1987). These characteristics take on particular importance in the brain, as the heterogeneity of angiogenic growth in glioblastoma can co-opt normal capillaries and disrupts BBB function, whereas the tumor–brain interface can retain an intact BBB in adjacent tumor areas.

32.5 Targeting of the Brain Tumors by Phage Display

Improvements in the understanding of glioblastoma and other brain tumors have brought the development and rational design of molecularly targeted agents for therapy. With a large number focused on inhibition of growth factor pathways, such as receptor tyrosine kinases, small molecule inhibitors and antibody-based therapies have only met with moderate success (reviewed in Sathornsumetee et al. 2007). These disappointments are in part due to the intrinsic multi-step targeting of these agents. Circulating agents, such as those mentioned above, would need to selectively target the brain, identify the tumor site in the brain, cross the endothelial lining of the tumor, and diffuse to the tumor cells. With the presence of the BBB and changes in blood flow within tumor blood vessels, it suggests that access from the circulation is a critical determinant of whether tumor-directed agents can reach and target brain tumors.

An alternative strategy for the development of targeted agents would be to selectively direct molecules to the highly prevalent angiogenic blood vessels in tumors. Phage display, among other approaches, brought to light the idea that molecular differences exist between blood vessels in different organs as well as between normal and angiogenic blood vessels (see above Section 32.2). This molecular heterogeneity of the endothelium permits ligand-directed targeting in an organ-specific and disease-specific manner. Furthermore, as the tumor vasculature responds to changes in the tumor microenvironment, stage-specific targeting of the vasculature in both early and late stages remains feasible (Hanahan and Folkman 1996; Joyce et al. 2003).

A number of screening methodologies have been explored that allow for the identification of vascular ligand–receptor systems specific to brain tumors. Profiling techniques, such as genome-wide gene expression analyses, give insight into potential changes in surface protein expression between normal and diseased tissue. Such analyses typically use tissue homogenates that contain an undefined mixture of cell types, including tumor, endothelium, and other stroma (DeRisi et al. 1996; Micallef et al. 2008). The complexity in tissue composition and the relative amounts of each component are particularly important concerns for the interpretation of the results derived from these methods. Cell separation techniques or microdissection have improved the ability to generate specific endothelial cell populations for gene profiling studies (St Croix et al. 2000). Once achieved, this comparative approach can yield a large list of candidate genes with differential expression rates in normal and diseased tissue. The investigator then identifies genes that correspond to cell surface molecules uniquely or differentially expressed in tumor cells and tumor blood vessels and validates such targets as lead candidates for targeted therapy.

Though genomic profiling is a promising methodology for the identification of surface molecules, one fundamental challenge with this approach is in the ability to identify with certainty cell surface proteins that are suitable for selective targeting. While it is generally trivial to determine in silico whether an overexpressed gene encodes a cell surface molecule, this is no guarantee that a suitable targeting epitope will be present. Epitope prediction software for immunological targeting has been developed in recent years and can help in this process (see Chapter 48). Furthermore, gene expression does not guarantee protein expression and proper cell surface routing. The tumor microenvironment and proangiogenic factors in particular can activate endothelial cells and, in this process, modify translational processing, protein trafficking, and degradation pathways (Hanahan and Folkman 1996; Carmeliet 2003). These factors alter the localization and configuration of proteins and of molecules with which proteins can interact. Thus, molecules that are either not known to be at the cell surface or present on intracellular sites may be overlooked in large-scale gene expression screens; these molecules could be essential to site-specific targeting. Moreover, study in the isolated setting of a single normal/diseased organ pair does not clearly identify whether blood vessel markers identified in the disease are unique to this organ or found in other non-diseased tissues and whether they are suitable for vascular targeting.

Phage display emerges as a different approach to identify candidate molecules for ligand-directed delivery, offering several unique advantages. In vitro screenings allow for interrogation of pure tumor cell populations and the identification of cell surface binding ligands. This has been successfully used for brain tumors, with the isolation of targeting peptides recognizing rat and human glioma cells (Spear et al. 2001; Ho, Lam and Hui 2004; Samoylova et al. 2003). In vivo screenings provide an improved methodology for target identification as an unbiased functional assay, i.e., involves no judgment in advance as to what molecules the investigator should seek and identifies molecular targets in a physiologically relevant context (i.e., complexed to co-receptors or supportive molecules). Sequential rounds of selection enrich for and isolate amino acid motif ligands mediating specific targeting, often recognizing protein binding sites or other functionally active sites of receptors present in either the endothelium or tumor cells (Schleusener and Xianglin 2004). Moreover, these vascular targeting peptide ligands are inherently accessible from the circulation, as they are systemically administered, and alleviate some concerns of endothelial permeability and interstitial pressures that can influence tumor cell targeting. Finally, phages have been approved for use in living cancer patients with safety guidelines established by the Food and Drug Administration (Krag et al. 2006). As such, phage should prove to be safe and acceptable vehicles for delivery of therapeutic and diagnostic agents.

32.6 Targeted Therapy and Imaging

The identification and validation of specific ligand–receptor systems for brain tumors could enable numerous applications for therapy and diagnostics. Several unique vascular receptors have been identified by in vivo phage display and represent viable candidates for therapeutic intervention (Sergeeva et al. 2006). Rational design of compounds that would have the capacity to bind and inhibit the function of targeted receptors could present a major advance for the treatment of brain tumors. Furthermore, depending on the nature of their binding site and properties, stand-alone peptidomimetics may inhibit specific receptor function and lead to modifications of tumor blood vessels or tumor cell physiology. Lastly, ligand-directed delivery of toxic agents or diagnostic compounds to brain tumors could be achieved through the addition of targeting peptides.

Notably, methods that efficiently and effectively combine therapeutics and diagnostics would provide steps toward more personalized medicine. In the setting of systemic targeting applications, treating physicians would be able to not only identify and assess the tumor but also treat and monitor therapeutic response non-invasively. This becomes particularly relevant with glioblastoma or other brain tumors, where the process of obtaining biopsies for diagnosis and staging is invasive and laborious.

32.6.1 AAVP, a Novel Hybrid Gene Delivery System

Molecular genetic imaging of transgenes delivered by gene therapy represents an ideal modality for the incorporation of both therapy and imaging. Ideally, a multi-functional gene delivery cassette, combining imaging and therapeutic gene products, would be selectively targeted to the site of interest and expressed at high levels once delivered. Many of the current gene delivery vectors, such as adeno-associated virus (AAV), natively target mammalian cells and have very high transduction efficiencies. However, a lack of targeting specificity of these vectors often limits systemic gene delivery and attempts to apply targeting moieties can disrupt transduction. Conversely, vectors such as phage can accommodate targeting moieties for ligand-directed delivery effectively but have very low transduction rates of mammalian cells.

Our group recently developed a hybrid gene delivery system, combining favorable attributes of both phage and recombinant AAV (termed AAVP), generating a new class of gene therapy vector (Hajitou et al. 2006b). As a proof of concept, using a phage displaying the double-cyclic peptide CDCRGDCFC (RGD-4C) as a genetic backbone, we inserted the *cis*-elements of recombinant AAV into an intergenomic region of the phage. The chimeric vector retained the binding properties intrinsic to the RGD-4C peptide, mediating specific binding to mammalian cells expressing αv integrins, as well as demonstrated successful gene delivery via GFP and ß-gal signal reporters. Of note, transgene persistence in cells exposed to AAVP lasted approximately 60 days, nearly 50 days longer than cells exposed to non-chimeric phage. Evaluation of the mechanism(s) by which the AAVP mediated superior gene persistence indicated several possible contributors, including integration of the entire gene cassette with the inverted terminal repeats (ITRs) and generation of head-to-tail concatemers (Hajitou et al. 2006b).

In vivo, the AAVP construct demonstrated systemic targeting to both endothelial and tumor cells consistent with the RGD-4C targeting ligand to several human tumor models in immunocompromised mice as well as to syngeneic tumors in immunocompetent mice. Furthermore, with addition of the firefly luciferase gene for bioluminescence imaging, the AAVP vector allowed for non-invasive monitoring of gene expression in living tumor-bearing animals. Transgene expression within the tumor was evident 3 days following AAVP administration and reached a maximum at day 10.

Lastly, as bioluminescence imaging has limited utility in clinical applications, we incorporated the herpes simplex virus thymidine kinase (*HSVtk*) gene, which can function both as a positron emission tomography (PET) reporter with phosphorylation of several nucleoside analogs ([^{18}F]FEAU, [^{124}I]FAIU, or [^{18}F]FHBG) and as a suicide gene when combined with ganciclovir (Hajitou et al. 2006b; Soghomonyan et al. 2007). Following a single injection of RGD-4C AAVP, serial PET imaging of tumor-bearing animals with [^{18}F]FEAU allowed for horizontal monitoring of *HSVtk* enzyme activity and spatial heterogeneity within the tumors. Moreover, this multi-modal gene cassette allowed for prediction of tumor response, and the loss of *HSVtk* correlated with tumor growth suppression following ganciclovir treatment (Hajitou et al. 2006b; Hajitou et al. 2008). Taken together, the AAVP vector presents a unique integration of targeted delivery, imaging, and therapy that is readily applicable to brain tumors and translatable to other gene therapy applications for tumors.

32.7 Conclusions

Targeted medicine presents a new paradigm for the management of tumors and overcomes some of the specificity limitations of current therapies. Vascular targeting strategies permit direct delivery of agents to tumors and circumvent issues of accessibility to the tumor cells, especially with respect to brain tumors "protected" from most circulating molecules by the BBB. However, selective targeting requires validation of viable cell surface molecules mediating delivery. In vivo phage display presents an elegant approach that simultaneously addresses accessibility with identification of ligand–receptor systems. Ultimately, peptide ligands can serve either as peptidomimetics for singular therapy or in combination with gene delivery systems for combination molecular genetic imaging and therapy.

Acknowledgments The authors thank Julianna K. Edwards for critical reading of the manuscript and David Bier for help with illustrations. This work was supported by grants from the NIH, the DOD, and by awards from the Marcus Foundation and the Gillson-Longenbaugh Foundation.

Conflict of interest The authors declare no competing interests.

References

Abbott NJ, Rönnbäck L, Hansson E (2006) Astrocyte-endothelial interactions at the blood-brain barrier. Nat Rev Neurosci 7:41–53.

Arap W, Kolonin MG, Trepel M, Lahdenranta J, Cardó-Vila M, Giordano RJ, Mintz PJ, Ardelt PU, Yao VJ, Vidal CI, Chen L, Flamm A, Valtanen H, Weavind LM, Hicks ME, Pollock RE, Botz GH, Bucana CD, Koivunen E, Cahill D, Troncoso P, Baggerly KA, Pentz RD, Do KA, Logothetis CJ, Pasqualini R (2002) Steps toward mapping the human vasculature by phage display. Nat Med 8:121–127.

Arap W, Pasqualini R, Ruoslahti E (1998) Cancer treatment by targeted drug delivery to tumor vasculature in a mouse model. Science 279:377–380.

Carmeliet P (2003) Angiogenesis in health and disease. Nat Med 9:653–660.

Cardó-Vila M, Zurita AJ, Giordano RJ, Sun J, Rangel R, Guzman-Rojas L, Anobom CD, Valente AP, Almeida FCL, Lahdenranta J, Kolonin MG, Arap W, Pasqualini R (2008) A ligand peptide motif selected from a cancer patient is a receptor-interacting site within human interleukin-11. PLoS ONE 3:e3452.

DeRisi J, Penland L, Brown PO, Bittner ML, Meltzer PS, Ray M, Chen Y, Su YA, Trent JM (1996) Use of cDNA microarray to analyse gene expression patterns in human cancer. Nat Genet 14:457–460.

Doorbar J and Winter G (1994) Isolation of a peptide antagonist to the thrombin receptor using phage display. J Mol Biol 244:361–369.

Friden PM, Walus LR, Musso GF, Taylor MA, Malfroy B, Starzyk RM (1991) Anti-transferrin receptor antibody and antibody-drug conjugates cross the blood-brain barrier. Proc Natl Acad Sci U S A 88:4771–4775.

Furnari FB, Fenton T, Bachoo RM, Mukasa A, Stommel JM, Stegh A, Hahn WC, Ligon KL, Louis DN, Brennan C, Chin L, DePinho RA, Cavenee WK (2007) Malignant astrocytic glioma: genetics, biology, and paths to treatment. Genes Devel 21:2683–2710.

Giordano RJ, Cardó-Vila M, Lahdenranta J, Pasqualini R, Arap W (2001) Biopanning and rapid analysis of selective interactive ligands. Nat Med 7:1249–53.

Goodson RJ, Doyle MV, Kaufman SE, Rosenberg S (1994) High-affinity urokinase receptor antagonists identified with bacteriophage peptide display. Proc Natl Acad Sci U S A 91:7129–7133.

Hajitou A, Lev DC, Hannay JA, Korchin B, Staquicini FI, Soghomonyan S, Alauddin MM, Benjamin RS, Pollock RE, Gelovani JG, Pasqualini R, Arap W (2008) A preclinical model for predicting drug response in soft-tissue sarcoma with targeted AAVP molecular imaging. Proc Natl Acad Sci U S A 105:4471–6.

Hajitou A, Pasqualini R, Arap W (2006a) Vascular targeting: recent advances and therapeutic perspectives. Trends Cardiovasc Med 16:80–88.

Hajitou A, Trepel M, Lilley CE, Soghomonyan S, Alauddin MM, Marini FC 3rd, Restel BH, Ozawa MG, Moya CA, Rangel R, Sun Y, Zaoui K, Schmidt M, von Kalle C, Weitzman MD, Gelovani JG, Pasqualini R, Arap W (2006b) A hybrid vector for ligand-directed tumor targeting and molecular imaging. Cell 125:385–398.

Hanahan D and Weinberg RA (2000) The hallmarks of cancer. Cell 100:57–70.

Hanahan D and Folkman J (1996) Patterns and emerging mechanisms of the angiogenic switch during tumorigenesis. Cell 86:353–364.

Ho IA, Lam PY, Hui KM (2004) Identification and characterization of novel human glioma-specific peptides to potentiate tumor-specific gene delivery. Hum Gene Ther 15:719–32.

Jain RK (1987) Transport of molecules in the tumor interstitium: a review. Cancer Res 47:3039–51.

Jain RK, di Tomaso E, Duda DG, Loeffler JS, Sorensen AG, Batchelor TT (2007) Angiogenesis in brain tumours. Nat Rev Neurosci 8:610–622.

Jemal A, Siegel R, Ward E, Hao Y, Xu J, Murray T, Thun MJ (2008) Cancer statistics, 2008. CA Cancer J Clin 58:71–96.

Joyce JA, Laakkonen P, Bernasconi M, Bergers G, Ruoslahti E, Hanahan D (2003) Stage-specific vascular markers revealed by phage display in a mouse model of pancreatic islet tumorigenesis. Cancer Cell 4:393–403.

Kaur B, Tan C, Brat DJ, Post DE, Van Meir EG (2004) Genetic and hypoxic regulation of angiogenesis in gliomas. J Neurooncol 70:229–243.

Kaur B, Khwaja FW, Severson EA, Matheny SL, Brat DJ, Van Meir EG (2005) Hypoxia and the hypoxia-inducible-factor pathway in glioma growth and angiogenesis. Neuro Oncol 7:134–153.

Kinzler KW and Vogelstein B (1997) Cancer-susceptibility genes. Gatekeepers and caretakers. Nature 386:761–763.

Koivunen E, Gay DA, Ruoslahti E (1993) Selection of peptides binding to the alpha 5 beta 1 integrin from phage display. J Biol Chem 268:20205–20210.

Koivunen E, Wang B, Ruoslahti E (1994) Isolation of a highly specific ligand for the alpha 5 beta 1 integrin from a phage display library. J Cell Biol 124:373–380.

Kolonin MG, Bover L, Sun J, Zurita AJ, Do KA, Lahdenranta J, Cardó-Vila M, Giordano RJ, Jaalouk DE, Ozawa MG, Moya CA, Souza GR, Staquicini FI, Kunyiasu A, Scudiero DA, Holbeck SL, Sausville EA, Arap W, Pasqualini R (2006) Ligand-directed surface profiling of human cancer cells with combinatorial peptide libraries. Cancer Res 66:34–40.

Krag DN, Shukla GS, Shen GP, Pero S, Ashikaga T, Fuller S, Weaver DL, Burdette-Radoux S, Thomas C (2006) Selection of tumor-binding ligands in cancer patients with phage display libraries. Cancer Res 66:7724–33.

McDonald DM and Foss AJ (2000). Endothelial cells of tumor vessels: abnormal but not absent. Cancer Metastasis Rev 19:109–20.

Micallef J, Gajadhar A, Wiley J, DeSouza LV, Michael Siu KW, Guha A (2008) Proteomics: present and future implications in neuro-oncology. Neurosurg 62:539–555.

Milano G, Spano JP, Leyland-Jones B (2008) EGFR-targeting drugs in combination with cytotoxic agents: from bench to bedside, a contrasted reality. Br J Cancer 99:1–5.

Mintz PJ, Kim J, Do KA, Wang X, Zinner RG, Cristofanilli M, Arap MA, Hong WK, Troncoso P, Logothetis CJ, Pasqualini R, Arap W (2003) Fingerprinting the circulating repertoire of antibodies from cancer patients. Nat Biotechnol 21:57–63.

Neri D and Bicknell R (2005) Tumor vascular targeting. Nat Rev Cancer 5:436–446.

Neuwelt E, Abbott NJ, Abrey L, Banks WA, Blakley B, Davis T, Engelhardt B, Grammas P, Nedergaard M, Nutt J, Pardridge W, Rosenberg GA, Smith Q, Drewes LR (2008) Strategies to advance translational research into brain barriers. Lancet Neurol 7:84–96.

Omuro AMP, Faivre S, Raymond E (2007) Lessons learned in the development of targeted therapy for malignant gliomas. Mol Cancer Ther 6:1909–1919.

Parmley SF and Smith GP (1988) Antibody-selectable filamentous fd phage vectors: affinity purification of target genes. Gene 73:305–18.

Pardridge WM (1998) CNS drug design based on principles of blood-brain barrier transport. J Neurochem 70:1781–1792.

Pardridge WM (2002) Drug and gene delivery to the brain: the vascular route. Neuron 36: 555–558.

Pardridge WM (2008) Re-engineering biopharmaceuticals for delivery to brain with molecular Trojan horses. Bioconjug Chem 19:1327–38.

Pasqualini R, Arap W, Rajotte D, Ruoslahti E (2001) in Phage Display: A Laboratory Manual, eds Barbas III CF, Burton DR, Scott JK et al Cold Spring Harbor Laboratory Press, NY 22.1–22.4.

Pasqualini R, Arap W, and McDonald DM (2002) Probing the structural and molecular diversity of tumor vasculature. Trends Mol Med 8:563–71.

Pasqualini R and Ruoslahti E (1996) Organ targeting in vivo using phage display peptide libraries. Nature 380:364–366.

Pentz RD, Flamm AL, Pasqualini R, Logothetis CJ, Arap W (2003) Revisiting ethical guidelines for research with terminal wean and brain-dead participants. Hastings Cent Rep 33:20–6

Rajotte D, Arap W, Hagedorn M, Koivunen E, Pasqualini R, Ruoslahti E (1998) Molecular heterogeneity of the vascular endothelium revealed by in vivo phage display. J Clin Invest 102:430–437.

Samoto K, Ikezaki K, Ono M, Shono T, Kohno K, Kuwano M, Fukui M (1995) Expression of vascular endothelial growth factor and its possible relation with neovascularization in human brain tumors. Cancer Res 55:1189–1193.

Samoylova TI, Petrenko VA, Morrison NE, Globa LP, Baker HJ, Cox NR (2003) Phage probes for malignant glial cells. Mol Cancer Ther 2:1129–37.

Sathornsumetee S, Reardon RA, Desjardins A, Quinn JA, Vredenburgh JJ, Rich JN (2007) Molecularly targeted therapy for malignant glioma. Cancer 110:13–24.

Schleusener HJ and Xianglin T (2004) Selection of recombinant phages binding to pathological endothelial and tumor cells of rat glioblastoma by in-vivo display. J Neurol Sci 224:77–82.

Scott JK and Smith GP (1990) Searching for peptide ligands with an epitope library. Science 249:386–390.

Sergeeva A, Kolonin MG, Molldrem JJ, Pasqualini R, Arap W (2006) Display technologies: application for the discovery of drug and gene delivery agents. Adv Drug Deliv Rev 58:1622–1654.

Sessa C, Guibal A, Del Conte G, Rüegg C (2008) Biomarkers of angiogenesis for the development of antiangiogenic therapies in oncology: tools or decorations? Nat Clin Practice Oncol 5:378–391.

Smith GP (1985) Filamentous fusion phage: novel expression vectors that display cloned antigens on the virion surface. Science 228:1315–7.

Soghomonyan S, Hajitou A, Rangel R, Trepel M, Pasqualini R, Arap W, Gelovani JG, Alauddin MM (2007) Molecular PET imaging of HSV1-tk reporter gene expression using [18F]FEAU. Nat Protocols 2:523–531.

Spear MA, Breakefield XO, Beltzer J, Schuback D, Weissleder R, Pardo FS, Ladner R (2001) Isolation, characterization, and recovery of small peptide phage display epitopes selected against viable malignant glioma cells. Cancer Gene Ther 8:506–11.

Spencer BJ and Verma IM (2007) Targeted delivery of proteins across the blood-brain barrier. Proc Natl Acad Sci U S A 104:7594–7599.

St Croix B, Rago C, Velculescu V, Traverso G, Romans KE, Montgomery E, Lal A, Riggins GJ, Lengauer C, Vogelstein B, Kinzler KW (2000) Genes expressed in human tumor endothelium. Science 289:1197–1202.

Stefanik DF, Rizkalla LR, Soi A, Goldblatt SA, Rizkalla WM (1991) Acidic and basic fibroblast growth factors are present in glioblastoma multiforme. Cancer Res 51:5760–5765.

Stupp R, Mason WP, van den Bent MJ, Weller M, Fisher B, Taphoorn MJ, Belanger K, Brandes AA, Marosi C, Bogdahn U, Curschmann J, Janzer RC, Ludwin SK, Gorlia T, Allgeier A, Lacombe D, Cairncross JG, Eisnehauer E, Mirimanoff RO, for the European Organisation for Research and Treatment of Cancer Brain Tumor and Radiotherapy Groups and the National Cancer Institute of Canada Clinical Trials Group (2005) Radiotherapy plus concomitant and adjuvant temozolomide for glioblastoma. N Engl J Med 352:987–996.

Szardenings M, Törnroth S, Mutulis F, Muceniece R, Keinänen K, Kuusinen A, Wikberg JE (1997) Phage display selection on whole cells yields a peptide specific for melanocortin receptor 1. J Biol Chem 272:27943–27948.

Wen PY and Kesari S (2008) Malignant gliomas in adults. N Engl J Med 359:492–507.

Yao VJ, Ozawa MG, Trepel M, Arap W, McDonald DM, Pasqualini R (2005) Targeting pancreatic islets with phage display assisted by laser pressure catapult microdissection. Am J Pathol 166:625–36.

Zurita AJ, Troncoso P, Cardó-Vila M, Logothetis CJ, Pasqualini R, Arap W (2004) Combinatorial screenings in patients: the interleukin-11 receptor alpha as a candidate target in the progression of human prostate cancer. Cancer Res 64:435–9.

Zlokovic BV (2008) The blood-brain barrier in health and chronic neurodegenerative disorders. Neuron 57:178–201.

Chapter 33
Impact of the Blood–Brain Barrier on Brain Tumor Imaging and Therapy

James Provenzale

Abstract The blood–brain barrier (BBB) figures importantly in detection and characterization of brain tumors using imaging as well as in understanding difficulties in providing chemotherapy for brain tumors. Importantly, new methods are being designed to tailor drugs for more efficient transit across the BBB, for alteration of the BBB to enhance drug effect, or to bypass the BBB when providing chemotherapy. Thus, it is important for investigators using neuroimaging techniques to study brain tumors and those providing brain tumor therapy to understand the structure and function of the BBB. This chapter provides a basic understanding of the BBB, explains its role in brain tumor imaging, and provides a review of recent trends to overcome the impediments to brain tumor therapy imposed by the BBB.

Contents

J. Provenzale (✉)
Department of Radiology, Biomedical Engineering and Oncology, Emory University School of Medicine, Atlanta, GA 30322, USA; Department of Radiology, Duke University Medical Center, Durham, NC 27710, USA
e-mail: jmprove@emory.edu

E.G. Van Meir (ed.), *CNS Cancer*, Cancer Drug Discovery and Development, DOI 10.1007/978-1-60327-553-8_33,
© Humana Press, a part of Springer Science+Business Media, LLC 2009

33.1 Introduction

The blood–brain barrier (BBB) is an organized complex network of many types of cells lining the vessels of the central nervous system (CNS) (Bart et al. 2000). This network serves to effectively isolate the CNS from the physiological variations that continuously occur outside the CNS and to provide only selective access to molecules that the normal CNS needs for effective homeostasis. Thus, the BBB provides benefits that are critical to maintaining neurophysiological function. The very efficiency of the BBB has long been recognized as an impediment to treatment of brain tumors, most notably in the case of administration of chemotherapy and the use of monoclonal antibodies. As a result, knowledge of the BBB, in both normal states and in the presence of a brain tumor, is important for individuals interested in treating CNS neoplasms. Such an understanding of the BBB allows one to comprehend the role of neuroradiological techniques for studying brain tumors and appreciate the many novel methods that are being developed to treat CNS neoplasms.

This chapter is intended to familiarize the reader with the microstructural organization of the BBB in order to explain circumstances in which the BBB is altered by brain tumors. The structure and function of the BBB is reviewed in the first part of this chapter with an emphasis on the impediments that the BBB imposes for treatment of brain tumors using chemotherapy. Interruption of the BBB by the presence of a brain tumor provides methods for using neuroradiological studies to detect tumors, characterize their degree of aggressiveness, and monitor response to therapy. Those topics are explained in the second part of this chapter. Finally, new techniques for optimizing therapeutics to overcome the obstacles provided by the BBB in the treatment of brain tumors are discussed in the third part of this chapter.

33.2 Historical Beginnings of the BBB Concept

The ability of the brain to remain impervious to various substances administered outside of the CNS was first noted by Paul Ehrlich in 1885 when he noted that, following parenteral administration of various dyes, almost all organs except the brain and spinal cord were stained (Ribatti et al., 2006). Subsequently,

Ehrlich also noted that intravenous infusion of aniline dyes was also followed by the same distribution of organ staining, although he did not generate the specific concept of a BBB at that time. Subsequently, other investigators, notably Bield and Kraus, in 1898, and Lewandowsky, in 1900, observed that intravenous infusion of some substances (e.g., sodium ferrocyanide) did not produce CNS effects after intravenous infusion but did produce CNS effects when infused into the brain ventricles (Ribatti). On this basis, they postulated that a barrier existed at the level of brain vessels preventing passage of some materials into the brain, with Lewandowsky first introducing the term "blood–-brain barrier." Thereafter, experiments by Goldmann (an associate of Ehrlich) in the early twentieth century showed that injection of the dye Trypan blue into the brain ventricles stained brain tissue but that intravenous infusion of the same dye stained all organs except the brain and spinal cord (although the choroid plexus also was stained). Such experiments showed that it was not a lack of affinity of the brain and spinal cord for the dye but, instead, a lack of access of the dye to the CNS that prevented staining of the brain and spine. Thus, the concept of a barrier between the blood and the brain as well as between the blood and the cerebrospinal fluid was formulated.

33.3 Structure and Function of the Blood–Brain Barrier

The BBB is an organized network of various types of cells (primarily endothelial cells but also including astroglia, pericytes, and perivascular macrophages) that serves to regulate passage of materials between the brain intravascular compartment and the extracellular and cellular compartments (Bart et al. 2000). In the normal brain, the BBB is intact and plays a very important role in brain homeostasis. The BBB functions to exclude large lipophilic molecules, except for some that are actively transported across the BBB (Fig. 33.1). Small lipophilic molecules can passively cross the BBB if they have specific physical properties (Bart et al. 2000). Most ionized water-soluble compounds larger than a certain molecular weight (essentially 180 Daltons) are excluded from the CNS (Bart et al. 2000; Kraemer et al. 2002). The BBB restricts passive diffusion (i.e., transport that is nonreceptor or noncarrier-mediated) of larger molecules into the CNS by a combination of endothelial tight junctions in combination with the absence of fenestrae between endothelial cells. As a result, the large majority of chemotherapeutic agents, which have molecular weights greater than 200 Da, are prevented from crossing across the BBB. In addition, astrocytic foot processes cover virtually the entire extent of the external surface of the endothelial cells, which adds to the barrier action (Bellavance et al. 2008). Finally, a further component of the BBB is the high electrical resistance of brain capillaries, which serves to exclude polar and ionic substances (Bart et al. 2000).

Based on the discussion above, many small lipophilic molecules should be able to cross the BBB. However, in fact, a number of these molecules face one additional barrier, i.e., efflux pumps that actively transport these molecules

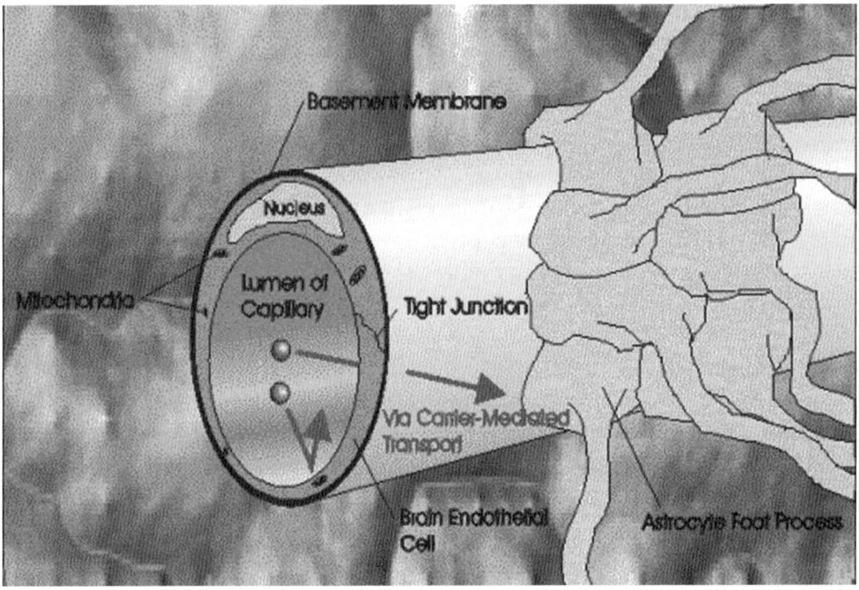

Fig. 33.1 Diagram depicting the structure of the blood–brain barrier shows tight junctions between vascular endothelial cells and close application of astrocytic foot processes against the outer wall of the blood vessel. Note that some molecules pass through the barrier via carrier-mediated transport, while others are retained in the vascular lumen (Image constructed by T.P. Davis and V. Hau and located on the following website: davislab.med.arizona.edu. Used with permission of T.P. Davis, Ph.D.)

back into the vascular compartment. These efflux pumps gained wide recognition among cancer biologists based on the fact that they are expressed in a number of multidrug-resistant tumors (Fojo et al. 1987). It is worthwhile to briefly mention two such efflux pump systems here; these systems are discussed in detail elsewhere (Bart et al. 2000). These two membrane efflux pumps are P-glycoprotein and those in the multidrug-resistance-associated protein family (Bart et al. 2000). P-glycoprotein is located at the luminal surface of endothelial cells in brain capillaries and serves to actively pump back into the vascular lumen lipophilic molecules that enter the endothelial cell (Higgins 1992). The MRP family has a number of homologues, of which some exist at the BBB (Bart et al. 2000). MRP appears to transport many drugs that are cotransported with glutathione (Bart et al. 2000). Some of the homologues of multidrug-resistance-associated protein are involved in the development of resistance to methotrexate, thereby limiting the effectiveness of a drug that is important in therapy of many types of brain tumors (Bart et al. 2000).

The BBB is typically altered to various degrees in the presence of a primary or metastatic brain tumor. At the mild end of the spectrum of changes, slight changes in the ultrastructural integrity of capillaries are seen in the form of loosening of tight junctions (Bart et al. 2000). These changes become more profound in the setting of a high-grade glial neoplasm, are manifested by more marked disruption of endothelium, tight junctions and basal lamina, increase in perivascular spaces, and proliferation of pinocytic vacuoles (Bart et al. 2000). On occasion, even low-grade tumors (e.g., pilocytic astrocytomas) are associated with substantial disruption of the BBB. One of the major effects of this BBB disruption is the development of vasogenic edema due to diffusion of water through the BBB into peritumoral tissue. Interruption of the BBB by tumors is likely mediated by a number of substances secreted by tumors, such as vascular endothelial growth factor (VEGF). It has long been recognized that corticosteroids stabilize the BBB and reduce vasogenic edema; recent evidence suggests that this effect may, in part, be due to the regulation of VEGF by corticosteroids (Kim et al. 2008). Furthermore, administration of an anti-VEGF antibody has been shown to normalize vasculature and decrease vasogenic edema adjacent to brain tumors (Batchelor et al., 2007).

The integrity (or lack thereof) of the BBB has long been recognized as a marker of degree of aggressiveness of tumors. Stated in simplistic terms, neuro-oncologists and other clinicians interested in categorizing tumors and measuring tumor response to therapy have viewed tumors that contrast-enhance as more aggressive than tumors that fail to contrast-enhance. In large part, that rationale is well founded because the presence or absence of contrast enhancement generally correlates with tumor grade. World Health Organization grade I and grade II tumors typically do not contrast-enhance and grade III and grade IV tumors almost always contrast-enhance. Grade III and grade IV tumors also often are found to have elevated relative cerebral blood volume (rCBV) (Fig. 33.2 and Color Plate 48). Nonetheless, in a busy clinical practice, enough exceptions occur to warrant caution on the part of the radiologist and the treating physician alike. On occasion, the degree of contrast enhancement is obvious but falsely attributed to another structure that normally contrast-enhances, e.g., choroid plexus. In other cases, degree of contrast enhancement is very subtle and, thus, overlooked. In unusual cases, despite close inspection of contrast-enhanced images, no contrast enhancement is present but the tumor is still found on biopsy to be a high-grade neoplasm (Fig. 33.3 and Color Plate 49) (Kondziolka et al, 1993).

It is also worth noting the role of contrast enhancement in the surgical resection of brain tumors. In many instances, the goal is removal of contrast-enhancing tumor on the premise that the enhancing portion is definitely tumor (as opposed to brain regions containing edema but not tumor, which is a distinction that is difficult on T2-weighted images) and that this portion of the tumor is the most aggressive region. The region of greatest relative cerebral blood volume (rCBV), which is the portion of tumor having greatest capillary density, is generally accepted to be the most aggressive region of the tumor. Typically, the region of greatest rCBV is, in fact, in a contrast-enhancing portion (Provenzale et al., 2006a) (Fig. 33.2). However, the region of greatest rCBV is often smaller than the region of contrast enhancement and greatest capillary permeability (Fig. 33.4 and Color Plate 50). Other contrast-enhancing regions may correspond to

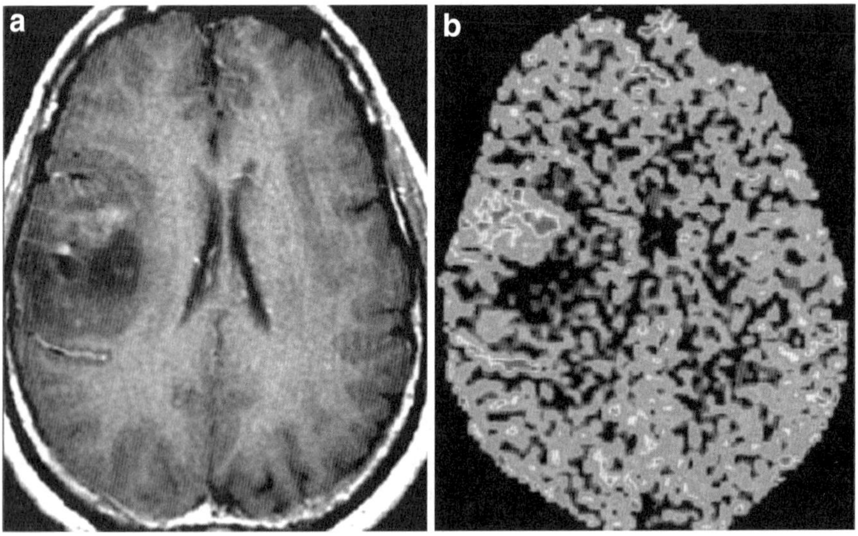

Fig. 33.2 Congruence of region of contrast enhancement and region of highest relative cerebral blood volume (rCBV), suggesting that contrast-enhancing region is the most aggressive portion of tumor, in a 37-year-old man with biopsy-proved World Health Organization grade III astrocytoma. (**a**) Axial contrast-enhanced T1-weighted image shows inhomogeneously enhancing mass in the right frontal lobe. Contrast enhancement is confined to the central portion of the mass. (**b**) rCBV map in which regions of high rCBV are depicted in *red* and *yellow* shows that the region of highest rCBV corresponds to the contrast-enhancing region shown in **a**. (Reprinted, with permission, from Provenzale et al. 2006) (*see* Color Plate 48)

regions of only mildly elevated rCBV or normal rCBV (Fig. 33.4); nonetheless, it is indeed appropriate to consider these regions as indicative of aggressive regions of tumor based on their increased permeability. However, it would be erroneous to believe that the contrast-enhancing portion of tumor is the sole region of brain involved by tumor. It is well established that high-grade brain tumors are infiltrative and often extend not only into adjacent regions that fail to contrast-enhance but even into unenhancing regions in the contralateral hemisphere. As stated earlier, on occasion, unenhancing tumor can contain regions of substantially elevated rCBV (Fig. 33.3).

33.3.1 Renewed Emphasis on Understanding of the Blood–Brain Barrier

As noted above, radiologists and treating physicians employ an elementary understanding of the BBB when they review contrast-enhanced imaging studies of brain tumor patients on a daily basis. However, due to the introduction of novel brain tumor therapies, a better understanding of the BBB is needed to

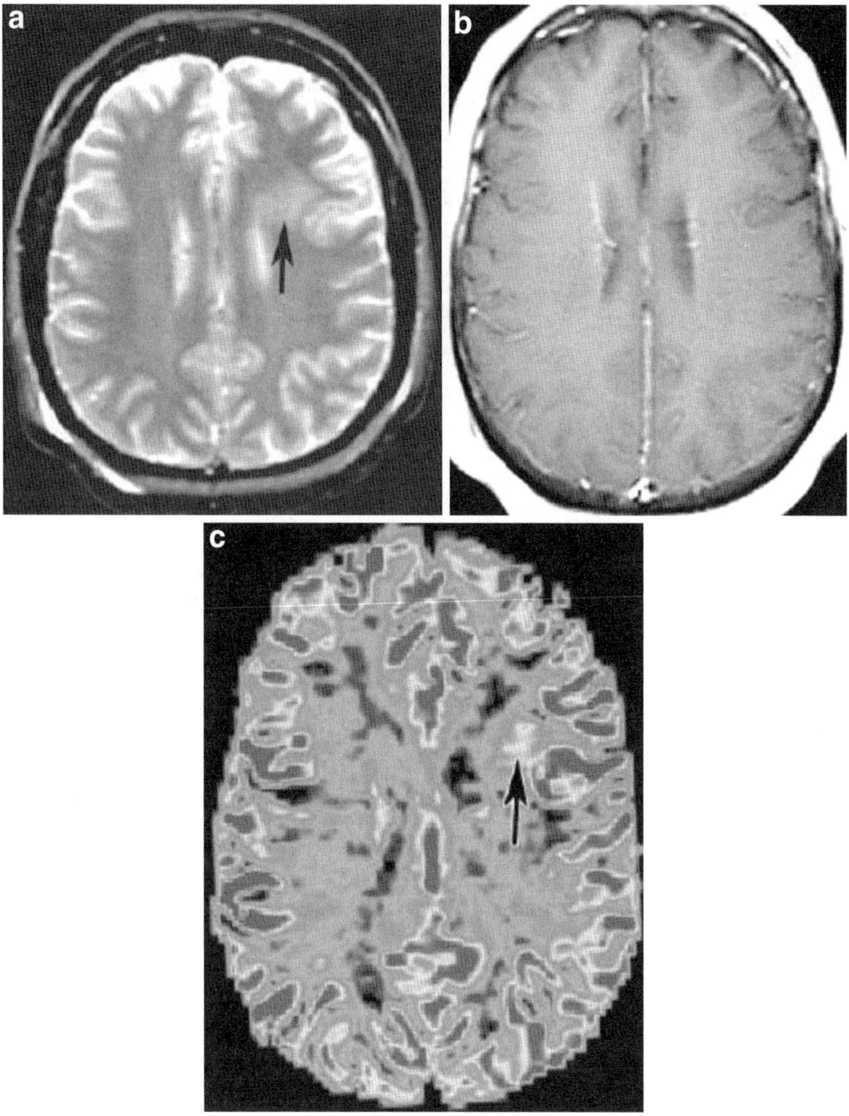

Fig. 33.3 Elevation of rCBV despite the absence of contrast enhancement (i.e., no evidence of elevated permeability) in a 44-year-old woman with World Health Organization grade III astrocytoma. (**a**) Axial T2-weighted MR image shows hyperintense region (*arrow*) consistent with a neoplasm in the left frontal lobe. (**b**) Axial contrast-enhanced T1-weighted MR image does not show any regions of contrast enhancement. On the basis of the T2-weighted image and the contrast-enhanced T1-weighted image, one might have assumed that the lesion is a low-grade neoplasm with no areas of elevated rCBV. (**c**) rCBV map in which *red* and *yellow* colors indicate areas of elevated rCBV shows a region of high rCBV area (*arrow*) corresponding to the region of hyperintense abnormality on the T2-weighted image. At biopsy, this region was shown to represent high-grade glioma (Reprinted, with permission, from Wong et al. 2000) (*see* Color Plate 49)

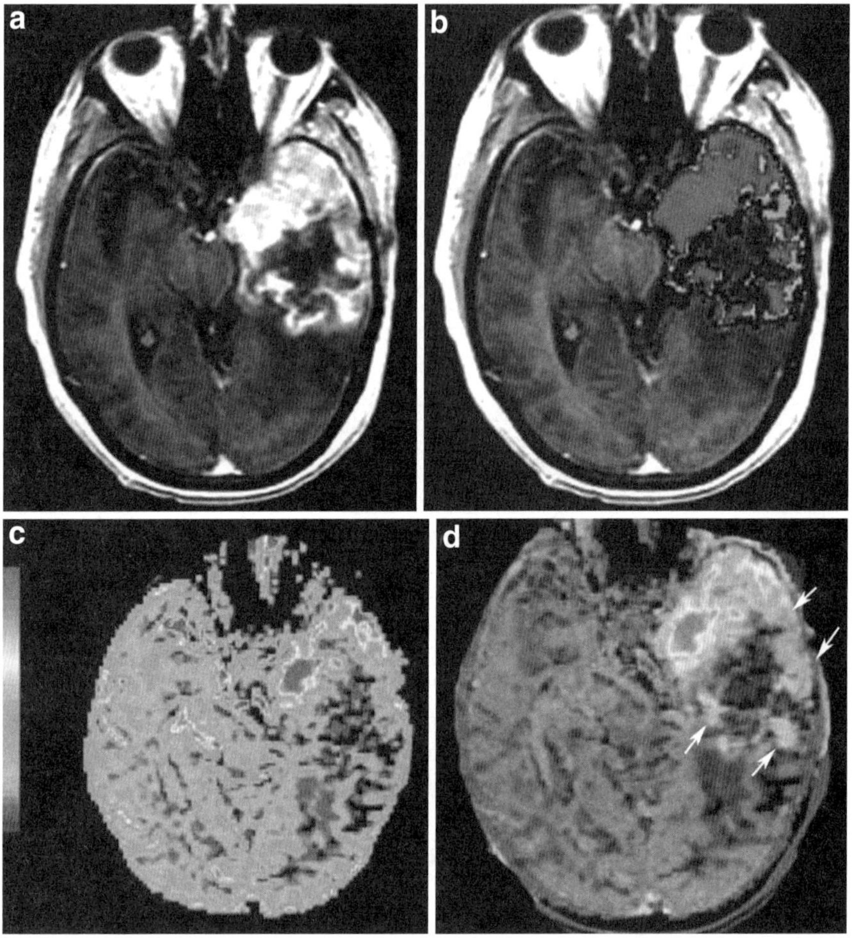

Fig. 33.4 Lack of correlation of all regions of elevated permeability with elevated rCBV in a 51-year-old man with biopsy-proven glioblastoma multiforme. (**a**) Axial contrast-enhanced T1-weighted image shows large enhancing mass in the left temporal lobe. (**b**) Color-coded relative permeability map obtained using dynamic contrast-enhanced imaging superimposed on the image shown in (**a**). The color-coded map shows pixels having one of the three different colors. Left hemisphere regions that have peak signal intensity values in the range of 3–5 standard deviations (SD) above mean signal intensity in the normal right hemisphere are depicted in *blue*. The pixels that are in the range of 5–7 SD above baseline are shown in *yellow* color and the *red* pixels are those in which the increased signal intensity is greater than 7 SD above baseline. Thus, a large area of the tumor has pixels in the highest range of permeability values. (**c**) Axial rCBV map derived from T2*-weighted dynamic susceptibility imaging sequence shows that regions of elevated rCBV (seen in *red* and *yellow* color) are essentially confined to medial and anterior aspects of the tumor. (**d**) Superimposition of rCBV map shown in **c** on permeability map shown in **b** depicts the fact that large portions of the contrast-enhancing regions showing marked permeability in (**a**) and (**b**) do not have elevated rCBV values (*arrows*). (Reprinted, with permission, from Provenzale et al. 2006b) (*see* Color Plate 50)

facilitate the development of methods for determining treatment response and improving efficacy of therapeutic agents. The degree of BBB permeability can serve as a surrogate marker for tumor aggressiveness and response to therapy. Knowledge of BBB dysfunction is important for tailoring the size, configuration, and electrical charge of molecules intended to cross the BBB as well as designing methods for manipulating the intact BBB to allow it to temporarily (and selectively) open in order to allow egress of therapeutic drugs from the brain vasculature into the tumor.

33.4 Importance of the BBB for Imaging of Brain Tumors

33.4.1 Angiogenesis and Permeability: Similarities and Differences

A fundamental concept that should be understood before proceeding to discussion of issues of the BBB is that angiogenesis and vascular permeability reflect two aspects of the same phenomenon within tumors. Thus, efforts to understand angiogenesis will indirectly lead to an understanding of vascular permeability; similarly, techniques to diminish angiogenesis within tumors may also contribute to decreasing vascular permeability. For instance, one of the major promoters of angiogenesis, i.e., vascular endothelial growth factor, is a potent promoter of permeability (Puduvalli and Sawaya 2000).

MR imaging in the first few days after antiangiogenesis therapy may show decrease in contrast enhancement (consistent with decreased vascular permeability) but not decreased capillary density, as reflected in lack of decrease in rCBV. Thus, one must be cautious in ascribing decreased contrast enhancement within a tumor after therapy (which primarily reflects vascular permeability) solely to a decrease in angiogenesis. Indeed, one would expect a decrease in tumor angiogenesis to require a longer period of time before an effect could reliably be noted using standard imaging techniques; changes in degree of contrast enhancement and degree of permeability in the first few days after antiangiogenesis therapy are much more likely to be due to BBB stabilization than to decreases in capillary density.

33.4.2 Permeability as a Surrogate Marker for Angiogenesis

One factor in the renewed interest in permeability from the standpoint of the radiologist is the potential use of imaging-based permeability measurements as a surrogate marker for response to antiangiogenesis therapy. In large part, this assumption that permeability measurements can serve as surrogate markers for degree of angiogenesis relies on data from non-CNS tumors. For instance, degree of permeability has been correlated with levels of vascular endothelial growth factor in breast cancer (Ikeda et al. 2004). Although more data with regard to correlation of angiogenesis factors and permeability indices in brain tumors (sheltered by the BBB) are indicated to further substantiate the role of permeability imaging in CNS tumors, the data from non-CNS tumors are certainly promising.

With this in mind, a number of methods for measuring permeability within tumors have been developed (Provenzale et al. 2005). Most of these techniques have employed T1-weighted imaging techniques that monitor rate and degree of increase in signal intensity following infusion of standard paramagnetic MR contrast material. These techniques may involve very fast imaging during the first minute after rapid infusion of contrast material or longer imaging times (on the order of many minutes) without the need for rapid infusion. However, permeability can also be inferred from T2*-weighted MR imaging techniques that are primarily designed to measure relative cerebral blood volume (rCBV) rather than permeability. These techniques will be discussed in turn.

33.4.3 T1-Weighted Imaging Techniques

The most commonly used techniques for measuring permeability use a T1-weighted pulse sequence that is essentially similar to the technique used in standard clinical MR imaging to measure contrast enhancement of tumors (Fig. 33.4). Unlike standard clinical T1-weighted imaging, however, sequences designed to measure permeability provide physiological information in addition to the routine anatomic information regarding size of enhancing tumor. Many of these T1-weighted pulse sequences are commonly referred to as dynamic contrast-enhanced techniques (Choyke et al. 2003). This technique is increasingly being used to assess effects of antiangiogenesis therapy (Fig. 33.5 and Color Plate 51). One of the more common techniques in use is a 3D spoiled gradient in the steady state that allows rapid imaging over the course of a few minutes. The data inherent in the time–signal intensity curve showing increase in signal intensity after infusion of contrast material can then be used to derive a number of hemodynamic parameters. Typical parameters studied include maximum enhancement index (expressing the relationship of signal intensity at any given time relative to baseline signal intensity), rise time (time to reach an arbitrary point on the uptake curve, e.g., half-maximum signal intensity), initial slope (derived soon after contrast material infusion), final slope (derived from curve within last few minutes of contrast enhancement), and area under the contrast enhancement curve (Pickles et al. 2008). Such a technique provides a rough calculation of degree of leakage of contrast material across the BBB and serves the needs of most investigators when a high degree of temporal resolution is not necessary (Tofts 1997). However, although the pharmacokinetic model that is the basis of analysis of such techniques has the benefit of being relatively simple compared to some analytical models, it depends on a number of assumptions that may not be valid in any particular

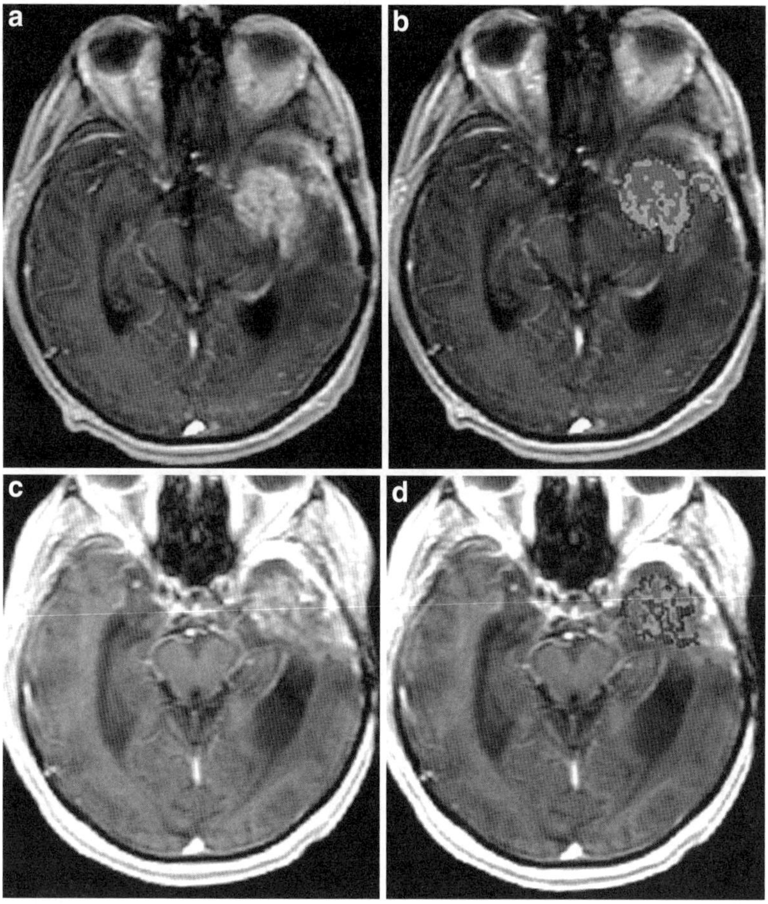

Fig. 33.5 A 62-year-old man with glioblastoma multiforme. Illustration of changes in contrast material leakage (a reflection of degree of blood–brain barrier disruption) after administration of an antiangiogenesis agent. This case is an example of the fact that decreases in permeability after angiogenesis therapy may be greater than changes in tumor size. (**a**) Axial contrast-enhanced T1-weighted image prior to therapy shows large contrast-enhancing left temporal lobe tumor. (**b**) Color-coded map derived from dynamic contrast-enhanced imaging sequence before therapy (performed during the same MR examination as in **a**) shows relative degrees of permeability in each pixel. Pixels having signal intensity that are 120–149% of normal tissue are shown in *blue*, those with signal intensity of 140–159% of normal tissue are shown in *green*, and those having signal intensity ≥160% of normal tissue are in *red*. The majority of pixels are in the >160% category, consistent with marked leakage of contrast material throughout the tumor and indicating widespread disruption of the blood–brain barrier. (**c**) Repeat imaging was performed 30 days after beginning therapy with antiangiogenesis therapy. Axial contrast-enhanced T1-weighted image shows mild decrease in size of contrast-enhancing mass. (**d**) Color-coded map derived from dynamic contrast-enhanced imaging data on imaging at 30 days after beginning therapy (during same MR examination as **c**) shows marked decrease in number of pixels associated with the highest degree of permeability (i.e., *green* and *red* pixels). Reprinted, with permission, from Provenzale (2007) (*see* Color Plate 51)

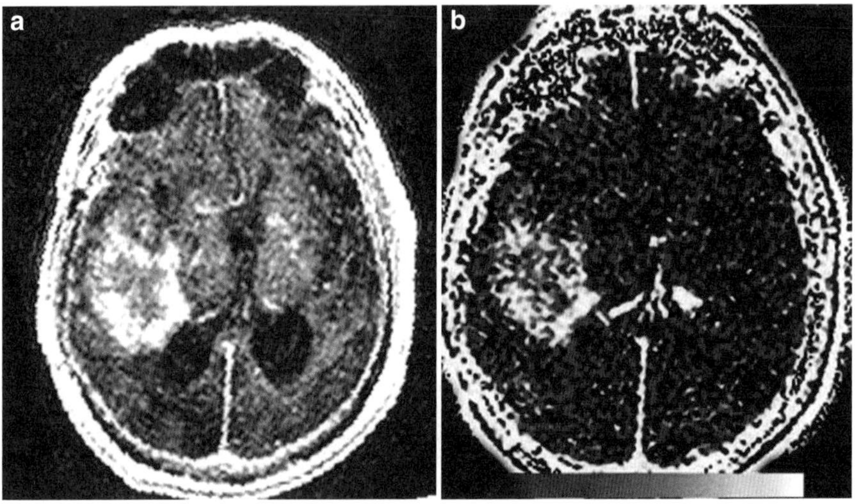

Fig. 33.6 Example of the use of T1-weighted dynamic contrast-enhanced imaging sequence to derive K^{trans} measurement of permeability. (**a**) Axial contrast-enhanced T1-weighted image obtained using spoiled gradient in the steady-state acquisition technique shows inhomogeneous enhancement of a right hemisphere neoplasm. (**b**) Color-coded K^{trans} map in which high degree of permeability is shown in *white* and *yellow* indicates that permeability in most of the periphery of the tumor is markedly increased. (Image provided courtesy of Daniel Barboriak, MD) Reprinted, with permission, from Provenzale et al. (2005)

study. For instance, the pharmacological model used in many T1-weighted techniques does not rigorously measure arterial input function or vascular volume of the tumor (Pickles et al. 2008). Such dynamic contrast-enhanced techniques have been shown to correspond relatively well with tumor grade (Roberts et al. 2000). Recently, using this technique, the degree of permeability increase prior to therapy has been shown to inversely correlate with disease-free survival and overall survival (Pickles et al. 2008).

Many investigators find that the assumptions inherent within the relatively simple pharmacological models outlined above are inadequate for the characterization of permeability needed for assessment of tumors. Thus, a number of models have been advanced for better representing the physiological characteristics of efflux of contrast material from the vascular compartment into tumors (Tofts 1997) (Fig. 33.6). One particular model, which is accepted by many investigators as best representing contrast material leakage into tumors, employs a two-compartment model in which the contrast material flux between the two compartments is proportional to the differences in the concentrations between compartments (Tofts 1999). The two compartments in this model are the intravascular compartment and the extravascular, extracellular compartment (EES). The intracellular compartment is (appropriately) deemed to be negligible. The model also assumes that the contrast material within the EES has arrived directly from nearby capillaries, rather than from other regions of the EES that receive contrast material from other, more distant capillaries. In addition, the model assumes that the increase in T1 relaxivity (which is the basic mechanism by which tissues gain increase in signal intensity after infusion of gadolinium-based contrast materials) is proportional to the concentration of the contrast agent and also that fast exchange of the contrast material takes place so that, in the case of MR imaging studies, the tissue of interest relaxes with a single T1 value (Tofts 1997). This imaging technique requires a number of unenhanced T1-weighted imaging pulse sequences using various flip angles in order to determine the intrinsic T1 value of tissue.

Some investigators are of the opinion that even these complex models of depicting permeability do not adequately take into account some tumor features. For instance, some argue that the degree of contrast enhancement within regions of a tumor depends not solely on delivery of contrast material and vascular leakiness but also on diffusion of contrast material within the tumor and that this factor must be taken into account in measuring permeability (Pellerin et al. 2007). Stated differently, some components of tumor contrast enhancement are derived from other areas within the EES, rather than directly from adjacent capillaries.

33.4.4 Dynamic Susceptibility Contrast MR Imaging in Brain Tumor Assessment

Another major form of hemodynamic imaging commonly performed for tumors is dynamic susceptibility contrast (DSC) MR imaging that relies on a T2*-weighted pulse sequence, as opposed to the T1-weighted dynamic contrast-enhanced pulse sequence discussed earlier (Petrella and Provenzale 2000). This form of imaging is predominantly oriented toward assessment of vascular density rather than degree of permeability. Because this discussion is directed toward permeability measurements, discussion of DSC imaging will be brief.

DSC imaging is typically performed using rapid bolus infusion of MR contrast material; in that respect it is similar to DCE (i.e., T1-weighted) imaging. However, unlike DCE imaging, DSC imaging is performed using an echo planar pulse sequence that is sensitive to signal intensity changes induced by passage of MR contrast material through vessels. Using this echo planar pulse sequence, a signal decrease (as opposed to signal increase) is induced in tissue that is proportional to the concentration of MR contrast material, which can then be used to generate an rCBV map. The concentration of contrast material (which is reflected in degree of signal intensity decrease) is proportional to the vascular density. As a result, the decrease in signal intensity is greater in tissues having a greater vascular density (e.g., gray matter structures, high-grade brain neoplasms) than in tissues with a lower vascular density (e.g., white matter). Thus, the change in signal intensity can be used as an indirect measure of tumor vascular density. By using a spin echo technique (rather than an alternative, a gradient echo technique), one can optimize the pulse sequence for detection of small vessels such as capillaries and thus obtain a measure of capillary density. Comparison of rCBV maps with permeability maps in the same patient during the same imaging examination often shows that some regions of elevated permeability do not have corresponding regions of highly elevated rCBV (Fig. 33.4), showing once again that, in the various regions of any particular tumor, a high degree of correspondence between permeability and elevated rCBV is not found.

The DSC imaging sequence has been widely used for assessment of degree of angiogenesis and response to antiangiogenesis therapy. For instance, the imaging technique has been used to not only reliably distinguish between high-grade tumors and low-grade tumors but also to distinguish high-grade tumors and other contrast-enhancing lesions such as abscesses and radiation necrosis (Holmes et al. 2004; Bruening et al. 1996; Aronen et al. 1995). DSC imaging can also be used to assess permeability because a component of contrast material leakage is also present during the first pass of contrast material used during T2*-weighted imaging (Weisskoff et al. 1994). Thus, one is able to derive both rCBV measurements and permeability measurements from a single infusion of contrast material. Studies using this form of permeability measurement have shown substantial differences between median permeability values in patients with high-grade brain neoplasms and low-grade brain neoplasms (Provenzale et al. 2002). Similarly, studies performed using DCE-based measurements of permeability and DSC-based measurements of rCBV have shown relatively good correlation (Provenzale et al. 2006b).

One study in which serial MR perfusion imaging of patients with low-grade gliomas was performed showed that this imaging technique can show significant rCBV increases before MR findings of tumor progression to high-grade neoplasm (as evidenced by new contrast enhancement) is seen (Danchaivijitr et al. 2008). Recently, the degree of elevation of rCBV has been shown to correlate with time to progression in patients with brain neoplasms (Law et al. 2008).

33.4.5 Correlation of MR Perfusion Imaging with Angiographic and Histological Tumor Features

In one study, the investigators compared hemodynamic features (in the form of rCBV within tumors) with angiographic blush seen at catheter angiography (Wetzel et al., 2002). The study showed good correlation between degree of elevation of rCBV and degree of vascularity seen at catheter angiography.

Although that study indicated good correlation between MR perfusion measurements and catheter angiography findings, it did not examine histological features indicative of tumor vascularity. However, such a correlation was performed in another study (Sugahara et al., 1998), which found a high degree of correlation between maximal rCBV values on MR perfusion imaging and vascularity within portions of surgically resected glial tumors of varying degrees of aggressiveness as well as between maximal rCBV measurements and degree of increased vascularity seen on catheter angiography. One limitation of that study is that it did not specifically attempt to directly correlate sites of maximal rCBV measurement on MR imaging and histological findings in the same region. In another study performed in mice in whom GL261 tumor cells were implanted within the brain and perfusion MR imaging was performed (Cha et al, 2003), mean vascular density was scored within histological sections of tumors after sacrifice of animals and correlated with maximal rCBV measurements. Tumors were seen to homogenously contrast-enhance on T1-weighted images in the first 2 weeks after tumor implantation but thereafter, during the stage of increasing tumor necrosis, tumors were seen to contrast-enhance in an inhomogeneous manner. Maximal rCBV values peaked during the phase of early inhomogeneous contrast enhancement (i.e., early tumor necrosis) and then decreased. Good correlation was seen between maximal rCBV values and scores of mean vascular density. Furthermore, during the late stage of necrosis, both maximal rCBV values and mean vascular density scores decreased. One interesting finding in this study was that contrast enhancement on T1-weighted images was seen before the onset of angiogenesis, indicating the role that leakage across the BBB, rather than increases in vascular density, may play in the early stages of contrast enhancement in tumors.

33.5 Importance of BBB for Therapy of Brain Tumors

33.5.1 Impact on Brain Tumor Therapy

Two important factors in the ability of a drug to cross the BBB are lipophilicity and hydrophilicity profiles of the drug in question (Kreuter 2001). An intact BBB is more effective at excluding water-soluble drugs (for which there is approximately 1% penetration of the BBB) from the CNS than lipid-soluble drugs (for which 30–40% penetration occurs) (Siegal and Zylber-Katz 2002). Even drugs with a favorable lipophilicity profile, which would be expected to readily cross the BBB, are excluded from the CNS by the multidrug resistance protein outlined earlier (Kreuter 2001). Furthermore, drugs that are effective in the laboratory setting are often not effective in human trials; in many instances, this fact is due to inadequate penetration of the drug across the BBB that was not encountered in laboratory experiments. For these reasons, many different methods have been explored to circumvent the hurdles to access the CNS imposed by an intact BBB. Some of the major strategies are outlined below.

33.5.2 Enhanced Transit of Agents across the Blood–Brain Barrier

Four major strategies have been developed to enhance the transit of chemotherapeutic agents across the BBB: (1) dose intensification, (2) altering the BBB to allow increased transport of standard chemotherapy drug formulations, (3) development of drugs that have increased transport across the BBB, and (4) bypass of the BBB by insertion of mechanical methods of drug delivery into the brain or the cerebrospinal fluid. The first three methods are primarily pharmacological in nature and can be considered as methods to increase uptake enhancement of intravascular drugs (Siegal and Zylber-Katz 2002). The fourth pathway is primarily surgical (Bellavance et al. 2008). It is worth exploring each in turn.

33.5.3 Drug Dose Intensification

One method to attempt to increase transport is by increasing the plasma concentration of drug plasma concentration, a process to which some refer as chemotherapeutic dose intensification (Kraemer et al. 2002; Siegal and Zylber-Katz 2002). Dose intensification has been defined as any regimen that delivers high-dose chemotherapy at the highest possible doses and for the shortest possible time, often in conjunction with chemoprotection methods to minimize toxicity (Kraemer et al. 2002). This strategy can also be employed with techniques to interrupt the BBB, which are discussed separately below. For instance, intra-arterial infusion of chemotherapy, which produces large increases in plasma concentration of chemotherapy at the site of the tumor, can be considered as one form of dose intensification therapy (Siegal and Zylber-Katz 2002; Kraemer et al. 2002).

33.5.4 BBB Alteration to Allow Increased Drug Transport

Modulation of the BBB, typically in combination of intra-arterial infusion of drug, provides another means of enhancing CNS drug delivery (Siegal and Zylber-Katz 2002). Increasing BBB permeability predominantly affects the penetration of water-soluble drugs. One technique that has been extensively studied is termed osmotic disruption of the BBB and is based on the principle that administration of a hyperosmolar solution, such as mannitol, greatly increases BBB permeability on a transient basis. The mechanism by which this occurs is not definitively known but a leading hypothesis is that the administration of a hyperosmolar solution causes retraction of the endothelial cell membrane, thereby opening tight junctions (Brightman et al. 1973). In rodent experiments, the percentage of methotrexate delivered to brain was markedly increased using this method (Remsen et al. 1995). Interestingly, radiation treatment prior to infusion markedly decreased drug delivery when radiation therapy was administered weeks before chemotherapy. The technique has been used with some success in humans, following a treatment paradigm that includes arterial catheterization under general anesthesia (which is administered in order to provide continuous stabilization of blood pressure and heart rate at levels that will optimize chemotherapy delivery). The degree of BBB disruption can be assessed immediately after the procedure by performing a contrast-enhanced CT or MR scan. This form of therapy has been employed in various brain tumors with varying degrees of success (Kraemer et al. 2002). In one study of primary CNS lymphoma patients, a statistically significant association between cumulative dose and survival was shown (Kraemer et al. 2001). Nonetheless, a number of limitations of this technique have been noted, which include relatively high cost, use of general anesthesia, invasive nature (based on need for intra-arterial catheterization), and risks of the catheterization procedure (Siegal and Zylber-Katz 2002). Furthermore, standardly the vascular territory of only one of the four major intracranial arteries is considered treatable in any one session (Bellavance et al. 2008). Thus, if the tumor is supplied by more than one major artery, then multiple treatment sessions are needed.

Another form of BBB disruption is that of receptor-mediated BBB opening (Siegal and Zylber-Katz 2002). Much of the work along these lines has been performed using bradykinin or receptor-mediated permeabilizier-7, which is the synthetic analogue of bradykinin. Both molecules provide a means to selectively open the BBB at the tumor site and thus provide targeted delivery, while only lesser degrees of drug are presented to adjacent brain regions (Siegal and Zylber-Katz 2002). One interesting application in an animal model involved preoperative application of a dye following receptor-mediated permeabilizier-7 infusion to more definitively outline surgical margins (Britz et al. 2002). Although therapy using these drugs to enhance drug transport to tumor, if effective, would provide clear advantages, recent small clinical trials have yet to show definite benefit (Warren et al. 2006).

33.5.5 Drugs with Increased Transport Capabilities Across the BBB

Another technique of increased transport is design of methods that enhance the permeability of a specific drug across the BBB (Pardridge 2002; Liu et al. 2006). This can be accomplished by provision of an inactive drug precursor (a so-called pro-drug) that has been modified to increase permeability across the BBB compared to the active form of the drug; the pro-drug can then be converted to an active form of the drug after passage across the BBB (Siegal and Zylber-Katz

2002). An example can be seen in the pro-drug temozolomide, which is lipid soluble and which is converted to an active metabolite at physiological pH within the CNS (Siegal and Zylber-Katz 2002).

33.5.6 Local Delivery Techniques

A wide variety of local delivery methods have been developed to enhance drug delivery without having to cross the BBB. One such strategy is direct infusion into the tumor of materials or substrates having sustained release capabilities. These substrates can range from placement of manufactured materials such as polymer wafers into surgical resection cavities (Chambers et al. 2007) to direct injection of viral-mediated therapies, such as drug-expressing adenovirus vectors, into the tumor itself (Chiocca et al. 2008). Monoclonal antibodies are another promising means of treatment of brain tumors but therapy is limited by a low degree of passage through the BBB. One method to bypass the BBB for monoclonal antibody therapy is infusion into a surgical resection cavity; substantial experience has been gained with this method of delivery using monoclonal antibodies bound to radionuclide materials that allows a means of targeted radiotherapy that directly treats the margins of the resection cavity but spares normal brain (Reardon et al. 2006). Yet another method of delivery of monoclonal antibodies is intrathecal infusion, which has been shown to substantially increase levels of antibodies to which tumor may be exposed (Wong 2005). Finally, another method of delivery attempted is intranasal delivery, which has shown promise in increased survival in small animal models (Hashizume et al. 2008).

33.5.7 Convection-Enhanced Delivery

An alternative method to deliver drug therapy to the CNS is to directly infuse agents into brain tissue. However, such infusions are limited by the fact that molecular weight and tissue clearance mechanisms impair diffusion of large amounts of drug from the infusion site. An alternative to direct infusion of drug, termed convection-enhanced delivery, has gained much attention in recent years. Convection-enhanced delivery is intended to use a fluid pressure gradient to instill therapeutic drug into interstitial spaces of a tumor using an indwelling catheter (Sampson et al. 2008). Drug diffusion produced by such infusions can be monitored by conventional MR imaging methods (Sampson et al. 2007).

33.5.8 Assessment of Drug Pharmacokinetics Within Brain Tissue

An important aspect of drug therapy for brain tumors is the assessment of actual drug delivery to the tumor. Various methods have been described to accomplish this goal. One especially promising method that has recently been optimized for brain tumor therapy is that of microdialysis (Benjamin et al. 2004). In one study, microdialysis was performed in brain tumor tissue in two patients and in brain tissue adjacent to tumor in another two patients during and after boron infusion for boron neutron capture therapy (Bergenheim et al. 2005). In all four patients, microdialysis was also performed in normal brain tissue. In the two patients in whom microdialysis was performed in tumor tissue, maximal drug level in tumor was approximately 50% of maximal boron level in blood in one patient (and 140% of that in normal brain) and approximately 80% of maximal boron level in blood (and 600% of that in normal brain) in the other patient. These findings were taken by the investigators to indicate that boron crossed the BBB adjacent to tumor in substantive amounts but at normal brain regions, in which the BBB is intact, brain levels are much lower. Among the two patients in whom boron levels in brain adjacent to tumor was measured, in one patient the maximal level was 75% of that of maximal blood levels (and 6 times that of levels in normal brain); in another patient, maximal level in brain adjacent to tumor was approximately 30% of the maximal level measured in blood.

33.6 Summary

This chapter has provided the basic information needed to understand the nature of the BBB and to comprehend the role of the BBB in CNS imaging and in new methods for providing therapy for CNS tumors. One may expect that, in the future, novel means of intermittently altering the BBB for therapeutic purposes will be developed. As those methods are developed, in parallel, better imaging techniques will be needed to monitor both BBB alteration and efflux of therapeutic agents across the BBB. Furthermore, more specific information will be required from neuroradiological studies to determine, at even earlier stages, whether therapy is effective so that changes in drug regimens can be made, as needed, early in the treatment course. With that in mind, the investigator who is involved in CNS tumor imaging or therapy is encouraged to read many excellent articles used in the preparation of this chapter with the intent of a more detailed understanding of the BBB.

Abbreviations

BBB Blood–brain barrier

DCE Dynamic contrast-enhanced imaging: a form of T1-weighted MR imaging that employs rapid infusion of MR contrast material followed by continuous imaging over a few minutes or many minutes to record increases in signal intensity

DSC Dynamic susceptibility contrast imaging: a form of T2*-weighted MR imaging in which rapid infusion of MR contrast material is followed by continuous imaging over a period of approximately 1 minute to monitor signal decrease. The signal decrease within tumors is measured as relative cerebral blood volume (rCBV)

EES Extracellular, extravascular space: the extracellular compartment between cells; essentially the same as the nonvascular interstitial space

MTT Mean transit time: the time taken for contrast material to pass through tissues, which is shortened in tumors that have a high degree of arteriovenous shunting

rCBV Relative cerebral blood volume: a measure of intravascular space within a volume of tissue. Within tumors, the rCBV is generally reflective of capillary density and is considered one measure of angiogenesis

References

Aronen HJ, Glass J, Pardo FS, Belliveau JW, Gruber ML, Buchbinder BR, Gazit IE, Lingood RM, Fischman AJ, Rosen BR. (1995) Echo-planar MR cerebral blood volume mapping of gliomas: clinical utility. *Acta Radiol* 36:520–528

Bart J, Groen HJM, Hendrikse NH, van der Graaf WTA, Vaalburg W, de Vries EGE. (2000) The blood-brain barrier and oncology: new insights into function and modulation. *Cancer Treat Rev* 26:449–462

Batchelor TT, Sorensen AG, di Tomaso E, Zhang WT, Duda DG, Cohen KS, Kozak KR, Cahill DP, Chen PJ, Zhu M, Ancukiewicz M, Mrugala MM, Plotkin S, Drappatz J, Louis DN, Ivy P, Scadden DT, Benner T, Loeffler JS, Wen PY, Jain RK. (2007) AZD2171, a pan-VEGF receptor tyrosine kinase inhibitor, normalizes tumor vasculature and alleviates edema in glioblastoma patients. *Cancer Cell* 11:83–95

Bellavance M-A, Blanchette M, Fortin D. (2008) Recent advances in blood–brain barrier disruption as a CNS delivery strategy. *AAPS J* 10:166–177

Benjamin RK, Hochberg FH, Fox E, Bungay PM, Elmquist WF, Stewart CF, Gallo JM, Collins JM, Pelletier RP, de Groot JF, Hickner RC, Cavus I, Grossman SA, Colvin OM. (2004) Review of microdialysis in brain tumors, from concept to application: First Annual Carolyn Frye-Halloran Symposium. *Neuro-Oncol* 6:65–74

Bergenheim AT, Capala J, Roslin M, Henriksson R. (2005) Distribution of BPA and metabolic assessment in glioblastoma patients during BNCT treatment: A microdialysis study. *J Neuro-Oncol* 71:287–293

Brightman MW, Hori M, Rapoport SI, Reese TS, Westergaard E. (1973) Osmotic opening of tight junctions in cerebral endothelium. *J Comp Neurol* 152:317–325

Britz GW, Ghatan S, Spence AM, Berger MS. Intracarotid RMP-7 enhanced indocyanine green staining of tumors in a rat glioma model. (2002) *J Neurooncol* 56:227–232

Bruening R, Kwong KK, Vevea MJ, Hochberg FH, Cher L, Harsh GR 4th, Niemi PT, Weisskoff RM, Rosen BR. (1996) Echo-planar MR determination of relative cerebral blood volume in human brain tumors: T1 versus T2 weighting. *AJNR Am J Neuroradiol* 17:831–840

Cha S, Johnson G, Wadghiri YZ, Jin O, Babb J, Zagzag D, Turnbull DH. (2003) Dynamic, contrast-enhanced perfusion MRI in mouse gliomas: correlation with histopathology. *Magn Reson Med* 49:848–855

Chambers A, Spithoff K, Laperriere N. (2007) Gliadel wafers in the treatment of malignant glioma: a systematic review. *Curr Oncol* 14:189–194
Chiocca EA, Smith KM, McKinney B, Palmer CA, Rosenfeld S, Lillehei K, Hamilton A, DeMasters BK, Judy K, Kirn D. (2008) A phase I trial of Ad.hIFN-beta gene therapy for glioma. *Mol Ther* 16:618–626
Choyke PL, Dwyer AJ, Knopp MV. (2003) Functional tumor imaging with dynamic contrast-enhanced magnetic resonance imaging. *J Magn Reson Imaging* 17:509–520
Danchaivijitr N, Waldman AD, Tozer DJ, Benton CE, Brasil Caseiras G, Tofts PS, Rees JH, Jäger HR. (2008) Low-grade gliomas: do changes in rCBV measurements at longitudinal perfusion-weighted MR imaging predict malignant transformation? *Radiology* 247: 170–178
Fojo AT, Ueda K, Slamon DJ, Poplack DG, Gottesman MM, Pastan I. (1987) Expression of a multidrug-resistance gene in human tumors and tissues. *Proc Natl Acad Sci USA* 84: 265–269
Hashizume R, Ozawa T, Gryaznov SM, Bollen AW, Lamborn KR, Frey WH 2nd, Deen DF. (2008) New therapeutic approach for brain tumors: Intranasal delivery of telomerase inhibitor GRN163. *Neuro Oncol* 10:112–120
Higgins CF. ABC transporters: from microorganisms to man. (1992) *Annu Rev Cell Biol* 8:67–113
Holmes TM, Petrella JR, Provenzale JM. (2004) Distinction between cerebral abscesses and high-grade neoplasms by dynamic susceptibility contrast MRI. *AJR Am J Roentgenol* 183:1247–1252
Ikeda O, Nishimura R, Miyayama H, Yasunaga T, Ozaki Y, Tuji A, Yamashita Y. (2004) Evaluation of tumor angiogenesis using dynamic enhanced magnetic resonance imaging: comparison of plasma vascular endothelial growth factor, hemodynamic, and pharmacokinetic parameters. *Acta Radiol* 45:446–452
Kim H, Lee JM, Park JS, Jo SA, Kim YO, Kim CW, Jo I. (2008) Dexamethasone coordinately regulates angiopoietin-1 and VEGF: a mechanism of glucocorticoid-induced stabilization of blood-brain barrier. *Biochem Biophys Res Commun* 372:243–248
Kondziolka D, Lunsford LD, Martinez AJ. (1993) Unreliability of contemporary neurodiagnostic imaging in evaluating suspected adult supratentorial (low-grade) astrocytoma. *J Neurosurg* 79:533–536
Kraemer DF, Fortin D, Doolittle ND, Neuwelt EA. (2001) Association of total dose intensity of chemotherapy in primary central nervous system lymphoma (human non-acquired immunodeficiency syndrome) and survival. *Neurosurgery* 48:1033–1040
Kraemer DF, Fortin D, Neuwelt EA. (2002) Chemotherapeutic dose intensification for treatment of malignant brain tumors: recent developments and future directions. *Curr Neurol Neurosci Rep* 2:216–224
Kreuter J. (2001) Nanoparticulate systems for brain delivery of drugs. *Advanced Drug Delivery Reviews* 47:65–81
Law M, Young RJ, Babb JS, Peccerelli N, Chheang S, Gruber ML, Miller DC, Golfinos JG, Zagzag D, Johnson G. (2008) Gliomas: predicting time to progression or survival with cerebral blood volume measurements at dynamic susceptibility-weighted contrast-enhanced perfusion MR imaging. *Radiology* 247:490–498
Liu HM, Liu XF, Yao JL, Wang CL, Yu Y, Wang R. (2006) Utilization of combined chemical modifications to enhance the blood-brain barrier permeability and pharmacological activity of endomorphin-1. *J Pharmacol Exp Ther* 319:308–316
Pardridge WM. (2002) Drug and gene targeting to the brain with molecular Trojan horses *Nature Reviews Drug Discovery* 1: 131–139
Pellerin M, Yankeelov TE, Lepage M. (2007) Incorporating contrast agent diffusion into the analysis of DCE-MRI data. *Magn Reson Med* 58:1124–1134
Petrella JR, Provenzale JM. (2000) MR Perfusion imaging of the brain: Techniques and applications. *AJR Am J Roentgenol* 175:207–220

Pickles MD, Manton DJ, Lowry M, Turnbull LW. (2008) Prognostic value of pre-treatment DCE-MRI parameters in predicting disease free and overall survival for breast cancer patients undergoing neoadjuvant chemotherapy. *Eur J Radiol* doi: 10.1016/j.ejrad.2008.05.007

Provenzale JM, Wang GR, Brenner T, Petrella JR, Sorensen AG. (2002) Comparison of permeability in high-grade and low-grade brain tumors using dynamic susceptibility contrast MR imaging. *AJR Am J Roentgenol* 178:711–716

Provenzale JM, Mukundan S, Dewhirst MW. (2005) The role of blood-brain barrier permeability in brain tumor imaging and therapeutics. *AJR Am J Roentgenol* 185:763–767

Provenzale JM, Mukundan S, Barboriak DP. (2006a) Diffusion-weighted and perfusion MR imaging for brain tumor characterization and assessment of treatment response. *Radiology* 239:632–649

Provenzale JM, York G, Moya MG, Parks L, Choma M, Kealey S, Cole P, Serajuddin H. (2006b) Correlation of relative permeability and relative cerebral blood volume in high-grade cerebral neoplasms. *AJR Am J Roentgenol* 187:1036–1042

Provenzale JM. Imaging of angiogenesis: Clinical techniques and novel imaging methods. *AJR Am J Roentgenol* 2007; 188:11–23

Puduvalli VK, Sawaya R. (2000) Antiangiogenesis – therapeutic strategies and clinical implications for brain tumors. *J Neuro-Oncol* 50:189–200

Reardon DA, Quinn JA, Akabani G, Coleman RE, Friedman AH, Friedman HS, Herndon JE II, McLendon RE, Pegram CN, Provenzale JM, Dowell JM, Rich JN, Vredenburgh JV, Desjardins A, Sampson JH, Gururangan S, Wong TZ, Badruddoja MA, Zhao XG, Bigner DD, Zalutsky MR. (2006) Novel human IgG2b/murine chimeric antitenascin monoclonal antibody construct radiolabeled with 131I and administered into the surgically created resection cavity of patients with malignant glioma: Phase I trial results. *J Nucl Med* 47:912–918

Remsen LG, McCormick CI, Sexton G, Pearse HD, Garcia R, Neuwelt EA. (1995) Decreased delivery and acute toxicity of cranial irradiation and chemotherapy given with osmotic blood-brain barrier disruption in a rodent model: the issue of sequence. *Clin Cancer Res* 1:731–739

Ribatti D, Nico B, Crivellato E, Artico M. (2006) Development of the blood-brain barrier: a historical perspective. *Anat Rec (Part B: New Anat)* 289B:3–8

Roberts HC, Roberts TPL, Brasch RC, Dillon WP. (2000) Measurement of microvascular permeability in human brain tumors achieved using dynamic contrast-enhanced MR imaging: correlation with histologic grade. *AJNR* 21:891–899

Sampson JH, Raghavan R, Provenzale JM, Croteau D, Reardon DA, Coleman RE, Rodríguez Ponce I, Pastan I, Puri RK, Pedain C. (2007) Induction of hyperintense signal on T2-weighted MR images correlates with infusion distribution from intracerebral convection-enhanced delivery of a tumor-targeted cytotoxin. *AJR Am J Roentgenol* 188:703–709

Sampson JH, Akabani G, Archer GE, Berger MS, Coleman RE, Friedman AH, Friedman HS, Greer K, Herndon JE 2nd, Kunwar S, McLendon RE, Paolino A, Petry NA, Provenzale JM, Reardon DA, Wong TZ, Zalutsky MR, Pastan I, Bigner DD. (2008) Intracerebral infusion of an EGFR-targeted toxin in recurrent malignant brain tumors. *Neuro-Oncol* 10:320–329

Siegal T, Zylber-Katz E. (2002) Strategies for increasing drug delivery to the brain. Focus on brain lymphoma. *Clin Pharmacokinet* 41:171–186

Sugahara T, Korogi Y, Kochi M, Ikushima I, Hiirai T, Okuda T, Sihigematsu Y, Liang L, Ge Y, Ushio Y, Takahashi M. (1998) Correlation of MR Imaging-determined cerebral blood volume maps with histologic and angiographic determination of vascularity of gliomas. *AJR* 171:1479–1486

Tofts PS. (1997) Modeling tracer kinetics in dynamic Gd-DTPA MR imaging. *J Magn Reson Imaging* 7:91–101

Tofts PS, Brix G, Evelhoch JL, Henderson E, Knopp MV, Larsson HB, Lee TY, Mayr NA, Parker GJ, Port RE, Taylor J, Weisskoff RM. (1999) Estimating kinetic parameters from dynamic contrast-enhanced T(1)-weighted MRI of a diffusible tracer: standardized quantities and symbols. *J Magn Reson Imaging* 10:223–232

Warren K, Jakacki R, Widemann B, Aikin A, Libucha M, Packer R, Vezina G, Reaman G, Shaw D, Krailo M, Osborne C, Cehelsky J, Caldwell D, Stanwood J, Steinberg SM, Balis FM. (2006) Phase II trial of intravenous lobradimil and carboplatin in childhood brain tumors: a report from the Children's Oncology Group. *Cancer Chemother Pharmacol* 58:343–347

Wetzel SG, Cha S, Law M, Johnson G, Golfinos J, Lee P, Nelson PK. (2002) Preoperative assessment of intracranial tumors with perfusion MR and a volumetric interpolated examination: A comparative study with DSA. *AJNR Am J Neuroradiol* 23:1767–1774

Weisskoff RM, Boxerman JL, Sorensen AG, Kulke SM, Campbell TA, Rosen BR. (1994) Simultaneous blood volume and permeability mapping using a single GD-based contrast injection. In: *Proceedings of the Society for Magnetic Resonance*. Berkeley, CA: Society for Magnetic Resonance. 1:279

Wong ET. (2005) Management of central nervous system lymphomas using monoclonal antibodies: challenges and opportunities. Clin Cancer Res 11:7151s–7157s

Wong JC, Provenzale JM, Petrella JR. Perfusion MR imaging of brain neoplasms. *AJR Am J Roentgenol* 2000; 174:1147–1157

Chapter 34
Targeting CXCR4 in Brain Tumors

Hyunsuk Shim

Abstract Chemokines (chemotactic cytokines) are a family of proteins associated with the trafficking and activation of leukocytes and other cell types in immune surveillance and inflammatory response. Besides their roles in the immune system, they play pleiotropic roles in tumor initiation, promotion, and progression. CXCL12, a chemokine that binds to CXCR4, has been frequently implicated in various cancers. Over the past several years, studies have increasingly shown that the CXCR4/CXCL12 axis plays critical roles in tumor progression, such as invasion, angiogenesis, survival, and homing to metastatic sites. This review focuses on the involvement of CXCR4/CXCL12 interaction in central and peripheral nervous system cancers. CXCR4 expression profiles can be utilized to determine different stages of malignancy in these cancers, which may lead to alternative prognostic markers for cancers and a plan to enhance both diagnostic and therapeutic strategies.

Contents

H. Shim (✉)
Department of Radiology, Winship Cancer Institute, Emory University School of Medicine, 1365C Clifton Road, N.E., C5008, Atlanta, GA 30322, USA
e-mail: hshim@emory.edu

E.G. Van Meir (ed.), *CNS Cancer*, Cancer Drug Discovery and Development, DOI 10.1007/978-1-60327-553-8_34,

© Humana Press, a part of Springer Science+Business Media, LLC 2009

34.1 Introduction

Chemokines are a superfamily of small secreted cytokines that, through their interaction with G protein-coupled receptors, induce cytoskeletal rearrangements and directional migration of several cell types (Butcher et al., 1999; Campbell and Butcher, 2000; Zlotnik and Yoshie, 2000). These secreted proteins act in a coordinated fashion with cell-surface proteins, including integrins, to direct the specific homing of various subsets of hematopoietic cells to specific anatomical sites (Forster et al., 1999; Homey et al., 2000; Morales et al., 1999; Peled et al., 1999). Chemokines are small peptidic ligands involved in the trafficking of leukocytes and other motile cells (Balabanian et al., 2005; Murphy et al., 2000).

Chemokines play a major role in regulating the migration of cells of the immune system, leading to modulation of immune responses. Their exact role depends on the expression pattern of receptors on specific leukocyte subsets (Murphy et al., 2000) but encompasses the regulation of lymphocyte trafficking, lymphoid tissue development, and the effecting of inflammatory reactions. Chemokine receptors are also found on other cell types and play a part in stem cell recruitment, angiogenesis, development, and wound healing (Rossi and Zlotnik, 2000).

Interest in chemokines and their receptors in the CNS has been rapidly increasing due to their involvement in a diverse range of neurological diseases. Concordantly, the volume of literature pertaining to their involvement in CNS development has been growing rapidly in recent years. Chemokines are also involved in neuronal and glial cell migration and patterning (Bajetto et al., 2001). For example, CXCL1–CXCR2 has been implicated in the migration and proliferation of oligodendrocyte progenitors (Tsai et al., 2002). In parallel to this implication in CNS patterning and developmental positioning, chemokines and their receptors act as physiological neuromodulators. Chemokines CXCL1, CXCL8, and CXCL12 regulate neurotransmitter release or modulate ion channel activity at both the presynaptic and postsynaptic levels (Giovannelli et al., 1998; Limatola et al., 2000). CXCL12–CXCR4 signaling controls the migration and survival of neural precursors (Dziembowska et al., 2005). CXCL12 is a potent neuromodulator of evoked excitatory synaptic transmission and is constitutively expressed in the CNS (Bertollini et al., 2006).

Beyond their role in the CNS under physiological conditions, chemokines and chemokine receptors are studied primarily as mediators of CNS pathologies, especially those with an inflammatory component such as multiple sclerosis. During neurological diseases, the expression of chemokines can be selectively induced or upregulated in a wide range of cells, including microglia, astrocytes, neurons, and endothelial cells (Charo and Ransohoff, 2006; Ubogu et al., 2006). Recent studies suggest that many cancers express an extensive network of chemokines and chemokine receptors (Balkwill and Mantovani, 2001; Vicari and Caux, 2002). These tumors are characterized by deregulation of chemokines and abnormal chemokine receptor expression. The role of chemokines and cytokines in the development of brain tumors has been previously reviewed (Dey et al., 2006; Van Meir, 1995, 1999).

As such, these molecules—both chemokines and their receptors—represent potential therapeutic targets. In this chapter, we will focus on the role of CXCR4 as a therapeutic target in brain tumors.

34.2 Classification of Chemokines and Their Receptors

Chemokines can be classified into four subfamilies of chemokines, CXC, CC, C, and CX3C, based on the number and spacing of conserved cysteine residues near the N-terminus (Balabanian et al., 2005; Mellado et al., 2001; Zlotnik and Yoshie, 2000) (Fig. 34.1A). CXC, CC, and CX3C chemokines all have four

a

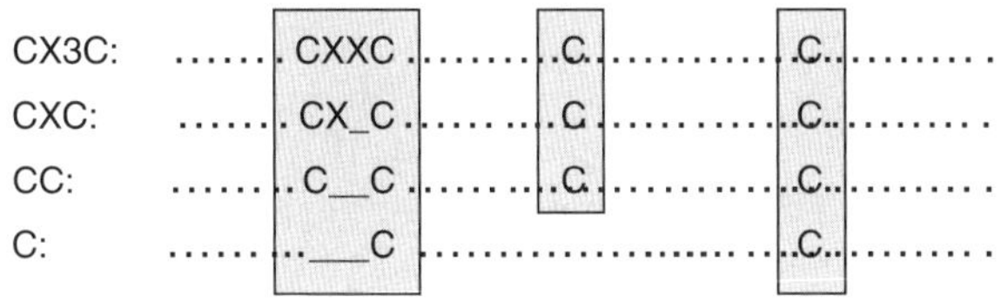

b

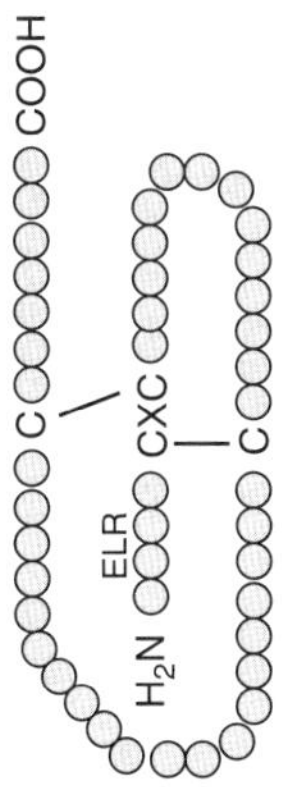

Subgroup	Nomenclature	Original name	Receptor
ELR+	CXCL1	GROα	CXCR2
	CXCL2	GROβ	CXCR2
	CXCL3	GROγ	CXCR2
	CXCL5	ENA-78	CXCR1, CXCR2
	CXCL6	GCP-2	CXCR1
	CXCL7	NAP-2	CXCR2
	CXCL8	IL-8	CXCR1, CXCR2
	CXCL15	Lungkine	CXCR2
ELR–	CXCL4	PF-4	
	CXCL9	MIG	CXCR3
	CXCL10	IP-10	CXCR3
	CXCL11	I-TAC	CXCR3, CXCR7
	CXCL12	SDF-1	CXCR4, CXCR7
	CXCL13	BCA-1	CXCR5
	CXCL14	BRAK	
	CXCL16	CXCL16	CXCR6

Fig. 34.1 (**a**) Chemokines are classified into four major subfamilies according to the configuration of the cysteine residues they contain (http://cytokine.medic.kumamoto-u.ac.jp/). (**b**) The CXC subfamily is further classified into two subgroups depending on the presence or absence of the sequence motif glutamate-leucine-arginine (ELR) at the N-terminus. Individual chemokines can bind more than one chemokine receptor

conserved cysteines, whereas C chemokines have only two. CXC and CX3C chemokines are distinguished by the presence of one (CXC) or three (CX3C) amino acids between the first and second cysteines, whereas the first two cysteines of CC chemokines are adjacent. The nomenclature of chemokines (e.g., "CXCL12") is comprised of their subclass (CXC, CC, etc.) followed by "L" for ligand and a specific number (Balabanian et al., 2005; Murphy et al., 2000). This CXC subfamily can be further subclassified into two groups, depending on the presence or absence of a tripeptide motif glutamic acid–leucine–arginine (ELR) in the N-terminal domain (Fig. 34.1B). The ELR presence has been proposed to relate to the functional correlation of structural characteristics of CXC chemokines, such as specificity for neutrophil chemotaxis and angiogenesis (Addison et al., 2000; Hebert et al., 1991; Moore et al., 1998; Strieter et al., 1995). The ELR-containing chemokines (such as IL-8, GRO, and ENA-78) have an apparent uniformity of function as a family of neutrophil chemoattractants and activators. They have also been reported to induce angiogenesis and to be chemotactic for endothelial cells. In contrast, the non-ELR-CXC chemokines (such as PF-4, IP-10, MIG, and CXCL12) show disparate activities. They are themselves nonangiogenic and are even known to possess antiangiogenic properties. One exception is CXCL12, which induces neovascularization (Salcedo et al., 1999). In general, the members of each chemokine subfamily show overlapping specificities. For instance, the CXC-ELR1 chemokines are chemoattractants for neutrophils, but not for monocytes. However, CXC-ELR2 chemokines attract lymphocytes and monocytes but are poor chemoattractants for neutrophils. Chemokine receptors are G protein-coupled receptors (GPCRs) with seven transmembrane domains that are highly conserved in evolution (DeVries et al., 2006; Fredriksson et al., 2003; Kawasawa et al., 2003). By binding to their corresponding receptors, chemokines activate a series of downstream signaling pathways to guide the movement of leukocytes to target tissues or organs (Rot and von Andrian, 2004). Directional movement of leukocytes through a concentration gradient of chemokine is defined as "chemotaxis." So far, 53 human chemokines and 23 chemokine receptors have been cloned or characterized (http://cytokine.medic.kumamoto-u.ac.jp/).

Chemokines bind within the extracellular domain of the chemokine receptor, which comprises the N-terminus and three extracellular loops (Mellado et al., 2001). The intracellular domain, which consists of three loops and the C-terminus, associates with G proteins that, upon activation, lead to events such as inhibition of adenylyl cyclase activity (Mellado et al., 2001). G proteins are then activated, driving dissociation of their heterotrimers into α and $\beta\gamma$ subunits. Next, various signaling effectors, such as G protein-sensitive phospholipase C isoforms, are activated resulting in inositol-3,4,5-trisphosphate generation. Some of the chemokines can also inhibit adenylate cyclase, activate MAP kinases or phosphatidyl inositol-3OH kinase (PI-3 K) (Cartier et al., 2005; Mellado et al., 2001), and stimulate the tyrosine phosphorylation of focal adhesion complex components (Fig. 34.2). Typical cellular consequences

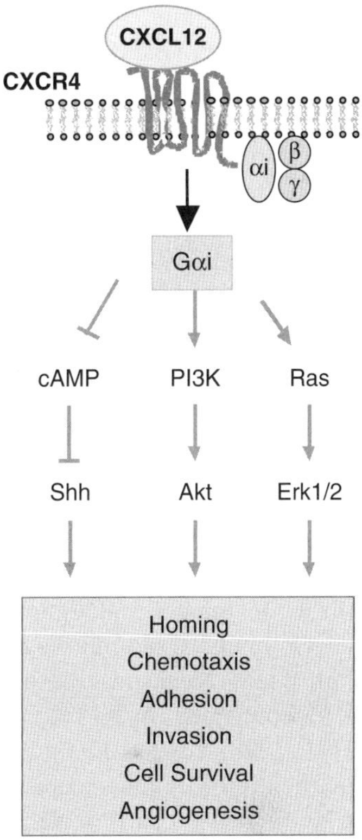

Fig. 34.2 CXCR4/CXCL12 (previously called stromal cell-derived factor-1 or SDF-1) signaling. Binding of CXCL12 to CXCR4 activates Gαi (pertussis toxin-sensitive) signaling pathways through which reduces cAMP signaling molecules in cells and leads to phosphatidylinositol 3-kinase (PI3K)/Akt and Ras/MAPK signaling pathways. These signaling pathways induce homing, chemotaxis, adhesion, invasion, cell survival, and angiogenesis in lymphocytes, macrophages, neutrophils, hematopoietic stem cells, and tumor cells

of chemokine binding include changes in gene expression, cell polarization, and chemotaxis (directed cell migration) (Kuang et al., 1996; Rossi and Zlotnik, 2000; Sozzani et al., 1993; Ward et al., 1998). When CXCL12 binds to CXCR4, the complex activates $G\alpha_i$ protein-mediated signaling (pertussis toxin-sensitive) (Chen et al., 1998), including downstream signal pathways such as Ras/MAP Kinases and PI-3 K/Akt in lymphocyte, megakaryocytes, and hematopoietic stem cells (Bleul et al., 1996; Deng et al., 1997; Kijowski et al., 2001; Majka et al., 2001; Sotsios et al., 1999; Vlahakis et al., 2002). The interaction of CXCR4 and CXCL12 has been shown to induce the activation of the PI-3 K/Akt signaling pathway. Also, PI-3 K activation is in turn closely correlated with cell motility and migration. Akt plays a critical role in promoting cell survival by phosphorylating and inactivating components of the apoptotic machinery, such as BAD, caspase-9, focal adhesion kinase (FAK), and FKHRL1.

34.3 History of CXCR4/CXCL12

A CXCL12 cDNA clone was first isolated by Tashiro et al. from a murine bone marrow stromal cell line by the signal sequence trap method and the gene was originally named stromal cell-derived factor-1 (SDF-1) (Tashiro et al., 1993).

A few years later, two groups identified its receptor, an orphan GPCR called LESTR/fusin (Bleul et al., 1996; Oberlin et al., 1996). LESTR/fusin was also identified as the coreceptor for human immunodeficiency virus (HIV-1) infection of CD4+ lymphocytes (Feng et al., 1996). CXCL12 was shown to inhibit infection by T-tropic HIV of HeLa-CD4 cells (Bleul et al., 1996; Oberlin et al., 1996). Because LESTR/fusin was found to bind to CXCL12, the nomenclature was revised and it was renamed CXCR4. The CXCL12/CXCR4 chemokine/receptor pair plays pleiotropic functions in the peripheral immune system. CXCL12 is a highly efficacious chemoattractant for lymphocytes and monocytes, but not neutrophils (Bleul et al., 1996). In addition, CXCL12/CXCR4 not only regulates the development of T and B lymphocytes but also contributes to the survival of mature lymphocytes and to the generation of memory T cells (Klein et al., 2001). Later studies have indicated that CXCL12/CXCR4 enhances the inflammatory infiltration of neutrophils or lymphocytes in diverse models and settings involving acute inflammation or fulminant infection (Ding et al., 2006; Petty et al., 2007; Wald et al., 2004). Most importantly, CXCL12 is a major regulator for the homing of hematopoietic progenitor cells (HPCs) to the bone marrow (BM) microenvironment (Lapidot et al., 2005). Deficient development of blood cells and the heart was also described in CXCL12 knockout mice (Nagasawa et al., 1996). Similar phenotypes were observed in knockout mice for its receptor, CXCR4, as well (Tachibana et al., 1998; Zou et al., 1998), suggesting that the interaction between CXCL12 and CXCR4 may be the major ligand/receptor pair relationship. Only recently, a new receptor, CXCR7, has been reported as an alternative nonsignaling CXCL12 receptor, suggesting that the CXCL12/CXCR4 relationship is not entirely exclusive (Burns et al., 2006). However, CXCR7, unlike CXCR4, is expressed only in limited tissue types.

34.4 Functions of CXCR4 in the Normal CNS

The interplay between CXCL12 and CXCR4 is critical to normal development. Unlike mice deficient in other chemokine/receptors, mice lacking CXCL12 or CXCR4 die in utero or shortly after birth (Balabanian et al., 2005; Nagasawa et al., 1996; Odemis et al., 2005; Tachibana et al., 1998; Zou et al., 1998). CXCL12/CXCR4 signaling is required during the development of the hematopoietic, cardiac, vascular, muscular, and nervous systems. Absence of this axis in embryonic life leads to defects in bone marrow myeloid cell formation, cardiac function due to impaired ventricular septum formation, and developmental defects in the cerebellum and in the vasculature of the gastrointestinal tract (Nagasawa et al., 1996; Tachibana et al., 1998; Zou et al., 1998). In the normal adult, CXCL12 and CXCR4 are involved in the homing and retention of hematopoietic progenitor cells in the bone marrow. These progenitor cells express high levels of CXCR4 and are attracted toward CXCL12 produced by stromal cells in specialized bone marrow niches. Mutations of the *CXCR4* gene lead to aberrant retention of myeloid cells within the bone marrow (Aiuti et al., 1997; Hernandez et al., 2003). In addition, CXCL12 acts as a major chemoattractant for stem cells and some differentiated cells in the pathological contexts of inflammation and tissue regeneration/repair (Gao and Li, 2007; Imitola et al., 2004; Kajiyama et al., 2007; Moyer et al., 2007).

The expression of CXCL12 and its receptor, CXCR4, has been described in neuronal, astroglial, and microglial cell populations in the CNS (Bajetto et al., 2001; Ohtani et al., 1998). CXCL12 exerts its chemotactic action to direct organogenesis and tissue structure in the developing brain. This is demonstrated by studies of both CXCL12–/– and CXCR4–/– knockout mice, in which gene deletion resulted in significant abnormalities in cerebellar and hippocampus development. These animals suffered from severe cerebellar abnormalities comprised of a misplaced external granule cell layer and clusters of proliferating granule cell precursors which had migrated inappropriately deep within the cerebellar anlagen (Bagri et al., 2002; Lu et al., 2002; Ma et al., 1998; Nagasawa et al., 1996; Reiss et al., 2002; Zhu et al., 2002; Zou et al., 1998). Thus, evidence is accumulating that the CXCR4 plays a crucial role in the normal development of the cerebellar cortex and in cell cycle control of neuronal precursors within the external granule cell layer (Fig. 34.3 and Color

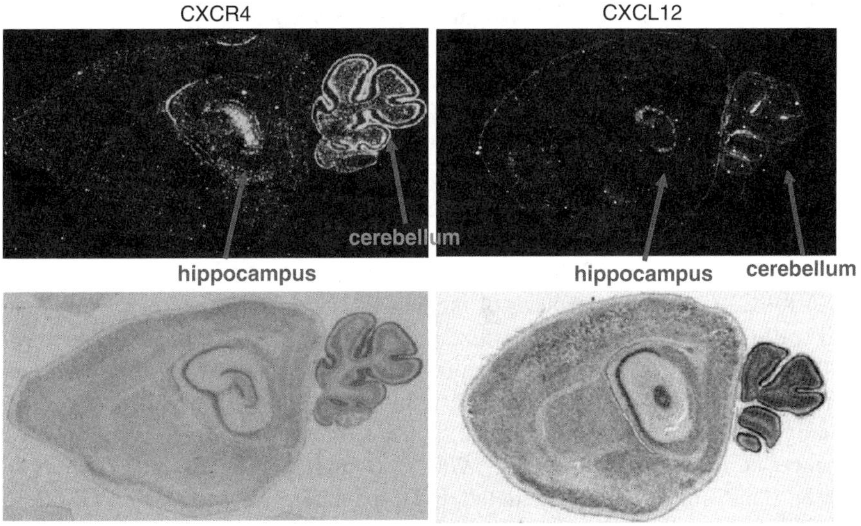

Fig. 34.3 Dark-field mRNA expression of CXCR4 (*upper left*) and CXCL12 (*upper right*) and bright-field (H&E) picture (*lower panels*) of adjacent brain sections from 7-day-old mouse brain by in situ hybridization (*sagittal view*). CXCR4 expression is significantly elevated in the cerebellum (external granular cell layer) and the hippocampus. CXCL12 expression is also notably high in the cerebellum and the hippocampus. The images are adapted from St. Jude Children's Research Hospital Brain gene expression map (http://www.stjudebgem.org/web/view/probe/viewProbeDetails.php?id = 53#more) (*see* Color Plate 52)

Plate 52). Additional cardinal features of the mutant animals were the mislocalization and failed proliferation of cerebellar granule precursor cells (GPCs). These phenotypic changes in GPCs reflect two effects of CXCL12: a chemotactic effect (Klein et al., 2001; Lu et al., 2001; Zhu et al., 2002) and the ability of CXCL12 to synergize with Sonic hedgehog (Shh) in the promotion of GPC proliferation (Klein et al., 2001). The capacity of CXCL12 and CXCR4 to regulate proliferation and migration of neural precursor cells raises the possibility that these molecules might be therapeutic targets in malignancies arising from CNS progenitors. It has also been reported that CXCL12 is synthesized and secreted by meningeal cells in the cerebellum and allows the stem cells of the external granule layer, which express CXCR4, to be attracted to the proliferating compartment. CXCR4 expression is absent in the postmitotic cells that migrate in the inner layer (Reiss et al., 2002; Zhu et al., 2002).

The entry of immune cells is tightly regulated in the central nervous system (CNS). Immune responses are not initiated within the CNS due to the absence of endogenous antigen-presenting cells (Ransohoff et al., 2003). Both CXCL12 and CXCR4 are constitutively expressed in the CNS but do not mediate leukocyte recruitment to that organ under normal physiological conditions (Banisadr et al., 2003; Tham et al., 2001; Tissir et al., 2004).

34.5 Involvement of CXCR4 in Non-CNS Cancers

CXCR4 is the most widely expressed chemokine receptor in many different cancers. The effects of CXCL12 on CXCR4-bearing tumor cells include a wide diversity of functions such as angiogenesis, invasion, locomotion, extravasation, directional migration, homing, and cell survival (see reviews: Ben-Baruch, 2008; Burger and Kipps, 2006; Vandercappellen et al., 2008; Zlotnik, 2006). Among these, the function of controlling cell migration and homing, which is the rate-limiting step of the multistep processes of metastasis, is unique for CXCR4/CXCL12. The process of metastasis is similar to leukocyte and stem cell trafficking, processes that utilize the CXCL12/CXCR4 axis (Kucia et al., 2005). The CXCR4 chemokine receptor mediates the migration of human stem cells to marrow and possibly peripheral blood cells to lymph nodes and spleen (Blades et al., 2002; Cashman et al., 2002; Kollet et al., 2001; Lapidot, 2001; Spencer et al., 2001; Vainchenker, 2001; Voermans et al., 2002; Wright et al., 2002). This migration is mediated by the binding of its ligand, CXCL12. In SCID mice transplanted with a human lymph node; CXCL12 induced CXCR4-positive cell migration specifically into the transplanted lymph node (Blades et al., 2002). These results imply that the CXCL12/CXCR4, "lock and key," directs cells to a specific home. Cancer cells that express CXCR4 exploit the same signaling pathway leading to homing and retention in tissues with enriched CXCL12. Metastasis is the result of several sequential steps and represents an organ-selective process (Nicolson, 1992). Although a number of mechanisms had been implicated in metastasis, the precise mechanisms determining the directional migration and invasion of tumor cells into specific organs remained elusive for a long time.

Muller et al. published a landmark study on the involvement of CXCR4 in breast cancer metastasis (Muller et al., 2001). In samples collected from various breast cancer patients, they found that the level of expression of CXCR4 is higher in primary tumors relative to normal mammary glands or mammary epithelial cells. By contrast, CXCL12 is highly expressed in the most common destinations of breast cancer metastasis, including the lymph nodes, lung, liver, and bone marrow. Current evidence suggests that the expression of CXCR4 on breast cancer cell surfaces leads to organ-specific metastasis by homing of circulating tumor cells to organs that express CXCL12. The treatment with CXCR4 antibodies inhibited metastasis to regional lymph nodes, while cells treated with isotype controls metastasized to the lymph nodes and lungs (Muller et al., 2001). These data indicated that neutralization of the interaction between CXCR4 and its ligand, CXCL12, by a CXCR4 antibody can significantly impair metastasis of breast cancer cells to the lymph nodes and lungs. Since that time, the CXCL12/CXCR4 pair has been demonstrated to play critical roles in the metastasis of various types of cancers. Two years later, by using an animal model of bone metastasis generated by the intracardiac injection of MDA-MB-231 breast cancer cells into female SCID (severe combined immunodeficient) mice, CXCR4 was demonstrated to be a key player in bone metastasis of breast cancer (Kang et al., 2003). A subsequent microarray analysis on a subpopulation of MDA-MB-231 cells with elevated metastatic activity isolated from the mice showed that one of the six genes responsible for the metastatic phenotype was CXCR4. Overexpression of CXCR4 alone in the original ATCC MDA-MB-231 cells significantly increased their metastatic activity. Two groups independently evaluated the efficacy of a CXCR4 antagonist 14-mer peptide (TN14003) in inhibiting metastasis in an animal model. They confirmed that blocking CXCR4 was effective in limiting metastasis of breast cancer (Liang et al., 2004; Tamamura et al., 2003). Liang et al. further demonstrated that silencing CXCR4 by RNA interference technology also prevented tumorigenesis in an animal model of breast cancer metastasis. They showed that blocking CXCR4 expression at the mRNA level with a combination of two small interfering RNAs impairs invasion of breast cancer cells in a matrigel invasion assay and inhibits breast cancer metastasis in an animal model (Liang et al., 2005). Furthermore, decreasing expression levels of CXCR4 by microRNA against CXCR4 also reduced migration and invasion in vitro and lung metastases in vivo (Liang et al., 2007b). MicroRNAs have been shown to function as regulatory molecules and to play an important role in cancer progression (for reviews, see Gartel and Kandel, 2008; Ma and Weinberg, 2008). These data support the possibility that small interfering RNAs or microRNAs against CXCR4 can serve as an alternative means of lowering CXCR4 expression to block subsequent invasion and metastasis. Both small interfering RNAs and microRNAs are gaining considerable attention in the pharmaceutical and biotechnology industries, as research has revealed their striking efficacy in knocking down the selected target genes. The capacity of small interfering RNAs to dramatically and specifically reduce the expression of targeted genes has gone into multiple clinical trials to establish the therapeutic potential of small RNAs targeting viral, cancer, and other disease-related genes (Pappas et al., 2008). Taken together, these studies confirm the necessity of CXCR4 in breast cancer metastasis and suggest a novel preventive and therapeutic strategy for cancer management.

Another intriguing report (Li et al., 2004) demonstrated that the receptor tyrosine kinase HER2 enhances the expression of CXCR4 and that there is a significant correlation between HER2 and CXCR4 expression in human breast tumor tissues. HER2, or human epidermal growth factor receptor 2, is overexpressed in 25% of hormone-refractory breast cancers. The same group reported that CXCR4 expression correlated with a poor overall survival rate in patients with breast cancer. They further demonstrated that anti-CXCR4 antibody blocked HER2-mediated invasion in vitro and lung metastasis in vivo. HER2-positive breast cancers are aggressive and, currently, anti-HER2 antibody (Trastuzumab, Genentech, Inc) is one of the most successful targeted therapies in recent years against hormone-refractory, HER2-positive breast cancer in patients. However, this therapy is extremely expensive due to the high cost of antibody production and limitation of bioavailability only by infusion. The above results provide a potential route of intervention for the inhibition of HER2-mediated breast cancer malignancy by blocking CXCR4 signaling pathways.

CXCR4 has been shown to be expressed at high levels on malignant tumor cells with high metastatic potential of other epithelial cancers. Table 34.1 summarizes the importance of the CXCR4/CXCL12 interaction in the malignant progression of numerous cancers. These CXCR4-positive tumor cells are able to home to other tissues in the presence of CXCL12 in the stroma of the target tissues. Various studies have shown significant CXCL12 concentrations in the fluid-filled cavities through which many cancers disseminate and at tissue locations in which metastases characteristically develop. In addition, CXCL12 has been shown to promote cancer cell growth along with other mitogenic factors. This has been demonstrated in cells from colorectal, prostate, and ovarian cancers (Oda et al., 2006; Oonakahara et al., 2004; Tang et al., 2008). In colorectal cancer, CXCR4 is abundantly expressed in various colorectal carcinoma cells (Alix-Panabieres et al., 2005; Hao et al., 2007). Interestingly, it was found that CXCR4 expression was not required for the migration of CT-26 colorectal tumor cells to the lungs, but rather for homing, e.g., tumor expansion at secondary sites (Ishibe et al., 2002; Zeelenberg et al., 2003). Others found that CXCR4 was overexpressed in human colorectal carcinoma tissues compared to normal tissues. Furthermore, elevated CXCR4 expression in colorectal cancer is associated with disease progression and reduced survival (Fukunaga et al., 2006; Ottaiano et al., 2005; Schimanski et al., 2005; Zeelenberg et al., 2003).

Table 34.1 Literatures on the involvement of CXCR4/CXCL12 in various cancers

Cancer type	References
Breast cancer	Muller et al. (2001); Bachelder et al. (2002); Chen et al. (2003); Tamamura et al. (2003); Lee et al. (2004); Li et al. (2004); Liang et al. (2004); Schmid et al. (2004); Cabioglu et al. (2005); Liang et al. (2005); Liang et al. (2006); Hao et al. (2007) and Liang et al. (2007b)
Cervical cancer	Kodama et al. (2007a)
Endometrial cancer	Kodama et al. (2007b)
Esophageal cancer	Kaifi et al. (2005); Koishi et al. (2006); Gockel et al. (2007) and Sasaki et al. (2008)
Gastrointestinal cancer	Tachibana et al. (1998); Zeelenberg et al. (2003); Kim et al. (2005) and Ottaiano et al. (2005)
Head and neck cancer	Samara et al. (2004) and Yoon et al. (2007)
Leukemia	Burger et al. (1999); Mohle et al. (1999); Ishibe et al. (2002); Barretina et al. (2003); Juarez et al. (2003); Dao-Ung et al. (2004); Ghobrial et al. (2004); Monaco et al. (2004); Tavor et al. (2004); Kalinkovich et al. (2006); Wu et al. (2006); Konoplev et al. (2007); Spoo et al. (2007); Fierro et al. (2009); Jin et al. (2008) and Scupoli et al. (2008)
Liver cancer	Begum et al. (1999); Shibuta et al. (2002); Schimanski et al. (2006) and Li et al. (2007)
Lung cancer	Kijima et al. (2002); Burger et al. (2003); Spano et al. (2004); Hartmann et al. (2005) and Phillips et al. (2005)
Lymphoma	Bertolini et al. (2002); Chan et al. (2003); Ghobrial et al. (2004) and Piovan et al. (2005)
Melanoma	Takenaga et al. (2004) and Scala et al. (2005)
Multiple myeloma	Alsayed et al. (2007)
Ovarian cancer	Porcile et al. (2004); Jiang et al. (2006) and Pils et al. (2007)
Pancreatic cancer	Koshiba et al. (2000) and Mori et al. (2004)
Prostate cancer	Taichman et al. (2002) and Sun et al. (2005)
Renal cancer	Schrader et al. (2002); Staller et al. (2003); Pan et al. (2006); Jones et al. (2007); Reckamp et al. (2008) and Struckmann et al. (2008)
Sarcoma	Libura et al. (2002); Laverdiere et al. (2005) and Oda et al. (2006)
Thyroid cancer	De Falco et al. (2007)

Another important function of CXCL12:CXCR4 is to promote cancer dissemination indirectly by enhancing the vascular supply, since the CXCL12/CXCR4 axis may also promote tumor angiogenesis. CXCL12 influences the interaction of CD34+ hematopoietic cells with the hematopoietic microenvironment by regulating their migration and adhesion as well as the secretion of vascular endothelial growth factor (VEGF) and matrix metalloproteinases (MMPs) (Majka et al., 2000a, b, c; Richard et al., 2006). On the other hand, CXCL12 has been shown to induce secretion of VEGF, but not matrix metalloproteinases in lymphohematopoietic CXCR4$^+$ cell lines (Kijowski et al., 2001). In this study, the authors showed that the VEGF protein levels increased in conditioned medium of cell lines treated with CXCL12. VEGF increased CXCL12 expression in endothelial cells (Salvucci et al., 2002), and anti-CXCR4 antibody disrupted extracellular matrix-dependent endothelial cell tube formation in vitro. This morphogenic process is closely associated with CXCR4 expression. Pertussis toxin (inhibitor of $G\alpha_i$) and neutralizing antibodies of CXCL12 inhibited bFGF (basic fibroblast growth factor) and VEGF-dependent neovascularization in vivo. The fact that blocking either CXCR4/CXCL12 interaction or the major G protein of the CXCR4/CXCL12 signaling pathway ($G\alpha_I$) inhibits VEGF-dependent neovascularization strongly suggests that CXCR4/CXCL12 indeed regulates VEGF-dependent angiogenesis. These results indicate that CXCL12/CXCR4 regulates VEGF-regulated paracrine signaling systems, which in turn are essential regulators of endothelial cell morphogenesis and angiogenesis (Fig. 34.4 and Color Plate 53). Numerous studies have shown that VEGF and MMPs actively contribute to cancer progression through angiogenesis and metastasis (Gontero et al., 2004; Kortylewski et al., 2005; Ribatti et al., 2004; Turner et al., 2003). This once again reinforces the attractiveness of the CXCR4/CXCL12 signaling cascade as a target for the intervention of neovascularization. The role of CXCR4/CXCL12 in tumor

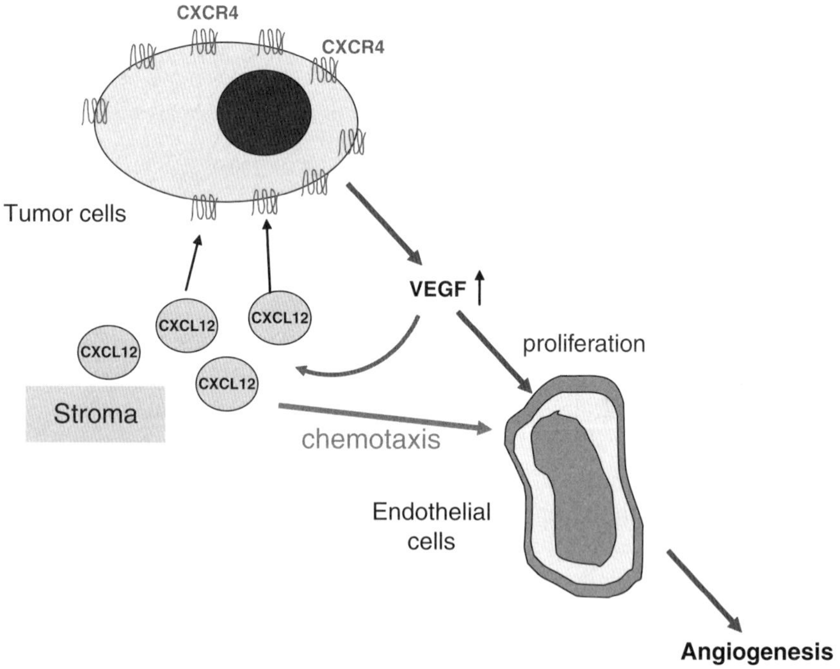

Fig. 34.4 Complex regulation of angiogenesis by CXCR4/CXCL12 via VEGF-dependent manner. VEGF increased CXCL12 expression in endothelial cells and its morphogenic process is closely associated with CXCR4 expression. Published results also suggest that CXCR4/CXCL12 regulates VEGF-dependent angiogenesis. These results indicate that CXCL12/CXCR4 regulates VEGF-regulated paracrine signaling systems, which in turn are essential regulators of endothelial cell morphogenesis and angiogenesis (*see* Color Plate 53)

angiogenesis in vivo was demonstrated in a squamous cell carcinoma of the head and neck (SCCHN) orthotopic animal model using highly metastatic subclones generated via in vivo selection of SCCHN cells through four rounds of serial metastases (Yoon et al., 2007). They showed that anti-CXCR4 treatment suppressed primary tumor growth by inhibiting tumor angiogenesis. Others reported that CXCR4/CXCL12 induced Akt phosphorylation, which resulted in upregulation of VEGF at both the mRNA and protein levels. Conversely, blocking the activation of Akt signaling led to a decrease in VEGF protein levels. Also, blocking CXCR4/CXCL12 interaction with a CXCR4 antagonist suppressed tumor angiogenesis and growth in vivo. Furthermore, VEGF mRNA levels correlated well with CXCR4 mRNA levels in patient tumor samples (Liang et al., 2007a). Thus, this study demonstrates that the CXCR4/CXCL12 signaling axis can induce angiogenesis and progression of tumors by increasing the expression of VEGF through the activation of the PI3K/Akt pathway.

Recently, CXCR4/CXCL12 became the focus of cancer stem cell because this pair is associated with stem cell recruitment. Cancer stem cells are a minority of tumor-initiating cells expressing a set of antigenic markers on their surface that is distinct from the majority of the population. This indicates that these two groups of cells are in different states of differentiation. In many normal tissues, stem cells are usually less differentiated, while their nonstem cell descendants enter states of increased differentiation. In addition, stem cells appear to have an essentially unlimited ability to regenerate. Because some of their progeny remain as stem cells, they are said to be "self-renewing" (Weinberg, 2006). It is therefore tempting to think that the same organization of cell behavior operates in human tumors, but definitive evidence of such a relationship is still missing. The heterogeneity observed in many types of human cancers may reflect the activation of specific genes and the different stem/progenitor cell populations in which these genetic or epigenetic events occur. Similarities have been observed in the pathways regulating stem cell homing and metastasis, and increasing evidence also suggests that treatment failure and the recurrence of human cancer may reflect the intrinsic quiescence and pro-survival of cancer stem cells (Zhang and Rosen, 2006). One of the intriguing reports demonstrating the critical role of CXCR4 of cancer stem cells in metastasis and pro-survival was in pancreatic cancer (Hermann et al., 2007). Pancreatic cancer has notorious fatality and the authors tempted to link its drug resistance and high metastatic potential to a distinct subpopulation of $CD133^+CXCR4^+$ cancer stem cells that are metastatic. This subpopulation was not only essential for tumor metastasis but also highly resistant to standard chemotherapy. Drug resistance can occur at several levels and is the main cause of treatment failure for oncology patients. The multidrug-resistant phenotype in highly migratory tumor cells becomes enhanced at metastatic sites. It is unknown how these cells, when tested with in vitro cell cultures, are not as resistant to chemotherapy as those tested in vivo. Thus, it has long been suspected that there must be an accomplice in the tumor microenvironment (tumor stroma) that promotes tumor cell survival. This speculation promoted a new generation of ideas to explain why chemotherapy causes transient tumor reduction followed by tumor recurrence, often at metastatic sites. It is proposed that drug resistance may evolve as a result of repeated cycles of chemotherapy (Gazitt, 2004). Following each cycle of chemotherapy, cancer stem cells lose adhesion molecules and CXCL12 signaling. Both adhesion molecules and CXCL12/CXCR4 signaling play key roles in homing and mobilization of hematopoietic progenitor and cancer stem cells. Surviving cells, released from tumor sites, circulate until re-expression of adhesion molecules and CXCR4 occurs, then home to stroma enriched with CXCL12, such as the lymph nodes, lungs, bones, and liver. CXCL12 secreted by cells in the new microenvironment at the metastatic site may induce proliferation and drug resistance of CXCR4-positive cancer stem cells. This process is amplified in each cycle of chemotherapy, resulting in disease progression.

In summary, CXCR4/CXCL12 provides a proliferative advantage to a subpopulation of CXCR4-positive cancer cells at multiple levels: (1) homing; (2) promoting cell survival; and (3) angiogenesis. These characteristics may be responsible for certain properties of cancer stem cells; essential for tumor metastasis as well as drug resistance to standard chemotherapy.

34.6 Involvement of CXCR4 in Glioma

Several studies have demonstrated the important role of CXCR4–CXCL12 in the biology of the most aggressive type of primary brain tumor, glioblastoma multiforme (GBM) (also known as WHO grade IV astrocytoma). GBM is the most common primary brain tumor and is uniformly fatal despite aggressive surgical and adjuvant therapies. One characteristic feature of GBM is the presence of hypoxic areas associated with increased angiogenesis. Hypoxia-inducible factor (HIF)-1 regulates the expression of target genes critical for the formation of new vasculature, such as VEGF and CXCR4, and provides a plausible explanation for the vascular hyperplasia seen in GBM (Kaur et al., 2004; Zagzag et al., 2005). Expression of CXCR4 has been shown in the endothelial cells of neovessels, with a high expression of its ligand in tumor cells adjacent to them. This suggests a role for CXCL12 in promoting angiogenesis (Rempel et al., 2000). Further observations suggest that the CXCR4/CXCL12 interaction plays a critical role in GBM progression (Zhou et al., 2002). Studies analyzing the cellular and genetic changes that occur during the genesis and progression of human gliomas have demonstrated the overexpression of CXCR4 in GBM tissue as compared with normal brain tissue and found a correlation between tumor grade and the expression of CXCR4 and its ligand CXCL12 (Rempel et al., 2000; Sehgal et al., 1998a, b). Using immunohistochemistry, they found low-level expression of CXCL12 and CXCR4 in low-grade gliomas and higher level expression in grade IV GBM, which are characterized by large regions of angiogenesis and necrosis. These data suggest that CXCL12 and CXCR4 expression could be useful biomarkers for gliomas. A relation between the expression of CXCL12 and a significantly shorter time to tumor progression in low-grade glioma in 50 patients (Salmaggi et al., 2005) suggests a potential role of CXCL12 as a marker of early disease progression.

Targeting of the CXCR4/CXCL12 ligand/receptor pair has confirmed its importance for glioma growth in preclinical models. Systemic administration of AMD3100, a small-molecule inhibitor of CXCR4 (Gerlach et al., 2001), decreased the growth of GBM in an orthotopic animal model. AMD3100 treatment reduced the activation of extracellular signal-regulated kinases 1 and 2 (Erk 1/2) as well as Akt and also increased rates of apoptosis. Their studies suggest that CXCR4 signaling is a critical component of brain tumor biology, which generated enthusiasm for the translation of this agent to the clinic for the treatment of brain tumor patients. However, AMD3100 has a partial agonistic activity and belongs to the class of metal-chelating bicyclams (Onuffer and Horuk, 2002; Trent et al., 2003). It was previously advanced as far as Phase II clinical evaluation as an HIV entry inhibitor (Donzella et al., 1998; Fujii et al., 2003; Hatse et al., 2002; Schols et al., 1997). However, it was withdrawn from that indication in response to adverse cardiac effects including cardiotoxicity (De Clercq, 2003). Currently, AMD3100 is being tested in the clinic for an indication of stem cell mobilization, which would require only a one time administration of the drug. Unfortunately, based on the experience of AMD3100 in the HIV trial, a safer drug is desired for the treatment of brain tumor patients.

Metastasis is not a major problem of GBM; it is rather fast proliferation and increased angiogenesis. In GBM, CXCR4/CXCL12 interaction promotes VEGF-dependent angiogenesis and cell survival against traditional chemotherapy.

34.7 Involvement of CXCR4 in Medulloblastoma

Medulloblastomas are the most common malignant brain tumors in childhood with a median age of onset at 9 years (Packer et al., 1999). Medulloblastomas are histologically divided into four major subgroups. While classic and desmoplastic tumors account for the vast majority of cases, medulloblastomas with extensive nodularity and large cell medulloblastomas are rare (Giangasparo et al., 2000). All medulloblastoma subtypes are believed to be originated from neural progenitors of the cerebellum, although the exact cellular origin remains to be elucidated in most cases.

CXCR4 is strongly expressed in proliferating granule cell precursors (Klein et al., 2001; Zhao et al., 2002). CXCL12, which is secreted by meningeal cells of the leptomeninx, significantly enhances granule cell proliferation (Zhao et al., 2002). This effect is reduced by blocking the CXCR4 receptor either by AMD 3100 or pertussis toxin. This indicates coupling of neuronal CXCR4 to Gαi, which has previously been demonstrated to be expressed in granule cell precursors (Rubin et al., 2003; Schuller et al., 2001). CXCR4 promoted survival, proliferation, and migration in a desmoplastic medulloblastoma cell line (Daoy) in vitro and in in vivo tumor models (Rubin et al., 2003). Whereas 18/20 classic MBs showed very low levels of CXCR4 mRNA, 17/18 desmoplastic and 6/7 extensively nodular MBs showed high levels (Schuller et al., 2005). This study also revealed that a small subset of medulloblastomas carry mutations in the gene encoding CXCR4. While overexpression of CXCR4 is common in most cases of cancers, CXCR4 mutation is rarely reported. The two mutations identified were located, respectively, in the first (A157C) and second (C414T) transmembrane regions of the receptor, the second being relatively close to the cell surface in a location possibly important for ligand binding (Brelot et al., 2000). They speculated that mutations within the transmembrane regions might contribute to pathologic receptor activity or to resistance to inhibitors such as AMD3100. Moreover, strong expression of CXCR4 mRNA was demonstrated in medulloblastomas that likely derive from the cerebellar external granule cell layer (Fig. 34.3). These data suggest that CXCR4 may be responsible for the development of specific medulloblastoma subtypes and that expression of CXCR4 mRNA could be an improved detection means of tumors derived from the cerebellar external granule cell layer over classical histology and silver staining.

CXCL12 could also contribute to the pattern of medulloblastoma spread. Medulloblastoma is distinctively different from other brain tumors because it often metastasizes to bone and liver tissues, which express CXCL12. Therefore, CXCR4 may play a critical role in this subtype of metastatic medulloblastomas for their growth and metastasis.

34.8 Involvement of CXCR4 in Meningioma

Meningiomas constitute about 20% of all primary intracranial tumors in adults. Meningothelial, fibrous, and transitional meningiomas are the most common meningiomas and are classified as grade I using the WHO system. They are slowly growing benign lesions with a good prognosis. Other subtypes, such as atypical (grade II) and anaplastic (grade III) meningiomas, are much more malignant with a high incidence of recurrence (Kleihues et al., 2002). CXCR4 plays an essential role in the development of the hippocampal dentate gyrus in which CXCL12, which is highly expressed in the meninges that overlay the hippocampus, has proliferative effects on dentate granule cell precursors and provides a guiding chemoattractant signal for CXCR4-expressing cells that migrate toward the dentate gyrus (Bagri et al., 2002; Lu et al., 2002). The expression of CXCR4 and CXCL12 was examined in 55 human meningioma specimens (Bajetto et al., 2007). CXCR4 mRNA was identified in 78% of the meningiomas, whereas CXCL12 mRNA was found in 53%. There was a significant relationship between the CXCR4 and CXCL12 mRNA expression, but no correlation with WHO tumor grade was found. This lack of correlation may potentially be due to the heterogeneous group of samples in the study, which included a large number of WHO grade I tumors (85%) and only a few cases of high-grade meningiomas, which corresponds to the real incidence of these tumors. The authors hypothesized that CXCR4 expression might represent an early factor regulating cell proliferation in benign tumor growth and concluded that CXCR4 could serve as a potential target to control the cell proliferation in the early stages of the disease. They also noted that CXCR4 does not play a key role in cell growth in the high-grade meningiomas (Bajetto et al., 2007).

The signaling mechanisms activated by the exclusive binding between CXCL12 and CXCR4 were examined in 12 primary cultures from meningioma tissues (Barbieri et al., 2006). CXCR4 was functionally coupled as demonstrated by the significant increase of DNA synthesis in meningioma cells in response to CXCL12. In three primary cultures, the CXCL12-dependent mitogenic activity was associated with a marked phosphorylation of extracellular signal-regulated kinase (ERK1/2). PD98059 (a MEK inhibitor) significantly reduced ERK1/2 activation, thus suggesting that an autocrine CXCL12/CXCR4 growth loop promotes meningioma cell proliferation via ERK1/2 signaling.

34.9 Involvement of CXCR4 in Neuroblastoma

Neuroblastoma is the second most common solid tumor found in children, originating from precursors derived from embryonic neural crest cells that form the peripheral sympathetic nervous system. About one-half of children have localized tumors that can be cured with surgery alone, while the remaining children have widespread metastatic disease or quite large, aggressive, localized tumors commonly in adrenal glands. The latter have a poor long-term survival rate of approximately 30%. Despite advances in combined therapies, the survival rate of patients with metastatic neuroblastoma has not significantly improved over the last decade. Therefore, there is an urgent need for genetic and biologic markers for the diverse clinical phenotypes observed in neuroblastoma patients. One of the emerging biomarkers in neuroblastoma is the overexpression of CXCR4 (Vasudevan et al., 2005). CXCR4 expression correlates with high-stage disease (Russell et al., 2004), and the interactions of CXCR4 with CXCL12 were shown to be necessary for the survival of several neuroblastoma cells in vitro (Meier et al., 2007). A higher expression of CXCR4 was found in primary neuroblastoma cells from patients with high-stage disease and in patients with bone and bone marrow metastases (Russell et al., 2004). Disease-free survival in patients with tumors expressing high levels of CXCR4 is significantly worse than in patients with low CXCR4 tumor expression.

The expression levels of CXCR4 were found in various NB cell lines and, using CXCR4-expressing SH-SY5Y cells, they found that CXCL12 induces the migration of CXCR4-expressing neuroblastoma cells in CXCR4- and G protein-dependent manners (Geminder et al., 2001). SH-SY5Y cells were found to interact at multiple levels with bone marrow components. Bone marrow-derived constituents were able to promote SH-SY5Y cell migration, adhesion to bone marrow stromal cells, and proliferation in vitro. These results suggest that SH-SY5Y neuroblastoma cells are capable of homing to the bone marrow and that the ability of neuroblastoma tumors to preferentially form metastases in the bone marrow may be influenced by CXCR4/CXCL12 interactions. Moreover, others screened chemokine/receptor profiles in different neuroblastoma cell lines and investigated the roles of CXCR4 in neuroblastoma tumor growth and progression using mouse xenograft models (Zhang et al., 2007). They demonstrated the important role of stromal cells in neuroblastoma metastasis and a potential regulatory tumor–host mechanism for CXCR4 in neuroblastoma in vitro transwell invasion assay. Several studies further demonstrated that CXCR4 expression can be regulated positively by cytokines such as TGF-β1, VEGF, and bFGF. CXCR4 expression can also be regulated negatively by cytokines such as IL-5 and IFN-α in leukocytes, endothelial cells, and neural cells (Franitza et al., 2002; Iikura et al., 2001; Rostasy et al., 2005; Salcedo et al., 1999; Schioppa et al., 2003). Overexpression of CXCR4 promoted neuroblastoma cell migration selectively toward bone marrow stromal cell-conditioned medium in vitro (Zhang et al., 2007). In a mouse xenograft model, bone marrow metastasis could be achieved by CXCR4 overexpression. Furthermore, Chen et al. (2006) suggested the regulation of angiogenesis by CXCR4 in neuroblastomas and that the dissemination of CXCR4-overexpressed neuroblastoma cells from primary tumors could result from increased neovasculatures.

In summary, these studies reveal critical roles for CXCR4 in NB metastasis and provide insights into the regulatory mechanism of chemokine receptors in NB and the importance of the tissue microenvironment in modulating tumor cell behavior. The ability of neuroblastoma tumors to preferentially form metastases in the bone marrow may be influenced by a set of complex CXCR4/CXCL12 interactions. Key events in this process may be increased adhesion to bone marrow cells, followed by proliferation of the tumor cells. Homing requires adhesion-mediated arrest of the cells on the bone marrow microvasculature. The homing of neuroblastoma cells to the bone marrow is mediated via an interaction between the CXCR4 receptor expressed by the tumor cells and the corresponding ligand, CXCL12, secreted by bone marrow stromal cells.

34.10 Concluding Remarks

Extensive evidence indicates that cancer cells express the CXCR4 chemokine receptor and that its interaction with CXCL12 is crucial for homing, tumor cell survival, and angiogenesis. CXCR4/CXCL12 appears to play a central role in the "seed-and-soil" hypothesis of Paget, which dates back to the 19th century (Mueller and Fusenig, 2004); CXCL12 is expressed by the "soil" organs and the "seed" cells in circulation will home to those organ sites. Therefore, modulating the CXCR4/CXCL12 homing interaction may provide an alternative target for cancer therapy by blocking cancer progression through distant metastases. In addition, CXCR4 expression profiles can be utilized to determine different stages of malignancy in various cancers, which may lead to alternative prognostic markers for cancers and a strategy to enhance both diagnostic and therapeutic strategies. Much research validates the notion of targeting the CXCR4/CXCL12 interaction in tumor progression as not only a therapeutic approach but also a chemopreventive strategy, blocking the development of more aggressive tumors (Balkwill, 2004). A better understanding of the role of CXCR4 and CXCL12 in brain tumors will enable improved manipulation of this important player of tumor progression to affect the outcome of brain tumors. Increased knowledge of the CXCR4 interaction with its ligand, and of the different signaling events resulting in CXCR4 functions, will also enhance future drug design.

References

Addison, C. L., Daniel, T. O., Burdick, M. D., Liu, H., Ehlert, J. E., Xue, Y. Y., Buechi, L., Walz, A., Richmond, A. and Strieter, R. M. 2000. The CXC chemokine receptor 2, CXCR2, is the putative receptor for ELR + CXC chemokine-induced angiogenic activity. Journal of Immunology 165: 5269–5277.

Aiuti, A., Webb, I. J., Bleul, C., Springer, T. and Gutierrez-Ramos, J. C. 1997. The chemokine SDF-1 is a chemoattractant for human CD34+ hematopoietic progenitor cells and provides a new mechanism to explain the mobilization of CD34+ progenitors to peripheral blood. The Journal of Experimental Medicine 185: 111–120.

Alix-Panabieres, C., Brouillet, J. P., Fabbro, M., Yssel, H., Rousset, T., Maudelonde, T., Choquet-Kastylevsky, G. and Vendrell, J. P. 2005. Characterization and enumeration of cells secreting tumor markers in the peripheral blood of breast cancer patients. Journal of Immunological Methods 299: 177–188.

Alsayed, Y., Ngo, H., Runnels, J., Leleu, X., Singha, U. K., Pitsillides, C. M., Spencer, J. A., Kimlinger, T., Ghobrial, J. M., Jia, X., Lu, G., Timm, M., Kumar, A., Cote, D., Veilleux, I., Hedin, K. E., Roodman, G. D., Witzig, T. E., Kung, A. L., Hideshima, T., Anderson, K. C., Lin, C. P. and Ghobrial, I. M. 2007. Mechanisms of regulation of CXCR4/SDF-1 (CXCL12)-dependent migration and homing in multiple myeloma. Blood 109: 2708–2717.

Bachelder, R. E., Wendt, M. A. and Mercurio, A. M. 2002. Vascular endothelial growth factor promotes breast carcinoma invasion in an autocrine manner by regulating the chemokine receptor CXCR4. Cancer Research 62: 7203–7206.

Bagri, A., Gurney, T., He, X., Zou, Y. R., Littman, D. R., Tessier-Lavigne, M. and Pleasure, S. J. 2002. The chemokine SDF1 regulates migration of dentate granule cells. Development (Cambridge, England) 129: 4249–4260.

Bajetto, A., Barbieri, F., Pattarozzi, A., Dorcaratto, A., Porcile, C., Ravetti, J. L., Zona, G., Spaziante, R., Schettini, G. and Florio, T. 2007. CXCR4 and SDF1 expression in human meningiomas: a proliferative role in tumoral meningothelial cells in vitro. Neuro-oncology 9: 3–11.

Bajetto, A., Bonavia, R., Barbero, S., Florio, T. and Schettini, G. 2001. Chemokines and their receptors in the central nervous system. Frontiers in Neuroendocrinology 22: 147–184.

Balabanian, K., Lagane, B., Infantino, S., Chow, K. Y., Harriague, J., Moepps, B., Arenzana-Seisdedos, F., Thelen, M. and Bachelerie, F. 2005. The chemokine SDF-1/CXCL12 binds to and signals through the orphan receptor RDC1 in T lymphocytes. The Journal of Biological Chemistry 280: 35760–35766.
Balkwill, F. 2004. The significance of cancer cell expression of the chemokine receptor CXCR4. Seminars in Cancer Biology 14: 171–179.
Balkwill, F. and Mantovani, A. 2001. Inflammation and cancer: back to Virchow? Lancet 357: 539–545.
Banisadr, G., Skrzydelski, D., Kitabgi, P., Rostene, W. and Parsadaniantz, S. M. 2003. Highly regionalized distribution of stromal cell-derived factor-1/CXCL12 in adult rat brain: constitutive expression in cholinergic, dopaminergic and vasopressinergic neurons. The European Journal of Neuroscience 18: 1593–1606.
Barbieri, F., Bajetto, A., Porcile, C., Pattarozzi, A., Massa, A., Lunardi, G., Zona, G., Dorcaratto, A., Ravetti, J. L., Spaziante, R., Schettini, G. and Florio, T. 2006. CXC receptor and chemokine expression in human meningioma: SDF1/CXCR4 signaling activates ERK1/2 and stimulates meningioma cell proliferation. Annals of the New York Academy of Sciences 1090: 332–343.
Barretina, J., Junca, J., Llano, A., Gutierrez, A., Flores, A., Blanco, J., Clotet, B. and Este, J. A. 2003. CXCR4 and SDF-1 expression in B-cell chronic lymphocytic leukemia and stage of the disease. Annals of hematology 82: 500–505.
Begum, N. A., Shibuta, K., Mori, M. and Barnard, G. F. 1999. Reduced expression of the CXCR4 receptor mRNA in hepatocellular carcinoma and lack of inducibility of its ligand alpha-chemokine hIRH/SDF1alpha/PBSF in vitro. International Journal of Oncology 14: 927–934.
Ben-Baruch, A. 2008. Organ selectivity in metastasis: regulation by chemokines and their receptors. Clinical & Experimental Metastasis 25: 345–356.
Bertolini, F., Dell'Agnola, C., Mancuso, P., Rabascio, C., Burlini, A., Monestiroli, S., Gobbi, A., Pruneri, G. and Martinelli, G. 2002. CXCR4 neutralization, a novel therapeutic approach for non-Hodgkin's lymphoma. Cancer Research 62: 3106–3112.
Bertollini, C., Ragozzino, D., Gross, C., Limatola, C. and Eusebi, F. 2006. Fractalkine/CX3CL1 depresses central synaptic transmission in mouse hippocampal slices. Neuropharmacology 51: 816–821.
Blades, M. C., Manzo, A., Ingegnoli, F., Taylor, P. R., Panayi, G. S., Irjala, H., Jalkanen, S., Haskard, D. O., Perretti, M. and Pitzalis, C. 2002. Stromal cell-derived factor 1 (CXCL12) induces human cell migration into human lymph nodes transplanted into SCID mice. J. Immunol. 168: 4308–4317.
Bleul, C. C., Farzan, M., Choe, H., Parolin, C., Clark-Lewis, I., Sodroski, J. and Springer, T. A. 1996. The lymphocyte chemoattractant SDF-1 is a ligand for LESTR/fusin and blocks HIV-1 entry. Nature 382: 829–833.
Brelot, A., Heveker, N., Montes, M. and Alizon, M. 2000. Identification of residues of CXCR4 critical for human immunodeficiency virus coreceptor and chemokine receptor activities. The Journal of Biological Chemistry 275: 23736–23744.
Burger, J. A., Burger, M. and Kipps, T. J. 1999. Chronic lymphocytic leukemia B cells express functional CXCR4 chemokine receptors that mediate spontaneous migration beneath bone marrow stromal cells. Blood 94: 3658–3667.
Burger, J. A. and Kipps, T. J. 2006. CXCR4: a key receptor in the crosstalk between tumor cells and their microenvironment. Blood 107: 1761–1767.
Burger, M., Glodek, A., Hartmann, T., Schmitt-Graff, A., Silberstein, L. E., Fujii, N., Kipps, T. J. and Burger, J. A. 2003. Functional expression of CXCR4 (CD184) on small-cell lung cancer cells mediates migration, integrin activation, and adhesion to stromal cells. Oncogene 22: 8093–8101.
Burns, J. M., Summers, B. C., Wang, Y., Melikian, A., Berahovich, R., Miao, Z., Penfold, M. E., Sunshine, M. J., Littman, D. R., Kuo, C. J., Wei, K., McMaster, B. E., Wright, K., Howard, M. C.

and Schall, T. J. 2006. A novel chemokine receptor for SDF-1 and I-TAC involved in cell survival, cell adhesion, and tumor development. The Journal of Experimental Medicine 203: 2201–2213.

Butcher, E. C., Williams, M., Youngman, K., Rott, L. and Briskin, M. 1999. Lymphocyte trafficking and regional immunity. Advances in Immunology 72: 209–253.

Cabioglu, N., Yazici, M. S., Arun, B., Broglio, K. R., Hortobagyi, G. N., Price, J. E. and Sahin, A. 2005. CCR7 and CXCR4 as novel biomarkers predicting axillary lymph node metastasis in T1 breast cancer. Clinical Cancer Research 11: 5686–5693.

Campbell, J. J. and Butcher, E. C. 2000. Chemokines in tissue-specific and micro-environment-specific lymphocyte homing. Current in Opinion Immunology 12: 336–341.

Cartier, L., Hartley, O., Dubois-Dauphin, M. and Krause, K. H. 2005. Chemokine receptors in the central nervous system: role in brain inflammation and neurodegenerative diseases. Brain Research. Brain Research Reviews 48: 16–42.

Cashman, J., Clark-Lewis, I., Eaves, A. and Eaves, C. 2002. Stromal-derived factor 1 inhibits the cycling of very primitive human hematopoietic cells in vitro and in NOD/SCID mice. Blood 99: 792–799.

Chan, C. C., Shen, D., Hackett, J. J., Buggage, R. R. and Tuaillon, N. 2003. Expression of chemokine receptors, CXCR4 and CXCR5, and chemokines, BLC and SDF-1, in the eyes of patients with primary intraocular lymphoma. Ophthalmology 110: 421–426.

Charo, I. F. and Ransohoff, R. M. 2006. The many roles of chemokines and chemokine receptors in inflammation. The New England Journal of Medicine 354: 610–621.

Chen, G. S., Yu, H. S., Lan, C. C., Chow, K. C., Lin, T. Y., Kok, L. F., Lu, M. P., Liu, C. H. and Wu, M. T. 2006. CXC chemokine receptor CXCR4 expression enhances tumorigenesis and angiogenesis of basal cell carcinoma. The British Journal of Dermatology 154: 910–918.

Chen, W. J., Jayawickreme, C., Watson, C., Wolfe, L., Holmes, W., Ferris, R., Armour, S., Dallas, W., Chen, G., Boone, L., Luther, M. and Kenakin, T. 1998. Recombinant human CXC-chemokine receptor-4 in melanophores are linked to Gi protein: seven transmembrane coreceptors for human immunodeficiency virus entry into cells. Molecular Pharmacology 53: 177–181.

Chen, Y., Stamatoyannopoulos, G. and Song, C. Z. 2003. Down-regulation of CXCR4 by inducible small interfering RNA inhibits breast cancer cell invasion in vitro. Cancer research 63: 4801–4804.

Dao-Ung, L. P., Sluyter, R., Fuller, S. J., Taper, J. and Wiley, J. S. 2004. CXCR4 but not CXCR3 expression correlates with lymphocyte counts in B-cell chronic lymphocytic leukemia. Annals of Hematology 83: 326–327.

De Clercq, E. 2003. The bicyclam AMD3100 story. Nature Reviews Drug Discovery 2: 581–587.

De Falco, V., Guarino, V., Avilla, E., Castellone, M. D., Salerno, P., Salvatore, G., Faviana, P., Basolo, F., Santoro, M. and Melillo, R. M. 2007. Biological role and potential therapeutic targeting of the chemokine receptor CXCR4 in undifferentiated thyroid cancer. Cancer Research 67: 11821–11829.

Deng, H. K., Unutmaz, D., KewalRamani, V. N. and Littman, D. R. 1997. Expression cloning of new receptors used by simian and human immunodeficiency viruses. Nature 388: 296–300.

DeVries, M. E., Kelvin, A. A., Xu, L., Ran, L., Robinson, J. and Kelvin, D. J. 2006. Defining the origins and evolution of the chemokine/chemokine receptor system. Journal of Immunology 176: 401–415.

Dey, N., Durden, D. L. and Van Meir, E. G. 2006. Cytokine expression and signaling in CNS tumors. In: *Cytokines and the CNS*. pp. 193–242. Eds. E. N. Benveniste, R. M. Ransohoff. CRS Press: San Francisco.

Ding, Z., Jia, S. H., Marshall, J. C., Downey, G. P. and Waddell, T. K. 2006. Up-regulation of functional CXCR4 expression on human lymphocytes in sepsis. Critical Care Medicine 34: 3011–3017.

Donzella, G. A., Schols, D., Lin, S. W., Este, J. A., Nagashima, K. A., Maddon, P. J., Allaway, G. P., Sakmar, T. P., Henson, G., De Clercq, E. and Moore, J. P. 1998. AMD3100, a small molecule inhibitor of HIV-1 entry via the CXCR4 co-receptor. Nature Medicine 4: 72–77.

Dziembowska, M., Tham, T. N., Lau, P., Vitry, S., Lazarini, F. and Dubois-Dalcq, M. 2005. A role for CXCR4 signaling in survival and migration of neural and oligodendrocyte precursors. Glia 50: 258–269.

Feng, Y., Broder, C. C., Kennedy, P. E. and Berger, E. A. 1996. HIV-1 entry cofactor: functional cDNA cloning of a seven-transmembrane, G protein-coupled receptor. Science 272: 872–877.

Fierro, F. A., Brenner, S., Oelschlaegel, U., Jacobi, A., Knoth, H., Ehninger, G., Illmer, T. and Bornhauser, M. 2009. Combining SDF-1/CXCR4 antagonism and chemotherapy in relapsed acute myeloid leukemia. Leukemia 23: 393–395.

Forster, R., Schubel, A., Breitfeld, D., Kremmer, E., Renner-Muller, I., Wolf, E. and Lipp, M. 1999. CCR7 coordinates the primary immune response by establishing functional microenvironments in secondary lymphoid organs. Cell 99: 23–33.

Franitza, S., Kollet, O., Brill, A., Vaday, G. G., Petit, I., Lapidot, T., Alon, R. and Lider, O. 2002. TGF-beta1 enhances SDF-1alpha-induced chemotaxis and homing of naive T cells by up-regulating CXCR4 expression and downstream cytoskeletal effector molecules. European Journal of Immunology 32: 193–202.

Fredriksson, R., Lagerstrom, M. C., Lundin, L. G. and Schioth, H. B. 2003. The G-protein-coupled receptors in the human genome form five main families. Phylogenetic analysis, paralogon groups, and fingerprints. Molecular Pharmacology 63: 1256–1272.

Fujii, N., Nakashima, H. and Tamamura, H. 2003. The therapeutic potential of CXCR4 antagonists in the treatment of HIV. Expert Opinion on Investigation Drugs 12: 185–195.

Fukunaga, S., Maeda, K., Noda, E., Inoue, T., Wada, K. and Hirakawa, K. 2006. Association between expression of vascular endothelial growth factor C, chemokine receptor CXCR4 and lymph node metastasis in colorectal cancer. Oncology 71: 204–211.

Gao, C. and Li, Y. 2007. SDF-1 plays a key role in the repairing and remodeling process on rat allo-orthotopic abdominal aorta grafts. Transplantation Proceedings 39: 268–272.

Gartel, A. L. and Kandel, E. S. 2008. miRNAs: Little known mediators of oncogenesis. Seminars in Cancer Biology 18: 103–110.

Gazitt, Y. 2004. Homing and mobilization of hematopoietic stem cells and hematopoietic cancer cells are mirror image processes, utilizing similar signaling pathways and occurring concurrently: circulating cancer cells constitute an ideal target for concurrent treatment with chemotherapy and antilineage-specific antibodies. Leukemia 18: 1–10.

Geminder, H., Sagi-Assif, O., Goldberg, L., Meshel, T., Rechavi, G., Witz, I. P. and Ben-Baruch, A. 2001. A possible role for CXCR4 and its ligand, the CXC chemokine stromal cell-derived factor-1, in the development of bone marrow metastases in neuroblastoma. Journal of Immunology 167: 4747–4757.

Gerlach, L. O., Skerlj, R. T., Bridger, G. J. and Schwartz, T. W. 2001. Molecular interactions of cyclam and bicyclam non-peptide antagonists with the CXCR4 chemokine receptor. The Journal of Biological Chemistry 276: 14153–14160.

Ghobrial, I. M., Bone, N. D., Stenson, M. J., Novak, A., Hedin, K. E., Kay, N. E. and Ansell, S. M. 2004. Expression of the chemokine receptors CXCR4 and CCR7 and disease progression in B-cell chronic lymphocytic leukemia/ small lymphocytic lymphoma. Mayo Clinic Proceedings 79: 318–325.

Giangasparo, F., Bigner, S. H., Kleinhues, P. K., Pietsch, T. and Trojanowsk, J. Q. 2000. Pathology and genetics of tumors of the nervous system. In: *Medulloblastoma*. pp. 129–137. Eds. P. Kleihues, W. K. Cavenee. IARC: Lyon.

Giovannelli, A., Limatola, C., Ragozzino, D., Mileo, A. M., Ruggieri, A., Ciotti, M. T., Mercanti, D., Santoni, A. and Eusebi, F. 1998. CXC chemokines interleukin-8 (IL-8) and growth-related gene product alpha (GROalpha) modulate Purkinje neuron activity in mouse cerebellum. Journal of Neuroimmunology 92: 122–132.

Gockel, I., Schimanski, C. C., Moehler, M. and Junginger, T. 2007. Novel therapeutic targets in esophageal cancer: impact of chemokine receptor CXCR4. Future oncology (London, England) 3: 119–122.

Gontero, P., Banisadr, S., Frea, B. and Brausi, M. 2004. Metastasis markers in bladder cancer: a review of the literature and clinical considerations. Eur Urol 46: 296–311.

Hao, L., Zhang, C., Qiu, Y., Wang, L., Luo, Y., Jin, M., Zhang, Y., Guo, T. B., Matsushima, K. and Zhang, Y. 2007. Recombination of CXCR4, VEGF, and MMP-9 predicting lymph node metastasis in human breast cancer. Cancer Letters 253: 34–42.

Hartmann, T. N., Burger, J. A., Glodek, A., Fujii, N. and Burger, M. 2005. CXCR4 chemokine receptor and integrin signaling co-operate in mediating adhesion and chemoresistance in small cell lung cancer (SCLC) cells. Oncogene 24: 4462–4471.

Hatse, S., Princen, K., Bridger, G., De Clercq, E. and Schols, D. 2002. Chemokine receptor inhibition by AMD3100 is strictly confined to CXCR4. FEBS Letters 527: 255–262.

Hebert, C. A., Vitangcol, R. V. and Baker, J. B. 1991. Scanning mutagenesis of interleukin-8 identifies a cluster of residues required for receptor binding. The Journal of Biological Chemistry 266: 18989–18994.

Hermann, P. C., Huber, S. L., Herrler, T., Aicher, A., Ellwart, J. W., Guba, M., Bruns, C. J. and Heeschen, C. 2007. Distinct populations of cancer stem cells determine tumor growth and metastatic activity in human pancreatic cancer. Cell Stem Cell 1: 313–323.

Hernandez, P. A., Gorlin, R. J., Lukens, J. N., Taniuchi, S., Bohinjec, J., Francois, F., Klotman, M. E. and Diaz, G. A. 2003. Mutations in the chemokine receptor gene CXCR4 are associated with WHIM syndrome, a combined immunodeficiency disease. Nature Genetics 34: 70–74.

Homey, B., Wang, W., Soto, H., Buchanan, M. E., Wiesenborn, A., Catron, D., Muller, A., McClanahan, T. K., Dieu-Nosjean, M. C., Orozco, R., Ruzicka, T., Lehmann, P., Oldham, E. and Zlotnik, A. 2000. Cutting edge: the orphan chemokine receptor G protein-coupled receptor- 2 (GPR-2, CCR10) binds the skin-associated chemokine CCL27 (CTACK/ALP/ILC). Journal of Immunology 164: 3465–3470.

Iikura, M., Miyamasu, M., Yamaguchi, M., Kawasaki, H., Matsushima, K., Kitaura, M., Morita, Y., Yoshie, O., Yamamoto, K. and Hirai, K. 2001. Chemokine receptors in human basophils: inducible expression of functional CXCR4. Journal of Leukocyte Biology 70: 113–120.

Imitola, J., Raddassi, K., Park, K. I., Mueller, F. J., Nieto, M., Teng, Y. D., Frenkel, D., Li, J., Sidman, R. L., Walsh, C. A., Snyder, E. Y. and Khoury, S. J. 2004. Directed migration of neural stem cells to sites of CNS injury by the stromal cell-derived factor 1alpha/CXC chemokine receptor 4 pathway. Proceedings of the National Academy of Sciences of the United States of America 101: 18117–18122.

Ishibe, N., Albitar, M., Jilani, I. B., Goldin, L. R., Marti, G. E. and Caporaso, N. E. 2002. CXCR4 expression is associated with survival in familial chronic lymphocytic leukemia, but CD38 expression is not. Blood 100: 1100–1101.

Jiang, Y. P., Wu, X. H., Shi, B., Wu, W. X. and Yin, G. R. 2006. Expression of chemokine CXCL12 and its receptor CXCR4 in human epithelial ovarian cancer: an independent prognostic factor for tumor progression. Gynecologic Oncology 103: 226–233.

Jin, L., Tabe, Y., Konoplev, S., Xu, Y., Leysath, C. E., Lu, H., Kimura, S., Ohsaka, A., Rios, M. B., Calvert, L., Kantarjian, H., Andreeff, M. and Konopleva, M. 2008. CXCR4 up-regulation by imatinib induces chronic myelogenous leukemia (CML) cell migration to bone marrow stroma and promotes survival of quiescent CML cells. Molecular Cancer Therapeutics 7: 48–58.

Jones, J., Marian, D., Weich, E., Engl, T., Wedel, S., Relja, B., Jonas, D. and Blaheta, R. A. 2007. CXCR4 chemokine receptor engagement modifies integrin dependent adhesion of renal carcinoma cells. Experimental Cell Research 313: 4051–4065.

Juarez, J., Bradstock, K. F., Gottlieb, D. J. and Bendall, L. J. 2003. Effects of inhibitors of the chemokine receptor CXCR4 on acute lymphoblastic leukemia cells in vitro. Leukemia 17: 1294–1300.

Kaifi, J. T., Yekebas, E. F., Schurr, P., Obonyo, D., Wachowiak, R., Busch, P., Heinecke, A., Pantel, K. and Izbicki, J. R. 2005. Tumor-cell homing to lymph nodes and bone marrow and CXCR4 expression in esophageal cancer. Journal of the National Cancer Institute 97: 1840–1847.

Kajiyama, H., Shibata, K., Ino, K., Nawa, A., Mizutani, S. and Kikkawa, F. 2007. Possible involvement of SDF-1alpha/CXCR4-DPPIV axis in TGF-beta1-induced enhancement of migratory potential in human peritoneal mesothelial cells. Cell and Tissue Research 330: 221–229.

Kalinkovich, A., Tavor, S., Avigdor, A., Kahn, J., Brill, A., Petit, I., Goichberg, P., Tesio, M., Netzer, N., Naparstek, E., Hardan, I., Nagler, A., Resnick, I., Tsimanis, A. and Lapidot, T. 2006. Functional CXCR4-expressing microparticles and SDF-1 correlate with circulating acute myelogenous leukemia cells. Cancer Research 66: 11013–11020.

Kang, Y., Siegel, P. M., Shu, W., Drobnjak, M., Kakonen, S. M., Cordon-Cardo, C., Guise, T. A. and Massague, J. 2003. A multigenic program mediating breast cancer metastasis to bone. Cancer Cell 3: 537–549.

Kaur, B., Tan, C., Brat, D. J., Post, D. E. and Van Meir, E. G. 2004. Genetic and hypoxic regulation of angiogenesis in gliomas. Journal of Neuro-Oncology 70: 229–243.

Kawasawa, Y., McKenzie, L. M., Hill, D. P., Bono, H. and Yanagisawa, M. 2003. G protein-coupled receptor genes in the FANTOM2 database. Genome Research 13: 1466–1477.

Kijima, T., Maulik, G., Ma, P. C., Tibaldi, E. V., Turner, R. E., Rollins, B., Sattler, M., Johnson, B. E. and Salgia, R. 2002. Regulation of cellular proliferation, cytoskeletal function, and signal transduction through CXCR4 and c-Kit in small cell lung cancer cells. Cancer Research 62: 6304–6311.

Kijowski, J., Baj-Krzyworzeka, M., Majka, M., Reca, R., Marquez, L. A., Christofidou-Solomidou, M., Janowska-Wieczorek, A. and Ratajczak, M. Z. 2001. The SDF-1-CXCR4 axis stimulates VEGF secretion and activates integrins but does not affect proliferation and survival in lymphohematopoietic cells. Stem Cells 19: 453–466.

Kim, J., Takeuchi, H., Lam, S. T., Turner, R. R., Wang, H. J., Kuo, C., Foshag, L., Bilchik, A. J. and Hoon, D. S. 2005. Chemokine receptor CXCR4 expression in colorectal cancer patients increases the risk for recurrence and for poor survival. Journal of Clinical Oncology 23: 2744–2753.

Kleihues, P., Louis, D. N., Scheithauer, B. W., Rorke, L. B., Reifenberger, G., Burger, P. C. and Cavenee, W. K. 2002. The WHO classification of tumors of the nervous system. Journal of Neuropathology and Experimental Neurology 61: 215–225; discussion 226–219.

Klein, R. S., Rubin, J. B., Gibson, H. D., DeHaan, E. N., Alvarez-Hernandez, X., Segal, R. A. and Luster, A. D. 2001. SDF-1 alpha induces chemotaxis and enhances Sonic hedgehog-induced proliferation of cerebellar granule cells. Development (Cambridge, England) 128: 1971–1981.

Kodama, J., Hasengaowa, Kusumoto, T., Seki, N., Matsuo, T., Ojima, Y., Nakamura, K., Hongo, A. and Hiramatsu, Y. 2007a. Association of CXCR4 and CCR7 chemokine receptor expression and lymph node metastasis in human cervical cancer. Annals of Oncology 18: 70–76.

Kodama, J., Hasengaowa, Seki, N., Kusumoto, T. and Hiramatsu, Y. 2007b. Expression of the CXCR4 and CCR7 chemokine receptors in human endometrial cancer. European Journal of Gynaecological Oncology 28: 370–375.

Koishi, K., Yoshikawa, R., Tsujimura, T., Hashimoto-Tamaoki, T., Kojima, S., Yanagi, H., Yamamura, T. and Fujiwara, Y. 2006. Persistent CXCR4 expression after preoperative chemoradiotherapy predicts early recurrence and poor prognosis in esophageal cancer. World Journal of Gastroenterology 12: 7585–7590.

Kollet, O., Spiegel, A., Peled, A., Petit, I., Byk, T., Hershkoviz, R., Guetta, E., Barkai, G., Nagler, A. and Lapidot, T. 2001. Rapid and efficient homing of human CD34(+)CD38(-/low)CXCR4(+) stem and progenitor cells to the bone marrow and spleen of NOD/SCID and NOD/SCID/B2m(null) mice. Blood 97: 3283–3291.

Konoplev, S., Rassidakis, G. Z., Estey, E., Kantarjian, H., Liakou, C. I., Huang, X., Xiao, L., Andreeff, M., Konopleva, M. and Medeiros, L. J. 2007. Overexpression of CXCR4 predicts adverse overall and event-free survival in patients with unmutated FLT3 acute myeloid leukemia with normal karyotype. Cancer 109: 1152–1156.

Kortylewski, M., Jove, R., Yu, H., Ribatti, D., Marimpietri, D., Pastorino, F., Brignole, C., Nico, B., Vacca, A., Ponzoni, M., Gontero, P., Banisadr, S., Frea, B., Brausi, M., Zhou, X. D., Turner, H. E., Harris, A. L., Melmed, S., Wass, J. A., Adhami, V. M., Ahmad, N., Mukhtar, H., Qin, L. X. and Tang, Z. Y. 2005. Targeting STAT3 affects melanoma on multiple fronts. Cancer and Metastasis Reviews 24: 315–327.

Koshiba, T., Hosotani, R., Miyamoto, Y., Ida, J., Tsuji, S., Nakajima, S., Kawaguchi, M., Kobayashi, H., Doi, R., Hori, T., Fujii, N. and Imamura, M. 2000. Expression of stromal cell-derived factor 1 and CXCR4 ligand receptor system in pancreatic cancer: a possible role for tumor progression. Clinical Cancer Research 6: 3530–3535.

Kuang, Y., Wu, Y., Jiang, H. and Wu, D. 1996. Selective G protein coupling by C-C chemokine receptors. The Journal of Biological Chemistry 271: 3975–3978.

Kucia, M., Reca, R., Miekus, K., Wanzeck, J., Wojakowski, W., Janowska-Wieczorek, A., Ratajczak, J. and Ratajczak, M. Z. 2005. Trafficking of normal stem cells and metastasis of cancer stem cells involve similar mechanisms: pivotal role of the SDF-1-CXCR4 axis. Stem Cells 23: 879–894.

Lapidot, T. 2001. Mechanism of human stem cell migration and repopulation of NOD/SCID and B2mnull NOD/SCID mice. The role of SDF-1/CXCR4 interactions. Annals of the New York Academy of Sciences 938: 83–95.

Lapidot, T., Dar, A. and Kollet, O. 2005. How do stem cells find their way home? Blood 106: 1901–1910.

Laverdiere, C., Hoang, B. H., Yang, R., Sowers, R., Qin, J., Meyers, P. A., Huvos, A. G., Healey, J. H. and Gorlick, R. 2005. Messenger RNA expression levels of CXCR4 correlate with metastatic behavior and outcome in patients with osteosarcoma. Clinical Cancer Research 11: 2561–2567.

Lee, B. C., Lee, T. H., Avraham, S. and Avraham, H. K. 2004. Involvement of the chemokine receptor CXCR4 and its ligand stromal cell-derived factor 1alpha in breast cancer cell migration through human brain microvascular endothelial cells. Molecular Cancer Research 2: 327–338.

Li, W., Gomez, E. and Zhang, Z. 2007. Immunohistochemical expression of stromal cell-derived factor-1 (SDF-1) and CXCR4 ligand receptor system in hepatocellular carcinoma. Journal of Experimental and Clinical Cancer Research 26: 527–533.

Li, Y. M., Pan, Y., Wei, Y., Cheng, X., Zhou, B. P., Tan, M., Zhou, X., Xia, W., Hortobagyi, G. N., Yu, D. and Hung, M. C. 2004. Upregulation of CXCR4 is essential for HER2-mediated tumor metastasis. Cancer Cell 6: 459–469.

Liang, Z., Brooks, J., Willard, M., Liang, K., Yoon, Y., Kang, S. and Shim, H. 2007a. CXCR4/CXCL12 axis promotes VEGF-mediated tumor angiogenesis through Akt signaling pathway. Biochemical and Biophysical Research Communications 359: 716–722.

Liang, Z., Lau, S. K., Devi, S., Yoon, Y., Cho, H. T. and Shim, H. 2006. Lower expression of CXCR4 in lymph node metastases than in primary breast cancer: Potential regulation by ligand-dependent degradation and HIF-1. Biochemical and Biophysical Research Communications 346: 252–258.

Liang, Z., Wu, H., Reddy, S., Zhu, A., Wang, S., Blevins, D., Yoon, Y., Zhang, Y. and Shim, H. 2007b. Blockade of invasion and metastasis of breast cancer cells via targeting CXCR4 with an artificial microRNA. Biochemical and Biophysical Research Communications 363: 542–546.

Liang, Z., Wu, T., Lou, H., Yu, X., Taichman, R. S., Lau, S. K., Nie, S., Umbreit, J. and Shim, H. 2004. Inhibition of breast cancer metastasis by selective synthetic polypeptide against CXCR4. Cancer Research 64: 4302–4308.

Liang, Z., Yoon, Y., Votaw, J., Goodman, M., William, L. and Shim, H. 2005. Silencing of CXCR4 blocks breast cancer metastasis. Cancer Research 65: 967–971.

Libura, J., Drukala, J., Majka, M., Tomescu, O., Navenot, J. M., Kucia, M., Marquez, L., Peiper, S. C., Barr, F. G., Janowska-Wieczorek, A. and Ratajczak, M. Z. 2002. CXCR4-SDF-1 signaling is active in rhabdomyosarcoma cells and regulates locomotion, chemotaxis, and adhesion. Blood 100: 2597–2606.

Limatola, C., Giovannelli, A., Maggi, L., Ragozzino, D., Castellani, L., Ciotti, M. T., Vacca, F., Mercanti, D., Santoni, A. and Eusebi, F. 2000. SDF-1alpha-mediated modulation of synaptic transmission in rat cerebellum. The European Journal of Neuroscience 12: 2497–2504.

Lu, M., Grove, E. A. and Miller, R. J. 2002. Abnormal development of the hippocampal dentate gyrus in mice lacking the CXCR4 chemokine receptor. Proceedings of the National Academy of Sciences of the United States of America 99: 7090–7095.

Lu, Q., Sun, E. E., Klein, R. S. and Flanagan, J. G. 2001. Ephrin-B reverse signaling is mediated by a novel PDZ-RGS protein and selectively inhibits G protein-coupled chemoattraction. Cell 105: 69–79.

Ma, L. and Weinberg, R. A. 2008. MicroRNAs in malignant progression. Cell Cycle (Georgetown, Tex) 7: 570–572.

Ma, Q., Jones, D., Borghesani, P. R., Segal, R. A., Nagasawa, T., Kishimoto, T., Bronson, R. T. and Springer, T. A. 1998. Impaired B-lymphopoiesis, myelopoiesis, and derailed cerebellar neuron migration in CXCR4- and SDF-1-deficient mice. Proceedings of the National Academy of Sciences of the United States of America 95: 9448–9453.

Majka, M., Janowska-Wieczorek, A., Ratajczak, J., Kowalska, M. A., Vilaire, G., Pan, Z. K., Honczarenko, M., Marquez, L. A., Poncz, M. and Ratajczak, M. Z. 2000a. Stromal-derived factor 1 and thrombopoietin regulate distinct aspects of human megakaryopoiesis. Blood 96: 4142–4151.

Majka, M., Ratajczak, J., Baj-Krzyworzek, M., Kijowski, J., Reca, R., Machalinski, B., Kubicze, K. and Ratajczak, M. Z. 2001. Biological significance of chemokine receptor expression by normal human megakaryoblasts. Folia. Histochemistry and Cytobiology 39: 235–244.

Majka, M., Ratajczak, J., Kowalska, M. A. and Ratajczak, M. Z. 2000b. Binding of stromal derived factor-1alpha (SDF-1alpha) to CXCR4 chemokine receptor in normal human megakaryoblasts but not in platelets induces phosphorylation of mitogen-activated protein kinase p42/44 (MAPK), ELK-1 transcription factor and serine/threonine kinase AKT. European Journal of Haematology 64: 164–172.

Majka, M., Ratajczak, J., Lee, B., Honczarenko, M., Douglas, R., Kowalska, M. A., Silberstein, L., Gewirtz, A. M. and Ratajczak, M. Z. 2000c. The role of HIV-related chemokine receptors and chemokines in human erythropoiesis in vitro. Stem Cells 18: 128–138.

Meier, R., Muhlethaler-Mottet, A., Flahaut, M., Coulon, A., Fusco, C., Louache, F., Auderset, K., Bourloud, K. B., Daudigeos, E., Ruegg, C., Vassal, G., Gross, N. and Joseph, J. M. 2007. The chemokine receptor CXCR4 strongly promotes neuroblastoma primary tumour and metastatic growth, but not invasion. PLoS ONE 2: e1016.

Mellado, M., Rodriguez-Frade, J. M., Manes, S. and Martinez, A. C. 2001. Chemokine signaling and functional responses: the role of receptor dimerization and TK pathway activation. Annual Review of Immunology 19: 397–421.

Mohle, R., Failenschmid, C., Bautz, F. and Kanz, L. 1999. Overexpression of the chemokine receptor CXCR4 in B cell chronic lymphocytic leukemia is associated with increased functional response to stromal cell-derived factor-1 (SDF-1). Leukemia 13: 1954–1959.

Monaco, G., Belmont, J. W., Konopleva, M., Andreeff, M., Tavor, S., Petit, I., Kollet, O. and Lapidot, T. 2004. Correlation between CXCR4 and homing or engraftment of acute myelogenous leukemia. Cancer Research 64: 6832 author reply 6832–6833.

Moore, B. B., Keane, M. P., Addison, C. L., Arenberg, D. A. and Strieter, R. M. 1998. CXC chemokine modulation of angiogenesis: the importance of balance between angiogenic and angiostatic members of the family. Journal of Investigation Medicine 46: 113–120.

Morales, J., Homey, B., Vicari, A. P., Hudak, S., Oldham, E., Hedrick, J., Orozco, R., Copeland, N. G., Jenkins, N. A., McEvoy, L. M. and Zlotnik, A. 1999. CTACK, a skin-associated chemokine that preferentially attracts skin- homing memory T cells. Proceedings of the National Academy of Sciences of the United States of America 96: 14470–14475.

Mori, T., Doi, R., Koizumi, M., Toyoda, E., Ito, D., Kami, K., Masui, T., Fujimoto, K., Tamamura, H., Hiramatsu, K., Fujii, N. and Imamura, M. 2004. CXCR4 antagonist inhibits stromal cell-derived factor 1-induced migration and invasion of human pancreatic cancer. Molecular Cancer Therapeutics 3: 29–37.

Moyer, R. A., Wendt, M. K., Johanesen, P. A., Turner, J. R. and Dwinell, M. B. 2007. Rho activation regulates CXCL12 chemokine stimulated actin rearrangement and restitution in model intestinal epithelia. Laboratory investigation; a Journal of Technical Methods and Pathology 87: 807–817.

Mueller, M. M. and Fusenig, N. E. 2004. Friends or foes – bipolar effects of the tumour stroma in cancer. Nature Reviews Cancer 4: 839–849.

Muller, A., Homey, B., Soto, H., Ge, N., Catron, D., Buchanan, M. E., McClanahan, T., Murphy, E., Yuan, W., Wagner, S. N., Barrera, J. L., Mohar, A., Verastegui, E. and Zlotnik, A. 2001. Involvement of chemokine receptors in breast cancer metastasis. Nature 410: 50–56.

Murphy, P. M., Baggiolini, M., Charo, I. F., Hebert, C. A., Horuk, R., Matsushima, K., Miller, L. H., Oppenheim, J. J. and Power, C. A. 2000. International union of pharmacology. XXII. Nomenclature for chemokine receptors. Pharmacological Reviews 52: 145–176.

Nagasawa, T., Nakajima, T., Tachibana, K., Iizasa, H., Bleul, C. C., Yoshie, O., Matsushima, K., Yoshida, N., Springer, T. A. and Kishimoto, T. 1996. Molecular cloning and characterization of a murine pre-B-cell growth-stimulating factor/stromal cell-derived factor 1 receptor, a murine homolog of the human immunodeficiency virus 1 entry coreceptor fusin. Proceedings of the National Academy of Sciences U S A 93: 14726–14729.

Nicolson, G. L. 1992. Paracrine/autocrine growth mechanisms in tumor metastasis. Oncology Research 4: 389–399.

Oberlin, E., Amara, A., Bachelerie, F., Bessia, C., Virelizier, J. L., Arenzana-Seisdedos, F., Schwartz, O., Heard, J. M., Clark-Lewis, I., Legler, D. F., Loetscher, M., Baggiolini, M. and Moser, B. 1996. The CXC chemokine SDF-1 is the ligand for LESTR/fusin and prevents infection by T-cell-line-adapted HIV-1. Nature 382: 833–835.

Oda, Y., Yamamoto, H., Tamiya, S., Matsuda, S., Tanaka, K., Yokoyama, R., Iwamoto, Y. and Tsuneyoshi, M. 2006. CXCR4 and VEGF expression in the primary site and the metastatic site of human osteosarcoma: analysis within a group of patients, all of whom developed lung metastasis. Modern Pathology 19: 738–745.

Odemis, V., Lamp, E., Pezeshki, G., Moepps, B., Schilling, K., Gierschik, P., Littman, D. R. and Engele, J. 2005. Mice deficient in the chemokine receptor CXCR4 exhibit impaired limb innervation and myogenesis. Molecular and Cellular Neurosciences 30: 494–505.

Ohtani, Y., Minami, M., Kawaguchi, N., Nishiyori, A., Yamamoto, J., Takami, S. and Satoh, M. 1998. Expression of stromal cell-derived factor-1 and CXCR4 chemokine receptor mRNAs in cultured rat glial and neuronal cells. Neuroscience Letters 249: 163–166.

Onuffer, J. J. and Horuk, R. 2002. Chemokines, chemokine receptors and small-molecule antagonists: recent developments. Trends in Pharmacological Sciences 23: 459–467.

Oonakahara, K., Matsuyama, W., Higashimoto, I., Kawabata, M., Arimura, K. and Osame, M. 2004. Stromal-derived factor-1alpha/CXCL12-CXCR 4 axis is involved in the dissemination of NSCLC cells into pleural space. American Journal of Respiratory Cell and Molecular Biology 30: 671–677.

Ottaiano, A., di Palma, A., Napolitano, M., Pisano, C., Pignata, S., Tatangelo, F., Botti, G., Acquaviva, A. M., Castello, G., Ascierto, P. A., Iaffaioli, R. V. and Scala, S. 2005. Inhibitory effects of anti-CXCR4 antibodies on human colon cancer cells. Cancer Immunology Immunotherapy 54: 781–791.

Packer, R. J., Goldwein, J., Nicholson, H. S., Vezina, L. G., Allen, J. C., Ris, M. D., Muraszko, K., Rorke, L. B., Wara, W. M., Cohen, B. H. and Boyett, J. M. 1999. Treatment of children with medulloblastomas with reduced-dose craniospinal radiation therapy and adjuvant chemotherapy: A Children's Cancer Group Study. Journal of Clinical Oncology 17: 2127–2136.

Pan, J., Mestas, J., Burdick, M. D., Phillips, R. J., Thomas, G. V., Reckamp, K., Belperio, J. A. and Strieter, R. M. 2006. Stromal derived factor-1 (SDF-1/CXCL12) and CXCR4 in renal cell carcinoma metastasis. Molecular Cancer 5: 56.

Pappas, T. C., Bader, A. G., Andruss, B. F., Brown, D. and Ford, L. P. 2008. Applying small RNA molecules to the directed treatment of human diseases: realizing the potential. Expert Opinion on Therapeutic Targets 12: 115–127.

Peled, A., Petit, I., Kollet, O., Magid, M., Ponomaryov, T., Byk, T., Nagler, A., Ben-Hur, H., Many, A., Shultz, L., Lider, O., Alon, R., Zipori, D. and Lapidot, T. 1999. Dependence of human stem cell engraftment and repopulation of NOD/SCID mice on CXCR4. Science 283: 845–848.

Petty, J. M., Sueblinvong, V., Lenox, C. C., Jones, C. C., Cosgrove, G. P., Cool, C. D., Rai, P. R., Brown, K. K., Weiss, D. J., Poynter, M. E. and Suratt, B. T. 2007. Pulmonary stromal-derived factor-1 expression and effect on neutrophil recruitment during acute lung injury. Journal of Immunology 178: 8148–8157.

Phillips, R. J., Mestas, J., Gharaee-Kermani, M., Burdick, M. D., Sica, A., Belperio, J. A., Keane, M. P. and Strieter, R. M. 2005. Epidermal growth factor and hypoxia-induced expression of CXC chemokine receptor 4 on non-small cell lung cancer cells is regulated by the phosphatidylinositol 3-kinase/PTEN/AKT/mammalian target of rapamycin signaling pathway and activation of hypoxia inducible factor-1alpha. The Journal of Biological Chemistry 280: 22473–22481.

Pils, D., Pinter, A., Reibenwein, J., Alfanz, A., Horak, P., Schmid, B. C., Hefler, L., Horvat, R., Reinthaller, A., Zeillinger, R. and Krainer, M. 2007. In ovarian cancer the prognostic influence of HER2/neu is not dependent on the CXCR4/SDF-1 signalling pathway. British Journal of Cancer 96: 485–491.

Piovan, E., Tosello, V., Indraccolo, S., Cabrelle, A., Baesso, I., Trentin, L., Zamarchi, R., Tamamura, H., Fujii, N., Semenzato, G., Chieco-Bianchi, L. and Amadori, A. 2005. Chemokine receptor expression in EBV-associated lymphoproliferation in hu/SCID mice: implications for CXCL12/CXCR4 axis in lymphoma generation. Blood 105: 931–939.

Porcile, C., Bajetto, A., Barbero, S., Pirani, P. and Schettini, G. 2004. CXCR4 activation induces epidermal growth factor receptor transactivation in an ovarian cancer cell line. Annals of the New York Academy of Sciences 1030: 162–169.

Ransohoff, R. M., Kivisakk, P. and Kidd, G. 2003. Three or more routes for leukocyte migration into the central nervous system. Nature Reviews 3: 569–581.

Reckamp, K. L., Strieter, R. M. and Figlin, R. A. 2008. Chemokines as therapeutic targets in renal cell carcinoma. Expert review of anticancer therapy 8: 887–893.

Reiss, K., Mentlein, R., Sievers, J. and Hartmann, D. 2002. Stromal cell-derived factor 1 is secreted by meningeal cells and acts as chemotactic factor on neuronal stem cells of the cerebellar external granular layer. Neuroscience 115: 295–305.

Rempel, S. A., Dudas, S., Ge, S. and Gutierrez, J. A. 2000. Identification and localization of the cytokine SDF1 and its receptor, CXC chemokine receptor 4, to regions of necrosis and angiogenesis in human glioblastoma. Clinical Cancer Research 6: 102–111.

Ribatti, D., Marimpietri, D., Pastorino, F., Brignole, C., Nico, B., Vacca, A. and Ponzoni, M. 2004. Angiogenesis in neuroblastoma. Annals of the New York Academy of Sciences 1028: 133–142.

Richard, C. L., Tan, E. Y. and Blay, J. 2006. Adenosine upregulates CXCR4 and enhances the proliferative and migratory responses of human carcinoma cells to CXCL12/SDF-1alpha. International Journal of Cancer 119: 2044–2053.

Rossi, D. and Zlotnik, A. 2000. The biology of chemokines and their receptors. Annual Review of Immunology 18: 217–242.

Rostasy, K., Gorgun, G., Kleyner, Y., Garcia, A., Kramer, M., Melanson, S. M., Mathys, J. M., Yiannoutsos, C., Skolnik, P. R. and Navia, B. A. 2005. Tumor necrosis factor alpha leads to increased cell surface expression of CXCR4 in SK-N-MC cells. Journal of Neurovirology 11: 247–255.

Rubin, J. B., Kung, A. L., Klein, R. S., Chan, J. A., Sun, Y., Schmidt, K., Kieran, M. W., Luster, A. D. and Segal, R. A. 2003. A small-molecule antagonist of CXCR4 inhibits intracranial growth of primary brain tumors. Proceedings of the National Academy of Sciences of the United States of America 100: 13513–13518.

Russell, H. V., Hicks, J., Okcu, M. F. and Nuchtern, J. G. 2004. CXCR4 expression in neuroblastoma primary tumors is associated with clinical presentation of bone and bone marrow metastases. Journal of Pediatric Surgery 39: 1506–1511.

Salcedo, R., Wasserman, K., Young, H. A., Grimm, M. C., Howard, O. M., Anver, M. R., Kleinman, H. K., Murphy, W. J. and Oppenheim, J. J. 1999. Vascular endothelial growth factor and basic fibroblast growth factor induce expression of CXCR4 on human endothelial cells: In vivo neovascularization induced by stromal-derived factor-1alpha. American Journal of Pathology 154: 1125–1135.

Salmaggi, A., Gelati, M., Pollo, B., Marras, C., Silvani, A., Balestrini, M. R., Eoli, M., Fariselli, L., Broggi, G. and Boiardi, A. 2005. CXCL12 expression is predictive of a shorter time to tumor progression in low-grade glioma: a single-institution study in 50 patients. Journal of Neuro-Oncology 74: 287–293.

Salvucci, O., Yao, L., Villalba, S., Sajewicz, A., Pittaluga, S. and Tosato, G. 2002. Regulation of endothelial cell branching morphogenesis by endogenous chemokine stromal-derived factor-1. Blood 99: 2703–2711.

Samara, G. J., Lawrence, D. M., Chiarelli, C. J., Valentino, M. D., Lyubsky, S., Zucker, S. and Vaday, G. G. 2004. CXCR4-mediated adhesion and MMP-9 secretion in head and neck squamous cell carcinoma. Cancer Letters 214: 231–241.

Sasaki, K., Natsugoe, S., Ishigami, S., Matsumoto, M., Okumura, H., Setoyama, T., Uchikado, Y., Kita, Y., Tamotsu, K., Sakurai, T., Owaki, T. and Aikou, T. 2008. Expression of CXCL12 and its receptor CXCR4 correlates with lymph node metastasis in submucosal esophageal cancer. Journal of Surgical Oncology 97: 433–438.

Scala, S., Ottaiano, A., Ascierto, P. A., Cavalli, M., Simeone, E., Giuliano, P., Napolitano, M., Franco, R., Botti, G. and Castello, G. 2005. Expression of CXCR4 predicts poor prognosis in patients with malignant melanoma. Clinical Cancer Research 11: 1835–1841.

Schimanski, C. C., Bahre, R., Gockel, I., Muller, A., Frerichs, K., Horner, V., Teufel, A., Simiantonaki, N., Biesterfeld, S., Wehler, T., Schuler, M., Achenbach, T., Junginger, T., Galle, P. R. and Moehler, M. 2006. Dissemination of hepatocellular carcinoma is mediated via chemokine receptor CXCR4. British Journal of Cancer 95: 210–217.

Schimanski, C. C., Schwald, S., Simiantonaki, N., Jayasinghe, C., Gonner, U., Wilsberg, V., Junginger, T., Berger, M. R., Galle, P. R. and Moehler, M. 2005. Effect of chemokine receptors CXCR4 and CCR7 on the metastatic behavior of human colorectal cancer. Clinical Cancer Research 11: 1743–1750.

Schioppa, T., Uranchimeg, B., Saccani, A., Biswas, S. K., Doni, A., Rapisarda, A., Bernasconi, S., Saccani, S., Nebuloni, M., Vago, L., Mantovani, A., Melillo, G. and Sica, A. 2003. Regulation of the chemokine receptor CXCR4 by hypoxia. The Journal of Experimental Medicine 198: 1391–1402.

Schmid, B. C., Rudas, M., Rezniczek, G. A., Leodolter, S. and Zeillinger, R. 2004. CXCR4 is expressed in ductal carcinoma in situ of the breast and in atypical ductal hyperplasia. Breast Cancer Research and Treatment 84: 247–250.

Schols, D., Este, J. A., Henson, G. and De Clercq, E. 1997. Bicyclams, a class of potent anti-HIV agents, are targeted at the HIV coreceptor fusin/CXCR-4. Antiviral Research 35: 147–156.

Schrader, A. J., Lechner, O., Templin, M., Dittmar, K. E., Machtens, S., Mengel, M., Probst-Kepper, M., Franzke, A., Wollensak, T., Gatzlaff, P., Atzpodien, J., Buer, J. and Lauber, J. 2002. CXCR4/CXCL12 expression and signalling in kidney cancer. British Journal of Cancer 86: 1250–1256.

Schuller, U., Koch, A., Hartmann, W., Garre, M. L., Goodyer, C. G., Cama, A., Sorensen, N., Wiestler, O. D. and Pietsch, T. 2005. Subtype-specific expression and genetic alterations of the chemokinereceptor gene CXCR4 in medulloblastomas. International Journal of Cancer 117: 82–89.

Schuller, U., Lamp, E. C. and Schilling, K. 2001. Developmental expression of heterotrimeric G-proteins in the murine cerebellar cortex. Histochemistry and Cell Biology 116: 149–159.

Scupoli, M. T., Donadelli, M., Cioffi, F., Rossi, M., Perbellini, O., Malpeli, G., Corbioli, S., Vinante, F., Krampera, M., Palmieri, M., Scarpa, A., Ariola, C., Foa, R. and Pizzolo, G. 2008. Bone marrow stromal cells and the upregulation of interleukin-8 production in human T-cell acute lymphoblastic leukemia through the CXCL12/CXCR4 axis and the NF-kappaB and JNK/AP-1 pathways. Haematologica 93: 524–532.

Sehgal, A., Keener, C., Boynton, A. L., Warrick, J. and Murphy, G. P. 1998a. CXCR-4, a chemokine receptor, is overexpressed in and required for proliferation of glioblastoma tumor cells. Journal of Surgery Oncology 69: 99–104.

Sehgal, A., Ricks, S., Boynton, A. L., Warrick, J. and Murphy, G. P. 1998b. Molecular characterization of CXCR-4: a potential brain tumor-associated gene. Journal of Surgery Oncology 69: 239–248.

Shibuta, K., Mori, M., Shimoda, K., Inoue, H., Mitra, P. and Barnard, G. F. 2002. Regional expression of CXCL12/CXCR4 in liver and hepatocellular carcinoma and cell-cycle variation during in vitro differentiation. Japan Journal of Cancer Research 93: 789–797.

Sotsios, Y., Whittaker, G. C., Westwick, J. and Ward, S. G. 1999. The CXC chemokine stromal cell-derived factor activates a Gi-coupled phosphoinositide 3-kinase in T lymphocytes. Journal of Immunology. 163: 5954–5963.

Sozzani, S., Molino, M., Locati, M., Luini, W., Cerletti, C., Vecchi, A. and Mantovani, A. 1993. Receptor-activated calcium influx in human monocytes exposed to monocyte chemotactic protein-1 and related cytokines. Journal of Immunology 150: 1544–1553.

Spano, J. P., Andre, F., Morat, L., Sabatier, L., Besse, B., Combadiere, C., Deterre, P., Martin, A., Azorin, J., Valeyre, D., Khayat, D., Le Chevalier, T. and Soria, J. C. 2004. Chemokine receptor CXCR4 and early-stage non-small cell lung cancer: attern of expression and correlation with outcome. Annals of Oncology 15: 613–617.

Spencer, A., Jackson, J. and Baulch-Brown, C. 2001. Enumeration of bone marrow 'homing' haemopoietic stem cells from G-CSF- mobilised normal donors and influence on engraftment following allogeneic transplantation. Bone Marrow Transplant 28: 1019–1022.

Spoo, A. C., Lubbert, M., Wierda, W. G. and Burger, J. A. 2007. CXCR4 is a prognostic marker in acute myelogenous leukemia. Blood 109: 786–791.

Staller, P., Sulitkova, J., Lisztwan, J., Moch, H., Oakeley, E. J. and Krek, W. 2003. Chemokine receptor CXCR4 downregulated by von Hippel-Lindau tumour suppressor pVHL. Nature 425: 307–311.

Strieter, R. M., Polverini, P. J., Kunkel, S. L., Arenberg, D. A., Burdick, M. D., Kasper, J., Dzuiba, J., Van Damme, J., Walz, A., Marriott, D. and et al. 1995. The functional role of the ELR motif in CXC chemokine-mediated angiogenesis. The Journal of Biological Chemistry 270: 27348–27357.

Struckmann, K., Mertz, K., Steu, S., Storz, M., Staller, P., Krek, W., Schraml, P. and Moch, H. 2008. pVHL co-ordinately regulates CXCR4/CXCL12 and MMP2/MMP9 expression in human clear-cell renal cell carcinoma. The Journal of Pathology 214: 464–471.

Sun, Y., Schneider, A., Jung, Y., Wang, J., Dia, J., Cook, K., Osman, N., Koh-Paige, A., Shim, H., Pienta, K., Keller, E., McCauley, L. and Taichman, R. S. 2005. Skeletal localization and neutralization of the SDF-1/CXCR4 axis blocks prostate cancer metastasis and growth in osseous sites in vivo. Journal of Bone Mineral Research 20: 318–329.

Tachibana, K., Hirota, S., Iizasa, H., Yoshida, H., Kawabata, K., Kataoka, Y., Kitamura, Y., Matsushima, K., Yoshida, N., Nishikawa, S., Kishimoto, T. and Nagasawa, T. 1998. The chemokine receptor CXCR4 is essential for vascularization of the gastrointestinal tract. Nature 393: 591–594.

Taichman, R. S., Cooper, C., Keller, E. T., Pienta, K. J., Taichman, N. S. and McCauley, L. K. 2002. Use of the stromal cell-derived factor-1/CXCR4 pathway in prostate cancer metastasis to bone. Cancer Research 62: 1832–1837.

Takenaga, M., Tamamura, H., Hiramatsu, K., Nakamura, N., Yamaguchi, Y., Kitagawa, A., Kawai, S., Nakashima, H., Fujii, N. and Igarashi, R. 2004. A single treatment with microcapsules containing a CXCR4 antagonist suppresses pulmonary metastasis of murine melanoma. Biochemical and Biophysical Research Communications 320: 226–232.

Tamamura, H., Hori, A., Kanzaki, N., Hiramatsu, K., Mizumoto, M., Nakashima, H., Yamamoto, N., Otaka, A. and Fujii, N. 2003. T140 analogs as CXCR4 antagonists identified as anti-metastatic agents in the treatment of breast cancer. FEBS Letters 550: 79–83.

Tang, C. H., Chuang, J. Y., Fong, Y. C., Maa, M. C., Way, T. D. and Hung, C. H. 2008. Bone-derived SDF-1 stimulates IL-6 Release via CXCR4, ERK and NF-κB pathways and promoting osteoclastogenesis in human oral cancer cells. Carcinogenesis 29: 1483–1492.

Tashiro, K., Tada, H., Heilker, R., Shirozu, M., Nakano, T. and Honjo, T. 1993. Signal sequence trap: a cloning strategy for secreted proteins and type I membrane proteins. Science 261: 600–603.

Tavor, S., Petit, I., Porozov, S., Avigdor, A., Dar, A., Leider-Trejo, L., Shemtov, N., Deutsch, V., Naparstek, E., Nagler, A. and Lapidot, T. 2004. CXCR4 regulates migration and development of human acute myelogenous leukemia stem cells in transplanted NOD/SCID mice. Cancer research 64: 2817–2824.

Tham, T. N., Lazarini, F., Franceschini, I. A., Lachapelle, F., Amara, A. and Dubois-Dalcq, M. 2001. Developmental pattern of expression of the alpha chemokine stromal cell-derived factor 1 in the rat central nervous system. The European Journal of Neuroscience 13: 845–856.

Tissir, F., Wang, C. E. and Goffinet, A. M. 2004. Expression of the chemokine receptor Cxcr4 mRNA during mouse brain development. Brain Research 149: 63–71.

Trent, J. O., Wang, Z. X., Murray, J. L., Shao, W., Tamamura, H., Fujii, N. and Peiper, S. C. 2003. Lipid bilayer simulations of CXCR4 with inverse agonists and weak partial agonists. The Journal of Biological Chemistry 278: 47136–47144.

Tsai, H. H., Frost, E., To, V., Robinson, S., Ffrench-Constant, C., Geertman, R., Ransohoff, R. M. and Miller, R. H. 2002. The chemokine receptor CXCR2 controls positioning of oligodendrocyte precursors in developing spinal cord by arresting their migration. Cell 110: 373–383.

Turner, H. E., Harris, A. L., Melmed, S. and Wass, J. A. 2003. Angiogenesis in endocrine tumors. Endocrines Reviews 24: 600–632.

Ubogu, E. E., Cossoy, M. B. and Ransohoff, R. M. 2006. The expression and function of chemokines involved in CNS inflammation. Trends in Pharmacological Sciences 27: 48–55.

Vainchenker, W. 2001. Hematopoietic stem cells. Therapie 56: 379–381.

Van Meir, E. G. 1995. Cytokines and tumors of the central nervous system. Glia 15: 264–288.

Van Meir, E. G. 1999. Cytokine expression in brain tumors: its role in tumor biology and tumor associated immune responses. In: *Inflammatory cells and mediators in CNS diseases*. pp. 169–244. Eds. R. R. Ruffolo, G. Z. Feuerstein, A. J. Hunter, G. Poste, B. W. Metcalf. Harwood Academic Publishers: London.

Vandercappellen, J., Van Damme, J. and Struyf, S. 2008. The role of CXC chemokines and their receptors in cancer. Cancer Letters 267: 226–244.

Vasudevan, S. A., Nuchtern, J. G. and Shohet, J. M. 2005. Gene profiling of high risk neuroblastoma. World Journal of Surgery 29: 317–324.

Vicari, A. P. and Caux, C. 2002. Chemokines in cancer. Cytokine & Growth Factor Reviews 13: 143–154.

Vlahakis, S. R., Villasis-Keever, A., Gomez, T., Vanegas, M., Vlahakis, N. and Paya, C. V. 2002. G protein-coupled chemokine receptors induce both survival and apoptotic signaling pathways. Journal of Immunology 169: 5546–5554.

Voermans, C., van Heese, W. P., de Jong, I., Gerritsen, W. R. and van Der Schoot, C. E. 2002. Migratory behavior of leukemic cells from acute myeloid leukemia patients. Leukemia 16: 650–657.

Wald, O., Pappo, O., Safadi, R., Dagan-Berger, M., Beider, K., Wald, H., Franitza, S., Weiss, I., Avniel, S., Boaz, P., Hanna, J., Zamir, G., Eid, A., Mandelboim, O., Spengler, U., Galun, E. and Peled, A. 2004. Involvement of the CXCL12/CXCR4 pathway in the advanced liver disease that is associated with hepatitis C virus or hepatitis B virus. European Journal of Immunology 34: 1164–1174.

Ward, S. G., Bacon, K. and Westwick, J. 1998. Chemokines and T lymphocytes: more than an attraction. Immunity 9: 1–11.

Weinberg, R. A. 2006. *Biology of Cancer*. Garland Science: New York.

Wright, D. E., Bowman, E. P., Wagers, A. J., Butcher, E. C. and Weissman, I. L. 2002. Hematopoietic stem cells are uniquely selective in their emigratory response to chemokines. Journal of Experimental Medicine 195: 1145–1154.

Wu, S., Gessner, R., Taube, T., Korte, A., von Stackelberg, A., Kirchner, R., Henze, G. and Seeger, K. 2006. Chemokine IL-8 and chemokine receptor CXCR3 and CXCR4 gene expression in childhood acute lymphoblastic leukemia at first relapse. Journal of Pediatr Hematology Oncology 28: 216–220.

Yoon, Y., Liang, Z., Zhang, X., Choe, M., Cho, H. T., Shin, D. M., Goodman, M., Chen, Z. and Shim, H. 2007. CXCR4 antagonist blocks both growth of primary tumor and metastasis of head and neck cancer in xenograft mouse models. Cancer Research 67: 7518–7524.

Zagzag, D., Krishnamachary, B., Yee, H., Okuyama, H., Chiriboga, L., Ali, M. A., Melamed, J. and Semenza, G. L. 2005. Stromal cell-derived factor-1alpha and CXCR4 expression in hemangioblastoma and clear cell-renal cell carcinoma: von Hippel-Lindau loss-of-function induces expression of a ligand and its receptor. Cancer Research 65: 6178–6188.

Zeelenberg, I. S., Ruuls-Van Stalle, L. and Roos, E. 2003. The chemokine receptor CXCR4 is required for outgrowth of colon carcinoma micrometastases. Cancer Research 63: 3833–3839.

Zhang, L., Yeger, H., Das, B., Irwin, M. S. and Baruchel, S. 2007. Tissue microenvironment modulates CXCR4 expression and tumor metastasis in neuroblastoma. Neoplasia 9: 36–46.

Zhang, M. and Rosen, J. M. 2006. Stem cells in the etiology and treatment of cancer. Current in Opinion Genetics Development 16: 60–64.

Zhao, Q., Kho, A., Kenney, A. M., Yuk Di, D. I., Kohane, I. and Rowitch, D. H. 2002. Identification of genes expressed with temporal–spatial restriction to developing cerebellar neuron precursors by a functional genomic approach. Proceedings of the National Academy of Sciences of the United States of America 99: 5704–5709.

Zhou, Y., Larsen, P. H., Hao, C. and Yong, V. W. 2002. CXCR4 is a major chemokine receptor on glioma cells and mediates their survival. The Journal of Biological Chemistry 277: 49481–49487.
Zhu, Y., Yu, T., Zhang, X. C., Nagasawa, T., Wu, J. Y. and Rao, Y. 2002. Role of the chemokine SDF-1 as the meningeal attractant for embryonic cerebellar neurons. Nature Neuroscience 5: 719–720.
Zlotnik, A. 2006. Chemokines and cancer. International Journal of Cancer 119: 2026–2029.
Zlotnik, A. and Yoshie, O. 2000. Chemokines: a new classification system and their role in immunity. Immunity 12: 121–127.
Zou, Y. R., Kottmann, A. H., Kuroda, M., Taniuchi, I. and Littman, D. R. 1998. Function of the chemokine receptor CXCR4 in haematopoiesis and in cerebellar development. Nature 393: 595–599.

Chapter 35
Molecular Targeting of IL-13Rα2 and EphA2 Receptor in GBM

Waldemar Debinski and Jill Wykosky

Abstract Finding widely overexpressed proteins specific to glioblastoma multiforme (GBM) was considered unlikely. Contrary to expectations, a number of such factors have been identified to be expressed in a majority of GBM but not in normal brain. These tumor-specific proteins are very attractive targets for novel, specific, rationally designed molecular therapies. Here we discuss the opportunities presented by two such factors, IL-13Rα2 and EphA2 receptor. IL-13Rα2 is a nonsignaling form of interleukin-13 receptor, which, in contrast to its physiological counterpart, is not bound by interleukin-4. IL-13Rα2 is overexpressed in 75% of GBM, and its presence in normal organs is very low or nonexistent, with the exception of the testes. EphA2 receptor belongs to the largest family of receptor tyrosine kinases. EphA2 is present in nearly all GBM, is highly overexpressed in 66% of them, is absent in normal brain, and is strongly associated with poor patient survival. Molecularly targeted cytotoxins that contain derivatives of bacterial toxins that specifically and potently kill GBM cells overexpressing either IL-13Rα2 or EphA2 receptor were produced. The first generation of an IL-13-based cytotoxin reached Phase III clinical trial, demonstrated safety of the approach in humans, improved progression-free survival of GBM patients in some centers, but did not modify mean survival of the whole cohort. The first EphA2-targeted cytotoxin has already demonstrated attractive features in recent preclinical examination. The overexpression of either IL-13Rα2 or EphA2 is seen in 95% of GBM, which means that by cotargeting these two receptors almost all patients will be eligible, making the need for pretherapy screening for marker expression unnecessary. The future efforts in exploiting potent cytotoxins for the treatment of GBM should focus

---

Financial support: 1 F31 NSO55533-01 to Jill Wykosky and RO1 CA 74145 to Waldemar Debinski

W. Debinski (✉)
Brain Tumor Center of Excellence, Wake Forest University School of Medicine, Medical Center Boulevard, Winston-Salem, NC 27157, USA
e-mail: debinski@wfubmc.edu

E.G. Van Meir (ed.), *CNS Cancer*, Cancer Drug Discovery and Development, DOI 10.1007/978-1-60327-553-8_35,
© Humana Press, a part of Springer Science+Business Media, LLC 2009

on combinatorial targeted therapy that involves either a multivalent approach or combination cocktails of the cytotoxins. In this way, multiple compartments of GBM tumors will be targeted benefiting all the patients.

Keywords IL-13Rα2 · EphA2 · Glioblastoma multiforme · Astrocytoma · Receptor · Recombinant cytotoxins

Contents

35.1 Molecularly Targeted Recombinant Cytotoxins for the Treatment of Brain Tumors

Virtually all patients with glioblastoma multiforme (GBM) are refractory to the treatment that includes surgery (Sanai et al. 2008), radiation therapy (Shaw et al. 2006), and various chemotherapeutic regimens (Stupp et al. 2005). This is best illustrated by the fact that during the last seven decades, one month per decade was added to the lives of patients with GBM. Thus, new and preferably molecularly specific methods of GBM treatment must be found.

A new approach in anti-GBM therapy utilizes recombinant chimera cytotoxic fusion proteins (Debinski 2002a, b, 2007, 2008; Laske et al. 1997) (Fig. 35.1). These cytotoxins are composed of two principal structural elements: (i) a targeting ligand/vector and (ii) an effector in a form of various derivatives

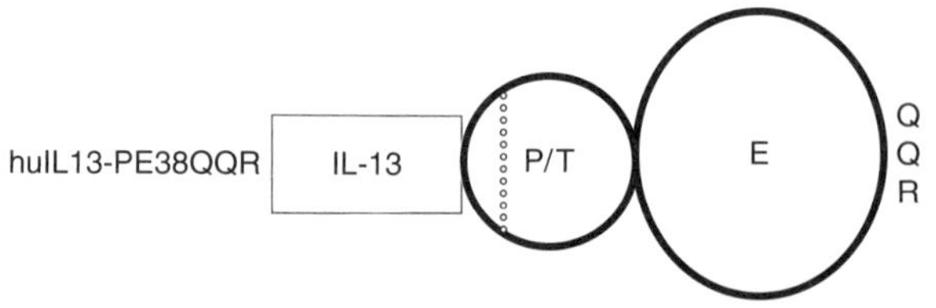

Fig. 35.1 Scheme of the first generation of interleukin-13 (IL-13)-based cytotoxin, huIL13-PE38QQR. Anticancer cytotoxins (recombinant fusion chimera protein) are composed of a carrier/ligand (in this case, wild-type IL-13) and an effector/catalyst (in this case, a derivative of *Pseudomonas* exotoxin A, PE38QQR). P/T, processing/translocation domain of PE; E, enzymatic, ADP-ribosylating enzyme in PE

of bacterial toxins preserving their catalytic activity (Fig. 35.1). Bacterial toxins are most frequently represented by Pseudomonas exotoxin A (PE) and Diphtheria toxin (DT) (Pastan et al. 1992), which are extremely potent and lethal to eukaryotic cells (Iglewski and Kabat 1975). PE and DT have been generated in a variety of genetically engineered forms with the general purpose of making the toxins inactive on eukaryotic cells either through the loss of receptor binding or enzymatic activity. However, in conjunction with a cell type-specific ligand/carrier, the toxins without receptor-binding domain can be delivered and are deadly only to targeted cells (Fig. 35.1).

Cytotoxins have a number of features that make them attractive for GBM therapy. They are relatively small compounds (less than 200 kDa), deliverable directly to the tumor site using an interstitial/intratumoral drug administration system termed convection-enhanced delivery (CED) (Laske et al. 1997; Wersall et al. 1997; Debinski 2002b; Raghavan et al. 2006), and extremely potent at killing GBM cells. Their IC_{50}s can reach even femtomolar ranges (Debinski 2002b). Cytotoxins do not produce resistance readily, since it is difficult to clone/propagate eukaryotic cells resistant against either PE or DT. Toxins work through an irreversible inhibition of de novo protein synthesis; hence, resistance to them can only be suicidal to the very cells because this would mean abolishing self-renewal functions (Carglia et al. 2000).

The molecularly targeted cytotoxins are one group of experimental drugs examined for the treatment of GBM that have been following the translational path from bench to the clinic relatively efficiently. The first cytotoxin that entered clinical trials was delivered directly into the tumor site by convection-enhanced delivery (CED) and targeted transferrin receptors overexpressed at the cell surface of GBM cells. The cytotoxin (DT.CRM107-Tf or TransMID, Celtic Pharma) consisted of human transferrin coupled with a modified diphtheria toxin as an effector (Laske et al. 1997; Weaver and Laske 2003). Phase I and Phase II trials demonstrated significant clinical responses in a large fraction of patients (Weaver and Laske 2003). Unfortunately, transferrin receptor is ubiquitous in the central nervous system (CNS), resulting in the possibility of normal tissue toxicity due to DT.CRM107-Tf killing nonmalignant cells as well as tumor cells (Connor and Fine 1986; Debinski et al. 1998b; Hulet et al. 1999; Debinski et al. 2000). Toxic side effects materialized in the clinical setting and the Phase III efficacy trial had to be interrupted prematurely (Celtic Pharma 2007).

cpIL4-PE38KDEL was another cytotoxin that entered clinical evaluation (Debinski et al. 1993, 1994; Weber et al. 2003). However, a small differential in the number of interleukin-4 (IL-4) receptors present on the surface of normal CNS cells and malignant brain tumor cells (Debinski et al. 1999b; Liu et al. 2000) was likely the reason for Phase I and II clinical trials demonstrating much less encouraging results from those seen with DT.CRM107-Tf. Another cytotoxin that entered the clinic, TGFα-PE38 (TP-38), targets the epidermal growth factor receptor (EGFR) that is abundantly overexpressed in less than 30% of patients with GBM and is naturally present in many normal organs (Debinski et al. 1999b; Ekstrand et al. 1991; Mizoguchi et al. 2006). Thus far, moderate responses were recorded in a marginal number of patients (Sampson et al. 2003), but more recent data demonstrated toxic events at very low doses of TP-38. Only 20% of patients retained the cytotoxin within the tumors by imaging, which correlates perfectly well with the overall number of GBM patients demonstrating significant overexpression of EGFR (Sampson et al. 2008).

35.2 Targetable Molecular Fingerprints in GBM

35.2.1 Overexpression of IL-13Rα2 in GBM

Previously identified markers/targets in GBM that were exploited for targeting with the cytotoxins were far from optimal for this particular therapeutic approach. EGFR or EGFRvIII proteins are found in less than 30% of patients with GBM, with EGFRvIII being overexpressed heterogeneously (Mizoguchi et al. 2006). IL-13Rα2 is an alternative molecular target that is richly overexpressed in GBM and that can be exploited uniquely for all three clinical purposes: diagnosis, imaging, and treatment (Debinski et al. 1999a). IL-13Rα2 is one of the two known receptors for interleukin-13 (IL-13). GBM cells express on their plasma membrane primarily IL-13Rα2, a monomeric protein to which IL-4, a homologue of IL-13, can neither bind nor transmit a signal through (Debinski et al. 1995b). IL-13Rα2 is one of the first factors ever documented to be overexpressed in a majority of patients with GBM and not in normal brain (Murphy et al. 1995; Rich et al. 1996). This discovery revealed that common molecular denominators of GBM do exist, a fact that is now generally acknowledged.

One of the most utilized approaches for molecular target discovery lies in the analysis of gene expression between normal and malignant cells, with the goal of finding differentially expressed genes that encode for proteins suitable for targeting. Interestingly, IL-13Rα2 would not have become a subject of our investigations had we based our approach solely on gene expression analysis using cDNA microarrays. The gene for the receptor using this methodology is expressed in ~30% of patients with GBM (Nutt et al. 2003). Some tumor specimens or established GBM cells overexpressing a large number of IL-13Rα2 as determined by various receptor-binding techniques and susceptibility to the targeted cytotoxins did not show the receptor's message in the gene arrays (Table 35.1). However, the gene expression of *IL-13Rα2* using RT-PCR is present in 100% of patients with GBM (Zhang et al. 2007, 2008). Experiments from a number of laboratories confirmed the notion that molecular targeting of IL-13Rα2 is an attractive strategy for molecular detection and treatment of GBM (Debinski et al. 1995b, 1998a, b, 1999a, b, 2000; Debinski and Gibo 2000;

Table 35.1 cDNA microarray analysis of *IL-13Rα2* mRNA expression in normal brain specimens, GBM specimens, established human GBM cell lines, and normal human cells (normal human astrocytes, NHA, and human umbilical vein endothelial cells, HUVEC)

Tissue/cells analyzed	*IL-13Rα2*	*AKT*	IL-13Rα2-binding sites per cell
G48a	+	+ + +	ND
U87MG	+	+	ND
U251MG	+	ND	28,000
A-172	–	ND	23,000
U373MG	–	ND	16,000
DBTRG	–	+	ND
HUVEC	–	ND	<200
NHA	ND	+ + +	<200
GBM 7	–	–	ND
GBM 21	–	ND	11,000
GBM 45	–	±	ND
Normal brain	–	ND	ND

The detection of *AKT* mRNA levels obtained in these assays is shown for comparison. Relative gene expression was scored on a scale from – (below detection limit) to ++++ (highly expressed). The third column presents the number of IL-13Rα2 receptors found on the cells using radiolabeled ligand-binding assays and Scatchard plots. For IL-13Rα2 1000 binding sites are enough for an IL-13-based cytotoxin to evoke potent, specific cell killing. ND, not done.

Jarboe et al. 2007; Liu et al. 2003c; Mintz and Debinski 2000; Mintz et al. 2002; Saikali et al. 2007; Wykosky et al. 2008a; Zhang et al. 2007, 2008).

The *IL-13Rα2* gene is located on the X chromosome, and the testes is the only normal tissue in which it is readily expressed, as determined by Northern blot (Debinski and Gibo 2000). This makes IL-13Rα2 a member of a group of antigens called cancer-testes tumor antigens (CTAs), for which gene expression by Northern blots was very low or absent in normal organs and was high only in the testes. IL-13Rα2 has been postulated to play the role of a decoy receptor for IL-13, as a number of laboratories could not demonstrate any downstream signaling associated with IL-13Rα2 (e.g., Rahaman et al. 2002), with the exception of a single report in which signaling was suspected in some specialized cells in vitro (Fichtner-Feigl et al. 2006). The examination of IL-13Rα2 expression first by autoradiography and then by immunohistochemistry found on average a 75% expression rate among GBM patient tumors (e.g., Mintz and Debinski 2000; Liu et al. 2003c; Saikali et al. 2007; Wykosky et al. 2008a). By autoradiography, 71% of 81 GBM specimens analyzed demonstrated overexpression of IL-13Rα2 (our unpublished data).

IL-13Rα2 is a direct gene target for EGFRvIII, a deletion mutant form of EGFR that signals constitutively (Lal et al. 2002). IL-13Rα2 is overexpressed in GBM cells, yet the activation of wild-type EGFR leads to further upregulation of the receptor, a process that is inhibited by both PI3-K and tyrosine kinase inhibitors (Hu et al. 2005) (Fig. 35.2 and Color Plate 54). The *IL-13Rα2* promoter contains AP-1 binding sites, among others, and a 64-base pair region

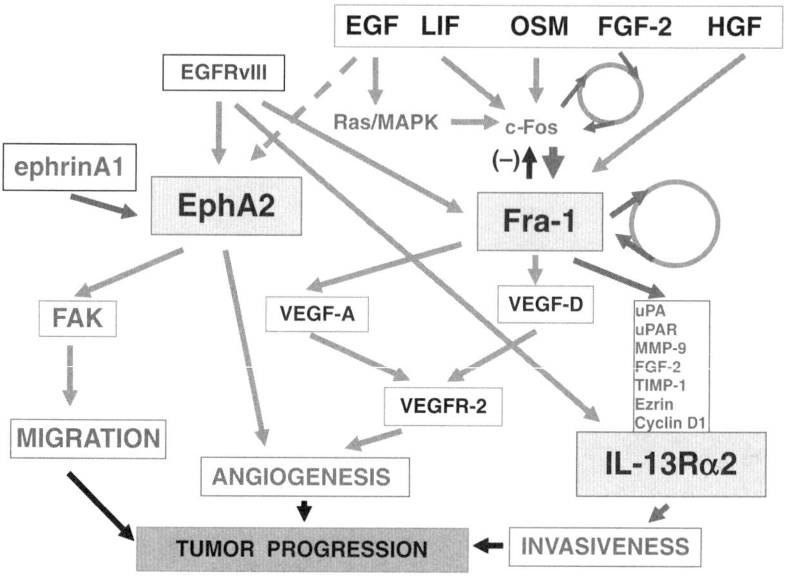

Fig. 35.2 Simplified scheme of EphA2, IL-13Rα2 and also fos-related antigen 1 (Fra-1) regulation of expression and role in GBM progression. Mitogenic/oncogenic/growth-promoting factors, such as EGF, LIF, OSM, FGF-2, and HGF, are all highly upregulated in GBM. They all activate c-Fos transiently, but they appear to stimulate Fra-1 stably and in a sustained manner (Debinski and Gibo 2005). EGFRvIII is a receptor that is constitutively activated in GBM. EphA2, Fra-1, and IL-13Rα2 belong to a selected group of factors that are its gene targets. EphA2, Fra-1, and IL-13Rα2 collectively contribute to tumor neovasculature, tumor cell migration and invasiveness, and thus tumor progression (*see* Color Plate 54)

that is necessary for promoter activity that contains AP-1, NFAT, and AP-2 *cis*-elements (David et al. 2003; Wu and Low 2003). In a simple association, the formation of and progression to GBM is paralleled by an increased AP-1 activity, which coincides with an overexpression of IL-13Rα2 (Fig. 35.2). It is also possible that epigenetics plays a role in the expression of IL-13Rα2 in GBM cells, since demethylation of DNA causes further upregulation of the gene for this receptor (Debinski et al. 2003).

35.2.2 Targeting IL-13Rα2 for Therapeutic Purposes

To target GBM cells expressing IL-13Rα2 an IL-13-based cytotoxin was developed and showed efficacy in preclinical GBM models, warranting clinical translation (Debinski et al. 1995a) (Fig. 35.1). A recombinant chimeric cytotoxin consisting of IL-13 and a truncated form of Pseudomonas exotoxin (PE38QQR) was designed and tested in the clinic under the name Cintredekin

Besudotox (CB or huIL13-PE38QQR; NeoPharm, Inc.). The CB cytotoxin was initially tested in three multicenter Phase I trials (Kunwar et al. 2007a). Convection-enhanced delivery (CED) was used as a locoregional delivery method to deliver the cytotoxin to ensure high tissue distribution and a large volume of distribution. The main objectives were to determine the maximum tolerated intraparenchymal dose at different infusion rates, tissue distribution of the cytotoxin, and optimization of delivery methods. Altogether 51 patients with malignant glioma were treated, 46 of which had GBM and enrollment did not take into account the status of IL-13Rα2 receptor expression. The MTD was determined at 0.5 μg/ml and infusions up to 6 days were well tolerated with only local adverse events. The trials also documented quite unprecedented efficacy of the cytotoxin: the overall mean survival for GBM patients was 42.7 weeks and extended to 55.6 weeks for patients with optimally positioned catheters, with several patients living beyond 5 years. These highly encouraging results led to a randomized Phase III trial (PRECISE trial) conducted in 52 centers that enrolled patients with GBM at first recurrence and the primary endpoint was overall survival from the time of 2:1 randomization (Kunwar et al. 2007b). Patients in the experimental arm of the trial received CB (huIL13-PE38QQR), while the control arm consisted of the standard of care, e.g., delivery of carmustine (BCNU) in Gliadel Wafers (Gallia et al. 2005). The median survival of the 184 patients in the CB arm was 36.4 weeks as compared to 35.3 weeks for the 92 patients in the control arm ($p = 0.476$). While this result did not meet expectations, the results were much more encouraging once the dataset was restricted to sites having enrolled more than six patients with confirmed drug delivery. In this case, the CB arm had an overall survival of 46.8 weeks versus 41.6 in the control arm ($p = 0.288$) and a hazard ratio of 0.77 ($p = 0.163$). More impressive was the finding that progression-free survival was 17.7 versus 11.4 weeks in favor of CB ($p = 0.008$). The trial evidenced that neurosurgeon training in the use of CED needs to be better monitored so that a more uniform method can be applied in different centers to ensure homogeneous drug delivery. Future trials may also benefit from using expression levels of IL-13Rα2 as a biological marker of enrollment and data analysis. The next generation of rationally designed cytotoxins will need to use reengineered IL-13-targeting motifs that bind specifically IL-13Rα2, but not the IL-13 physiological receptor, so as to be better suited for specific molecular-targeted treatment of GBM (Debinski et al. 1998a; Mintz et al. 2002).

Multiple molecular therapies targeting IL-13Rα2 in addition to huIL13-PE38QQR have been generated. Targeted cytotoxic therapy, targeted gene therapy, targeted radiation therapy, and targeted chemotherapy all have the potential of being applied to patients with GBM. Among them are vaccines, already in the clinic (Okano et al. 2002; Eguchi et al. 2006; Mintz et al. 2008), targeted viruses (Zhou et al. 2002), retargeted cytotoxic T cells, already in the clinic (Kahlon et al. 2004), and new rationally designed IL-13-based cytotoxins (Li et al. 2002; Mintz et al. 2003). Additionally, novel IL-13Rα2-targeted adenoviral constructs have been developed and could potentially be used as gene therapy vectors for the treatment of gliomas (Ulasov et al. 2007; Curtin et al. 2008). Thus, IL-13Rα2 is a truly attractive molecular target overexpressed in a majority, but not all patients with GBM (Wykosky et al. 2008a).

35.2.3 EphA2 Receptor in GBM

In search for additional specific molecular targets in GBM, we and others came across the EphA2 receptor (Wykosky et al. 2005; Hatano et al. 2005). Unlike *IL-13Rα2*, the *EphA2* gene was overexpressed prominently and frequently in GBM using cDNA microarrays (Debinski et al. 2001; Wykosky et al. 2005). This prompted a further investigation of EphA2 protein expression in GBM. Eph receptors comprise the largest family of receptor tyrosine kinases (RTKs), a group of transmembrane proteins that are crucial in mediating signal transduction pathways in cells such as those controlling growth, migration, and differentiation (Pasquale 2008; Wykosky and Debinski 2008) (Fig. 35.3 and Color Plate 55). Ephs have been extensively studied for their important functions in CNS development, and more recently several have been found to play a role in the pathogenesis of cancer. Eph receptors are unique among the RTKs in that their endogenous ligands, the ephrins, have been shown to be cell surface-anchored proteins rather than soluble factors. We have provided evidence, however, that this model might not fully depict the situation in cancer (Wykosky et al. 2008b). Namely, ephrinA1, the primary ligand for EphA2, is released from the plasma membrane of GBM cells and is, indeed, functional as a soluble ligand (Fig. 35.3). This suggests that in addition to mediating juxtacrine signaling, ephrinA1 may function in a paracrine manner in tumors.

Interestingly, EphA2 protein is upregulated by EGFR-mediated signaling in GBM cells (Larsen et al. 2007), and the gene is a direct transcriptional target of the Ras-MAPK pathway (Macrae et al. 2005). *EphA2*, similar to *IL-13Rα2*, has been shown to be part of a small group of genes that are EGFRvIII gene targets

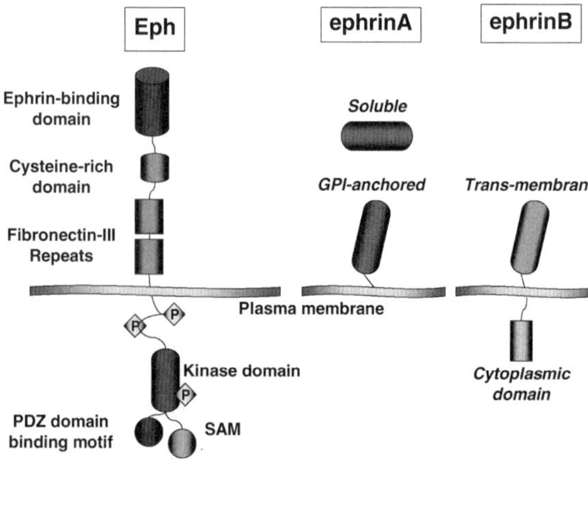

Fig. 35.3 Eph receptors and ephrin ligands. Each color represents a functionally or structurally distinct domain or motif. EphrinA ligands exist as GPI-anchored or soluble proteins, while ephrinB ligands are transmembrane proteins with a cytoplasmic domain. Tyrosine phosphorylation sites within Eph receptor are denoted by "P." SAM, sterile alpha motif (*see* Color Plate 55)

in GBM (Lal et al. 2002; Ramnarain et al. 2006) (Fig. 35.2). Thus, both EphA2 and IL-13Rα2 share a direct relationship to a receptor, which is considered to be important in contributing to the pathogenesis of GBM in those tumors in which it is expressed (Ekstrand et al. 1991; Liu et al. 2005) (Fig. 35.2).

35.2.3.1 EphA2 Protein Expression in GBM Cells and Tumors

Western blotting analysis was used to examine the expression of the EphA2 protein, and seven different GBM cell lines displayed elevated levels of EphA2. The only cell line that did not abundantly overexpress the receptor was U87MG (Wykosky et al. 2005). In GBM tumor specimens, immunoreactive EphA2 was elevated in 13 of 14 tumors, and 6 of these exhibited abundant overexpression of the receptor (Wykosky et al. 2008a). Importantly, Western blot analysis of two different commercially purchased normal human brain protein medleys and tissue isolated in-house from the frontal lobe of a normal human brain revealed no specific EphA2-immunoreactive band. The expression of EphA2 in stem cells from the CNS has not yet been determined, but due to its well-defined role in nervous system embryonic development, an elevated level of EphA2 in this specific cell population would not be unexpected. Confocal microscopy revealed the plasma membrane localization of EphA2 in GBM cells (Fig. 35.4

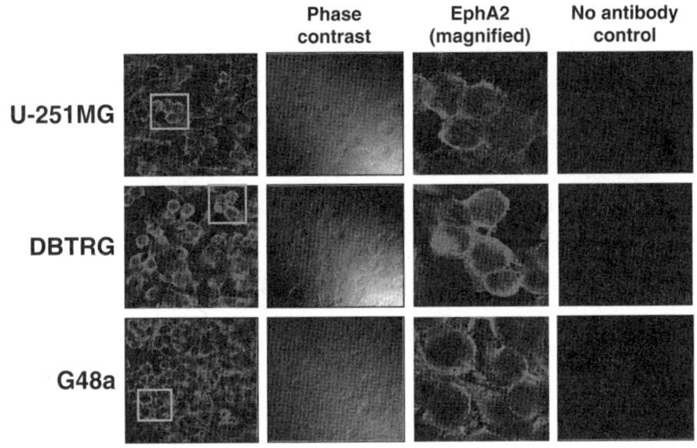

Fig. 35.4 EphA2 staining in GBM cells. Glioblastoma cell lines (U-251 MG, DBTRG-MG, G48a) were grown on sterile glass slides and fixed in acetone for 2 min at –20°C, washed in PBS, and either used immediately or stored at –80°C. Slides were blocked for 1 h in 10% normal goat serum (NGS) at RT. Primary EphA2 monoclonal antibody B208 (1:200; MedImmune) was diluted in 1.5× NGS and incubated overnight at 4°C. Slides were incubated with secondary antibody for 45 min at RT. The secondary antibody was a goat antimouse IgG Oregon Green (1:200) (Molecular Probes, Eugene, OR). Control slides without primary antibody were also used as negative controls for nonspecific binding of the secondary antibody. Confocal microscopy analysis of samples stained with monoclonal EphA2 antibody was performed using a Zeiss LSM 510 Laser Scanning Confocal Microscope with a 63× lens. Photomicrographs were taken with a 40× magnification objective lens in all cases with a Retiga EXi digital camera. Images were processed with Jasc Paint Shop Pro v6.0 (*see* Color Plate 56)

and Color Plate 56), which was confirmed by flow cytometry analysis (Wykosky et al. 2005, 2007).

A further assessment of EphA2 expression by immunostaining of human GBM tissue and nonmalignant brain demonstrated dense, specific EphA2 staining throughout the GBM tumor sections, including astrocytoma cells as well as tumor vascular endothelial cells. EphA2 staining was again near the detection limit or absent in nonmalignant brain (Wykosky et al. 2005, 2008a). Interestingly, unlike the high degree of specific staining observed for EphA2, the ephrinA1 ligand was found at low levels throughout the GBM specimens. In nonmalignant brain, we observed ephrinA1 staining specifically and intensely localized to the endothelial cells of vessels (Wykosky et al. 2005, 2008a). Interestingly, this specific vascular endothelial cell localization of ephrinA1 in normal brain is less intense in GBM specimens.

EphA2 expression has also been extensively analyzed in normal brain and tumor tissue from patients with grade II and III astrocytoma compared to those with grade IV GBM (Wykosky et al. 2008a). EphA2 staining in grade IV GBM was significantly higher than that in lower grade astrocytomas. The percent of specimens which presented with the highest frequency of EphA2-positive tumor cells was 91% for grade IV, 7% for grade III, and 2% for grade II (Wykosky et al. 2008a). In addition, 29% of grade IV, 15% of grade III, and 56% of grade II specimens were positive for EGFR, which is similar to previously observed patterns of expression for this receptor (Ekstrand et al. 1991; Mizoguchi et al. 2006). A similar abundance of EphA2 expression was observed by Western blotting of human GBM tumor tissue, human GBM xenograft tissues and cell lines, and primary GBM explant cells (Wykosky et al. 2008a). Importantly, it has also been documented that high expression of the EphA2 receptor correlates with poor survival of GBM patients (Liu et al. 2006; Wang et al. 2008). Thus, EphA2 is expressed in abundance in the majority of GBM tumors, and in the majority of individual cells within these tumors.

To further explore EphA2 expression in addition to that of IL-13Rα2 in GBM, we analyzed explanted human GBM tumors that have been serially passaged in nude mice and more closely resemble characteristics of the original tumor (Pandita et al. 2004; Sarkaria et al. 2006). These tumors have been previously characterized for *EGFR* amplification and protein expression, and it has been shown that the EGFR status of the tumors has a tendency to change upon establishment in culture (Sarkaria et al. 2006), which may also hold true for the markers of interest here. Interestingly, some tumors without *EGFR* amplification had no detectable EphA2 or IL-13Rα2 (Wykosky et al. 2008a). In contrast, EphA2 and IL-13Rα2 were found to be overexpressed in some *EGFR*-amplified tumors, one of which had amplified *EGFRvIII*, the others which overexpressed wild-type EGFR. Thus, there is a general trend for correlation of EphA2 and IL-13Rα2 expression with the expression of EGFR in these tumors (Fig. 35.2). Of importance, however, these receptors can also be overexpressed independently of EGFR, indicative of other mechanisms likely involved in their upregulation.

35.2.3.2 Function of EphA2 in GBM

We next investigated the possibility that EphA2 is playing a functional role in affecting the pathobiology of GBM, specifically in the context of its relationship with the ephrinA1 ligand. We found a significant dose-dependent inhibitory effect of ephrinA1 on the anchorage-independent growth of U251MG and A-172 GBM cells that was absent or much less pronounced in H4 and U87MG cells, which express very low levels of EphA2 (Wykosky et al. 2005). The U251MG and A-172 cells are high overexpressors of EphA2 and also exhibited a substantial dose-dependent decrease in invasiveness in response to increasing concentrations of ephrinA1 (Wykosky et al. 2005). Despite the abundance of EphA2 in GBM cell lines and tumors, we detected little to no tyrosine phosphorylated EphA2. Upon treatment of GBM cells with ephrinA1, however, the levels of tyrosine phosphorylated EphA2 increased dramatically over time. The ephrinA1-induced activation of the receptor was transient, as phosphorylated EphA2 was found to occur as early as 10 min and was no longer detected 2 h following treatment with ephrinA1 (Wykosky et al. 2005). In addition, the levels of total immunoreactive EphA2 in ephrinA1-treated cell lysates began to decrease after 60 min, as expected due to the fact that ligand binding induces internalization and degradation of the receptor in epithelial cells (Walker-Daniels et al. 2002). Moreover, ephrinA1 induced changes in GBM cell morphology within the immediate time frame of receptor phosphorylation. Specifically, profound cell rounding occurred, which was associated with a dramatic loss of cellular processes and polarity (Wykosky et al. 2005, 2008b). Overall, ephrinA1 imparts tumor-suppressing properties on GBM cells by inducing phosphorylation and subsequent downregulation of the EphA2 receptor (Fig. 35.2). Most other RTK–ligand pairs that have been investigated in the context of cancer positively influence malignancy as a result of ligand stimulation or constitutive receptor activation, making the function of the EphA2–ephrinA1 system in affecting GBM pathobiology different and unique (Wykosky and Debinski 2008).

35.2.3.3 Targeting EphA2 in GBM with EphrinA1-Based Cytotoxins

The expression of EphA2 in both vascular endothelial cells and GBM tumor cells highlights the important role that EphA2 plays in tumor angiogenesis (Cheng et al. 2002). This unique dual function of the EphA2/ephrinA1 system in tumorigenesis and angiogenesis provides a rarely seen opportunity to target such a system therapeutically in a variety of ways. One approach would be taking advantage of the tumor-suppressing function of ephrinA1 to modulate the behavior of EphA2-expressing tumor cells. Alternatively, direct knockdown of EphA2 throughout a tumor could provide a way to suppress the function of this oncoprotein in tumor cells and endothelial cells simultaneously. Of note,

EphA2-deficient mice in an ErbB2-overexpressing model of mammary carcinoma had impaired tumor progression and metastasis (Brantley-Sieders et al. 2008). Yet another approach, and one that is of interest in the context of molecularly based cytotoxins, involves targeting EphA2 to deliver agents specifically to tumor cells and tumor vasculature.

An EphA2-targeted cytotoxin was created by conjugating ephrinA1-Fc to a derivative of PE, PE38QQR, and provided a proof of principle for the possibility of generating effective ephrinA1-based cytotoxins (Wykosky et al. 2007). To the best of our knowledge, this is the first EphA2-targeted toxin conjugate based on an ephrin. The ephrinA1-PE38QQR conjugate potently killed U251MG, SNB-19, DBTRG-05 MG, G48a, and U373MG GBM cells in vitro, which are all abundant EphA2 overexpressors (Wykosky et al. 2007). The observed cytotoxic effect was highly specific, because it was blocked by an excess of the ephrinA1 ligand alone. In further support of the specificity of ephrinA1-PE38QQR, either natural or forced nonoverexpressors of EphA2, including normal cells, were not susceptible to the cytotoxic effects of the conjugate. In a pilot in vivo experiment, ephrinA1-PE38QQR delivered by intratumoral injection caused more than 50% reduction in tumor burden in nu/nu mice bearing subcutaneous flank U-251 MG xenograft tumors (unpublished).

EphrinA1-PE38QQR exhibited very potent and specific killing of GBM cells expressing EphA2, which was comparable to the activity of an IL-13-based cytotoxin (Wykosky et al. 2007). It is noteworthy that on a molar basis ephrinA1-PE38QQR was as active in vitro on GBM cells as hIL13.E13K-PE38QQR, which is one of the most potent antiglioma agents known. However, one of the primary explant GBM cell lines generated in our Center, BTCOE-4536, responded very well to hIL13.E13K-PE38QQR, but was much less susceptible to ephrinA1-PE38QQR (Wykosky et al. 2007). The reason for this result lays in the fact that these cells expressed abundant IL-13Rα2 and much less EphA2 receptor. This finding emphasizes the notion that treatment with an individual cytotoxin will likely not be applicable to all patients with GBM and that the ideal approach will involve a combinatorial strategy against multiple targets simultaneously (Liu et al. 2003a, b; Stish et al. 2008) (Fig. 35.2).

In a GBM cohort, the profile of EphA2 expression is different from the one for IL-13Rα2, although they expectedly somewhat overlap due to the high prevalence of the two receptors (Wykosky et al. 2008a). EphrinA1-based cytotoxins are attractive drug candidates when considered alone but are even more attractive when considered as part of a cocktail with IL-13-based cytotoxins for future clinical applications (Figs. 35.1 and 35.2). Such a multitargeted therapy would represent the first molecular-based cytotoxin therapy that targets nearly 100% of patients with GBM despite the heterogeneity of this aggressive disease and without the need for expensive and time-consuming molecular profiling of patient tumors (Debinski 2008). This combinatorial approach could also be utilized in various forms of anticancer immunotherapy (Debinski 2005). In fact, mice immunized with an EphA2-derived peptide mounted an epitope-specific cytotoxic T lymphocyte response, and the EphA2 receptor has thus become a target that is being used in the development of anti-GBM vaccines (Hatano et al. 2004).

35.3 Summary

IL-13Rα2 and EphA2 are two cell surface receptors found to be abundantly expressed in malignant gliomas, but not in normal brain. IL-13Rα2 and EphA2 are overexpressed in the tumor compartment and EphA2 is additionally expressed in the neovascular bed. These properties make them attractive targets for the development of novel therapies and as molecular markers. Despite the fact that IL-13Rα2 and EphA2 are each overexpressed in a large fraction of GBM, none of them is overexpressed in all patient GBMs as expected for this heterogeneous disease. Therefore, it is desirable to develop a specific combinatorial therapy to simultaneously target multiple markers so that it is suitable for the treatment of the majority of GBM patients. Virtually all patients with GBM express either IL-13Rα2 or EphA2 or both, making a cocktail of cytotoxins directed at these two cell surface markers an attractive new therapeutic regimen that can be administered without the knowledge of individual marker expression in individual patients. Their expression profile in healthy brain tissue is low or absent, suggesting that collateral toxicity will be limited even though their presence on rare cell populations in the brain, such as stem cells, is currently unknown. Being that the heterogeneity of GBM is one of the factors hampering the outcome of treatment, the possibility of targeting simultaneously two specific molecular targets, which differ in their inter- and intratumoral distributions is of high promise for effective molecular targeted therapies (Fig. 35.2).

Conflict of Interest Dr. Debinski is an inventor of multiple issued patents that may be pertinent to the content of this chapter. Many of these patents have been licensed by industry. Dr. Debinski does not own any of the patents nor does he license them. No work discussed in the chapter was supported by industry. Dr. Debinski owns stock and consults to Targepeutics, Inc. Dr. Wykosky is a coinventor of a couple of patent applications related to the subject of this chapter.

References

Carglia M, Budillon A, Vitale G (2000) Modulation of molecular mechanisms involved in protein synthesis machinery as a new tool for the control of cell proliferation. Eur J Biochem 267:3919–3936.
Celtic Pharma press release (2007) Celtic Pharma terminates TransmidTM trial KSB311R/CIII/001. Bermuda, London, NY, February 7.
Cheng N, Brantley DM, Chen J (2002) The ephrins and Eph receptors in angiogenesis. Cytokine Growth Factor Rev 13:75–85.

Connor, JR, and Fine, RE (1986) The distribution of transferrin immunoreactivity in the rat central nervous system. Brain Res 368:319–328.
Curtin JF, Candolfi M, Xiong W et al (2008) Turning the gene tap off; implications of regulating gene expression for cancer therapeutics. Mol Cancer Ther 7:439–448.
Brantley-Sieders DM et al (2008). The receptor tyrosine kinase EphA2 promotes mammary adenocarcinoma tumorigenesis and metastatic progression in mice by amplifying ErbB2 signaling. J Clin Invest 118:64–78.
David MD, Bertoglio J and Pierre J (2003) Functional characterization of IL13 receptor a2 gene promoter: a critical role of the transcription factor STAT6 for regulated expression. Oncogene 22:3386–3394.
Debinski W, Puri RK, Kreitman RJ et al (1993) A wide range of human cancers express interleukin-4 receptors that can be targeted with a chimeric toxin containing Pseudomonas exotoxin A. J Biol Chem 268:14065–14070.
Debinski W, Puri RK, Pastan I (1994) Interleukin-4 receptors expressed on tumor cells may serve as a target for anticancer therapy using chimeric Pseudomonas exotoxin. Int J Cancer 58:744–751.
Debinski W, Obiri NI, Pastan I et al (1995a) A novel chimeric protein composed of interleukin 13 (IL13) and *Pseudomonas* exotoxin is highly cytotoxic to human carcinoma cells expressing receptors for IL 13 and IL4. J Biol Chem 270:16775–16780.
Debinski W, Obiri NI, Powers SK et al (1995b) Human glioma cells overexpress receptor for interleukin 13 and are extremely sensitive to a novel chimeric protein composed of interleukin 13 and Pseudomonas exotoxin. Clin Cancer Res 1:1253–1258.
Debinski W, Gibo DM, Kealiher A et al (1998a) Novel anti-brain tumor cytotoxins specific for cancer cells. Nature Biotech 16:449–453.
Debinski W, Gibo DM, Puri RK (1998b) Novel way to increase targeting specificity to a human glioblastoma-associated receptor for interleukin 13. Int J Cancer 76:547–51.
Debinski W, Gibo DM, Hulet SW et al (1999a) Receptor for interleukin 13 is a marker and therapeutic target for human high grade gliomas. Clin Cancer Res 5:985–990.
Debinski W, Gibo DM, Slagle B et al (1999b) Receptor for interleukin 13 is abundantly and specifically over-expressed in patients with glioblastoma multiforme. Int J Oncol 15:481–486.
Debinski W, Slagle B, Gibo DM et al (2000) Expression of a restrictive receptor for interleukin 13 is associated with glial transformation. J Neuro-Oncol 48:103–111.
Debinski W, Gibo DM (2000) Molecular expression analysis of restrictive receptor for interleukin 13, a brain tumor-associated cancer/testis antigen. Mol Med 6:440–449.
Debinski W, Slagle-Webb B, Achen M et al (2001) VEGF-D is an X-linked/AP-1 regulated putative onco-angiogen in human glioblastoma multiforme. Mol Med 7:598–608.
Debinski W (2002a) Molecular Targeting of Brain Tumors with Cytotoxins. In: "Chimeric Toxins" eds. Lorberboum-Galski, H. and Lazarovici, P. (Newark, Harwood Academic Publishers), pp. 222–246.
Debinski W (2002b) Local treatment of brain tumors with targeted chimera cytotoxic proteins. Cancer Invest 20:801–809.
Debinski W, Gibo DM and Mintz A (2003) Epigenetics in high-grade astrocytomas: Opportunities for prevention and detection of brain tumors. Ann NY Acad Sci 983:232–242.
Debinski W (2005) Personalized, multivalent, and more affordable: the globalization of vaccines. Clin Cancer Res 11:5663–5664.
Debinski W, Gibo DM (2005) Fos-related antigen 1 modulates malignant features of glioma cells. Mol Cancer Res 3:237–249.
Debinski W (2007) Molecular targeting of brain tumors with recombinant cytotoxins. Res Adv in Cancer 7:155–165.
Debinski W (2008) Drug cocktails for effective treatment of GBM. Exp Rev Neurotherapeut 8:515–518.

Eguchi J, Hatano M, Nishimura F et al (2006) Identification of interleukin-13 receptor alpha2 peptide analogues capable of inducing improved antiglioma CTL responses. Cancer Res 66:5883–5891.
Ekstrand AJ, James CD, Cavenee WK et al (1991) Genes for epidermal growth factor receptor, transforming growth factor alpha, and epidermal growth factor and their expression in human gliomas in vivo. Cancer Res 51:2164–2172.
Fichtner-Feigl S, Strober W, Kawakami K, Puri RK et al (2006) IL-13 signaling through the IL-13alpha2 receptor is involved in induction of TGF-beta1 production and fibrosis. Nat Med 12:99–106.
Gallia GL, Brem S, Brem H. (2005) Local treatment of malignant brain tumors using implantable chemotherapeutic polymers. J Natl Compreh Cancer Network 3:721–728.
Hatano M, Eguchi J, Tatsumi T et al (2005) EphA2 as a Glioma-Associated Antigen: A Novel Target for Glioma Vaccines. Neoplasia 7:717–22.
Hatano M, Kuwashima N, Tatsumi T et al (2004) Vaccination with EphA2-derived T cell-epitopes promotes immunity against both EphA2-expressing and EphA2-negative tumors. J Transl Med 2:40.
Hu N, Gibo DM, Debinski W (2005) Cytokine up-regulation of IL13R-alpha2 in GBM cells leads to an increased potency of recombinant IL13 cytotoxin. Cancer Therapy 3:531–542.
Hulet SW, Powers S, Connor JR (1999) Distribution of transferrin and ferritin binding in normal and multiple sclerotic human brains. J Neurol Sci 165:48–55.
Iglewski BH, Kabat D (1975) NAD-dependent inhibition of protein synthesis by Pseudomonas aeruginosa toxin. Proc Natl Acad Sci USA 72:2284–2288.
Jarboe JS, Johnson KR, Choi Y et al (2007) Expression of Interleukin-13 receptor α2 in glioblastoma multiforme: Implications for targeted therapies. Cancer Res 67:7983–7896.
Kahlon KS, Brown C, Cooper LJN et al (2004) Specific recognition and killing of glioblastoma multiforme by interleukin 13-zetakine redirected cytolytic T cells. Cancer Res 64:9160–9167.
Kunwar S, Prados MD, Chang SM et al (2007a) Direct intracerebral delivery of cintredekin besudotox (IL13-PE38QQR) in recurrent malignant glioma: a report by the Cintredekin Besudotox Intraparenchymal Study Group. J Clin Oncol 25:837–844.
Kunwar S, Westphal M, Medhorn M et al (2007b) Results from PRECISE: A randomized Phase 3 study in patients with first recurrent GBM comparing Cintredekin Besudotox administered via convection-enhanced delivery with Gliadel wafers. Neuro-Oncology 9, p. 531.
Lal A, Glazer CA, Martinson HM et al. (2002) Mutant epidermal growth factor receptor up-regulates molecular effectors of tumor invasion. Cancer Res 62:3335–3339.
Larsen AB, Pedersen MW, Stockhausen MT et al (2007) Activation of the EGFR Gene Target EphA2 Inhibits Epidermal Growth Factor-Induced Cancer Cell Motility. Mol Cancer Res 5:283–293.
Laske DW, Youle RJ, Oldfield EH (1997) Tumor regression with regional distribution of the targeted toxin TF-CRM107 in patients with malignant brain tumors. Nature Med 3:1362–1368.
Li Chunbin, Hall WA, Jin N et al (2002) Targeting glioblastoma multiforme with an IL-13 / diphtheria toxin fusion protein in vitro and in vivo in nude mice. Prot Engin 15:419–427.
Liu F, Park PJ, Lai W et al (2006) A genome-wide screen reveals functional gene clusters in the cancer genome and identifies EphA2 as a mitogen in glioblastoma. Cancer Res 66:10815–10823.
Liu H, Jacobs BS, Liu J (2000) Interleukin-13 sensitivity and receptor phenotypes of human glial cell lines: non-neoplastic glia and low-grade astrocytoma differ from malignant glioma. Cancer Immunol Immunother 49:319–24.
Liu L, Backlund LM, Nilsson BR et al (2005) Clinical significance of EGFR amplification and the aberrant EGFRvIII transcript in conventionally treated astrocytic gliomas. J Mol Med 83:917–926.
Liu TF, Cai J, Gibo D et al (2006) Variant IL13-directed *diphtheria* toxin fusion recombinant cytotoxin for the treatment of malignant gliomas. Neuro-Oncology 8:429.

Liu TF, Willingham MC, Tatter SB et al (2003a) Combination fusion protein therapy of refractory brain tumors: demonstration of efficacy in cell culture. J Neurooncol 65:77–85.
Liu TF, Willingham MC, Tatter SB et al (2003b) Diphtheria toxin-epidermal growth factor fusion protein and Pseudomonas exotoxin–interleukin 13 fusion protein exert synergistic toxicity against human glioblastoma multiforme cells. Bioconjug Chem 14:1107–1114.
Liu TF, Tatter SB, Willingham MC et al (2003c) Growth factor receptor expression varies among high-grade glioma and normal brain: epidermal growth factor receptor has excellent properties for interstitial fusion protein therapy. Mol Cancer Ther 2:783–787.
Macrae M, Neve RM, Rodriguez-Viciana P et al (2005) A conditional feedback loop regulates Ras activity through EphA2. Cancer Cell 8:111–118.
Mintz A, Debinski W (2000) Cancer genetics/epigenetics and the X chromosome: Possible new links for malignant glioma pathogenesis and immune-based therapies. Critic Rev Oncogen 11:77–95.
Mintz A, Gibo DM, Webb (Slagle) B, Debinski W (2002) IL13Rα2 is a glioma-restricted receptor for IL13. Neoplasia 4:388–399.
Mintz A, Gibo DM, Madhankumar AB et al (2003) Molecular targeting with recombinant cytotoxins of interleukin-13 receptor alpha-2-expressing glioma. J Neuro-Oncol 64:117–123.
MintzA, Gibo DM, Madhankumar AB et al. (2008) Protein and DNA-based active immunotherapy targeting interleukin 13 receptor alpha 2. Cancer Biother Radiopharm, 23:581–589, 2008.
Mizoguchi M, Betensky RA, Batchelor TT et al (2006) Activation of STAT3, MAPK, and AKT in malignant astrocytic gliomas: correlation with EGFR status, tumor grade, and survival. J Neuropathol Exp Neurol 65:1181–1188.
Murphy EV, Zhang Y, Zhu W et al (1995) The human glioma pathogensis-related protein is structurally related to plant pathogenesis-related proteins and its gene is expressed specifically in brain tumors. Gene 159:131–135.
Nutt CL, Mani DR, Betensky RA et al. (2003) Gene expression-based classification of malignant gliomas correlated better with survival than histological classification. Cancer Res 63:1602–1607.
Okano F, Storkus WJ, Chambers WH et al (2002) Identification of a novel HLA-A*0201-restricted, cytotoxic T lymphocyte epitope in a human glioma-associated antigen, interleukin 13 receptor α2 chain. Clin Cancer Res 8:2851–2855.
Pandita A, Aldape KD, Zadeh G (2004) Contrasting in vivo and in vitro fates of glioblastoma cell subpopulations with amplified EGFR. Genes Chromosomes Cancer 39:29–36.
Pasquale EB (2008) Eph-ephrin bidirectional signaling in physiology and disease. Cell 133:38–52.
Pastan I, Chaudhary VK, and Fitzgerald D (1992) Recombinant toxins as novel therapeutic agents. Ann Rev Biochem 61:331–354.
Raghavan R, Brady ML, Rodriguez-Ponce MI et al (2006) Convection-enhanced delivery of therapeutics for brain disease, and its optimization. Neurosurg Focus 20(4):E12.
Rahaman SO, Sharma P, Harbor PC et al (2002) IL-13R(alpha)2, a decoy receptor for IL-13 acts as an inhibitor of IL-4-dependent signal transduction in glioblastoma cells. Cancer Res 62:1103–1109.
Ramnarain DB, Park S, Lee DY et al (2006) Differential gene expression analysis reveals generation of an autocrine loop by a mutant epidermal growth factor receptor in glioma cells. Cancer Res 66:867–874.
Rich T, Chen P, Furman F et al (1996) RTVP-1, a novel human gene with sequence similarity to genes of diverse species, is expressed in tumor cell lines of glial but not neuronal origin. Gene 180:125–130.
Saikali S, Avril T, Collet B et al (2007) Expression of nine tumour antigens in a series of human glioblastoma multiforme: interest of EGFRvIII, IL-13Ralpha2, gp100 and TRP-2 for immunotherapy. J Neurooncol 81:139–148.
Sampson JH, Akabani G, Archer GE et al (2003) Progress report of a Phase I study of the intracerebral microinfusion of a recombinant protein composed of transforming growth

factor (TGF)-alpha and a mutated form of Pseudomonas exotoxin termed PE-38 (TP-38) for the treatment of malignant brain tumors. J Neuro-Oncol 65:27–35.

Sampson JH, Akabani G, Archer GE, et al (2008) Intracerebral infusion of an EGFR-targeted toxin in recurrent malignant brain tumors. Neuro Oncol. 10:320–329.

Sanai N, Mirzadeh Z, Berger MS (2008) Functional outcome after language mapping for glioma resection. N Engl J Med. 2008 358:18–27.

Sarkaria JN, Carlson BL, Schroeder MA et al (2006) Use of an orthotopic xenograft model for assessing the effect of epidermal growth factor receptor amplification on glioblastoma radiation response. Clin Cancer Res 12:2264–2271.

Shaw EG, Debinski W, Robbins, R. Clinical Radiation Oncology, In: "Central Nervous System Tumors – Overview" eds. Gunderson, L.L. and Tepper, J.E. Second Edition (Elsevier, Churchill Livingstone), pp. 459–491, 2006.

Stish BJ, Chen H, Shu Y, Panoskaltsis-Mortari A, Vallera DA (2008) Anti-glioblastoma effect of a recombinant bi-specific cytotoxin co-targeting human IL-13 and EGF receptors in a mouse xenograft model. J Neurooncol 87:51–61.

Stupp R, Mason WP, van den Bent MJ, et al. (2005) Radiotherapy plus concomitant and adjuvant temozolomide for glioblastoma. N Engl J Med 352:987–96.

Ulasov IV, Tyler MA, Han Y et al (2007) Novel recombinant adenoviral vector that targets the interleukin-13 receptor alpha2 chain permits effective gene transfer to malignant glioma. Hum Gene Ther 18:118–129.

Walker-Daniels J, Riese DJ, Kinch MS (2002) c-Cbl-dependent EphA2 protein degradation is induced by ligand binding. Mol Cancer Res 1:79–87.

Wang LF, Fokas E, Bieker M et al (2008) Increased expression of EphA2 correlates with adverse outcome in primary and recurrent glioblastoma multiforme patients. Oncol Rep 19:151–156.

Weaver M, Laske DW (2003) Transferrin receptor ligand-targeted toxin conjugate (Tf-CRM107) for therapy of malignant gliomas. J Neurooncol 65:3–13.

Weber F et al (2003) Safety, tolerability, and tumor response of IL4-Pseudomonas exotoxin (NBI-3001) in patients with recurrent malignant glioma. J Neuro-Oncol 64:125–137.

Wersall P, Ohlsson I, Biberfeld P et al (1997) Intratumoral infusion of the monoclonal antibody, mAb 425, against the epidermal-growth-factor receptor in patients with advanced malignant glioma. Cancer Immunol Immunother 44:157–164.

Wu AH, Low WC (2003) Molecular cloning and identification of the human interleukin 13 alpha 2 receptor (IL-13Rα2) promoter. Neuro-oncol. 5:179–87.

Wykosky J, Gibo DM, Stanton C et al (2005) EphA2 as a novel molecular marker and target in glioblastoma multiforme. Mol Cancer Res 3:541–551.

Wykosky J, Gibo DM, Debinski W (2007) A novel, potent, and specific ephrinA1-based cytotoxin against EphA2 receptor-expressing tumor cells. Mol Cancer Ther 6:3208–3218.

Wykosky J, Gibo DM, Stanton C et al (2008a) IL-13 Receptor alpha-2, EphA2, and Fra-1 as molecular denominators of high-grade astrocytomas and specific targets for combinatorial therapy. Clin Cancer Res 14:199–208.

WykoskyJ, Palma E, Gibo DM et al (2008b). Soluble monomeric ephrinA1 is released from tumor cells and is a functional ligand for the EphA2 receptor. Oncogene, 27:7260–7273, 2008.

Wykosky J, Debinski W (2008) The EphA2 receptor and ephrinA1 ligand in solid tumors: Function and therapeutic targeting. Mol Cancer Res, 6:1795–1806, 2008.

Zhang JG, Eguchi J, Kruse C et al (2007) Antigenic profiling of glioma cells to generate allogeneic vaccines or dendritic cell-based therapeutics. Clin Cancer Res 13:566–575.

Zhang JG, Kruse CA, Driggers L et al (2008) Tumor antigen precursor protein profiles of adult and pediatric brain tumors identify potential targets for immunotherapy. Neurooncol 88:65–76.

Zhou G, Ye G-J, Debinski W et al (2002) Genetic engineering of a herpes virus 1 vector dependent on the IL-13Rα2 receptor for entry into cells: interaction of glycoprotein D with its receptors is independent of the fusion of the envelope and the plasma membrane. Proc Natl Acad Sci 99:15124–15129.

Chapter 36
Molecular Targets for Antibody-Mediated Immunotherapy of Malignant Glioma

Joanne E. Ayriss, Chien-Tsun Kuan, Susan T. Boulton, David A. Reardon, and Darell D. Bigner

Abstract Despite advances in surgical and radiation therapy over the past two decades, the prognosis for many brain-tumor patients remains dismal. Novel antibody-mediated immunotherapeutics are emerging in the next generation of targeted therapeutic drugs for cancer treatment, and at least nine have been approved by the FDA to date. In this chapter we review the identification and validation of appropriate CNS tumor-associated antigens and the current status of antibody-mediated therapies under development and those that are already showing encouraging promise in the clinical setting.

Contents

36.1 Introduction

Immunotherapy has been explored since the beginning of the nineteenth century when Emil von Behring, Erich Wernicke, and Shibasaburo Kitasato observed and described the "anti-toxin" in response to diphtheria and tetanus

J.E. Ayriss (✉)
Department of Pathology, 181A Medical Sciences Research Building, Duke University Medical Center, Box 3156, Durham, NC 27710, USA
e-mail: joanne.ayriss@duke.edu

E.G. Van Meir (ed.), *CNS Cancer*, Cancer Drug Discovery and Development, DOI 10.1007/978-1-60327-553-8_36,
© Humana Press, a part of Springer Science+Business Media, LLC 2009

toxins (Kantha, 1991). They developed effective therapeutic serums and proposed the theory of humoral immunity, describing that a mediator in serum could react with a foreign antigen (Gronski et al., 1991). This work prompted Paul Ehrlich to propose the "side chain theory" for antibody and antigen interaction in 1897. Ehrlich hypothesized that receptors (described as side chains), present on the surface of cells, could specifically bind to toxins via a "lock-and-key" interaction and subsequently initiate the production of antibodies. He went on to describe the concept of using antibodies (Abs) as "magic bullets" to specifically bind and kill microbes or tumor cells (Ehrlich, 1906). Both Emil von Behring and Paul Ehrlich received the Nobel Prize in physiology or medicine for their work in 1901 and 1908, respectively. Since then, several important technological advances have made the use of specific tumor-targeting Abs feasible. The invention of hybridoma technology by Nobel laureates Georges Köhler, César Milstein, and Niels Jerne (Kohler and Milstein, 1975; Raju, 2000) allowed unlimited generation, isolation, and subsequent purification of monoclonal Abs (mAbs) with monospecific and high-affinity properties. Furthermore, development of phage display techniques (Smith, 1985) enabled mAbs to be selected and engineered in vitro (McCafferty et al., 1990). In an attempt to overcome the anti-antibody response observed with non-human-derived-antibody therapies (Shawler et al., 1985), DNA technologies were developed to create human–mouse chimeric antibodies, including those that combine the constant domains of the human immunoglobulin G (IgG) molecule with the murine variable regions in order to remove the immunogenic portion of the mAb (Boulianne et al., 1984; Morrison et al., 1984). In another approach, mAbs were humanized by grafting murine complementarity-determining regions (CDRs) into the human antibody backbone (Jones et al., 1986; Riechmann et al., 1988). Fully human therapeutic antibodies have been developed from mice that have had their endogenous immunoglobulin genes inactivated and replaced with the human counterparts (Green et al., 1994), and fully human variable domains have been isolated from phage display libraries and converted into whole mAbs (Krebs et al., 2001). The different mAb formats used as antibody therapeutics are schematically represented in Fig. 36.1, and the advantages or disadvantages of their use as therapeutic agents are described in Table 36.1.

There are many strategies that utilize mAbs for immunotherapy. Monoclonal antibodies may be armed or unarmed and exert their therapeutic effect by eliciting or enhancing an immune response, disrupting tumor cellular processes, or targeting drugs directly to tumor cells. To be effective as a naked, or "unarmed," therapeutic agent, the antibody must directly affect the tumor's growth and/or survival. This can occur when the antibody, upon tumor binding, initiates the recruitment and activation of immune effector mechanisms, such as antibody-dependent cell-mediated cytotoxicity (ADCC) and/or complement-dependent cytotoxicity (CDC), or when it blocks growth factor receptor activation, or when it transduces negative signals that impair tumor cell growth or survival. Monoclonal antibodies can be armed for targeted delivery by conjugation with radionuclides (Brechbiel, 2007; Zalutsky et al., 2007), cytotoxic drugs,

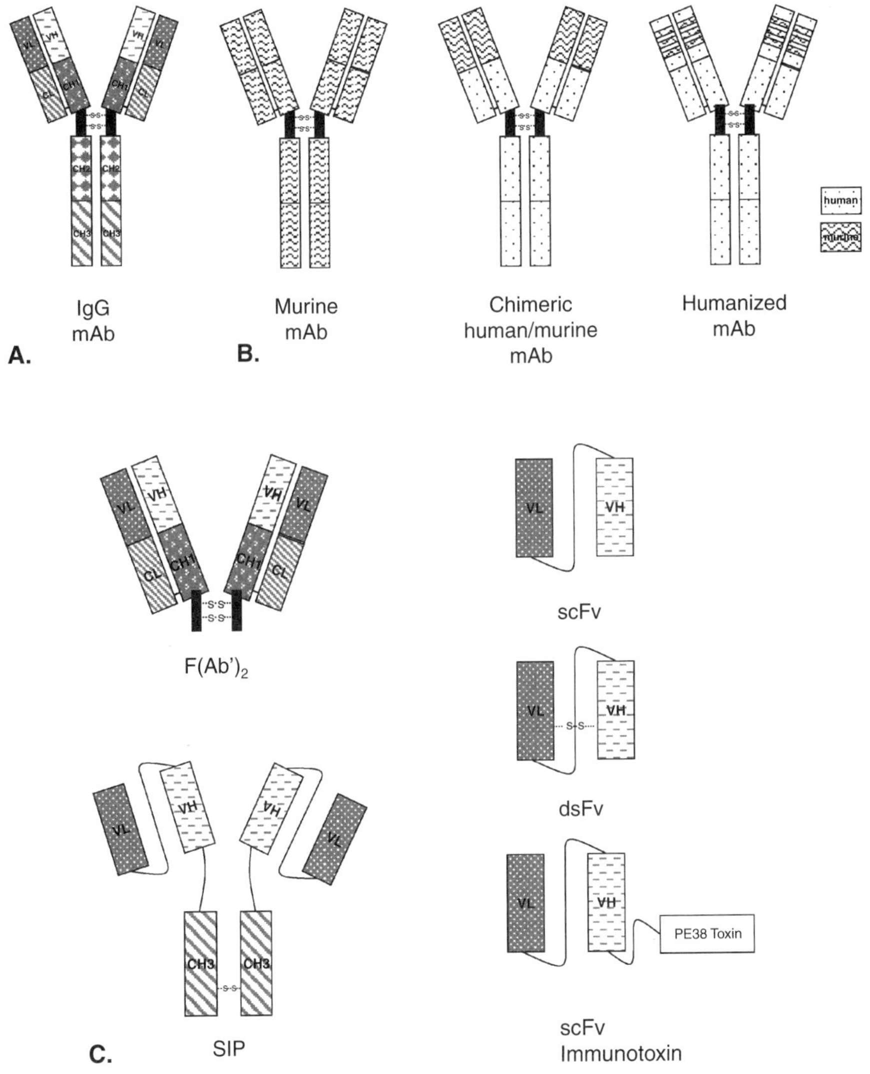

Fig. 36.1 Different monoclonal antibody (mAb) formats used as antibody therapeutics. (**A**) Schematic structure and legend of intact IgG mAb; (**B**) Schematic structure of murine mAb, chimeric human/murine mAb with hybridization of domains of human and murine origin, and humanized mAb grafted with murine complementary determining regions; (**C**) Schematic structure of mAb fragments including F(ab')2, single-chain variable fragment (scFv), disulfide-stabilized scFv (dsFv), scFv genetically conjugated to immunotoxin (scFv immunotoxin) and small immunoprotein (SIP) also known as scFv-CH3 minibody

cytokines, or biological toxins (Schrama et al., 2006; see also Chapter 35). Therapeutic efficacy is dependent on the format, affinity, and stability of the targeting mAb and its kinetics within the tumor environment, which includes tumor vascularity, vascular permeability, extracellular fluid dynamics, and

Table 36.1 Characteristics, description, and advantages of intact and fragment IgG monoclonal antibodies

	Molecule (size)	Description	Advantage/disadvantage
Intact antibody	Murine mAb (150 kDa)	Whole IgG isolated from mouse	Reference standard **D**: immunogenicity (HAMA) in human; size limits permeability
	Chimeric human/murine mAb (150 kDa)	IgG with murine variable and human constant regions	**A**: full antigen-binding capacity with reduced immunogenicity **D**: size limits permeability
	Humanized mAb (150 kDa)	IgG with murine CDR regions grafted in the human variable regions	**A**: full antigen-binding capacity with reduced immunogenicity **D**: size limits permeability
Fragment antibody	$F(ab')_2$ (110 kDa)	IgG without Fc portion (constant regions CH2 and CH3)	**A:** intermediate size, retains bivalent binding capacity of whole IgG with slightly reduced immunogenicity **D:** no effector functions
	scFv (26 kDa)	VH and VL domains connected with a polypeptide linker	**A:** small size, lower immunogenicity, and better tumor penetration **D:** monovalent, very rapid clearance, and possibility of aggregation
	dsFv (26 kDa)	VH and VL domains connected with a polypeptide linker and further stabilized with inter-molecular disulfide bond	**A:** small size, lower immunogenicity, and better tumor penetration **D:** monovalent, very rapid clearance, and reduced possibility of aggregation
	scFv PE38 Immunotoxin (64 kDa)	VH and VL domains connected with a polypeptide linker and genetically fused to Pseudomonas exotoxin A.	**A:** small size, lower immunogenicity, better tumor penetration and toxin delivery. **D:** monovalent, very rapid clearance, and reduced possibility of aggregation
	Small Immunoprotein (SIP) (80 kDa)	Two scFv units, hinge region and IgG1 CH3 domain (to promote dimerization)	**A:** intermediate size, bivalent, chimeric, and single-chain construct with reduced immunogenicity **D:** no effector functions

A: ***Advantage***; **D:** ***Disadvantage***.

interstitial pressure. In order to determine therapeutic efficacy, pharmacokinetic (PK), pharmacodynamic (PD), and biodistribution studies are performed. Pharmacokinetics concern the time course study of a drug's concentration within the body, in relation to absorption, distribution, metabolism, and elimination processes that take place after administration. Pharmacodynamics describe the efficacy and toxicity of the drug through the mechanisms of drug action, the relationship between drug concentration and effect, and the relationship of the drug concentration to the biochemical and physiological effects on the body, ultimately determining whether the therapeutic drug reaches the target site in vivo and mediates the anticipated effect. Biodistribution studies concern the description of the in vivo distribution of a drug present in various organs, as a function of time, following its administration. Herein we describe brain-tumor-associated molecular targets that are being investigated for antibody-mediated immunotherapy.

36.2 Brain-Tumor Targets and Immunotherapeutic Antibodies

The identification and validation of appropriate tumor-associated antigens is a key challenge for antibody-mediated immunotherapeutic approaches in the targeted treatment of CNS tumors. The antigen must be accessible (located upon the cellular membrane, be a secreted protein, or be present within the extracellular matrix), stable (low shedding profile and/or internalization), expressed at sufficient density, and ideally, tumor specific (Wikstrand et al., 2001). An ideal tumor-specific antigen is one that would be produced only by the tumor and not by any other cell type, for example, epidermal growth factor variant III (EGFRvIII; see below). However, many molecular targets that are targeted for immunotherapy such as EGFR and Glycoprotein Nonmetastatic Melanoma Protein B (GPNMB; see below), are present within other tissue types but are targeted because they are significantly overexpressed by the tumor cells. The administration route must be carefully selected to ensure optimal delivery of the immunotherapeutic because of the limited permeability of the blood– brain barrier. The impact of the blood–brain barrier on brain-tumor imaging and therapy is reviewed in more detail in Chapter 33.

Several brain-tumor target antigens have been identified and antibodies specific to six of them tested in clinical trials over the past 15 years (Table 36.2). Following is a description of some of these antigens, along with their corresponding antibodies.

36.2.1 Tenascin

Tenascin-C (Tn-C) is a multidomain, extracellular matrix glycoprotein that is composed of six monomers that form a highly symmetrical, spider-like structure, called a hexabrachion (Erickson and Inglesias, 1984). Each monomeric

Table 36.2 Brain-tumor therapeutic antibodies evaluated in clinical trials

Antibody	Original isotype	Antibody format	Therapeutic format	Molecular target	Tumor type	Phase	Reference
81C6 (Neuradiab™)	IgG_{2b}	Murine mAb	^{131}I-labeled	Tenascin	Malignant glioma	II	Reardon et al. (2008)
Bevacizumab (Avastin®)	IgG_1	Humanized mAb	+ Irinotecan	VEGF	Malignant glioma	II	Vredenburgh et al. (2007a, b)
Cetuximab (Erbitux®)	IgG_1	Chimeric murine/human mAb	Naked	EGFRwt	GBM	II	Combs et al. (2006)
Nimotuzumab	IgG_1	Humanized mAb	Naked	EGFRwt	GBM	II	Ramos et al. (2006)
Trastuzumab (Herceptin®)	IgG_1	Humanized mAb	Naked	HER2	GBM	I/II	www.virtualtrials.com
Mel-14	IgG_{2a}	$F(ab')_2$	^{131}I-labeled	CSPG	GBM/Neoplastic meningitis	I	Cokgor et al. (2001)
BC-2	IgG_1	Murine mAb	^{131}I-labeled	Tenascin	Malignant glioma	II	Riva et al. (2000)
BC-4	IgG_1	Murine mAb	^{131}I-labeled	Tenascin	Malignant glioma	II	Riva et al. (2000)
ERIC-1	IgG_1	Murine mAb	^{90}Y-labeled	NCAM	Malignant glioma	I	Hopkins et al. (1995)
ERIC-1	IgG_1	Murine mAb	^{131}I-labeled	NCAM	Malignant glioma	I	Papanastassiou et al. (1993)
UJ13a	IgG_{2a}	Murine mAb	^{131}I-labeled	NCAM	Malignant meningitis	I	Kemshead et al. (1987)

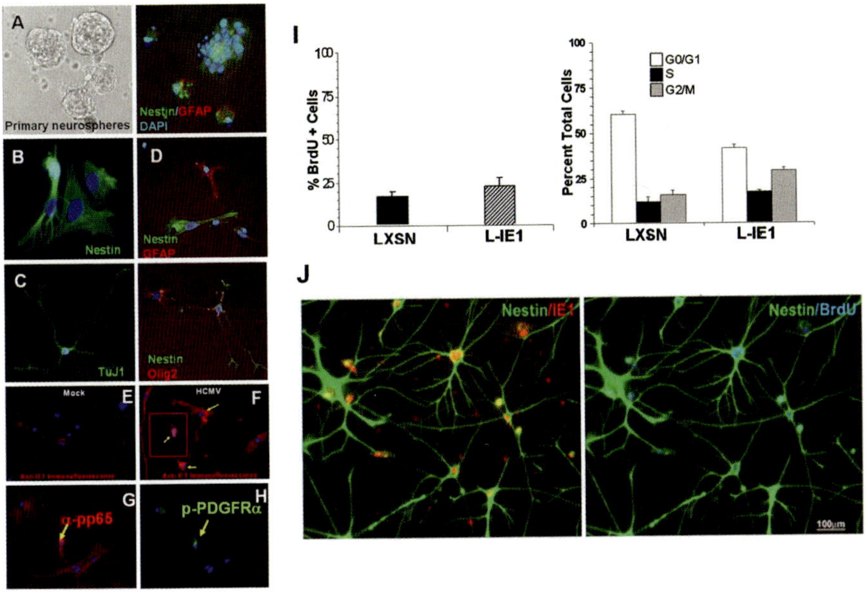

Color Plate 31. Adult human normal NPCs can be grown as neurospheres and are permissive to HCMV infection (Chapter 19, Fig. 4; *see* complete caption on p. 432 and discussion on p. 431).

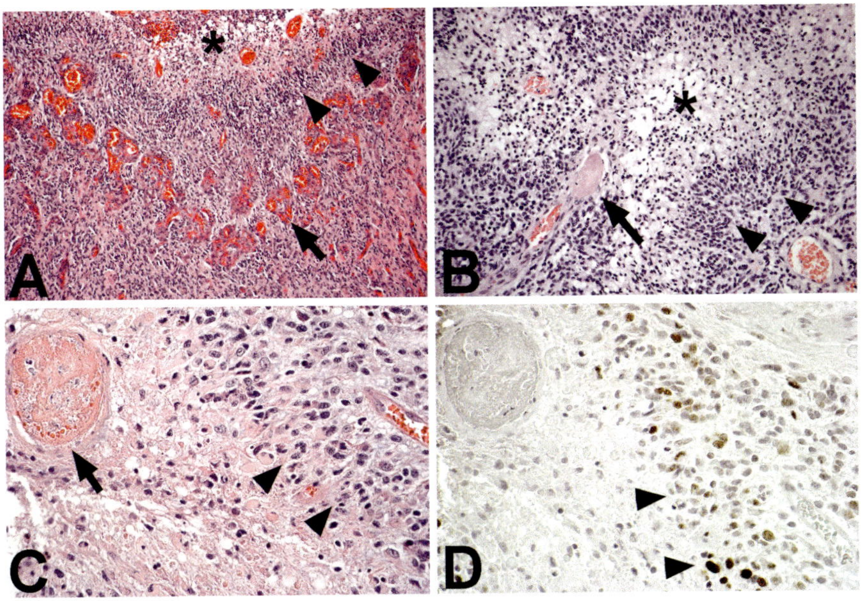

Color Plate 32. Pathologic features of glioblastoma (Chapter 22, Fig. 2; *see* complete caption on p. 510 and discussion on p. 509).

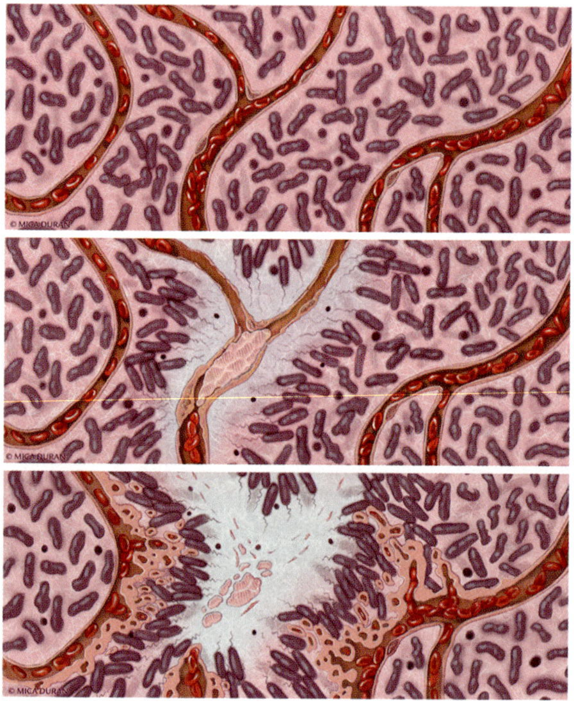

Color Plate 33. Potential mechanism of pseudopalisade formation (Chapter 22, Fig. 3; *see* complete caption on p. 511 and discussion on p. 510).

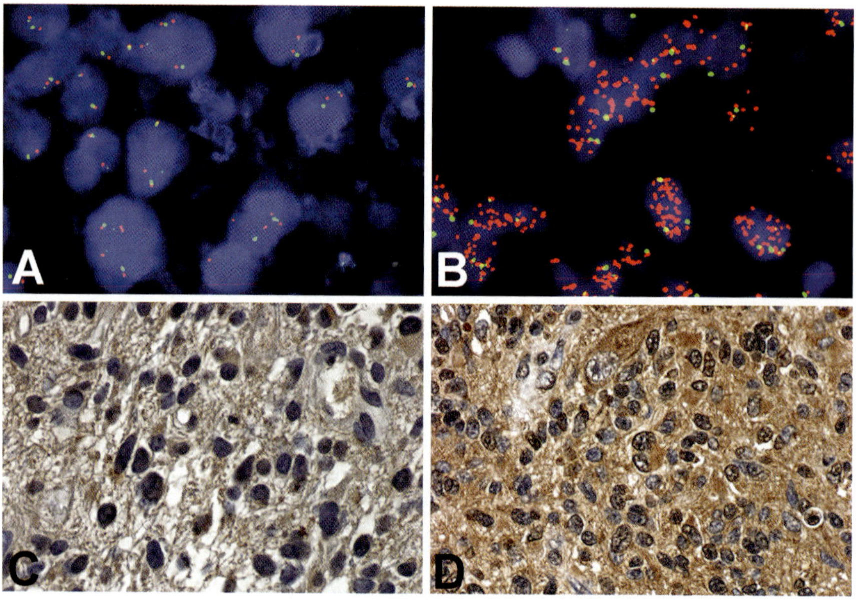

Color Plate 34. Fluorescence in situ hybridization (FISH) analysis of *EGFR* gene status and IHC analysis of EGFR and TF protein in human GBM and AA specimens (Chapter 22, Fig. 5; *see* complete caption on p. 519 and discussion on p. 517).

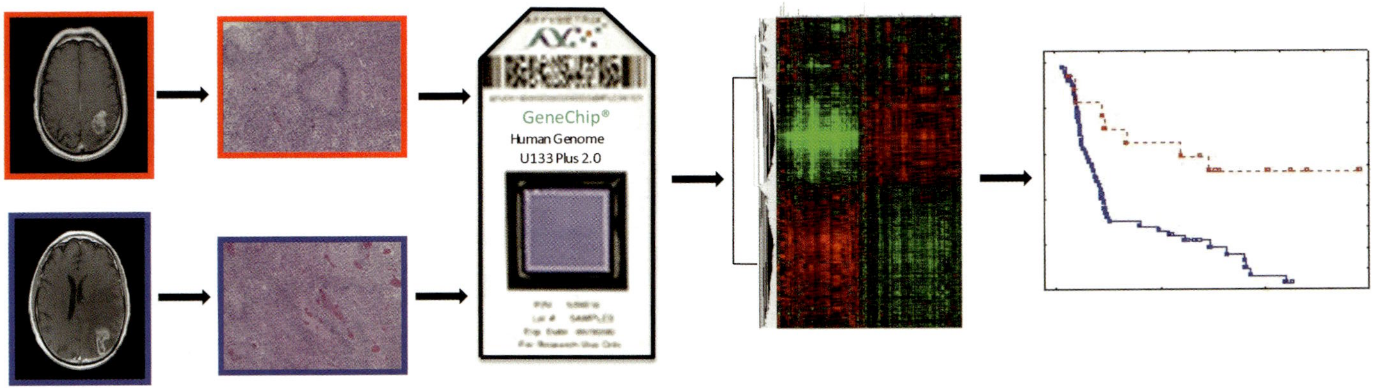

Color Plate 35. Gene expression profiling in brain tumors. Tumor-specific, such as tumor imaging and histopathology, as well as patient-specific information, such as age and sex, is used to provide prognostic information. Tissue obtained at diagnosis, either from biopsy or from surgical resection, is utilized to develop a complex profile of gene expression in the tumor. Labeled (typically fluorescently) target samples are made from total RNA that is enzymatically processed into complementary DNA (or RNA) and represent relative messenger RNA (mRNA) abundance within the tumor for all expressed genes. This is hybridized to filter-, glass slide-, or silicon chip-based arrays of cDNA or oligonucleotide probes and the signals are measured and normalized. Clustering provides a means to identify sets of genes with similar expression and group tumors based on these clusters (unsupervised), thus identifying unique molecular signatures or group genes based on known characteristics of the tumors (supervised). Gene signatures identified may have prognostic significance. Tumors that appear similar on imaging and histologic examination may be shown to exhibit differing molecular profiles and therefore different clinical outcomes using microarray technologies (Chapter 23, Fig. 1; *see* discussion on p. 530).

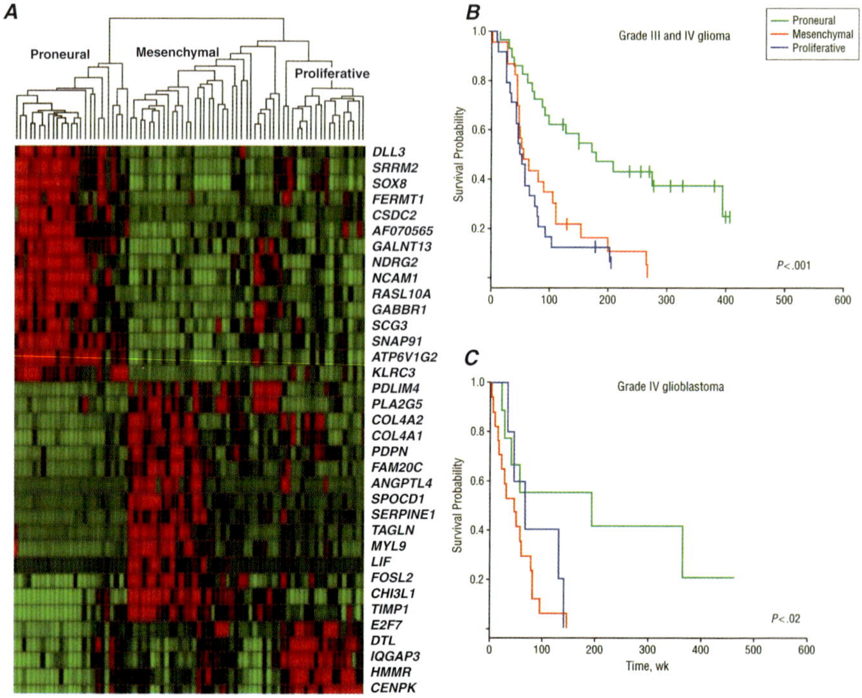

Color Plate 36. A mesenchymal molecular signature in GBM is prognostic for poor survival. (**A**) Identification of distinct molecular subtypes of malignant gliomas from gene expression profiling consisting of proneural, mesenchymal, and proliferative phenotypes (Phillips et al. 2006). Genes with high expression are shown in *red*, while those with low expression are shown in *green*. The proneural, mesenchymal, and proliferative subtypes demonstrate statistically significant associations with patient outcome in both grade III and IV glioma (**B**) and in an independent data set consisting only of grade IV GBM with necrosis (**C**). Adapted with permission from Elsevier Limited (Chapter 23, Fig. 2; *see* discussion on p. 539).

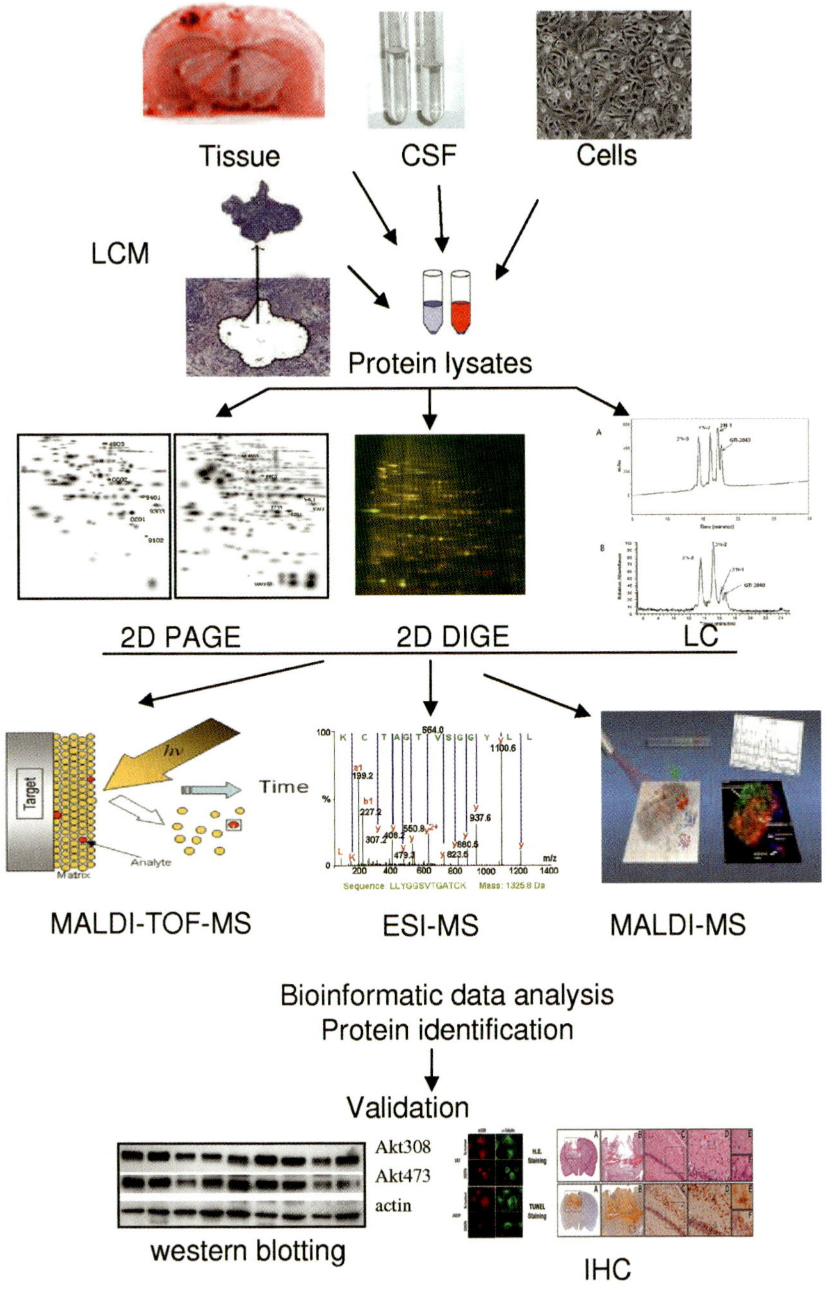

Color Plate 37. Summary of the protein separation and the MS-based protein identification (Chapter 24, Fig. 1; *see* complete caption on p. 563 and discussion on p. 561).

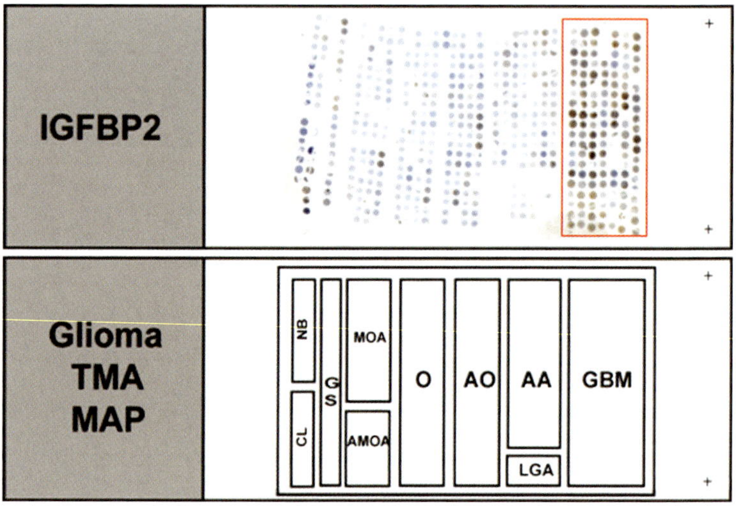

Color Plate 38. Detection of IGFBP2 expression in a glioma TMA. GBM, glioblastoma; AA, anaplastic astrocytoma; LGA, low grade astrocytoma; AO, anaplastic oligodendroglioma; O, oligodendroglioma; MOA, mixed oligoastrocytoma; AMOA, anaplastic mixed oligoastrocytoma; GS, gliosarcoma; NB, normal brain; CL, cell lines (Chapter 24, Fig. 2; *see* discussion on p. 563).

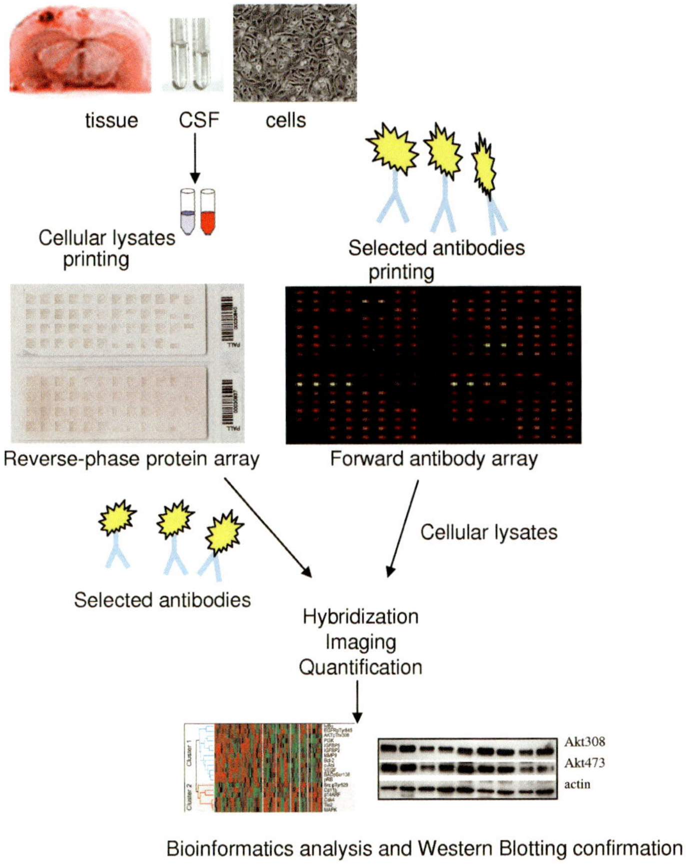

Color Plate 39. Protein arrays. Antibody array (forward-phase protein array) is formatted by printing the selective antibodies on a slide, while the reverse-phase protein array is printed with the cellular lysate extracted from tissue, cerebral spinal fluid, or cell lines (Chapter 24, Fig. 3; *see* complete caption and discussion on p. 565).

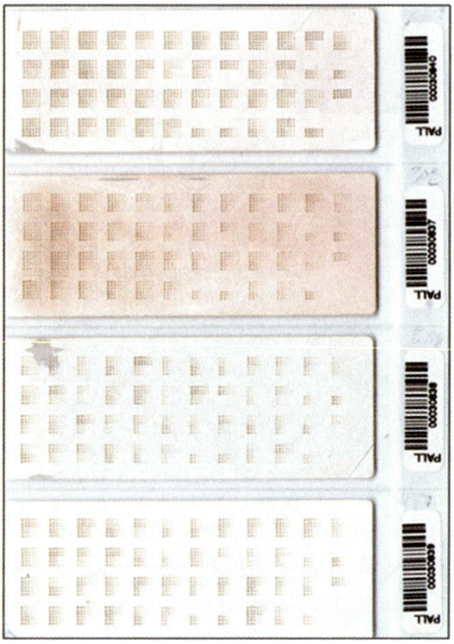

Color Plate 40. Glioma protein lysate array. Protein was isolated from frozen glioma tissues and adjusted to 20 mg/mL with lysis buffer tissue. The serially diluted protein lysates were printed on PVDF-coated glass slides in triplicate using a robotic spotter (G3, Genomics Solutions). Detection was conducted with a DakoCytomation-catalyzed signal amplification system kit. Individual glass slide can be hybridized with antibodies against β-actin, pThr308 AKT, pSer473 AKT, total AKT, or other proteins; β-actin served as a positive control. The hybridized slides were scanned at an optical resolution of 1200 dpi and saved as uncompressed TIFF files (Chapter 24, Fig. 4; *see* discussion on p. 567).

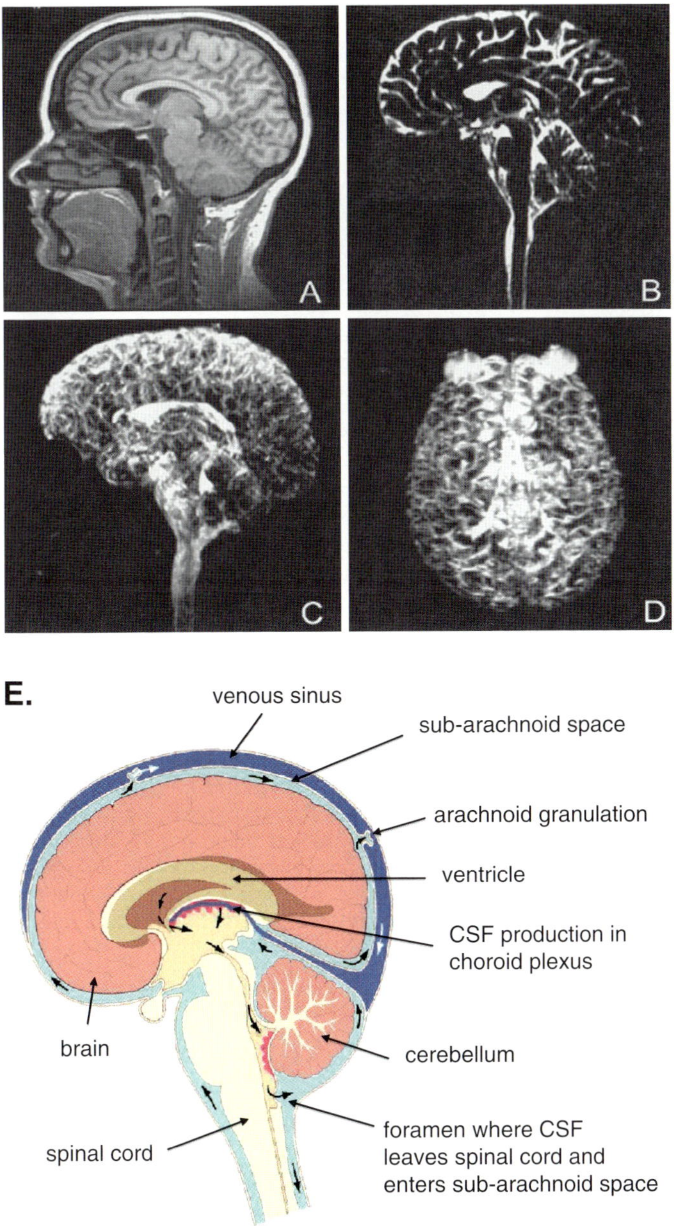

Color Plate 41. Magnetic resonance imaging enables to noninvasively visualize whole brain structures and CSF at high resolution and sharp contrast (Chapter 25, Fig. 1; *see* complete caption on p. 581 and discussion on p. 579).

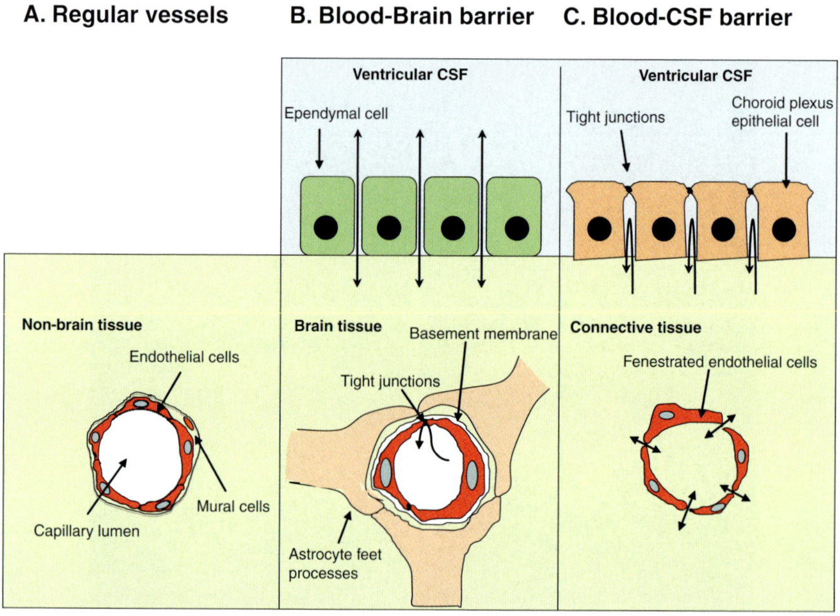

Color Plate 42. Blood–brain barrier and blood–CSF barrier. **A.** Simplified structure of normal blood vessel not present in the brain. In normal blood vessels, the endothelial cells (shown in *pink*) are surrounded by mural cells such as pericytes and smooth muscle cells. **B.** Blood–brain barrier: In normal brain, the endothelial cells of the capillaries contain tight junctions creating a strong barrier that prevents diffusion of hydrophilic substances from CNS capillaries into the surrounding tissues and vice versa. However, necessary nutrients and metabolites such as glucose are transported with the aid of specific transport mechanisms. **C.** Blood–CSF barrier: In the choroid plexus, the blood–brain barrier is absent as the capillary endothelial cells here are fenestrated. This allows substances to pass freely from the bloodstream into the brain tissue and also in the opposite direction. However, here, tight junctions are present in the overlying ependyma (choroid plexus epithelium), thus creating a two-way barrier between brain tissue and ventricular CSF (Chapter 25, Fig. 2; *see* discussion on p. 582).

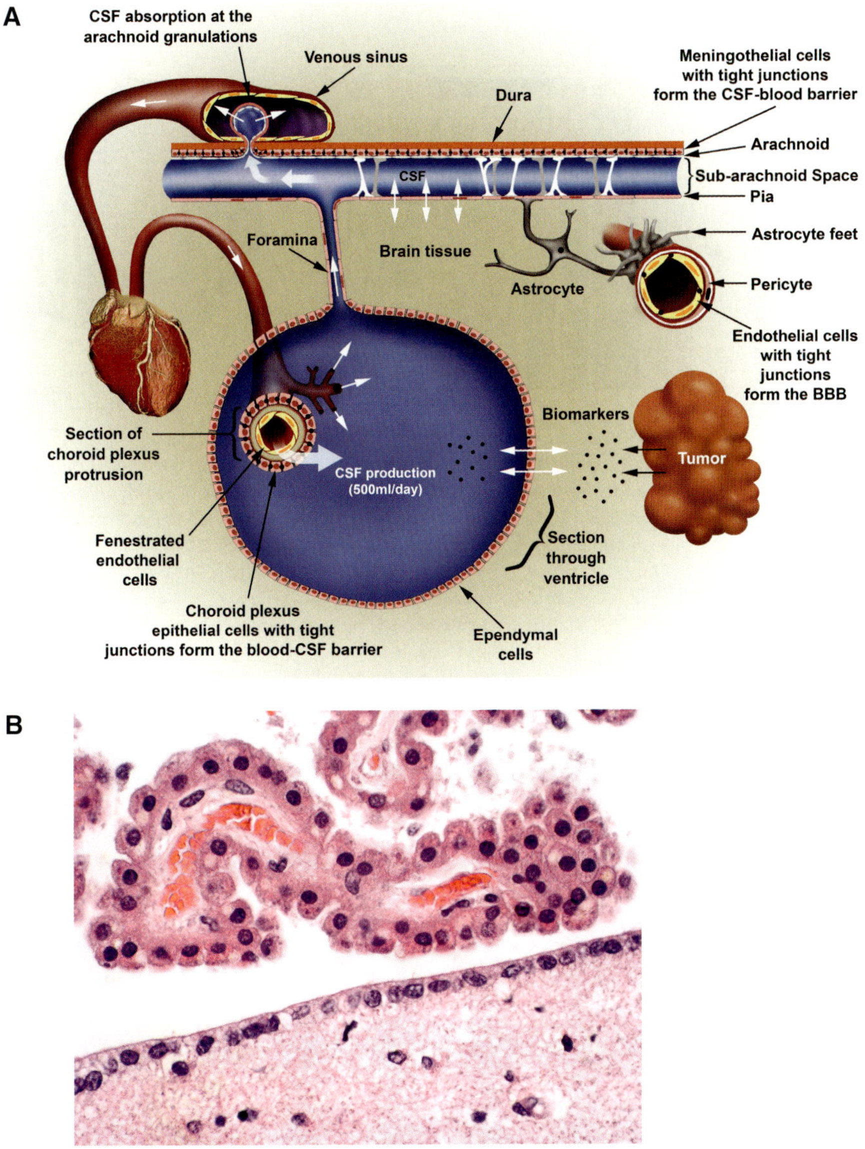

Color Plate 43. A. Schematic illustration of the flow of CSF in the brain and the different cellular structures that create the blood–CSF barrier. This representation is not intended to be entirely anatomically correct and does not show many ultrastructural details. Incoming arterial blood flow from the heart connects to the choroid plexus, a cauliflower-shaped organ where blood is "filtered" through a double cellular layer, endothelial cells lining the arterial capillary and the choroid plexus epithelial cells that are connected through tight junctions. This constitutes the first component of the blood–CSF barrier. Note that the endothelial cells in the choroid plexus are not connected by tight junctions (Chapter 25, Fig. 3; *see* complete caption on p. 587 and discussion on p. 585).

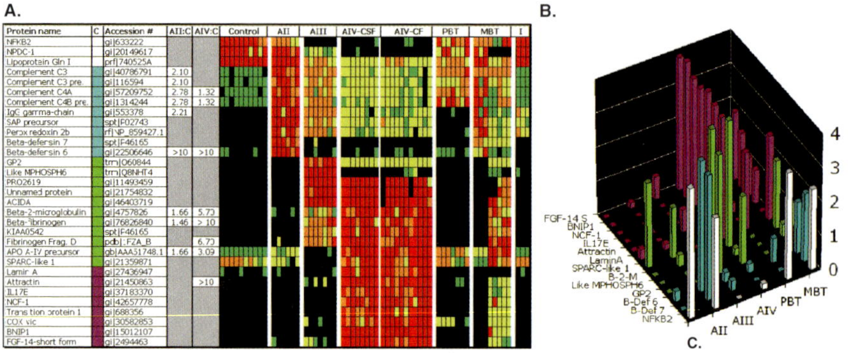

Color Plate 44. Potential biomarker panels differentiate between astrocytoma grades using CSF. **A.** Panel of 32 proteins that can be used to differentiate between AII–IV patients, nontumoral controls, and other forms of brain tumors. *Black* = no expression, *yellow* = low expression, *orange* = moderate expression, and *red* = high expression level as determined from ImageMaster analysis of 2-DE gels. C = Biomarker class; *white* = control specific, *light blue* = AII, *green* = AIII, and *pink* = AIV biomarker. **B.** Restricted panel containing top 13 proteins from panel **A**. *White* = control, *light blue* = AII, *green* = AIII, and *purple* = AIV biomarkers. Vertical axis represents relative level (0–4) of each protein as estimated from 2-DE (Reproduced from Khwaja et al. Journal of Proteome Research 2007.) (Chapter 25, Fig. 6; *see* discussion on p. 596).

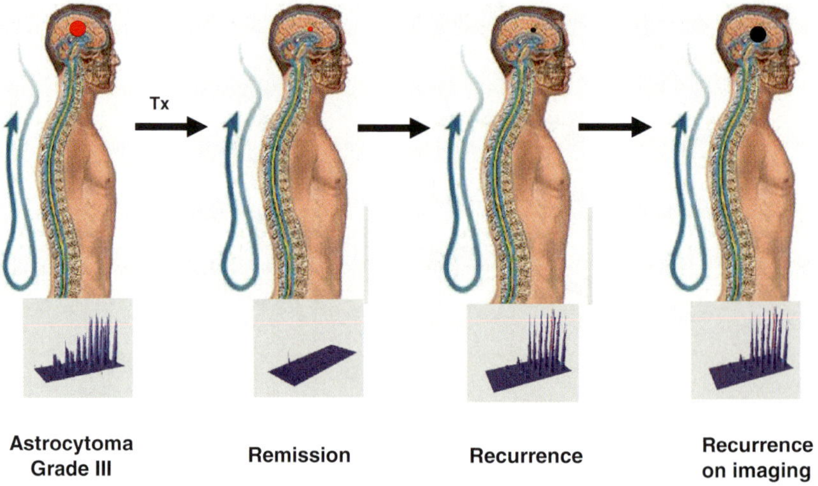

Color Plate 45. Possible future applications of CSF biomarkers. Protein markers found in the CSF through a spinal tap could be used individually or in combination in a biomarker panel to diagnose CNS malignancies. A protein or an antibody array developed using identified biomarkers would allow for personalized medicine based on the unique limited protein profile. These markers could also allow for early detection of original, residual, or recurrent disease in a minimally invasive procedure compared to biopsy or surgery (Chapter 25, Fig. 7; *see* complete caption on p. 597 and discussion on p. 596).

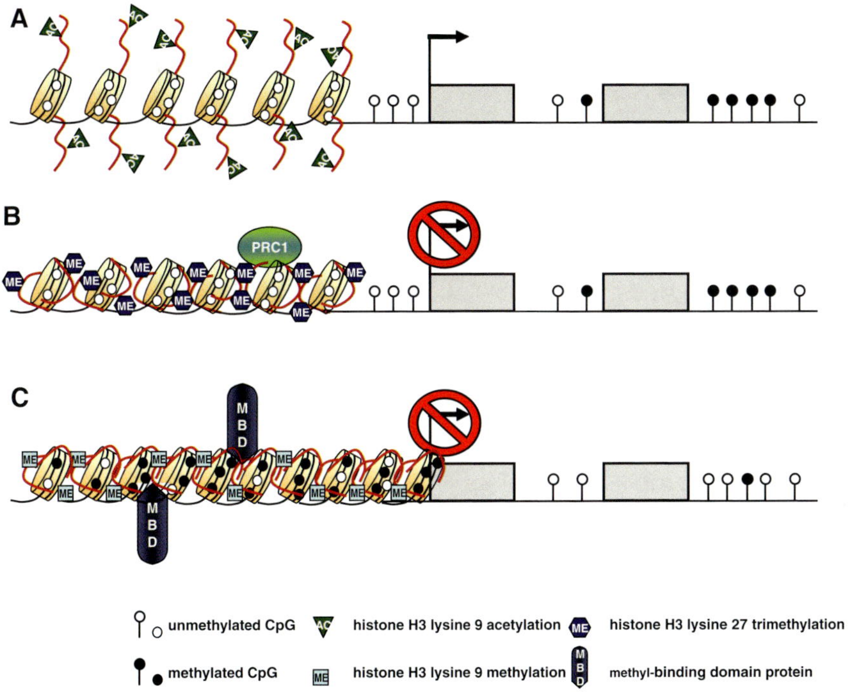

Color Plate 46. Role of DNA methylation and histone modifications at promoter CpG islands in normal cells and cancer. In normal cells, most promoter CpG islands do not exhibit DNA methylation. Thus the expression status of CpG island-containing genes is primarily determined by the presence or absence of transcription factors and by histone modifications around the promoters of such genes. **(A)** In general, transcriptionally active CpG island loci exhibit unmethylated DNA and high levels of histone H3 lysine 9 acetylation, which are accompanied by an open chromatin configuration. **(B)** Transcriptionally silent genes, however, are marked by histone H3 lysine 27 trimethylation, a modification catalyzed by EZH2 (enhancer of zeste 2), a member of the Polycomb repressor complex 2 (PRC2). Following H3 lysine 27 trimethylation, these promoters can be bound by members of the Polycomb repressor complex 1 (PRC1), which blocks transcription initiation by RNA polymerase II. This is also a mechanism of abnormal gene silencing in cancer, in the absence of aberrant DNA methylation. **(C)** In cancer, a large number of CpG islands are hypermethylated at their DNA, which generally correlates with transcriptional repression of the associated genes. These CpG islands generally exhibit a closed chromatin configuration, marked by histone H3 lysine 9 methylation, loss of acetylation, nucleosome occupancy around the transcription start site and various types of methyl-binding domain proteins. Altogether, these modifications render the chromatin non-permissive for transcription initiation (Chapter 26, Fig. 1; *see* discussion on p. 619).

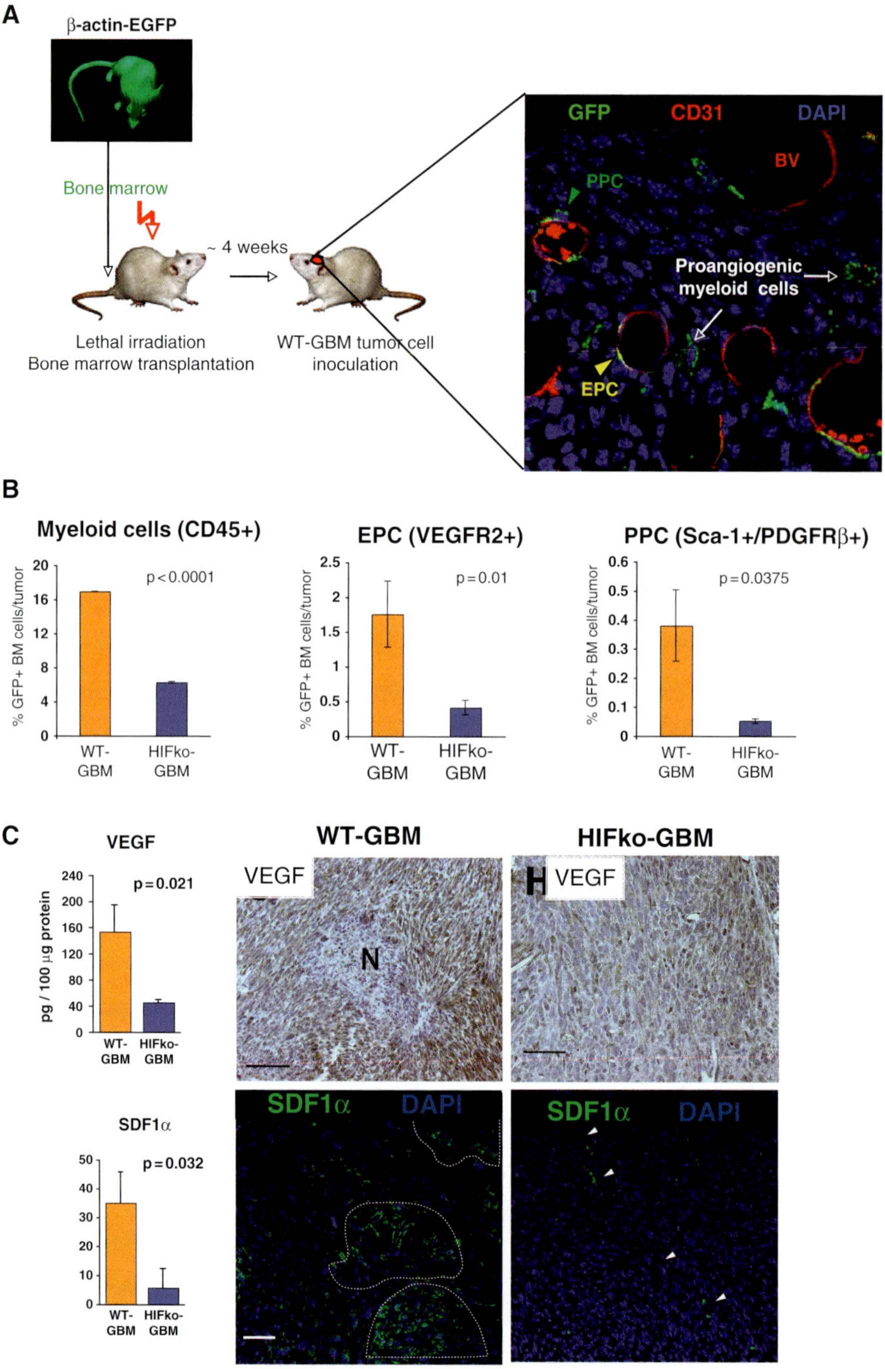

Color Plate 47. HIF1 recruits bone marrow-derived cells (BMDC) to orthotopic glioblastomas (GBM) (Chapter 31, Fig. 1; *see* complete caption on p. 754 and discussion on p. 752).

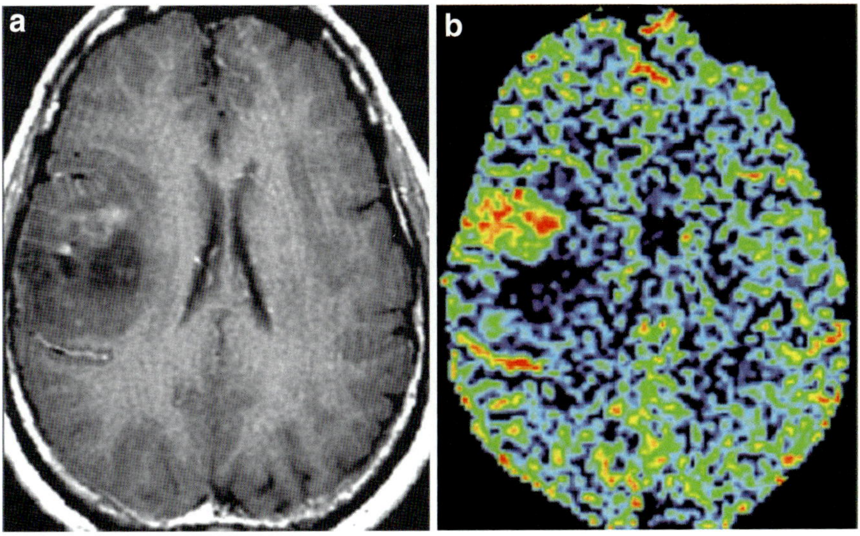

Color Plate 48. Congruence of region of contrast enhancement and region of highest relative cerebral blood volume (rCBV), suggesting that contrast-enhancing region is the most aggressive portion of tumor, in a 37-year-old man with biopsy-proved World Health Organization grade III astrocytoma. (**a**) Axial contrast-enhanced T1-weighted image shows inhomogeneously enhancing mass in the right frontal lobe. Contrast enhancement is confined to the central portion of the mass. (**b**) rCBV map in which regions of high rCBV are depicted in *red* and *yellow* shows that the region of highest rCBV corresponds to the contrast-enhancing region shown in **a**. (Reprinted, with permission, from Provenzale et al. 2006) (Chapter 33, Fig. 2; *see* discussion on p. 793).

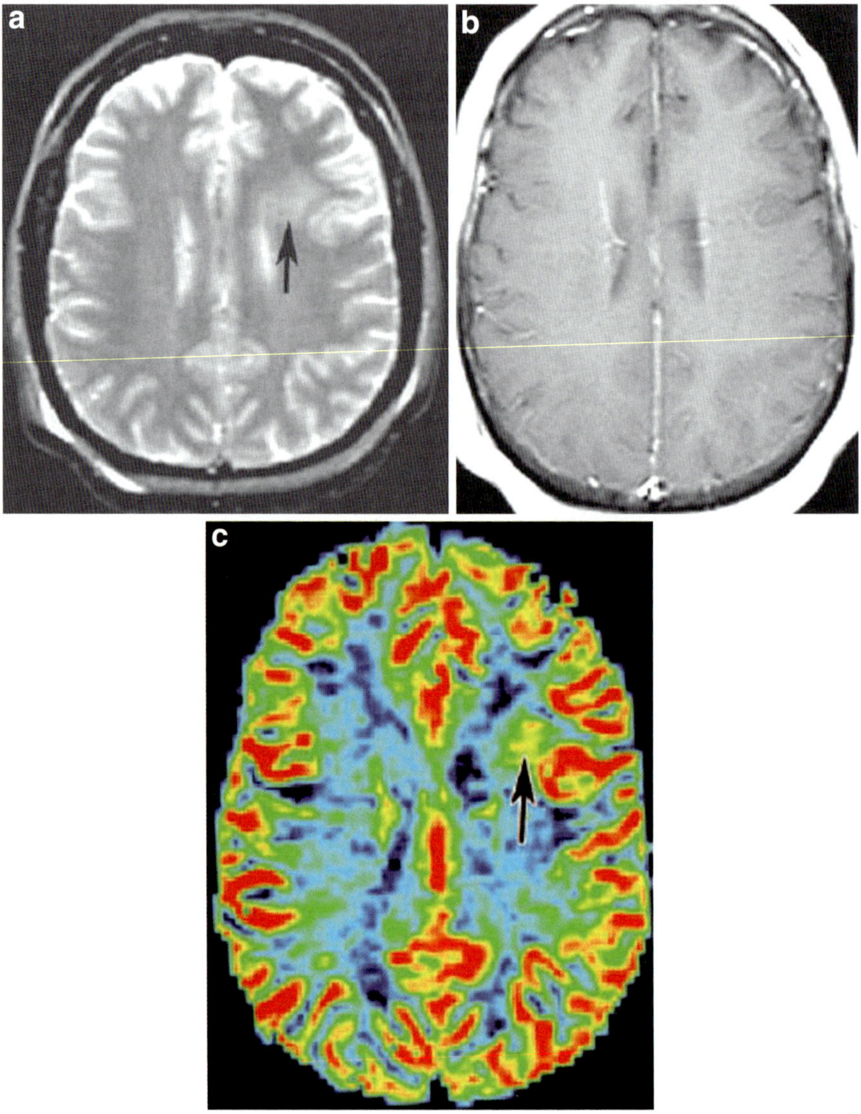

Color Plate 49. Elevation of rCBV despite the absence of contrast enhancement (i.e., no evidence of elevated permeability) in a 44-year-old woman with World Health Organization grade III astrocytoma. (**a**) Axial T2-weighted MR image shows hyperintense region (*arrow*) consistent with a neoplasm in the left frontal lobe. (**b**) Axial contrast-enhanced T1-weighted MR image does not show any regions of contrast enhancement. On the basis of the T2-weighted image and the contrast-enhanced T1-weighted image, one might have assumed that the lesion is a low-grade neoplasm with no areas of elevated rCBV. (**c**) rCBV map in which *red* and *yellow* colors indicate areas of elevated rCBV shows a region of high rCBV area (*arrow*) corresponding to the region of hyperintense abnormality on the T2-weighted image. At biopsy, this region was shown to represent high-grade glioma (Reprinted, with permission, from Wong et al. 2000) (Chapter 33, Fig. 3; *see* discussion on p. 793).

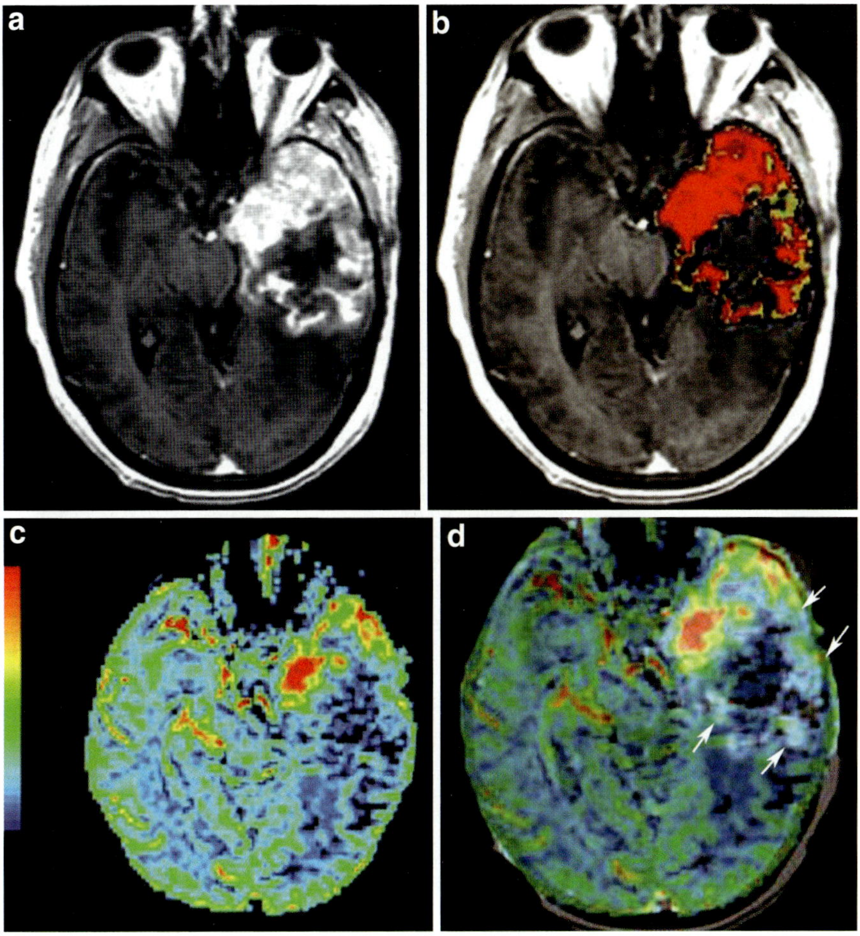

Color Plate 50. Lack of correlation of all regions of elevated permeability with elevated rCBV in a 51-year-old man with biopsy-proven glioblastoma multiforme. (**a**) Axial contrast-enhanced T1-weighted image shows large enhancing mass in the left temporal lobe. (**b**) Color-coded relative permeability map obtained using dynamic contrast-enhanced imaging superimposed on the image shown in (**a**). The color-coded map shows pixels having one of the three different colors. Left hemisphere regions that have peak signal intensity values in the range of 3–5 standard deviations (SD) above mean signal intensity in the normal right hemisphere are depicted in *blue*. The pixels that are in the range of 5–7 SD above baseline are shown in *yellow* color and the *red* pixels are those in which the increased signal intensity is greater than 7 SD above baseline. Thus, a large area of the tumor has pixels in the highest range of permeability values. (**c**) Axial rCBV map derived from T2*-weighted dynamic susceptibility imaging sequence shows that regions of elevated rCBV (seen in *red* and *yellow* color) are essentially confined to medial and anterior aspects of the tumor. (**d**) Superimposition of rCBV map shown in **c** on permeability map shown in **b** depicts the fact that large portions of the contrast-enhancing regions showing marked permeability in (**a**) and (**b**) do not have elevated rCBV values (*arrows*). (Reprinted, with permission, from Provenzale et al. 2006b) (Chapter 33, Fig. 4; *see* discussion on p. 793).

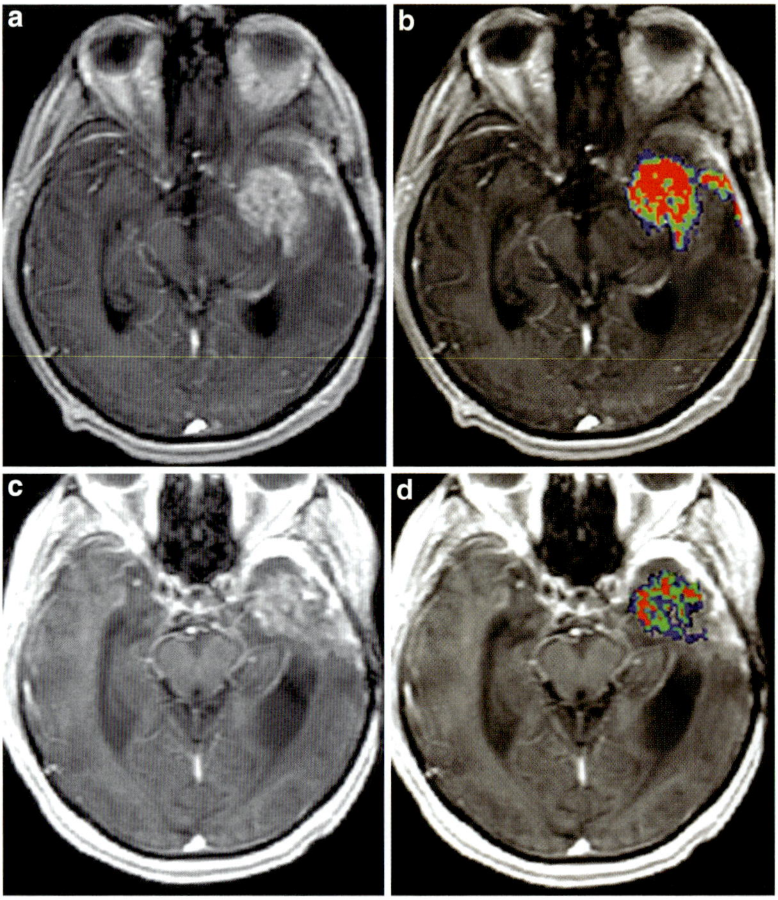

Color Plate 51. A 62-year-old man with glioblastoma multiforme. Illustration of changes in contrast material leakage (a reflection of degree of blood–brain barrier disruption) after administration of an antiangiogenesis agent. This case is an example of the fact that decreases in permeability after angiogenesis therapy may be greater than changes in tumor size. (**a**) Axial contrast-enhanced T1-weighted image prior to therapy shows large contrast-enhancing left temporal lobe tumor. (**b**) Color-coded map derived from dynamic contrast-enhanced imaging sequence before therapy (performed during the same MR examination as in **a**) shows relative degrees of permeability in each pixel. Pixels having signal intensity that are 120–149% of normal tissue are shown in *blue*, those with signal intensity of 140–159% of normal tissue are shown in *green*, and those having signal intensity ≥160% of normal tissue are in *red*. The majority of pixels are in the >160% category, consistent with marked leakage of contrast material throughout the tumor and indicating widespread disruption of the blood–brain barrier. (**c**) Repeat imaging was performed 30 days after beginning therapy with antiangiogenesis therapy. Axial contrast-enhanced T1-weighted image shows mild decrease in size of contrast-enhancing mass. (**d**) Color-coded map derived from dynamic contrast-enhanced imaging data on imaging at 30 days after beginning therapy (during same MR examination as **c**) shows marked decrease in number of pixels associated with the highest degree of permeability (i.e., *green* and *red* pixels). Reprinted, with permission, from Provenzale (2007) (Chapter 33, Fig. 5; *see* discussion on p. 798).

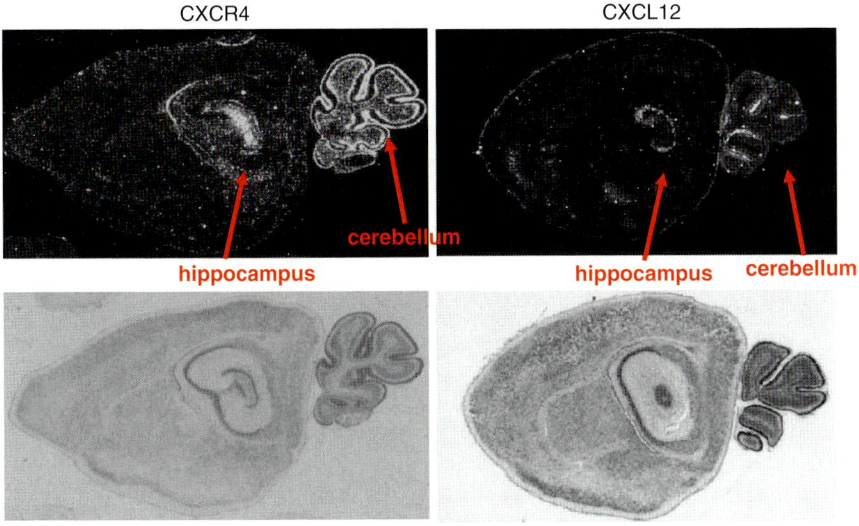

Color Plate 52. Dark-field mRNA expression of CXCR4 (*upper left*) and CXCL12 (*upper right*) and bright-field (H&E) picture (*lower panels*) of adjacent brain sections from 7-day-old mouse brain by in situ hybridization (*sagittal view*). (Chapter 34, Fig. 3; *see* complete caption and discussion on p. 819).

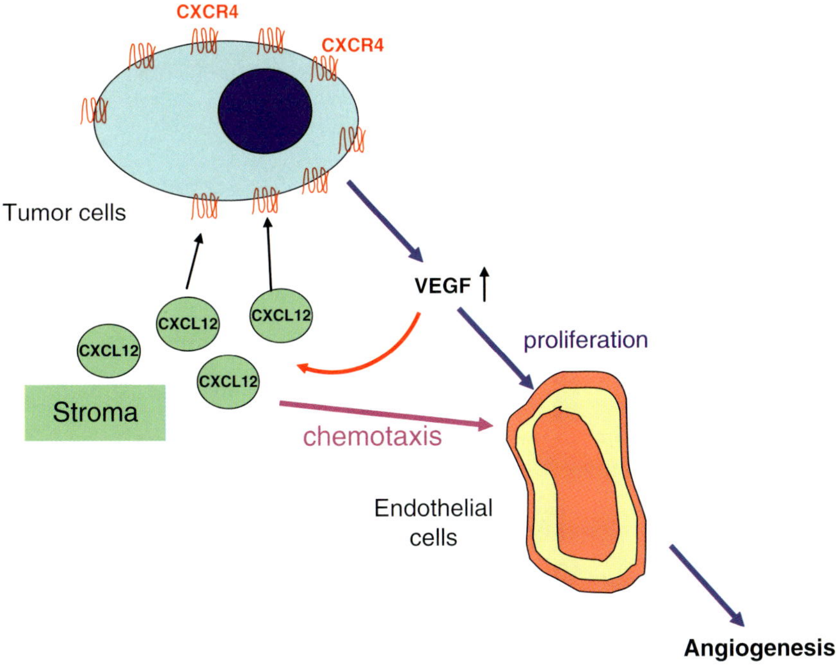

Color Plate 53. Complex regulation of angiogenesis by CXCR4/CXCL12 via VEGF-dependent manner (Chapter 34, Fig. 4; *see* complete caption and discussion on p. 824).

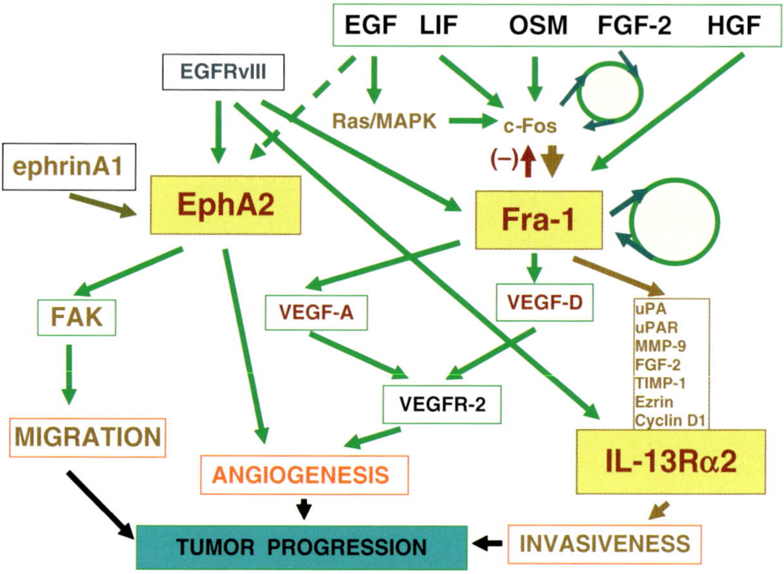

Color Plate 54. Simplified scheme of EphA2, IL-13Rα2 and also fos-related antigen 1 (Fra-1) regulation of expression and role in GBM progression. Mitogenic/oncogenic/growth-promoting factors, such as EGF, LIF, OSM, FGF-2, and HGF, are all highly upregulated in GBM. They all activate c-Fos transiently, but they appear to stimulate Fra-1 stably and in a sustained manner (Debinski and Gibo 2005). EGFRvIII is a receptor that is constitutively activated in GBM. EphA2, Fra-1, and IL-13Rα2 belong to a selected group of factors that are its gene targets. EphA2, Fra-1, and IL-13Rα2 collectively contribute to tumor neovasculature, tumor cell migration and invasiveness, and thus tumor progression (Chapter 35, Fig. 2; *see* discussion on p. 851).

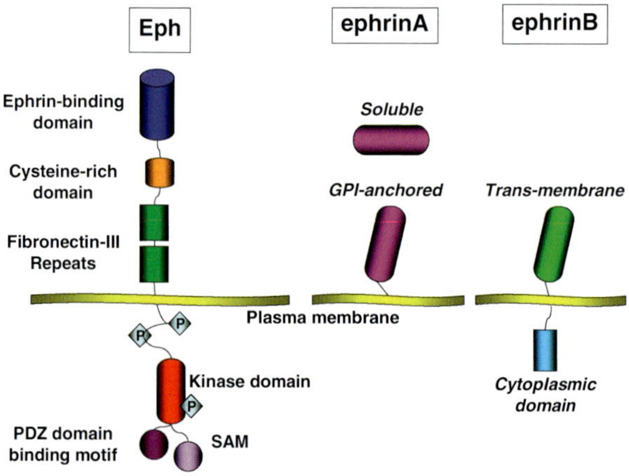

Color Plate 55. Eph receptors and ephrin ligands. Each color represents a functionally or structurally distinct domain or motif. EphrinA ligands exist as GPI-anchored or soluble proteins, while ephrinB ligands are transmembrane proteins with a cytoplasmic domain. Tyrosine phosphorylation sites within Eph receptor are denoted by "P." SAM, sterile alpha motif (Chapter 35, Fig. 3; *see* discussion on p. 854).

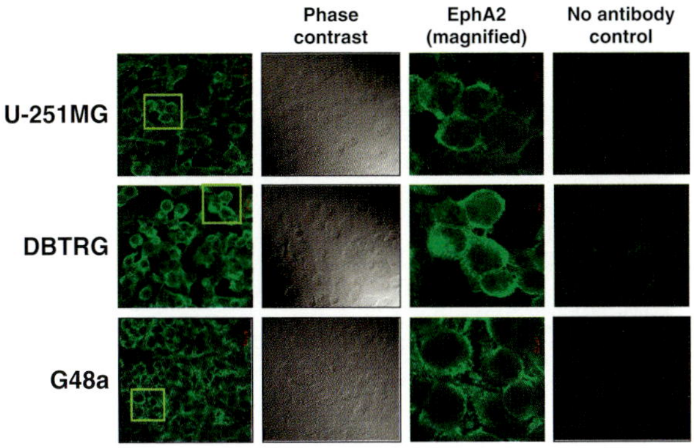

Color Plate 56. EphA2 staining in GBM cells. Glioblastoma cell lines (U-251 MG, DBTRG-MG, G48a) were grown on sterile glass slides and fixed in acetone for 2 min at –20°C, washed in PBS, and either used immediately or stored at –80°C. Slides were blocked for 1 h in 10% normal goat serum (NGS) at RT. Primary EphA2 monoclonal antibody B208 (1:200; MedImmune) was diluted in 1.5× NGS and incubated overnight at 4°C. Slides were incubated with secondary antibody for 45 min at RT. The secondary antibody was a goat antimouse IgG Oregon Green (1:200) (Molecular Probes, Eugene, OR). Control slides without primary antibody were also used as negative controls for nonspecific binding of the secondary antibody. Confocal microscopy analysis of samples stained with monoclonal EphA2 antibody was performed using a Zeiss LSM 510 Laser Scanning Confocal Microscope with a 63× lens. Photomicrographs were taken with a 40× magnification objective lens in all cases with a Retiga EXi digital camera. Images were processed with Jasc Paint Shop Pro v6.0 (Chapter 35, Fig. 4; *see* discussion on p. 855).

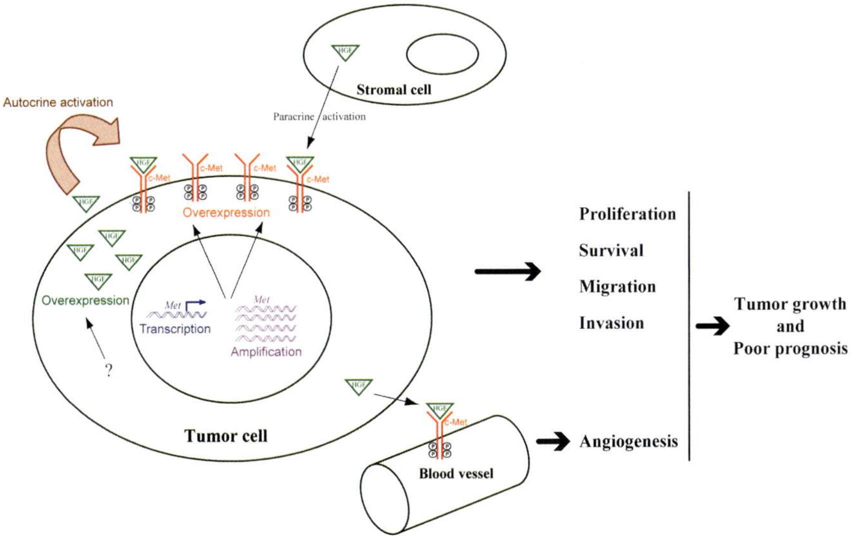

Color Plate 57. HGF/c-Met deregulation and oncogenic effects (Chapter 39, Fig. 3; *see* discussion on p. 937).

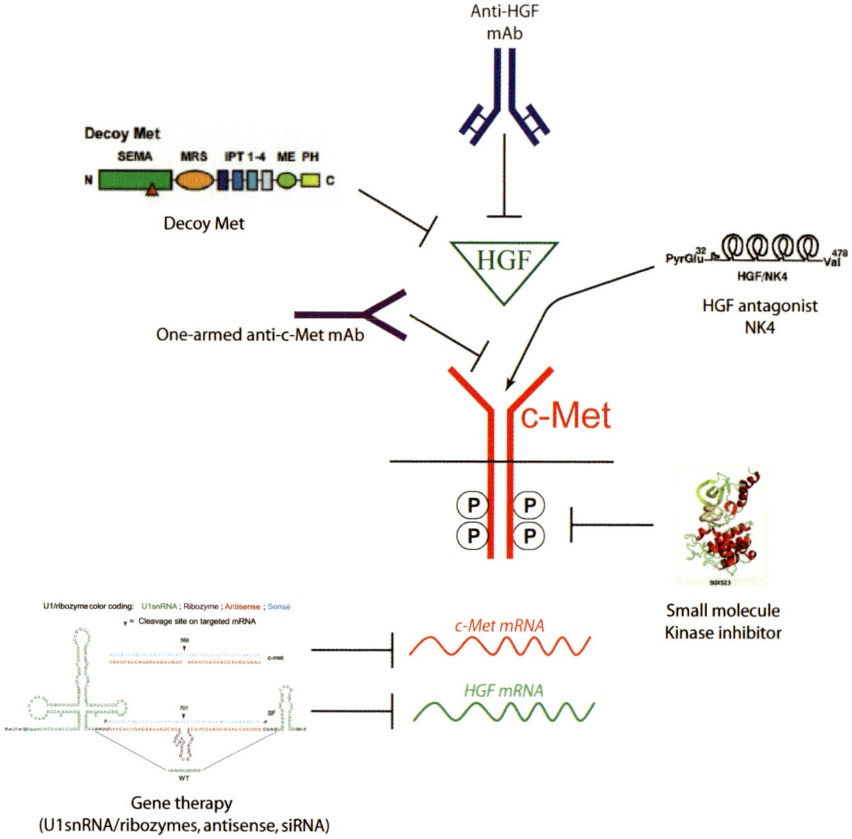

Color Plate 58. Therapeutic targeting strategies of HGF/c-Met (Chapter 39, Fig. 4; *see* discussion on p. 943).

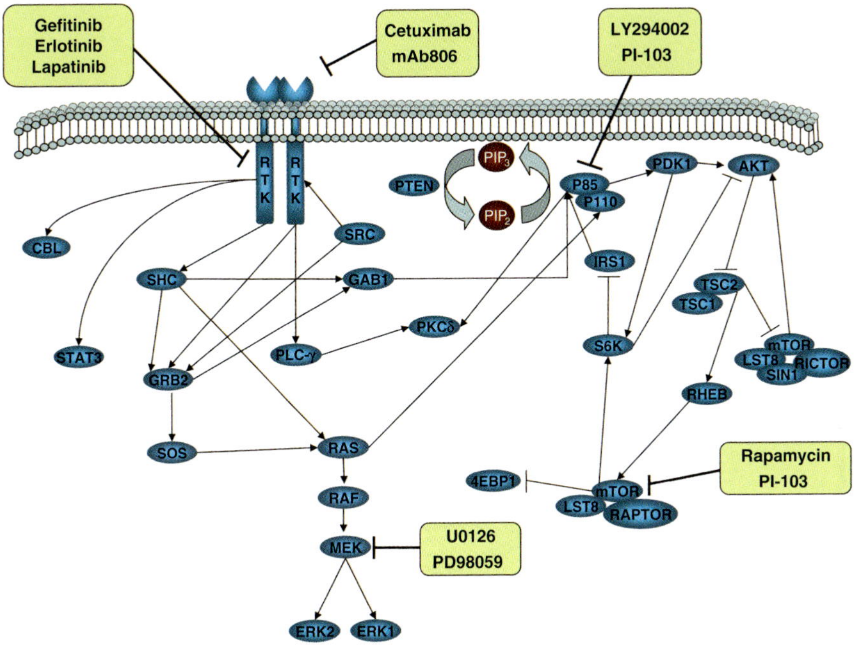

Color Plate 59. Oncogenic signaling networks in glioblastoma (Chapter 40, Fig. 1; *see* complete caption on p. 955 and discussion on p. 954).

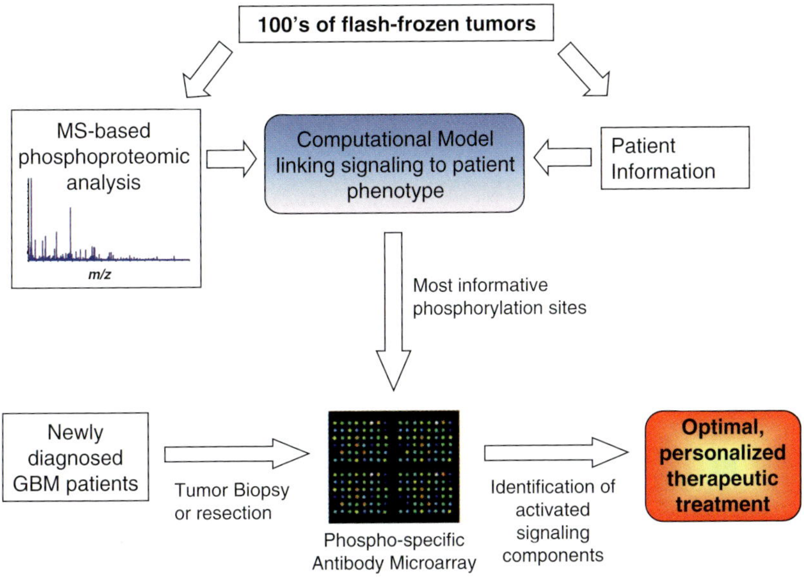

Color Plate 60. Bench-to-bedside strategy for personalized therapeutic treatment of glioblastoma patients (Chapter 40, Fig. 4; *see* complete caption on p. 969 and discussion on p. 968).

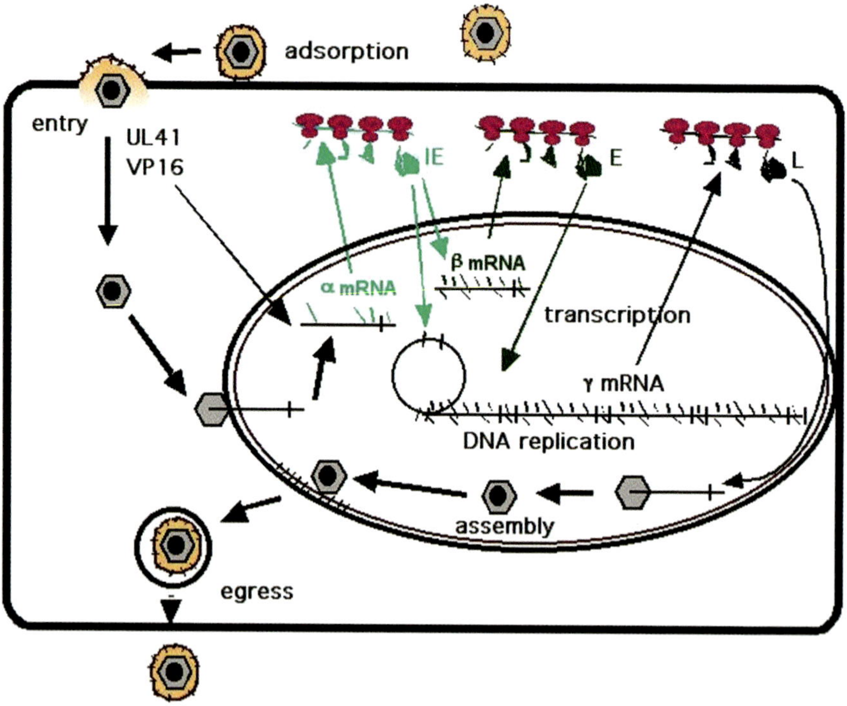

Color Plate 61. HSV-1 productive infection. HSV-1 cell attachment and entry, gene expression, DNA replication, assembly, and release are shown (Chapter 46, Fig. 3; *see* discussion on p. 1108).

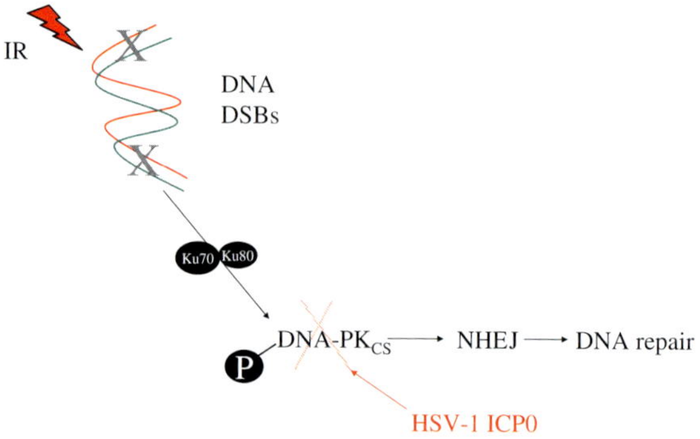

Color Plate 62. Diagram of DNA DSB production by IR and inhibition of NHEJ DNA repair pathway by ICP0 through degradation of DNA-PK$_{CS}$. IR, ionizing radiation; DSB, double-strand break; NHEJ, non-homologous end joining (Chapter 46, Fig. 4; *see* discussion on p. 1118).

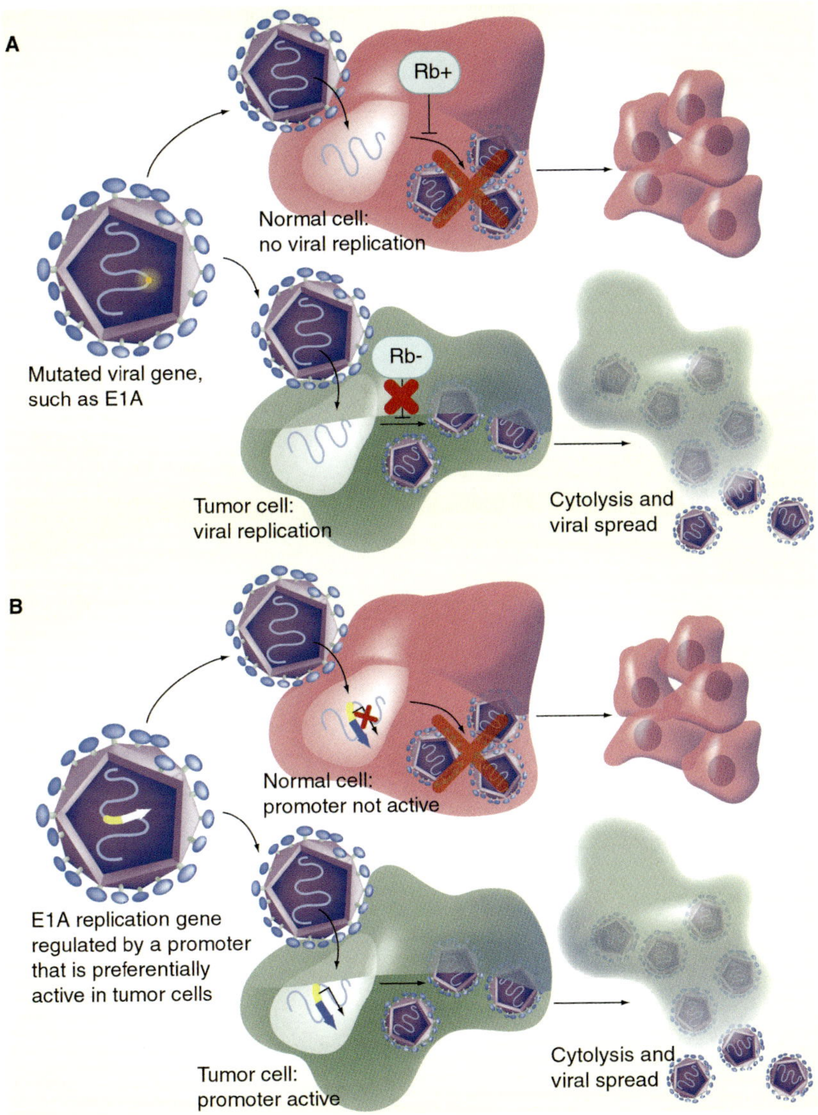

Color Plate 63. Strategies used to target Ad replication specifically to tumor cells. (**A**) Targeting Ad replication to tumor cells by viral gene mutation. Specific mutations within the Ad *E1A*, *E1B*, or viral-associated RNA-coding sequences that abrogate protein function have been shown to result in the selective replication of the mutant Ad in tumor cells that contain dysfunctional pRb, p53, or Ras pathways, respectively (Chapter 47, Fig. 2; *see* complete caption on p. 1142 and discussion on p. 1140).

subunit has a molecular mass of 180–250 kDa and comprises four main parts: the globular N-terminal domain; 14.5 epidermal growth factor (EGF)-like repeats, 8–15 fibronectin type III (FNIII)-like repeats, and a fibrinogen-like domain at the carboxy terminus (Gulcher et al., 1991). Alternate splicing occurs frequently within the FNIII repeats, resulting in both small and large isoforms (Gulcher et al., 1989) that have distinct biological functions. A diagrammatic representation of one structural subunit of Tn-C is shown in Fig. 36.2a. Tn-C expression is virtually undetectable in healthy adult tissue but is expressed during embryogenesis (Jones and Jones, 2000a) and in adult tissues undergoing tissue remodeling, including wound healing, infection, inflammation, and neoplasia (Jones and Jones, 2000b). Tenascin-C is localized in the stroma in a

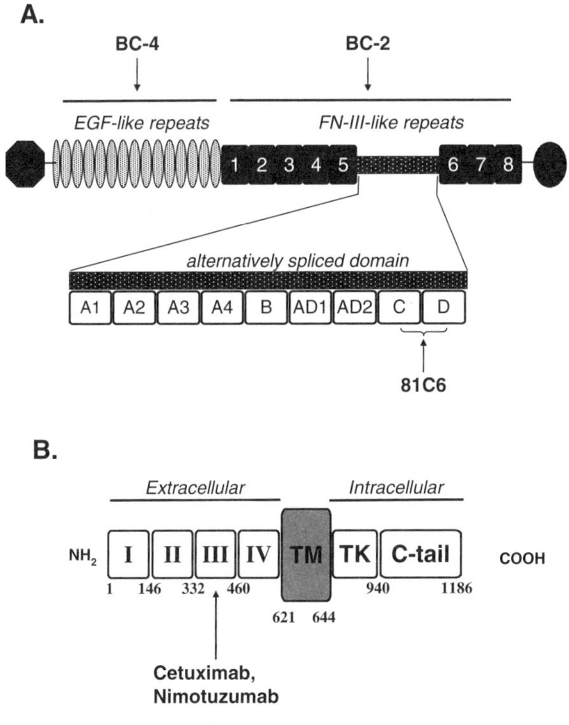

Fig. 36.2 Clinical antibodies against molecular targets tenacin-c and wild-type epidermal growth factor (EGFRwt) (**A**) Diagrammatic representation of one structural subunit of tenascin-C. Structural domains include a globular N-terminal domain (*Hexagon*), epidermal growth factor (EGF)-like repeats (*Ovals*), fibronectin type III (FN-III)-like repeats (*black squares*), alternatively spliced FN-III-like domains (*black oblong* inset with *white squares*), fibrinogen terminal globe (*circle*). *Arrows* indicate the site of mAbs BC-4, BC-2, and 81C6 interaction. (**B**) Schematic representation of EGFRwt. NH_2, amino terminus of EGFR-WT; extracellular portion consisting of four domains (I-IV); TM, transmembrane domain; TK, tyrosine kinase domain; C-tail, the carboxyl terminus of the intracellular domain; COOH, carboxyl terminus of EGFRwt. Arrows indicate the binding reactivity of the two clinical antibodies cetuximab and nimotuzumab

variety of tumor types including breast carcinoma (Borsi et al., 1992), oral squamous cell carcinoma (Hindermann et al., 1999), lung cancer (Kusagawa et al., 1998), prostate carcinoma (Katenkamp et al., 2004; Kusagawa et al., 1998), and melanoma (Ilmonen et al., 2004). Tn-C was originally discovered as a glioma mesenchymal extracellular matrix antigen (Bourdon et al., 1983) and is highly expressed in astrocytoma but not in normal brain (Ventimiglia et al., 1992). More than 90% of glioblastoma multiforme (GBM, WHO grade IV) patients exhibit high levels of Tn-C expression (Wikstrand et al., 1998a), which correlates with advancing astrocytoma tumor grade and angiogenesis (Herold-Mende et al., 2002; Zagzag et al., 1995), indicators of poor prognosis.

Many anti-tenascin mAbs have been generated to date (Bourdon et al., 1983; Brack et al., 2006; De Santis et al., 2003; Petronzelli et al., 2005; Silacci et al., 2006; Siri et al., 1991), and several have been introduced into clinical trials in both the USA and Europe (Goetz et al., 2003). One promising application of anti-Tn-C mAbs is radioimmunotherapy, which provides localized radiation by specifically delivering a radioisotope to the tumor site for treatment of newly diagnosed and recurrent GBM patients. Riva and colleagues have conducted several clinical trials evaluating the loco-regional administration of several anti-tenascin mAbs. BC-4 and ST2146 mAbs bind to an epitope within the EGF-like repeat region that is present on all tenascin-C isoforms (Balza et al., 1993; De Santis et al., 2003). In contrast, BC-2 and ST2485 react with an epitope found on alternatively spliced FNIII A1 and A4 repeats (Balza et al., 1993). A diagram indicating the sites of BC-4 and BC-2 interaction with Tn-C is shown in Fig. 36.2a. Of note, it was discovered that the BC-4 mAb hybridoma clone also generated an additional nonfunctional light chain. ST2146 was developed as a BC-4 replacement to overcome this problem (De Santis et al., 2003). In addition, ST2485, which exhibits an enhanced affinity to Tn-C compared with BC-2, was subsequently developed to combine with ST2146 to augment tumor targeting (Petronzelli et al., 2005). While clinical trials with ST2146 and ST2485 have yet to be reported, outcome with BC-2 and BC-4 labeled with either ^{131}I or ^{90}Y have been described for the treatment of patients with malignant glioma (Riva et al., 1995; Riva et al., 1999). Unfortunately, it was impossible to discern which tenascin-C binding epitope played any role in therapeutic efficacy or normal tissue toxicity because no distinction was made between the two mAbs in these protocols. Furthermore, differentiation of response results for newly diagnosed and recurrent patients also was not done.

^{131}I-labeled anti-tenascin-C BC-2 and BC-4 mAbs were also evaluated in a phase II study of 91 patients (GBM, n = 74; AA, n = 9; AO, n = 7; oligodendroglioma, n = 1) (Riva et al., 2000). Among these patients, 52 (57%) had small (defined as less than 2 cm^3) or undetectable residual tumor, while larger tumors were present in the remaining patients. The patient population was nearly equally divided into two groups: 47 patients (52%) had newly diagnosed tumors while 44 patients (48%) were recurrent. Three to ten loco-regional injections of ^{131}I-labeled mAb with cumulative activities of up to 2035 MBq were administered. The half-life clearance from the tumor cavity of ^{131}I was 57.1 h while a mean of 150 Gy was delivered to the surgically created resection cavity (SCRC) perimeter. On this study, patients with GBM, AA, and AO achieved median survivals of 19, >46, and 23 months, respectively. GBM patients with smaller volume disease had a more favorable response rate (56.7%) compared to those with larger tumors (17.8%).

The Italian group also performed a similar study with ^{90}Y-labeled BC-2 and BC-4 mAbs (Riva et al., 2000). Forty-three patients (35 GBM, 6 AA, 2 O) were evaluated including 16 (37%) with small or undetected residual tumor and 19 (44%) with larger lesions. Sixteen patients (37%) in this study had newly diagnosed tumors while 19 patients (44%) were treated following recurrence. The treatment protocol consisted of between 3 and 5 cycles of ^{90}Y-labeled anti-tenascin-C mAb up to a cumulative activity of 3145 MBq. Dosimetry analyses revealed that the median effective half-life of ^{90}Y in the tumor cavity was 43.2 h while the mean radiation dose delivered to the SCRC interface was 280 Gy, a value nearly twice that observed for ^{131}I. Median overall survival from initial diagnosis was 90 months for the AA patients and 20 months for the GBM patients. Interestingly, the response rate among larger tumor patients following ^{90}Y-labeled mAb treatment was somewhat higher that that observed with ^{131}I-labeled mAb treatment (26.3% vs. 17.8%), which might reflect the longer β-particle range of ^{90}Y, while among patients with smaller volume disease, the response rate for ^{90}Y-labeled mAb treatment, 56.3%, was nearly identical to that observed with ^{131}I-labeled mAb treatment.

A more recent two-institution study in Italy (Maurizio Bufalini Hospital, Cesena) and Munich (Ludwig-Maximilians-Universität München) included 37 patients with malignant brain tumors (13 AA, 24 GBM) that received loco-regional injections of either ^{131}I-labeled or ^{90}Y-labeled BC-4 (Goetz et al., 2003). Multiple cycles (mean 3, maximum 8) of labeled mAbs were administered in Italy at intervals of 6–8 weeks, while treatment in Munich was limited to a single injection of 1100 MBq ^{131}I-labeled BC-4. Unfortunately, the whole-group estimated median survival time was not reached. However, the median survival for all GBM patients was 17 months and the 5-year survival probability for AA patients was approximately 85%. In addition a low incidence of side effects, even following multiple injections of labeled mAbs, was reported.

81C6 (Neuradiab^{TM}) is a murine immunoglobulin (Ig)G_{2b} that reacts within domains C and D of the FNIII-like CDR region of tenascin and that is ubiquitously expressed within malignant glioma (Bourdon et al., 1983). A diagram indicating the site of 81C6 interaction with Tenascin-C is shown in Fig. 36.2a. Preclinical studies demonstrated preferential localization of ^{131}I-labeled 81C6 for Tn-C-expressing subcutaneous and intracranial human xenografts in mice (Bourdon et al., 1984). Additional preclinical studies showed that intravenous (IV) administration of ^{131}I-labeled 81C6 in athymic mice bearing subcutaneous and intracranial D54MG human glioma xenografts caused significant tumor growth delay and regression (Lee et al., 1988a, b) and, in addition, prolonged median survival for athymic rats bearing intracranial tumors (Lee et al., 1987). Specificity of tumor localization was confirmed in glioma patients treated with 5–50 mg of ^{131}I-labeled 81C6 in whom tissue obtained at surgery revealed an average tumor:normal brain localization ratio of 25:1, with values as high as 200:1 in some samples (Zalutsky et al., 1989). Despite the success of ^{131}I-labeled 81C6 localization, the study revealed that only 0.001–0.005% per gram of the injected dose of radiolabeled 81C6 mAb localized to the intracranial tumor of the patients following IV or intra-arterial administration (Zalutsky et al., 1990). Although the precise factors responsible for limiting intratumoral uptake following systemic administration are not clear; potential factors include the blood–brain barrier and elevated interstitial pressure within the tumor.

Furthermore, radiation dosimetry calculations indicated the possibility of administering more than 700 cGy of ^{131}I-labeled 81C6 to intracranial glioma, under optimal conditions, without causing significant organ toxicity (Schold et al., 1993). Further Phase I studies were performed to determine the maximum tolerated dose (MTD) following regional administration into the surgically created resection cavity (SCRC) in order to achieve high local ^{131}I-labeled 81C6 concentrations and avoid systemic toxicity by circumventing the blood–brain barrier and overcoming the high intratumoral interstitial pressures. The MTD for three subgroups of patients with CNS tumors was determined to be (1) 80 mCi for adult patients with leptomeningeal neoplasms or brain-tumor resection cavities that communicate with the subarachnoid space (Bigner et al., 1995), (2) 100 mCi for patients with recurrent malignant gliomas who received prior radiation therapy with or without chemotherapy (Bigner et al., 1998a), and (3) 120 mCi for previously untreated, newly diagnosed GBM patients (Cokgor et al., 2000). In the latter group, delayed neurotoxicity was dose limiting, and the median survival for all patients and those with GBM was 79 and 69 weeks, respectively (Cokgor et al., 2000). In a follow-up Phase II trial, 33 patients with newly diagnosed glioma receiving an administered dose of 120 mCi into the SCRC had prolonged overall survival compared to that achieved with conventional therapy or interstitial chemotherapy. Overall, median survival achieved for all 33 patients and the subset of 27 with GBM was 86.7 and 79.4 weeks, respectively (Reardon et al., 2002).

Dosimetry analysis performed on our Phase I study revealed a significant range of absorbed doses to the 2-cm cavity margin that depended on cavity volume and residence time (Akabani et al., 2000). Specifically, the average absorbed doses of ^{131}I-81C6 to the SCRC interface and 2-cm SCRC perimeter were 1435 Gy (range, 46-9531 Gy) and 32 Gy (range, 3–59 Gy), respectively. In addition, the average SCRC volume was 21 cm^3 (range, 2–81 cm^3), and the average SCRC residence time was 79 hours (range, 10–113 hours). We therefore examined the relationship between absorbed dose to the 2-cm cavity margin and histopathology results among 16 patients with progressive changes on serial MRI scans following ^{131}I-81C6 administration. The average absorbed dose to the 2-cm cavity margin among five patients with solely recurrent tumor noted on stereotactic biopsy was 25 Gy (range, 12–44 Gy). Of note, none of these five patients developed any type of neurotoxicity. In contrast, biopsy results of five additional patients demonstrated solely radionecrosis. The average absorbed dose to the 2-cm shell among these patients was 47 Gy (range,

34–55 Gy). Furthermore, two of these patients also developed delayed neurotoxicity, and one developed both acute and delayed neurotoxicity. These findings suggest a quantitative relationship between absorbed dose to the 2-cm cavity margin and clinicopathologic outcome. Specifically, patients who received less than 44 Gy to the 2-cm cavity margin were most likely to develop tumor recurrence with no radionecrosis or treatment-related toxicity. On the other hand, patients who received more than 44 Gy to the 2-cm cavity margin were most likely to develop radionecrosis with possible signs of clinical neurotoxicity. With these findings, we determined the optimal radiation boost dose to the 2-cm shell from ^{131}I-81C6 for patients with newly diagnosed malignant glioma to be 44 Gy.

We therefore performed a pilot study using a novel, patient-specific dosing strategy of ^{131}I-81C6 designed to achieve a 44-Gy boost to the 2-cm SCRC margin (Reardon et al., 2008). The primary objective of this study was to determine the feasibility, efficacy, and toxicity of administering ^{131}I-81C6 into the SCRC to achieve a 44-Gy boost to the 2-cm SCRC margin in adult newly diagnosed malignant glioma patients. A 1–3-mCi dose of ^{131}I-81C6 was administered into the resection cavity 3–7 days postoperatively to determine the amount of ^{131}I-81C6 required to achieve a 44-Gy boost to the 2-cm SCRC perimeter. Gamma camera images were obtained immediately, and 2, 24, and 48 hours later, to calculate the effective half-life and biological clearance half-life of murine 81C6. By correcting for the physical half-life of ^{131}I, ^{131}I-81C6 residence time was calculated. The SCRC volume was calculated from a three-dimensional reconstruction of the head and SCRC derived from postoperative MRI images to a 2-mm depth (refer to Fig. 36.3). By using the measured ^{131}I-81C6 residence time and SCRC volume, the radioactivity dose of ^{131}I-81C6 predicted to achieve a 44-Gy boost to the SCRC margin was calculated and administered into the SCRC, followed by conventional external beam radiotherapy and chemotherapy. Twenty-one patients were enrolled, including 16 with GBM and 5 with anaplastic astrocytoma (AA).

Only one patient failed to achieve the targeted 44-Gy boost $\pm 10\%$ to the SCRC. The amount of ^{131}I-mu81C6 was deliberately diminished in this patient, due to technical factors affecting fluid aspiration at the time of mAb administration. Attributable toxicity was mild and limited to reversible grade 3 neutropenia or thrombocytopenia ($n = 3$; 14%), CNS wound infections ($n = 3$; 14%), and headache ($n = 2$; 10%). With a median follow-up of 151 weeks, 87% of the GBM patients were alive at 1 year, while the median overall survival for all patients and those with GBM was 96.6 and 90.6 weeks, respectively. These results confirm that patient-specific dosing of ^{131}I-81C6 is feasible and can consistently achieve a 44-Gy boost dose to the SCRC margin. Furthermore, this approach, followed by conventional radiotherapy (XRT) and systemic chemotherapy, was well tolerated and associated with a median survival that exceeds that of historical controls treated with surgery plus carmustine-impregnated biodegradable wafers, as well as that associated with current standard of care incorporating temozolomide (TMZ) and external beam radiotherapy (Stupp et al., 2005). The latest adaptation of XRT involving patient-specific

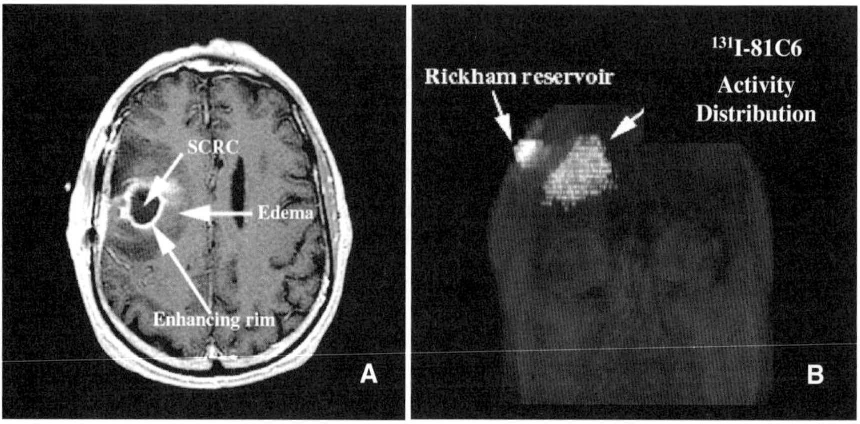

Fig. 36.3 Radioimmunotherapy with ^{131}I-81C6 surgically created resection cavity (SCRC). (**A**) Gadolinium-enhanced T1-weighted axial image demonstrating SCRC following tumor resection; (**B**) Three-dimensional view of registered MRI and SPECT images of a patient immediately after ^{131}I-81C6 administered into the SCRC. Notice the well-defined Rickham reservoir over the skull surface. Reprinted from Int J Radiat Oncol Biol Phys, 46/4, Akabani et al. (2000), with permission from Elsevier (license number 2053641366863)

^{131}I-81C6 dosing and achieving a targeted 44-Gy boost to the 2-cm SCRC perimeter (Reardon et al., 2008) is a significant achievement in radiotherapy treatment. As a result, a multi-institutional Phase III study, known as the GLASS-ART (http://www.glassarttrial.com/), has been initiated that will randomize newly diagnosed GBM patients to a regimen of TMZ/XRT plus adjuvant TMZ vs. that regimen plus patient-specific ^{131}I-81C6. Approximately 750 patients will enroll and the primary endpoint of this study is overall survival.

36.2.2 Epidermal Growth Factor Receptor and Its Variant III Form

The epidermal growth factor receptor (EGFR) is a 170-kDa transmembrane glycoprotein that is composed of three functional domains – an extracellular ligand-binding domain, an anchoring membrane-spanning region, and an intracellular catalytic domain that functions as a tyrosine kinase receptor (Fig. 36.2b). EGFR is activated following binding of either epidermal growth factor (EGF) or transforming growth factor alpha (TGF-α) ligand; the receptor dimerizes, which leads to kinase activation and autophosphorylation, triggering subsequent signal transduction, receptor internalization, and downregulation (Arteaga, 2001; see also Chapter 20). The involvement of increased and/or aberrant EGFR activity has been documented in human cancers including 25–77% of colorectal tumors (Goodin, 2008; Messa et al., 1998), 14–91% of breast cancer, 40–80%, of non-small-lung carcinoma, 35–70% of ovarian tumors, 31–48% of bladder cancer, 30–50% of pancreatic cancer, and 50–90% of renal carcinoma (Herbst and Shin, 2002). EGFR expression also occurs in 80–100% of squamous cell carcinomas of the head and neck (Santini et al., 1991; Shin et al., 1994). The incidence of EGFR in malignant glioma has been shown to increase with tumor grade: 27–57% for astrocytoma (WHO grade II), 71–94% for AA (grade III), and 68–90% for GBM (grade IV) (Wikstrand et al., 1998a). *EGFR* gene amplification is one of the underlying mechanisms of EGFR protein overexpression, associated with high levels of EGFR messenger RNA. *EGFR* gene amplification is primarily associated with GBM and not with pilocytic astrocytomas (WHO grade I) or astrocytomas of WHO grades II/III (Agosti et al., 1992), as estimates of the frequency of EGFR gene amplification, by genetic analysis, in GBM and AA are 36–60% and 10–22%, respectively. Furthermore, *EGFR* gene amplification or EGFR protein expression is common (>63%) within primary, or de novo GBM but rare in secondary, or progressive GBM (<0%) (Wikstrand and Bigner, 2008). However, studies have found that EGFR protein overexpression without *EGFR* gene amplification occurs in 12–38% of GBM tumors (Chaffanet et al., 1992; Schlegel et al., 1994), suggesting that multiple systems of deregulation, in EGFR expression, may exist at translational and post-translational levels.

Most cases of gene amplification are accompanied by gene rearrangements (Wikstrand et al., 1998b) and mutations (Kuan et al., 2001) that result in simultaneous expression of both wild-type and truncated receptor proteins on the cell surface (Wikstrand et al., 1997). Seven different types of naturally occurring *EGFR* genomic variants have been identified (Bigner et al., 1998a), including the most frequently observed EGFR mutation, EGFR variant III (EGFRvIII). The *EGFRvIII* gene has an in-frame deletion of 801 bp (exons 2–7) that results in removal of amino acid residues 6–273 within the extracellular binding domain of intact EGFR, producing a 145-kDa EGFRvIII protein that contains a unique glycine residue at the fusion point (Batra et al., 1995). EGFRvIII has not been observed in normal tissue but is overexpressed in 42% of head and neck squamous cell carcinoma tumors (Sok et al., 2006), 15–39% of non-small-lung cancer (Garcia de Palazzo et al., 1993; Okamoto et al., 2003), 40% of primary invasive breast tumors, and 29% of non-invasive ductal carcinoma in situ (Yu et al., 2008), as well as in 41–54% of GBM tumors exhibiting *EGFR wild-type* (*EGFRwt*) gene amplification (Aldape et al., 2004; Barker et al., 2001; Biernat et al., 2004). The real prognostic significance remains unclear to date, as the correlation between amplification of either *EGFRwt* and/or *EGFRvIII* has resulted in many inconclusive or contradictory reports (Wikstrand, 2008). In a recent analysis, with a large patient cohort, there was no significant association found between *EGFR* amplification or rearrangement and GBM patient survival. However, *EGFR* aberrations in AA were associated with shorter survival (Liu et al., 2005). Another retrospective series of GBM patients demonstrated that *EGFRvIII* negative patients fared better than those with detectable EGFRvIII expression. In fact, established clinical prognostic factors were not predictive of outcome among the cohort of EGFRvIII positive patients (Pelloski et al., 2007).

Many different mAbs have been developed that target EGFRwt for cancer immunotherapy (Friedlander et al., 2008). Two of these antibodies, cetuximab (Erbitux®, ImClone Systems, NY) and nimotuzumab (also referred to as h-R3, YM Biosciences), are currently being investigated for the treatment of malignant glioma (Combs et al., 2006; Ramos et al., 2006). The interaction of the two antibodies with EGFRwt is shown in Fig. 36.2a.

Both EGFRwt and EGFRvIII are co-expressed within malignant glioma, and generally only a fraction of tumor cells, within a given EGFRvIII positive tumor, express the mutant protein. Immunohistochemistry analysis routinely shows that EGFRvIII-containing cells are clustered and scattered diffusely within tumor tissue, ranging from relatively small numbers to occasional complete homogeneous staining (Nishikawa et al., 2004). Unlike EGFR, EGFRvIII is EGF and TGF-α ligand independent and is constitutively phosphorylated (Huang et al., 1997). As a result, EGFRvIII does not trigger the ligand-dependent signal transduction pathways that initiate receptor internalization and subsequent downregulation (Huang et al., 1997). EGFRvIII is a tumorigenic factor (Batra et al., 1995; Nishikawa et al., 1994) and promotes tumorigenesis of GBM cells in vivo through increased cellular proliferation (Narita et al., 2002), decreased cellular apoptosis (Nagane et al., 1996), and promotion of tumor cell invasion (Lal et al., 2002). Therefore, EGFRvIII is a desirable target for therapeutic intervention, and as a result several anti-EGFRvIII mAbs have been investigated including L8A4 (Reist et al., 1997), H10 (Pelloski et al., 2007; Wikstrand et al., 1995), Y10 (Sampson et al., 2000), and MR1 (Lorimer et al., 1996). The therapeutic potential of L8A4, Y10, and H10 has been demonstrated by direct conjugation with Pseudomonas exotoxin A (Lorimer et al., 1995), with radioiodination (Reist et al., 1995), and through development of chimeric L8A4 (Reist et al., 1997). All three immunotoxins were cytotoxic (with 50% inhibition of protein synthesis occurring in the 15–50-pM range), all radiolabeled antibodies internalized, and in vivo biodistribution studies demonstrated that radiolabeled L8A4 and H10 specifically localized to EGFRvIII-expressing tumor xenografts that had been established in nude mice. The in vitro binding and internalization activity of chimeric L8A4 was identical to that of its murine counterpart, and comparative tissue distribution studies of the chimeric construct showed that it is superior to the murine mAb as a targeting agent in vivo (Reist et al., 1997). Preclinical studies have determined that boronated ^{125}I-L8A4 (^{125}I-BD) in combination with anti-EGFRwt antibody, cetuximab, resulted in almost twice as much ^{125}I being localized in the composite tumors compared with ^{125}I-BD-cetuximab or ^{125}I-BD-L8A4 alone. In addition, the mean survival time of animals bearing composite tumors, which received both mAbs, was 55 days ($P < 0.0001$) compared with 36 days for BD-L8A4 and 38 days for BD-C225 alone (Yang et al., 2008).

MR1-1 (Beers et al., 2000) is a very promising scFv antibody therapeutic for EGFRvIII-expressing tumors. MR1-1 was produced from the parental antibody clone, MR1, by affinity maturation in order to generate a higher affinity clone. MR1-1 differs from parental MR1 by 3 amino acid residues; one residue change from phenylalanine to tryptophan at amino acid position 92 [F92W] in CDR3 of the variable light chain and two residue changes in CDR3 of the heavy chain [S98P, T99Y]. The resulting protein has a 15-fold higher K_d (1.5×10^{-9}M) for EGFRvIII. Compared to ^{125}I-MR1, the higher affinity clone, ^{131}I-MR1-1 exhibited levels of both cell surface retention and internalization up to five times higher than the parent molecule, and biodistribution studies in mice demonstrated improved tumor retention and rapid clearance from normal tissues, as well as higher tumor:normal organ ratios (Kuan et al., 2000). Preclinical studies have also investigated the potential use of MR1-1 for radiotherapy (Shankar et al., 2006) and determined that therapeutic treatment using MR1-1 (dsFv) immunotoxin (MR1-1 was fused at the genetic level to Pseudomonas exotoxin domains II and III to form the MR1-1 immunotoxin) enhanced antitumor immunity (Ochiai et al., 2008). An FDA-approved Investigational New Drug Permit was issued in 2007, and a clinical trial of MR1-1 delivered intratumorally, via convection enhanced delivery, was initiated in the USA (Duke University, NC), in 2008. The clinical trial is currently in progress for patients with recurrent primary malignant brain tumors whose tumor cells test positive for expression of EGFRvIII, as detected by immunohistochemistry. The first two patients have been treated, and approximately 20 patients are expected to accrue.

36.2.3 Chondroitin Sulfate Proteoglycans

Chondroitin sulfate proteoglycans (CSPGs) consist of a large variety of core glycosylated proteins that are covalently attached to long, unbranched polysaccharides (glycosaminoglycans), comprising sulfated glucuronic acid and N-acetyl galactosamine disaccharide unit repeats. The four major groups of CSPGs are (1) lecticans (a family including aggrecan, versican, neurocan, and brevican), (2) phosphacan/receptor-type protein–tyrosine phosphatase β, (3) small leucine-rich proteoglycans (e.g., decorin and biglycan), and (4) others including neuroglycan-C and NG2. In the normal CNS, CSPGs have a role in development and plasticity during postnatal development (Galtrey and Fawcett, 2007). Increased production of CSPGs is a well-characterized phenomenon in a variety of malignant tumors including melanoma (Touab et al., 2002), colon carcinoma (Adany et al., 1990), breast cancer (Suwiwat et al., 2004), and cervical cancer (Kodama et al., 2007). Expressions of NG2 (Chekenya et al., 1999), brevican (Viapiano et al., 2005), and versican (Paulus et al., 1996) have been demonstrated on malignant glioma and correlate with tumor grade (Chekenya et al., 1999; Schrappe et al., 1991). Thus, they are potential molecular targets for the development of antibody therapeutics.

Very few antibodies to CSPGs have been characterized to date. The very first CSPG hybridoma antibodies, Mel-5 and Mel-14, were developed at the Swiss Institute for Experimental Cancer Research (Carrel et al., 1980) following an investigation into melanoma-associated antigens. Additional studies revealed that both antibodies react with glioma cell lines (Carrel et al., 1982) and localize to subcutaneous D54MG xenografts (Wikstrand et al., 1987), warranting their continued investigation for brain-tumor diagnosis and therapy. Tumor uptake of radioiodinated Mel-14 $F(ab')_2$ into subcutaneous and intracranial xenografts out-performed the whole IgG with respect to higher tumor:normal tissue ratios in evaluation of biodistribution and radiation delivery (Colapinto et al., 1988). ^{131}I-radiolabeled Mel-14 $F(ab')_2$ has been approved by the FDA as an investigational new drug (BB-IND-3344). Phase I dose escalation studies produced encouraging results including disease stabilization (less than 50% reduction in tumor size and no clinical progression) or partial response (greater than 50% reduction in tumor size) in five of eight evaluable patients (1 with GBM, 1 with oligodendroglioma and 3 with neoplastic meningitis). Furthermore, administration of ^{131}I-Mel-14 $F(ab')_2$ into the SCRC was associated with a lack of neurotoxicity (Bigner et al., 1995). In one case, a patient with neoplastic meningitis underwent a complete clinical response following treatment with ^{131}I-Mel-14 $F(ab')_2$ (Cokgor et al., 2001). Studies are currently taking place in the USA (Duke University, NC), to further develop Mel-14 as a single-chain variable-fragment (scFv) antibody immunotherapeutic with the aim of minimizing immunogenicity while maintaining binding specificity, affinity, and localization for both Mel-14 IgG_{2a} and chimeric Mel-14 (Batra et al., 1994).

The IgG_{2a} murine monoclonal antibody 9.2.27 is another candidate being investigated by our group for the treatment of malignant brain tumors. As with Mel-14, the 9.2.27 antibody was originally identified following reactivity with a melanoma-associated glycoprotein (Morgan et al., 1981), which was further identified as a CSPG (Bumol and Reisfeld, 1982). It was shown that 9.2.27 reacts with CSPG on glioma cells and proliferating brain endothelial cells, but not with the white or grey matter from the medulla oblongata, cerebellum, or spinal cord of normal human adult (Schrappe et al., 1991). Further studies demonstrated that 9.2.27 chemo-immuno-conjugates retained full binding capacity in vitro and delayed tumor growth in human glioma xenografts for 130 days, compared to 30 and 40 days for the control and unconjugated drug, respectively (Schrappe et al., 1992). In addition, intratumoral administration of 9.2.27 IgG_2a immunotoxin delayed tumor progression and prolonged survival among rats with intracranial GBM xenografts in a study (Hjortland et al., 2004) confirming 9.2.27 immunotoxin to be a promising therapeutic for malignant glioma. Currently, we are preparing the scFv antibody from 9.2.27 hybridoma (provided by Dr. Reisfeld) and will carry out studies to determine the therapeutic properties for treatment of malignant glioma.

36.2.4 *Other Molecular Targets of Interest*

The molecular targets described earlier in this review are well characterized, and the therapeutic potential of their corresponding therapeutic antibodies is already being investigated in the clinical setting. There are a number of other molecular targets that have been identified (Table 36.3), and the following section describes those that are currently undergoing validation as potential targets for immunotherapy.

36.2.4.1 Gangliosides

Gangliosides are sialic-acid-containing glycosphingolipids found on the outer surface of most cell membranes and are concentrated within gray matter and synaptic junctions in the CNS, especially during brain development (Rodden et al., 1991). They are promising therapeutic targets for cancer therapy because all tumors exhibit aberrant ganglioside expression. Presently, ganglioside vaccination strategies are dominating clinical trials for melanoma (Chapman, 2007), small-cell lung cancer (Manjili, 2007), breast carcinoma (Diaz et al., 2003), and neuroblastoma (Modak and Cheung, 2007), targeting N-glycolyl-GM3, GD1-3, and GD2 gangliosides. However, ganglioside-based vaccination studies for malignant brain tumor therapy are in the very early stages of development. One original study demonstrated that vaccination of seven patients with recurrent or progressive gliomas with a GD2-conjugate was safe but did not elicit an immune response; accordingly no tumor regression was observed (Becker et al., 2002). The ganglioside-rich environment of the CNS prompted the initiation of studies to identify tumor-associated gangliosides with no detectable expression within the normal brain. As a result, the oncofetal gangliosides 3′-isoLM1 and 3′, 6′-isoLD1 were identified (Fredman et al., 1988), characterized (Svennerholm et al., 1989), and subsequently validated as glioma-associated antigens (Wikstrand et al., 1991). Monoclonal antibodies SL-50 and DmAb22 produced against the respective gangliosides 3′-isoLM1 and 3′,6′-isoLD1 (Wikstrand et al., 1991) have proved to be useful research tools but were never optimized for in vivo studies because of their IgM class. Currently, new immunotherapeutic antibodies with reactivity to 3′-isoLM1 and 3′,6′-isoLD1 gangliosides are being developed in the USA (Duke University, NC).

36.2.4.2 Glycoprotein Nonmetastatic Melanoma Protein B

Glycoprotein Nonmetastatic Melanoma Protein B (GPNMB) is a type I transmembrane protein that was originally identified as a potential GBM antigen by using SAGE genetic analysis (Loging et al., 2000). The human GPNMB gene encodes a predicted 560-amino-acid protein consisting of three domains, including a long extracellular domain, preceded by a signal peptide, a single

Table 36.3 Brain tumor therapeutic antibodies currently undergoing preclinical development

Molecular target	Tumor type	Antibody	Original isotype	Antibody format	Therapeutic format	Reference
Tenascin	U87 GBM	F16	–	scFv & SIP	^{125}I-labeled	Brack et al. (2006)
Tenascin	U87 GBM	P12	–	scFv & SIP	^{125}I-labeled	Brack et al. (2006)
Tenascin	U118 GBM	ST2146	IgG_{2b}	Murine mAb	^{125}I-labeled	De Santis et al. (2006)
Podoplanin	Astrocytic tumors	NZ-1	IgG_{2a}	Rat mAb	N/A	Kato et al. (2006)
Tenascin	U87 GBM	G11	–	scFv & SIP	^{125}I-labeled	Silacci et al. (2006)
Tenascin	Colon carcinoma	ST2485	IgG_1	Murine mAb	^{125}I-labeled	Petronzelli et al. (2005)
CSPG	GBM	9.2.27	IgG_{2a}	Murine mAb	Immunotoxin	Hjortland et al. (2004)
EGFRvIII	Brain melanoma	Y10	IgG_{2a}	Murine mAb	Naked	Sampson et al. (2000)
EGFRvIII	NR6M cells	MR1-1	–	dsFv	Naked	Beers et al. (2000)
EGFRvIII	U87 GBM	L8A4	IgG_1	Chimeric murine /human mAb	^{131}I-labeled	Reist et al. (1997)
EGFRvIII	Glioma	H10	IgG_1	Murine mAb	Naked	Wikstrand et al. (1995)
3'-isoLM1 Ganglioside	GBM	SL50	IgM	Murine mAb	Naked	Wikstrand et al. (1991)
3'6'-isoLD1 Ganglioside	GBM	DmAb22	IgM	Murine mAb	Naked	Wikstrand et al. (1991)
GPNMB	GBM	F6V	–		Immunotoxin	Kuan et al. (unpublished data)

scFv = single-chain variable-fragment antibody; SIP = small immunoprotein; dsFv = disulfide stabilized scFv.

transmembrane region, and a relatively short cytoplasmic domain (Kuan et al., 2006). GPNMB has been shown to correlate with tumor invasion and metastasis (Rich et al., 2001). Seventy percent of GBM patient samples were positive for *GPNMB* transcripts, and 38% of GBM tumors showed a >10-fold increase in *GPNMB* mRNA expression over normal brain (Kuan et al., 2006). Our group has developed scFv antibody F6V that targets GPNMB-expressing malignant gliomas. An F6V-immunotoxin that has been prepared by fusion to the gene encoding Pseudomonas exotoxin A (Kreitman et al., 1993) has demonstrated internalization and cytotoxicity in vitro. Studies are continuing to validate F6V scFv as an antibody-mediated immunotherapeutic (Kuan et al., unpublished data).

36.2.4.3 Multidrug Resistance Protein 3

The multidrug resistance protein (MRP) family comprises nine (MRP1-9) related ABC transporters that are able to transport structurally diverse lipophilic anions and function as drug efflux pumps. All members are structurally homologous to MRP1, a 190-kDa transmembrane protein, with MRP3 having the highest degree of structural resemblance (58%) (Kruh and Belinsky, 2003). The MRP3 transporter is involved in resistance to several anti-cancer drugs, including methotrexate, etoposide, and teniposide (Kool et al., 1999), all three of which are used for treatment of CNS neoplasms, including GBM (Bredel, 2001). Additional studies have demonstrated that MRP3 protein is not involved in resistance to taxol, anthracyclines, or mitoxantrone (Zeng et al., 1999). No publications demonstrating the relationship between the MRP3 protein and temozolomide resistance have been reported to date. MRP3 protein is highly expressed in the intestine and kidney and is also present at lower levels within the liver, bile duct, and pancreas (Scheffer et al., 2002), but not in normal brain (Nies et al., 2004). It will be important to also assess whether MRP3 might be expressed by normal stem cells. Studies have shown that MRP3 protein expression is higher in low-grade astrocytomas as compared to high-grade gliomas, medulloblastomas/primitive neuroectodermal tumors (PNETs), ependymomas, and oligodendrogliomas (Calatozzolo et al., 2005; Valera et al., 2007). Although specific MRP3 mAbs have been reported (Scheffer et al., 2000) and are available from several commercial sources, they have not currently been developed as therapeutic drugs. Our group has used phage display techniques to generate anti-MRP3 scFv antibodies that are currently being evaluated for therapeutic potential.

36.2.4.4 Podoplanin

Human podoplanin is a 36-kDa, type I transmembrane sialoglycoprotein that comprises an extracellular domain with abundant Ser and Thr residues as potential *O*-glycosylation sites, a single transmembrane portion, and a short cytoplasmic tail with putative sites for protein kinase C and cAMP phosphorylation (Kato et al., 2003). In normal human tissue, podoplanin is expressed in kidney podocytes (Breiteneder-Geleff et al., 1999), skeletal muscle, placenta, heart, lung (Martin-Villar et al., 2005), and myofibroblasts of the breast and salivary glands (Ordonez, 2006). Podoplanin is specifically expressed in the endothelium of lymphatic capillaries (Breiteneder-Geleff et al., 1999) and aggregate platelets, through interaction with a CLEC-2 (C-type lectin-like receptor 2) (Kato et al., 2008). It is putatively involved in cancer cell migration, invasion, and metastasis (Wicki et al., 2006) and is overexpressed in several neoplasms, including squamous cell carcinoma of the larynx, lung, cervix, skin, and esophagus (Kato et al., 2005); testicular seminoma (Kato et al., 2004); and mesothelioma (Kimura and Kimura, 2005). Recent work demonstrated that podoplanin is a molecular marker of malignant progression in astrocytic tumors (Mishima et al., 2006b), and further immunohistochemical analysis revealed that podoplanin expression was present on 98% (40/41) of CNS germinomas tested (Mishima et al., 2006a) and was highly expressed on numerous CNS tumors, including GBM (29/35, 82.9%), ependymoma (28/29, 96.6%), and pilocytic astrocytoma (12/12, 100%) (Shibahara et al., 2006). Several anti-podoplanin mAbs have been developed, including D2-40 (Dako) (Marks et al., 1999), gp36 (Abcam) (Zimmer et al., 1999), YM-1 (MBL) (Kaneko et al., 2004), and NZ-1 (AngioBio). (Kato et al., 2006), and have been used to investigate the identity, biological role, and incidence of podoplanin within both normal and cancerous human tissue. These antibodies have the potential to be further developed and engineered for therapeutic treatment of podoplanin-expressing tumors of the CNS.

36.2.4.5 Neural Cell Adhesion Molecule

Neural Cell Adhesion Molecule (NCAM) is a glycoprotein member of the immunoglobulin (Ig) superfamily that is considered to be a signal-transducing receptor molecule, able to modulate diverse biological properties, such as adhesion, migration, proliferation, differentiation, and synaptic plasticity (Panicker et al., 2003). A single gene encodes NCAM, but alternate splicing results in three major isoforms, whose molecular weights are 120, 140, and 180 kDa. NCAM 140 and 180 are predominantly expressed during embryonic development, whereas the glycosyl-phosphatidylinositol (GPI)-anchored 120-kDa isoform is found in many different adult tissues (Jensen and Berthold, 2007). During tumor development NCAM often undergoes an isoform switch from the adult GPI-linked 120-kDa isoform to the embryonic, transmembrane isoforms of 140 kDa or 180 kDa (Cavallaro and Christofori, 2004). All three isoforms of NCAM are expressed on early-stage astrocytic tumors, but expression of the molecule decreases with progression toward malignant glioma. In advanced glioma, the loss of NCAM correlates with a more aggressive phenotype and with poor prognosis (Sasaki et al., 1998). In contrast, NCAM is highly expressed on medulloblastoma (He et al., 1991) and other primitive neuroectodermal tumors (Molenaar et al., 1991) and is associated with cancer progression in neuroblastoma (Gluer et al., 1998). NCAM is thus a molecular target for immunotherapy of medulloblastoma and other PNETs and an indicator of tumor progression in astrocytic tumors.

36.2.4.6 Vascular Endothelial Growth Factor

The structure and expression profile of the vascular endothelial growth factor (VEGF), along with current clinical agents used to target brain-tumor vasculature, are described in Chapters 21 and 30. Malignant gliomas are remarkably angiogenic, and VEGF is the dominant pro-angiogenic factor. Recent clinical trials targeting VEGF signaling have achieved dramatic rates of durable radiographic and clinical response, while also confirming adequate safety among recurrent malignant glioma patients. Specifically, over half of heavily pretreated recurrent malignant glioma patients achieved a radiographic response following treatment with bevacizumab, a humanized VEGF mAb, combined with irinotecan, a topoisomerase-1 inhibitor. In addition, progression-free and overall survival rates were significantly increased in these patients as compared to those observed with historical salvage therapies (Vredenburgh et al., 2007a, b).

36.3 Perspective

Development of new treatments for any type of malignant glioma has been notoriously difficult. There have been only two new treatments approved by the FDA for glioblastoma in the last 30–40 years, those treatments being Gliadel (nitrosourea released with biodegradable polymers) and temozolomide. The earliest attempts at developing antibody treatments of glioma took place in the USA (Duke University, NC) under the aegis of Drs. Steven Mahaley and Eugene Day in 1965. They used polyclonal rabbit antisera to effectively image brain tumors, but the amount of uptake was so small that treatment could not be carried out. Also, the mixture of polyclonal antisera raised against glioma tissue crude-extract made it impossible to know what antigens the polyclonal antisera were detecting. With the advent of monoclonal antibody technology, new molecular targets have been identified, and new mAb treatment strategies against malignant gliomas have been developed.

At the present time, there are two monoclonal antibody treatments for glioblastoma that are in a registered trial for approval by the FDA. The most advanced is bevacizumab (Avastin®), which is a fully human antibody that neutralizes VEGF. Because it is not necessary for Avastin to cross the blood–brain barrier, it can be given systemically, and there have been very promising clinical and radiographic responses and durable survival increases observed in multi-institutional trials currently being evaluated by the FDA for approval in patients with recurrent glioblastoma multiforme. A second registration trial is currently underway with the anti-tenascin monoclonal antibody 81C6, radiolabeled with ^{131}I (Neuradiab^{TM}). This multi-institutional trial is randomized with resection-cavity-administered Neuradiab^{TM} compared to standard of care, with external beam therapy and temozolomide.

With modern genomic technology, many additional molecular targets have been identified, and there are many antibody constructs currently under development, such as those against GPNMB, CSPG, MRP3, 3′-isoLM1, and 3′,6′-isoLD1 gangliosides, and other molecular targets discussed in the body of this chapter. One might ask "Why are so many molecular targets necessary?" The answer to that lies in the innate heterogeneity of glioblastoma multiforme. There is no single molecular target that is expressed on all the cells in malignant gliomas, and although the FDA will require initial trials to be done with single agents, ultimately, a cocktail of multiple antibody constructs targeting up to three or four different molecular targets may be necessary for eradication of all cells in malignant gliomas. However, there are promising results with some constructs, such as the clinical trial with TP38, a transforming growth factor α Pseudomonas exotoxin construct, which apparently invoked a secondary immune reaction against the contents of tumor cells killed with the primary construct. Such bystander effects could have the result of greatly expanding the effects of a single molecularly targeted construct.

The necessity for carefully identifying patients whose tumors express the molecular target present is illustrated by the failure of the large multi-institutional IL-13 Pseudomonas toxin construct trial in recurrent glioblastoma patients (see trial details in Chapter 35). Although there are many potential reasons for the trial not meeting the expected endpoint of increased overall survival, it has been postulated by some that the lack of establishing eligibility for the trial with only patients whose tumors expressed the molecular target was one of the primary reasons for failure of the trial.

The difficult problem of drug delivery is likely to be overcome by using convection-enhanced delivery with multiple catheters placed either within or around a resected tumor, guided by computer algorithms in which accurate catheter placement can be made so that delivery is achieved to the target areas. A group at the University of California at San Francisco, in preclinical animal models, is also piloting a non-invasive convection approach with nasal delivery of large molecules, such as monoclonal antibodies and their different therapeutic formats.

The future looks brighter for brain-tumor patients, as together, all of these findings indicate that there is a high likelihood for a number of mAb constructs to be approved for the successful treatment of malignant gliomas in the next 5–10 years. Moreover, these approaches with mAbs will also likely be part of a multi-modality treatment of these tumors, and they will likely be used in combination with small-molecule therapeutics targeting key oncogenic pathways. Overall, these are wonderful developments and provide hope for patients with brain tumors, which have proved so difficult to treat in the past.

An exciting future area of investigation will be identifying which existing mAbs will react with brain-tumor stem cells and determining whether such cells might harbor new cancer-specific epitopes that can be exploited to design antibodies specifically targeting them. Such studies are underway in several laboratories. Such approaches will have to be taken with caution so as to not deplete normal stem cell populations in the brain and obtain cures at the cost of severe neural deficits.

36.4 Conclusion

The concept envisioned by Paul Ehrlich at the turn of the last century of specifically targeting disease with antibodies as precise "bullets" has now been implemented, and antibody-mediated therapeutics are gaining a prominent place among the next generation of targeted drugs for the treatment of neoplasia. Advances in the identification of brain-tumor-associated antigens, combined with monoclonal antibody production and engineering, have enabled potential therapeutics to be developed. These candidates are now making their way into the clinic and are providing hope for brain-tumor patients who desperately need some of the promised dream to come true. Clearly, while the translation of antibodies for cancer therapy into clinical practice is an exciting development and the fruit of decades of research, it is important to realize that these agents are no miracle cures and are yet to be integrated into a multi-modal therapy approach. The future is bright but there are still obstacles on the horizon.

Abbreviations

AA	anaplastic astrocytoma
BD	boronated polyamidoamine dendrimer
CDC	complement-dependent cytotoxicity
CDR	complementarity-determining region
CSPG	chondroitin sulfate proteoglycan
ds/scFv	disulfide-linked scFv
EGF	epidermal growth factor
EGFR	epidermal growth factor receptor
EGFRvIII	EGFR variant III
EGFRwt	EGFR wild type
FNIII	fibronectin type III
GBM	glioblastoma multiforme
GPI	glycosyl-phosphatidylinositol
GPNMB	glycoprotein nonmetastatic melanoma protein B
Ig	immunoglobulin
IV	intravenous
mAb	monoclonal antibody

MRP	multidrug resistance protein
MTD	maximum tolerated dose
NCAM	neural cell adhesion molecule
PNET	primitive neuroectodermal tumor
scFv	single-chain variable-fragment antibody
SCRC	surgically created resection cavity
SIP	small immunoprotein
TMZ	temozolomide
Tn-C	tenascin-C
VEGF	vascular endothelial growth factor
XRT	radioimmunotherapy

Acknowledgements We would like to thank Paul Walker for reading this manuscript and providing constructive comments and feedback. Also, we thank Dr. Yukinari Kato for suggesting amendments to the section describing podoplanin. The research of Dr. Bigner is supported by NINDS Grant 5P50-NS20023-25, NIH Merit Award R37 CA 011898-38, NIH SPORE Grant 5P50 CA108786-4, and a Pediatric Brain Tumor Foundation Institute Grant. Darell D. Bigner is a paid consultant or receives royalties or holds stock in Amgen, Bradmer Pharmaceuticals, and Avant.

References

Adany, R., R. Heimer, B. Caterson, J.M. Sorrell, and R.V. Iozzo. 1990. Altered expression of chondroitin sulfate proteoglycan in the stroma of human colon carcinoma. Hypomethylation of PG-40 gene correlates with increased PG-40 content and mRNA levels. *J Biol Chem*. 265:11389–96.

Agosti, R.M., M. Leuthold, W.J. Gullick, M.G. Yasargil, and O.D. Wiestler. 1992. Expression of the epidermal growth factor receptor in astrocytic tumours is specifically associated with glioblastoma multiforme. *Virchows Arch A Pathol Anat Histopathol*. 420:321–5.

Akabani, G., I. Cokgor, R.E. Coleman, D. Gonzalez Trotter, T.Z. Wong, H.S. Friedman, A.H. Friedman, A. Garcia-Turner, J.E. Herndon, D. DeLong, R.E. McLendon, X.G. Zhao, C.N. Pegram, J.M. Provenzale, D.D. Bigner, and M.R. Zalutsky. 2000. Dosimetry and dose-response relationships in newly diagnosed patients with malignant gliomas treated with iodine-131-labeled anti-tenascin monoclonal antibody 81C6 therapy. *Int J Radiat Oncol Biol Phys*. 46:947–58.

Aldape, K.D., K. Ballman, A. Furth, J.C. Buckner, C. Giannini, P.C. Burger, B.W. Scheithauer, R.B. Jenkins, and C.D. James. 2004. Immunohistochemical detection of EGFRvIII in high malignancy grade astrocytomas and evaluation of prognostic significance. *J Neuropathol Exp Neurol*. 63:700–7.

Arteaga, C.L. 2001. The epidermal growth factor receptor: from mutant oncogene in nonhuman cancers to therapeutic target in human neoplasia. *J Clin Oncol*. 19:32S–40S.

Balza, E., A. Siri, M. Ponassi, F. Caocci, A. Linnala, I. Virtanen, and L. Zardi. 1993. Production and characterization of monoclonal antibodies specific for different epitopes of human tenascin. *FEBS Lett*. 332:39–43.

Barker, F.G., 2nd, M.L. Simmons, S.M. Chang, M.D. Prados, D.A. Larson, P.K. Sneed, W.M. Wara, M.S. Berger, P. Chen, M.A. Israel, and K.D. Aldape. 2001. EGFR overexpression and radiation response in glioblastoma multiforme. *Int J Radiat Oncol Biol pyhs*. 51:410–8.

Batra, S.K., S. Castelino-Prabhu, C.J. Wikstrand, X. Zhu, P.A. Humphrey, H.S. Friedman, and D.D. Bigner. 1995. Epidermal growth factor ligand-independent, unregulated, cell-transforming potential of a naturally occurring human mutant EGFRvIII gene. *Cell Growth Differ*. 6:1251–9.

Batra, S.K., M.L. Niswonger, C.J. Wikstrand, C.N. Pegram, M.R. Zalutsky, S.L. Morrison, and D.D. Bigner. 1994. Mouse/human chimeric Mel-14 antibody: genomic cloning of the variable region genes, linkage to human constant region genes, expression, and characterization. *Hybridoma*. 13:87–97.

Becker, R., M.K. Eichler, R. Jennemann, and H. Bertalanffy. 2002. Phase I clinical trial on adjuvant active immunotherapy of human gliomas with GD2-conjugate. *Br J Neurosurg*. 16:269–75.

Beers, R., P. Chowdhury, D. Bigner, and I. Pastan. 2000. Immunotoxins with increased activity against epidermal growth factor receptor vIII-expressing cells produced by antibody phage display. *Clin Cancer Res*. 6:2835–43.

Biernat, W., H. Hung, H. Yokoo, P. Kleilues, and H. Ohgaki. 2004. Predominant expression of mutant EGFR (EGFRvIII) is rare in primary glioblastomas. *Brain Pathol*. 14:131–6.

Bigner, D.D., M. Brown, R.E. Coleman, A.H. Friedman, H.S. Friedman, R.E. McLendon, S.H. Bigner, X.G. Zhao, C.J. Wikstrand, C.N. Pegram, T. Kerby, and M.R. Zalutsky. 1995. Phase I studies of treatment of malignant gliomas and neoplastic meningitis with 131I-radiolabeled monoclonal antibodies anti-tenascin 81C6 and anti-chondroitin proteoglycan sulfate Mel-14 F (ab′)2 – a preliminary report. *J Neurooncol*. 24:109–22.

Bigner, D.D., M.T. Brown, A.H. Friedman, R.E. Coleman, G. Akabani, H.S. Friedman, W.L. Thorstad, R.E. McLendon, S.H. Bigner, X.G. Zhao, C.N. Pegram, C.J. Wikstrand, J.E. Herndon, 2nd, N.A. Vick, N. Paleologos, I. Cokgor, J.M. Provenzale, and M.R. Zalutsky. 1998a. Iodine-131-labeled antitenascin monoclonal antibody 81C6 treatment of patients with recurrent malignant gliomas: phase I trial results. *J Clin Oncol*. 16: 2202–12.

Bigner, S.H., S.K. Batra, and B.K.A. Rasheed. 1998b. Mechanisms of altered growth control. Cytogenetics, oncogenes and suppressor genes. In Russell and Rubinstein's Pathology of the Nervous System, 6th ed., pp 47–82. D.D. Bigner, R.E. McLendon, and J.M. Bruner, Eds. Arnold Publishing, London.

Borsi, L., B. Carnemolla, G. Nicolo, B. Spina, G. Tanara, and L. Zardi. 1992. Expression of different tenascin isoforms in normal, hyperplastic and neoplastic human breast tissues. *Int J Cancer*. 52:688–92.

Boulianne, G.L., N. Hozumi, and M.J. Shulman. 1984. Production of functional chimaeric mouse/human antibody. *Nature*. 312:643–6.

Bourdon, M.A., R.E. Coleman, R.G. Blasberg, D.R. Groothuis, and D.D. Bigner. 1984. Monoclonal antibody localization in subcutaneous and intracranial human glioma xenografts: paired-label and imaging analysis. *Anticancer Res*. 4:133–40.

Bourdon, M.A., C.J. Wikstrand, H. Furthmayr, T.J. Matthews, and D.D. Bigner. 1983. Human glioma-mesenchymal extracellular matrix antigen defined by monoclonal antibody. *Cancer Res*. 43:2796–805.

Brack, S.S., M. Silacci, M. Birchler, and D. Neri. 2006. Tumor-targeting properties of novel antibodies specific to the large isoform of tenascin-C. *Clin Cancer Res*. 12:3200–8.

Brechbiel, M.W. 2007. Targeted alpha-therapy: past, present, future? *Dalton Trans*: 4918–28.

Bredel, M. 2001. Anticancer drug resistance in primary human brain tumors. *Brain Res Brain Res Rev*. 35:161–204.

Breiteneder-Geleff, S., A. Soleiman, H. Kowalski, R. Horvat, G. Amann, E. Kriehuber, K. Diem, W. Weninger, E. Tschachler, K. Alitalo, and D. Kerjaschki. 1999. Angiosarcomas express mixed endothelial phenotypes of blood and lymphatic capillaries: podoplanin as a specific marker for lymphatic endothelium. *Am J Pathol*. 154:385–94.

Bumol, T.F., and R.A. Reisfeld. 1982. Unique glycoprotein-proteoglycan complex defined by monoclonal antibody on human melanoma cells. *Proc Natl Acad Sci U S A*. 79:1245–9.

Calatozzolo, C., M. Gelati, E. Ciusani, F.L. Sciacca, B. Pollo, L. Cajola, C. Marras, A. Silvani, L. Vitellaro-Zuccarello, D. Croci, A. Boiardi, and A. Salmaggi. 2005. Expression of drug resistance proteins Pgp, MRP1, MRP3, MRP5 and GST-pi in human glioma. *J Neurooncol*. 74:113–21.

Carrel, S., R.S. Accolla, A.L. Carmagnola, and J.P. Mach. 1980. Common human melanoma-associated antigen(s) detected by monoclonal antibodies. *Cancer Res.* 40:2523–8.
Carrel, S., N. de Tribolet, and J.P. Mach. 1982. Expression of neuroectodermal antigens common to melanomas, gliomas, and neuroblastomas. I. Identification by monoclonal anti-melanoma and anti- glioma antibodies. *Acta Neuropathol.* 57:158–64.
Cavallaro, U., and G. Christofori. 2004. Cell adhesion and signalling by cadherins and Ig-CAMs in cancer. *Nat Rev Cancer.* 4:118–32.
Chaffanet, M., C. Chauvin, M. Laine, F. Berger, M. Chedin, N. Rost, M.F. Nissou, and A.L. Benabid. 1992. EGF receptor amplification and expression in human brain tumours. *Eur J Cancer.* 28:11–7.
Chapman, P.B. 2007. Melanoma vaccines. *Semin Oncol.* 34:516–23.
Chekenya, M., H.K. Rooprai, D. Davies, J.M. Levine, A.M. Butt, and G.J. Pilkington. 1999. The NG2 chondroitin sulfate proteoglycan: role in malignant progression of human brain tumours. *Int J Dev Neurosci.* 17:421–35.
Cokgor, I., G. Akabani, H.S. Friedman, A.H. Friedman, M.R. Zalutsky, L.M. Zehngebot, J.M. Provenzale, C.D. Guy, C.J. Wikstrand, and D.D. Bigner. 2001. Long term response in a patient with neoplastic meningitis secondary to melanoma treated with (131)I-radiolabeled antichondroitin proteoglycan sulfate Mel-14 F(ab′)(2): a case study. *Cancer.* 91:1809–13.
Cokgor, I., G. Akabani, C.T. Kuan, H.S. Friedman, A.H. Friedman, R.E. Coleman, R.E. McLendon, S.H. Bigner, X.G. Zhao, A.M. Garcia-Turner, C.N. Pegram, C.J. Wikstrand, T.D. Shafman, J.E. Herndon, 2nd, J.M. Provenzale, M.R. Zalutsky, and D.D. Bigner. 2000. Phase I trial results of iodine-131-labeled antitenascin monoclonal antibody 81C6 treatment of patients with newly diagnosed malignant gliomas. *J Clin Oncol.* 18:3862–72.
Colapinto, E.V., P.A. Humphrey, M.R. Zalutsky, D.R. Groothuis, H.S. Friedman, N. de Tribolet, S. Carrel, and D.D. Bigner. 1988. Comparative localization of murine monoclonal antibody Me1-14 F(ab')2 fragment and whole IgG2a in human glioma xenografts. *Cancer Res.* 48:5701–7.
Combs, S.E., S. Heeger, R. Haselmann, L. Edler, J. Debus, and D. Schulz-Ertner. 2006. Treatment of primary glioblastoma multiforme with cetuximab, radiotherapy and temozolomide (GERT) – phase I/II trial: study protocol. *BMC Cancer.* 6:133.
De Santis, R., C. Albertoni, F. Petronzelli, S. Campo, V. D'Alessio, A. Rosi, A.M. Anastasi, R. Lindstedt, N. Caroni, B. Arseni, P. Chiodi, A. Verdoliva, G. Cassani, M. Chinol, G. Paganelli, and P. Carminati. 2006. Low and high tenascin-expressing tumors are efficiently targeted by ST2146 monoclonal antibody. *Clin Cancer Res.* 12:2191–6.
De Santis, R., A.M. Anastasi, V. D'Alessio, A. Pelliccia, C. Albertoni, A. Rosi, B. Leoni, R. Lindstedt, F. Petronzelli, M. Dani, A. Verdoliva, A. Ippolito, N. Campanile, V. Manfredi, A. Esposito, G. Cassani, M. Chinol, G. Paganelli, and P. Carminati. 2003. Novel antitenascin antibody with increased tumour localisation for Pretargeted Antibody-Guided RadioImmunoTherapy (PAGRIT). *Br J Cancer.* 88:996–1003.
Diaz, A., M. Alfonso, R. Alonso, G. Saurez, M. Troche, M. Catala, R.M. Diaz, R. Perez, and A.M. Vazquez. 2003. Immune responses in breast cancer patients immunized with an anti-idiotype antibody mimicking NeuGc-containing gangliosides. *Clin Immunol.* 107:80–9.
Ehrlich, P. 1906. Collected Studies on Immunity. John Wiley and Sons, New York.
Erickson, H.P., and J.L. Inglesias. 1984. A six-armed oligomer isolated from cell surface fibronectin preparations. *Nature.* 311:267–9.
Fredman, P., H. von Holst, V.P. Collins, L. Granholm, and L. Svennerholm. 1988. Sialyllactotetraosylceramide, a ganglioside marker for human malignant gliomas. *J Neurochem.* 50:912–9.
Friedlander, E., M. Barok, J. Szollosi, and G. Vereb. 2008. ErbB-directed immunotherapy: antibodies in current practice and promising new agents. *Immunol Lett.* 116:126–40.
Galtrey, C.M., and J.W. Fawcett. 2007. The role of chondroitin sulfate proteoglycans in regeneration and plasticity in the central nervous system. *Brain Res Rev.* 54:1–18.

Garcia de Palazzo, I.E., G.P. Adams, P. Sundareshan, A.J. Wong, J.R. Testa, D.D. Bigner, and L.M. Weiner. 1993. Expression of mutated epidermal growth factor receptor by non-small cell lung carcinomas. *Cancer Res.* 53:3217–20.

Gluer, S., M. Zense, E. Radtke, and D. von Schweinitz. 1998. Polysialylated neural cell adhesion molecule in childhood ganglioneuroma and neuroblastoma of different histological grade and clinical stage. *Langenbecks Arch Surg.* 383:340–4.

Goetz, C., P. Riva, G. Poepperl, F.J. Gildehaus, A. Hischa, K. Tatsch, and H.J. Reulen. 2003. Locoregional radioimmunotherapy in selected patients with malignant glioma: experiences, side effects and survival times. *J Neurooncol.* 62:321–8.

Goodin, S. 2008. Development of monoclonal antibodies for the treatment of colorectal cancer. *Am J Health Syst Pharm.* 65:S3–7; quiz S22–4.

Green, L.L., M.C. Hardy, C.E. Maynard-Currie, H. Tsuda, D.M. Louie, M.J. Mendez, H. Abderrahim, M. Noguchi, D.H. Smith, Y. Zeng, N.E. David, H. Sasai, D. Garza, D.G. Brenner, J.F. Hales, R.P. McGuinness, D.J. Capon, S. Klapholz, and A. Jakobovits. 1994. Antigen-specific human monoclonal antibodies from mice engineered with human Ig heavy and light chain YACs. *Nat Genet.* 7:13–21.

Gronski, P., F.R. Seiler, and H.G. Schwick. 1991. Discovery of antitoxins and development of antibody preparations for clinical uses from 1890 to 1990. *Mol Immunol.* 28:1321–32.

Gulcher, J.R., D.E. Nies, M.J. Alexakos, N.A. Ravikant, M.E. Sturgill, L.S. Marton, and K. Stefansson. 1991. Structure of the human hexabrachion (tenascin) gene. *Proc Natl Acad Sci U S A.* 88:9438–42.

Gulcher, J.R., D.E. Nies, L.S. Marton, and K. Stefansson. 1989. An alternatively spliced region of the human hexabrachion contains a repeat of potential N-glycosylation sites. *Proc Natl Acad Sci U S A.* 86:1588–92.

He, X.M., C.J. Wikstrand, H.S. Friedman, S.H. Bigner, S. Pleasure, J.Q. Trojanowski, and D.D. Bigner. 1991. Differentiation characteristics of newly established medulloblastoma cell lines (D384 Med, D425 Med, and D458 Med) and their transplantable xenografts. *Lab Invest.* 64:833–43.

Herbst, R.S., and D.M. Shin. 2002. Monoclonal antibodies to target epidermal growth factor receptor-positive tumors: a new paradigm for cancer therapy. *Cancer.* 94:1593–611.

Herold-Mende, C., M.M. Mueller, M.M. Bonsanto, H.P. Schmitt, S. Kunze, and H.H. Steiner. 2002. Clinical impact and functional aspects of tenascin-C expression during glioma progression. *Int J Cancer.* 98:362–9.

Hindermann, W., A. Berndt, L. Borsi, X. Luo, P. Hyckel, D. Katenkamp, and H. Kosmehl. 1999. Synthesis and protein distribution of the unspliced large tenascin-C isoform in oral squamous cell carcinoma. *J Pathol.* 189:475–80.

Hjortland, G.O., S.S. Garman-Vik, S. Juell, O.E. Olsen, H. Hirschberg, O. Fodstad, and O. Engebraaten. 2004. Immunotoxin treatment targeted to the high-molecular-weight melanoma-associated antigen prolonging the survival of immunodeficient rats with invasive intracranial human glioblastoma multiforme. *J Neurosurg.* 100:320–7.

Hopkins, K., C. Chandler, J. Bullimore, D. Sandeman, H. Coakham, and J.T. Kemshead. 1995. A pilot study of the treatment of patients with recurrent malignant gliomas with intratumoral yttrium-90 radioimmunoconjugates. *Radiother Oncol.* 34:121–31.

Ilmonen, S., T. Jahkola, J.P. Turunen, T. Muhonen, and S. Asko-Seljavaara. 2004. Tenascin-C in primary malignant melanoma of the skin. *Histopathology.* 45:405–11.

Jensen, M., and F. Berthold. 2007. Targeting the neural cell adhesion molecule in cancer. *Cancer Lett.* 258:9–21.

Jones, F.S., and P.L. Jones. 2000a. The tenascin family of ECM glycoproteins: structure, function, and regulation during embryonic development and tissue remodeling. *Dev Dyn.* 218:235–59.

Jones, P.L., and F.S. Jones. 2000b. Tenascin-C in development and disease: gene regulation and cell function. *Matrix Biol.* 19:581–96.

Jones, P.T., P.H. Dear, J. Foote, M.S. Neuberger, and G. Winter. 1986. Replacing the complementarity-determining regions in a human antibody with those from a mouse. *Nature.* 321:522–5.

Kaneko, M., Y. Kato, A. Kunita, N. Fujita, T. Tsuruo, and M. Osawa. 2004. Functional sialylated O-glycan to platelet aggregation on Aggrus (T1alpha/podoplanin) molecules expressed in Chinese hamster ovary cells. *J Biol Chem*. 279:38838–43.

Kantha, S.S. 1991. A centennial review; the 1890 tetanus antitoxin paper of von Behring and Kitasato and the related developments. *Keio J Med*. 40:35–9.

Katenkamp, K., A. Berndt, W. Hindermann, H. Wunderlich, K.M. Haas, L. Borsi, L. Zardi, and H. Kosmehl. 2004. mRNA expression and protein distribution of the unspliced tenascin-C isoform in prostatic adenocarcinoma. *J Pathol*. 203:771–9.

Kato, Y., N. Fujita, A. Kunita, S. Sato, M. Kaneko, M. Osawa, and T. Tsuruo. 2003. Molecular identification of Aggrus/T1alpha as a platelet aggregation-inducing factor expressed in colorectal tumors. *J Biol Chem*. 278:51599–605.

Kato, Y., M. Kaneko, M. Sata, N. Fujita, T. Tsuruo, and M. Osawa. 2005. Enhanced expression of Aggrus (T1alpha/ podoplanin), a platelet-aggregation-inducing factor in lung squamous cell carcinoma. *Tumour Biol*. 26:195–200.

Kato, Y., M.K. Kaneko, A. Kunita, H. Ito, A. Kameyama, S. Ogasawara, N. Matsuura, Y. Hasegawa, K. Suzuki-Inoue, O. Inoue, Y. Ozaki, and H. Narimatsu. 2008. Molecular analysis of the pathophysiological binding of the platelet aggregation-inducing factor podoplanin to the C-type lectin-like receptor CLEC-2. *Cancer Sci*. 99:54–61.

Kato, Y., M.K. Kaneko, A. Kuno, N. Uchiyama, K. Amano, Y. Chiba, Y. Hasegawa, J. Hirabayashi, H. Narimatsu, K. Mishima, and M. Osawa. 2006. Inhibition of tumor cell-induced platelet aggregation using a novel anti-podoplanin antibody reacting with its platelet-aggregation-stimulating domain. *Biochem Biophys Res Commun*. 349:1301–7.

Kato, Y., I. Sasagawa, M. Kaneko, M. Osawa, N. Fujita, and T. Tsuruo. 2004. Aggrus: a diagnostic marker that distinguishes seminoma from embryonal carcinoma in testicular germ cell tumors. *Oncogene*. 23:8552–6.

Kemshead, J.T., L.S. Lashford, D.H. Jones, and H.B. Coakham. 1987. Diagnosis and therapy of neuroectodermally associated tumours using targeted radiation. *Dev Neurosci*. 9:69–83.

Kimura, N., and I. Kimura. 2005. Podoplanin as a marker for mesothelioma. *Pathol Int*. 55:83–6.

Kodama, J., Hasengaowa, T. Kusumoto, N. Seki, T. Matsuo, K. Nakamura, A. Hongo, and Y. Hiramatsu. 2007. Versican expression in human cervical cancer. *Eur J Cancer*. 43:1460–6.

Kohler, G., and C. Milstein. 1975. Continuous cultures of fused cells secreting antibody of predefined specificity. *Nature*. 256:495–7.

Kool, M., M. van der Linden, M. de Haas, G.L. Scheffer, J.M. de Vree, A.J. Smith, G. Jansen, G.J. Peters, N. Ponne, R.J. Scheper, R.P. Elferink, F. Baas, and P. Borst. 1999. MRP3, an organic anion transporter able to transport anti-cancer drugs. *Proc Natl Acad Sci U S A*. 96:6914–9.

Krebs, B., R. Rauchenberger, S. Reiffert, C. Rothe, M. Tesar, E. Thomassen, M. Cao, T. Dreier, D. Fischer, A. Hoss, L. Inge, A. Knappik, M. Marget, P. Pack, X.Q. Meng, R. Schier, P. Sohlemann, J. Winter, J. Wolle, and T. Kretzschmar. 2001. High-throughput generation and engineering of recombinant human antibodies. *J Immunol Methods*. 254:67–84.

Kreitman, R.J., J.K. Batra, S. Seetharam, V.K. Chaudhary, D.J. FitzGerald, and I. Pastan. 1993. Single-chain immunotoxin fusions between anti-Tac and Pseudomonas exotoxin: relative importance of the two toxin disulfide bonds. *Bioconjug Chem*. 4:112–20.

Kruh, G.D., and M.G. Belinsky. 2003. The MRP family of drug efflux pumps. *Oncogene*. 22:7537–52.

Kuan, C.T., K. Wakiya, J.M. Dowell, J.E. Herndon, 2nd, D.A. Reardon, M.W. Graner, G.J. Riggins, C.J. Wikstrand, and D.D. Bigner. 2006. Glycoprotein nonmetastatic melanoma protein B, a potential molecular therapeutic target in patients with glioblastoma multiforme. *Clin Cancer Res*. 12:1970–82.

Kuan, C.T., C.J. Wikstrand, G. Archer, R. Beers, I. Pastan, M.R. Zalutsky, and D.D. Bigner. 2000. Increased binding affinity enhances targeting of glioma xenografts by EGFRvIII-specific scFv. *Int J Cancer*. 88:962–9.

Kuan, C.T., C.J. Wikstrand, and D.D. Bigner. 2001. EGF mutant receptor vIII as a molecular target in cancer therapy. *Endocr Relat Cancer*. 8:83–96.
Kusagawa, H., K. Onoda, S. Namikawa, I. Yada, A. Okada, T. Yoshida, and T. Sakakura. 1998. Expression and degeneration of tenascin-C in human lung cancers. *Br J Cancer*. 77:98–102.
Lal, A., C.A. Glazer, H.M. Martinson, H.S. Friedman, G.E. Archer, J.H. Sampson, and G.J. Riggins. 2002. Mutant epidermal growth factor receptor up-regulates molecular effectors of tumor invasion. *Cancer Res*. 62:3335–9.
Lee, Y., D.E. Bullard, P.A. Humphrey, E.V. Colapinto, H.S. Friedman, M.R. Zalutsky, R.E. Coleman, and D.D. Bigner. 1988a. Treatment of intracranial human glioma xenografts with 131I-labeled anti-tenascin monoclonal antibody 81C6. *Cancer Res*. 48:2904–10.
Lee, Y.S., D.E. Bullard, C.J. Wikstrand, M.R. Zalutsky, L.H. Muhlbaier, and D.D. Bigner. 1987. Comparison of monoclonal antibody delivery to intracranial glioma xenografts by intravenous and intracarotid administration. *Cancer Res*. 47:1941–6.
Lee, Y.S., D.E. Bullard, M.R. Zalutsky, R.E. Coleman, C.J. Wikstrand, H.S. Friedman, E.V. Colapinto, and D.D. Bigner. 1988b. Therapeutic efficacy of antiglioma mesenchymal extracellular matrix 131I-radiolabeled murine monoclonal antibody in a human glioma xenograft model. *Cancer Res*. 48:559–66.
Liu, L., L.M. Backlund, B.R. Nilsson, D. Grander, K. Ichimura, H.M. Goike, and V.P. Collins. 2005. Clinical significance of EGFR amplification and the aberrant EGFRvIII transcript in conventionally treated astrocytic gliomas. *J Mol Med*. 83:917–26.
Loging, W.T., A. Lal, I.M. Siu, T.L. Loney, C.J. Wikstrand, M.A. Marra, C. Prange, D.D. Bigner, R.L. Strausberg, and G.J. Riggins. 2000. Identifying potential tumor markers and antigens by database mining and rapid expression screening. *Genome Res*. 10:1393–402.
Lorimer, I.A., A. Keppler-Hafkemeyer, R.A. Beers, C.N. Pegram, D.D. Bigner, and I. Pastan. 1996. Recombinant immunotoxins specific for a mutant epidermal growth factor receptor: targeting with a single chain antibody variable domain isolated by phage display. *Proc Natl Acad Sci U S A*. 93:14815–20.
Lorimer, I.A., C.J. Wikstrand, S.K. Batra, D.D. Bigner, and I. Pastan. 1995. Immunotoxins that target an oncogenic mutant epidermal growth factor receptor expressed in human tumors. *Clin Cancer Res*. 1:859–64.
Manjili, M.H. 2007. Come forth 1E10 anti-idiotype vaccine: delivering the promise to immunotherapy of small cell lung cancer. *Cancer Biol Ther*. 6:151–2.
Marks, A., D.R. Sutherland, D. Bailey, J. Iglesias, J. Law, M. Lei, H. Yeger, D. Banerjee, and R. Baumal. 1999. Characterization and distribution of an oncofetal antigen (M2A antigen) expressed on testicular germ cell tumours. *Br J Cancer*. 80:569–78.
Martin-Villar, E., F.G. Scholl, C. Gamallo, M.M. Yurrita, M. Munoz-Guerra, J. Cruces, and M. Quintanilla. 2005. Characterization of human PA2.26 antigen (T1alpha-2, podoplanin), a small membrane mucin induced in oral squamous cell carcinomas. *Int J Cancer*. 113:899–910.
McCafferty, J., A.D. Griffiths, G. Winter, and D.J. Chiswell. 1990. Phage antibodies: filamentous phage displaying antibody variable domains. *Nature*. 348:552–4.
Messa, C., F. Russo, M.G. Caruso, and A. Di Leo. 1998. EGF, TGF-alpha, and EGF-R in human colorectal adenocarcinoma. *Acta Oncol*. 37:285–9.
Mishima, K., Y. Kato, M.K. Kaneko, Y. Nakazawa, A. Kunita, N. Fujita, T. Tsuruo, R. Nishikawa, T. Hirose, and M. Matsutani. 2006a. Podoplanin expression in primary central nervous system germ cell tumors: a useful histological marker for the diagnosis of germinoma. *Acta Neuropathol*. 111:563–8.
Mishima, K., Y. Kato, M.K. Kaneko, R. Nishikawa, T. Hirose, and M. Matsutani. 2006b. Increased expression of podoplanin in malignant astrocytic tumors as a novel molecular marker of malignant progression. *Acta Neuropathol*. 111:483–8.
Modak, S., and N.K. Cheung. 2007. Disialoganglioside directed immunotherapy of neuroblastoma. *Cancer Invest*. 25:67–77.

Molenaar, W.M., L. de Leij, and J.Q. Trojanowski. 1991. Neuroectodermal tumors of the peripheral and the central nervous system share neuroendocrine N-CAM-related antigens with small cell lung carcinomas. *Acta Neuropathol.* 83:46–54.

Morgan, A.C., Jr., D.R. Galloway, and R.A. Reisfeld. 1981. Production and characterization of monoclonal antibody to a melanoma specific glycoprotein. *Hybridoma.* 1:27–36.

Morrison, S.L., M.J. Johnson, L.A. Herzenberg, and V.T. Oi. 1984. Chimeric human antibody molecules: mouse antigen-binding domains with human constant region domains. *Proc Natl Acad Sci U S A.* 81:6851–5.

Nagane, M., F. Coufal, H. Lin, O. Bogler, W.K. Cavenee, and H.J. Huang. 1996. A common mutant epidermal growth factor receptor confers enhanced tumorigenicity on human glioblastoma cells by increasing proliferation and reducing apoptosis. *Cancer Res.* 56:5079–86.

Narita, Y., M. Nagane, K. Mishima, H.J. Huang, F.B. Furnari, and W.K. Cavenee. 2002. Mutant epidermal growth factor receptor signaling down-regulates p27 through activation of the phosphatidylinositol 3-kinase/Akt pathway in glioblastomas. *Cancer Res.* 62:6764–9.

Nies, A.T., G. Jedlitschky, J. Konig, C. Herold-Mende, H.H. Steiner, H.P. Schmitt, and D. Keppler. 2004. Expression and immunolocalization of the multidrug resistance proteins, MRP1–MRP6 (ABCC1–ABCC6), in human brain. *Neuroscience.* 129:349–60.

Nishikawa, R., X.D. Ji, R.C. Harmon, C.S. Lazar, G.N. Gill, W.K. Cavenee, and H.J. Huang. 1994. A mutant epidermal growth factor receptor common in human glioma confers enhanced tumorigenicity. *Proc Natl Acad Sci U S A.* 91:7727–31.

Nishikawa, R., T. Sugiyama, Y. Narita, F. Furnari, W.K. Cavenee, and M. Matsutani. 2004. Immunohistochemical analysis of the mutant epidermal growth factor, deltaEGFR, in glioblastoma. *Brain Tumor Pathol.* 21:53–6.

Ochiai, H., G.E. Archer, J.E. Herndon, 2nd, C.T. Kuan, D.A. Mitchell, D.D. Bigner, I.H. Pastan, and J.H. Sampson. 2008. EGFRvIII-targeted immunotoxin induces antitumor immunity that is inhibited in the absence of CD4+ and CD8+ T cells. *Cancer Immunol Immunother.* 57:115–21.

Okamoto, I., L.C. Kenyon, D.R. Emlet, T. Mori, J. Sasaki, S. Hirosako, Y. Ichikawa, H. Kishi, A.K. Godwin, M. Yoshioka, M. Suga, M. Matsumoto, and A.J. Wong. 2003. Expression of constitutively activated EGFRvIII in non-small cell lung cancer. *Cancer Sci.* 94:50–6.

Ordonez, N.G. 2006. Podoplanin: a novel diagnostic immunohistochemical marker. *Adv Anat Pathol.* 13:83–8.

Panicker, A.K., M. Buhusi, K. Thelen, and P.F. Maness. 2003. Cellular signalling mechanisms of neural cell adhesion molecules. *Front Biosci.* 8:d900–11.

Papanastassiou, V., B.L. Pizer, H.B. Coakham, J. Bullimore, T. Zananiri, and J.T. Kemshead. 1993. Treatment of recurrent and cystic malignant gliomas by a single intracavity injection of 131I monoclonal antibody: feasibility, pharmacokinetics and dosimetry. *Br J Cancer.* 67:144–51.

Paulus, W., I. Baur, M.T. Dours-Zimmermann, and D.R. Zimmermann. 1996. Differential expression of versican isoforms in brain tumors. *J Neuropathol Exp Neurol.* 55:528–33.

Pelloski, C.E., K.V. Ballman, A.F. Furth, L. Zhang, E. Lin, E.P. Sulman, K. Bhat, J.M. McDonald, W.K. Yung, H. Colman, S.Y. Woo, A.B. Heimberger, D. Suki, M.D. Prados, S.M. Chang, F.G. Barker, 2nd, J.C. Buckner, C.D. James, and K. Aldape. 2007. Epidermal growth factor receptor variant III status defines clinically distinct subtypes of glioblastoma. *J Clin Oncol.* 25:2288–94.

Petronzelli, F., A. Pelliccia, A.M. Anastasi, V. D'Alessio, C. Albertoni, A. Rosi, B. Leoni, C. De Angelis, G. Paganelli, G. Palombo, M. Dani, P. Carminati, and R. De Santis. 2005. Improved tumor targeting by combined use of two antitenascin antibodies. *Clin Cancer Res.* 11:7137s-7145s.

Raju, T.N. 2000. The Nobel chronicles. 1984: Niels Kai Jerne, (1911–94); Cesar Milstein (b 1926); and Georges Jean Franz Kohler (1946–95). *Lancet.* 355:75.

Ramos, T.C., J. Figueredo, M. Catala, S. Gonzalez, J.C. Selva, T.M. Cruz, C. Toledo, S. Silva, Y. Pestano, M. Ramos, I. Leonard, O. Torres, P. Marinello, R. Perez, and A. Lage. 2006. Treatment of high-grade glioma patients with the humanized anti-epidermal growth factor receptor (EGFR) antibody h-R3: report from a phase I/II trial. *Cancer Biol Ther*. 5:375–9.

Reardon, D.A., G. Akabani, R.E. Coleman, A.H. Friedman, H.S. Friedman, J.E. Herndon, 2nd, I. Cokgor, R.E. McLendon, C.N. Pegram, J.M. Provenzale, J.A. Quinn, J.N. Rich, L.V. Regalado, J.H. Sampson, T.D. Shafman, C.J. Wikstrand, T.Z. Wong, X.G. Zhao, M.R. Zalutsky, and D.D. Bigner. 2002. Phase II trial of murine (131)I-labeled antitenascin monoclonal antibody 81C6 administered into surgically created resection cavities of patients with newly diagnosed malignant gliomas. *J Clin Oncol*. 20:1389–97.

Reardon, D.A., M.R. Zalutsky, G. Akabani, R.E. Coleman, A.H. Friedman, J.E. Herndon, 2nd, R.E. McLendon, C.N. Pegram, J.A. Quinn, J.N. Rich, J.J. Vredenburgh, A. Desjardins, S. Guruangan, S. Boulton, R.H. Raynor, J.M. Dowell, T.Z. Wong, X.G. Zhao, H.S. Friedman, and D.D. Bigner. 2008. A pilot study: 131I-antitenascin monoclonal antibody 81c6 to deliver a 44-Gy resection cavity boost. *Neuro Oncol*. 10:182–9.

Reist, C.J., G.E. Archer, S.N. Kurpad, C.J. Wikstrand, G. Vaidyanathan, M.C. Willingham, D.K. Moscatello, A.J. Wong, D.D. Bigner, and M.R. Zalutsky. 1995. Tumor-specific anti-epidermal growth factor receptor variant III monoclonal antibodies: use of the tyramine-cellobiose radioiodination method enhances cellular retention and uptake in tumor xenografts. *Cancer Res*. 55:4375–82.

Reist, C.J., S.K. Batra, C.N. Pegram, D.D. Bigner, and M.R. Zalutsky. 1997. In vitro and in vivo behavior of radiolabeled chimeric anti-EGFRvIII monoclonal antibody: comparison with its murine parent. *Nucl Med Biol*. 24:639–47.

Rich, J.N., C. Guo, R.E. McLendon, D.D. Bigner, X.F. Wang, and C.M. Counter. 2001. A genetically tractable model of human glioma formation. *Cancer Res*. 61:3556–60.

Riechmann, L., M. Clark, H. Waldmann, and G. Winter. 1988. Reshaping human antibodies for therapy. *Nature*. 332:323–7.

Riva, P., A. Arista, G. Franceschi, M. Frattarelli, C. Sturiale, N. Riva, M. Casi, and R. Rossitti. 1995. Local treatment of malignant gliomas by direct infusion of specific monoclonal antibodies labeled with 131I: comparison of the results obtained in recurrent and newly diagnosed tumors. *Cancer Res*. 55:5952s–5956s.

Riva, P., G. Franceschi, M. Frattarelli, N. Riva, G. Guiducci, A.M. Cremonini, G. Giuliani, M. Casi, R. Gentile, A.A. Jekunen, and K.J. Kairemo. 1999. 131I radioconjugated antibodies for the locoregional radioimmunotherapy of high-grade malignant glioma – phase I and II study. *Acta Oncol*. 38:351–9.

Riva, P., G. Franceschi, N. Riva, M. Casi, M. Santimaria, and M. Adamo. 2000. Role of nuclear medicine in the treatment of malignant gliomas: the locoregional radioimmunotherapy approach. *Eur J Nucl Med*. 27:601–9.

Rodden, F.A., H. Wiegandt, and B.L. Bauer. 1991. Gangliosides: the relevance of current research to neurosurgery. *J Neurosurg*. 74:606–19.

Sampson, J.H., L.E. Crotty, S. Lee, G.E. Archer, D.M. Ashley, C.J. Wikstrand, L.P. Hale, C. Small, G. Dranoff, A.H. Friedman, H.S. Friedman, and D.D. Bigner. 2000. Unarmed, tumor-specific monoclonal antibody effectively treats brain tumors. *Proc Natl Acad Sci USA*. 97:7503–8.

Santini, J., J.L. Formento, M. Francoual, G. Milano, M. Schneider, O. Dassonville, and F. Demard. 1991. Characterization, quantification, and potential clinical value of the epidermal growth factor receptor in head and neck squamous cell carcinomas. *Head Neck*. 13:132–9.

Sasaki, H., K. Yoshida, E. Ikeda, H. Asou, M. Inaba, M. Otani, and T. Kawase. 1998. Expression of the neural cell adhesion molecule in astrocytic tumors: an inverse correlation with malignancy. *Cancer*. 82:1921–31.

Scheffer, G.L., M. Kool, M. de Haas, J.M. de Vree, A.C. Pijnenborg, D.K. Bosman, R.P. Elferink, P. van der Valk, P. Borst, and R.J. Scheper. 2002. Tissue distribution and induction of human multidrug resistant protein 3. *Lab Invest*. 82:193–201.

Scheffer, G.L., M. Kool, M. Heijn, M. de Haas, A.C. Pijnenborg, J. Wijnholds, A. van Helvoort, M.C. de Jong, J.H. Hooijberg, C.A. Mol, M. van der Linden, J.M. de Vree, P. van der Valk, R.P. Elferink, P. Borst, and R.J. Scheper. 2000. Specific detection of multidrug resistance proteins MRP1, MRP2, MRP3, MRP5, and MDR3 P-glycoprotein with a panel of monoclonal antibodies. *Cancer Res.* 60:5269–77.

Schold, S.C., Jr., M.R. Zalutsky, R.E. Coleman, M.J. Glantz, A.H. Friedman, R.J. Jaszczak, S.H. Bigner, and D.D. Bigner. 1993. Distribution and dosimetry of I-123-labeled monoclonal antibody 81C6 in patients with anaplastic glioma. *Invest Radiol.* 28:488–96.

Schrama, D., R.A. Reisfeld, and J.C. Becker. 2006. Antibody targeted drugs as cancer therapeutics. *Nat Rev Drug Discov.* 5:147–59.

Schrappe, M., T.F. Bumol, L.D. Apelgren, S.L. Briggs, G.A. Koppel, D.D. Markowitz, B.M. Mueller, and R.A. Reisfeld. 1992. Long-term growth suppression of human glioma xenografts by chemoimmunoconjugates of 4-desacetylvinblastine-3-carboxyhydrazide and monoclonal antibody 9.2.27. *Cancer Res.* 52:3838–44.

Schrappe, M., F.G. Klier, R.C. Spiro, T.A. Waltz, R.A. Reisfeld, and C.L. Gladson. 1991. Correlation of chondroitin sulfate proteoglycan expression on proliferating brain capillary endothelial cells with the malignant phenotype of astroglial cells. *Cancer Res.* 51:4986–93.

Shankar, S., G. Vaidyanathan, C.T. Kuan, D.D. Bigner, and M.R. Zalutsky. 2006. Anti-epidermal growth factor variant III scFv fragment: effect of radioiodination method on tumor targeting and normal tissue clearance. *Nucl Med Biol.* 33:101–10.

Shawler, D.L., R.M. Bartholomew, L.M. Smith, and R.O. Dillman. 1985. Human immune response to multiple injections of murine monoclonal IgG. *J Immunol.* 135:1530–5.

Shibahara, J., T. Kashima, Y. Kikuchi, A. Kunita, and M. Fukayama. 2006. Podoplanin is expressed in subsets of tumors of the central nervous system. *Virchows Arch.* 448:493–9.

Shin, D.M., J.Y. Ro, W.K. Hong, and W.N. Hittelman. 1994. Dysregulation of epidermal growth factor receptor expression in premalignant lesions during head and neck tumorigenesis. *Cancer Res.* 54:3153–9.

Silacci, M., S.S. Brack, N. Spath, A. Buck, S. Hillinger, S. Arni, W. Weder, L. Zardi, and D. Neri. 2006. Human monoclonal antibodies to domain C of tenascin-C selectively target solid tumors in vivo. *Protein Eng Des Sel.* 19:471–8.

Siri, A., B. Carnemolla, M. Saginati, A. Leprini, G. Casari, F. Baralle, and L. Zardi. 1991. Human tenascin: primary structure, pre-mRNA splicing patterns and localization of the epitopes recognized by two monoclonal antibodies. *Nucleic Acids Res.* 19:525–31.

Smith, G.P. 1985. Filamentous fusion phage: novel expression vectors that display cloned antigens on the virion surface. *Science.* 228:1315–7.

Sok, J.C., F.M. Coppelli, S.M. Thomas, M.N. Lango, S. Xi, J.L. Hunt, M.L. Freilino, M.W. Graner, C.J. Wikstrand, D.D. Bigner, W.E. Gooding, F.B. Furnari, and J.R. Grandis. 2006. Mutant epidermal growth factor receptor (EGFRvIII) contributes to head and neck cancer growth and resistance to EGFR targeting. *Clin Cancer Res.* 12:5064–73.

Stupp, R., W.P. Mason, M.J. van den Bent, M. Weller, B. Fisher, M.J. Taphoorn, K. Belanger, A.A. Brandes, C. Marosi, U. Bogdahn, J. Curschmann, R.C. Janzer, S.K. Ludwin, T. Gorlia, A. Allgeier, D. Lacombe, J.G. Cairncross, E. Eisenhauer, and R.O. Mirimanoff. 2005. Radiotherapy plus concomitant and adjuvant temozolomide for glioblastoma. *N Engl J Med.* 352:987–96.

Suwiwat, S., C. Ricciardelli, R. Tammi, M. Tammi, P. Auvinen, V.M. Kosma, R.G. LeBaron, W.A. Raymond, W.D. Tilley, and D.J. Horsfall. 2004. Expression of extracellular matrix components versican, chondroitin sulfate, tenascin, and hyaluronan, and their association with disease outcome in node-negative breast cancer. *Clin Cancer Res.* 10: 2491–8.

Svennerholm, L., K. Bostrom, P. Fredman, J.E. Mansson, B. Rosengren, and B.M. Rynmark. 1989. Human brain gangliosides: developmental changes from early fetal stage to advanced age. *Biochim Biophys Acta.* 1005:109–17.

Touab, M., J. Villena, C. Barranco, M. Arumi-Uria, and A. Bassols. 2002. Versican is differentially expressed in human melanoma and may play a role in tumor development. *Am J Pathol.* 160:549–57.

Valera, E.T., A.K. Lucio-Eterovic, L. Neder, C.A. Scrideli, H.R. Machado, C.G. Carlotti-Junior, R.G. Queiroz, F.J. Motta, and L.G. Tone. 2007. Quantitative PCR analysis of the expression profile of genes related to multiple drug resistance in tumors of the central nervous system. *J Neurooncol.* 85:1–10.

Ventimiglia, J.B., C.J. Wikstrand, L.E. Ostrowski, M.A. Bourdon, V.A. Lightner, and D.D. Bigner. 1992. Tenascin expression in human glioma cell lines and normal tissues. *J Neuroimmunol.* 36:41–55.

Viapiano, M.S., W.L. Bi, J. Piepmeier, S. Hockfield, and R.T. Matthews. 2005. Novel tumor-specific isoforms of BEHAB/brevican identified in human malignant gliomas. *Cancer Res.* 65:6726–33.

Vredenburgh, J.J., A. Desjardins, J.E. Herndon, 2nd, J.M. Dowell, D.A. Reardon, J.A. Quinn, J.N. Rich, S. Sathornsumetee, S. Gururangan, M. Wagner, D.D. Bigner, A.H. Friedman, and H.S. Friedman. 2007a. Phase II trial of bevacizumab and irinotecan in recurrent malignant glioma. *Clin Cancer Res.* 13:1253–9.

Vredenburgh, J.J., A. Desjardins, J.E. Herndon, 2nd, J. Marcello, D.A. Reardon, J.A. Quinn, J.N. Rich, S. Sathornsumetee, S. Gururangan, J. Sampson, M. Wagner, L. Bailey, D.D. Bigner, A.H. Friedman, and H.S. Friedman. 2007b. Bevacizumab plus irinotecan in recurrent glioblastoma multiforme. *J Clin Oncol.* 25:4722–9.

Wicki, A., F. Lehembre, N. Wick, B. Hantusch, D. Kerjaschki, and G. Christofori. 2006. Tumor invasion in the absence of epithelial-mesenchymal transition: podoplanin-mediated remodeling of the actin cytoskeleton. *Cancer Cell.* 9:261–72.

Wikstrand, C.J., and D.D. Bigner. 2009. Constitutive activation of truncated EGF receptors in glioblastoma. Chapter 19 in EGFR Signaling Networks in Cancer Therapy (Series: Cancer Drug Discovery and Development), J.D. Haley and W.J. Gullick, Eds. Springer-Humana, Totowa, New Jersey.

Wikstrand, C.J., K.M. Fung, J.Q. Trojanowski, R.E. McLendon, and D.D. Bigner. 1998a. Antibodies and molecular immunology: Immunohistochemistry and antigens of diagnostic significance. *In* Russell and Rubinstein's Pathology of the Nervous System. D.D. Bigner, R. E. McLendon and J.M. Bruner, Eds. Oxford University Press, New York. 251–304.

Wikstrand, C.J., L.P. Hale, S.K. Batra, M.L. Hill, P.A. Humphrey, S.N. Kurpad, R.E. McLendon, D. Moscatello, C.N. Pegram, C.J. Reist, S.T. Traweek, A.J. Wong, M.R. Zalutsky, and D.D. Bigner. 1995. Monoclonal antibodies against EGFRvIII are tumor specific and react with breast and lung carcinomas and malignant gliomas. *Cancer Res.* 55:3140–8.

Wikstrand, C.J., X.M. He, G.N. Fuller, S.H. Bigner, P. Fredman, L. Svennerholm, and D.D. Bigner. 1991. Occurrence of lacto series gangliosides 3′-isoLM1 and 3′,6′-isoLD1 in human gliomas in vitro and in vivo. *J Neuropathol Exp Neurol.* 50:756–69.

Wikstrand, C.J., R.E. McLendon, S. Carrel, J.T. Kemshead, J.P. Mach, H.B. Coakham, N. de Tribolet, D.E. Bullard, M.R. Zalutsky, and D.D. Bigner. 1987. Comparative localization of glioma-reactive monoclonal antibodies in vivo in an athymic mouse human glioma xenograft model. *J Neuroimmunol.* 15:37–56.

Wikstrand, C.J., R.E. McLendon, A.H. Friedman, and D.D. Bigner. 1997. Cell surface localization and density of the tumor-associated variant of the epidermal growth factor receptor, EGFRvIII. *Cancer Res.* 57:4130–40.

Wikstrand, C.J., C.J. Reist, G.E. Archer, M.R. Zalutsky, and D.D. Bigner. 1998b. The class III variant of the epidermal growth factor receptor (EGFRvIII): characterization and utilization as an immunotherapeutic target. *J Neurovirol.* 4:148–58.

Wikstrand, C.J., M.R. Zalutsky, and D.D. Bigner. 2001. Radiolabeled antibodies for therapy of brain tumors. *In* Brain Tumor Immunotherapy. L.M. Liau, D.P. Becker, T.F. Cloughesy, and D.D. Bigner. Eds. Humana Press, Totowa, NJ, USA.

Yang, W., G. Wu, R.F. Barth, M.R. Swindall, A.K. Bandyopadhyaya, W. Tjarks, K. Tordoff, M. Moeschberger, T.J. Sferra, P.J. Binns, K.J. Riley, M.J. Ciesielski, R.A. Fenstermaker, and C.J. Wikstrand. 2008. Molecular targeting and treatment of composite EGFR and EGFRvIII-positive gliomas using boronated monoclonal antibodies. *Clin Cancer Res*. 14:883–91.

Yu, H., X. Gong, X. Luo, W. Han, G. Hong, B. Singh, and C.K. Tang. 2008. Co-expression of EGFRvIII with ErbB-2 enhances tumorigenesis: EGFRvIII mediated constitutively activated and sustained signaling pathways, whereas EGF-induced a transient effect on EGFR-mediated signaling pathways. *Cancer Biol Ther*. 7:1818–28.

Zagzag, D., D.R. Friedlander, D.C. Miller, J. Dosik, J. Cangiarella, M. Kostianovsky, H. Cohen, M. Grumet, and M.A. Greco. 1995. Tenascin expression in astrocytomas correlates with angiogenesis. *Cancer Res*. 55:907–14.

Zalutsky, M.R., R.P. Moseley, J.C. Benjamin, E.V. Colapinto, G.N. Fuller, H.P. Coakham, and D.D. Bigner. 1990. Monoclonal antibody and F(ab')2 fragment delivery to tumor in patients with glioma: comparison of intracarotid and intravenous administration. *Cancer Res*. 50:4105–10.

Zalutsky, M.R., R.P. Moseley, H.B. Coakham, R.E. Coleman, and D.D. Bigner. 1989. Pharmacokinetics and tumor localization of 131I-labeled anti-tenascin monoclonal antibody 81C6 in patients with gliomas and other intracranial malignancies. *Cancer Res*. 49:2807–13.

Zalutsky, M.R., D.A. Reardon, O.R. Pozzi, G. Vaidyanathan, and D.D. Bigner. 2007. Targeted alpha-particle radiotherapy with 211At-labeled monoclonal antibodies. *Nucl Med Biol*. 34:779–85.

Zeng, H., L.J. Bain, M.G. Belinsky, and G.D. Kruh. 1999. Expression of multidrug resistance protein-3 (multispecific organic anion transporter-D) in human embryonic kidney 293 cells confers resistance to anticancer agents. *Cancer Res*. 59:5964–7.

Zimmer, G., F. Oeffner, V. Von Messling, T. Tschernig, H.J. Groness, H.D. Klenk, and G. Herrler. 1999. Cloning and characterization of gp36, a human mucin-type glycoprotein preferentially expressed in vascular endothelium. *Biochem J*. 341 (Pt 2):277–84.

Chapter 37
Stat3 Oncogenic Signaling in Glioblastoma Multiforme

Saikh Jaharul Haque and Pankaj Sharma

Abstract Glioblastoma multiforme (GBM) is the most common and devastating malignancy of the central nervous system. Many growth factor and cytokine signaling pathways are deregulated in GBM, which aberrantly activate the signal transducer and the activator of transcription (Stat)3. Activated Stat3, in turn, exhibits a number of protumor activities that include induction of proliferation and suppression of programmed death of GBM cells, induction of tumor angiogenesis, and suppression of antitumor immunity. Paradoxically, it also acts as a tumor suppressor presumably by inducing the differentiation of GBM-initiating stem cells. In this review, we discuss these roles of activated Stat3 in the pathogenesis of GBM.

Contents

S.J. Haque (✉)
Department of Cancer Biology, Lerner Research Institute; Brain Tumor and Neuro-Oncology Center, Division of Neurosciences, Cleveland Clinic, Cleveland, OH 44195, USA
e-mail: haquej@ccf.org

E.G. Van Meir (ed.), *CNS Cancer*, Cancer Drug Discovery and Development, DOI 10.1007/978-1-60327-553-8_37,
© Humana Press, a part of Springer Science+Business Media, LLC 2009

37.1 Introduction

Stat proteins execute dual functions in the cell: transduction of cytokine and growth factor signals from plasma membrane to the nucleus and subsequent transcriptional activation of cognate genes (Darnell, 1997; Haque and Sharma, 2006; Stark et al., 1998). Mammalian genomes encode seven Stats (Stat1 through Stat4, Stat5A, Stat5B, and Stat6) which are differentially activated by a variety of cytokines and growth factors (Darnell, 1997). Stat3 was initially identified as an IL-6 inducible acute phase response factor that binds to the promoters of hepatic acute phase protein-encoding genes (Wegenka et al., 1993). The *Stat3* cDNA was subsequently cloned from both mouse (Akira et al., 1994; Zhong et al., 1994) and humans (Yoshimura et al., 1995). While mice deficient in other Stats are viable, deletion of *Stat3* in mice leads to embryonic lethality at E6.5–7.5 (Akira, 1999; Takeda et al., 1997), underscoring its essential, non-redundant functions during development.

Stat3 shares a striking amino acid sequence homology with other Stats except at its carboxy-terminal region (Darnell, 1997). Stat3 has three alternatively spliced variants. The longest form, Stat3a, contains 770 amino acids, while another variant lacks a segment in the 5' UTR, and three nucleotides within the Stat3a coding region resulting in a protein of 769 amino acids. The shortest variant, Stat3b, is due to a 50 bp deletion and consequent frame-shift in the transcript, encoding a protein with 722 amino acids and a unique 7-amino acid carboxy-terminus (Schaefer et al., 1995). Stat3a and Stat3b have unique and specific functions, as revealed by specific deletion of individual isoforms (Maritano et al., 2004). Stat3a, however, remains the predominantly expressed isoform. Hereafter, Stat3a will be referred to as Stat3, unless otherwise mentioned.

Like other Stats, Stat3 contains a number of modular domains (Fig. 37.1). Stat3 has an amino-terminal oligomerization domain, followed by a coiled-coil domain likely involved in nuclear translocation, a DNA-binding domain critical for binding to cognate DNA sequences ($TTN_{4/5}AA$), and a short linker region of unknown function. Adjacent to the linker is an SH2 domain responsible for the dimerization of $tyrosine_{705}$-phosphorylated Stat3 molecules, which is mediated by an intermolecular interaction between the SH2 domain of one Stat3 molecule and the phospho-$tyrosine_{705}$ residue located in the short tail region immediately following the SH2 domain of another Stat3 molecule (Darnell, 1997). This is followed by the carboxy-terminal transactivation domain involved in the transcriptional activation of Stat3-responsive genes.

Stat3 is ubiquitously expressed in mammalian cells in a latent form and activated by the IL-6 family cytokines that include IL-6 itself, ciliary neurotrophic factor (CNTF), oncostatin M (OSM), and leukemia inhibitory factor (LIF) and by a variety of growth factors including epidermal growth factor (EGF), transforming growth factor (TGF)-α, and platelet-derived growth factor (PDGF) (Darnell et al., 1994; Haque and Sharma, 2006; Heinrich et al., 1998; Zhong et al., 1994). Phosphorylation of $tyrosine_{705}$ is essential for Stat3

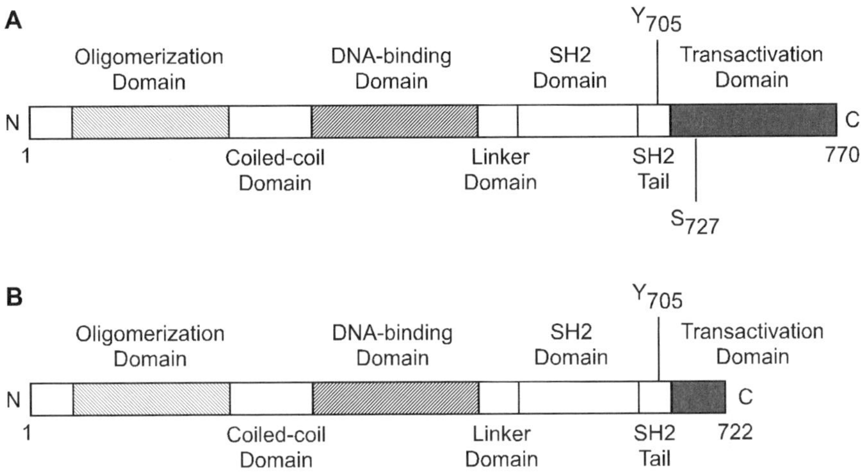

Fig. 37.1 Schematic representation of Stat3 structure and functional domains. (**A**) Stat3a is a 91 kDa protein comprised of 770 amino acids. It interacts with other proteins (including Stat3 itself) via the N-terminal oligomerization domain that is followed by the coiled-coil domain. The DNA-binding domain that recognizes the cognate DNA sequences is followed by a short linker region of unknown function. The SH2 domain and its short tail containing a conserved tyrosine residue (at position 705) are responsible for Stat3 activation, and the C-terminal transactivation domain (including the conserved serine residue at position 727) facilitates the transcription of Stat3-responsive genes. (**B**) Stat3b is an 86 kDa protein comprised of 722 amino acids. It results from an alternatively spliced transcript with a 50 bp deletion and consequent frame-shift. Compared with Stat3a, Stat3b has unique seven amino acids in its C-terminal transactivation domain that lacks the conserved serine residue at position 727 in Stat3a

activation (Zhong et al., 1994). Since the receptors of the IL-6 family cytokines do not possess intrinsic tyrosine kinase activity, members of the Janus family of tyrosine kinases including Jak1, Jak2, and Tyk2 associate with the receptors and phosphorylate Stat3 (Haque and Sharma, 2006; Heinrich et al., 1998). A canonical Jak-Stat pathway that activates Stat3 in response to IL-6 stimulation is illustrated in Fig. 37.2.

Stat3 activation and consequent gene activation are transient in normal cells (Haque et al., 2000; Haque and Sharma, 2006). However, persistent activation of Stat3 is detected in a variety of human cancers including GBM (Catlett-Falcone et al., 1999; Garcia and Jove, 1998; Rahaman et al., 2002a). The objective of this chapter is to draw a comprehensive portrait that reflects our current understanding of the roles of activated Stat3 in the pathogenesis of GBM.

37.2 Biology of Malignant Gliomas

Malignant gliomas are the most common primary tumors of the central nervous system (Holland, 2000; Kleihues et al., 1993; Maher et al., 2001; Weissenberger et al., 1997). Patients with GBM, the most malignant form (WHO grade IV), live

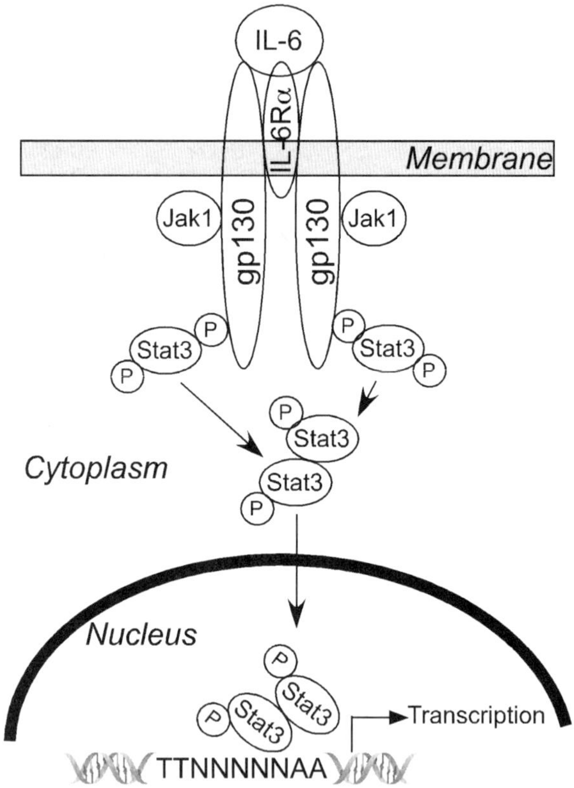

Fig. 37.2 A canonical pathway of Stat3 activation. Binding of IL-6 to its high-affinity receptor IL-6Rα recruits two molecules of gp130, a transmembrane-signaling receptor, which are constitutively associated with the tyrosine kinase Jak1. The two Jak1 molecules trans-phosphorylate each other which is followed by phosphorylation of the gp130 molecules on multiple tyrosine residues in its cytoplasmic region. Stat3 docks on the gp130 molecules by binding to these phosphotyrosine residues via its SH2 domain and is phosphorylated (on Y_{705}) by Jak1. It is then released from gp130 and forms a dimer with another Y_{705}-phosphorylated Stat3 molecule. The Stat3-dimer translocates to the nucleus where it binds to cognate DNA sequences located in the promoters of Stat3-responsive genes via its DNA-binding domain and activates their transcription through its transactivation domain

on an average less than 1 year despite surgery, radiation, and chemotherapy (Maher et al., 2001). There are two categories of GBM tumors: the de novo or primary GBM that arises spontaneously and the progressive or secondary GBM that progresses from low-grade tumors (Maher et al., 2001). Primary and secondary GBMs have distinct and overlapping genetic alterations, although pathologically the two groups are indistinguishable (Maher et al., 2001). Both categories of GBM are highly proliferative, aggressively invasive, and invariably angiogenic in character (Maher et al., 2001).

37.3 Activated Stat3 Acts as an Oncoprotein

Enhanced activation of Stat3 in Src-transformed cells was first reported in 1995 by Richard Jove's laboratory, raising the possibility that Stat3 may contribute to Src-induced carcinogenesis (Yu et al., 1995). Of note, one of the first mouse models for astrocytoma was based on astrocyte-specific overexpression of v-Src (Weissenberger et al., 1997) that induced an activation of Stat3 (Weissenberger et al., 2004). Subsequent studies from this laboratory have shown that a number of human tumor-derived cell lines contain constitutively activated Stat3, providing a growth advantage to cancer cells (Catlett-Falcone et al., 1999; Garcia and Jove, 1998). In 1999, Bromberg and Darnell reported that a constitutively active Stat3 engineered by substitution of two cysteine residues within the carboxy-terminal loop of the SH2 domain induced the oncogenic transformation of immortalized fibroblasts, as assessed by colony formation in soft agar and tumor formation in immune-compromised mice, underscoring the significance of constitutive Stat3 activation in human tumors (Bromberg et al., 1999).

37.4 Stat3 Signaling Is Activated in GBM and Other Brain Tumors

Initial studies have found that in a number of human brain tumors including astrocytoma, anaplastic astrocytoma, GBM, medulloblastoma, ependymoma, and meningioma, steady-state levels of Stat3 protein are higher than those in control peritumoral brain tissues (Cattaneo et al., 1998; Magrassi et al., 1999). Previously a number of studies have shown that GBM cells secrete IL-6 and/or respond to it (Goswami et al., 1998; Rolhion et al., 2001; Tchirkov et al., 2001; Van Meir et al., 1990). However, little was known about IL-6-dependent signal transduction and subsequent gene expression in the pathogenesis of GBM. Subsequently, over 90% of GBM tumors and all GBM-derived cell lines examined have been found to contain high levels of constitutively activated Stat3 compared with normal astrocytes cultured in vitro, white matter derived from epilepsy patients, and normal brain tissues adjacent to tumors (Rahaman et al., 2002a). In fact, the frequency of aberrant, constitutive activation of Stat3 is one of the highest among the molecules frequently deregulated in GBM (Furnari et al., 2007; Maher et al., 2001; Rahaman et al., 2002a; Shervington et al., 2006; Wechsler-Reya and Scott, 2001) (Table 37.1). These observations raise an obvious question: How does Stat3 become activated in GBM cells?

Some GBM cell lines like U251MG express both IL-6 and functional IL-6 receptor, supporting an autocrine activation of Stat3 which is blocked by incubation of cells with IL-6 neutralizing antibodies (Rahaman et al., 2002a). In contrast, others (U87MG and D54MG) do not express the IL-6 receptor, but show Stat3 activation in response to autocrine EGF and TGF-α signaling (Ghosh et al., 2005). Further, a number of glioma cell lines express the receptors for the IL-6 family cytokines OSM and LIF, and Stat1, Stat3, and Stat5B are

Table 37.1 Frequency of different molecular alterations in GBM

Molecular alterations	Frequency (%)	References
Activation of Stat3	94	Rahaman et al. (2002a)
Overexpression of c-Myc	80	Shervington et al. (2006)
Activation of EGFR	45	TCGA (2008)
Activation of CDK4	14	Parsons et al. (2008)
Amplification of MDM2	14	TCGA (2008)
Inactivation of p16	52	TCGA (2008)
Inactivation of ARF	49	TCGA (2008)
Inactivation of PTEN	36	TCGA (2008)
Inactivation of p53	55	Parsons et al. (2008)
Inactivation of Rb	14	Parsons et al. (2008)

activated in these cell lines by OSM, and at least in part by LIF, in an autocrine manner (Halfter et al., 2000a). Surprisingly, IL-4, which normally activates Stat6 in almost all cell types including normal astrocytes, does not activate Stat6 but Stat3 in several GBM cell lines. Fibroblast growth factor (FGF) also is found to further activate Stat3 in C6 rat glioma cell line (Cuevas et al., 2006). Recent genomic analyses reveal that a number of receptor tyrosine kinases (RTKs) including EGFR, ERBB2, PDGFRA, and MET are activated in GBM (TCGA, 2008; Parsons et al., 2008). These RTKs are known to induce Stat3 activation in a variety of normal and cancer cells (Cramer et al., 2005; Ghosh et al., 2005; Wang et al., 2000; Yuan et al., 2008).

37.5 Activated Stat3 Induces Proliferation and Survival of GBM Cells

Stat3 has been found persistently activated in bone marrow mononuclear cells of patients with multiple myeloma. In an IL-6-dependent human myeloma cell line U266, Stat3 contributes to the pathogenesis of multiple myeloma by inducing the expression of the prosurvival protein Bcl-$_{XL}$, thereby preventing their spontaneous apoptosis (Catlett-Falcone et al., 1999). In agreement with these studies, Stat3 is found to bind to the promoter of the *Bcl-$_X$* gene as well as to the promoters of two other *Bcl-2* family antiapoptotic genes, *Bcl-2* itself and *Mcl-1* (Rahaman et al., 2005). Treatment of U251MG cells with Jak inhibitor AG490 significantly reduces the activation of Stat3 and induces spontaneous apoptosis with a concomitant reduction in the steady-state levels of Bcl-2, Bcl-$_{XL}$, and Mcl-1. Moreover, expression of a dominant negative mutant Stat3 (DN-Stat3) protein or treatment with AG490 markedly reduces the proliferation of U251MG cells by inhibiting the constitutive activation of Stat3 (Rahaman et al., 2002a). In D54MG and U87MG cell lines, suppression of EGFR-activated Stat3 by PD153035 or AG1478 reduces the expression of Mcl-1 but not Bcl-2 or Bcl-$_{XL}$ (Ghosh et al., 2005). IL-4 inhibits the proliferation of cells derived from human normal cortex and low-grade gliomas but not high-grade tumors, which is associated with cyclin-dependent kinase inhibitor (CDKI) p21-dependent elevation of the expression of another CDKI, p27 (Liu et al., 2000). Interestingly, we have found that IL-4-activated Stat3 provides the growth advantage of GBM cells (Rahaman et al., 2002b; Rahaman et al., 2005). The aberrant activation of Stat3 is likely mediated by the tumor antigen IL-13Rα2 (Rahaman et al., 2002b) expressed in anaplastic astrocytoma and GBM but not normal astrocytes or low-grade astrocytoma (Joshi et al., 2000). IL-13Rα2 was initially identified as a high-affinity decoy receptor for IL-13 in renal cell carcinoma cell lines and subsequently was detected in high grades of malignant gliomas but not normal astrocytes or low-grade gliomas (see also Chapter 35). Of note, IL-13Rα2 is a high-affinity IL-13-binding transmembrane protein that acts as a decoy receptor for IL-13 and inhibits IL-4-dependent Stat6 activation in GBM and other cells (Rahaman et al., 2002b, 2005). FGF causes activation of Stat3 in a variety of cells (Deo et al., 2002; Udayakumar et al., 2002). Dobesilate, a synthetic inhibitor of FGF, blocks Stat3 activation in C6 glioma cells concomitant with the inhibition of cyclin D1 and Bcl-$_{XL}$ expression, suggesting that activated Stat3 induces proliferation and suppresses spontaneous apoptosis of these GBM cells (Cuevas et al., 2006). An AG490-related compound WP1066 is found to be a more effective inducer of apoptosis of GBM cells in vitro and in vivo in mice; it activates Bax and inhibits the expression of Myc and Bcl-$_{XL}$ (Iwamaru et al., 2007). Moreover, RNAi-mediated inhibition of Stat3 expression induces

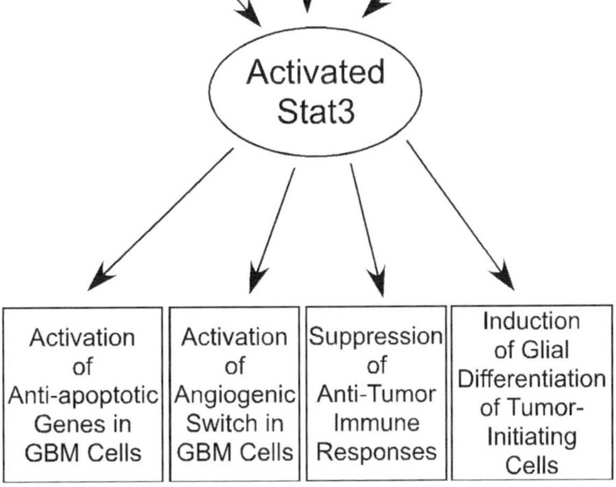

Fig. 37.3 Roles of Stat3 in GBM. Stat3 is activated in GBM by multiple cytokines and growth factors. In GBM, activated Stat3 plays tumor-promoting roles by (i) inducing the transcription of prosurvival genes in tumor cells, (ii) activating the neo-angiogenesis in GBM tumor tissue, and (iii) suppressing antitumor immune responses. Paradoxically, Stat3 also acts as a tumor suppressor in GBM by inducing the differentiation of tumor-initiating cells to the astrocytic lineage

apoptosis in a number of GBM cell lines (Konnikova et al., 2003; Ren et al., 2008). Telomere 3' overhang-specific DNA oligonucleotide that inhibits proliferation of GBM cells (presumably by mimicking telomere loop disruption) is found to induce non-apoptotic, autophagic cell death concomitant with the inhibition of Stat3- and mTOR signaling (Aoki et al., 2007; Yokoyama et al., 2007). Interestingly, retinoic acid (at low concentrations: 0.01–1.0 μM) is also found to induce Stat3 activation and proliferation of a human glioblastoma cell line, GL-15 (Paillaud et al., 2002). Taken together, these studies reveal that Stat3 is the converging point for a variety of cytokines and growth factor-activated signaling pathways, and plays critical roles in promoting the proliferation and survival of GBM cells (Fig. 37.3).

37.6 Proangiogenic Activity of Stat3 in GBM

Outgrowth of GBM tumors is associated with hypoxia, necrosis, and neoangiogenesis (Brat and Van Meir, 2004; Rong et al., 2006) (see also Chapter 22). The mechanisms leading to the occurrence of large areas of necrosis in GBM are not completely understood, but may be linked to the tumor outgrowing its blood supply. Micronecrotic areas surrounded by pseudo-palisading cells are a characteristic of a subset of GBM (Brat and Van Meir, 2004; Rong et al., 2006) and may occur in part due to vaso-occlusion caused by intravascular thrombosis and/or angiopoietin-2-mediated apoptosis of endothelial cells of the intratumoral blood vessels (Bergers and Benjamin, 2003; Brat and Van Meir, 2004; Holash et al., 1999). Hypoxia acts as a major inducer of proangiogenic genes (Bergers and Benjamin, 2003; Naumov et al., 2006). Hypoxia-induced gene expression is mediated by hypoxia-inducible factor (HIF), a helix–loop–helix transcription factor made of a heterodimer of α and β subunits. The HIF-dimer binds to the hypoxia-responsive element (HRE) located in the enhancers of a variety of hypoxia-regulated genes and activates transcription (Bergers and Benjamin, 2003; Fong, 2008; Harris, 2002). HIF activates the expression of over 100 genes which control a variety of biological mechanisms that ensure cell survival under hypoxia. One of these encodes vascular endothelial growth factor (VEGF), a major proangiogenic mediator in GBM and other tumors (Fischer et al., 2005; Plate et al., 1992; Shweiki et al., 1992).

Stat3 has been implicated in the transcription of *VEGF* in a variety of cancer cells (Gray et al., 2005; Jung et al., 2005; Niu et al., 2002; Xu et al., 2005b). In malignant glioma and medulloblastoma, Stat3 activation is persistent in endothelial cells of intratumoral blood vessels, which is likely the result of paracrine activation of VEGFR2 signaling following secretion of VEGF by tumor cells in response to hypoxia and other factors (Schaefer et al., 2002). Cytokines such as OSM and IL-6 are produced by glioma cells and both can induce VEGF production by the tumor (Loeffler et al., 2005; Repovic et al., 2003). IL-6 also activates *VEGF* transcription in normal astrocytes and GBM cells via a direct physical interaction between Stat3 and Sp1. This study shows that there is no functional Stat3-binding site in the *VEGF* promoter and that the Sp1–Stat3 complex occupies the GC-boxes in the promoter (Loeffler et al., 2005).

Because Stat3 and HIF can cooperate in the activation of *VEGF*, we have expressed DN-Stat3 in U87MG cell line in a hypoxia/HIF-1-inducible manner using a bidirectional expression vector (Post and Van Meir, 2001) and found that DN-Stat3 reduces U87MG-derived tumor volume by inhibiting tumor cell survival as well as tumor angiogenesis, suggesting that Stat3 activation is required by hypoxic U87MG cells to suppress apoptosis and induce neo-angiogenesis. Furthermore, persistent activation of Stat3 is upregulated by hypoxia, which in turn induces the transcription of the *VEGF* gene in U87MG cells (Dasgupta et al., 2008). These studies suggest that activated Stat3 acts as a potent inducer of neo-angiogenesis in GBM tumors.

37.7 Immune Suppression by Stat3 in GBM

Malignant glioma patients as well as rodents bearing experimental gliomas suffer from the suppression of cell-mediated and humoral arms of both systemic and local immunity (Cserr and Knopf, 1992; Gordon et al., 1997; Roszman et al., 1991). This may largely be attributable to the production of immune-suppressant molecules including TGF-β2, prostaglandin E2, and IL-10 by GBM cells (Benedetti et al., 1999; Giezeman-Smits et al., 2000; Hishii et al., 1995). Of note, IL-10 activates Stat3 in a variety of immune cells leading to the expression of genes responsible for antitumor immune responses (Yu et al., 2007). Therefore, growth of malignant gliomas is privileged by the immune-compromised microenvironments of the tumor. This notion is supported by the results of an international population-based case–control study which reveals an inverse association between gliomas and allergic diseases that result from aberrant activation of the immune system (Schlehofer et al., 1999). In consistence with this study, several immune-modulating cytokines including IL-2, IL-4, IL-12, and granulocyte monocytes colony-stimulating factor (GM-CSF) have been shown to induce antitumor immune responses in glioma-bearing rodents (Benedetti et al., 2000; Bennett et al., 1997; Dey et al., 2006; Iwadate et al., 2001; Jean et al., 2004) .

Recently, WP1066, a novel inhibitor of Stat3 is found to reverse systemic tolerance of immune cells isolated from human GBM patients. WP1066 enhances the expression of co-stimulatory molecules on peripheral macrophages and tumor-infiltrating microglia and induces the production of cytokines like IL-2, IL-4, IL-12, and IL-15 by macrophages, which stimulate T-cell effector functions (Hussain et al., 2007). Systemic administration of another Stat3 inhibitor, JSI-124, to mice-bearing syngenic GL261 glioma in the brain promotes antitumor activities of tumor-infiltrating immune cells by inducing the production of CXCL-10 and IL-15. This leads to an enhanced efficacy of the adoptive transfer therapy of type 1 cytotoxic T lymphocytes in these GL261 glioma-bearing mice (Fujita et al., 2008). Collectively, these findings clearly indicate that activated Stat3 acts as an immune suppressor in malignant gliomas.

37.8 Antitumor Activity of Stat3 in GBM

There is now compelling evidence that virtually every cancer is derived from a single cell; therefore, all neoplastic cells in a cancer tissue, including GBM, represent the progeny of that cell. Thus, a given tumor tissue is comprised of a population of cancer cells which are homogenous with respect to the genetic alterations that have transformed the cell in which the tumor is initiated. Therefore, in accordance with the stochastic model, each cancer cell in a tumor tissue should be able to initiate a new tumor when implanted into an appropriate host, like immune-suppressed rodents (Dick, 2003). In reality, however, a single cancer cell is unable to initiate a tumor in vivo; about a million cancer cells are required for new tumor initiation in immune-compromised rodents (Dick, 2003). Studies have suggested that a cancer cell must acquire a mitogenic signal to enter the cell cycle and divide, which are the first criteria to initiate a new tumor (Hanahan and Weinberg, 2000). However, mitogenic signals also induce either spontaneous apoptosis or death receptor-mediated apoptosis (Green and Evan, 2002). Therefore, the tumor-initiating cell must need survival signals along with the mitogenic signals (Hanahan and Weinberg, 2000).

The third signal a cell must acquire to initiate a tumor is an antidifferentiation or de-differentiation signal that confers the 'stemness' (stem cell properties) to the tumor-initiating cell (Blau et al., 2001; Gurdon, 2006; Gurdon et al., 2003; Gurdon et al., 2005). This is consistent with the emerging cancer stem cell hypothesis that growth of cancers including GBM is maintained not by the major population of cancer cells which are differentiated, but by a minor population of cancer cells called 'cancer stem cells' which possess stem cell-like properties (Bao et al., 2006; Gilbertson and Rich, 2007; Singh et al., 2004a; Singh et al., 2003; Singh et al., 2004b).

In the developing brain, neural progenitor cells (NPCs), also called neural stem cells (NSCs), differentiate into neurons, astrocytes, and oligodendrocytes (Temple, 2001). Recent studies have shown that FGF2-activated Stat3 is required to maintain the undifferentiated state of NPCs, and this is mediated by Stat3-dependent expression of Notch ligand Delta-like1; consistently, conditional deletion of Stat3 in NPCs promotes neuronal differentiation (Yoshimatsu et al., 2006). On the other hand, Stat3 activated by the IL-6 family of cytokines in collaboration with the bone morphogenetic protein (BMP) family-activated

Smad1–Smad4 complex induces astrocytic differentiation of NPCs (Nakashima et al., 1999; Taga and Fukuda, 2005). Another report claims that OSM induces growth inhibition and the astrocytic differentiation of GBM cells, which are not significantly blocked by the expression of a dominant negative mutant Stat3 protein, suggesting that activated Stat3 may not be required for the differentiation of GBM cells (Halfter et al., 2000b). However, overexpression of DN-Stat3 in the C6 rat glioma cell line results in the suppression of c-AMP-induced IL-6-mediated differentiation as revealed by the repression of *glial fibrillary acidic protein (GFAP)* promoter activity, suggesting that Stat3 activation is required for the differentiation of C6 cells (Takanaga et al., 2004). Therefore, the role of activated Stat3 in the differentiation of GBM cells remains unclear, although it is established that Stat3 activation is required for the astrocytic differentiation of normal NPCs (Nakashima et al., 1999).

A recent study shows that BMP- and CNTF-mediated astrocytic differentiation is compromised by enhancer of zeste homolog (EZH2)-dependent epigenetic silencing of the BMP receptor 1B gene in a subset of GBM-initiating cells (Lee et al., 2008). It is apparent from these studies that Stat3 plays multiple roles in CNS development as well as in brain tumor formation. On the one hand, Stat3 maintains the pluripotency of NPCs by inducing the Notch signaling pathway (Yoshimatsu et al., 2006); on the other hand, Stat3 in cooperation with Smad1–Smad4 complex induces glial differentiation (Nakashima et al., 1999), thereby acting as a tumor suppressor. In agreement with this notion, activation of AKT due to loss of PTEN function results in the phosphorylation and inactivation of FOXO3, leading to an inhibition of FOXO3-dependent expression of LIFRβ. This in turn compromises the LIF-mediated activation of Stat3 and subsequent astrocytic differentiation of NPCs (de la Iglesia et al., 2008b). These authors have further shown that Stat3 forms a complex with mutant EGFR (EGFRvIII) in the nucleus and acts as an oncoprotein in gliomagenesis (de la Iglesia et al., 2008b). In a recent report, activated Stat3 was shown to occupy the *IL-8* promoter and suppress its activation suggesting that Stat3 may also inhibit angiogenesis under some circumstances (de la Iglesia et al., 2008a).

Although the findings discussed above suggest that activated Stat3 may play a role in the differentiation of GBM-initiating cells, further genetic and epigenetic studies are necessary for unfolding the role of activated Stat3 as a tumor suppressor in GBM.

37.9 Physiologic and Pharmacologic Inhibitors of Stat3

Under normal physiological conditions, Stat3 activation is limited in both duration and magnitude by a variety of negative regulators acting at different steps in the signaling pathways through distinct mechanisms (Haque and Sharma, 2006). The protein inhibitors of activated Stats (PIAS) family proteins are identified as inhibitors of Stat binding to DNA. PIAS3 is shown to specifically block the DNA-binding activity of Stat3 (Chung et al., 1997). Reduced expression of PIAS3 is found in a variety of human cancers including GBM (Wang and Banerjee, 2004). A recent study has shown that PIAS3 is expressed at significantly lower levels in GBM compared with control brain tissues. Moreover, overexpression and silencing of the PIAS3 gene reveal that PIS3 expression inversely correlates with the proliferation of GBM cells (Brantley et al., 2008).

We have found that DN-Stat3, in which $tyrosine_{705}$ is replaced by phenylalanine, inhibits the proliferation and induces apoptosis of U87MG and U251MG cells, by compromising the constitutive activation of endogenous Stat3 (Ghosh et al., 2005; Rahaman et al., 2002a). The Jak inhibitor AG490 inhibits Stat3 activation in U251MG cells but not in U87MG cells in which Stat3 activation is inhibited by EGFR inhibitors PD153035 and AG1478 (Ghosh et al., 2005; Rahaman et al., 2002a). The *c-Fos* promoter contains an enhancer element that binds to activated Stat3 (Wagner et al., 1990). Transfection of U251MG and A172 cells with a 15-mer oligonucleotide duplex encompassing the Stat3-binding site significantly inhibits Stat3 activation (Gu et al., 2008). Further, treatment of these cells with JSI-124, an inhibitor of Jak/Stat3 pathway, causes a marked reduction of Stat3 activation (Su et al., 2008). JSI-124 also induces apoptosis in both medulloblastoma and glioblastoma cells and sensitizes the cells to conventional chemotherapeutic agents (Lo et al., 2008). Another recent study finds that treatment of GBM cells with purified peptide aptamers markedly compromises constitutive activation of Stat3 (Borghouts et al., 2008). Suppression of Stat3 expression by RNAi and subsequent induction of apoptosis are demonstrated in a number of GBM cell lines (Konnikova et al., 2003; Ren et al., 2008).

Aberrant activation of Stat3 is found in a variety of cancers including GBM which contribute to the expression of genes involved in cancer cell proliferation and survival, induction of tumor angiogenesis, and suppression of immune surveillance (Yu and Jove, 2004). Based on these findings, Stat3 can be considered as an ideal target for cancer therapy (Darnell, 2002; Yu and Jove, 2004). To this end, different strategies for targeting Stat3 in a variety of cancers have been evaluated in a recent review (Al Zaid Siddiquee and Turkson, 2008). Because Stat3 is activated by growth factor receptor intrinsic or cytokine receptor-associated tyrosine kinases, antagonizing receptor function and targeting the relevant kinase(s) are promising strategies that have been validated in a number of cancers (Kamath and Buolamwini, 2006; Xu et al., 2005a). Further, direct inhibition of Stat3 function such as interference of physical interactions of Stat3 with other proteins (including itself) or DNA by small molecules is an ideal strategy (Darnell, 2002). Phase I clinical trials of ZD 1839, an inhibitor of EGFR in head and neck squamous carcinoma, gastric and breast adenocarcinoma (Albanell et al., 2001), and non-small cell lung cancer (Han et al., 2005), have used the reduction of Stat3 activation (among others) as a surrogate marker for monitoring the drug efficacy.

37.10 Perspectives

A large number of intracellular signaling pathways activated by a variety of extracellular signaling molecules including cytokines and growth factors converge to a limited number of transcription factors that induce the expression of specific sets of intracellular and secretary proteins which execute many essential cellular and physiological functions in higher organisms (Haque and Sharma, 2006). Stat3 is one of these transcription factors whose deficiency leads to embryonic lethality (Takeda et al., 1997), and in GBM, Stat3 is aberrantly activated by multiple, deregulated intracellular signaling pathways and activates genes that are essentially involved in tumor promotion as well as tumor suppression (Fig. 37.3). These apparently paradoxical functions of Stat3 may depend on the specific set of genes it activates in collaboration with other transcription factors and cofactors and on the epigenetic status of the target promoters. For example, a recent study suggests that whether Stat3 will play a pro-oncogenic or tumor-suppressive role depends on the mutational profile of the tumor (de la Iglesia et al., 2008b).

Activated Stat3 can induce its own expression by transcriptional activation, which explains why steady-state levels of Stat3 are relatively higher in a variety of cancer cells (including GBM cells) than normal cells (Yang et al., 2007). A recent study shows the accumulation of unphosphorylated (unactivated) Stat3 in IL-6 treated cells, which activates a distinct set of genes including IL-6 and IL-8 that are not induced by activated Stat3 (Yang and Stark, 2008). Thus, Stat3 appears to contribute to the pathogenesis of many human cancers including GBM by acting through a complex network of molecular mechanisms.

Therefore, further studies are necessary for unfolding the complexity of Stat3 functions in malignant gliomas and other human malignancies. Though numerous studies have provided compelling proof-of-concept evidence for targeting aberrant Stat3 activity in numerous tumors, any therapeutic intervention should take into account the specific targeting of tumor cells as Stat3 plays important roles in multiple, normal physiological processes.

Acknowledgments This work is supported by NIH grant CA095006 to SJH. We thank Etty N Benveniste and Erwin G Van Meir for critical reading of the manuscript.

References

Akira, S. (1999). Functional roles of STAT family proteins: lessons from knockout mice. Stem Cells *17*, 138–146.

Akira, S., Nishio, Y., Inoue, M., Wang, X. J., Wei, S., Matsusaka, T., Yoshida, K., Sudo, T., Naruto, M., and Kishimoto, T. (1994). Molecular cloning of APRF, a novel IFN-stimulated gene factor 3 p91-related transcription factor involved in the gp130-mediated signaling pathway. Cell *77*, 63–71.

Al Zaid Siddiquee, K., and Turkson, J. (2008). STAT3 as a target for inducing apoptosis in solid and hematological tumors. Cell Res *18*, 254–267.

Albanell, J., Rojo, F., and Baselga, J. (2001). Pharmacodynamic studies with the epidermal growth factor receptor tyrosine kinase inhibitor ZD1839. Semin Oncol *28*, 56–66.

Aoki, H., Iwado, E., Eller, M. S., Kondo, Y., Fujiwara, K., Li, G. Z., Hess, K. R., Siwak, D. R., Sawaya, R., Mills, G. B., et al. (2007). Telomere 3' overhang-specific DNA oligonucleotides induce autophagy in malignant glioma cells. Faseb J *21*, 2918–2930.

Bao, S., Wu, Q., McLendon, R. E., Hao, Y., Shi, Q., Hjelmeland, A. B., Dewhirst, M. W., Bigner, D. D., and Rich, J. N. (2006). Glioma stem cells promote radioresistance by preferential activation of the DNA damage response. Nature *444*, 756–760.

Benedetti, S., Bruzzone, M. G., Pollo, B., DiMeco, F., Magrassi, L., Pirola, B., Cirenei, N., Colombo, M. P., and Finocchiaro, G. (1999). Eradication of rat malignant gliomas by retroviral-mediated, in vivo delivery of the interleukin 4 gene. Cancer Res *59*, 645–652.

Benedetti, S., Pirola, B., Pollo, B., Magrassi, L., Bruzzone, M. G., Rigamonti, D., Galli, R., Selleri, S., Di Meco, F., De Fraja, C., et al. (2000). Gene therapy of experimental brain tumors using neural progenitor cells. Nat Med *6*, 447–450.

Bennett, B. L., Cruz, R., Lacson, R. G., and Manning, A. M. (1997). Interleukin-4 suppression of tumor necrosis factor alpha-stimulated E-selectin gene transcription is mediated by STAT6 antagonism of NF-kappaB. J Biol Chem *272*, 10212–10219.

Bergers, G., and Benjamin, L. E. (2003). Tumorigenesis and the angiogenic switch. Nat Rev Cancer *3*, 401–410.

Blau, H. M., Brazelton, T. R., and Weimann, J. M. (2001). The evolving concept of a stem cell: entity or function? Cell *105*, 829–841.

Borghouts, C., Kunz, C., Delis, N., and Groner, B. (2008). Monomeric recombinant peptide aptamers are required for efficient intracellular uptake and target inhibition. Mol Cancer Res *6*, 267–281.

Brantley, E. C., Nabors, L. B., Gillespie, G. Y., Choi, Y. H., Palmer, C. A., Harrison, K., Roarty, K., and Benveniste, E. N. (2008). Loss of protein inhibitors of activated STAT-3 expression in glioblastoma multiforme tumors: implications for STAT-3 activation and gene expression. Clin Cancer Res *14*, 4694–4704.

Brat, D. J., and Van Meir, E. G. (2004). Vaso-occlusive and prothrombotic mechanisms associated with tumor hypoxia, necrosis, and accelerated growth in glioblastoma. Lab Invest *84*, 397–405.

Bromberg, J. F., Wrzeszczynska, M. H., Devgan, G., Zhao, Y., Pestell, R. G., Albanese, C., and Darnell, J. E., Jr. (1999). Stat3 as an oncogene. Cell *98*, 295–303.

Catlett-Falcone, R., Landowski, T. H., Oshiro, M. M., Turkson, J., Levitzki, A., Savino, R., Ciliberto, G., Moscinski, L., Fernandez-Luna, J. L., Nunez, G., et al. (1999). Constitutive activation of Stat3 signaling confers resistance to apoptosis in human U266 myeloma cells. Immunity *10*, 105–115.

Cattaneo, E., Magrassi, L., De-Fraja, C., Conti, L., Di Gennaro, I., Butti, G., and Govoni, S. (1998). Variations in the levels of the JAK/STAT and ShcA proteins in human brain tumors. Anticancer Res *18*, 2381–2387.

Chung, C. D., Liao, J., Liu, B., Rao, X., Jay, P., Berta, P., and Shuai, K. (1997). Specific inhibition of Stat3 signal transduction by PIAS3. Science *278*, 1803–1805.

Cramer, A., Kleiner, S., Westermann, M., Meissner, A., Lange, A., and Friedrich, K. (2005). Activation of the c-Met receptor complex in fibroblasts drives invasive cell behavior by signaling through transcription factor STAT3. J Cell Biochem *95*, 805–816.

Cserr, H. F., and Knopf, P. M. (1992). Cervical lymphatics, the blood-brain barrier and the immunoreactivity of the brain: a new view. Immunol Today *13*, 507–512.

Cuevas, P., Diaz-Gonzalez, D., Sanchez, I., Lozano, R. M., Gimenez-Gallego, G., and Dujovny, M. (2006). Dobesilate inhibits the activation of signal transducer and activator of transcription 3, and the expression of cyclin D1 and bcl-XL in glioma cells. Neurol Res *28*, 127–130.

Darnell, J. E., Jr. (1997). STATs and gene regulation. Science *277*, 1630–1635.

Darnell, J. E., Jr. (2002). Transcription factors as targets for cancer therapy. Nat Rev Cancer *2*, 740–749.

Darnell, J. E., Jr., Kerr, I. M., and Stark, G. R. (1994). Jak-STAT pathways and transcriptional activation in response to IFNs and other extracellular signaling proteins. Science *264*, 1415–1421.

Dasgupta, A., Raychaudhuri, B., Haqqi, T., Prayson, R., Van Meir, E. G., Vogelbaum, M., and Haque, S. J. (2008). Stat3 activation is required for the progression of the growth of glioblastoma multiforme. Eur J Cancer *45*, 677–684.

de la Iglesia, N., Konopka, G., Lim, K. L., Nutt, C. L., Bromberg, J. F., Frank, D. A., Mischel, P. S., Louis, D. N., and Bonni, A. (2008a). Deregulation of a STAT3-interleukin 8 signaling pathway promotes human glioblastoma cell proliferation and invasiveness. J Neurosci *28*, 5870–5878.

de la Iglesia, N., Konopka, G., Puram, S. V., Chan, J. A., Bachoo, R. M., You, M. J., Levy, D. E., Depinho, R. A., and Bonni, A. (2008b). Identification of a PTEN-regulated STAT3 brain tumor suppressor pathway. Genes Dev *22*, 449–462.

Deo, D. D., Axelrad, T. W., Robert, E. G., Marcheselli, V., Bazan, N. G., and Hunt, J. D. (2002). Phosphorylation of STAT-3 in response to basic fibroblast growth factor occurs through a mechanism involving platelet-activating factor, JAK-2, and Src in human umbilical vein endothelial cells. Evidence for a dual kinase mechanism. J Biol Chem *277*, 21237–21245.

Dey, N., Durden, D. L., and Van Meir, E. G. (2006). Cytokine Expression and Signaling in Brain Tumors. In Cytokines and the CNS II, R. M. Ransohoff, and E. N. Benveniste, eds. (Boca Raton, FL, CRC Press), pp. 193–242.

Dick, J. E. (2003). Breast cancer stem cells revealed. Proc Natl Acad Sci U S A *100*, 3547–3549.

Fischer, I., Gagner, J. P., Law, M., Newcomb, E. W., and Zagzag, D. (2005). Angiogenesis in gliomas: biology and molecular pathophysiology. Brain Pathol *15*, 297–310.

Fong, G. H. (2008). Mechanisms of adaptive angiogenesis to tissue hypoxia. Angiogenesis *11*, 121–140.

Fujita, M., Zhu, X., Sasaki, K., Ueda, R., Low, K. L., Pollack, I. F., and Okada, H. (2008). Inhibition of STAT3 promotes the efficacy of adoptive transfer therapy using type-1 CTLs by modulation of the immunological microenvironment in a murine intracranial glioma. J Immunol *180*, 2089–2098.

Furnari, F. B., Fenton, T., Bachoo, R. M., Mukasa, A., Stommel, J. M., Stegh, A., Hahn, W. C., Ligon, K. L., Louis, D. N., Brennan, C., et al. (2007). Malignant astrocytic glioma: genetics, biology, and paths to treatment. Genes Dev *21*, 2683–2710.

Garcia, R., and Jove, R. (1998). Activation of STAT transcription factors in oncogenic tyrosine kinase signaling. J Biomed Sci *5*, 79–85.

Ghosh, M. K., Sharma, P., Harbor, P. C., Rahaman, S. O., and Haque, S. J. (2005). PI3K-AKT pathway negatively controls EGFR-dependent DNA-binding activity of Stat3 in glioblastoma multiforme cells. Oncogene *24*, 7290–7300.

Giezeman-Smits, K. M., Okada, H., Brissette-Storkus, C. S., Villa, L. A., Attanucci, J., Lotze, M. T., Pollack, I. F., Bozik, M. E., and Chambers, W. H. (2000). Cytokine gene therapy of gliomas: induction of reactive CD4+ T cells by interleukin-4-transfected 9L gliosarcoma is essential for protective immunity. Cancer Res *60*, 2449–2457.

Gilbertson, R. J., and Rich, J. N. (2007). Making a tumour's bed: glioblastoma stem cells and the vascular niche. Nat Rev Cancer *7*, 733–736.

Gordon, L. B., Nolan, S. C., Cserr, H. F., Knopf, P. M., and Harling-Berg, C. J. (1997). Growth of P511 mastocytoma cells in BALB/c mouse brain elicits CTL response without tumor elimination: a new tumor model for regional central nervous system immunity. J Immunol *159*, 2399–2408.

Goswami, S., Gupta, A., and Sharma, S. K. (1998). Interleukin-6-mediated autocrine growth promotion in human glioblastoma multiforme cell line U87MG. J Neurochem *71*, 1837–1845.

Gray, M. J., Zhang, J., Ellis, L. M., Semenza, G. L., Evans, D. B., Watowich, S. S., and Gallick, G. E. (2005). HIF-1alpha, STAT3, CBP/p300 and Ref-1/APE are components of a transcriptional complex that regulates Src-dependent hypoxia-induced expression of VEGF in pancreatic and prostate carcinomas. Oncogene *24*, 3110–3120.

Green, D. R., and Evan, G. I. (2002). A matter of life and death. Cancer Cell *1*, 19–30.

Gu, J., Li, G., Sun, T., Su, Y., Zhang, X., Shen, J., Tian, Z., and Zhang, J. (2008). Blockage of the STAT3 signaling pathway with a decoy oligonucleotide suppresses growth of human malignant glioma cells. J Neurooncol.

Gurdon, J. B. (2006). From Nuclear Transfer to Nuclear Reprogramming: The Reversal of Cell Differentiation. Annu Rev Cell Dev Biol.

Gurdon, J. B., Byrne, J. A., and Simonsson, S. (2003). Nuclear reprogramming and stem cell creation. Proc Natl Acad Sci U S A *100 Suppl 1*, 11819–11822.

Gurdon, J. B., Byrne, J. A., and Simonsson, S. (2005). Nuclear reprogramming by xenopus oocytes. Novartis Found Symp *265*, 129–136; discussion 136–141, 204–111.

Halfter, H., Postert, C., Friedrich, M., Ringelstein, E. B., and Stogbauer, F. (2000a). Activation of the Jak-Stat- and MAPK-pathways by oncostatin M is not sufficient to cause growth inhibition of human glioma cells. Brain Res Mol Brain Res *80*, 198–206.

Halfter, H., Stogbauer, F., Friedrich, M., Serve, S., Serve, H., and Ringelstein, E. B. (2000b). Oncostatin M-mediated growth inhibition of human glioblastoma cells does not depend on stat3 or on mitogen-activated protein kinase activation. J Neurochem *75*, 973–981.

Han, S. W., Hwang, P. G., Chung, D. H., Kim, D. W., Im, S. A., Kim, Y. T., Kim, T. Y., Heo, D. S., Bang, Y. J., and Kim, N. K. (2005). Epidermal growth factor receptor (EGFR) downstream molecules as response predictive markers for gefitinib (Iressa, ZD1839) in chemotherapy-resistant non-small cell lung cancer. Int J Cancer *113*, 109–115.

Hanahan, D., and Weinberg, R. A. (2000). The hallmarks of cancer. Cell *100*, 57–70.

Haque, S. J., Harbor, P. C., and Williams, B. R. (2000). Identification of critical residues required for suppressor of cytokine signaling-specific regulation of interleukin-4 signaling. J Biol Chem *275*, 26500–26506.

Haque, S. J., and Sharma, P. (2006). Interleukins and STAT Signaling. Vitam Horm *74C*, 165–206.

Harris, A. L. (2002). Hypoxia – a key regulatory factor in tumour growth. Nat Rev Cancer *2*, 38–47.

Heinrich, P. C., Behrmann, I., Muller-Newen, G., Schaper, F., and Graeve, L. (1998). Interleukin-6-type cytokine signalling through the gp130/Jak/STAT pathway. Biochem J *334 (Pt 2)*, 297–314.

Hishii, M., Nitta, T., Ishida, H., Ebato, M., Kurosu, A., Yagita, H., Sato, K., and Okumura, K. (1995). Human glioma-derived interleukin-10 inhibits antitumor immune responses in vitro. Neurosurgery *37*, 1160–1166; discussion 1166–1167.

Holash, J., Wiegand, S. J., and Yancopoulos, G. D. (1999). New model of tumor angiogenesis: dynamic balance between vessel regression and growth mediated by angiopoietins and VEGF. Oncogene *18*, 5356–5362.

Holland, E. C. (2000). Glioblastoma multiforme: the terminator. Proc Natl Acad Sci U S A *97*, 6242–6244.

Hussain, S. F., Kong, L. Y., Jordan, J., Conrad, C., Madden, T., Fokt, I., Priebe, W., and Heimberger, A. B. (2007). A novel small molecule inhibitor of signal transducers and activators of transcription 3 reverses immune tolerance in malignant glioma patients. Cancer Res *67*, 9630–9636.

Iwadate, Y., Yamaura, A., Sato, Y., Sakiyama, S., and Tagawa, M. (2001). Induction of immunity in peripheral tissues combined with intracerebral transplantation of interleukin-2-producing cells eliminates established brain tumors. Cancer Res *61*, 8769–8774.

Iwamaru, A., Szymanski, S., Iwado, E., Aoki, H., Yokoyama, T., Fokt, I., Hess, K., Conrad, C., Madden, T., Sawaya, R., et al. (2007). A novel inhibitor of the STAT3 pathway induces apoptosis in malignant glioma cells both in vitro and in vivo. Oncogene *26*, 2435–2444.

Jean, W. C., Spellman, S. R., Wallenfriedman, M. A., Flores, C. T., Kurtz, B. P., Hall, W. A., and Low, W. C. (2004). Effects of combined granulocyte-macrophage colony-stimulating factor (GM-CSF), interleukin-2, and interleukin-12 based immunotherapy against intracranial glioma in the rat. J Neurooncol *66*, 39–49.

Joshi, B. H., Plautz, G. E., and Puri, R. K. (2000). Interleukin-13 receptor alpha chain: a novel tumor-associated transmembrane protein in primary explants of human malignant gliomas. Cancer Res *60*, 1168–1172.

Jung, J. E., Lee, H. G., Cho, I. H., Chung, D. H., Yoon, S. H., Yang, Y. M., Lee, J. W., Choi, S., Park, J. W., Ye, S. K., and Chung, M. H. (2005). STAT3 is a potential modulator of HIF-1-mediated VEGF expression in human renal carcinoma cells. Faseb J *19*, 1296–1298.

Kamath, S., and Buolamwini, J. K. (2006). Targeting EGFR and HER-2 receptor tyrosine kinases for cancer drug discovery and development. Med Res Rev *26*, 569–594.

Kleihues, P., Burger, P. C., and Scheithauer, B. W. (1993). The new WHO classification of brain tumours. Brain Pathol *3*, 255–268.

Konnikova, L., Kotecki, M., Kruger, M. M., and Cochran, B. H. (2003). Knockdown of STAT3 expression by RNAi induces apoptosis in astrocytoma cells. BMC Cancer *3*, 23.

Lee, J., Son, M. J., Woolard, K., Donin, N. M., Li, A., Cheng, C. H., Kotliarova, S., Kotliarov, Y., Walling, J., Ahn, S., et al. (2008). Epigenetic-mediated dysfunction of the bone morphogenetic protein pathway inhibits differentiation of glioblastoma-initiating cells. Cancer Cell *13*, 69–80.

Liu, J., Estes, M. L., Drazba, J. A., Liu, H., Prayson, R., Kondo, S., Jacobs, B. S., Barnett, G. H., and Barna, B. P. (2000). Anti-sense oligonucleotide of p21(waf1/cip1) prevents interleukin 4-mediated elevation of p27(kip1) in low grade astrocytoma cells. Oncogene *19*, 661–669.

Lo, H. W., Cao, X., Zhu, H., and Ali-Osman, F. (2008). Constitutively activated STAT3 frequently coexpresses with epidermal growth factor receptor in high-grade gliomas and targeting STAT3 sensitizes them to Iressa and alkylators. Clin Cancer Res *14*, 6042–6054.

Loeffler, S., Fayard, B., Weis, J., and Weissenberger, J. (2005). Interleukin-6 induces transcriptional activation of vascular endothelial growth factor (VEGF) in astrocytes in vivo and regulates VEGF promoter activity in glioblastoma cells via direct interaction between STAT3 and Sp1. Int J Cancer *115*, 202–213.

Magrassi, L., De-Fraja, C., Conti, L., Butti, G., Infuso, L., Govoni, S., and Cattaneo, E. (1999). Expression of the JAK and STAT superfamilies in human meningiomas. J Neurosurg *91*, 440–446.

Maher, E. A., Furnari, F. B., Bachoo, R. M., Rowitch, D. H., Louis, D. N., Cavenee, W. K., and DePinho, R. A. (2001). Malignant glioma: genetics and biology of a grave matter. Genes Dev *15*, 1311–1333.

Maritano, D., Sugrue, M. L., Tininini, S., Dewilde, S., Strobl, B., Fu, X., Murray-Tait, V., Chiarle, R., and Poli, V. (2004). The STAT3 isoforms alpha and beta have unique and specific functions. Nat Immunol *5*, 401–409.

Nakashima, K., Yanagisawa, M., Arakawa, H., Kimura, N., Hisatsune, T., Kawabata, M., Miyazono, K., and Taga, T. (1999). Synergistic signaling in fetal brain by STAT3-Smad1 complex bridged by p300. Science *284*, 479–482.

Naumov, G. N., Bender, E., Zurakowski, D., Kang, S. Y., Sampson, D., Flynn, E., Watnick, R. S., Straume, O., Akslen, L. A., Folkman, J., and Almog, N. (2006). A model of human tumor dormancy: an angiogenic switch from the nonangiogenic phenotype. J Natl Cancer Inst *98*, 316–325.

Niu, G., Wright, K. L., Huang, M., Song, L., Haura, E., Turkson, J., Zhang, S., Wang, T., Sinibaldi, D., Coppola, D., et al. (2002). Constitutive Stat3 activity up-regulates VEGF expression and tumor angiogenesis. Oncogene *21*, 2000–2008.

Paillaud, E., Costa, S., Fages, C., Plassat, J. L., Rochette-Egly, C., Monville, C., and Tardy, M. (2002). Retinoic acid increases proliferation rate of GL-15 glioma cells, involving activation of STAT-3 transcription factor. J Neurosci Res *67*, 670–679.

Parsons, D. W., Jones, S., Zhang, X., Lin, J. C., Leary, R. J., Angenendt, P., Mankoo, P., Carter, H., Siu, I. M., Gallia, G. L., et al. (2008). An integrated genomic analysis of human glioblastoma multiforme. Science *321*, 1807–1812.

Plate, K. H., Breier, G., Weich, H. A., and Risau, W. (1992). Vascular endothelial growth factor is a potential tumour angiogenesis factor in human gliomas in vivo. Nature *359*, 845–848.

Post, D. E., and Van Meir, E. G. (2001). Generation of bidirectional hypoxia/HIF-responsive expression vectors to target gene expression to hypoxic cells. Gene Ther *8*, 1801–1807.

Rahaman, S. O., Harbor, P. C., Chernova, O., Barnett, G. H., Vogelbaum, M. A., and Haque, S. J. (2002a). Inhibition of constitutively active Stat3 suppresses proliferation and induces apoptosis in glioblastoma multiforme cells. Oncogene *21*, 8404–8413.

Rahaman, S. O., Sharma, P., Harbor, P. C., Aman, M. J., Vogelbaum, M. A., and Haque, S. J. (2002b). IL-13R(alpha)2, a decoy receptor for IL-13 acts as an inhibitor of IL-4-dependent signal transduction in glioblastoma cells. Cancer Res *62*, 1103–1109.

Rahaman, S. O., Vogelbaum, M. A., and Haque, S. J. (2005). Aberrant Stat3 signaling by interleukin-4 in malignant glioma cells: involvement of IL-13Ralpha2. Cancer Res *65*, 2956–2963.

Ren, W., Duan, Y., Yang, Y., Ji, Y., and Chen, F. (2008). Down-regulation of Stat3 induces apoptosis of human glioma cell: a potential method to treat brain cancer. Neurol Res *30*, 297–301.

Repovic, P., Fears, C. Y., Gladson, C. L., and Benveniste, E. N. (2003). Oncostatin-M induction of vascular endothelial growth factor expression in astroglioma cells. Oncogene *22*, 8117–8124.

Rolhion, C., Penault-Llorca, F., Kemeny, J. L., Lemaire, J. J., Jullien, C., Labit-Bouvier, C., Finat-Duclos, F., and Verrelle, P. (2001). Interleukin-6 overexpression as a marker of malignancy in human gliomas. J Neurosurg *94*, 97–101.

Rong, Y., Durden, D. L., Van Meir, E. G., and Brat, D. J. (2006). 'Pseudopalisading' necrosis in glioblastoma: a familiar morphologic feature that links vascular pathology, hypoxia, and angiogenesis. J Neuropathol Exp Neurol *65*, 529–539.

Roszman, T., Elliott, L., and Brooks, W. (1991). Modulation of T-cell function by gliomas. Immunol Today *12*, 370–374.

Schaefer, L. K., Ren, Z., Fuller, G. N., and Schaefer, T. S. (2002). Constitutive activation of Stat3alpha in brain tumors: localization to tumor endothelial cells and activation by the endothelial tyrosine kinase receptor (VEGFR-2). Oncogene *21*, 2058–2065.

Schaefer, T. S., Sanders, L. K., and Nathans, D. (1995). Cooperative transcriptional activity of Jun and Stat3 beta, a short form of Stat3. Proc Natl Acad Sci U S A *92*, 9097–9101.

Schlehofer, B., Blettner, M., Preston-Martin, S., Niehoff, D., Wahrendorf, J., Arslan, A., Ahlbom, A., Choi, W. N., Giles, G. G., Howe, G. R., et al. (1999). Role of medical history in brain tumour development. Results from the international adult brain tumour study. Int J Cancer *82*, 155–160.

Shervington, A., Cruickshanks, N., Wright, H., Atkinson-Dell, R., Lea, R., Roberts, G., and Shervington, L. (2006). Glioma: what is the role of c-Myc, hsp90 and telomerase? Mol Cell Biochem *283*, 1–9.

Shweiki, D., Itin, A., Soffer, D., and Keshet, E. (1992). Vascular endothelial growth factor induced by hypoxia may mediate hypoxia-initiated angiogenesis. Nature *359*, 843–845.

Singh, S. K., Clarke, I. D., Hide, T., and Dirks, P. B. (2004a). Cancer stem cells in nervous system tumors. Oncogene *23*, 7267–7273.

Singh, S. K., Clarke, I. D., Terasaki, M., Bonn, V. E., Hawkins, C., Squire, J., and Dirks, P. B. (2003). Identification of a cancer stem cell in human brain tumors. Cancer Res *63*, 5821–5828.

Singh, S. K., Hawkins, C., Clarke, I. D., Squire, J. A., Bayani, J., Hide, T., Henkelman, R. M., Cusimano, M. D., and Dirks, P. B. (2004b). Identification of human brain tumour initiating cells. Nature *432*, 396–401.

Stark, G. R., Kerr, I. M., Williams, B. R., Silverman, R. H., and Schreiber, R. D. (1998). How cells respond to interferons. Annu Rev Biochem *67*, 227–264.

Su, Y., Li, G., Zhang, X., Gu, J., Zhang, C., Tian, Z., and Zhang, J. (2008). JSI-124 Inhibits Glioblastoma Multiforme Cell Proliferation through G2/M Cell Cycle Arrest and Apoptosis Augment. Cancer Biol Ther *7*, 1243–1249.

Taga, T., and Fukuda, S. (2005). Role of IL-6 in the neural stem cell differentiation. Clin Rev Allergy Immunol *28*, 249–256.

Takanaga, H., Yoshitake, T., Hara, S., Yamasaki, C., and Kunimoto, M. (2004). cAMP-induced astrocytic differentiation of C6 glioma cells is mediated by autocrine interleukin-6. J Biol Chem *279*, 15441–15447.

Takeda, K., Noguchi, K., Shi, W., Tanaka, T., Matsumoto, M., Yoshida, N., Kishimoto, T., and Akira, S. (1997). Targeted disruption of the mouse Stat3 gene leads to early embryonic lethality. Proc Natl Acad Sci U S A *94*, 3801–3804.

Tchirkov, A., Rolhion, C., Bertrand, S., Dore, J. F., Dubost, J. J., and Verrelle, P. (2001). IL-6 gene amplification and expression in human glioblastomas. Br J Cancer *85*, 518–522.

Temple, S. (2001). The development of neural stem cells. Nature *414*, 112–117.

The Cancer Genome Atlas Research Network, McLendon, R., Friedman, A., Bigner, D., Van Meir, E. G., Brat, D. J., Mastrogianakis, M., Olson, J. J., Mikkelsen, T., Lehman, N., Aldape, K., et al. (2008). Comprehensive genomic characterization defines human glioblastoma genes and core pathways. Nature.

Udayakumar, T. S., Stratton, M. S., Nagle, R. B., and Bowden, G. T. (2002). Fibroblast growth factor-1 induced promatrilysin expression through the activation of extracellular-regulated kinases and STAT3. Neoplasia *4*, 60–67.

Van Meir, E., Sawamura, Y., Diserens, A. C., Hamou, M. F., and de Tribolet, N. (1990). Human glioblastoma cells release interleukin 6 in vivo and in vitro. Cancer Res *50*, 6683–6688.

Wagner, B. J., Hayes, T. E., Hoban, C. J., and Cochran, B. H. (1990). The SIF binding element confers sis/PDGF inducibility onto the c-fos promoter. Embo J *9*, 4477–4484.

Wang, L., and Banerjee, S. (2004). Differential PIAS3 expression in human malignancy. Oncol Rep *11*, 1319–1324.

Wang, Y. Z., Wharton, W., Garcia, R., Kraker, A., Jove, R., and Pledger, W. J. (2000). Activation of Stat3 preassembled with platelet-derived growth factor beta receptors requires Src kinase activity. Oncogene *19*, 2075–2085.

Wechsler-Reya, R., and Scott, M. P. (2001). The developmental biology of brain tumors. Annu Rev Neurosci *24*, 385–428.

Wegenka, U. M., Buschmann, J., Lutticken, C., Heinrich, P. C., and Horn, F. (1993). Acute-phase response factor, a nuclear factor binding to acute-phase response elements, is rapidly activated by interleukin-6 at the posttranslational level. Mol Cell Biol *13*, 276–288.

Weissenberger, J., Loeffler, S., Kappeler, A., Kopf, M., Lukes, A., Afanasieva, T. A., Aguzzi, A., and Weis, J. (2004). IL-6 is required for glioma development in a mouse model. Oncogene *23*, 3308–3316.

Weissenberger, J., Steinbach, J. P., Malin, G., Spada, S., Rulicke, T., and Aguzzi, A. (1997). Development and malignant progression of astrocytomas in GFAP-v-src transgenic mice. Oncogene *14*, 2005–2013.

Xu, H., Yu, Y., Marciniak, D., Rishi, A. K., Sarkar, F. H., Kucuk, O., and Majumdar, A. P. (2005a). Epidermal growth factor receptor (EGFR)-related protein inhibits multiple members of the EGFR family in colon and breast cancer cells. Mol Cancer Ther *4*, 435–442.

Xu, Q., Briggs, J., Park, S., Niu, G., Kortylewski, M., Zhang, S., Gritsko, T., Turkson, J., Kay, H., Semenza, G. L., et al. (2005b). Targeting Stat3 blocks both HIF-1 and VEGF expression induced by multiple oncogenic growth signaling pathways. Oncogene *24*, 5552–5560.

Yang, J., Liao, X., Agarwal, M. K., Barnes, L., Auron, P. E., and Stark, G. R. (2007). Unphosphorylated STAT3 accumulates in response to IL-6 and activates transcription by binding to NFkappaB. Genes Dev *21*, 1396–1408.

Yang, J., and Stark, G. R. (2008). Roles of unphosphorylated STATs in signaling. Cell Res *18*, 443–451.

Yokoyama, T., Kondo, Y., and Kondo, S. (2007). Roles of mTOR and STAT3 in autophagy induced by telomere 3' overhang-specific DNA oligonucleotides. Autophagy *3*, 496–498.

Yoshimatsu, T., Kawaguchi, D., Oishi, K., Takeda, K., Akira, S., Masuyama, N., and Gotoh, Y. (2006). Non-cell-autonomous action of STAT3 in maintenance of neural precursor cells in the mouse neocortex. Development *133*, 2553–2563.

Yoshimura, A., Ohkubo, T., Kiguchi, T., Jenkins, N. A., Gilbert, D. J., Copeland, N. G., Hara, T., and Miyajima, A. (1995). A novel cytokine-inducible gene CIS encodes an SH2-containing protein that binds to tyrosine-phosphorylated interleukin 3 and erythropoietin receptors. Embo J *14*, 2816–2826.

Yu, C. L., Meyer, D. J., Campbell, G. S., Larner, A. C., Carter-Su, C., Schwartz, J., and Jove, R. (1995). Enhanced DNA-binding activity of a Stat3-related protein in cells transformed by the Src oncoprotein. Science *269*, 81–83.

Yu, H., and Jove, R. (2004). The STATs of cancer – new molecular targets come of age. Nat Rev Cancer *4*, 97–105.

Yu, H., Kortylewski, M., and Pardoll, D. (2007). Crosstalk between cancer and immune cells: role of STAT3 in the tumour microenvironment. Nat Rev Immunol *7*, 41–51.

Yuan, G., Qian, L., Shi, M., Lu, F., Li, D., Hu, M., Yu, M., Shen, B., and Guo, N. (2008). HER2-dependent MMP-7 expression is mediated by activated STAT3. Cell Signal *20*, 1284–1291.

Zhong, Z., Wen, Z., and Darnell, J. E., Jr. (1994). Stat3: a STAT family member activated by tyrosine phosphorylation in response to epidermal growth factor and interleukin-6. Science *264*, 95–98.

Chapter 38
Inhibition of Ras Signaling for Brain Tumor Therapy

Sameer Agnihotri, Diana Munoz, and Abhijit Guha

Abstract Overactive p21-Ras signaling is a major contributing factor in the initiation and progression of glioblastoma multiforme (GBM). Thirty percent of all cancers exhibit mutations in the *p21-Ras* gene. Elevated levels of p21-Ras activity can also arise through abnormal receptor expression as is the case in GBM. Hence, development of p21-Ras inhibitors such as farnesyltransferase inhibitors (FTIs) or other targets of p21-Ras signaling is a promising but unproven antitumor strategy. p21-Ras is a member of the small guanine nucleotide-binding protein family and plays a pivotal role in signal transduction. Activated p21-Ras and its downstream signaling cascades are involved in a variety of biological processes including cell proliferation, cell cycle progression, survival, development, and differentiation. Although mutations in *p21-Ras* are rare in GBM, elevated levels of activated p21-Ras are consistently seen in GBM. Current data suggest that activation of p21-Ras is a consequence of aberrant tyrosine kinase receptor activation (EGFR, PDGFR, Met, etc.), which are frequent events in GBM. Targeting p21-Ras in gliomas has not been fully exploited and a better understanding of p21-Ras and its function may lead to novel therapies that can be synergistic with other conventional and biological modalities.

Contents

S. Agnihotri (✉)
University of Toronto, Toronto, ONT, Canada
e-mail: Abhijit.Guha@uhn.on.ca

E.G. Van Meir (ed.), *CNS Cancer*, Cancer Drug Discovery and Development, DOI 10.1007/978-1-60327-553-8_38,
© Humana Press, a part of Springer Science+Business Media, LLC 2009

38.1 Introduction

Glioblastoma multiforme (GBM) is the most common and lethal of all gliomas and is defined by several hallmark features such as hypercellularity, resistance to apoptosis, genomic instability, extensive angiogenesis, necrosis, and robust invasion. GBM is a highly heterogeneous tumor broadly characterized by several gain-of-function and loss-of-function alterations, epigenetic reprogramming, and germline and somatic mutations (TCGA, 2008). Emerging biologically relevant targeted therapies depend on an enhanced understanding of the underlying mechanisms that drive the malignant phenotype. Amongst these targets is p21-Ras, and it has attracted much attention due to its central role in normal and cancer cell intracellular signaling pathways. The primary mechanism for the activation of p21-Ras in cancer is through point mutations in the *p21-ras* gene, yielding constitutively active p21-Ras protein expression and this occurs in ~30% of cancers. A number of cancers including breast cancer and gliomas also show p21-Ras activation by secondary mechanisms, such as aberrant receptor signaling of EGFR, PDGFR, and mutations in Ras-GAP proteins such as NF1, which serve to inactivate p21-Ras.

Targeting of p21-Ras and effectors of p21-Ras signaling is therefore a rationale and an attractive strategy for novel therapeutic intervention in many cancers, including brain tumors such as gliomas and perhaps other CNS tumors (see subsequent sections). While the *p21-Ras* gene is rarely mutated in GBM and other primary brain tumors, its elevated activity and that of the multiple downstream effectors of p21-Ras signaling can be targeted. In this chapter, we highlight how p21-Ras contributes to GBM and other primary CNS tumor biology, review the prior strategies to target this pathway that have not worked so effectively, and present future targeting approaches.

38.2 p21-Ras Structure and Processing

p21-Ras is a member of the Ras protein family, which is small guanine nucleotide-binding protein (G proteins) that cycles between an inactive guanosine diphosphate (GDP)-bound form and an active guanosine triphosphate (GTP)-bound form (Sprang 1997a, b) (Fig. 38.1A). p21-Ras plays a fundamental role in signal transduction and can be modulated by a diversity of cytokines and growth factors. There are three mammalian *p21-Ras* genes that encode four closely related GTPases of K-RasB (188 amino acids), H-RasA, K-RasA, and N-RasA (189 amino acids). K-RasA and K-RasB arise from alternative splicing of K-Ras gene products. High sequence homology exists between the Ras isoforms, where the first 86 amino acids are identical, the next 79 are 78% homologous, and the last 24 amino acids are highly variable (Boguski and McCormick 1993a; Ellis et al. 1981; Lowy and Willumsen 1993; Lowy et al. 1993) (Fig. 38.1B).

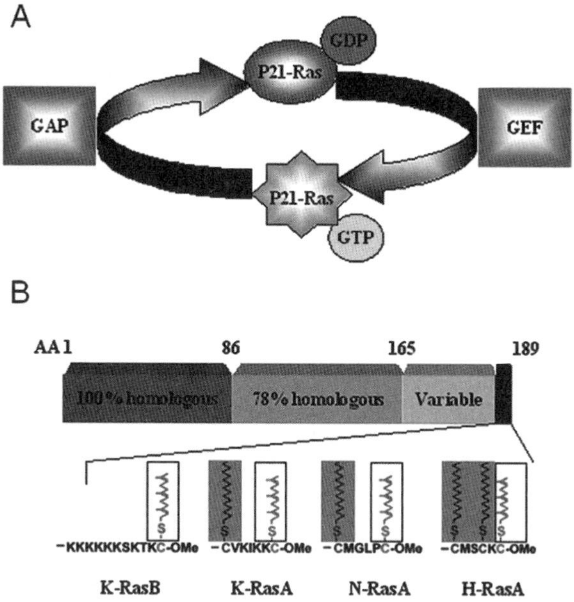

Fig. 38.1 Ras activation and various isoforms of p21-Ras. p21-Ras family proteins are small guanine nucleotide-binding proteins. They are inactive when bound to GDP and active when bound to GTP. This molecular switch occurs through a GDP–GTP cycle that is regulated by the opposing functions of guanine nucleotide-exchange factors (GEFs), which catalyze the exchange of GDP for GTP, and GTPase-activating proteins (GAPs), which increase the rate of GTP hydrolysis to GDP. p21-Ras and its family members interact through a variety of effector proteins, which influence cell processes such as cell cycle progression, proliferation, and survival. (**1A**)*Top*. Sequence conservation between p21-Ras proteins. Amino acids (AA) 1–86 of the p21-Ras proteins are 100% homologous. AA 87–165 have 78% identity and the remaining AAs are variable. (**1B**)*Bottom*. p21-Ras proteins are shown with their respective posttranslational modifications. The farnesylated cysteine residue which is conserved in all p21-Ras proteins is shown in open boxes. Palmitoylated cysteine residues in N- and H-Ras proteins are shown in shaded boxes

Activated p21-Ras or mutated Ras undergoes several posttranslational modifications (PTMs) that are vital for the attachment and activation at the inner plasma membrane. The first and most critical modification is the addition of a farnesyl isoprenoid moiety to the C-terminus of p21-Ras, which is facilitated by the enzyme farnesyltransferase (FTase), a member of the prenyltransferase family that includes geranylgeranyl transferases (GGTase). FTase is a heterodimeric enzyme that catalyzes the addition of a 15-carbon farnesyl moiety from farnesyl pyrophosphate (FPP) in a thioester covalent linkage to cysteine in the C-terminal CAAX motif of p21-Ras (Gelb 1997; Zhang and Casey 1996; Glomset and Farnsworth 1994). Similarly, with K-Ras a GGTase adds a geranylgeranyl moiety from geranylgeranyl pyrophosphate (GGPP). Of the four isoforms of p21-Ras, Ha-Ras is fully dependent on FTase for its activation, while other isoforms and cancer mutants can undergo geranylation if farnesylation is inhibited. FTase inhibitors (FTIs) have become of clinical relevance and will be discussed in the subsequent sections. After farnesylation, there is endoproteolytic cleavage and removal of the three carboxyl terminal amino acids (AAX) by a CAAX-specific endoprotease (PPSEP) at the endoplasmic reticulum. p21-Ras is further modified by the addition of a methyl group from *S*-adenosylmethionine (SAM) to the carboxyl group of the prenylated cysteine residue by an uncharacterized methyltransferase (PPSMTase) (Park et al. 1997; Trueblood et al. 1997; Trueblood et al. 1997; Pellicena et al. 1996). Ha-Ras and N-Ras further undergo palmitylation at 1–2 cysteines near the farnesylated C-terminus by a prenyl protein-specific palmitoyltransferase. Although each of these PTMs increase hydrophobicity of p21-Ras to promote membrane association, the initial farnesylation is sufficient to promote membrane association. In addition to FTase, GGTase-I and GGTase-II can also prenylate the C-terminal ends like FTase by attaching either one or two 20-carbon geranylgeranyl isoprenyl moieties (Gibbs et al. 1993; McCormick 1993b; Casey et al. 1989). Figures 38.1B (bottom panel) and 38.2 depict the PTM modifications that the p21-Ras isoforms are subjected to.

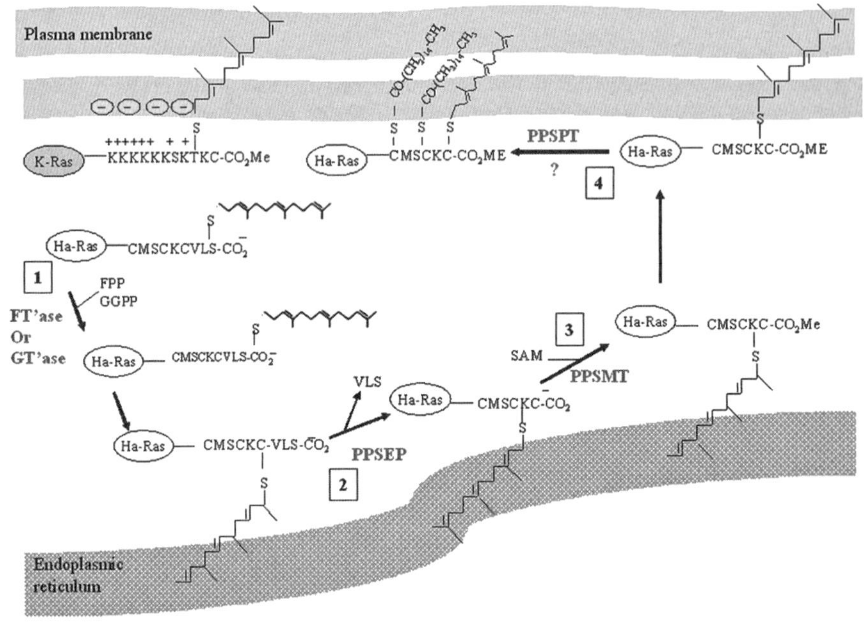

Fig. 38.2 Posttranslational modification of p21-Ras. p21-Ras is synthesized as a pro-peptide, which undergoes a series of posttranslational modifications, resulting in attachment to the inner surface of the plasma membrane, where it can be cycled from inactive GDP- to active GTP-bound state. 1. First FTase or GGTase transfers a farnesyl or a geranylgeranyl group from FPP or GGPP to the thiol group of the cysteine residue in the CAAX motif of p21-Ras. 2. The C-terminal tri-peptide is then removed by a CAAX-specific endoprotease (PPSEP) in the endoplasmic reticulum. 3. A PPSMTase attaches the methyl group from *S*-adenosylmethionine (SAM) to the C-terminal cysteine. 4. Finally, a prenyl protein-specific palmitoyltranferase (PPSPTase) attaches palmitoyl groups to cysteines near the farnesylated C-terminus

38.3 Activation and p21-Ras Signaling

p21-Ras serves as a membrane-bound biological switch that relays signals from stimulated receptors to initiate effector signaling cascades (Fig. 38.3). In general, ligand binding to the extracellular domain of receptor tyrosine kinases (RTKs) causes dimerization, stimulating tyrosine kinase activity leading to auto-phosphorylation of the receptor. These intracellular phosphorylated tyrosine residues serve as docking sites to recruit adapter proteins, such as Grb2 and Shc to the membrane–receptor complex. These proteins have phosphotyrosine-binding (PTB) domain and SH2 domains, which facilitate the interaction and binding of these adapter proteins to the receptor. Grb2 is complexed with an enzyme called Sos that serves as a p21-Ras guanine exchange factor or Ras-GEF, an interaction mediated by the SH3 domain of Grb2 and the proline-rich region of Sos (McCormick 1993a; Marshall 1995; Schlessinger 1993). The Grb2–Sos complex can interact with p21-Ras, effectively targeting it to the cellular membrane and resulting in the inactive GDP of Ras being exchanged for GTP. Ras activation is not exclusive to RTKs as non-RTK such as Lyn, Jak2, and Fes can recruit Grb2–Sos complexes and activate Ras signaling cascades. Inactivation of Ras occurs when p21-Ras-GTP becomes p21-Ras-GDP through a hydrolysis reaction catalyzed by GTPase. p21-Ras and other small G protein have intrinsic GTPase activity but it is slow, and more efficient GTPase activity is carried out by another family of proteins known as Ras-GAPs (GTPase-activating proteins) (Buhring et al. 1993; Marshall 1995). Two well-studied Ras-GAPs include p120GAP and NF1, the latter being the protein product inactivated in the cancer predisposition syndrome neurofibromatosis-1 (NF-1) (see also Chapters 3 and 6).

Active p21-Ras-GTP can then trigger several downstream signaling cascades including the Ras-MAPK pathway through activation of the serine threonine kinase Raf-1 (Marshall 1996; Pawson and Saxton 1999; Kolch et al. 1991; Cowley et al. 1994; Mansour et al. 1994; Stokoe et al. 1994; Leevers et al. 1994; Pritchard and McMahon 1997; Tamada et al. 1997; Jaaro et al. 1997). PI(3)K signaling cascades and activation of Rho and Rac are also transduced through p21-Ras activation (Fig. 38.3). Ras-Raf-MAPK signaling is the best studied signaling cascade of Ras activation and frequently aberrantly expressed in several cancers. Activation of Raf occurs when it is recruited to the cell membrane but the mechanism by which p21-Ras activates Raf is under investigation. Activated Raf will phosphorylate the ser-thr kinases MEK1 and MEK2 which then activate downstream the MAPKs ERK1 and ERK2. ERK1 and ERK2 phosphorylate a multitude of cytoplasmic and nuclear proteins including S6 kinases and ELK-1, a transcription factor responsible for the transcription of p21-Ras signaling induced genes.

p21-Ras can also activate the PI(3) kinase signaling cascade by binding to the catalytic p110 subunit of PI(3)K leading to activation of PDK-1 and PDK-2, which are responsible for activation of AKT and non-conventional protein kinase C family members (ncPKCs) (see also Chapter 15).

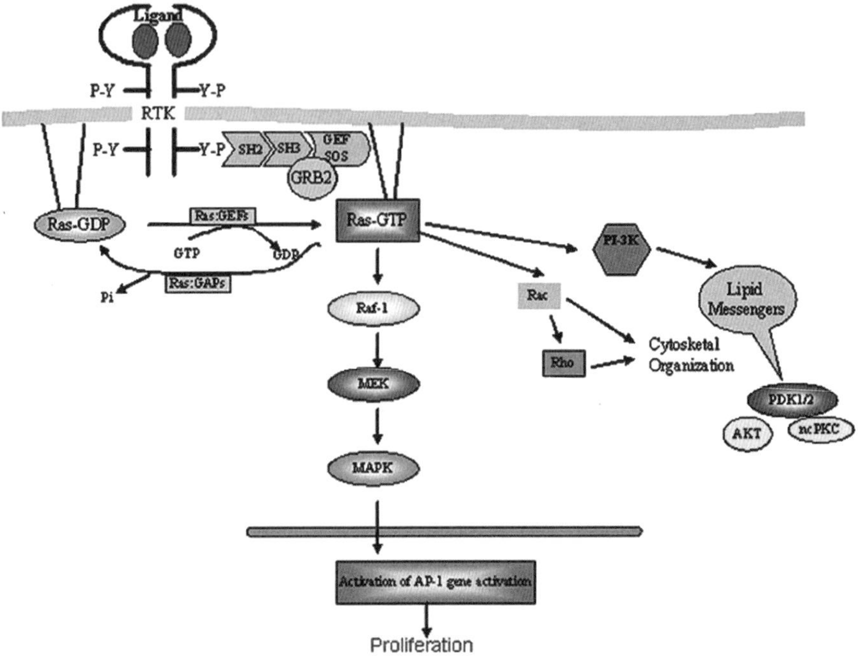

Fig. 38.3 Activation of p21-Ras signaling. In response to growth factor receptor activation and tyrosine (Y) phosphorylation, Grb2 which is complexed to p21-Ras guanine nucleotide exchange factor sos is recruited in proximity to mature p21-Ras attached to the inner cell membrane. Sos catalyzes exchange of GTP for GDP to form activated p21-Ras-GTP. Activated p21-Ras-GTP interacts and activates several effector pathways, including Raf:-MAPK/ERK pathway, PI-3 K, Rac and Rho, to transmit signals to other cytoplasmic regions and the nucleus. Although there is a small intrinsic GTPase activity to revert activated p21-Ras-GTP into inactive p21-Ras-GDP, this hydrolysis is further catalyzed by a family of proteins termed Ras:GAPs (GTPase activating proteins). Y-P represents a phosphorylated tyrosine residue

Activated p21-Ras can also regulate other small G proteins such as Rho, Rac, and CDC42, which are involved in regulating cell morphology, motility, and invasion. Like p21-Ras, these small G proteins also cycle between an active GTP state by GEFs and an inactive GDP state when acted upon GAP proteins. Rho modulates actin cytoskeleton that regulates membrane ruffling, formation of stress fibers, cell shape, cell invasion, formation of filopodia, and focal adhesions.

38.4 Mutated and Activated p21-Ras in Brain Tumors

Mutated p21-Ras oncogenes were first identified by their ability to transform NIH-3T3 cells (Bos 1989; Perucho et al. 1981). The majority of p21-Ras mutations in humans occur in K-Ras, some in N-Ras and rarely in Ha-Ras. Common mutations occur in amino acids numbers 12, 13, or 61 making p21-Ras-GTP unable to bind and thus rendering them insensitive to Ras-GAPs. Mutations at amino acid number 12, with glycine mutated to serine, arginine, alanine, or valine, are the most common (Boguski and McCormick 1993b; Bos 1989). Of therapeutic concern is that activated levels of p21-Ras, in addition to their transformation ability, contribute to radiation and chemotherapy resistance in several tumors including GBM. Inhibition of p21-Ras by expressing dominant negative mutants leads to GBM tumor cells being more sensitive to the chemotherapeutic agent cisplatin in vivo and in vitro (Messina et al. 2004).

Although oncogenic mutations in p21-Ras are rare in GBM, several direct and indirect pieces of evidence demonstrate that activation of p21-Ras and its downstream targets are critical for contributing to GBM malignancy. First our group and others have shown that p21-Ras levels are higher in malignant glioma cell lines and operative samples compared to normal brain and normal astrocytes (Feldkamp et al. 1999a; Guha et al. 1997), comparison between p21-Ras levels in GBM cells that behave like progenitor cells and normal stem cells has not been extensively researched. Secondly, sequencing of *p21-Ras* genes from these samples revealed no primary mutations, suggesting that activation of p21-Ras was due to aberrantly activated upstream receptor signaling in these tumors (Guha et al. 1997). Thirdly, p21-Ras is essential for glioma proliferation and angiogenesis in vivo and in vitro (Feldkamp et al. 1999a, b). Fourthly, increased p21-activated levels correlate with reduced NF-1 GAP activity (Gutmann et al. 1993). The latter notion is further supported by the sequencing analysis undertaken by The Cancer Genome Atlas (TCGA) project, where NF-1 mutations were seen in 30% of primary the GBM operative samples (TCGA, 2008) (see also Chapters 3 and 6). Current investigation of microRNAs (miRNA) has led to the interesting observation that loss or reduced expression of Let-7 miRNA leads to elevated levels of Ras. Let-7 control of Ras expression is through its targeting of the 3'-untranslated regions of N-Ras, Ha-Ras, and K-Ras mRNAs (Johnson et al. 2005) (see also Chapter 27) whether all forms of Ras are equally effected remains unanswered. Lastly, we have developed a germline transgenic mouse model that expresses a ^{12}*V-Ha-Ras* gene under the regulation of the *GFAP* astrocyte-specific promoter (see Chapter 4). These mice are born normally but develop high-grade astrocytomas that are pathologically similar to human tumors at 3–4 months (Ding et al. 2001; Shannon et al. 2005), suggesting that high levels of Ras can create an unstable genetic background in which additional alterations or mutations can lead to tumor development.

38.5 Farnesyltransferase Inhibitors (FTIs) and Preclinical Studies

The importance of farnesylation for the proper function of p21-Ras has been discussed in the prior section. In addition to p21-Ras, there are over 200 other proteins that are also farnesylated, some of which are also involved in the p21-Ras signaling pathway (Tamanoi et al. 2001b, a). One such protein is

RhoB which is processed by farnesylation and geranylgeranylation and is involved in a negative role tumorigenesis and is often deleted in several cancers (Du and Prendergast 1999). Another farnesylated protein and family member of p21-Ras is Rig (Ras-related inhibitor of cell growth). Rig plays a negative role by inhibiting cell growth and transformation and is frequently lost in primary gliomas (Ellis et al. 2002). Since farnesylation is a common PTM, it was feared that the use of FTase inhibitors to target p21-Ras may generate unwanted cytotoxic effects as other important biological processes would be disturbed. Interestingly, such cytotoxic effects were not found in animals and lead to human clinical trials (Nagasu et al. 1995; Sepp-Lorenzino et al. 1995). The lack of toxicity of FTase maybe due to the fact that several proteins that are farnesylated can also be geranylgeranylated, suggesting some functional redundancy between FTase and GTase.

FTIs can be broadly categorized into three groups.

1. Analogs of farnesyl pyrophosphate (FPP) substrate such as (-hydroxyl farnesyl) phosphonic acid and -ketophosphonic acid derivatives.
2. CAAX peptide analogs and non-peptide tricyclic FTIs.
3. Substrate inhibitors such as phosphonic acid and hydroxylamine acid analogs.

Preclinical studies using FTIs on transgenic mouse models or xenograft mouse tumor models have yielded interesting observations. First, MMTV-^{12}VHa Ras mice that develop mammary and salivary tumors were sensitive to FTIs, whereas tumors with mice harboring mutations in N-Ras or K-Ras were resistant (Kohl et al. 1995; Mangues et al. 1998). Inhibiting p21-Ras in glioma cell lines and xenografts results in an antiproliferation effect using dominant negative Ras mutants and FTIs (Feldkamp et al. 1999b; Nagasu et al. 1995). GBM cell lines with abnormal levels of mutant epidermal growth factor receptor (EGFR), which are prevalent in GBM, were more sensitive to FTIs in vitro and in vivo. The antitumor effects that were observed were not limited to reduced proliferation but included increased apoptosis and reduced tumor vasculature (Feldkamp et al. 2001). Since only a subset of tumors was sensitive to FTIs, tumor xenografts were measured for isospecific forms of p21-Ras. In vivo and in vitro experiments revealed that there was a close relationship between FTI sensitivity and tumors that expressed high levels of Ha-Ras versus those that expressed high levels of N-Ras and K-Ras.

The above preclinical data lead to the early phase I/II clinical trial of FTIs that are currently under investigation. The FTI, R115777 (Tipifarnib/Zarnestra), was evaluated in phase I/II trials of recurrent glioma. Phase I data defined the maximal tolerable dose (MTD), while phase II evaluations in the same patient population using the defined MTD showed promising results with 23% of patients progression free at 6 months (Cloughesy et al. 2006). In addition to specific FTIs, non-specific FTIs such as lovastatin (blocks geranylgeranylation, PI3K signaling, interferes with RhoB recruitment to the membrane) and manumycin (an antibiotic that inhibits selective FTases) have shown efficacy against gliomas in vitro (Bouterfa et al. 2000; Wang and Macaulay 1999). Even though FTIs inhibit farnesylation, N-Ras and K-Ras can switch to geranylgeranylation diminishing the effectiveness of FTIs in most human cancers. Xenograft models of mice with brain tumors treated with farnesylation inhibitors exhibited a switch in Ras processing from farnesylation to geranylgeranylation with respect to N-Ras and K-Ras, suggesting a switch in posttranslational modification preventing FTIs from eliminating the tumor. Therefore, FTIs may not be the "magic bullet" or used as a single agent but their low neurotoxicity and positive effect in a subset of GBM patients may make them ideal in combination with other therapies. Additional FTI clinical trials in combination with other GBM-relevant drugs such as temozolomide will be of great interest. Due to the heterogeneity of GBM, biological tailoring to subset of patients will be invaluable, and FTIs and other therapeutics may be used in specific situations depending on the molecular profile of the patient's tumor.

38.6 Alternative Methods to Target p21-Ras Signaling

In addition to FTIs, geranyl (GGTIs), and dual prenylation inhibitors (DPIs) have also been investigated for their antitumor effects. GGTIs have shown to exhibit antitumor effects primarily by blocking cells from entering the S phase of cell cycle. This is supported by the evidence that GGTIs induce the cell cycle inhibitor p21-WAF1. However, these promising results are in vitro, and GGTIs unlike FTIs exhibit greater toxicity, therefore putting into question their therapeutic benefit (Lobell et al. 2001).

Raf is another component of the Ras pathway that has attracted a vast interest as a therapeutic target. As previously mentioned, p21-Ras activates the serine threonine kinase Raf (Fig. 38.3). B-Raf phosphorylates MEK1 and MEK2 which in turn phosphorylate the ERK1 and ERK2 MAPKs. Activated ERK1/2 then translocate to the nucleus to phosphorylate several transcription factors such as Elk1 and Ets-2, causing a variety of genes to be activated or expression of other genes to be repressed. Recent studies on B-Raf in pediatric gliomas have shown that the B-Raf gene is often amplified in pediatric gliomas leading to elevated levels of B-Raf. In addition, somatic mutations in *B-Raf* genes were identified in pediatric glioma patients leading to the constitutive activation of B-Raf and Ras-MAPK signaling (Pfister et al. 2008). Therefore, MEK and B-Raf inhibitors are of potential promise in glioma treatment. Sorafenib (Nexavar) by Bayer/Onyx is a B-Raf inhibitor that has been approved to treat patients with renal cell carcinoma (RCC). Although its mechanism has not been fully elucidated, sorafenib may act as an antiangiogenic agent by targeting VEGFR2. RAF265, an orally administered Raf inhibitor, has been shown to inhibit all three isoforms of Raf in vitro and is now in phase I trials for patients with metastatic melanoma (Roberts and Der 2007).

Although direct targeting of p21-Ras may not be the most effective therapeutic, targeting downstream effectors of Ras that were previously mentioned remains an attractive and viable option for future antitumor targeting. For example AZD6244 and AZ4318 by Array BioPharma, targeting MEK and MEK2, have entered phase II and phase I clinical trials, respectively (Roberts and Der 2007). Another example results from the observation that activated p21-Ras leads to increased levels of PI(3)K/AKT/mTOR signaling and hence could be another potential therapeutic target. Rapamycin, an inhibitor of mTOR, has shown to reduce proliferation and tumor vasculature in vitro and in xenograft models (Cloughesy et al. 2008).

38.7 p21-Ras Signaling in Non-glioma CNS Tumors

Ras-MAPK signaling has been extensively studied in gliomas including oligodendrogliomas and astrocytomas such as GBM. The research in non-glioma primary CNS tumors is sparse. Primary CNS tumors such as ependymoma, neuroblastoma, and medulloblastoma have not been studied in detail for p21-Ras signaling. Sequencing of the p21-Ras family members in medulloblastoma, ependymoma, and neuroblastoma revealed no significant mutations in p21-Ras, which is similar to observations in GBM (MacDonald et al. 2001; Ballas et al. 1988; Cruz III et al. 2003). p21-Ras mutation is approximately under 7–10% in medulloblastoma, and some evidence suggests that elevated levels of Ras in medulloblastoma arise through aberrant expression of the PDGF receptors (Ballas et al. 1988; Gilbertson et al. 2006). Stimulation of medulloblastoma cell lines such as the malignant Daoy cell line with PDGF causes hyper-activation of Ras-MAPK signaling and increases cell proliferation in vitro (MacDonald et al. 2001). Therefore, investigation of p21-Ras inhibitors and effects on medulloblastoma may be warranted. The cause of elevated levels of p21-Ras and its role in neuroblastoma and ependymomas is still sparse and further investigation is required to determine if aberrant activation of p21-RAS has a significant role in these tumors.

38.8 Conclusion

Activated p21-Ras and its downstream signaling effects are critical in GBM biology and provide a key target for novel therapeutic strategies. However, the complexity of p21-Ras signaling demonstrates the immense crosstalk between p21-Ras signaling pathways and other prevalent signaling pathways in gliomas such as PI3K signaling. This crosstalk of signaling pathways also leads to the notion that single targeting of one molecule in the p21-Ras pathway or any pathway will be likely ineffective. FTIs are effective against Ha-Ras but not

K-Ras and N-Ras since the latter two can be geranylgeranylated when farnesylation is abolished, making FTIs ineffective by themselves. Combinatorial therapeutics with FTIs and other novel small molecule inhibitors are likely to be more effective in targeting the multiple pathways abnormally activated in malignant gliomas.

References

Ballas K, Lyons J, Janssen JW, Bartram CR (1988) Incidence of *ras* gene mutations in neuroblastoma. *Eur. J. Pediatr.*, **147:** 313–314.

Boguski MS, McCormick F (1993) Proteins regulating Ras and its relatives. *Nature*, **366:** 643–654.

Bos JL (1989) Ras oncogenes in human cancer: a review. *Cancer Res.*, **49:** 4682–4689.

Bouterfa HL, Sattelmeyer V, Czub S, Vordermark D, Roosen K, Tonn JC (2000) Inhibition of Ras farnesylation by lovastatin leads to downregulation of proliferation and migration in primary cultured human glioblastoma cells. *Anticancer Res.*, **20:** 2761–2771.

Buhring HJ, Herbst R, Kostka G, Bossenmaier B, Bartke I, Kropshofer H, Kalbacher H, Busch FW, Muller CA, Schlessinger J (1993) Modulation of p145c-kit function in cells of patients with acute myeloblastic leukemia. *Cancer Res.*, **53:** 4424–4431.

Casey PJ, Solski PA, Der CJ, Buss JE (1989) p21ras is modified by a farnesyl isoprenoid. *Proc. Natl. Acad. Sci. U. S. A*, **86:** 8323–8327.

Cloughesy TF, Wen PY, Robins HI, Chang SM, Groves MD, Fink KL, Junck L, Schiff D, Abrey L, Gilbert MR, Lieberman F, Kuhn J, DeAngelis LM, Mehta M, Raizer JJ, Yung WK, Aldape K, Wright J, Lamborn KR, Prados MD (2006) Phase II trial of tipifarnib in patients with recurrent malignant glioma either receiving or not receiving enzyme-inducing antiepileptic drugs: a North American Brain tumor consortium study. *J. Clin. Oncol.*, **24:** 3651–3656.

Cloughesy TF, Yoshimoto K, Nghiemphu P, Brown K, Dang J, Zhu S, Hsueh T, Chen Y, Wang W, Youngkin D, Liau L, Martin N, Becker D, Bergsneider M, Lai A, Green R, Oglesby T, Koleto M, Trent J, Horvath S, Mischel PS, Mellinghoff IK, Sawyers CL (2008) Antitumor activity of rapamycin in a Phase I trial for patients with recurrent PTEN-deficient glioblastoma. *PLoS. Med.*, **5:** e8.

Cowley S, Paterson H, Kemp P, Marshall CJ (1994) Activation of MAP kinase kinase is necessary and sufficient for PC12 differentiation and for transformation of NIH 3T3 cells. *Cell*, **77:** 841–852.

Cruz F, III, Rubin BP, Wilson D, Town A, Schroeder A, Haley A, Bainbridge T, Heinrich MC, Corless CL (2003) Absence of BRAF and NRAS mutations in uveal melanoma. *Cancer Res.*, **63:** 5761–5766.

Ding H, Roncari L, Shannon P, Wu X, Lau N, Karaskova J, Gutmann DH, Squire JA, Nagy A, Guha A (2001) Astrocyte-specific expression of activated p21-ras results in malignant astrocytoma formation in a transgenic mouse model of human gliomas. *Cancer Res.*, **61:** 3826–3836.

Du W, Prendergast GC (1999) Geranylgeranylated RhoB mediates suppression of human tumor cell growth by farnesyltransferase inhibitors. *Cancer Res.*, **59:** 5492–5496.

Ellis CA, Vos MD, Howell H, Vallecorsa T, Fults DW, Clark GJ (2002) Rig is a novel Ras-related protein and potential neural tumor suppressor. *Proc. Natl. Acad. Sci. U. S. A*, **99:** 9876–9881.

Ellis RW, Defeo D, Shih TY, Gonda MA, Young HA, Tsuchida N, Lowy DR, Scolnick EM (1981) The p21 src genes of Harvey and Kirsten sarcoma viruses originate from divergent members of a family of normal vertebrate genes. *Nature*, **292:** 506–511.

Feldkamp MM, Lau N, Guha A (1999a) Growth inhibition of astrocytoma cells by farnesyl transferase inhibitors is mediated by a combination of anti-proliferative, pro-apoptotic and anti-angiogenic effects. *Oncogene*, **18:** 7514–7526.

Feldkamp MM, Lau N, Guha A (1999a) Growth inhibition of astrocytoma cells by farnesyl transferase inhibitors is mediated by a combination of anti-proliferative, pro-apoptotic and anti-angiogenic effects. *Oncogene*, **18:** 7514–7526.

Feldkamp MM, Lau N, Rak J, Kerbel RS, Guha A (1999b) Normoxic and hypoxic regulation of vascular endothelial growth factor (VEGF) by astrocytoma cells is mediated by Ras. *Int. J. Cancer*, **81:** 118–124.

Feldkamp MM, Lau N, Roncari L, Guha A (2001) Isotype-specific Ras.GTP-levels predict the efficacy of farnesyl transferase inhibitors against human astrocytomas regardless of Ras mutational status. *Cancer Res.*, **61:** 4425–4431.

Gelb MH (1997) Protein prenylation, et cetera: signal transduction in two dimensions. *Science*, **275:** 1750–1751.

Gibbs JB, Pompliano DL, Mosser SD, Rands E, Lingham RB, Singh SB, Scolnick EM, Kohl NE, Oliff A (1993) Selective inhibition of farnesyl-protein transferase blocks ras processing in vivo. *J. Biol. Chem.*, **268:** 7617–7620.

Gilbertson RJ, Langdon JA, Hollander A, Hernan R, Hogg TL, Gajjar A, Fuller C, Clifford SC (2006) Mutational analysis of PDGFR-RAS/MAPK pathway activation in childhood medulloblastoma. *Eur. J. Cancer*, **42:** 646–649.

Glomset JA, Farnsworth CC (1994) Role of protein modification reactions in programming interactions between ras-related GTPases and cell membranes. *Annu. Rev. Cell Biol.*, **10:** 181–205.

Guha A, Feldkamp MM, Lau N, Boss G, Pawson A (1997) Proliferation of human malignant astrocytomas is dependent on Ras activation. *Oncogene*, **15:** 2755–2765.

Gutmann DH, Boguski M, Marchuk D, Wigler M, Collins FS, Ballester R (1993) Analysis of the neurofibromatosis type 1 (NF1) GAP-related domain by site-directed mutagenesis. *Oncogene*, **8:** 761–769.

Jaaro H, Rubinfeld H, Hanoch T, Seger R (1997) Nuclear translocation of mitogen-activated protein kinase kinase (MEK1) in response to mitogenic stimulation. *Proc. Natl. Acad. Sci. U. S. A*, **94:** 3742–3747.

Johnson SM, Grosshans H, Shingara J, Byrom M, Jarvis R, Cheng A, Labourier E, Reinert KL, Brown D, Slack FJ (2005) RAS is regulated by the let-7 microRNA family. *Cell*, **120:** 635–647.

Kohl NE, Omer CA, Conner MW, Anthony NJ, Davide JP, deSolms SJ, Giuliani EA, Gomez RP, Graham SL, Hamilton K (1995) Inhibition of farnesyltransferase induces regression of mammary and salivary carcinomas in ras transgenic mice. *Nat. Med.*, **1:** 792–797.

Kolch W, Heidecker G, Lloyd P, Rapp UR (1991) Raf-1 protein kinase is required for growth of induced NIH/3T3 cells. *Nature*, **349:** 426–428.

Leevers SJ, Paterson HF, Marshall CJ (1994) Requirement for Ras in Raf activation is overcome by targeting Raf to the plasma membrane. *Nature*, **369:** 411–414.

Lobell RB, Omer CA, Abrams MT, Bhimnathwala HG, Brucker MJ, Buser CA, Davide JP, deSolms SJ, Dinsmore CJ, Ellis-Hutchings MS, Kral AM, Liu D, Lumma WC, Machotka SV, Rands E, Williams TM, Graham SL, Hartman GD, Oliff AI, Heimbrook DC, Kohl NE (2001) Evaluation of farnesyl:protein transferase and geranylgeranyl:protein transferase inhibitor combinations in preclinical models. *Cancer Res.*, **61:** 8758–8768.

Lowy DR, Johnson MR, DeClue JE, Cen H, Zhang K, Papageorge AG, Vass WC, Willumsen BM, Valentine MB, Look AT (1993) Cell transformation by ras and regulation of its protein product. *Ciba Found. Symp.*, **176:** 67–80.

Lowy DR, Willumsen BM (1993) Function and regulation of ras. *Annu. Rev. Biochem.*, **62:** 851–891.

MacDonald TJ, Brown KM, LaFleur B, Peterson K, Lawlor C, Chen Y, Packer RJ, Cogen P, Stephan DA (2001) Expression profiling of medulloblastoma: PDGFRA and the RAS/MAPK pathway as therapeutic targets for metastatic disease. *Nat. Genet.*, **29:** 143–152.

Mangues R, Corral T, Kohl NE, Symmans WF, Lu S, Malumbres M, Gibbs JB, Oliff A, Pellicer A (1998) Antitumor effect of a farnesyl protein transferase inhibitor in mammary and lymphoid tumors overexpressing N-ras in transgenic mice. *Cancer Res.*, **58:** 1253–1259.

Mansour SJ, Matten WT, Hermann AS, Candia JM, Rong S, Fukasawa K, Vande Woude GF, Ahn NG (1994) Transformation of mammalian cells by constitutively active MAP kinase kinase. *Science*, **265:** 966–970.

Marshall CJ (1995) Specificity of receptor tyrosine kinase signaling: transient versus sustained extracellular signal-regulated kinase activation. *Cell*, **80:** 179–185.

Marshall CJ (1996) Cell signalling. Raf gets it together. *Nature*, **383:** 127–128.

McCormick F (1993b) Signal transduction. How receptors turn Ras on. *Nature*, **363:** 15–16.

McCormick F (1993a) Signal transduction. How receptors turn Ras on. *Nature*, **363:** 15–16.

Messina S, Leonetti C, De Gregorio G, Affatigato V, Ragona G, Frati L, Zupi G, Santoni A, Porcellini A (2004) Ras inhibition amplifies cisplatin sensitivity of human glioblastoma. *Biochem. Biophys. Res. Commun.*, **320:** 493–500.

Nagasu T, Yoshimatsu K, Rowell C, Lewis MD, Garcia AM (1995) Inhibition of human tumor xenograft growth by treatment with the farnesyl transferase inhibitor B956. *Cancer Res.*, **55:** 5310–5314.

Park HW, Boduluri SR, Moomaw JF, Casey PJ, Beese LS (1997) Crystal structure of protein farnesyltransferase at 2.25 angstrom resolution. *Science*, **275:** 1800–1804.

Pawson T, Saxton TM (1999) Signaling networks – do all roads lead to the same genes? *Cell*, **97:** 675–678.

Pellicena P, Scholten JD, Zimmerman K, Creswell M, Huang CC, Miller WT (1996) Involvement of the alpha subunit of farnesyl-protein transferase in substrate recognition. *Biochemistry*, **35:** 13494–13500.

Perucho M, Goldfarb M, Shimizu K, Lama C, Fogh J, Wigler M (1981) Human-tumor-derived cell lines contain common and different transforming genes. *Cell*, **27:** 467–476.

Pfister S, Janzarik WG, Remke M, Ernst A, Werft W, Becker N, Toedt G, Wittmann A, Kratz C, Olbrich H, Ahmadi R, Thieme B, Joos S, Radlwimmer B, Kulozik A, Pietsch T, Herold-Mende C, Gnekow A, Reifenberger G, Korshunov A, Scheurlen W, Omran H, Lichter P (2008) BRAF gene duplication constitutes a mechanism of MAPK pathway activation in low-grade astrocytomas. *J. Clin. Invest*, **118:** 1739–1749.

Pritchard C, McMahon M (1997) Raf revealed in life-or-death decisions. *Nat. Genet.*, **16:** 214–215.

Roberts PJ, Der CJ (2007) Targeting the Raf-MEK-ERK mitogen-activated protein kinase cascade for the treatment of cancer. *Oncogene*, **26:** 3291–3310.

Schlessinger J (1993) Cellular signaling by receptor tyrosine kinases. *Harvey Lect.*, **89:** 105–123.

Sepp-Lorenzino L, Ma Z, Rands E, Kohl NE, Gibbs JB, Oliff A, Rosen N (1995) A peptidomimetic inhibitor of farnesyl:protein transferase blocks the anchorage-dependent and -independent growth of human tumor cell lines. *Cancer Res.*, **55:** 5302–5309.

Shannon P, Sabha N, Lau N, Kamnasaran D, Gutmann DH, Guha A (2005) Pathological and molecular progression of astrocytomas in a GFAP: 12 V-Ha-Ras mouse astrocytoma model. *Am. J. Pathol.*, **167:** 859–867.

Sprang SR (1997a) G protein mechanisms: insights from structural analysis. *Annu. Rev. Biochem.*, **66:** 639–678.

Sprang SR (1997b) G proteins, effectors and GAPs: structure and mechanism. *Curr. Opin. Struct. Biol.*, **7:** 849–856.

Stokoe D, Macdonald SG, Cadwallader K, Symons M, Hancock JF (1994) Activation of Raf as a result of recruitment to the plasma membrane. *Science*, **264:** 1463–1467.

Tamada M, Hu CD, Kariya K, Okada T, Kataoka T (1997) Membrane recruitment of Raf-1 is not the only function of Ras in Raf-1 activation. *Oncogene*, **15:** 2959–2964.

Tamanoi F, Gau CL, Jiang C, Edamatsu H, Kato-Stankiewicz J (2001a) Protein farnesylation in mammalian cells: effects of farnesyltransferase inhibitors on cancer cells. *Cell Mol. Life Sci.*, **58:** 1636–1649.

Tamanoi F, Kato-Stankiewicz J, Jiang C, Machado I, Thapar N (2001b) Farnesylated proteins and cell cycle progression. *J. Cell Biochem. Suppl*, **Suppl 37:** 64–70.

The Cancer Genome Atlas Research Network, McLendon R, Friedman A, Bigner D, Van Meir EG, Brat DJ, Mastrogianakis M, Olson JJ, Mikkelsen T, Lehman N, Aldape K, et al. (2008) Comprehensive genomic characterization defines human glioblastoma genes and core pathways. Cancer Genome Atlas Research Network. *Nature*, **455**(7216): 1061–1068.

Trueblood CE, Boyartchuk VL, Rine J (1997) Substrate specificity determinants in the farnesyltransferase beta-subunit. *Proc. Natl. Acad. Sci. U. S. A*, **94:** 10774–10779.

Wang W, Macaulay RJ (1999) Apoptosis of medulloblastoma cells in vitro follows inhibition of farnesylation using manumycin A. *Int. J. Cancer*, **82:** 430–434.

Zhang FL, Casey PJ (1996) Protein prenylation: molecular mechanisms and functional consequences. *Annu. Rev. Biochem.*, **65:** 241–269.

Chapter 39
HGF/c-Met Signaling and Targeted Therapeutics in Brain Tumors

Roger Abounader and John Laterra

Abstract The receptor tyrosine kinase c-Met and its ligand the growth factor hepatocyte growth factor [HGF] are key determinants of malignancy of human cancers including brain tumors. c-Met is often aberrantly activated in high-grade gliomas, embryonal brain tumors, ependymomas, and meningiomas. c-Met activation in brain tumors is associated with poor clinical outcomes and is mostly caused by transcriptional overexpression of receptor and ligand and autocrine loop formation. c-Met activation in brain tumors enhances malignancy and tumor growth by inducing cell proliferation, inhibiting cell death, inducing cell migration and cell invasion, and promoting tumor angiogenesis. The oncogenic effects of HGF/c-Met are mediated by a complex downstream signaling network, the most prominent components of which are the Ras/MAPK and PI3K/Akt pathways. Based on their widespread and profound involvement in human cancer, HGF and c-Met have emerged as attractive targets for cancer therapy. Different approaches to inhibiting HGF and c-Met have been developed. These include HGF and *c-Met* gene expression inhibition with ribozymes and antisense oligonucleotides, receptor antagonism with HGF fragments such as NK4, competitive ligand binding with soluble Met receptors, neutralizing antibodies to HGF or c-Met, and small-molecule inhibitors of c-Met kinase.

Contents

Supported by NIH grants NS045209 [RA], CA129192 [JL], and NS43987 [JL].

R. Abounader (✉)
University of Virginia Health System, 21 Hospital Drive, Room 4813, Charlottesville, VA 22908, USA
e-mail: ra6u@virginia.edu

E.G. Van Meir (ed.), *CNS Cancer*, Cancer Drug Discovery and Development, DOI 10.1007/978-1-60327-553-8_39,
© Humana Press, a part of Springer Science+Business Media, LLC 2009

39.1 Introduction

The receptor tyrosine kinase c-Met and its ligand the growth factor hepatocyte growth factor [HGF] also known as scatter factor [SF] are key determinants of malignancy of human cancers including brain tumors. c-Met is often aberrantly activated in high-grade gliomas, embryonal brain tumors, ependymomas, and meningiomas, and receptor activation is associated with poor clinical outcomes. c-Met activation in brain tumors enhances malignancy and tumor growth by inducing cell proliferation, inhibiting cell death, inducing cell migration and cell invasion, and promoting tumor angiogenesis. Inhibiting endogenous HGF and/or c-Met in experimental brain tumor models leads to tumor growth inhibition and tumor regression. The oncogenic effects of HGF/c-Met are mediated by a complex downstream signaling network, the most prominent components of which are the Ras/MAPK and PI3K/Akt pathways. Based on the pathway's widespread involvement in human cancer, HGF and c-Met have emerged as promising therapeutic targets, and several clinically translatable agents that target HGF/c-Met signaling are under development. While some of these agents have already entered clinical trials, their successful application will require a better understanding of the factors that determine HGF/c-Met pathway dependency in human tumors. The present chapter reviews our current knowledge of HGF/c-Met pathway deregulation in brain tumors, its functional and molecular involvement in malignancy, and the emerging therapeutic approaches to target this pathway.

39.2 c-Met and HGF Structure and Signal Transduction

39.2.1 Structure of HGF and c-Met

The human *c-Met* gene is located on chromosome 7q21–q31. c-Met is synthesized as a 170-kDa glycosylated precursor that is cleaved into a 50-kDa α-chain and a 140-kDa β-chain that are linked by a disulfide bridge (Giordano et al.,

1989). The α-chain is extracellular and, along with the first 212 residues of the transmembraneous β-chain, binds to HGF. The β-chain contains the cytoplasmic kinase domain and a protein docking site in the carboxy-terminal that are essential for downstream signaling (Birchmeier et al., 2003; Gherardi et al., 2003). The docking site contains two tyrosines, Y1349 and Y1356, which are phosphorylated by the c-Met kinase domain upon HGF ligand binding (Ponzetto et al., 1994) (Fig. 39.1). The gene encoding the c-Met ligand *HGF* is located on chromosome 7q21.1 (Seki et al., 1991). It produces a single-chain inactive precursor that is cleaved by serine proteases into two chains that are linked by a disulfide bond (Miyazawa et al., 1993). Biologically active HGF is a heterodimer composed of a 69-kDa α-chain and a 34-kDa β-chain (Nakamura et al., 1989). The α-chain contains an N-terminal hairpin domain followed by four kringle domains, and the β-chain contains a serine protease-like domain with no enzymatic activity (Fig. 39.1).

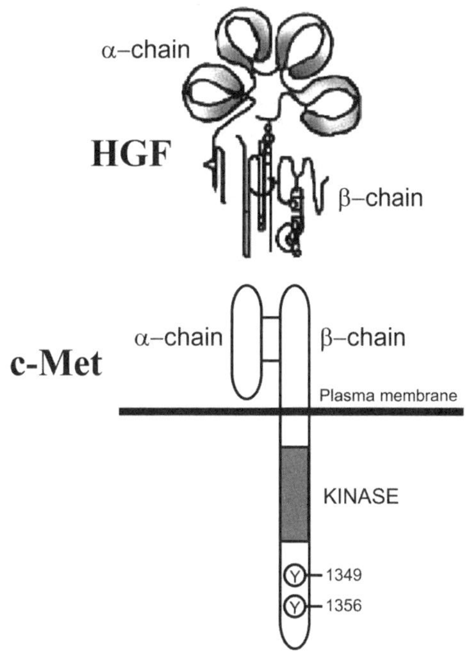

Fig. 39.1 Structures of HGF and c-Met (modified, with permission, from Fig. 1 in Matsumoto and Nakamura, 2003)

39.2.2 c-Met-Dependent Signal Transduction

Binding of HGF to c-Met leads to the phosphorylation of multiple residues in the receptor's intracellular domain. When tyrosines Y1349 and Y1356 are phosphorylated, numerous substrates are recruited and bind to the c-Met docking site, including Gab1, Grb2, PI3K, and others (Ponzetto et al., 1994;

Weidner et al., 1996; Lock et al., 2000). This leads to the activation of downstream signaling pathways including the Ras/MAPK, PI3K/Akt, and STAT pathways, which mediate the various functions of HGF/c-Met (Fig. 39.2). Activation of Ras and of ERK/MAPK alters the expression/activation of cell cycle regulators [including p27, cdk2, pRb, and others] leading to changes in cell proliferation (Walter et al., 2002; Li et al., 2005). Ras/MAPK activation by HGF/c-Met also alters the expression of matrix metalloproteinases (MMPs) and urokinase plasminogen activator (uPA) and cytoskeletal functions that control cell migration and invasion. HGF activates a cell survival signaling pathway through PI3K, Akt, Pak1, and NFκB that mediates resistance to apoptosis through multiple downstream mediators, including inhibition of caspase-9 and Bad (Bowers et al., 2000; Xiao et al., 2001) (Fan et al., 2001; Fan et al., 2007; Li et al., 2008). Both Ras/MAPK activation and PI3K/Akt activation are required for the complex morphogenic phenomenon of tubule formation induced by c-Met activation (Birchmeier et al., 2003). The STAT signaling pathway has been implicated in epithelial tubule morphogenesis and in endothelial cell proliferation and might, therefore, contribute to

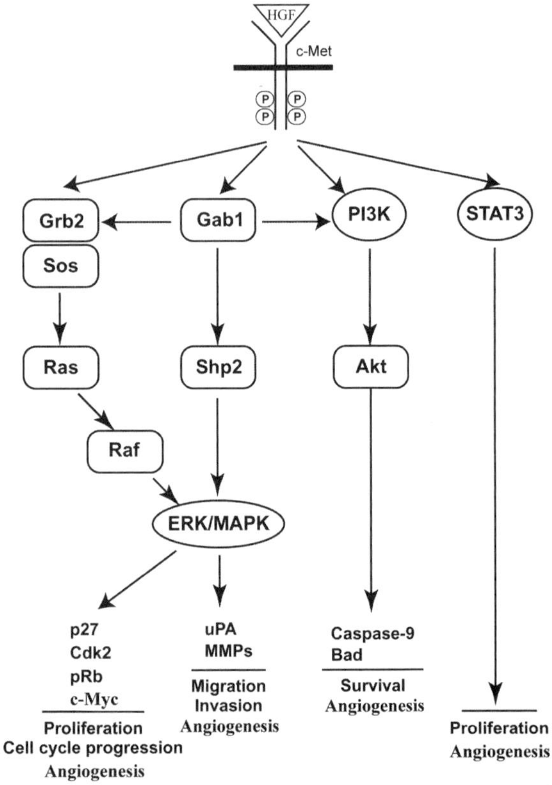

Fig. 39.2 c-Met-dependent signaling (modified, with permission, from Fig. 6 in Birchmeier et al., 2003)

c-Met-induced angiogenesis (Boccaccio et al., 1998; Nakagami et al., 2001) (Fig. 39.2). HGF also has the capacity to indirectly activate alternative receptor tyrosine kinases such as EGFR by upregulating expression of EGFR ligands TGF-α and HB-EGFL (Reznik et al., 2008).

39.3 Involvement of HGF/c-Met in Brain Tumors

The involvement of the HGF/c-Met pathway in brain tumor malignancy is demonstrated by the following: (1) HGF and c-Met are deregulated in human brain tumors, (2) activation of the pathway in cells and animal models induces malignancy, and (3) inhibition of endogenous HGF or c-Met leads to inhibition of several malignancy parameters and in vivo brain tumor growth. The following sections review the evidence that implicates the HGF/c-Met pathway in brain tumor malignancy (Fig. 39.3 and Color Plate 57).

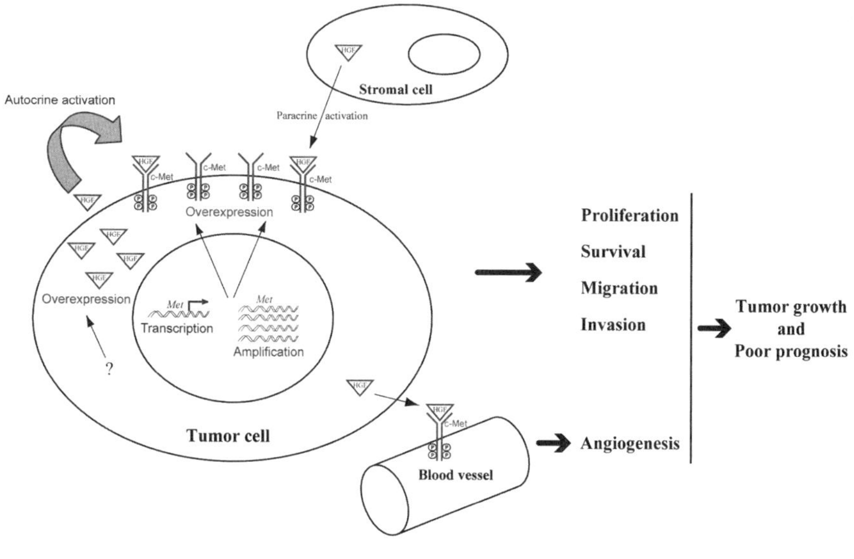

Fig. 39.3 HGF/c-Met deregulation and oncogenic effects (*see* Color Plate 57)

39.3.1 Deregulation of HGF and c-Met in Brain Tumors

39.3.1.1 Mechanisms of HGF and c-Met Deregulation in Brain Tumors

HGF and c-Met are frequently deregulated in human brain tumors including gliomas, embryonal brain tumors, meningiomas, ependymomas, and schwannomas. Various mechanisms of deregulation of HGF and c-Met have been described in human cancer. These include overexpression of ligand and/or receptor, autocrine activation of c-Met by HGF expressed in the same cell, activating mutations of c-Met, and receptor transactivation by other membrane receptors (Corso et al., 2005). Overexpression and autocrine loop formation are the most frequent mechanisms of HGF and c-Met deregulation in brain tumors. Activating mutations appear to represent a less frequent mechanism of c-Met deregulation in brain tumors. Receptor transactivation by other transmembrane receptors in brain tumors is not well understood to date. Overexpression of HGF and c-Met in brain tumors is mostly caused by transcriptional upregulation. There is a positive feedback loop from the c-Met receptor upon HGF binding that leads to transcriptional activation of the *c-Met* gene via a mechanism that involves Ras, MAPK, and the transcription factor AP-1 (Abounader et al., 2001). Autocrine activation of c-Met by HGF also represents a major mechanism of pathway activation in brain tumors and has been associated with increased malignancy and advanced tumor grades (Koochekpour et al., 1997). *c-Met* gene amplification has also been reported and may be a mechanism for ligand-independent receptor activation (Wullich et al., 1994; Tong et al., 2004).

39.3.1.2 HGF and c-Met Expression in Brain Tumors

c-Met receptor expression has been detected in all gliomas, medulloblastoma, ependymoma, and schwannoma tumors, and cell lines examined to date (Koochekpour et al., 1997; Moriyama et al., 1998a; Hecht et al., 2004). Several studies found that HGF and c-Met are expressed in human gliomas and that expression levels correlate with tumor grade (Rosen et al., 1996; Koochekpour et al., 1997; Moriyama et al., 1998a). HGF content was measured in 74 clinical samples obtained from human low-grade and high-grade gliomas. HGF expression in high-grade [WHO grade III–IV] tumors was significantly higher than in low-grade [I–II] tumors (Lamszus et al., 1998). Similarly, co-expression of HGF and c-Met is observed more frequently in grade IV glioblastoma than in low-grade glioma, consistent with the contribution of an HGF/c-Met autocrine loop to malignant progression in these tumors (Koochekpour et al., 1997; Moriyama et al., 1998a). The expression of c-Met and HGF was also assessed in several medulloblastoma cell lines and 32 clinical samples of human embryonal brain tumors including medulloblastoma. All cell lines and tumors expressed c-Met. All cell lines and all but two tumors expressed HGF. Importantly, c-Met expression levels in embryonal brain tumors significantly correlated with poor patient survival (Li et al., 2005). Some evidence also suggests that c-Met activation in medulloblastoma is associated with the most malignant large cell anaplastic medulloblastoma subtype (Li et al., 2005; Li et al., 2008). One study found that c-Met was amplified in 38.5% of 14 human medulloblastoma tumors analyzed (Tong et al., 2004). Elevated HGF levels and co-expression of HGF and c-Met were also found to correlate with meningioma recurrence and poor prognosis (Arrieta et al., 2002; Martinez-Rumayor et al., 2004).

39.3.1.3 HGF and c-Met Expression in Brain Tumor Endothelial Cells

In addition to their expression in brain tumor cells, HGF and c-Met are also overexpressed in brain tumor endothelial cells, consistent with the well described role of HGF as a potent angiogenic factor. Several studies have shown that c-Met and HGF are expressed and functional in neuromicrovascular and brain tumor vascular cells. Moderate to high levels of immunoreactive and biologically active HGF were found in cultured brain-derived microvascular endothelial cells (Rosen et al., 1996). Using double immunofluorescence staining and quantitative confocal laser scanning microscopy, it was also shown that the intensity of HGF and c-Met staining in human primary brain tumors is prevalent in both the infiltrating tumor cells and hyperplastic endothelium. Additionally, prominent HGF and c-Met immunostaining was observed in the vasculature of glioblastoma, whereas less intense c-Met and HGF immunostaining was observed in areas of neovascularization within low-grade astrocytoma [WHO grade I and II] and anaplastic astrocytoma [WHO grade III] (Koochekpour et al., 1997). Using in situ hybridization, strong HGF mRNA expression was also detected in the majority of tumor cells and in vascular endothelial cells in glioblastoma specimens but was less prevalent in anaplastic astrocytoma, diffuse astrocytoma, pilocytic astrocytoma, and normal brain. c-Met immunoreactivity was also observed in GFAP-expressing astrocytic tumor cells and endothelial cells as well as in a subset of microglia/macrophages. Other experimental evidence points to autocrine and paracrine endothelium c-Met activation as a contributor to tumor angiogenesis (Kunkel et al., 2001).

In summary, there is substantial evidence from human tissue specimens that HGF and c-Met are deregulated via multiple mechanisms in brain tumor cells and brain tumor endothelial cells. HGF and c-Met deregulation in brain tumors lead to c-Met activation and are associated with increased malignancy and poor prognosis.

39.3.2 Oncogenic Effects of c-Met Activation in Brain Tumors

Activation of c-Met in brain tumors enhances several oncogenic mechanisms including cell proliferation and cell cycle progression, cell survival and resistance to cytotoxic therapies, cell migration and invasion, and tumor angiogenesis. This section reviews the oncogenic effects of c-Met activation in brain tumors and the cell signaling and molecular mechanisms that mediate them.

39.3.2.1 Cell Proliferation

Activation of c-Met induces brain tumor cell and brain tumor endothelial cell proliferation. Treatment of glioma and medulloblastoma cells with exogenous recombinant HGF or forced expression of HGF in glioma and medulloblastoma cells induces tumor cell and tumor endothelial cell DNA synthesis and proliferation (Rosen et al., 1996; Laterra et al., 1997a; Lamszus et al., 1999; Li et al., 2005). Conversely, inhibiting endogenous HGF or c-Met expression in glioma cells with U1snRNA/ribozymes, the HGF antagonist NK4, or an anti-HGF neutralizing monoclonal antibody inhibits tumor cell proliferation (Brockmann et al., 2003a; Kim et al., 2006). Also, inhibiting HGF and c-Met expression in human glioma xenografts reduces tumor cell proliferation as assessed by Ki-67 immunostaining (Abounader et al., 1999, 2002). HGF/c-Met-induced cell proliferation in brain tumor cells is [at least partially] due to HGF/c-Met-induced G1/S cell cycle progression. Treating glioblastoma as well as medulloblastoma cells with HGF induces G1/S cell cycle progression (Walter et al., 2002; Li et al., 2005). The signal transduction pathways and molecular mechanisms that mediate HGF/c-Met-induced brain tumor cell proliferation and cell cycle progression have not been fully investigated to date. Evidence implicates mechanisms involving p27 inhibition, Cdk2 kinase activation, transcriptional and posttranscriptional mechanisms of c-Myc activation in medulloblastoma cells (Li et al., 2005, 2008). c-Myc was also found to mediate HGF-induced cell proliferation and cell cycle progression in glioblastoma cells (Walter et al., 2002).

39.3.2.2 Cell Survival

HGF is a potent inhibitor of apoptosis and chemotherapy- and radiotherapy-induced cell death in brain tumor cells. Treating human glioblastoma cells with recombinant HGF partially inhibits the cytotoxic effects of gamma irradiation, cisplatin, camptothecin, adriamycin, and taxol (Bowers et al., 2000). Similarly, forced expression of HGF in rat intracranial gliosarcomas reduces tumor cell sensitivity to in vivo gamma irradiation (Bowers et al., 2000). Conversely, inhibiting endogenous HGF in either glioma cells or glioma xenografts leads to induction of apoptosis and cell death with increased cleaved caspase-3 expression in cells and in xenografts (Bowers et al., 2000; Abounader et al., 2002). Inhibiting endogenous HGF and c-Met synergizes with radiation therapy in inhibiting the in vivo growth of glioblastoma xenografts. This provides a rationale for using anti-HGF/c-Met therapies to sensitize brain tumors to radiation therapy (Lal et al., 2005). Forced expression of both HGF and Sonic Hedgehog [Shh] in nestin-expressing cerebellar neural progenitor cells in newborn mice was found to increase spontaneous medulloblastoma formation, ~2-fold over animals expressing Shh alone. Treating these HGF + Shh transgenic mice with an HGF pathway inhibitor increased medulloblastoma cell apoptosis as evidenced by caspase-3 activation and prolonged animal survival. While HGF inhibits cell death and apoptosis in some established human medulloblastoma cell lines, it can enhance apoptotic cell death in other medulloblastoma cell lines (Li et al., 2008). The factor[s] that determines HGF-mediated inhibition vs. induction of apoptosis in brain tumors and cancer in general is not known. The cytoprotective effects of HGF/c-Met in glioma and medulloblastoma are mediated by the PI3K/Akt pathway. Inhibiting either

PI3K or Akt with pharmacological agents and dominant negative constructs abrogates HGF-induced inhibition of apoptosis in glioblastoma cells (Bowers et al., 2000). Similarly, pharmacological inhibition of PI3K in medulloblastoma cells in which c-Met activation is anti-apoptotic completely inhibits HGF-induced tumor cell survival (Li et al., 2005). In medulloblastoma cell subtypes where HGF exerts pro-apoptotic effects, c-Myc mediates these effects (Li et al., 2008). Altogether, the above findings indicate that the HGF/c-Met pathway is a promising target for sensitizing selected brain tumors to cytotoxic therapies.

39.3.2.3 Cell Migration and Cell Invasion

HGF induces tumor cell motility and invasion. The effects of HGF, EGF, bFGF, PDGF-BB, and TGF-beta 1 on the motility and invasion of seven primary glioma cultures were compared. The results revealed that HGF promotes cell motility with chemokinetic and strong chemotactic activities. Concentric circle assays showed that HGF was the strongest promoter of two-dimensional expansion [proliferation and motility] among the five growth factors studied. HGF also stimulates cerebral microvascular endothelial cell motility and significantly stimulates chemotaxis of both glioma and cerebral microvascular endothelial cells (Brockmann et al., 2003b). Treating glioma cells with HGF enhances invasiveness (Welch et al., 1999). HGF was also found to markedly stimulate the chemotactic migration of 10/10 glioma cell lines as well as 3/3 neural microvascular endothelial cell lines (Lamszus et al., 1998). HGF and c-Met expression inhibition by U1snRNA/ribozymes inhibited glioblastoma cell migration in a two-dimensional scratch assay (Abounader et al., 2002). In medulloblastoma, forced expression of HGF alters the phenotype of intracranial medulloblastoma xenografts increasing tumor cell infiltration into the surrounding brain and spread to the subarachnoid space (Li et al., 2005). The molecular mechanisms of HGF-induced brain tumor cell migration and invasion have not been thoroughly investigated to date. Two studies showed that HGF induces MMP-2 and uPA expression in glioblastoma cells, but a causal link between protease induction and tumor cell migration and invasion was not established (Hamasuna et al., 1999; Moriyama et al., 1999).

39.3.2.4 Angiogenesis

HGF and c-Met also contribute to brain tumor malignancy by promoting tumor angiogenesis. The potential contributions of VEGF, HGF, and basic fibroblast growth factor [bFGF] to glioma angiogenesis were examined. Growth factor levels were quantified in extracts of 71 gliomas by enzyme-linked immunoabsorbent assay. The levels of bFGF in low-grade gliomas [WHO grade II] were only marginally different from high-grade gliomas [WHO grades III and IV]. In contrast, the mean concentrations of VEGF and HGF were 11-fold and 7-fold higher, respectively, in the high-grade lesions. Both HGF and VEGF but not bFGF highly significantly correlated with microvessel density as determined by immunostaining for factor VIII-related antigen. Multiple regression analysis indicated that HGF and VEGF are independent predictors of glioma microvessel density and presumably angiogenesis (Schmidt et al., 1999).

HGF promotes glioma angiogenesis by enhancing brain tumor endothelial cell proliferation, motility, and invasion as described in the previous sections. The organization of endothelial cells into tube-like structures is an essential step in blood vessel formation. One study analyzed the capacity of bFGF, VEGF, and HGF to induce endothelial tube formation in collagen gels. Both HGF and VEGF independently synergized with bFGF, an essential angiogenic cofactor. As predicted by tissue levels of angiogenic factors, extracts from high-grade gliomas were significantly more potent than extracts from low-grade tumors in stimulating endothelial cell tube formation. Neutralizing antibodies to bFGF, VEGF, or HGF inhibited extract-induced tube formation by up to 98, 62, and 54%, respectively. Taken together, these in vitro and in vivo findings suggest a model of tumor angiogenesis whereby increasing levels of VEGF and/or HGF typically seen with malignant glioma progression synergize with bFGF, which is already elevated in poorly vascularized low-grade tumors (Schmidt et al., 1999). Another study found that macro- and microvascular endothelial cells formed tubular structures when cultured within a three-dimensional fibrin matrix and that this process was enhanced by HGF. Also, endothelial tubulogenesis was found to be increased in co-cultures of endothelial cells and glioma tumor cells that secrete angiogenic factors, including HGF, but not with non-tumorigenic cell types such as MDCK [Madin–Darby canine kidney] epithelial cells (Lafleur et al., 2002). VEGF induction might also contribute to HGF-induced brain tumor angiogenesis (Moriyama et al., 1998b).

Gain-of-function and loss-of-function approaches provide additional in vivo evidence for HGF-induced glioma angiogenesis. Forced HGF expression in HGF^{-}/c-Met^{+} rat and human glioma cell lines increases tumor xenograft angiogenesis as measured by microvascular density determinations (Laterra et al., 1997a, b). In HGF^{+}/c-Met^{+} cells, knocking down either HGF or c-Met expression with ribozyme-based approaches or inhibiting c-Met activation with functional inhibitors reduces xenograft angiogenesis (Abounader et al., 1999, 2002; Burgess et al., 2006; Kim et al., 2006).

In summary, there is substantial evidence that the HGF/c-Met pathway strongly promotes brain tumor progression by directly inducing several biological parameters of malignancy. Targeting this pathway in brain tumors, as will be discussed in the following sections, therefore constitutes a promising approach for brain tumor therapy.

39.4 HGF and c-Met as Targets for Brain Tumor Therapy

Based on their widespread and profound involvement in human cancer, HGF and c-Met have emerged as attractive targets for cancer therapy. Different approaches to inhibiting HGF and c-Met have been developed. These include

HGF and *c-Met* gene expression inhibition with ribozymes and antisense oligonucleotides, receptor antagonism with HGF fragments such as NK4, competitive ligand binding with soluble Met receptors, neutralizing antibodies to HGF or c-Met, and small-molecule inhibitors of c-Met kinase (Fig. 39.4 and Color Plate 58).

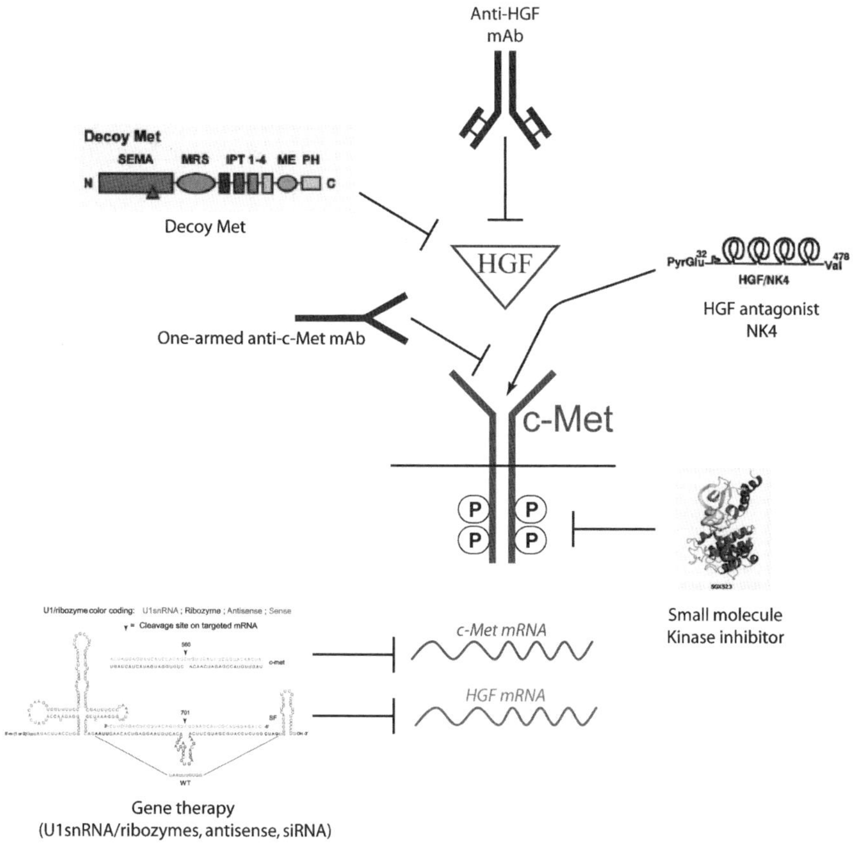

Fig. 39.4 Therapeutic targeting strategies of HGF/c-Met (*see* Color Plate 58)

39.4.1 U1snRNA/Ribozymes and Antisense

Gene therapy approaches to inhibit HGF and/or c-Met have been used to inhibit HGF and c-Met expressions in experimental brain tumor animal models. Chimeric U1snRNA/ribozyme transgenes were the first agents used to inhibit HGF and c-Met expression in human cancer (Abounader et al., 1999, 2002, 2004). Delivery of these U1snRNA/ribozymes to pre-established subcutaneous and intracranial glioma xenografts via liposome–DNA complexes and adenoviruses significantly inhibited tumor growth as well as tumor HGF and c-Met expression levels. Histologic analysis of tumors treated with U1snRNA/ribozymes showed a significant increase in brain tumor cell apoptosis and a significant decrease in tumor blood vessel density (Abounader et al., 1999, 2002). U1snRNA/ribozyme-mediated in vivo inhibition of HGF and c-Met was later tested in combination with hypofractionated γ-radiation administered every 5 days at 300 cGy per fraction and achieved synergistic inhibition of intracranial glioblastoma xenograft growth. Ionizing radiation therapy and U1snRNA/ribozyme therapy had additive effects on angiogenesis inhibition demonstrating the value of applying ionizing radiation in conjunction with HGF/c-Met pathway inhibition to target glioma blood vessel formation (Lal et al., 2005). c-Met antisense oligonucleotides were also tested in a glioma xenograft animal model. The uptake of therapeutic concentrations of these c-Met antisense oligonucleotides in vivo in rats bearing glioma xenografts was demonstrated but their effects on tumor growth was not assessed (Chu et al., 2007). These molecular approaches have been critical in providing proof of principle that inhibiting HGF and c-Met in brain tumors can have therapeutic value. However, the clinical translation of such approaches must overcome numerous hurdles. Other agents described below [e.g., small-molecule kinase inhibitors and neutralizing mAbs] have a much clearer path to clinical translation.

39.4.2 NK4

NK4 is a synthetic molecule that comprises the NH_2-terminal hairpin domain and subsequent four kringle domains of HGF, but it lacks the entire α-chain. NK4 inhibits the specific binding of HGF to its receptor c-Met in a competitive fashion and inhibits HGF-induced effects on tumor cells and endothelial cells. In one study, mice bearing intracranial glioma xenografts received daily intratumoral injections of NK4 or buffer, beginning 1–7 days after tumor cell implantation. Tumor volumes were reduced by 61% in the NK4-treated mice. Intratumoral microvessel densities were reduced by 65 and 37%, when treatment started on day 1 or day 7, respectively (Brockmann et al., 2003a). The proliferative activity of the tumor cells was reduced by >30% regardless of when NK4 treatment was initiated. The apoptotic fraction of tumor cells was increased up to 2-fold. In vitro, NK4 inhibited HGF-induced glioblastoma and endothelial cell migration and proliferation in a dose-dependent fashion (Brockmann et al., 2003a). Interestingly, NK4 was also able to inhibit angiogenesis independently of c-Met (Matsumoto and Nakamura, 2003). This effect is thought to be caused by NK4's remarkable structural homology with the anti-angiogenic protein angiostatin and its potential to inhibit other kringle-dependent angiogenic protein–protein interactions (O'Reilly et al., 1994). NK4 is currently being developed for clinical use by Kringle Pharmaceuticals.

39.4.3 Soluble Met

A soluble decoy c-Met receptor has been generated consisting of recombinant protein corresponding to the entire c-Met extracellular domain, truncated before the transmembrane domain (Michieli et al., 2004). Lentiviral-based delivery of decoy c-Met inhibited ligand-dependent and ligand-independent c-Met activation in various in vitro and in vivo cancer models. Decoy c-Met impaired HGF-induced endothelial cell migration and branching. Decoy c-Met also inhibited the growth and dissemination of established mammary tumor xenografts. In these tumors, c-Met inhibition reduced tumor vessel arborization. Using ex vivo studies, the authors subsequently showed that optimal tumor growth inhibition results from the actions of decoy c-Met expressed by both tumor cells and endothelial cells. Systemic administration of decoy c-Met prevented tumor growth, metastasis, and angiogenesis without substantially affecting housekeeping physiological functions of normal tissues. To our knowledge, decoy c-Met has not been tested in a brain tumor model.

39.4.4 Small-Molecule Inhibitors

Small-molecule kinase inhibitors are one of the most promising classes of targeted therapeutics for interfering with oncogenic pathway activation. These small molecules have the potential for excellent bioavailability following systemic delivery and have been clinically validated against other targets. There has been a recent surge in the development of small-molecule c-Met inhibitors with at least 10 compounds in various phases of development (Comoglio et al., 2008). The first c-Met kinase inhibitor with respectable specificity was developed by Sugen/Pfizer and designated PHA-665752 (Christensen et al., 2003). PHA-665752 is a small-molecule, ATP-competitive, active site inhibitor of the catalytic activity of c-Met kinase with an IC_{50} of 9 nM. PHA-665752 exhibits >50-fold selectivity for c-Met as compared with a panel of diverse tyrosine and serine–threonine kinases including the epidermal growth factor receptor. In cellular studies in vitro, PHA-665752 potently inhibits constitutive and HGF-stimulated c-Met phosphorylation, as well as HGF-driven responses such as cell growth [proliferation and survival], cell motility, invasion, and/or morphogenesis in a variety of tumor cell types. PHA-665752 inhibits HGF-stimulated and constitutive phosphorylation of c-Met signal transduction messengers including Gab-1, extracellular regulated kinase, Akt, STAT3, phospholipase C gamma, and focal adhesion kinase, in multiple cell lines. A single dose of PHA-665752 inhibited c-Met phosphorylation in tumor xenografts for up to 12 h. Inhibition of c-Met phosphorylation was associated with dose-dependent tumor xenograft growth inhibition or growth delay over a repeated administration schedule at well-tolerated doses. Potent cytoreductive activity was demonstrated in a gastric carcinoma xenograft model. Collectively, these results were a breakthrough in demonstrating preclinically the feasibility of selectively targeting c-Met with ATP-competitive small molecules and suggested the therapeutic potential of targeting c-Met in human cancers. Pfizer has since developed a second-generation orally bioavailable, ATP-competitive small-molecule inhibitor of c-Met kinase, which is currently in clinical trial for systemic cancers. PF-2341066 has improved specificity [twice as selective than PHA-665752] and activity profiles [enzymatic IC_{50} = 4 nM] against c-Met, although anaplastic lymphoma kinase [ALK] is also targeted. PF-2341066 inhibits c-Met-dependent cell responses including endothelial "angiogenic" behaviors in vitro with biological IC_{50} values between 5 and 20 nM. Preclinical therapeutic responses indicate that the antitumor activity of PF-2341066 may be mediated by direct effects on tumor cell growth/survival and anti-angiogenic mechanisms (Zou et al., 2007).

Other small-molecule inhibitors of c-Met with varying selectivity are currently in the preclinical or clinical developmental stage. Two of these with a high degree of selectivity and activity are SGX523 from SGX Pharmaceuticals and JNJ38877605 from Johnson & Johnson. In vivo evaluation of SGX523 demonstrated that it is orally bioavailable and has good pharmacokinetic properties in mice, rats, and dogs. SGX523 demonstrated potent antitumor activity when dosed orally in a human gastric tumor xenograft model with no overt toxicity. Orally administered SGX523 and JNJ38877605 have been shown to induce the regression of pre-established U87MG glioma xenografts. ARQ197 [ArQule] stands out as a non-ATP-competitive c-Met-specific inhibitor with an excellent selectivity profile. IC_{50} values for c-Met inhibition and for multiple c-Met-driven cell responses are in the 50–100 nM range. ARQ197 is currently in phase I and II trials for various systemic cancers. Inhibitors that are somewhat less specific but have the potential to simultaneously target multiple oncogenic kinases relevant to brain cancers include MP470 from SuperGen [also inhibits PDGFR, FLT3] and XL880 from Exelixis [also inhibits VEGFR2].

39.4.5 Neutralizing Monoclonal Antibodies

Together with small-molecule inhibitors, monoclonal antibodies [mAb] presently constitute the most clinically applicable HGF/c-Met pathway inhibitors. Monoclonal Abs have the advantage of very high target specificity and long biological half-life. Their high molecular weight raises questions regarding their ultimate clinical efficacy in CNS malignancies. Monoclonal Abs have the potential to chelate diffusible targets out of the brain and tumor parenchyma even if the blood–brain barrier limits mAb tumor levels. It was originally reported that HGF possesses a minimum of three distinct epitopes that must be blocked using multiple mAb idiotypes to prevent c-Met activation (Cao et al., 2001). This idea was overturned by two contemporaneous reports of neutralizing anti-HGF mAbs with excellent preclinical activity against HGF-dependent processes. AMGEN has generated and characterized five distinct fully human mAbs, each of which binds and neutralizes human HGF. Antibodies with subnanomolar affinities for HGF blocked binding of human HGF to c-Met and inhibited HGF-mediated c-Met phosphorylation, cell proliferation, survival, and invasion. Using a series of human–mouse chimeric HGF proteins, it was shown that the neutralizing antibodies bind to a unique epitope in the β-chain of human HGF. Each of these antibodies inhibited HGF-dependent autocrine-driven tumor growth and caused significant regression of established subcutaneous glioblastoma tumor xenografts. Treatment with anti-HGF antibody rapidly inhibited tumor cell proliferation and significantly increased the proportion of apoptotic glioblastoma tumor cells in vivo (Burgess et al., 2006). These data suggested that an antibody to an epitope in the ß-chain of HGF has potential as a novel therapeutic agent for treating patients with HGF-dependent tumors. One of these mAbs [AMG102] is currently in phase II clinical trial for recurrent glioblastoma. Interpretation of available results from 40 patients showing at most modest efficacy as a single agent awaits biomarker analyses for tumor levels of HGF and c-Met activation in trial subjects. Galaxy Biotech developed a murine anti-HGF mAb [L2G7] that similarly blocks c-Met activation by inhibiting HGF binding to c-Met. Anti-HGF L2G7 strongly inhibits all biological activities of HGF measured in vitro, including cell proliferation, cell scattering, and endothelial tubule formation. Systemic L2G7 completely inhibited the growth of two established HGF^{+}/c-Met^{+} subcutaneous glioma xenograft models [U118MG and U87MG] without affecting the growth of an HGF^{-} glioma xenograft. Moreover, systemic administration of L2G7 induced the regression of intracranial U87MG xenografts and prolonged the survival of tumor-bearing mice from a median of 39 to >90 days (Kim et al., 2006). Systemic L2G7 has recently been found to prolong the survival of immune competent mice that spontaneously develop cerebellar medulloblastoma induced by HGF + Shh. These findings show that blocking the HGF–Met interaction with systemically administered anti-HGF mAb can have profound antitumor effects even within the central nervous system, a site previously believed to be resistant to systemic antibody-based therapeutics. This antibody has been humanized and is planned to enter clinical trials in the near future.

It has not been possible to inhibit c-Met using bivalent anti-Met antibodies since antibody-mediated receptor dimerization can induce receptor activation. Novel one-armed [monovalent] anti-c-Met antibody [OA-5D5] has been developed that inhibits c-Met activation and glioblastoma xenograft growth (Martens et al., 2006). Infusing the OA-5D5 anti-c-Met antibody directly into intracranial tumor xenografts inhibited the growth of HGF^{+}/c-Met^{+} U87MG gliomas and did not affect HGF^{-}/c-Met^{+} G55 gliomas. In OA-5D5-treated U87MG tumors, cell proliferation was reduced >75%, microvessel density was reduced >90%, and apoptosis was increased >60%. Furthermore, OA-5D5 treatment decreased tumor cell density >2-fold, with an apparent increase in deposition of matrix proteins laminin, fibronectin, and tenascin. Gene expression microarray analyses showed no expression change in these ECM factors and downregulation of urokinase-type plasminogen activator and matrix metalloproteinase 16 in glioblastoma cells treated with OA-5D5. This study demonstrates the feasibility and effectiveness of local intracranial delivery for brain tumor therapy. Tumor responses to systemic OA-5D5 have not been reported.

39.5 Therapeutic Considerations

Brain tumors are extremely heterogeneous with numerous histopathologically distinct entities. Even the most common malignant brain tumor in adults, glioblastoma, displays considerable histopathological, and genetic heterogeneity. Due to this complexity, it is most likely that only a subset of patients will benefit from HGF/c-Met pathway inhibition alone. To achieve greater therapeutic efficiency from HGF/c-Met targeting, it will be important to better understand the molecular determinants of HGF/c-Met pathway dependency. This will require that the clinical testing of pathway inhibitors includes the rigorous analysis of HGF and c-Met expression levels, c-Met activation levels, autocrine loop formation, c-Met mutations, PTEN status, and the co-expression and co-activation of other receptor tyrosine kinases commonly active in malignant brain tumors [e.g., EGFR, EGFRvIII, PDFGR]. Knowledge of the factors that determine HGF/c-Met sensitivity and dependence and the development of tests for determining such factors will hopefully identify patient subsets most likely to respond to pathway inhibitors. It is also likely that HGF/c-Met pathway targeting will be most useful in combination with other existing and emerging therapies. Basic and translational research has provided a rationale for combining anti-HGF/c-Met therapies with traditional cytotoxic therapies such as radiotherapy and chemotherapy (Lal et al., 2005). New therapeutically relevant interrelationships between EGFR and c-Met have been discovered [e.g., cross activation, pathway switching] in glioma models and systemic human cancers, raising the prospect for considerable therapeutic benefit by simultaneously targeting these pathways (Engelman et al., 2007; Stommel et al., 2007).

In summary, the HGF/c-Met pathway has emerged as an important contributor to brain tumor malignancy and is recognized to be a promising target for brain tumor therapy. Recent advances have led to the development of very promising HGF/c-Met inhibitors for translation to the clinical setting. Considerable preclinical and clinical work is needed for their successful application.

References

Abounader R, Montgomery R, Dietz H, Laterra J (2004) Design and expression of chimeric U1/ribozyme transgenes. Methods Mol Biol 252:209–219.

Abounader R, Ranganathan S, Kim BY, Nichols C, Laterra J (2001) Signaling pathways in the induction of c-met receptor expression by its ligand scatter factor/hepatocyte growth factor in human glioblastoma. J Neurochem 76:1497–1508.

Abounader R, Lal B, Luddy C, Koe G, Davidson B, Rosen EM, Laterra J (2002) In vivo targeting of SF/HGF and c-met expression via U1snRNA/ribozymes inhibits glioma growth and angiogenesis and promotes apoptosis. Faseb J 16:108–110.

Abounader R, Ranganathan S, Lal B, Fielding K, Book A, Dietz H, Burger P, Laterra J (1999) Reversion of human glioblastoma malignancy by U1 small nuclear RNA/ribozyme targeting of scatter factor/hepatocyte growth factor and c- met expression. J Natl Cancer Inst 91:1548–1556.

Arrieta O, Garcia E, Guevara P, Garcia-Navarrete R, Ondarza R, Rembao D, Sotelo J (2002) Hepatocyte growth factor is associated with poor prognosis of malignant gliomas and is a predictor for recurrence of meningioma. Cancer 94:3210–3218.

Birchmeier C, Birchmeier W, Gherardi E, Vande Woude GF (2003) Met, metastasis, motility and more. Nat Rev Mol Cell Biol 4:915–925.

Boccaccio C, Ando M, Tamagnone L, Bardelli A, Michieli P, Battistini C, Comoglio PM (1998) Induction of epithelial tubules by growth factor HGF depends on the STAT pathway. Nature 391:285–288.

Bowers DC, Fan S, Walter K, Abounader R, Williams JA, Rosen EM, Laterra J (2000) Scatter factor/hepatocyte growth factor activates AKT and protects against cytotoxic death in human glioblastoma via PI3-kinase and AKT-dependent pathways. Cancer Res 60:4277–4283.

Brockmann MA, Papadimitriou A, Brandt M, Fillbrandt R, Westphal M, Lamszus K (2003a) Inhibition of intracerebral glioblastoma growth by local treatment with the scatter factor/hepatocyte growth factor-antagonist NK4. Clin Cancer Res 9:4578–4585.

Brockmann MA, Ulbricht U, Gruner K, Fillbrandt R, Westphal M, Lamszus K (2003b) Glioblastoma and cerebral microvascular endothelial cell migration in response to tumor-associated growth factors. Neurosurgery 52:1391– 1399; discussion 1399.

Burgess T, Coxon A, Meyer S, Sun J, Rex K, Tsuruda T, Chen Q, Ho SY, Li L, Kaufman S, McDorman K, Cattley RC, Sun J, Elliott G, Zhang K, Feng X, Jia XC, Green L, Radinsky R, Kendall R (2006) Fully human monoclonal antibodies to hepatocyte growth factor with therapeutic potential against hepatocyte growth factor/c-Met-dependent human tumors. Cancer Res 66:1721–1729.

Cao B, Su Y, Oskarsson M, Zhao P, Kort EJ, Fisher RJ, Wang LM, Vande Woude GF (2001) Neutralizing monoclonal antibodies to hepatocyte growth factor/scatter factor (HGF/SF) display antitumor activity in animal models. Proc Natl Acad Sci U S A 98:7443–7448.

Christensen JG, Schreck R, Burrows J, Kuruganti P, Chan E, Le P, Chen J, Wang X, Ruslim L, Blake R, Lipson KE, Ramphal J, Do S, Cui JJ, Cherrington JM, Mendel DB (2003) A selective small molecule inhibitor of c-Met kinase inhibits c-Met-dependent phenotypes in vitro and exhibits cytoreductive antitumor activity in vivo. Cancer Res 63:7345–7355.

Chu SH, Zhang H, Ma YB, Feng DF, Zhu ZA, Yuan XH, Li ZQ (2007) c-Met antisense oligodeoxynucleotides as a novel therapeutic agent for glioma: in vitro and in vivo studies of uptake, effects, and toxicity. J Surg Res 141:284–288.

Comoglio PM, Giordano S, Trusolino L (2008) Drug development of MET inhibitors: targeting oncogene addiction and expedience. Nat Rev Drug Discov 7:504–516.

Corso S, Comoglio PM, Giordano S (2005) Cancer therapy: can the challenge be MET? Trends Mol Med 11:284–292.

Engelman JA, Zejnullahu K, Mitsudomi T, Song Y, Hyland C, Park JO, Lindeman N, Gale CM, Zhao X, Christensen J, Kosaka T, Holmes AJ, Rogers AM, Cappuzzo F, Mok T, Lee C, Johnson BE, Cantley LC, Janne PA (2007) MET amplification leads to gefitinib resistance in lung cancer by activating ERBB3 signaling. Science 316:1039–1043.

Fan S, Meng Q, Laterra JJ, Rosen EM (2007) Ras effector pathways modulate scatter factor-stimulated NF-kappaB signaling and protection against DNA damage. Oncogene 26:4774–4796.

Fan S, Ma YX, Gao M, Yuan RQ, Meng Q, Goldberg ID, Rosen EM (2001) The multisubstrate adapter Gab1 regulates hepatocyte growth factor (scatter factor)-c-Met signaling for cell survival and DNA repair. Mol Cell Biol 21:4968–4984.

Gherardi E, Youles ME, Miguel RN, Blundell TL, Iamele L, Gough J, Bandyopadhyay A, Hartmann G, Butler PJ (2003) Functional map and domain structure of MET, the product of the c-met protooncogene and receptor for hepatocyte growth factor/scatter factor. Proc Natl Acad Sci U S A 100:12039–12044.

Giordano S, Ponzetto C, Di Renzo MF, Cooper CS, Comoglio PM (1989) Tyrosine kinase receptor indistinguishable from the c-met protein. Nature 339:155–156.

Hamasuna R, Kataoka H, Moriyama T, Itoh H, Seiki M, Koono M (1999) Regulation of matrix metalloproteinase-2 (MMP-2) by hepatocyte growth factor/scatter factor (HGF/SF) in human glioma cells: HGF/SF enhances MMP-2 expression and activation accompanying up-regulation of membrane type-1 MMP. Int J Cancer 82:274–281.

Hecht M, Papoutsi M, Tran HD, Wilting J, Schweigerer L (2004) Hepatocyte growth factor/c-Met signaling promotes the progression of experimental human neuroblastomas. Cancer Res 64:6109–6118.

Kim KJ, Wang L, Su YC, Gillespie GY, Salhotra A, Lal B, Laterra J (2006) Systemic antihepatocyte growth factor monoclonal antibody therapy induces the regression of intracranial glioma xenografts. Clin Cancer Res 12:1292–1298.

Koochekpour S, Jeffers M, Rulong S, Taylor G, Klineberg E, Hudson EA, Resau JH, Vande Woude GF (1997) Met and hepatocyte growth factor/scatter factor expression in human gliomas. Cancer Res 57:5391–5398.

Kunkel P, Muller S, Schirmacher P, Stavrou D, Fillbrandt R, Westphal M, Lamszus K (2001) Expression and localization of scatter factor/hepatocyte growth factor in human astrocytomas. Neuro-oncol 3:82–88.

Lafleur MA, Handsley MM, Knauper V, Murphy G, Edwards DR (2002) Endothelial tubulogenesis within fibrin gels specifically requires the activity of membrane-type-matrix metalloproteinases (MT-MMPs). J Cell Sci 115:3427–3438.

Lal B, Xia S, Abounader R, Laterra J (2005) Targeting the c-Met pathway potentiates glioblastoma responses to gamma-radiation. Clin Cancer Res 11:4479–4486.

Lamszus K, Laterra J, Westphol M, Rosen EM (1999) Scatter factor/hepatocyte growth factor content and function in human gliomas. Intl J Dev Neuroosci 17:517–530.

Lamszus K, Liang J, Laterra J, Zagzag D, Way D, Witte M, Goldberg ID, Rosen EM (1998) Scatter factor promotes motility of human glioma and neuromicrovascular endothelial cells. Intl J Cancer 75:19–28.

Laterra J, Nam M, Rosen E, Rao JS, Johnston P (1997a) Scatter factor/hepatocyte growth factor gene transfer to 9L glioma cells enhances glioma growth and angiogenesis in vivo. Lab Invest 76:565–577.

Laterra J, Rosen EM, Nam M, Ranganathan S, Fielding K, Johnston P (1997b) Scatter factor/hepatocyte growth factor expression enhances human glioblastoma tumorigenicity and growth. Biochem Biophys Res Comm 235:743–747.

Li Y, Lal B, Kwon S, Fan X, Saldanha U, Reznik TE, Kuchner EB, Eberhart C, Laterra J, Abounader R (2005) The scatter factor/hepatocyte growth factor: c-met pathway in human embryonal central nervous system tumor malignancy. Cancer Res 65:9355–9362.

Li Y, Guessous F, Johnson EB, Eberhart CG, Li XN, Shu Q, Fan S, Lal B, Laterra J, Schiff D, Abounader R (2008) Functional and molecular interactions between the HGF/c-Met pathway and c-Myc in large-cell medulloblastoma. Lab Invest 88:98–111.

Lock LS, Royal I, Naujokas MA, Park M (2000) Identification of an atypical Grb2 carboxyl-terminal SH3 domain binding site in Gab docking proteins reveals Grb2-dependent and -independent recruitment of Gab1 to receptor tyrosine kinases. J Biol Chem 275:31536–31545.

Martens T, Schmidt NO, Eckerich C, Fillbrandt R, Merchant M, Schwall R, Westphal M, Lamszus K (2006) A novel one-armed anti-c-Met antibody inhibits glioblastoma growth in vivo. Clin Cancer Res 12:6144–6152.

Martinez-Rumayor A, Arrieta O, Guevara P, Escobar E, Rembao D, Salina C, Sotelo J (2004) Coexpression of hepatocyte growth factor/scatter factor (HGF/SF) and its receptor cMET predict recurrence of meningiomas. Cancer Lett 213:117–124.

Matsumoto K, Nakamura T (2003) NK4 (HGF-antagonist/angiogenesis inhibitor) in cancer biology and therapeutics. Cancer Sci 94:321–327.

Michieli P, Mazzone M, Basilico C, Cavassa S, Sottile A, Naldini L, Comoglio PM (2004) Targeting the tumor and its microenvironment by a dual-function decoy Met receptor. Cancer Cell 6:61–73.

Miyazawa K, Shimomura T, Kitamura A, Kondo J, Morimoto Y, Kitamura N (1993) Molecular cloning and sequence analysis of the cDNA for a human serine protease reponsible for activation of hepatocyte growth factor. Structural similarity of the protease precursor to blood coagulation factor XII. J Biol Chem 268:10024–10028.

Moriyama T, Kataoka H, Kawano Y, Yokogami K, Nakano S, Goya T, Uchino H, Koono M, Wakisaka S (1998a) Comparative analysis of expression of hepatocyte growth factor and its receptor, c-met, in gliomas, meningiomas and schwannomas. Canc Lett 124: 149–155.

Moriyama T, Kataoka H, Hamasuna R, Yokogami K, Uehara H, Kawano H, Goya T, Tsubouchi H, Koono M, Wakisaka S (1998b) Up-regulation of vascular endothelial growth factor induced by hepatocyte growth factor scatter factor stimulation in human glioma cells. Biochem Biophys Res Commun 249:73–77.

Moriyama T, Kataoka H, Hamasuna R, Yoshida E, Sameshima T, Iseda T, Yokogami K, Nakano S, Koono M, Wakisaka S (1999) Simultaneous up-regulation of urokinase-type plasminogen activator (uPA) and uPA receptor by hepatocyte growth factor/scatter factor in human glioma cells. Clin Exp Metastasis 17:873–879.

Nakagami H, Morishita R, Yamamoto K, Taniyama Y, Aoki M, Matsumoto K, Nakamura T, Kaneda Y, Horiuchi M, Ogihara T (2001) Mitogenic and antiapoptotic actions of hepatocyte growth factor through ERK, STAT3, and AKT in endothelial cells. Hypertension 37:581–586.

Nakamura T, Nishizawa T, Hagiya M, Seki T, Shimonishi M, Sugimura A, Tashiro K, Shimizu S (1989) Molecular cloning and expression of human hepatocyte growth factor. Nature 342:440–443.

O'Reilly MS, Holmgren L, Shing Y, Chen C, Rosenthal RA, Moses M, Lane WS, Cao Y, Sage EH, Folkman J (1994) Angiostatin: a novel angiogenesis inhibitor that mediates the suppression of metastases by a Lewis lung carcinoma [see comments]. Cell 79:315–328.

Ponzetto C, Bardelli A, Zhen Z, Maina F, Zonca P, Giordano S, Graziani A, Panayoyou G, Comoglio PM (1994) A multifunctional docking site mediates signalling and transformation by the HGF/SF receptor family. Cell 77:261–271.

Reznik TE, Sang Y, Ma Y, Abounader R, Rosen EM, Xia S, Laterra J (2008) Transcription-dependent epidermal growth factor receptor activation by hepatocyte growth factor. Mol Cancer Res 6:139–150.

Rosen EM, Laterra J, Joseph A, Jin L, Fuchs A, Witte M, Weinarnd M, Goldberg ID (1996) Scatter factor expression and regulation in human glial tumors. Intl J Cancer 67:248–255.

Schmidt MO, Westphal M, Hagel C, Ergun S, Stavrou D, Rosen EM, Lamszus K (1999) Levels of vascular endothelial growth factor, hepatocyte growth factor/scatter factor and basic fibroblast growth factor in human gliomas and their relationship to angiogenesis. Intl J Cancer 84:10–18.

Seki T, Hagiya M, Shimonishi M, Nakamura T, Shimizu S (1991) Organization of the human hepatocyte growth factor-encoding gene. Gene 102:213–219.

Stommel JM, Kimmelman AC, Ying H, Nabioullin R, Ponugoti AH, Wiedemeyer R, Stegh AH, Bradner JE, Ligon KL, Brennan C, Chin L, DePinho RA (2007) Coactivation of receptor tyrosine kinases affects the response of tumor cells to targeted therapies. Science 318:287–290.

Tong CY, Hui AB, Yin XL, Pang JC, Zhu XL, Poon WS, Ng HK (2004) Detection of oncogene amplifications in medulloblastomas by comparative genomic hybridization and array-based comparative genomic hybridization. J Neurosurg 100:187–193.

Walter KA, Hossain MD, Luddy C, Goel N, Reznick TE, Laterra J (2002) Scatter factor/hepatocyte growth factor stimulation of glioblastoma cell cycle progression through G1 c-Myc dependent, and independent of p27 suppression cdk2 activation, or E2F1-dependent transcription. Mol Cell Biol 22: 2703–2715.

Weidner KM, Di Cesare S, Sachs M, Brinkmann V, Behrens J, Birchmeier W (1996) Interaction between Gab1 and the c-Met receptor tyrosine kinase is responsible for epithelial morphogenesis. Nature 384:173–176.

Welch WC, Kornblith PL, Michalopoulos GK, Petersen BE, Beedle A, Gollin SM, Goldfarb RH (1999) Hepatocyte growth factor (HGF) and receptor (c-met) in normal and malignant astrocytic cells. Anticancer Res 19:1635–1640.

Wullich B, Sattler HP, Fischer U, Meese E (1994) Two independent amplification events on chromosome 7 in glioma: Amplification of the epidermal growth factor receptor gene and amplification of the oncogene met. Anticancer Res 14:577–579.

Xiao GH, Jeffers M, Bellacosa A, Mitsuuchi Y, Vande Woude GF, Testa JR (2001) Anti-apoptotic signaling by hepatocyte growth factor/Met via the phosphatidylinositol 3-kinase/Akt and mitogen-activated protein kinase pathways. Proc Natl Acad Sci U S A 98:247–252.

Zou HY, Li Q, Lee JH, Arango ME, McDonnell SR, Yamazaki S, Koudriakova TB, Alton G, Cui JJ, Kung PP, Nambu MD, Los G, Bender SL, Mroczkowski B, Christensen JG (2007) An orally available small-molecule inhibitor of c-Met, PF-2341 066, exhibits cytoreductive antitumor efficacy through antiproliferative and antiangiogenic mechanisms. Cancer Res 67:4408–4417.

Chapter 40
Combinatorial Therapeutic Strategies for Blocking Kinase Pathways in Brain Tumors

Paul H. Huang and Forest M. White

Abstract Recent studies have demonstrated that robustness in oncogenic signaling networks is a key contributor of resistance to kinase inhibitor monotherapy in glioblastoma patients. In this chapter, we will review several examples where combinatorial kinase inhibition has been employed as a means to overcome chemoresistance in the laboratory setting. Additionally, we will summarize approaches by which systems-level phosphoproteomic platforms, in combination with computational tools, can be employed to develop better combinatorial therapeutic strategies and translate such discoveries from the bench to the bedside.

Contents

F.M. White (✉)
Department of Biological Engineering, Massachusetts Institute of Technology, Room 56-754, Cambridge, MA 02139, USA
e-mail: fwhite@mit.edu

E.G. Van Meir (ed.), *CNS Cancer*, Cancer Drug Discovery and Development, DOI 10.1007/978-1-60327-553-8_40,
© Humana Press, a part of Springer Science+Business Media, LLC 2009

40.1 Introduction: From Single Genes to Biological Networks

Glioblastoma (GBM, WHO grade IV) is a complex disease driven by an interplay of multiple genetic aberrations, each contributing in a somewhat enigmatic manner to the initiation and propagation of the disease. Decades of genetics and molecular pathology research have revealed many of the genes commonly found to be deregulated in GBMs, including important regulators of cell cycle progression such as INK4A/ARF and p53, as well as oncogenic signaling components including PTEN, PDGFR, and EGFR (Furnari et al. 2007) (see also Chapters 14, 15, and 20). While the focus on individual genes has undoubtedly led to advances in the molecular understanding of this disease, the complexity of inherent, intricate biological networks has, in most cases, inhibited successful therapeutic treatment of the disease state.

In fact, several recent studies have suggested that it is the deregulation of signaling networks rather than individual genes that are ultimately responsible for many of the classical features associated with GBM tumors, in particular, chemoresistance to both conventional cytotoxics and newer targeted therapeutics that are currently in clinical trials. These discoveries have resulted in the development of a number of combinatorial approaches for the treatment of GBM with the explicit aim of simultaneously targeting multiple components of oncogenic signaling networks. In this chapter, we will summarize recent examples where combinatorial approaches such as multi-kinase inhibition have demonstrated efficacy in the laboratory. In addition, we will elaborate on contemporary phosphoproteomic techniques available to probe for deregulated oncogenic networks and how the use of such approaches in combination with computational predictions could allow one to translate current laboratory successes into the clinic.

40.2 Robustness in Oncogenic Signaling Networks

Many of the aberrant signaling pathways in GBMs have been extensively discussed in prior chapters in this book. These pathways are classically initiated by either the constitutive activation/overexpression of a dominant oncogene (e.g., EGFR) or the inactivation/deletion of a tumor suppressor (e.g., PTEN). These initiator events are then propagated by downstream signaling processes (primarily comprised of protein and lipid phosphorylation events) into several key pathways including the PI3K/Akt/mTOR and the RAS/RAF/MEK/MAPK signaling cascades (Fig. 40.1 and Color Plate 59. It is important to emphasize that these signaling pathways are dynamic in nature, responding to intra- and extracellular perturbations. Furthermore, signaling pathways are often interconnected into networks and have evolved mechanisms to adapt to changes in network structure and utilization (Amit et al. 2007). In

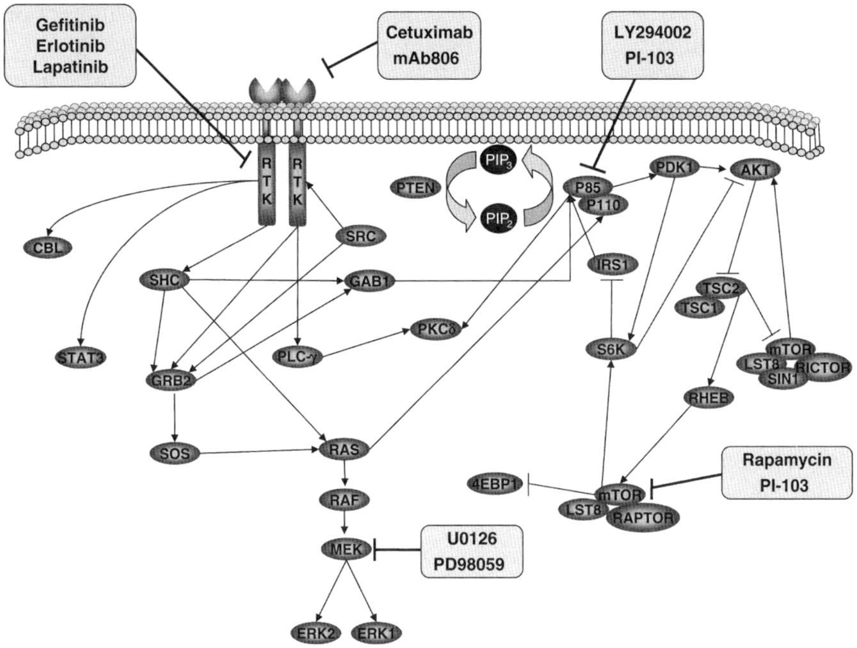

Fig. 40.1 Oncogenic signaling networks in glioblastoma. Growth factor signaling is initiated by the phosphorylation and activation of receptor tyrosine kinases (RTKs). Signal transduction is propagated by protein and lipid phosphorylation events into several key pathways including the RAS/RAF/MEK/MAPK and PI3K/Akt/mTOR pathways. There is a variety of feedback and crosstalk mechanisms by which signaling networks maintain robustness (see text for details). Currently available inhibitors of key signaling network components are highlighted in *yellow* (*see* Color Plate 59)

this section, we highlight three examples of how such robustness in oncogenic networks contributes to chemoresistance in GBM patients.

40.2.1 The Akt–mTOR Feedback Loop

In response to growth factor signaling, the class Ia phosphoinositide 3-kinases (PI3K) are activated to convert plasma membrane phosphatidylinositol-4,5-bisphosphate [PI(4,5)P_2] to phosphatidylinositol-3,4,5-trisphosphate [PI(3,4,5)P_3] (Cantley 2002). The formation of PI(3,4,5)P_3 triggers the recruitment of a number of critical signaling proteins via direct lipid binding to the pleckstrin homology (PH) domain, including the kinases PDK1 and Akt (Cantley 2002). PDK1 phosphorylates Akt on T308 and the mTORC2 complex phosphorylates Akt on S473, resulting in full kinase activity (Sarbassov et al. 2005) (Fig. 40.1). Upon activation, Akt phosphorylates a large number of substrates at the consensus RxRxxS/T motif

(Alessi et al. 1996). These substrates play important roles in the regulation of cell survival, growth, cell cycle, and metabolism (Manning and Cantley 2007).

Constitutive activation of the PI3K/Akt/mTOR pathway in GBM tumors occurs through a variety of mechanisms. For instance, the phosphatase and tensin homolog (PTEN), a negative regulator of the PI3K pathway, is a tumor suppressor that is mutated or deleted in 50% of GBMs (Furnari et al. 2007; Ohgaki and Kleihues 2007). PTEN loss of function upsets the PI3K–PTEN balance which results in elevated $PI(3,4,5)P_3$, thereby activating Akt promoting anti-apoptotic pathways (Chapter 15). Additionally, mutations in the PIK3CA gene, which encodes the alpha isoform of the p110 catalytic subunit of the PI3K complex, have been found in 5–15% of GBM tumors, some of which have been shown to confer oncogenic gain of function (Broderick et al. 2004; Hartmann et al. 2005; Gallia et al. 2006; TCGA, 2008).

Intuitively, GBM tumors represent prime candidates for treatment with single agents targeting components of the PI3K/Akt pathway. In particular, the availability of small molecule inhibitors to the mammalian target of rapamycin (mTOR), a downstream effector of the PI3K/Akt cascade, has made targeting this pathway especially attractive. mTOR is indirectly activated by Akt via the phosphorylation of its inhibitor, tuberous sclerosis complex 2 (TSC2). Activation of mTOR promotes the formation of a complex with raptor (regulatory-associated protein mTOR), known as mTORC1. The mTORC1 complex is associated with cell growth and proliferation, primarily acting through activation of the S6-kinase (Hay 2005). Since this complex is sensitive to rapamycin, the use of this compound and its analogs has been proposed as a possible form of treatment in GBM patients. Indeed, in a recent phase I clinical trial in which 14 patients with PTEN-null recurrent GBM were administered with a rapamycin regimen, 2 patients showed a reduction in tumor mass with 5 other patients demonstrating a decrease in mitotic index (Cloughesy et al. 2008). However, in a subset of patients (7 patients, 50% of the cohort), inhibition of mTORC1 complex by rapamycin resulted in an increase in Akt phosphorylation which was correlated with a shorter time-to-progression after surgery.

The authors proposed that the observed increase in Akt activation can be attributed to a negative feedback loop exerted by the mTORC1 complex on Akt, in which phosphorylation of the insulin receptor subtrate-1 (IRS-1) by the mTORC1 effector S6K inhibits Akt function (Cloughesy et al. 2008). This effect is also seen in $TSC2^{-/-}$ cells, where loss of the TSC2 tumor suppressor results in the constitutive activation of mTOR and inhibition of Akt. Conversely, inhibition of the mTORC1 complex disrupts the negative feedback loop via IRS-1 and leads to an increase in Akt pro-survival signals (Radimerski et al. 2002; Hay 2005). As a consequence of these observations, it has been proposed that a combination of PI3K/Akt inhibitors and rapamycin may be required to simultaneously target both components of the pathway and overcome the feedback loop. This hypothesis has been validated in a GBM xenograft model where the use of PI-103 (a dual inhibitor of PI3K and mTOR) was superior to monotherapy with either PI3K inhibitors or rapamycin (Wang et al. 2006; Fan et al.

2007). Further trials are required to determine if this combinatorial approach will be efficacious in the clinic.

While this negative feedback loop provides an explanation for those patients that did not respond well to rapamycin monotherapy, there must be additional molecular determinants that enabled some patients to respond favorably to monotherapy despite the presence of this negative feedback loop. Supplementary molecular analyses of GBM tumors need to be performed in order to better understand the molecular basis of this selective sensitivity to rapamycin monotherapy. A greater understanding of such network features will facilitate patient stratification and selection of the proper combinatorial regimens in the future.

40.2.2 EGFRvIII–PTEN Connection

Aberrations in epidermal growth factor receptor (EGFR) expression levels are common in GBMs, with 40–70% of primary GBMs exhibiting amplification of the *EGFR gene* (Ekstrand et al. 1992; Ohgaki et al. 2004). In addition to receptor amplification, activating mutants of EGFR have also been found in GBMs, with the type III EGFR variant deletion mutant (EGFRvIII) being the most common (Chapter 20). In fact, approximately 50% of GBMs that overexpress wildtype EGFR concurrently express EGFRvIII (20% of all GBMs) (Sugawa et al. 1990; Frederick et al. 2000). EGFRvIII is a truncated mutant which lacks exons 2–7 of the EGFR gene (Wong et al. 1992) and is constitutively active despite lacking a ligand-binding domain. Clinical studies have shown a correlation between EGFRvIII expression and poor prognosis in glioma patients (Feldkamp et al. 1999). These data suggest that EGFRvIII may be an effective candidate for single-agent therapeutic intervention, especially given that three tyrosine kinase inhibitors (TKIs) targeting EGFR (gefitinib, erlotinib, and lapatinib) have already been approved for use in the clinic, to treat lung, breast, and pancreatic cancers (Nyati et al. 2006).

Intriguingly, despite ectopic expression of EGFRvIII, several GBM cell line and xenograft models are resistant to both gefitinib and erlotinib treatments (Learn et al. 2004; Mellinghoff et al. 2005; Pedersen et al. 2005; Ji et al. 2006). AG1478, a tyrphostin small molecule inhibitor that showed higher specificity for EGFRvIII over wildtype EGFR in vitro, also had no efficacy as a single agent in xenograft models (Han et al. 1996; Johns et al. 2003). Several phase II clinical trials employing gefitinib and erlotinib as single-agent treatments in newly diagnosed or recurrent GBM have also failed to show a clinical benefit compared to previous treatment protocols (Rich et al. 2004; Omuro et al. 2007).

The observed resistance to EGFR TKIs is somewhat puzzling considering that these drugs shut down EGFRvIII activity in in vitro assays and are presumed to have similar efficacy in patients. Interestingly, a study in 2005 identified a correlation between EGFRvIII and PTEN co-expression and favorable response to treatment with EGFR TKIs (Mellinghoff et al. 2005). More recently, it has been proposed that the apparent resistance to EGFR TKIs in the EGFRvIII-positive, PTEN-null patient subpopulation is a consequence of the uncoupling of the PI3K/Akt/mTOR pathway (due to the loss of PTEN) from EGFRvIII upstream signals (Mellinghoff et al. 2007). In other words, without an active negative regulator in the pathway, simply turning off the upstream signal does not eliminate the downstream activation of the PI3K/Akt/mTOR pathway. Conceptually, this situation appears to be ideal for combinatorial treatment with EGFR TKIs in conjunction with PI3K/Akt/mTOR pathway inhibitors, thereby blocking upstream and downstream aspects of the pathway simultaneously. In vitro experiments in GBM cell lines reinforce this hypothesis, and treatment of EGFRvIII-positive, PTEN-null cells with erlotinib in combination with rapamycin or PI-103 led to a decrease in tumor cell proliferation compared to administration of either drug alone (Wang et al. 2006; Fan et al. 2007). Multiple ongoing clinical trials of EGFR kinase inhibitor together with rapamycin/rapamycin analogs are currently being conducted to determine if this preclinical efficacy materializes in the clinic (Omuro et al. 2007).

40.2.3 The RAS–PI3K Crosstalk

The mitogen-activated protein kinase (MAPK) pathway comprised of RAS/RAF/MEK/MAPK is another critical mediator of the biological effects of EGFR (Chapters 4 and 38). Upon ligand binding and receptor dimerization, EGFR becomes phosphorylated at multiple tyrosine sites in its cytoplasmic tail. Growth factor receptor-bound protein 2 (Grb2) recruitment to tyrosyl-phosphorylated EGFR sets off a canonical signaling cascade in which son-of-sevenless (Sos) converts inactive Ras-GDP to active Ras-GTP. Activated Ras then binds to and activates Raf-1, a serine/threonine kinase that phosphorylates MEK, a dual-specificity kinase that phosphorylates and activates MAP kinases Erk1 and Erk2 (Fig. 40.1). Activation of Erk1/2 results in the phosphorylation, typically at a PXS/TP motif, of a large number of substrates, including multiple latent transcription factors (e.g., c-Fos, Elk-1, and c-Jun) and kinases (RSK and MNK) (Chen et al. 2001).

The PI3K and MAPK signaling pathways undergo bidirectional crosstalk at several levels, adding a significant amount of complexity and robustness to the signaling network. For instance, binding of RAS to the PI3K p110α subunit potentiates EGFR-mediated phosphorylation of Akt both in vitro and in vivo (Downward 2003; Gupta et al. 2007). In this manner, oncogenic activation of RAS, either by the deregulation of the RAS/RAF/MEK/MAPK pathway (rare in GBMs) or by the action of upstream components such as growth factor receptor signaling, induces rapid proliferation characteristic of the RAS pathway while also initiating pro-survival signals via the action of PI3K.

In another example, a recent study showed that the PI3K pathway also stimulates the Erk1/2 MAP kinase cascade and that this cross-activation was dependent on EGFR signal strength (Sampaio et al. 2008). In GBM cells that overexpress EGFR, activation of Erk1/2 occurs primarily through the binding of the GAB-1 adaptor protein to phosphorylated EGFR via Grb2, independent of PI3K activation status. Interestingly, activation of Erk1/2 in cells that express low EGFR levels was shown to be dependent on the binding of GAB-1 through its PH domain to PIP_3, a downstream product of PI3K. In this study, the authors demonstrate that inhibition of EGFR activation with an EGFR tyrosine kinase inhibitor (TKI) had little effect on Erk1/2 activation, and that a combinatorial inhibition of both EGFR and PI3K was required to observe a dramatic decrease in Erk1/2 activation (Sampaio et al. 2008). These data suggest that the clinically observed resistance of EGFR positive GBM patients to EGFR TKIs may be due in part to the incomplete inhibition of EGFR and the continuous activation of the Erk1/2 pathway as a result of the compensatory PI3K mechanism. These studies would once again suggest that a therapeutic combination of EGFR TKI with PI3K/Akt and/or MAPK inhibitors may be beneficial in overcoming EGFR TKI resistance.

40.3 Tools to Survey Signaling Networks in GBM

It is apparent from the three examples described above that plasticity in pathway utilization and multiple layers of cross-activation contribute to the robustness of oncogenic signaling networks. GBM tumor cells take advantage of this complexity and robustness, utilizing these contingency mechanisms to overcome single-target inhibition. All of the examples discussed in the previous section have for the most part relied on logical combinations of conventional, canonical signaling targets such as EGFR and components of the PI3K/Akt/mTOR pathways (Fig. 40.1). However, given the complexity of the networks and the cross-activation implicit in these pathways, it is likely that additional, non-canonical, nodes will be prime targets for combinatorial therapeutic intervention in GBM signaling networks. Unfortunately, identification of non-intuitive nodes that are critical for the maintenance of oncogenic signaling networks still remains a significant challenge. In this section, we will describe several systems-wide tools that have been developed to address this challenge and are now capable of surveying phosphorylation-mediated signaling networks (the "phosphoproteome") in tumor cells.

40.3.1 Revealing Novel Network Connections Through Mass Spectrometry

Of the multiple platforms available for quantitatively surveying signaling networks, mass spectrometry (MS) stands out in its ability to sequence novel proteins and phosphorylation sites in an unbiased fashion. Although it is not a high-throughput approach, new enrichment techniques and instrumentation allow for high-sensitivity phosphoprotein detection over a large dynamic range (Schmelzle and White 2006). Because of the combination of sensitivity, detection dynamic range, and identification of novel phosphorylation sites, MS has become the tool of choice to measure both established and novel signaling network components in a system-wide fashion. This approach was highlighted in a recent study in which MS was employed to investigate the effects of EGFRvIII receptor expression levels on downstream network phosphorylation in U87MG GBM cells (Huang et al. 2007b). Consistent with prior reports (Montgomery et al. 1995; Moscatello et al. 1998; de la Iglesia et al. 2008), increased titration of EGFRvIII levels resulted in a dramatic increase in PI3K pathway activation while the MAPK and STAT3 pathways remain relatively unchanged. Similar to the examples described above, these observations support the use of EGFR kinase inhibitors in combination with PI3K pathway inhibitors to shut down oncogenic signaling in EGFRvIII-positive GBM cells.

In addition to quantification of the canonical EGFR signaling network pathways, a previously unappreciated complexity in signaling networks was also uncovered, in which multiple receptor tyrosine kinases (RTKs), such as c-Met and Axl, are co-activated by EGFRvIII in GBMs (Huang et al. 2007a, b). Interestingly, c-Met and Axl expression levels have been correlated with glioma grade, indicating the potential clinical relevance of EGFRvIII–c-Met or EGFRvIII–Axl cross-activation (Koochekpour et al. 1997; Hutterer et al. 2008). Upon further interrogation of the EGFRvIII–c-Met crosstalk, it was determined that the c-Met receptor pathway is important in tumor maintenance in glioma and that co-inhibition of EGFRvIII and c-Met is sufficient to overcome resistance to EGFR TKI monotherapy in vitro. Importantly, these experiments were performed in the PTEN-null U87 glioma cell line, indicating that this combinatorial strategy may work well on gliomas regardless of PTEN status. Furthermore, resistance to classical cytotoxics (e.g., cisplatin), a phenotype previously attributed to the action of EGFRvIII, could be overcome by the administration of c-Met kinase inhibitors, suggesting that c-Met activation may account for a significant proportion of EGFRvIII-mediated chemoresistance. It is therefore likely that many of the tumor-associated phenotypes functionally ascribed to EGFRvIII may be due in part to cross-activation with multiple RTKs.

Already from this initial foray, MS-based phosphoproteomics, depicted schematically in Fig. 40.2, has revealed a novel therapeutic approach in which c-Met kinase inhibitors, when used in combination with either EGFR TKIs or standard chemotherapeutics, may overcome the clinically observed chemoresistance in EGFRvIII-positive GBM patients. It is likely that additional MS-based analysis of GBM signaling networks will reveal additional nodes that may be targeted, alone or in combination, both in vitro in GBM cell lines and eventually in the clinic.

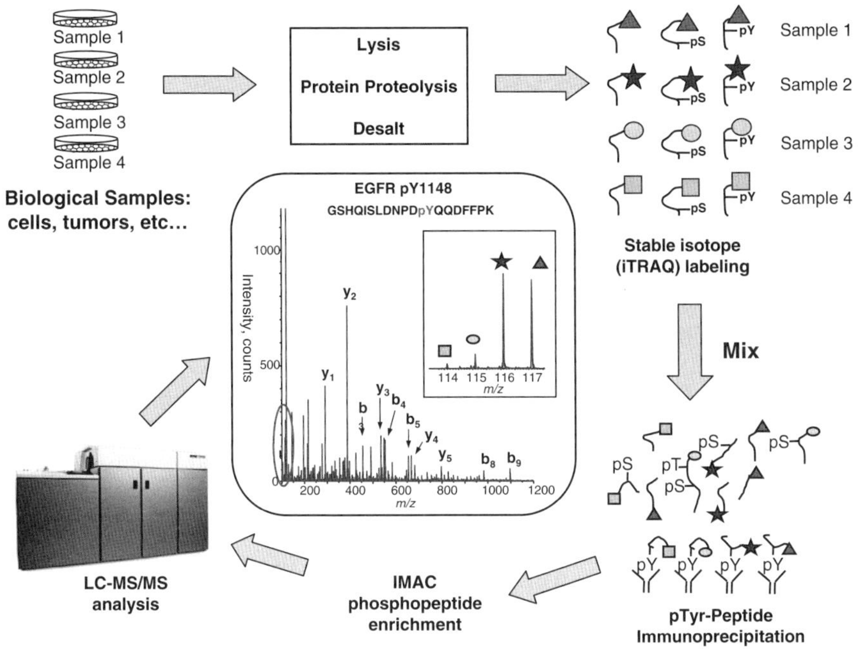

Fig. 40.2 Quantitative mass spectrometry-based proteomic analysis of phosphorylation-mediated signaling networks. Biological samples (e.g., cells, tissues, tumors) are lyzed or homogenized, typically with 8 M urea, and proteins are enzymatically proteolyzed to peptides. Stable isotope labeling of peptides from each of the samples enables downstream relative quantification across the biological samples. Following stable isotope labeling, tyrosine phosphorylated peptides are enriched by immunoprecipitation with pan-specific anti-phosphotyrosine antibodies. To remove nonspecifically retained non-phosphorylated peptides, immobilized metal affinity chromatography (IMAC) is used as a second-stage enrichment for phosphorylated peptides, which are subsequently passed to a liquid chromatography column and analyzed by LC-MS/MS. Several thousand MS/MS spectra are obtained per analysis, providing identification (y- and b-type fragment ions) and relative quantification (stable isotope ions) for hundreds of phosphorylated peptides across multiple biological samples

40.3.2 Understanding Chemoresistance Through the Use of Antibody Microarrays

In contrast to mass spectrometry, antibody microarrays feature increased throughput with minimal sample/reagent consumption, while simultaneously measuring tens of phosphorylation sites in a targeted fashion. Such arrays are particularly useful in determining how signaling networks adapt to TKI monotherapy and to establish which signaling pathways confer resistance in tumors. In a recent study of EGFR TKI resistance in non-small cell lung cancer (NSCLC), RTK-directed antibody arrays were utilized to examine the effect of gefitinib on the activation status of 42 RTKs in NSCLC cells that were either resistant or sensitive to gefitinib (Engelman et al. 2007). The authors discovered an "oncogene switching" mechanism in which gefitinib resistant cells compensated for EGFR inhibition by the upregulation and activation of c-Met, resulting in a persistent activation of the PI3K pathway. It was thus proposed that concurrent inhibition of EGFR and c-Met may be efficacious in overcoming the oncogene switch in NSCLC cells.

Using a similar RTK-directed antibody microarray, Stommel et al. screened a large number of GBM cell lines and xenografts and found that in all the lines examined, different combinations of RTKs, including EGFR, c-Met, and PDGFR, were simultaneously tyrosine phosphorylated at any one time (Stommel et al. 2007). They went on to show that inhibition of at least three RTKs (EGFR, c-Met, and PDGFR) was required to optimally kill GBM cells in vitro. Interestingly, as with the EGFR and c-Met combined inhibition above, this triple inhibitor combination appeared to work in both PTEN-wt and PTEN-null cells. Taken together, both the MS and microarray studies point to RTK co-activation as an important means of conferring chemoresistance in GBM patients and that the screening of resected tumors for RTK co-activity may provide intriguing combinatorial therapeutic strategies for future clinical treatment options.

40.3.3 Multiparameter Flow Cytometry as a Tool for Determining Oncogenic Networks in Cancer Stem Cell Populations

Multiparameter flow cytometry is an approach in which phosphorylation levels in proteins are measured by labeling fixed, permeabilized cells with fluorophore-conjugated phospho-specific antibodies. These cells are subjected to flow cytometry to quantify fluorescence intensity that is directly proportional to the amount of phospho-antigen in each cell (Perez and Nolan 2006). Current state-of-the-art flow cytometers allow for analysis of up to 13 different emission wavelengths (colors), greatly enhancing the ability to measure several parameters simultaneously. In a landmark study using this technique, Irish and coworkers stimulated leukemia cells from 30 acute myeloid leukemia (AML) patients with a panel of 6 cytokines and followed the phosphorylation changes in 6 different phosphoproteins important in the JAK/STAT and MAPK pathways (Irish et al. 2004). Subjecting the data to unsupervised hierarchical clustering, the authors demonstrated that tumors from individual cancer patients can be categorized by their molecular response to cytokine inputs and that this classification can discern genetic mutations and disease outcomes.

A major advantage of this approach is that the measurement occurs at the single cell level and has the potential of isolating subpopulations of cells that have distinct phosphorylation profiles that would otherwise have been lost in averaged cell population data (Irish et al. 2004). While this technique has yet to be applied to GBM, it is conceivable that it could be used to probe oncogenic signaling networks in brain tumor stem cell populations. Recent studies have demonstrated that brain tumor stem cell-enriched populations have distinct characteristics compared to cells from the bulk of the tumor, including increased chemo- and radioresistance (Chapter 29). It is thought that this stem cell population is responsible for tumor recurrence, clinically observed in GBM patients' post-surgery and chemo-/radiotherapy (Eyler and Rich 2008). One can envisage the use of antibodies for stem cell identification markers (e.g., CD133) in combination with antibodies for phosphoproteins to simultaneously monitor the phosphorylation profiles in such cells. This approach should allow one to determine if the signaling pathways thought to confer chemoresistance in the bulk tumor, for instance RTK co-activation, are also dominant in the brain tumor stem cell population. Developing combination protocols based on stem cell-specific signaling networks may ultimately be useful in preventing GBM tumor recurrence post-surgery.

40.4 Combinatorial Targets from GBM Signaling Networks Through Integrative Analysis

As described, there are multiple methods to obtain quantitative information regarding the phosphorylation status of components within a signaling network, either individually or in ensemble. However, using this quantitative data to derive optimum therapeutic targets or biological insight regarding the mechanistic regulation of complex biological phenotypes remains challenging. For all data types, the knowledge that a particular protein is phosphorylated is not sufficient to establish that protein as a good drug target for mono- or combinatorial inhibition. The situation is perhaps worse for MS-based signaling network data, where the inability to derive biological insight is often due to a lack of knowledge regarding the biological function of most phosphorylation sites within the network. In fact, due to the poor characterization of many, if not most, of the phosphorylation sites within these datasets, these large-scale analyses are typically simplified to the level of activation/inhibition of several well-characterized pathways (e.g., PI3K/Akt, MAPK pathways, or selected RTKs (as in Huang et al. 2007a, b)), while the remainder of the data is largely ignored. As a result, most of the therapeutic avenues are targeted at well-established, centralized nodes in the network, despite a vast amount of additional information describing potentially thousands of additional phosphorylation events. Since there is such a dizzying array of uncharacterized sites, it is non-trivial to distinguish which sites are likely to be associated with any given biological process, and which sites/proteins should be targeted to have maximal impact on a given biological phenotype. Faced with these challenging problems, in order to access the bulk of the phosphoproteomic data and begin to propose functional association for given phosphorylation sites, it is necessary to link cellular phenotypic information with quantitative phosphoproteomic information acquired under the same conditions. To state it more generally, to understand regulatory signaling networks from a systems-level perspective and to predict which nodes or combinations of nodes might be optimal therapeutic targets, computational techniques should be used to integrate quantitative phosphoproteomics datasets with additional data types.

Perhaps the most informative datasets to combine with phosphoproteomic measurements are quantitative phenotypic assays regarding cellular response to perturbation. This information provides a direct measurement of the effect of cellular perturbation and ensures that the phosphorylation data has been acquired under biologically relevant conditions. As an example, to determine the signaling networks affected by treatment of GBM cells with temozolomide (TMZ, the standard of care for GBM patients), one might wish to treat cells with multiple concentrations of TMZ while measuring DNA damage, cell cycle arrest, apoptosis, and perhaps proliferation. Each of these measurements could then be correlated to quantitative phosphoproteomic data obtained from cells treated with the same concentrations of TMZ, providing a tentative association between phosphorylation sites and cellular phenotype. Moreover, resistant and sensitive cells could be compared with this technique to uncover the regulatory signaling networks responsible for chemoresistance in selected GBM cell lines. Integration of phosphoproteomic and phenotypic data from these studies should then highlight proteins that could be targeted in combination with TMZ to overcome resistance to this treatment. The general scheme for the integrative analysis approach is demonstrated in Fig. 40.3. While these experiments require a significant amount of effort, there is now precedence in the literature for this approach.

For instance, Wolf-Yadlin et al. treated human mammary epithelial cells (HMECs) expressing low or high levels of HER2 (ErbB2) with either epidermal growth factor (EGF) or heregulin (HRG) to activate EGFR or HER3, respectively (Wolf-Yadlin et al. 2006). Since activation of the EGFR family of receptor tyrosine kinases is known to stimulate a large network of protein tyrosine phosphorylation sites (Zhang et al. 2005; Olsen et al. 2006; Wolf-Yadlin et al. 2007), the authors utilized MS-based phosphoproteomics to quantify temporal phosphorylation profiles of 322 tyrosine phosphorylation sites from each treatment condition. To quantify the downstream biological effect of these stimulation conditions, proliferation was assayed by ^{3}[H]-incorporation, and scratch wounding assays were performed to measure migration. Partial least-squares regression (PLSR) was performed to correlate these datasets, thereby generating a quantitative correlation metric for each phosphorylation site relative to each phenotype. Gratifyingly, this computational analysis correctly associated several well-characterized phosphorylation sites with their known biological function, including HER2 Y1248 with migration and EGFR Y1173 with proliferation (Okabayashi et al. 1994; Dittmar et al. 2002). Even more interesting were some of the unexpected findings, including strong correlation of hypothetical protein KIAA1217 Y393, a previously uncharacterized phosphorylation site on a novel protein within the network, with migration.

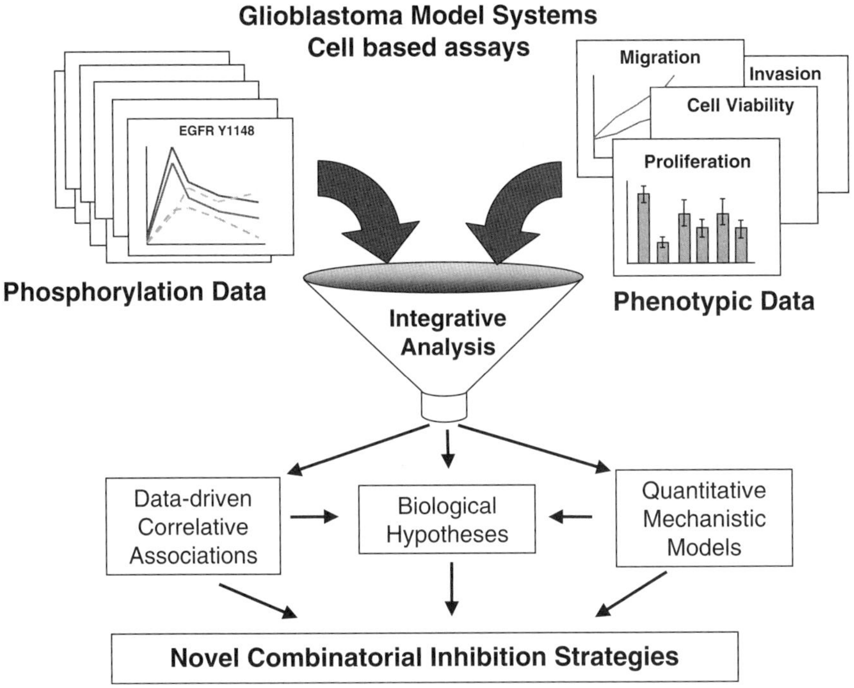

Fig. 40.3 Integrative analysis leads to novel combinatorial therapeutic strategies. By combining phosphoproteomic datasets with phenotypic datasets and additional data from the literature, it is possible to derive novel biological insight into activated signaling networks. This insight could take the form of novel hypotheses, correlative associations between phosphorylation sites and phenotypic outcome, or mechanistic computational models. Novel combinatorial therapeutic strategies can be realized from information derived from this combination of biological insights into a given activated network

Other functional assignments, such as Annexin A2 Y23 and Y237, which were also strongly correlated with migration, have now been validated by several additional studies (Falsey et al. 2006; Rescher et al. 2008). Although this study was performed in HMECs, the tools and techniques are obviously extensible to GBM cell lines.

It is worth noting that integrative studies are not limited to mass spectrometry-based phosphoproteomics and can be effectively applied to other quantitative signaling measurement techniques and phenotypic assays. For instance, Janes et al. used a combination of western blots, kinase activity assays, and antibody microarrays to quantify temporal changes of 11 key nodes in HT29 colon carcinoma cells stimulated with TNFa, insulin, and EGF, individually or in combination (Janes et al. 2005). This data was then correlated with five different apoptosis assays to determine the intracellular signals that were most strongly correlated with apoptosis under these conditions. Through this integrative approach, a novel role for the MAPK-activated protein kinase 2

(MK2) was revealed: at early time points, MK2 is strongly positively correlated with apoptosis, while at later time points, MK2 is strongly anti-correlated with apoptosis. Based on this finding, the authors tested the effect of inhibiting MK2 either throughout the study or only at late time points and were able to validate the hypothesis that MK2 is a pro-survival kinase at late time points.

40.5 Mechanistic Models and Computational Approaches to Drug Targets

While these correlative studies provide association between signaling molecules and downstream biological outcome, they do not provide direct information as to the mechanism by which these phosphorylation events regulate biological response to perturbation. Additionally, it is not necessarily straightforward to use correlative information to identify optimum drug targets with which to perturb the phenotype. Many signaling molecules might be correlated with a given response, but only a fraction of these will be responsible for controlling the phenotype, while the others may be simply phosphorylated as a result of the cellular response. In order to select optimum therapeutic targets or combinations of targets, a more detailed mechanistic mathematical model is often required. Several examples of these models have been generated over the past several years, including a detailed model of the EGFR signaling network (Hornberg et al. 2005), receptor tyrosine kinase endocytosis and trafficking network (Shankaran et al. 2007), and *Dictyostelium* chemosensing (Meier-Schellersheim et al. 2006). With these kinetic, mechanistic models, it is possible to vary the parameter values and determine which parameters are most sensitive to the selected biological outcome. Sensitivity analysis (Savageau 1971) highlights the optimum nodes in the network that will most significantly change the biological response. This approach should be directly extensible to selecting optimum targets for therapeutic treatment of GBM. For instance, following quantitative analysis of signaling networks, perhaps via multiple analytical techniques (e.g., MS and antibody microarrays), one would be able to identify the phosphorylated nodes in the network and determine their response to cellular perturbation. This information, when combined with canonical pathways from the literature, protein–protein interaction, and known kinase–substrate interactions, could be used to build a mechanistic model of the signaling networks activated in response to TMZ treatment of chemoresistant GBM. Sensitivity analysis of this mechanistic model would then predict the nodes in the network that, when inhibited, would have the greatest effect on the entire network; these nodes would therefore be the optimum drug targets, assuming they were "targetable" proteins. Since, as described above, many of these networks are remarkably robust to single-point interventions, sensitivity analysis can be employed to predict which combinations are likely to have the greatest effect on the network, eliminating much of the guesswork and trial-and-error associated with combinatorial strategies. Through computational modeling of the network, it is also possible to determine the optimal inhibition level for maximal effect. Especially in the case of combinatorial treatment strategies, it is often not necessary, and many times not desirable, to completely ablate all of the targets. Simulating the effect of partial inhibition on multiple nodes in the network provides a rapid, in silico approach to predict optimal combinatorial strategies before in vivo validation of these predictions.

Many of these same concepts can also be applied to uncover mechanisms underlying resistance that develops following mono-therapeutic treatment. Since intracellular signaling networks tend to be robust, initial strong positive response to therapy is often followed by recurrence associated with a resistant population of cells, as has been documented for gefitinib-sensitive non-small cell lung cancer (NSCLC), imatinib-sensitive chronic myeloid leukemia (CML), and tamoxifen-sensitive breast cancer. Phosphoproteomic analysis of the sensitive and resistant populations may identify pathways which are activated in the resistant state (Engelman et al. 2007), potentially highlighting further combinatorial therapeutic targets to overcome resistance. However, these analyses can also be misleading, as the optimal drug targets are not always the most phosphorylated, most modified, or most activated proteins. Here again computational analysis can be employed in silico not only to predict resistance and the resulting activation of given pathways but also to understand the mechanism by which resistance occurred, by predicting network adaptations to therapeutic intervention. Through sensitivity analysis of the adapted networks, these models can also be used to identify the optimum drug targets to avoid resistance altogether, before it occurs in the clinic. Of course, this level of modeling requires a significant amount of a priori knowledge of feedback, crosstalk, and network complexity that is just now being uncovered experimentally. However, with this knowledge in hand, over the next several years there should be rapid advances in the quality and complexity of the models, resulting in significantly enhanced predictions for complex phenotypes such as chemoresistance.

40.6 Bench to Bedside – Can Integrative Strategies Be Extended to the Clinic?

Integrative examples in the literature to date have largely dealt with model systems based on mammalian cell culture, since these systems are fairly well defined, are easily manipulated, have quantifiable phenotypes, and while complex, are still much less complex than in vivo systems (either murine models or human tumors). One of the principle challenges facing the field of systems biology is to extend these integrative studies out of these model systems in the lab to study in vivo systems, thereby increasing the direct impact in the clinic. While this is a daunting task given the biological variability and complexity represented by in vivo systems, there is good reason to be optimistic, as many of the analysis techniques can be directly applied to clinical samples.

How can integrative approaches be transferred to the clinic and applied to brain cancers? First, it is necessary to start with large-scale data acquisition to define the network status of human tumors. Much as genomic strategies have recently defined a spectrum and frequency of mutations associated with GBM (TCGA, 2008; Parsons et al. 2008), similar proteomic strategies can be applied to define the phosphorylated/activated pathways and networks in these same samples. On the surface, this information will provide a quantitative catalog of the various phosphorylation events, pathways, and networks found in human brain tumors. When coupled with patient phenotypic information, this quantitative phosphoproteomic data will identify novel biomarkers, proteins, and phosphorylation sites associated with disease progression, survival time, and, perhaps most importantly, sensitivity and resistance to various therapeutic treatment options. This correlative data, by itself, will enable better diagnoses and improved prognosis for brain cancer patients, all based on the phosphorylation status of multiple key biomarkers in the resected tumor section. More importantly, the phosphoproteomic data from clinical samples can be overlaid on signaling networks defined in cell culture model systems, thereby identifying the key nodes and most sensitive proteins to target therapeutically. As mentioned above, these optimal therapeutic targets will not necessarily be the most phosphorylated or most activated proteins in the sample, but instead will be those whose inhibition most drastically affects the remainder of the network, resulting in network failure and cell death. As highlighted in Fig. 40.4 and Color Plate 60, given the future combination of computational models and large-scale clinical data, it is possible to imagine that small samples obtained from patients diagnosed with brain cancer will be analyzed to determine the phosphorylation status of $\sim$10–50 proteins; this information will then enable the selection of therapeutic options specifically selected to provide optimal therapeutic benefit for the patient.

While this vision of integrative biology for personalized medicine sounds very promising, there remains a significant amount of work to be done before it can be realized. First, additional studies of cell culture model systems must be performed (1) to understand the complexity inherent in the signaling networks and (2) to uncover the feedback loops, crosstalk, and network–phenotype relationships. These studies will have to be performed in a variety of cell lines under a variety of culture and stimulation conditions, to provide a degree of robustness to the data encoded in the model. Second, the information from these studies will need to be encoded in large-scale mechanistic and correlative (data-driven) computational models to predict response to cellular perturbation. These models will need to be validated to ascertain their prediction accuracy to multiple stimuli, alone and in combination. Third, as mentioned above, large-scale data acquisition efforts will need to begin to quantify signaling networks in human brain tumors and to correlate this data with patient phenotypic information. In this phase, multiple complementary analysis

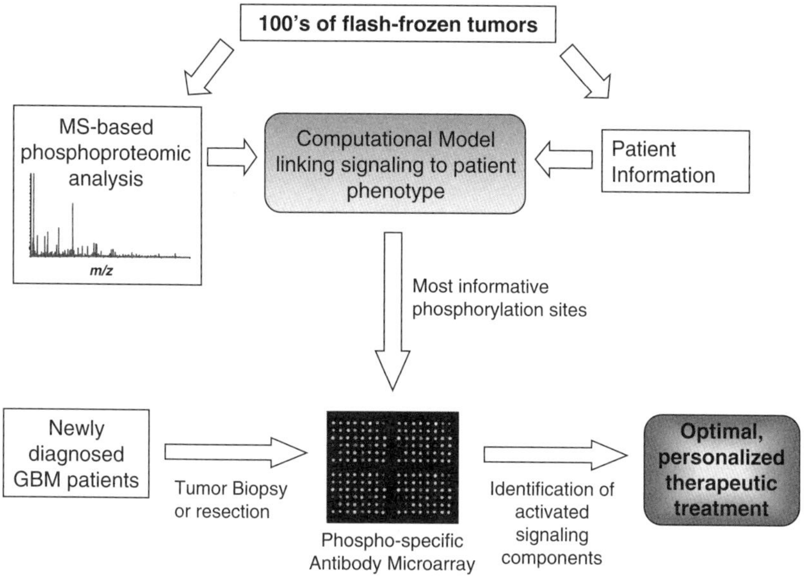

Fig. 40.4 Bench-to-bedside strategy for personalized therapeutic treatment of glioblastoma patients. Hundreds of flash-frozen tumors will be analyzed by mass spectrometry to define signaling networks in these samples. Patient information (e.g., prognosis, genotype, sensitivity to selected agents) for these tumors will be incorporated in an integrative analysis to identify phosphorylation sites that best correlate with the patient phenotypic information. Phospho-specific antibodies will be raised against these selected sites. These antibodies can then be used on an antibody microarray to screen additional human tumors, thereby identifying activated signaling networks in these new tumors. This information, when coupled with the cell-based computational model, will facilitate the identification of novel, personalized, combinatorial therapeutic treatment strategies for each patient (*see* Color Plate 60)

methods should be applied to obtain the most accurate and comprehensive coverage of the signaling networks in these samples. Finally, this clinical proteomic data must be incorporated in the models to determine which nodes/pathways/networks are activated in given samples; model predictions will then identify the most sensitive nodes to be targeted with combinatorial therapeutics.

40.7 Conclusions

Recent efforts to quantify signaling network activation in human GBM cell line model systems have uncovered connectivity between various pathways and kinases within GBM signaling networks. Combinatorial targeting of some of these kinases has provided promising results in cell culture model systems and murine xenografts, and it will hopefully have a positive impact in the clinic in the near future. While these results are intriguing and may have clinical impact, the optimum combinatorial treatment strategies are still undetermined. As a community, we are just beginning to uncover the network complexity associated with GBM and other human pathologies (Parsons et al. 2008). For instance, as described above, increased EGFRvIII expression also leads to increased phosphorylation of the activating phosphorylation site on multiple additional RTKs, but it is not clear yet how these other points of crosstalk affect the phenotype. Will these RTKs represent additional targets for combinatorial inhibition, or will they alter the phenotype in a more discrete fashion, potentially by regulating chemoresistance, proliferation, invasion, or through transcriptional regulation? At this point in time, there is simply not enough known about the complexity of the signaling networks to begin to assign function to these recently discovered nodes in the EGFRvIII network. Clearly, additional integrative studies need to be performed to uncover the network–phenotype relationship for this and other oncogenic systems. These integrative studies, when coupled to computational models of signaling networks, will facilitate the identification of the optimal combinatorial therapeutic strategies for GBM in the future.

References

Alessi, D. R., Caudwell, F. B., Andjelkovic, M., Hemmings, B. A. and Cohen, P. (1996). "Molecular basis for the substrate specificity of protein kinase B; comparison with MAP-KAP kinase-1 and p70 S6 kinase." *FEBS Lett* **399**(3): 333–8.

Amit, I., Wides, R. and Yarden, Y. (2007). "Evolvable signaling networks of receptor tyrosine kinases: relevance of robustness to malignancy and to cancer therapy." *Mol Syst Biol* **3**: 151.

Broderick, D. K., Di, C., Parrett, T. J., Samuels, Y. R., Cummins, J. M., McLendon, R. E., Fults, D. W., Velculescu, V. E., Bigner, D. D. and Yan, H. (2004). "Mutations of PIK3CA in anaplastic oligodendrogliomas, high-grade astrocytomas, and medulloblastomas." *Cancer Res* **64**(15): 5048–50.

Cantley, L. C. (2002). "The phosphoinositide 3-kinase pathway." *Science* **296**(5573): 1655–7.

Chen, Z., Gibson, T. B., Robinson, F., Silvestro, L., Pearson, G., Xu, B., Wright, A., Vanderbilt, C. and Cobb, M. H. (2001). "MAP kinases." *Chem Rev* **101**(8): 2449–76.

Cloughesy, T. F., Yoshimoto, K., Nghiemphu, P., Brown, K., Dang, J., Zhu, S., Hsueh, T., Chen, Y., Wang, W., Youngkin, D., Liau, L., Martin, N., Becker, D., Bergsneider, M., Lai, A., Green, R., Oglesby, T., Koleto, M., Trent, J., Horvath, S., Mischel, P. S., Mellinghoff, I. K. and Sawyers, C. L. (2008). "Antitumor activity of rapamycin in a Phase I trial for patients with recurrent PTEN-deficient glioblastoma." *PLoS Med* **5**(1): e8.

de la Iglesia, N., Konopka, G., Puram, S. V., Chan, J. A., Bachoo, R. M., You, M. J., Levy, D. E., Depinho, R. A. and Bonni, A. (2008). "Identification of a PTEN-regulated STAT3 brain tumor suppressor pathway." *Genes Dev* **22**(4): 449–62.

Dittmar, T., Husemann, A., Schewe, Y., Nofer, J. R., Niggemann, B., Zanker, K. S. and Brandt, B. H. (2002). "Induction of cancer cell migration by epidermal growth factor is initiated by specific phosphorylation of tyrosine 1248 of c-erbB-2 receptor via EGFR." *Faseb J* **16**(13): 1823–5.

Downward, J. (2003). "Targeting RAS signalling pathways in cancer therapy." *Nat Rev Cancer* **3**(1): 11–22.

Ekstrand, A. J., Sugawa, N., James, C. D. and Collins, V. P. (1992). "Amplified and rearranged epidermal growth factor receptor genes in human glioblastomas reveal deletions of sequences encoding portions of the N- and/or C-terminal tails." *Proc Natl Acad Sci U S A* **89**(10): 4309–13.

Engelman, J. A., Zejnullahu, K., Mitsudomi, T., Song, Y., Hyland, C., Park, J. O., Lindeman, N., Gale, C. M., Zhao, X., Christensen, J., Kosaka, T., Holmes, A. J., Rogers, A. M., Cappuzzo, F., Mok, T., Lee, C., Johnson, B. E., Cantley, L. C. and Janne, P. A. (2007). "MET amplification leads to gefitinib resistance in lung cancer by activating ERBB3 signaling." *Science* **316**(5827): 1039–43.

Eyler, C. E. and Rich, J. N. (2008). "Survival of the fittest: cancer stem cells in therapeutic resistance and angiogenesis." *J Clin Oncol* **26**(17): 2839–45.

Falsey, R. R., Marron, M. T., Gunaherath, G. M., Shirahatti, N., Mahadevan, D., Gunatilaka, A. A. and Whitesell, L. (2006). "Actin microfilament aggregation induced by withaferin A is mediated by annexin II." *Nat Chem Biol* **2**(1): 33–8.

Fan, Q. W., Cheng, C. K., Nicolaides, T. P., Hackett, C. S., Knight, Z. A., Shokat, K. M. and Weiss, W. A. (2007). "A dual phosphoinositide-3-kinase alpha/mTOR inhibitor cooperates with blockade of epidermal growth factor receptor in PTEN-mutant glioma." *Cancer Res* **67**(17): 7960–5.

Feldkamp, M. M., Lala, P., Lau, N., Roncari, L. and Guha, A. (1999). "Expression of activated epidermal growth factor receptors, Ras-guanosine triphosphate, and mitogen-activated protein kinase in human glioblastoma multiforme specimens." *Neurosurgery* **45**(6): 1442–53.

Frederick, L., Wang, X. Y., Eley, G. and James, C. D. (2000). "Diversity and frequency of epidermal growth factor receptor mutations in human glioblastomas." *Cancer Res* **60**(5): 1383–7.

Furnari, F. B., Fenton, T., Bachoo, R. M., Mukasa, A., Stommel, J. M., Stegh, A., Hahn, W. C., Ligon, K. L., Louis, D. N., Brennan, C., Chin, L., DePinho, R. A. and Cavenee, W. K. (2007). "Malignant astrocytic glioma: genetics, biology, and paths to treatment." *Genes Dev* **21**(21): 2683–710.

Gallia, G. L., Rand, V., Siu, I. M., Eberhart, C. G., James, C. D., Marie, S. K., Oba-Shinjo, S. M., Carlotti, C. G., Caballero, O. L., Simpson, A. J., Brock, M. V., Massion, P. P., Carson, B. S., Sr. and Riggins, G. J. (2006). "PIK3CA gene mutations in pediatric and adult glioblastoma multiforme." *Mol Cancer Res* **4**(10): 709–14.

Gupta, S., Ramjaun, A. R., Haiko, P., Wang, Y., Warne, P. H., Nicke, B., Nye, E., Stamp, G., Alitalo, K. and Downward, J. (2007). "Binding of ras to phosphoinositide 3-kinase p110alpha is required for ras-driven tumorigenesis in mice." *Cell* **129**(5): 957–68.

Han, Y., Caday, C. G., Nanda, A., Cavenee, W. K. and Huang, H. J. (1996). "Tyrphostin AG 1478 preferentially inhibits human glioma cells expressing truncated rather than wild-type epidermal growth factor receptors." *Cancer Res* **56**(17): 3859–61.

Hartmann, C., Bartels, G., Gehlhaar, C., Holtkamp, N. and von Deimling, A. (2005). "PIK3CA mutations in glioblastoma multiforme." *Acta Neuropathol* **109**(6): 639–42.

Hay, N. (2005). "The Akt-mTOR tango and its relevance to cancer." *Cancer Cell* **8**(3): 179–83.

Hornberg, J. J., Binder, B., Bruggeman, F. J., Schoeberl, B., Heinrich, R. and Westerhoff, H. V. (2005). "Control of MAPK signalling: from complexity to what really matters." *Oncogene* **24**(36): 5533–42.

Huang, P. H., Cavenee, W. K., Furnari, F. B. and White, F. M. (2007a). "Uncovering therapeutic targets for glioblastoma: a systems biology approach." *Cell Cycle* **6**(22): 2750–4.

Huang, P. H., Mukasa, A., Bonavia, R., Flynn, R. A., Brewer, Z. E., Cavenee, W. K., Furnari, F. B. and White, F. M. (2007b). "Quantitative analysis of EGFRvIII cellular signaling networks reveals a combinatorial therapeutic strategy for glioblastoma." *Proc Natl Acad Sci U S A* **104**(31): 12867–72.

Hutterer, M., Knyazev, P., Abate, A., Reschke, M., Maier, H., Stefanova, N., Knyazeva, T., Barbieri, V., Reindl, M., Muigg, A., Kostron, H., Stockhammer, G. and Ullrich, A.

(2008). "Axl and growth arrest-specific gene 6 are frequently overexpressed in human gliomas and predict poor prognosis in patients with glioblastoma multiforme." *Clin Cancer Res* **14**(1): 130–8.

Irish, J. M., Hovland, R., Krutzik, P. O., Perez, O. D., Bruserud, O., Gjertsen, B. T. and Nolan, G. P. (2004). "Single cell profiling of potentiated phospho-protein networks in cancer cells." *Cell* **118**(2): 217–28.

Janes, K. A., Albeck, J. G., Gaudet, S., Sorger, P. K., Lauffenburger, D. A. and Yaffe, M. B. (2005). "A systems model of signaling identifies a molecular basis set for cytokine-induced apoptosis." *Science* **310**(5754): 1646–53.

Ji, H., Zhao, X., Yuza, Y., Shimamura, T., Li, D., Protopopov, A., Jung, B. L., McNamara, K., Xia, H., Glatt, K. A., Thomas, R. K., Sasaki, H., Horner, J. W., Eck, M., Mitchell, A., Sun, Y., Al-Hashem, R., Bronson, R. T., Rabindran, S. K., Discafani, C. M., Maher, E., Shapiro, G. I., Meyerson, M. and Wong, K. K. (2006). "Epidermal growth factor receptor variant III mutations in lung tumorigenesis and sensitivity to tyrosine kinase inhibitors." *Proc Natl Acad Sci U S A* **103**(20): 7817–22.

Johns, T. G., Luwor, R. B., Murone, C., Walker, F., Weinstock, J., Vitali, A. A., Perera, R. M., Jungbluth, A. A., Stockert, E., Old, L. J., Nice, E. C., Burgess, A. W. and Scott, A. M. (2003). "Antitumor efficacy of cytotoxic drugs and the monoclonal antibody 806 is enhanced by the EGF receptor inhibitor AG1478." *Proc Natl Acad Sci U S A* **100**(26): 15871–6.

Koochekpour, S., Jeffers, M., Rulong, S., Taylor, G., Klineberg, E., Hudson, E. A., Resau, J. H. and Vande Woude, G. F. (1997). "Met and hepatocyte growth factor/scatter factor expression in human gliomas." *Cancer Res* **57**(23): 5391–8.

Learn, C. A., Hartzell, T. L., Wikstrand, C. J., Archer, G. E., Rich, J. N., Friedman, A. H., Friedman, H. S., Bigner, D. D. and Sampson, J. H. (2004). "Resistance to tyrosine kinase inhibition by mutant epidermal growth factor receptor variant III contributes to the neoplastic phenotype of glioblastoma multiforme." *Clin Cancer Res* **10**(9): 3216–24.

Manning, B. D. and Cantley, L. C. (2007). "AKT/PKB signaling: navigating downstream." *Cell* **129**(7): 1261–74.

Meier-Schellersheim, M., Xu, X., Angermann, B., Kunkel, E. J., Jin, T. and Germain, R. N. (2006). "Key role of local regulation in chemosensing revealed by a new molecular interaction-based modeling method." *PLoS Comput Biol* **2**(7): e82.

Mellinghoff, I. K., Cloughesy, T. F. and Mischel, P. S. (2007). "PTEN-mediated resistance to epidermal growth factor receptor kinase inhibitors." *Clin Cancer Res* **13**(2 Pt 1): 378–81.

Mellinghoff, I. K., Wang, M. Y., Vivanco, I., Haas-Kogan, D. A., Zhu, S., Dia, E. Q., Lu, K. V., Yoshimoto, K., Huang, J. H., Chute, D. J., Riggs, B. L., Horvath, S., Liau, L. M., Cavenee, W. K., Rao, P. N., Beroukhim, R., Peck, T. C., Lee, J. C., Sellers, W. R., Stokoe, D., Prados, M., Cloughesy, T. F., Sawyers, C. L. and Mischel, P. S. (2005). "Molecular determinants of the response of glioblastomas to EGFR kinase inhibitors." *N Engl J Med* **353**(19): 2012–24.

Montgomery, R. B., Moscatello, D. K., Wong, A. J., Cooper, J. A. and Stahl, W. L. (1995). "Differential modulation of mitogen-activated protein (MAP) kinase/extracellular signal-related kinase kinase and MAP kinase activities by a mutant epidermal growth factor receptor." *J Biol Chem* **270**(51): 30562–6.

Moscatello, D. K., Holgado-Madruga, M., Emlet, D. R., Montgomery, R. B. and Wong, A. J. (1998). "Constitutive activation of phosphatidylinositol 3-kinase by a naturally occurring mutant epidermal growth factor receptor." *J Biol Chem* **273**(1): 200–6.

Nyati, M. K., Morgan, M. A., Feng, F. Y. and Lawrence, T. S. (2006). "Integration of EGFR inhibitors with radiochemotherapy." *Nat Rev Cancer* **6**(11): 876–85.

Ohgaki, H., Dessen, P., Jourde, B., Horstmann, S., Nishikawa, T., Di Patre, P. L., Burkhard, C., Schuler, D., Probst-Hensch, N. M., Maiorka, P. C., Baeza, N., Pisani, P., Yonekawa, Y.,

Yasargil, M. G., Lutolf, U. M. and Kleihues, P. (2004). "Genetic pathways to glioblastoma: a population-based study." *Cancer Res* **64**(19): 6892–9.

Ohgaki, H. and Kleihues, P. (2007). "Genetic pathways to primary and secondary glioblastoma." *Am J Pathol* **170**(5): 1445–53.

Okabayashi, Y., Kido, Y., Okutani, T., Sugimoto, Y., Sakaguchi, K. and Kasuga, M. (1994). "Tyrosines 1148 and 1173 of activated human epidermal growth factor receptors are binding sites of Shc in intact cells." *J Biol Chem* **269**(28): 18674–8.

Olsen, J. V., Blagoev, B., Gnad, F., Macek, B., Kumar, C., Mortensen, P. and Mann, M. (2006). "Global, in vivo, and site-specific phosphorylation dynamics in signaling networks." *Cell* **127**(3): 635–48.

Omuro, A. M., Faivre, S. and Raymond, E. (2007). "Lessons learned in the development of targeted therapy for malignant gliomas." *Mol Cancer Ther* **6**(7): 1909–19.

Parsons, D. W., Jones, S., Zhang, X., Lin, J. C., Leary, R. J., Angenendt, P., Mankoo, P., Carter, H., Siu, I. M., Gallia, G. L., Olivi, A., McLendon, R., Rasheed, B. A., Keir, S., Nikolskaya, T., Nikolsky, Y., Busam, D. A., Tekleab, H., Diaz, L. A., Jr., Hartigan, J., Smith, D. R., Strausberg, R. L., Marie, S. K., Shinjo, S. M., Yan, H., Riggins, G. J., Bigner, D. D., Karchin, R., Papadopoulos, N., Parmigiani, G., Vogelstein, B., Velculescu, V. E. and Kinzler, K. W. (2008). "An Integrated Genomic Analysis of Human Glioblastoma Multiforme." *Science* **321**(5897): 1807–12.

Pedersen, M. W., Pedersen, N., Ottesen, L. H. and Poulsen, H. S. (2005). "Differential response to gefitinib of cells expressing normal EGFR and the mutant EGFRvIII." *Br J Cancer* **93**(8): 915–23.

Perez, O. D. and Nolan, G. P. (2006). "Phospho-proteomic immune analysis by flow cytometry: from mechanism to translational medicine at the single-cell level." *Immunol Rev* **210**: 208–28.

Radimerski, T., Montagne, J., Hemmings-Mieszczak, M. and Thomas, G. (2002). "Lethality of Drosophila lacking TSC tumor suppressor function rescued by reducing dS6K signaling." *Genes Dev* **16**(20): 2627–32.

Rescher, U., Ludwig, C., Konietzko, V., Kharitonenkov, A. and Gerke, V. (2008). "Tyrosine phosphorylation of annexin A2 regulates Rho-mediated actin rearrangement and cell adhesion." *J Cell Sci* **121**(Pt 13): 2177–85.

Rich, J. N., Reardon, D. A., Peery, T., Dowell, J. M., Quinn, J. A., Penne, K. L., Wikstrand, C. J., Van Duyn, L. B., Dancey, J. E., McLendon, R. E., Kao, J. C., Stenzel, T. T., Ahmed Rasheed, B. K., Tourt-Uhlig, S. E., Herndon, J. E., 2nd, Vredenburgh, J. J., Sampson, J. H., Friedman, A. H., Bigner, D. D. and Friedman, H. S. (2004). "Phase II trial of gefitinib in recurrent glioblastoma." *J Clin Oncol* **22**(1): 133–42.

Sampaio, C., Dance, M., Montagner, A., Edouard, T., Malet, N., Perret, B., Yart, A., Salles, J. P. and Raynal, P. (2008). "Signal strength dictates phosphoinositide 3-kinase contribution to Ras/extracellular signal-regulated kinase 1 and 2 activation via differential Gab1/Shp2 recruitment: consequences for resistance to epidermal growth factor receptor inhibition." *Mol Cell Biol* **28**(2): 587–600.

Sarbassov, D. D., Guertin, D. A., Ali, S. M. and Sabatini, D. M. (2005). "Phosphorylation and regulation of Akt/PKB by the rictor-mTOR complex." *Science* **307**(5712): 1098–101.

Savageau, M. A. (1971). "Parameter sensitivity as a criterion for evaluating and comparing the performance of biochemical systems." *Nature* **229**(5286): 542–4.

Schmelzle, K. and White, F. M. (2006). "Phosphoproteomic approaches to elucidate cellular signaling networks." *Curr Opin Biotechnol* **17**(4): 406–14.

Shankaran, H., Wiley, H. S. and Resat, H. (2007). "Receptor downregulation and desensitization enhance the information processing ability of signalling receptors." *BMC Syst Biol* **1**: 48.

Stommel, J. M., Kimmelman, A. C., Ying, H., Nabioullin, R., Ponugoti, A. H., Wiedemeyer, R., Stegh, A. H., Bradner, J. E., Ligon, K. L., Brennan, C., Chin, L. and DePinho, R. A. (2007).

"Coactivation of receptor tyrosine kinases affects the response of tumor cells to targeted therapies." *Science* **318**(5848): 287–90.

Sugawa, N., Ekstrand, A. J., James, C. D. and Collins, V. P. (1990). "Identical splicing of aberrant epidermal growth factor receptor transcripts from amplified rearranged genes in human glioblastomas." *Proc Natl Acad Sci U S A* **87**(21): 8602–6.

The Cancer Genome Atlas Research Network, McLendon, R., Friedman, A., Bigner, D., Van Meir, E. G., Brat, D. J., Mastrogianakis, M., Olson, J. J., Mikkelsen, T., Lehman, N., Aldape, K., Alfred Yung, W. K., Bogler, O., Vandenberg, S., Berger, M., Prados, M., Muzny, D., Morgan, M., Scherer, S., Sabo, A., Nazareth, L., Lewis, L., Hall, O., Zhu, Y., Ren, Y., Alvi, O., Yao, J., Hawes, A., Jhangiani, S., Fowler, G., San Lucas, A., Kovar, C., Cree, A., Dinh, H., Santibanez, J., Joshi, V., Gonzalez-Garay, M. L., Miller, C. A., Milosavljevic, A., Donehower, L., Wheeler, D. A., Gibbs, R. A., Cibulskis, K., Sougnez, C., Fennell, T., Mahan, S., Wilkinson, J., Ziaugra, L., Onofrio, R., Bloom, T., Nicol, R., Ardlie, K., Baldwin, J., Gabriel, S., Lander, E. S., Ding, L., Fulton, R. S., McLellan, M. D., Wallis, J., Larson, D. E., Shi, X., Abbott, R., Fulton, L., Chen, K., Koboldt, D. C., Wendl, M. C., Meyer, R., Tang, Y., Lin, L., Osborne, J. R., Dunford-Shore, B. H., Miner, T. L., Delehaunty, K., Markovic, C., Swift, G., Courtney, W., Pohl, C., Abbott, S., Hawkins, A., Leong, S., Haipek, C., Schmidt, H., Wiechert, M., Vickery, T., Scott, S., Dooling, D. J., Chinwalla, A., Weinstock, G. M., Mardis, E. R., Wilson, R. K., Getz, G., Winckler, W., Verhaak, R. G., Lawrence, M. S., O'Kelly, M., Robinson, J., Alexe, G., Beroukhim, R., Carter, S., Chiang, D., Gould, J., Gupta, S., Korn, J., Mermel, C., Mesirov, J., Monti, S., Nguyen, H., Parkin, M., Reich, M., Stransky, N., Weir, B. A., Garraway, L., Golub, T., Meyerson, M., Chin, L., Protopopov, A., Zhang, J., Perna, I., Aronson, S., Sathiamoorthy, N., Ren, G., Yao, J., Wiedemeyer, W. R., Kim, H., Won Kong, S., Xiao, Y., Kohane, I. S., Seidman, J., Park, P. J., Kucherlapati, R., Laird, P. W., Cope, L., Herman, J. G., Weisenberger, D. J., Pan, F., Van Den Berg, D., Van Neste, L., Mi Yi, J., Schuebel, K. E., Baylin, S. B., Absher, D. M., Li, J. Z., Southwick, A., Brady, S., Aggarwal, A., Chung, T. , Sherlock, G., Brooks, J. D., Myers, R. M., Spellman, P. T., Purdom, E., Jakkula, L. R., Lapuk, A. V., Marr, H., Dorton, S., Gi Choi, Y., Han, J., Ray, A., Wang, V., Durinck, S., Robinson, M., Wang, N. J., Vranizan, K., Peng, V., Van Name, E., Fontenay, G. V., Ngai, J., Conboy, J. G., Parvin, B., Feiler, H. S., Speed, T. P., Gray, J. W., Brennan, C., Socci, N. D., Olshen, A., Taylor, B. S., Lash, A., Schultz, N., Reva, B., Antipin, Y., Stukalov, A., Gross, B., Cerami, E., Qing Wang, W., Qin, L. X., Seshan, V. E., Villafania, L., Cavatore, M., Borsu, L., Viale, A., Gerald, W., Sander, C., Ladanyi, M., Perou, C. M., Neil Hayes, D., Topal, M. D., Hoadley, K. A., Qi, Y., Balu, S., Shi, Y., Wu, J., Penny, R., Bittner, M., Shelton, T., Lenkiewicz, E., Morris, S., Beasley, D., Sanders, S., Kahn, A., Sfeir, R., Chen, J., Nassau, D., Feng, L., Hickey, E., Zhang, J., Weinstein, J. N., Barker, A., Gerhard, D. S., Vockley, J., Compton, C., Vaught, J., Fielding, P., Ferguson, M. L., Schaefer, C., Madhavan, S., Buetow, K. H., Collins, F., Good, P., Guyer, M., Ozenberger, B., Peterson, J. and Thomson, E. (2008). "Comprehensive genomic characterization defines human glioblastoma genes and core pathways." *Nature* **455**(7216): 1061–8.

Wang, M. Y., Lu, K. V., Zhu, S., Dia, E. Q., Vivanco, I., Shackleford, G. M., Cavenee, W. K., Mellinghoff, I. K., Cloughesy, T. F., Sawyers, C. L. and Mischel, P. S. (2006). "Mammalian target of rapamycin inhibition promotes response to epidermal growth factor receptor kinase inhibitors in PTEN-deficient and PTEN-intact glioblastoma cells." *Cancer Res* **66**(16): 7864–9.

Wolf-Yadlin, A., Hautaniemi, S., Lauffenburger, D. A. and White, F. M. (2007). "Multiple reaction monitoring for robust quantitative proteomic analysis of cellular signaling networks." *Proc Natl Acad Sci U S A* **104**(14): 5860–5.

Wolf-Yadlin, A., Kumar, N., Zhang, Y., Hautaniemi, S., Zaman, M., Kim, H. D., Grantcharova, V., Lauffenburger, D. A. and White, F. M. (2006). "Effects of HER2 overexpression on cell signaling networks governing proliferation and migration." *Mol Syst Biol* **2**: 54.

Wong, A. J., Ruppert, J. M., Bigner, S. H., Grzeschik, C. H., Humphrey, P. A., Bigner, D. S. and Vogelstein, B. (1992). "Structural alterations of the epidermal growth factor receptor gene in human gliomas." *Proc Natl Acad Sci U S A* **89**(7): 2965–9.

Zhang, Y., Wolf-Yadlin, A., Ross, P. L., Pappin, D. J., Rush, J., Lauffenburger, D. A. and White, F. M. (2005). "Time-resolved mass spectrometry of tyrosine phosphorylation sites in the epidermal growth factor receptor signaling network reveals dynamic modules." *Mol Cell Proteomics* **4**(9): 1240–50.

Chapter 41
Targeting of TRAIL Apoptotic Pathways for Glioblastoma Therapies

Anita C. Bellail, Patrick Mulligan, and Chunhai Hao

Abstract Recent advances in cancer biology have generated novel cancer therapeutics that can activate apoptotic pathways in human cancers. Among the apoptotic therapeutics, tumor necrosis factor-related apoptosis-inducing ligand (TRAIL) has received much attention because it can selectively induce apoptosis in cancer cells. Preclinical studies in glioblastoma cell lines, primary cultures, and xenografts have resulted in the development of TRAIL-based therapeutic modalities for the treatment of glioblastoma. These include recombinant human TRAIL (rhTRAIL), agonistic antibodies against TRAIL death receptors, DR4 and DR5, TRAIL-producing neural stem cells, TRAIL-expressing oncolytic vectors, and nanoparticles conjugated with TRAIL-expressing vectors. Although rhTRAIL and DR4 and DR5 agonistic antibodies have entered clinical trials in patients with solid cancers and hematological malignancies, many challenges remain before any of these therapeutic modalities can be successfully developed into clinical treatments for glioblastoma. It remains to be seen whether and how the therapeutics can be effectively distributed through glioblastoma that is diffusely infiltrating through the human brain. In addition, the vast majority of the tumors are resistant to TRAIL and thus require combination treatments that can overcome the resistance. Finally, genetic analysis of human glioblastomas is required to identify the genetic defects in apoptotic genes that could be used as biomarkers to predict the responsiveness of the tumors to TRAIL-based therapies.

Contents

C. Hao (✉)
Department of Pathology & Laboratory Medicine, Winship Cancer Institute, Emory University School of Medicine, 1365-C Clifton Road, Atlanta, GA 30322, USA
e-mail: chao@emory.edu

E.G. Van Meir (ed.), *CNS Cancer*, Cancer Drug Discovery and Development, DOI 10.1007/978-1-60327-553-8_41,
© Humana Press, a part of Springer Science+Business Media, LLC 2009

41.1 Introduction

Primary diffuse astrocytic gliomas are the most common brain tumors and are classified into astrocytoma, anaplastic astrocytoma, and glioblastoma. Glioblastoma is the most common and lethal glioma and current therapeutic modalities including surgical resection, radiation therapy, and temozolomide chemotherapy provide no cure. In the last three decades, researchers have gained significant insight into signaling pathways involved in the generation of the tumors and their malignant progression. As a result, novel therapeutic agents have been generated specifically targeting the signaling pathways activated in the tumors (Rich and Bigner, 2004). Cancers such as glioblastomas are genetic diseases in which genomic alterations result in the deregulation of cell growth and death signaling pathways, which leads to the relentless cancer cell growth at the expense of cancer cell death (Vogelstein and Kinzler, 2004). Many novel therapeutic agents have been generated targeting cancer growth pathways, but there is an increasing interest in the development of therapeutics that can trigger cancer cell death pathways. The ultimate goal of cell death pathways-targeted therapies is to restore endogenous death pathways and thus drive cancer cells into self-destruction (Letai, 2008). Several cell death pathways have been reported including apoptosis, necrosis, autophagy, and mitotic catastrophe. Of these death pathways, apoptosis is the best characterized, and a number of therapeutic agents targeting the pathways are currently in clinical trials (Reed, 2006).

Apoptosis is a genetically programmed biochemical process that removes unwanted cells and maintains tissue homeostasis under physiological and pathological conditions. In principle, there are two pathways that control the initiation of apoptosis: the death receptors-mediated extrinsic pathway and the mitochondria-involved intrinsic pathway. Death receptors belong to the tumor necrosis factor receptor (TNFR) family and can engage intracellular apoptotic pathways upon binding of the ligands. Ligands of the tumor necrosis factor (TNF) family can trigger the intracellular apoptotic process through binding of their cognate death receptors. TRAIL is a TNF family ligand that can trigger intracellular apoptotic pathways through binding on one of the two death receptors, DR4 and DR5. In this chapter, we will first provide a historic review of the development of cancer therapeutics targeting the death receptors of the TNF family. We will then discuss the signaling pathways in TRAIL-induced apoptosis, the development of novel cancer therapeutics targeting DR4 and DR5, and the resistance of cancer cells to these therapeutics. Finally, we will review the advances in the TRAIL-based therapies in glioblastomas and the challenges faced in the development of such therapies in the clinical treatment of glioblastomas.

41.2 Development of TNF Family Death Receptors Targeted Cancer Therapies

TNFα, the prototype of TNF family ligands, was first reported for its antitumor activity in mice treated with endotoxin in 1975 (Carswell et al., 1975). Eighteen ligands and 28 death receptors have been identified since (Ashkenazi, 2002), but the following three sets of ligands and their cognate death receptors have been well studied for their cancer therapeutic potentials: TNFα (Beutler et al., 1985; Carswell et al., 1975; Pennica et al., 1984) and TNFR 1 (p55, CD120a) (Lewis et al., 1991); Fas ligand (FasL, CD95L) (Suda et al., 1993) and Fas (CD95) (Itoh et al., 1991); and TRAIL (Pitti et al., 1996; Wiley et al., 1995) and DR4/TRAIL-R1 (Pan et al., 1997; Schneider et al., 1997a) and DR5/TRAIL-R2 (Chaudhary et al., 1997; Schneider et al., 1997a; Walczak et al., 1997; Wu et al., 1997).

41.2.1 Toxicity in TNFR and Fas-Targeted Therapies

In 1984, TNFα was cloned from human (Pennica et al., 1984) and, subsequently, recombinant human TNFα (rhTNFα) was generated targeting TNFR and shown to have antitumor activity and toxicity in tumor xenograft mice (Tracey et al., 1986). Despite the toxicity of rhTNFα observed in mice, phase I and II clinical trials of rhTNFα were launched and, unfortunately, revealed dose-limiting side effects of hypotension and hepatotoxicity in patients (Creagan et al., 1988; Creaven et al., 1989; Lenk et al., 1989; Schiller et al., 1991; Skillings et al., 1992). The systemic use of rhTNFα as a therapeutic agent has therefore been abandoned since the 1990s. In 1989, an agonistic antibody against death receptor, Fas, was generated (Trauth et al., 1989). Systemic injection of the Fas agonistic antibody in mice, however, caused profound hepatotoxicity (Ogasawara et al., 1993) so that clinical trials of Fas agonistic antibodies have never been considered. Current antitumor strategies using rhTNFα or agonistic Fas antibody are limited to local delivery to avoid the systemic side effects (ElOjeimy et al., 2006; Grunhagen et al., 2006).

41.2.2 Controversy in TRAIL-Induced Toxicity

TRAIL was identified in the middle 1990s (Pitti et al., 1996; Wiley et al., 1995) and rhTRAIL was subsequently generated as a cancer therapeutic (Ashkenazi et al., 1999; Walczak et al., 1999). Studies of various forms of rhTRAIL, however, created a controversy with regard to toxicity to normal human cells. A leucine zipper-fused rhTRAIL killed isolated human astrocytes (Walczak et al., 1999), a polyhistidine-tagged rhTRAIL was toxic to isolated human hepatocytes (Jo et al., 2000), and a flag-tagged rhTRAIL-induced apoptotic cell death of human brain cells in brain slice culture (Nitsch et al., 2000). These in vitro studies raised the same safety concern as those expressed with rhTNFα and Fas agonistic antibody (Nagata, 2000). In 2001, however, it was reported that non-tagged soluble rhTRAIL (amino acids 114–281) was non-toxic to isolated human astrocytes (Hao et al., 2001), human hepatocytes, and normal cells in non-human primates (Lawrence et al., 2001). In the same year, a mouse monoclonal antibody (mAb) against human DR5 (TRA-8) was reported, exhibiting antitumor activity without hepatotoxicity (Ichikawa et al., 2001). In 2004, it was further shown that systemic injection of non-tagged rhTRAIL inhibited cancer xenograft growth without causing injury to human hepatocytes in chimeric mice reconstituted with human livers (Hao et al., 2004).

Preclinical findings that soluble rhTRAIL and TRAIL agonistic antibodies are non-toxic to normal human cells have provided renewed impetus for the launch of clinical trials of rhTRAIL and its agonistic antibodies for the treatment of cancer. In 2005, phase I trials of human DR4 (HGS-ETR1) and DR5 agonistic antibody (HGS-ETR2) were first presented at the 96th Annual Meeting of the American Association for Cancer Research (AACR) and demonstrated the safety and tolerability of the antibodies in patients. In 2006, a phase I trial of rhTRAIL (Apo2L/TRAIL) was reported at the 42nd Annual Meeting of the American Society of Clinical Oncology (ASCO) and showed that rhTRAIL was safe and well tolerated in patients. While the question remains why targeting TNFR and Fas but not DR4/DR5 damages normal human cells, these preclinical and clinical studies have finally put the TRAIL toxicity issue behind us. Currently, phase II trials are evaluating the therapeutic efficacy of these TRAIL agonists in patients with solid cancers and hematological malignancies. There is a great expectation that the results of clinical trials with these new agents will lead to the genesis of a new class of anticancer therapeutics activating apoptotic pathways in human cancer cells.

41.3 TRAIL-Induced Apoptotic Pathways in Human Cancer Cells

TRAIL and its death receptors were identified in the 1990s (Chaudhary et al., 1997; Pan et al., 1997; Pitti et al., 1996; Schneider et al., 1997a; Walczak et al., 1997; Wiley et al., 1995; Wu et al., 1997) and subsequent studies of mice revealed the physiological functions of TRAIL in innate and adaptive immunity. Studies of mice treated with TRAIL-neutralizing antibody showed that TRAIL is required for natural killer (NK) cell-mediated immunosurveillance against tumor progression and metastasis (Takeda et al., 2001, 2002). Studies of TRAIL-deficient mice confirmed the role of TRAIL in innate immunosurveillance against tumorigenesis (Cretney et al., 2002). Additional studies showed that TRAIL contributes to T lymphocyte and dendritic cell-mediated innate and adaptive immunity in suppression of tumor progression (Schmaltz et al., 2002; Taieb et al., 2006). These studies have, therefore, established TRAIL as a natural cancer killer that can drive cancer cells into self-destruction through the activation of apoptotic pathways (Smyth et al., 2003).

41.3.1 TRAIL-Induced DISC and Extrinsic Apoptotic Pathway

TRAIL-induced apoptosis occurs through its binding of the cell surface death receptors, leading to the activation of the extrinsic apoptotic pathway (Fig. 41.1). TRAIL has two death receptors, DR4 (Pan et al., 1997; Schneider et al., 1997a) and DR5 (Chaudhary et al., 1997; Walczak et al., 1997; Wu et al., 1997); both are type I transmembrane proteins with two extracellular cysteine-rich domains and a cytoplasmic death domain (DD). DR4 and DR5 exist either as homotrimers or heterotrimers linked through an interaction between the pre-ligand assembly domains in the extracellular termini (Clancy et al., 2005). Upon TRAIL ligation, DR4 and DR5 recruit the intracellular adaptor, Fas-associated death domain (FADD) (Schneider et al., 1997b; Walczak et al., 1997). FADD contains a carboxy-terminal DD and an amino-terminal death effector domain (DED) (Chinnaiyan et al., 1995). Through the DED, FADD recruits DED-containing caspase-8 (Bodmer et al., 2000; Kischkel et al., 2000; Xiao et al., 2002) and caspase-10 (Kischkel et al., 2001; Sprick et al., 2002; Wang et al., 2001; Xiao et al., 2002) to the receptors for the formation of a death-inducing signaling complex (DISC), similar to the one reported in the Fas

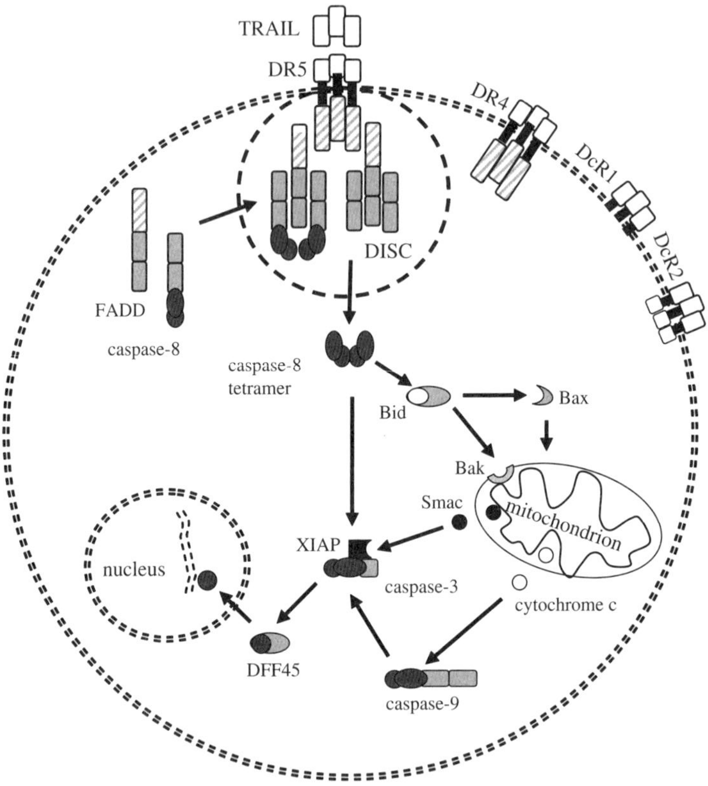

Fig. 41.1 TRAIL-induced apoptosis through the extrinsic and intrinsic pathways

apoptotic pathway (Kischkel et al., 1995; Muzio et al., 1996). In the DISC, the apoptosis initiators, caspase-8 and -10 are proteolytically cleaved, thus becoming enzymatically active, and then cleave effectors caspase-3 and -7 in the execution of apoptotic cell death (Boldin et al., 1996).

41.3.2 TRAIL-Induced Intrinsic Apoptotic Pathway

The intrinsic mitochondrial pathway is required for TRAIL-induced apoptosis (Fig. 41.1). Once cleaved and enzymatically activated in the DISC, caspase-8 cleaves Bcl-2 inhibitory BH3-domain-containing protein (Bid) (Li et al., 1998). The truncated Bid (tBid) interacts with Bax and Bak and induces the oligomerization of Bax and Bak in the mitochondrial membrane, leading to the change of the membrane potential and subsequent release from the mitochondria of cytochrome *c* (Luo et al., 1998) and second mitochondria-derived activator of caspase (Smac) or direct inhibitor of apoptosis binding protein with low p*I*

(DIABLO) (Du et al., 2000; Verhagen et al., 2000). In the cytosol, cytochrome *c* binds to Apaf1 and recruits dATP and caspase-9 to form the apoptosome. Herein caspase-9 is cleaved through autoproteolysis and further cleaves downstream caspase-3 (Li et al., 1997). The caspase-3 cleavage, however, is inhibited in many human cancers due to the expression of X-linked inhibitor of apoptosis (XIAP), which interacts with caspase-3 and inhibits its cleavage (Wagenknecht et al., 1999). Rescue of the TRAIL-induced extrinsic pathway is accomplished by Smac which, once released from mitochondria, interacts with XIAP and releases its inhibition of caspase-3 cleavage (Deng et al., 2002).

41.3.3 Caspase-8 in TRAIL-Induced Apoptosis

Caspase-8 is an apoptosis-initiating caspase that is synthesized as a zymogen and exists in two isoforms (p55, p53); each consists of two DED domains and a protease domain made of two subunits, p18 and p12 (Scaffidi et al., 1997). Through its DEDs, caspase-8 zymogens are recruited to the DISC and cleaved through a two-step autoproteolytic processes: the first intramolecular/*cis* cleavage generates the p12 subunit (Walker et al., 1994; Wilson et al., 1994) and the second cleavage results in the release of the p18 subunit from DED and p10 from the p12 subunit (Medema et al., 1997; Yang et al., 1998). The caspase-8 p18 and p10 active subunits in turn cleave downstream caspase-3 and caspase-7 (Boldin et al., 1996). Caspase-3 and caspase-7 are effector caspases and each of them consists of a protease domain with a large and small subunit. Once cleaved, caspase-3 further cleaves downstream DNA fragmentation factor 45 (DFF45), resulting in the execution of apoptotic cell death (Liu et al., 1997).

How can a caspase-8 zymogen be cleaved when there is no protease above it? An induced proximity model initially suggested that caspase-8 zymogens were brought into close proximity in the DISC for the autoproteolytic cleavage (Muzio et al., 1998; Salvesen and Dixit, 1999). Further in vitro biochemical studies proposed the dimerization model that caspase-8 zymogens first form dimers through an interaction of alanine 397 residues (based on caspase-3 nomenclature) of their protease domains and become proteolytically active and cleaved to form the enzymatically active p18 and p10 tetramers (Boatright et al., 2003; Chang et al., 2003; Donepudi et al., 2003). However, this model of caspase-8 activation remains to be established in vivo in normal or cancerous cells. In addition, the question remains why there are two apoptosis initiators, caspase-8 and -10 in TRAIL-induced apoptosis.

41.3.4 TRAIL-Induced Apoptosis in Glioblastoma Cells

The cytotoxicity of rhTRAIL was first reported in glioblastoma cells (Ashkenazi et al., 1999) and its antitumor activity in mouse glioblastoma xenografts

(Roth et al., 1999). In 2001, rhTRAIL and its agonistic DR5 agonistic antibody TRA-8 were reported to be able to trigger apoptotic cell death in glioblastoma cell lines (Hao et al., 2001; Ichikawa et al., 2001; Knight et al., 2001; Pollack et al., 2001). TRAIL-induced apoptosis was further shown to involve the DISC assembly through DR5-mediated recruitment of FADD, caspase-8 and -10 (Xiao et al., 2002). In the DISC, caspase-8 and -10 are cleaved through autoproteolysis, releasing the enzymatically active subunits. In the cytoplasm, the enzymatically active caspase-8 and -10 cleave Bid and the tBid in turn induces mitochondrial release of cytochrome *c* and Smac, leading to the cleavage of XIAP and caspase-3 in TRAIL-induced apoptosis (Song et al., 2003b). These studies have revealed TRAIL apoptotic pathways in glioblastoma cells and thus provided the basis for the development of TRAIL-based therapies for glioblastomas.

41.4 TRAIL Resistance in Human Cancers

Studies of TRAIL-deficient mice suggest that TRAIL plays a physiologic role in cancer immunosurveillance and, therefore, targeting of TRAIL apoptotic pathways may provide novel therapeutic strategies in cancer therapies (Smyth et al., 2003). On the other hand, however, this notion predicts that cancer may occur in patients with compromised immunosurveillance, or by evasion of immunosurveillance. In support of these possibilities, studies of human cancer cell lines and primary cultures have identified TRAIL-sensitive and -resistant cancer cells. These studies have further illustrated the molecular mechanisms that control TRAIL-induced apoptotic pathways. While much effort has been devoted to the investigation of the cell-intrinsic molecular mechanisms by which cancer cells evade TRAIL-induced apoptotic pathways, little is known regarding the role of TRAIL in immunosurveillance against cancer in human.

41.4.1 Decoy Receptors

In addition to death receptors, TRAIL has two membrane-associated decoy receptors, DcR1 (TRAIL-R3) (Degli-Esposti et al., 1997b; Mongkolsapaya et al., 1998; Sheridan et al., 1997) and DcR2 (TRAIL-R4) (Degli-Esposti et al., 1997a; Marsters et al., 1997; Pan et al., 1998). DcR1 is a glycosyl phosphatidylinositol (GPI)-anchored membrane protein with cysteine-rich extracellular domains but no cytoplasmic truncated DD. DcR2 is a type I transmembrane protein with extracellular domains and a cytoplasmic DD. Through their extracellular domains, DcR1 and DcR2 interact with TRAIL and inhibit TRAIL-induced apoptosis either by competing with death receptors for TRAIL binding (Liu et al., 2005; Sheikh et al., 1999) or by interrupting the homotrimeric formation of death receptors (Merino et al., 2006). Studies also show that the interaction of TRAIL and DcR2 activates cell survival nuclear factor-κB (NF-κB) signal (Degli-Esposti et al., 1997a). These studies have established DcR1 and DcR2 as TRAIL inhibitors and therefore raise concerns about the usefulness of rhTRAIL as compared to DR4 and DR5 agonistic antibodies. This notion, however, is mainly based on the studies in transfectants, and the biological functions of endogenous DcR1 and DcR2 are largely unknown.

41.4.2 DISC Modifications

The DISC can be modified by intracellular adaptor proteins, leading to the inhibition of caspase-8 cleavage and the activation of cell survival pathways (Fig. 41.2). Receptor-interacting protein (RIP) and TNFR1-associated death domain (TRADD), first identified as DD adaptor proteins in the TNFR1- and Fas-DISC (Hsu et al., 1996a; Hsu et al., 1996b; Stanger et al., 1995), can be

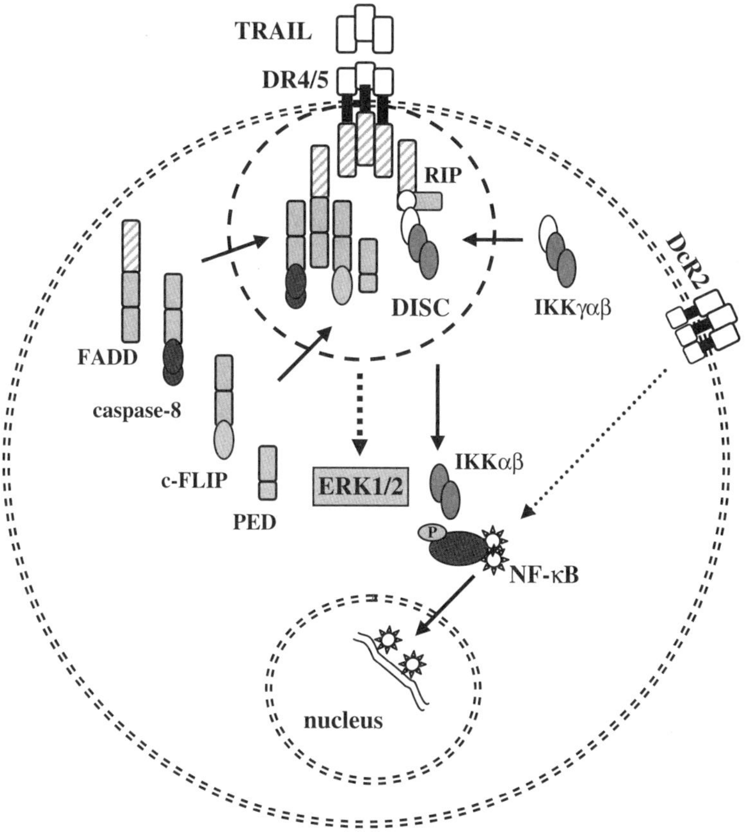

Fig. 41.2 The DISC modification in TRAIL-induced non-apoptotic signals

recruited by DR4/DR5 to the DISC through their DD–DD interaction (Chaudhary et al., 1997). Studies of cancer cell lines detected RIP in the DISC and showed that RIP recruits an inhibitor of κB (IκB) kinase γ (IKKγ), through which IKKα and IKKβ are subsequently recruited to the DISC. This leads to the activation of IKKα/β kinases, the phosphorylation of IκB, and the activation of nuclear factor-κB (NF-κB) (Harper et al., 2001; Lin et al., 2000; Varfolomeev et al., 2005).

Through its DED, FADD can recruit two DED adaptor proteins to the DISC, cellular FADD-like interleukin-1β-converting enzyme [FLICE]-inhibitory protein (c-FLIP) (Irmler et al., 1997) and phosphoprotein enriched in diabetes (PED) or phosphoprotein enriched in astrocytes-15 kDa (PEA-15) (Condorelli et al., 1998). The c-FLIP exists at least in two isoforms, including a short form (c-$FLIP_S$) consisting of two DEDs and a long form (c-$FLIP_L$) that has two DEDs and a caspase-like domain that lacks catalytic activity (Irmler et al., 1997; Scaffidi et al., 1999). PED possess a DED but not a caspase-like domain (Condorelli et al., 1999; Condorelli et al., 1998). Through the DED, c-FLIP and PED/PEA-15 can be recruited by FADD to the DISC where they may interact with caspase-8 through DED–DED interaction and thus inhibit caspase-8 cleavage (Xiao et al., 2002; Yang et al., 2003). Recent studies further showed that c-FLIP and PED/PEA-15 may interact with RIP and TNFR-associated factor 2 (TRAF2) and link the DISC to NF-κB and extracellular signal-regulated kinase 1/2 (ERK1/2) pathway (Kataoka et al., 2000; Kataoka and Tschopp, 2004; Krueger et al., 2005). It remains to be illustrated how these proteins interact with each other in the DISC for the dual functions: inhibition of caspase-8 cleavage and linkage to NF-κB and ERK1/2 pathways.

41.4.3 NF-κB and ERK1/2 Pathways

Studies have demonstrated that TRAIL can activate NF-κB and ERK1/2 signaling pathways; however, the question then is whether NF-κB and ERK1/2 activities in cancer cells lead to the cell resistance to TRAIL. Some have reported that NF-κB activity inhibits TRAIL-induced apoptosis in lymphoid cells (Jeremias et al., 1998) and promotes the growth of ductal carcinoma cells (Trauzold et al., 2006), thus raising concern about the therapeutic use of TRAIL agonists (Malhi and Gores, 2006). These effects might be cell type dependent as no such effects were observed in other cancer cells such as non-small cell lung carcinoma (NSCLC) (Song et al., 2007). NF-κB activity has been shown to upregulate anti-apoptotic genes such as *c-FLIP*, *Mcl-1*, and *cIAP2* (Kreuz et al., 2001; Micheau et al., 2001; Ricci et al., 2007) as well as apoptotic genes such as *TRAIL* and *DR5* (Baetu et al., 2001; Shetty et al., 2005). TRAIL-induced NF-κB activity requires IκB phosphorylation and NF-κB nuclear translocation; however, targeting these steps affects neither c-FLIP expression nor TRAIL resistance (Song et al., 2007; Steele et al., 2006). In contrast, knockdown of RIP, c-FLIP, and PED releases the inhibition of caspase-8 cleavage and converts TRAIL-resistant cells to the sensitive phenotype (Sharp et al., 2005; Song et al., 2007). These studies suggest that the DISC is the molecular switch that controls caspase-8 cleavage and thereby the intracellular cell death and survival machinery. Current research effort focuses on the identification of the proteins and their interactions in the DISC that control the dimerization and cleavage of caspase-8 and thus define the cell death or survival in the response to TRAIL.

41.4.4 Bcl-2 and IAP Family Proteins

TRAIL-induced apoptosis requires the activation of the intrinsic mitochondrial pathway, which is modulated by the Bcl-2 family proteins. The Bcl-2 family can be further divided into Bcl-2, Bax, and BH3-only protein subfamily (Cory and Adams, 2002). Bid is a BH3-only protein and once cleaved by caspase-8, truncated Bid (tBid) interacts with Bax and Bak of the Bax subfamily. This induces the oligomerization of Bax and Bak at the mitochondrial membrane and a subsequent change of mitochondrial membrane potential (Gross et al., 1998; Wei et al., 2000). Bcl-2 and Bcl-X_L of the Bcl-2 subfamily interact with Bax and Bak to maintain the mitochondrial membrane potential. Overexpression of either Bcl-2 or Bcl-X_L blocks TRAIL-induced apoptosis (Hinz et al., 2000; Munshi et al., 2001), and inactivation of Bax leads to the cell resistance to TRAIL (LeBlanc et al., 2002). However, it is largely unknown how these Bcl-2 family proteins are expressed in cancers and consequently how they interact with each other in control of the mitochondrial pathway.

The family of inhibitors of apoptosis proteins (IAP) consists of XIAP, cellular IAP1 (cIAP1), cIAP2, survivin, and livin. IAPs interact with caspase-3 and caspase-7 to prevent their cleavage and enzymatic activation (Salvesen and Duckett, 2002). XIAP, cIAP1, and cIAP2 have been shown to be highly expressed in various human cancer cell lines and tissues in correlation with poor clinical prognosis (Bockbrader et al., 2005; Karikari et al., 2007; Mizutani et al., 2007; Wagenknecht et al., 1999). Inhibition of the expression of XIAP and survivin enhances TRAIL-induced apoptosis in cancer cells (Chawla-Sarkar et al., 2004; Cummins et al., 2004). These studies consistently prove that Bcl-2 and IAP family proteins inhibit TRAIL-induced apoptosis; however, it is unclear whether Bcl-2 and/or IAP constitute the check points that block TRAIL apoptotic pathway in any given human cancers.

41.4.5 Cancer Genomics

Genomic studies have identified genetic mutations, epigenetic silencing, and chromosomal alterations that result in the loss or silencing of apoptotic genes involved in TRAIL apoptotic pathways in human cancers. Somatic inactive mutations of the *Bax* gene were first identified (Rampino et al., 1997) and resulted in TRAIL resistance in colon cancer cells (LeBlanc et al., 2002). Somatic inactive mutations of *DR4* and *DR5* were then reported in NHL, lung, head, neck, gastric, and breast cancers (Fisher et al., 2001; Lee et al., 1999, 2001; Park et al., 2001; Shin et al., 2001). The mutations occur mainly in the DD of DR4/DR5 and thus block DR4/DR5-mediated intracellular signal transduction (Bin et al., 2007; McDonald et al., 2001). *DR4* and *DR5* genes map to human chromosome 8p12–23 and cytogenetic analysis revealed loss of chromosome 8p12–23 in TRAIL-resistant glioblastoma cell lines (Li et al., 2006).

Caspase-8 is silenced in neuroblastoma by DNA methylation, leading to TRAIL resistance (Eggert et al., 2001; Hopkins-Donaldson et al., 2000). Somatic inactive mutations of *caspase-8* were further reported in colorectal and gastric carcinomas (Kim et al., 2003; Soung et al., 2005) and loss of the caspase 8 locus on chromosome 2q33–34 was identified in TRAIL-resistant glioblastoma cell lines (Li et al., 2006). Loss of these genes related to TRAIL-induced apoptosis plays a role not only in tumorigenesis but also in the tumor resistance to TRAIL treatment. Therefore, genetic analysis of these genes should accompany clinical trials, as the genetic defects in TRAIL apoptotic pathways could be used as biomarkers to predict the responsiveness of cancers to TRAIL-based treatments.

41.4.6 TRAIL Resistance in Glioblastomas

Studies of glioblastoma cell lines and cultures, unfortunately, have also demonstrated TRAIL resistance in the majority of the cells (Hao et al., 2001; Knight et al., 2001; Song et al., 2003b). Except a few cells that have been shown to lose *DR4*/*DR5* and *caspase-8* chromosomal loci (Li et al., 2006), the vast majority of the resistant cells express DR4/5, DcR1/2, FADD, and caspase-8/-10. TRAIL resistance does not correlate as well with the expression of Bcl-2 family and IAP proteins, although overexpression of Bcl-2 was reported to inhibit TRAIL-induced apoptosis (Fulda et al., 2002a). Instead, studies have shown that c-FLIP (c-FLIP$_L$ and c-FLIP$_S$) and PED/PEA-15 are highly expressed (Hao et al., 2001; Song et al., 2003b) and recruited to the DISC. This recruitment is responsible for the inhibition of caspase-8 and -10 in TRAIL-resistant glioblastoma cell lines (Xiao et al., 2002). In addition, XIAP is highly expressed in glioblastomas (Wagenknecht et al., 1999) and interacts with caspase-3 to inhibit its cleavage (Deng et al., 2002). Targeting of XIAP by Smac peptide (Fulda et al., 2002b), Smac mimic (Li et al., 2004), and XIAP antisense RNA (Naumann et al., 2007) therefore enhances TRAIL-induced apoptosis in already sensitive glioblastoma cells, although their ability to convert resistant cells to the sensitive phenotype remains to be seen.

Mutations and/or deletions of *TP53*, $p14^{ARF}/p16^{INK4A}$ and *PTEN* genes are commonly seen in glioblastomas and their derived cell lines (Ishii et al., 1999), but the status of these genes does not correlate with TRAIL resistance (Hao et al., 2001; Song et al., 2003b). One study, however, reported that a p53 rescue compound can induce the expression of DR5 (a p53 target gene) (Wu et al., 1997) and enhance TRAIL killing of glioblastoma cells (Weinmann et al., 2008). Another study has shown that rhTRAIL and DR5 agnostic antibody TRA-8 can activate NF-κB signaling in glioblastoma cells (Choi et al., 2002). Other studies, however, show that inhibition of NF-κB activity does not sensitize glioblastoma cells to TRAIL (La Ferla-Bruhl et al., 2007). Several other mechanisms have also been reported to contribute to TRAIL resistance in glioblastomas. These include calcium/calmodulin-dependent protein kinase II (CaMK II), which mediates the phosphorylation of c-$FLIP_L$ (Yang et al., 2003); mTOR, which controls c-$FLIP_S$ expression (Panner et al., 2005); DNA methyltransferases, which upregulate PED/PEA-15 (Eramo et al., 2005); heat shock protein 90α, which is required for c-$FLIP_S$ recruitment to the DISC (Panner et al., 2007); microRNA-21, levels of which are elevated in glioblastomas and whose knockdown potentiates TRAIL killing of the tumor cells (Corsten et al., 2007); and lastly, the ubiquitin-proteasome pathway, which may control the expression of c-$FLIP_S$ and thus TRAIL resistance in glioblastomas (Koschny et al., 2007).

41.5 Development of TRAIL-Based Combination Therapies

The genetic defects in TRAIL apoptotic genes have been detected only in a small fraction of human cancers. The vast majority of cancers have been shown to have intact TRAIL apoptotic pathways, which, unfortunately, are inhibited at multiple levels, from upstream DISC modulations to the IAP inhibition of caspase-3 cleavage. Cancer therapeutic agents targeting these resistance mechanisms have been developed in preclinical studies for the combination therapies with TRAIL agonists. Moreover, studies have shown that cancer-addicted oncogenes drive cancer cell growth and inhibit cancer cell death simultaneously and, therefore, therapeutic agents targeting oncogene-driven signaling pathways are currently under preclinical studies for their synergistic antitumor activity with TRAIL agonists. Finally, chemotherapy remains the standard clinical treatment of human cancers and has synergistic antitumor activity with TRAIL agonists.

41.5.1 Targeting of TRAIL Resistance in the DISC and Mitochondrial Pathway

A number of therapeutic agents that target c-FLIP, Bcl-2, and XIAP have been developed for cancer treatment, either as single agents or in combination with

TRAIL agonists. 2-Cyano-3,12-dioxooleana-1,9-dien-28-oic acid (CDDO) a synthetic oleanane triterpenoid (Honda et al., 2000) and its derivatives, CDDO-methyl ester (CDDO-Me) and CDDO-imidazolide (CDDO-Im), can inhibit c-FLIP expression and thus promote TRAIL-induced apoptosis in cancer cells (Hyer et al., 2005; Zou et al., 2004). CDDO compounds are currently in phase I trials as single agents sponsored by Reata Pharmaceuticals in collaboration with the National Cancer Institute. Antisense oligodeoxynucleotides targeting Bcl-2 (Genasense®, Genta Inc., Berkeley Heights, NJ) (Klasa et al., 2002), survivin (ISIS-23722, ISIS Pharmaceuticals, Inc., Carlsbad, CA and Eli Lilly & Company, Indianapolis, IN) (Altieri, 2003; Chen et al., 2000), and XIAP (AEG-35156, Aegera Therapeutics Inc. Montreal, Canada) (Cummings et al., 2005) have also advanced to the level of phase I safety and pharmacokinetic analysis. In addition, a number of Smac mimetics with a high affinity for XIAP including synthetic Smac N-terminal peptide (Fulda et al., 2002b), small molecule Smac mimic (Li et al., 2004), and Smac peptidomimetic (LBW242, Novartis, Cambridge, MA) (Chauhan et al., 2007) have been generated and are currently in preclinical studies.

41.5.2 Targeting Oncogene-Driven Signaling Pathways

Cancers are genetic diseases in which mutations in oncogenes result in the activation of cell growth pathways and the inhibition of cell death pathways (Vogelstein and Kinzler, 2004). Therapeutic agents targeting oncogene-driven signaling pathways have been developed to be used in clinical treatments of cancers. These therapeutic agents are currently under preclinical evaluation for their synergistic antitumor activity in combination with TRAIL agonists. They include proteasome inhibitor bortezomib (Mitsiades et al., 2001), epidermal growth factor receptor inhibitors (Gibson et al., 2002), histone deacetylase inhibitor (Guo et al., 2004), DNA methylation inhibitor (Eramo et al., 2005), cyclooxygenase 2 inhibitors (Liu et al., 2004; Martin et al., 2005), Akt-mammalian target of rapamycin (mTOR) inhibitor (Panner et al., 2005), phosphatidylinositide-3-kinase (PI3K) inhibitor (Poh et al., 2007), Myc and multikinase inhibitor sorafenib (Ricci et al., 2007), and CD29 antibody Rituximab (Daniel et al., 2007). The molecular mechanisms by which these therapeutic agents can overcome the cancer resistance to TRAIL are currently under the investigation.

41.5.3 Combination of TRAIL and Chemotherapy

Chemotherapeutic agents can interact with DNA and form intra-strand cross-links that activate several intracellular signal pathways including apoptosis (Siddik, 2003). Unfortunately, human cancers eventually become resistant to chemotherapy. In addition, chemotherapy non-specifically targets both cancer and normal cells and thus causes a broad range of unwanted side effects at therapeutic doses. Recent studies have shown that chemotherapy agents at non-toxic doses appear to target key regulatory proteins in TRAIL signaling pathway and thus enhance TRAIL-induced apoptosis of human cancer cells (Asakuma et al., 2003; Ferreira et al., 2000; Gibson et al., 2000; Keane et al., 1999; Lacour et al., 2001; Nagane et al., 2000; Nimmanapalli et al., 2001; Ohtsuka et al., 2003; Singh et al., 2003; Song et al., 2003a). The molecular mechanisms by which TRAIL synergizes with chemotherapeutic agents remain controversial. Some studies suggest that cisplatin and etoposide upregulate DR4 and DR5 mRNA (Lacour et al., 2001), but others indicate that cisplatin treatment has no effect on the expression of DR4 and DR5 protein (Ferreira et al., 2000). In addition, studies also suggest that camptothecin upregulates Bax (Song et al., 2003a), that cisplatin activates JNK/p38 (Ohtsuka et al., 2003), and that cisplatin inhibits c-FLIP$_S$ expression (Song et al., 2003a). While the molecular mechanisms remain controversial, there is no doubt that chemotherapy can enhance TRAIL apoptotic effects on cancers. Chemotherapy is currently under clinical trials in combination with TRAIL agonists for cancer therapies.

41.5.4 TRAIL-Based Combination Therapies for Glioblastomas

In 2000, chemotherapeutic agents CDDP and etoposide were reported to upregulate DR5 and enhance TRAIL cytotoxicity in glioblastoma cells (Nagane et al., 2000). It was then reported that 1-(2-chloroethyl)-3-cyclohexyl-1-nitrosourea (CCNU), temozolomide, and topotecan have the synergistic cytotoxicity with TRAIL (Rohn et al., 2001). Further studies reported the synergistic effect of cisplatin and camptothecin on TRAIL-induced apoptosis but demonstrated that the synergistic effect is due to the downregulation of c-FLIP$_S$ in glioblastoma cells (Song et al., 2003b). Systemic injection of TRAIL and temozolomide increases the survival of the xenograft mice (Saito et al., 2004). Unfortunately, genomic loss of *DR4*/*DR5* and *caspase-8* gene has been identified in a few glioblastoma cell lines and results in the resistance of glioblastoma cells to the combination treatment (Li et al., 2006).

Recent studies have shown the synergistic cytotoxic effects of radiation with rhTRAIL and DR5 agonistic antibodies on glioblastomas. Combination treatment with rhTRAIL and ionizing radiation has been shown to kill human glioblastoma cells through activation of the extrinsic and intrinsic apoptotic pathways (Nagane et al., 2007). Radiation treatment can upregulate caspase-8 (Tsurushima et al., 2008) and DR5 (Fiveash et al., 2008) and combination treatment of radiation and TRA-8 antibody increases the survival of mice with intracranial glioblastoma xenografts (Fiveash et al., 2008). Clearly, the combination treatment of TRAIL agonists with radiation requires the presence of the TRAIL death machinery.

41.6 Clinical Development of TRAIL Agonists for Cancer Therapies

The unraveling of TRAIL apoptotic pathways in cancer cells has resulted in a rapid development of TRAIL-based cancer therapies. TRAIL apoptotic pathways have been targeted mainly by two approaches: rhTRAIL ligands and DR4 and DR5 agonistic antibodies. Monoclonal antibodies (mAb) have proven to be effective clinical cancer therapeutics because they selectively target specific cancer antigens and have a much longer half-life than recombinant proteins. Two categories of monoclonal antibodies targeting DR4 and DR5 are currently under clinical development as TRAIL agonistic therapeutics: humanized mouse mAb and fully human mAb. These DR4 and DR5 agonistic antibodies and rhTRAIL are currently in phase I–II studies to evaluate their safety, pharmacokinetics, and therapeutic efficacy (Table 41.1).

Table 41.1 TRAIL agonistic therapeutic agents

Target	Reagent	Principle	Sponsoring company	Clinical trial
DR4/5	Apo2L/TRAIL	rhTRAIL	Amgen/Genentech	Phase I/II
DR4	HGS-ETR1	Human mAb	Human genome sciences	Phase I/II
DR5	HGS-ETR2	Human mAb	Human genome sciences	Phase I/II
DR5	HGS-TR2J	Human mAb	Human genome sciences	Phase I
DR5	CS-1008	Humanized mAb	Daiichi Sankyo	Phase I
DR5	AMG 655	Human mAb	Amgen	Phase I/II
DR5	Apomab	Human mAb	Genentech	Phase I/II
DR5	LBY135	Humanized mAb	Novartis	Phase I

The preliminary data of phase I trials of rhTRAIL and DR4/DR5 agonistic antibodies have been reported recently and demonstrated the safety and tolerability of theses TRAIL agonists in patients (Gajewski, 2007). The best tumor response, however, observed in patients from these phase I trials of these TRAIL agonistics is a stable disease. This clinical observation seems to confirm the finding from preclinical studies that the vast majority of human cancers are TRAIL resistant (Thorburn et al., 2008). Many therapeutic agents have been developed targeting TRAIL resistance mechanisms and some of them have entered clinical trials either as single agents or in combination with TRAIL agonists.

41.6.1 Clinical Trials of rhTRAIL

TRAIL is a type II transmembrane protein with a short intracellular amino-terminal tail and a long extracellular carboxy-terminal tail (Pitti et al., 1996; Wiley et al., 1995). The extracellular carboxy-terminal region contains the receptor-binding domain (Cha et al., 1999) and can be cleaved by metalloproteinases to yield a biologically active soluble protein containing amino acids 114–281 of the full TRAIL protein (Mariani and Krammer, 1998). Therefore, rhTRAIL has been generated mainly from the extracellular domain of amino acids 114–281 (Ashkenazi et al., 1999; Hao et al., 2001; Walczak et al., 1999). While epitope-tagged forms of rhTRAIL were shown to be toxic to normal human cells (Nagata, 2000), non-tagged rhTRAIL of amino acids 114–281 proved to be non-toxic to normal human cells in vitro and in vivo (Hao et al., 2001, 2004; Lawrence et al., 2001). These preclinical studies have further shown that rhTRAIL has a half-life of approximately 30 min in non-human primates (Lawrence et al., 2001) and have also demonstrated its therapeutic potential in treating tumor xenografts in mice as a signal agent (Hao et al., 2004) or in combination with chemotherapy (Jin et al., 2004).

A soluble form of rhTRAIL (Apo2L/TRAIL) is currently under co-development by Genentech and Amgen for the clinical treatment of solid and hematological malignancies (Ashkenazi et al., 2008). Preliminary data of phase I safety and pharmacokinetic studies of Apo2L/TRAIL were reported at the 42nd ASCO Annual Meeting in 2006: 41 patients with advanced solid cancers and non-Hodgkin lymphoma (NHL) were enrolled and treated with up to 15 mg/kg Apo2L/TRAIL. The Apo2L/TRAIL treatment was well tolerated and no-dose-limiting toxicity was seen in patients. Of 36 patients whose tumors could be evaluated, 21 had stable disease and 1 showed a significant tumor shrinkage at 8 weeks of treatment. Pharmacokinetic results from a phase Ia trial were also reported at the meeting and indicated that as in non-human primates, Apo2L/TRAIL has a short half-life. A phase Ib/II trial of the Apo2L/TRAIL and Rituximab combination has recently been launched for the treatment of Rituximab refractory NHL.

41.6.2 Clinical Trials of DR4 and DR5 Agonistic Antibodies

In 2001, a mouse mAb against human DR5 (TRA-8) was generated by immunizing mice with a fusion protein of DR5 extracellular domain and IgG (Ichikawa et al., 2001). This mouse mAb was recently humanized through a complementarity-determining region grafting method by Daiichi Sankyo (Yada et al., 2008). The humanized DR5 mAb (CS-1008) is currently being evaluated in a phase I safety and pharmacokinetic study. In 2002 at the 93rd AACR Annual Meeting, Human Genome Sciences in collaboration with Cambridge Antibody Technology reported the generation of fully human monoclonal antibodies against human DR4 and DR5 through phage display. HGS-ETR1 (mapatumumab), DR4 agonistic mAb, and HGS-ETR2 (lexatumumab) and HGS-TR2J (KMTR2), both DR5 agonistic mAb, have entered clinical trials in patients with solid cancer and NHL (Humphreys and Halpern, 2008).

In 2007, the results of a phase I trial of HGS-ETR1 were reported in patients with advanced solid cancer (Tolcher et al., 2007): 49 patients were enrolled and all tolerated HGS-ETR1 treatment as a single agent up to 20 mg/kg; 19 patients had stable disease; and the half-life of HGS-ETR1 was approximately 18 days. A phase II trial of HGS-ETR1 as single therapeutic agent is currently ongoing in patients with NHL, NSCLC, and colorectal cancer. A phase Ib trial has also been launched for combination therapy of HGS-ETR1 with the chemotherapeutic agents gemcitabine, cisplatin, paclitaxel, or carboplatin. A phase I trial of HGS-ETR2 in patients with advanced solid cancer was also reported in 2007 (Plummer et al., 2007). In this study, 37 patients were enrolled; the 10 mg/kg dose was identified as the maximum tolerated dose and the mAb had a half-life of approximately 16 days. Dose-limiting toxicity of asymptomatic elevations of serum amylase, transaminases, and bilirubin was reached at 20 mg/kg and 12 of the patients had stable disease. HGS-ETR2 is currently in phase II therapeutic efficacy trials in combination with chemotherapy. HGS-TR2J is currently in phase I safety and pharmacokinetic studies.

Very recently, several other humanized and fully human DR5 antibodies have been reported. At the 43rd ASCO Annual Meeting in 2007, Genentech reported the data from a phase I trial of a fully human DR5 mAB, Apomab, which was generated through phage display (Adams et al., 2008). Apomab is currently in phase I/II trials as single agent in patients with advanced solid cancers and in combination with Rituximab in patients with advanced NHL. At the AACR Centennial Annual Meeting in 2008, Amgen reported its preclinical study of a fully human DR5 agonistic mAb, AMG 655. AMG 655 is currently in phase II trials in combination with gemcitabine in patients with pancreatic cancer and in combination with mFOLFOX6 and bevacizumab in treating patients with metastatic colorectal cancers. At the 44th ASCO Annual Meeting in 2008, Novartis presented the data from a phase I trial of a humanized mouse mAb, LYB135, alone and in combination with capecitabine in advanced solid cancers: LBY135 was well tolerated in 56 patients enrolled and showed signs of clinical activity.

41.7 Development of TRAIL-Based Treatments of Glioblastomas

Glioblastoma is one of the most challenging tumors to treat due to its unique location in the brain and its diffuse infiltrative nature. Human brain is protected by the blood brain barrier (BBB) that separates the brain from systemic blood circulation and thus prevents blood toxic substances from entering the brain (see also Chapter 33). The BBB forms a physiologic impediment to the systemic delivery of therapeutic agents in glioblastoma patients. It seems that the BBB is either not formed properly or leaky in the bulk of glioblastoma and may therefore allow therapeutic agents to enter the tumors. In nature, glioblastoma diffusely infiltrates through the normal brain tissue where the BBB is intact and thus prevents the entry of therapeutic agents. Several TRAIL modalities have been developed to distribute TRAIL agonists into the tumors through local and systemic delivery in murine intracerebral xenograft models (Table 41.2).

Table 41. 2 TRAIL therapeutic modalities in glioblastoma cell line xenografts

Reagent	Delivery	Xenograft	References
rhTRAIL	i.t.	U87MG	Roth et al. (1999)
rhTRAIL + CDDP	i.p.	U87MG	Nagane et al. (2000)
rhTRAIL	Convection	U87MG	Saito et al. (2004)
TRAIL-neural stem cell	i.t.	U343MG	Ehtesham et al. (2002)
TRAIL-adenovirus vector	i.t.	U87MG	Wohlfahrt et al. (2007)
TRAIL-vector-CBSA-NP	i.v.	C6	Lu et al. (2006)
TRA-8 + temozolomid	i.v.	D54MG	Fiveash et al. (2008)

41.7.1 TRAIL-Based Therapeutic Modalities

Intratumoral (i.t.) injection of rhTRAIL was shown to be able to eradicate mouse intracranial xenografts generated from the TRAIL-resistant U87MG glioblastoma cell line (Roth et al., 1999). A local convection-enhanced delivery can effectively distribute TRAIL throughout U87MG xenografts and normal brain tissue in rats (Saito et al., 2004). Neural stem cells are able to track glioblastoma cells and i.t. injection of TRAIL-secreting neural stem cells inhibits the growth of U343MG glioblastoma xenografts in mice (Ehtesham et al., 2002). Furthermore, an adenovirus vector that specifically replicates in tumor cells and expresses TRAIL has been generated and i.t. injection of this oncolytic vector significantly inhibits the growth of U87MG xenografts in mice (Wohlfahrt et al., 2007).

Systemic administration by intraperitoneal (i.p.) and intravenous (i.v) injection of rhTRAIL and chemotherapeutic agent CDDP significantly extends the survival of mice bearing U87MG xenografts (Nagane et al., 2000). Systemic i.v. injection of cationic albumin-conjugated pegylated nanoparticles (CBSA-NP) containing a TRAIL-expressing vector can lead to their accumulation in murine C6 xenografts through absorptive-mediated transcytosis and cause significant delays in the xenograft growth (Lu et al., 2006). Studies have further shown that systemic delivery of DR5 agonistic antibody TRA-8 and chemotherapeutic agent temozolomide increases the survival of mice with intracerebral D54MG xenografts (Fiveash et al., 2008). While these therapeutic modalities can distribute TRAIL and its agonistic antibodies to the tumor in murine models, it remains to be established whether these therapeutic modalities can effectively distribute TRAIL agonists into the tumor mass and the tumor infiltrating areas of the brain.

41.7.2 Evaluation of Patient Glioblastomas in TRAIL-Based Treatments

Studies of glioblastoma cell lines and xenografts have provided a solid basis in our understanding of TRAIL cancer biology and therapeutic potential. The question, however, remains how patients' glioblastomas will respond to TRAIL-based therapies. While clinical trials are the ultimate test, several groups have started to examine this issue using patient's glioblastoma-derived and xenografts-derived cultures. Study of three primary cultures showed that one was TRAIL-sensitive and the other two resistant and resistant cultures became sensitive to TRAIL in the presence of the chemotherapeutic agent, camptothecin (Song et al., 2003b). In another study, six glioblastoma-xenograft-derived short-term cultures were examined, revealing three to be TRAIL sensitive. The remaining three cultures were TRAIL resistant, but were sensitized by an mTOR inhibitor (Panner et al., 2005). In a study of 13 short-term primary cultures of grade II to grade IV astrocytic gliomas, the cultures were found resistant to TRAIL, but this resistance could be overcome by the proteasome inhibitor, bortezomib (Koschny et al., 2007). Additional studies of 17 minimally cultured and 5 uncultured gliomas further confirmed TRAIL resistance in these tumors and demonstrated that only a small fraction of the tumors become sensitive to TRAIL in the presence of various chemotherapeutic agents (Ashley et al., 2008). These preclinical studies indicate that the vast majority of patients' glioblastoma are TRAIL-resistant, but that TRAIL-based combination therapies may benefit some glioblastoma patients.

41.8 Conclusions and Future Directions

A vast amount of research in glioblastoma cell lines has demonstrated the ability of TRAIL to activate extrinsic and intrinsic apoptotic pathways in the cell lines and thus drive cancer cells into self-destruction. However, these studies have also shown that the majority of the cell lines are resistant to TRAIL-induced cytotoxicity. From a therapeutic point of view, the resistant cells can be classified into two groups: the cell lines that can be sensitized by combination treatment and the cell lines that are completely resistant to TRAIL-based therapies. In the first group, TRAIL apoptotic pathways are inhibited either by anti-apoptotic proteins such as c-FLIP, PED/PEA-15, XIAP, or oncogene-driven signal pathways. The cell lines in the second group have genomic loss of TRAIL pathway apoptotic proteins such as DR4, DR5, and caspase-8 and thus are resistant to any type of TRAIL-based therapies.

Recent studies of patients' glioblastoma-derived cultures have confirmed that the majority of the tumors are resistant to TRAIL-induced cytotoxicity. However, these studies have also indicated that a fraction of the tumors can be treated by TRAIL-based therapeutics alone or in combination with other therapeutic agents. The question then is how this fraction of patients can be identified and effectively treated through TRAIL-based therapies. To address this issue, studies of patients' glioblastomas-derived cultures and tissues should be performed to assess the loss of apoptotic genes required for TRAIL-induced apoptosis. Glioblastoma is a genetically heterogeneous disease among patients and within each patient. These studies should help determine whether genetically defective TRAIL-resistant clones exist in any given tumor. Future clinical trials of TRAIL-based therapies may consider genomic analyses of the tumor tissues to identify genomic alterations that may be used as biomarkers to predict the responsiveness of the tumors to TRAIL-targeted therapies.

Several therapeutic modalities targeting TRAIL apoptotic pathways have been developed for glioblastoma including rhTRAIL, DR4 and DR5 agonistic antibodies, TRAIL-secreting neural stem cells, TRAIL-expressing oncolytic vectors, and TRAIL vector-conjugated nanoparticles. Local or systemic administration of the therapeutics can either inhibit or eliminate the growth of glioblastoma xenografts in murine models. However, it remains to be demonstrated whether and how these therapeutic agents can be effectively distributed to glioblastomas. It is unclear whether and how the locally injected neural stem cells and viral vectors can track down and kill the glioblastoma cells in human brain. Local convection-enhanced delivery is a promising approach in the distribution of rhTRAIL through the BBB. Yet it needs to be demonstrated in human brain that this approach can deliver therapeutic agents into the tumors at a therapeutic dose. It is difficult if not impossible to systemically administer the larger therapeutic agents such as rhTRAIL and DR4/DR5 agonistic antibodies due to the presence of the BBB in brain. Can a small TRAIL mimetic be developed to cross the BBB? This is the type of challenging question that needs to be answered before effective TRAIL apoptotic pathways-targeted therapies can become reality.

Acknowledgments We thank Dr. Russell O. Pieper for critically reading this manuscript. The work in our laboratory has been supported in part by grants from the Alberta Heritage Foundation for Medical Research, Canadian Institutes of Health Research, National Cancer Institute of Canada, Georgia Cancer Coalition, and Southeastern Brain Tumor Foundation. C.H. is a Georgia Cancer Coalition Distinguished Cancer Scholar.

References

Adams, C., Totpal, K., Lawrence, D., Marsters, S., Pitti, R., Yee, S., Ross, S., Deforge, L., Koeppen, H., Sagolla, M., et al. (2008). Structural and functional analysis of the interaction between the agonistic monoclonal antibody Apomab and the proapoptotic receptor DR5. Cell Death Differ *15*, 751–761.

Altieri, D. C. (2003). Blocking survivin to kill cancer cells. Methods Mol Biol *223*, 533–542.

Asakuma, J., Sumitomo, M., Asano, T., and Hayakawa, M. (2003). Selective Akt inactivation and tumor necrosis actor-related apoptosis-inducing ligand sensitization of renal cancer cells by low concentrations of paclitaxel. Cancer Res *63*, 1365–1370.

Ashkenazi, A. (2002). Targeting death and decoy receptors of the tumour-necrosis factor superfamily. Nat Rev Cancer *2*, 420–430.

Ashkenazi, A., Holland, P., and Eckhardt, S. G. (2008). Ligand-based targeting of apoptosis in cancer: the potential of recombinant human apoptosis ligand 2/Tumor necrosis factor-related apoptosis-inducing ligand (rhApo2L/TRAIL). J Clin Oncol *26*, 3621–3630.

Ashkenazi, A., Pai, R. C., Fong, S., Leung, S., Lawrence, D. A., Marsters, S. A., Blackie, C., Chang, L., McMurtrey, A. E., Hebert, A., et al. (1999). Safety and antitumor activity of recombinant soluble Apo2 ligand. J Clin Invest *104*, 155–162.

Ashley, D. M., Riffkin, C. D., Lovric, M. M., Mikeska, T., Dobrovic, A., Maxwell, J. A., Friedman, H. S., Drummond, K. J., Kaye, A. H., Gan, H. K., et al. (2008). In vitro sensitivity testing of minimally passaged and uncultured gliomas with TRAIL and/or chemotherapy drugs. Br J Cancer *99*, 294–304.

Baetu, T. M., Kwon, H., Sharma, S., Grandvaux, N., and Hiscott, J. (2001). Disruption of NF-kappaB signaling reveals a novel role for NF-kappaB in the regulation of TNF-related apoptosis-inducing ligand expression. J Immunol *167*, 3164–3173.

Beutler, B., Greenwald, D., Hulmes, J. D., Chang, M., Pan, Y. C., Mathison, J., Ulevitch, R., and Cerami, A. (1985). Identity of tumour necrosis factor and the macrophage-secreted factor cachectin. Nature *316*, 552–554.

Bin, L., Thorburn, J., Thomas, L. R., Clark, P. E., Humphreys, R., and Thorburn, A. (2007). Tumor-derived mutations in the TRAIL receptor DR5 inhibit TRAIL signaling through the DR4 receptor by competing for ligand binding. J Biol Chem *282*, 28189–28194.

Boatright, K. M., Renatus, M., Scott, F. L., Sperandio, S., Shin, H., Pedersen, I. M., Ricci, J. E., Edris, W. A., Sutherlin, D. P., Green, D. R., and Salvesen, G. S. (2003). A unified model for apical caspase activation. Mol Cell *11*, 529–541.

Bockbrader, K. M., Tan, M., and Sun, Y. (2005). A small molecule Smac-mimic compound induces apoptosis and sensitizes TRAIL- and etoposide-induced apoptosis in breast cancer cells. Oncogene *24*, 7381–7388.

Bodmer, J. L., Holler, N., Reynard, S., Vinciguerra, P., Schneider, P., Juo, P., Blenis, J., and Tschopp, J. (2000). TRAIL receptor-2 signals apoptosis through FADD and caspase-8. Nat Cell Biol *2*, 241–243.

Boldin, M. P., Goncharov, T. M., Goltsev, Y. V., and Wallach, D. (1996). Involvement of MACH, a novel MORT1/FADD-interacting protease, in Fas/APO-1- and TNF receptor-induced cell death. Cell *85*, 803–815.

Carswell, E. A., Old, L. J., Kassel, R. L., Green, S., Fiore, N., and Williamson, B. (1975). An endotoxin-induced serum factor that causes necrosis of tumors. Proc Natl Acad Sci U S A *72*, 3666–3670.

Cha, S. S., Kim, M. S., Choi, Y. H., Sung, B. J., Shin, N. K., Shin, H. C., Sung, Y. C., and Oh, B. H. (1999). 2.8 A resolution crystal structure of human TRAIL, a cytokine with selective antitumor activity. Immunity *11*, 253–261.

Chang, D. W., Xing, Z., Capacio, V. L., Peter, M. E., and Yang, X. (2003). Interdimer processing mechanism of procaspase-8 activation. Embo J *22*, 4132–4142.

Chaudhary, P. M., Eby, M., Jasmin, A., Bookwalter, A., Murray, J., and Hood, L. (1997). Death receptor 5, a new member of the TNFR family, and DR4 induce FADD-dependent apoptosis and activate the NF-kappaB pathway. Immunity *7*, 821–830.

Chauhan, D., Neri, P., Velankar, M., Podar, K., Hideshima, T., Fulciniti, M., Tassone, P., Raje, N., Mitsiades, C., Mitsiades, N., et al. (2007). Targeting mitochondrial factor Smac/DIABLO as therapy for multiple myeloma (MM). Blood *109*, 1220–1227.

Chawla-Sarkar, M., Bae, S. I., Reu, F. J., Jacobs, B. S., Lindner, D. J., and Borden, E. C. (2004). Downregulation of Bcl-2, FLIP or IAPs (XIAP and survivin) by siRNAs sensitizes resistant melanoma cells to Apo2L/TRAIL-induced apoptosis. Cell Death Differ *11*, 915–923.

Chen, J., Wu, W., Tahir, S. K., Kroeger, P. E., Rosenberg, S. H., Cowsert, L. M., Bennett, F., Krajewski, S., Krajewska, M., Welsh, K., et al. (2000). Down-regulation of survivin by antisense oligonucleotides increases apoptosis, inhibits cytokinesis and anchorage-independent growth. Neoplasia *2*, 235–241.

Chinnaiyan, A. M., O'Rourke, K., Tewari, M., and Dixit, V. M. (1995). FADD, a novel death domain-containing protein, interacts with the death domain of Fas and initiates apoptosis. Cell *81*, 505–512.

Choi, C., Kutsch, O., Park, J., Zhou, T., Seol, D. W., and Benveniste, E. N. (2002). Tumor necrosis factor-related apoptosis-inducing ligand induces caspase-dependent interleukin-8 expression and apoptosis in human astroglioma cells. Mol Cell Biol *22*, 724–736.

Clancy, L., Mruk, K., Archer, K., Woelfel, M., Mongkolsapaya, J., Screaton, G., Lenardo, M. J., and Chan, F. K. (2005). Preligand assembly domain-mediated ligand-independent association between TRAIL receptor 4 (TR4) and TR2 regulates TRAIL-induced apoptosis. Proc Natl Acad Sci U S A *102*, 18099–18104.

Condorelli, G., Vigliotta, G., Cafieri, A., Trencia, A., Andalo, P., Oriente, F., Miele, C., Caruso, M., Formisano, P., and Beguinot, F. (1999). PED/PEA-15: an anti-apoptotic molecule that regulates FAS/TNFR1-induced apoptosis. Oncogene *18*, 4409–4415.

Condorelli, G., Vigliotta, G., Iavarone, C., Caruso, M., Tocchetti, C. G., Andreozzi, F., Cafieri, A., Tecce, M. F., Formisano, P., Beguinot, L., and Beguinot, F. (1998). PED/PEA-15 gene controls glucose transport and is overexpressed in type 2 diabetes mellitus. Embo J *17*, 3858–3866.

Corsten, M. F., Miranda, R., Kasmieh, R., Krichevsky, A. M., Weissleder, R., and Shah, K. (2007). MicroRNA-21 knockdown disrupts glioma growth in vivo and displays synergistic cytotoxicity with neural precursor cell delivered S-TRAIL in human gliomas. Cancer Res *67*, 8994–9000.

Cory, S., and Adams, J. M. (2002). The Bcl2 family: regulators of the cellular life-or-death switch. Nat Rev Cancer *2*, 647–656.

Creagan, E. T., Kovach, J. S., Moertel, C. G., Frytak, S., and Kvols, L. K. (1988). A phase I clinical trial of recombinant human tumor necrosis factor. Cancer *62*, 2467–2471.

Creaven, P. J., Brenner, D. E., Cowens, J. W., Huben, R. P., Wolf, R. M., Takita, H., Arbuck, S. G., Razack, M. S., and Proefrock, A. D. (1989). A phase I clinical trial of recombinant human tumor necrosis factor given daily for five days. Cancer Chemother Pharmacol *23*, 186–191.

Cretney, E., Takeda, K., Yagita, H., Glaccum, M., Peschon, J. J., and Smyth, M. J. (2002). Increased susceptibility to tumor initiation and metastasis in TNF-related apoptosis-inducing ligand-deficient mice. J Immunol *168*, 1356–1361.

Cummings, J., Ward, T. H., LaCasse, E., Lefebvre, C., St-Jean, M., Durkin, J., Ranson, M., and Dive, C. (2005). Validation of pharmacodynamic assays to evaluate the clinical efficacy of an antisense compound (AEG 35156) targeted to the X-linked inhibitor of apoptosis protein XIAP. Br J Cancer *92*, 532–538.

Cummins, J. M., Kohli, M., Rago, C., Kinzler, K. W., Vogelstein, B., and Bunz, F. (2004). X-linked inhibitor of apoptosis protein (XIAP) is a nonredundant modulator of tumor necrosis factor-related apoptosis-inducing ligand (TRAIL)-mediated apoptosis in human cancer cells. Cancer Res *64*, 3006–3008.

Daniel, D., Yang, B., Lawrence, D. A., Totpal, K., Balter, I., Lee, W. P., Gogineni, A., Cole, M. J., Yee, S. F., Ross, S., and Ashkenazi, A. (2007). Cooperation of the proapoptotic receptor agonist rhApo2L/TRAIL with the CD20 antibody rituximab against non-Hodgkin lymphoma xenografts. Blood *110*, 4037–4046.

Degli-Esposti, M. A., Dougall, W. C., Smolak, P. J., Waugh, J. Y., Smith, C. A., and Goodwin, R. G. (1997a). The novel receptor TRAIL-R4 induces NF-kappaB and protects against TRAIL-mediated apoptosis, yet retains an incomplete death domain. Immunity *7*, 813–820.

Degli-Esposti, M. A., Smolak, P. J., Walczak, H., Waugh, J., Huang, C. P., DuBose, R. F., Goodwin, R. G., and Smith, C. A. (1997b). Cloning and characterization of TRAIL-R3, a novel member of the emerging TRAIL receptor family. J Exp Med *186*, 1165–1170.

Deng, Y., Lin, Y., and Wu, X. (2002). TRAIL-induced apoptosis requires Bax-dependent mitochondrial release of Smac/DIABLO. Genes Dev *16*, 33–45.
Donepudi, M., Mac Sweeney, A., Briand, C., and Grutter, M. G. (2003). Insights into the regulatory mechanism for caspase-8 activation. Mol Cell *11*, 543–549.
Du, C., Fang, M., Li, Y., Li, L., and Wang, X. (2000). Smac, a mitochondrial protein that promotes cytochrome c-dependent caspase activation by eliminating IAP inhibition. Cell *102*, 33–42.
Eggert, A., Grotzer, M. A., Zuzak, T. J., Wiewrodt, B. R., Ho, R., Ikegaki, N., and Brodeur, G. M. (2001). Resistance to tumor necrosis factor-related apoptosis-inducing ligand (TRAIL)-induced apoptosis in neuroblastoma cells correlates with a loss of caspase-8 expression. Cancer Res *61*, 1314–1319.
Ehtesham, M., Kabos, P., Gutierrez, M. A., Chung, N. H., Griffith, T. S., Black, K. L., and Yu, J. S. (2002). Induction of glioblastoma apoptosis using neural stem cell-mediated delivery of tumor necrosis factor-related apoptosis-inducing ligand. Cancer Res *62*, 7170–7174.
ElOjeimy, S., McKillop, J. C., El-Zawahry, A. M., Holman, D. H., Liu, X., Schwartz, D. A., Day, T. A., Dong, J. Y., and Norris, J. S. (2006). FasL gene therapy: a new therapeutic modality for head and neck cancer. Cancer Gene Ther *13*, 739–745.
Eramo, A., Pallini, R., Lotti, F., Sette, G., Patti, M., Bartucci, M., Ricci-Vitiani, L., Signore, M., Stassi, G., Larocca, L. M., *et al.* (2005). Inhibition of DNA methylation sensitizes glioblastoma for tumor necrosis factor-related apoptosis-inducing ligand-mediated destruction. Cancer Res *65*, 11469–11477.
Ferreira, C. G., Span, S. W., Peters, G. J., Kruyt, F. A., and Giaccone, G. (2000). Chemotherapy triggers apoptosis in a caspase-8-dependent and mitochondria-controlled manner in the non-small cell lung cancer cell line NCI-H460. Cancer Res *60*, 7133–7141.
Fisher, M. J., Virmani, A. K., Wu, L., Aplenc, R., Harper, J. C., Powell, S. M., Rebbeck, T. R., Sidransky, D., Gazdar, A. F., and El-Deiry, W. S. (2001). Nucleotide substitution in the ectodomain of trail receptor DR4 is associated with lung cancer and head and neck cancer. Clin Cancer Res *7*, 1688–1697.
Fiveash, J. B., Gillespie, G. Y., Oliver, P. G., Zhou, T., Belenky, M. L., and Buchsbaum, D. J. (2008). Enhancement of glioma radiotherapy and chemotherapy response with targeted antibody therapy against death receptor 5. Int J Radiat Oncol Biol Phys *71*, 507–516.
Fulda, S., Meyer, E., and Debatin, K. M. (2002a). Inhibition of TRAIL-induced apoptosis by Bcl-2 overexpression. Oncogene *21*, 2283–2294.
Fulda, S., Wick, W., Weller, M., and Debatin, K. M. (2002b). Smac agonists sensitize for Apo2L/TRAIL- or anticancer drug-induced apoptosis and induce regression of malignant glioma in vivo. Nat Med *8*, 808–815.
Gajewski, T. F. (2007). On the TRAIL toward death receptor-based cancer therapeutics. J Clin Oncol *25*, 1305–1307.
Gibson, E. M., Henson, E. S., Haney, N., Villanueva, J., and Gibson, S. B. (2002). Epidermal growth factor protects epithelial-derived cells from tumor necrosis factor-related apoptosis-inducing ligand-induced apoptosis by inhibiting cytochrome c release. Cancer Res *62*, 488–496.
Gibson, S. B., Oyer, R., Spalding, A. C., Anderson, S. M., and Johnson, G. L. (2000). Increased expression of death receptors 4 and 5 synergizes the apoptosis response to combined treatment with etoposide and TRAIL. Mol Cell Biol *20*, 205–212.
Gross, A., Jockel, J., Wei, M. C., and Korsmeyer, S. J. (1998). Enforced dimerization of BAX results in its translocation, mitochondrial dysfunction and apoptosis. Embo J *17*, 3878–3885.
Grunhagen, D. J., de Wilt, J. H., ten Hagen, T. L., and Eggermont, A. M. (2006). Technology insight: Utility of TNF-alpha-based isolated limb perfusion to avoid amputation of irresectable tumors of the extremities. Nat Clin Pract Oncol *3*, 94–103.

Guo, F., Sigua, C., Tao, J., Bali, P., George, P., Li, Y., Wittmann, S., Moscinski, L., Atadja, P., and Bhalla, K. (2004). Cotreatment with histone deacetylase inhibitor LAQ824 enhances Apo-2L/tumor necrosis factor-related apoptosis inducing ligand-induced death inducing signaling complex activity and apoptosis of human acute leukemia cells. Cancer Res *64*, 2580–2589.

Hao, C., Beguinot, F., Condorelli, G., Trencia, A., Van Meir, E. G., Yong, V. W., Parney, I. F., Roa, W. H., and Petruk, K. C. (2001). Induction and intracellular regulation of tumor necrosis factor-related apoptosis-inducing ligand (TRAIL) mediated apoptosis in human malignant glioma cells. Cancer Res *61*, 1162–1170.

Hao, C., Song, J. H., Hsi, B., Lewis, J., Song, D. K., Petruk, K. C., Tyrrell, D. L., and Kneteman, N. M. (2004). TRAIL inhibits tumor growth but is nontoxic to human hepatocytes in chimeric mice. Cancer Res *64*, 8502–8506.

Harper, N., Farrow, S. N., Kaptein, A., Cohen, G. M., and MacFarlane, M. (2001). Modulation of tumor necrosis factor apoptosis-inducing ligand- induced NF-kappa B activation by inhibition of apical caspases. J Biol Chem *276*, 34743–34752.

Hinz, S., Trauzold, A., Boenicke, L., Sandberg, C., Beckmann, S., Bayer, E., Walczak, H., Kalthoff, H., and Ungefroren, H. (2000). Bcl-XL protects pancreatic adenocarcinoma cells against CD95- and TRAIL-receptor-mediated apoptosis. Oncogene *19*, 5477–5486.

Honda, T., Rounds, B. V., Bore, L., Finlay, H. J., Favaloro, F. G., Jr., Suh, N., Wang, Y., Sporn, M. B., and Gribble, G. W. (2000). Synthetic oleanane and ursane triterpenoids with modified rings A and C: a series of highly active inhibitors of nitric oxide production in mouse macrophages. J Med Chem *43*, 4233–4246.

Hopkins-Donaldson, S., Bodmer, J. L., Bourloud, K. B., Brognara, C. B., Tschopp, J., and Gross, N. (2000). Loss of caspase-8 expression in highly malignant human neuroblastoma cells correlates with resistance to tumor necrosis factor-related apoptosis-inducing ligand-induced apoptosis. Cancer Res *60*, 4315–4319.

Hsu, H., Huang, J., Shu, H. B., Baichwal, V., and Goeddel, D. V. (1996a). TNF-dependent recruitment of the protein kinase RIP to the TNF receptor-1 signaling complex. Immunity *4*, 387–396.

Hsu, H., Shu, H. B., Pan, M. G., and Goeddel, D. V. (1996b). TRADD-TRAF2 and TRADD-FADD interactions define two distinct TNF receptor 1 signal transduction pathways. Cell *84*, 299–308.

Humphreys, R. C., and Halpern, W. (2008). Trail receptors: targets for cancer therapy. Adv Exp Med Biol *615*, 127–158.

Hyer, M. L., Croxton, R., Krajewska, M., Krajewski, S., Kress, C. L., Lu, M., Suh, N., Sporn, M. B., Cryns, V. L., Zapata, J. M., and Reed, J. C. (2005). Synthetic triterpenoids cooperate with tumor necrosis factor-related apoptosis-inducing ligand to induce apoptosis of breast cancer cells. Cancer Res *65*, 4799–4808.

Ichikawa, K., Liu, W., Zhao, L., Wang, Z., Liu, D., Ohtsuka, T., Zhang, H., Mountz, J. D., Koopman, W. J., Kimberly, R. P., and Zhou, T. (2001). Tumoricidal activity of a novel anti-human DR5 monoclonal antibody without hepatocyte cytotoxicity. Nat Med *7*, 954–960.

Irmler, M., Thome, M., Hahne, M., Schneider, P., Hofmann, K., Steiner, V., Bodmer, J. L., Schroter, M., Burns, K., Mattmann, C., et al. (1997). Inhibition of death receptor signals by cellular FLIP. Nature *388*, 190–195.

Ishii, N., Maier, D., Merlo, A., Tada, M., Sawamura, Y., Diserens, A. C., and Van Meir, E. G. (1999). Frequent co-alterations of TP53, p16/CDKN2A, p14ARF, PTEN tumor suppressor genes in human glioma cell lines. Brain Pathol *9*, 469–479.

Itoh, N., Yonehara, S., Ishii, A., Yonehara, M., Mizushima, S., Sameshima, M., Hase, A., Seto, Y., and Nagata, S. (1991). The polypeptide encoded by the cDNA for human cell surface antigen Fas can mediate apoptosis. Cell *66*, 233–243.

Jeremias, I., Kupatt, C., Baumann, B., Herr, I., Wirth, T., and Debatin, K. M. (1998). Inhibition of nuclear factor kappaB activation attenuates apoptosis resistance in lymphoid cells. Blood *91*, 4624–4631.

Jin, H., Yang, R., Fong, S., Totpal, K., Lawrence, D., Zheng, Z., Ross, J., Koeppen, H., Schwall, R., and Ashkenazi, A. (2004). Apo2 ligand/tumor necrosis factor-related apoptosis-inducing ligand cooperates with chemotherapy to inhibit orthotopic lung tumor growth and improve survival. Cancer Res *64*, 4900–4905.

Jo, M., Kim, T. H., Seol, D. W., Esplen, J. E., Dorko, K., Billiar, T. R., and Strom, S. C. (2000). Apoptosis induced in normal human hepatocytes by tumor necrosis factor-related apoptosis-inducing ligand. Nat Med *6*, 564–567.

Karikari, C. A., Roy, I., Tryggestad, E., Feldmann, G., Pinilla, C., Welsh, K., Reed, J. C., Armour, E. P., Wong, J., Herman, J., et al. (2007). Targeting the apoptotic machinery in pancreatic cancers using small-molecule antagonists of the X-linked inhibitor of apoptosis protein. Mol Cancer Ther *6*, 957–966.

Kataoka, T., Budd, R. C., Holler, N., Thome, M., Martinon, F., Irmler, M., Burns, K., Hahne, M., Kennedy, N., Kovacsovics, M., and Tschopp, J. (2000). The caspase-8 inhibitor FLIP promotes activation of NF-kappaB and Erk signaling pathways. Curr Biol *10*, 640–648.

Kataoka, T., and Tschopp, J. (2004). N-terminal fragment of c-FLIP(L) processed by caspase 8 specifically interacts with TRAF2 and induces activation of the NF-kappaB signaling pathway. Mol Cell Biol *24*, 2627–2636.

Keane, M. M., Ettenberg, S. A., Nau, M. M., Russell, E. K., and Lipkowitz, S. (1999). Chemotherapy augments TRAIL-induced apoptosis in breast cell lines. Cancer Res *59*, 734–741.

Kim, H. S., Lee, J. W., Soung, Y. H., Park, W. S., Kim, S. Y., Lee, J. H., Park, J. Y., Cho, Y. G., Kim, C. J., Jeong, S. W., et al. (2003). Inactivating mutations of caspase-8 gene in colorectal carcinomas. Gastroenterology *125*, 708–715.

Kischkel, F. C., Hellbardt, S., Behrmann, I., Germer, M., Pawlita, M., Krammer, P. H., and Peter, M. E. (1995). Cytotoxicity-dependent APO-1 (Fas/CD95)-associated proteins form a death-inducing signaling complex (DISC) with the receptor. Embo J *14*, 5579–5588.

Kischkel, F. C., Lawrence, D. A., Chuntharapai, A., Schow, P., Kim, K. J., and Ashkenazi, A. (2000). Apo2L/TRAIL-dependent recruitment of endogenous FADD and caspase-8 to death receptors 4 and 5. Immunity *12*, 611–620.

Kischkel, F. C., Lawrence, D. A., Tinel, A., LeBlanc, H., Virmani, A., Schow, P., Gazdar, A., Blenis, J., Arnott, D., and Ashkenazi, A. (2001). Death receptor recruitment of endogenous caspase-10 and apoptosis initiation in the absence of caspase-8. J Biol Chem *276*, 46639–46646.

Klasa, R. J., Gillum, A. M., Klem, R. E., and Frankel, S. R. (2002). Oblimersen Bcl-2 antisense: facilitating apoptosis in anticancer treatment. Antisense Nucleic Acid Drug Dev *12*, 193–213.

Knight, M. J., Riffkin, C. D., Muscat, A. M., Ashley, D. M., and Hawkins, C. J. (2001). Analysis of FasL and TRAIL induced apoptosis pathways in glioma cells. Oncogene *20*, 5789–5798.

Koschny, R., Holland, H., Sykora, J., Haas, T. L., Sprick, M. R., Ganten, T. M., Krupp, W., Bauer, M., Ahnert, P., Meixensberger, J., and Walczak, H. (2007). Bortezomib sensitizes primary human astrocytoma cells of WHO grades I to IV for tumor necrosis factor-related apoptosis-inducing ligand-induced apoptosis. Clin Cancer Res *13*, 3403–3412.

Kreuz, S., Siegmund, D., Scheurich, P., and Wajant, H. (2001). NF-kappaB inducers upregulate cFLIP, a cycloheximide-sensitive inhibitor of death receptor signaling. Mol Cell Biol *21*, 3964–3973.

Krueger, J., Chou, F. L., Glading, A., Schaefer, E., and Ginsberg, M. H. (2005). Phosphorylation of phosphoprotein enriched in astrocytes (PEA-15) regulates extracellular signal-regulated kinase-dependent transcription and cell proliferation. Mol Biol Cell *16*, 3552–3561.

La Ferla-Bruhl, K., Westhoff, M. A., Karl, S., Kasperczyk, H., Zwacka, R. M., Debatin, K. M., and Fulda, S. (2007). NF-kappaB-independent sensitization of glioblastoma cells for TRAIL-induced apoptosis by proteasome inhibition. Oncogene *26*, 571–582.

Lacour, S., Hammann, A., Wotawa, A., Corcos, L., Solary, E., and Dimanche-Boitrel, M. T. (2001). Anticancer agents sensitize tumor cells to tumor necrosis factor-related apoptosis-inducing ligand-mediated caspase-8 activation and apoptosis. Cancer Res *61*, 1645–1651.

Lawrence, D., Shahrokh, Z., Marsters, S., Achilles, K., Shih, D., Mounho, B., Hillan, K., Totpal, K., DeForge, L., Schow, P., et al. (2001). Differential hepatocyte toxicity of recombinant Apo2L/TRAIL versions. Nat Med *7*, 383–385.

LeBlanc, H., Lawrence, D., Varfolomeev, E., Totpal, K., Morlan, J., Schow, P., Fong, S., Schwall, R., Sinicropi, D., and Ashkenazi, A. (2002). Tumor-cell resistance to death receptor–induced apoptosis through mutational inactivation of the proapoptotic Bcl-2 homolog Bax. Nat Med *8*, 274–281.

Lee, S. H., Shin, M. S., Kim, H. S., Lee, H. K., Park, W. S., Kim, S. Y., Lee, J. H., Han, S. Y., Park, J. Y., Oh, R. R., et al. (1999). Alterations of the DR5/TRAIL receptor 2 gene in non-small cell lung cancers. Cancer Res *59*, 5683–5686.

Lee, S. H., Shin, M. S., Kim, H. S., Lee, H. K., Park, W. S., Kim, S. Y., Lee, J. H., Han, S. Y., Park, J. Y., Oh, R. R., et al. (2001). Somatic mutations of TRAIL-receptor 1 and TRAIL-receptor 2 genes in non-Hodgkin's lymphoma. Oncogene *20*, 399–403.

Lenk, H., Tanneberger, S., Muller, U., Ebert, J., and Shiga, T. (1989). Phase II clinical trial of high-dose recombinant human tumor necrosis factor. Cancer Chemother Pharmacol *24*, 391–392.

Letai, A. G. (2008). Diagnosing and exploiting cancer's addiction to blocks in apoptosis. Nat Rev Cancer *8*, 121–132.

Lewis, M., Tartaglia, L. A., Lee, A., Bennett, G. L., Rice, G. C., Wong, G. H., Chen, E. Y., and Goeddel, D. V. (1991). Cloning and expression of cDNAs for two distinct murine tumor necrosis factor receptors demonstrate one receptor is species specific. Proc Natl Acad Sci U S A *88*, 2830–2834.

Li, H., Zhu, H., Xu, C. J., and Yuan, J. (1998). Cleavage of BID by caspase 8 mediates the mitochondrial damage in the Fas pathway of apoptosis. Cell *94*, 491–501.

Li, L., Thomas, R. M., Suzuki, H., De Brabander, J. K., Wang, X., and Harran, P. G. (2004). A small molecule Smac mimic potentiates TRAIL- and TNFalpha-mediated cell death. Science *305*, 1471–1474.

Li, P., Nijhawan, D., Budihardjo, I., Srinivasula, S. M., Ahmad, M., Alnemri, E. S., and Wang, X. (1997). Cytochrome c and dATP-dependent formation of Apaf-1/caspase-9 complex initiates an apoptotic protease cascade. Cell *91*, 479–489.

Li, Y. C., Tzeng, C. C., Song, J. H., Tsia, F. J., Hsieh, L. J., Liao, S. J., Tsai, C. H., Van Meir, E. G., Hao, C., and Lin, C. C. (2006). Genomic alterations in human malignant glioma cells associate with the cell resistance to the combination treatment with tumor necrosis factor-related apoptosis-inducing ligand and chemotherapy. Clin Cancer Res *12*, 2716–2729.

Lin, Y., Devin, A., Cook, A., Keane, M. M., Kelliher, M., Lipkowitz, S., and Liu, Z. G. (2000). The death domain kinase RIP is essential for TRAIL (Apo2L)-induced activation of IkappaB kinase and c-Jun N-terminal kinase. Mol Cell Biol *20*, 6638–6645.

Liu, X., Yue, P., Khuri, F. R., and Sun, S. Y. (2005). Decoy receptor 2 (DcR2) is a p53 target gene and regulates chemosensitivity. Cancer Res *65*, 9169–9175.

Liu, X., Yue, P., Zhou, Z., Khuri, F. R., and Sun, S. Y. (2004). Death receptor regulation and celecoxib-induced apoptosis in human lung cancer cells. J Natl Cancer Inst *96*, 1769–1780.

Liu, X., Zou, H., Slaughter, C., and Wang, X. (1997). DFF, a heterodimeric protein that functions downstream of caspase-3 to trigger DNA fragmentation during apoptosis. Cell *89*, 175–184.

Lu, W., Sun, Q., Wan, J., She, Z., and Jiang, X. G. (2006). Cationic albumin-conjugated pegylated nanoparticles allow gene delivery into brain tumors via intravenous administration. Cancer Res *66*, 11878–11887.
Luo, X., Budihardjo, I., Zou, H., Slaughter, C., and Wang, X. (1998). Bid, a Bcl2 interacting protein, mediates cytochrome c release from mitochondria in response to activation of cell surface death receptors. Cell *94*, 481–490.
Malhi, H., and Gores, G. J. (2006). TRAIL resistance results in cancer progression: a TRAIL to perdition? Oncogene *25*, 7333–7335.
Mariani, S. M., and Krammer, P. H. (1998). Differential regulation of TRAIL and CD95 ligand in transformed cells of the T and B lymphocyte lineage. Eur J Immunol *28*, 973–982.
Marsters, S. A., Sheridan, J. P., Pitti, R. M., Huang, A., Skubatch, M., Baldwin, D., Yuan, J., Gurney, A., Goddard, A. D., Godowski, P., and Ashkenazi, A. (1997). A novel receptor for Apo2L/TRAIL contains a truncated death domain. Curr Biol *7*, 1003–1006.
Martin, S., Phillips, D. C., Szekely-Szucs, K., Elghazi, L., Desmots, F., and Houghton, J. A. (2005). Cyclooxygenase-2 inhibition sensitizes human colon carcinoma cells to TRAIL-induced apoptosis through clustering of DR5 and concentrating death-inducing signaling complex components into ceramide-enriched caveolae. Cancer Res *65*, 11447–11458.
McDonald, E. R., 3rd, Chui, P. C., Martelli, P. F., Dicker, D. T., and El-Deiry, W. S. (2001). Death domain mutagenesis of KILLER/DR5 reveals residues critical for apoptotic signaling. J Biol Chem *276*, 14939–14945.
Medema, J. P., Scaffidi, C., Kischkel, F. C., Shevchenko, A., Mann, M., Krammer, P. H., and Peter, M. E. (1997). FLICE is activated by association with the CD95 death-inducing signaling complex (DISC). Embo J *16*, 2794–2804.
Merino, D., Lalaoui, N., Morizot, A., Schneider, P., Solary, E., and Micheau, O. (2006). Differential inhibition of TRAIL-mediated DR5-DISC formation by decoy receptors 1 and 2. Mol Cell Biol *26*, 7046–7055.
Micheau, O., Lens, S., Gaide, O., Alevizopoulos, K., and Tschopp, J. (2001). NF-kappaB signals induce the expression of c-FLIP. Mol Cell Biol *21*, 5299–5305.
Mitsiades, C. S., Treon, S. P., Mitsiades, N., Shima, Y., Richardson, P., Schlossman, R., Hideshima, T., and Anderson, K. C. (2001). TRAIL/Apo2L ligand selectively induces apoptosis and overcomes drug resistance in multiple myeloma: therapeutic applications. Blood *98*, 795–804.
Mizutani, Y., Nakanishi, H., Li, Y. N., Matsubara, H., Yamamoto, K., Sato, N., Shiraishi, T., Nakamura, T., Mikami, K., Okihara, K., et al. (2007). Overexpression of XIAP expression in renal cell carcinoma predicts a worse prognosis. Int J Oncol *30*, 919–925.
Mongkolsapaya, J., Cowper, A. E., Xu, X. N., Morris, G., McMichael, A. J., Bell, J. I., and Screaton, G. R. (1998). Lymphocyte inhibitor of TRAIL (TNF-related apoptosis-inducing ligand): a new receptor protecting lymphocytes from the death ligand TRAIL. J Immunol *160*, 3–6.
Munshi, A., Pappas, G., Honda, T., McDonnell, T. J., Younes, A., Li, Y., and Meyn, R. E. (2001). TRAIL (APO-2L) induces apoptosis in human prostate cancer cells that is inhibitable by Bcl-2. Oncogene *20*, 3757–3765.
Muzio, M., Chinnaiyan, A. M., Kischkel, F. C., O'Rourke, K., Shevchenko, A., Ni, J., Scaffidi, C., Bretz, J. D., Zhang, M., Gentz, R., et al. (1996). FLICE, a novel FADD-homologous ICE/CED-3-like protease, is recruited to the CD95 (Fas/APO-1) death–inducing signaling complex. Cell *85*, 817–827.
Muzio, M., Stockwell, B. R., Stennicke, H. R., Salvesen, G. S., and Dixit, V. M. (1998). An induced proximity model for caspase-8 activation. J Biol Chem *273*, 2926–2930.
Nagane, M., Cavenee, W. K., and Shiokawa, Y. (2007). Synergistic cytotoxicity through the activation of multiple apoptosis pathways in human glioma cells induced by combined treatment with ionizing radiation and tumor necrosis factor-related apoptosis-inducing ligand. J Neurosurg *106*, 407–416.

Nagane, M., Pan, G., Weddle, J. J., Dixit, V. M., Cavenee, W. K., and Huang, H. J. (2000). Increased death receptor 5 expression by chemotherapeutic agents in human gliomas causes synergistic cytotoxicity with tumor necrosis factor-related apoptosis-inducing ligand in vitro and in vivo. Cancer Res *60*, 847–853.

Nagata, S. (2000). Steering anti-cancer drugs away from the TRAIL. Nat Med *6*, 502–503.

Naumann, U., Bahr, O., Wolburg, H., Altenberend, S., Wick, W., Liston, P., Ashkenazi, A., and Weller, M. (2007). Adenoviral expression of XIAP antisense RNA induces apoptosis in glioma cells and suppresses the growth of xenografts in nude mice. Gene Ther *14*, 147–161.

Nimmanapalli, R., Perkins, C. L., Orlando, M., O'Bryan, E., Nguyen, D., and Bhalla, K. N. (2001). Pretreatment with paclitaxel enhances apo-2 ligand/tumor necrosis factor-related apoptosis-inducing ligand-induced apoptosis of prostate cancer cells by inducing death receptors 4 and 5 protein levels. Cancer Res *61*, 759–763.

Nitsch, R., Bechmann, I., Deisz, R. A., Haas, D., Lehmann, T. N., Wendling, U., and Zipp, F. (2000). Human brain-cell death induced by tumour-necrosis-factor-related apoptosis-inducing ligand (TRAIL). Lancet *356*, 827–828.

Ogasawara, J., Watanabe-Fukunaga, R., Adachi, M., Matsuzawa, A., Kasugai, T., Kitamura, Y., Itoh, N., Suda, T., and Nagata, S. (1993). Lethal effect of the anti-Fas antibody in mice. Nature *364*, 806–809.

Ohtsuka, T., Buchsbaum, D., Oliver, P., Makhija, S., Kimberly, R., and Zhou, T. (2003). Synergistic induction of tumor cell apoptosis by death receptor antibody and chemotherapy agent through JNK/p38 and mitochondrial death pathway. Oncogene *22*, 2034–2044.

Pan, G., Ni, J., Yu, G., Wei, Y. F., and Dixit, V. M. (1998). TRUNDD, a new member of the TRAIL receptor family that antagonizes TRAIL signalling. FEBS Lett *424*, 41–45.

Pan, G., O'Rourke, K., Chinnaiyan, A. M., Gentz, R., Ebner, R., Ni, J., and Dixit, V. M. (1997). The receptor for the cytotoxic ligand TRAIL. Science *276*, 111–113.

Panner, A., James, C. D., Berger, M. S., and Pieper, R. O. (2005). mTOR controls FLIPS translation and TRAIL sensitivity in glioblastoma multiforme cells. Mol Cell Biol *25*, 8809–8823.

Panner, A., Murray, J. C., Berger, M. S., and Pieper, R. O. (2007). Heat shock protein 90alpha recruits FLIPS to the death-inducing signaling complex and contributes to TRAIL resistance in human glioma. Cancer Res *67*, 9482–9489.

Park, W. S., Lee, J. H., Shin, M. S., Park, J. Y., Kim, H. S., Kim, Y. S., Park, C. H., Lee, S. K., Lee, S. H., Lee, S. N., et al. (2001). Inactivating mutations of KILLER/DR5 gene in gastric cancers. Gastroenterology *121*, 1219–1225.

Pennica, D., Nedwin, G. E., Hayflick, J. S., Seeburg, P. H., Derynck, R., Palladino, M. A., Kohr, W. J., Aggarwal, B. B., and Goeddel, D. V. (1984). Human tumour necrosis factor: precursor structure, expression and homology to lymphotoxin. Nature *312*, 724–729.

Pitti, R. M., Marsters, S. A., Ruppert, S., Donahue, C. J., Moore, A., and Ashkenazi, A. (1996). Induction of apoptosis by Apo-2 ligand, a new member of the tumor necrosis factor cytokine family. J Biol Chem *271*, 12687–12690.

Plummer, R., Attard, G., Pacey, S., Li, L., Razak, A., Perrett, R., Barrett, M., Judson, I., Kaye, S., Fox, N. L., et al. (2007). Phase 1 and pharmacokinetic study of lexatumumab in patients with advanced cancers. Clin Cancer Res *13*, 6187–6194.

Poh, T. W., Huang, S., Hirpara, J. L., and Pervaiz, S. (2007). LY303511 amplifies TRAIL-induced apoptosis in tumor cells by enhancing DR5 oligomerization, DISC assembly, and mitochondrial permeabilization. Cell Death Differ *14*, 1813–1825.

Pollack, I. F., Erff, M., and Ashkenazi, A. (2001). Direct stimulation of apoptotic signaling by soluble Apo2l/tumor necrosis factor-related apoptosis-inducing ligand leads to selective killing of glioma cells. Clin Cancer Res *7*, 1362–1369.

Rampino, N., Yamamoto, H., Ionov, Y., Li, Y., Sawai, H., Reed, J. C., and Perucho, M. (1997). Somatic frameshift mutations in the BAX gene in colon cancers of the microsatellite mutator phenotype. Science *275*, 967–969.

Reed, J. C. (2006). Drug insight: cancer therapy strategies based on restoration of endogenous cell death mechanisms. Nat Clin Pract Oncol *3*, 388–398.

Ricci, M. S., Kim, S. H., Ogi, K., Plastaras, J. P., Ling, J., Wang, W., Jin, Z., Liu, Y. Y., Dicker, D. T., Chiao, P. J., et al. (2007). Reduction of TRAIL-induced Mcl-1 and cIAP2 by c-Myc or sorafenib sensitizes resistant human cancer cells to TRAIL-induced death. Cancer Cell *12*, 66–80.

Rich, J. N., and Bigner, D. D. (2004). Development of novel targeted therapies in the treatment of malignant glioma. Nat Rev Drug Discov *3*, 430–446.

Rohn, T. A., Wagenknecht, B., Roth, W., Naumann, U., Gulbins, E., Krammer, P. H., Walczak, H., and Weller, M. (2001). CCNU-dependent potentiation of TRAIL/Apo2L-induced apoptosis in human glioma cells is p53-independent but may involve enhanced cytochrome c release. Oncogene *20*, 4128–4137.

Roth, W., Isenmann, S., Naumann, U., Kugler, S., Bahr, M., Dichgans, J., Ashkenazi, A., and Weller, M. (1999). Locoregional Apo2L/TRAIL eradicates intracranial human malignant glioma xenografts in athymic mice in the absence of neurotoxicity. Biochem Biophys Res Commun *265*, 479–483.

Saito, R., Bringas, J. R., Panner, A., Tamas, M., Pieper, R. O., Berger, M. S., and Bankiewicz, K. S. (2004). Convection-enhanced delivery of tumor necrosis factor-related apoptosis-inducing ligand with systemic administration of temozolomide prolongs survival in an intracranial glioblastoma xenograft model. Cancer Res *64*, 6858–6862.

Salvesen, G. S., and Dixit, V. M. (1999). Caspase activation: the induced-proximity model. Proc Natl Acad Sci U S A *96*, 10964–10967.

Salvesen, G. S., and Duckett, C. S. (2002). IAP proteins: blocking the road to death's door. Nat Rev Mol Cell Biol *3*, 401–410.

Scaffidi, C., Medema, J. P., Krammer, P. H., and Peter, M. E. (1997). FLICE is predominantly expressed as two functionally active isoforms, caspase-8/a and caspase-8/b. J Biol Chem *272*, 26953–26958.

Scaffidi, C., Schmitz, I., Krammer, P. H., and Peter, M. E. (1999). The role of c-FLIP in modulation of CD95-induced apoptosis. J Biol Chem *274*, 1541–1548.

Schiller, J. H., Storer, B. E., Witt, P. L., Alberti, D., Tombes, M. B., Arzoomanian, R., Proctor, R. A., McCarthy, D., Brown, R. R., Voss, S. D., and et al. (1991). Biological and clinical effects of intravenous tumor necrosis factor-alpha administered three times weekly. Cancer Res *51*, 1651–1658.

Schmaltz, C., Alpdogan, O., Kappel, B. J., Muriglan, S. J., Rotolo, J. A., Ongchin, J., Willis, L. M., Greenberg, A. S., Eng, J. M., Crawford, J. M., et al. (2002). T cells require TRAIL for optimal graft-versus-tumor activity. Nat Med *8*, 1433–1437.

Schneider, P., Bodmer, J. L., Thome, M., Hofmann, K., Holler, N., and Tschopp, J. (1997a). Characterization of two receptors for TRAIL. FEBS Lett *416*, 329–334.

Schneider, P., Thome, M., Burns, K., Bodmer, J. L., Hofmann, K., Kataoka, T., Holler, N., and Tschopp, J. (1997b). TRAIL receptors 1 (DR4) and 2 (DR5) signal FADD-dependent apoptosis and activate NF-kappaB. Immunity *7*, 831–836.

Sharp, D. A., Lawrence, D. A., and Ashkenazi, A. (2005). Selective Knockdown of the Long Variant of Cellular FLICE Inhibitory Protein Augments Death Receptor-mediated Caspase-8 Activation and Apoptosis. J Biol Chem *280*, 19401–19409.

Sheikh, M. S., Huang, Y., Fernandez-Salas, E. A., El-Deiry, W. S., Friess, H., Amundson, S., Yin, J., Meltzer, S. J., Holbrook, N. J., and Fornace, A. J., Jr. (1999). The antiapoptotic decoy receptor TRID/TRAIL-R3 is a p53-regulated DNA damage-inducible gene that is overexpressed in primary tumors of the gastrointestinal tract. Oncogene *18*, 4153–4159.

Sheridan, J. P., Marsters, S. A., Pitti, R. M., Gurney, A., Skubatch, M., Baldwin, D., Ramakrishnan, L., Gray, C. L., Baker, K., Wood, W. I., et al. (1997). Control of TRAIL-induced apoptosis by a family of signaling and decoy receptors. Science *277*, 818–821.

Shetty, S., Graham, B. A., Brown, J. G., Hu, X., Vegh-Yarema, N., Harding, G., Paul, J. T., and Gibson, S. B. (2005). Transcription factor NF-kappaB differentially regulates death receptor 5 expression involving histone deacetylase 1. Mol Cell Biol *25*, 5404–5416.

Shin, M. S., Kim, H. S., Lee, S. H., Park, W. S., Kim, S. Y., Park, J. Y., Lee, J. H., Lee, S. K., Lee, S. N., Jung, S. S., et al. (2001). Mutations of tumor necrosis factor-related apoptosis-inducing ligand receptor 1 (TRAIL-R1) and receptor 2 (TRAIL-R2) genes in metastatic breast cancers. Cancer Res *61*, 4942–4946.

Siddik, Z. H. (2003). Cisplatin: mode of cytotoxic action and molecular basis of resistance. Oncogene *22*, 7265–7279.

Singh, T. R., Shankar, S., Chen, X., Asim, M., and Srivastava, R. K. (2003). Synergistic interactions of chemotherapeutic drugs and tumor necrosis factor-related apoptosis-inducing ligand/Apo-2 ligand on apoptosis and on regression of breast carcinoma in vivo. Cancer Res *63*, 5390–5400.

Skillings, J., Wierzbicki, R., Eisenhauer, E., Venner, P., Letendre, F., Stewart, D., and Weinerman, B. (1992). A phase II study of recombinant tumor necrosis factor in renal cell carcinoma: a study of the National Cancer Institute of Canada Clinical Trials Group. J Immunother (1991) *11*, 67–70.

Smyth, M. J., Takeda, K., Hayakawa, Y., Peschon, J. J., van den Brink, M. R., and Yagita, H. (2003). Nature's TRAIL–on a path to cancer immunotherapy. Immunity *18*, 1–6.

Song, J. H., Song, D. K., Herlyn, M., Petruk, K. C., and Hao, C. (2003a). Cisplatin down-regulation of cellular Fas-associated death domain-like interleukin-1beta-converting enzyme-like inhibitory proteins to restore tumor necrosis factor-related apoptosis-inducing ligand-induced apoptosis in human melanoma cells. Clin Cancer Res *9*, 4255–4266.

Song, J. H., Song, D. K., Pyrzynska, B., Petruk, K. C., Van Meir, E. G., and Hao, C. (2003b). TRAIL triggers apoptosis in malignant glioma cells through extrinsic and intrinsic pathways. Brain Pathol *13*, 539–553.

Song, J. H., Tse, M. C. L., Bellail, A., Khuri, F. R., Phuphanich, S., Kneteman, N. M., and Hao, C. (2007). Lipid rafts and non-rafts mediate TRAIL-induced apoptotic and non-apoptotic signals in non-small cell lung carcinoma cells. Cancer Res *67*, 1–10.

Soung, Y. H., Lee, J. W., Kim, S. Y., Jang, J., Park, Y. G., Park, W. S., Nam, S. W., Lee, J. Y., Yoo, N. J., and Lee, S. H. (2005). CASPASE-8 gene is inactivated by somatic mutations in gastric carcinomas. Cancer Res *65*, 815–821.

Sprick, M. R., Rieser, E., Stahl, H., Grosse-Wilde, A., Weigand, M. A., and Walczak, H. (2002). Caspase-10 is recruited to and activated at the native TRAIL and CD95 death-inducing signalling complexes in a FADD-dependent manner but can not functionally substitute caspase-8. Embo J *21*, 4520–4530.

Stanger, B. Z., Leder, P., Lee, T. H., Kim, E., and Seed, B. (1995). RIP: a novel protein containing a death domain that interacts with Fas/APO-1 (CD95) in yeast and causes cell death. Cell *81*, 513–523.

Steele, L. P., Georgopoulos, N. T., Southgate, J., Selby, P. J., and Trejdosiewicz, L. K. (2006). Differential susceptibility to TRAIL of normal versus malignant human urothelial cells. Cell Death Differ *13*, 1564–1576.

Suda, T., Takahashi, T., Golstein, P., and Nagata, S. (1993). Molecular cloning and expression of the Fas ligand, a novel member of the tumor necrosis factor family. Cell *75*, 1169–1178.

Taieb, J., Chaput, N., Menard, C., Apetoh, L., Ullrich, E., Bonmort, M., Pequignot, M., Casares, N., Terme, M., Flament, C., et al. (2006). A novel dendritic cell subset involved in tumor immunosurveillance. Nat Med *12*, 214–219.

Takeda, K., Hayakawa, Y., Smyth, M. J., Kayagaki, N., Yamaguchi, N., Kakuta, S., Iwakura, Y., Yagita, H., and Okumura, K. (2001). Involvement of tumor necrosis factor-related apoptosis-inducing ligand in surveillance of tumor metastasis by liver natural killer cells. Nat Med *7*, 94–100.

Takeda, K., Smyth, M. J., Cretney, E., Hayakawa, Y., Kayagaki, N., Yagita, H., and Okumura, K. (2002). Critical role for tumor necrosis factor-related apoptosis-inducing ligand in immune surveillance against tumor development. J Exp Med *195*, 161–169.

Thorburn, A., Behbakht, K., and Ford, H. (2008). TRAIL receptor-targeted therapeutics: resistance mechanisms and strategies to avoid them. Drug Resist Updat *11*, 17–24.

Tolcher, A. W., Mita, M., Meropol, N. J., von Mehren, M., Patnaik, A., Padavic, K., Hill, M., Mays, T., McCoy, T., Fox, N. L., et al. (2007). Phase I pharmacokinetic and biologic correlative study of mapatumumab, a fully human monoclonal antibody with agonist activity to tumor necrosis factor-related apoptosis-inducing ligand receptor-1. J Clin Oncol *25*, 1390–1395.

Tracey, K. J., Beutler, B., Lowry, S. F., Merryweather, J., Wolpe, S., Milsark, I. W., Hariri, R. J., Fahey, T. J., 3rd, Zentella, A., Albert, J. D., and et al. (1986). Shock and tissue injury induced by recombinant human cachectin. Science *234*, 470–474.

Trauth, B. C., Klas, C., Peters, A. M., Matzku, S., Moller, P., Falk, W., Debatin, K. M., and Krammer, P. H. (1989). Monoclonal antibody-mediated tumor regression by induction of apoptosis. Science *245*, 301–305.

Trauzold, A., Siegmund, D., Schniewind, B., Sipos, B., Egberts, J., Zorenkov, D., Emme, D., Roder, C., Kalthoff, H., and Wajant, H. (2006). TRAIL promotes metastasis of human pancreatic ductal adenocarcinoma. Oncogene.

Tsurushima, H., Yuan, X., Dillehay, L. E., and Leong, K. W. (2008). Radiation-inducible caspase-8 gene therapy for malignant brain tumors. Int J Radiat Oncol Biol Phys *71*, 517–525.

Varfolomeev, E., Maecker, H., Sharp, D., Lawrence, D., Renz, M., Vucic, D., and Ashkenazi, A. (2005). Molecular determinants of kinase pathway activation by Apo2 ligand/tumor necrosis factor-related apoptosis-inducing ligand. J Biol Chem *280*, 40599–40608.

Verhagen, A. M., Ekert, P. G., Pakusch, M., Silke, J., Connolly, L. M., Reid, G. E., Moritz, R. L., Simpson, R. J., and Vaux, D. L. (2000). Identification of DIABLO, a mammalian protein that promotes apoptosis by binding to and antagonizing IAP proteins. Cell *102*, 43–53.

Vogelstein, B., and Kinzler, K. W. (2004). Cancer genes and the pathways they control. Nat Med *10*, 789–799.

Wagenknecht, B., Glaser, T., Naumann, U., Kugler, S., Isenmann, S., Bahr, M., Korneluk, R., Liston, P., and Weller, M. (1999). Expression and biological activity of X-linked inhibitor of apoptosis (XIAP) in human malignant glioma. Cell Death Differ *6*, 370–376.

Walczak, H., Degli-Esposti, M. A., Johnson, R. S., Smolak, P. J., Waugh, J. Y., Boiani, N., Timour, M. S., Gerhart, M. J., Schooley, K. A., Smith, C. A., et al. (1997). TRAIL-R2: a novel apoptosis-mediating receptor for TRAIL. Embo J *16*, 5386–5397.

Walczak, H., Miller, R. E., Ariail, K., Gliniak, B., Griffith, T. S., Kubin, M., Chin, W., Jones, J., Woodward, A., Le, T., et al. (1999). Tumoricidal activity of tumor necrosis factor-related apoptosis-inducing ligand in vivo. Nat Med *5*, 157–163.

Walker, N. P., Talanian, R. V., Brady, K. D., Dang, L. C., Bump, N. J., Ferenz, C. R., Franklin, S., Ghayur, T., Hackett, M. C., Hammill, L. D., and et al. (1994). Crystal structure of the cysteine protease interleukin-1 beta-converting enzyme: a (p20/p10)2 homodimer. Cell *78*, 343–352.

Wang, J., Chun, H. J., Wong, W., Spencer, D. M., and Lenardo, M. J. (2001). Caspase-10 is an initiator caspase in death receptor signaling. Proc Natl Acad Sci U S A *98*, 13884–13888.

Wei, M. C., Lindsten, T., Mootha, V. K., Weiler, S., Gross, A., Ashiya, M., Thompson, C. B., and Korsmeyer, S. J. (2000). tBID, a membrane-targeted death ligand, oligomerizes BAK to release cytochrome c. Genes Dev *14*, 2060–2071.

Weinmann, L., Wischhusen, J., Demma, M. J., Naumann, U., Roth, P., Dasmahapatra, B., and Weller, M. (2008). A novel p53 rescue compound induces p53-dependent growth arrest and sensitises glioma cells to Apo2L/TRAIL-induced apoptosis. Cell Death Differ *15*, 718–729.

Wiley, S. R., Schooley, K., Smolak, P. J., Din, W. S., Huang, C. P., Nicholl, J. K., Sutherland, G. R., Smith, T. D., Rauch, C., Smith, C. A., and et al. (1995). Identification and characterization of a new member of the TNF family that induces apoptosis. Immunity *3*, 673–682.

Wilson, K. P., Black, J. A., Thomson, J. A., Kim, E. E., Griffith, J. P., Navia, M. A., Murcko, M. A., Chambers, S. P., Aldape, R. A., Raybuck, S. A., and et al. (1994). Structure and mechanism of interleukin-1 beta converting enzyme. Nature *370*, 270–275.

Wohlfahrt, M. E., Beard, B. C., Lieber, A., and Kiem, H. P. (2007). A capsid-modified, conditionally replicating oncolytic adenovirus vector expressing TRAIL Leads to enhanced cancer cell killing in human glioblastoma models. Cancer Res *67*, 8783–8790.

Wu, G. S., Burns, T. F., McDonald, E. R., 3rd, Jiang, W., Meng, R., Krantz, I. D., Kao, G., Gan, D. D., Zhou, J. Y., Muschel, R., et al. (1997). KILLER/DR5 is a DNA damage-inducible p53-regulated death receptor gene. Nat Genet *17*, 141–143.

Xiao, C., Yang, B. F., Asadi, N., Beguinot, F., and Hao, C. (2002). Tumor necrosis factor-related apoptosis-inducing ligand-induced death-inducing signaling complex and its modulation by c-FLIP and PED/PEA-15 in glioma cells. J Biol Chem *277*, 25020–25025.

Yada, A., Yazawa, M., Ishida, S., Yoshida, H., Ichikawa, K., Kurakata, S., and Fujiwara, K. (2008). A novel humanized anti-human death receptor 5 antibody CS-1008 induces apoptosis in tumor cells without toxicity in hepatocytes. Ann Oncol *19*, 1060–1067.

Yang, B. F., Xiao, C., Roa, W. H., Krammer, P. H., and Hao, C. (2003). Calcium/Calmodulin-dependent Protein Kinase II Regulation of c-FLIP Expression and Phosphorylation in Modulation of Fas-mediated Signaling in Malignant Glioma Cells. J Biol Chem *278*, 7043–7050.

Yang, X., Chang, H. Y., and Baltimore, D. (1998). Autoproteolytic activation of pro-caspases by oligomerization. Mol Cell *1*, 319–325.

Zou, W., Liu, X., Yue, P., Zhou, Z., Sporn, M. B., Lotan, R., Khuri, F. R., and Sun, S. Y. (2004). c-Jun NH2-terminal kinase-mediated up-regulation of death receptor 5 contributes to induction of apoptosis by the novel synthetic triterpenoid methyl-2-cyano-3,12-dioxooleana-1,9-dien-28-oate in human lung cancer cells. Cancer Res *64*, 7570–7578.

Chapter 42
The NF-κB Signaling Pathway in GBMs: Implications for Apoptotic and Inflammatory Responses and Exploitation for Therapy

Travis Laver, Susan Nozell, and Etty N. Benveniste

Abstract Malignant gliomas are diffusively infiltrative and remain among the deadliest of all cancers. The NF-κB transcription factor family is an important mediator of immune and inflammatory responses. Through its ability to induce gene expression, NF-κB can regulate the processes of cell growth, migration and invasion, angiogenesis, and resistance to apoptosis. In gliomas, NF-κB is constitutively activated, the levels of NF-κB- regulated genes are elevated, and these circumstances are inversely correlated with patient prognosis. Herein, we discuss the contributions made by NF-κB and its target genes in mediating facets of glioma behavior, mechanisms that might explain how NF-κB becomes activated in these tumors, and current strategies to antagonize this pathway in gliomas.

Keywords NF-κB · Gliomas · Signaling · Apoptosis

Contents

Travis Laver and Susan Nozell contributed equally to this book chapter.

S. Nozell (✉)
Department of Cell Biology, University of Alabama at Birmingham, Birmingham, 1530 3rd Ave S, MCLM 310, AL 35294-0004, USA
e-mail: snozell@uab.edu

E.G. Van Meir (ed.), *CNS Cancer*, Cancer Drug Discovery and Development, DOI 10.1007/978-1-60327-553-8_42,
© Humana Press, a part of Springer Science+Business Media, LLC 2009

42.1 NF-κB Family and Signaling Pathway

NF-κB is a five-member family of transcription factors consisting of RelA (p65), c-Rel, RelB NFκB1 (p105/p50), and NFκB2 (p100/p52) (Ghosh and Karin, 2002; Hayden and Ghosh, 2008). These proteins are capable of transducing signals from over 500 stimuli, in order to induce changes in gene expression, and NF-κB can be activated by diverse cellular processes including inflammation, development, growth, and apoptosis (Gilmore, 2008). The unifying feature of this family is the presence of the N-terminal Rel homology domain (RHD), which enables these proteins to bind DNA and form numerous hetero- and homodimers with other family members (Fig. 42.1). Of the five NF-κB family members, only

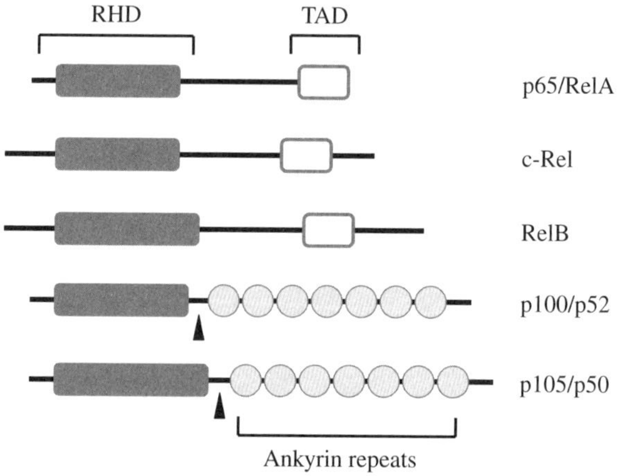

Fig. 42.1 The NF-κB family of transcription factors. The NF-κB family contains five members, p65/RelA, c-Rel, RelB, p105/p50 (NFKB1), and p100/p52 (NFKB2). Each member contains an N-terminal Rel homology domain (RHD), which enables homo- and heterodimeric interactions with other family members. p65/RelA, c-Rel, and RelB each contain a C-terminal transactivation domain (TAD). The remaining family members are each initially synthesized in their long forms (p100 and p105) and inactivated through their own C-terminal ankyrin repeat motifs, which bind to the RHD. Proteolytic removal of these portions reveals the mature short family members (p50 and p52)

p65/RelA, c-Rel, and RelB have a transactivation domain (TAD) within their C-terminus. Therefore, while all NF-κB molecules are competent to bind DNA, only those containing p65, c-Rel, or RelB are able to positively affect gene expression. The remaining two family members (NFκB1 and NFκB2) are each synthesized as long forms (p105 and p100) that are inactivated through interactions with their own C-terminal ankyrin repeat motifs, which bind to the RHD. Proteolytic removal of the ankyrin repeats reveals the mature short family members p50 and p52, respectively. While p105 is constitutively processed to produce p50, proteolytic activation of p100/p52 requires activation of the alternative pathway. Although functionally silent in most cells, once activated, NF-κB isoforms can induce the expression of as many as 100 genes (Gilmore, 2008). It is the collective body of NF-κB-regulated genes that ultimately mediates the cellular outcomes and consequences of NF-κB activation.

NF-κB is a key regulator of numerous cellular processes and therefore its activity is tightly controlled. NF-κB activation may be induced via three distinct pathways: the canonical or classical, non-canonical or alternative, and atypical pathways (Fig. 42.2). The canonical or classical pathway describes activation of

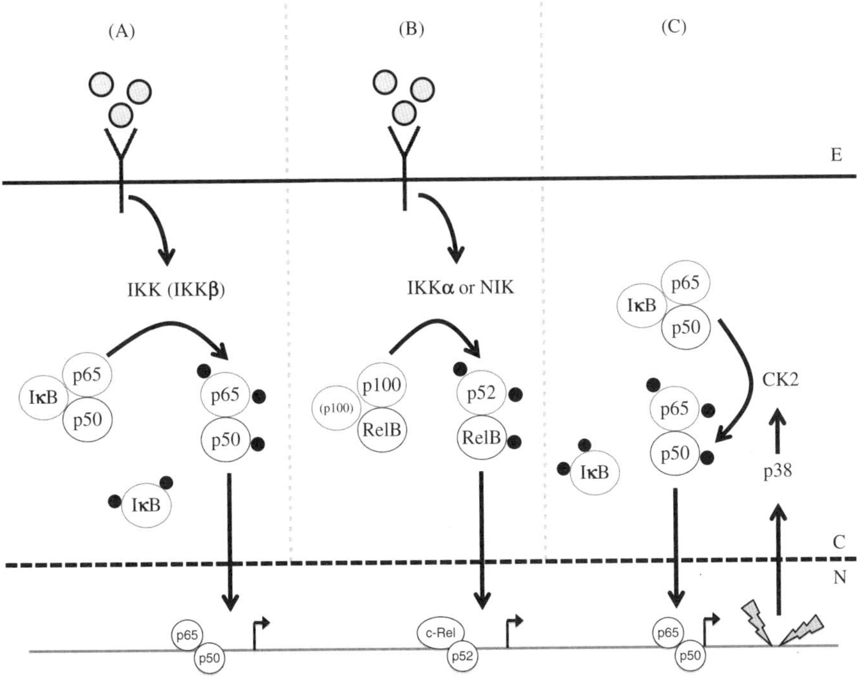

Fig. 42.2 Activation of the NF-κB proteins. The NF-κB proteins can be activated by three distinct signaling pathways: (**A**) canonical or classical, (**B**) non-canonical or nonclassical, and (**C**) alternative. Key: extracellular (**E**), cytosolic (**C**), and nuclear (**N**); *black circles* represent phosphorylated amino acids. See text for details

an NF-κB molecule containing p65/RelA, c-Rel, and/or p50 proteins, which are held in the cytoplasm through interactions with the inhibitor of NF-κB proteins (IκB) family of proteins (Fig. 42.2A). The IκB proteins bind to and block the DNA binding domain of NF-κB and the nuclear localization signal (NLS) of p65. However, p65/p50 heterodimers bound to IκB can still oscillate into and out of the nucleus due to an NLS on p50. In the canonical pathway, activation is mediated primarily through the IκB kinase (IKK) complex, which consists of IKKα, IKKβ, and IKKγ (NEMO) and is activated in response to extracellular or intracellular signaling. Once activated, IKKβ phosphorylates IκB, which is then rapidly ubiquitinated and targeted for degradation by the proteasome. The newly liberated NF-κB dimers are phosphorylated and accumulate in the nucleus, where they bind to NF-κB responsive elements in the promoter regions of numerous target genes, including IκBα (Ghosh and Karin, 2002; Gilmore, 2008; Hayden and Ghosh, 2008). Once new IκBα is resynthesized, it binds to NF-κB dimers, thus reshielding their DNA-binding domain and effectively silencing their activities.

In the non-canonical or alternative pathway, NF-κB dimers containing RelB/p100 are activated to become RelB/p52 (Fig. 42.2B) (Xiao et al., 2006). These heterodimers are inactivated by interactions with the C-terminal portion of p100, which functions analogously to the IκB proteins in the canonical pathway. Like the canonical pathway, the IKK complex mediates NF-κB activation but this event largely relies on the IKKα subunit, which phosphorylates p100 to promote its cleavage and removal of the inhibitory C-terminal ankyrin repeat portion. Additionally, in contrast to the classical and atypical pathways, which can promote NF-κB activation in all cell types, the alternative pathway is mostly involved in the development of lymphoid cells.

Finally, the atypical pathway refers to the DNA-damage-induced activation of NF-κB dimers containing p65/RelA, c-Rel, and p50 (Fig. 42.2C) (Wu and Miyamoto, 2007). Unlike the other pathways, NF-κB activation in the atypical pathway is independent of the IKK complex and relies on alternative kinases. In particular, p38 MAPK is activated and signals to casein kinase 2 (CK2), which, in turn, phosphorylates IκB leading to its degradation and activation of NF-κB molecules. Additionally, this pathway may be activated in response to viral or bacterial pathogens or physical or chemical stresses. Herein, we will focus on the classical and atypical pathways leading to NF-κB activation.

While there is some evidence that NF-κB may be able to directly transform cells as an oncogene, the greater evidence points to a role for NF-κB as an accessory to tumorigenesis. Specifically, NF-κB is activated in a number of cancers, and those genes activated by NF-κB are collectively responsible for mediating diverse processes such as angiogenesis, apoptosis, and invasion/metastasis, which promote tumorigenesis (Fig. 42.3) (Bharti and Aggarwal, 2002; Kim et al., 2006; Lee et al., 2007; Nakanishi and Toi, 2005; Nozell et al., 2008; Olivier et al., 2006; Ravi and Bedi, 2004; Sethi et al., 2008; Van Waes, 2007; Wang et al., 1996).

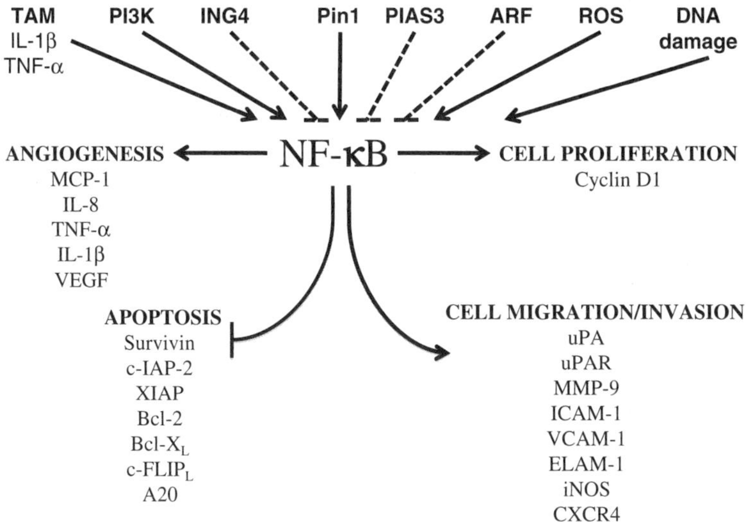

Fig. 42.3 NF-κB activation in GBM, its target genes, and the hallmarks of cancer. NF-κB is constitutively activated in gliomas. While no single mechanism is likely responsible for this phenomenon, in gliomas, NF-κB may be inappropriately activated in numerous ways. These mechanisms include elevated immune cell filtration (TAM) and cytokine secretion (IL-1β and TNF-α), the absence (*dashed lines*) of intracellular negative regulators (ING4, PIAS3, ARF), or the presence of elevated levels of positive regulators of NF-κB (Pin1). Additionally, numerous growth factors are elevated and/or their receptors are amplified and positively affect the PI3K pathway, which activates NF-κB. Once activated, NF-κB induces the expression of genes whose products regulate processes involved in cancer formation and progression. These processes include promoting cell growth, angiogenesis and cell migration and invasion, and inhibiting apoptosis. See text for more details

42.2 NF-κB and Angiogenesis

Because rapidly growing tumors quickly outgrow their blood supply, angiogenesis is critical for growth and progression of solid tumors (Bogler and Mikkelsen, 2005; Brat et al., 2005). As such, tumors must be able to induce the production of new vasculature in order to import and export necessary materials. NF-κB may contribute to angiogenesis by inducing the expression of monocyte chemoattractant protein-1 (MCP-1), interleukin-8 (IL-8), tumor necrosis factor-α (TNF-α), interleukin-1β (IL-1β), and vascular endothelial growth factor (VEGF) (Desbaillets et al., 1999, 1994). Constitutive activation of NF-κB may, therefore, be a driving force for these processes in many types of tumors. In fact, inhibition of NF-κB has been shown to decrease the expression of IL-8 and VEGF, resulting in decreased vascularization and correspondingly smaller tumors in an in vivo model of ovarian cancer (Bogler and Mikkelsen, 2005; Brat et al., 2005; Huang et al., 2000; Nozell et al., 2006).

42.3 NF-κB and Cell Migration and Invasion

One of the most destructive aspects of tumors, especially of gliomas, is their ability to invade into and destroy nearby healthy tissue (Tsunoda et al., 2005; Van Waes, 2007). The aggressiveness of many tumors is greatly enhanced by NF-κB through the activation of genes, including those encoding urokinase plasminogen activator (uPA) and the uPA receptor (uPAR), matrix metalloproteinase-9 (MMP-9), intercellular adhesion molecule-1 (ICAM-1), vascular cellular adhesion molecule-1 (VCAM-1), endothelial–leukocyte adhesion molecule-1 (ELAM-1), inducible nitric oxide synthetase (iNOS), and the chemokine receptor CXCR4 (Aggarwal, 2004; Bharti and Aggarwal, 2002; Kim et al., 2006; Lee et al., 2007; Li et al., 2007; Pacifico and Leonardi, 2006; Psaila et al., 2006; Sethi et al., 2008; Tsunoda et al., 2005). Activation of these genes gives tumor cells the ability to break down the extracellular matrix and create a path for movement into nearby and distant tissues (Yan and Boyd, 2007). Additionally, some of the proteins involved in allowing tumor cells to hone to specific distant sites are NF-κB-regulated gene products such as CXCR4 and VEGF (Sawyer et al., 2006; Tsunoda et al., 2005).

42.4 NF-κB and Cellular Proliferation

Through the regulation of genes such as cyclin D1, cyclin E, cyclin-dependent kinase 2 (CDK2), c-Myc, and interleukin-6 (IL-6), NF-κB can regulate cellular proliferation and apoptosis (Kim et al., 2006; Lee et al., 2007; Sethi et al., 2008; Van Waes, 2007).

42.4.1 Cyclin D1, E, and CDK2

Cyclin D1 is a protein that binds to and activates CDK2, which regulates cell cycle progression from the G1 phase into the S phase, while cyclin E promotes DNA synthesis (Baudino et al., 2003; Roberts and Sherr, 2003; Sherr, 2000; Sherr and Roberts, 2004). While *cyclin D1* is only amplified in a small fraction of gliomas, the protein levels of both cyclin D1 and cyclin E are elevated in the majority of GBMs (Abdullah et al., 2007; Arato-Ohshima and Sawa, 1999; Buschges et al., 1999; Cavalla et al., 1998; Zhang et al., 2005). Additionally, the levels of cyclin D1 are positively correlated with high cell proliferation activity, aggressive behavior, increased invasiveness, and the onset and progression of gliomas (Abdullah et al., 2007; Arato-Ohshima and Sawa, 1999; Buschges et al., 1999; Cavalla et al., 1998; Zhang et al., 2005). Interestingly, a small eight amino acid peptide (PVKRRLFG), termed the LFG peptide, designed to represent the minimal amino acids needed by a CDK inhibitor (CKI) to bind and abrogate CDK activity was shown to induce apoptosis in human glioma cells, although the mechanism remains unclear (Chen et al., 2004). Moreover, glioma cells treated with bortezomib, a proteasome inhibitor that blocks degradation of IκBα and other proteins, showed reduced activation of NF-κB, decreased CDK expression, and enhanced apoptosis as induced by TNF-α or TRAIL (Lashinger et al., 2005).

42.4.2 c-Myc

c-Myc is a transcription factor that is believed to influence the expression of nearly 20% of the human transcriptome (Liao et al., 2007; Robson et al., 2006). In particular, c-Myc can induce the expression of numerous cyclins and CDK proteins, and inhibits the expression of several CKI proteins. Because of the proliferative potential bestowed by c-Myc, its activity is normally monitored by the tumor suppressor proteins alternative reading frame (ARF) and p53 (Dai et al., 2006). In normal cells, deregulated c-Myc can induce apoptosis through the activation of these proteins (Sherr, 2006). However, c-Myc activity is elevated in 73% of gliomas, and many gliomas also lack ARF and p53 activities due to mutations or deletions (Bigner et al., 1988; Bigner and Vogelstein, 1990; Fulci et al., 2000; Ishii et al., 1999; LaRocca et al., 1989; Rasheed and Bigner, 1991; Wasson et al., 1990).

42.4.3 Interleukin-6

Interleukin-6 is a cytokine that activates the signal transducer and activator of transcription (STAT)-3 protein (Brantley and Benveniste, 2008). Like NF-κB, STAT-3 is a transcription factor that induces the expression of genes that promote cell proliferation and inhibit apoptosis (Brantley and Benveniste, 2008) (see also Chapter 37). Several studies have shown that the levels of IL-6 mRNA and protein are elevated in GBM when compared to other gliomas or normal tissues, and that the levels of IL-6 correlate with constitutively activated STAT-3 and inversely correlate with patient survival (Black et al., 1992; Cinque et al., 1992; Schneider et al., 1992; Van Meir et al., 1990). Recent data suggest that IL-6 may play a critical role during the progression from pre-neoplastic to gliomagenic in a murine model of spontaneous gliomas (Weissenberger et al., 2004). In particular, transgenic mice expressing the v-src protein under the regulation of the *GFAP* gene promoter, which are predisposed to forming spontaneous gliomas, developed pre-neoplastic astrogliosis that did not progress to gliomas if the mice were also null for IL-6 (Weissenberger et al., 2004). As such, IL-6 is also an attractive target for therapeutic intervention. Indeed, human glioma cells treated with antisense oligonucleotides specific for IL-6 or IL-6 antibodies demonstrated reduced cell growth (Goswami et al., 1998).

42.5 NF-κB and Apoptosis

Perhaps the most immediate pro-tumorigenic effect of NF-κB activation is the inhibition of apoptosis. Apoptosis, or programed cell death, is a process characterized by the ordered breakdown of cellular contents into membrane-bound vesicles that are removed by phagocytes (Green, 2003). This process is mediated by the proteolytic activation of a group of proteins known as caspases (cysteinal aspartate proteases), in response to either extracellular (TNF-α, FasL, etc.) or intracellular (release of cytochrome *c*, DNA damage, etc.) signals. Synthesized as zymogens, caspases become activated upon removal of their N-terminal pro-domains (Conti et al., 2005; Green, 2003; Okada and Mak, 2004). Apoptosis begins when initiator caspases (e.g., caspase-8, -9, and -10) activate downstream effector caspases (e.g., caspase-3, -6, and -7) (Green, 2003; Okada and Mak, 2004). Once activated, effector caspases then cleave components of the actin cytoskeleton, protein kinases, nuclear lamins, and other key cellular components. Additionally, caspases activate the processes leading to DNA degradation and chromatin condensation (Green, 2003). Under normal conditions, the apoptotic process removes cells that are not needed or are damaged. However, despite the presence of stimuli that induce apoptosis in the tumor microenvironment, most tumor cells have undergone genetic alterations and/or adopted mechanisms that allow these cells to evade programed cell death. One mechanism by which tumor cells evade apoptosis is via activation of NF-κB. In most cell types, NF-κB is a key mediator of pro-survival (Ghosh and Karin, 2002; Hayden and Ghosh, 2008). For example, fibroblasts and macrophages from RelA-deficient mice are sensitive to TNF-α-induced apoptosis, while their wild-type counterparts are insensitive (Beg and Baltimore, 1996).

Caspase cleavage and hence apoptosis may be initiated via two distinct pathways: the extrinsic and the intrinsic pathways (Fig. 42.4) (Green, 2003; Okada and Mak, 2004). In the *extrinsic* pathway, extracellular death-inducing signaling molecules such as TNF-α or FasL bind to the TNF-α receptor (TNFR) and Fas receptor, respectively. These death receptors contain an intracellular protein-interaction domain called the death domain (DD). Upon ligand binding, the death receptors trimerize and use their DD to recruit adapter molecules that also contain DD domains (Green, 2003). In particular, Fas binds Fas-associated DD (FADD), while TNFR first recruits TNF-α receptor associated DD (TRADD) and then FADD (Green, 2003; Okada and Mak, 2004). Through a second domain, the death effector domain (DED), FADD recruits and binds to the DED within procaspase-8 and pro-caspase-10. This complex of proteins is called the death-induced signaling complex (DISC), and its formation results in the activation of the initiator caspases. Once activated, initiator caspases then cleave downstream effector caspases, leading to the full apoptotic process (Green, 2003; Levine, 1997; Okada and Mak, 2004) (for more detail see Chapter 41).

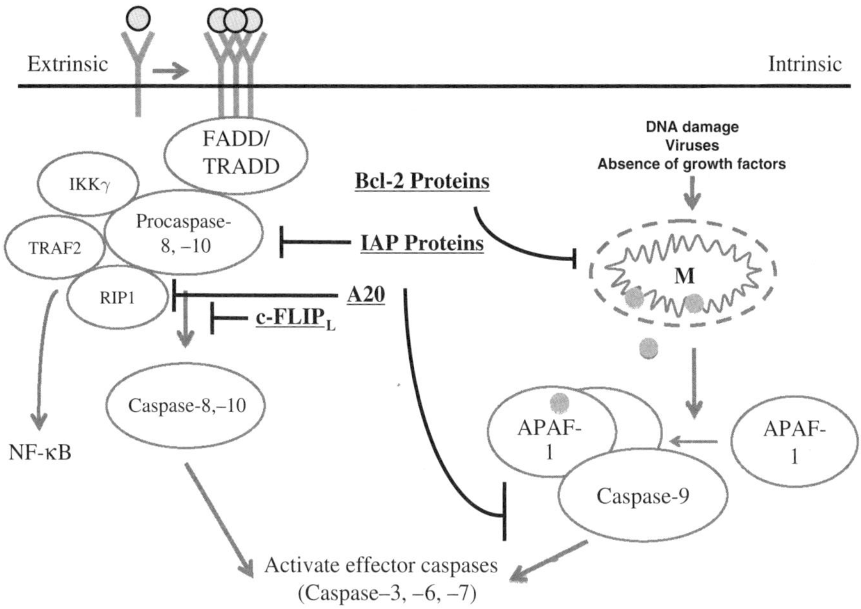

Fig. 42.4 NF-κB and its target genes mediate apoptotic resistance. Apoptosis may be induced through extracellular stimuli (extrinsic pathway) or intracellular insults (intrinsic pathway). In each pathway, these stimuli activate a caspase cascade that culminates in cell death. Through the induction of IAPs, Bcl-2 family members, A20, and c-FLIP$_L$, NF-κB can inhibit the initiation and/or progression of apoptosis. Key: mitochondria (M), small *grey circles* represent cytochrome c. See text for details

In the *intrinsic* pathway, apoptosis is initiated in response to DNA damage, ultraviolet (UV) radiation, viral infection, or the absence of growth factors (Green, 2003; Okada and Mak, 2004). In contrast to the extrinsic pathway, which transduces extracellular apoptotic stimuli to intracellular death-inducing machinery through the use of membrane-bound receptors, the intrinsic pathway relies heavily on the mitochondria and proteins that lie therein (Fig. 42.4). During apoptosis as induced by the intrinsic pathway, the mitochondrial outer membrane becomes permeabilized and leads to the release of holocytochrome c, a key protein in the electron transport chain. In the cytosol, cytochrome c binds to apoptotic-protease activating factor (APAF-1), which normally exists as a monomer in living cells. However, upon binding to cytochrome c, APAF-1 is activated, oligomerizes, and exposes a caspase-recruitment domain (CARD). Once exposed, the CARD domain of APAF-1 binds to procaspase-9 through a similar CARD motif, yielding the formation of the apoptosome and activation of caspase-9. Like other initiator caspases, caspase-9 proteolytically activates effector caspases to initiate the apoptotic cascade. Importantly, NF-κB can be activated by apoptotic stimuli and can inhibit apoptosis in both the extrinsic and intrinsic pathways (Lamkanfi et al.,

2006). In the extrinsic pathway, the pro-domains of caspase-2, -8, and -10 can recruit TNFR-associated factor 2 (TRAF2), receptor interacting protein 1 (RIP1), and NEMO/IKKγ. TRAF2, an E3-ubiquitin ligase, and RIP1, a kinase, promote the activation of IKK and consequently NF-κB. Interestingly, elevated levels of TRAF2 mRNA and protein have been detected in gliomas and are positively correlated with tumor grade (Conti et al., 2005).

Once activated, NF-κB inhibits apoptosis through the expression of target genes. In particular, NF-κB induces the expression of members of the inhibitor of apoptosis (IAP) family such as c-IAP2, XIAP, and survivin (Fig. 42.3) (Angileri et al., 2008; Hunter et al., 2007; Wang et al., 1998; Wei et al., 2008). IAP proteins interact with and inhibit the activity of active caspases to antagonize cell death and serve as the cell's final fail safe before committing to apoptosis (Hunter et al., 2007; Wei et al., 2008) (Fig. 42.4). In gliomas, IAP proteins are over-expressed, correlate with aberrant NF-κB transcriptional activity, and are associated with refractory disease and poor disease prognosis (Angileri et al., 2008; Conti et al., 2005; Steinbach and Weller, 2004; Weaver et al., 2003). In work from our own laboratory, we found that reducing p65 expression through the use of *shRNA* abrogated the induction of c-IAP2, and re-sensitized glioma cells to TNF-α-induced apoptosis (unpublished observation). Strikingly, one study developed a small-molecule antagonist of IAP proteins that promoted auto-ubiquitination and degradation of IAPs within minutes of its application and induced TNF-α mediated cell death in several cell lines, including breast, colorectal, and fibrosarcoma (Li et al., 2004). At present, antagonists of the IAP proteins are being evaluated as therapeutic targets in several tumor types. Second mitochondria-derived activator of caspase (Smac)/direct IAP binding protein with low pI (DIABLO) is a protein secreted from the mitochondria. Smac/DIABLO is a physiological negative regulator of IAPs that binds to and antagonizes IAP proteins during apoptosis (Fulda et al., 2002; Li et al., 2004), suggesting that it can be exploited to sensitize cells to apoptosis. Indeed, expression of a small, cell-permeable peptide portion of Smac/DIABLO was sufficient to inhibit IAPs and promote caspase activation in human glioma cell lines. It was also shown to enhance the cytotoxicity of TRAIL and TNF-α in human glioma xenograft models.

To specifically inhibit apoptosis mediated through the intrinsic pathway, NF-κB induces the expression of Bcl-2 and Bcl-X_L (Lamkanfi et al., 2006). These proteins reside in the outer mitochondrial membrane and can prevent its permeabilization and thus assembly and activation of the apoptosome (Angileri et al., 2008; Ehrmann et al., 1997; Green, 2003; Krajewski et al., 1997; Rieger et al., 2007, 1998). In gliomas, Bcl-2 and Bcl-X_L are over-expressed, and this inversely correlates with patient survival (Angileri et al., 2008; Cusack et al., 2001; Ehrmann et al., 1997; Julien et al., 2000; Rieger et al., 1998). In human glioma cell lines, the use of Bcl-2 antisense oligonucleotides induced growth arrest and apoptosis in human glioma cell lines, while forced over-expression of Bcl-2 rendered them more resistant to the cytotoxic effects of chemotherapies and gamma irradiation (Angileri et al., 2008; Cusack et al., 2001; Ehrmann et al., 1997; Julien et al., 2000; Rieger et al., 1998).

c-FLIP$_L$, another NF-κB target gene, is a structural homolog of caspase-8 that lacks the caspase activity (Lamkanfi et al., 2006). When present at elevated levels, c-FLIP$_L$ prevented full processing and release of active caspase-8 from the DISC complex, and prevented apoptosis in human glioma cells (Koschny et al., 2007; Panner et al., 2005). The expression of c-FLIP is transcriptionally regulated by NF-κB. c-FLIP is expressed in a number of human glioma cell lines, and the levels of c-FLIP are correlated with TRAIL resistance in glioma cells (Xiao et al., 2002).

A20/TNF-α–induced protein 3 (TNFAIP3), another NF-κB-regulated gene, is an important factor in mediating cell survival in gliomas (Bredel et al., 2006). A20 is a zinc finger protein that contains two ubiquitin-editing domains, which can modify ubiquitination of RIP and target this protein for degradation by the proteasome (Bredel et al., 2006; Lamkanfi et al., 2006). In this manner, A20 can indirectly inhibit NF-κB activation. However, A20 is consistently down-regulated in resistant glioblastomas, and the levels of A20 are inversely correlated with patient response to chemotherapy (Bredel et al., 2006). Indeed, one study determined that A20 was one of only four genes identified in an optimized outcome predictor of patient survival and resistance to O^6-alkylating agents (Bredel et al., 2006).

42.6 Activation of NF-κB in Gliomas

As reported in the literature, the levels of NF-κB activity are much higher in GBM compared to non-GBM tissue (Ito et al., 1994; Wang et al., 2004). Additionally, the levels of NF-κB activation correspond with increasing tumor grade in astrocytic tumors. While the mechanism of NF-κB activation in GBM is largely undefined, the heterogeneity of human GBMs makes identifying a single NF-κB activating factor difficult. Instead, the activation of NF-κB may be an inevitable consequence of the tumor microenvironment and the numerous proteins and pathways that are dysregulated in gliomas (Fig. 42.4).

42.6.1 Immune Cell Infiltration

A characteristic feature of many solid tumors, including GBMs, is the presence of immune infiltrates. In some tumors, macrophages and other infiltrating immune cells make up 50% of the total tumor mass (Hussain et al., 2006). These cells may be recruited in part by MCP-1, a chemokine whose levels are elevated in gliomas, possibly through gene activation by NF-κB (Desbaillets et al., 1994; Leung et al., 1997). Once recruited and activated, tumor-associated macrophages (TAMs) secrete cytokines such as TNF-α and IL-1β, both of which can activate NF-κB (Hussain et al., 2006). In gliomas, the levels of TNF-α and IL-1β are elevated (Cinque et al., 1992; Munoz-Fernandez et al., 1991). Moreover, in 1321N1 astrocytoma cells, IL-1β stimulation resulted in persistent, long-term activation of NF-κB, which was relatively unaffected by the re-synthesis of IκBα, the inhibitor of NF-κB (Xu et al., 2006). A more detailed review of NF-κB-activated cytokines and their role in gliomas is provided elsewhere (Dey et al., 2006).

42.6.2 The PI3K Pathway

One pathway that is commonly activated in GBM and can lead to NF-κB activation is the PI3K pathway (Fan et al., 2002; Mischel and Cloughesy, 2003). Normally, the PI3K pathway is activated in response to numerous growth factors, which bind their respective receptors and activate their intrinsic kinase or receptor-associated Jak activities. Receptors that can activate PI3K include epidermal growth factor receptor (EGFR), platelet-derived growth factor receptor (PDGFR), fibroblast growth factor receptor (FGFR), insulin-like growth factor 1 receptor (IGF-1R), interleukin receptors, vascular endothelial growth factor receptor (VEGFR), interferon receptors, and integrin receptors (Mischel and Cloughesy, 2003; Ren et al., 2007). In GBM, many of these growth factors are elevated and/or the receptors are constitutively activated. For example, amplification, over-expression, and mutation of EGFR is one of the most common genetic abnormalities associated with GBM, with approximately 36% of GBMs showing some abnormality in EGFR (see also Chapter 20) (TCGA, 2008). Once activated, PI3K signals to Akt/protein kinase B, which then phosphorylates and activates IKK, thus ultimately promoting NF-κB activation. Within this pathway, PI3K suppressor phosphatase and tensin homolog deleted on chromosome 10 (PTEN) serves as an antagonist of PI3K, in order to attenuate signaling downstream of PI3K (Fan et al., 2002; Jiang and Liu, 2008; Mischel and Cloughesy, 2003; Ohgaki and Kleihues, 2007). However, PTEN is commonly deleted in GBM (TCGA, 2008). Moreover, activating mutations in Akt or in the catalytic subunit of PI3K have been documented in GBM (Beyaert et al., 2000; Bredel et al., 2006; Danial and Korsmeyer, 2004; Lee et al., 2007; TCGA, 2008) (see also Chapter 15). Thus, genetic abnormalities leading to activation of the PI3K pathway may contribute to NF-κB activation in gliomas.

42.6.3 ING4

Inhibitor of growth 4 (ING4) is a recently identified tumor suppressor protein (Kim, 2005). Although the functions of ING4 remain largely uncharacterized, this protein contains motifs that enable it to interact with and regulate the activity of many proteins associated with transcription (Doyon et al., 2006; Shiseki et al., 2003). In particular, ING4 has been shown to positively regulate the activity of p53, another tumor suppressor, and negatively regulate the activity of NF-κB (Garkavtsev et al., 2004; Kim et al., 2004; Shiseki et al., 2003; Zhang et al., 2004). Interestingly, one report demonstrated that ING4 expression was reduced and/or the *ING4* gene was mutated in gliomas, and that this correlated with increasing tumor grade (Garkavtsev et al., 2004). Work from our own laboratory has determined that ING4 can negatively regulate the activity of NF-κB while it is bound to a target gene promoter (Nozell et al., 2008). In particular, ING4 may be necessary for inactivating nuclear and DNA-bound NF-κB, in order to attenuate the expression of NF-κB-regulated genes. Therefore, the absence of functional ING4 activity may allow NF-κB, once activated, to perpetually induce the expression of pro-tumorigenic genes in gliomas.

42.6.4 Pin1

Another protein shown to regulate the activity of NF-κB is Pin1 (Lu et al., 2006; Ryo et al., 2003b). Pin1 is a member of the peptidyl-prolyl isomerase family with the unique ability to isomerize peptide bonds that are present between proline residues and phosphorylated threonine or serine residues (Lu et al., 2006). In this manner, Pin1 can regulate the post-post-translational activity of a protein (Lu et al., 2006). To date, Pin1 has been shown to interact with and influence the activity of many proteins, including p53, p73, c-Jun, and β-catenin. One report has determined that Pin1 can interact with and promote the activity of NF-κB (Ryo et al., 2003b). In particular, Pin1 was shown to associate with the NF-κB p65 subunit through residue threonine 254 and lead to stabilization of p65 (Ryo et al., 2003b). In the absence of Pin1, p65 is ubiquitinated in a SOCS-1-dependent manner, and subsequently degraded (Ryo et al., 2007). In gliomas, Pin1 protein levels are elevated, and thus it may stabilize and prolong NF-κB protein levels and activity (Ryo et al., 2003b). Pin1 has also been shown to inhibit Daxx-mediated cellular apoptosis by hydrogen peroxide or Fas antibodies (Ryo et al., 2007). Additionally, reductions in Pin1 protein levels through the use of siRNA significantly reduced tumor growth and migration while increasing their sensitivity to apoptotic stimuli (Ding et al., 2008). In other studies, over-expression of Pin1 can confer transforming properties to normal cells, or even enhance the transformed phenotype of other oncogenes including Ras and Neu (Ryo et al., 2003a, 2002). For these reasons, Pin1 raised interest as a potentially attractive anticancer target. Unfortunately, Pin1 knockout mice develop testicular atrophy, retinal atrophy, and neurodegeneration, indicating that antagonizing Pin1 activity may have non-desirable side effects, especially in the brain (Liou et al., 2002; Takahashi et al., 2007).

42.6.5 PIAS Family

Members of the protein inhibitor of activated STAT (PIAS) family were initially identified as negative regulators of the STAT proteins (Shuai, 2006; Shuai and Liu, 2005). At present, these proteins are capable of positively and negatively regulating the activity of more than 60 proteins, many of which are transcription factors (Shuai, 2006; Shuai and Liu, 2005). One member, PIAS3, can interact with and negatively regulate the activity of NF-κB p65 (Jang et al., 2004). In particular, in cells stimulated with TNF-α, a nuclear PIAS3-NF-κB p65 interaction was detected, and this was shown to inhibit NF-κB's ability to bind to CBP, a histone acetyltransferase (HAT) required for the expression of many NF-κB target genes. Work from our laboratory has demonstrated that in gliomas, the expression of PIAS3 protein is reduced or absent, although *PIAS3* mRNA is present. While it is currently unclear why or how this protein is not expressed, the absence of PIAS3 may promote nuclear NF-κB activities (Brantley et al., 2008). Indeed, the over-expression of PIAS3 in glioma cells inhibits transcription of the *MMP-9* promoter, linking PIAS3 expression to inhibition of NF-κB signaling (Brantley et al., 2008).

42.6.6 Alternative Reading Frame (ARF)

The activity of NF-κB can also be regulated by ARF (Ivanchuk et al., 2001). ARF is a tumor suppressor protein that most notably prevents tumor formation by antagonizing Mdm2-mediated ubiquitination of p53. However, ARF also promotes ATR- and Chk-1-induced phosphorylation of p65 at a residue that inhibits NF-κB transactivation (Perkins, 2004; Rocha et al., 2005; Rocha and Perkins, 2005). In gliomas, the ARF gene is hyper-methylated and/or absent in approximately 25% of grade II fibrillary astrocytomas, which later underwent progression or recurrence, and the loss of ARF expression is one of the most common abnormalities in high-grade gliomas (Esteller et al., 2001). Moreover, 10% of ARF knockout mice develop spontaneous gliomas (Fulci et al., 2000; Holland, 2000; Uhrbom et al., 2002). Thus, the absence of ARF may also contribute to persistent activation of NF-κB and the chronic expression of pro-tumorigenic genes.

42.6.7 DNA Damage and Reactive Oxygen Species (ROS)

Finally, NF-κB can be activated by spontaneous and/or chemotherapy-induced DNA damage, reactive oxygen species (ROS), and cytotoxic treatments (Bharti and Aggarwal, 2002; Wu and Miyamoto, 2007). Many of these insults mediate their cellular response through ataxia-telangiectasia mutated (ATM) protein kinase (Wu and Miyamoto, 2007). In response to DNA damage and other cellular stresses, ATM is activated and phosphorylates p53, BRCA1, and Chk2 to promote the repair of DNA. Unfortunately, ATM also phosphorylates NF-κB at a residue that leads to its activation. In cells that contain both p53 and NF-κB, the ultimate choice between NF-κB-mediated cell survival and p53-induced cell death is complex and influenced by ATM and other proteins (Wu and Miyamoto, 2007). However, in gliomas, which often lack p53 activity, activation of ATM ensures that NF-κB is activated and promotes cell survival and proliferation. Additionally, NF-κB induces the expression of multidrug resistance protein 1 (MDR1), which expels cytotoxic agents from the intracellular compartment, and O6-methylguanine-DNA methyltransferase (MGMT), which can repair numerous types of DNA damage, including those induced by alkylating agents used for anti-glioma therapy (Kuo et al., 2002; Wu and Miyamoto, 2007). Collectively, the tumor microenvironment, the incidence of numerous aberrant signaling pathways, and perhaps even the therapeutic approaches in treating gliomas, may ultimately ensure that NF-κB becomes or remains activated in these tumors.

42.7 Targeting NF-κB in Gliomas

NF-κB is intimately involved in the fundamental processes of tumor survival and growth and thus is a logical therapeutic target. Moreover, because NF-κB mediates resistance to chemo- and radiotherapy in many tumors, it may become necessary to design and implement approaches to inhibit the NF-κB pathway. Indeed, in our studies, the use of shRNA molecules to reduce NF-κB p65 expression re-sensitized glioma cells to the pro-apoptotic effects of TNF-α (unpublished observation). Unfortunately in gliomas, the blood–brain barrier complicates the administration of many drugs and chemotherapy since this semipermeable barrier may not allow all molecules to access the brain and reach the tumor cells to be targeted (see Chapter 33). Therefore, current and future chemotherapies targeting the NF-κB pathway in gliomas must consider accessibility to the target site as well as specifically, but not globally, inhibiting the NF-κB pathway. Currently, strategies have been designed to inhibit NF-κB directly or indirectly via signaling components upstream (Kim et al., 2006; Nakanishi and Toi, 2005; Olivier et al., 2006; Ravi and Bedi, 2004; Weaver et al., 2003). Those strategies designed to directly block the activities of NF-κB include the use of decoy oligonucleotides (ODNs) containing the NF-κB response element, glucocorticoids that target NF-κB transactivation, and antisense oligonucleotides (ASO) targeting NF-κB mRNA. Corticosteroids such as dexamethasone are frequently used to treat gliomal peritumoral edema and therefore will not be discussed further herein. Additionally, the use of ODN remains in its infancy and the remaining strategies are only being tested in other tumor types and are not currently under examination in gliomas (Gill et al., 2002). As such, we will focus herein on therapies that are currently being considered and that indirectly inhibit NF-κB activation (Fig. 42.5). The list of

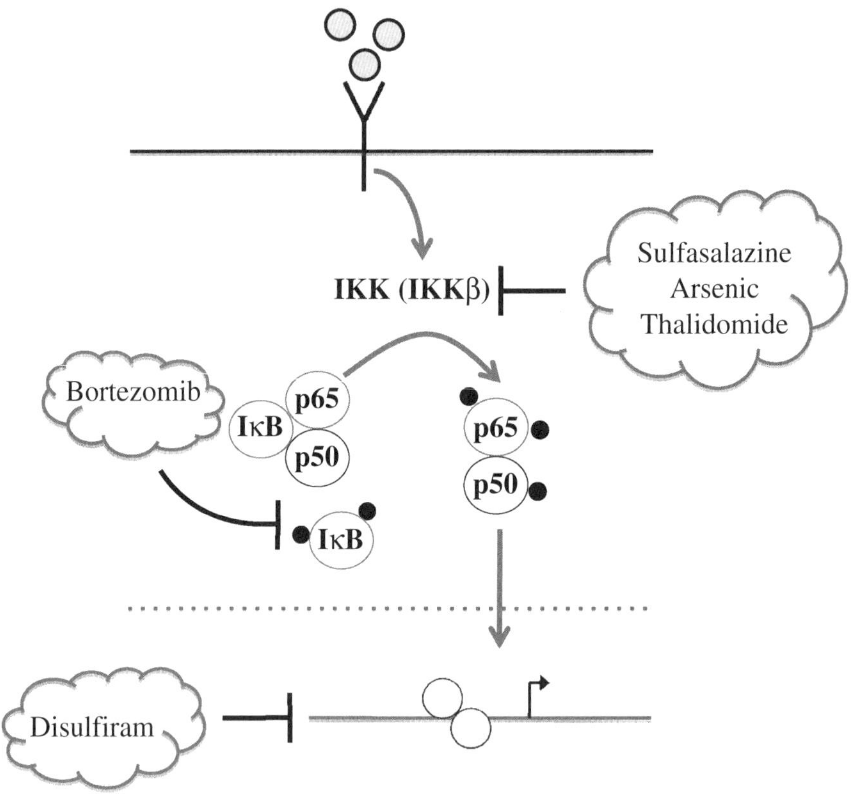

Fig. 42.5 Targeting NF-κB in gliomas. IKK activation following growth factor binding to cell surface receptors is shown to free the p65/p50 NF-κB isoforms and lead to activation of transcription. Several steps of this activation of the NF-κB pathway are being targeted in current and ongoing clinical trials and therapies in gliomas. See text for details

therapeutic candidates includes (**a**) proteasome inhibitors, (**b**) IKK inhibitors, and (**c**) antioxidants.

42.7.1 Proteasome Inhibitors

The proteasome plays a critical role in regulating the proteolysis of most nuclear and cytosolic proteins, many of which are short-lived proteins that govern growth, activation, and signaling. Within the NF-κB pathway, IκBα binds to and inhibits NF-κB activation (Ghosh and Karin, 2002; Hayden and Ghosh, 2008). However, phosphorylation of IκBα leads to its proteasomal-mediated degradation and NF-κB activation (Ghosh and Karin, 2002; Hayden and Ghosh, 2008) (Fig. 42.2). Therefore, the use of proteasomal inhibitors would prevent the degradation of proteins such as IκBα. Bortezomib (Velcade,

PS-341) is a dipeptidyl boronic acid that specifically inhibits the 26S proteasome (Yin et al., 2005). Recently approved for use in multiple myeloma, bortezomib has also shown anti-tumoral activity in numerous solid tumors including carcinomas of the breast, lung, colon, bladder, ovary, pancreas, and prostate (Yin et al., 2005; Yu et al., 2006). Like other proteasome inhibitors, including lactacystin, MG132 and AcLLNa1, bortezomib can inhibit glioma cell growth in vitro, presumably by stabilizing the levels of IκBα and reducing NF-κB activity (Koschny et al., 2007). When combined with TNF-α or TRAIL, several GBM cell lines demonstrated marked increases in sensitivity to apoptosis, suggesting that bortezomib may be a clinically useful adjunctive therapy in human gliomas (Cusack et al., 2001; Yin et al., 2005). Indeed, when used in combination with TRAIL, several TRAIL-resistant primary glioma cells were re-sensitized to the apoptotic effects of TRAIL, perhaps by increasing the expression of TRAIL-R1/DR4 and TRAIL-R2/DR5 (Kardosh et al., 2008). Additional reports also demonstrate increased cytotoxicity in human glioma cell lines through the combined use of bortezomib and celecoxib (Celebrex), an inhibitor of cyclooxygenase-2 (COX-2), although the mechanism may depend on the induction of aggravated endoplasmic reticulum stress (Fribley and Wang, 2006; Nawrocki et al., 2005a, b).

42.7.2 IKK Inhibitors

Several compounds that inhibit IKK are currently under consideration for use in glioma chemotherapy. These include sulfasalazine, arsenic trioxide, and thalidomide (Bode and Dong, 2002; Lin et al., 2008; Robe et al., 2004). Sulfasalazine is an anti-inflammatory drug used to treat inflammatory bowel disease and severe, resistant rheumatoid arthritis (Robe et al., 2004). This drug consists of an antibiotic (sulfapyridine) and an anti-inflammatory reagent (5-aminosalicylic acid) that is absorbed unchanged and then degraded by colonic bacteria into the two separate components. In vitro, sulfasalazine inhibited NF-κB activity and glioma cell proliferation in a dose-dependent manner, while having no effect on cell survival in primary rat and human normal astrocytes (Koschny et al., 2007; Lawson et al., 2007; Robe et al., 2004). When used in a mouse model with intracranially implanted U87MG human glioblastoma cells, sulfasalazine reduced mean tumor volume. Currently, the prospects of sulfasalazine use in gliomas are being explored in a phase 1–2 prospective clinical trial for its safety and efficacy in treating recurrent malignant gliomas (Robe et al., 2006).

The chemical element arsenic and many of its compounds are especially potent poisons, a property epitomized in the classic 1944 movie "Arsenic and Old Lace," by director Frank Capra. Arsenic is particularly lethal since it interferes with ATP production by inhibiting pyruvate dehydrogenase and by uncoupling electron transport from ATP synthesis. Additionally, arsenic elevates hydrogen peroxide production, which may increase the formation of reactive oxygen species and cause oxidative stress. Paradoxically, both scientists and physicians have been harnessing the therapeutic potential of arsenic long before they even understood its lethality. In particular, Paul Ehrlich treated syphilis in the early 1900s with an arsenic derivative, while later, Thomas Fowler used a 1% potassium arsenite solution to successfully treat psoriasis. More recently, the U.S. Food and Drug Administration (FDA) approved the use of arsenic trioxide for the treatment of patients with relapsed/refractory acute promyelocytic leukemia (APL) that is resistant to ATRA (Kitamura et al., 1997). One of the first molecular targets of arsenic identified was IKKβ, wherein arsenic binds to IKKβ at cysteine 179 and inhibits IKKβ's ability to activate NF-κB (Bode and Dong, 2002; Lin et al., 2008). Interestingly, depending on the dose and duration of exposure, arsenic can have differential effects on the activity of NF-κB. In particular, acute exposure or low doses of arsenic can lead to NF-κB activation, while either chronic exposure or higher doses of arsenic can reduce the basal levels of NF-κB and inhibit NF-κB activity.

Thalidomide is another example of how a dangerous compound can be used therapeutically with adequate precautions and procedures. First distributed from 1957 to 1961 as a sedative and anti-nausea remedy to pregnant women, thalidomide quickly garnered unwanted attention as a potent teratogen, generating phocomelia or atrophied limbs in over 10,000 children worldwide (Keifer et al., 2001). Although removed from the market, thalidomide reappeared in the late 1990s as a clinically relevant drug that harbors both immunomodulatory and anti-angiogenic properties. In 1998, the FDA approved the use of thalidomide for the treatment of leprosy, and in 2006 for multiple myeloma under the name Thalomid. Thalidomide in combination with bortezomib changed the treatment of multiple myeloma, reducing the need for stem cell transplants and showing better efficacy than standard chemotherapy. Thalidomide appears to have multiple mechanisms of action and inhibits the production of TNF-α, IKK activity and prevents TNF-α–induced NF-κB activation (Keifer et al., 2001; Kirsch et al., 2000; Majumdar et al., 2002; Sampaio et al., 1991). While thalidomide inhibits endothelial cell proliferation and tumor cell migration in vitro, its ability to inhibit tumor cell growth and migration has been variable (Puduvalli et al., 2008). Early results of a phase II clinical trial investigating thalidomide in patients with high-grade gliomas demonstrated low toxicity but unfortunately minimal responses to treatment. However, more recent phase II clinical trials investigating combinatorial use of thalidomide and other cytotoxic agents, such as irinotecan, cisplatin, and temozolomide, have shown both promising and disappointing results (Sampaio et al., 1991; Sauna et al., 2005; Zustovich et al., 2007).

42.7.3 Antioxidants

For nearly half a century, tetraethylthiuramdisulfide (disulfiram; DTDS) has been used to treat alcohol dependency. Now, disulfiram and its major metabolite, diethyldithiocarbamate (DDTC), are demonstrating significant potential in the treatment of human cancers (Liu et al., 1998). In experimental studies, disulfiram protected rats against alkylating carcinogens and neoplastic agents, while in cultured cells, DDTC inhibited the ability of NF-κB to bind DNA and induced cell death (Marikovsky et al., 2002). Additional studies demonstrated that DDTC inhibited neovascularization in vivo and proliferation of C6 glioma cells in culture (Lamkanfi et al., 2006). Currently, disulfiram is being investigated alone or in combination in several clinical trials of human gliomas.

42.8 Conclusions

By traditional standards, NF-κB is an unconventional therapeutic target. In cancers, it is neither amplified nor mutated; it is neither an oncogene nor a tumor suppressor. Instead, NF-κB is a transcription factor that induces genes that mediate nearly every facet of the formation and progression of gliomas and other cancers. Normally kept in check by numerous mechanisms, it is the breakdown of these mechanisms that ultimately leads to deregulated NF-κB activity and enables this family of proteins to inadvertently function as tumor promoters. While inhibiting these proteins may seem a straightforward approach, their role as key mediators of immune and inflammatory processes complicates the situation since global suppression of NF-κB is not a suitable option. As such, understanding the molecular events that lead to deregulated NF-κB activity and gene expression in gliomas remains an area in glioma biology that needs exploration. Recent advances in these areas and in targeting the NF-κB pathway have yielded promising results and suggest that exploration of this family and its role in glioma biology will continue to provide much needed insights about gliomas and potential future therapeutic interventions.

Acknowledgments This work was supported in part by NIH grants CA-97247 and NS-54158, IRG-60-001-47 from the American Cancer Society, and CA-13148 from the NCI. T. L. was supported by NIH T32 AI-07051.

References

Abdullah, J.M., Ahmad, F., Ahmad, K.A., Ghazali, M.M., Jaafar, H., Ideris, A., Ali, A.M., Omar, A.R., Yusoff, K., Lila, M.A., et al. 2007. Molecular genetic analysis of BAX and cyclin D1 genes in patients with malignant glioma. Neurol Res 29, 239–242.

Aggarwal, B.B. 2004. NF-κB: the enemy within. Cancer Cell 6, 203–208.

Angileri, F.F., Aguennouz, M., Conti, A., La Torre, D., Cardali, S., Crupi, R., Tomasello, C., Germano, A., Vita, G., and Tomasello, F. 2008. NF-κB activation and differential expression of survivin and Bcl-2 in human grade 2–4 astrocytomas. Cancer 112, 2258–2266.

Arato-Ohshima, T., and Sawa, H. 1999. Over-expression of cyclin D1 induces glioma invasion by increasing matrix metalloproteinase activity and cell motility. Int J Cancer 83, 387–392.

Baudino, T.A., Maclean, K.H., Brennan, J., Parganas, E., Yang, C., Aslanian, A., Lees, J.A., Sherr, C.J., Roussel, M.F., and Cleveland, J.L. 2003. Myc-mediated proliferation and lymphomagenesis, but not apoptosis, are compromised by E2F1 loss. Mol Cell 11, 905–914.

Beg, A.A., and Baltimore, D. 1996. An essential role for NF-κB in preventing TNF-alpha-induced cell death. Science 274, 782–784.

Beyaert, R., Heyninck, K., and Van Huffel, S. 2000. A20 and A20-binding proteins as cellular inhibitors of NF-κB-dependent gene expression and apoptosis. Biochem Pharmacol 60, 1143–1151.

Bharti, A.C., and Aggarwal, B.B. 2002. NF-κB and cancer: its role in prevention and therapy. Biochem Pharmacol 64, 883–888.

Bigner, S.H., Burger, P.C., Wong, A.J., Werner, M.H., Hamilton, S.R., Muhlbaier, L.H., Vogelstein, B., and Bigner, D.D. 1988. Gene amplification in malignant human gliomas: clinical and histopathologic aspects. J Neuropathol Exp Neurol 47, 191–205.

Bigner, S.H., and Vogelstein, B. 1990. Cytogenetics and molecular genetics of malignant gliomas and medulloblastoma. Brain Pathol 1, 12–18.

Black, K.L., Chen, K., Becker, D.P., and Merrill, J.E. 1992. Inflammatory leukocytes associated with increased immunosuppression by glioblastoma. J Neurosurg 77, 120–126.

Bode, A.M., and Dong, Z. 2002. The paradox of arsenic: molecular mechanisms of cell transformation and chemotherapeutic effects. Crit Rev Oncol Hematol 42, 5–24.

Bogler, O., and Mikkelsen, T. 2005. Angiogenesis and apoptosis in glioma: two arenas for promising new therapies. J Cell Biochem 96, 16–24.

Brantley, E.C., and Benveniste, E.N. 2008. Signal transducer and activator of transcription-3: a molecular hub for signaling pathways in gliomas. Mol Cancer Res 6, 675–684.

Brantley, E.C., Nabors, L.B., Gillespie, G.Y., Choi, Y.H., Palmer, C.A., Harrison, K., Roarty, K., and Benveniste, E.N. 2008. Loss of protein inhibitors of activated STAT-3 expression in glioblastoma multiforme tumors: implications for STAT-3 activation and gene expression. Clin Cancer Res 14, 4694–4704.

Brat, D.J., Bellail, A.C., and Van Meir, E.G. 2005. The role of interleukin-8 and its receptors in gliomagenesis and tumoral angiogenesis. Neuro Oncol 7, 122–133.

Bredel, M., Bredel, C., Juric, D., Duran, G.E., Yu, R.X., Harsh, G.R., Vogel, H., Recht, L.D., Scheck, A.C., and Sikic, B.I. 2006. Tumor necrosis factor-alpha-induced protein 3 as a putative regulator of nuclear factor-kappaB-mediated resistance to O6-alkylating agents in human glioblastomas. J Clin Oncol 24, 274–287.

Buschges, R., Weber, R.G., Actor, B., Lichter, P., Collins, V.P., and Reifenberger, G. 1999. Amplification and expression of cyclin D genes (CCND1, CCND2 and CCND3) in human malignant gliomas. Brain Pathol 9, 435–442; discussion 432–433.

Cavalla, P., Dutto, A., Piva, R., Richiardi, P., Grosso, R., and Schiffer, D. 1998. Cyclin D1 expression in gliomas. Acta Neuropathol 95, 131–135.

Chen, W., Lee, J., Cho, S.Y., and Fine, H.A. 2004. Proteasome-mediated destruction of the cyclin a/cyclin-dependent kinase 2 complex suppresses tumor cell growth in vitro and in vivo. Cancer Res 64, 3949–3957.

Cinque, S., Willems, J., Depraetere, S., Vermeire, L., and Joniau, M. 1992. "In vitro" effect of interleukin-1 beta on human glioma cell lines: regulation of cell proliferation and IL-6 production. Immunol Lett 34, 267–271.

Conti, A., Ageunnouz, M., La Torre, D., Cardali, S., Angileri, F.F., Buemi, C., Tomasello, C., Iacopino, D.G., D'Avella, D., Vita, G., et al. 2005. Expression of the tumor necrosis factor receptor-associated factors 1 and 2 and regulation of the NF-κB antiapoptotic activity in human gliomas. J Neurosurg 103, 873–881.

Cusack, J.C., Jr., Liu, R., Houston, M., Abendroth, K., Elliott, P.J., Adams, J., and Baldwin, A.S., Jr. 2001. Enhanced chemosensitivity to CPT-11 with proteasome inhibitor PS-341: implications for systemic NF-κB inhibition. Cancer Res 61, 3535–3540.

Dai, M.S., Jin, Y., Gallegos, J.R., and Lu, H. 2006. Balance of Yin and Yang: ubiquitylation-mediated regulation of p53 and c-Myc. Neoplasia 8, 630–644.

Danial, N.N., and Korsmeyer, S.J. 2004. Cell death: critical control points. Cell 116, 205–219.
Desbaillets, I., Diserens, A.C., de Tribolet, N., Hamou, M.F., and Van Meir, E.G. 1999. Regulation of interleukin-8 expression by reduced oxygen pressure in human glioblastoma. Oncogene 18, 1447–1456.
Desbaillets, I., Tada, M., de Tribolet, N., Diserens, A.C., Hamou, M.F., and Van Meir, E.G. 1994. Human astrocytomas and glioblastomas express monocyte chemoattractant protein-1 (MCP-1) in vivo and in vitro. Int J Cancer 58, 240–247.
Dey, N., Durden, D.L., and Van Meir, E.G. (2006). Cytokine expression and signaling in CNS tumors. *Cytokines and the CNS II*, (E.N. Benveniste, and R.M. Ransohoff, Editors) (CRC Press), pp. 193–242.
Ding, Q., Huo, L., Yang, J.Y., Xia, W., Wei, Y., Liao, Y., Chang, C.J., Yang, Y., Lai, C.C., Lee, D.F., et al. 2008. Down-regulation of myeloid cell leukemia-1 through inhibiting Erk/Pin 1 pathway by sorafenib facilitates chemosensitization in breast cancer. Cancer Res 68, 6109–6117.
Doyon, Y., Cayrou, C., Ullah, M., Landry, A.J., Cote, V., Selleck, W., Lane, W.S., Tan, S., Yang, X.J., and Cote, J. 2006. ING tumor suppressor proteins are critical regulators of chromatin acetylation required for genome expression and perpetuation. Mol Cell 21, 51–64.
Ehrmann, J., Jr., Kolar, Z., Vojtesek, B., Kala, M., Komenda, S., and Oulton, A. 1997. Prognostic factors in astrocytomas: relationship of p53, MDM-2, BCL-2 and PCNA immunohistochemical expression to tumor grade and overall patient survival. Neoplasma 44, 299–304.
Esteller, M., Cordon-Cardo, C., Corn, P.G., Meltzer, S.J., Pohar, K.S., Watkins, D.N., Capella, G., Peinado, M.A., Matias-Guiu, X., Prat, J., et al. 2001. p14ARF silencing by promoter hypermethylation mediates abnormal intracellular localization of MDM2. Cancer Res 61, 2816–2821.
Fan, X., Aalto, Y., Sanko, S.G., Knuutila, S., Klatzmann, D., and Castresana, J.S. 2002. Genetic profile, PTEN mutation and therapeutic role of PTEN in glioblastomas. Int J Oncol 21, 1141–1150.
Fribley, A., and Wang, C.Y. 2006. Proteasome inhibitor induces apoptosis through induction of endoplasmic reticulum stress. Cancer Biol Ther 5, 745–748.
Fulci, G., Labuhn, M., Maier, D., Lachat, Y., Hausmann, O., Hegi, M.E., Janzer, R.C., Merlo, A., and Van Meir, E.G. 2000. p53 gene mutation and ink4a-arf deletion appear to be two mutually exclusive events in human glioblastoma. Oncogene 19, 3816–3822.
Fulda, S., Wick, W., Weller, M., and Debatin, K.M. 2002. Smac agonists sensitize for Apo2L/TRAIL- or anticancer drug-induced apoptosis and induce regression of malignant glioma in vivo. Nat Med 8, 808–815.
Garkavtsev, I., Kozin, S.V., Chernova, O., Xu, L., Winkler, F., Brown, E., Barnett, G.H., and Jain, R.K. 2004. The candidate tumour suppressor protein ING4 regulates brain tumour growth and angiogenesis. Nature 428, 328–332.
Ghosh, S., and Karin, M. 2002. Missing pieces in the NF-κB puzzle. Cell 109 Suppl, S81–96.
Gill, J.S., Zhu, X., Moore, M.J., Lu, L., Yaszemski, M.J., and Windebank, A.J. 2002. Effects of NFkappaB decoy oligonucleotides released from biodegradable polymer microparticles on a glioblastoma cell line. Biomaterials 23, 2773–2781.
Gilmore, T. 2008. www.NF-kB.org.
Goswami, S., Gupta, A., and Sharma, S.K. 1998. Interleukin-6-mediated autocrine growth promotion in human glioblastoma multiforme cell line U87MG. J Neurochem 71, 1837–1845.
Green, D.R. 2003. Overview: apoptotic signaling pathways in the immune system. Immunol Rev 193, 5–9.
Hayden, M.S., and Ghosh, S. 2008. Shared principles in NF-κB signaling. Cell 132, 344–362.
Holland, E.C. 2000. A mouse model for glioma: biology, pathology, and therapeutic opportunities. Toxicol Pathol 28, 171–177.

Huang, S., Robinson, J.B., Deguzman, A., Bucana, C.D., and Fidler, I.J. 2000. Blockade of NF-κB signaling inhibits angiogenesis and tumorigenicity of human ovarian cancer cells by suppressing expression of vascular endothelial growth factor and interleukin 8. Cancer Res 60, 5334–5339.

Hunter, A.M., LaCasse, E.C., and Korneluk, R.G. 2007. The inhibitors of apoptosis (IAPs) as cancer targets. Apoptosis 12, 1543–1568.

Hussain, S.F., Yang, D., Suki, D., Aldape, K., Grimm, E., and Heimberger, A.B. 2006. The role of human glioma-infiltrating microglia/macrophages in mediating antitumor immune responses. Neuro Oncol 8, 261–279.

Ishii, N., Maier, D., Merlo, A., Tada, M., Sawamura, Y., Diserens, A.C., and Van Meir, E.G. 1999. Frequent co-alterations of TP53, p16/CDKN2A, p14ARF, PTEN tumor suppressor genes in human glioma cell lines. Brain Pathol 9, 469–479.

Ito, C.Y., Kazantsev, A.G., and Baldwin, A.S., Jr. 1994. Three NF-κB sites in the IκB-alpha promoter are required for induction of gene expression by TNF alpha. Nucleic Acids Res 22, 3787–3792.

Ivanchuk, S.M., Mondal, S., Dirks, P.B., and Rutka, J.T. 2001. The INK4A/ARF locus: role in cell cycle control and apoptosis and implications for glioma growth. J Neurooncol 51, 219–229.

Jang, H.D., Yoon, K., Shin, Y.J., Kim, J., and Lee, S.Y. 2004. PIAS3 suppresses NF-κB-mediated transcription by interacting with the p65/RelA subunit. J Biol Chem 279, 24873–24880.

Jiang, B.H., and Liu, L.Z. 2008. PI3K/PTEN signaling in tumorigenesis and angiogenesis. Biochim Biophys Acta 1784, 150–158.

Julien, T., Frankel, B., Longo, S., Kyle, M., Gibson, S., Shillitoe, E., and Ryken, T. 2000. Antisense-mediated inhibition of the bcl-2 gene induces apoptosis in human malignant glioma. Surg Neurol 53, 360–368; discussion 368–369.

Kardosh, A., Golden, E.B., Pyrko, P., Uddin, J., Hofman, F.M., Chen, T.C., Louie, S.G., Petasis, N.A., and Schonthal, A.H. 2008. Aggravated endoplasmic reticulum stress as a basis for enhanced glioblastoma cell killing by bortezomib in combination with celecoxib or its non-coxib analogue, 2,5-dimethyl-celecoxib. Cancer Res 68, 843–851.

Keifer, J.A., Guttridge, D.C., Ashburner, B.P., and Baldwin, A.S., Jr. 2001. Inhibition of NF-κB activity by thalidomide through suppression of IκB kinase activity. J Biol Chem 276, 22382–22387.

Kim, H.J., Hawke, N., and Baldwin, A.S. 2006. NF-κB and IKK as therapeutic targets in cancer. Cell Death Differ 13, 738–747.

Kim, S. 2005. HuntING4 new tumor suppressors. Cell Cycle 4, 516–517.

Kim, S., Chin, K., Gray, J.W., and Bishop, J.M. 2004. A screen for genes that suppress loss of contact inhibition: identification of ING4 as a candidate tumor suppressor gene in human cancer. Proc Natl Acad Sci U S A 101, 16251–16256.

Kirsch, M., Schackert, G., and Black, P.M. 2000. Anti-angiogenic treatment strategies for malignant brain tumors. J Neurooncol 50, 149–163.

Kitamura, K., Kiyoi, H., Yoshida, H., Tobita, T., Takeshita, A., Ohno, R., and Naoe, T. 1997. New retinoids and arsenic compounds for the treatment of refractory acute promyelocytic leukemia: clinical and basic studies for the next generation. Cancer Chemother Pharmacol 40 Suppl, S36–41.

Koschny, R., Holland, H., Sykora, J., Haas, T.L., Sprick, M.R., Ganten, T.M., Krupp, W., Bauer, M., Ahnert, P., Meixensberger, J., et al. 2007. Bortezomib sensitizes primary human astrocytoma cells of WHO grades I to IV for tumor necrosis factor-related apoptosis-inducing ligand-induced apoptosis. Clin Cancer Res 13, 3403–3412.

Krajewski, S., Krajewska, M., Ehrmann, J., Sikorska, M., Lach, B., Chatten, J., and Reed, J.C. 1997. Immunohistochemical analysis of Bcl-2, Bcl-X, Mcl-1, and Bax in tumors of central and peripheral nervous system origin. Am J Pathol 150, 805–814.

Kuo, M.T., Liu, Z., Wei, Y., Lin-Lee, Y.C., Tatebe, S., Mills, G.B., and Unate, H. 2002. Induction of human MDR1 gene expression by 2-acetylaminofluorene is mediated by

effectors of the phosphoinositide 3-kinase pathway that activate NF-kappaB signaling. Oncogene 21, 1945–1954.
Lamkanfi, M., Declercq, W., Vanden Berghe, T., and Vandenabeele, P. 2006. Caspases leave the beaten track: caspase-mediated activation of NF-κB. J Cell Biol 173, 165–171.
LaRocca, R.V., Rosenblum, M., Westermark, B., and Israel, M.A. 1989. Patterns of proto-oncogene expression in human glioma cell lines. J Neurosci Res 24, 97–106.
Lashinger, L.M., Zhu, K., Williams, S.A., Shrader, M., Dinney, C.P., and McConkey, D.J. 2005. Bortezomib abolishes tumor necrosis factor-related apoptosis-inducing ligand resistance via a p21-dependent mechanism in human bladder and prostate cancer cells. Cancer Res 65, 4902–4908.
Lawson, H.C., Sampath, P., Bohan, E., Park, M.C., Hussain, N., Olivi, A., Weingart, J., Kleinberg, L., and Brem, H. 2007. Interstitial chemotherapy for malignant gliomas: the Johns Hopkins experience. J Neurooncol 83, 61–70.
Lee, C.H., Jeon, Y.T., Kim, S.H., and Song, Y.S. 2007. NF-κB as a potential molecular target for cancer therapy. Biofactors 29, 19–35.
Leung, S.Y., Wong, M.P., Chung, L.P., Chan, A.S., and Yuen, S.T. 1997. Monocyte chemoattractant protein-1 expression and macrophage infiltration in gliomas. Acta Neuropathol 93, 518–527.
Levine, A.J. 1997. p53, the cellular gatekeeper for growth and division. Cell 88, 323–331.
Li, L., Gondi, C.S., Dinh, D.H., Olivero, W.C., Gujrati, M., and Rao, J.S. 2007. Transfection with anti-p65 intrabody suppresses invasion and angiogenesis in glioma cells by blocking NF-κB transcriptional activity. Clin Cancer Res 13, 2178–2190.
Li, L., Thomas, R.M., Suzuki, H., De Brabander, J.K., Wang, X., and Harran, P.G. 2004. A small molecule Smac mimic potentiates TRAIL- and TNFalpha-mediated cell death. Science 305, 1471–1474.
Liao, D.J., Thakur, A., Wu, J., Biliran, H., and Sarkar, F.H. 2007. Perspectives on c-Myc, Cyclin D1, and their interaction in cancer formation, progression, and response to chemotherapy. Crit Rev Oncog 13, 93–158.
Lin, T.H., Kuo, H.C., Chou, F.P., and Lu, F.J. 2008. Berberine enhances inhibition of glioma tumor cell migration and invasiveness mediated by arsenic trioxide. BMC Cancer 8, 58.
Liou, Y.C., Ryo, A., Huang, H.K., Lu, P.J., Bronson, R., Fujimori, F., Uchida, T., Hunter, T., and Lu, K.P. 2002. Loss of Pin1 function in the mouse causes phenotypes resembling cyclin D1-null phenotypes. Proc Natl Acad Sci U S A 99, 1335–1340.
Liu, G.Y., Frank, N., Bartsch, H., and Lin, J.K. 1998. Induction of apoptosis by thiuramdisulfides, the reactive metabolites of dithiocarbamates, through coordinative modulation of NF-κB, c-fos/c-jun, and p53 proteins. Mol Carcinog 22, 235–246.
Lu, K.P., Suizu, F., Zhou, X.Z., Finn, G., Lam, P., and Wulf, G. 2006. Targeting carcinogenesis: a role for the prolyl isomerase Pin1? Mol Carcinog 45, 397–402.
Majumdar, S., Lamothe, B., and Aggarwal, B.B. 2002. Thalidomide suppresses NF-κB activation induced by TNF and H2O2, but not that activated by ceramide, lipopolysaccharides, or phorbol ester. J Immunol 168, 2644–2651.
Marikovsky, M., Nevo, N., Vadai, E., and Harris-Cerruti, C. 2002. Cu/Zn superoxide dismutase plays a role in angiogenesis. Int J Cancer 97, 34–41.
Mischel, P.S., and Cloughesy, T.F. 2003. Targeted molecular therapy of GBM. Brain Pathol 13, 52–61.
Munoz-Fernandez, M.A., Armas-Portela, R., Diaz-Nido, J., Alonso, J.L., Fresno, M., and Avila, J. 1991. Differential effects of tumor necrosis factor on the growth and differentiation of neuroblastoma and glioma cells. Exp Cell Res 194, 161–164.
Nakanishi, C., and Toi, M. 2005. NF-κB inhibitors as sensitizers to anticancer drugs. Nat Rev Cancer 5, 297–309.
Nawrocki, S.T., Carew, J.S., Dunner, K., Jr., Boise, L.H., Chiao, P.J., Huang, P., Abbruzzese, J.L., and McConkey, D.J. 2005a. Bortezomib inhibits PKR-like endoplasmic reticulum

(ER) kinase and induces apoptosis via ER stress in human pancreatic cancer cells. Cancer Res 65, 11510–11519.

Nawrocki, S.T., Carew, J.S., Pino, M.S., Highshaw, R.A., Dunner, K., Jr., Huang, P., Abbruzzese, J.L., and McConkey, D.J. 2005b. Bortezomib sensitizes pancreatic cancer cells to endoplasmic reticulum stress-mediated apoptosis. Cancer Res 65, 11658–11666.

Nozell, S., Laver, T., Moseley, D., Nowoslawski, L., DeVos, M., Atkinson, G.P., Harrison, K., Nabors, L.B., and Benveniste, E.N. 2008. The ING4 tumor suppressor attenuates NF-κB activity at the promoter of target genes. Mol Cell Biol 28, 6632–6645.

Nozell, S., Laver, T., Patel, K., and Benveniste, E.N. 2006. Mechanism of IFN-beta-mediated inhibition of IL-8 gene expression in astroglioma cells. J Immunol 177, 822–830.

Ohgaki, H., and Kleihues, P. 2007. Genetic pathways to primary and secondary glioblastoma. Am J Pathol 170, 1445–1453.

Okada, H., and Mak, T.W. 2004. Pathways of apoptotic and non-apoptotic death in tumour cells. Nat Rev Cancer 4, 592–603.

Olivier, S., Robe, P., and Bours, V. 2006. Can NF-κB be a target for novel and efficient anti-cancer agents? Biochem Pharmacol 72, 1054–1068.

Pacifico, F., and Leonardi, A. 2006. NF-κB in solid tumors. Biochem Pharmacol 72, 1142–1152.

Panner, A., James, C.D., Berger, M.S., and Pieper, R.O. 2005. mTOR controls FLIPS translation and TRAIL sensitivity in glioblastoma multiforme cells. Mol Cell Biol 25, 8809–8823.

Perkins, N.D. 2004. Regulation of NF-κB by atypical activators and tumour suppressors. Biochem Soc Trans 32, 936–939.

Psaila, B., Kaplan, R.N., Port, E.R., and Lyden, D. 2006. Priming the 'soil' for breast cancer metastasis: the pre-metastatic niche. Breast Dis 26, 65–74.

Puduvalli, V.K., Giglio, P., Groves, M.D., Hess, K.R., Gilbert, M.R., Mahankali, S., Jackson, E.F., Levin, V.A., Conrad, C.A., Hsu, S.H., et al. 2008. Phase II trial of irinotecan and thalidomide in adults with recurrent glioblastoma multiforme. Neuro Oncol 10, 216–222.

Rasheed, B.K., and Bigner, S.H. 1991. Genetic alterations in glioma and medulloblastoma. Cancer Metastasis Rev 10, 289–299.

Ravi, R., and Bedi, A. 2004. NF-κB in cancer–a friend turned foe. Drug Resist Updat 7, 53–67.

Ren, H., Yang, B.F., and Rainov, N.G. 2007. Receptor tyrosine kinases as therapeutic targets in malignant glioma. Rev Recent Clin Trials 2, 87–101.

Rieger, J., Frank, B., Weller, M., and Wick, W. 2007. Mechanisms of resistance of human glioma cells to Apo2 ligand/TNF-related apoptosis-inducing ligand. Cell Physiol Biochem 20, 23–34.

Rieger, L., Weller, M., Bornemann, A., Schabet, M., Dichgans, J., and Meyermann, R. 1998. BCL-2 family protein expression in human malignant glioma: a clinical-pathological correlative study. J Neurol Sci 155, 68–75.

Robe, P.A., Bentires-Alj, M., Bonif, M., Rogister, B., Deprez, M., Haddada, H., Khac, M.T., Jolois, O., Erkmen, K., Merville, M.P., et al. 2004. In vitro and in vivo activity of the NF-κB inhibitor sulfasalazine in human glioblastomas. Clin Cancer Res 10, 5595–5603.

Robe, P.A., Martin, D., Albert, A., Deprez, M., Chariot, A., and Bours, V. 2006. A phase 1–2, prospective, double blind, randomized study of the safety and efficacy of Sulfasalazine for the treatment of progressing malignant gliomas: study protocol of [ISRCTN45828668]. BMC Cancer 6, 29.

Roberts, J.M., and Sherr, C.J. 2003. Bared essentials of CDK2 and cyclin E. Nat Genet 35, 9–10.

Robson, S., Pelengaris, S., and Khan, M. 2006. c-Myc and downstream targets in the pathogenesis and treatment of cancer. Recent Patents Anticancer Drug Discov 1, 305–326.

Rocha, S., Garrett, M.D., Campbell, K.J., Schumm, K., and Perkins, N.D. 2005. Regulation of NF-κB and p53 through activation of ATR and Chk1 by the ARF tumour suppressor. Embo J 24, 1157–1169.

Rocha, S., and Perkins, N.D. 2005. ARF the integrator: linking NF-κB, p53 and checkpoint kinases. Cell Cycle 4, 756–759.
Ryo, A., Hirai, A., Nishi, M., Liou, Y.C., Perrem, K., Lin, S.C., Hirano, H., Lee, S.W., and Aoki, I. 2007. A suppressive role of the prolyl isomerase Pin1 in cellular apoptosis mediated by the death-associated protein Daxx. J Biol Chem 282, 36671–36681.
Ryo, A., Liou, Y.C., Lu, K.P., and Wulf, G. 2003a. Prolyl isomerase Pin1: a catalyst for oncogenesis and a potential therapeutic target in cancer. J Cell Sci 116, 773–783.
Ryo, A., Liou, Y.C., Wulf, G., Nakamura, M., Lee, S.W., and Lu, K.P. 2002. PIN1 is an E2F target gene essential for Neu/Ras-induced transformation of mammary epithelial cells. Mol Cell Biol 22, 5281–5295.
Ryo, A., Suizu, F., Yoshida, Y., Perrem, K., Liou, Y.C., Wulf, G., Rottapel, R., Yamaoka, S., and Lu, K.P. 2003b. Regulation of NF-κB signaling by Pin1-dependent prolyl isomerization and ubiquitin-mediated proteolysis of p65/RelA. Mol Cell 12, 1413–1426.
Sampaio, E.P., Sarno, E.N., Galilly, R., Cohn, Z.A., and Kaplan, G. 1991. Thalidomide selectively inhibits tumor necrosis factor alpha production by stimulated human monocytes. J Exp Med 173, 699–703.
Sauna, Z.E., Shukla, S., and Ambudkar, S.V. 2005. Disulfiram, an old drug with new potential therapeutic uses for human cancers and fungal infections. Mol Biosyst 1, 127–134.
Sawyer, A.J., Piepmeier, J.M., and Saltzman, W.M. 2006. New methods for direct delivery of chemotherapy for treating brain tumors. Yale J Biol Med 79, 141–152.
Schneider, J., Hofman, F.M., Apuzzo, M.L., and Hinton, D.R. 1992. Cytokines and immunoregulatory molecules in malignant glial neoplasms. J Neurosurg 77, 265–273.
Sethi, G., Sung, B., and Aggarwal, B.B. 2008. NF-κB activation: from bench to bedside. Exp Biol Med (Maywood) 233, 21–31.
Sherr, C.J. 2000. Cell cycle control and cancer. Harvey Lect 96, 73–92.
Sherr, C.J. 2006. Divorcing ARF and p53: an unsettled case. Nat Rev Cancer 6, 663–673.
Sherr, C.J., and Roberts, J.M. 2004. Living with or without cyclins and cyclin-dependent kinases. Genes Dev 18, 2699–2711.
Shiseki, M., Nagashima, M., Pedeux, R.M., Kitahama-Shiseki, M., Miura, K., Okamura, S., Onogi, H., Higashimoto, Y., Appella, E., Yokota, J., et al. 2003. p29ING4 and p28ING5 bind to p53 and p300, and enhance p53 activity. Cancer Res 63, 2373–2378.
Shuai, K. 2006. Regulation of cytokine signaling pathways by PIAS proteins. Cell Res 16, 196–202.
Shuai, K., and Liu, B. 2005. Regulation of gene-activation pathways by PIAS proteins in the immune system. Nat Rev Immunol 5, 593–605.
Steinbach, J.P., and Weller, M. 2004. Apoptosis in gliomas: molecular mechanisms and therapeutic implications. J Neurooncol 70, 245–254.
Takahashi, K., Akiyama, H., Shimazaki, K., Uchida, C., Akiyama-Okunuki, H., Tomita, M., Fukumoto, M., and Uchida, T. 2007. Ablation of a peptidyl prolyl isomerase Pin1 from p53-null mice accelerated thymic hyperplasia by increasing the level of the intracellular form of Notch1. Oncogene 26, 3835–3845.
The Cancer Genome Atlas Research Network, McLendon, R., Friedman, A., Bigner, D., Van Meir, E.G., Brat, D.J., Mastrogianakis, M., Olson, J.J., Mikkelsen, T., Lehman, N., Aldape, K., et al. 2008. Comprehensive genomic characterization defines human glioblastoma genes and core pathways. Nature.
Tsunoda, K., Kitange, G., Anda, T., Shabani, H.K., Kaminogo, M., Shibata, S., and Nagata, I. 2005. Expression of the constitutively activated RelA/NF-κB in human astrocytic tumors and the in vitro implication in the regulation of urokinase-type plasminogen activator, migration, and invasion. Brain Tumor Pathol 22, 79–87.
Uhrbom, L., Dai, C., Celestino, J.C., Rosenblum, M.K., Fuller, G.N., and Holland, E.C. 2002. Ink4a-Arf loss cooperates with KRas activation in astrocytes and neural progenitors to generate glioblastomas of various morphologies depending on activated Akt. Cancer Res 62, 5551–5558.

Van Meir, E., Sawamura, Y., Diserens, A.C., Hamou, M.F., and de Tribolet, N. 1990. Human glioblastoma cells release interleukin 6 in vivo and in vitro. Cancer Res 50, 6683–6688.

Van Waes, C. 2007. NF-κB in development, prevention, and therapy of cancer. Clin Cancer Res 13, 1076–1082.

Wang, C.Y., Mayo, M.W., and Baldwin, A.S., Jr. 1996. TNF- and cancer therapy-induced apoptosis: potentiation by inhibition of NF-κB. Science 274, 784–787.

Wang, C.Y., Mayo, M.W., Korneluk, R.G., Goeddel, D.V., and Baldwin, A.S., Jr. 1998. NF-κB antiapoptosis: induction of TRAF1 and TRAF2 and c-IAP1 and c-IAP2 to suppress caspase-8 activation. Science 281, 1680–1683.

Wang, H., Zhang, W., Huang, H.J., Liao, W.S., and Fuller, G.N. 2004. Analysis of the activation status of Akt, NF-κB, and Stat3 in human diffuse gliomas. Lab Invest 84, 941–951.

Wasson, J.C., Saylors, R.L., 3rd, Zeltzer, P., Friedman, H.S., Bigner, S.H., Burger, P.C., Bigner, D.D., Look, A.T., Douglass, E.C., and Brodeur, G.M. 1990. Oncogene amplification in pediatric brain tumors. Cancer Res 50, 2987–2990.

Weaver, K.D., Yeyeodu, S., Cusack, J.C., Jr., Baldwin, A.S., Jr., and Ewend, M.G. 2003. Potentiation of chemotherapeutic agents following antagonism of NF-κB in human gliomas. J Neurooncol 61, 187–196.

Wei, Y., Fan, T., and Yu, M. 2008. Inhibitor of apoptosis proteins and apoptosis. Acta Biochim Biophys Sin (Shanghai) 40, 278–288.

Weissenberger, J., Loeffler, S., Kappeler, A., Kopf, M., Lukes, A., Afanasieva, T.A., Aguzzi, A., and Weis, J. 2004. IL-6 is required for glioma development in a mouse model. Oncogene 23, 3308–3316.

Wu, Z.H., and Miyamoto, S. 2007. Many faces of NF-κB signaling induced by genotoxic stress. J Mol Med 85, 1187–1202.

Xiao, C., Yang, B.F., Asadi, N., Beguinot, F., and Hao, C. 2002. Tumor necrosis factor-related apoptosis-inducing ligand-induced death-inducing signaling complex and its modulation by c-FLIP and PED/PEA-15 in glioma cells. J Biol Chem 277, 25020–25025.

Xiao, G., Rabson, A.B., Young, W., Qing, G., and Qu, Z. 2006. Alternative pathways of NF-κB activation: a double-edged sword in health and disease. Cytokine Growth Factor Rev 17, 281–293.

Xu, S., Bayat, H., Hou, X., and Jiang, B. 2006. Ribosomal S6 kinase-1 modulates interleukin-1beta-induced persistent activation of NF-κB through phosphorylation of IκBbeta. Am J Physiol Cell Physiol 291, C1336–1345.

Yan, C., and Boyd, D.D. 2007. Regulation of matrix metalloproteinase gene expression. J Cell Physiol 211, 19–26.

Yin, D., Zhou, H., Kumagai, T., Liu, G., Ong, J.M., Black, K.L., and Koeffler, H.P. 2005. Proteasome inhibitor PS-341 causes cell growth arrest and apoptosis in human glioblastoma multiforme (GBM). Oncogene 24, 344–354.

Yu, C., Friday, B.B., Lai, J.P., Yang, L., Sarkaria, J., Kay, N.E., Carter, C.A., Roberts, L.R., Kaufmann, S.H., and Adjei, A.A. 2006. Cytotoxic synergy between the multikinase inhibitor sorafenib and the proteasome inhibitor bortezomib in vitro: induction of apoptosis through Akt and c-Jun NH2-terminal kinase pathways. Mol Cancer Ther 5, 2378–2387.

Zhang, X., Xu, L.S., Wang, Z.Q., Wang, K.S., Li, N., Cheng, Z.H., Huang, S.Z., Wei, D.Z., and Han, Z.G. 2004. ING4 induces G2/M cell cycle arrest and enhances the chemosensitivity to DNA-damage agents in HepG2 cells. FEBS Lett 570, 7–12.

Zhang, X., Zhao, M., Huang, A.Y., Fei, Z., Zhang, W., and Wang, X.L. 2005. The effect of cyclin D expression on cell proliferation in human gliomas. J Clin Neurosci 12, 166–168.

Zustovich, F., Cartei, G., Ceravolo, R., Zovato, S., Della Puppa, A., Pastorelli, D., Mattiazzi, M., Bertorelle, R., and Gardiman, M.P. 2007. A phase I study of cisplatin, temozolomide and thalidomide in patients with malignant brain tumors. Anticancer Res 27, 1019–1024.

Chapter 43
Targeting Endoplasmic Reticulum Stress for Malignant Glioma Therapy

Peter Pyrko, Axel H. Schönthal, and Thomas C. Chen

Abstract The endoplasmic reticulum stress response (ESR) is essential for maintaining cellular homeostasis in response to noxious internal and external stimuli. In malignant gliomas, ESR is induced by a low nutrient, hypoxic microenvironment, compounded by external chemotherapy and radiation therapy. Powerful protective mechanisms, including induction of the ER chaperone glucose-regulated protein 78 (GRP78), protect the glioma cells from undergoing apoptosis. This chapter reviews the ESR and how it may be modulated to induce apoptosis in malignant gliomas. Downregulation of protective mechanisms such as GRP78 may be obtained with drugs such as the green tea extract epigallocatechin gallate (EGCG), leading to increased apoptosis when glioma cells are treated with the chemotherapeutic agent temozolomide (TMZ). Conversely, glioma apoptosis may also be induced by increasing ER stress to overwhelming levels with inhibitors of sarcoplasmic/ER calcium ATPase (SERCA) such as celecoxib and dimethyl-celecoxib. Protease inhibitors such as nelfinavir also inhibit proteasome activity, leading to accumulation of misfolded proteins, triggering ER stress. These modulations of the ESR may thus lead to chemotherapy or radiation sensitization of malignant gliomas. Further understanding of the ESR in glioma cells may lead to new treatments for this currently incurable cancer.

Keywords Endoplasmic reticulum · Malignant gliomas · Celecoxib · DMC · Protease inhibitors · CHOP · GRP78

Contents

T.C. Chen (✉)
Department of Neurosurgery, University of Southern California Keck School of Medicine, 1200 N State St #5046, Los Angeles, CA 90033, USA
e-mail: tchen68670@aol.com

E.G. Van Meir (ed.), *CNS Cancer*, Cancer Drug Discovery and Development, DOI 10.1007/978-1-60327-553-8_43,

© Humana Press, a part of Springer Science+Business Media, LLC 2009

43.1 Introduction

Malignant gliomas are the most commonly diagnosed malignant adult primary brain tumors and include anaplastic astrocytoma (WHO Grade III) as well as glioblastoma multiforme (GBM; Grade IV). Median survival for GBM is approximately 12–15 months. Surgical resection or diagnostic biopsy is usually the first step of therapy, followed by adjuvant radiation and chemotherapy (Stupp et al., 2006). Despite significant improvements in surgical treatments, a complete resection is difficult to achieve secondary to diffuse brain invasion by tumor cells, which may be found at great distances from the site of the primary tumor, including the contralateral hemisphere (Hentschel and Lang, 2003). Chemotherapy with methylating agents, i.e., nitrosoureas and temozolomide, has only a slight impact on survival and is usually more effective in patients whose tumors show epigenetic silencing of the gene encoding O^6-methylguanine DNA-methyltransferase (MGMT). Lack of MGMT activity leads to compromised DNA repair and sensitivity to alkylating agents (van den Bent et al., 2006). Radiation treatment of the tumor and the tumor resection cavity by itself increases patients' survival, albeit only by a few months (Friedman and Bigner, 2005). Even the combination of radiation therapy with temozolomide for newly diagnosed GBM adds only 2 months to the median patient survival (Stupp et al., 2005). While these treatments constitute a significant improvement in the fight against this deadly cancer, new therapies targeting novel treatment sites are highly desirable. This review summarizes experimental studies examining the role of endoplasmic reticulum (ER) stress modulation in the treatment of malignant gliomas.

43.2 ER Stress Response (ESR)

The endoplasmic reticulum (ER) is a membranous organelle, in which synthesis and modification of proteins destined for either extracellular secretion or cytoplasmic organelles (i.e., lysosomes, Golgi body) occur under an optimal environment. The ER is also an important organelle for the synthesis of lipids and sterols necessary for cell functioning, as well as storage of cellular calcium (Kaufman, 1999). The ER stress response evolved in all eukaryotic cells to ameliorate various problems that can arise within the ER during the process of protein, lipid, and sterol synthesis. It consists of a set of adaptive pathways that can be triggered by disparate perturbations in normal ER function, i.e., accumulation of misfolded proteins, lipid or glycolipid imbalances, or changes in the ionic conditions of the ER lumen (Boyce and Yuan, 2006; Wu and Kaufman, 2006). The primary purpose of the ER stress response is to restore proper ER homeostasis. In the case of intense, overwhelming, or persistent ER stress, however, these pathways may trigger programed cell death/apoptosis. Usually, early ER stress events occur at the translational apparatus (like inhibition of cellular protein synthesis), while later events consist of modifications at the gene expression level and often result in long-term adaptation or apoptosis.

One of the central pro-survival regulators of the ER stress is glucose-regulated protein 78 (GRP78 or BiP), an ER chaperone, which has important roles in protein folding and assembly, in targeting misfolded proteins for degradation, in ER Ca^{2+}-binding, and in controlling the activation of transmembrane ER stress sensors. Elevation of GRP78/BiP has been observed and described in many cancer cell lines and patient biopsy samples, correlating to cell protection from various chemotherapeutic regimens (9). The transmembrane ER stress sensors include the proteins PERK, IRE1, and ATF6. PERK [PKR (double-stranded-RNA-dependent protein kinase)-like ER kinase] is an ER transmembrane protein, which in conjunction with IRE1 (inositol-requiring enzyme 1), a type I transmembrane serine/threonine kinase/endoribonuclease, senses unfolded protein levels within the ER. ATF6 is a transcription factor, which is essential for a pro-survival response to ER perturbation from the external microenvironment. All three transmembrane proteins are regulated by GRP78, which in an unstressed ER binds to them and inhibits their activity. In response to stressful stimuli, GRP78 dissociates from these transmembrane sensors, activating them, leading to induction of the eukaryotic translation inhibition factor 2 (eIF2a), leading to inhibition of global protein synthesis (Boyce and Yuan, 2006; Wu and Kaufman, 2006). If balance within the ER can be restored, cell survival ensues. However, prolonged or overwhelming stress can lead to apoptosis with induction of CHOP (CCAAT/enhancer binding protein transcription factor), caspase 4, and caspase 7, critical executioners of the pro-apoptotic arm of the ER stress response (10, 11) (Fig. 43.1).

In this review, we will discuss how balance in the ER can be shifted from survival to death by modulating various components of the ER stress response, leading to new targets for anti-glioma therapy. First, we show how sensitivity of glioma cells to temozolomide (TMZ, Temodar) can be increased by down-regulating the ER chaperone GRP78/BiP. Second, we explore how the ER stress response can modulate calcium homeostasis, increasing death of various cancer cell lines, including malignant gliomas. Third, we demonstrate how prevention of the glioma cells' ability to degrade and synthesize proteins via protease inhibitors can be used for malignant glioma chemotherapy. Finally, we

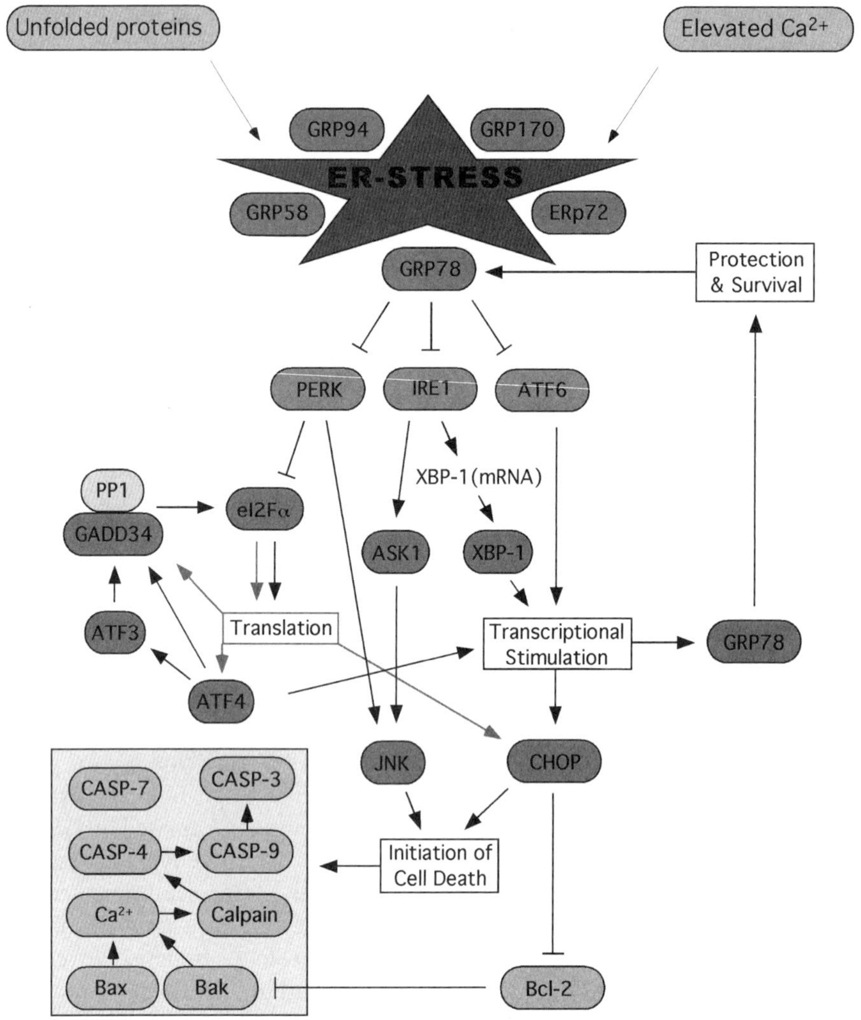

Fig. 43.1 ER stress response (ESR). The figure shows major players within the ER and their interactions. Many different stimuli activate ESR including ionic disturbances and accumulation of misfolded proteins. ER chaperones (glucose regulated proteins (GRPs) and ERp72) respond first by binding misfolded proteins and ions. Among those chaperones, GRP78 plays a crucial role in directing activation of ESR genes and modulation of protein synthesis (inhibition of general protein synthesis and activation of synthesis of ESR proteins). In an unstressed ER, GRP78 binds to transmembrane ER sensors (PERK, IRE1, ATF6) and inhibits them. In response to stressful stimuli, GRP78 dissociates from transmembrane ER sensors, which activates them. Multiple downstream pathways are turned on including eIF2a, which is responsible for inhibiting protein synthesis. Chaperones including GRP78 and other ER proteins can escape the protein synthesis inhibition and are synthesized. If balance within the ER can be restored, cell survival ensues. If the stress persists ER stress pro-apoptotic arm is activated, which includes CHOP, Caspase4 and 7. Once apoptosis is activated the cell dies. (For more detailed ER stress review see Boyce, 2006 and Wu, 2006 (Boyce and Yuan, 2006; Wu and Kaufman, 2006))

demonstrate how simultaneous targeting of various components of the ER stress response results in increased glioma cell death.

43.3 Downregulation of the ER Chaperone GRP78 Results in Increased Glioma Cell Sensitivity to Temozolomide (TMZ)

Figure 43.2 illustrates the central role of GRP78 in ESR activation (Lee, 2001). More than just a chaperone, GRP78/BiP sits on the crossroads of life and death signaling from the ER. Its actions within the ER are analogous to the function of p53 protein in regulating apoptosis due to DNA damage in the nucleus. Just like p53 is able to recognize DNA damage, inhibit DNA synthesis, and induce various genes necessary for DNA repair, GRP78/BiP senses Ca^{2+} disturbances and misfolded proteins within the ER and responds by activating mechanisms that lead to inhibition of protein synthesis and induction of transcriptional events that lead to restoration of proper ER

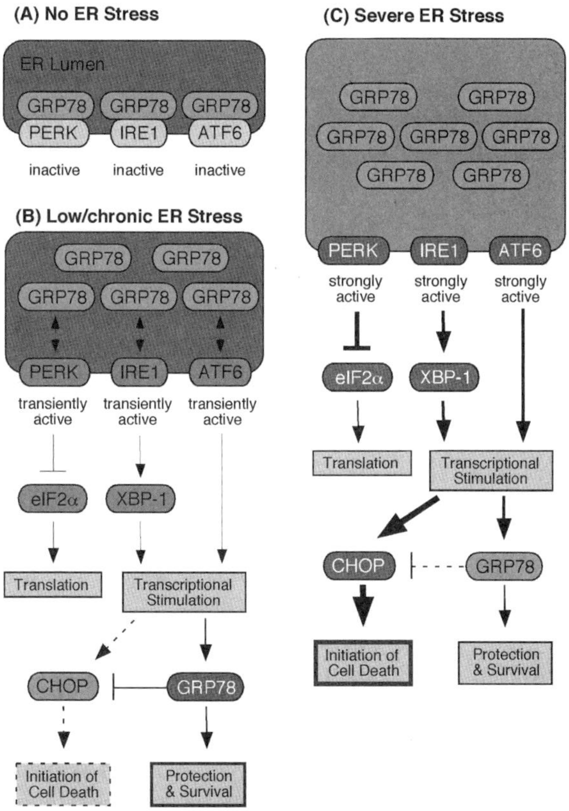

Fig. 43.2 GRP78 plays a central role in ESR activation. In a healthy cell, GRP78 is bound to ER transmembrane sensors and inhibits their function (**A**). During a low level, chronic stress GRP78 dissociates from transmembrane sensors allowing their transient activation. Translation is temporarily halted and ER stress gene activation results in cell survival (**B**). In case of severe ER stress **(C)**, GRP78 permanently dissociates from transmembrane sensors. When the protective action of ER stress response is overwhelmed, apoptosis is mediated through CHOP activation and cell death results

functioning. GRP78/BiP represents a pro-survival arm of the ER stress response. Several different studies have demonstrated that downregulating GRP78/BiP results in increased chemosensitivity. In lung cancer, increased GRP78 correlated with resistance to doxorubicin and taxol (Koomagi et al., 1999). In breast cancer, increased GRP78 correlated with resistance to doxorubicin, etoposide, and taxol (Dong et al., 2005). Similarly, we have recently demonstrated that downregulation of GRP78/BiP in glioma cells results in increased sensitivity of these cells to TMZ and may have important prognostic and therapeutic applications for glioma treatment (Pyrko et al., 2007c).

In a survey of several malignant glioma cell lines, GRP78/BiP overexpression was demonstrated, independent of p53 or PTEN status. Glioma cell lines with the fastest proliferation rates had the highest levels of GRP78 expression, and downregulation of GRP78 in two glioma cell lines with siRNA specific for GRP78 resulted in decreased proliferation rates for both cell lines. Elevation of GRP78 expression was also detected in patients' biopsies prior to adjuvant treatment. These results raise the possibility that the levels of GRP78 in patient biopsies could be used as a predictive factor of aggressiveness for GBMs, independent of their p53 and PTEN status. These findings also suggest that tumors with low GRP78 levels represent slow growing, less aggressive tumors, while those with high GRP78 are rapidly proliferating, aggressive tumors.

TMZ is currently the standard of care for treatment of both newly diagnosed and recurrent malignant gliomas. This well-tolerated drug has been shown to increase the time to tumor progression, and to prolong patient survival in patients with malignant gliomas, including GBM (Dehdashti et al., 2006). The mechanism of TMZ activity is thought to be DNA methylation on cytosines and subsequent substitution of cytosine by thymidine. This leads to activation of the mismatch repair (MMR) mechanism, which if unsuccessful in DNA repair, triggers apoptosis (Nagasubramanian and Dolan, 2003). Because chemotherapy such as TMZ induces intense cell perturbation, the ESR is triggered. We have recently demonstrated that TMZ augments the levels of GRP78 and CHOP in a concentration-dependent manner. In the same study, downregulation of GRP78 in glioma cell lines resulted in significant increase in glioma cell death in response to TMZ treatment. In addition, treatment of glioma cells with the green tea extract epigallocatechin gallate (EGCG), a known inhibitor of GRP78 function (but which does not affect GRP78 levels), also sensitized glioma cells to TMZ (Pyrko et al., 2007c). The latter discovery has important implications as EGCG is readily available as an oral supplement, allowing possible combination therapy with TMZ. Downregulation of GRP78 with siGRP78 also increased chemosensitivity of gliomas to 5-fluorouracil (5-FU) and irinotecan (CPT-11)—two chemotherapeutic agents that have been used for malignant glioma therapy in clinical trials, raising the possibility that protection by GRP78 is not TMZ specific but could constitute a general mechanism, by which glioma cells achieve protection from ER stress induced by various chemotherapeutic agents.

43.4 ER Stress Modulation of Intracellular Calcium in Malignant Gliomas

The well-balanced maintenance of intracellular calcium levels is critical for efficient cell functioning, and the fine-tuned control of various pumps and channels affecting calcium transport is important to maintain proper homeostasis (Clapham, 2007). Several avenues of investigation have explored the possibility of manipulating calcium levels pharmacologically as a means toward enhanced glioma cell killing (Yin et al., 2007). One of these approaches is being aimed at the ER, which represents the main storage space for intracellular calcium. Three major regulators of calcium flow span the ER membrane: inositol (1,4,5) trisphosphate (IP3) receptors and ryanodine receptors are primarily responsible for controlled calcium release, whereas sarcoplasmic/ER calcium ATPase (SERCA) is responsible for returning calcium back into the ER. This latter pump constitutes the critical force that establishes and maintains the steep gradient of the ion between the ER and the cytosol (Fig. 43.3).

Thapsigargin, a naturally occurring sesquiterpene lactone, is an extremely potent SERCA inhibitor, and exposure of cells to this compound causes rapid

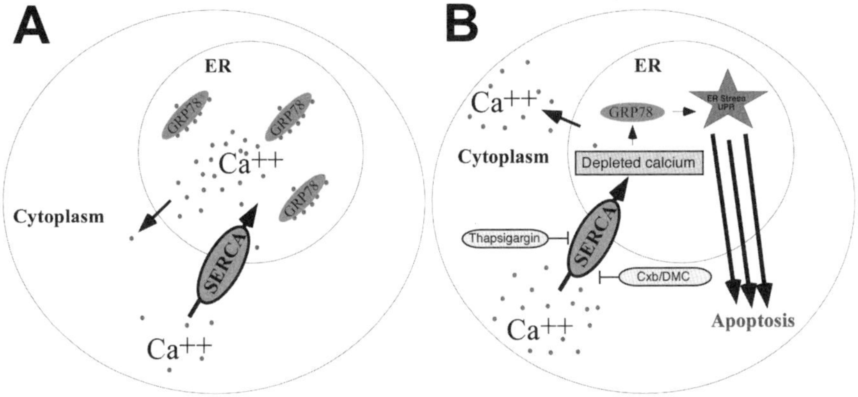

Fig. 43.3 Activation of ER stress response through inhibition of SERCA (sarcoplasmic/ER calcium ATPase). In a non-stressed cell (**A**) majority of calcium is stored in the ER. Calcium is continuously pumped into the ER by SERCA and other calcium channels. At the same time, calcium leaks out of the ER through other channels into the cytoplasm down its concentration gradient but SERCA is able to maintain high calcium concentration in the ER and low calcium concentration in the cytoplasm. In the ER, the concentration of calcium is sensed by GRP78 while it is bound to this protein. Inhibition of SERCA (**B**) leads to depletion of calcium in the ER, which when sensed by GRP78 initiates ER stress response, which when overwhelmed results in apoptosis

leakage of calcium from the ER into the cytosol (Treiman et al., 1998). This efficient depletion of ER-stored calcium represents a well-known trigger of severe ER stress and eventually leads to cell death. Studies have shown that thapsigargin evokes a much larger and faster calcium release in glioblastoma cells than in normal astrocytes, indicating the presence of a therapeutic window for glioblastoma therapy (Kovacs et al., 2005). Because thapsigargin in general is rather toxic and therefore not suitable for systemic use, pro-drug versions have been developed that allow tumor-targeted activation of this compound. Although not yet studied in glioma, such pro-drugs have shown promise in other types of cancer (Chandran et al., 2007; Denmeade et al., 2003).

Another type of SERCA inhibitor, celecoxib (Celebrex®) (Fig. 43.4), has shown efficacy in preclinical glioblastoma models and, at the same time, appears to be well tolerated. Although originally described as a selective inhibitor of cyclooxygenase-2 (COX-2) (Penning et al., 1997), celecoxib has revealed several additional biological activities that are independent of its COX-2-inhibitory quality (Schönthal, 2007). Prime among the COX-2-independent activities of this drug appears to be its ability to inhibit SERCA (Johnson et al., 2002; Pyrko et al., 2007a) (Figs. 43.3 and 43.4), and this surprising feature seems to play a critical role in the documented anti-glioma activity of celecoxib in vitro and in vivo (Chuang et al., 2008; Kang et al., 2006; Kardosh et al., 2004; Wang et al., 2006). Intriguingly, the inhibition of SERCA by celecoxib is entirely independent of the COX-2-inhibitory function, and in fact, celecoxib analogs have been synthesized that display potent SERCA inhibition in the absence of COX-2 inhibition. One such compound is 2,5-dimethyl-celecoxib (DMC) (Fig. 43.4), which faithfully mimics the SERCA-inhibitory activity of celecoxib, but does not inhibit COX-2 (Schönthal, 2006). Just like celecoxib, DMC has been shown to cause calcium leakage from the ER, which results in severe ER stress and subsequent tumor cell death (Pyrko et al., 2007a, 2008). However, because these agents are only moderately potent inhibitors of SERCA, systemic toxicity is greatly reduced and tumor-specific

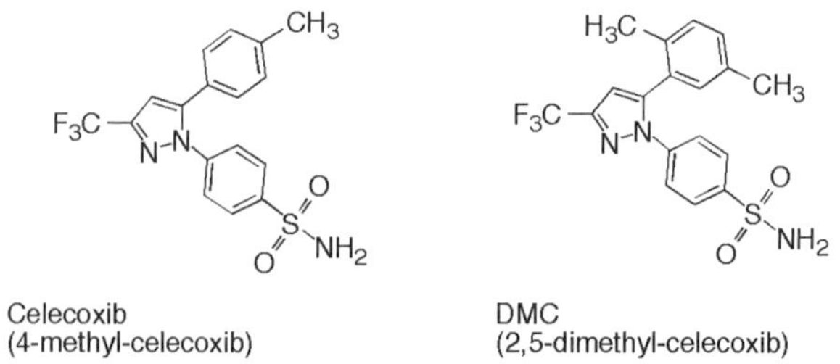

Fig. 43.4 Molecular structures of celecoxib and its non-COX-2-inhibitory analog DMC. DMC was created by adding second methyl group to the benzene ring of celecoxib. This extra group prohibits binding to COX-2 enzyme and results in a molecule, which is capable of binding SERCA but which is not a COX-2 inhibitor

characteristics of the ER stress response system can be exploited for therapeutic advantage (Schönthal, 2008). Thus, in brain tumor animal models, celecoxib and DMC have demonstrated antitumor efficacy in the absence of obvious side effects (Kardosh et al., 2008; Pyrko et al., 2007a, 2008).

When used in humans, the application of high dosages of celecoxib for extended periods of time—as would be necessitated during cancer chemotherapy—has uncovered emerging side effects that can be life-threatening, such as cardiac events, stroke, or kidney failure. It appears that these problems are due to the long-term inhibition of COX-2 and represent a "class effect" of several selective COX-2 inhibitors, including rofecoxib (Vioxx®) and valdecoxib (Bextra®) (Brophy, 2007). While this increased risk is relatively small and, considering the dire situation of cancer patients, perhaps acceptable, there might be an alternative, which comes in the form of DMC. DMC has not yet been investigated in clinical trials; however, its activity profile perhaps may be superior to celecoxib. DMC has displayed stronger antitumor effects when compared to celecoxib in various in vitro or in vivo models, and this increased potency appears to be due to its somewhat stronger inhibition of SERCA, which results in more severe ER stress and a higher rate of tumor cell death (Chuang et al., 2008; Kardosh et al., 2008; Pyrko et al., 2007a, 2008). In addition, because DMC does not inhibit COX-2, the use of this drug might avoid those side effects that are due to the long-term inhibition of this enzyme. However, this optimistic expectation is not certain and needs to be confirmed in appropriate clinical trials.

Besides SERCA, the ER transmembrane IP3 receptor has been found to be involved in the regulation of glioblastoma growth and survival. For instance, lipid-activated protein kinase B (PKB)/Akt, an antiapoptotic signaling protein that provides chemo- and radio-resistance to tumor cells, is able to phosphorylate IP3 receptors, which results in diminished calcium release activity and reduced cellular susceptibility to apoptotic stimuli (Szado et al., 2008). Because PKB/Akt is frequently found overly active in glioblastoma cells due to PTEN loss or activating mutations in PI3 kinase, this newly discovered ability to manipulate calcium levels is thought to be responsible for the recognized resistance of glioblastoma cells to various forms of therapy.

In addition to the regulation of calcium levels by PKB/Akt, there are indications of a reverse control loop where calcium levels may affect the activity of PKB/Akt. In this regard, it was demonstrated that transfection and overexpression of calreticulin, a multifunctional calcium-binding protein in the ER that is involved in intracellular signaling (Gelebart et al., 2005), was able to downregulate survival signaling of PKB/Akt, resulting in pronounced radiosensitization of glioblastoma cells (Okunaga et al., 2006). Because alterations in calcium levels may trigger ER stress, it will be important to determine whether the interdependence of PKB/Akt activity and calcium levels contributes to the low level, chronic ER stress conditions that are frequently observed in tumor cells.

43.5 Induction of ER Stress by Affecting Protein Balance in the ER

Several of the human immunodeficiency virus type 1 (HIV-1) protease inhibitors (PIs) have been shown to have anticancer activity in non-HIV-associated human cancer cells. The underlying mechanism of this effect is unclear. In a recent study (Pyrko et al., 2007b), we demonstrated that the PIs nelfinavir and atazanavir cause efficient cell death in various malignant glioma cell lines in vitro independent of the cell line's PTEN or p53 status. The underlying mechanism of this antitumor effect involves the potent induction of the ER stress response as indicated by increased expression of two ER stress markers, GRP78 and CHOP, and activation of ER stress-associated caspase 4. Induction of ER stress appears to play a central role in PI-induced cell death because siRNA-mediated knockdown of the protective ER chaperone GRP78 sensitizes cells; whereas, knockdown of pro-apoptotic caspase 4 protects cells from PI-induced cell death. Furthermore, the treatment of glioma cells with PIs leads to accumulation of polyubiquitinated proteins and aggresome formation (aggresome is an intracellular structure composed of aggregated polyubiquitinated proteins), implying proteasome inhibition (Fig. 43.5). These results support a model whereby PIs cause tumor cell death through inhibition of human proteasome activity (not to be confused with viral protease activity) and subsequent accumulation of misfolded proteins, which triggers ER stress response. Induction of glioma cell death via ER stress takes place in the in vivo setting as well, as nelfinavir inhibits the growth of xenografted human malignant glioma, with concomitant induction of the pro-apoptotic ER stress marker CHOP in animal tumor tissues. The induction of CHOP is paralleled by the increase of apoptotic cells within tumor tissue. Because ER stress has also been reported as the mechanism for insulin resistance and diabetes, our ER stress model of PI function may also explain why these drugs may induce insulin resistance as one of its most common side effects.

The use of PIs in gliomas has a number of potential advantages and disadvantages. PIs are small molecules that should cross the blood–brain barrier (BBB) readily. They have already been demonstrated (albeit, indirectly) to have activity in the CNS, as the number of HIV patients with CNS lymphomas has decreased significantly since initiation of the current HIV multi-prong treatment protocol (HAART: highly active anti-retroviral therapy) (Sgadari et al., 2002). Laurent et al. have demonstrated that ritonavir penetrated across the BBB and achieved adequate concentrations in the CNS in an intracranial glioma model (Laurent et al., 2004). Yilmaz et al. have measured cerebrospinal fluid (CSF) levels of both nelfinavir and saquinavir, with better CSF concentrations of nelfinavir, compared to saquinavir (Yilmaz et al., 2006). PIs are oral agents, which are well tolerated, even by AIDS patients. Whether PIs can be used as a stand-alone agent is not known; combination therapy with other cytotoxic agents is a possibility. Furthermore, the data demonstrating that both nelfinavir and atazanavir are effective in glioma cell lines with different p53 and

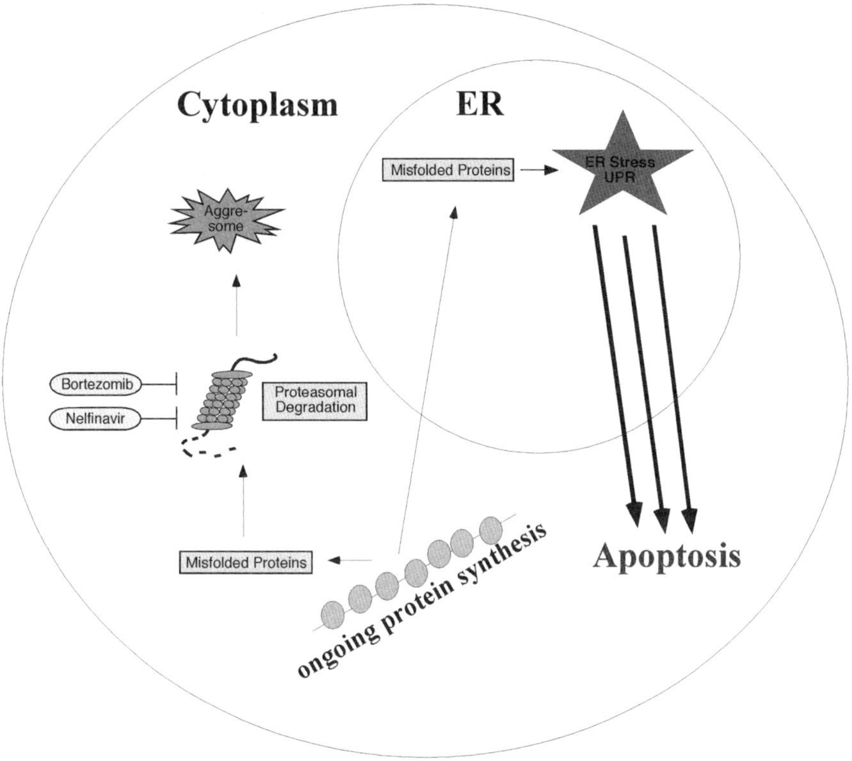

Fig. 43.5 ER stress response as a mechanism of action of protease inhibitors. PIs inhibit the proteasome, which prevents the degradation of proteins; at the same time, general protein synthesis continues to proceed, which results in the accumulation of unfolded/misfolded proteins and appearance of the aggresome (an aggregate of polyubiquitinated proteins). This in turn triggers ESR as the cells attempt to neutralize impending proteotoxicity. Because proteins cannot be degraded due to constant inhibition of the proteasome in the continued presence of the drug, the protective arm of the ESR eventually is overwhelmed, and the balance is shifted toward its pro-apoptotic components (CHOP and caspase 4), which initiates cell death

PTEN status are encouraging, as PIs may potentially be effective in treating all glioma patients, irrespective of their tumor's genetic makeup. Lastly, PIs have been demonstrated by Gupta et al. to act as radiation sensitizers via both in vitro and in vivo models (Gupta et al., 2005). The value of radiation sensitization for the treatment of malignant gliomas has been clearly demonstrated by Stupp et al. who showed that patients treated with both low dose temozolomide and radiation had better outcomes than patients treated with radiation alone (Stupp et al., 2005). In addition, PIs have minimal effect on the induction of myelotoxicity, which can be seen in all cytotoxic agents, including temozolomide.

43.6 Combination Therapy by Affecting Multiple Targets Within the ER

Very recent studies have indicated that efficient glioma cell death can be achieved by the combination of drugs that trigger severe ER stress via different mechanisms (Fig. 43.6). For example, the above-mentioned SERCA inhibitors cause ER stress via the depletion of calcium from the ER, whereas proteasome inhibitors trigger ER stress due to the resulting accumulation of misfolded and other waste proteins. Intriguingly, the combination of celecoxib or DMC (i.e., SERCA inhibitors) with either bortezomib (a proteasome inhibitor (Nawrocki et al., 2005)) or HIV protease inhibitors (which also act as proteasome inhibitors (Pyrko et al., 2007b)) resulted in greatly enhanced killing of glioblastoma

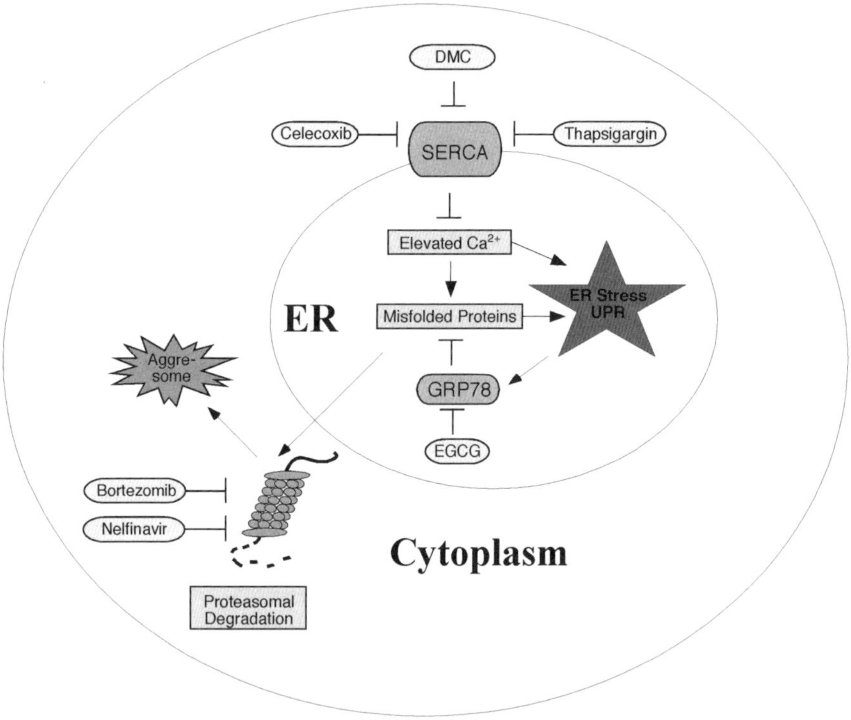

Fig. 43.6 Possible cancer therapy targets within the ER. Within the ER of a cancer cell SERCA can be inhibited by celecoxib, DMC, and thapsigargin, while the function of GRP78 can be inhibited by EGCG (similar effects are possible by decreasing the amount of GRP78 protein with GRP78 siRNAs when delivery of such siRNA becomes feasible). Inhibition of the cytoplasmic proteasome (with protease inhibitors or specific proteasome inhibitors) results in a backlog of unfolded proteins in the ER and ER stress. Since death results from the overwhelmed ESR affecting multiple targets within ER is more effective than single target therapy

and other tumor cells (Kardosh et al., 2008). The underlying mechanism of this synergy could be ascribed to aggravated ER stress, i.e., ER stress and resulting cell death were much greater in combination drug treatments than in individual drug treatments. Importantly, these decisive events could also be verified in tumors of drug-treated animals. For example, the expression of CHOP, the critical pro-apoptotic marker protein for severe ER stress (Oyadomari and Mori, 2004), was strongly elevated in tumors from animals that received combination drug treatment, but it was only moderately increased in tumors from animals receiving monotherapy (Kardosh et al., 2008). In comparison, tumors from non-treated control animals did not display detectable levels of CHOP. In parallel, and mirroring the in vitro events, the amount of cell death closely correlated with the observed CHOP levels; i.e., the tumors with the highest amount of CHOP protein also exhibited the greatest number of apoptotic cells (Kardosh et al., 2008).

Combination drug treatments aimed at different components of the ER stress response system represent a little-explored, yet potentially promising approach toward improved brain cancer therapy. However, a possible obstacle with some of the mentioned agents could be posed by the blood–brain barrier. Bortezomib (Velcade®), for example, does not efficiently cross the BBB and therefore cannot be effectively delivered via its conventional intravenous administration. In this case, intratumoral injections or slow release from intracranially implanted devices may be an alternative.

43.7 Potential Clinical Applications of ER Stress Modulation in Malignant Glioma Treatment

Our data demonstrating that GRP78 is elevated in malignant gliomas and that increased GRP78 is associated with resistance to TMZ are potentially clinically important. Agents capable of downregulating GRP78 levels or functionally inactivating it may be used as TMZ chemosensitizers (Wilke et al., 1994). Further, the level of GRP78 may be used as a predictor of malignant glioma aggressiveness and response to therapy. Other investigators have reported similar results in different malignancies. For example, elevation of GRP78 was shown to be correlated with lymph node metastasis and poor prognosis for patients with gastric carcinoma (Zhang et al., 2006). Increased GRP78 expression was also associated with the development of hormone refractory prostate cancer (Pootrakul et al., 2006). In breast cancer, the levels of GRP78 were found higher in malignant and lower in non-malignant breast lesions (Fernandez et al., 2000), and GRP78 was used as a predictor of breast cancer's responsiveness to chemotherapy (Lee et al., 2006). The use of GRP78 as a novel predictor of malignant glioma aggressiveness should be further investigated. Our data correlating increased GRP78 levels with cell proliferation may be a useful marker for response to therapy. Moreover, downregulation or inactivation of GRP78 (i.e., by EGCG) holds great promise for combination therapy with TMZ, as EGCG is a well-tolerated extract commonly found in green tea and is sold over the counter in vitamin stores. Future studies should examine the downregulation of GRP78 systematically in an in vivo setting with the ultimate goal of downregulating GRP78 levels in malignant gliomas and to determine if such downregulation results in increased response to TMZ.

The action of temozolomide (TMZ) is usually attributed to its ability to damage DNA (Ma et al., 2002). TMZ has been demonstrated to be effective in combination therapy with radiation (Stupp et al., 2005). Zhai et al. have reported that downregulation of GRP78 increased sensitivity of transformed human fibroblasts to UVC radiation (Zhai et al., 2005). This discovery might turn out very important for malignant glioma research if it turns out to be also true for ionizing radiation. Studies aimed at GRP78's role in sensitivity to ionizing radiation should be undertaken in malignant gliomas.

In one of the studies described here we proposed two new possible candidates: celecoxib and DMC. An important clinical aspect of our study is the elucidation of the non-COX-2 mode of action of celecoxib. While the celecoxib molecule displays two separate functions, i.e., inhibition of COX-2 and induction of apoptosis, the DMC molecule is a "pure" apoptosis inducer that lacks coxib activity. While it shall remain undisputed that the inhibition of COX-2, as exerted by celecoxib, has clinically relevant anti-neoplastic applications, we propose that DMC might have antitumor effects in its own right—perhaps under conditions where the carcinogenic process is not dominated by elevated levels of prostaglandins. In this case, the absence of COX-2-inhibitory potential in DMC might turn out to be advantageous, as it is conceivable that the antitumor results might be achieved with less of the coxib-associated side effects. In terms of malignant glioma therapy, celecoxib and DMC's effects should be further investigated in combination with TMZ, radiation, and other agents used against malignant glioma. TMZ, celecoxib, and DMC all induce ER stress but via different mechanisms. Therefore, combination of TMZ and DMC or celecoxib holds potential for clinical usage as we have previously demonstrated in preclinical models (Kardosh et al., 2004). In support of our data, a study of CXB and TMZ in patients with melanoma has shown a potential benefit of such combination therapy (Gogas et al., 2006). It is conceivable that adding a calcium-modulating drug like celecoxib or DMC to TMZ treatment might overwhelm the antiapoptotic arm of the ER (GRP78) and overcome such resistance leading to chemosensitization of glioma cells to TMZ. An animal study in a C6 glioma model has recently demonstrated a significant decrease in tumor size in the TMZ with celecoxib combination group as compared to TMZ alone (Kang et al., 2006). Celecoxib crosses the blood–brain barrier (BBB) and was previously used in studies involving glioma patients (Giglio and Levin, 2004; Levin et al., 2006). The ability of DMC to cross the BBB, a property necessary for every effective anti-brain tumor agent, has not been quantified. We are currently undertaking studies in animals aimed at determining, at least indirectly, if DMC has the capacity to cross the BBB. The results of these studies will have to be further confirmed in human trials in the future.

Our demonstration that human immunodeficiency virus type-1 (HIV-1) protease inhibitors (PIs) can induce ER stress may also find clinical applicability in the treatment of malignant gliomas. While PIs have been developed to combat HIV, the treatment with ritonavir, indinavir, or sequinavir has had an unexpected additional consequence—the regression of Kaposi's sarcoma and primary CNS lymphomas (Pati et al., 2002; Sgadari et al., 2002). Since then PIs have been evaluated in various other cancer models including hepatic carcinoma, multiple myeloma, and prostate cancer (Esposito et al., 2006; Ikezoe et al., 2004; Yang et al., 2005). The effects of PIs in malignant glioma have been unclear. In a study using an established glioblastoma cell line, ritonavir had in vitro effects but no effect was observed in vivo (Laurent et al., 2004). In our study, we demonstrated that nelfinavir and atazanavir inhibit proliferation and cause cell death in three different glioblastoma cell lines. We also documented that nelfinavir caused a significant decrease in U87MG tumor growth in a subcutaneous in vivo xenograft model. Thus we propose that PIs are potential candidates for malignant glioma treatment; however, the use of PIs in gliomas has a number of possible advantages and disadvantages. PIs are small molecules that should cross the blood–brain barrier (BBB) readily. They have already been demonstrated (albeit, indirectly) to have activity in the CNS, as the number of HIV patients with CNS lymphomas has decreased significantly since initiation of HAART (Sgadari et al., 2002). Ritonavir was shown to cross the BBB, and it achieved adequate concentrations in the CNS in an intracranial glioma model (Laurent et al., 2004). Measurements in cerebrospinal fluid (CSF) showed better CSF concentrations of nelfinavir, compared to saquinavir (Yilmaz et al., 2006). Whether the levels achieved in the CNS for nelfinavir or saquinavir would be sufficient for treatment of gliomas remains to be determined. PIs are oral agents, which are well tolerated, even by AIDS patients. Whether PIs can be used as a stand-alone agent is not known; combination therapy with other cytotoxic agents including TMZ is a possibility and should be explored. Furthermore, our data demonstrating that both nelfinavir and atazanavir are effective in glioma cell lines with different p53 and PTEN status are encouraging, as PIs may potentially be effective in treating all glioma patients, irrespective of their tumor's genetic makeup (Gupta et al., 2005; Pajonk et al., 2002). The possibility of PIs as radiation sensitizers presents an intriguing treatment algorithm. In terms of side effects, PIs have minimal effect on induction of myelotoxicity. One commonly observed side effect of PIs, insulin resistance (Nolan, 2003; Rudich et al., 2005), may be explained by the fact that PIs induce ER stress which was recently linked to insulin resistance and diabetes (Ozcan et al., 2004, 2006). The development of insulin resistance may be problematic in brain tumor patients who are often on systemic steroids. Glucocorticoids, like dexamethasone (Decadron), which is often used in glioma patients, have been shown to increase blood sugar levels

(Hirsch and Paauw, 1997). Combination of decadron with PIs may be detrimental to glioma patients through its potential impact on blood glucose levels; how significant this elevation might be will need to be determined.

Finally, since celecoxib, DMC, and PIs all result in chemo- and radio-sensitization, it is possible to stipulate that tipping the balance in the ER toward death may in general have a chemo- and radio-sensitizing effect. For instance, radio-sensitization may occur because abrogation of protein synthesis, which has a general protective effect in ER stress, may have a deleterious effect when DNA repair is undertaken by the cell following radiation treatment. Such inhibition of protein synthesis (even though transient) may lead to the absence of synthesis of DNA repair proteins, which in turn may close the window of time allowed for the cell to recover. In such way, a protective mechanism in the ER may tip the balance toward death in the nucleus or other parts of the cell. We show here that DNA-damaging agent TMZ causes stress in the ER. Similar effect was observed with a platinum compound cisplatin, which also causes DNA damage (Mandic et al., 2003). These two observations may suggest that DNA damage in itself may lead to ER stress. Such connection of the nuclear and ER processes should be investigated in greater detail.

43.8 Conclusion

We have demonstrated that modulation of ER stress is an important new treatment modality for malignant gliomas. We have reported recently that downregulation of GRP78 is associated with increased chemosensitivity to TMZ. Moreover, the use of celecoxib and DMC to modulate intracellular calcium levels to increase ER stress is a novel mechanism that may be further enhanced with more potent analogs of either drug. Our demonstration that protease inhibitors may be used to induce ER stress suggests that these agents may also be useful as potential combination agents with other chemotherapeutic agents. Lastly, we emphasize the importance of combination therapy, not only with other cytotoxic agents but with different pathways that affect ER stress.

References

Boyce, M., and Yuan, J. (2006). Cellular response to endoplasmic reticulum stress: a matter of life or death. Cell Death Differ *13*, 363–373.

Brophy, J. M. (2007). Cardiovascular effects of cyclooxygenase-2 inhibitors. Curr Opin Gastroenterol *23*, 617–624.

Chandran, S. S., Nan, A., Rosen, D. M., Ghandehari, H., and Denmeade, S. R. (2007). A prostate-specific antigen activated N-(2-hydroxypropyl) methacrylamide copolymer prodrug as dual-targeted therapy for prostate cancer. Mol Cancer Ther *6*, 2928–2937.

Chuang, H.-C., Kardosh, A., Gaffney, K. J., Petasis, N. A., and Schönthal, A. H. (2008). COX-2 inhibition is neither necessary nor sufficient for celecoxib to suppress tumor cell proliferation and focus formation in vitro. Mol Cancer, *7*, 38.

Clapham, D. E. (2007). Calcium signaling. Cell *131*, 1047–1058.

Dehdashti, A. R., Hegi, M. E., Regli, L., Pica, A., and Stupp, R. (2006). New trends in the medical management of glioblastoma multiforme: the role of temozolomide chemotherapy. Neurosurg Focus *20*, E6.

Denmeade, S. R., Jakobsen, C. M., Janssen, S., Khan, S. R., Garrett, E. S., Lilja, H., Christensen, S. B., and Isaacs, J. T. (2003). Prostate-specific antigen-activated thapsigargin prodrug as targeted therapy for prostate cancer. J Natl Cancer Inst *95*, 990–1000.

Dong, D., Ko, B., Baumeister, P., Swenson, S., Costa, F., Markland, F., Stiles, C., Patterson, J. B., Bates, S. E., and Lee, A. S. (2005). Vascular targeting and antiangiogenesis agents induce drug resistance effector GRP78 within the tumor microenvironment. Cancer Res *65*, 5785–5791.

Esposito, V., Palescandolo, E., Spugnini, E. P., Montesarchio, V., De Luca, A., Cardillo, I., Cortese, G., Baldi, A., and Chirianni, A. (2006). Evaluation of antitumoral properties of the protease inhibitor indinavir in a murine model of hepatocarcinoma. Clin Cancer Res *12*, 2634–2639.

Fernandez, P. M., Tabbara, S. O., Jacobs, L. K., Manning, F. C., Tsangaris, T. N., Schwartz, A. M., Kennedy, K. A., and Patierno, S. R. (2000). Overexpression of the glucose-regulated stress gene GRP78 in malignant but not benign human breast lesions. Breast Cancer Res Treat *59*, 15–26.

Friedman, H. S., and Bigner, D. D. (2005). Glioblastoma multiforme and the epidermal growth factor receptor. N Engl J Med *353*, 1997–1999.

Gelebart, P., Opas, M., and Michalak, M. (2005). Calreticulin, a Ca2 + -binding chaperone of the endoplasmic reticulum. Int J Biochem Cell Biol *37*, 260–266.

Giglio, P., and Levin, V. (2004). Cyclooxygenase-2 inhibitors in glioma therapy. Am J Ther *11*, 141–143.

Gogas, H., Polyzos, A., Stavrinidis, I., Frangia, K., Tsoutsos, D., Panagiotou, P., Markopoulos, C., Papadopoulos, O., Pectasides, D., Mantzourani, M., et al. (2006). Temozolomide in combination with celecoxib in patients with advanced melanoma. A phase II study of the Hellenic Cooperative Oncology Group. Ann Oncol *17*, 1835–1841.

Gupta, A. K., Cerniglia, G. J., Mick, R., McKenna, W. G., and Muschel, R. J. (2005). HIV protease inhibitors block Akt signaling and radiosensitize tumor cells both in vitro and in vivo. Cancer Res *65*, 8256–8265.

Hentschel, S. J., and Lang, F. F. (2003). Current surgical management of glioblastoma. Cancer J *9*, 113–125.

Hirsch, I. B., and Paauw, D. S. (1997). Diabetes management in special situations. Endocrinol Metab Clin North Am *26*, 631–645.

Ikezoe, T., Saito, T., Bandobashi, K., Yang, Y., Koeffler, H. P., and Taguchi, H. (2004). HIV-1 protease inhibitor induces growth arrest and apoptosis of human multiple myeloma cells via inactivation of signal transducer and activator of transcription 3 and extracellular signal-regulated kinase 1/2. Mol Cancer Ther *3*, 473–479.

Johnson, A. J., Hsu, A. L., Lin, H. P., Song, X., and Chen, C. S. (2002). The cyclo-oxygenase-2 inhibitor celecoxib perturbs intracellular calcium by inhibiting endoplasmic reticulum Ca2 + -ATPases: a plausible link with its anti-tumour effect and cardiovascular risks. Biochem J *366*, 831–837.

Kang, S. G., Kim, J. S., Park, K., Kim, J. S., Groves, M. D., and Nam, D. H. (2006). Combination celecoxib and temozolomide in C6 rat glioma orthotopic model. Oncol Rep *15*, 7–13.

Kardosh, A., Blumenthal, M., Wang, W. J., Chen, T. C., and Schönthal, A. H. (2004). Differential effects of selective COX-2 inhibitors on cell cycle regulation and proliferation of glioblastoma cell lines. Cancer Biol Ther *3*, 9–16.

Kardosh, A., Golden, E. B., Pyrko, P., Uddin, J., Hofman, F. M., Chen, C. T., Louie, S. G., Petasis, N. A., and Schönthal, A. H. (2008). Aggravated endoplasmic reticulum (ER) stress as a basis for enhanced glioblastoma cell killing by bortezomib in combination with celecoxib or its non-coxib analog, 2,5-dimethyl-celecoxib. Cancer Research *68*, 843–851.

Kaufman, R. J. (1999). Stress signaling from the lumen of the endoplasmic reticulum: coordination of gene transcriptional and translational controls. Genes Dev *13*, 1211–1233.

Koomagi, R., Mattern, J., and Volm, M. (1999). Glucose-related protein (GRP78) and its relationship to the drug-resistance proteins P170, GST-pi, LRP56 and angiogenesis in non-small cell lung carcinomas. Anticancer Res *19*, 4333–4336.

Kovacs, G. G., Zsembery, A., Anderson, S. J., Komlosi, P., Gillespie, G. Y., Bell, P. D., Benos, D. J., and Fuller, C. M. (2005). Changes in intracellular Ca2+ and pH in response to thapsigargin in human glioblastoma cells and normal astrocytes. Am J Physiol Cell Physiol *289*, C361–371.

Laurent, N., de Bouard, S., Guillamo, J. S., Christov, C., Zini, R., Jouault, H., Andre, P., Lotteau, V., and Peschanski, M. (2004). Effects of the proteasome inhibitor ritonavir on glioma growth in vitro and in vivo. Mol Cancer Ther *3*, 129–136.

Lee, A. S. (2001). The glucose-regulated proteins: stress induction and clinical applications. Trends Biochem Sci *26*, 504–510.

Lee, E., Nichols, P., Spicer, D., Groshen, S., Yu, M. C., and Lee, A. S. (2006). GRP78 as a Novel Predictor of Responsiveness to Chemotherapy in Breast Cancer. Cancer Res *66*, 7849–7853.

Levin, V. A., Giglio, P., Puduvalli, V. K., Jochec, J., Groves, M. D., Yung, W. K., and Hess, K. (2006). Combination chemotherapy with 13-cis-retinoic acid and celecoxib in the treatment of glioblastoma multiforme. J Neurooncol *78*, 85–90.

Ma, J., Murphy, M., O'Dwyer, P. J., Berman, E., Reed, K., and Gallo, J. M. (2002). Biochemical changes associated with a multidrug-resistant phenotype of a human glioma cell line with temozolomide-acquired resistance. Biochem Pharmacol *63*, 1219–1228.

Mandic, A., Hansson, J., Linder, S., and Shoshan, M. C. (2003). Cisplatin induces endoplasmic reticulum stress and nucleus-independent apoptotic signaling. J Biol Chem *278*, 9100–9106.

Nagasubramanian, R., and Dolan, M. E. (2003). Temozolomide: realizing the promise and potential. Curr Opin Oncol *15*, 412–418.

Nawrocki, S. T., Carew, J. S., Dunner, K., Jr., Boise, L. H., Chiao, P. J., Huang, P., Abbruzzese, J. L., and McConkey, D. J. (2005). Bortezomib inhibits PKR-like endoplasmic reticulum (ER) kinase and induces apoptosis via ER stress in human pancreatic cancer cells. Cancer Res *65*, 11510–11519.

Nolan, D. (2003). Metabolic complications associated with HIV protease inhibitor therapy. Drugs *63*, 2555–2574.

Okunaga, T., Urata, Y., Goto, S., Matsuo, T., Mizota, S., Tsutsumi, K., Nagata, I., Kondo, T., and Ihara, Y. (2006). Calreticulin, a molecular chaperone in the endoplasmic reticulum, modulates radiosensitivity of human glioblastoma U251MG cells. Cancer Res *66*, 8662–8671.

Oyadomari, S., and Mori, M. (2004). Roles of CHOP/GADD153 in endoplasmic reticulum stress. Cell Death Differ *11*, 381–389.

Ozcan, U., Cao, Q., Yilmaz, E., Lee, A. H., Iwakoshi, N. N., Ozdelen, E., Tuncman, G., Gorgun, C., Glimcher, L. H., and Hotamisligil, G. S. (2004). Endoplasmic reticulum stress links obesity, insulin action, and type 2 diabetes. Science *306*, 457–461.

Ozcan, U., Yilmaz, E., Ozcan, L., Furuhashi, M., Vaillancourt, E., Smith, R. O., Gorgun, C. Z., and Hotamisligil, G. S. (2006). Chemical chaperones reduce ER stress and restore glucose homeostasis in a mouse model of type 2 diabetes. Science *313*, 1137–1140.

Pajonk, F., Himmelsbach, J., Riess, K., Sommer, A., and McBride, W. H. (2002). The human immunodeficiency virus (HIV)-1 protease inhibitor saquinavir inhibits proteasome function and causes apoptosis and radiosensitization in non-HIV-associated human cancer cells. Cancer Res *62*, 5230–5235.

Pati, S., Pelser, C. B., Dufraine, J., Bryant, J. L., Reitz, M. S., Jr., and Weichold, F. F. (2002). Antitumorigenic effects of HIV protease inhibitor ritonavir: inhibition of Kaposi sarcoma. Blood *99*, 3771–3779.

Penning, T. D., Talley, J. J., Bertenshaw, S. R., Carter, J. S., Collins, P. W., Docter, S., Graneto, M. J., Lee, L. F., Malecha, J. W., Miyashiro, J. M., et al. (1997). Synthesis and biological evaluation of the 1,5-diarylpyrazole class of cyclooxygenase-2 inhibitors: identification of 4-[5-(4-methylphenyl)-3-(trifluoromethyl)-1H-pyrazol-1-yl]benze nesulfonamide (SC-58635, celecoxib). J Med Chem *40*, 1347–1365.

Pootrakul, L., Datar, R. H., Shi, S. R., Cai, J., Hawes, D., Groshen, S. G., Lee, A. S., and Cote, R. J. (2006). Expression of stress response protein Grp78 is associated with the development of castration-resistant prostate cancer. Clin Cancer Res *12*, 5987–5993.

Pryko, P., Kardosh, A., Liu, Y. T., Soriano, N., Xiong, W., Chow, R. H., Uddin, J., 20Petasis, N. A., Mircheff, A. K., Farley, R. A., Louie, S. G., Chen, T. C., and Schonthal, A. H. (2007a). Calcium-activated endoplasmic reticulum stress as a major component of tumor cell death induced by 2,5-dimethyl-celecoxib, a non-coxib analogue of celecoxib. Mol Cancer Ther *6*(4): 1262–1275.

Pyrko, P., Kardosh, A., Wang, W., Xiong, W., Schonthal, A. H., and Chen, T. C. (2007b). HIV-1 protease inhibitors nelfinavir and atazanavir induce malignant glioma death by triggering endoplasmic reticulum stress. Cancer Res *67*(22): 10920–10928.

Pyrko, P., Kardosh, A., and Schönthal, A. H. (2008). Celecoxib transiently inhibits protein synthesis. Biochem Pharmacol *75*, 395–404.

Pyrko, P., Schönthal, A. H., Hofman, F. M., Chen, T. C., and Lee, A. S. (2007c). The unfolded protein response regulator GRP78/BiP as a novel target for increasing chemosensitivity in malignant gliomas. Cancer Res *67*, 9809–9816.

Rudich, A., Ben-Romano, R., Etzion, S., and Bashan, N. (2005). Cellular mechanisms of insulin resistance, lipodystrophy and atherosclerosis induced by HIV protease inhibitors. Acta Physiol Scand *183*, 75–88.

Schönthal, A. H. (2006). Antitumor properties of dimethyl-celecoxib, a derivative of celecoxib that does not inhibit cyclooxygenase-2: implications for glioblastoma therapy. Neurosurgical Focus 20, *E21*, 21–10.

Schönthal, A. H. (2007). Direct non-cyclooxygenase-2 targets of celecoxib and their potential relevance for cancer therapy. Br J Cancer *97*, 1465–1468.

Schönthal, A. H. (2009). Endoplasmic reticulum stress and autophagy as targets for cancer therapy. Cancer Lett *275*(2), 163–169.

Sgadari, C., Barillari, G., Toschi, E., Carlei, D., Bacigalupo, I., Baccarini, S., Palladino, C., Leone, P., Bugarini, R., Malavasi, L., et al. (2002). HIV protease inhibitors are potent anti-angiogenic molecules and promote regression of Kaposi sarcoma. Nat Med *8*, 225–232.

Stupp, R., Hegi, M. E., van den Bent, M. J., Mason, W. P., Weller, M., Mirimanoff, R. O., and Cairncross, J. G. (2006). Changing paradigms–an update on the multidisciplinary management of malignant glioma. Oncologist *11*, 165–180.

Stupp, R., Mason, W. P., van den Bent, M. J., Weller, M., Fisher, B., Taphoorn, M. J., Belanger, K., Brandes, A. A., Marosi, C., Bogdahn, U., et al. (2005). Radiotherapy plus concomitant and adjuvant temozolomide for glioblastoma. N Engl J Med *352*, 987–996.

Szado, T., Vanderheyden, V., Parys, J. B., De Smedt, H., Rietdorf, K., Kotelevets, L., Chastre, E., Khan, F., Landegren, U., Soderberg, O., et al. (2008). Phosphorylation of inositol 1,4,5-trisphosphate receptors by protein kinase B/Akt inhibits Ca2+ release and apoptosis. Proc Natl Acad Sci U S A *105*, 2427–2432.

Treiman, M., Caspersen, C., and Christensen, S. B. (1998). A tool coming of age: thapsigargin as an inhibitor of sarco-endoplasmic reticulum Ca(2+)-ATPases. Trends Pharmacol Sci *19*, 131–135.

van den Bent, M. J., Hegi, M. E., and Stupp, R. (2006). Recent developments in the use of chemotherapy in brain tumours. Eur J Cancer *42*, 582–588.

Wang, W., Kardosh, A., Su, Y. S., Schonthal, A. H., and Chen, T. C. (2006). Efficacy of celecoxib in the treatment of CNS lymphomas: an in vivo model. Neurosurg Focus *21*, E14.

Wilke, N., Sganga, M., Barhite, S., and Miles, M. F. (1994). Effects of alcohol on gene expression in neural cells. Exs *71*, 49–59.

Wu, J., and Kaufman, R. J. (2006). From acute ER stress to physiological roles of the unfolded protein response. Cell Death Differ *13*, 374–384.

Yang, Y., Ikezoe, T., Takeuchi, T., Adachi, Y., Ohtsuki, Y., Takeuchi, S., Koeffler, H. P., and Taguchi, H. (2005). HIV-1 protease inhibitor induces growth arrest and apoptosis of human prostate cancer LNCaP cells in vitro and in vivo in conjunction with blockade of androgen receptor STAT3 and AKT signaling. Cancer Sci *96*, 425–433.

Yilmaz, A., Fuchs, D., Hagberg, L., Nillroth, U., Stahle, L., Svensson, J. O., and Gisslen, M. (2006). Cerebrospinal fluid HIV-1 RNA, intrathecal immunoactivation, and drug concentrations after treatment with a combination of saquinavir, nelfinavir, and two nucleoside analogues: the M61022 study. BMC Infect Dis *6*, 63.

Yin, L. T., Fu, Y. J., Xu, Q. L., Yang, J., Liu, Z. L., Liang, A. H., Fan, X. J., and Xu, C. G. (2007). Potential biochemical therapy of glioma cancer. Biochem Biophys Res Commun *362*, 225–229.

Zhai, L., Kita, K., Wano, C., Wu, Y., Sugaya, S., and Suzuki, N. (2005). Decreased cell survival and DNA repair capacity after UVC irradiation in association with down-regulation of GRP78/BiP in human RSa cells. Exp Cell Res *305*, 244–252.

Zhang, J., Jiang, Y., Jia, Z., Li, Q., Gong, W., Wang, L., Wei, D., Yao, J., Fang, S., and Xie, K. (2006). Association of elevated GRP78 expression with increased lymph node metastasis and poor prognosis in patients with gastric cancer. Clin Exp Metastasis *23*, 401–410.

Chapter 44
Brain Cancer Stem Cells as Targets of Novel Therapies

Jennifer M. Atkinson, Richard J. Gilbertson, and Jeremy N. Rich

Abstract The cancer stem cell hypothesis posits that tumors are heterogeneous in their cell composition and contain a population of neoplastic cells that display sustained self-renewal, proliferative potential, and the capacity for tumor propagation. The significance of cancer stem cells in clinical practice remains undefined but laboratory studies have identified specific cancer stem cell signaling pathways and niches that may offer new therapeutic avenues. Characterizing cancer stem cells may also inform improved brain tumor prognosis and imaging.

Contents

J.N. Rich (✉)
Department of Stem Cell Biology and Regenerative Medicine, Cleveland Clinic, 9500 Euclid Avenue / NE30, Cleveland, OH 44195, USA
e-mail: richj@ccf.org

E.G. Van Meir (ed.), *CNS Cancer*, Cancer Drug Discovery and Development, DOI 10.1007/978-1-60327-553-8_44,
© Humana Press, a part of Springer Science+Business Media, LLC 2009

44.1 Introduction

Brain tumors comprise heterogeneous collections of cells that include small subsets that are strikingly similar to normal neural stem and progenitor cells. These so-called cancer stem cells (CSC) have the capacity to self-renew (generate identical daughter cells) indefinitely, undergo multi-lineage differentiation, and are both sufficient and required to propagate the disease as xenotransplants in immunocompromised mice. CSC have been variously termed tumor-initiating cells or tumor-propagating cells and are best defined through specific functional assays. The terminology engenders some confusion as the cell of origin is distinguished as the normal cell that undergoes malignant transformation. The tumor-initiating cell would presumably be the initial transformed cell but this term has been used for cells that propagate tumors. Since these cells are thought to drive tumor maintenance, spread, and resistance, they are emerging as an important focus in the development of new treatments.

44.2 Defining Cancer Stem Cells

Tumors, including those arising in the brain, are complex tissues that include a neoplastic compartment, associated vasculature, inflammatory cells, and reactive cellular and extracellular components (Furnari et al. 2007) (see also Chapters 21, 22, 31, and 48). Regional variance is also observed within the population of neoplastic cells and includes variable patterns of tumor cell differentiation, gene expression, and response to therapy. Studies conducted over the last several years in systemic cancers suggest that this heterogeneity may be explained by a hierarchal model of tumorigenesis (Lapidot et al. 1994; Bonnet and Dick 1997; Al-Hajj et al. 2003; Hope et al. 2004; Li et al. 2007; O'Brien et al. 2007; Ricci-Vitiani et al. 2007; Dalerba et al. 2007), known as the CSC hypothesis (Reya et al. 2001). This theory proposes that the neoplastic transformation of tissue-specific cells (that might include the stem or precursor cells themselves) results in the formation of a minority population of CSC that adopt or maintain a stem cell phenotype. CSC are thought to undergo asymmetric division that maintains the CSC fraction while generating a cellular hierarchy that includes the disease bulk and mimics partly the normal host tissue. CSC displaying these properties have been isolated from all major types of brain tumor including gliomas, medulloblastomas, and ependymomas (Ignatova et al. 2002; Hemmati et al. 2003; Singh et al. 2003; Galli et al. 2004; Singh et al. 2004; Yuan et al. 2004; Taylor et al. 2005).

Normal tissue stem cells are defined functionally by their ability to self-renew as well as generate the full cellular constituents of their host tissue (multipotency). For example, in the central nervous system (CNS), neural stem cells generate the oligodendrocytes, neurons, astrocytes, and ependymal cells that populate the brain (Uchida et al. 2000; Rietze et al. 2001; Sanai et al. 2004). Specialized culture systems have been developed that provide some measure of stem cell properties. In certain cell culture systems that lack serum but contain fibroblast growth factor (FGF) and epidermal growth factor (EGF), neural progenitor cells form three-dimensional non-adherent structures called neurospheres (Uchida et al. 2000). Of note, these culture conditions appear to maintain the gene expression profile of glioma cells better than serum-containing conditions (Lee et al. 2006). Complex neuronal processes may be formed in these structures and cultures may be assessed for self-renewal through the sequential clonal passage of neurospheres. Assessment of multipotency can be made by forcing the differentiation of these cultures and observing the cell phenotypes that form. However, caution must be exercised in interpreting the significance of sphere assays, which may be subject to tissue culture artifacts (Singec et al. 2006). The gold-standard assay of a normal tissue stem cell remains lineage tracing of those cells in vivo.

The requirements for identifying CSC are no less stringent and demand the demonstration that CSC are able and required to generate the entire tumor cell population in vivo. The current preferred assay for this purpose is the limiting dilution assay in which progressively smaller numbers of a defined fraction of tumor cells (usually sorted based on cell surface markers) are implanted in an orthotopic location to demonstrate the minimal number of cells required to form tumors (Singh et al. 2004). These results are usually contrasted with the numbers of marker-negative cells able (or not) to form tumors under identical conditions. A range of markers have been used to identify CSC and these vary between different tumors including breast ($CD44^+$ and $CD24^-$) (Al-Hajj et al. 2003), colorectal ($CD133^+$) (O'Brien et al. 2007), ependymoma ($CD133^+$, $Nestin^+$, $BLBP^+$) (Taylor et al. 2005), glioblastoma, and medulloblastoma ($CD133^+$) (Singh et al. 2004). CD133 (Prominin-1) was initially discovered as an antigen on $CD34^+$ hematopoietic stem cells (Yin et al. 1997), then was found to be useful in the isolation of neural stem cells (Uchida et al. 2000) and to isolate cancer stem cells from human brain tumors (Singh et al. 2004).

44.3 Signaling Pathways as Drug Targets in Cancer Stem Cells

Since CSC might be especially critical in the generation of tumors they offer an important new avenue of research in the hunt for new cancer treatments. Key signaling pathways essential for development and regulation of neural stem cell fate and differentiation – PTEN, Olig2, sonic hedgehog, Notch, Wnt, BMI-1, bone morphogenic proteins (BMPs), maternal embryonic leucine zipper kinase

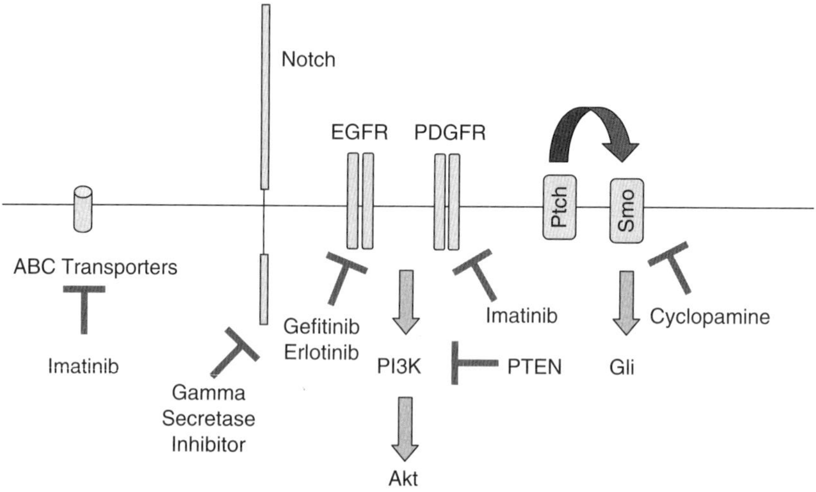

Fig. 44.1 Key cancer stem cell signaling. Several regulatory pathways for cancer stem cells (CSC) have been elucidated. Notch binds to the Delta and Serrate ligands on adjacent cells. Epidermal growth factor and platelet-derived growth factor receptors (EGFR and PDGFR, respectively) may be activated by ligand or mutation to initiate tumors and promote CSC maintenance. A key intracellular pathway downstream from growth factor receptors is PI3K-Akt-mammalian target of rapamycin (TOR). PI3K signaling activates cell survival mechanisms in addition to promoting angiogenesis and invasion. The PTEN tumor suppressor is frequently mutated in gliomas and counteracts PI3K signaling. Patched receptors (Ptch) inhibit Smoothened (Smo) transmembrane proteins in the absence of the hedgehog ligands. If sonic hedgehog (Shh) is present (and binds Ptch) or Ptch receptors are not expressed due to mutations, Smo will signal unopposed to drive cellular proliferation through Gli proteins. Inhibitors to each pathway are shown. The ATP-binding cassette (ABC) transporters are expressed by many stem cells and may contribute to CSC chemoresistance

(MELK) – have been shown to be active in brain tumors (Fig. 44.1). For example, a number of studies have highlighted considerable overlap between the gene expression signatures detected in human brain tumors (such as glioblastoma and ependymoma) and progenitor cells in the CNS (Taylor et al. 2005; Phillips et al. 2006). Examples include the transcription factor OLIG2 which promotes the proliferation of both neural progenitors and glioblastoma stem cells (Ligon et al. 2007). Better understanding of the mechanisms that regulate and dysregulate these signaling systems in normal and malignant neural stem cells, respectively, could lead to the development of effective therapeutic strategies.

44.3.1 Epidermal Growth Factor and PI(3)K Signaling

The epithelial growth factor receptor (EGFR) pathway is a key intracellular regulator that is upregulated in a number of human tumors including malignant gliomas. Since EGF is required for cancer stem cells to grow as self-renewing, multipotent cultures in vitro (Lee et al. 2006), it follows that this signaling pathway is likely crucial for the maintenance of CSC. Indeed recent studies suggest that EGFR kinase inhibitors might suppress the proliferation and self-renewal of these cells, reducing the $CD133^{+}$ population by inducing apoptosis (Soeda et al. 2008). Erlotinib and gefitinib, both EGFR inhibitors, have been used clinically to treat brain tumors although only $<20\%$ of patients showed a response to these agents (Rich et al. 2004; Prados et al. 2006). The poor response to EGFR inhibitors observed clinically may be due to loss of the tumor suppressor PTEN which is frequently deleted or mutated in brain tumors and leads to PI3K activation, a downstream event in variant EGFR signaling. PTEN plays an important role in regulating neural progenitor cells and evidence suggests that PTEN negatively regulates neural stem cell proliferation by activating mTOR through the PI(3)K pathway (Groszer et al. 2001). Loss of PTEN, seen frequently in high-grade gliomas results in activation of mTOR, increasing translation of a range of proteins required for cell cycle progression. A number of clinical studies of rapamycin, sirolimus, and CCI-779 have been reported in high-grade glioma patients in either unselected cohorts or with defects in PTEN and all studies point to the need for combination therapy to achieve a significant clinical impact (Chang et al. 2005; Galanis et al. 2005; Reardon et al. 2006; Doherty et al. 2006; Cloughesy et al. 2008). Leukemic CSC display a specific dependence on PTEN activity and are sensitive to mTOR antagonists (Yilmaz et al. 2006) but glioma CSC appear less sensitive (Eyler et al. 2008).

44.3.2 Hedgehog Signaling

Sonic hedgehog (SHH) signaling that plays a central role in the formation of the cerebellar medulloblastoma (Goodrich et al. 1997; Vorechovský et al. 1997) has been demonstrated to be a critical regulator of granule neuron progenitor cells in the cerebellum (Wechsler-Reya and Scott 1999). Blockade of the SHH pathway in brain tumors can reduce sphere formation, deplete $CD133^{+}$ cells, reduce xenograft tumor take rates, and cure mice harboring $Ptch1^{+/-}$ medulloblastoma suggesting a key role for this signaling pathway in the biology of cancer stem cells (Romer et al. 2004; Bar et al. 2007; Clement et al. 2007). Whilst the use of hedgehog signaling inhibitors has not yet reached the clinic there are a number of active drug discovery projects underway to identify agents which may affect this signaling pathway which would potentially be of therapeutic significance in brain tumors (Williams et al. 2003; Feldmann et al. 2008).

A number of other signaling pathways have been interrogated in brain CSC studies. Many of these are based on defined roles in normal stem cell biology, but others may be cancer specific.

44.3.3 Bone Morphogenic Protein Signaling

The BMPs induce neural stem cell differentiation and BMP receptor expression may be negatively regulated in glioblastoma CSC through epigenetic mechanisms (Lee et al. 2008). Further, emerging data suggest that BMPs may be useful for inhibiting brain CSC tumor growth through the induction of a differentiated state (Piccirillo et al. 2006).

44.3.4 Notch Signaling

The Notch signaling pathway is a highly conserved cell–cell communication pathway originally discovered due to the presence of notched wings in *Drosophila* mutants. There are four Notch proteins that are single-pass receptors for the Delta and Serrate ligands. Upon binding of Notch with the appropriate ligands, two sequential cleavage events of the Notch protein are required for the intracellular domain of Notch to become liberated and regulate transcription. The second Notch cleavage event is catalyzed by gamma secretase. Notch is frequently expressed by stem cells and by CSCs (Fan et al. 2006). Therefore, gamma secretase inhibitors (originally developed for Alzheimer's disease) can attenuate Notch activity to decrease CSC function both in culture and in vivo (Fan et al. 2006). These inhibitors have entered into early clinical trials for a number of tumor types, primarily leukemias.

44.3.5 Platelet-Derived Growth Factor Signaling

The platelet-derived growth factor (PDGF) pathways can be activated in neural stem and progenitor cells to form gliomas (Dai et al. 2001; Jackson et al. 2006; Assanah et al. 2006). Imatinib mesylate targets several pathways including PDGF signaling and can inhibit glioma neurosphere growth in culture (Gal et al. 2008) but has demonstrated very limited efficacy in clinical trials, even in combination with cytotoxic therapies.

44.3.6 Additional CSC Regulators

Other CSC targets include maternal embryonic leucine zipper kinase (MELK), a serine–threonine kinase that regulates cell survival under stress (Nakano et al. 2008), and L1 cell adhesion molecule (L1CAM), a transmembrane cell adhesion molecule originally described as a promigratory molecule in the developing nervous system (Bao et al. 2008). Several additional selective therapies have been tested against brain CSC with preliminary evidence of activity, including AKT inhibitors (Eyler et al. 2008), the HSP90 inhibitor

17-AAG (Sauvageot et al. 2008), and cannabinoids (Aguado et al. 2007). In studies interrogating PI3K/AKT signaling, brain tumor stem cells display lower pathway activation but display greater sensitivity to PI3K and AKT inhibitors in induction of apoptosis and inhibition of invasion/motility (Eyler et al. 2008).

While a number of signaling pathways important in the regulation and survival of both neural and cancer stem cells have been identified, the specific role of these pathways and the true extent of how successful pharmacological intervention will be remain to be determined.

44.4 Targeting the Perivascular Stem Cell Niche

Stem cells reside within specialized microenvironments termed stem cell niches (Fuchs et al. 2004; Moore and Lemischka 2006; Scheres 2007). Stem cell niches are not merely repositories for stem cells, but are complex dynamic entities that actively regulate stem cell function (Scadden 2006). The central structural element of the neural stem cell niche is provided by capillaries that generate regulatory signals to influence neural stem cell fate (Leventhal et al. 1999; Palmer et al. 2000; Shen et al. 2004; Shen et al. 2008; Tavazoie et al. 2008). The precise cocktail of vascular-derived factors that regulate neural stem cells remains to be determined, but brain-derived neurotrophic factor (BDNF), vascular endothelial growth factor (VEGF) C, and pigment epithelium-derived factor (PEDF) are likely candidates (Li et al. 2006; Ramírez-Castillejo et al. 2006; Le Bras et al. 2006). This communication is not unidirectional, and there is evidence that stem cells can modulate the microenvironments that nurture and sustain them (Scadden 2006). For example, co-culture experiments have shown that neural stem cells can maintain brain-derived endothelial cells in culture and induce these to form vascular tubes. This appears to be mediated by VEGF and BDNF secreted from neural stem cells (Li et al. 2006).

As stem cell niches have such a crucial role in regulating stem cell self-renewal and fate, it is not surprising that these microanatomical units are emerging as participants in disease states. A series of recently published studies have shown that aberrant vascular stem cell niches, reminiscent of those observed in the normal brain, exist in glioblastoma and other types of brain tumor and support the CSC (Bao et al. 2006a, b; Calabrese et al. 2007).

Aberrant vascularity is a well-established feature of many brain tumors (Jain et al. 2007) and was presumed to be important for satisfying the voracious demands for nutrients of the rapidly growing tumor. However, the discovery of brain CSC and vascular stem cell niches in the normal brain suggests a further sinister role for the tumor vascular bed: the formation of abnormal stem cell niches that maintain the CSC. Evidence of a functional relationship between the tumor vasculature and brain CSC was first provided in a study showing that high-level production of VEGF by $CD133^{+}$ human glioblastoma cells might contribute to their tumor-generative capacity (Bao et al. 2006a, b). The authors demonstrated that freshly resected $CD133^+$, but not $CD133^-$, human glioblastoma cells readily formed highly vascular and hemorrhagic tumors in the brains of immunocompromised mice. Further, treating $CD133^+$ glioblastoma cells with the VEGF-neutralizing antibody Bevacizumab blocked their ability to induce endothelial cell migration and tube formation in culture and to initiate tumors in vivo. Thus, similar to normal neural stem cells, glioblastoma stem cells appear to possess potent angiogenic properties and recruit vessels during tumorigenesis.

Although glioblastoma stem cells may recruit blood vessels, communication between these two elements should be bidirectional if capillaries participate in a cancer stem cell niche. Compelling data were provided showing that stem cells from a variety of brain tumors, including glioblastoma, are maintained within vascular niches that mimic the neural stem cell niche (Calabrese et al. 2007). They showed that $CD133^+$, $Nestin^+$ cells within sections of human glioblastomas, medulloblastomas, ependymomas, and oligodendrogliomas are located in close proximity to tumor capillaries. They then demonstrated that $CD133^+$ and $Nestin^+$ cells but not other cells isolated from these tumors interact intimately with the vascular tubes that are formed by endothelial cells in three-dimensional cultures. The self-renewal and proliferation of these CSC in culture were maintained by factors secreted by endothelial cells. Importantly, by co-transplanting brain tumor stem cells and endothelial cells into immunocompromised mice, the investigators showed that endothelial-derived factors also accelerate the initiation and growth of tumors in the brain. Similar perivascular tumor cell niches were subsequently described in mouse models of medulloblastoma (Hambardzumyan et al. 2008). The use of CD133 as a CSC marker is complicated by the presence of tumor propagation in CD133-negative cells (Beier et al. 2007; Ogden et al. 2008). CD133 is also regulated by the cell cycle (Jaksch et al. 2008) and through promoter methylation (Tabu et al. 2008; Yi et al. 2008).

The observation that brain CSC reside in perivascular niches raises the intriguing possibility that these malignant microenvironments might be targeted by antiangiogenic therapies. Clinical trials of the antiangiogenic drugs Bevacizumab, an anti-VEGF antibody (Vredenburgh et al. 2007a, b), and Cediranib (AZD2171), a small molecule inhibitor of the VEGFR signaling (Batchelor et al. 2007), have demonstrated encouraging efficacy in patients with glioblastoma (see also Chapter 30). This anti-tumor effect could be the result of 'normalization' of the tumor vasculature or depletion of the tumor blood supply that are proposed mechanisms of action of antiangiogenic drugs. However, the presence of a glioblastoma stem cell niche would imply that these drugs may function also to disrupt stem cell maintenance. In this regard, Bevacizumab depletes brain tumor blood vessels to cause a dramatic reduction in the number of CSC and inhibition of tumor growth (Calabrese et al. 2007). This treatment did not impact the proliferation or survival of most of the cells in the tumor, consistent with the speculation that the drugs might have specifically acted on CSC. Similar data were obtained using a rat C6 glioma model, and these studies provided evidence that antiangiogenic strategies combined with conventional cytotoxic drugs might prove especially effective (Folkins et al. 2007).

44.5 Cancer Stem Cells and Niches in Therapeutic Resistance

44.5.1 Cancer Stem Cells Are Resistant to Conventional Therapy

Although radiation and cytotoxic chemotherapy remain the mainstay of brain cancer adjuvant treatments, these treatments fail to cure the majority of patients (Stupp et al. 2005). Many mechanisms may contribute to the development of therapeutic resistance including cell intrinsic factors, selection of resistant genetic subclones, and microenvironmental factors. Several groups have demonstrated that cells expressing stem cell markers are resistant to conventional cancer therapies (Eramo et al. 2006; Bao et al. 2006a, b; Liu et al. 2006; Blazek et al. 2007). If cancer is, as the cancer stem cell theory postulates (Reya et al. 2001), maintained by a small number of CSC characterized by low rates of division and proliferation, it is clear that therapies such as radiation and chemotherapy, which target rapidly proliferating cells, are likely ineffective at eradicating the tumor stem cell population. The rate of CSC proliferation in solid tumors remains to be determined. In addition to their quiescence, CSC may also be resistant to chemotherapy due to their enhanced capacity for DNA repair and ABC-transporter expression. One group found that CSC from gliomas display marked resistance to several chemotherapeutic agents including temozolomide, carboplatin, etoposide, and paclitaxel (Liu et al. 2006).

44.5.2 Cancer Stem Cells Express High Levels of ABC Drug Transporters

Both normal neural stem cells and CSC express high levels of (ATP-binding cassette) ABC drug transporters, which are transmembrane proteins that utilize ATP hydrolysis to transport substrates including drugs from the intracellular to the extracellular compartments. The transporters which have been most extensively studied in stem cells are ABCB1 which encodes p-glycoprotein and ABCC1 and ABCG2 which are the principle multidrug resistance genes in tumor cells and encode promiscuous drug efflux pumps which recognize both hydrophobic and hydrophilic agents (Dean et al. 2005). Knock-out mice lacking one of these transporters have normal stem cell compartments but crucially are more susceptible to cytotoxic agents such as vinblastine and topotecan suggesting a role for these proteins in protecting cells from toxins (Schinkel et al. 1994). The identification of potent, specific, and non-toxic inhibitors of

ABCB1, ABCG2, and ABCC1 is required in order to assess the feasibility of targeting drug efflux pumps to sensitize cancer stem cells to cytotoxic agents. This may of course be difficult to accomplish without destruction of normal stem cells that depend on the expression of transporters to survive drug therapy, such as those in the hematopoietic system. It must not be forgotten that stem cell-driven tissue repopulation is found not only in tumors but also in regrowth of normal tissues including the bone marrow, gastrointestinal tract, and hair follicles. It remains to be seen for both targeting of drug transporters and signaling pathways whether a sufficient therapeutic window exists between normal stem cells and CSC. It is also important to consider that the role of CSC in tumor resistance has not been validated in human brain tumor subjects and that any agent to be utilized in the management of brain tumors must be able to permeate though the blood–brain barrier.

44.5.3 Cancer Stem Cells Have Augmented DNA Damage Repair Capacity

While the high expression of ABC-transporters by cancer stem cells could render them insensitive to cytotoxics, the DNA repair capacity of cells is also likely to play a role in their resistance to chemotherapy and radiotherapy. Preclinical glioma models have been used to demonstrate that CSC (identified as human glioblastoma-derived $CD133^+$ populations) preferentially activate DNA damage checkpoint responses and have an increased capacity for DNA repair, relative to $CD133^-$ glioma cells (Bao et al. 2006a, b). Radiation of glioma cells in culture and in allograft models resulted in an enrichment of the $CD133^+$ cell population, which demonstrated high-level repair of radiation-induced DNA damage relative to $CD133^-$ cells. Furthermore, this radioresistance of $CD133^+$ cells could be reversed with a specific inhibitor of Chk1 and Chk2 kinases, suggesting that therapeutic strategies targeted toward DNA damage checkpoint response may sensitize cancer stem cells to radiotherapy. It is currently unclear if mechanisms of cancer stem cell therapeutic resistance are shared across cancer types. Indeed if the cell of origin varies among and between brain tumors, it is probable that the response to therapy of CSC will vary accordingly.

44.5.4 The Perivascular Niche Contributes to Cancer Stem Cell Resistance to Therapy

Recent data have also implicated the perivascular CSC niche in the resistance of brain tumors to conventional therapies (Hambardzumyan et al. 2008). Using a number of mouse models of medulloblastoma this study demonstrated that the great majority of proliferating cells in brain tumors undergo radiation-induced, p53-dependent apoptotic cell death. In contrast, the fraction of nestin-expressing perivascular CSC survive radiation, activate PI3K/Akt pathway, undergo p53-dependent cell cycle arrest, and re-enter the cell cycle 72 hours later. Remarkably, inhibition of Akt signaling sensitized these cells in the perivascular region to radiation-induced apoptosis. Therefore, these data implicate the CSC niche in promoting therapy resistance and suggest that appropriate molecular therapies might circumvent this clinical problem.

44.6 Cancer Stem Cells as Markers of Prognosis

Oncologists have difficulties in predicting individual patient survival because apparently identical cancers can behave with strikingly different outcomes. Current prognosis (and thus clinical management) of brain tumor patients utilizes patient characteristics (age, performance status, etc.) and tumor characteristics (histology, grade, extent of resection, and presence of metastasis in some tumor types). To date, molecular testing of tumor specimens has contributed only modestly to brain tumor patient management. If CSC contribute disproportionately to the progression of cancer, then these cells might offer a more accurate indicator for predicting outcome. Encouragingly, a recent study found that CSC gene expression profiles derived from breast cancers predicted patient survival, perhaps indicating that CSC prevalence can dictate both gene expression and tumor growth (Liu et al. 2007). While similar studies are not yet published in brain tumor patient populations, studies have found that the percentage of glioblastoma cells that express CD133, a potential glioma stem cell marker, correlates with patient survival and risk of tumor regrowth (Zeppernick et al. 2008; Beier et al. 2008). It remains possible that prognostic models may be strengthened if cancer stem cell populations are directly characterized. Characterizing cancer stem cells at diagnosis and during treatment may yield novel cancer markers that more closely predict the clinical course of cancer patients.

44.7 Imaging of Cancer Stem Cells

Current imaging techniques utilized in brain tumor patient management frequently quantify tumor burden indirectly through edema, vascular integrity (i.e., contrast enhancement), or metabolic activity. The newfound importance of CSC in tumor growth suggests that the development of novel imaging modalities to visualize these cells non-invasively in patients is a priority. Small numbers of brain tumor cells present formidable challenges to detect in live subjects. As brain tumor stem cells may occur at low density and exhibit early propensity toward dissemination (a key behavior of brain tumors that underlies the need to identify these cells), imaging cancer stem cells is likely to present severe technical challenges. Potential methodologies under development for cancer stem cell identification are based on the expression of specific channels/pumps (e.g., the side population), enzymatic activity (aldehyde dehydrogenase, ALDH), or marker expression. As these aspects may be shared with normal stem cells, interpretation of CSC imaging modalities will face anatomic restrictions near high-density areas of normal stem cells. CSC imaging may have implications in the evaluation of clinical outcome. The FDA has required improved survival as the endpoint for approval of most cancer therapies. Surrogate endpoints, such as radiographic tumor response, are attractive for clinical trials, but tumor response (i.e., shrinkage of tumor) may not correlate with overall survival (Sorensen et al. 2008) (of note, progression-free survival is a better predictor of survival) (Lamborn et al. 2008). Non-stem tumor cells account for the bulk of the tumor and may display preferential sensitivity to some cancer therapies while CSC may represent restricted subsets of tumor populations but contribute to tumor progression and recurrence – and thus, tumor lethality. Based on this model, the majority of the tumor may respond to treatment, but survival may be determined by the residual CSC. If this assumption is correct, imaging of CSC becomes of even greater importance.

44.8 Perspectives

Although the concept of brain tumor heterogeneity dates back at least to Bailey and Cushing in the 1920s, the CSC hypothesis in neuro-oncology has only gained attention very recently. It remains to be seen how CSC and stochastic models of tumor initiation and progression will be integrated to improve our understanding of brain tumor biology. Many unresolved questions must be answered in the CSC field. The true frequency of CSC is uncertain. Because the current definition of CSC is functional, the relative fraction of CSC may change as the assays currently used are improved. For example, tumor formation assays will change as new immunocompromised models are developed with additional conditioning of the microenvironment (including humanized surrounding cells). The current CSC marker panel needs improvement. Only a subset of marker-positive cells are functional CSC and some tumors have CSC despite an absence of CSC markers. Other researchers argue that CSC are still an unproven entity and may be a product of the weakness in our cancer models. If CSC are more fully validated in human tumors, many more studies will be required to better understand how CSC are formed and maintained with a hope to identify potential therapies against this tumor compartment. Implicit in the selection of CSC targeting is a desire to minimize toxicity against normal stem cells. We remain ignorant of the role of some organ-specific stem cells in adults, e.g., neural stem cells. However, it is hoped that the CSC hypothesis will inform improved brain cancer diagnosis, prognosis, and therapy.

44.9 Summary

Brain tumors are formed from heterogeneous neoplastic cells as well as immune, neural, and vascular components. New models of tumor initiation and maintenance suggest that tumor cells may variably contribute to tumor biology. Cancer stem cells (CSC) are tumor populations with shared characteristics with adult stem cells, including sustained self-renewal, proliferation potential, and differentiation. CSC are currently defined through functional assays but cell surface markers have been identified that can prospectively enrich for CSC from tumors. These advances have permitted the direct study of CSC with resulting insights of CSC resistance to therapy and promotion of angiogenesis. Not only are CSC signaling pathways becoming elucidated but CSC also reside in specific physiologic niches that are essential for tumor growth. Therefore, it may become possible that the study of CSC will provide improved brain tumor therapy.

Acknowledgments We thank Dr. Constantinos Hadjipanayis for commenting on the manuscript.

References

Aguado T, Carracedo A, Julien B, Velasco G, Milman G, Mechoulam R, Alvarez L, Guzmán M, Galve-Roperh I (2007) Cannabinoids induce glioma stem-like cell differentiation and inhibit gliomagenesis. J Biol Chem 282:6854–6862

Al-Hajj M, Wicha MS, Benito-Hernandez A, Morrison SJ, Clarke MF (2003) Prospective identification of tumorigenic breast cancer cells. Proc Natl Acad Sci U S A 100:3983–3988

Ali SA, McHayleh WM, Ahmad A, Sehgal R, Braffet M, Rahman M, Bejjani G, Friedland DM (2008). Bevacizumab and irinotecan therapy in glioblastoma multiforme: a series of 13 cases. J Neurosurg 109:268–272

Assanah M, Lochhead R, Ogden A, Bruce J, Goldman J, Canoll P (2006) Glial progenitors in adult white matter are driven to form malignant gliomas by platelet-derived growth factor-expressing retroviruses. J Neurosci 26:6781–6790

Bailey OT (1985) Genesis of the percival Bailey-Cushing classification of gliomas. Pediatr Neurosci 12:261–265

Bao S, Wu Q, Sathornsumetee S, Hao Y, Li Z, Hjelmeland AB, Shi Q, McLendon RE, Bigner DD, Rich JN (2006a) Stem cell-like glioma cells promote tumor angiogenesis through vascular endothelial growth factor. Cancer Res 66:7843–7848

Bao S, Wu Q, McLendon RE, Hao Y, Shi Q, Hjelmeland AB, Dewhirst MW, Bigner DD, Rich JN (2006b) Glioma stem cells promote radioresistance by preferential activation of the DNA damage response. Nature 444:756–760

Bao S, Wu Q, Li Z, Sathornsumetee S, Wang H, McLendon RE, Hjelmeland AB, Rich JN (2008) Targeting cancer stem cells through L1CAM suppresses glioma growth. Cancer Res 68:6043–6048

Bar EE, Chaudhry A, Lin A, Fan X, Schreck K, Matsui W, Piccirillo S, Vescovi AL, DiMeco F, Olivi A, Eberhart CG (2007) Cyclopamine-mediated hedgehog pathway inhibition depletes stem-like cancer cells in glioblastoma. Stem Cells 25:2524–2533

Batchelor TT, Sorensen AG, di Tomaso E, Zhang WT, Duda DG, Cohen KS, Kozak KR, Cahill DP, Chen PJ, Zhu M, Ancukiewicz M, Mrugala MM, Plotkin S, Drappatz J, Louis

DN, Ivy P, Scadden DT, Benner T, Loeffler JS, Wen PY, Jain RK (2007) AZD2171, a pan-VEGF receptor tyrosine kinase inhibitor, normalizes tumor vasculature and alleviates edema in glioblastoma patients. Cancer Cell 11:83–95

Beier D, Hau P, Proescholdt M, Lohmeier A, Wischhusen J, Oefner PJ, Aigner L, Brawanski A, Bogdahn U, Beier CP (2007) CD133(+) and CD133(-) glioblastoma-derived cancer stem cells show differential growth characteristics and molecular profiles. Cancer Res 67:4010–4015

Beier D, Wischhusen J, Dietmaier W, Hau P, Proescholdt M, Brawanski A, Bogdahn U, Beier CP (2008) CD133 expression and cancer stem cells predict prognosis in high-grade oligodendroglial tumors. Brain Pathol 18:370–377

Blazek ER, Foutch JL, Maki G (2007) Daoy medulloblastoma cells that express CD133 are radioresistant relative to CD133- cells, and the CD133 + sector is enlarged by hypoxia. Int J Radiat Oncol Biol Phys 67:1–5

Bonnet D, Dick JE (1997) Human acute myeloid leukemia is organized as a hierarchy that originates from a primitive hematopoietic cell. Nature Med 3:730–737

Calabrese C, Poppleton H, Kocak M, Hogg TL, Fuller C, Hamner B, Oh EY, Gaber MW, Finklestein D, Allen M, Frank A, Bayazitov IT, Zakharenko SS, Gajjar A, Davidoff A, Gilbertson RJ (2007) A perivascular niche for brain tumor stem cells. Cancer Cell 11:69–82

Chang SM, Wen P, Cloughesy T, Greenberg H, Schiff D, Conrad C, Fink K, Robins HI, De Angelis L, Raizer J, Hess K, Aldape K, Lamborn KR, Kuhn J, Dancey J, Prados MD; North American Brain Tumor Consortium and the National Cancer Institute (2005) Phase II study of CCI-779 in patients with recurrent glioblastoma multiforme. Invest New Drugs 23:357–361

Clark PA, Treisman DM, Ebben J, Kuo JS (2007) Developmental signaling pathways in brain tumor-derived stem-like cells. Dev Dyn 236:3297–3308

Clement V, Sanchez P, de Tribolet N, Radovanovic I, Ruiz i Altaba A (2007) HEDGEHOG-GLI1 signaling regulates human glioma growth, cancer stem cell self-renewal, and tumorigenicity. Curr Biol 17:165–172

Cloughesy TF, Yoshimoto K, Nghiemphu P, Brown K, Dang J, Zhu S, Hsueh T, Chen Y, Wang W, Youngkin D, Liau L, Martin N, Becker D, Bergsneider M, Lai A, Green R, Oglesby T, Koleto M, Trent J, Horvath S, Mischel PS, Mellinghoff IK, Sawyers CL (2008) Antitumor activity of rapamycin in a Phase I trial for patients with recurrent PTEN-deficient glioblastoma. PLoS Med 5:e8

Dalerba P, Dylla SJ, Park IK, Liu R, Wang X, Cho RW, Hoey T, Gurney A, Huang EH, Simeone DM, Shelton AA, Parmiani G, Castelli C, Clarke MF (2007) Phenotypic characterization of human colorectal cancer stem cells. Proc Natl Acad Sci U S A 104: 10158–10163

Dai C, Celestino JC, Okada Y, Louis DN, Fuller GN, Holland EC (2001) PDGF autocrine stimulation dedifferentiates cultured astrocytes and induces oligodendrogliomas and oligoastrocytomas from neural progenitors and astrocytes in vivo. Genes Dev 15:1913–1925

Dean M, Fojo T, Bates S (2005) Tumour stem cells and drug resistance. Nat Rev Cancer 5:275–284

Doherty L, Gigas DC, Kesari S, Drappatz J, Kim R, Zimmerman J, Ostrowsky L, Wen PY (2006) Pilot study of the combination of EGFR and mTOR inhibitors in recurrent malignant gliomas. Neurology 67:156–158

Eramo A, Ricci-Vitiani L, Zeuner A, Pallini R, Lotti F, Sette G, Pilozzi E, Larocca LM, Peschle C, De Maria R (2006) Chemotherapy resistance of glioblastoma stem cells. Cell Death Differ 13:1238–1241

Eyler CE, Foo WC, Lafiura KM, McLendon RE, Hjelmeland AB, Rich JN (2008) Brain Cancer Stem Cells Display Preferential Sensitivity to Akt Inhibition. Stem Cells [Epub ahead of print]

Fan X, Matsui W, Khaki L, Stearns D, Chun J, Li YM, Eberhart CG (2006) Notch pathway inhibition depletes stem-like cells and blocks engraftment in embryonal brain tumors. Cancer Res 66:7445–7452

Feldmann G, Fendrich V, McGovern K, Bedja D, Bisht S, Alvarez H, Koorstra JB, Habbe N, Karikari C, Mullendore M, Gabrielson KL, Sharma R, Matsui W, Maitra A F (2008) An orally bioavailable small-molecule inhibitor of Hedgehog signaling inhibits tumor initiation and metastasis in pancreatic cancer. Mol Cancer Ther 7:2725–2735

Fischer I, Cunliffe CH, Bollo RJ, Raza S, Monoky D, Chiriboga L, Parker EC, Golfinos JG, Kelly PJ, Knopp EA, Gruber ML, Zagzag D, Narayana A. (2008) High-grade glioma before and after treatment with radiation and Avastin: Initial observations. Neuro Oncol 10:700–8

Folkins C, Man S, Xu P, Shaked Y, Hicklin DJ, Kerbel RS (2007) Anticancer therapies combining antiangiogenic and tumor cell cytotoxic effects reduce the tumor stem-like cell fraction in glioma xenograft tumors. Cancer Res 67:3560–3564

Fuchs E, Tumbar T, Guasch G (2004) Socializing with the neighbors: stem cells and their niche. Cell 116:769–778

Furnari FB, Fenton T, Bachoo RM, Mukasa A, Stommel JM, Stegh A, Hahn WC, Ligon KL, Louis DN, Brennan C, Chin L, DePinho RA, Cavenee WK 1 (2007) Malignant astrocytic glioma: genetics, biology, and paths to treatment. Genes Dev 21:2683–2710

Gal H, Pandi G, Kanner AA, Ram Z, Lithwick-Yanai G, Amariglio N, Rechavi G, Givol D (2008) MIR-451 and Imatinib mesylate inhibit tumor growth of Glioblastoma stem cells. Biochem Biophys Res Commun [Epub ahead of print]

Galanis E, Buckner JC, Maurer MJ, Kreisberg JI, Ballman K, Boni J, Peralba JM, Jenkins RB, Dakhil SR, Morton RF, Jaeckle KA, Scheithauer BW, Dancey J, Hidalgo M, Walsh DJ; North Central Cancer Treatment Group (2005) Phase II trial of temsirolimus (CCI-779) in recurrent glioblastoma multiforme: a North Central Cancer Treatment Group Study. J Clin Oncol 23:5294–5304

Galli R, Binda E, Orfanelli U, Cipelletti B, Gritti A, De Vitis S, Fiocco R, Foroni C, Dimeco F, Vescovi A (2004) Isolation and characterization of tumorigenic, stem-like neural precursors from human glioblastoma. Cancer Res 64:7011–7021

Goodrich LV, Milenković L, Higgins KM, Scott MP (1997) Altered neural cell fates and medulloblastoma in mouse patched mutants. Science 277:1109–1113

Groszer M, Erickson R, Scripture-Adams DD, Dougherty JD, Le Belle J, Zack JA, Geschwind DH, Liu X, Kornblum HI, Wu H (2001) Negative regulation of neural stem/progenitor cell proliferation by the Pten tumor suppressor gene in vivo. Science 294: 2186–2189

Hambardzumyan D, Becher OJ, Rosenblum MK, Pandolfi PP, Manova-Todorova K, Holland EC (2008) PI3K pathway regulates survival of cancer stem cells residing in the perivascular niche following radiation in medulloblastoma in vivo. Genes Dev 22:436–448

Hemmati HD, Nakano I, Lazareff JA, Masterman-Smith M, Geschwind DH, Bronner-Fraser M, Kornblum HI (2003) Cancerous stem cells can arise from pediatric brain tumors. Proc Natl Acad Sci U S A 100:15178–15183

Hope KJ, Jin L, Dick JE (2004) Acute myeloid leukemia originates from a hierarchy of leukemic stem cell classes that differ in self-renewal capacity. Nat Immunol 5:738–743

Ignatova TN, Kukekov VG, Laywell ED, Suslov ON, Vrionis FD, Steindler DA (2002) Human cortical glial tumors contain neural stem-like cells expressing astroglial and neuronal markers in vitro. Glia 39:193–206

Jackson EL, Garcia-Verdugo JM, Gil-Perotin S, Roy M, Quinones-Hinojosa A, VandenBerg S, Alvarez-Buylla A (2006) PDGFR alpha-positive B cells are neural stem cells in the adult SVZ that form glioma-like growths in response to increased PDGF signaling. Neuron 51:187–199

Jain RK, di Tomaso E, Duda DG, Loeffler JS, Sorensen AG, Batchelor TT (2007) Angiogenesis in brain tumours. Nat Rev Neurosci 8:610–622

Jaksch M, Múnera J, Bajpai R, Terskikh A, Oshima RG (2008) Cell cycle-dependent variation of a CD133 epitope in human embryonic stem cell, colon cancer, and melanoma cell lines. Cancer Res 68:7882–7886.

Lamborn KR, Yung WK, Chang SM, Wen PY, Cloughesy TF, DeAngelis LM, Robins HI, Lieberman FS, Fine HA, Fink KL, Junck L, Abrey L, Gilbert MR, Mehta M, Kuhn JG, Aldape KD, Hibberts J, Peterson PM, Prados MD; North American Brain Tumor Consortium (2008) Progression-free survival: an important end point in evaluating therapy for recurrent high-grade gliomas. Neuro Oncol 10:162–170

Lapidot T, Sirard C, Vormoor J, Murdoch B, Hoang T, Caceres-Cortes J, Minden M, Paterson B, Caligiuri MA, Dick JE (1994) A cell initiating human acute myeloid leukaemia after transplantation into SCID mice. Nature 367:645–648

Le Bras B, Barallobre MJ, Homman-Ludiye J, Ny A, Wyns S, Tammela T, Haiko P, Karkkainen MJ, Yuan L, Muriel MP, Chatzopoulou E, Bréant C, Zalc B, Carmeliet P, Alitalo K, Eichmann A, Thomas JL (2006) VEGF-C is a trophic factor for neural progenitors in the vertebrate embryonic brain. Nat Neurosci 9:340–348

Lee J, Kotliarova S, Kotliarov Y, Li A, Su Q, Donin NM, Pastorino S, Purow BW, Christopher N, Zhang W, Park JK, Fine HA (2006) Tumor stem cells derived from glioblastomas cultured in bFGF and EGF more closely mirror the phenotype and genotype of primary tumors than do serum-cultured cell lines. Cancer Cell 9:391–403

Lee J, Son MJ, Woolard K, Donin NM, Li A, Cheng CH, Kotliarova S, Kotliarov Y, Walling J, Ahn S, Kim M, Totonchy M, Cusack T, Ene C, Ma H, Su Q, Zenklusen JC, Zhang W, Maric D, Fine HA (2008) Epigenetic-mediated dysfunction of the bone morphogenetic protein pathway inhibits differentiation of glioblastoma-initiating cells. Cancer Cell 13:69–80

Leventhal C, Rafii S, Rafii D, Shahar A, Goldman SA (1999) Endothelial Trophic Support of Neuronal Production and Recruitment from the Adult Mammalian Subependyma. Mol Cell Neurosci 13:450–464

Li C, Heidt DG, Dalerba P, Burant CF, Zhang L, Adsay V, Wicha M, Clarke MF, Simeone DM (2007) Identification of pancreatic cancer stem cells. Cancer Res 67:1030–1037

Li Q, Ford MC, Lavik EB, Madri JA (2006) Modeling the neurovascular niche: VEGF- and BDNF-mediated cross-talk between neural stem cells and endothelial cells: an in vitro study. J Neurosci Res 84:1656–1668

Ligon KL, Huillard E, Mehta S, Kesari S, Liu H, Alberta JA, Bachoo RM, Kane M, Louis DN, Depinho RA, Anderson DJ, Stiles CD, Rowitch DH (2007) Olig2-regulated lineage-restricted pathway controls replication competence in neural stem cells and malignant glioma. Neuron 53: 503–517

Liu G, Yuan X, Zeng Z, Tunici P, Ng H, Abdulkadir IR, Lu L, Irvin D, Black KL, Yu JS (2006) Analysis of gene expression and chemoresistance of CD133+ cancer stem cells in glioblastoma. Mol Cancer 5:67

Liu R, Wang X, Chen GY, Dalerba P, Gurney A, Hoey T, Sherlock G, Lewicki J, Shedden K, Clarke MF (2007) The prognostic role of a gene signature from tumorigenic breast-cancer cells. N Engl J Med 356:217–226

Melchior K, Weiss J, Zaehres H, Kim YM, Lutzko C, Roosta N, Hescheler J, Müschen M (2008) The WNT receptor FZD7 contributes to self-renewal signaling of human embryonic stem cells. Biol Chem 389:897–903

Moore KA, Lemischka IR (2006) Stem cells and their niches. Science 311:1880–1885

Nakano I, Masterman-Smith M, Saigusa K, Paucar AA, Horvath S, Shoemaker L, Watanabe M, Negro A, Bajpai R, Howes A, Lelievre V, Waschek JA, Lazareff JA, Freije WA, Liau LM, Gilbertson RJ, Cloughesy TF, Geschwind DH, Nelson SF, Mischel PS, Terskikh AV, Kornblum HI (2008) Maternal embryonic leucine zipper kinase is a key regulator of the proliferation of malignant brain tumors, including brain tumor stem cells. J Neurosci Res 86:48–60

Narayana A, Golfinos JG, Fischer I, Raza S, Kelly P, Parker E, Knopp EA, Medabalmi P, Zagzag D, Eagan P, Gruber ML (2008) Feasibility of using bevacizumab with radiation therapy and temozolomide in newly diagnosed high-grade glioma. Int J Radiat Oncol Biol Phys 72:383–389

O'Brien CA, Pollett A, Gallinger S, Dick JE (2007) A human colon cancer cell capable of initiating tumour growth in immunodeficient mice. Nature 445:106–110

Ogden AT, Waziri AE, Lochhead RA, Fusco D, Lopez K, Ellis JA, Kang J, Assanah M, McKhann GM, Sisti MB, McCormick PC, Canoll P, Bruce JN (2008) Identification of A2B5 + CD133- tumor-initiating cells in adult human gliomas. Neurosurgery 62:505–514

Palmer TD, Willhoite AR, Gage FH (2000) Vascular niche for adult hippocampal neurogenesis. J Comp Neurol 425:479–494

Phillips HS, Kharbanda S, Chen R, Forrest WF, Soriano RH, Wu TD, Misra A, Nigro JM, Colman H, Soroceanu L, Williams PM, Modrusan Z, Feuerstein BG, Aldape K (2006) Molecular subclasses of high-grade glioma predict prognosis, delineate a pattern of disease progression, and resemble stages in neurogenesis. Cancer Cell 9:157–173

Piccirillo SG, Reynolds BA, Zanetti N, Lamorte G, Binda E, Broggi G, Brem H, Olivi A, Dimeco F, Vescovi AL (2006) Bone morphogenetic proteins inhibit the tumorigenic potential of human brain tumour-initiating cells. Nature 444:761–765

Prados MD, Lamborn KR, Chang S, Burton E, Butowski N, Malec M, Kapadia A, Rabbitt J, Page MS, Fedoroff A, Xie D, Kelley SK (2006) Phase 1 study of erlotinib HCl alone and combined with temozolomide in patients with stable or recurrent malignant glioma. Neuro Oncol 8:67–78

Ramírez-Castillejo C, Sánchez-Sánchez F, Andreu-Agulló C, Ferrón SR, Aroca-Aguilar JD, Sánchez P, Mira H, Escribano J, Fariñas I (2006) Pigment epithelium-derived factor is a niche signal for neural stem cell renewal. Nat Neurosci 9:331–339

Reardon DA, Quinn JA, Vredenburgh JJ, Gururangan S, Friedman AH, Desjardins A, Sathornsumetee S, Herndon JE 2nd, Dowell JM, McLendon RE, Provenzale JM, Sampson JH, Smith RP, Swaisland AJ, Ochs JS, Lyons P, Tourt-Uhlig S, Bigner DD, Friedman HS, Rich JN (2006) Phase 1 trial of gefitinib plus sirolimus in adults with recurrent malignant glioma. Clin Cancer Res 12:860–868

Reya T and Clevers H (2005) Wnt signalling in stem cells and cancer. Nature 434:843–850

Reya T, Morrison SJ, Clarke MF, Weissman IL (2001) Stem cells, cancer, and cancer stem cells. Nature 414:105–111

Ricci-Vitiani L, Lombardi DG, Pilozzi E, Biffoni M, Todaro M, Peschle C, De Maria R (2007) Identification and expansion of human colon-cancer initiating cells. Nature 445:111–115

Rich JN, Reardon DA, Peery T, Dowell JM, Quinn JA, Penne KL, Wikstrand CJ, Van Duyn LB, Dancey JE, McLendon RE, Kao JC, Stenzel TT, Ahmed Rasheed BK, Tourt-Uhlig SE, Herndon JE 2nd, Vredenburgh JJ, Sampson JH, Friedman AH, Bigner DD, Friedman HS (2004) Phase II trial of gefitinib in recurrent glioblastoma. J Clin Oncol 22:133–142

Rietze RL, Valcanis H, Brooker GF, Thomas T, Voss AK, Bartlett PF (2001) Purification of a pluripotent neural stem cell from the adult mouse brain. Nature 412:736–739

Romer JT, Kimura H, Magdaleno S, Sasai K, Fuller C, Baines H, Connelly M, Stewart CF, Gould S, Rubin LL, Curran T (2004) Suppression of the Shh pathway using a small molecule inhibitor eliminates medulloblastoma in Ptc1(+/-)p53(-/-) mice. Cancer Cell 6:229–240

Sanai N, Tramontin AD, Quiñones-Hinojosa A, Barbaro NM, Gupta N, Kunwar S, Lawton MT, McDermott MW, Parsa AT, Manuel-García Verdugo J, Berger MS, Alvarez-Buylla A (2004) Unique astrocyte ribbon in adult human brain contains neural stem cells but lacks chain migration. Nature 427:740–744

Sauvageot CM, Weatherbee JL, Kesari S, Winters SE, Barnes J, Dellagatta J, Ramakrishna NR, Stiles CD, Kung AL, Kieran MW, Wen PY (2008) Efficacy of the HSP90 inhibitor 17-AAG in human glioma cell lines and tumorigenic glioma stem cells. Neuro Oncol [Epub ahead of print]

Scadden DT (2006) The stem-cell niche as an entity of action. Nature 441:1075–1079

Scheres B (2007) Stem-cell niches: nursery rhymes across kingdoms. Nat Rev Mol Cell Biol 8:345–354

Schinkel AH, Smit JJ, van Tellingen O, Beijnen JH, Wagenaar E, van Deemter L, Mol CA, van der Valk MA, Robanus-Maandag EC, te Riele HP, Berns AJM, Borst P (1994) Disruption of the mouse mdr1a P-glycoprotein gene leads to a deficiency in the blood-brain barrier and to increased sensitivity to drugs. Cell 77:491–502

Shen Q, Goderie SK, Jin L, Karanth N, Sun Y, Abramova N, Vincent P, Pumiglia K, Temple S (2004) Endothelial cells stimulate self-renewal and expand neurogenesis of neural stem cells. Science 304:1338–1340

Shen Q, Wang Y, Kokovay E, Lin G, Chuang SM, Goderie SK, Roysam B, Temple S (2008) Adult SVZ stem cells lie in a vascular niche: a quantitative analysis of niche cell-cell interactions. Cell Stem Cell 3:289–300

Shih AH, Holland EC (2006) Notch signaling enhances nestin expression in gliomas. Neoplasia 8:1072–1082

Singec I, Knoth R, Meyer RP, Maciaczyk J, Volk B, Nikkhah G, Frotscher M, Snyder EY (2006) Defining the actual sensitivity and specificity of the neurosphere assay in stem cell biology. Nat Methods 3:801–806

Singh SK, Clarke ID, Terasaki M, Bonn VE, Hawkins C, Squire J, Dirks PB (2003) Identification of a cancer stem cell in human brain tumors. Cancer Res 63:5821–5828

Singh SK, Hawkins C, Clarke ID, Squire JA, Bayani J, Hide T, Henkelman RM, Cusimano MD, Dirks PB (2004) Identification of human brain tumour initiating cells. Nature 432:396–401

Soeda A, Inagaki A, Oka N, Ikegame Y, Aoki H, Yoshimura S, Nakashima S, Kunisada T, Iwama T (2008) Epidermal growth factor plays a crucial role in mitogenic regulation of human brain tumor stem cells. J Biol Chem 283:10958–10966

Sorensen AG, Batchelor TT, Wen PY, Zhang WT, Jain RK (2008) Response criteria for glioma. Nat Clin Pract Oncol [Epub ahead of print]

Stupp R, Mason WP, van den Bent MJ, Weller M, Fisher B, Taphoorn MJ, Belanger K, Brandes AA, Marosi C, Bogdahn U, Curschmann J, Janzer RC, Ludwin SK, Gorlia T, Allgeier A, Lacombe D, Cairncross JG, Eisenhauer E, Mirimanoff RO; European Organisation for Research and Treatment of Cancer Brain Tumor and Radiotherapy Groups; National Cancer Institute of Canada Clinical Trials Group (2005) Radiotherapy plus concomitant and adjuvant temozolomide for glioblastoma. N Engl J Med 352: 987–996

Tabu K, Sasai K, Kimura T, Wang L, Aoyanagi E, Kohsaka S, Tanino M, Nishihara H, Tanaka S (2008) Promoter hypomethylation regulates CD133 expression in human gliomas. Cell Res 18:1037–1046

Tavazoie M, Van der Veken L, Silva-Vargas V, Louissaint M, Colonna L, Zaidi B, Garcia-Verdugo JM, Doetsch F (2008) A specialized vascular niche for adult neural stem cells. Cell Stem Cell 3:279–288

Taylor MD, Poppleton H, Fuller C, Su X, Liu Y, Jensen P, Magdaleno S, Dalton J, Calabrese C, Board J, Macdonald T, Rutka J, Guha A, Gajjar A, Curran T, Gilbertson RJ (2005) Radial glia cells are candidate stem cells of ependymoma. Cancer Cell 8:323–335

Uchida N, Buck DW, He D, Reitsma MJ, Masek M, Phan TV, Tsukamoto AS, Gage FH, Weissman IL (2000) Direct isolation of human central nervous system stem cells. Proc Natl Acad Sci U S A 97:14720–14725

Vorechovský I, Tingby O, Hartman M, Strömberg B, Nister M, Collins VP, Toftgård R (1997) Somatic mutations in the human homologue of Drosophila patched in primitive neuroectodermal tumours. Oncogene 15:361–366

Vredenburgh JJ, Desjardins A, Herndon JE 2nd, Dowell JM, Reardon DA, Quinn JA, Rich JN, Sathornsumetee S, Gururangan S, Wagner M, Bigner DD, Friedman AH, Friedman HS (2007a) Phase II trial of bevacizumab and irinotecan in recurrent malignant glioma. Clin Cancer Res 13:1253–1259

Vredenburgh JJ, Desjardins A, Herndon JE 2nd, Marcello J, Reardon DA, Quinn JA, Rich JN, Sathornsumetee S, Gururangan S, Sampson J, Wagner M, Bailey L, Bigner DD,

Friedman AH, Friedman HS (2007b) Bevacizumab plus irinotecan in recurrent glioblastoma multiforme. J Clin Oncol 25:4722–4729

Wechsler-Reya RJ, Scott MP (1999) Control of neuronal precursor proliferation in the cerebellum by Sonic Hedgehog. Neuron 22:103–114

Williams JA, Guicherit OM, Zaharian BI, Xu Y, Chai L, Wichterle H, Kon C, Gatchalian C, Porter JA, Rubin LL, Wang FY (2003) Identification of a small molecule inhibitor of the hedgehog signaling pathway: effects on basal cell carcinoma-like lesions. Proc Natl Acad Sci U S A 100:4616–4621

Yi JM, Tsai HC, Glöckner SC, Lin S, Ohm JE, Easwaran H, James CD, Costello JF, Riggins G, Eberhart CG, Laterra J, Vescovi AL, Ahuja N, Herman JG, Schuebel KE, Baylin SB (2008) Abnormal DNA methylation of CD133 in colorectal and glioblastoma tumors. Cancer Res 68:8094–8103

Yilmaz OH, Valdez R, Theisen BK, Guo W, Ferguson DO, Wu H, Morrison SJ (2006) Pten dependence distinguishes haematopoietic stem cells from leukaemia-initiating cells. Nature 441:475–482

Yin AH, Miraglia S, Zanjani ED, Almeida-Porada G, Ogawa M, Leary AG, Olweus J, Kearney J, Buck DW (1997) AC133, a novel marker for human hematopoietic stem and progenitor cells. Blood 90:5002–5012

Yuan X, Curtin J, Xiong Y, Liu G, Waschsmann-Hogiu S, Farkas DL, Black KL, Yu JS (2004) Isolation of cancer stem cells from adult glioblastoma multiforme. Oncogene 23:9392–9400

Zeppernick F, Ahmadi R, Campos B, Dictus C, Helmke BM, Becker N, Lichter P, Unterberg A, Radlwimmer B, Herold-Mende CC (2008) Stem cell marker CD133 affects clinical outcome in glioma patients. Clin Cancer Res 14:123–129

Chapter 45
The Use of Retinoids as Differentiation Agents Against Medulloblastoma

Matthew Wortham and Hai Yan

Abstract Medulloblastoma (MB) therapy—resection, chemotherapy, and radiation—results in admirable survival rates (70–85% 5-year survival of medium- to high-risk cases) but unacceptable chronic toxicities, including endocrine dysfunction and cognitive impairment. The limited efficacy of the current therapeutic regimen may be linked to the recently discovered MB cancer stem cells, which may regenerate tumors after bulk mass reduction. Nonetheless, the discovery of tumor stem cells as a new target has suggested a potential new approach for improving upon conventional cytotoxic chemotherapy. Differentiation agents that would specifically target tumor stem cells without being universally cytotoxic to proliferating cells could reduce systemic toxicity as well as deplete cell populations responsible for tumor maintenance. All-*trans* retinoic acid (ATRA) is the first and only differentiation agent that has proven effective in the clinical setting, inducing a 90% remission rate of acute promyelocytic leukemia (APL) when used as adjuvant to chemotherapy. Retinoids have also proven effective against a large fraction of MB cell lines and primary tumors. MB is an embryonal tumor that, like APL, relies upon the circumvention of endogenous differentiation pathways for tumorigenesis. Retinoid resistance in some MB cell lines has hindered its development as a universally applicable therapeutic. It has been shown that retinoid-resistant cell lines can be responsive to downstream targets of retinoid activity, suggesting that retinoid resistance occurs via disruption of upstream components of the pathway. Functional intermediates of retinoid activity have been identified; however, the ultimate targets of such intermediates remain elusive. Some studies have shown that retinoids exert their antitumor effect against MB in part by inducing Bmp2 production and subsequent activation of the TGFβ pathway. Other studies have demonstrated that ATRA silences the OTX2 oncogene, whose expression correlates with ATRA responsiveness of MB cell lines. Alternative pathways

M. Wortham (✉)
Department of Pathology, Duke University Medical Center,
189 Medical Sciences Research Building, Box 3156, Durham, NC 27710, USA
e-mail: matthew.wortham@duke.edu

E.G. Van Meir (ed.), *CNS Cancer*, Cancer Drug Discovery and Development, DOI 10.1007/978-1-60327-553-8_45,
© Humana Press, a part of Springer Science+Business Media, LLC 2009

accounting for the full effect of retinoids against MB (independent of Bmp2 and OTX2) as well as final targets of known pathways have yet to be identified. Delineation of the pathways through which ATRA exerts its pleiotropic effects could reveal potential therapeutic targets that recapitulate differentiation or apoptosis in both retinoid-sensitive and retinoid-resistant cell lines and thus serve as a more broadly applicable therapy.

Contents

45.1 Introduction—Medulloblastoma (MB) as a Lapse of Proper Development

The majority of tumor types develop from clonal expansion of cells that have undergone a succession of highly improbable initiator and promoter mutations over time, ultimately inactivating sufficient regulatory pathways to acquire oncogenic properties (Vogelstein and Kinzler 1993). However, some tumors predominantly manifest at younger ages, violating the paradigm that cancer incidence as a whole increases with age due to the requirement for multiple, rare events. Such pediatric tumors are considered developmental aberrations, and the progenitor cell lineages from which these tumors originate are presumably more susceptible to transformation than their differentiated counterparts (Grimmer and Weiss 2006; Wechsler-Reya and Scott 2001). MB is one such disease, manifesting as a tumor of the cerebellum and occurring in children at a peak age of 7 (Louis et al. 2007). The theory that progenitor cells are uniquely susceptible to tumorigenesis has been demonstrated in one subset of MBs that are induced by aberrant activation of the Sonic Hedgehog (Shh) pathway. In this model, mice harbor a heterozygous deletion of the *ptc1* gene, whose product antagonizes oncogenic Shh signaling, and 7.7% develop MB (Pazzaglia et al. 2002). Irradiation of these mice during cerebellum development (P4) increases MB incidence to 51%, while this treatment has no such effect in adult mice.

It should not be surprising that progenitor cells are particularly amenable to taking on oncogenic properties. Indeed, in order for a terminally differentiated cell to transform, it must take on many properties of progenitor cells, such as cell cycle entry, self-renewal, loss of lineage-specific markers, and, in metastatic tumors, the ability to migrate and survive in the absence of tissue architecture. Accordingly, a progenitor cell that is already self-renewing and capable of migration would require perturbation of fewer pathways to acquire oncogenic properties (Fan and Eberhart 2008). Thus, it is conceivable that during particular intervals of development, the disruption of the specific signal(s) that direct the transition from a progenitor to a terminally differentiated cell would greatly accelerate tumor promotion. Sustained proliferation naturally increases the probability of mutations, which are particularly risky in cells requiring fewer subsequent "hits" for transformation.

Much of what is known about cerebellar development has been gleaned from studies of MB which are currently classified by histology (Louis et al. 2007). Classic MBs are composed of tightly packed cells of dense nuclei and limited cytoplasm and are typically of neural differentiation. Desmoplastic/nodular MB is characterized by neurally differentiated nodules surrounded by dense, reticulum-interwoven proliferative cells. Anaplastic MB is the most aggressive and least treatable form, identified by the presence of nuclear heterogeneity, cell wrapping, and high indices of apoptotic and mitotic activities. Based upon morphology, gene expression data, and animal models of tumorigenesis, mounting evidence suggests that different classes of MBs arise from different cell origins. Thus, transformation of particular cell lineages may ultimately dictate the morphology and gene expression patterns of the resulting tumor (Gilbertson and Ellison 2008).

45.1.1 Normal Cerebellum Development

To understand the developmental programs that go awry during MB tumorigenesis, it is important to comprehend the networks regulating proper cerebellum development. The mature cerebellum develops via a network of morphogens and growth factors coordinating the fate and function of three main lineages (Gilbertson and Ellison 2008). First, at E10.5–E12.5, glutamatergic progenitors arise from the rhombic lip and migrate rostrally to form deep nuclei neurons. Subsequently, GABAergic neuron precursors arise from progenitor cells at the roof of the fourth ventricle. This lineage then migrates deep into the cerebellum and will ultimately form Purkinje cells, Golgi neurons, interneurons, and the deep nuclei. Bone morphogenic proteins (Bmps) produced by GABAergic progenitors target progenitor lineages of the rhombic lip to induce production of granule cell precursors (GCPs). GCPs then migrate to the outer edge of the developing cerebellum to form the external granular layer at birth. At this stage, Purkinje neurons adjacent to the external granular layer produce high levels of the morphogen Shh, which drives GCP proliferation. From birth to P21, GCPs undergo waves of proliferation, cell cycle exit, and inward migration, ultimately constituting a large proportion of cerebellar gray matter (Wechsler-Reya and Scott 2001). At P21, cells of the external granular layer have completely migrated inward, composing the internal granular layer adjacent to the Purkinje cell layer. In the adult, cerebellar tissue replenishment may occur via stem cells of the white matter that are capable of differentiating into multiple CNS lineages (Lee et al. 2005).

45.1.2 Mice with Dysregulated Shh Signaling Develop Desmoplastic/Nodular MB

The identification of an increased incidence of MBs in patients with Gorlin's syndrome, caused by germ-line mutations of the *PTCH1* gene (Gorlin 1987), first revealed that the cerebellum is exquisitely sensitive to tumorigenesis driven by dysregulated Shh signaling. Mice with heterozygous deletion of *ptc1* develop MBs resembling human desmoplastic/nodular MB at an incidence of 7–14% (Goodrich et al. 1997; Hahn et al. 1998). Low penetrance of this phenotype suggests that although these mice are genetically susceptible to MB, subsequent events, including silencing of the remaining *ptc1* allele (Oliver et al. 2005), are required for transformation. Indeed, a large proportion of mice that do not develop MB have sustained ectopic populations of proliferating granule cell precursors that resemble early neoplastic lesions. Transgenic mice expressing constitutively active Smoothened (which is normally inhibited by the *ptc1* gene product) in GCPs develop MBs at a frequency of 48% with one copy (Hallahan et al. 2004) or 94% with two copies (Hatton et al. 2008). Furthermore, inactivation of *ptc1* gene function is a frequent secondary event in mouse models of anaplastic MB (Zindy et al. 2007; Shakhova et al. 2006).

Mutations of the Shh pathway regulators *PTCH1* and *SUFU* have been identified in a subset of sporadic desmoplastic/nodular MBs exhibiting similar gene expression patterns indicative of Shh activation (Thompson et al. 2006). That study implicates Shh activation in 20% (9/46) of sporadic MBs.

45.1.3 Wnt Pathway Activation in Classic MBs

Mutation analysis of primary human tumors has implicated dysregulation of the Wnt pathway in classic MBs. Wnt signaling is required for proper cerebellum development. Deletion of β-catenin in nestin-expressing cells at E14.5 in mice results in premature commitment of multipotent cells and ultimately a failure to form the cerebellar vermis (Schuller and Rowitch 2007). A subset of classic primary MBs that exhibited similar gene expression patterns was found to have *CTNBB1* mutations and enhanced Wnt pathway target signatures (Thompson et al. 2006); this subset accounted for 13% (6/46) of MBs studied. Classic MBs generally do not express GCP lineage markers (Buhren et al. 2000), and Wnt pathway activation does not enhance proliferation in GCPs, which suggests that classic MBs deficient in Wnt regulation arise from a cell of origin distinct from GCPs (Gilbertson and Ellison 2008). The ability of Wnt activation to transform other cerebellar lineages, such as GABAergic precursors and white matter stem cells, remains to be determined.

45.1.4 Notch Amplification and Overexpression in MBs

The *Notch2* gene has been shown to be amplified in 15% of MBs (Fan et al. 2004) and is also involved in gliomagenesis (see Chapter 44). *Notch* is required for the maintenance of neural progenitors during development (Swiatek et al. 1994; de la Pompa et al. 1997). In the cerebellum, Notch activity is detected in the key germinal centers, the ventricular zone (Gaiano et al. 2000) and the rhombic lip (Machold et al. 2007). Overexpression of Notch results in sustained neural progenitor populations (Gaiano and Fishell 2002), and Notch activation promotes proliferation and inhibits differentiation of GCPs (Solecki et al. 2001). Notch signaling is required for the maintenance of $CD133^+$ stem-like cell populations in MB cell lines, whereas some cell lines apoptose or differentiate in response to Notch inhibition (Fan et al. 2006). Finally, Notch pathway activation is induced by constitutive Shh signaling (Hallahan et al. 2004).

45.1.5 OTX2 Amplification and Overexpression in Anaplastic MBs

Orthodenticle homolog 2, or *OTX2*, has been identified by digital karyotyping, SNP array, and FISH to be the most frequently amplified gene in MBs (Taylor M, personal communication). *OTX2* exhibited copy number gain in 20% of MB samples (out of 11 cell lines and 201 primary tumors), and it was overexpressed in 67% (73/109) of primary MB samples (Taylor M, personal communication). In addition, *OTX2* amplification was associated with the anaplastic subtype of MBs, being overexpressed in 93% (14/15) of primary anaplastic tumors and in 20% (2/10) of tumors of other histological subtypes (Di et al. 2005; Yan H, unpublished results). OTX2 is a homeobox transcription factor vital to anteroposterior patterning of the early embryo, development of the eye, regionalization of the midbrain/hindbrain threshold, and subsequent development of the cerebellum (Matsuo et al. 1995; Acampora and Simeone 1999; Broccoli et al. 1999; Vernay et al. 2005). Homozygous deletion of *OTX2* in nestin-expressing cells results in posterior truncation of the cerebellum as well as development of an ectopic cerebellar structure anterior to the cerebellum proper (Vernay et al. 2005). Functional studies support an oncogenic function of OTX2: forced OTX2 expression is sufficient to drive MB cell line proliferation, and OTX2 is required for the survival of OTX2-expressing MB cells (Yan H, unpublished results). In addition, ChIP-chip promoter arrays, in which DNA fragments bound by OTX2 in an MB cell line were quantified by microarray hybridization, revealed that OTX2 predominantly regulates genes involved in proliferation, cell cycle, and differentiation. siRNA knockdown of OTX2 inhibits proliferation and anchorage-independent growth of OTX2-expressing MB cell lines, resulting in apoptosis or differentiation (Yan H, unpublished results).

45.2 Endogenous Retinoid Function

45.2.1 An Introduction to Retinoid Metabolism and Signal Regulation

Retinoids comprise a class of natural and synthetic derivatives of vitamin A, of which all-*trans* retinoic acid, or ATRA, functions as the endogenously produced, active form. Retinoids play vital roles in development, gametogenesis, and phototransduction (Niederreither and Dolle 2008). They are derived from dietary carotenoids, which are abundant in cruciferous vegetables. Hepatic stellate cells are the site of retinol storage in the adult, maintaining retinyl esters within lipid droplets to be hydrolyzed and released to maintain 1–2 μM serum retinol concentrations (Blomhoff and Blomhoff 2006). Retinol can cross the plasma membrane from the circulation to enter the cytoplasm. Within cells, retinol is oxidized to retinaldehyde (retinal) by alcohol dehydrogenases (Adh1-4), which collectively are expressed in all tissues. Retinal is oxidized again to ATRA, its biologically active metabolite, by Raldh enzymes (Raldh1–4). Raldh2 is expressed dynamically and specifically in the developing embryo, regionalizing endogenous retinoid signaling during development (Niederreither et al. 1999). ATRA catabolic enzymes (CYP26A1, CYP26B1, and CYP26C1) are also dynamically expressed, providing regulation of retinoic acid activity at the cellular level. Collectively broad expression of retinoic acid receptor (RAR) isoforms suggests that retinoid signaling is not regionalized by expression of its receptors. Hence, the activity of retinoids is mainly controlled by (1) the synthesis of ATRA from retinol, which is maintained at 1–2 μM in the serum, and (2) the degradation of ATRA within cells by expression of catabolic enzymes.

45.2.2 Retinoids Function by Activating Ligand-Activated Transcription Factors

Retinoids exert their effects through the nuclear receptors RAR and the retinoid X receptor (RXR), which function as heterodimers bound to DNA. RAR and RXR belong to the steroid hormone nuclear receptor superfamily

(Mangelsdorf et al. 1995). RAR and RXR are both expressed as three subtypes, α, β, and γ, each of which has unique spatiotemporal expression patterns (Germain et al. 2006b; Germain et al. 2006a). Knockout of individual RAR or RXR subtypes in mice does not result in overt phenotypes (Mark et al. 2006), which suggests for some level of functional redundancy among receptor subtypes. However, the identification of more subtle phenotypes, such as altered drug metabolism in hepatocyte RXRα knockout mice (Wan et al. 2000), suggests that phenotypes of knockouts may be concealed in the conventional laboratory animal environment. As this review is not intended to discuss functional differences among retinoid receptor subtypes, RAR and RXR subtypes will hereafter be collectively referred to as RAR and RXR, respectively. The main pathway through which endogenous ATRA functions is activation of RAR/RXR heterodimers by binding to the RAR ligand-binding domain (Germain et al. 2006a). RAR/RXR heterodimers bind DNA on retinoic acid response elements [RAREs, direct repeats of (A/G)G(G/T)TCA separated by 1, 2, or 5 nucleotides] in the absence or presence of ligand. When unbound by ligand, RAR and RXR recruit corepressors such as NCoR and SMRT, as well as HDACs, to inhibit transcription. Ligand binding induces the dissociation of corepressors and recruitment of coactivators, such as p300/CBP and HATs, to activate transcription of target genes. By repressing transcription in the absence of ligand and activating transcription in the presence of ligand, nuclear receptors exert a dynamic range of control upon target genes.

45.2.3 Endogenous Function of Retinoids During Embryonic Development

ATRA signaling plays vital roles in the regionalization of the early embryo and in coordinating differentiation of progenitor cells during organogenesis (Reviewed in: Niederreither and Dolle 2008). ATRA is also involved in eye development and in establishing germ cell meiosis cycles. The diversity of ATRA function is a result of signal cooperativity between ATRA and other morphogens acting upon target cells; the response depends upon the integration of signals of variable intensity as well as the responsive pathways present in the target cell. Knockout of Raldh2 is lethal to the mouse embryo, and knockdown of combinations of RAR subtypes results in an assortment of developmental defects (Niederreither et al. 1999; Mark et al. 2006). Teratogenicity experiments reveal that mislocalized or excessive ATRA exposure interferes with proper development, most notably resulting in caudalization of the neural tube (Niederreither et al. 2008).

The mechanistic rationale for investigating antitumor effects of retinoids stems from the well-established function of ATRA serving as a differentiation signal for a variety of target sites during development. The role of ATRA at the retreating edge of the primitive streak is a well-characterized example of

ATRA-induced differentiation during vertebrate development (Niederreither et al. 2008). During early somitogenesis, the edge of the retracting primitive streak marks a mutual boundary of fibroblast growth factor 8 and ATRA production, which induce "stemness" and differentiation, respectively. ATRA is particularly vital to neural differentiation, as quail embryos deficient in vitamin A exhibit markedly reduced neurofilament staining (Maden et al. 1996). Additionally, *Xenopus* embryos expressing a dominant negative RARα also exhibit diminished populations of primary neurons (Blumberg et al. 1997), whereas forced expression of RARα/RXRβ results in ectopic neuron populations (Sharpe and Goldstone 1997).

ATRA is a remarkable differentiation agent of cultured multipotent cells, including embryonal carcinomas, stem cells, teratocarcinomas, and neuroblastomas (Edwards and McBurney 1983; Maden 2001). The concentration of ATRA exposure dictates the lineage induced, ranging from cardiac and skeletal muscle to neurons and glia. Differentiation treatment of a single multipotent culture can produce a variety of cell types within the lineage, as neuron-differentiating populations generate a diverse population of neurons, each responsive to different neurotransmitters (Berger et al. 1997).

Microarray analysis of differentiating embryonal carcinoma cells has revealed potential functional targets (79 upregulated and 10 downregulated genes) of ATRA-induced differentiation (Satoh and Kuroda 2000). A multitude of publications have functionally characterized such genes as those whose ATRA-induced regulation partially mimics the ATRA effect (Maden 2001). Accordingly, ATRA activates many parallel pathways that each contribute to collectively induce differentiation. Such targets represent a variety of gene products, including transcription factors, cytoskeletal proteins, and signaling molecules.

45.2.4 A Focus upon ATRA Function in Cerebellar Development

Recent studies suggest that ATRA may play a role in the development of the cerebellum, in particular on granule cell migration and neurite outgrowth (Yamamoto et al. 1999). Endogenous ATRA is synthesized in the meninges adjacent to the cerebellum as well as in the choroid plexus of the fourth ventricle under the regulation of Raldh2 expression, peaking just before birth and again just after birth (Yamamoto et al. 1996; Zhang et al. 2003). Interestingly, neurite extension can be induced by ATRA treatment of explanted embryonic rat cerebellum, and co-culture with the choroid plexus induces the same effect. The importance of ATRA to regionalization and development of prospective brain structures, including the cerebellum, has precluded study of the effect of ATRA-signaling deficiency in cerebellar development. Administration of ATRA to neonatal rats at birth results in ectopic undifferentiated granule cell precursors in the molecular layer (Yamamoto et al. 1999). Although teratogenic effects of morphogens are frequently the result of a disrupted signaling gradient at sites of endogenous morphogen activity, a role for ATRA in the development of cerebellar architecture in vivo has not been conclusively demonstrated.

45.3 Therapeutic Application of Retinoids

45.3.1 A Link Between Vitamin A Deficiency and Cancer

Evidence for the potential role of vitamin A in cancer prevention comes from three main findings—first, that VAD (vitamin A-deficient) mice have higher rates of spontaneous and carcinogen-induced tumors (Saffiotti et al. 1967); second, that epidemiological studies have identified an inverse correlation between vitamin A/β-carotene intake and cancer incidence (Bjelke 1975; Szarka et al. 1994); and finally, that dosing of adult mice with vitamin A at supraphysiological levels reduces the incidence of carcinogen-induced tumors (Bollag 1972; Sporn et al. 1976; Harisiadis et al. 1978). Unfortunately, clinical trials utilizing β-carotene for chemoprevention have generally been unsuccessful at replicating the effects found in animal models, so the potential of vitamin supplementation as a chemopreventive is uncertain (Vainio 2003). However, metabolites and derivates of β-carotene have shown promise as chemopreventive agents, as summarized in Table 45.1.

The importance of properly regulated retinoid signaling is clearly demonstrated by the tumorigenic effect of RARα dysfunction in acute promyelocytic leukemia (APL) due to fusion between *RARα* and *PML* genes (de The et al. 1990). *RARα* fusion results in the constitutive recruitment of corepressors at RARE sites on DNA, resulting in the negation of retinoid signaling effector gene expression at physiological retinoid levels and thus failure to induce cellular differentiation.

The well-established differentiation effect of ATRA may be the underlying molecular mechanism explaining improved survival in tumor prevention studies, as forced differentiation of early neoplasms would presumably reduce their likelihood to progress into full blown tumors. Vitamin A deficiency may not be clinically relevant in developed countries; however, three million preschool-aged children worldwide show clinically deficient levels (Clugston et al. 1995). In addition to systemic deficiency in vitamin A levels leading to a lack of RAR differentiation signals, tumors can locally evade the action of retinoids. The circumvention of retinoid signaling specifically in tumors has been shown to occur via upregulation of ATRA catabolic enzymes (Shelton et al. 2006) and reduced ATRA levels (Pasquali et al. 1996; Guo et al. 2001) as well as downregulation of retinoid receptors (Sun and Lotan 2002). These findings have therapeutic implications for tumors that have circumvented ATRA signaling, as targeting intact downstream components of the pathway could induce differentiation in otherwise resistant tumors.

Table 45.1 Promising clinical results of retinoid activity for prevention, adjuvant therapy, and primary therapy for a variety of tumors

Tumor target*	Retinoid#	Source
Chemoprevention		
Cervical neoplasia	ATRA	Meyskens et al. (1994)
Oral neoplasia	13-*cis* RA	Hong et al. (1986) and Lippman et al. (2006)
Bronchial epithelium neoplasia in smokers	Etretinate	Misset et al. (1986)
Cutaneous actinic keratoses	Fenretinide, etretinate, ATRA	Bavinck et al. (1995), Rook et al. (1995), and Moglia et al. (1996)
Adjuvant therapy		
Breast cancer	Fenretinide	Veronesi et al. (2006)
Neuroblastoma	13-*cis* RA†	Matthay et al. (1999)
Stage I NSCLC	RP, 13-*cis* RA	Pastorino et al. (1993) and Lippman et al. (2001)
Hepatocellular carcinoma	Polyprenoic acid†	Muto et al. (1996)
Bladder cancer	Etretinate	Studer et al. (1984) and Studer et al. (1995)
Skin SCC	Retinol	Moon et al. (1997)
Dysplastic nevi	ATRA	Edwards and Jaffe (1990) and Halpern et al. (1994)
BCC, SCC in Xeroderma Pigmentosa patients	13-*cis* RA	Kraemer et al. (1988)
Primary therapy		
Acute promyelocytic leukemia	ATRA†	Degos et al. (1995)
Head and neck SCC	13-*cis* RA†	Gravis et al. (1999)
Renal cell carcinoma	ATRA†	Goldberg et al. (2002) and Boorjian et al. (2007)
Skin SCC	13-*cis* RA†	Shin et al. (2002)
BCC	13-*cis* RA†	Sankowski et al. (1987)
Cervical SCC	13-*cis* RA†	Lippman et al. (1992)

Abbreviations: ATRA = all-*trans* retinoic acid, BCC = basal cell carcinoma, RA = retinoic acid, RP = retinyl palmate; SCC = squamous cell carcinoma.

*Chemoprevention designates treatment during precancerous stages. Adjuvant therapy designates treatment after resection or curative therapy. Primary therapy designates treatment in the absence of resection or curative therapy.

#Etretinate is a synthetic retinoid. Polyprenoic acid is an acyclic retinoid. Fenretinide is a synthetic retinoid that exerts effects independent of RA receptors.

†Indicates retinoid is used in combination therapy.

45.3.2 Clinical Application of Retinoids

In the clinical setting, retinoids have shown promise in chemoprevention, adjuvant treatment, and as a primary therapy (in combination with other agents) against a variety of tumors (Table 45.1). APL treatment is the model example of successful tumor differentiation therapy. Treatment of APL patients with pharmacological levels of ATRA results in activation of the PML/RARα protein chimera, and combination of ATRA treatment and chemotherapy results in full remission of 90% of patients (Fenaux et al. 1995). Retinoids have also proven clinically effective against neuroblastoma, a poorly differentiated pediatric tumor related to MB that arises from primitive undifferentiated cells derived from the neural crest (Louis et al. 2007). Treatment of pediatric neuroblastoma patients with 13-*cis* retinoic acid (13-*cis* RA) after surgical resection, radiotherapy, and either autologous bone marrow transplant or chemotherapy increased 3-year event-free survival from 29 ± 5 to 46 ± 6%, with a low frequency (2%) of skin toxicity as the most common side effect (Matthay et al. 1999). The most positive responses were seen in patients with minimal residual disease, which suggests that retinoids could prevent expansion of micrometastases and tumor remnants after initial tumor mass reduction. Indeed, a survey of clinical results (Table 45.1) leaves the impression that retinoid therapy is most effective in the context of minimal disease.

Development of synthetic retinoids such as 13-*cis* RA for clinical application is a result of the discordance between achievable serum ATRA concentrations (0.1–1 μM) and optimal ATRA activity in vitro (5–10 μM). Phase I trials utilizing 13-*cis* RA have achieved serum concentrations of 7 μM in pediatric neuroblastoma patients (Khan et al. 1996). Compared to ATRA, 13-*cis* RA has a lower affinity for RAR and is less effective than ATRA against APL cell lines, leading some groups to propose that 13-*cis* RA functions as a prodrug to all-*trans* RA (Reynolds 2000), being metabolized within cells to ATRA. Accordingly, the following discussion of ATRA activity against MB cell lines at concentrations beyond those clinically achievable for ATRA reflects a potential for 13-*cis* RA to emulate such effects, which have been described in preclinical studies of medulloblastoma xenografts (Hallahan et al. 2003, described below).

45.3.3 Mechanisms of Retinoid Antitumor Activity

In vitro studies of retinoid activity against a variety of tumors have identified three main responses of tumor-derived cell lines: differentiation, growth inhibition, and apoptosis. Retinoids are active against a diversity of tumor types, and the pathways involved vary considerably. It is likely that cell type of origin dictates the mechanism of tumor response, as literature reviews reveal that tumors of epithelial origin (breast carcinoma, squamous cell carcinoma, lung carcinoma) activate distinct pathways following retinoid treatment relative to those originating from cells derived from the neural crest (neuroblastoma and melanoma; Niles 2004). Altogether, retinoids have been shown to modulate their effects via a tremendous diversity of signaling pathways, including ERK1/2, JNK, PI3K, PKC, AP-1, TGFβ, p38 MAPK, TNFα, Wnt, Notch, and Shh. Furthermore, retinoids have been shown to affect the cell cycle by directly modulating expression and activity of cyclins, cyclin-dependent kinases

(CDKs), and CDK inhibitors (Ink4a family and Waf/Cip family), and retinoids can modulate the apoptotic response via upregulation of caspases (Garattini et al. 2007). The differentiation effect of ATRA upon neuroblastomas is similar to that on embryonic carcinoma and embryonic stem cells (described below), and it is possible that analogous genes may be activated in other tumors that differentiate in response to ATRA.

45.3.4 Retinoid Therapy Targets Pathways Implicated in MB Tumorigenesis

The standard of care for medium- to high-risk pediatric MB is resection followed by craniospinal radiation and cyclophosphamide-based chemotherapy (Gajjar et al. 2006; Gajjar 2008) with admirable 5-year overall survival rates for both medium-risk (85%) and high-risk (70%) cases. However, such treatment results in significant cognitive impairment (Hoppe-Hirsch et al. 1990; Ris et al. 2001) and endocrine defects (Xu et al. 2004). Indeed radio- and chemotherapies generally targeting proliferating cells invariably exert off-target effects and may not deplete cancer stem cell populations. Tumor stem cells uniquely resistant to cytotoxins can regenerate the tumor after conventional therapy, possibly accounting for relapse after bulk mass reduction (Singh et al. 2004; Bao et al. 2006). There is hope that with a better understanding of the differentiation machinery, it may be possible to implement differentiation agents to deplete both the bulk of the tumor and the cancer stem cells. Such approach would circumvent the toxicity associated with the traditional chemotherapy and could prove more effective against recurrence by specifically targeting cytotoxic-resistant tumor stem cells (refer to Chapter 44 for a review of stem cell-targeting therapeutics).

It is becoming increasingly apparent that MBs hijack normal developmental pathways to maintain proliferative competence, resulting in self-renewing cell populations and maintenance of the tumor mass (Discussed in Section 45.1; Singh et al. 2004; Fan and Eberhart 2008). Gene expression studies have identified similarities between MBs and progenitor or stem cells (Lee et al. 2003). Progenitor cells in the cerebellum are capable of taking on neoplastic phenotypes when these cell types are deficient in functional p53 and Ink4c (Zindy et al. 2007). Finally, a substantial proportion of primary MBs harbor genetic lesions of developmental pathway genes, such as *Shh*, *Wnt*, and *Notch* (discussed above), that are involved in stem cell renewal and progenitor maintenance.

Characterization of the mechanisms of retinoid activity against MB is a recently emerging field, in which there is limited consensus. Cell line heterogeneity and lack of clinically relevant mouse models for some tumor subtypes may underlie contradictory results. Regardless, a collection of 12 published studies of retinoid activity against MB has implicated four potential mechanisms (Fig. 45.1): (1) direct modulation of the apoptotic machinery, i.e., caspase upregulation (Jiang et al. 2008) or Fas translocation to the plasma membrane (Liu et al. 2000a); (2) a paracrine-mediated apoptotic effect via enhanced Bmp2 secretion and activation of the TGFβ pathway (Hallahan et al. 2003); (3) the induction of differentiation as evidenced by neurite outgrowth (Hallahan et al. 2003), expression of lineage-specific markers (Gumireddy et al. 2003), and exit of the cell cycle by an unknown mechanism perhaps involving Bmp2 (Zhao et al. 2008); and finally (4) downregulation of the oncogene *OTX2*, which drives proliferation and inhibits differentiation (Di et al. 2005; Yan H, unpublished results). It is important to note that these effects are not exclusive of one another. There is evidence that endogenous differentiation agents require activation of parallel pathways of growth inhibition and morphological differentiation, whereas cell cycle blockade in the absence of a differentiation program results in apoptosis (Alvarez-Rodriguez et al. 2007). Furthermore, the role of Bmp2 in modulation of the apoptotic machinery, such as caspase upregulation or Fas translocation, is unknown. The notable apoptotic effect of retinoids is encouraging, as MBs are particularly sensitive to activation of apoptotic pathways relative to neighboring cerebellar tissue or mature granule cell neurons (Johnson et al. 2007).

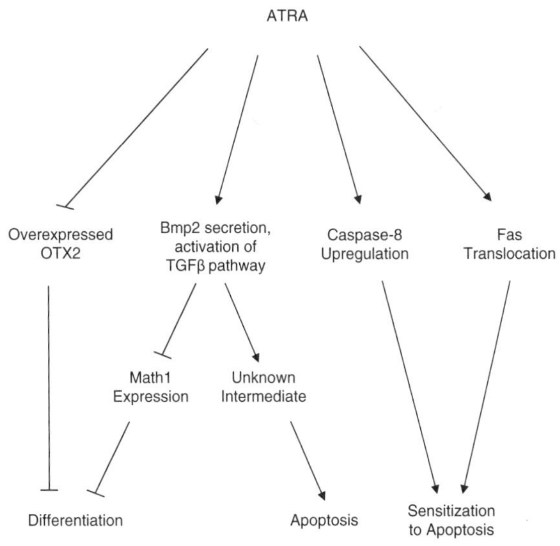

Fig. 45.1 Proposed mechanisms whereby ATRA chemosensitizes or induces differentiation/apoptosis in MB cell lines and cultured primary tumors. The relationships among parallel pathways have yet to be determined. Data are summarized from Liu et al. (2000a), Gumireddy et al. (2003), Hallahan et al. (2003), Di et al. (2005), Jiang et al. (2008), Zhao et al. (2008), and unpublished data (Yan H)

Although non-canonical retinoid signaling has been implicated in differentiation therapy of other tumor types (Garattini et al. 2007), the currently identified effects of ATRA against MB have been shown in some cell lines (D283, D341) to be mediated through canonical retinoid signaling, functioning through RAR/RXR heterodimers and exhibiting sensitivity to RAR/RXR antagonists (Hallahan et al. 2003). When tested, primary MBs and MB cell lines express functional subtypes of RAR and RXR (Gumireddy et al. 2003; Hallahan et al. 2003). A known exception to an RAR-dependent effect is that of fenretinide, which is a potent inducer of apoptosis in some MB cell lines in spite of its greatly reduced affinity for RARs (discussed below; Damodar Reddy et al. 2006).

45.3.4.1 Variability of Retinoid Responsiveness Among MB Cell Lines Resulted in Disproportionately Negative Results in Early Studies

Results of early attempts to induce differentiation in medulloblastoma cell lines foretold variable ATRA sensitivity among MBs (Table 45.2). Disappointingly, the application of ATRA to some of the first established MB cell lines (RB2, UW228, UW443, and MCD-1) did not affect viability and only induced very subtle morphological changes in one cell line (UW228; Maria et al. 1989; Keles et al. 1993; Moore et al. 1996).

Table 45.2 Retinoid responses of established MB cell lines and association with OTX2 expression level

Cell line	OTX2 expression*	Retinoid response
D487	128.0	V, AI
D721	90.6	V, AI
D425	72.2	A#, D, AI
D283	56.8	A#, D, AI
D384	42.83	V, AI
D556	35.59	V, AI
D458	35.03	A#, D, AI
D341	13.1	A
D581	0.91	None
D324	0.1	None
MHH1	0.01	NS
MCD-1	0.01	None
UW228	0	None
Daoy	0	Minimal C, AI
RB2	NS	Minimal V
Med-3	NS	V, D

Abbreviations: AI = inhibition of anchorage-independent growth, A = apoptosis, C = cell cycle blockade D = differentiation, V = reduction in viability (undetermined mechanism), NS = not studied.

* OTX2 expression data were obtained from Q-PCR expression relative to normal cerebellum (Di et al. 2005).

#Indicates predominant response (refer to Section 45.3.4).

45.3.4.2 ATRA Can Induce Reversible Differentiation and Chemosensitize MB Cells

The growing cohort of established MB cell lines revealed that a substantial proportion of cell lines were in fact responsive to retinoid treatment (Table 45.2). Retinoid-induced differentiation coupled to growth inhibition has been described as the major response in an MB cell line (Med-3) (Liu et al. 2000b), whereas treatment with 5–10 μM ATRA for 3 days inhibited proliferation and telomerase activity and induced striking neurite outgrowth and cell body elongation (Liu et al. 2000b). Retinoid-induced differentiation was reversible upon ATRA withdrawal. This finding was proof of principle that an endogenous differentiation signal could force transient differentiation in an MB cell line. It is important to note that although 5 μM ATRA exceeds clinically achievable serum concentrations, such results reflect a potential for synthetic retinoids, which can be maintained at higher serum concentrations than ATRA, to exert such effects (discussed above).

Combination therapy of ATRA with a genotoxic agent, cisplatin, induced apoptosis in this model (Liu et al. 2000a), suggesting that ATRA sensitizes cells to apoptosis induced by genotoxic agents. It was found that ATRA treatment resulted in Fas translocation from the cytosol to the plasma membrane. Accordingly, it was proposed that increased Fas responsiveness to its ligand, FasL, which was shown to be expressed in both untreated and treated cells, was responsible for the increased sensitivity to cisplatin. Direct modulation of apoptotic pathways by ATRA has been described elsewhere, as caspase-8 protein expression has been shown to be induced by ATRA in other MB cell lines (BT-3 and BT-14), suggesting another potential mechanism of ATRA-induced sensitization. However, the concentration of retinoids used (100 μM) greatly exceeded clinically achievable serum concentrations of either ATRA or synthetic retinoids (Jiang et al. 2008).

45.3.4.3 ATRA Can Introduce a Cell Cycle Blockade in an MB Cell Line

ATRA has also been shown to introduce a cell cycle blockade in an MB cell line (Daoy; Chang et al. 2007) that is generally considered to be minimally responsive to ATRA (Gumireddy et al. 2003; Hallahan et al. 2003; Di et al. 2005). This group found that 3 days of ATRA treatment (10 μM) increased G_0/G_1 phase cells from 55 to 75%. This effect was presumably induced by suppression of c-myc and cyclin D1 expression.

45.3.4.4 Identifying a Predominantly Apoptotic Response to ATRA in Some MB Cell Lines

A predominantly apoptotic response to ATRA treatment alone has since been described in a number of cell lines (D283, D425, D458), whereas low concentrations of ATRA (as low as 200 nM) greatly reduced cell viability (Gumireddy et al. 2003). Comparably low concentrations (100 nM) of ATRA massively reduced anchorage-independent colony formation and inhibited DNA synthesis in these cell lines. ATRA treatment induced signs of apoptotic cell death, including release of nucleosome-associated DNA fragments and induction of caspase-3 activity. Morphological differentiation was not appreciably induced at these concentrations (up to 500 nM) during 2 weeks of treatment. However, the neurofilament protein and neural differentiation marker neurofilament-L was induced after 3 days treatment, suggesting that in some cell subpopulations, a program of differentiation is at least partially initiated by low concentrations of ATRA.

45.3.4.5 Bmp2 Is a Functional Downstream Target of Retinoid Treatment in MB Cell Lines and Surgically Derived Primary Tumors

One mechanism of ATRA-induced apoptotic cell death in sensitive lines is the upregulation of the secreted TGFβ pathway activator, Bmp2 (Hallahan et al. 2003). Bmp2 was identified by gene expression analysis to be a candidate intermediate of retinoid-induced apoptosis by the following criteria: (1) agonists of different RAR subtypes (which independently induce apoptosis) activated its expression; (2) its induction occurred in ATRA-sensitive cell lines (D283, D341) but not in ATRA-resistant cell lines (UW228, Daoy); and (3) it has been implicated to play a role in apoptosis of a cell line derived from a different tumor type, myeloma (Kawamura et al. 2000). Bmp2 plays an endogenous role in differentiation of GCPs during cerebellar development by suppressing the proliferative Shh signal as GCPs migrate inward (Rios et al. 2004; Alvarez-Rodriguez et al. 2007). Addition of Bmp2 to the media of retinoid-sensitive cells recapitulates apoptosis (76% of that of ATRA treatment), and a Bmp2-specific inhibitor, noggin, blocks this activity (Hallahan et al. 2003). Bmp2 treatment induced canonical TGFβ effects such as phosphorylation of Smad1 and p38 MAPK. Intriguingly, ATRA-resistant cells were also sensitive to Bmp2-induced apoptosis. This finding suggests that the mechanism of retinoid resistance in some MB cell lines (Daoy and UW228) lies upstream of Bmp2 transcriptional upregulation and that direct Bmp2 induction or treatment may yield more consistent therapeutic outcomes. However, sensitivity to TGFβ pathway activation is not a universal trait of MB cell lines, as MCD-1 cells are not responsive to TGFβ (Moore et al. 1996).

Intriguingly, a differentiation effect was described in the cells that did not undergo apoptosis following ATRA exposure (30% of the culture; Hallahan et al. 2003). Surviving cells underwent striking morphological changes including neurite outgrowth, cell body elongation, and expression of neural-specific markers. This effect is compatible with the previous findings that while apoptosis is the predominant ATRA response of some MB cell lines, the neural differentiation marker neurofilament-L can be induced in surviving cells (Gumireddy et al. 2003). That Bmp2 treatment alone did not induce differentiation in either ATRA-resistant or ATRA-sensitive cell lines suggests that the differentiation effect of ATRA requires a Bmp2-independent mechanism.

Retinoids were also shown to be effective against alternative and perhaps more clinically relevant models of MB. First, ATRA sensitivity was described in primary cultures of surgically derived MBs, whereas seven out of nine primary MBs underwent apoptosis in response to ATRA exposure. As in retinoid-sensitive cell lines, the population of primary MB cells that did not undergo apoptosis following ATRA treatment grew neurites and expressed neural differentiation markers, which suggests that all MB cells of retinoid-sensitive tumors will undergo either apoptosis or differentiation. Furthermore, 13-*cis* RA was shown to be effective in inhibiting growth of flank xenografts (D283 cells) representative of solid MB tumors.

Characterization of the Bmp2-mediated effect was followed up in a study of Bmp2 and Bmp4 effects upon primary GCPs of wild-type mice as well as primary MBs isolated from either *Ink4c*$^{-/-}$ *ptc1*$^{+/-}$ mice or *Ink4c*$^{-/-}$ mice lacking *p53* in nestin-expressing cells (Zhao et al. 2008). In contrast to findings described previously, Bmp2 or Bmp4 treatment of primary GCPs (cultured in the presence of Shh to induce proliferation) or primary mouse MBs resulted in G_0/G_1 cell cycle arrest and expression of neuronal lineage markers. Bmp2 and Bmp4 are both expressed in granular layers of the developing cerebellum with distinct spatiotemporal expression patterns that vary among species (Rios et al. 2004; Angley et al. 2003). Bmp2-induced differentiation of primary mouse GCPs has been documented elsewhere (Alvarez-Rodriguez et al. 2007). Bmp2 or Bmp4 treatment resulted in activation of the canonical TGFβ pathway. The differentiation effect of Bmp proteins upon GCPs and primary mouse MB was attributed to proteasome-mediated degradation of the Math1/Atoh1 transcription factor. Math1/Atoh1 is expressed in proliferating GCPs but is shut down as GCPs exit the cell cycle and migrate inward, and in both mouse models of MB and in clinical tumors, Math1/Atoh1 expression is frequently maintained (Oliver et al. 2005; Salsano et al. 2007). Forced expression of Math1/Atoh1 completely circumvented Bmp-induced cell cycle arrest of primary GCPs (Zhao et al. 2008). Pretreatment of primary mouse tumor cells with Bmp4 or forced expression of Bmp4 prevented xenograft tumor growth. Finally, the effect of Bmp4 expression upon xenograft tumor growth was completely circumvented by forced expression of Math1/Atoh1.

The discrepancies between the findings regarding the mechanism of antitumor activity of Bmp proteins may reflect differences in cells and tumors studied as models. While human MB cell lines and cultured primary human MBs exclusively underwent apoptosis in response to ATRA, primary GCPs from wild-type mice and tumor cells derived from MB-prone mice (resulting from activation of specific pathways) underwent differentiation (Zhao et al. 2008). However, the findings of the two groups may not seem so incompatible considering the more recent finding that in cultured GCP's TIEG-1, a downstream target of Bmp2, induces cell cycle arrest that leads to differentiation in the presence of differentiating signals or, alternatively, leads to apoptosis in the absence of differentiation signals (Alvarez-Rodriguez et al. 2007).

45.3.4.6 ATRA Treatment Silences the Oncogene *OTX2*, Which Is Distinctly Expressed in Retinoid-Sensitive Cell Lines

It has been reported that expression of the *OTX2* oncogene (described above) is a consistent predictive marker for retinoid sensitivity in MB cell lines. ATRA serves as an endogenous posteriorizing signal that inhibits OTX2 expression at the anteroposterior border of the early embryo via a *cis*-acting element (Simeone et al. 1995). It has been shown that ATRA inhibits OTX2 expression in MB cell lines, which results in reduction of cell viability, inhibition of anchorage-independent growth, and ultimately, either apoptosis or senescence (Di et al. 2005; Yan H, unpublished results). OTX2-expressing MB cell lines are distinctly sensitive to ATRA treatment (2 μM), whereas cell lines not expressing OTX2 do not respond to ATRA. This result is consistent among all cell lines studied (Table 45.2), including seven cell lines expressing OTX2 (D283, D458, D384, D425, D487, D556, and D721) and four cell lines not expressing OTX2 (D324, D581, MCD1, and UW228).

Studies are currently underway to determine if the antineoplastic effect of ATRA is in fact mediated by OTX2 and, if so, whether this effect occurs via the same pathways as Bmp2-induced apoptosis/differentiation. It is important to note that ATRA-resistant cell lines that do not express OTX2 (UW228, Daoy) are sensitive to Bmp2 treatment (Hallahan et al. 2003).

45.3.4.7 Development of Retinoid-Based Therapeutic Strategies in Preclinical Models

In vitro studies of ATRA-mediated apoptosis in cultured primary MBs and cell lines have led to investigation of combination treatment strategies in preclinical xenograft models. A rational approach has been taken to pursue synergistic therapeutic effects of retinoids, which activate RAR/RXR heterodimers bound to RAREs, and histone deacetylase inhibitors (HDIs), which nonspecifically induce histone hyperacetylation to relax chromatin conformation and facilitate transcription (Spiller et al. 2008). The premise for such a study is that coupling a specific transcriptional activator with a general activator of transcription will result in enhanced activation of specific genes, in this case, those harboring RAREs. Additionally, synergistic effects of drugs used in combination therapy allow for dosing at concentrations well below those that induce off-target toxicity. In cultured D283 cells, 13-*cis* RA and SAHA synergistically induce Bmp2 mRNA expression (over sevenfold). Treatment regimens of 13-*cis* RA (100 mg/kg/day, alternating 7 days on and 7 days off), SAHA (200 mg/kg/day), or both drugs were applied to established D283 xenograft tumors. After 3 weeks of therapy, retinoid treatment neither significantly reduced tumor volume relative to control tumors nor exerted an additive effect when combined with SAHA. Additionally, 13-*cis* RA + SAHA combination therapy was not more effective than SAHA only in inducing caspase-3 activation in tumors of ND2:SmoA1 mice, and 13-*cis* RA itself did not induce caspase-3 activity (Spiller et al. 2008). The lack of retinoid responsiveness of the D283 xenograft is in conflict with the observed retinoid effect described previously by the same group (Hallahan et al. 2003), who described a twofold reduction of tumor mass in mice treated with 13-*cis* RA (200 mg/kg/day, the highest tolerable dose) after 23 days of treatment. Inconsistent retinoid sensitivity of flank xenografts could reflect differences in dosing regimes or in tumor size at the onset of retinoid treatment. Indeed, it has been noted in a phase III clinical study of neuroblastoma that 13-*cis* RA was most beneficial in patients with minimal residual disease, which suggests that retinoids are more effective in preventing the growth of recurrent tumors than in reducing the bulk mass of established tumors (Matthay et al. 1999).

45.3.4.8 A Synthetic Retinoid, Fenretinide, Induces Apoptosis in MBs via an RAR-Independent Effect

Fenretinide, a synthetic retinoid, has emerged as a promising chemopreventive agent active in a number of clinical trials (Table 45.1). Fenretinide was originally developed to circumvent toxicity of other clinically available retinoids. Although the structural modifications introduced to the pharmacophore resulted in greatly reduced affinity for RARs, fenretinide has demonstrated potent antitumor effects. Fenretinide commonly induces apoptosis in tumor cell lines by inducing reactive oxygen species, ceramide, and ganglioside GD3 (Hail et al. 2006). In many cell types, these signaling intermediates appear to be induced by mechanisms that are independent of RAR activation and to function via activation of the intrinsic apoptotic pathway. Fenretinide has proven effective against a number of MB cell lines, as 5-μM treatment greatly reduces viability of the ATRA-sensitive cell lines D425, D458, D283, and D341 (Damodar Reddy et al. 2006). This effect is dependent on induction of oxidative intermediates. Fenretinide treatment induced caspase-3 activity and apoptotic body formation in the four cell lines, confirming an apoptotic response. The unique mechanism of this synthetic retinoid suggests it may be applicable to retinoid-resistant MBs.

45.3.4.9 Overview of Known Retinoid Targets in MB

Thus far there has been only one unbiased study to identify the functional targets of retinoids in MB; this study utilized microarrays of 5,800 transcripts to identify functional targets (Hallahan et al. 2003). The functional target identified (Bmp2) induces apoptosis in some MB models (clinically derived primary cultures and cell lines; Hallahan et al. 2003) and differentiation in others (primary GCPs, primary tumors from mouse models; Zhao et al. 2008). The proportion of available MB cell lines that are sensitive to Bmp2 is unknown. An understanding of Bmp2 effects across MB cell lines and other MB models could determine the extent of Bmp2 sensitivity as well as identify the predominant response. Although the mechanistic basis is debated, it is clear that enhanced secretion of Bmp2 is a functional downstream target of retinoids that exert antitumor effects upon a collection of MB models.

Aside from Bmp2, the functional intermediates of ATRA treatment remain elusive. Although observational data show that ATRA can induce expression of caspases (Jiang et al. 2008) and translocate the Fas receptor (Jiang et al. 2008;

Liu et al. 2000a, b), the functional significance of each of these changes to the overall ATRA response is not known. A lack of longitudinal studies of available MB cell lines precludes the identification of these effects as either general or unique to particular cell lines. It is important that characterization of the mechanistic basis for therapeutic response of a heterogeneous disease such as MB is proven to be consistent across samples.

The perfect association between OTX2 expression and retinoid sensitivity merits functional investigation (Di et al. 2005). Although *OTX2* has been implicated as an oncogene by genetics of clinical samples and in vitro studies (Di et al. 2005; Taylor M, personal communication; Yan H, unpublished results), the requirement for its downregulation during ATRA-induced apoptosis or differentiation has yet to be characterized.

45.3.4.10 Strategies to Identify Mechanisms of Retinoid Resistance in MB Cell Lines

The variation of responses among different cell lines to retinoid treatment is notable; such variation speaks to the heterogeneity of MBs. Although a systematic study of the genetic changes in each line has not been carried out, genetic studies have revealed heterogeneity among cell lines regarding copy number changes and epigenetic events (Taylor M, personal communication, Yan H, unpublished data). No doubt this is also the case for mutations. Thus, as with any therapeutic strategy, characterization of the ATRA response requires either (1) identification of pathways that can be targeted by chemotherapeutic agents and are consistently responsive among all MBs or (2) the use of definitive biomarkers to facilitate implementation of personalized therapy in the clinic.

To understand the molecular mechanisms underlying retinoid resistance, it is first necessary to characterize (1) the kinetics of intracellular retinoid concentrations during treatment and (2) the level of activation of RARs among retinoid-resistant and retinoid-sensitive cell lines. Such a study is necessary to ensure that retinoid signaling is not circumvented altogether (mechanisms discussed above) in resistant cell lines before characterization of other mechanisms is pursued.

Differential retinoid receptor expression among MB cell lines (D283, D425, D558, and Daoy) has been described (Gumireddy et al. 2003). These cell lines express RARα, RXRα, and RXRγ as the functional subtypes of retinoid receptors. Resistant cell lines expressed the lowest levels of RXRα and RXRγ, and the retinoid-responsive cell lines expressed similar, high levels of RXRα and RXRγ. Identifying a functional link between retinoid receptor expression levels and RARE activity in MB cell lines will reveal whether or not reduced RAR expression is a mechanism of retinoid resistance.

As a morphogen, ATRA exhibits endogenous effects that are cell type dependent (Chytil and Sherman 1987), and it is tempting to suggest that different cell origins underlay differential retinoid sensitivity in MB cell lines. However, most available MB cell lines express neural lineage markers; this includes cell lines sensitive to retinoids (D283, D384, D425, D458) as well as retinoid-resistant cell lines (MCD-1, UW228). Therefore, it seems unlikely that cell origin is a definitive indicator of retinoid sensitivity unless more subtle cell origin phenotypes underlay resistance.

It is possible that mechanisms of retinoid resistance may be more subtle among cell lines. For example, if we assume that RARE activation upon retinoid treatment is consistent among cell lines, the widespread sensitivity of cell lines to Bmp2 treatment suggests that RAR activation is somehow uncoupled from Bmp2 upregulation in resistant cell lines.

45.3.4.11 Clinical Trials Utilizing Retinoid Treatment for MB

Phase II (Gardner 2005) and Phase III (Olson and Packer 2006) clinical trials implementing 13-*cis* RA as an adjuvant therapy following radiation and chemotherapy against MB are currently recruiting patients. Additionally, a Phase I trial investigating dose tolerance and preliminary efficacy of 13-*cis* RA and suberoylanilide hydroxamic acid (SAHA, discussed above) combination treatment for adjuvant MB therapy is underway (Fouladi 2005). Time will tell whether or not retinoids can improve upon adjuvant therapy of MB. Concurrent preclinical studies will be of benefit to understanding the mechanism of retinoid activity against this tumor type. The synthesis of laboratory and clinical studies will be informative regarding the development of rational combination therapies and the identification of criteria to stratify patients into proper treatment groups.

45.4 Overview of Retinoid-Mediated Differentiation Therapy of MB

In sum, MB is a tumor of aberrant development, occurring at a young age and frequently resulting from constitutively active developmental pathways conferring properties of progenitor or stem cells such as self-renewal, proliferative competence, and migration (Singh et al. 2004; Bao et al. 2006). Histological MB classifications often reflect distinct pathways contributing to MB development, suggesting characteristic genetic changes contributing to tumorigenesis of each subtype. Well-known aberrations include activation of the Shh, Wnt, and Notch pathways, and there is increasing evidence for activation of the OTX2 transcriptional network in anaplastic MBs. As with other poorly differentiated tumors, MBs are sensitive to differentiation/apoptosis therapy such as retinoid treatment. Retinoid-induced differentiation of MB, which may involve Bmp2, is variable among cell lines and poorly understood; thus, characterization of the networks involved is of keen interest. Retinoid-induced apoptosis may function via direct modulation of the apoptotic machinery or by upregulation of the secreted factor Bmp2. Identification of intermediates of retinoid-induced apoptosis that could therapeutically circumvent the uncoupling of retinoid exposure to apoptosis/differentiation in resistant MBs is of considerable value to the development of broadly applicable MB therapeutics.

Abbreviations

13-*cis* RA	13-*cis* retinoic acid
AP-1	activator protein 1
APL	acute promyelocytic leukemia
ATRA	all-*trans* retinoic acid
Bmp2	bone morphogenetic protein-2
Bmp4	bone morphogenic protein-4
CNS	central nervous system
ERK	extracellular signal-regulated kinase
FISH	fluorescence in situ hybridization
GCP	granule cell precursor
HAT	histone acetyltransferase
HDAC	histone deacetylase
JNK	JUN *N*-terminal kinase
MAPK	mitogen-activated protein kinase
MB	medulloblastoma
NCoR	nuclear receptor corepressor
OTX2	orthodenticle homolog 2
PI3K	phosphatidylinositol 3 kinase
PKC	protein kinase C
RARE	retinoic acid responsive element
Shh	Sonic Hedgehog
SNP	single nucleotide polymorphism
SMRT	silencing mediator for retinoid and thyroid hormone receptors
TGFβ	transforming growth factor β
TNFα	tumor necrosis factor α
Wnt	wingless-type MMTV integration site family

References

Acampora D, Simeone A (1999) The tins lecture. Understanding the roles of otx1 and otx2 in the control of brain morphogenesis. Trends Neurosci 22(3):116–22

Alvarez-Rodriguez R, Barzi M, Berenguer J et al (2007) Bone morphogenetic protein 2 opposes shh-mediated proliferation in cerebellar granule cells through a tieg-1-based regulation of nmyc. J Biol Chem 282(51):37170–80

Angley C, Kumar M, Dinsio KJ, Hall AK, Siegel RE (2003) Signaling by bone morphogenic proteins and Smad1 modulates the postnatal differentiation of cerebellar cells. J Neurosci 23(1):260–8

Bao S, Wu Q, McLendon RE et al (2006) Glioma stem cells promote radioresistance by preferential activation of the DNA damage response. Nature 444(7120):756–60

Bavinck JN, Tieben LM, Van der Woude FJ et al (1995) Prevention of skin cancer and reduction of keratotic skin lesions during acitretin therapy in renal transplant recipients: A double-blind, placebo-controlled study. J Clin Oncol 13(8):1933–8
Berger C, Reinhardt S, Rentrop M et al (1997) De novo acquisition of neuronal polarity in retinoic acid-induced embryonal carcinoma cells. Eur J Cell Biol 74(3):230–45
Bjelke E (1975) Dietary vitamin a and human lung cancer. Int J Cancer 15(4):561–5
Blomhoff R, Blomhoff HK (2006) Overview of retinoid metabolism and function. J Neurobiol 66(7):606–30
Blumberg B, Bolado J Jr., Moreno TA et al (1997) An essential role for retinoid signaling in anteroposterior neural patterning. Development 124(2):373–9
Bollag W (1972) Prophylaxis of chemically induced papillomas and carcinomas of mouse skin by vitamin a-acid. Experientia 28(10):1219–20
Boorjian SA, Milowsky MI, Kaplan J et al (2007) Phase 1/2 clinical trial of interferon alpha2b and weekly liposome-encapsulated all-trans retinoic acid in patients with advanced renal cell carcinoma. J Immunother 30(6):655–62
Broccoli V, Boncinelli E, Wurst W (1999) The caudal limit of otx2 expression positions the isthmic organizer. Nature 401(6749):164–8
Buhren J, Christoph AH, Buslei R et al (2000) Expression of the neurotrophin receptor p75ntr in MBs is correlated with distinct histological and clinical features: Evidence for a MB subtype derived from the external granule cell layer. J Neuropathol Exp Neurol 59(3):229–40
Chang Q, Chen Z, You J et al (2007) All-trans-retinoic acid induces cell growth arrest in a human MB cell line. J Neurooncol 84(3):263–7
Chytil F, Sherman DR (1987) How do retinoids work? Dermatologica 175 Suppl 1:8–12
Clugston G, Underwood b, Gorstein J (1995) Global prevalence of Vitamin A Deficiency. Micronutrient Deficiency Information System Working Paper No. 2. World Health Organization, Geneva
Damodar Reddy C, Guttapalli A, Adamson PC et al (2006) Anticancer effects of fenretinide in human MB. Cancer Lett 231(2):262–9
de la Pompa JL, Wakeham A, Correia KM et al (1997) Conservation of the notch signalling pathway in mammalian neurogenesis. Development 124(6):1139–48
de The H, Chomienne C, Lanotte M et al (1990) The t(15;17) translocation of acute promyelocytic leukaemia fuses the retinoic acid receptor alpha gene to a novel transcribed locus. Nature 347(6293):558–61
Degos L, Dombret H, Chomienne C et al (1995) All-trans-retinoic acid as a differentiating agent in the treatment of acute promyelocytic leukemia. Blood 85(10):2643–53
Di C, Liao S, Adamson DC et al (2005) Identification of otx2 as a MB oncogene whose product can be targeted by all-trans retinoic acid. Cancer Res 65(3):919–24
Edwards L, Jaffe P (1990) The effect of topical tretinoin on dysplastic nevi. A preliminary trial. Arch Dermatol 126(4):494–9
Edwards MK, McBurney MW (1983) The concentration of retinoic acid determines the differentiated cell types formed by a teratocarcinoma cell line. Dev Biol 98(1):187–91
Fan X, Mikolaenko I, Elhassan I et al (2004) Notch1 and notch2 have opposite effects on embryonal brain tumor growth. Cancer Res 64(21):7787–93
Fan X, Matsui W, Khaki L et al (2006) Notch pathway inhibition depletes stem-like cells and blocks engraftment in embryonal brain tumors. Cancer Res 66(15):7445–52
Fan X, Eberhart CG (2008) MB stem cells. J Clin Oncol 26(17):2821–7
Fenaux P, Chastang C, Chomienne C et al (1995) Treatment of newly diagnosed acute promyelocytic leukemia (APL) by all trans retinoic acid (ATRA) combined with chemotherapy: The European experience. European APL Group. Leuk Lymphoma 16(5–6):431–7
Fouladi (2005) Vorinostat With or Without Isotretinoin in Treating Young Patients With Recurrent or Refractory Solid Tumors, Lymphoma, or Leukemia. ClinicalTrials.gov. http://clinicaltrials.gov/ct2/show/NCT00217412. Accessed 24 July 2008

Gaiano N, Nye JS, Fishell G (2000) Radial glial identity is promoted by notch1 signaling in the murine forebrain. Neuron 26(2):395–404

Gaiano N, Fishell G (2002) The role of notch in promoting glial and neural stem cell fates. Annu Rev Neurosci 25:471–90

Gajjar A, Chintagumpala M, Ashley D et al (2006) Risk-adapted craniospinal radiotherapy followed by high-dose chemotherapy and stem-cell rescue in children with newly diagnosed MB (St Jude MB-96): Long-term results from a prospective, multicentre trial. Lancet Oncol 7(10):813–20

Gajjar A (2008) High-dose chemotherapy for recurrent MB: Time for a reappraisal. Cancer 112(8):1643–5

Garattini E, Gianni M, Terao M (2007) Retinoids as differentiating agents in oncology: A network of interactions with intracellular pathways as the basis for rational therapeutic combinations. Curr Pharm Des 13(13):1375–400

Gardner (2005) Temozolomide, Thiotepa and Carboplatin with Autologous Stem Cell Rescue Followed by 13-Cis-Retinoic Acid in Patients with Recurrent/Refractory Malignant Brain Tumors. ClinicalTrials.gov. http://clinicaltrials.gov/ct2/show/NCT00528437. Accessed 24 July 2008

Germain P, Chambon P, Eichele G et al (2006a) International Union of Pharmacology. LX. Retinoic acid receptors. Pharmacol Rev 58(4):712–25

Germain P, Chambon P, Eichele G et al (2006b) International union of pharmacology. LXIII. Retinoid X receptors. Pharmacol Rev 58(4):760–72

Gilbertson RJ, Ellison DW (2008) The origins of MB subtypes. Annu Rev Pathol 3:341–65

Goldberg JS, Vargas M, Rosmarin AS et al (2002) Phase I trial of interferon alpha2b and liposome-encapsulated all-trans retinoic acid in the treatment of patients with advanced renal cell carcinoma. Cancer 95(6):1220–7

Goodrich LV, Milenkovic L, Higgins KM et al (1997) Altered neural cell fates and MB in mouse patched mutants. Science 277(5329):1109–13

Gorlin RJ (1987) Nevoid basal-cell carcinoma syndrome. Medicine (Baltimore) 66(2):98–113

Gravis G, Pech-Gourgh F, Viens P et al (1999) Phase II study of a combination of low-dose cisplatin with 13-cis-retinoic acid and interferon-alpha in patients with advanced head and neck squamous cell carcinoma. Anticancer Drugs 10(4):369–74

Grimmer MR, Weiss WA (2006) Childhood tumors of the nervous system as disorders of normal development. Curr Opin Pediatr 18(6):634–8

Gumireddy K, Sutton LN, Phillips PC et al (2003) All-*trans*-retinoic acid-induced apoptosis in human MB: Activation of caspase-3/poly(ADP-ribose) polymerase 1 pathway. Clin Cancer Res 9(11):4052–9

Guo X, Nanus DM, Ruiz A et al (2001) Reduced levels of retinyl esters and vitamin a in human renal cancers. Cancer Res 61(6):2774–81

Hahn H, Wojnowski L, Zimmer AM et al (1998) Rhabdomyosarcomas and radiation hypersensitivity in a mouse model of Gorlin syndrome. Nat Med 4(5):619–22

Hail N, Kim HJ, Lotan R (2006) Mechanisms of fenretinide-induced apoptosis. Apoptosis 11(10):1677–94

Hallahan AR, Pritchard JI, Chandraratna RA et al (2003) Bmp-2 mediates retinoid-induced apoptosis in MB cells through a paracrine effect. Nat Med 9(8):1033–8

Hallahan AR, Pritchard JI, Hansen S et al (2004) The smoa1 mouse model reveals that notch signaling is critical for the growth and survival of sonic hedgehog-induced MBs. Cancer Res 64(21):7794–800

Halpern AC, Schuchter LM, Elder DE et al (1994) Effects of topical tretinoin on dysplastic nevi. J Clin Oncol 12(5):1028–35

Harisiadis L, Miller RC, Hall EJ et al (1978) A vitamin a analogue inhibits radiation-induced oncogenic transformation. Nature 274(5670):486–7

Hatton BA, Villavicencio EH, Tsuchiya KD et al (2008) The smo/smo model: Hedgehog-induced MB with 90% incidence and leptomeningeal spread. Cancer Res 68(6):1768–76

Hong WK, Endicott J, Itri LM et al (1986) 13-cis-retinoic acid in the treatment of oral leukoplakia. N Engl J Med 315(24):1501–5
Hoppe-Hirsch E, Renier D, Lellouch-Tubiana A et al (1990) MB in childhood: Progressive intellectual deterioration. Childs Nerv Syst 6(2):60–5
Jiang M, Zhu K, Grenet J et al (2008) Retinoic acid induces caspase-8 transcription via phospho-creb and increases apoptotic responses to death stimuli in neuroblastoma cells. Biochim Biophys Acta 1783(6):1055–67
Johnson CE, Huang YY, Parrish AB et al (2007) Differential apaf-1 levels allow cytochrome c to induce apoptosis in brain tumors but not in normal neural tissues. Proc Natl Acad Sci U S A 104(52):20820–5
Kawamura C, Kizaki M, Yamato K et al (2000) Bone morphogenetic protein-2 induces apoptosis in human myeloma cells with modulation of stat3. Blood 96(6):2005–11
Keles GE, Berger MS, Schofield D et al (1993) Nerve growth factor receptor expression in MBs and the potential role of nerve growth factor as a differentiating agent in MB cell lines. Neurosurgery 32(2):274–80; discussion 280
Khan AA, Villablanca JG, Reynolds CP, Avramis VI (1996) Pharmacokinetic studies of 13-*cis* retinoic acid in pediatric patients with neuroblastoma following bone marrow transplantation. Cancer Chemother Pharmacol 39:34–41
Kraemer KH, DiGiovanna JJ, Moshell AN et al (1988) Prevention of skin cancer in xeroderma pigmentosum with the use of oral isotretinoin. N Engl J Med 318(25):1633–7
Lee A, Kessler JD, Read TA et al (2005) Isolation of neural stem cells from the postnatal cerebellum. Nat Neurosci 8(6):723–9
Lee Y, Miller HL, Jensen P et al (2003) A molecular fingerprint for MB. Cancer Res 63(17):5428–37
Lippman SM, Kavanagh JJ, Paredes-Espinoza M et al (1992) 13-cis-retinoic acid plus interferon alpha-2a: Highly active systemic therapy for squamous cell carcinoma of the cervix. J Natl Cancer Inst 84(4):241–5
Lippman SM, Lee JJ, Karp DD et al (2001) Randomized phase III intergroup trial of isotretinoin to prevent second primary tumors in stage I non-small-cell lung cancer. J Natl Cancer Inst 93(8):605–18
Lippman SM, Lee JJ, Martin JW et al (2006) Fenretinide activity in retinoid-resistant oral leukoplakia. Clin Cancer Res 12(10):3109–14
Liu J, Guo L, Jun-Wei L et al (2000a) All-*trans* retinoic acid modulates Fas expression and enhances chemosensitivity of human MB cells. Int J Mol Med 5(2):145–9
Liu J, Guo L, Luo Y et al (2000b) All *trans*-retinoic acid suppresses in vitro growth and down-regulates LIF gene expression as well as telomerase activity of human MB cells. Anticancer Res 20(4):2659–64
Louis D, Ohgaki H, Wiestler O et al (2007) WHO Classification of Tumours of the Central Nervous System. IARC, Lyon, France.
Machold RP, Kittell DJ Fishell GJ (2007) Antagonism between notch and bone morphogenetic protein receptor signaling regulates neurogenesis in the cerebellar rhombic lip. Neural Develop 2:5
Maden M, Gale E, Kostetskii I et al (1996) Vitamin a-deficient quail embryos have half a hindbrain and other neural defects. Curr Biol 6(4):417–26
Maden M (2001) Role and distribution of retinoic acid during CNS development. Int Rev Cytol 209:1–77
Mangelsdorf DJ, Thummel C, Beato M et al (1995) The nuclear receptor superfamily: The second decade. Cell 83(6):835–9
Maria BL, Steck PA, Yung WK et al (1989) The modulation of astrocytic differentiation in cells derived from a MB surgical specimen. J Neurooncol 7(4):329–38
Mark M, Ghyselinck NB, Chambon P (2006) Function of retinoid nuclear receptors: Lessons from genetic and pharmacological dissections of the retinoic acid signaling pathway during mouse embryogenesis. Annu Rev Pharmacol Toxicol 46:451–80

Matsuo I, Kuratani S, Kimura C et al (1995) Mouse otx2 functions in the formation and patterning of rostral head. Genes Dev 9(21):2646–58
Matthay KK, Villablanca JG, Seeger RC et al (1999) Treatment of high-risk neuroblastoma with intensive chemotherapy, radiotherapy, autologous bone marrow transplantation, and 13-cis-retinoic acid. Children's Cancer Group. N Engl J Med 341(16):1165–73
Meyskens FL, Jr., Surwit E, Moon TE et al (1994) Enhancement of regression of cervical intraepithelial neoplasia ii (moderate dysplasia) with topically applied all-*trans*-retinoic acid: A randomized trial. J Natl Cancer Inst 86(7):539–43
Misset JL, Mathe G, Santelli G et al (1986) Regression of bronchial epidermoid metaplasia in heavy smokers with etretinate treatment. Cancer Detect Prev 9(1–2):167–70
Moglia D, Formelli F, Baliva G et al (1996) Effects of topical treatment with fenretinide (4-hpr) and plasma vitamin a levels in patients with actinic keratoses. Cancer Lett 110(1–2):87–91
Moon TE, Levine N, Cartmel B et al (1997) Retinoids in prevention of skin cancer. Cancer Lett 114(1–2):203–5
Moore KD, Dillon-Carter O, Conejero C et al (1996) In vitro properties of a newly established MB cell line, MCD-1. Mol Chem Neuropathol 29(2–3):107–26
Muto Y, Moriwaki H, Ninomiya M et al (1996) Prevention of second primary tumors by an acyclic retinoid, polyprenoic acid, in patients with hepatocellular carcinoma. Hepatoma Prevention Study Group. N Engl J Med 334(24):1561–7
Niederreither K, Subbarayan V, Dolle P et al. (1999) Embryonic retinoic acid synthesis is essential for early mouse post-implantation development. Nat Genet 21(4):444–8
Niederreither K, Dolle P (2008) Retinoic acid in development: Towards an integrated view. Nat Rev Genet 9(7):541–53
Niles RM (2004) Signaling pathways in retinoid chemoprevention and treatment of cancer. Mutat Res 555(1–2):81–96
Oliver TG, Read TA, Kessler JD et al (2005) Loss of patched and disruption of granule cell development in a pre-neoplastic stage of MB. Development 132(10):2425–39
Olson J, Packer R (2006) Chemotherapy and Radiation Therapy in Treating Young Patients With Newly Diagnosed, Previously Untreated, High-Risk MB or Supratentorial Primitive Neuroectodermal Tumor. http://clinicaltrials.gov/show/NCT00392327.
Pasquali D, Thaller C, Eichele G (1996) Abnormal level of retinoic acid in prostate cancer tissues. J Clin Endocrinol Metab 81(6):2186–91
Pastorino U, Infante M, Maioli M et al (1993) Adjuvant treatment of stage I lung cancer with high-dose vitamin A. J Clin Oncol 11(7):1216–22
Pazzaglia S, Mancuso M, Atkinson MJ et al (2002) High incidence of MB following X-ray-irradiation of newborn Ptc1 heterozygous mice. Oncogene 21(49):7580–4
Reynolds CP (2000) Differentiation agents in pediatric malignancies: retinoids in neuroblastoma. Curr Oncol Rep 2(6)511–8
Rios I, Alvarez-Rodriguez R, Marti E et al (2004) Bmp2 antagonizes sonic hedgehog-mediated proliferation of cerebellar granule neurones through Smad5 signalling. Development 131(13):3159–68
Ris MD, Packer R, Goldwein J et al (2001) Intellectual outcome after reduced-dose radiation therapy plus adjuvant chemotherapy for MB: A Children's Cancer Group study. J Clin Oncol 19(15):3470–6
Rook AH, Jaworsky C, Nguyen T et al (1995) Beneficial effect of low-dose systemic retinoid in combination with topical tretinoin for the treatment and prophylaxis of premalignant and malignant skin lesions in renal transplant recipients. Transplantation 59(5):714–9
Saffiotti U, Montesano R, Sellakumar AR et al (1967) Experimental cancer of the lung. Inhibition by vitamin A of the induction of tracheobronchial squamous metaplasia and squamous cell tumors. Cancer 20(5):857–64
Salsano E, Croci L, Maderna E et al (2007) Expression of the neurogenic basic helix-loop-helix transcription factor *NEUROG1* identifies a subgroup of MBs not expressing *ATOH1*. Neuro Oncol 9(3):298–307

Sankowski A, Janik P, Jeziorska M et al (1987) The results of topical application of 13-cis-retinoic acid on basal cell carcinoma. A correlation of the clinical effect with histopathological examination and serum retinol level. Neoplasma 34(4):485–9

Satoh J, Kuroda Y (2000) Differential gene expression between human neurons and neuronal progenitor cells in culture: An analysis of arrayed cDNA clones in NTera2 human embryonal carcinoma cell line as a model system. J Neurosci Methods 94(2):155–64

Schuller U, Rowitch DH (2007) Beta-catenin function is required for cerebellar morphogenesis. Brain Res 1140:161–9

Shakhova O, Leung C, van Montfort E et al (2006) Lack of Rb and p53 delays cerebellar development and predisposes to large cell anaplastic MB through amplification of *N-Myc* and *Ptch2*. Cancer Res 66(10):5190–200

Sharpe CR, Goldstone K (1997) Retinoid receptors promote primary neurogenesis in *Xenopus*. Development 124(2):515–23

Shelton DN, Sandoval IT, Eisinger A et al (2006) Up-regulation of cyp26a1 in adenomatous polyposis coli-deficient vertebrates via a WNT-dependent mechanism: Implications for intestinal cell differentiation and colon tumor development. Cancer Res 66(15):7571–7

Shin DM, Glisson BS, Khuri FR et al (2002) Phase II and biologic study of interferon alfa, retinoic acid, and cisplatin in advanced squamous skin cancer. J Clin Oncol 20(2):364–70

Simeone A, Avantaggiato V, Moroni MC et al (1995) Retinoic acid induces stage-specific antero-posterior transformation of rostral central nervous system. Mech Dev 51(1):83–98

Singh SK, Hawkins C, Clarke ID et al (2004) Identification of human brain tumour initiating cells. Nature 432(7015):396–401

Solecki DJ, Liu XL, Tomoda T et al (2001) Activated *Notch2* signaling inhibits differentiation of cerebellar granule neuron precursors by maintaining proliferation. Neuron 31(4):557–68

Spiller SE, Ditzler SH, Pullar BJ et al (2008) Response of preclinical MB models to combination therapy with 13-cis retinoic acid and suberoylanilide hydroxamic acid (SAHA). J Neurooncol 87(2):133–41

Sporn MB, Dunlop NM, Newton DL et al (1976) Prevention of chemical carcinogenesis by vitamin A and its synthetic analogs (retinoids). Fed Proc 35(6):1332–8

Studer UE, Biedermann C, Chollet D et al (1984) Prevention of recurrent superficial bladder tumors by oral etretinate: Preliminary results of a randomized, double blind multicenter trial in Switzerland. J Urol 131(1):47–9

Studer UE, Jenzer S, Biedermann C et al (1995) Adjuvant treatment with a vitamin a analogue (etretinate) after transurethral resection of superficial bladder tumors. Final analysis of a prospective, randomized multicenter trial in Switzerland. Eur Urol 28(4):284–90

Sun SY, Lotan R (2002) Retinoids and their receptors in cancer development and chemoprevention. Crit Rev Oncol Hematol 41(1):41–55

Swiatek PJ, Lindsell CE, del Amo FF et al (1994) *Notch1* is essential for postimplantation development in mice. Genes Dev 8(6):707–19

Szarka CE, Grana G, Engstrom PF (1994) Chemoprevention of cancer. Curr Probl Cancer 18(1):6–79

Thompson MC, Fuller C, Hogg TL et al (2006) Genomics identifies MB subgroups that are enriched for specific genetic alterations. J Clin Oncol 24(12):1924–31

Vainio H (2003) Chemoprevention. In: Stewart BW, Kleihues P (eds) World Cancer Report. IARC, Lyon, France.

Vernay B, Koch M, Vaccarino F et al (2005) Otx2 regulates subtype specification and neurogenesis in the midbrain. J Neurosci 25(19):4856–67

Veronesi U, Mariani L, Decensi A et al (2006) Fifteen-year results of a randomized phase III trial of fenretinide to prevent second breast cancer. Ann Oncol 17(7):1065–71

Vogelstein B, Kinzler KW (1993) The multistep nature of cancer. Trends Genet 9(4):138–141

Wan YJ, An D, Cai Y et al (2000) Hepatocyte-specific mutation establishes retinoid X receptor alpha as a heterodimeric integrator of multiple physiological processes in the liver. Mol Cell Biol 20(12):4436–44

Wechsler-Reya R, Scott MP (2001) The developmental biology of brain tumors. Annu Rev Neurosci 24:385–428
Xu W, Janss A, Packer RJ et al (2004) Endocrine outcome in children with MB treated with 18 Gy of craniospinal radiation therapy. Neuro Oncol 6(2):113–8
Yamamoto M, McCaffery P, Drager UC (1996) Influence of the choroid plexus on cerebellar development: Analysis of retinoic acid synthesis. Brain Res Dev Brain Res 93(1–2):182–90
Yamamoto M, Ullman D, Drager UC et al (1999) Postnatal effects of retinoic acid on cerebellar development. Neurotoxicol Teratol 21(2):141–6
Zhang J, Smith D, Yamamoto M et al (2003) The meninges is a source of retinoic acid for the late-developing hindbrain. J Neurosci 23(20):7610–20
Zhao H, Ayrault O, Zindy F et al (2008) Post-transcriptional down-regulation of Atoh1/Math1 by bone morphogenic proteins suppresses MB development. Genes Dev 22(6):722–7
Zindy F, Uziel T, Ayrault O et al (2007) Genetic alterations in mouse MBs and generation of tumors de novo from primary cerebellar granule neuron precursors. Cancer Res 67(6):2676–84

Chapter 46
Herpes Simplex Virus 1 (HSV-1) for Glioblastoma Multiforme Therapy

Costas G. Hadjipanayis

Abstract Herpes simplex virus 1 (HSV-1) is a double-stranded DNA virus that has been studied for use in the treatment of malignant gliomas. Various HSV-1 recombinants have been used to target malignant gliomas by direct intratumoral or peritumoral delivery, and most recently convection-enhanced delivery (CED). The basic biology of HSV-1 is reviewed for understanding the two main categories of HSV-1 constructs used, either replication-defective or conditionally replicative (oncolytic) viruses. The potential for HSV-1 as a gene therapy vector is discussed and the human clinical trials that have been conducted utilizing HSV-1 are reviewed. Current limitations of HSV-mediated therapy of gliomas, new perspectives on further targeting of HSV-1 against malignant gliomas, and combination therapies will be highlighted.

Keywords Herpes simplex virus 1 (HSV-1) · Malignant glioma · Glioblastoma multiforme (GBM) · Replication-defective virus · Oncolytic virus · Gene therapy · DNA repair · Convection-enhanced delivery

Contents

Financial support: This work was supported in part by grants from the NIH (NS053454), American Brain Tumor Association, and the Georgia Cancer Coalition (GCC), Distinguished Cancer Clinicians and Scientists Program. C. G. Hadjipanayis is a Georgia Cancer Coalition Distinguished Cancer Scholar.

C.G. Hadjipanayis (✉)
Department of Neurological Surgery, Winship Cancer Institute, Emory University School of Medicine, 1365B Clifton Rd., Suite 6200, Atlanta, GA 30322, USA
e-mail: chadjip@emory.edu

E.G. Van Meir (ed.), *CNS Cancer*, Cancer Drug Discovery and Development, DOI 10.1007/978-1-60327-553-8_46,
© Humana Press, a part of Springer Science+Business Media, LLC 2009

46.1 Introduction

Current malignant glioma treatment remains challenged by the inability to properly target tumor cells that infiltrate normal brain and withstand current therapeutic modalities such as surgery, ionizing radiation (IR), and chemotherapy. Neovascularization, tumor genetic heterogeneity (epidermal growth factor (EGFR) overexpression/amplification, p53 mutation, etc.), invasiveness, and tumor initiating cells (TICs) that have stem cell properties (multipotency, self-renewal, and proliferation) all define glioblastoma multiforme (GBM) tumors, the most common malignant glioma (Furnari et al., 2007; Singh et al., 2004).

Herpes simplex virus 1 (HSV-1) is a double-stranded DNA virus that has been studied for use in the treatment of malignant gliomas (Harrow et al., 2004; Markert et al., 2000b; Papanastassiou et al., 2002; Rampling et al., 2000). Malignant gliomas are a potential target for HSV-1 infection and tumor lysis in the central nervous system. HSV-1 constructs can infect rapidly dividing tumor cells but spare surrounding quiescent, non-dividing neurons and other supporting cells in the brain. HSV-1 recombinants have been used to target malignant gliomas. Viral administration has been performed by direct intratumoral or peritumoral injection in the brain, and most recently convection-enhanced delivery (CED) (Hadjipanayis et al., 2008b). Two main categories of HSV-1 constructs have been used, either replication-defective or conditionally replicative (oncolytic) viruses. The replication-defective viruses deliver transgenes to cells whose expression can result in tumor cell death

(Hadjipanayis and DeLuca, 2005; Miyatake et al., 1997; Moriuchi et al., 2002; Niranjan et al., 2000). Oncolytic viruses have been shown to selectively replicate in dividing tumor cells causing cell lysis and tumor death (Martuza et al., 1991; Mineta et al., 1995; Parker et al., 2000; Todo et al., 2001).

The potential for HSV-1 as a gene therapy vector will be presented and a review of both replication-defective and oncolytic HSV-1 constructs as therapeutic agents for malignant gliomas will be discussed. The human clinical trials that have been conducted utilizing HSV-1 will be reviewed. Current limitations of HSV-mediated therapy of gliomas will be discussed in regards to delivery, spread through tumors, transgene expression, as well as the host response to viral infection. Finally, new perspectives on further targeting of HSV-1 against GBM and combination therapies will be highlighted.

46.2 Basic Biology of HSV-1

HSV-1 is a well-adapted pathogen, demonstrated by its widespread prevalence in human, its only known natural host. There are two types of HSV, type 1 and type 2 (HSV-1 and HSV-2) and both belong to the Herpesviridae family, Alphaherpesvirinae subfamily. Over 75% of all adults in the United States have antibodies to HSV-1. Approximately 40 million infected individuals will experience recurrent herpes disease due to reactivation of their own "personal" viruses sometime in their lifetime. HSV initially gains access to the host via infection of epithelial cells at skin and/or mucosal surfaces leading to the production of characteristic painful vesicular lesions. HSV-1 is associated with oral infection and is transmitted via oral and respiratory secretions. HSV-2 is associated with genital area infection and associated sexually transmitted diseases.

HSV-1 infection can result in other infectious processes, including herpes keratitis and encephalitis. Herpes keratitis can result in corneal blindness. Due to HSV-1 neurotropism and its ability to replicate in neurons and glia, access to the CNS can cause encephalitis. Herpes simplex encephalitis (HSE) occurs relatively infrequently, with an incidence of 1 case per 250,000 population/year in the United States (Whitley and Roizman, 2001).

46.2.1 HSV-1 Structure and Genome

HSV-1 consists of linear double-stranded DNA packaged into an icosadeltahedral capsid (Furlong et al., 1972; Homa and Brown, 1997) (Fig. 46.1). The capsid is surrounded by an amorphous tegument layer that is held within a trilaminar envelope containing glycoprotein spikes (Haarr and Skulstad, 1994) (Batterson and Roizman, 1983; Spear, 1993). Glycoproteins are embedded in the trilaminar envelope of the mature virion (Roizman and Sears, 1996). HSV-1 particle size ranges from 150 to 200 nm.

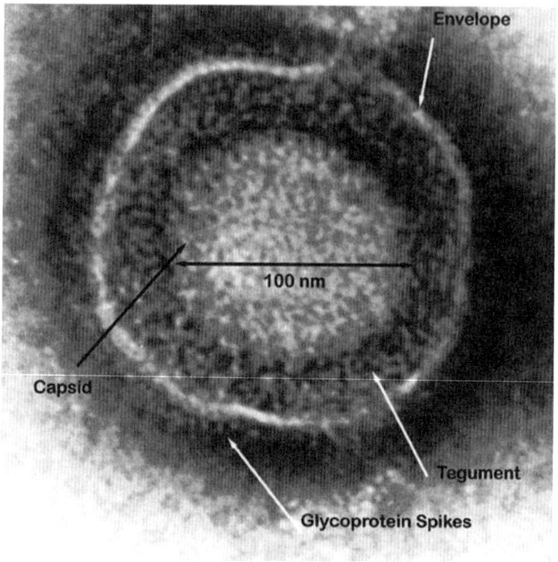

Fig. 46.1 Transmission electron micrograph of HSV-1 particle

The HSV-1 genome consists of 152 kb pairs comprising 84 genes and an excess of 90 open reading frames (ORFs) (Becker et al., 1968; Kieff et al., 1971; Weir, 2001). This genome encodes proteins that regulate the coordinated expression of viral genes that permit viral replication as well as structural proteins that constitute the envelope of HSV-1. The viral genome is separated by a unique long (U_L) and unique short (U_S) sequence flanked on each end by terminal inverted repeat sequences (McGeoch et al., 1988; McGeoch et al., 1986) (Fig. 46.2). The U_L and U_S sequences are covalently joined by internal repeat sequences. The U_L and U_S sequences can randomly invert relative to each other so the HSV-1 genome actually can exist in four equimolar isomers (Hayward et al., 1975).

46.2.2 HSV-1 Cell Entry

HSV-1 infection involves virus attachment to the cell surface, fusion of the viral envelope with the plasma membrane, and entry of the viral capsid into the cytoplasm (Fig. 46.3 and Color Plate 61) (Morgan et al., 1968; Spear, 1993). The initial binding of HSV-1 to the cell surface occurs by heparan sulfate (HS) proteoglycans present on the membrane of most types of vertebrate cells (WuDunn and Spear, 1989). HSV-1 glycoproteins, B (gB) and C (gC), have been shown to be involved in the initial attachment phase through the interaction of positively charged glycoprotein structures with negatively charged HS moieties located on cell surface proteoglycans (Laquerre et al., 1998). Removal of HS from the cell surface, either by enzymatic treatment or by selection of cell lines defective in the HS pathway, renders cells partially resistant to HSV infection (Gruenheid et al., 1993; Shieh et al., 1992).

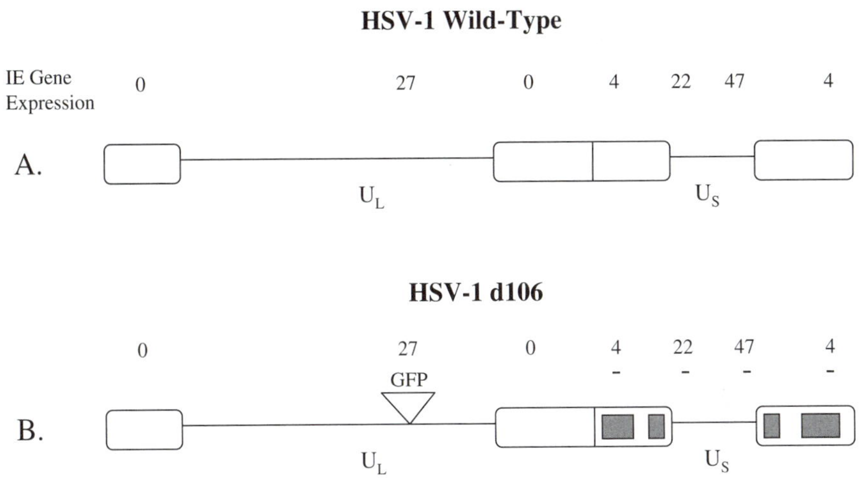

Fig. 46.2 Diagram of HSV-1 genome. (**A**) Wild-type HSV-1 genome. (**B**) Replication-defective genome of d106 indicating sites of mutations (ICP 4, 22, 47) and trangene (GFP) insertion (ICP27). U_S (unique short sequence), U_L (unique long sequence), GFP (green fluorescent protein)

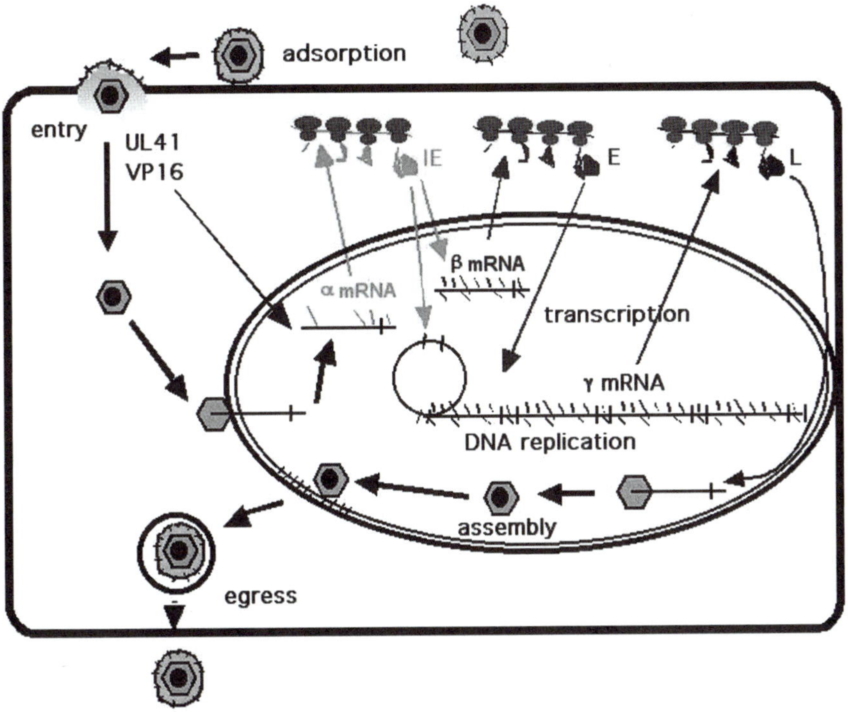

Fig. 46.3 HSV-1 productive infection. HSV-1 cell attachment and entry, gene expression, DNA replication, assembly, and release are shown (*see* Color Plate 61)

Following the initial adsorption event, a secondary binding event occurs between viral glycoprotein D and cellular receptors identified as herpesviral entry mediators, or HVEMs (Geraghty et al., 1998; Montgomery et al., 1996). These include HveA, HveB (nectin-2), and HveC (nectin-1). Fusion of the viral envelope with the cell membrane occurs after the binding of gD to its cognate cell surface receptor (Morgan et al., 1968). Three other HSV-1 glycoproteins are implicated in the fusion process, gB, gH, and gL (DeLuca et al., 1982; Desai et al., 1988; Roop et al., 1993). Once fusion occurs, the nucleocapsid is released into the cell cytoplasm and viral capsids are transported to nuclear pores where DNA is released into the nucleus and gene expression can occur. In certain cell types, HSV-1 entry is dependent on endocytosis and exposure to a low pH (Nicola et al., 2003). Inhibition of endocytosis has been shown to prevent uptake of HSV-1 from HeLa and Chinese hamster ovary cells.

46.2.3 HSV-1 Pathogenesis

Initial infection results in productive viral replication in cells of the epidermis and dermis (Roizman and Sears, 1996). HSV-1 may gain access to nerve termini of sensory neurons and is transmitted to the neuronal cell body by retrograde transport (Cook and Stevens, 1973). HSV can cause a latent infection in which the viral genome adopts a persistent, quiescent state. Establishment of latency occurs predominantly in terminally differentiated, non-dividing neurons of the peripheral nervous system that innervate the initial site of infection. Neurons of sensory and autonomic ganglia are infected following primary rounds of replication in cells of mucosal or epidermal surfaces. HSV-1 latent infection of peripheral neurons is an effective survival mechanism, as there are no vaccines or antiviral agents that can clear the virus once it has reached the latent infection stage. Consequently, once the host is infected with HSV-1, the host is infected for life.

46.2.4 HSV-1 Gene Expression

If lytic infection occurs after HSV nuclear entry, viral genes are expressed in a tightly regulated temporal cascade in which three classes of viral genes are sequentially expressed: immediate-early (IE) or α, early (E) or β, and late (L) or γ (Fig. 46.3) (Honess and Roizman, 1974; Honess and Roizman, 1975). All viral genes are expressed as cellular RNA polymerase II transcription units utilizing the host cellular transcription machinery. Each class of genes differs with respect to its promoter structure, which decreases in complexity from IE to L genes (Weir, 2001) (Table 46.1).

Table 46.1 Summary of important HSV-1 genes and respective proteins

HSV-1 gene	Gene class (IE, E, or L)	Protein	Protein function
ICP0	IE	ICP0	Transactivator of viral and cellular genes. Promotes lytic infection and inhibits latency. Implicated in the inhibition of host DNA repair and targets degradation of specific host proteins by functioning as an E3 ubiquitin ligase
ICP4	IE	ICP4	Required for viral replication. Transcriptional activator of E and L genes. Interacts with host transcriptional machinery
ICP22	IE	ICP22	Facilitates L gene expression promoting switch from E to L gene expression
ICP27	IE	ICP27	Required for viral replication. Can block RNA splicing and affect the shut-off of host protein synthesis
ICP47	IE	ICP47	Responsible for downregulation of host immune response by inhibition of TAP
HSV-tk	E	tk	Enzyme necessary for viral DNA synthesis
U_L39	E	RR (ICP6)	Enzyme necessary for viral DNA synthesis.
$\gamma_1 34.5$	E	ICP34.5	Responsible for the neurovirulence elicited by HSV infection.

The IE genes are the first viral genes expressed upon infection and possess the main regulatory activities of viral gene expression. The resultant IE proteins are necessary for the subsequent expression of the E and L gene classes. The E genes encode proteins involved in viral DNA synthesis such as viral ribonucleotide reductase (RR) and herpes simplex virus type 1 thymidine kinase (HSV-tk). HSV encodes its own DNA replication machinery. The third class of viral genes expressed, the L genes, encode mainly structural components of the virus particle.

46.2.5 HSV-1 Latency

Latency occurs when the cell represses immediate-early (IE) viral gene expression, inhibiting the cascade of early (E) and late (L) viral gene expression that leads to lytic infection (Everett, 2000). In the latent state, the HSV viral genome circularizes (Garber et al., 1993; Jackson and DeLuca, 2003; Poffenberger et al., 1983), becomes associated with nucleosomes in a chromatin structure (Deshmane and Fraser, 1989), and persists extrachromosomally (Mellerick and Fraser, 1987). Viral gene expression during latency is limited to a set of non-translated RNA species, the latency-associated transcripts (LATs), which are expressed as stable lariat intron RNA molecules and are detectable in the nuclei of latently infected neurons (Croen et al., 1987; Spivack and Fraser, 1987;

Stevens et al., 1987). Viral genomes can remain in this state in the nucleus of neurons for the lifetime of the host. Alterations in the host–virus interaction may cause "reactivation" of the viral infection from a quiescent state to a productive, lytic cycle of viral replication. Expression of ICP0 and various types of stress can trigger reactivation (Cai et al., 1993; Gordon et al., 1990; Halford et al., 2001; Halford and Schaffer, 2001; Leib et al., 1989; Russell et al., 1987). During latency, however, ICP0 is not expressed, and reactivation is thought to occur when stress stimuli derepress ICP0, promoting viral gene expression and lytic infection (Everett, 2000). Productive infection results in a lytic cascade of viral gene expression and the production of mature virions, which can then travel back down the nerve axon via anterograde transport and establish infection at mucocutaneous surfaces innervated by the infected neuron (Cook and Stevens, 1973). At least 76 of the total 84 HSV-1 genes are expressed during lytic infection (McGeoch et al., 1993). Cell lysis and release of mature virions allow for spread of the virus. Recurrent cutaneous infections occur due to reactivation of the virus from latency in neurons at different time points throughout the life of the individual.

46.2.6 HSV-1 Immediate-Early (IE) Proteins

There are five HSV-1 IE proteins expressed, which are designated infected cell polypeptide 0 (ICP0), ICP4, ICP22, ICP27, and ICP47 (Fig. 46.2). The IE (α) genes are expressed in the absence of de novo viral protein synthesis. During HSV lytic infection, the viral transactivator, VP16, enters the cell as a component of the virion tegument (Fig. 46.3) (Triezenberg et al., 1988a). VP16 complexes with host cellular factors, Oct-1 and host cell factor (HCF), and binds TAATGARRAT motifs present in all HSV-1 immediate-early (IE) promoters (Flint and Shenk, 1997; Kristie et al., 1989; Kristie and Roizman, 1987; O'Hare et al., 1988; Preston, 2000; Triezenberg et al., 1988b). This complex recruits transcriptional activators and RNA polymerase II to IE promoters, which subsequently express the five infected cell polypeptides (ICP). In addition to a TATA box and TAATGARAT elements, sites exist for several cellular *cis*-acting factors such as Sp1 and others that contribute to enhanced transcription or transcription in the absence of VP16 (Gelman and Silverstein, 1987).

Gene expression during lytic infection progresses in a regulated cascade in which the five IE gene products, ICP0, ICP4, ICP22, ICP27, and ICP47, are the first viral proteins synthesized upon infection. With the exception of ICP47, they encode the primary regulatory functions of the virus necessary for the efficient and timely expression of early and late gene expression (Clements et al., 1977; Honess and Roizman, 1975; Pereira et al., 1977). Of the five IE proteins, only ICP4 and ICP27 are absolutely essential for productive viral replication (DeLuca et al., 1985; Dixon and Schaffer, 1980; McCarthy et al., 1989). The remaining IE proteins ICP0, ICP22, and ICP47 fulfill accessory roles to optimize viral replication.

46.2.7 HSV-1 DNA Replication and Recombination

Replication of HSV-1 occurs within the nucleus of the infected cell (Fig. 46.3). HSV encodes over 80 gene products that contribute to viral replication in either cultured cells or animal hosts that include viral RR, HSV-tk, DNA polymerase, and helicase (Roizman and Sears, 1996). Due to the limited size of the HSV-1 genome, the virus cannot code for every function required for its propagation. HSV-1 must rely upon factors supplied by the host cell for replication. For example, HSV-1 exclusively uses the host cell RNA polymerase II for transcription of viral genes (Costanzo et al., 1977).

Viral DNA synthesis takes place within globular domains called replication compartments (Quinlan et al., 1984), which contain the seven essential viral DNA replication proteins: the origin-binding protein (UL9), the single-stranded DNA-binding protein (UL29 or ICP8), the helicase–primase heterotrimer (UL5/UL8/UL52), the viral polymerase (UL30), and its processivity factor (UL42) (Weller, 1995). Other viral proteins that are found in the replication centers include ICP4, ICP27, and the major capsid protein VP5 (de Bruyn Kops et al., 1998; Knipe et al., 1987; Liptak et al., 1996; Phelan et al., 1997). Cellular proteins that have been shown to localize within replication compartments include p53, Rb, and the DNA-binding replication protein A (RPA) (Wilcock and Lane, 1991). Recently, various cellular proteins involved in DNA recombination/repair have also been shown to localize within replication compartments such as DNA-PK_{CS}, Ku86, BLM, Nbs1, PCNA, BRCA1, MSH2, Rad50, Rad51, and WRN (Taylor and Knipe, 2004; Wilkinson and Weller, 2004).

46.2.8 HSV-1 Assembly and Release

The replication of HSV-1 does not produce genomic DNA molecules, but rather concatemers containing many head-to-tail copies of the viral genome (Fig. 46.3). Individual genomes are subsequently liberated from the concatemers by cleavage of the viral DNA at terminal repeat sequences, producing genome length segments that can then be packaged into preformed capsids (Mettenleiter, 2002). These particles, or nucleocapsids, are non-infectious and unstable until they acquire an envelope. The mature nucleocapsid that is assembled within the nucleus initially acquires an envelope by budding through the inner nuclear membrane (Flint et al., 2004). Upon fusion with the outer nuclear membrane, this membrane is lost as unenveloped nucleocapsids are released from the cytoplasm (Mettenleiter, 2002). Envelope glycoproteins are initially added in the first stage of the secretory pathway, the endoplasmic reticulum. The final envelope is acquired upon budding of tegument-containing structures into a late compartment of the secretory pathway in the trans-Golgi network. The viral particles then reach the cellular plasma membrane and are released into the extracellular space via cellular secretory and trafficking pathways in which the capsids may exchange envelope moieties with other cellular membrane-bound compartments.

46.3 HSV-1 as a Gene Therapy Vector Against Malignant Gliomas

A number of important facts support the use of HSV-1 for therapy against malignant gliomas: (1) HSV-1 is a neurotropic virus that is able to infect a wide range of cells. (2) HSV-1 is susceptible to medical therapy with acyclovir and gancyclovir, providing a safety mechanism when administering HSV-1 to the brain. (3) The inability of the HSV-1 genome to integrate into the host cellular genome eliminates the potential for insertional mutagenesis found with other viruses (retrovirus and adeno-associated virus (AAV)). (4) HSV-1 mutants can be designed with deletions that minimize neurotoxicity in the brain, while permitting viral replication in tumor cells. (5) Large portions of the HSV-1 genome can be deleted to allow for replacement with therapeutic transgenes. As much as 30 kb of the HSV genome can be deleted and replaced by transgenes in replication-defective or conditionally replicative viruses. Examples of transgenes used include HSV-1 thymidine kinase, connexin, tumor necrosis factor alpha (TNFα), and cytokines (IL-2, IL-4, IL-12, GB-CSF).

46.3.1 HSV-1 Replication-Defective Mutants

46.3.1.1 Generation of Replication-Deficient HSV-1 Viruses

Recombinant HSV-1 mutants have been constructed with deletions in IE genes to reduce cell toxicity, permit transgene expression, and inhibit viral replication (Samaniego et al., 1998; Wu et al., 1996). In ICP4 recombinant viruses, expression of viral early and late genes is dramatically reduced, inhibiting viral replication (DeLuca et al., 1985). This has led to the consideration of such attenuated viruses as starting points for the construction of replication-incompetent HSV-1 gene transfer vehicles. Despite the limited expression of the HSV genome in ICP4 mutant backgrounds, such mutants are very toxic to cells. This is due to the overexpression of the remaining IE proteins in the absence of ICP4 (DeLuca et al., 1985). Improved cell survival has been shown by further reduction in IE gene expression after deletion of other IE genes in the HSV-1 genome (Johnson et al., 1994; Samaniego et al., 1998, 1997). Both ICP0 and ICP22 contribute to toxicity, as demonstrated by the improved survival of infected cells when either is deleted in viruses already deficient in ICP4 and ICP27 expression (Samaniego et al., 1997; Wu et al., 1996). At high multiplicities of infection (MOI), both of these triple mutants remain toxic to cells. Elimination of all IE gene and protein expression (ICP 0, 4, 22, 27, and 47) results in a virus that is non-toxic at high MOI and is capable of long-term persistence in non-neuronal cells.

The degree of transgene expression in different IE-deficient HSV mutants has been shown to be dependent on the ICP0 protein (Samaniego et al., 1998). Green fluorescent protein (GFP) transgene expression has been shown to be abundant in cells infected with a recombinant HSV-1 virus that expresses only ICP0. In the absence of all of the HSV IE proteins, the level of GFP transgene expression is low. Transgene expression of cells infected by a complete IE-deficient virus can be stimulated by ICP0.

46.3.1.2 Replication-Defective HSV-1 in Malignant Glioma Therapy

Cancer gene therapy mediated by replication-defective HSV-1 vectors has largely focused on the delivery of suicide genes (Spencer, 2000). Suicide gene delivery allows for the viral transfer of a suicide gene into tumor cells, which renders these and their clonal progeny sensitive to treatment with a prodrug (Moolten, 1986). One transgene used in the past against malignant gliomas was the early gene, HSV-tk (Table 46.1) (Miyatake et al., 1997; Moriuchi et al., 1998). Tumor cell transduction with HSV-tk in conjunction with gancyclovir (GCV) administration allows for tk phosphorylation of gancyclovir to form a toxic nucleotide analog that is incorporated into replicating DNA causing strand termination and cell death by apoptosis (Beltinger et al., 1999). Terminally differentiated cells, such as neurons in the brain, are spared because their DNA does not replicate. HSV-tk/gancyclovir treatment is particularly efficacious because it elicits a "bystander effect", e.g., the spreading of the toxic effect to non-infected cells. Activated gancyclovir within infected cells can be transmitted across cell gap junctions to destroy neighboring uninfected tumor cells, a phenomenon known as the "bystander effect" (Freeman et al., 1993; Wu et al., 1994). To maximize the bystander effect in malignant gliomas, a transgene expressing connexin-43 has been added to the HSV-tk virus for improved efficacy (Marconi et al., 2000). Connexin molecules form the intercellular channels that comprise gap junctions, and addition of connexin-43, a key component, resulted in a synergistic antineoplastic effect.

Replication-defective HSV constructs have been engineered to express other therapeutic genes for the treatment of malignant gliomas. These include metallo-proteinases-2 (TIMP-2) (Hoshi et al., 2000), IL-12 (Toda et al., 1998), IFN-γ (Kanno et al., 1999), and granulocyte-macrophage colony-stimulating factor (GM-CSF) (Toda et al., 2000). Therapeutic genes have been used singly or in combination: coexpression of HSV-tk and TNF-α (Moriuchi et al., 1998; Niranjan et al., 2000), HSV-tk, connexin-43, and TNF-α (Niranjan et al., 2003), HSV-tk and IL-12 (Toda et al., 2001), and HSV-tk and IκBα (Moriuchi et al., 2005) have all shown greater antitumor effects than with single transgene expression. The expression of multiple suicide genes does not always allow for greater efficacy against malignant gliomas. Coexpression of the *Escherichia coli* cytosine deaminase (CD) and HSV-tk genes, followed by exposure to their respective prodrugs (5-FC and GCV), was shown to be inferior in tumor cell killing than with constructs expressing single genes (Moriuchi et al., 2002).

46.3.2 HSV-1 Replication-Conditional (Oncolytic) Viruses

Conditionally replicating HSV-1 viruses, also known as oncolytic viruses, have been genetically engineered to replicate and grow in tumor cells and cause their demise (Chiocca, 2002; Fulci and Chiocca, 2007; Lin and Nemunaitis, 2004). A number of different genetically engineered oncolytic HSV viruses have been constructed with genetic alterations in one or more HSV genes ($\gamma_1$34.5, U_L39 (RR), tk, UTPase, and α47) (Table 46.1). Deletion or mutation in these viral genes decreases the toxicity of the recombinant HSV to the CNS and renders the virus dependent upon complementation by host cell factors for its replication (Chou et al., 1990; Chou and Roizman, 1990; Coen et al., 1989; Hunter et al., 1999; Kramm et al., 1997; Martuza et al., 1991; Mineta et al., 1995; Pyles et al., 1997; Todo et al., 2001). The rationale for targeting malignant glioma cells compared with normal brain tissue rests on the fact that in order for oncolytic HSV-1 constructs to replicate, nucleotide precursors are required. Wild-type HSV-1 can infect and replicate in dividing tumor cells as well as non-dividing normal brain cells (neurons) since it encodes multiple enzymes necessary for viral DNA synthesis (e.g., HSV-tk and RR). Deletion of viral genes, which encode the enzymes needed for viral DNA synthesis, results in limiting viral replication to cells that can substitute them with cellular homologues and provide nucleotide pools. The surrounding non-dividing neurons, in contrast, have low nucleotide pools and do not support efficient viral DNA synthesis, resulting in selective killing of tumor cells.

The first study of a genetically engineered virus used as an oncolytic agent was performed with an *HSV-tk* deletion mutant, dlsptk (Martuza et al., 1991). This virus had been previously constructed, and determined to lack neurovirulence (Coen et al., 1989). In a mouse xenograft glioma model, dlsptk demonstrated anti-glioma effects with tumor growth inhibition in the brain and increases in animal median survival. Shortcomings of the dlsptk virus included acyclovir resistance, due to the *HSV-tk* deletion, and long-term surviving animals had evidence of low-grade encephalitis. Another HSV-1 oncolytic virus (R3616) was generated containing a 1 kb deletion in both genomic copies of the $\gamma_1 34.5$ viral gene ($\Delta\gamma$34.5), which is located in the terminal α repeats of the U_L segment and encodes the ICP34.5 protein (Chou et al., 1990). ICP34.5 is responsible for the neurovirulence elicited by HSV infection and has been termed the neurovirulence factor. The carboxy terminus of this protein is responsible for evading a stereotypical antiviral response of the host cell that normally triggers the shutdown of all protein synthesis in the cell to prevent further spread of viral infection to other cells in the host organism (Chou and Roizman, 1994). This is mediated by the inactivation of a critical mRNA translation factor called eukaryotic initiation factor 2α (eIF2a), which gets inactivated by phosphorylation in response to viral infection. The ICP34.5 protein has been shown to recruit protein phosphatase-1 to dephosphorylate the inactivated eIF2a and reactivate viral mRNA translation, thus allowing for viral protein synthesis to occur. Replication of viral DNA can occur in non-replicating cells such as postmitotic neurons, contributing to HSV-1 neurovirulence. As anticipated following the deletion of the $\gamma_1 34.5$ viral genes, R3616 was found to be aneurovirulent at the highest achievable doses upon intracerebral inoculation in susceptible mouse species and had an antitumor effect (Chou and Roizman, 1990). HSV1716 was also developed which had both copies of the $\gamma_1 34.5$ gene (Rampling et al., 2000). Other oncolytic constructs have been subsequently... generated with double mutations of the $\gamma_1 34.5$ gene (Samoto et al., 2002).

Second-generation HSV-1 oncolytic viruses have been developed based on further modification of the parent R3616 virus (Mineta et al., 1995; Parker et al., 2000). G207 was created by inactivating the $U_L 39$ gene locus through the introduction of a *lacZ* reporter gene (Mineta et al., 1995). $U_L 39$ encodes for the large unit of HSV's ribonucleotide reductase (RR), ICP6, which is necessary for the replication of the viral DNA in non-replicating cells. G207 has demonstrated an adequate safety profile in cell culture as well as in animal models and is efficacious in vivo with human clinical trials (Markert et al., 2000b; Martuza, 2000; Sundaresan et al., 2000). A third-generation HSV-1 oncolytic vector derived from G207, G47Δ, has been constructed after deletion of the *α47* (ICP47) gene and the promoter region of *US11* (Todo et al., 2001). The ICP47 protein is responsible for inhibiting the TAP host cell protein, a transporter associated with antigen presentation. Cells infected with G47Δ have increased MHC class I expression. G47Δ is significantly more efficacious in vivo than its parent G207 at inhibiting tumor growth in both immune-competent and immune-deficient animal models.

Further attempts at harnessing the immune system for the augmentation of the tumoricidal capacity of oncolytic HSVs have been made with viral constructs expressing cytokines such as IL-4 and IL-12 (Andreansky et al., 1998; Parker et al., 2000). A synergistic antitumor effect was obtained with these viruses in animal models, which was mediated in part by induction of tumor-specific cytotoxic T-lymphocytes and inhibition of angiogenesis.

46.4 Combination Therapies with HSV-1 for Malignant Gliomas

The combination of ionizing radiation (IR) and temozolomide (TMZ), both DNA-damaging agents, has demonstrated a survival benefit in patients with glioblastoma multiforme (GBM) and is now standard of care (Stupp et al., 2005). Chemoradiation confers some survival advantage, but resistance of the tumor cells to the effects of chemoradiation limits the success of treatment.

Combining the effects of IR and HSV-1 in the therapy of GBM has been well documented (Advani et al., 2006, 1998; Bradley et al., 1999; Markert et al., 2000a). Viral replication and tumor kill are increased with HSV-1 oncolytic viruses in conjunction with IR (20 and 25 Gy) (Advani et al., 1998; Bradley et al., 1999). Low doses of external beam irradiation were shown to significantly enhance the infectivity and spread of $\Delta\gamma34.5$ HSV constructs (Advani et al., 2006). The mitogen-activated protein kinase, p38, has been implicated in the increase in viral replication upon IR exposure. Activated p38 enhances HSV-1 replication by increasing late viral gene expression (Zachos et al., 1999, 2001). In the case of replication-defective HSV-1 constructs, greater animal survival has been shown with the addition of radiosurgery (margin dose of 15 Gy; center dose of 21.4 Gy) (Niranjan et al., 2000, 2003).

The use of TMZ and HSV-1 therapy of GBM has also been described and demonstrated a synergistic interaction (Aghi et al., 2006). Use of the oncolytic HSV-1 construct, G207, demonstrated a significant increase in animal survival when combined with TMZ. In this study, mutations that enable gliomas to express DNA repair genes after TMZ treatment were used to improve viral oncolysis. Both cellular GADD34 and ribonucleotide reductase (RR) proteins are upregulated following DNA damage induced by IR in mammalian cells. GADD34 is a cellular protein involved in DNA repair. GADD34 shares significant homology with the carboxyl half of ICP34.5 and can restore viral protein translation when substituted for the carboxy terminus of ICP34.5 (He et al., 1996). Increased tumor cell expression of GADD34 and ribonucleotide reductase (RR) after TMZ treatment reduced TMZ-induced DNA damage in glioma cell lines, irrespective of the DNA repair enzyme, O^6 -methylguanine DNA methyltransferase (MGMT) status, and enhanced replication of $\Delta\gamma34.5$ and RR-mutated HSV constructs.

46.4.1 HSV-1 d106-Mediated Chemoradiosensitivity Enhancement in GBM

Inhibiting DNA repair mechanisms may improve the chemoradiosensitivity of GBM. Recently, the replication-defective HSV-1 vector, d106, has been shown to inhibit DNA repair and enhance the radiosensitivity of human GBM cells (Hadjipanayis and DeLuca, 2005) (Fig. 46.2). The mutant virus, d106, is defective in the expression of all of the immediate-early (IE) viral genes except that which encodes ICP0 (Samaniego et al., 1998). Besides ICP0, the only viral protein product readily detected in d106-infected cells is RR, which has been previously shown to have no cytotoxic effect on the host cell (Johnson et al., 1994). The ICP0 protein naturally inhibits the repair of DNA double-strand breaks (DSBs) after IR treatment of human GBM cells leading to decreased cell survival and induction of apoptosis in vitro (Hadjipanayis and DeLuca, 2005) (Fig. 46.4 and Color Plate 62). The ICP0 protein has been shown to cause the degradation of the catalytic subunit of DNA-dependent protein kinase (DNA-PK_{cs}) in human glioblastoma cells. DNA-PK_{cs} is a component of the DNA-PK holoenzyme, which includes the Ku heterodimer, and is responsible for the DNA repair process of non-homologous end joining (NHEJ). NHEJ is a key DNA double-strand repair pathway in eukaryotic cells.

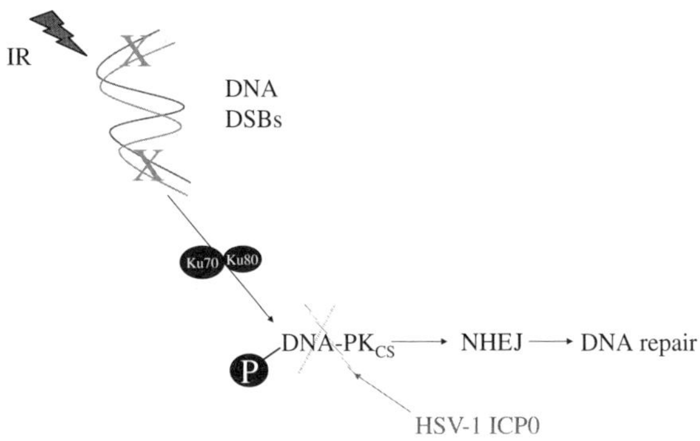

Fig. 46.4 Diagram of DNA DSB production by IR and inhibition of NHEJ DNA repair pathway by ICP0 through degradation of DNA-PK$_{CS}$. IR, ionizing radiation; DSB, double-strand break; NHEJ, non-homologous end joining (*see* Color Plate 62)

Intracerebral convection-enhanced delivery (CED) of d106 in combination with whole-brain irradiation or TMZ enhanced the survival of animals implanted with human GBM xenografts (Hadjipanayis et al., 2008b). This was achieved using a 50% lower radiation dose (10 Gy) than in other studies (Advani et al., 1998; Niranjan et al., 2000) and a subtherapeutic total dose of TMZ (20 mg/kg) as compared to another study (Aghi et al., 2006). Optimal intracerebral d106 delivery by CED was demonstrated to allow for adequate xenograft infection, transduction, and ultimate tumor cell demise by chemo- or radiosensitivity enhancement. CED of the replication-defective d106 construct was also shown to be safe in the mouse.

46.4.1.1 ICP0 and Effects on Cell Metabolism

The ICP0 protein has other effects on cell metabolism that have been described. (Gu et al., 2005; Lomonte et al., 2004). ICP0 has been shown to function as an E3 ubiquitin ligase (Boutell et al., 2002; Everett, 2000) conjugating ubiquitin onto proteins, in a RING finger-dependent manner, and targeting them for degradation by the ubiquitin-dependent proteosome degradation pathway (Everett et al., 1998). ICP0 is thought to target cellular proteins that repress viral gene expression (Everett, 2000; Everett et al., 2006). Proteins targeted by ICP0 include promyelocytic leukemia protein (PML) and Sp100, which are major constituents of nuclear structures called ND10 bodies (Everett et al., 1998). ND10 bodies are discrete nuclear foci where HSV-1 genomes may localize early during infection (Maul et al., 1996). Recent studies have suggested that these foci are sites of DNA double-strand break (DSB) repair and inhibition of HSV genome circularization by ICP0 (Carbone et al., 2002; Jackson and DeLuca, 2003). Other proteins targeted for degradation include centromere proteins, CENP-A (Lomonte et al., 2001) and CENP-C (Everett et al., 1999b; Lomonte and Everett, 1999), the E2 ubiquitin-conjugating enzyme cdc34 (UbcH3) (Hagglund and Roizman, 2004), ubiquitin-specific protease (USP7) (Boutell et al., 2005), and the catalytic subunit of DNA-dependent protein kinase (DNA-PK$_{cs}$) as shown in Fig. 46.4 (Lees-Miller et al., 1996; Parkinson et al., 1999). Disruption of centromeres by ICP0 degradation of CENP-C and CENP-A has been shown to cause cell cycle arrest at both G1/S and G2/M checkpoints (Everett et al., 1999a; Lomonte and Everett, 1999; Lomonte et al., 2001) independently of p53 (Hobbs and DeLuca, 1999). More recently, ICP0 gene expression has been implicated in triggering apoptosis during viral infection of human cells (Sanfilippo and Blaho, 2006).

46.5 Clinical Trials with HSV-1 Based Viruses for Malignant Glioma Therapy

Phase I clinical studies in humans with malignant gliomas have demonstrated modest antitumor effects with the HSV-1 oncolytic viruses G207 and 1716 (Harrow et al., 2004; Markert et al., 2000b; Rampling et al., 2000) (Table 46.2). These trials established the safety of injecting these viruses directly into the brains of patients with malignant gliomas at concentrations up to 3×10^9 PFU.

Three Phase I clinical trials have been conducted with G207. A Phase I dose-escalating safety trial for patients with recurrent malignant gliomas (WHO grade III and IV), who had failed standard therapy, and whose lesion had become greater than 1 cm in diameter was performed (Markert et al., 2000b). A total of 21 patients were recruited and cohorts of three patients received multiple (up to five) stereotactic intratumoral injections of G207 in escalating doses beginning at 1×10^6 PFU and concluding with a final dose of 3×10^9 PFU. Adverse events were noted in several patients but no toxicity or adverse event was ascribed to G207 administration. No patient developed herpes simplex encephalitis, and host seroconversion to HSV was documented in only one of five seronegative volunteers. Two participants were long-term survivors (5.5 and 7.5 years). A Phase IB trial was performed in six patients with recurrent glioma. Stereotactic infusion of the G207 virus was performed followed by surgical excision of the injected tumor 2–5 days later. The patients received additional freehand viral injection into the remaining tumor cavity wall. A third Phase I trial of G207 combined with radiation therapy has also been performed. This trial was carried out based on the observation that a single low dose (5 Gy) of radiation administered within 24 h of virus injection produced an increase in viral replication and spread in experimental tumors. Nine patients have been enrolled in this trial.

An HSV-1 construct deleted in both copies of the $\gamma_1 34.5$ gene, 1716, and expressing lacZ under the control of the latency-associated transcripts has been studied in Scotland in patients with recurrent malignant gliomas. A total of nine patients were evaluated at one of three doses of virus, beginning at 1×10^3 PFU and escalating by a factor of 10 to 1×10^5 PFU (Papanastassiou et al., 2002; Rampling et al., 2000). No reports of significant adverse events directly attributable to intracerebral virus administration occurred. Four of the nine patients were alive 12–24 months after injection. In a follow-up trial, six patients with recurrent tumor and six patients with newly diagnosed malignant

Table 46.2 Summary of HSV-1 human clinical trials for malignant gliomas

HSV-1 vector and methodology	Newly diagnosed or recurrent	Phase	Dose PFU	Patients treated	Adverse events (serious)	Long-term survival	Encephalitis, reactivation, seroconversion
G207 intratumoral injection (Markert et al., 2000b)	Recurrent	I	1×10^6 to 3×10^9	21	Yes (none)	2 patients (5.5 and 7.5 y)	None, not reported, 1/21
G207 intratumoral infusion and subsequent resection followed by injection of resection cavity	Recurrent	IB	1.5×10^8 then 8.5×10^8	6	Not reported	Not reported	Not reported, not reported, not reported
G207 intratumoral injection + ionizing radiation (5 Gy)	Recurrent	I	Not given	9	Not reported	Not reported	Not reported, not reported, not reported
1716 intratumoral injection (Papanastassiou et al., 2002; Rampling et al., 2000)	Recurrent	I	1×10^3 to 1×10^5	9	None	4 patients alive at 14–24 mos.	None, none, none
1716 injection of resection cavity (Harrow et al., 2004)	Both	I	1×10^5	12 (6 + 6)	None	3 patients alive 15–22 mos.	Not reported, not reported, 2/12

glioma underwent injection of virus into several sites after tumor resection. The promising results of the trials in Scotland and the United States have led to Phase II trials in the United Kingdom, the results of which are expected in the near future.

46.6 Limitations in the Treatment of Malignant Gliomas with HSV-Mediated Therapy

46.6.1 Delivery

Delivery of HSV-1 vectors in all clinical trials has been by multiple stereotactic intratumoral or peritumoral injections after surgical resection (Harrow et al., 2004; Markert et al., 2000b). Such techniques are problematic as viral delivery is unable to produce widespread and uniform distribution within tumors. Viral particles accumulate adjacent to the needle tract, and limited dispersal of particles occurs by diffusion. The binding of viral particles to the heparan sulfate proteoglycans found abundantly in the extracellular matrix and glycocalyx in the brain may contribute to limited dispersal (WuDunn and Spear, 1989).

Convection-enhanced delivery (CED) is an approach developed to overcome the obstacles associated with current CNS agent delivery (Bobo et al., 1994; Morrison et al., 1994) and is increasingly used to distribute therapeutic agents for treatment of malignant gliomas. Currently, multiple clinical trials involve CED for the treatment of recurrent GBM (Kunwar et al., 2003; Voges et al., 2003; Weaver and Laske, 2003; Weingart et al., 2002). In CED, a small hydrostatic pressure differential, imposed by a syringe pump to distribute the infusate directly to small or large regions of the CNS, is used in a safe, reliable, targeted, and homogeneous manner (Croteau et al., 2005). CED relies on bulk flow that is driven by a small gradient to distribute molecules within the interstitial spaces of the CNS. Convection is not limited by the infusate's molecular weight, concentration, or diffusivity (Bobo et al., 1994; Morrison et al., 1994; Strasser et al., 1995).

Limited use of CED for viral vector delivery to the rodent brain has been reported, mainly with the adeno-associated virus type 2 (AAV-2) (Bankiewicz et al., 2000; Cunningham et al., 2000; Nguyen et al., 2001). In one study, the authors suggested heparin co-infusion significantly increased the volume of distribution of AAV-2 by blocking the binding of virus to heparan sulfate proteoglycans in the extracellular matrix (Nguyen et al., 2001). Recently, CED of a replication-defective HSV-1 construct was shown to be effective at intracerebral distribution of virus and human GBM xenograft tumor lysis in a mouse model when combined with ionizing radiation or chemotherapy (Hadjipanayis et al., 2008b). A comparison between stereotactic manual injection and CED of HSV-1 confirmed greater viral distribution and more homogeneous viral infection of the brain.

46.6.2 Host Immune Response

Current evidence supports the fact that cells of the innate immune system in the brain may react to viral vectors and limit the efficacy of HSV-1 against malignant gliomas (Friedman et al., 2006; Ikeda et al., 1999; Wakimoto et al., 2003). Due to the large exposure of the human population to HSV-1, the immune system is primed for a rapid anti-HSV immune response. Both replication-defective and oncolytic viruses are able to generate an HSV-specific immune response in rodents (Brehm et al., 1999, 1997; Fulci et al., 2006). Replication-defective viruses have been reported to generate a cytotoxic T-lymphocyte response (CTL). Oncolytic viruses have been associated with a rapid increase in natural killer cells, microglia/macrophages (CD68+ and CD163+), and IFN-γ that limit viral replication and spread within tumors generated in rodents. In animal model data, generated host humoral immune responses have not limited virus replication but have reduced gene transfer into brain tumors (Herrlinger et al., 1998).

Since the capacity of oncolytic viruses to replicate and spread within malignant gliomas is compromised by the innate immune system, immunomodulation tactics have been employed to overcome this problem. The use of immunosuppressive agents, such as cyclophosphamide, has been shown to inhibit the innate immune response and allow for greater oncolytic viral replication and spread within tumors in preclinical animal models (Fulci et al., 2006; Ikeda et al., 1999).

Use of immunosuppression may allow for increased oncolytic viral replication and spread within brain tumors; however, activation of an anti-cancer immune response by HSV-1 has also been shown to be important in the recruitment of immune cells and tumor cell lysis (Davis and Fang, 2005; Kurozumi et al., 2007; Wakimoto et al., 2004). Therefore, virotherapy that involves the initial use of immunosuppressive agents for enhanced viral replication and spread followed by termination of immunosuppression to allow for HSV-1 to elicit an antitumoral immune response may be required to optimize the tumoricidal effect. Furthermore, the expression of proinflammatory cytokines in HSV-1 constructs, such as IL-4 or IL-12, has not diminished the antitumor effect but has consistently demonstrated an enhanced survival benefit in preclinical models (Andreansky et al., 1998; Hellums et al., 2005; Parker et al., 2000).

46.6.3 Safety

The ability of HSV-1 to infect a wide range of human cells raises the possibility of viral toxicity onto normal tissues in the brain. Despite the established safety of HSV-1 oncolytic constructs in human patients with malignant gliomas, development of herpes encephalitis remains a concern with intracerebral delivery of the virus. Because of the widespread exposure of the human population to HSV-1, the possibility of homologous recombination of a viral construct with a latent wild-type virus harbored by a cell can in theory result in the generation of a fully virulent wild-type virus that could result in encephalitis. Animal studies have not been able to show a significant risk of wild-type virus reactivation (Sundaresan et al., 2000; Wang et al., 1997). Furthermore, unwanted HSV-1 replication may be controlled by the use of antiviral medications such as acyclovir (Villarreal, 2003).

46.7 Perspectives

46.7.1 Tumor Targeting of HSV-1

The design and construction of novel HSV-1 vectors that specifically target cell surface molecules expressed by malignant glioma cells and not normal cells may increase antitumor efficacy while reducing unwanted toxicity in the brain. Viral mutants may be constructed to express ligands that bind to receptors which are overexpressed by malignant glioma cells such as IL-13Rα2 (Debinski et al., 1999a, b) (see also Chapter 35), uPAR (Gladson et al., 1995), or epidermal growth factor receptor (EGFR) (Nakamura, 2007). HSV-1 constructs have been designed to bind to these receptors in vitro and may be candidates for trial in humans (Kamiyama et al., 2006; Zhou and Roizman, 2005; Zhou et al., 2002).

Several HSV-1 constructs have been constructed to contain tumor-specific promoters for glioma-selective oncolysis (Kambara et al., 2005; Kanai et al., 2006). One oncolytic HSV-1 mutant has been constructed to express ICP34.5 under the control of the *nestin* gene promoter. Nestin is a type IV intermediate filament protein widely expressed in the neuronal precursor cells of the subventricular zone of the brain and has also been shown as a molecular marker of malignant gliomas. Selective expression of ICP34.5 in glioma cells can prevent host cell shut-off of protein synthesis caused by hyperphosphorylation of eIF2a and a significant antitumor effect.

Another important targeting scheme may be to generate HSV-1 mutants which selectively bind to or replicate within tumor initiating cells (TICs), also known as cancer stem cells, present in malignant gliomas. These are rare subpopulations of cancer cells, which share canonical properties with neural stem cells, and may be integral to the development and perpetuation of malignant gliomas (Galli et al., 2004; Singh et al., 2004). TICs have the ability to self-renew, develop into any cell in the overall tumor population (multipotency), and proliferate. They have been shown to initiate new tumors in vivo when transplanted into immunocompromised mice with efficiencies of 100–1,000 fold that of the bulk of cells in the tumor. Currently, these cells are characterized by a cell surface protein known at CD133 (Prominin-1). An adenovirus has already been constructed based on directing the expression of replication factor E1A under the *CD133* gene promoter (Nandi et al., 2008). Other cell surface targets on TICs will be discovered which may allow for HSV-1 targeting.

46.7.2 Chemo/Radiotherapy-Activated Transcriptional Targeting of Malignant Gliomas

Enhancing and targeting the effects of chemoradiation may provide for a further increase in progression-free and overall survival in patients with malignant gliomas. Chemo/radiotherapy-activated gene therapy is a developing treatment paradigm that attempts to improve the therapeutic index of a variety of potentially therapeutic compounds. Genetically engineered promoters that respond to IR, chemotherapy, and hypoxia have been developed and used in adenoviral vectors for malignant gliomas (Weichselbaum et al., 2002; Yamini et al., 2007; Post et al., 2007) (see also Chapter 47).

46.7.3 Imaging

The ability to non-invasively image the location of HSV-1 delivery and transgene expression in vivo remains an area of extreme importance in determining the efficacy of various viral constructs. Current therapeutic HSV-1 viruses lack the ability to be detected in the brain by magnetic resonance imaging (MRI). Only edema or inflammation can be determined by MRI. As delivery of the virus improves to the brain, such as with CED, determining the location and infection of tumor cells within the brain will help provide answers on whether the HSV-1 construct reaches tumor cells. A viral marker gene whose protein product may be detected robustly by MRI after cell infection may be the one method of localization. Recently, a replication-defective adenoviral vector has been constructed to express metalloproteins from the ferritin family which can be detected robustly in the brain in vitro and in vivo with MRI (Genove et al., 2005). Magnetic nanotechnology may also permit more effective in vivo imaging of HSV-1 distribution in the brain and optimal targeting of tumor tissues (Hadjipanayis et al., 2008a).

46.8 Summary

HSV-1 remains an attractive biologic agent for the therapy of malignant gliomas. Both replication-defective and oncolytic constructs have shown antitumor efficacy in preclinical animal models. Human clinical trials of several oncolytic viruses have established safety and a modest increase in patient survival. HSV-1 delivery to the brain remains an important limiting factor in the use of HSV-1 as a therapeutic agent. Convection-enhanced delivery (CED) may be the most effective method currently used for distribution of the virus in the brain and maximizing the efficacy of various HSV-1 constructs. Combination therapies with temozolomide and IR can further enhance the antitumor effect of HSV-1. New targeting schemes and imaging are needed to further increase progression-free and overall survival in patients with malignant gliomas.

Acknowledgments The author would like to thank Giulia Fulci for her critical review of the chapter and her thoughtful comments. The author would also like to thank Neal Deluca for providing the transmission electron micrograph of the HSV-1 particle.

References

Advani, S. J., Mezhir, J. J., Roizman, B., and Weichselbaum, R. R. (2006). ReVOLT: radiation-enhanced viral oncolytic therapy. Int J Radiat Oncol Biol Phys *66*, 637–646.

Advani, S. J., Sibley, G. S., Song, P. Y., Hallahan, D. E., Kataoka, Y., Roizman, B., and Weichselbaum, R. R. (1998). Enhancement of replication of genetically engineered herpes simplex viruses by ionizing radiation: a new paradigm for destruction of therapeutically intractable tumors. Gene Ther *5*, 160–165.

Aghi, M., Rabkin, S., and Martuza, R. L. (2006). Effect of chemotherapy-induced DNA repair on oncolytic herpes simplex viral replication. J Natl Cancer Inst *98*, 38–50.

Andreansky, S., He, B., van Cott, J., McGhee, J., Markert, J. M., Gillespie, G. Y., Roizman, B., and Whitley, R. J. (1998). Treatment of intracranial gliomas in immunocompetent mice using herpes simplex viruses that express murine interleukins. Gene Ther *5*, 121–130.

Bankiewicz, K. S., Eberling, J. L., Kohutnicka, M., Jagust, W., Pivirotto, P., Bringas, J., Cunningham, J., Budinger, T. F., and Harvey-White, J. (2000). Convection-enhanced delivery of AAV vector in parkinsonian monkeys; in vivo detection of gene expression and restoration of dopaminergic function using pro-drug approach. Exp Neurol *164*, 2–14.

Batterson, W., and Roizman, B. (1983). Characterization of the herpes simplex virion-associated factor responsible for the induction of alpha genes. J Virol *46*, 371–377.

Becker, Y., Dym, H., and Sarov, I. (1968). Herpes simplex virus DNA. Virology *36*, 184–192.

Beltinger, C., Fulda, S., Kammertoens, T., Meyer, E., Uckert, W., and Debatin, K. M. (1999). Herpes simplex virus thymidine kinase/ganciclovir-induced apoptosis involves ligand-independent death receptor aggregation and activation of caspases. Proc Natl Acad Sci U S A *96*, 8699–8704.

Bobo, R. H., Laske, D. W., Akbasak, A., Morrison, P. F., Dedrick, R. L., and Oldfield, E. H. (1994). Convection-enhanced delivery of macromolecules in the brain. Proc Natl Acad Sci U S A *91*, 2076–2080.

Boutell, C., Canning, M., Orr, A., and Everett, R. D. (2005). Reciprocal activities between herpes simplex virus type 1 regulatory protein ICP0, a ubiquitin E3 ligase, and ubiquitin-specific protease USP7. J Virol *79*, 12342–12354.

Boutell, C., Sadis, S., and Everett, R. D. (2002). Herpes simplex virus type 1 immediate-early protein ICP0 and is isolated RING finger domain act as ubiquitin E3 ligases in vitro. J Virol *76*, 841–850.

Bradley, J. D., Kataoka, Y., Advani, S., Chung, S. M., Arani, R. B., Gillespie, G. Y., Whitley, R. J., Markert, J. M., Roizman, B., and Weichselbaum, R. R. (1999). Ionizing radiation improves survival in mice bearing intracranial high-grade gliomas injected with genetically modified herpes simplex virus. Clin Cancer Res *5*, 1517–1522.

Brehm, M., Samaniego, L. A., Bonneau, R. H., DeLuca, N. A., and Tevethia, S. S. (1999). Immunogenicity of herpes simplex virus type 1 mutants containing deletions in one or more alpha-genes: ICP4, ICP27, ICP22, and ICP0. Virology *256*, 258–269.

Brehm, M. A., Bonneau, R. H., Knipe, D. M., and Tevethia, S. S. (1997). Immunization with a replication-deficient mutant of herpes simplex virus type 1 (HSV-1) induces a CD8+ cytotoxic T-lymphocyte response and confers a level of protection comparable to that of wild-type HSV-1. J Virol *71*, 3534–3544.

Cai, W., Astor, T. L., Liptak, L. M., Cho, C., Coen, D. M., and Schaffer, P. A. (1993). The herpes simplex virus type 1 regulatory protein ICP0 enhances virus replication during acute infection and reactivation from latency. J Virol *67*, 7501–7512.

Carbone, R., Pearson, M., Minucci, S., and Pelicci, P. G. (2002). PML NBs associate with the hMre11 complex and p53 at sites of irradiation induced DNA damage. Oncogene *21*, 1633–1640.

Chiocca, E. A. (2002). Oncolytic viruses. Nat Rev Cancer *2*, 938–950.

Chou, J., Kern, E. R., Whitley, R. J., and Roizman, B. (1990). Mapping of herpes simplex virus-1 neurovirulence to gamma 134.5, a gene nonessential for growth in culture. Science *250*, 1262–1266.

Chou, J., and Roizman, B. (1990). The herpes simplex virus 1 gene for ICP34.5, which maps in inverted repeats, is conserved in several limited-passage isolates but not in strain 17syn+. J Virol *64*, 1014–1020.

Chou, J., and Roizman, B. (1994). Herpes simplex virus 1 gamma(1)34.5 gene function, which blocks the host response to infection, maps in the homologous domain of the genes expressed during growth arrest and DNA damage. Proc Natl Acad Sci U S A *91*, 5247–5251.

Clements, J. B., Watson, R. J., and Wilkie, N. M. (1977). Temporal regulation of herpes simplex virus type 1 transcription: location of transcripts on the viral genome. Cell *12*, 275–285.

Coen, D. M., Kosz-Vnenchak, M., Jacobson, J. G., Leib, D. A., Bogard, C. L., Schaffer, P. A. , Tyler, K. L., and Knipe, D. M. (1989). Thymidine kinase-negative herpes simplex virus mutants establish latency in mouse trigeminal ganglia but do not reactivate. Proc Natl Acad Sci U S A *86*, 4736–4740.

Cook, M. L., and Stevens, J. G. (1973). Pathogenesis of herpetic neuritis and ganglionitis in mice: evidence for intra-axonal transport of infection. Infect Immun *7*, 272–288.

Costanzo, F., Campadelli-Fiume, G., Foa-Tomasi, L., and Cassai, E. (1977). Evidence that herpes simplex virus DNA is transcribed by cellular RNA polymerase B. J Virol *21*, 996–1001.

Croen, K. D., Ostrove, J. M., Dragovic, L. J., Smialek, J. E., and Straus, S. E. (1987). Latent herpes simplex virus in human trigeminal ganglia. Detection of an immediate early gene "anti-sense" transcript by in situ hybridization. N Engl J Med *317*, 1427–1432.

Croteau, D., Walbridge, S., Morrison, P. F., Butman, J. A., Vortmeyer, A. O., Johnson, D., Oldfield, E. H., and Lonser, R. R. (2005). Real-time in vivo imaging of the convective distribution of a low-molecular-weight tracer. J Neurosurg *102*, 90–97.

Cunningham, J., Oiwa, Y., Nagy, D., Podsakoff, G., Colosi, P., and Bankiewicz, K. S. (2000). Distribution of AAV-TK following intracranial convection-enhanced delivery into rats. Cell Transplant *9*, 585–594.

Davis, J. J., and Fang, B. (2005). Oncolytic virotherapy for cancer treatment: challenges and solutions. J Gene Med *7*, 1380–1389.

de Bruyn Kops, A., Uprichard, S. L., Chen, M., and Knipe, D. M. (1998). Comparison of the intranuclear distributions of herpes simplex virus proteins involved in various viral functions. Virology *252*, 162–178.

Debinski, W., Gibo, D. M., Hulet, S. W., Connor, J. R., and Gillespie, G. Y. (1999a). Receptor for interleukin 13 is a marker and therapeutic target for human high-grade gliomas. Clin Cancer Res *5*, 985–990.

Debinski, W., Gibo, D. M., Slagle, B., Powers, S. K., and Gillespie, G. Y. (1999b). Receptor for interleukin 13 is abundantly and specifically over-expressed in patients with glioblastoma multiforme. Int J Oncol *15*, 481–486.
DeLuca, N., Bzik, D. J., Bond, V. C., Person, S., and Snipes, W. (1982). Nucleotide sequences of herpes simplex virus type 1 (HSV-1) affecting virus entry, cell fusion, and production of glycoprotein gb (VP7). Virology *122*, 411–423.
DeLuca, N. A., McCarthy, A. M., and Schaffer, P. A. (1985). Isolation and characterization of deletion mutants of herpes simplex virus type 1 in the gene encoding immediate-early regulatory protein ICP4. J Virol *56*, 558–570.
Desai, P. J., Schaffer, P. A., and Minson, A. C. (1988). Excretion of non-infectious virus particles lacking glycoprotein H by a temperature-sensitive mutant of herpes simplex virus type 1: evidence that gH is essential for virion infectivity. J Gen Virol *69 (Pt 6)*, 1147–1156.
Deshmane, S. L., and Fraser, N. W. (1989). During latency, herpes simplex virus type 1 DNA is associated with nucleosomes in a chromatin structure. J Virol *63*, 943–947.
Dixon, R. A., and Schaffer, P. A. (1980). Fine-structure mapping and functional analysis of temperature-sensitive mutants in the gene encoding the herpes simplex virus type 1 immediate early protein VP175. J Virol *36*, 189–203.
Everett, R. D. (2000). ICP0, a regulator of herpes simplex virus during lytic and latent infection. Bioessays *22*, 761–770.
Everett, R. D., Earnshaw, W. C., Findlay, J., and Lomonte, P. (1999a). Specific destruction of kinetochore protein CENP-C and disruption of cell division by herpes simplex virus immediate-early protein Vmw110. Embo J *18*, 1526–1538.
Everett, R. D., Earnshaw, W. C., Pluta, A. F., Sternsdorf, T., Ainsztein, A. M., Carmena, M., Ruchaud, S., Hsu, W. L., and Orr, A. (1999b). A dynamic connection between centromeres and ND10 proteins. J Cell Sci *112 (Pt 20)*, 3443–3454.
Everett, R. D., Freemont, P., Saitoh, H., Dasso, M., Orr, A., Kathoria, M., and Parkinson, J. (1998). The disruption of ND10 during herpes simplex virus infection correlates with the Vmw110- and proteasome-dependent loss of several PML isoforms. J Virol *72*, 6581–6591.
Everett, R. D., Rechter, S., Papior, P., Tavalai, N., Stamminger, T., and Orr, A. (2006). PML contributes to a cellular mechanism of repression of herpes simplex virus type 1 infection that is inactivated by ICP0. J Virol *80*, 7995–8005.
Flint, J., and Shenk, T. (1997). Viral transactivating proteins. Annu Rev Genet *31*, 177–212.
Flint, S. J., Enquist, L. W., Racaniello, V. R., and Skalka, A. M. (2004). Principles of Virology, Second edn (Washington D. C.: ASM Press).
Freeman, S. M., Abboud, C. N., Whartenby, K. A., Packman, C. H., Koeplin, D. S., Moolten, F. L., and Abraham, G. N. (1993). The "bystander effect": tumor regression when a fraction of the tumor mass is genetically modified. Cancer Res *53*, 5274–5283.
Friedman, A., Tian, J. P., Fulci, G., Chiocca, E. A., and Wang, J. (2006). Glioma virotherapy: effects of innate immune suppression and increased viral replication capacity. Cancer Res *66*, 2314–2319.
Fulci, G., Breymann, L., Gianni, D., Kurozomi, K., Rhee, S. S., Yu, J., Kaur, B., Louis, D. N., Weissleder, R., Caligiuri, M. A., and Chiocca, E. A. (2006). Cyclophosphamide enhances glioma virotherapy by inhibiting innate immune responses. Proc Natl Acad Sci U S A *103*, 12873–12878.
Fulci, G., and Chiocca, E. A. (2007). The status of gene therapy for brain tumors. Expert Opin Biol Ther *7*, 197–208.
Furlong, D., Swift, H., and Roizman, B. (1972). Arrangement of herpesvirus deoxyribonucleic acid in the core. J Virol *10*, 1071–1074.
Furnari, F. B., Fenton, T., Bachoo, R. M., Mukasa, A., Stommel, J. M., Stegh, A., Hahn, W. C., Ligon, K. L., Louis, D. N., Brennan, C., *et al.* (2007). Malignant astrocytic glioma: genetics, biology, and paths to treatment. Genes Dev *21*, 2683–2710.
Galli, R., Binda, E., Orfanelli, U., Cipelletti, B., Gritti, A., De Vitis, S., Fiocco, R., Foroni, C., Dimeco, F., and Vescovi, A. (2004). Isolation and characterization of tumorigenic, stem-like neural precursors from human glioblastoma. Cancer Res *64*, 7011–7021.

Garber, D. A., Beverley, S. M., and Coen, D. M. (1993). Demonstration of circularization of herpes simplex virus DNA following infection using pulsed field gel electrophoresis. Virology *197*, 459–462.

Gelman, I. H., and Silverstein, S. (1987). Dissection of immediate-early gene promoters from herpes simplex virus: sequences that respond to the virus transcriptional activators. J Virol *61*, 3167–3172.

Genove, G., DeMarco, U., Xu, H., Goins, W. F., and Ahrens, E. T. (2005). A new transgene reporter for in vivo magnetic resonance imaging. Nat Med *11*, 450–454.

Geraghty, R. J., Krummenacher, C., Cohen, G. H., Eisenberg, R. J., and Spear, P. G. (1998). Entry of alphaherpesviruses mediated by poliovirus receptor-related protein 1 and poliovirus receptor. Science *280*, 1618–1620.

Gladson, C. L., Pijuan-Thompson, V., Olman, M. A., Gillespie, G. Y., and Yacoub, I. Z. (1995). Up-regulation of urokinase and urokinase receptor genes in malignant astrocytoma. Am J Pathol *146*, 1150–1160.

Gordon, Y. J., McKnight, J. L., Ostrove, J. M., Romanowski, E., and Araullo-Cruz, T. (1990). Host species and strain differences affect the ability of an HSV-1 ICP0 deletion mutant to establish latency and spontaneously reactivate in vivo. Virology *178*, 469–477.

Gruenheid, S., Gatzke, L., Meadows, H., and Tufaro, F. (1993). Herpes simplex virus infection and propagation in a mouse L cell mutant lacking heparan sulfate proteoglycans. J Virol *67*, 93–100.

Gu, H., Liang, Y., Mandel, G., and Roizman, B. (2005). Components of the REST/CoREST/histone deacetylase repressor complex are disrupted, modified, and translocated in HSV-1-infected cells. Proc Natl Acad Sci U S A *102*, 7571–7576.

Haarr, L., and Skulstad, S. (1994). The herpes simplex virus type 1 particle: structure and molecular functions. Review article. APMIS *102*, 321–346.

Hadjipanayis, C. G., Bonder, M. J., Balakrishnan, S., Wang, X., Mao, H., and Hadjipanayis, G. C. (2008a). Metallic iron nanoparticles for MRI contrast enhancement and local hyperthermia. Small.

Hadjipanayis, C. G., and DeLuca, N. A. (2005). Inhibition of DNA repair by a herpes simplex virus vector enhances the radiosensitivity of human glioblastoma cells. Cancer Res *65*, 5310–5316.

Hadjipanayis, C. G., Fellows-Mayle, W., and Deluca, N. A. (2008b). Therapeutic efficacy of a herpes simplex virus in combination with radiation or temozolomide for intracranial glioblastoma after convection-enhanced delivery. Mol Ther.

Hagglund, R., and Roizman, B. (2004). Role of ICP0 in the strategy of conquest of the host cell by herpes simplex virus 1. J Virol *78*, 2169–2178.

Halford, W. P., Kemp, C. D., Isler, J. A., Davido, D. J., and Schaffer, P. A. (2001). ICP0, ICP4, or VP16 expressed from adenovirus vectors induces reactivation of latent herpes simplex virus type 1 in primary cultures of latently infected trigeminal ganglion cells. J Virol *75*, 6143–6153.

Halford, W. P., and Schaffer, P. A. (2001). ICP0 is required for efficient reactivation of herpes simplex virus type 1 from neuronal latency. J Virol *75*, 3240–3249.

Harrow, S., Papanastassiou, V., Harland, J., Mabbs, R., Petty, R., Fraser, M., Hadley, D., Patterson, J., Brown, S. M., and Rampling, R. (2004). HSV1716 injection into the brain adjacent to tumour following surgical resection of high-grade glioma: safety data and long-term survival. Gene Ther *11*, 1648–1658.

Hayward, G. S., Jacob, R. J., Wadsworth, S. C., and Roizman, B. (1975). Anatomy of herpes simplex virus DNA: evidence for four populations of molecules that differ in the relative orientations of their long and short components. Proc Natl Acad Sci U S A *72*, 4243–4247.

He, B., Chou, J., Liebermann, D. A., Hoffman, B., and Roizman, B. (1996). The carboxyl terminus of the murine MyD116 gene substitutes for the corresponding domain of the gamma(1)34.5 gene of herpes simplex virus to preclude the premature shutoff of total protein synthesis in infected human cells. J Virol *70*, 84–90.

Hellums, E. K., Markert, J. M., Parker, J. N., He, B., Perbal, B., Roizman, B., Whitley, R. J., Langford, C. P., Bharara, S., and Gillespie, G. Y. (2005). Increased efficacy of an interleukin-12-secreting herpes simplex virus in a syngeneic intracranial murine glioma model. Neurooncology *7*, 213–224.

Herrlinger, U., Kramm, C. M., Aboody-Guterman, K. S., Silver, J. S., Ikeda, K., Johnston, K. M., Pechan, P. A., Barth, R. F., Finkelstein, D., Chiocca, E. A., *et al.* (1998). Pre-existing herpes simplex virus 1 (HSV-1) immunity decreases, but does not abolish, gene transfer to experimental brain tumors by a HSV-1 vector. Gene Ther *5*, 809–819.

Hobbs, W. E., 2nd, and DeLuca, N. A. (1999). Perturbation of cell cycle progression and cellular gene expression as a function of herpes simplex virus ICP0. J Virol *73*, 8245–8255.

Homa, F. L., and Brown, J. C. (1997). Capsid assembly and DNA packaging in herpes simplex virus. Rev Med Virol *7*, 107–122.

Honess, R. W., and Roizman, B. (1974). Regulation of herpesvirus macromolecular synthesis. I. Cascade regulation of the synthesis of three groups of viral proteins. J Virol *14*, 8–19.

Honess, R. W., and Roizman, B. (1975). Regulation of herpesvirus macromolecular synthesis: sequential transition of polypeptide synthesis requires functional viral polypeptides. Proc Natl Acad Sci U S A *72*, 1276–1280.

Hoshi, M., Harada, A., Kawase, T., Uyemura, K., and Yazaki, T. (2000). Antitumoral effects of defective herpes simplex virus-mediated transfer of tissue inhibitor of metalloproteinases-2 gene in malignant glioma U87 in vitro: consequences for anti-cancer gene therapy. Cancer Gene Ther *7*, 799–805.

Hunter, W. D., Martuza, R. L., Feigenbaum, F., Todo, T., Mineta, T., Yazaki, T., Toda, M., Newsome, J. T., Platenberg, R. C., Manz, H. J., and Rabkin, S. D. (1999). Attenuated, replication-competent herpes simplex virus type 1 mutant G207: safety evaluation of intracerebral injection in nonhuman primates. J Virol *73*, 6319–6326.

Ikeda, K., Ichikawa, T., Wakimoto, H., Silver, J. S., Deisboeck, T. S., Finkelstein, D., Harsh, G. R. t., Louis, D. N., Bartus, R. T., Hochberg, F. H., and Chiocca, E. A. (1999). Oncolytic virus therapy of multiple tumors in the brain requires suppression of innate and elicited antiviral responses. Nat Med *5*, 881–887.

Jackson, S. A., and DeLuca, N. A. (2003). Relationship of herpes simplex virus genome configuration to productive and persistent infections. Proc Natl Acad Sci U S A *100*, 7871–7876.

Johnson, P. A., Wang, M. J., and Friedmann, T. (1994). Improved cell survival by the reduction of immediate-early gene expression in replication-defective mutants of herpes simplex virus type 1 but not by mutation of the virion host shutoff function. J Virol *68*, 6347–6362.

Kambara, H., Okano, H., Chiocca, E. A., and Saeki, Y. (2005). An oncolytic HSV-1 mutant expressing ICP34.5 under control of a nestin promoter increases survival of animals even when symptomatic from a brain tumor. Cancer Res *65*, 2832–2839.

Kamiyama, H., Zhou, G., and Roizman, B. (2006). Herpes simplex virus 1 recombinant virions exhibiting the amino terminal fragment of urokinase-type plasminogen activator can enter cells via the cognate receptor. Gene Ther *13*, 621–629.

Kanai, R., Tomita, H., Shinoda, A., Takahashi, M., Goldman, S., Okano, H., Kawase, T., and Yazaki, T. (2006). Enhanced therapeutic efficacy of G207 for the treatment of glioma through Musashi1 promoter retargeting of gamma34.5-mediated virulence. Gene Ther *13*, 106–116.

Kanno, H., Hattori, S., Sato, H., Murata, H., Huang, F. H., Hayashi, A., Suzuki, N., Yamamoto, I., Kawamoto, S., Minami, M., *et al.* (1999). Experimental gene therapy against subcutaneously implanted glioma with a herpes simplex virus-defective vector expressing interferon-gamma. Cancer Gene Ther *6*, 147–154.

Kieff, E. D., Bachenheimer, S. L., and Roizman, B. (1971). Size, composition, and structure of the deoxyribonucleic acid of herpes simplex virus subtypes 1 and 2. J Virol *8*, 125–132.

Knipe, D. M., Senechek, D., Rice, S. A., and Smith, J. L. (1987). Stages in the nuclear association of the herpes simplex virus transcriptional activator protein ICP4. J Virol *61*, 276–284.

Kramm, C. M., Chase, M., Herrlinger, U., Jacobs, A., Pechan, P. A., Rainov, N. G., Sena-Esteves, M., Aghi, M., Barnett, F. H., Chiocca, E. A., and Breakefield, X. O. (1997). Therapeutic efficiency and safety of a second-generation replication-conditional HSV1 vector for brain tumor gene therapy. Hum Gene Ther *8*, 2057–2068.

Kristie, T. M., LeBowitz, J. H., and Sharp, P. A. (1989). The octamer-binding proteins form multi-protein–DNA complexes with the HSV alpha TIF regulatory protein. Embo J *8*, 4229–4238.

Kristie, T. M., and Roizman, B. (1987). Host cell proteins bind to the cis-acting site required for virion-mediated induction of herpes simplex virus 1 alpha genes. Proc Natl Acad Sci U S A *84*, 71–75.

Kunwar, S., Prados, M. D., and Lang, F. F. (2003). Pre and post-operative infusion of IL13-pE38QQR cytotoxin by convection-enhanced delivery (CED) in recurrent malignant glioma: a phase I study. Proc Am Soc Clin Oncol *22*, 119 (Abstract).

Kurozumi, K., Hardcastle, J., Thakur, R., Yang, M., Christoforidis, G., Fulci, G., Hochberg, F. H., Weissleder, R., Carson, W., Chiocca, E. A., and Kaur, B. (2007). Effect of tumor microenvironment modulation on the efficacy of oncolytic virus therapy. J Natl Cancer Inst *99*, 1768–1781.

Laquerre, S., Argnani, R., Anderson, D. B., Zucchini, S., Manservigi, R., and Glorioso, J. C. (1998). Heparan sulfate proteoglycan binding by herpes simplex virus type 1 glycoproteins B and C, which differ in their contributions to virus attachment, penetration, and cell-to-cell spread. J Virol *72*, 6119–6130.

Lees-Miller, S. P., Long, M. C., Kilvert, M. A., Lam, V., Rice, S. A., and Spencer, C. A. (1996). Attenuation of DNA-dependent protein kinase activity and its catalytic subunit by the herpes simplex virus type 1 transactivator ICP0. J Virol *70*, 7471–7477.

Leib, D. A., Coen, D. M., Bogard, C. L., Hicks, K. A., Yager, D. R., Knipe, D. M., Tyler, K. L., and Schaffer, P. A. (1989). Immediate-early regulatory gene mutants define different stages in the establishment and reactivation of herpes simplex virus latency. J Virol *63*, 759–768.

Lin, E., and Nemunaitis, J. (2004). Oncolytic viral therapies. Cancer Gene Ther *11*, 643–664.

Liptak, L. M., Uprichard, S. L., and Knipe, D. M. (1996). Functional order of assembly of herpes simplex virus DNA replication proteins into prereplicative site structures. J Virol *70*, 1759–1767.

Lomonte, P., and Everett, R. D. (1999). Herpes simplex virus type 1 immediate-early protein Vmw110 inhibits progression of cells through mitosis and from G(1) into S phase of the cell cycle. J Virol *73*, 9456–9467.

Lomonte, P., Sullivan, K. F., and Everett, R. D. (2001). Degradation of nucleosome-associated centromeric histone H3-like protein CENP-A induced by herpes simplex virus type 1 protein ICP0. J Biol Chem *276*, 5829–5835.

Lomonte, P., Thomas, J., Texier, P., Caron, C., Khochbin, S., and Epstein, A. L. (2004). Functional interaction between class II histone deacetylases and ICP0 of herpes simplex virus type 1. J Virol *78*, 6744–6757.

Marconi, P., Tamura, M., Moriuchi, S., Krisky, D. M., Niranjan, A., Goins, W. F., Cohen, J. B., and Glorioso, J. C. (2000). Connexin 43-enhanced suicide gene therapy using herpesviral vectors. Mol Ther *1*, 71–81.

Markert, J. M., Gillespie, G. Y., Weichselbaum, R. R., Roizman, B., and Whitley, R. J. (2000a). Genetically engineered HSV in the treatment of glioma: a review. Rev Med Virol *10*, 17–30.

Markert, J. M., Medlock, M. D., Rabkin, S. D., Gillespie, G. Y., Todo, T., Hunter, W. D., Palmer, C. A., Feigenbaum, F., Tornatore, C., Tufaro, F., and Martuza, R. L. (2000b). Conditionally replicating herpes simplex virus mutant, G207 for the treatment of malignant glioma: results of a phase I trial. Gene Ther *7*, 867–874.

Martuza, R. L. (2000). Conditionally replicating herpes vectors for cancer therapy. J Clin Invest *105*, 841–846.

Martuza, R. L., Malick, A., Markert, J. M., Ruffner, K. L., and Coen, D. M. (1991). Experimental therapy of human glioma by means of a genetically engineered virus mutant. Science *252*, 854–856.

Maul, G. G., Ishov, A. M., and Everett, R. D. (1996). Nuclear domain 10 as preexisting potential replication start sites of herpes simplex virus type-1. Virology *217*, 67–75.

McCarthy, A. M., McMahan, L., and Schaffer, P. A. (1989). Herpes simplex virus type 1 ICP27 deletion mutants exhibit altered patterns of transcription and are DNA deficient. J Virol *63*, 18–27.

McGeoch, D. J., Barnett, B. C., and MacLean, C. A. (1993). Emerging functions ofalpha-herpesvirus genes. Semin Virol *4*, 125–134.

McGeoch, D. J., Dalrymple, M. A., Davison, A. J., Dolan, A., Frame, M. C., McNab, D., Perry, L. J., Scott, J. E., and Taylor, P. (1988). The complete DNA sequence of the long unique region in the genome of herpes simplex virus type 1. J Gen Virol *69 (Pt 7)*, 1531–1574.

McGeoch, D. J., Dolan, A., Donald, S., and Brauer, D. H. (1986). Complete DNA sequence of the short repeat region in the genome of herpes simplex virus type 1. Nucleic Acids Res *14*, 1727–1745.

Mellerick, D. M., and Fraser, N. W. (1987). Physical state of the latent herpes simplex virus genome in a mouse model system: evidence suggesting an episomal state. Virology *158*, 265–275.

Mettenleiter, T. C. (2002). Herpesvirus assembly and egress. J Virol *76*, 1537–1547.

Mineta, T., Rabkin, S. D., Yazaki, T., Hunter, W. D., and Martuza, R. L. (1995). Attenuated multi-mutated herpes simplex virus-1 for the treatment of malignant gliomas. Nat Med *1*, 938–943.

Miyatake, S., Martuza, R. L., and Rabkin, S. D. (1997). Defective herpes simplex virus vectors expressing thymidine kinase for the treatment of malignant glioma. Cancer Gene Ther *4*, 222–228.

Montgomery, R. I., Warner, M. S., Lum, B. J., and Spear, P. G. (1996). Herpes simplex virus-1 entry into cells mediated by a novel member of the TNF/NGF receptor family. Cell *87*, 427–436.

Moolten, F. L. (1986). Tumor chemosensitivity conferred by inserted herpes thymidine kinase genes: paradigm for a prospective cancer control strategy. Cancer Res *46*, 5276–5281.

Morgan, C., Rose, H. M., and Mednis, B. (1968). Electron microscopy of herpes simplex virus. I. Entry. J Virol *2*, 507–516.

Moriuchi, S., Glorioso, J. C., Maruno, M., Izumoto, S., Wolfe, D., Huang, S., Cohen, J. B., and Yoshimine, T. (2005). Combination gene therapy for glioblastoma involving herpes simplex virus vector-mediated codelivery of mutant IkappaBalpha and HSV thymidine kinase. Cancer Gene Ther *12*, 487–496.

Moriuchi, S., Oligino, T., Krisky, D., Marconi, P., Fink, D., Cohen, J., and Glorioso, J. C. (1998). Enhanced tumor cell killing in the presence of ganciclovir by herpes simplex virus type 1 vector-directed coexpression of human tumor necrosis factor-alpha and herpes simplex virus thymidine kinase. Cancer Res *58*, 5731–5737.

Moriuchi, S., Wolfe, D., Tamura, M., Yoshimine, T., Miura, F., Cohen, J. B., and Glorioso, J. C. (2002). Double suicide gene therapy using a replication defective herpes simplex virus vector reveals reciprocal interference in a malignant glioma model. Gene Ther *9*, 584–591.

Morrison, P. F., Laske, D. W., Bobo, H., Oldfield, E. H., and Dedrick, R. L. (1994). High-flow microinfusion: tissue penetration and pharmacodynamics. Am J Physiol *266*, R292–305.

Nakamura, J. L. (2007). The epidermal growth factor receptor in malignant gliomas: pathogenesis and therapeutic implications. Expert Opin Ther Targets *11*, 463–472.

Nandi, S., Ulasov, I. V., Tyler, M. A., Sugihara, A. Q., Molinero, L., Han, Y., Zhu, Z. B., and Lesniak, M. S. (2008). Low-dose radiation enhances survivin-mediated virotherapy against malignant glioma stem cells. Cancer Res *68*, 5778–5784.

Nguyen, J. B., Sanchez-Pernaute, R., Cunningham, J., and Bankiewicz, K. S. (2001). Convection-enhanced delivery of AAV-2 combined with heparin increases TK gene transfer in the rat brain. Neuroreport *12*, 1961–1964.

Nicola, A. V., McEvoy, A. M., and Straus, S. E. (2003). Roles for endocytosis and low pH in herpes simplex virus entry into HeLa and Chinese hamster ovary cells. J Virol *77*, 5324–5332.

Niranjan, A., Moriuchi, S., Lunsford, L. D., Kondziolka, D., Flickinger, J. C., Fellows, W., Rajendiran, S., Tamura, M., Cohen, J. B., and Glorioso, J. C. (2000). Effective treatment of experimental glioblastoma by HSV vector-mediated TNF alpha and HSV-tk gene transfer in combination with radiosurgery and ganciclovir administration. Mol Ther *2*, 114–120.

Niranjan, A., Wolfe, D., Tamura, M., Soares, M. K., Krisky, D. M., Lunsford, L. D., Li, S., Fellows-Mayle, W., DeLuca, N. A., Cohen, J. B., and Glorioso, J. C. (2003). Treatment of rat gliosarcoma brain tumors by HSV-based multigene therapy combined with radiosurgery. Mol Ther *8*, 530–542.

O'Hare, P., Goding, C. R., and Haigh, A. (1988). Direct combinatorial interaction between a herpes simplex virus regulatory protein and a cellular octamer-binding factor mediates specific induction of virus immediate-early gene expression. Embo J *7*, 4231–4238.

Papanastassiou, V., Rampling, R., Fraser, M., Petty, R., Hadley, D., Nicoll, J., Harland, J., Mabbs, R., and Brown, M. (2002). The potential for efficacy of the modified (ICP 34.5(-)) herpes simplex virus HSV1716 following intratumoural injection into human malignant glioma: a proof of principle study. Gene Ther *9*, 398–406.

Parker, J. N., Gillespie, G. Y., Love, C. E., Randall, S., Whitley, R. J., and Markert, J. M. (2000). Engineered herpes simplex virus expressing IL-12 in the treatment of experimental murine brain tumors. Proc Natl Acad Sci U S A *97*, 2208–2213.

Parkinson, J., Lees-Miller, S. P., and Everett, R. D. (1999). Herpes simplex virus type 1 immediate-early protein vmw110 induces the proteasome-dependent degradation of the catalytic subunit of DNA-dependent protein kinase. J Virol *73*, 650–657.

Pereira, L., Wolff, M. H., Fenwick, M., and Roizman, B. (1977). Regulation of herpesvirus macromolecular synthesis. V. Properties of alpha polypeptides made in HSV-1 and HSV-2 infected cells. Virology *77*, 733–749.

Phelan, A., Dunlop, J., Patel, A. H., Stow, N. D., and Clements, J. B. (1997). Nuclear sites of herpes simplex virus type 1 DNA replication and transcription colocalize at early times postinfection and are largely distinct from RNA processing factors. J Virol *71*, 1124–1132.

Poffenberger, K. L., Tabares, E., and Roizman, B. (1983). Characterization of a viable, noninverting herpes simplex virus 1 genome derived by insertion and deletion of sequences at the junction of components L and S. Proc Natl Acad Sci U S A *80*, 2690–2694.

Post, D. E., Sandberg, E. M., Kyle, M. M., Devi, N. S., Brat, D. J., Xu, Z., Tighiouart, M., and Van Meir, E. G. (2007). Targeted cancer gene therapy using a hypoxia inducible factor dependent oncolytic adenovirus armed with interleukin-4. Cancer Res *67*, 6872–6881.

Preston, C. M. (2000). Repression of viral transcription during herpes simplex virus latency. J Gen Virol *81*, 1–19.

Pyles, R. B., Warnick, R. E., Chalk, C. L., Szanti, B. E., and Parysek, L. M. (1997). A novel multiply-mutated HSV-1 strain for the treatment of human brain tumors. Hum Gene Ther *8*, 533–544.

Quinlan, M. P., Chen, L. B., and Knipe, D. M. (1984). The intranuclear location of a herpes simplex virus DNA-binding protein is determined by the status of viral DNA replication. Cell *36*, 857–868.

Rampling, R., Cruickshank, G., Papanastassiou, V., Nicoll, J., Hadley, D., Brennan, D., Petty, R., MacLean, A., Harland, J., McKie, E., *et al.* (2000). Toxicity evaluation of replication-competent herpes simplex virus (ICP 34.5 null mutant 1716) in patients with recurrent malignant glioma. Gene Ther *7*, 859–866.

Roizman, B., and Sears, A. E., eds. (1996). Herpes simplex viruses and their replication, (Philadelphia, PA: Lippincott-Raven Publishers).

Roop, C., Hutchinson, L., and Johnson, D. C. (1993). A mutant herpes simplex virus type 1 unable to express glycoprotein L cannot enter cells, and its particles lack glycoprotein H. J Virol *67*, 2285–2297.

Russell, J., Stow, N. D., Stow, E. C., and Preston, C. M. (1987). Herpes simplex virus genes involved in latency in vitro. J Gen Virol *68 (Pt 12)*, 3009–3018.

Samaniego, L. A., Neiderhiser, L., and DeLuca, N. A. (1998). Persistence and expression of the herpes simplex virus genome in the absence of immediate-early proteins. J Virol *72*, 3307–3320.

Samaniego, L. A., Wu, N., and DeLuca, N. A. (1997). The herpes simplex virus immediate-early protein ICP0 affects transcription from the viral genome and infected-cell survival in the absence of ICP4 and ICP27. J Virol *71*, 4614–4625.

Samoto, K., Ehtesham, M., Perng, G. C., Hashizume, K., Wechsler, S. L., Nesburn, A. B., Black, K. L., and Yu, J. S. (2002). A herpes simplex virus type 1 mutant with gamma 34.5 and LAT deletions effectively oncolyses human U87 glioblastomas in nude mice. Neurosurgery *50*, 599–605; discussion 605–596.

Sanfilippo, C. M., and Blaho, J. A. (2006). ICP0 gene expression is a herpes simplex virus type 1 apoptotic trigger. J Virol *80*, 6810–6821.

Shieh, M. T., WuDunn, D., Montgomery, R. I., Esko, J. D., and Spear, P. G. (1992). Cell surface receptors for herpes simplex virus are heparan sulfate proteoglycans. J Cell Biol *116*, 1273–1281.

Singh, S. K., Hawkins, C., Clarke, I. D., Squire, J. A., Bayani, J., Hide, T., Henkelman, R. M., Cusimano, M. D., and Dirks, P. B. (2004). Identification of human brain tumour initiating cells. Nature *432*, 396–401.

Spear, P. G. (1993). Entry of alphaherpesviruses into cells. Semin Virol *4*, 167–180.

Spencer, D. M. (2000). Developments in suicide genes for preclinical and clinical applications. Curr Opin Mol Ther *2*, 433–440.

Spivack, J. G., and Fraser, N. W. (1987). Detection of herpes simplex virus type 1 transcripts during latent infection in mice. J Virol *61*, 3841–3847.

Stevens, J. G., Wagner, E. K., Devi-Rao, G. B., Cook, M. L., and Feldman, L. T. (1987). RNA complementary to a herpesvirus alpha gene mRNA is prominent in latently infected neurons. Science *235*, 1056–1059.

Strasser, J. F., Fung, L. K., Eller, S., Grossman, S. A., and Saltzman, W. M. (1995). Distribution of 1,3-bis(2-chloroethyl)-1-nitrosourea and tracers in the rabbit brain after interstitial delivery by biodegradable polymer implants. J Pharmacol Exp Ther *275*, 1647–1655.

Stupp, R., Mason, W. P., van den Bent, M. J., Weller, M., Fisher, B., Taphoorn, M. J., Belanger, K., Brandes, A. A., Marosi, C., Bogdahn, U., et al. (2005). Radiotherapy plus concomitant and adjuvant temozolomide for glioblastoma. N Engl J Med *352*, 987–996.

Sundaresan, P., Hunter, W. D., Martuza, R. L., and Rabkin, S. D. (2000). Attenuated, replication-competent herpes simplex virus type 1 mutant G207: safety evaluation in mice. J Virol *74*, 3832–3841.

Taylor, T. J., and Knipe, D. M. (2004). Proteomics of herpes simplex virus replication compartments: association of cellular DNA replication, repair, recombination, and chromatin remodeling proteins with ICP8. J Virol *78*, 5856–5866.

Toda, M., Martuza, R. L., Kojima, H., and Rabkin, S. D. (1998). In situ cancer vaccination: an IL-12 defective vector/replication-competent herpes simplex virus combination induces local and systemic antitumor activity. J Immunol *160*, 4457–4464.

Toda, M., Martuza, R. L., and Rabkin, S. D. (2000). Tumor growth inhibition by intratumoral inoculation of defective herpes simplex virus vectors expressing granulocyte-macrophage colony-stimulating factor. Mol Ther *2*, 324–329.

Toda, M., Martuza, R. L., and Rabkin, S. D. (2001). Combination suicide/cytokine gene therapy as adjuvants to a defective herpes simplex virus-based cancer vaccine. Gene Ther *8*, 332–339.

Todo, T., Martuza, R. L., Rabkin, S. D., and Johnson, P. A. (2001). Oncolytic herpes simplex virus vector with enhanced MHC class I presentation and tumor cell killing. Proc Natl Acad Sci U S A *98*, 6396–6401.

Triezenberg, S. J., Kingsbury, R. C., and McKnight, S. L. (1988a). Functional dissection of VP16, the trans-activator of herpes simplex virus immediate early gene expression. Genes Dev *2*, 718–729.

Triezenberg, S. J., LaMarco, K. L., and McKnight, S. L. (1988b). Evidence of DNA: protein interactions that mediate HSV-1 immediate early gene activation by VP16. Genes Dev *2*, 730–742.

Villarreal, E. C. (2003). Current and potential therapies for the treatment of herpes-virus infections. Prog Drug Res *60*, 263–307.

Voges, J., Reszka, R., Gossmann, A., Dittmar, C., Richter, R., Garlip, G., Kracht, L., Coenen, H. H., Sturm, V., Wienhard, K., *et al.* (2003). Imaging-guided convection-enhanced delivery and gene therapy of glioblastoma. Ann Neurol *54*, 479–487.

Wakimoto, H., Fulci, G., Tyminski, E., and Chiocca, E. A. (2004). Altered expression of antiviral cytokine mRNAs associated with cyclophosphamide's enhancement of viral oncolysis. Gene Ther *11*, 214–223.

Wakimoto, H., Johnson, P. R., Knipe, D. M., and Chiocca, E. A. (2003). Effects of innate immunity on herpes simplex virus and its ability to kill tumor cells. Gene Ther *10*, 983–990.

Wang, Q., Guo, J., and Jia, W. (1997). Intracerebral recombinant HSV-1 vector does not reactivate latent HSV-1. Gene Ther *4*, 1300–1304.

Weaver, M., and Laske, D. W. (2003). Transferrin receptor ligand-targeted toxin conjugate (Tf-CRM107) for therapy of malignant gliomas. J Neurooncol *65*, 3–13.

Weichselbaum, R. R., Kufe, D. W., Hellman, S., Rasmussen, H. S., King, C. R., Fischer, P. H., and Mauceri, H. J. (2002). Radiation-induced tumour necrosis factor-alpha expression: clinical application of transcriptional and physical targeting of gene therapy. Lancet Oncol *3*, 665–671.

Weingart, J., Strauss, L. C., and Grossman, S. A. (2002). Phase I/II study: intra-tumoral infusion of IL13-pE38QQR cytotoxin for recurrent supratentorial malignant glioma. Neuro-oncol *4*, 379 (Abstract).

Weir, J. P. (2001). Regulation of herpes simplex virus gene expression. Gene *271*, 117–130.

Weller, S. K. e. (1995). Herpes simplex virus DNA replication and genome maturation, (Washington, D.C.: ASM Press).

Whitley, R. J., and Roizman, B. (2001). Herpes simplex virus infections. Lancet *357*, 1513–1518.

Wilcock, D., and Lane, D. P. (1991). Localization of p53, retinoblastoma and host replication proteins at sites of viral replication in herpes-infected cells. Nature *349*, 429–431.

Wilkinson, D. E., and Weller, S. K. (2004). Recruitment of cellular recombination and repair proteins to sites of herpes simplex virus type 1 DNA replication is dependent on the composition of viral proteins within prereplicative sites and correlates with the induction of the DNA damage response. J Virol *78*, 4783–4796.

Wu, J. K., Cano, W. G., Meylaerts, S. A., Qi, P., Vrionis, F., and Cherington, V. (1994). Bystander tumoricidal effect in the treatment of experimental brain tumors. Neurosurgery *35*, 1094–1102; discussion 1102–1093.

Wu, N., Watkins, S. C., Schaffer, P. A., and DeLuca, N. A. (1996). Prolonged gene expression and cell survival after infection by a herpes simplex virus mutant defective in the immediate-early genes encoding ICP4, ICP27, and ICP22. J Virol *70*, 6358–6369.

WuDunn, D., and Spear, P. G. (1989). Initial interaction of herpes simplex virus with cells is binding to heparan sulfate. J Virol *63*, 52–58.

Yamini, B., Yu, X., Pytel, P., Galanopoulos, N., Rawlani, V., Veerapong, J., Bickenbach, K., and Weichselbaum, R. R. (2007). Adenovirally delivered tumor necrosis factor-alpha improves the antiglioma efficacy of concomitant radiation and temozolomide therapy. Clin Cancer Res *13*, 6217–6223.

Zachos, G., Clements, B., and Conner, J. (1999). Herpes simplex virus type 1 infection stimulates p38/c-Jun N-terminal mitogen-activated protein kinase pathways and activates transcription factor AP-1. J Biol Chem *274*, 5097–5103.

Zachos, G., Koffa, M., Preston, C. M., Clements, J. B., and Conner, J. (2001). Herpes simplex virus type 1 blocks the apoptotic host cell defense mechanisms that target Bcl-2 and manipulates activation of p38 mitogen-activated protein kinase to improve viral replication. J Virol *75*, 2710–2728.

Zhou, G., and Roizman, B. (2005). Characterization of a recombinant herpes simplex virus 1 designed to enter cells via the IL13Ralpha2 receptor of malignant glioma cells. J Virol *79*, 5272–5277.

Zhou, G., Ye, G. J., Debinski, W., and Roizman, B. (2002). Engineered herpes simplex virus 1 is dependent on IL13Ralpha 2 receptor for cell entry and independent of glycoprotein D receptor interaction. Proc Natl Acad Sci U S A *99*, 15124–15129.

Chapter 47
The Development of Targeted Cancer Gene-Therapy Adenoviruses for High-Grade Glioma Treatment

Dawn E. Post and Erwin G. Van Meir

Abstract The replication cycle of many viruses kills the host cell, and this property is an attractive feature for the development of anticancer viral therapy. The challenge resides in modifying the viral genome so that it will direct the formation of viral particles that can preferentially replicate in and destroy tumor cells while sparing normal tissue. In this review, we will discuss the different strategies that have been developed to engineer cancer-targeted adenoviruses, both replication-deficient gene-therapy vectors and replication-competent oncolytic vectors. Their specific application to the targeting of malignant gliomas in preclinical studies and the results of the first eight clinical trials are presented. Lastly, new ongoing developments in the design, imaging, and replication potency of new generations of therapeutic viruses are discussed.

Contents

D.E. Post (✉)
Department of Neurosurgery and Microbiology & Immunology,
State University of New York Upstate Medical University, 750 East Adams St,
IHP Bldg., Rm 4117, Syracuse, NY 13210, USA
e-mail: postd@upstate.edu

E.G. Van Meir (ed.), *CNS Cancer*, Cancer Drug Discovery
and Development, DOI 10.1007/978-1-60327-553-8_47,

© Humana Press, a part of Springer Science+Business Media, LLC 2009

47.1 Historic Background

The adenovirus (Ad) is currently being evaluated as a cancer therapy agent for a wide variety of tumor types, including brain tumors. Shortly after its isolation in the 1950s, it was demonstrated that the Ad has in vitro oncolytic activity and induces a relatively mild pathogenesis of limited duration in normal healthy subjects (Kelly and Russell 2007, Sinkovics and Horvath 1993). Based on these findings, the testing of this virus as an oncolytic agent in cancer patients rapidly ensued. In an initial study, 30 patients with cervical cancer were administered an Ad preparation of unknown titer directly into the tumor mass, intra-arterially, or intravenously (Huebner et al. 1956). While this clinical study was crude compared to modern standards, it provided the first evidence that direct inoculation of cancer patients with an Ad is safe and leads to destruction of tumor tissue. However, a major drawback to the use of a wild-type Ad for anticancer therapy is its lack of tumor specificity and therefore the potential for toxicity to normal tissue. Overcoming this limitation required increased knowledge of the molecular biology of the Ad replication cycle and the advent of sophisticated recombinant DNA technologies for the direct modification of the Ad genome. This led to a number of strategies to improve its tumor specificity and the ability to introduce into the viral genome adjuvant therapeutic genes that have antitumor activity. Ads that have been developed by genetic engineering can be grouped into two categories: replication-deficient and conditionally replication-competent Ads. This chapter summarizes the development of genetically modified replication-deficient and conditionally replication-competent Ads for cancer therapy and their clinical trial testing in patients with malignant glioma. Current obstacles that must be addressed to improve the therapeutic benefit of these viruses in cancer patients will also be discussed.

47.2 The Ad as a Cancer Therapy Agent

The Ad family contains over 45 serotypes that infect humans and cause a variety of illnesses affecting the eye, respiratory and gastrointestinal tracts [reviewed in (Flint et al., 2004)]. These viruses are nonenveloped and contain a linear, double-stranded DNA genome that is 36–38 kb in size. The Ad replication cycle is a highly complex sequence of co-ordinated events in which viral proteins activate or repress numerous cellular pathways to ensure efficient viral DNA replication and progeny production. The molecular analysis of viral protein function(s) and their interactions with cellular factors has provided opportunities for the design of genetically engineered Ads for cancer therapy, with serotype 5 being the major subtype used for this purpose (Fig. 47.1).

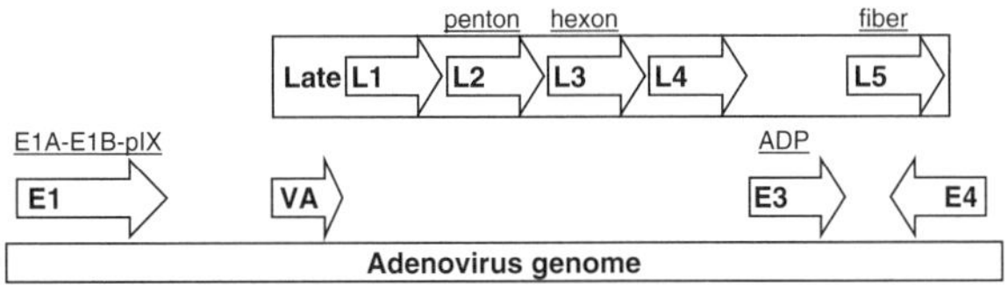

Fig. 47.1 Schematic of adenovirus genome. Regions of the Ad genome pertinent to this chapter are shown (not drawn to scale). Specific Ad genes discussed in this text are underlined and shown above the corresponding gene transcription region. See text for details

47.2.1 Replication-Deficient Ads

All replication-deficient Ads are designed to be viral vectors that deliver gene therapy without the risks associated with viral propagation in the patient. This is achieved through genetically engineering a deletion of the viral *E1* gene region, which contains the essential *E1A* replication gene. These viruses are then further modified to function as adjuvant therapeutic gene delivery vehicles. To accomplish this, a DNA expression cassette containing the gene of interest under the transcriptional control of an exogenous promoter is introduced into the viral genome at the deleted *E1* locus. Infectious viral particles are then produced in Ad packaging cells, which complement *in trans* the E1A protein. These are typically human embryonic neuronal 293 cells, which were immortalized by stably expressing the adenoviral *E1* gene. Deletion of the *E1* gene region provides a cloning capacity up to approximately 3.5 kb in the viral genome. To accommodate larger inserts, the *E1* and *E3* gene regions can be deleted providing a cloning capacity up to 6.2 kb. The *E3* gene region is also an alternative exogenous DNA insertion site.

The antitumor action of replication-deficient Ads is conferred by the gene therapy. There are a large number of potential adjuvant therapeutic candidates that could be utilized for gene therapy of malignant glioma such as genes that (i) inhibit cell growth by modulating intrinsic cell properties, typically the cell cycle, senescence or apoptosis and (ii) genes that exert cell extrinsic effects, triggering a bystander effect. The latter include angiogenesis inhibitors, immune response modulators (immunogene therapy), or suicide genes that work in conjunction with a prodrug system. For the treatment of malignant gliomas, replication-deficient Ads that express the p53 tumor suppressor, interferon beta (INFβ) immune modulator, and herpes simplex virus thymidine kinase (HSV-TK) gene/ganciclovir (GCV) prodrug systems have been generated. In preclinical studies using malignant glioma models, it was demonstrated that transduction of tumor cells with Ad-HSV-TK (Chen et al. 1994, Culver et al. 1992, Vile et al. 1997), Ad-p53 (Kock et al. 1996, Lang et al. 1999, Li et al. 1999), or Ad-INFβ (Qin et al. 1998, 2001) leads to a potent antitumor effect. The therapeutic potential of these replication-deficient viruses was subsequently evaluated in clinical trials in patients with malignant glioma (see Section 47.3).

47.2.2 Tumor-Specific Replication-Competent Ads

Tumor-specific replication-competent Ads (also called oncolytic adenoviruses or conditionally replicating adenoviruses) are distinct from replication-deficient Ads in that viral replication genes are present, viral-replication preferentially occurs in tumor cells, and the cytolytic replication cycle of the virus causes tumor cell death. Two strategies have been used to genetically engineer the replication of the Ad specifically to tumor cells: (i) viral gene mutation/deletion and (ii) transcriptional regulation of viral replication genes (Fig. 47.2 and Color Plate 63). These viruses can be further engineered to deliver gene therapy, thereby increasing their antitumor activity [reviewed in (Chu et al. 2004)].

In the first tumor-targeting approach, Ad genes that are essential for viral replication are mutated or deleted resulting in the absence of the corresponding viral protein function (Fig. 47.2A). The absence of this viral protein leads to an abortive replication cycle in normal cells. In contrast, the mutant virus can selectively replicate in tumor cells because the missing viral protein function is compensated by the presence of tumor-specific genetic alterations. To date, three genetically mutated Ads have been created using this approach. Abrogation of Ad *E1A*, *E1B-55K*, or viral-associated (VA) RNA-coding sequences' function by gene deletion or mutation leads to conditional replication of the mutated Ad in tumor cells that contain a dysregulated retinoblastoma (Rb), p53, or Ras pathway, respectively [reviewed in (Chu et al. 2004)]. However, further analysis of the Ad E1B-55K mutant would reveal that this tumor-targeting approach is more complicated than initially expected. The Ad E1B-55K protein has a dual role in the Ad replication cycle: (i) bind and inactivate p53, thereby circumventing a p53-dependent antiviral apoptotic response and (ii) nuclear export of viral transcripts. Initial preclinical studies with the E1B-55K mutant Ad (*dl*1520, also known as ONYX-015) suggested that replication of this virus was targeted to tumor cells lacking p53 function (Bischoff et al. 1996). Further studies would reveal that the tumor selectivity of *dl*1520 is determined by the ability of tumor cells to compensate for the late viral RNA export function of E1B-55K, rather than p53 inactivation (O'Shea et al. 2004).

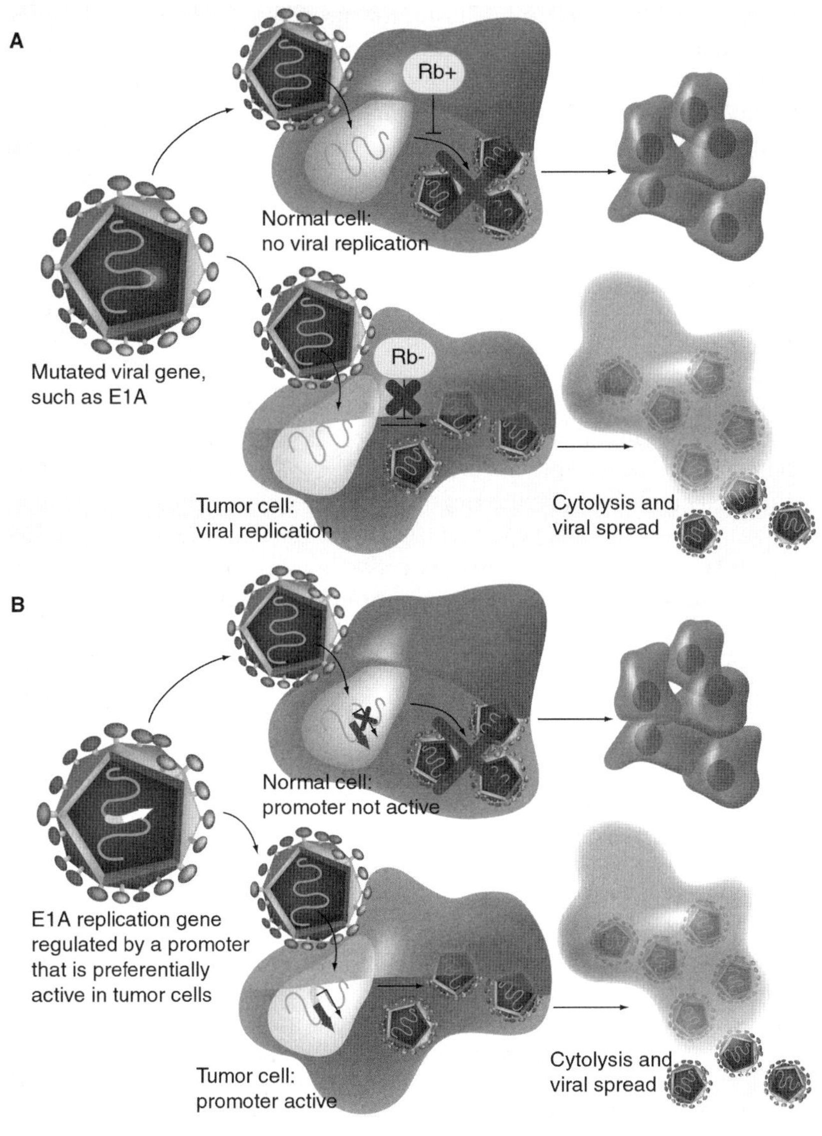

Fig. 47.2 Strategies used to target Ad replication specifically to tumor cells. (**A**) Targeting Ad replication to tumor cells by viral gene mutation. Specific mutations within the Ad *E1A*, *E1B*, or viral-associated RNA-coding sequences that abrogate protein function have been shown to result in the selective replication of the mutant Ad in tumor cells that contain dysfunctional pRb, p53, or Ras pathways, respectively. In the example shown here, a small deletion in conserved region 2 (CR-2) of *E1A* abrogates its interaction with the pRb family of proteins. While this E1A-mutant Ad can infect both normal (pRb-functional) and tumor (pRb-deficient) cells, its replication is restricted to cells with a dysregulated Rb pathway. After lysis of permissive host cells, viral progeny infect nearby tumor cells, thereby propagating the viral infection and host cell lysis cycle throughout the tumor mass. In contrast, normal cells do not support replication of the *E1A* mutant Ad. (**B**) Targeting Ad replication to tumor cells by

Regardless, *dl*1520 demonstrates antitumor specificity. In clinical trial testing in cancer patients, *dl*1520 demonstrated overall safety and modest antitumor efficacy following diverse delivery routes and in combination with several chemotherapy drugs (Post et al. 2005). Importantly, a similar E1B-55K-deleted Ad (H101) was recently approved for cancer treatment in China (Garber 2006).

In the second tumor-targeting approach, Ad genes that are essential for viral replication (*E1A* and *E4*) are placed under the transcriptional regulation of promoters that are predominantly active in tumor cells relative to normal cells [Fig. 47.2B, reviewed in (Chu et al. 2004)]. For this, tissue-specific promoters have been used to target Ad replication to one tumor type such as brain, breast, prostate, liver, melanoma, lung, colon, neuroblastoma, and ovarian cancer. Alternatively, to target viral replication to a broad range of tumor types, promoters that are responsive to tetracycline, telomerase reverse transcriptase (TERT), hypoxia-inducible factor (HIF), or E2F-1 have been utilized.

There are a large number of tumor-specific replication-competent Ads that are potential candidates for the treatment of malignant glioma. This includes the Ads that contain viral gene mutations/deletions and the transcriptionally regulated Ads with promoters that are active in a broad range of tumor types. The tissue-specific glial fibrillary acidic protein (GFAP) promoter has been used to generate a glioma-specific oncolytic Ad (Horst et al. 2007). This virus demonstrated specificity for GFAP-positive, but not GFAP-negative, tumor cells. However, its potential toxicity to normal glial tissue which is GFAP positive was not experimentally addressed. Infection of these permissive cells is expected to result in viral replication and death of the normal cells. Additionally, the identification of promoters that are active in cancer stem cells, such as CD133-positive brain tumor stem cells, will enable the development of oncolytic Ads for the specific killing of this clinically important tumor cell population (Singh et al. 2004, Bauerschmitz et al. 2008). Of significance is the finding that CD133-positive brain tumor stem cells are susceptible to Ad infection due to high levels of Ad cell surface receptors (Jiang et al. 2007). Moreover, infection of these cells with an oncolytic Ad that is active in cells with a defective Rb pathway (delta-24-RGD) leads to efficient viral replication and oncolysis (Jiang et al. 2007). This demonstrates the potential clinical application of oncolytic Ads for the specific killing of brain tumor stem cells. To date, only the E1B-55K-deleted Ad has undergone phase I clinical trial testing in malignant glioma patients (see Section 47.3.4).

Fig. 47.2 (continued) transcriptional regulation of viral replication genes. The Ad *E1A* gene (*gray arrow*) encodes a protein that is essential for viral replication and its absence leads to a replication-deficient virus. Transcriptional regulation of *E1A* by a promoter (*dashed rectangle*) that is preferentially overactive in tumor cells will result in tumor-selective Ad replication. The use of a promoter that is not active in normal cells will result in an inability of the virus to express E1A and replicate in these cells. Figure reproduced from Future Oncology (2005) 1(2), 1–12 with permission from Future Medicine Ltd (Post et al. 2005) (*see* Color Plate 63)

The antitumor efficacy of tumor-specific replication-competent Ads is dependent on their ability to kill infected tumor cells and spread to nearby tumor cells at high efficiency. However, the mechanism underlying how adenovirus induces host cell lysis is currently unknown and available data are contradictory. The adenovirus death protein (ADP) located in the *E3* gene region appears to play a role in host cell lysis and viral egress at the completion of the viral replicative cycle by an unknown mechanism (Lichtenstein et al. 2004). Caspase-dependent (apoptosis) and caspase-independent cell death pathways appear to play a role in ADP-mediated host cell death (Zou et al. 2004). This contrasts with studies showing that classical apoptosis does not occur during a productive Ad infection (Baird et al. 2008, Ito et al. 2006). The autophagy pathway has been implicated to mediate caspase-independent cell death by Ads (Alonso et al. 2008, Jiang et al. 2007, Ito et al. 2006). However, another study indicates that the autophagy pathway functions as a cell survival, rather than cell death, response during the Ad replication cycle (Baird et al. 2008). These contradictions may be due to the dual role of the autophagy pathway in cell survival and cell death and its ability to directly interact with the classical apoptosis pathway (Thorburn 2008). Additionally, the tumor cell lines used in these studies may contain genetic alterations within the autophagy and apoptosis pathways, making it difficult to interpret the relative contribution of each. Therefore, future studies should include a series of normal cell lines and inhibitors that are specific for each pathway. In conclusion, a more thorough understanding of the mechanisms underlying Ad-mediated cytolysis may stimulate the development of strategies to increase the oncolytic potential of this virus.

47.2.3 Advantages and Disadvantages of Using the Ad as a Cancer Therapy Agent

The Ad offers several advantages for the purpose of cancer therapy, including (1) a high transduction efficiency of a wide range of cell types, (2) infects both proliferating and quiescent cells, (3) genetic modification of viral capsid proteins enables retargeted infection to tumor cells and reduced infection of normal cells, (4) can be easily modified to express transgenes, (5) can be manufactured to high viral titers (10^{10}–10^{13} plaque-forming units/ml) for clinical applications, (6) episomal viral genome location circumvents problems of integration into cellular genome, (7) genetically stable following the introduction of various transgenes and/or genetic modification of viral genes, (8) infection leads to tolerable clinical symptoms, and (9) its cytolytic replication cycle can be conditionally targeted to tumor cells thereby minimizing toxicity to normal cells.

These benefits must be balanced with some disadvantages of the Ad such as (1) systemic intravenous delivery to tumors is inefficient due to rapid liver-mediated clearance, (2) lack of a specific anti-Ad drug to inhibit viral replication, and (3) the induction of an inflammatory response following virus administration. The latter drawback is a serious safety concern that was realized following the death of a patient on a gene-therapy clinical trial (Marshall 1999). This patient received hepatic intra-arterial infusion of 4×10^{13} particles of a replication-deficient adenovirus for the treatment of ornithine transcarbamylase deficiency. Within 4 days of virus administration, the patient suffered a fatal systemic inflammatory response syndrome that was attributable to administration of the Ad vector. The NIH Recombinant DNA Advisory Committee (RAC) reviewed the preclinical and clinical data from this trial and concluded that Ad-based clinical trials should continue with caution (NIH Recombinant DNA Advisory Committee 2002). The committee also proposed a number of recommendations to improve the design and conduct of clinical trials using Ad-based vectors as a means to increase the safety of patients.

47.3 Clinical Trials of Cancer Therapy Ads for Glioma Therapy

There have been eight published clinical trial studies utilizing replication-deficient or tumor-specific conditionally replication-competent Ads in patients with malignant brain tumors (Table 47.1). Seven of the studies used replication-deficient Ads which express HSV-TK, p53, or IFNβ, and one study used a conditionally replication-competent oncolytic Ad (*dl*1520, ONYX-015) which contains a deletion of the E1B-55K viral protein. Clinical trial studies with these cancer therapy Ads have yielded important insights into the safety and effectiveness of this therapeutic strategy for the treatment of malignant brain tumors.

47.3.1 Ad-HSV-TK Clinical Trials

HSV-TK is an enzyme that phosphorylates the nucleoside analog prodrug ganciclovir (GCV) into its triphosphate form, a cytotoxic agent that inhibits DNA synthesis resulting in apoptotic cell death [reviewed in (Eck et al. 1996)]. Gene therapy with HSV-TK also leads to death of non-transduced cells. This "bystander killing effect" is mediated by intercellular movement of GCV triphosphate from transduced to non-transduced cells through gap junctions (Touraine et al. 1998, Elshami et al. 1996), induction of apoptosis (Hamel et al. 1996), and the host immune response (Vile et al. 1997). GCV has been widely used in the clinic as an antiviral drug for CMV infections. Following intravenous administration, GCV is widely distributed to all tissues, including the brain. Its clinical use is associated with several toxic side effects in humans such as neutrophilia, thrombocytopenia, hepatic and renal impairment, fever, rash, headaches, and confusion (Eck et al. 1996).

Table 47.1 Clinical trials of cancer gene-therapy Ads in malignant glioma patients

Virus	Promoter	Tumor (n = patients)	n	Objectives	Virus delivery	Virus dose	Adverse events[a]	NA response	Virus dissemination	References
HSV-TK	RSV	recurrent	13	toxicity MTD	intratumoral	2×10^{9}VP 2×10^{10} VP 2×10^{11} VP 2×10^{12} VP	2	10/12	serum-neg urine-neg nasal-neg	Trask et al. (2000)
HSV-TK	RSV	recurrent	11	toxicity MTD	resected tumor cavity margin	2.5×10^{11} VP 3.0×10^{11} VP 9.0×10^{11} VP	1	ND	blood-neg urine-neg nasal-neg	Germano et al. (2003)
HSV-TK	Ad major late	recurrent	14	toxicity MTD	resected tumor cavity margin	4.6×10^{8} VP 4.6×10^{9} VP 4.6×10^{10} VP 4.6×10^{11} VP	0	ND	blood-neg urine-neg nasal-neg stool-neg	Smitt et al. (2003)
HSV-TK	CMV	recurrent (4) primary (3)	7	toxicity efficacy	resected tumor cavity margin	3×10^{10} PFU	4	4/7	plasma-neg urine-neg	Sandmair et al. (2000)
HSV-TK	CMV	recurrent (12) primary (24)	36	toxicity efficacy (randomized)	resected tumor cavity margin	3×10^{10} PFU	5	6/17	plasma-pos (n = 2/17)	Immonen et al. (2004)
p53	CMV	recurrent	15	toxicity MTD molecular endpoints	intratumoral followed by resected tumor cavity margin	3×10^{10} VP 3×10^{11} VP 1×10^{12} VP 3×10^{12} VP	45	10/12	plasma-neg urine-neg sputum-neg rectal-neg	Lang et al. (2003)

Table 47.1 (continued)

Virus	Promoter	Tumor (n = patients)	n	Objectives	Virus delivery	Virus dose	Adverse events[a]	NA response	Virus dissemination	References
IFNβ	CMV	recurrent	11	toxicity MTD molecular endpoints	intratumoral followed by resected tumor cavity margin	2×10^{10} VP 6×10^{10} VP 2×10^{11} VP	1	5/11	blood-pos (n = 2/11) nasal-pos (n = 5/11) CSF-pos (n = 2/2)	Chiocca et al. (2008)
ONYX-015 (E1B mutant)	NA	recurrent	24	toxicity MTD efficacy	resected tumor cavity margin	1×10^{7} PFU 1×10^{8} PFU 1×10^{9} PFU 1×10^{10} PFU	0	2/24	ND	Chiocca et al. (2004)

Abbreviations: n: number of patients; NA: neutralizing antibody; RSV: rous sarcoma virus; CMV: cytomegalovirus; VP: virus particle; ND: not determined; MTD: maximum tolerated dose; pos: positive; neg: negative

[a]Number of adverse events judged as related or possibly related to the virus treatment are listed.

The safety and maximum tolerated dose (MTD) of Ad-HSV-TK/GCV therapy in patients with recurrent malignant glioma was initially evaluated following a single intratumoral virus injection (Trask et al. 2000). The starting viral dose was 2×10^9 virus particles (VP) and was increased by one-log increments to 2×10^{12} VP. The treatment was safely tolerated in the 2×10^8 to 2×10^{11} VP groups with no adverse events attributable to the gene therapy. Treatment with 2×10^{12} VP led to toxicities of confusion, hyponatremia, and seizures in two patients that were related to the virus/GCV treatment. In one of these patients, the adverse event was possibly due to virus entry into the CSF by unintentional intraventricular injection. The dose level for the subsequent four patients was reduced to 2×10^{11} VP with no adverse events attributable to the gene therapy. Two subsequent clinical trials evaluated the safety and MTD of Ad-HSV-TK/GCV therapy following virus injection into the resected tumor cavity margins (Germano et al. 2003, Smitt et al. 2003). The ranges of virus doses used in these studies were 2.5×10^{11} to 9.0×10^{11} VP and 4.6×10^8 to 4.6×10^{11} VP, respectively. In the 25 treated patients, one adverse event of status epilepticus occurred following administration of 2.5×10^{11} VP that was possibly related to the gene therapy (Germano et al. 2003). All other adverse events were judged as not related to the gene-therapy virus. Thus, these studies established an MTD of 2×10^{11} VP for intratumoral Ad-HSV-TK/GCV therapy, while an MTD for virus administration into the resected tumor cavity margins was not reached.

There were two clinical trials published by the same group that evaluated efficacy as well as toxicity of Ad-HSV-TK/GCV therapy in patients with primary and recurrent malignant glioma (Sandmair et al. 2000, Immonen et al. 2004). In both studies, 3×10^{10} plaque-forming units (pfu) of virus were injected into the resected tumor cavity margin. In study 1, two patients who had epileptic seizures prior to the gene therapy experienced an increased frequency of seizures following virus administration (Sandmair et al. 2000). Additionally, two patients experienced a short-term fever reaction following Ad-HSV-TK delivery that correlated with opening of the ventricular system during surgery. Of the seven treated patients in study 1, three showed evidence of stable disease by MRI at 3-months post-treatment. The survival time of these patients was 8 (recurrent), 20 (recurrent), and 21 (primary) months. These data were encouraging and led to a second study in which 36 patients with primary or recurrent malignant glioma were randomized to receive tumor debulking followed by Ad-HSV-TK/GCV therapy or standard of care consisting of tumor debulking followed by radiotherapy in those patients with primary tumors (Immonen et al. 2004). Overall, Ad-HSV-TK/GCV therapy was well tolerated and no significant safety issues arose. Three patients developed a transient elevation of liver enzymes starting 5–7 days after GCV treatment. Additionally, two patients developed localized intracerebral edema during GCV treatment, one with an associated hemiparesis, which required additional surgery. In this study, survival was measured as the date of surgery/gene-therapy administration to death or surgery for recurrence. It was found that AdHSV-TK/GCV treatment led to a mean survival of 70.6 ± 52.9 (SD) weeks which was significant, greater than the mean survival of the standard of care group [39 ± 19.7 (SD), $p = 0.0095$]. These data are promising and will need to be further investigated in a randomized efficacy study using a larger study group.

47.3.2 Ad-p53 Clinical Trial

The p53 tumor suppressor is a transcription factor that regulates the cell cycle and apoptosis pathways in response to cellular stress or DNA damage (Vousden and Lu 2002). Consistent with its central role as "guardian of the genome," p53 is frequently inactivated in human gliomas by a variety of mechanisms (see Chapter 14). Thus it was logical to evaluate whether reintroduction of p53 using a virus-based gene-therapy approach would be beneficial for the treatment of malignant gliomas. The replication-deficient Ad-p53 was intratumorally injected at increasing doses via catheter into 15 patients with recurrent malignant glioma (Lang et al. 2003). Three days later the tumor was removed and additional virus was injected into the resected tumor cavity margins. This two-stage study design allowed for biological endpoint analysis and evaluation of clinical toxicity. Comparative analysis of pretreatment vs. posttreatment tumor specimens indicated that Ad-p53 treatment led to the expression of functionally active p53 protein in the tumor. This was based on nuclear and cytoplasmic p53 expression, induction of the p53 transcriptional target $p21^{CIP/WAF}$, and induction of apoptosis in the area immediately surrounding the catheter site where p53 expression was high. Disappointingly, the mean distance of Ad-p53-transduced cells from the catheter was 4.9 ± 1.7 mm (range 1–8 mm), and the distance of transduced cells did not expand as the viral dose was increased. The limited intratumoral distribution of Ad-p53 is consistent with a previous study using a replication-deficient Ad that expresses β-galactosidase and a similar viral administration procedure (Puumalainen et al. 1998). The clinical toxicity of Ad-p53 therapy was described as minimal with 45 adverse events possibly or probably/definitely related to the treatment. The most common adverse events potentially attributable to Ad-p53 were headache (53% of patients), fatigue (40%), and fever (27%). Other adverse events related to Ad-p53 treatment included one incident of grade 3 hemiparesis in the 3×10^{11} VP group and grade 2–3 aphasia in two patients in the 1×10^{12} VP group. Three additional patients at the 1×10^{12} VP dose level did not experience significant neurologic toxicity. Thus, a maximum tolerated dose was not defined and additional dose escalation was not possible due to manufacturing and virus storage limitations.

47.3.3 Ad-IFNβ Clinical Trial

The IFNβ cytokine elicits multimodal antitumor effects associated with its antiproliferative, anti-angiogenic, and immunomodulatory activities [reviewed in (Eck et al. 2001, Chiocca et al. 2008)]. However, its clinical use is limited by toxicities of myelosuppression, transaminitis, seizures, and encephalopathy.

To circumvent this issue, a local IFNβ gene-delivery strategy was evaluated using a replication-deficient Ad (Chiocca et al. 2008). Eleven patients with recurrent malignant glioma were intratumorally injected into five sites with Ad-IFNβ at increasing doses by stereotactic needle passes. Eight (cohort 1) or four (cohorts 2 and 3) days later, the tumor was removed and additional virus was injected into the resected tumor cavity margins. Similar to the Ad-p53 trial described above, the two-stage study design allowed for molecular endpoint and clinical toxicity assessment. Biologically active hIFNβ expression from the injected virus was indicated by intratumoral hIFNβ expression, a dose-dependent increase of the IFN-inducible markers neopterin and IL-10, and a dose-dependent induction of intratumoral apoptosis and necrosis. Areas of necrosis were associated with inflammatory infiltrates composed of neutrophils, macrophages, and monocytes. However, it cannot be determined from these studies whether the inflammatory infiltrate is due to a specific hINFβ-mediated response or a generalized innate immune response to the virus. All of the clinical adverse events were judged as unrelated to virus treatment, with one exception. One patient in the highest viral dose group (2×10^{11} VP) experienced a dose limiting toxicity of grade 4 confusion. This event was classified as related to virus treatment and was associated with virus extravasation into the CSF during virus injection into the resected tumor cavity margin. While a maximum tolerated dose was not defined, the authors recommend a dose limit of $<2\times10^{11}$ virus particles for future studies because of potential patient safety and toxicity issues.

47.3.4 *E1B-55K-Deleted Oncolytic Ad (dl1520, ONYX-015) Clinical Trial*

ONYX-015, which lacks E1B-55K expression due to gene-specific mutations, is the first oncolytic Ad that was tested in malignant glioma patients (Chiocca et al. 2004). The toxicity and potential efficacy of ONYX-015 was evaluated in 24 patients with recurrent high-grade glioma following viral administration into the resected tumor cavity margin. The starting viral dose was 1×10^{7} pfu and was increased by one-log increments to 1×10^{10} pfu. All of the clinical adverse events were judged as unrelated to virus treatment. Therefore, this study demonstrated that ONYX-015 therapy was safely tolerated and did not result in clinical or radiologic evidence of neurologic or systemic toxicity when injected into the resected tumor cavity margins at doses up to 10^{10} pfu.

47.3.5 *Clinical Trial Data: Anti-Ad Neutralizing Antibody Levels*

The presence or induction of anti-Ad neutralizing antibodies is a potential issue that may negatively impact the therapeutic efficacy of cancer therapy Ads. The levels of systemic anti-Ad neutralizing antibodies before and after intracranial injection of virus were measured in six of the clinical studies described above (Table 47.1). Forty-five percent (37/83) of assessable patients had an increase in anti-Ad neutralizing antibodies following virus injection. A more detailed timeline of the neutralizing antibody response was evaluated in the Ad-p53 clinical trial (Lang et al. 2003). In this study, antibody titers increased 1–2 weeks after virus injection, reached maximal levels at 1–2 months, and then returned to pretreatment levels by 4–6 months. The impact of anti-Ad neutralizing antibodies on the therapeutic efficacy of the viruses was not discussed in the published reports. Overall, intracerebral injection of Ads appears to result in a lower incidence of a neutralizing antibody response compared to non-CNS viral administration [45% vs. 92–100%, respectively, (Post et al. 2005)]. This may result from the relatively immunocompromised state of malignant glioma patients due to steroid medication, radiation, and chemotherapy and/or the relatively immunoprivileged status of the brain (Chiocca et al. 2004).

47.3.6 Clinical Trial Data: Regional and Systemic Virus Dissemination

Virus dissemination beyond the injection site is a serious concern as it could potentially lead to toxic side effects, as evidenced by the development of serious adverse events in two patients, which was attributable to virus entry into the CSF (Trask et al. 2000, Chiocca et al. 2008). Seven of the clinical trials described above evaluated virus dissemination (Table 47.1). In five studies, virus was not detected in blood, serum, plasma, urine, stool/rectal, sputum, or nasal swab specimens, indicating a lack of systemic virus dissemination. In contrast, viral spread beyond the injection site was detected in plasma, blood, nasal swab, and CSF samples in a subset of patients in two studies. The presence of virus in the plasma and blood was detectable for 2–7 days post-treatment, but not thereafter. The amount of virus in nasal swabs was highly variable between patients and did result in clinical symptoms. The discrepancy in virus dissemination between the clinical studies may be due to differences in sample collection schedules or unintentional injection of the virus into blood vessels or brain ventricles during surgery. Clearly, intracerebral injection of a replication-deficient cancer therapy Ad has the potential to spread into the CSF and systemically.

47.3.7 Clinical Trial Data: Antitumor Efficacy

Evidence of antitumor efficacy was monitored in all of the studies described above. In each study, there were isolated patients who appeared to respond to the viral-mediated gene therapy based on long-term survival compared to historical controls. However, in the majority of cases, this was associated with the presence of one or more favorable prognostic factors for longer survival such as younger age, higher functional status, shorter duration of symptoms, presence of a WHO grade III and not IV glioma, total vs. partial surgical resection, or smaller tumor size. The Ad-HSV-TK study published by Immonen et al. (2004) provides the strongest evidence of antitumor efficacy. However, it must be emphasized that all of these studies are early stage clinical trials with primary objectives of toxicity and MTD assessment and which contain a low number of patients at each viral dose level. The relative safety and low toxicity of the cancer gene therapy and oncolytic Ads tested to date strongly support the continued investigation of these agents as antitumor therapies for malignant glioma patients.

47.4 Future Directions to Improve the Safety and Efficacy of Cancer Gene-Therapy and Oncolytic Ads for Glioma Therapy

Clinical trial studies using replication-deficient and conditionally replication-competent Ads in cancer patients, including those with malignant glioma, have demonstrated the overall safety of this therapeutic approach. However, clinical evidence of antitumor efficacy has been disappointing and there is a discord with preclinical laboratory studies in which viral treatment results in potent antitumor responses including complete tumor regressions. Below we highlight some factors that may explain these findings and avenues being explored to improve the efficacy of cancer therapy Ads in cancer patients without compromising safety.

47.4.1 Preclinical Brain Tumor Models

Currently available preclinical brain tumor models do not faithfully recapitulate the origin, histopathology, biology, or treatment of human malignant brain tumors in the clinical setting (Barth 1998) (see Chapters 1–13). It is also critically important to note that human Ads only replicate at high efficiency in human cells and not most murine cells. This creates a challenge with extrapolating antitumor efficacy and safety obtained with these models to that which may be achieved in a human cancer patient. First, preclinical tumor models utilize homogenous tumor cell lines, whereas the tumor mass in a patient consists of a heterogenous mix of tumor cells. Second, the tumor mass present in a patient is relatively larger compared to the preclinical tumors established in rodents, which oftentimes are a maximum diameter close to the 5-mm diffusion limit observed in human trials. Third, many preclinical models are performed in immunocompromised mice due to xenografting of human tumor cells, which may avoid immune-mediated neutralization of viral replication. Fourth, the limited replication potential afforded by mouse tissues precludes safety testing. Finally, many of the preclinical tumor studies utilize a multiple virus injection protocol that is not feasible in patients.

Cancer therapy Ads have predominantly been evaluated using human glioma xenografts in immunocompromised (athymic *nu*/*nu*, SCID) mice or syngeneic rodent brain tumor models that were originally established by chemical induction (Barth 1998, Szatmari et al. 2006, Fomchenko and Holland 2006). The former model is applicable for the evaluation of both replication-deficient and conditionally replication-competent Ads. However, the use of an immunocompromised animal tumor model is severely limited in that it precludes the evaluation of these viruses in the context of a fully functional host immune response, a setting that more closely emulates the clinical situation. The latter tumor models offer the advantage of an immunocompetent host and are useful for the evaluation of the replication-deficient Ads. At least one of the syngeneic rodent brain tumor models, GL261, appears to support human Ad replication and therefore will be useful for the preclinical evaluation of oncolytic Ads (Ulasov et al. 2007a) (see Chapter 12). Furthermore, some of the cell lines derived from chemically induced models show spontaneous immunogenicity, likely because they were generated on outbred rodents strains (C6 glioma for example) or because the mutation load from the chemical treatment created new epitopes (not formally proven but 9L could be an example) (see Chapter 10). Alternative immunocompetent models are the use of spontaneous brain tumors in genetically engineered mice which are created by germline modification or somatic cell gene transfer (Fomchenko and Holland 2006). The utility of these genetically engineered glioma models for the preclinical testing of cancer therapy Ads has not yet been evaluated. Several non-glioma rodent tumor cell lines that support human Ad replication have recently been identified (Toth et al. 2005, Hallden et al. 2003, Wang et al. 2003, Guo et al. 2006). These syngeneic rodent tumor models are valuable tools that can also be used to assess the antitumor potential of oncolytic Ads in the context of a fully functional host immune response. However, these studies may be restricted to subcutaneous tumor models as it is currently unknown whether any of these non-glioma cell lines can establish a tumor when implanted intracerebrally. The canine J3T glioma model which can be established in immunotolerant allogeneic Beagle dogs is a useful large animal model (Candolfi et al. 2007b, a, Rainov et al. 2000). The substantial cost of this large animal glioma model restricts its use to late-stage preclinical testing (see Chapter 13). Clearly, continued research is needed in the further development and characterization of syngeneic brain tumor models for the preclinical testing of cancer therapy Ads. A better understanding of the Ad replication cycle may also engender transgenic mice that will be competent for Ad replication (Tallone et al. 2001).

It will also be important to develop a set of universal standards for the preclinical testing of replication-deficient and oncolytic Ads for malignant glioma therapy. This should include testing in normal human cells such as astrocytes and in tumor models (specific cell lines, s.c. vs. i.c. tumor implantation), virus injection schedule, virus injection dose, and the incorporation of appropriate control Ads such as a replication-deficient AdLacZ or AdGFP or a replication-competent wild-type Ad. This will facilitate virus-to-virus comparison and the identification of the most promising cancer therapy Ads for subsequent clinical trial testing.

47.4.2 Improving the Virus Vectors

A number of current cancer therapy Ads contain deficiencies including (i) lack of the Ad *E3* gene region, (ii) lack of the adenovirus death protein (ADP) gene, and (iii) attenuated replication even in permissive tumor cells. As described below, it is essential to develop cancer therapy Ads in which these deficiencies are not present or have been minimized.

A large number of cancer therapy Ads contain a partial or complete deletion of the *E3* gene region which is nonessential for viral replication in cell culture. In many cases, deletion of the *E3* gene region is needed to accommodate the exogenous transgene or promoter DNA insert. The Ad *E3* gene region encodes a set of immunomodulatory proteins which function to counteract the host antiviral immune response (Lichtenstein et al. 2004). Consistent with this, Ads that lack all or part of the *E3* gene region show accelerated virus clearance in vivo in both athymic (*nu*/*nu*) and immunocompetent tumor-bearing mice compared to Ads that retain this gene region (Wang et al. 2003, Suzuki et al. 2002). Another important gene located in the *E3* gene region is *ADP* which plays a role in host cell lysis and viral egress at the completion of the viral replication cycle. Oncolytic Ads that lack *ADP* display a delay in these processes (Lichtenstein et al. 2004). Given the vital in vivo roles of the genes located within the *E3* region, it is important to minimize deletion of this region.

Another potential concern that is specific for the oncolytic Ads is the presence of attenuated viral replication. It is important that the replication of these tumor-specific viruses is similar to or greater than a wild-type Ad to ensure a maximal oncolytic response. At least two oncolytic Ads have been identified that exhibit attenuated replication relative to a wild-type Ad. One contains a deletion of the *E1B-55K* gene (Bischoff et al. 1996, Rothmann et al. 1998, Goodrum and Ornelles 1998) and the other contains a hypoxia-inducible promoter to regulate expression of the Ad *E1A* replication gene (Post et al. 2007). A large number of oncolytic Ad studies do not include a wild-type Ad for comparison. Therefore, it is difficult to determine how widespread the issue of attenuated replication is and to identify causative factors, such as the use of a particular Ad backbone vector. The issue of attenuated viral replication needs to be carefully evaluated prior to clinical trial testing as it directly impacts the antitumor potency of these viruses.

Finally, it will be important to exploit scientific advances for the design of new cancer gene-therapy and oncolytic Ads. For example, recent advances have uncovered the critical role played by microRNAs in many aspects of biology and have already identified their involvement in cancer development, including brain cancer (see Chapter 27). MicroRNAs are 21–22 base RNA oligonucleotides that bind to and block the translation of mRNAs which have sites in their 3'-untranslated regions (3'-UTR) that are complementary to the microRNA (Ha et al. 1996). It has been demonstrated that expression of certain microRNAs is missing in tumor cells (for example let-7), while being active in surrounding normal tissues. This has led some investigators to design virotherapy that would be specifically active in the tumor cells. In one approach, replication-deficient viruses carry a transgene engineered to contain an artificial 3'-UTR-containing complementary sites for that microRNA. As a result, the transgene will be expressed in tumor cells but not in normal tissue (Brown et al. 2007b, a, c). The same concept can be used to control the expression of a gene necessary for viral replication, thus generating a miRNA-dependent conditional replicative oncolytic virus, the proof of concept which was recently demonstrated in a vesicular stomatitis virus (Edge et al. 2008). This new concept has not yet been applied in the design of an oncolytic adenoviruses adapted for exclusive replication in tumors expressing certain microRNAs.

47.4.3 Improving Virus Delivery, Intratumoral Dispersion, and Transduction of Tumor Cells

Clinical trial studies have revealed the severely restricted distribution of cancer therapy Ads following intracranial administration (Puumalainen et al. 1998, Lang et al. 2003). One strategy to improve virus distribution is the use of convection enhanced delivery (CED), which is virus infusion under high pressure using intracranial catheters (ter Horst et al. 2006, Oh et al. 2007, Chen et al. 2005). While promising, the use of CED for intracranial drug delivery in the clinic requires further optimization and validation (Sampson et al. 2008). Factors that will need to be addressed are virus stability during the infusion process and entry of the virus into the CSF. The latter is an important toxicity and patient safety issue given the results of the clinical studies described above. An alternative approach that is in the early stages of investigation is the use of mesenchymal stem cells to deliver oncolytic Ads to intracranial tumors (Sonabend et al. 2008). A third strategy to improve virus delivery as well as intratumoral dispersion of oncolytic Ads following in situ viral replication is to degrade extracellular matrix components using proteolytic enzymes such as trypsin, collagenase, hyaluronidase, or relaxin (Kuriyama et al. 2001, Ganesh et al. 2008, 2007).

The success of cancer therapy Ads for anti-glioma therapy is critically dependent on the ability of these viruses to efficiently and specifically infect tumor cells. Ad infection of permissive cells is a rapid process ($\approx$ 30 min) that occurs by receptor-mediated endocytosis (Flint et al., 2004). Cell surface binding of Ad serotype 5 occurs by direct interaction between the viral fiber capsid protein and the cellular coxsackie-adenovirus receptor (CAR). Subsequent internalization of the virus by endocytosis results from the interaction of the viral penton capsid protein with the cellular integrin $\alpha_v\beta_3$ and $\alpha_v\beta_5$ receptors. There are two potential issues regarding virus infection during Ad-based therapy of malignant brain tumors. First, the expression of CAR by numerous normal cell types within the brain may result in sequestration of the virus by non-neoplastic cells and clinical toxicity (Fueyo et al. 2003, Persson et al. 2007, 2006). Second, CAR expression in human gliomas is highly variable, with tumor cells expressing negligible to high levels of the receptor (Fueyo et al. 2003, Fuxe et al. 2003, Miller et al. 1998). It is anticipated that CAR-negative glioma cells would be resistant to the Ad-based cancer therapy. One possible explanation for the reduced expression of CAR in malignant gliomas is its ability to function as a tumor suppressor (Kim et al. 2003). These issues are not unique to the treatment of gliomas but appear more universal (Post et al. 2003). To overcome these potential issues, a large number of genetically engineered Ads that contain modified capsid proteins have been created as a strategy to decrease infection of normal cells, reduce viral clearance by Kupffer cells of the liver, and increase transduction of tumor cells [reviewed in (Glasgow et al. 2004)]. Capsid modifications that have been evaluated include fiber pseudotyping (genetic replacement of the entire fiber or knob domain with its structural counterpart from another serotype) and incorporation of targeting ligands in the fiber, hexon, and pIX capsid proteins. Numerous proof-of-principle studies have demonstrated that various capsid modifications lead to improved transduction of tumor cells in vitro and in vivo, including glioma tumor models. Importantly, further evidence that these Ad capsid modifications translate into augmented antitumor activity against glioma xenografts has also been demonstrated (Ulasov et al. 2007b, Hoffmann et al. 2007, Fueyo et al. 2003, Shinoura et al. 1999). To facilitate identification of tumor-specific targeting ligands, Miura et al. (2007) created a library of Ads that display random peptides on the fiber knob domain. This library was then screened against a low-CAR expressing glioma cell line. From this, a targeting peptide that mediated high infectivity was identified (Miura et al. 2007). These studies have the potential to identify a large repertoire of peptides fitting in the capsid that can be tailored to the compendium of cell surface molecules present on tumor cells but not normal tissue. A further extension of these studies forecasts the development of personalized viruses that will be tailored to the cell surface of the patient's specific tumors. These studies are promising and warrant continued development of capsid-modified cancer therapy Ads toward clinical trial testing.

47.4.4 Local and Systemic Host Immune Response

The role of the host immune response following cancer therapy Ad treatment is largely unknown, especially in the context of the relatively immunosuppressed state of the brain tumor microenvironment (Stanford et al. 2008, Weller and Fontana 1995). Clearance of the injected virus by innate and adaptive antiviral immune responses may limit the time during which the virus can elicit an antitumor effect (Wang et al. 2003). On the other hand, stimulation of a local inflammatory response following virus treatment, either by the virus vector or by the expression of immunomodulatory transgenes, may lead to the development of an antitumor response (Lee et al. 2006, Hu et al. 2007). Importantly, the induction of an inflammatory response in the brain will need to be weighed against the potential toxicity to normal brain tissue, especially neurons (Zipp and Aktas 2006). These issues will need to be first addressed preclinically, using syngeneic, immunocompetent rodent brain tumor models, and then clinically, by the addition of biological endpoint analysis in the study design.

47.4.5 Tracking Viral Replication in the Patient

An important area of investigation for the successful use of adenovirotherapy in patients will be the development of viruses that can be monitored non-invasively through imaging procedures (Raty et al. 2007). Ideally, one would like to be able to track viral replication at the injected site or viral seeding in tissues upon systemic injection and monitor replication at unwanted sites. Furthermore, one may want to monitor the biodistribution and pharmacokinetics of the virus to examine the rate of clearance as well as trapping in the reticuloendothelial system. While in rodent models fluorescence and bioluminescence imaging technologies have been used to track viral spread (Rehemtulla et al. 2002), these techniques are not amenable for use in patients. Magnetic resonance imaging (MRI), single photon emission tomography (SPECT), and positron emission tomography (PET) are the current imaging modalities used for viral tracking in patients.

The detection of viruses by MRI has been achieved using two different approaches. The first approach necessitates the delivery of contrast agents that will specifically bind to viral particles, infected cells, or be activated by virally encoded enzymes (Allen et al. 2005, Louie et al. 2000). The use of paramagnetic nanoparticles coupled to various ligands specific for virus coat proteins or infected cell surface receptors have been used successfully in rodent models (Raty et al. 2006, Ichikawa et al. 2002). The second more recent approach circumvents the need for a contrast agent by using viruses that are pre-conjugated with paramagnetic lanthanide ions or nanoparticles (Vasalatiy et al. 2008, Perez et al. 2003). Alternatively, the use of virally encoded gene products that will directly augment the magnetic status of infected cells can be used. For example, viral vectors encoding transferrin receptors lead to body iron accumulation in infected cells (Genove et al. 2005, Cohen et al. 2005). More recently, genes derived from bacteria, such as MagA, have been shown to directly confer a magnetic signature, and these could be incorporated in the viral genome (Zurkiya et al. 2008).

A number of radioactive substrates have been developed which can reveal by SPECT or PET the enzymatic activity of specific genes (thymidine kinase and sodium iodide transporter) carried by genetically engineered viruses (Tjuvajev et al. 2002, Min et al. 2003, Buchmann et al. 2007, Barton et al. 2003). While most of these studies have been proof of principle in animal models, the first phase I studies have been completed and demonstrated safety and feasibility in patients (Penuelas et al. 2005, Barton et al. 2008, Dempsey et al. 2006).

47.5 Summary

The potential of cancer therapy Ads for anti-glioma therapy remains high. Clinical trial testing of four cancer therapy Ads in malignant glioma patients has demonstrated the relative safety and low toxicity of these viruses when injected intratumorally or in the resected tumor cavity margin. Additionally, local intracerebral injection of these viruses can, in some cases, lead to regional and/or systemic virus dissemination. For the full antitumor potential of cancer therapy Ads to be realized, it will be necessary to improve the antitumor potency of these viruses, virus delivery, and intratumoral virus dispersion. This will require refinements to the preclinical brain tumor models and the virus vectors. Furthermore, it will be important to gain a better understanding of the complex interactions between the virus and the host immune system within the tumor microenvironment as it may lead to new strategies to increase the antitumor capabilities of these viruses. Given the high cost of clinical trial testing, it will be essential to identify in future preclinical studies those viruses that have the greatest potential of inducing an antitumor response and improving the survival of patients with malignant brain tumors. Moreover, the continued inclusion of biological endpoint analysis in clinical trial studies will provide valuable information about efficacy and also draw attention to issues that need further refinement. The evaluation of the safety and efficacy of these viruses is still in the early stages of investigation, and there is a continued need for further basic research and clinical trial testing.

Acknowledgments DEP received research support from the NIH (grant NS49300), Bayer Schering Pharmaceuticals, and the Department of Neurosurgery at SUNY Upstate Medical University. EGVM received research support from the NIH (grants CA86335, CA87830, and CA116804) and the Brain Tumor Society.

References

Allen, M., Bulte, J.W., Liepold, L., Basu, G., Zywicke, H.A., Frank, J.A., Young, M., and Douglas, T. 2005. Paramagnetic viral nanoparticles as potential high-relaxivity magnetic resonance contrast agents. *Magn Reson Med* 54: 807–812.

Alonso, M.M., Jiang, H., Yokoyama, T., Xu, J., Bekele, N.B., Lang, F.F., Kondo, S., Gomez-Manzano, C., and Fueyo, J. 2008. Delta-24-RGD in combination with RAD001 induces enhanced anti-glioma effect via autophagic cell death. *Mol Ther* 16: 487–493.

Baird, S.K., Aerts, J.L., Eddaoudi, A., Lockley, M., Lemoine, N.R., and McNeish, I.A. 2008. Oncolytic adenoviral mutants induce a novel mode of programmed cell death in ovarian cancer. *Oncogene* 27: 3081–3090.

Barth, R.F. 1998. Rat brain tumor models in experimental neuro-oncology: The 9L, C6, T9, F98, RG2 (D74), RT-2 and CNS-1 gliomas. *J Neurooncol* 36: 91–102.

Barton, K.N., Stricker, H., Brown, S.L., Elshaikh, M., Aref, I., Lu, M., Pegg, J., Zhang, Y., Karvelis, K.C., Siddiqui, F., Kim, J.H., Freytag, S.O., and Movsas, B. 2008. Phase I study of noninvasive imaging of adenovirus-mediated gene expression in the human prostate. *Mol Ther* 16: 1761–1769.

Barton, K.N., Tyson, D., Stricker, H., Lew, Y.S., Heisey, G., Koul, S., de la, Z.A., Yin, F.F., Yan, H., Nagaraja, T.N., Randall, K.A., Jin, G.K., Fenstermacher, J.D., Jhiang, S., Ho, K.J., Freytag, S.O., and Brown, S.L. 2003. GENIS: gene expression of sodium iodide symporter for noninvasive imaging of gene therapy vectors and quantification of gene expression in vivo. *Mol Ther* 8: 508–518.

Bauerschmitz, G.J., Ranki, T., Kangasniemi, L., Ribacka, C., Eriksson, M., Porten, M., Herrmann, I., Ristimaki, A., Virkkunen, P., Tarkkanen, M., Hakkarainen, T., Kanerva, A., Rein, D., Pesonen, S., and Hemminki, A. 2008. Tissue-specific promoters active in CD44 + CD24-/low breast cancer cells. *Cancer Res* 68: 5533–5539.

Bischoff, J.R., Kirn, D.H., Williams, A., Heise, C., Horn, S., Muna, M., Ng, L., Nye, J.A., Sampson-Johannes, A., Fattaey, A., and McCormick, F. 1996. An adenovirus mutant that replicates selectively in p53-deficient human tumor cells. *Science* 274: 373–376.

Brown, B.D., Cantore, A., Annoni, A., Sergi, L.S., Lombardo, A., Della, V.P., D'Angelo, A., and Naldini, L. 2007a. A microRNA-regulated lentiviral vector mediates stable correction of hemophilia B mice. *Blood* 110: 4144–4152.

Brown, B.D., Gentner, B., Cantore, A., Colleoni, S., Amendola, M., Zingale, A., Baccarini, A., Lazzari, G., Galli, C., and Naldini, L. 2007b. Endogenous microRNA can be broadly exploited to regulate transgene expression according to tissue, lineage and differentiation state. *Nat Biotechnol* 25: 1457–1467.

Brown, B.D., Sitia, G., Annoni, A., Hauben, E., Sergi, L.S., Zingale, A., Roncarolo, M.G., Guidotti, L.G., and Naldini, L. 2007c. In vivo administration of lentiviral vectors triggers a type I interferon response that restricts hepatocyte gene transfer and promotes vector clearance. *Blood* 109: 2797–2805.

Buchmann, I., Riedmuller, K., Hoffner, S., Mack, U., Aulmann, S., and Haberkorn, U. 2007. Comparison of 99mtechnetium-pertechnetate and 123iodide SPECT with FDG-PET in patients suspicious for breast cancer. *Cancer Biother Radiopharm* 22: 779–789.

Candolfi, M., Kroeger, K.M., Pluhar, G.E., Bergeron, J., Puntel, M., Curtin, J.F., McNiel, E. A., Freese, A.B., Ohlfest, J.R., Moore, P., Lowenstein, P.R., and Castro, M.G. 2007a. Adenoviral-mediated gene transfer into the canine brain in vivo. *Neurosurgery* 60: 167–177.

Candolfi, M., Pluhar, G.E., Kroeger, K., Puntel, M., Curtin, J., Barcia, C., Muhammad, A.K., Xiong, W., Liu, C., Mondkar, S., Kuoy, W., Kang, T., McNeil, E.A., Freese, A.B., Ohlfest, J.R., Moore, P., Palmer, D., Ng, P., Young, J.D., Lowenstein, P.R., and Castro, M.G. 2007b. Optimization of adenoviral vector-mediated transgene expression in the canine brain in vivo, and in canine glioma cells in vitro. *Neuro Oncol* 9: 245–258.

Chen, M.Y., Hoffer, A., Morrison, P.F., Hamilton, J.F., Hughes, J., Schlageter, K.S., Lee, J., Kelly, B.R., and Oldfield, E.H. 2005. Surface properties, more than size, limiting convective distribution of virus-sized particles and viruses in the central nervous system. *J Neurosurg* 103: 311–319.

Chen, S.H., Shine, H.D., Goodman, J.C., Grossman, R.G., and Woo, S.L. 1994. Gene therapy for brain tumors: regression of experimental gliomas by adenovirus-mediated gene transfer in vivo. *Proc Natl Acad Sci U S A* 91: 3054–3057.

Chiocca, E.A., Abbed, K.M., Tatter, S., Louis, D.N., Hochberg, F.H., Barker, F., Kracher, J., Grossman, S.A., Fisher, J.D., Carson, K., Rosenblum, M., Mikkelsen, T., Olson, J.,

Markert, J., Rosenfeld, S., Nabors, L.B., Brem, S., Phuphanich, S., Freeman, S., Kaplan, R., and Zwiebel, J. 2004. A phase I open-label, dose-escalation, multi-institutional trial of injection with an E1B-Attenuated adenovirus, ONYX-015, into the peritumoral region of recurrent malignant gliomas, in the adjuvant setting. *Mol Ther* 10: 958–966.

Chiocca, E.A., Smith, K.M., McKinney, B., Palmer, C.A., Rosenfeld, S., Lillehei, K., Hamilton, A., DeMasters, B.K., Judy, K., and Kirn, D. 2008. A phase I trial of Ad.hIFN-beta gene therapy for glioma. *Mol Ther* 16: 618–626.

Chu, R.L., Post, D.E., Khuri, F.R., and Van Meir, E.G. 2004. Use of replicating oncolytic adenoviruses in combination therapy for cancer. *Clin Cancer Res* 10: 5299–5312.

Cohen, B., Dafni, H., Meir, G., Harmelin, A., and Neeman, M. 2005. Ferritin as an endogenous MRI reporter for noninvasive imaging of gene expression in C6 glioma tumors. *Neoplasia* 7: 109–117.

Culver, K.W., Ram, Z., Wallbridge, S., Ishii, H., Oldfield, E.H., and Blaese, R.M. 1992. In vivo gene transfer with retroviral vector-producer cells for treatment of experimental brain tumors. *Science* 256: 1550–1552.

Dempsey, M.F., Wyper, D., Owens, J., Pimlott, S., Papanastassiou, V., Patterson, J., Hadley, D.M., Nicol, A., Rampling, R., and Brown, S.M. 2006. Assessment of 123I-FIAU imaging of herpes simplex viral gene expression in the treatment of glioma. *Nucl Med Commun* 27: 611–617.

Eck, S.L., Alavi, J.B., Alavi, A., Davis, A., Hackney, D., Judy, K., Mollman, J., Phillips, P.C., Wheeldon, E.B., and Wilson, J.M. 1996. Treatment of advanced CNS malignancies with the recombinant adenovirus H5.010RSVTK: a phase I trial. *Hum Gene Ther* 7: 1465–1482.

Eck, S.L., Alavi, J.B., Judy, K., Phillips, P., Alavi, A., Hackney, D., Cross, P., Hughes, J., Gao, G., Wilson, J.M., and Propert, K. 2001. Treatment of recurrent or progressive malignant glioma with a recombinant adenovirus expressing human interferon-beta (H5.010CMVhIFN-beta): a phase I trial. *Hum Gene Ther* 12: 97–113.

Edge, R.E., Falls, T.J., Brown, C.W., Lichty, B.D., Atkins, H., and Bell, J.C. 2008. A let-7 MicroRNA-sensitive vesicular stomatitis virus demonstrates tumor-specific replication. *Mol Ther* 16: 1437–1443.

Elshami, A.A., Saavedra, A., Zhang, H., Kucharczuk, J.C., Spray, D.C., Fishman, G.I., Amin, K.M., Kaiser, L.R., and Albelda, S.M. 1996. Gap junctions play a role in the 'bystander effect' of the herpes simplex virus thymidine kinase/ganciclovir system in vitro. *Gene Ther* 3: 85–92.

Flint, S.J., Enquist, L.W., Racaniello, V.R., and Skalka, A.M. (2004). Principles of virology: molecular biology, pathogenesis, and control of animal viruses. (Washington D.C.: ASM Press).

Fomchenko, E.I. and Holland, E.C. 2006. Mouse models of brain tumors and their applications in preclinical trials. *Clin Cancer Res* 12: 5288–5297.

Fueyo, J., Alemany, R., Gomez-Manzano, C., Fuller, G.N., Khan, A., Conrad, C.A., Liu, T. J., Jiang, H., Lemoine, M.G., Suzuki, K., Sawaya, R., Curiel, D.T., Yung, W.K., and Lang, F.F. 2003. Preclinical characterization of the antiglioma activity of a tropism-enhanced adenovirus targeted to the retinoblastoma pathway. *J Natl Cancer Inst* 95: 652–660.

Fuxe, J., Liu, L., Malin, S., Philipson, L., Collins, V.P., and Pettersson, R.F. 2003. Expression of the coxsackie and adenovirus receptor in human astrocytic tumors and xenografts. *Int J Cancer* 103: 723–729.

Ganesh, S., Gonzalez, E.M., Idamakanti, N., Abramova, M., Vanroey, M., Robinson, M., Yun, C.O., and Jooss, K. 2007. Relaxin-expressing, fiber chimeric oncolytic adenovirus prolongs survival of tumor-bearing mice. *Cancer Res* 67: 4399–4407.

Ganesh, S., Gonzalez-Edick, M., Gibbons, D., Van, R.M., and Jooss, K. 2008. Intratumoral coadministration of hyaluronidase enzyme and oncolytic adenoviruses enhances virus potency in metastatic tumor models. *Clin Cancer Res* 14: 3933–3941.

Garber, K. 2006. China approves world's first oncolytic virus therapy for cancer treatment. *J Natl Cancer Inst* 98: 298–300.

Genove, G., DeMarco, U., Xu, H., Goins, W.F., and Ahrens, E.T. 2005. A new transgene reporter for in vivo magnetic resonance imaging. *Nat Med* 11: 450–454.
Germano, I.M., Fable, J., Gultekin, S.H., and Silvers, A. 2003. Adenovirus/herpes simplex-thymidine kinase/ganciclovir complex: preliminary results of a phase I trial in patients with recurrent malignant gliomas. *J Neurooncol* 65: 279–289.
Glasgow, J.N., Bauerschmitz, G.J., Curiel, D.T., and Hemminki, A. 2004. Transductional and transcriptional targeting of adenovirus for clinical applications. *Curr Gene Ther* 4: 1–14.
Goodrum, F.D. and Ornelles, D.A. 1998. p53 status does not determine outcome of E1B 55-kilodalton mutant adenovirus lytic infection. *J Virol* 72: 9479–9490.
Guo, W., Zhu, H., Zhang, L., Davis, J., Teraishi, F., Roth, J.A., Stephens, C., Fueyo, J., Jiang, H., Conrad, C., and Fang, B. 2006. Combination effect of oncolytic adenovirotherapy and TRAIL gene therapy in syngeneic murine breast cancer models. *Cancer Gene Ther* 13: 82–90.
Ha, I., Wightman, B., and Ruvkun, G. 1996. A bulged lin-4/lin-14 RNA duplex is sufficient for Caenorhabditis elegans lin-14 temporal gradient formation. *Genes Dev* 10: 3041–3050.
Hallden, G., Hill, R., Wang, Y., Anand, A., Liu, T.C., Lemoine, N.R., Francis, J., Hawkins, L., and Kirn, D. 2003. Novel immunocompetent murine tumor models for the assessment of replication-competent oncolytic adenovirus efficacy. *Mol Ther* 8: 412–424.
Hamel, W., Magnelli, L., Chiarugi, V.P., and Israel, M.A. 1996. Herpes simplex virus thymidine kinase/ganciclovir-mediated apoptotic death of bystander cells. *Cancer Res* 56: 2697–2702.
Hoffmann, D., Meyer, B., and Wildner, O. 2007. Improved glioblastoma treatment with Ad5/35 fiber chimeric conditionally replicating adenoviruses. *J Gene Med* 9: 764–778.
Horst, M., Brouwer, E., Verwijnen, S., Rodijk, M., de, J.M., Hoeben, R., de, L.B., and Smitt, P.S. 2007. Targeting malignant gliomas with a glial fibrillary acidic protein (GFAP)-selective oncolytic adenovirus. *J Gene Med* 9: 1071–1079.
Hu, W., Davis, J.J., Zhu, H., Dong, F., Guo, W., Ang, J., Peng, H., Guo, Z.S., Bartlett, D.L., Swisher, S.G., and Fang, B. 2007. Redirecting adaptive immunity against foreign antigens to tumors for cancer therapy. *Cancer Biol Ther* 6: 1773–1779.
Huebner, R.J., Rowe, W.P., Schatten, W.E., Smith, R.R., and Thomas, L.B. 1956. Studies on the use of viruses in the treatment of carcinoma of the cervix. *Cancer* 9: 1211–1218.
Ichikawa, T., Hogemann, D., Saeki, Y., Tyminski, E., Terada, K., Weissleder, R., Chiocca, E. A., and Basilion, J.P. 2002. MRI of transgene expression: correlation to therapeutic gene expression. *Neoplasia* 4: 523–530.
Immonen, A., Vapalahti, M., Tyynela, K., Hurskainen, H., Sandmair, A., Vanninen, R., Langford, G., Murray, N., and yla-herttuala, S. 2004. AdvHSV-tk gene therapy with intravenous ganciclovir improves survival in human malignant glioma: a randomised, controlled study. *Mol Ther* 10: 967–972.
Ito, H., Aoki, H., Kuhnel, F., Kondo, Y., Kubicka, S., Wirth, T., Iwado, E., Iwamaru, A., Fujiwara, K., Hess, K.R., Lang, F.F., Sawaya, R., and Kondo, S. 2006. Autophagic cell death of malignant glioma cells induced by a conditionally replicating adenovirus. *J Natl Cancer Inst* 98: 625–636.
Jiang, H., Gomez-Manzano, C., Aoki, H., Alonso, M.M., Kondo, S., McCormick, F., Xu, J., Kondo, Y., Bekele, B.N., Colman, H., Lang, F.F., and Fueyo, J. 2007. Examination of the therapeutic potential of Delta-24-RGD in brain tumor stem cells: role of autophagic cell death. *J Natl Cancer Inst* 99: 1410–1414.
Kelly, E. and Russell, S.J. 2007. History of oncolytic viruses: genesis to genetic engineering. *Mol Ther* 15: 651–659.
Kim, M., Sumerel, L.A., Belousova, N., Lyons, G.R., Carey, D.E., Krasnykh, V., and Douglas, J.T. 2003. The coxsackievirus and adenovirus receptor acts as a tumour suppressor in malignant glioma cells. *Br J Cancer* 88: 1411–1416.
Kock, H., Harris, M.P., Anderson, S.C., Machemer, T., Hancock, W., Sutjipto, S., Wills, K.N., Gregory, R.J., Shepard, H.M., Westphal, M., and Maneval, D.C. 1996. Adenovirus-mediated

p53 gene transfer suppresses growth of human glioblastoma cells in vitro and in vivo. *Int J Cancer* 67: 808–815.

Kuriyama, N., Kuriyama, H., Julin, C.M., Lamborn, K.R., and Israel, M.A. 2001. Protease pretreatment increases the efficacy of adenovirus-mediated gene therapy for the treatment of an experimental glioblastoma model. *Cancer Res* 61: 1805–1809.

Lang, F.F., Bruner, J.M., Fuller, G.N., Aldape, K., Prados, M.D., Chang, S., Berger, M.S., McDermott, M.W., Kunwar, S.M., Junck, L.R., Chandler, W., Zwiebel, J.A., Kaplan, R. S., and Yung, W.K. 2003. Phase I trial of adenovirus-mediated p53 gene therapy for recurrent glioma: biological and clinical results. *J Clin Oncol* 21: 2508–2518.

Lang, F.F., Yung, W.K., Sawaya, R., and Tofilon, P.J. 1999. Adenovirus-mediated p53 gene therapy for human gliomas. *Neurosurgery* 45: 1093–1104.

Lee, Y.S., Kim, J.H., Choi, K.J., Choi, I.K., Kim, H., Cho, S., Cho, B.C., and Yun, C.O. 2006. Enhanced antitumor effect of oncolytic adenovirus expressing interleukin-12 and B7-1 in an immunocompetent murine model. *Clin Cancer Res* 12: 5859–5868.

Li, H., onso-Vanegas, M., Colicos, M.A., Jung, S.S., Lochmuller, H., Sadikot, A.F., Snipes, G.J., Seth, P., Karpati, G., and Nalbantoglu, J. 1999. Intracerebral adenovirus-mediated p53 tumor suppressor gene therapy for experimental human glioma. *Clin Cancer Res* 5: 637–642.

Lichtenstein, D.L., Toth, K., Doronin, K., Tollefson, A.E., and Wold, W.S. 2004. Functions and mechanisms of action of the adenovirus E3 proteins. *Int Rev Immunol* 23: 75–111.

Louie, A.Y., Huber, M.M., Ahrens, E.T., Rothbacher, U., Moats, R., Jacobs, R.E., Fraser, S. E., and Meade, T.J. 2000. In vivo visualization of gene expression using magnetic resonance imaging. *Nat Biotechnol* 18: 321–325.

Marshall, E. 1999. Gene therapy death prompts review of adenovirus vector. *Science* 286: 2244–2245.

Miller, C.R., Buchsbaum, D.J., Reynolds, P.N., Douglas, J.T., Gillespie, G.Y., Mayo, M.S., Raben, D., and Curiel, D.T. 1998. Differential susceptibility of primary and established human glioma cells to adenovirus infection: Targeting via the epidermal growth factor receptor achieves fiber receptor-independent gene transfer. *Cancer Res* 58: 5738–5748.

Min, J.J., Iyer, M., and Gambhir, S.S. 2003. Comparison of [18F]FHBG and [14C]FIAU for imaging of HSV1-tk reporter gene expression: adenoviral infection vs stable transfection. *Eur J Nucl Med Mol Imaging* 30: 1547–1560.

Miura, Y., Yoshida, K., Nishimoto, T., Hatanaka, K., Ohnami, S., Asaka, M., Douglas, J.T., Curiel, D.T., Yoshida, T., and Aoki, K. 2007. Direct selection of targeted adenovirus vectors by random peptide display on the fiber knob. *Gene Ther* 14: 1448–1460.

NIH Recombinant DNA Advisory Committee. 2002. Assessment of adenoviral vector safety and toxicity: report of the National Institutes of Health Recombinant DNA Advisory Committee. *Hum Gene Ther* 13: 3–13.

O'Shea, C.C., Johnson, L., Bagus, B., Choi, S., Nicholas, C., Shen, A., Boyle, L., Pandey, K., Soria, C., Kunich, J., Shen, Y., Habets, G., Ginzinger, D., and McCormick, F. 2004. Late viral RNA export, rather than p53 inactivation, determines ONYX-015 tumor selectivity. *Cancer Cell* 6: 611–623.

Oh, S., Odland, R., Wilson, S.R., Kroeger, K.M., Liu, C., Lowenstein, P.R., Castro, M. G., Hall, W.A., and Ohlfest, J.R. 2007. Improved distribution of small molecules and viral vectors in the murine brain using a hollow fiber catheter. *J Neurosurg* 107: 568–577.

Penuelas, I., Mazzolini, G., Boan, J.F., Sangro, B., Marti-Climent, J., Ruiz, M., Ruiz, J., Satyamurthy, N., Qian, C., Barrio, J.R., Phelps, M.E., Richter, J.A., Gambhir, S.S., and Prieto, J. 2005. Positron emission tomography imaging of adenoviral-mediated transgene expression in liver cancer patients. *Gastroenterology* 128: 1787–1795.

Perez, J.M., Simeone, F.J., Saeki, Y., Josephson, L., and Weissleder, R. 2003. Viral-induced self-assembly of magnetic nanoparticles allows the detection of viral particles in biological media. *J Am Chem Soc* 125: 10192–10193.

Persson, A., Fan, X., Salford, L.G., Widegren, B., and Englund, E. 2007. Neuroblastomas and medulloblastomas exhibit more Coxsackie adenovirus receptor expression than gliomas and other brain tumors. *Neuropathology* 27: 233–236.
Persson, A., Fan, X., Widegren, B., and Englund, E. 2006. Cell type- and region-dependent coxsackie adenovirus receptor expression in the central nervous system. *J Neurooncol* 78: 1–6.
Post, D.E., Khuri, F.R., Simons, J.W., and Van Meir, E.G. 2003. Replicative oncolytic adenoviruses in multimodal cancer regimens. *Hum Gene Ther* 14: 933–946.
Post, D.E., Sandberg, E.M., Kyle, M.M., Devi, N.S., Brat, D.J., Xu, Z., Tighiouart, M., and Van Meir, E.G. 2007. Targeted Cancer Gene Therapy Using a Hypoxia Inducible Factor Dependent Oncolytic Adenovirus Armed with Interleukin-4. *Cancer Res* 67: 6872–6881.
Post, D.E., Shim, H., Toussaint-Smith, E., and Van Meir, E.G. 2005. Cancer scene investigation: how a cold virus became a tumor killer. *Future Oncol* 1: 247–258.
Puumalainen, A.M., Vapalahti, M., Agrawal, R.S., Kossila, M., Laurence, J., Lehtolainen, P., Viita, H., Paljärvi, L., Vanninen, R., and Yla-herttuala, S. 1998. B-galactosidase gene transfer to human malignant glioma in vitro using replication- deficient retroviruses and adenoviruses. *Hum Gene Ther* 9: 1769–1774.
Qin, X.Q., Beckham, C., Brown, J.L., Lukashev, M., and Barsoum, J. 2001. Human and mouse IFN-beta gene therapy exhibits different anti-tumor mechanisms in mouse models. *Mol Ther* 4: 356–364.
Qin, X.Q., Tao, N., Dergay, A., Moy, P., Fawell, S., Davis, A., Wilson, J.M., and Barsoum, J. 1998. Interferon-beta gene therapy inhibits tumor formation and causes regression of established tumors in immune-deficient mice. *Proc Natl Acad Sci U S A* 95: 14411–14416.
Rainov, N.G., Koch, S., Sena-Esteves, M., and Berens, M.E. 2000. Characterization of a canine glioma cell line as related to established experimental brain tumor models. *J Neuropathol Exp Neurol* 59: 607–613.
Raty, J.K., Liimatainen, T., Unelma, K.M., Grohn, O., Airenne, K.J., and yla-herttuala, S. 2007. Non-invasive Imaging in Gene Therapy. *Mol Ther* 15: 1579–1586.
Raty, J.K., Liimatainen, T., Wirth, T., Airenne, K.J., Ihalainen, T.O., Huhtala, T., Hamerlynck, E., Vihinen-Ranta, M., Narvanen, A., yla-herttuala, S., and Hakumaki, J.M. 2006. Magnetic resonance imaging of viral particle biodistribution in vivo. *Gene Ther* 13: 1440–1446.
Rehemtulla, A., Hall, D.E., Stegman, L.D., Prasad, U., Chen, G., Bhojani, M.S., Chenevert, T.L., and Ross, B.D. 2002. Molecular imaging of gene expression and efficacy following adenoviral-mediated brain tumor gene therapy. *Mol Imaging* 1: 43–55.
Rothmann, T., Hengstermann, A., Whitaker, N.J., Scheffner, M., and zur, H.H. 1998. Replication of ONYX-015, a potential anticancer adenovirus, is independent of p53 status in tumor cells. *J Virol* 72: 9470–9478.
Sampson, J.H., Akabani, G., Archer, G.E., Berger, M.S., Coleman, R.E., Friedman, A.H., Friedman, H.S., Greer, K., Herndon Ii, J.E., Kunwar, S., McLendon, R.E., Paolino, A., Petry, N.A., Provenzale, J.M., Reardon, D.A., Wong, T.Z., Zalutsky, M.R., Pastan, I., and Bigner, D.D. 2008. Intracerebral infusion of an EGFR-targeted toxin in recurrent malignant brain tumors. *Neuro Oncol* 10: 320–329.
Sandmair, A.M., Loimas, S., Puranen, P., Immonen, A., Kossila, M., Puranen, M., Hurskainen, H., Tyynelä, K., Turunen, M., Vanninen, R., lehtolainen, P., Paljärvi, L., Johansson, R., Vapalahti, M., and Ylä-Herttuala, S. 2000. Thymidine kinase gene therapy for human malignant glioma, using replication-deficient retroviruses or adenoviruses. *Hum Gene Ther* 11: 2197–2205.
Shinoura, N., Yoshida, Y., Tsunoda, R., Ohashi, M., Zhang, W.P., Asai, A., Kirino, T., and Hamada, H. 1999. Highly augmented cytopathic effect of a fiber-mutant E1B-defective adenovirus for gene therapy of gliomas. *Cancer Res* 59: 3411–3416.
Singh, S.K., Hawkins, C., Clarke, I.D., Squire, J.A., Bayani, J., Hide, T., Henkelman, R.M., Cusimano, M.D., and Dirks, P.B. 2004. Identification of human brain tumour initiating cells. *Nature* 432: 396–401.

Sinkovics, J. and Horvath, J. 1993. New developments in the virus therapy of cancer: a historical review. *Intervirology* 36: 193–214.

Smitt, P.S., Driesse, M., Wolbers, J., Kros, M., and Avezaat, C. 2003. Treatment of relapsed malignant glioma with an adenoviral vector containing the herpes simplex thymidine kinase gene followed by ganciclovir. *Mol Ther* 7: 851–858.

Sonabend, A.M., Ulasov, I.V., Tyler, M.A., Rivera, A.A., Mathis, J.M., and Lesniak, M.S. 2008. Mesenchymal stem cells effectively deliver an oncolytic adenovirus to intracranial glioma. *Stem Cells* 26: 831–841.

Stanford, M.M., Breitbach, C.J., Bell, J.C., and McFadden, G. 2008. Innate immunity, tumor microenvironment and oncolytic virus therapy: friends or foes? *Curr Opin Mol Ther* 10: 32–37.

Suzuki, K., Alemany, R., Yamamoto, M., and Curiel, D.T. 2002. The presence of the adenovirus E3 region improves the oncolytic potency of conditionally replicative adenoviruses. *Clin Cancer Res* 8: 3348–3359.

Szatmari, T., Lumniczky, K., Desaknai, S., Trajcevski, S., Hidvegi, E.J., Hamada, H., and Safrany, G. 2006. Detailed characterization of the mouse glioma 261 tumor model for experimental glioblastoma therapy. *Cancer Sci* 97: 546–553.

Tallone, T., Malin, S., Samuelsson, A., Wilbertz, J., Miyahara, M., Okamoto, K., Poellinger, L., Philipson, L., and Pettersson, S. 2001. A mouse model for adenovirus gene delivery. *Proc Natl Acad Sci U S A* 98: 7910–7915.

ter Horst, M., Verwijnen, S.M., Brouwer, E., Hoeben, R.C., de, J.M., de Leeuw, B.H., and Sillevis Smitt, P.A. 2006. Locoregional delivery of adenoviral vectors. *J Nucl Med* 47: 1483–1489.

Thorburn, A. 2008. Apoptosis and autophagy: regulatory connections between two supposedly different processes. *Apoptosis* 13: 1–9.

Tjuvajev, J.G., Doubrovin, M., Akhurst, T., Cai, S., Balatoni, J., Alauddin, M.M., Finn, R., Bornmann, W., Thaler, H., Conti, P.S., and Blasberg, R.G. 2002. Comparison of radiolabeled nucleoside probes (FIAU, FHBG, and FHPG) for PET imaging of HSV1-tk gene expression. *J Nucl Med* 43: 1072–1083.

Toth, K., Spencer, J.F., Tollefson, A.E., Kuppuswamy, M., Doronin, K., Lichtenstein, D.L., La Regina, M.C., Prince, G.A., and Wold, W.S. 2005. Cotton rat tumor model for the evaluation of oncolytic adenoviruses. *Hum Gene Ther* 16: 139–146.

Touraine, R.L., Ishii-Morita, H., Ramsey, W.J., and Blaese, R.M. 1998. The bystander effect in the HSVtk/ganciclovir system and its relationship to gap junctional communication. *Gene Ther* 5: 1705–1711.

Trask, T.W., Trask, R.P., guilar-Cordova, E., Shine, H.D., Wyde, P.R., Goodman, J.C., Hamilton, W.J., Rojas-Martinez, A., Chen, S.H., Woo, S.L., and Grossman, R.G. 2000. Phase I study of adenoviral delivery of the HSV-tk gene and ganciclovir administration in patients with current malignant brain tumors. *Mol Ther* 1: 195–203.

Ulasov, I.V., Rivera, A.A., Nettelbeck, D.M., Rivera, L.B., Mathis, J.M., Sonabend, A.M., Tyler, M., Wang, M., Douglas, J.T., and Lesniak, M.S. 2007a. An oncolytic adenoviral vector carrying the tyrosinase promoter for glioma gene therapy. *Int J Oncol* 31: 1177–1185.

Ulasov, I.V., Zhu, Z.B., Tyler, M.A., Han, Y., Rivera, A.A., Khramtsov, A., Curiel, D.T., and Lesniak, M.S. 2007b. Survivin-driven and fiber-modified oncolytic adenovirus exhibits potent antitumor activity in established intracranial glioma. *Hum Gene Ther* 18: 589–602.

Vasalatiy, O., Gerard, R.D., Zhao, P., Sun, X., and Sherry, A.D. 2008. Labeling of adenovirus particles with PARACEST agents. *Bioconjug Chem* 19: 598–606.

Vile, R.G., Castleden, S., Marshall, J., Camplejohn, R., Upton, C., and Chong, H. 1997. Generation of an anti-tumour immune response in a non-immunogenic tumour: HSVtk killing in vivo stimulates a mononuclear cell infiltrate and a Th1-like profile of intratumoural cytokine expression. *Int J Cancer* 71: 267–274.

Vousden, K.H. and Lu, X. 2002. Live or let die: the cell's response to p53. *Nat Rev Cancer* 2: 594–604.
Wang, Y., Hallden, G., Hill, R., Anand, A., Liu, T.C., Francis, J., Brooks, G., Lemoine, N., and Kirn, D. 2003. E3 gene manipulations affect oncolytic adenovirus activity in immunocompetent tumor models. *Nat Biotechnol* 21: 1328–1335.
Weller, M. and Fontana, A. 1995. The failure of current immunotherapy for malignant glioma. Tumor-derived TGF-B, T-cell apoptosis, and the immune privilege of the brain. *Brain Res Rev* 21: 128–151.
Zipp, F. and Aktas, O. 2006. The brain as a target of inflammation: common pathways link inflammatory and neurodegenerative diseases. *Trends Neurosci* 29: 518–527.
Zou, A., Atencio, I., Huang, W.M., Horn, M., and Ramachandra, M. 2004. Overexpression of adenovirus E3-11.6K protein induces cell killing by both caspase-dependent and caspase-independent mechanisms. *Virology* 326: 240–249.
Zurkiya, O., Chan, A.W., and Hu, X. 2008. MagA is sufficient for producing magnetic nanoparticles in mammalian cells, making it an MRI reporter. *Magn Reson Med* 59: 1225–1231.

Chapter 48
Harnessing T-Cell Immunity to Target Brain Tumors

Paul R. Walker, Robert M. Prins, Pierre-Yves Dietrich, and Linda M. Liau

Abstract T-cell mediated immunotherapy is a conceptually attractive treatment option to envisage for glioma, since T lymphocytes can actively seek out neoplastic cells in the brain, and they have the potential to safely and specifically eliminate tumor. Some antigenic targets on glioma cells are already defined, and we can be optimistic that more will be discovered from progress in T-cell epitope identification and gene expression profiling of brain tumors. In parallel, advances in immunology (regional immunology, neuroimmunology, tumor immunology) now equip us to build upon the results from current immunotherapy trials in which the safety and feasibility of brain tumor immunotherapy have already been confirmed. We can now look to the next phase of immunotherapy, in which we must harness the most promising basic science advances and existing clinical expertise, and apply these to randomized clinical trials to determine the real clinical impact and applicability of these approaches for treating patients with currently incurable malignant brain tumors.

Contents

P.R. Walker (✉)
Centre of Oncology, Geneva University Hospitals and University of Geneva, rue Micheli-du-Crest 24, 1211 Geneva 14, Switzerland
e-mail: Paul.Walker@hcuge.ch

E.G. Van Meir (ed.), *CNS Cancer*, Cancer Drug Discovery and Development, DOI 10.1007/978-1-60327-553-8_48,
© Humana Press, a part of Springer Science+Business Media, LLC 2009

48.1 Introductory Remarks

Is our immune system capable of recognizing and destroying tumor cells in the brain, either spontaneously or after "doping" by some immunotherapeutic strategy? After some decades of uncertainties concerning tumor immunity and its applicability to the CNS, the answer in the twenty-first century is yes, but with a number of caveats that can best be summarized as "under certain conditions." The aim of this chapter is to overview the science that may help us to understand the particular circumstances under which elements of the immune system can recognize and destroy tumor in the brain, and then to assess how this information has been put to the test in current clinical trials.

48.2 Immune Privilege and Cancer Immunosurveillance

The dialogue between the immune system and brain tumors has been strongly influenced by two key hypotheses, *immune privilege* and *cancer immunosurveillance*, both of which originated more than 50 ago. In the 1940s, Medawar reported that allografts in the CNS survived longer than those in other tissues (Medewar, 1948), which led Barker and Billingham to coin the term *immune privilege* to describe such sites (Barker and Billingham, 1977). The concept of limited immune responsiveness in the brain was interpreted as being consistent with the overriding need to control inflammatory reactions and their potentially damaging consequences to neuronal networks with low regenerative capacity. The absence of a lymphatic system within the CNS and the presence of a specialized blood-brain barrier (BBB) in most CNS compartments suggested immune isolation achieved by restricting entry of blood-born molecules such as immunoglobulins, as well as leukocytes, albeit by mechanisms that are under constant revision (Bechmann et al., 2007). With several decades of more detailed observations of immune responses in the CNS, it is now clear that both protective (e.g., antiviral) and pathogenic (e.g., autoimmune) immune responses can and do occur in the CNS, but these may be quantitatively and qualitatively different to those occurring in other sites. In a reappraisal of CNS immune privilege (Bechmann et al., 2007), many compelling arguments were made for a redefinition of privilege, underlining that it is a *relative* state, and only applicable to the parenchyma of the intact, noninflamed brain.

Moreover, perhaps in view of the longstanding, oversimplistic interpretations of immune privilege, one of the cornerstones of modern tumor immunology, the *cancer immunosurveillance hypothesis* of Burnet and Thomas (Burnet, 1970) was not immediately seen to directly concern brain tumors. The theory proposes that the immune system continually surveys the organism and recognizes and destroys abnormal cells. Recognition of cancer certainly occurs, but it is now clear that the outcome of such detection is not always protective immunosurveillance. This led to a refined theory of *immunoediting* (Dunn et al., 2006) in which different outcomes are described following cancer and immune system interaction: namely, elimination, equilibrium, and tumor escape. Analysis of mouse models with clearly defined immunodeficiencies shows that both innate and adaptive immune responses influence tumor outgrowth: mice lacking T lymphocytes, B lymphocytes, natural killer (NK) cells, and those with deficiencies in Type 1 or Type 2 interferons (IFNs) have higher tumor incidence. Moreover, analyses of large cohorts of immunosuppressed patients show that incidence of not only virally associated cancers but also cancers with no known association with infection is increased. However, to date, brain tumors have not been among the tumors noted to occur more frequently. This is likely due to the lower expected frequency of these malignancies, but it may also be because brain tumors are rarely eliminated spontaneously, and more likely persist in equilibrium with the host. Or else they rapidly escape immune control, as would appear to be the case once malignant gliomas are detected. In this case, the notion of immunoediting predicts that outgrowing tumors will have been sculpted by interaction with the immune system, for example, by selection of tumors able to neutralize immune effector mechanisms, as will be discussed (see below).

It should be noted that these ideas are in the context of *spontaneous* immunity against *spontaneous* cancers. When this occurs, and when we can study it, we should do so. Indeed, naturally occurring immune mechanisms endowed by millennia of selection and evolution may provide precious information for rational immunotherapy design.

48.3 The Stages of Tumor Immunity

Spontaneous tumor immunity can be conveniently divided into a minimum of three chronologically distinct events (innate immune activation, induction of adaptive immunity, and effector phase of adaptive immunity) that occur in two

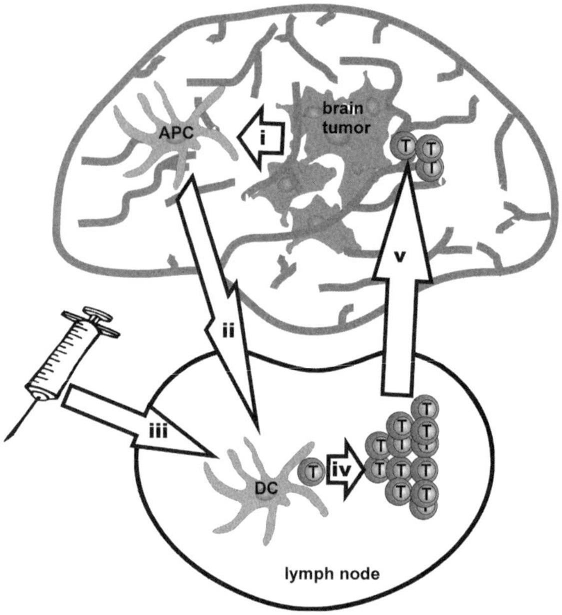

Fig. 48.1 The stages of T-cell mediated tumor immunity. The tissue damage and stress associated with tumor growth will alert cells of the innate immune system, including microglia. Resident or recruited APC (i) phagocytose tumor-derived antigen (e.g., cellular debris) and transport it to LNs (ii). Tumor antigens can also arrive in the LN following peripheral vaccination (iii). Immigrant DC or LN resident DC presents antigen to naïve T cells, leading to their activation and clonal expansion (iv). Activated T cells exit the LN and infiltrate the site of tumor growth (v) to exert their effector functions

distinct anatomical sites: the tumor site and secondary lymphoid tissue (Fig. 48.1). Immunotherapies must reinforce, reproduce, or substitute for each of these phases. We will outline the general features of how and where the stages of an idealized spontaneous antitumor immune response occur, indicating the particularities of the CNS.

48.3.1 The Tumor First Stimulates Innate Immune Sentinels, at the Site of the Malignancy

48.3.1.1 Detection

The first step in tumor immunity is alerting the immune system to the presence of tumor; this is achieved by innate immunity. The innate immune system comprises soluble factors such as components of the complement system, but more important for tumor immunity are the cells, such as the macrophages/ microglia, granulocytes, NK cells, and dendritic cells (DCs). These cells efficiently detect pathogen-associated molecular patterns by means of germline-encoded pathogen-recognition receptors (PRRs) that include the toll-like receptors (TLRs). However, their role is now understood to be wider than merely detecting infection by a pathogen; they can also detect perturbations to the organism that can be considered "dangerous" (Matzinger, 1994), and PRR can also be viewed as "pattern" recognition receptors able to deliver danger signals. For example, endogenous ligands have been identified for all human TLRs except for TLRs 5 and 10. These include the heat shock proteins (HSPs) upregulated by stressed cells (binding to TLRs 2 and 4) and nucleic acids released by dying tumor cells (binding to TLRs 3, 7, and 9) (Barrat and Coffman, 2008; Barton and Medzhitov, 2002; Pulendran, 2005).

Detection of cancer will be initially mediated by tissue-resident sentinel cells of the innate immune system, which for most tissues are the DCs and the macrophages. But for the brain, DCs are not resident in the parenchyma (although they may appear at later stages of a response), and the most important endogenous sentinels are the microglial cells (Hanisch and Kettenmann, 2007). These specialized brain macrophages are widely distributed throughout the brain parenchyma and may actually be recruited to the site of glioma occurrence, where they can represent up to a third of the cells composing the tumor (Graeber et al., 2002). Microglia express several TLRs, including TLR 4 that is proposed to bind several factors produced by dying cells in the glioma microenvironment (Hussain et al., 2006). If TLR ligation leads to full activation of the microglial cell, subsequent functions potentially include phagocytosis, chemokine and cytokine release, antigen presentation, and even tumor cell killing. However, other less useful outcomes have been suggested, including neurotoxicity and enhancement of tumor invasiveness through the upregulation of metalloproteinases. These contrasting functions may be attributed to the extreme plasticity of microglia in response to their local milieu. Indeed, the brain microenvironment in which they must function is also comprised of astroglial cells which exhibit characteristics of innate immune function, including PRR expression, activation to a reactive state, and secretion of cytokines and chemokines (Farina et al., 2007). Furthermore, in the case of malignancy, microglial function will also be subject to modulation by the local tumor microenvironment (Hussain et al., 2006; Markovic et al., 2005).

48.3.1.2 Innate Immune Functions

In a protective antitumor immune response, once the endogenous sentinels of innate immunity are alerted, there are two subsequent events: to limit (or eliminate) the source of danger by innate effector functions of resident cells and to recruit further resources (particularly T cells, as discussed in the next section). For glioma, there is little in vivo evidence to suggest that tumoricidal microglia spontaneously restrain brain tumor growth (Graeber et al., 2002). The other innate effector cell that has the potential to recognize and kill tumor cells is the NK cell, which has been the subject of intensive investigations to characterize the receptors that regulate its function. In order to mediate cytolysis, NK cells must receive a signal through one of their activating receptors such as NKG2D, but to result in activation, there must be an absence of signaling through inhibitory receptors (e.g., members of the CD158 family of receptors) (Lanier, 2008). Expression of ligands for NKG2D is low on normal cells, but upregulated on cells subjected to genotoxic stress, as occurs in neoplastic transformation. Indeed, certain human glioma fulfill the requirements for NK cell recognition and activation, with expression of the NKG2D ligands MICA/B (major histocompatibility complex (MHC) class I-chain-related molecules A and B) and UL16-binding proteins (ULBP) 1–3 (Eisele et al., 2006), and a downregulation of some HLA molecules which are ligands for the CD158 inhibitory receptors (Facoetti et al., 2005). NK cells are not only cytotoxic but also an early source of IFN-γ, which can be angiostatic and can amplify T-cell mediated tumor immunity. However, little is known about the NK cells or their potential impact at the tumor site in human glioma; although in a murine intracranial tumor model (B16 melanoma), interactions between DCs, NK cells, and T cells facilitated protective tumor immunity (Prins et al., 2006c).

48.3.2 The Induction of Adaptive Immune Responses Against Brain Tumors: From the Brain to the Lymph Node

Although macrophages and microglia are the major components of the immune infiltrate in brain tumors at every stage of the response, after initial detection of the malignancy they will be joined by T lymphocytes, which are responsible for the cell-mediated immune responses of adaptive immunity. The B lymphocytes, giving rise to antibody-secreting plasma cells and the humoral arm of adaptive immunity, are probably not a major component of spontaneous immunity to brain tumors. On the other hand, antibodies administered therapeutically have important applications in glioma therapy and will be covered elsewhere in this book (see Chapter 36). In this chapter, the focus is on T cells (both CD4 and CD8 subsets), which once activated have the potential to infiltrate tumors and mediate potent effector functions including cytotoxicity and local cytokine release. It will become clear that while these potentially useful effector functions may be T-cell mediated, their initiation is totally dependent on innate immune cooperation.

48.3.2.1 Generation of Naïve CD4 and CD8 T Cells

T cells that are mature and naïve (i.e., cells not yet stimulated by their cognate antigen) are generated in the thymus, and then travel in the blood and lymph to recirculate between secondary lymphoid organs such as the spleen and LNs. Although the majority of naïve T cells do not efficiently enter nonlymphoid tissues, including the CNS, exceptions have been reported (Brabb et al., 2000). Such atypical T-cell trafficking probably does not account for a significant proportion of T cells under normal conditions and may even be associated with tolerance induction rather than induction of efficient antitumor immunity. Therefore, for understanding the generation of efficacious tumor immunity, the "conventional" trafficking and activation of T cells in LNs will be considered here.

A large number of T cells are generated in each individual, with each bearing clonally distributed antigen receptors that are generated by somatic rearrangement of a limited number of gene segments. These encode a heterodimeric T-cell receptor for antigen (TCR) comprised of α and β chains for the main T-cell population that will be discussed here, and of γ and δ chains for receptors used by a minority $\gamma\delta$ T-cell population. The ligands for the TCR of CD8 T cells are short peptides of around 8–10 amino acids bound to class I MHC molecules, whereas CD4 T cells recognize slightly longer peptides (~13–17 amino acids) bound to MHC class II molecules. Since TCR are randomly generated, the repertoire potentially includes receptors of any conceivable specificity, but the frequencies of naïve T cells expressing a TCR of a given specificity in the whole T cell population are very low (in the order of 1 in 10^6 cells), necessitating significant clonal expansion in order for T cells to achieve a biological effect in vivo.

48.3.2.2 Naïve T-Cell Activation Requires Two Signals

If naïve T cells receive only a single signal via ligation of their TCR by an MHC/peptide complex, they may become anergic, i.e., without effector function and refractory to further stimulation. Full activation of naïve T cells to become effector cells requires a second signal, which is usually delivered by costimulatory molecules such as members of the B7 family (particularly CD80 and CD86) expressed by antigen presenting cells (APCs) of the innate immune system, the most efficient of which are the DCs (Fig. 48.2). Activation of naïve T cells (priming) by APCs within the secondary lymphoid tissue triggers clonal expansion of T cells and a differentiation program that will influence the magnitude and quality of the antitumor immune response, i.e., T-cell effector functions (cytotoxicity, cytokine release, suppression), tissue tropism, and persistence as T effector or T memory cells. Although this is occurring in the LN, these factors are principally predetermined by the innate immune reaction, upstream at the tumor site (or at a vaccination site). The resulting clonally expanded T cells (now highly enriched for tumor antigen specificity) can then exit the LN via the efferent lymph, enter the bloodstream, and traffic more or less efficiently to the tumor site, depending upon the pattern of adhesion molecules and chemokine receptors (their "homing phenotype") with which they have been programed to express by the DC.

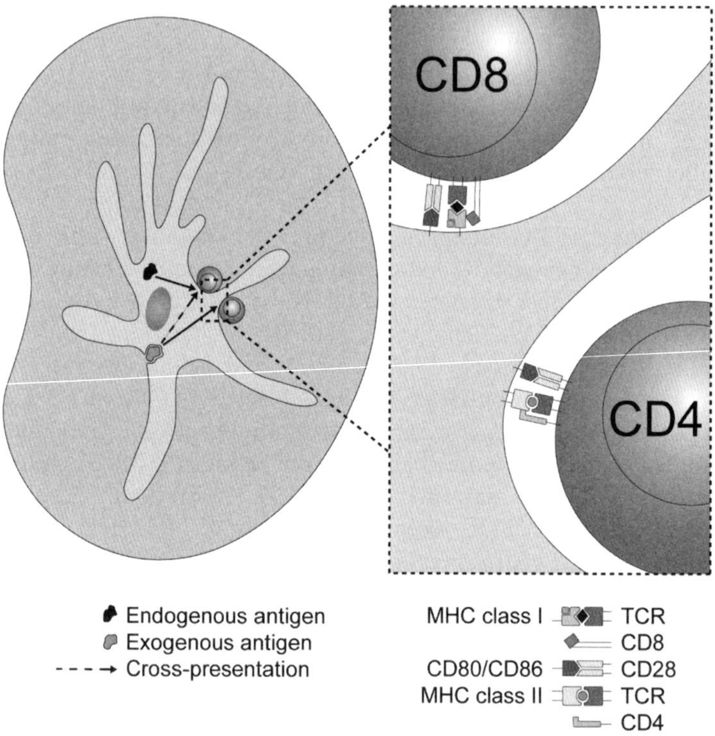

Fig. 48.2 T-cell activation in the lymph node. Naïve T cells are activated (primed) in secondary lymphoid tissue by DCs that are able to present tumor antigens (i.e., exogenous antigens) on MHC class I (cross-presentation) and MHC class II molecules to CD8 and CD4 T cells, respectively. In addition, all DCs present endogenous antigens to CD8 T cells. The DCs also express costimulatory molecules (e.g., CD80/CD86) that deliver a second signal to receptors on the T cells, ensuring T-cell activation rather than tolerance (see text)

48.3.2.3 How Does Antigen from the Tumor Site Reach the Naïve T Cells in the Lymph Node?

The best understood route for antigen transport to the LN is via DCs, which are able to phagocytose tumor-derived antigens, then migrate via lymphatic vessels to the T-cell zones of draining LN, wherein they can await encounter with a recirculating naïve T cell with specificity for the captured antigen bound to an MHC molecule. For brain tumors, this scenario is complicated by the particularities of CNS cellular composition and anatomy: there are no lymphatic vessels in the brain, and there are no resident DCs in the healthy brain parenchyma. Nevertheless, several different experimental approaches all now confirm that functional antigen drainage from the brain parenchyma to lymphoid tissues occurs, principally to the cervical LNs (Cserr and Knopf, 1992).

48.3.2.4 Cell-Free Drainage of Antigen

Early studies examined transport of soluble products which flow with interstitial tissue fluid via the perivascular spaces, to drain either into the subarachnoid space or to lymphatics via arachnoid sheaths of certain cranial nerves and spinal nerve roots to reach the cervical LNs (Bechmann et al., 2007). More recently, particulate material was also shown to reach cervical and submandibular LN after intracerebral injection (Walter and Albert, 2007). These studies confirm functional drainage in the absence of lymphatics, but they do not adequately explain the initiation of adaptive immunity. For this to occur without induction of immune tolerance, there must be not only antigen presented to T cells in the cervical LN but also a second signal indicating danger or infection. The best understood source of such a second signal is an APC that has sensed danger at its source, i.e., at the tumor site in the brain.

48.3.2.5 Cell-Mediated Transport of Antigen from the Brain to the Lymph Node

A cell able to transport brain tumor-derived antigenic material to LNs and stimulate T cells therein should have the following properties: it should be phagocytic; it should be able to process and present tumor antigens on MHC class I and class II molecules; it should express costimulatory molecules; and it should be migratory. The microglia are the most abundant phagocytes in the brain, and they can be induced to express costimulatory molecules, and they can present antigens to MHC class II restricted CD4 T cells in vitro (Aloisi et al., 2000). The more demanding function of cross-presentation, i.e., uptake of exogenous antigens and presentation of processed peptides derived therefrom on MHC class I molecules, has only been reported in one in vitro study using ovalbumin as antigen (Beauvillain et al., 2008). Whether these in vitro results apply to microglia in vivo is debatable, partly because of the criteria used to define microglia, such as morphology, anatomic location, and level of expression of macrophage associated markers, and even function (Davoust et al., 2008). Indeed, efficient antigen presentation in vitro requires a phenotype and function of a reactive, or activated microglial cell, which is virtually indistinguishable from any activated macrophage. The final function necessary for in vivo initiation of T-cell immunity is migration to the LN. Expression of the chemokine receptor CCR7 is associated with migration to LN and has been reported for murine microglia (Dijkstra et al., 2006), but functional LN homing experiments were not performed.

In vivo studies suggest that brain APC function for presentation of peptides to CD4 T cells resides in a population of perivascular cells originally characterized by their radiosensitivity (Platten and Steinman, 2005). In fact, these cells may represent "differentiated" microglia that can express the DC marker CD11c and that morphologically resemble DCs (Fischer and Reichmann, 2001). However, phenotypic studies do not always allow extrapolation to function, and in different mouse models, CNS DC interactions with T cells have been defined as either stimulatory (Fischer and Reichmann, 2001; Ling et al., 2008) or inhibitory (Suter et al., 2003). Overall, these studies confirm that the plasticity of microglial cells may give rise to cells that resemble macrophages or DCs, but they do not give definitive answers for the origins and identity of the cell that is ultimately able to form the link between innate immune detection of malignancy in the brain and the induction of adaptive immunity in the LN. This could still be a conventional DC or a precursor recruited either from peripheral brain regions rich in CD11c-expressing cells (choroid plexus, meninges) or from venous blood in response to initial microglial and astroglial activation.

An alternative approach to address the issue of CNS to LN APC migration has been to inject labeled DCs in the brain and track their subsequent migration. Such approaches have in some cases confirmed migration to cervical LNs (Carson et al., 1999; Ehtesham et al., 2003; Karman et al., 2004; Kuwashima et al., 2005), although there may be limitations to the interpretation of such systems. First, the migratory behavior of injected DCs may not accurately reflect endogenous pathways, and second, the volume and site of injection within the CNS (brain parenchyma vs. ventricles) may influence the migration pattern (Bechmann et al., 2007; Hatterer et al., 2006; Thomas et al., 2008). However, despite these considerations, T-cell activation and expansion is observed in the cervical LNs in brain tumor models reliant on endogenous APCs (Calzascia et al., 2005; Prins et al., 2008b; Walter and Albert, 2007).

48.3.3 The Effector Phase of the T-Cell Mediated Antitumor Response: From the Lymph Node to the Brain

Activated T cells enriched for tumor specificity can be primed in various ways: in a spontaneous immune response, after vaccination, or even in vitro. But in all cases, to impact on the tumor, they need to enter the site harboring the malignancy, infiltrate the tumor bed, and exert their effector functions in the local tumor microenvironment. Although certain general properties of effector T cells apply to any tumor in any site, optimal antitumor function in the context of a cerebral malignancy requires specific features in the T-cell response.

48.3.3.1 T-Cell Entry to the Brain and Antigen Specificity

Most reports suggest that the principle factors influencing entry of T cells to the brain are the activation or differentiation status of the T cell, and the activation status of the vasculature. Nevertheless, an antigen-specific component of CD8 T-cell recruitment to brain was proposed in a study in which peptide was injected intracerebrally, then subsequently presented on the luminal surface of endothelial cells (Galea et al., 2007). However, it is currently unclear whether endothelial cells would be as efficient in phagocytosing and cross-presenting tumor-derived antigens as they are in presenting soluble peptide, and so it remains to be determined whether such a mechanism will have relevance for tumor immunity. Generally, there are considered to be more opportunities for T cells to interact with their specific antigen once they traverse the endothelium barrier, as demonstrated by the preferential retention in the brain of autoreactive and virus-specific CD4 T cells (Hickey, 1999) and of tumor specific CD8 T cells (Calzascia et al., 2003).

48.3.3.2 Antigen-Independent T-Cell Extravasation to the Brain

General features of leukocyte extravasation are common to all tissues because of similar hemodynamic constraints. The enormous velocity of the T cell in the bloodstream relative to the static endothelial cell forming the vessel structure is initially reduced by transient adhesive interactions between the T cell and the endothelium. Selectins (e.g., E-selectin, P-selectin) on the endothelium engage their ligands on T cells, slowing the flow of the T cells so that they begin to roll along the vessel wall. This facilitates contact between chemokine receptors on the T cell (such as CCR5) and corresponding immobilized chemokines on the luminal face of the endothelial cell (such as CCL5). Chemokine receptor signaling leads to conformational changes in T-cell-expressed integrins, allowing firm adhesion to the cell adhesion molecules on the endothelium, arrest, and diapedesis (Butcher et al., 1999). Tissue-specific combinations of adhesion molecules and chemokines allow selective recruitment of particular T-cell populations (Luster et al., 2005).

Many of the underlying concepts of immune cell entry into the CNS are based on CNS autoimmune conditions, principally multiple sclerosis (MS) in patients and experimental autoimmune encephalomyelitis (EAE) in mice (Engelhardt, 2006). This precious information may also apply to cerebral malignancies but will require validation. Indeed, there is a preponderance of information on CD4 T cells in EAE, but less on CD8 T cells, and furthermore, certain molecular considerations of homing are proposed to be influenced by the mouse strain, and the precise CNS region, factors that have not yet been addressed for tumors. Nevertheless, several key findings do now appear to apply to different strains, species, and neuropathologies (Table 48.1).

Table 48.1 Key adhesion molecules and chemokine receptors proposed for T-cell extravasation to the CNS

Receptor/molecule on T cell	Ligand/counterreceptor
Adhesion molecules*	
LFA-1 ($\alpha_L\beta_2$ integrin, CD11a/CD18)	ICAM-1, ICAM-2, JAM-A
$\alpha_4\beta_1$ integrin (VLA-4, CD49d/CD29)	VCAM-1, JAM-B
E- and P-selectin ligands (several, contain sialo-fucosylated Lewis carbohydrates)	E-selectin, P-selectin
CD6	ALCAM (CD166)
Chemokine receptors*	
CXCR3	CXCL9, CXCL10, CXCL11
CCR5	CCL3, CCL4, CCL5, CCL8, CCL3L1
CCR7	CCL19, CCL21

*Non-exhaustive listing, referring only to molecules discussed in text.

48.3.3.3 Role of Integrins in CNS Tropism

The adhesion molecule that is consistently implicated in T-cell entry to the CNS in most species and models tested is α_4 integrin (CD49d). Integrins are expressed as heterodimers and α_4 partners with either β_1 (CD29) or β_7 integrin chains. For the CNS, the $\alpha_4\beta_1$ integrin (also called VLA-4) and its interaction with VCAM-1 on endothelial cells are central. In EAE, $\alpha_4\beta_1$ may facilitate both lower affinity rolling interactions and higher affinity arrest, according to the particular CNS microvasculature involved (Engelhardt, 2006). In mouse brain tumor models, $\alpha_4\beta_1$ integrin was also shown to be a key molecule for T-cell entry to the tumor site. We found that high levels of $\alpha_4\beta_1$ integrin are induced on tumor-specific CD4 T cells (PRW and PYD unpublished data) and CD8 T cells (Calzascia et al., 2005), when they are primed by endogenous APC in the cervical LN of brain tumor-bearing mice. This was functionally relevant since α_4-specific blocking antibody significantly reduced brain entry of these T cells. Further exploration of the role of integrins in brain tropism has been performed on CD8 T cells polarized toward different cytokine-secreting profiles. Mouse CD8 T cells with a type 1 profile (IFN-γ-secreting) expressed higher levels of $\alpha_4\beta_1$ integrin and trafficked to the brain more efficiently than type 2, interleukin (IL)-4 secreting CD8 T cells (Sasaki et al., 2007). This finding is particularly relevant for brain tumor immunotherapy, since T cells receiving the same in vitro or in vivo stimuli can manifest two key characteristics for efficacious antitumor function: appropriate tissue tropism and cytokine expression. The same key $\alpha_4\beta_1$ integrin is also implicated in CNS entry of T cells in humans. Patients with MS receiving a novel treatment in which α_4 integrins were targeted using the humanized antibody natalizumab had reduced levels of inflammatory leukocytes in the cerebrospinal fluid, and generally showed some clinical improvement (Stuve et al., 2006). Taken together, the results from these different studies unequivocally establish an important role for $\alpha_4\beta_1$ integrin in T-cell homing to the CNS. However, this should not be interpreted to mean that $\alpha_4\beta_1$ specifically targets T cells to the brain, since most of the studies have analyzed a single tissue, the brain. Rather, it is likely that if $\alpha_4\beta_1$ integrin is abundantly expressed by a T cell; this molecule can facilitate entry to the CNS. Nevertheless, since the inhibition or blocking of $\alpha_4\beta_1$ does not totally abrogate T cell entry to the CNS, other molecules are probably also involved and may either substitute for or synergize with $\alpha_4\beta_1$.

48.3.3.4 Role of Non-integrin Adhesion Molecules

To date, there are mixed findings for the involvement of non-integrin adhesion molecules in T-cell entry to the CNS. Nearly all of this data derives from studies on EAE and MS, with findings that are often specific for particular CNS regions and specific stages of the disease. Roles in T-cell extravasation to brain tumors, either in spontaneous immunity or in immunotherapy applications, cannot be excluded. An induction of E- and P-selectin ligands on tumor-specific CD8 T cells dividing in the cervical LN was observed in mice harboring intracranial tumors, but the functional significance of this observation was not analyzed (Calzascia et al., 2005). P-selectin (and to a lesser extent, E-selectin) and their ligands were found to contribute to T-cell rolling on certain inflamed CNS microvessels using intravital microscopy and in vitro studies. This study concluded that CD8 T cells from MS patients preferentially rolled via P-selectin, whereas CD4 T cells rolled via α_4 integrin (Battistini et al., 2003). However, others have found that CNS inflammation was not altered following genetic ablation or overexpression of E- and P-selectins or their ligands, or after antibody blocking (Engelhardt, 2006). Therefore, the real in vivo significance of the selectins, at least in EAE, has been difficult to establish.

A further adhesion molecule that may influence T-cell adhesion to endothelium is lymphocyte function-associated antigen-1 (LFA-1), which is expressed by naïve and activated T cells. Intercellular adhesion molecules 1 and 2 (ICAM-1, ICAM-2) are the ligands for LFA-1 and are present either constitutively or after activation on CNS microvessels, including those of human glioma (Engelhardt, 2006; Kuppner et al., 1990). In vitro studies in EAE suggested potential roles for LFA-1 particularly during the transendothelial migration of T cells. In vivo experiments have been difficult to interpret, probably because LFA-1 and ICAM interactions are also critical for the immunological synapse that facilitates the antigen-specific interactions between T cells and APC or target cells.

A recent observation highlighted the role of activated leukocyte cell adhesion molecule (ALCAM) in facilitating CNS infiltration of T cells and monocytes (Cayrol et al., 2008). Expression of ALCAM was noted to be higher on BBB endothelial cells than endothelium from other organs, and it was upregulated in inflamed vasculature. Antibody blockade experiments showed that CD4 T cell and monocyte transmigration across brain endothelial cells was partially ALCAM dependent, and ALCAM neutralization in vivo reduced EAE severity. It was noteworthy that among the T cells, only the CD4 T-cell subset appears to use ALCAM during transmigration, since CD8 T cells were totally unaffected, even though they express similar levels of the CD6 ALCAM receptor. These findings, if confirmed in the context of brain tumor immunity, may open up future possibilities to modulate T-cell subset brain infiltration in future immunotherapies.

48.3.3.5 Role of Chemokines and Chemokine Receptors

Chemokines are low molecular weight chemoattractant cytokines that function by binding to G-protein coupled receptors expressed on a wide range of cells, including leukocytes. Unraveling the roles of individual chemokines (~50) and their receptors (~20) is complex because chemokines can bind multiple receptors, and receptors can bind multiple chemokines. Furthermore, in the context of brain tumors, the tumor itself is a source of chemokines which may influence the quantity and quality of the resulting immune infiltrate (Van Meir, 1999, Dey et al., 2006, Brown et al., 2007; Jordan et al., 2008). Chemokines are proposed to influence multiple steps of CNS infiltration, from the blood to migration within the brain parenchyma, although not all steps have been validated in vivo in the CNS (Rebenko-Moll et al., 2006). In the lumen of CNS microvessels, chemokines immobilized on endothelial cells can trigger integrin activation of tethered leukocytes (particularly $\alpha_4\beta_1$ in the context of brain tropic T cells) and facilitate high-affinity interactions and arrest. Diapedesis can then be promoted by chemokines mediating locomotion to interendothelial junctions. T cells may then sample abluminal chemokines by extending processes through intercellular junctions. And finally, chemokine gradients exist within the brain parenchyma to attract T cells to the tumor site.

Concerning the role of specific chemokines in T-cell infiltration of brain tumors, very few in vivo studies have been performed, and conclusions are mostly based on EAE, MS, or infection with neurotropic viruses (Rebenko-Moll et al., 2006). The proportion of T cells expressing CXCR3 is enhanced among T cells present in the cerebrospinal fluid of patients with MS and in EAE, and the levels of two of its ligands, CXCL9 and CXCL10, are elevated in the CSF during acute phase of MS. However, in vivo experiments with blocking antibodies and CXCR3 deficient mice have yielded conflicting results, probably because CXCR3 influences EAE at multiple levels (e.g., IFN-γ production) and not just at the level of trafficking. Similar considerations exist for CCR5 and its ligand CCL5, which are suggested to have roles in CNS viral infection (including West Nile virus, HIV, and coronavirus) but probably relate to T-cell function rather than trafficking. Another chemokine receptor expressed on T cells, CCR7, and its ligands CCL19 and CCL21 may have multiple roles in CNS pathologies. The cerebrospinal fluid of patients with MS and brain lesions of mice with progressive EAE accumulate CCR7-expressing T cells. Moreover, in addition, two ligands of CCR7, CCL19 and CCL21, are expressed at the BBB in brain of mice with EAE and at least in vitro, can mediate adhesion of $CCR7^+$ T cells. However, studying the in vivo functional significance of this is difficult when using blocking antibodies or gene deficient mice, since naïve T cells, a subset of memory T cells (Tcm), as well as some DCs, all express CCR7.

48.3.3.6 Suboptimal Trafficking of T Cells to Brain Tumors May Lead to Suboptimal Tumor Therapies

As the previous sections indicate, there is little direct data about the properties of protective T cells able to traffic efficiently to brain tumors. Nevertheless, the level of infiltration of tumor-specific T cells will be a factor that will limit the efficacy of immunotherapies. Many current tumor T-cell immunotherapy protocols are adapted directly from therapies being tested for tumors in other sites, and yet the tumor pathology is fundamentally different. The lethality of most extracranial tumors is due to metastases, and the goal of T-cell immunotherapy will be that therapeutic T cells can reach the many sites of tumor dissemination. For primary CNS malignancies such as malignant glioma, the situation is different; these tumors are unique in oncology because they very rarely metastasize from their tissue of origin. The immunological problem for such tumors is thus strictly one of regional immunity. Thus, promoting efficient brain tropism of *protective* immune cells will undoubtedly benefit future glioma immunotherapies. For this it will be necessary to not only understand and induce the key molecules for T cell-entry to the CNS but also avoid induction of a homing phenotype that may lead to their entrapment elsewhere (for example, the mucosal surfaces if there is high $\alpha_4\beta_7$ and CCR9 expression). In this regard, preclinical models in which multiple sites are studied will be helpful (Calzascia et al., 2005), for which the emerging technology of whole body imaging will be particularly appropriate (Prins et al., 2008b). A further refinement would be to ensure infiltration of only protective T cells, since a gross augmentation of any inflammatory infiltrate will be inappropriate and dangerous for the brain. An understanding of how subset-specific trafficking can be achieved would be a useful objective in the optimization of therapies.

48.3.4 The Effector Phase of the T-Cell Mediated Antitumor Response: At the Tumor Site

48.3.4.1 CD8 T Cells

In an idealized antitumor immune response, tumor-specific $CD8^+$ cytotoxic T lymphocytes (CTLs) that have penetrated the brain parenchyma and made contact with the tumor will kill malignant cells by direct cell-mediated cytotoxicity. This occurs in some preclinical brain tumor models, and to date, possibly for a minority of malignant cells forming the intracranial tumor mass in patients with glioma. If the CD8 T cell has been fully activated in the periphery, the tumor cell needs only to express MHC class I/peptide (costimulatory molecules are not essential at the effector stage) for it to become a CTL target. Cytotoxicity occurs by the polarized exocytosis of the contents of cytotoxic granules into the immunological synapse formed between the CTL and the tumor target, and it is exquisitely specific, with no bystander killing. The granule contents include perforin and granulysin that perturb the tumor cell membrane and serine proteases known as granzymes that induce tumor cell death mainly through caspase-dependent pathways. Secondary cytotoxic mechanisms also exist, through cell-associated or cell-secreted cytotoxic molecules, including Fas ligand (CD95L), tumor necrosis factor (TNF), and lymphotoxins (LTs).

Antitumor effects can also be mediated by CD8 T cells after indirect recognition of tumor derived antigenic peptides on MHC class I molecules of an APC, i.e., by cross-presentation. As already discussed, the role of APCs in priming CD8 T-cell responses in the LN is essential, but they may also have a role at the effector stage of the response. Indeed, local APCs can potentially amplify T-cell-mediated antitumor effects occurring at a low level after direct T cell-tumor cell contact (Karman et al., 2006; Masson et al., 2007), or they may substitute for this contact in the absence of direct antigen presentation by the tumor cell, for example, because of MHC downregulation. One of the key factors proposed for an indirect antitumor effect is IFN-γ, which impedes tumor growth by acting on IFN-γ receptor expressing tumor stroma and inhibiting angiogenesis (Qin et al., 2003).

Cross-presentation of antigen to CD8 T cells has been demonstrated in vitro by microglial cells (Beauvillain et al., 2008), but the principle cross-presenting APC in vivo is most likely to be the DC (Jung et al., 2002). Cross-presenting DCs in the brain have not yet been reported, to our knowledge, for human malignant glioma. One consequence of cross-presentation of antigen is that antigen-specific T cells will be retained at the site of this cellular interaction. Indeed, we observed retention of tumor-specific CD8 T cells in the brain in a mouse model designed to address the issue of cross-presentation (Calzascia et al., 2003). In this model, intracranially implanted MT539MG astrocytoma cells were unable to directly present a defined tumor antigen, and so the presentation of this tumor antigen to T cells in the brain was occurring solely through cross-presentation, although the identity of the APC in this study was not determined. In several other experimental situations, indirect stimulation of CD8 T cells at the tumor site has been achieved by intracranial injection of DCs (Ehtesham et al., 2003; Kikuchi et al., 2002; Masson et al., 2007; Nishimura et al., 2006; Pellegatta et al., 2006). The local functions of these cells may be to enhance T-cell proliferation at the tumor site, promote T-cell retention in the brain, and/or to amplify effector functions such as IFN-γ release.

48.3.4.2 CD4 T Cells

The role of CD4 T cells in brain tumor immunity is complex, because CD4 T cells can differentiate toward at least four different subsets (T_h1, T_h2, T_h17, and T_{reg}) that are difficult to identify phenotypically and that can have either pro- or antitumor effects. Moreover, very few (if any) glioma antigens recognized by CD4 T cells have been identified. Nevertheless, it is assumed that an IFN-γ-secreting CD4 Th1 cell component of brain tumor immunity may have antitumor activity and potentially aid CD8 T-cell accumulation, survival, and function, as has been demonstrated in certain (but not all) rodent models (Ciesielski et al., 2008; Wang et al., 2007).

48.4 Glioma Immune Escape

The inevitable progressive growth of malignant glioma indicates that the idealized T-cell mediated antitumor response does not occur spontaneously or that it is neutralized by the time high-grade gliomas are clinically detectable. There are a multitude of passive and active immune escape mechanisms that are proposed to explain this and which may have contributed to the impaired cellular immune function in glioma patients that has been reported for decades (Walker et al., 2003). However, these are putative mechanisms that have not yet been validated in vivo for malignant glioma in patients, with the exception of transforming growth factor (TGF)-β, as will be discussed. Arguably, what may be equally important is the low-level induction of spontaneous antitumor immunity and the non-immunological treatments (radiotherapy, chemotherapy, steroidal anti-inflammatory drugs) that may antagonize any nascent protective immune response.

48.4.1 Passive Immune Escape Mechanisms

Gliomas may attempt to passively escape immune detection by downregulation of MHC expression or of molecules associated with antigen presentation to CD8 T cells. Interestingly, these characteristics are associated with higher grade astrocytomas (Facoetti et al., 2005; Mehling et al., 2007). Of importance for future immunotherapy strategies are the in vitro observations that MHC can be upregulated on glioblastoma cell lines by IFN-γ or IFN-α (Yang et al., 2004). Tumor cells escaping T-cell mediated immunity by downregulating MHC expression may risk attack by NK cells, which are normally inactive if their inhibitory receptors are ligated by MHC. However, several adaptations of malignant glioma may guard against this. Expression of MICA and ULBP2, ligands for the NKGD activating receptors on NK cells, was low or absent for WHO grade III and IV astrocytomas (Eisele et al., 2006), whereas an array of ligands (HLA-E, HLA-G, lectin-like transcript-1) for inhibitory NK receptors was overexpressed (Roth et al., 2007; Wischhusen et al., 2007). A further major consideration that can be considered as a factor leading to immune escape is the presence of areas of hypoxia, well documented in human glioma (Louis, 2006). These areas of tumor will be a particularly hostile microenvironment for immune cells, and the function and survival of T cells may be particularly sensitive to low oxygen tension (Sitkovsky and Lukashev, 2005).

48.4.2 Active Immune Escape

Caution should be exercised in interpreting the role of "immunosuppressive" molecules. Immunosuppressive effects have often been established in vitro or in some cases in vivo with ectopic overexpression of the molecule under test. The ultimate in vivo role will depend upon the microenvironmental context, and the level of expression, which may be very different in the human pathology and in animal models. Much ingenuity will be needed to determine whether these molecules will really influence human glioma pathogenesis and response to treatment, and in the meantime, our conclusions must remain provisional.

48.4.2.1 Soluble Immunosuppresive Molecules

Soluble factors can act either directly on the effector T cell or through recruitment of a third party "immunosuppressive" cell. In some cases, the same molecule may function in multiple ways, the most notorious example of which is TGF-β. This multifunctional cytokine not only directly suppresses NK and T-cell proliferation and antitumor functions (including granzyme, FasL and IFN-γ expression) but also promotes other suppressive cells (see below), angiogenesis, and tumor invasion (Wrzesinski et al., 2007). TGF-β (and in particular the TGF-β_2 isoform) is produced by glioma cell lines and by glioblastoma in vivo (Bodmer et al., 1989; Liau et al., 2005). Moreover, in a phase I DC vaccination trial for glioblastoma, we noted increased intratumoral infiltration by CTLs in four of eight patients who underwent reoperation after vaccination, which was inversely correlated with TGF-β_2 expression within the tumor and positively correlated with clinical survival ($P = 0.047$) (Liau et al., 2005). Consequently, TGF-β or its effects have become attractive targets, and novel therapeutic approaches with inhibitors and antisense oligonucleotides are being actively explored. Other soluble factors of astrocytoma origin that may have immunosuppressive potential include prostaglandin E_2, gangliosides, and IL-10 (Walker et al., 2003), but the real in vivo concentration and impact of these factors has yet to be firmly established.

48.4.2.2 Cell Surface Immunosuppressive Factors

A candidate immunosuppressive molecule is Fas ligand (CD95L), which is involved in immune homeostasis and cytotoxicity by inducing apoptosis in target cells. Gliomas express Fas ligand in vitro and in vivo. In vitro, Fas ligand expressing glioma cell lines can kill Fas (CD95) expressing CD4 and CD8 T cell lines from the autologous donor, but in vivo, the role of Fas ligand expressing tumor cells is controversial (Walker et al., 2003, 1997). Gliomas also express B7-H1 (also called PD-L1), a member of the B7 family that is able to interact with T-cell expressed programed death-1 (PD-1) receptor expressed by T cells (Wilmotte et al., 2005; Wintterle et al., 2003), an interaction which negatively regulates T-cell activation. Interestingly, the expression of B7-H1 has been associated with a genetic event in gliomas, the loss of the tumor suppressor PTEN, which activates the PI3 kinase pathway (Parsa et al., 2007). The immunosuppressive potential of PD-1-B7-H1 interactions in vivo has yet to be explored in intracranial tumors. CD70 is another cell surface molecule proposed to facilitate glioma immune escape as it can engage the counterreceptor on immune cells and induce apoptosis. CD70 is expressed by glioma in vitro and can indeed trigger apoptosis of immune cells (reviewed by (Walker et al., 2003)). However, the first in vivo studies of gliomas transfected with CD70 indicated an immune stimulatory role, and the authors even suggested exploiting the CD70–CD27 axis in immunotherapy (Aulwurm et al., 2006). The role of CD70 expressed by non-manipulated human glioma in vivo therefore awaits clarification.

48.4.2.3 Immunosuppressive Cells

In recent years, there has been a major resurgence in the interest and understanding of cellular-based mechanisms that may regulate or suppress tumor immunity. Cells of different origin (see below) can be involved in suppressing immune responses and have valuable roles in regulating autimmmunity and controlling inflammation. However, these functions may also blunt spontaneous or vaccine-induced tumor immunity. Furthermore, immunosuppressive cells can in some cases be recruited or induced by factors (e.g., cytokines such as TGF-β) produced by tumor cells. Mesenchymal stem cells have strong anti-inflammatory or antiproliferative effects on immune cells but may increase glioma cell proliferation. They are attracted by glioma culture supernatant and purified factors including IL-8, VEGF, and TGF-β (Birnbaum et al., 2007), but in vivo immunosuppressive roles in glioma remain to be determined. Myeloid-derived suppressor cells are another potentially immunosuppressive cell type receiving increasing attention in the context of cancer, and it is noteworthy that they are stimulated by prostaglandin E_2, which can be secreted by glioma cells (Marx, 2008). Myeloid-derived suppressor cells have also been studied in the context of brain tumor models (Prins et al., 2002), although little is known about their presence at the brain tumor site in patients.

The cellular mediator of immune suppression that is currently the most studied in cancer is the $CD4^+CD25^+$ regulatory T cell (T_{reg}), which is the best-defined T suppressor cell (Sakaguchi et al., 2008). Either T_{regs} are produced as a functionally mature T-cell subset in the thymus (natural Tregs) or other naïve CD4 T cells can differentiate into induced T_{regs} under the influence of certain cytokines including TGF-β and IL-2. The role of T_{regs} in immune homeostasis is now well defined. They maintain immunological tolerance to self-antigens, and mutations leading to their absence in animals (Scurfy mice) or patients (IPEX), or their inhibition or ablation, leads to autoimmune and inflammatory disease. T_{regs} function by an array of cell contact and cytokine-mediated mechanisms to suppress T cells, B cells, NK cells, macrophages, and DCs at both the induction and effector stages of immune responses. In the context of malignancy, T_{regs} accumulate in many tumors, including human glioma (El Andaloussi and Lesniak, 2007; Fecci et al., 2006a; Hussain et al., 2006), and T_{reg} depletion or inhibition in murine brain tumor models can reveal spontaneous tumor immunity, or enhance induced immunity (Curtin et al., 2008; El Andaloussi et al., 2006; Fecci et al., 2006b; Grauer et al., 2007). While the importance of T_{reg} in the antiglioma immune response is widely accepted, there are many challenges in identifying and modulating these cells. Foremost is the lack of a unique marker to identify T_{regs}. Most markers are shared with activated effector T cells (e.g., CD25), and the best specific T_{reg} marker in mice (the transcription factor Foxp3) is intracellular (and so inaccessible to antibodies in vivo), and expression is not restricted to T_{reg} in human T cells.

48.5 Identification of Glioma-Associated Antigens

Advancing our understanding of the mechanisms underlying the induction of an immune effector response against the tumor, and how it may sometimes be compromised, is only possible if we are able to define the specificity of tumor immunity. This is a major and ongoing challenge for human glioma.

48.5.1 Identifying Tumor-Associated-Antigens ("Reverse Immunology")

Significant progress in defining the nature of the antitumor response has been made by the discovery and characterization of TAAs, beginning with the report of the first melanoma antigen (MAGE) in 1991 (Van den Eynde et al., 1995; van der Bruggen et al., 1991). Intensive research is underway into the use of TAAs as potential targets of immune-based cancer treatments. The key TAAs under investigation are MAGE-3, MART-1, tyrosinase, TRP-2, and gp100 for melanoma (Panelli et al., 2000; Parkhurst et al., 1998, 1996; Ribas, 2006; Ribas et al., 2000); PSA and PAP for prostate cancer (Murphy et al., 1996 1999); survivin for many solid tumors (Katoh et al., 2003); and HER-2/neu for breast and ovarian cancers (Disis et al., 2002, 2004; Knutson and Disis, 2001; Knutson et al., 2001). A prominent issue that distinguishes cerebral malignancies from other tumors, such as melanoma, is the paucity of well-defined tumor-specific antigens. Indeed, the difficulties of immune response monitoring are particularly acute in patients with malignant gliomas because, in contrast to patients with melanoma, there are few extensively characterized tumor antigens that can be recognized by T cells. Unless advances in this domain occur, rational advances in immune-based brain tumor therapy may be significantly hampered.

In recent years, genome-wide techniques have dramatically accelerated our ability to obtain molecular profiles of gene defects in gliomas, resulting in a more readily accessible source of information on the genes and gene products that produce antigens (TCGA, 2008). Advances in brain tumor "immunomics" have led to the recent identification of several TAAs expressed by human gliomas. These include tumor-specific antigens unique to the oncogenic transformation process (EGFRvIII) or overexpressed following activation of oncogenic pathways (EphA2, IL-13Rα) (Husain et al., 2001; Kuwashima et al., 2005; Okano et al., 2002; Saikali et al., 2007; Shimato et al., 2008; Wu et al., 2006) (see also Chapter 35), cancer-testes antigens normally expressed only during development (cancer-testes antigens; NY-ESO-1, MAGE, GAGE, SART, SSX) (Bodey et al., 2008; Chi et al., 1997; Sahin et al., 2000), neuroectodermal antigens involved in pigment synthesis (e.g., melanoma-associated antigens; gp100, tyrosinase, TRP-1, TRP-2) (Liu et al., 2004a, b; Saikali et al., 2007; Zhang et al., 2008), and other antigens associated with proliferation and cell survival (hTERT, Survivin, B-cyclin, Her-2/neu) (Katoh et al., 2003; Liu et al.,

2004a; Saikali et al., 2007; Ueda et al., 2007; Zhang et al., 2008). Recent studies have additionally suggested that many human gliomas are latently infected with human cytomegalovirus (CMV) (Cobbs et al., 2002; Mitchell et al., 2008), and that CMV may be a clinically relevant target for immune-based therapies (Prins et al., 2008a).

Many TAAs were originally identified via serological analysis of tumor antigens by recombinant cDNA expression cloning (SEREX) in immunogenic solid tumors such as melanoma (Chen et al., 1997). A similar attempt to identify antigens recognized by the immune system in an IL-4-secreting rat 9L glioma immunization successfully identified mouse Id-associated protein 1 (MIDA) as an antigen that could induce antitumor immunity (Okada et al., 2001). In human gliomas, however, attempts to identify T-cell antigens have been less successful (Pallasch et al., 2005; Schmits et al., 2002). Nevertheless, some recent studies have demonstrated that many established human glioma cell lines express well-characterized TAAs that can be recognized by antigen-specific $CD8^+$ T cells (Zhang et al., 2007). Interestingly, the pattern of antigen expression seems to differ between adult and pediatric human gliomas (Okada et al., 2008; Zhang et al., 2008).

48.5.2 Microarray Technology and Tumor-Associated-Antigens

With the rapid advances provided by high throughput microarray chip technology, the entire compendium of genes showing elevated expression in tumors will soon be established, and the repertoire of potential glioma-specific antigens defined (Horvath et al., 2006; Liau et al., 2000; Mischel et al., 2003a, b). Furthermore, recent progress in our understanding of tumor immunology can link the information generated from gene-expression profiling of CNS tumors to the identification of precise immunogenic epitopes that can serve as useful targets for specific immunotherapy (Freije et al., 2004). For instance, since T cells can only recognize antigens in the context of MHC, tumor-associated genes can be scrutinized for amino acid sequences that can interact with relevant MHC molecules and efficiently bind via the proteosomal degradation system. Candidate tumor-specific peptide epitopes for CTLs can now be identified using available computer algorithms that predict the MHC binding affinities of specific peptide and epitope sequences (http://bimas.dcrt.nih.gov/molbio/hla_bind/, http://www.uni-tuebingen.de/uni/kxi/). By subsequently testing the stability of MHC molecules with candidate tumor-specific peptides in vitro, an estimation of the potential immunogenicity of an in silico-identified antigen can be determined (Maecker et al., 2001). The immunogenicity of human cancer genes or their predicted CTL peptide epitopes can also be assessed in animal models using HLA transgenic mice (Butterfield et al., 2001), providing even better estimates for immunotherapy targets in vivo. Recently, experiments involving the screening of human tumor samples for CTL reactivity have identified human glioma-associated antigen epitopes to EphA2 and IL13Rα specifically recognized by the immune system and associated with extended survival (Okano et al., 2002; Ueda et al., 2007). Based on these recent advances, it is suggested that cancer genomics can be directly linked to tumor immunotherapy by "reverse immunology," which paves the way for the design of new, more specific targets for brain tumor immunotherapy.

48.6 Preclinical Studies of T-Cell Immunity to Target Brain Tumors

48.6.1 Passive Immunotherapy

48.6.1.1 Adoptive Transfer

Adoptive transfer of immune cells is the introduction (adoption) into the patient of either autologous or allogeneic immune cells that may, or may not, have been stimulated in vitro with tumor antigens (Mitchell et al., 2003). Sometimes, these cells are injected into the tumor cavity to maximize the exposure of the infused cells to tumor cells, while other strategies call for systemic infusion. Cytolytic effector cells are cultured in vitro with cytokines to activate them to attack tumor tissue in vivo. This approach was not clinically applicable until the discovery of IL-2 and other cytokines that modulate T-cell growth and survival. Before that time, it was not possible to obtain sufficient numbers of immune cells and maintain them in culture during the in vitro sensitization period. IL-2, originally called T-cell growth factor, is a cytokine that mediates lymphocyte activation and stimulates division.

In recent years, the ability to adoptively transfer defined tumor antigen-specific T cells has greatly increased our knowledge of critical homing markers, cytokine dependence and in vivo trafficking patterns necessary to target and eradicate tumors in the brain. Preclinical studies in rat and murine glioma models first demonstrated that polyclonal, glioma-specific T cells could eradicate CNS gliomas (Baldwin et al., 1997; Kruse et al., 1990; Plautz et al., 1997; Rice et al., 1997) and was associated with enhanced trafficking of these lymphocytes to the brain (Hazelrigg et al., 2002). Subsequent work demonstrated that the draining LN population, from which these lymphocytes are isolated, also includes suppressor populations that can impair the efficacy of the adoptively transferred population (Peng et al., 2002). Removal of the CD62L^{high} population enriched the lymphocyte population with enhanced antitumor activity (Plautz et al., 1997). This contrasts with other recent studies on adoptive immunity, in which clonally derived CD8$^+$ T lymphocytes were used. In this case, the CD62L$^+$ population identified CD8$^+$ T cells of the central memory phenotype that possess enhanced trafficking, expansion, and survival (Klebanoff et al., 2005). Different models may account for the differences observed but suggest that careful characterization of the cellular infusate is critical for antitumor activity.

48.6.1.2 Cytokines

Cytokines can influence the priming of tumor antigen-specific T cells prior to adoptive transfer and subsequently alter their homing patterns, survival, and antitumor activity. In an adoptive transfer model where antigen-specific $CD8^+$ T cells were polarized to a type 1 (Tc1) cytokine profile using IL-12 and blocking antibodies to IL-4 (Nishimura et al., 2006), the T cells showed preferential homing to intracranial tumors (probably due to high expression of VLA-4/$\alpha_4\beta_1$ integrin, as discussed above) and enhanced antitumor efficacy (Sasaki et al., 2007). Other work has demonstrated that chemokines, such as tumor-derived monocyte chemotactic protein-1 (MCP-1) (Desbaillets et al., 1999), can be sufficient to mediate the tropism of tumor-specific T cells to intracranial tumors (Brown et al., 2007). Most recent studies have also demonstrated that tumor-specific $CD8^+$ T cells primed with antigen, IL-2, and IL-15 can lead to enhanced trafficking to intracranial tumors and migration through the cervical LNs, spleen, and bone marrow (Prins et al., 2008b). In this adoptive transfer setting, endogenous host cytokines are also important for the survival and effector functions of the transferred cells. Host lymphodepletion, via whole body radiation or cytotoxic chemotherapy, can facilitate the homeostatic expansion of adoptively transferred T cells by improved competition for endogenous cytokines (Gattinoni et al., 2005), such as IL-7 and IL-15, eliminating endogenous regulatory T cells (Chang et al., 1986) and/or enhancing the intratumoral accumulation of the transferred cells (Wang et al., 2005).

48.6.1.3 Toll- Like Receptor Agonists

More recent work has demonstrated that TLR agonists, such as imiquimod (Prins et al., 2006b) and STAT-3 inhibitors (Fujita et al., 2008) can increase serum cytokines and enhance the antitumor activity of adoptively transferred T cells in intracranial tumor-bearing mice. Such studies collectively suggest that the cytokine microenvironment can impose phenotypic changes on tumor-specific T cells that can alter their in vivo trafficking patterns, function, and tropism for tumors growing in anatomically distinct compartments.

48.6.2 Active Immunotherapy (Tumor Vaccines)

Active immunotherapy strategies (tumor vaccines) require administration of the antigenic material to induce an (primary) immune response, in effect, a vaccination. Most tumor antigens are poor immunogens, and thus active immunotherapy usually includes the use of an “adjuvant” (e.g., *Bacille*

Calmette-Guerin or cytokines) that enhances the immune response by prolonging the time of exposure to antigen and by increasing the activity of APCs. DC-based therapies are one type of active immunotherapy (Liau et al., 1999). Other approaches have included irradiated whole tumor cell vaccines and cytokine immuno-gene therapy strategies (Glick et al., 2001; Okada et al., 2003).

48.6.2.1 Dendritic Cell-Based Vaccines

As discussed earlier, DCs are the most potent APCs in the body, due in part to their high expression of MHC class I and II, and costimulatory molecules, and their secretion of cytokines that promote T cell priming (e.g., IL-12). Immune activation by DCs facilitates engagement of all effector mechanisms of the immune system, such as CTLs and $CD4^+$ helper T cells (T_h), as well as NK cells and antibodies. The use of DCs for cancer immunotherapy became feasible a decade ago with the advent of new techniques to grow these cells from bone marrow precursors in animals (Thurner et al., 1999) and from $CD14^+$ monocytes in human peripheral blood (Kiertscher and Roth, 1996). These advantages prompted a wide array of preclinical studies to define the constraints and mechanisms by which DC can prime tumor-specific T-cell responses.

DC-based immunotherapy can accommodate many different forms of antigen, but chief among them is the use of materials derived from autologous tumor cells. DC pulsed with tumor-eluted peptides (Liau et al., 1999), apoptotic/necrotic tumor cells (Siesjo et al., 1996), tumor lysates (Aoki et al., 2001; Ni et al., 2001; Pellegatta et al., 2006), tumor-derived RNA (Insug et al., 2002), and even glioma neurospheres (Pellegatta et al., 2006) can induce relevant antitumor immunity for tumors in the brain. The advantage of using such materials is that this approach is applicable against neoplasms for which immunogenic tumor-specific or tumor-associated antigens are unknown. The disadvantages, however, are that such autologous tumor extracts may be heterogeneous and are therefore difficult to characterize and quantitate. Also, the use of unfractionated tumor material may lead to relatively low concentrations of effective immunogens in the mixture, as antigenic tumor peptides may conceivably be diluted by relatively non-immunogenic proteins and thereby lower the immunogenicity of the vaccine. Furthermore, a risk for inducing immunity against self-antigens that may lead to autoimmune encephalitis is real (Bigner et al., 1981).

Alternative forms of antigen loading for DC-based vaccines include the use of defined peptides and genetic transfection (Morse et al., 2005; Ribas, 2006). As such, it was demonstrated that tumor-specific, MHC class I-restricted peptides can be pulsed onto DCs and used to induce significant antitumor immunity to intracranial tumors (Ciesielski et al., 2008; Hatano et al., 2004; Heimberger et al., 2002, 2003; Prins et al., 2003). Similarly, viral transduction of DCs with tumor antigens (Broder et al., 2003), cytokines (Kim et al., 2006; Tsugawa et al., 2004; Yamanaka et al., 2003b), and/or fusions of DCs and tumor cells (Kjaergaard et al., 2005) has generated antitumor immunity that is being translated into clinical trials. Currently, DCs are recognized as a promising vehicle for active immunotherapy of cancer. Numerous animal experiments have demonstrated the potential of DC-based immunotherapy in both protecting mice from tumor formation and eliminating established tumors. However, other work has shown that DC vaccination is more effective at priming tumor-specific T-cell responses but relatively inefficient for boosting the same response (Jouanneau et al., 2006). Thus, there is a rationale for incorporating DC vaccination with chemotherapy, adjuvants, and/or viral vectors that may synergize to induce therapeutic antitumor immunity.

48.6.2.2 Adjuvants

It is becoming clear from preclinical studies and human trials that enhancement of DC vaccines with adjuvants will be required to generate an antitumor immune response that is both reproducibly effective and long lasting. DCs express numerous TLRs (see above) that are important in host defense against bacteria and other microbial pathogens (Barrat and Coffman, 2008; Barton and Medzhitov, 2002; Pulendran, 2005). Stimulation of TLRs ultimately results in gene expression profiles that lead to the production of cytokines including TNF-α, IL-1, IL-6, and IL-12 as well as type I and type II IFNs (IFN-α and IFN-γ) (Barton and Medzhitov, 2002; Pulendran, 2005). TLR ligation on DC induces a maturational signal that can up-regulate MHC and costimulatory molecule expression, induce migration to LNs, and induce expression of cytokines that can promote and enhance T-cell priming against tumors (Steinman and Banchereau, 2007). Since it is commonly believed that activated DCs can prime T-cell responses more effectively (Steinman and Banchereau, 2007), numerous groups have utilized adjuvants to effectively mature DCs for cancer immunotherapy. For example, the TLR-7 agonist, imiquimod (Aldara®), could synergize with peptide-pulsed DC vaccination paradigms to induce effective antitumor immunity to intracranial tumors (Prins et al., 2006b). Imiquimod enhanced not only DC survival and trafficking to LNs but also the priming of self, tumor antigen-specific T cells (Prins et al., 2006b). Similar findings were reported with poly-ICLC, a TLR-3 agonist (Zhu et al., 2007), and CpG, a TLR-9 agonist (Wu et al., 2007).

48.6.2.3 Blocking Regulatory T Cells (T_{regs})

The blockade of immuno-inhibitory molecules can also generate antitumor immunity and/or synergize with active vaccination approaches for the treatment of CNS tumors. T_{regs} (see above) have recently been shown to accumulate in the peripheral blood and tumors of mice (Grauer et al., 2007) and patients (El Andaloussi and Lesniak, 2007; Fecci et al., 2006a) with malignant glioma, and this was associated with the degree of malignancy and immune competency (El Andaloussi and Lesniak, 2007; Fecci et al., 2006a; Heimberger et al., 2008; Learn et al., 2006). These data suggest that a tumor-derived factor may influence this type of immune evasion so as to prevent proper immune surveillance of tumors arising in the CNS. As such, recent studies have demonstrated that blockade of the negative costimulatory molecule, CTLA-4, can ameliorate changes to the $CD4^+$ T-cell compartment and confer long-term survival in intracranial tumor-bearing animals (Fecci et al., 2007). Similarly, others have recently demonstrated that functional blockade of T_{regs} with in vivo CD25 mAb administration can enhance the antitumor immunity to vaccines in a prophylactic setting (Fecci et al., 2006b; Grauer et al., 2008). However, these studies highlight the difficulties of T_{reg} depletion, since the CD25 mAb (PC61) used therein can also bind and inhibit activated T cells, completely removing any beneficial effect of an active vaccination immunotherapy in established intracranial tumor-bearing mice (Curtin et al., 2008). Such studies highlight the importance of the T-cell compartment in CNS tumor immunity. New methodologies are being explored to functionally reverse the T_{reg} influence in combination with antitumor vaccination strategies.

48.6.2.4 Immune Gene Therapy

Other studies of cancer vaccines have used irradiated whole tumor cells modified with cytokine genes (reviewed in (Okada and Pollack, 2004)), viral vectors (reviewed in (Curtin et al., 2005)), or even live, attenuated bacterial vectors (Liau et al., 2002; Prins et al., 2006a) to generate antitumor immunity. The pioneering cytokine gene therapy studies performed over a decade ago demonstrated that cytokine-secreting tumor cells could induce antitumor immunity. With CNS tumor models, cytokine-gene therapy studies have been able to demonstrate efficacious antitumor immunity to intracranial gliomas by induction of IL-2, IL-4, IL-6, IL-7, IL-12, GM-CSF, mM-CSF, and IFN-$\alpha/\beta/\gamma$ (Glick et al., 2001, Dey et al., 2006). Such cytokine-secreting tumors revealed that multiple facets of the cellular immune response could be mobilized to induce antitumor immunity. Other groups have utilized intracranial injections of viral vectors, which encode cytokines and/or conditional cytotoxicity (HSV-TK) (Ali et al., 2005; Curtin et al., 2005) (see also Chapters 46 and 47).

48.6.2.5 Bacterial/Viral-Based Vaccines

Live bacteria and/or viruses may also serve as the basis for active immunotherapies against brain tumors (Chabalgoity et al., 2002). Viral/bacterial infections and the resulting tissue damage can also provide the appropriate "danger signals" (Matzinger, 1994) to attract professional APC necessary for adequate antigen presentation. CTL-mediated immunity can be induced using live, attenuated bacterial or viral vectors that both stimulate the innate immune system and simultaneously deliver antigens (Chabalgoity et al., 2002).

For instance, *Listeria monocytogenes (LM)* is a facultative, gram-positive intracellular bacterium that is able to enter host cells, escape from the endocytic vesicle, multiply within the cytoplasm, and spread directly from cell to cell without encountering the extracellular milieu. Antigens expressed by *LM* can access both MHC class I and class II processing pathways and are presented to both $CD8^+$ and $CD4^+$ T cells. Additionally, *LM* has been shown to stimulate TLRs (Barton and Medzhitov, 2002) on the surface of APC and activate internal pattern recognition molecules, which may contribute to its immuno-stimulatory action (Ulevitch, 2004). In published studies, it has been demonstrated that immunization with an attenuated, recombinant *Listeria monocytogenes (rLM)* expressing the lymphocytic choriomeningitis virus nucleoprotein (LCMV-NP) led to the rejection of a glioma expressing the heterologous NP antigen (Liau et al., 2002). Interestingly, animals clearing these tumors were subsequently immune to re-challenge with subcutaneous and intracranial glioma cells that did not express NP, suggesting that epitope spreading had occurred, which is a phenomenon whereby T cells can recognize other endogenous glioma epitopes along with the targeted antigen(s) (Liau et al., 2002). Given the heterogeneity of human brain tumors and the possibility for the immune escape, exploiting the process of epitope spreading will be valuable in the clinical context of future tumor vaccine design. These studies reveal the complexity of the multiple mechanisms by which antitumor immunity can be generated.

48.7 Clinical Trials of Cellular Immunotherapy for Brain Tumors

48.7.1 Lymphokine-Activated Killer Cells

The majority of previous clinical adoptive immunotherapy trials for brain tumors have employed lymphokine-activated killer (LAK) or mitogen-activated killer cells. LAK cells are peripheral blood lymphocytes functionally defined by their ability to lyse NK-resistant tumor targets in vitro following stimulation with IL-2 and/or mitogens. LAK cells have been implanted into the resection cavity during surgery (Dillman et al., 2004; Hayes et al., 1995; Merchant et al., 1988a, b), and sporadic clinical responses were observed. However, LAK cell therapy is nonspecific in that the cells are not stimulated in vitro with any glioma-specific antigens. The limitations of LAK cell adoptive transfer to eradicate tumor cells in clinical trials may be due to its inherent non-specificity, the fact that cells do not migrate efficiently to tumor sites, and/or the induction of diffuse cerebral edema from IL-2 and other cytokines.

48.7.2 Cytotoxic T Lymphocytes

One refinement to the previous adoptive transfer approaches is to stimulate lymphocytes in vivo with autologous tumor cells to generate MHC class I-restricted CTLs that are then expanded in vitro and re-infused into patients

(Kruse et al., 1997; Merchant et al., 1997). The theory is that antigen-stimulated CTLs would be more specific than LAK cells. Clinical trials using adoptive transfer of activated CTLs have produced somewhat encouraging initial results (Kruse et al., 1997; Plautz et al., 2000; Wood et al., 2000). However, because these pilot phase I trials were designed primarily to demonstrate feasibility and safety, definitive evaluation of efficacy will require further study.

Often, pilot trials of adoptive immunotherapy have suggested efficacy (Ishikawa et al., 2004; Quattrocchi et al., 1999), but they have not been followed up with phase II or III larger trials designed to show true improvement in survival. Adoptive transfer studies in melanoma have been particularly encouraging, and currently ~50% of treated patients will have an objective clinical response by RECIST criteria (Dudley et al., 2005). However, the ability to clone and expand high-affinity tumor-infiltrating lymphocytes is currently restricted to a few centers.

A newer option that may become feasible in the future, when glioma-specific TCRs are cloned, will be to use genetic engineering to specifically confer tumor recognition to normal lymphocytes (Morgan et al., 2006). Alternatively, the use of bispecific antibodies, which have the potential to engage all CTLs in patients for lysis of cancer cells, may have therapeutic potential for the treatment of malignant diseases. Contrary to other antibody-based approaches, which call for injection of massive doses of purified antibodies, a recent study has shown tumor regression in non-Hodgkin's lymphoma patients by treating patients with very low doses of recombinant bispecific antibodies (blinatumomab), which render the cancer cells sensitive to almost all CTLs that they may encounter (Bargou et al., 2008). Conceivably, such bispecific single-chain antibodies, where one variable region recognizes an antigen on tumor cells and the other variable region binds to CD3, may be engineered for solid tumors, such as malignant gliomas.

Overall, it appears that adoptive immunotherapy may offer certain advantages that active vaccination strategies cannot provide: (1) T cells are expanded in the absence of tumor-derived soluble factors and (2) CTLs can be grown to extremely large numbers sufficient for infusion (Wang et al., 2004). A summary of recently published clinical trials of adoptive cellular immunotherapy for malignant gliomas is presented in Table 48.2.

48.7.3 Dendritic Cell Vaccination Trials

Approaches that combine adoptive transfer of antigen-pulsed DCs for tumor vaccination in malignant glioma patients are currently under active investigation at several different centers around the world (Caruso et al., 2004; De Vleeschouwer et al., 2008; Kikuchi et al., 2004, 2001; Liau et al., 2005; Yamanaka et al., 2003a, 2005; Yu et al., 2004; Yu et al., 2001). This strategy involves ex vivo exposure of a patient's DCs to their tumor antigen followed by their in vivo infusion to stimulate an endogenous immune response (Liau et al., 1999; Prins et al., 2003). The theory behind this therapeutic strategy is based

Table 48.2 Summary of clinical trials of *adoptive* cellular immunotherapy for malignant gliomas

Therapy	Phase	Tumor HISTOLOGY	Responses	Survival	References
Allo-CTL + IL-2	Phase I ($n = 5$)	GBM (2); AA (1); AO (2) [recurrent]	NR	AA/AO patients with SD > 28 months	Kruse et al. (1997)
TILs + IL-2	Phase I ($n = 6$)	GBM; AA [recurrent]	1 CR; 2 PR	NR	Quattrocchi et al. (1999)
Activated CTL from lymph nodes	Phase I ($n = 12$)	GBM (6); AA(4); LGA (2) [newly diagnosed]	4 PR	3 patients > 2 yr	Plautz et al. (2000)
Activated CTL from PBMC	Phase I ($n = 9$)	GBM; AA [recurrent]	3 PR	2/9 patients > 4 yr	Wood et al. (2000)
LAK cells + IL-2	Phase I ($n = 28$)	GBM; AA [recurrent]	Lymphocytic infiltration; locally ↑ IL-2 & IFN-γ	6/28 patients > 2 yr	Hayes et al. (2001)
NK cells	Phase I ($n = 9$)	GBM (3); AA (6) [recurrent]	3 PR; 2 MR	NR	Ishikawa et al. (2004)
LAK cells	Phase I ($n = 40$)	GBM [recurrent]	NR	34% 1-yr survival; Median OS = 17.5 months	Dillman et al. (2004)

TIL = tumor-infiltrating lymphocyte; GBM = glioblastoma multiforme; AA = anaplastic astrocytoma; AO = anaplastic oligodendroglioma; LGA = low-grade (grade II) astrocytoma; PFS = progression-free survival; CR = complete response; PR = partial response; MR = minimal response; OS = overall survival; NR = not reported.

upon evidence that tumor cells are poor APCs, and do not adequately stimulate endogenous professional APCs. The lack of immune activation may affect not only $CD8^+$ T cells but also the $CD4^+$ "helper" T cells (T_h) that require antigen presentation in association with MHC class II. Unless tumor antigens are secreted as soluble proteins and can be processed by professional APCs, the CTL response will be handicapped by the lack of critical T_h function such as cytokine secretion and full DC activation. Soluble antigen may be released by tumor cells in later stages with the development of necrotic areas; but by this time, the tumor may be past the threshold from which its growth can be impeded by immune activity. To circumvent this, investigators are using ex vivo cytokine stimulation of DC and antigen exposure of autologous DCs with autologous tumor lysate, tumor peptides, or tumor cell fusions (Table 48.3).

Table 48.3 Summary of clinical trials of *active* immunotherapy (tumor vaccines) for adult malignant gliomas

Therapy	Phase	Tumor histology	Responses	Survival	References
Tumor cells modified with Newcastle disease virus (NDV)	Phase I ($n=11$)	GBM [newly diagnosed]	Local skin reaction	Median OS = 46 wks	Schneider et al. (2001)
DC pulsed with acid-eluted tumor peptides	Phase I ($n=9$)	GBM (7); AA (2) [recurrent]	2/4 patients with ↑ lymphocytic infiltration		Yu et al. (2001)
DC-glioma cell fusions	Phase I ($n=8$)	GBM; AA	4/5 patients with ↑ CD16+ & CD56+ cells; ↑ IFN-γ in peripheral blood	NR	Kikuchi et al. (2001)
Tumor cell + IL4-transfected fibroblasts	Phase I ($n=1$)	GBM	Local CD4+, CD8+, and CD1a+ T cells ↑ with IL-4 produced at injection site	Patient survived 10 months	Okada et al. (2003)
DC pulsed with tumor lysate (intradermal + intratumoral via Ommaya reservoir)	Phase I/II ($n=10$)	GBM (7); AA (3)	2/5 patients with ↑ELISPOT activity; 3/10 with ↑DTH; 2 with ↑lymphocytic infiltration	NR	Yamanaka et al. (2003a)
DC pulsed with tumor lysate	Phase I ($n=14$)	GBM (8); AA (6) [recurrent]	6/10 with ↑IFN-γ in peripheral blood; 3/6 with ↑lymphocytic infiltration	Median OS = 133 wks	Yu et al. (2004)
DC-glioma cell fusion + IL-12	Phase I ($n=15$)	GBM; AA	4/15 with >50% ↓tumor size	NR	Kikuchi et al. (2004)
Tumor cell modified with Newcastle disease virus (NVD)	Phase II ($n=23$)	GBM	↑DTH; ↑tumor-infiltrating lymphocytes	Median OS = 100 weeks (vs. 49 weeks in controls, $n=87$); 39% 2-yr survival rate	Steiner et al. (2004)
DC pulsed with acid-eluted tumor peptides	Phase I ($n=12$)	GBM (12) [7 newly diagnosed; 5 recurrent]	6/12 with ↑CTL activity; 4/8 ↑tumor-infiltrating lymphocytes	Median OS = 23.4 months; 50% 2-yr survival rate	Liau et al. (2005)

Table 48.3 (continued)

Therapy	Phase	Tumor histology	Responses	Survival	References
DC pulsed with tumor lysate	Phase II ($n = 32$)	GBM [11 newly diagnosed, 23 recurrent]	14/26 with >1.5-fold ↑ in IFN-γ levels	Mean OS = 21.4 months; 41% 2-yr survival rate for vaccine responders	Wheeler et al. (2008)
DC pulsed with tumor lysate	Phase I/II ($n = 56$)	GBM [recurrent]	9/17 with pos. DTH post-vaccination	Median OS = 9.6 months; 14.8% 2-yr survival rate	De Vleeschouwer et al. (2008)

GBM = glioblastoma multiforme; AA = anaplastic astrocytoma; DTH = delayed-type hypersensitivity; PR = partial response; OS = overall survival; NR = not reported.

In a recent phase I clinical trial with 5-year follow-up, 12 patients with newly diagnosed ($n = 7$) or recurrent ($n = 5$) glioblastoma were enrolled. Patients received standard of care, which included surgery followed by external beam radiation therapy. Glioma cells were dissociated from the tumor specimen and cultured in vitro. After approximately 5 weeks in culture, MHC-bound tumor peptides were eluted from the surface of the tumor cells using an acid-elution protocol (Liau et al., 1999). The patient's own autologous DCs were then harvested from peripheral blood mononuclear cells and subsequently loaded with the autologous acid-eluted tumor peptides. The patients then received three intradermal injections of peptide-pulsed DCs at 2-week intervals. Although this phase I study was not powered to detect clinical efficacy, it provided further evidence on the feasibility, safety, and in vivo bioactivity of autologous peptide-pulsed DCs in patients with glioblastoma, as did other similar studies (Kikuchi et al., 2004, 2001; Liau et al., 2005; Yajima et al., 2005; Yamanaka et al., 2003a; Yu et al., 2004, 2001). Although admittedly a select population of patients, prolonged survival times and significant immunological responses were observed in some of these patients, which supports the possibility of an immune-related effect on tumor control. A recent study correlated quantitative T-cell immune responses, as measured by IFN-γ enhancement, with clinical time to tumor progression (TTP) and survival (Wheeler et al., 2008). Proof of clinical benefit from DC-based vaccines remains to be established in future multi-center phase II clinical trials for malignant glioma patients, which are currently underway.

The following conclusions can be drawn from these DC-based clinical trial data to date. First, DC therapy appears to be relatively safe and well tolerated. For the most part, no serious side effects have been observed with any of these trials. Second, many of these trials report induction of cellular immunity, humoral immunity, or both, against vaccine components. Most importantly, some of these trials report complete/partial response rates or prolonged survival, which suggest that DC-based immunotherapy can significantly impact disease-free and overall survival. The true benefit of these therapies still needs to be assessed in rigorously controlled randomized trials, some of which are underway.

48.7.4 Bacterial and Viral Tumor Vaccine Trials for Malignant Glioma

Salmonella typhimurium is a gram-negative enterobacterium that causes typhoid fever. These are motile bacteria that have an anaerobic metabolism and, therefore, will thrive in hypoxic environments such as those occurring in tumors. *Salmonella typhimurium*, attenuated by genetically modifying the *purI* and *msbB* genes responsible for virulence and innate immune recognition, respectively, were found to specifically target and localize to transplantable murine tumors and partially inhibit tumor growth in vivo (Clairmont et al., 2000; Rosenberg et al., 2002). These preclinical results led to a phase I clinical trial of the intravenous administration of attenuated *Salmonella typhimurium* (VNP20009) to patients with metastatic melanoma (Rosenberg et al., 2002). This clinical study showed that the VNP20009 strain of *Salmonella typhimurium* could be safely administered to patients and that some tumor colonization by *Salmonella* was observed at the highest tolerated dose. However, no antitumor effects were seen (Toso et al., 2002).

Viral vaccines have also been investigated for the treatment of malignant gliomas (Schneider et al., 2001). More recently, a Newcastle disease virus vaccine (MTH-68/H) was used in four patients with advanced high-grade glioma, with purported survival times of 5–9 years (Csatary et al., 2004). In a similar, expanded study, a vaccine prepared from patients' tumor cell cultures infected with Newcastle disease virus was used and followed by gamma-irradiation. This was a non-randomized study of 23 vaccinated patients compared with 87 non-vaccinated controls. The 2-year survival rate in the vaccinated patients was 39% as compared with 11% for the controls ($p<0.001$). This viral-based vaccine appeared to be feasible and safe, and the improved prognosis of the vaccinated patients was substantiated by observed antitumor immune responses (Steiner et al., 2004).

Each of the immune-based therapies outlined above utilizes principles of basic immunology to find a strategy that hopefully brings us closer to the goal of killing the residual microscopic tumor cells that lead to inevitable recurrence of malignant gliomas. Major improvements in our understanding of glioma molecular biology and tumor immunology are now being translated into innovative clinical trials that provide new hope for patients with this devastating disease (see Tables 48.2 and 48.3).

48.8 Conclusion

There is challenging work being done today to take basic immunology into the clinical realm. To date, clinical trials of immunotherapy for CNS gliomas have not yet demonstrated objective proof of clinical efficacy in rigorous multicenter phase II and III studies. Nevertheless, such trials should be pursued because of encouraging results in many phase I studies (Salgaller and Liau, 2006). As future testing in this field continues, our ability to design effective, targeted immune therapies will mature and hopefully yield increased therapeutic success.

With this in mind, the priority areas of research and scientific investigation that appear to be most critical at this time involve (1) developing techniques of new antigen identification, based on readily available sources of information on the genes and gene products that are abnormally expressed by primary tumor cells (Ryu et al., 2006) and by examining which of them produce immunogenic antigens (Andersen et al., 2001); (2) characterizing both CNS and systemic immune responses in patients with brain tumors; (3) developing immunotherapies that are optimized for the particularities of the brain (efficient homing of effector cells and acceptable levels of local inflammation); and (4) considering the problems and challenges posed by patient and tumor heterogeneity. It should be noted that as with any other targeted treatment modality for brain tumors, immunotherapy trials might only realize significant potential clinical efficacy if given to the appropriate subgroup of patients and/or if administered in combination with other therapies. With the current experience in cancer treatments, it appears that simultaneously targeting several components essential to the neoplastic process should provide maximal chances of tumor control. Therefore, therapies based on immuno-enhancement and cancer vaccines could be combined with the traditional surgery, radiation, and chemotherapies, along with molecularly targeted biological agents. Such integrated treatment strategies may prove to be of low toxicity and should be synergistic. In addition, the combined use of conventional treatments within the context of clinical trials of immunotherapy will allow evaluation of efficacy, yet retain the ethical requirements for human investigation.

Over the next decade, the concept of stimulating a patient's natural immunity to produce antitumor responses may lead to the approach of "customized immunotherapy" (Salgaller, 2000) for patients with malignant glioma. Such "personalized immunotherapeutics" may be a potential solution to deal with the important observations of patient and tumor hetereogeneity. However, there are still significant obstacles for developing highly patient-selective treatments – the patient accrual on clinical trials is slower, the potential market for an approved product is lower, and so development times to clinical applications are prolonged.

Furthermore, there are significant manufacturing challenges that face the clinical development of many immunotherapeutics, especially with regard to patient-specific vaccines. This is arguably the greatest technical (and financial) hurdle to getting these types of treatments into large-scale, pivotal trials. Because so-called GMP-level facilities on many academic campuses do not meet the stricter regulations of the FDA for non-pilot studies, further clinical development of cellular therapies and biologic agents for brain tumors will require partnerships between international academic medical centers, government agencies, and biotechnology companies in order to overcome the manufacturing challenges that currently impede large-scale, multi-center phase III clinical trials.

As we have pointed out above, there is already a plethora of small-scale phase I/II brain tumor immunotherapy trials that still await confirmation of clinical efficacy. In order to obtain meaningful biological and clinical data from more complicated trials of customized immunotherapy in selected patient groups, larger multi-institutional studies need to be performed with more structured collaborations from academic and community medical centers, the biotechnology industry, and patient advocacy groups.

Currently, immunotherapy is cautiously and deliberately making its way to the patient bedside, as adjuncts to standard modalities of surgery, radiotherapy, and chemotherapy. While the number of clinical trials evaluating such immunotherapeutic strategies is still limited, current advances in the high-throughput production of clinical-grade cellular/biologic therapeutics and molecular/genetic target identification will hopefully spur future clinical development.

Abbreviations

APC	antigen presenting cell
BBB	blood–brain barrier
CTL	cytotoxic T lymphocyte
DC	dendritic cell
EAE	experimental autoimmune encephalomyelitis
IFN	interferon
LAK	lymphokine activated killer (cell)
LN	lymph node
MHC	major histocompatibility complex
MS	multiple sclerosis
NK	natural killer (cell)
TAA	tumor-associated antigen
TCR	T-cell receptor (for antigen)
TGF	transforming growth factor
TLR	toll-like receptors

Acknowledgements We thank Dr Nhu Nam Tran Thang for help in preparing the figures.

Glossary of Key Immunological Terms

Autologous The cells, tissues, and molecules derived from self, as opposed to another individual (cf. syngeneic, allogeneic).

Adaptive Immunity Immunity mediated by antigen-specific T and B lymphocytes, so called because it adapts to become more efficient upon repeated exposure to antigens (cf. innate immunity), and can provide immunological memory once the initial source of antigen has been eliminated.

Adoptive Transfer The introduction into the patient or animal of biological material (usually cells) of autologous, syngeneic, or allogeneic origin. For tumor immunotherapy, adoptive transfer offers the possibility of administering cells enriched for specific cell types (e.g., CTLs) or specificities (e.g., for tumor-specific or tumor-associated antigens) by appropriate in vitro stimulation and expansion.

T-cell activation Resting T cells do not proliferate and exert their immunological functions (cytotoxicity, cytokine release) until their TCRs engage their cognate ligand (antigenic peptide associated with an MHC molecule). The initial antigen-specific activation of mature T cells is referred to as priming and requires particularly stringent conditions to occur. These are generally only achieved by professional APCs (e.g., DCs) which express costimulatory molecules in addition to MHC–peptide complexes. The optimal and most clearly understood conditions for T cell priming are in secondary lymphoid tissues. The conditions for subsequent activation of a T cell that has already been primed (i.e., in a secondary immune response, sometimes referred to as re-activation or re-stimulation) are less demanding and can be achieved by various cell types (including tumor cells) that express the appropriate MHC–peptide complex, without costimulation, and in nonlymphoid tissues including the CNS.

Allogeneic The cells, tissues, and histocompatibility molecules derived from a genetically different individual (cf. syngeneic, allogeneic).

Anergy A T cell (or a B cell) that is unable to respond to its specific antigen. One way in which this may occur is when antigen is initially presented in the absence of costimulatory molecules; this can limit autoimmune reactions but may also limit antitumor reactions.

Antigens Material that can be recognized by the T and B lymphocytes of the adaptive immune system via their antigen receptors. The portion of the material that bound by the antigen receptors is the epitope (see also tumor-specific and tumor-associated antigens)

Antigen processing and presentation Antigen processing and presentation are divided into three major categories. In the first, exogenous antigens in the extracellular milieu such as cellular debris and opsonised microbes are taken up by antigen presenting cells (APCs), then degraded within acidic endosomes to generate short peptides, certain of which bind to MHC class II molecules and reach the cell surface to be recognized by CD4 T cells. In the second major route, endogenous antigens (i.e., normal, viral, or aberrant proteins synthesized within the cell) are degraded by the proteasome within the cytosol then transported into the endoplasmic reticulum wherein peptide binding to MHC class I molecules can occur, followed by transport to the cell surface for recognition by CD8 T cells. A third category of antigen presentation called cross-presentation is important in tumor immunology and immunotherapy. Cross-presentation is the pathway in which exogenous antigen is taken up by professional APCs, then processed (degraded into short peptides) and presented at the cell surface bound to MHC class I molecules. The most important cell responsible for cross-presentation is the DC. Cross-presentation is particularly important when malignant transformation occurs in parenchymal cells, rather than in professional APCs. For CD8 T cells to be alerted to such threats requires the intervention of an adjacent professional APC such as a DC, which can acquire material derived from the transformed cell (e.g., from dying cells or cellular debris) and cross-present this exogenous antigen to activate naïve CD8 T cells. Tumor vaccines used in immunotherapy need to exploit the cross-presentation pathway in order to activate tumor-specific CD8 T cells.

Antigen Presenting Cells (APCs) Cells capable of presenting peptide antigens bound to MHC molecules to T cells. The so-called professional APCs (DCs, macrophages, B cells) also express costimulatory molecules and are capable of activating naïve T cells. The most potent professional APCs are the DCs which (unlike the other professional APCs) have no other major biological function.

Autoimmunity A T- or B-cell mediated response directed against antigens of the individuals own body.

B cells or B-lymphocytes Lymphocytes of the adaptive immune system that develop in the bone marrow, which express clonally distributed antigen receptors, and which are stimulated by antigen in secondary lymphoid organs to differentiate into plasma cells that secrete antibodies.

Costimulatory molecules and signals For activation of naïve T cells, they must receive a first signal from MHC-peptide antigen, and a second costimulatory signal delivered by costimulatory molecules on the APC. CD80 and CD86 are major costimulatory molecules on APC, which bind to CD28 on T cells, which then transduces a costimulatory signal to the cell.

Cytotoxic T lymphocytes (CTLs) Fully activated CD8 T cells able to kill target cells expressing their cognate MHC-peptide antigen. A major cytotoxic mechanism (shared by NK cells) is the polarized release of the contents of lytic granules stored within the effector cell directly onto a target cell (e.g., a tumor cell). The principle cytotoxic molecules are perforin, granzymes, and granulysin, and they function by inducing apoptosis in the target cell. Other cytotoxic mechanisms can include cell surface molecules such as Fas ligand, and cytokines such as tumor necrosis factor.

Dendritic Cells (DCs) The most efficient professional APCs, of bone marrow origin, which have a branched, dendritic morphology. They fulfill different functions according to their differentiation state. In nonlymphoid tissues, DCs are efficient at phagocytosing and processing antigens and are termed immature. Upon activation via receptors such as TLRs, DCs become mature and migrate to secondary lymphoid tissue, they express high levels of costimulatory and MHC molecules, and they efficiently activate naïve T cells.

Epitope The part of an antigen that is bound by an antibody molecule (a B-cell epitope), or that can bind to an MHC molecule and stimulate T cells (a T-cell epitope).

HLA transgenic mice Transgenic mice that express a human histocompatibility molecule. These models allow in vivo studies of mouse T-cell immune responses specific for antigens defined in humans of the same HLA-type.

Immunological Synapse The immunological synapse is the stable interface between a T cell and target cell presenting cognate MHC peptide. It forms through cell–cell interaction of adhesion and signaling molecules. Polarized release of cytokines or cytotoxic molecules into the space formed at the synapse can ensure antigen specificity of T-cell effector function even when mediated by antigen non-specific molecules.

Innate Immunity Host immune defenses that react rapidly to infection or danger by means of germline-encoded pattern or pathogen recognition receptors. In contrast to adaptive immune responses, innate improve responses do not become more efficient upon repeat exposure to the original stimulus.

Lymphocytes A class of mononuclear leukocytes capable of migrating in blood, lymph, lymphoid, and nonlymphoid tissues according to their state of activation or differention. The small lymphocytes of the blood encompass the B and T cells of the adaptive immune system, which bear clonally distributed antigen receptors. Mature lymphocytes are termed naïve before they are stimulated by antigen. Large granular lymphocytes are the NK cells of the innate immune system.

Lymphoid Organs Primary lymphoid organs are the organized tissues where lymphocytes are formed, i.e., the bone marrow (for B cells) and the thymus (for T cells). The secondary lymphoid organs are the main site of encounter between APC and naïve T and B lymphocytes, and subsequent lymphocyte activation. The principal secondary lymphoid tissues are the spleen, lymph nodes (LNs), and the mucosa-associated lymphoid tissues (such as the tonsils and Peyer's patches).

Major Histocompatibility Complex (MHC) A cluster of genes encoding MHC molecules, a family of polymorphic cell surface glycoproteins called HLA molecules in humans, which are responsible for presenting peptide antigens to T cells. MHC class I molecules present peptides to CD8 T cells and are constitutively expressed on most cells of the body (but notably, are absent or at low levels on astrocytes, oligodendrocytes, and neurons). MHC class II molecules are mainly expressed on professional APCs and present peptide antigens to CD4 T cells.

Macrophages and microglial cells Macrophages are a family of large mononuclear phagocytes that can exist in many forms in different tissues and pathologies. They derive from blood monocytes which are in turn derived from the bone marrow. They can function as APCs (although they do not migrate to lymphoid tissue like DCs), they can exert effector functions against pathogens and tumors, but they can also promote tumor invasion and angiogenesis. Macrophages associated with the CNS can be distinguished according to the compartment in which they are found. Macrophages in the perivascular space, the leptomeninges, and the choroid plexus are phenotypically very similar to other tissue macrophages. Macrophages of the brain parenchyma on the other hand express only low levels of most classical macrophage markers under non-inflammatory conditions and have a ramified morphology. These cells are referred to as microglial cells, and upon activation they can differentiate to acquire macrophage phenotype and function and may even express the DC marker CD11c under some conditions.

Natural Killer (NK) Cells These cells are large, granular, cytotoxic lymphocytes, but unlike the T and B lymphocytes, they mediate innate immune responses. Their most important functions are cytotoxicity and IFN-γ

secretion, which are regulated by the balance of signals transduced through activating and inhibitory receptors expressed at the NK cell surface.

Pathogen/Pattern Recognition Receptors These receptors are germline encoded and detect conserved patterns present on pathogens, as well as material from stressed or dying cells. Cells of the innate immune system always express some of these receptors, but they are present on other cell types as well. They include the toll-like receptors (TLRs).

Serological Identification of Antigens by Expression Cloning (SEREX) A technique by which patient antibodies from serum can be used to screen tumor cell proteins for those which elicit immune responses. A cDNA expression library is initially made of a tumor. This library is subsequently probed in an unbiased fashion with autologous patient serum to search for tumor proteins that elicit host immune responses.

Syngeneic The cells, tissues, and histocompatibility molecules derived from a genetically identical individual (cf. syngeneic, allogeneic), such as an identical twin, or fully inbred strains of laboratory animals.

T Cells or T lymphocytes Lymphocytes of the adaptive immune system that mature in the thymus from bone marrow-derived progenitors, which express clonally distributed antigen receptors, and which are stimulated by APC in secondary lymphoid organs to express different effector functions. The two major populations of T cells are based on the expression of CD4 or CD8 cell surface glycoproteins. CD4 T cells recognize peptide antigen associated with MHC class II molecules and are subdivided into subsets based largely on cytokine secretion profiles for the T-helper cells: T_h1 (IFN-γ), T_h2 (IL-4), and T_h17 (IL-17). For T_{reg}, the definition is based on a range of phenotypic markers (including Foxp3) and function (suppression of other immune cells). CD8 T cells recognize peptides bound to MHC class I molecules and generally have cytotoxic potential (see CTLs) but can also secrete cytokines (especially IFN-γ).

T-Cell Receptor for antigen (TCR) A highly variable receptor expressed exclusively by T cells, in a clonally distributed manner. It is not germline encoded but is generated by somatic rearrangement of gene segments. The ligand is a short peptide epitope bound to an MHC molecule expressed at the surface of another cell.

Tolerance Immunological tolerance refers to the unresponsiveness of T and B cells to a particular antigen. Central tolerance is established in the bone marrow for B cells and in the thymus for T cells, wherein cell highly reactive with self-antigens (autoreactive cells) can be eliminated. Residual populations of autoreactive cells that escape deletion are restrained by different mechanisms of peripheral tolerance. Tumor immunotherapy often aims to exploit these cells that may react to tumor expressed TAAs and may thus need to attempt to "break" tolerance.

Tumor-associated antigens (TAAs). These antigens are expressed by malignant cells but also by normal cells. They may still be useful targets for immunotherapy because tumor cells may express the TAA at a higher level than normal tissue, or because normal cells express the TAA only at a certain stage of development, or in specific sites that may be shielded from immune attack (e.g., the so-called cancer-testis antigens). These antigens may be common to many patients, facilitating defined targeting and immune monitoring. However, since TAAs are self-antigens, it may be difficult to induce effective immune responses because of partial or complete immunological tolerance, and if this is overcome, there is a risk of inducing autoimmune pathology.

Tumor-specific antigens (TSAs) These antigens are only expressed by malignant cells (e.g., following mutations). They present advantages for immunotherapy because the patient should have no central tolerance to these antigens, and there is no risk of immune effector mechanisms damaging normal tissues because they do not express the antigen. However, many of these antigens are unique to individual patients, meaning that defined targeting and immune monitoring would need to be personalized.

References

Ali, S., King, G.D., Curtin, J.F., Candolfi, M., Xiong, W., Liu, C., Puntel, M., Cheng, Q., Prieto, J., Ribas, A., Kupiec-Weglinski, J., van Rooijen, N., Lassmann, H., Lowenstein, P.R., and Castro, M.G. (2005). Combined immunostimulation and conditional cytotoxic gene therapy provide long-term survival in a large glioma model. Cancer Res 65, 7194–204.

Aloisi, F., Ria, F., and Adorini, L. (2000). Regulation of T-cell responses by CNS antigen-presenting cells: different roles for microglia and astrocytes. Immunol Today 21, 141–7.

Andersen, M.H., Pedersen, L.O., Capeller, B., Brocker, E.B., Becker, J.C., and Thor, S.P. (2001). Spontaneous cytotoxic T-cell responses against survivin-derived MHC class I-restricted T-cell epitopes in situ as well as ex vivo in cancer patients. Cancer Res 61, 5964–68.

Aoki, H., Mizuno, M., Natsume, A., Tsugawa, T., Tsujimura, K., Takahashi, T., and Yoshida, J. (2001). Dendritic cells pulsed with tumor extract-cationic liposome complex increase the induction of cytotoxic T lymphocytes in mouse brain tumor. Cancer Immunol Immunother 50, 463–8.

Aulwurm, S., Wischhusen, J., Friese, M., Borst, J., and Weller, M. (2006). Immune stimulatory effects of CD70 override CD70-mediated immune cell apoptosis in rodent glioma models and confer long-lasting antiglioma immunity in vivo. Int J Cancer 118, 1728–35.

Baldwin, N.G., Rice, C.D., Tuttle, T.M., Bear, H.D., Hirsch, J.I., and Merchant, R.E. (1997). Ex vivo expansion of tumor-draining lymph node cells using compounds which activate intracellular signal transduction. I. Characterization and in vivo anti-tumor activity of glioma-sensitized lymphocytes. J Neurooncol 32, 19–28.

Bargou, R., Leo, E., Zugmaier, G., Klinger, M., Goebeler, M., Knop, S., Noppeney, R., Viardot, A., Hess, G., Schuler, M., Einsele, H., Brandl, C., Wolf, A., Kirchinger, P., Klappers, P., Schmidt, M., Riethmuller, G., Reinhardt, C., Baeuerle, P.A., and Kufer, P. (2008). Tumor regression in cancer patients by very low doses of a T cell-engaging antibody. Science 321, 974–7.

Barker, C.F. and Billingham, R.E. (1977). Immunologically privileged sites. Adv Immunol 25, 1–54.

Barrat, F.J. and Coffman, R.L. (2008). Development of TLR inhibitors for the treatment of autoimmune diseases. Immunol Rev 223, 271–83.

Barton, G.M. and Medzhitov, R. (2002). Toll-like receptors and their ligands. Curr Top Microbiol Immunol 270, 81–92.

Battistini, L., Piccio, L., Rossi, B., Bach, S., Galgani, S., Gasperini, C., Ottoboni, L., Ciabini, D., Caramia, M.D., Bernardi, G., Laudanna, C., Scarpini, E., McEver, R.P., Butcher, E.C., Borsellino, G., and Constantin, G. (2003). CD8+ T cells from patients with acute multiple sclerosis display selective increase of adhesiveness in brain venules: a critical role for P-selectin glycoprotein ligand-1. Blood 101, 4775–82.

Beauvillain, C., Donnou, S., Jarry, U., Scotet, M., Gascan, H., Delneste, Y., Guermonprez, P., Jeannin, P., and Couez, D. (2008). Neonatal and adult microglia cross-present exogenous antigens. Glia 56, 69–77.

Bechmann, I., Galea, I., and Perry, V.H. (2007). What is the blood-brain barrier (not)? Trends Immunol 28, 5–11.

Bigner, D.D., Pitts, O.M., and Wikstrand, C.J. (1981). Induction of lethal experimental allergic encephalomyelitis in nonhuman primates and guinea pigs with human glioblastoma multiforme tissue. J Neurosurg 55, 32–42.

Birnbaum, T., Roider, J., Schankin, C.J., Padovan, C.S., Schichor, C., Goldbrunner, R., and Straube, A. (2007). Malignant gliomas actively recruit bone marrow stromal cells by secreting angiogenic cytokines. J Neurooncol 83, 241–7.

Bodey, B., Bodey, V., and Siegel, S.E. (2008). Expression in childhood primary brain tumors of NY-ESO-1, a cancer/testis antigen: an immunohistochemical study. In Vivo 22, 83–7.

Bodmer, S., Strommer, K., Frei, K., Siepl, C., de Tribolet, N., Heid, I., and Fontana, A. (1989). Immunosuppression and transforming growth factor-beta in glioblastoma. Preferential production of transforming growth factor-beta 2. J Immunol 143, 3222–9.

Brabb, T., von Dassow, P., Ordonez, N., Schnabel, B., Duke, B., and Goverman, J. (2000). In situ tolerance within the central nervous system as a mechanism for preventing autoimmunity. J Exp Med 192, 871–80.

Broder, H., Anderson, A., Kremen, T.J., Odesa, S.K., and Liau, L.M. (2003). MART-1 adenovirus-transduced dendritic cell immunization in a murine model of metastatic central nervous system tumor. J Neurooncol 64, 21–30.

Brown, C.E., Vishwanath, R.P., Aguilar, B., Starr, R., Najbauer, J., Aboody, K.S., and Jensen, M.C. (2007). Tumor-derived chemokine MCP-1/CCL2 is sufficient for mediating tumor tropism of adoptively transferred T cells. J Immunol 179, 3332–41.

Burnet F.M., (1970). The concept of immunological surveillance. Prog Exp Tumor Res 13, 1–27.

Butcher, E.C., Williams, M., Youngman, K., Rott, L., and Briskin, M. (1999). Lymphocyte trafficking and regional immunity. Adv Immunol 72, 209–53.

Butterfield, L.H., Meng, W.S., Koh, A., Vollmer, C.M., Ribas, A., Dissette, V.B., Faull, K., Glaspy, J.A., McBride, W.H., and Economou, J.S. (2001). T cell responses to HLA-A*0201-restricted peptides derived from human alpha fetoprotein. J Immunol 166, 5300–8.

Calzascia, T., Di Berardino-Besson, W., Wilmotte, R., Masson, F., de Tribolet, N., Dietrich, P.Y., and Walker, P.R. (2003). Cutting edge: cross-presentation as a mechanism for efficient recruitment of tumor-specific CTL to the brain. J Immunol 171, 2187–91.

Calzascia, T., Masson, F., Di Berardino-Besson, W., Contassot, E., Wilmotte, R., Aurrand-Lions, M., Ruegg, C., Dietrich, P.Y., and Walker, P.R. (2005). Homing phenotypes of tumor-specific CD8 T cells are predetermined at the tumor site by crosspresenting APCs. Immunity 22, 175–84.

Carson, M.J., Reilly, C.R., Sutcliffe, J.G., and Lo, D. (1999). Disproportionate recruitment of CD8+ T cells into the central nervous system by professional antigen-presenting cells. Am J Pathol 154, 481–94.

Caruso, D.A., Orme, L.M., Neale, A.M., Radcliff, F.J., Amor, G.M., Maixner, W., Downie, P., Hassall, T.E., Tang, L.K., and Ashley, D.M. (2004). Results of a phase 1 study utilizing monocyte-derived dendritic cells pulsed with tumor RNA in children and young adults with brain cancer. Neuro-Oncology 6, 236–46.

Cayrol, R., Wosik, K., Berard, J.L., Dodelet-Devillers, A., Ifergan, I., Kebir, H., Haqqani, A.S., Kreymborg, K., Krug, S., Moumdjian, R., Bouthillier, A., Becher, B., Arbour, N., David, S., Stanimirovic, D., and Prat, A. (2008). Activated leukocyte cell adhesion molecule promotes leukocyte trafficking into the central nervous system. Nat Immunol 9, 137–45.

Chabalgoity, J.A., Dougan, G., Mastroeni, P., and Aspinall, R.J. (2002). Live bacteria as the basis for immunotherapies against cancer. Expert Rev Vaccines 1, 495–505.

Chang, A.E., Shu, S.Y., Chou, T., Lafreniere, R., and Rosenberg, S.A. (1986). Differences in the effects of host suppression on the adoptive immunotherapy of subcutaneous and visceral tumors. Cancer Res 46, 3426–30.

Chen, Y.T., Scanlan, M.J., Sahin, U., Tureci, O., Gure, A.O., Tsang, S., Williamson, B., Stockert, E., Pfreundschuh, M., and Old, L.J. (1997). A testicular antigen aberrantly expressed in human cancers detected by autologous antibody screening. Proc Natl Acad Sci U S A 94, 1914–8.

Chi, D.D., Merchant, R.E., Rand, R., Conrad, A.J., Garrison, D., Turner, R., Morton, D.L., and Hoon, D.S. (1997). Molecular detection of tumor-associated antigens shared by human cutaneous melanomas and gliomas. Am J Pathol 150, 2143–52.

Ciesielski, M.J., Kozbor, D., Castanaro, C.A., Barone, T.A., and Fenstermaker, R.A. (2008). Therapeutic effect of a T helper cell supported CTL response induced by a survivin peptide vaccine against murine cerebral glioma. Cancer Immunol Immunother.

Clairmont, C., Lee, K.C., Pike, J., Ittensohn, M., Low, K.B., Pawelek, J., Bermudes, D., Brecher, S.M., Margitich, D., Turnier, J., Li, Z., Luo, X., King, I., and Zheng, L.M. (2000). Biodistribution and genetic stability of the novel antitumor agent VNP20009, a genetically modified strain of Salmonella typhimurium. J Infect Dis 181, 1996–2002.

Cobbs, C.S., Harkins, L., Samanta, M., Gillespie, G.Y., Bharara, S., King, P.H., Nabors, L.B., Cobbs, C.G., and Britt, W.J. (2002). Human cytomegalovirus infection and expression in human malignant glioma. Cancer Res 62, 3347–50.

Csatary, L.K., Gosztonyi, G., Szeberenyi, J., Fabian, Z., Liszka, V., Bodey, B., and Csatary, C.M. (2004). MTH-68/H oncolytic viral treatment in human high-grade gliomas. J Neurooncol 67, 83–93.

Cserr, H.F. and Knopf, P.M. (1992). Cervical lymphatics, the blood-brain barrier and the immunoreactivity of the brain: a new view. Immunol Today 13, 507–12.

Curtin, J.F., Candolfi, M., Fakhouri, T.M., Liu, C., Alden, A., Edwards, M., Lowenstein, P.R., and Castro, M.G. (2008). Treg depletion inhibits efficacy of cancer immunotherapy: implications for clinical trials. PLoS ONE 3, e1983.

Curtin, J.F., King, G.D., Candolfi, M., Greeno, R.B., Kroeger, K.M., Lowenstein, P.R., and Castro, M.G. (2005). Combining cytotoxic and immune-mediated gene therapy to treat brain tumors. Curr Top Med Chem 5, 1151–70.

Davoust, N., Vuaillat, C., Androdias, G., and Nataf, S. (2008). From bone marrow to microglia: barriers and avenues. Trends Immunol 29, 227–34.

Desbaillets, I., Tada, M., de Tribolet, N., Diserens, A-C., Hamou, M-F., and Van Meir, E.G. (1994). Human astrocytomas and glioblastomas express Monocyte Chemoattractant Protein-1 (MCP-1) in vivo and in vitro. Int J Cancer, 58, 240–7.

De Vleeschouwer, S., Fieuws, S., Rutkowski, S., Van Calenbergh, F., Van Loon, J., Goffin, J., Sciot, R., Wilms, G., Demaerel, P., Warmuth-Metz, M., Soerensen, N., Wolff, J.E., Wagner, S., Kaempgen, E., and Van Gool, S.W. (2008). Postoperative adjuvant dendritic cell-based immunotherapy in patients with relapsed glioblastoma multiforme. Clin Cancer Res 14, 3098–104.

Dey, N., Durden, D.L., and Van Meir, E.G. (2006). Cytokine expression and signaling in CNS tumors. In Cytokines and the CNS II. Benveniste, E.N. and Ransohoff, R.M. (eds.), CRC Press. pp.193–242.

Dijkstra, I.M., de Haas, A.H., Brouwer, N., Boddeke, H.W., and Biber, K. (2006). Challenge with innate and protein antigens induces CCR7 expression by microglia in vitro and in vivo. Glia 54, 861–72.

Dillman, R.O., Duma, C.M., Schiltz, P.M., DePriest, C., Ellis, R.A., Okamoto, K., Beutel, L.D., De Leon, C., and Chico, S. (2004). Intracavitary placement of autologous lymphokine-activated killer (LAK) cells after resection of recurrent glioblastoma. J Immunother 27, 398–404.

Disis, M.L., Gooley, T.A., Rinn, K., Davis, D., Piepkorn, M., Cheever, M.A., Knutson, K.L., and Schiffman, K. (2002). Generation of T-cell immunity to the HER-2/neu protein after active immunization with HER-2/neu peptide-based vaccines. J Clin Oncol 20, 2624–32.

Disis, M.L., Schiffman, K., Guthrie, K., Salazar, L.G., Knutson, K.L., Goodell, V., dela Rosa, C., and Cheever, M.A. (2004). Effect of dose on immune response in patients vaccinated with an her-2/neu intracellular domain protein–based vaccine. J Clin Oncol 22, 1916–25.

Dudley, M.E., Wunderlich, J.R., Yang, J.C., Sherry, R.M., Topalian, S.L., Restifo, N.P., Royal, R.E., Kammula, U., White, D.E., Mavroukakis, S.A., Rogers, L.J., Gracia, G.J., Jones, S.A., Mangiameli, D.P., Pelletier, M.M., Gea-Banacloche, J., Robinson, M.R., Berman, D.M., Filie, A.C., Abati, A., and Rosenberg, S.A. (2005). Adoptive cell transfer therapy following non-myeloablative but lymphodepleting chemotherapy for the treatment of patients with refractory metastatic melanoma. J Clin Oncol 23, 2346–57.

Dunn, G.P., Koebel, C.M., and Schreiber, R.D. (2006). Interferons, immunity and cancer immunoediting. Nat Rev Immunol 6, 836–48.

Ehtesham, M., Kabos, P., Gutierrez, M.A., Samoto, K., Black, K.L., and Yu, J.S. (2003). Intratumoral dendritic cell vaccination elicits potent tumoricidal immunity against malignant glioma in rats. J Immunother 26, 107–16.

Eisele, G., Wischhusen, J., Mittelbronn, M., Meyermann, R., Waldhauer, I., Steinle, A., Weller, M., and Friese, M.A. (2006). TGF-beta and metalloproteinases differentially suppress NKG2D ligand surface expression on malignant glioma cells. Brain 129, 2416–25.

El Andaloussi, A., Han, Y., and Lesniak, M.S. (2006). Prolongation of survival following depletion of CD4 + CD25 + regulatory T cells in mice with experimental brain tumors. J Neurosurg 105, 430–7.

El Andaloussi, A. and Lesniak, M.S. (2007). CD4 + CD25 + FoxP3 + T-cell infiltration and heme oxygenase-1 expression correlate with tumor grade in human gliomas. J Neurooncol 83, 145–52.

Engelhardt B. (2006). Molecular mechanisms involved in T cell migration across the blood-brain barrier. J Neural Transm 113, 477–85.

Facoetti, A., Nano, R., Zelini, P., Morbini, P., Benericetti, E., Ceroni, M., Campoli, M., and Ferrone, S. (2005). Human leukocyte antigen and antigen processing machinery component defects in astrocytic tumors. Clin Cancer Res 11, 8304–11.

Farina, C., Aloisi, F., and Meinl, E. (2007). Astrocytes are active players in cerebral innate immunity. Trends Immunol 28, 138–45.

Fecci, P.E., Mitchell, D.A., Whitesides, J.F., Xie, W., Friedman, A.H., Archer, G.E., Herndon, J.E., 2nd, Bigner, D.D., Dranoff, G., and Sampson, J.H. (2006a). Increased regulatory T-cell fraction amidst a diminished CD4 compartment explains cellular immune defects in patients with malignant glioma. Cancer Res 66, 3294–302.

Fecci, P.E., Ochiai, H., Mitchell, D.A., Grossi, P.M., Sweeney, A.E., Archer, G.E., Cummings, T., Allison, J.P., Bigner, D.D., and Sampson, J.H. (2007). Systemic CTLA-4 blockade ameliorates glioma-induced changes to the CD4 + T cell compartment without affecting regulatory T-cell function. Clin Cancer Res 13, 2158–67.

Fecci, P.E., Sweeney, A.E., Grossi, P.M., Nair, S.K., Learn, C.A., Mitchell, D.A., Cui, X., Cummings, T.J., Bigner, D.D., Gilboa, E., and Sampson, J.H. (2006b). Systemic anti-CD25 monoclonal antibody administration safely enhances immunity in murine glioma without eliminating regulatory T cells. Clin Cancer Res 12, 4294–305.

Fischer, H.G. and Reichmann, G. (2001). Brain dendritic cells and macrophages/microglia in central nervous system inflammation. J Immunol 166, 2717–26.

Freije, W.A., Castro-Vargas, F.E., Fang, Z., Horvath, S., Cloughesy, T., Liau, L.M., Mischel, P.S., and Nelson, S.F. (2004). Gene expression profiling of gliomas strongly predicts survival. Cancer Res 64, 6503–10.

Fujita, M., Zhu, X., Sasaki, K., Ueda, R., Low, K.L., Pollack, I.F., and Okada, H. (2008). Inhibition of STAT3 promotes the efficacy of adoptive transfer therapy using type-1 CTLs by modulation of the immunological microenvironment in a murine intracranial glioma. J Immunol 180, 2089–98.

Galea, I., Bernardes-Silva, M., Forse, P.A., van Rooijen, N., Liblau, R.S., and Perry, V.H. (2007). An antigen-specific pathway for CD8 T cells across the blood-brain barrier. J Exp Med 204, 2023–30.

Gattinoni, L., Finkelstein, S.E., Klebanoff, C.A., Antony, P.A., Palmer, D.C., Spiess, P.J., Hwang, L.N., Yu, Z., Wrzesinski, C., Heimann, D.M., Surh, C.D., Rosenberg, S.A., and Restifo, N.P. (2005). Removal of homeostatic cytokine sinks by lymphodepletion enhances the efficacy of adoptively transferred tumor-specific CD8+ T cells. J Exp Med 202, 907–12.

Glick, R.P., Lichtor, T., and Cohen, E.P. (2001). Cytokine-based immuno-gene therapy for brain tumors. In Brain Tumor Immunotherapy, L.M. Liau, Becker, D.P., Cloughesy, T.F., and Bigner, D.D., eds. (Totowa, New Jersey: Humana Press), pp. 273–88.

Graeber, M.B., Scheithauer, B.W., and Kreutzberg, G.W. (2002). Microglia in brain tumors. Glia 40, 252–9.

Grauer, O.M., Nierkens, S., Bennink, E., Toonen, L.W., Boon, L., Wesseling, P., Sutmuller, R.P., and Adema, G.J. (2007). CD4+FoxP3+ regulatory T cells gradually accumulate in gliomas during tumor growth and efficiently suppress antiglioma immune responses in vivo. Int J Cancer 121, 95–105.

Grauer, O.M., Sutmuller, R.P., van Maren, W., Jacobs, J.F., Bennink, E., Toonen, L.W., Nierkens, S., and Adema, G.J. (2008). Elimination of regulatory T cells is essential for an effective vaccination with tumor lysate-pulsed dendritic cells in a murine glioma model. Int J Cancer 122, 1794–802.

Hanisch, U.K. and Kettenmann, H. (2007). Microglia: active sensor and versatile effector cells in the normal and pathologic brain. Nat Neurosci 10, 1387–94.

Hatano, M., Kuwashima, N., Tatsumi, T., Dusak, J.E., Nishimura, F., Reilly, K.M., Storkus, W.J., and Okada, H. (2004). Vaccination with EphA2-derived T cell-epitopes promotes immunity against both EphA2-expressing and EphA2-negative tumors. J Transl Med 2, 40.

Hatterer, E., Davoust, N., Didier-Bazes, M., Vuaillat, C., Malcus, C., Belin, M.F., and Nataf, S. (2006). How to drain without lymphatics? Dendritic cells migrate from the cerebrospinal fluid to the B-cell follicles of cervical lymph nodes. Blood 107, 806–12.

Hayes, R.L., Koslow, M., Hiesiger, E.M., Hymes, K.B., Hochster, H.S., Moore, E.J., Pierz, D.M., Chen, D.K., Budzilovich, G.N., and Ransohoff, J. (1995). Improved long term survival after intracavitary interleukin-2 and lymphokine-activated killer cells for adults with recurrent malignant glioma. Cancer 76, 840–52.

Hazelrigg, M.R., Hirsch, J.I., and Merchant, R.E. (2002). Distribution of adoptively transferred, tumor-sensitized lymphocytes in the glioma-bearing rat. J Neurooncol 60, 143–50.

Heimberger, A.B., Abou-Ghazal, M., Reina-Ortiz, C., Yang, D.S., Sun, W., Qiao, W., Hiraoka, N., and Fuller, G.N. (2008). Incidence and Prognostic Impact of FoxP3+ Regulatory T Cells in Human Gliomas. Clin Cancer Res 14, 5166–72.

Heimberger, A.B., Archer, G.E., Crotty, L.E., McLendon, R.E., Friedman, A.H., Friedman, H.S., Bigner, D.D., and Sampson, J.H. (2002). Dendritic cells pulsed with a tumor-specific peptide induce long-lasting immunity and are effective against murine intracerebral melanoma. Neurosurgery 50, 158–64; discussion 64–6.

Heimberger, A.B., Crotty, L.E., Archer, G.E., Hess, K.R., Wikstrand, C.J., Friedman, A.H., Friedman, H.S., Bigner, D.D., and Sampson, J.H. (2003). Epidermal growth factor receptor VIII peptide vaccination is efficacious against established intracerebral tumors. Clin Cancer Res 9, 4247–54.

Hickey W.F. (1999). Leukocyte traffic in the central nervous system: the participants and their roles. Semin Immunol 11, 125–37.

Horvath, S., Zhang, B., Carlson, M., Lu, K.V., Zhu, S., Felciano, R.M., Laurance, M.F., Zhao, W., Qi, S., Chen, Z., Lee, Y., Scheck, A.C., Liau, L.M., Wu, H., Geschwind, D.H., Febbo, P.G., Kornblum, H.I., Cloughesy, T.F., Nelson, S.F., and Mischel, P.S. (2006). Analysis of oncogenic signaling networks in glioblastoma identifies ASPM as a molecular target. Proc Natl Acad Sci U S A 103, 17402–7.

Husain, S.R., Joshi, B.H., and Puri, R.K. (2001). Interleukin-13 receptor as a unique target for anti-glioblastoma therapy. Int J Cancer 92, 168–75.

Hussain, S.F., Yang, D., Suki, D., Aldape, K., Grimm, E., and Heimberger, A.B. (2006). The role of human glioma-infiltrating microglia/macrophages in mediating antitumor immune responses. Neuro Oncol 8, 261–79.

Insug, O., Ku, G., Ertl, H.C., and Blaszczyk-Thurin, M. (2002). A dendritic cell vaccine induces protective immunity to intracranial growth of glioma. Anticancer Res 22, 613–21.

Ishikawa, E., Tsuboi, K., Saijo, K., Harada, H., Takano, S., Nose, T., and Ohno, T. (2004). Autologous natural killer cell therapy for human recurrent malignant glioma. Anticancer Res 24, 1861–71.

Jordan, J.T., Sun, W., Hussain, S.F., DeAngulo, G., Prabhu, S.S., and Heimberger, A.B. (2008). Preferential migration of regulatory T cells mediated by glioma-secreted chemokines can be blocked with chemotherapy. Cancer Immunol Immunother 57, 123–31.

Jouanneau, E., Poujol, D., Gulia, S., Le Mercier, I., Blay, J.Y., Belin, M.F., and Puisieux, I. (2006). Dendritic cells are essential for priming but inefficient for boosting antitumour immune response in an orthotopic murine glioma model. Cancer Immunol Immunother 55, 254–67.

Jung, S., Unutmaz, D., Wong, P., Sano, G., De los Santos, K., Sparwasser, T., Wu, S., Vuthoori, S., Ko, K., Zavala, F., Pamer, E.G., Littman, D.R., and Lang, R.A. (2002). In vivo depletion of CD11c(+) dendritic cells abrogates priming of CD8(+) T cells by exogenous cell-associated antigens. Immunity 17, 211–20.

Karman, J., Chu, H.H., Co, D.O., Seroogy, C.M., Sandor, M., and Fabry, Z. (2006). Dendritic cells amplify T cell-mediated immune responses in the central nervous system. J Immunol 177, 7750–60.

Karman, J., Ling, C., Sandor, M., and Fabry, Z. (2004). Initiation of immune responses in brain is promoted by local dendritic cells. J Immunol 173, 2353–61.

Katoh, M., Wilmotte, R., Belkouch, M.C., de Tribolet, N., Pizzolato, G., and Dietrich, P.Y. (2003). Survivin in brain tumors: an attractive target for immunotherapy. J Neurooncol 64, 71–6.

Kiertscher, S.M. and Roth, M.D. (1996). Human CD14+ leukocytes acquire the phenotype and function of antigen-presenting dendritic cells when cultured in GM-CSF and IL-4. J Leukoc Biol 59, 208–18.

Kikuchi, T., Akasaki, Y., Abe, T., Fukuda, T., Saotome, H., Ryan, J.L., Kufe, D.W., and Ohno, T. (2004). Vaccination of glioma patients with fusions of dendritic and glioma cells and recombinant human interleukin 12. J Immunother 27, 452–9.

Kikuchi, T., Akasaki, Y., Abe, T., and Ohno, T. (2002). Intratumoral injection of dendritic and irradiated glioma cells induces anti-tumor effects in a mouse brain tumor model. Cancer Immunol Immunother 51, 424–30.

Kikuchi, T., Akasaki, Y., Irie, M., Homma, S., Abe, T., and Ohno, T. (2001). Results of a phase I clinical trial of vaccination of glioma patients with fusions of dendritic and glioma cells. Cancer Immunol Immunother 50, 337–44.

Kim, C.H., Hong, M.J., Park, S.D., Kim, C.K., Park, M.Y., Sohn, H.J., Cho, H.I., Kim, T.G., and Hong, Y.K. (2006). Enhancement of anti-tumor immunity specific to murine glioma by vaccination with tumor cell lysate-pulsed dendritic cells engineered to produce interleukin-12. Cancer Immunol Immunother 55, 1309–19.

Kjaergaard, J., Wang, L.X., Kuriyama, H., Shu, S., and Plautz, G.E. (2005). Active immunotherapy for advanced intracranial murine tumors by using dendritic cell-tumor cell fusion vaccines. J Neurosurg 103, 156–64.

Klebanoff, C.A., Gattinoni, L., Torabi-Parizi, P., Kerstann, K., Cardones, A.R., Finkelstein, S.E., Palmer, D.C., Antony, P.A., Hwang, S.T., Rosenberg, S.A., Waldmann, T.A., and Restifo, N.P. (2005). Central memory self/tumor-reactive CD8+ T cells confer superior antitumor immunity compared with effector memory T cells. Proc Natl Acad Sci U S A 102, 9571–6.

Knutson, K.L. and Disis, M.L. (2001). Expansion of HER2/neu-specific T cells ex vivo following immunization with a HER2/neu peptide-based vaccine. Clin Breast Cancer 2, 73–9.

Knutson, K.L., Schiffman, K., and Disis, M.L. (2001). Immunization with a HER-2/neu helper peptide vaccine generates HER-2/neu CD8 T-cell immunity in cancer patients. J Clin Invest 107, 477–84.

Kruse, C.A., Cepeda, L., Owens, B., Johnson, S.D., Stears, J., and Lillehei, K.O. (1997). Treatment of recurrent glioma with intracavitary alloreactive cytotoxic T lymphocytes and interleukin-2. Cancer Immunol Immunother 45, 77–87.

Kruse, C.A., Lillehei, K.O., Mitchell, D.H., Kleinschmidt-DeMasters, B., and Bellgrau, D. (1990). Analysis of interleukin 2 and various effector cell populations in adoptive immunotherapy of 9L rat gliosarcoma: allogeneic cytotoxic T lymphocytes prevent tumor take. Proc Natl Acad Sci U S A 87, 9577–81.

Kuppner, M.C., Hamou, M.F., and de Tribolet, N. (1990). Activation and adhesion molecule expression on lymphoid infiltrates in human glioblastomas. J Neuroimmunol 29, 229–38.

Kuwashima, N., Nishimura, F., Eguchi, J., Sato, H., Hatano, M., Tsugawa, T., Sakaida, T., Dusak, J.E., Fellows-Mayle, W.K., Papworth, G.D., Watkins, S.C., Gambotto, A., Pollack, I.F., Storkus, W.J., and Okada, H. (2005). Delivery of dendritic cells engineered to secrete IFN-alpha into central nervous system tumors enhances the efficacy of peripheral tumor cell vaccines: dependence on apoptotic pathways. J Immunol 175, 2730–40.

Lanier L.L., (2008). Up on the tightrope: natural killer cell activation and inhibition. Nat Immunol 9, 495–502.

Learn, C.A., Fecci, P.E., Schmittling, R.J., Xie, W., Karikari, I., Mitchell, D.A., Archer, G.E., Wei, Z., Dressman, H., and Sampson, J.H. (2006). Profiling of CD4+, CD8+, and CD4+CD25+CD45RO+FoxP3+ T cells in patients with malignant glioma reveals differential expression of the immunologic transcriptome compared with T cells from healthy volunteers. Clin Cancer Res 12, 7306–15.

Liau, L.M., Black, K.L., Prins, R.M., Sykes, S.N., DiPatre, P.L., Cloughesy, T.F., Becker, D.P., and Bronstein, J.M. (1999). Treatment of intracranial gliomas with bone marrow-derived dendritic cells pulsed with tumor antigens. J Neurosurg 90, 1115–24.

Liau, L.M., Jensen, E.R., Kremen, T.J., Odesa, S.K., Sykes, S.N., Soung, M.C., Miller, J.F., and Bronstein, J.M. (2002). Tumor immunity within the central nervous system stimulated by recombinant Listeria monocytogenes vaccination. Cancer Res 62, 2287–93.

Liau, L.M., Lallone, R.L., Seitz, R.S., Buznikov, A., Gregg, J.P., Kornblum, H.I., Nelson, S.F., and Bronstein, J.M. (2000). Identification of a human glioma-associated growth factor gene, granulin, using differential immuno-absorption. Cancer Res 60, 1353–60.

Liau, L.M., Prins, R.M., Kiertscher, S.M., Odesa, S.K., Kremen, T.J., Giovannone, A.J., Lin, J.W., Chute, D.J., Mischel, P.S., Cloughesy, T.F., and Roth, M.D. (2005). Dendritic cell vaccination in glioblastoma patients induces systemic and intracranial T-cell responses modulated by the local central nervous system tumor microenvironment. Clin Cancer Res 11, 5515–25.

Ling, C., Verbny, Y.I., Banks, M.I., Sandor, M., and Fabry, Z. (2008). In situ activation of antigen-specific CD8(+) T cells in the presence of antigen in organotypic brain slices. J Immunol 180, 8393–9.

Liu, G., Ying, H., Zeng, G., Wheeler, C.J., Black, K.L., and Yu, J.S. (2004a). HER-2, gp100, and MAGE-1 are expressed in human glioblastoma and recognized by cytotoxic T cells. Cancer Res 64, 4980–6.

Liu, G., Yu, J.S., Zeng, G., Yin, D., Xie, D., Black, K.L., and Ying, H. (2004b). AIM-2: a novel tumor antigen is expressed and presented by human glioma cells. J Immunother 27, 220–6.
Louis D.N. (2006). Molecular pathology of malignant gliomas. Annu Rev Pathol 1, 97–117.
Luster, A.D., Alon, R., and von Andrian, U.H. (2005). Immune cell migration in inflammation: present and future therapeutic targets. Nat Immunol 6, 1182–90.
Maecker, B., von, B.-B., Anderson, K.S., Vonderheide, R.H., and Schultze, J.L. (2001). Linking genomics to immunotherapy by reverse immunology–'immunomics' in the new millennium. Curr Mol Med 1, 609–19.
Markovic, D.S., Glass, R., Synowitz, M., Rooijen, N., and Kettenmann, H. (2005). Microglia stimulate the invasiveness of glioma cells by increasing the activity of metalloprotease-2. J Neuropathol Exp Neurol 64, 754–62.
Marx J. (2008). Cancer immunology. Cancer's bulwark against immune attack: MDS cells. Science 319, 154–6.
Masson, F., Calzascia, T., Di Berardino-Besson, W., de Tribolet, N., Dietrich, P.Y., and Walker, P.R. (2007). Brain microenvironment promotes the final functional maturation of tumor-specific effector CD8+ T cells. J Immunol 179, 845–53.
Matzinger P. (1994). Tolerance, danger, and the extended family. Annu Rev Immunol 12, 991–1045.
Medewar P.B. (1948). Immunity to homologous grafted skin. III. The fate of skin homografts transplanted to the brain, to subcutaneous tissue and to the anterior chamber of the eye. Br J Exp Pathol 29, 58–69.
Mehling, M., Simon, P., Mittelbronn, M., Meyermann, R., Ferrone, S., Weller, M., and Wiendl, H. (2007). WHO grade associated downregulation of MHC class I antigen-processing machinery components in human astrocytomas: does it reflect a potential immune escape mechanism? Acta Neuropathol 114, 111–9.
Merchant, R.E., Baldwin, N.G., Rice, C.D., and Bear, H.D. (1997). Adoptive immunotherapy of malignant glioma using tumor-sensitized T lymphocytes. Neurol Res 19, 145–52.
Merchant, R.E., Grant, A.J., Merchant, L.H., and Young, H.F. (1988a). Adoptive immunotherapy for recurrent glioblastoma multiforme using lymphokine activated killer cells and recombinant interleukin-2. Cancer 62, 665–71.
Merchant, R.E., Merchant, L.H., Cook, S.H., McVicar, D.W., and Young, H.F. (1988b). Intralesional infusion of lymphokine-activated killer (LAK) cells and recombinant interleukin-2 (rIL-2) for the treatment of patients with malignant brain tumor. Neurosurgery 23, 725–32.
Mischel, P.S., Nelson, S.F., and Cloughesy, T.F. (2003a). Molecular analysis of glioblastoma: pathway profiling and its implications for patient therapy. Cancer Biol Ther 2, 242–7.
Mischel, P.S., Shai, R., Shi, T., Horvath, S., Lu, K.V., Choe, G., Seligson, D., Kremen, T.J., Palotie, A., Liau, L.M., Cloughesy, T.F., and Nelson, S.F. (2003b). Identification of molecular subtypes of glioblastoma by gene expression profiling. Oncogene 22, 2361–73.
Mitchell, D.A., Fecci, P.E., and Sampson, J.H. (2003). Adoptive immunotherapy for malignant glioma. Cancer J 9, 157–66.
Mitchell, D.A., Xie, W., Schmittling, R., Learn, C., Friedman, A., McLendon, R.E., and Sampson, J.H. (2008). Sensitive detection of human cytomegalovirus in tumors and peripheral blood of patients diagnosed with glioblastoma. Neuro Oncol 10, 10–8.
Morgan, R.A., Dudley, M.E., Wunderlich, J.R., Hughes, M.S., Yang, J.C., Sherry, R.M., Royal, R.E., Topalian, S.L., Kammula, U.S., Restifo, N.P., Zheng, Z., Nahvi, A., de Vries, C.R., Rogers-Freezer, L.J., Mavroukakis, S.A., and Rosenberg, S.A. (2006). Cancer regression in patients after transfer of genetically engineered lymphocytes. Science 314, 126–9.
Morse, M.A., Clay, T.M., Hobeika, A.C., Osada, T., Khan, S., Chui, S., Niedzwiecki, D., Panicali, D., Schlom, J., and Lyerly, H.K. (2005). Phase I study of immunization with dendritic cells modified with fowlpox encoding carcinoembryonic antigen and costimulatory molecules. Clin Cancer Res 11, 3017–24.

Murphy, G.P., Barren, R.J., Erickson, S.J., Bowes, V.A., Wolfert, R.L., Bartsch, G., Klocker, H., Pointner, J., Reissigl, A., McLeod, D.G., Douglas, T., Morgan, T., Kenny, G.M., Ragde, H., Boynton, A.L., and Holmes, E.H. (1996). Evaluation and comparison of two new prostate carcinoma markers. Free-prostate specific antigen and prostate specific membrane antigen. Cancer 78, 809–18.

Murphy, G.P., Tjoa, B.A., Simmons, S.J., Jarisch, J., Bowes, V.A., Ragde, H., Rogers, M., Elgamal, A., Kenny, G.M., Cobb, O.E., Ireton, R.C., Troychak, M.J., Salgaller, M.L., and Boynton, A.L. (1999). Infusion of dendritic cells pulsed with HLA-A2-specific prostate-specific membrane antigen peptides: a phase II prostate cancer vaccine trial involving patients with hormone-refractory metastatic disease. Prostate 38, 73–8.

Ni, H.T., Spellman, S.R., Jean, W.C., Hall, W.A., and Low, W.C. (2001). Immunization with dendritic cells pulsed with tumor extract increases survival of mice bearing intracranial gliomas. J Neurooncol 51, 1–9.

Nishimura, F., Dusak, J.E., Eguchi, J., Zhu, X., Gambotto, A., Storkus, W.J., and Okada, H. (2006). Adoptive transfer of type 1 CTL mediates effective anti-central nervous system tumor response: critical roles of IFN-inducible protein-10. Cancer Res 66, 4478–87.

Okada, H., Attanucci, J., Giezeman-Smits, K.M., Brissette-Storkus, C., Fellows, W.K., Gambotto, A., Pollack, L.F., Pogue-Geile, K., Lotze, M.T., Bozik, M.E., and Chambers, W.H. (2001). Immunization with an antigen identified by cytokine tumor vaccine-assisted SEREX (CAS) suppressed growth of the rat 9L glioma in vivo. Cancer Res 61, 2625–31.

Okada, H., Lieberman, F.S., Edington, H.D., Witham, T.F., Wargo, M.J., Cai, Q., Elder, E.H., Whiteside, T.L., Schold, S.C., Jr., and Pollack, I.F. (2003). Autologous glioma cell vaccine admixed with interleukin-4 gene transfected fibroblasts in the treatment of recurrent glioblastoma: preliminary observations in a patient with a favorable response to therapy. J Neurooncol 64, 13–20.

Okada, H., Low, K.L., Kohanbash, G., McDonald, H.A., Hamilton, R.L., and Pollack, I.F. (2008). Expression of glioma-associated antigens in pediatric brain stem and non-brain stem gliomas. J Neurooncol 88, 245–50.

Okada, H. and Pollack, I.F. (2004). Cytokine gene therapy for malignant glioma. Expert Opin Biol Ther 4, 1609–20.

Okano, F., Storkus, W.J., Chambers, W.H., Pollack, I.F., and Okada, H. (2002). Identification of a novel HLA-A*0201-restricted, cytotoxic T lymphocyte epitope in a human glioma-associated antigen, interleukin 13 receptor alpha2 chain. Clin Cancer Res 8, 2851–5.

Pallasch, C.P., Struss, A.K., Munnia, A., Konig, J., Steudel, W.I., Fischer, U., and Meese, E. (2005). Autoantibodies against GLEA2 and PHF3 in glioblastoma: tumor-associated autoantibodies correlated with prolonged survival. Int J Cancer 117, 456–9.

Panelli, M.C., Wunderlich, J., Jeffries, J., Wang, E., Mixon, A., Rosenberg, S.A., and Marincola, F.M. (2000). Phase 1 study in patients with metastatic melanoma of immunization with dendritic cells presenting epitopes derived from the melanoma-associated antigens MART-1 and gp100. J Immunother 23, 487–98.

Parkhurst, M.R., Fitzgerald, E.B., Southwood, S., Sette, A., Rosenberg, S.A., and Kawakami, Y. (1998). Identification of a shared HLA-A*0201-restricted T-cell epitope from the melanoma antigen tyrosinase-related protein 2 (TRP2). Cancer Res 58, 4895–901.

Parkhurst, M.R., Salgaller, M.L., Southwood, S., Robbins, P.F., Sette, A., Rosenberg, S.A., and Kawakami, Y. (1996). Improved induction of melanoma-reactive CTL with peptides from the melanoma antigen gp100 modified at HLA-A*0201-binding residues. J Immunol 157, 2539–48.

Parsa, A.T., Waldron, J.S., Panner, A., Crane, C.A., Parney, I.F., Barry, J.J., Cachola, K.E., Murray, J.C., Tihan, T., Jensen, M.C., Mischel, P.S., Stokoe, D., and Pieper, R.O. (2007). Loss of tumor suppressor PTEN function increases B7-H1 expression and immunoresistance in glioma. Nat Med 13, 84–8.

Pellegatta, S., Poliani, P.L., Corno, D., Grisoli, M., Cusimano, M., Ubiali, F., Baggi, F., Bruzzone, M.G., and Finocchiaro, G. (2006). Dendritic cells pulsed with glioma lysates induce immunity against syngeneic intracranial gliomas and increase survival of tumor-bearing mice. Neurol Res 28, 527–31.

Peng, L., Kjaergaard, J., Plautz, G.E., Awad, M., Drazba, J.A., Shu, S., and Cohen, P.A. (2002). Tumor-induced L-selectinhigh suppressor T cells mediate potent effector T cell blockade and cause failure of otherwise curative adoptive immunotherapy. J Immunol 169, 4811–21.

Platten, M. and Steinman, L. (2005). Multiple sclerosis: trapped in deadly glue. Nat Med 11, 252–3.

Plautz, G.E., Miller, D.W., Barnett, G.H., Stevens, G.H., Maffett, S., Kim, J., Cohen, P.A., and Shu, S. (2000). T cell adoptive immunotherapy of newly diagnosed gliomas. Clin Cancer Res 6, 2209–18.

Plautz, G.E., Touhalisky, J.E., and Shu, S. (1997). Treatment of murine gliomas by adoptive transfer of ex vivo activated tumor-draining lymph node cells. Cell Immunol 178, 101–7.

Prins, R.M., Bruhn, K.W., Craft, N., Lin, J.W., Kim, C.H., Odesa, S.K., Miller, J.F., and Liau, L.M. (2006a). Central nervous system tumor immunity generated by a recombinant listeria monocytogenes vaccine targeting tyrosinase related protein-2 and real-time imaging of intracranial tumor burden. Neurosurgery 58, 169–78; discussion 69–78.

Prins, R.M., Cloughesy, T.F., and Liau, L.M. (2008a). Cytomegalovirus immunity after vaccination with autologous glioblastoma lysate. N Engl J Med 359, 539–41.

Prins, R.M., Craft, N., Bruhn, K.W., Khan-Farooqi, H., Koya, R.C., Stripecke, R., Miller, J.F., and Liau, L.M. (2006b). The TLR-7 agonist, imiquimod, enhances dendritic cell survival and promotes tumor antigen-specific T cell priming: relation to central nervous system antitumor immunity. J Immunol 176, 157–64.

Prins, R.M., Odesa, S.K., and Liau, L.M. (2003). Immunotherapeutic targeting of shared melanoma-associated antigens in a murine glioma model. Cancer Res 63, 8487–91.

Prins, R.M., Scott, G.P., Merchant, R.E., and Graf, M.R. (2002). Irradiated tumor cell vaccine for treatment of an established glioma. II. Expansion of myeloid suppressor cells that promote tumor progression. Cancer Immunol Immunother 51, 190–9.

Prins, R.M., Shu, C.J., Radu, C.G., Vo, D.D., Khan-Farooqi, H., Soto, H., Yang, M.Y., Lin, M.S., Shelly, S., Witte, O.N., Ribas, A., and Liau, L.M. (2008b). Anti-tumor activity and trafficking of self, tumor-specific T cells against tumors located in the brain. Cancer Immunol Immunother 57, 1279–89.

Prins, R.M., Vo, D.D., Khan-Farooqi, H., Yang, M.Y., Soto, H., Economou, J.S., Liau, L.M., and Ribas, A. (2006c). NK and CD4 cells collaborate to protect against melanoma tumor formation in the brain. J Immunol 177, 8448–55.

Pulendran B., (2005). Variegation of the immune response with dendritic cells and pathogen recognition receptors. J Immunol 174, 2457–65.

Qin, Z., Schwartzkopff, J., Pradera, F., Kammertoens, T., Seliger, B., Pircher, H., and Blankenstein, T. (2003). A critical requirement of interferon gamma-mediated angiostasis for tumor rejection by CD8 + T cells. Cancer Res 63, 4095–100.

Quattrocchi, K.B., Miller, C.H., Cush, S., Bernard, S.A., Dull, S.T., Smith, M., Gudeman, S., and Varia, M.A. (1999). Pilot study of local autologous tumor infiltrating lymphocytes for the treatment of recurrent malignant gliomas. J Neurooncol 45, 141–57.

Rebenko-Moll, N.M., Liu, L., Cardona, A., and Ransohoff, R.M. (2006). Chemokines, mononuclear cells and the nervous system: heaven (or hell) is in the details. Curr Opin Immunol 18, 683–9.

Ribas, A., (2006). Update on immunotherapy for melanoma. J Natl Compr Canc Netw 4, 687–94.

Ribas, A., Butterfield, L.H., Hu, B., Dissette, V.B., Chen, A.Y., Koh, A., Amarnani, S.N., Glaspy, J.A., McBride, W.H., and Economou, J.S. (2000). Generation of T-cell immunity to a murine melanoma using MART-1-engineered dendritic cells. J Immunother 23, 59–66.

Rice, C.D., Baldwin, N.G., Biron, R.T., Bear, H.D., and Merchant, R.E. (1997). Ex vivo expansion of tumor-draining lymph node cells using compounds which activate intracellular signal transduction. II. Cytokine production and in vivo efficacy of glioma-sensitized lymphocytes. J Neurooncol 32, 29–38.

Rosenberg, S.A., Spiess, P.J., and Kleiner, D.E. (2002). Antitumor effects in mice of the intravenous injection of attenuated Salmonella typhimurium. J Immunother 25, 218–25.

Roth, P., Mittelbronn, M., Wick, W., Meyermann, R., Tatagiba, M., and Weller, M. (2007). Malignant glioma cells counteract antitumor immune responses through expression of lectin-like transcript-1. Cancer Res 67, 3540–4.

Ryu, J., Kim, C., Cheong, J., Bak, K., Kim, J., and Oh, S. (2006). Co-expression of survivin and Bcl-2 in primary brain tumors: their potential effect on anti-apoptosis. J Korean Neurosurg Soc 40, 1–5.

Sahin, U., Koslowski, M., Tureci, O., Eberle, T., Zwick, C., Romeike, B., Moringlane, J.R., Schwechheimer, K., Feiden, W., and Pfreundschuh, M. (2000). Expression of cancer testis genes in human brain tumors. Clin Cancer Res 6, 3916–22.

Saikali, S., Avril, T., Collet, B., Hamlat, A., Bansard, J.Y., Drenou, B., Guegan, Y., and Quillien, V. (2007). Expression of nine tumour antigens in a series of human glioblastoma multiforme: interest of EGFRvIII, IL-13Ralpha2, gp100 and TRP-2 for immunotherapy. J Neurooncol 81, 139–48.

Sakaguchi, S., Yamaguchi, T., Nomura, T., and Ono, M. (2008). Regulatory T cells and immune tolerance. Cell 133, 775–87.

Salgaller, M.L. (2000). American Association for Cancer Research: dendritic cells: strategies and vaccines. April 1–5, 2000, San Francisco, CA, USA. Expert Opin Investig Drugs 9, 1407–12.

Salgaller, M.L. and Liau, L.M. (2006). Current status of clinical trials for glioblastoma. Reviews on Recent Clinical Trials 1, 265–81.

Sasaki, K., Zhu, X., Vasquez, C., Nishimura, F., Dusak, J.E., Huang, J., Fujita, M., Wesa, A., Potter, D.M., Walker, P.R., Storkus, W.J., and Okada, H. (2007). Preferential expression of very late antigen-4 on type 1 CTL cells plays a critical role in trafficking into central nervous system tumors. Cancer Res 67, 6451–8.

Schmits, R., Cochlovius, B., Treitz, G., Regitz, E., Ketter, R., Preuss, K.D., Romeike, B.F., and Pfreundschuh, M. (2002). Analysis of the antibody repertoire of astrocytoma patients against antigens expressed by gliomas. Int J Cancer 98, 73–7.

Schneider, T., Gerhards, R., Kirches, E., and Firsching, R. (2001). Preliminary results of active specific immunization with modified tumor cell vaccine in glioblastoma multiforme. J Neurooncol 53, 39–46.

Shimato, S., Natsume, A., Wakabayashi, T., Tsujimura, K., Nakahara, N., Ishii, J., Ito, M., Akatsuka, Y., Kuzushima, K., and Yoshida, J. (2008). Identification of a human leukocyte antigen-A24-restricted T-cell epitope derived from interleukin-13 receptor alpha2 chain, a glioma-associated antigen. J Neurosurg 109, 117–22.

Siesjo, P., Visse, E., and Sjogren, H.O. (1996). Cure of established, intracerebral rat gliomas induced by therapeutic immunizations with tumor cells and purified APC or adjuvant IFN-gamma treatment. J Immunother Emphasis Tumor Immunol 19, 334–45.

Sitkovsky, M. and Lukashev, D. (2005). Regulation of immune cells by local-tissue oxygen tension: HIF1 alpha and adenosine receptors. Nat Rev Immunol 5, 712–21.

Steiner, H.H., Bonsanto, M.M., Beckhove, P., Brysch, M., Geletneky, K., Ahmadi, R., Schuele-Freyer, R., Kremer, P., Ranaie, G., Matejic, D., Bauer, H., Kiessling, M., Kunze, S., Schirrmacher, V., and Herold-Mende, C. (2004). Antitumor vaccination of patients with glioblastoma multiforme: a pilot study to assess feasibility, safety, and clinical benefit. J Clin Oncol 22, 4272–81.

Steinman, R.M. and Banchereau, J. (2007). Taking dendritic cells into medicine. Nature 449, 419–26.

Stuve, O., Marra, C.M., Bar-Or, A., Niino, M., Cravens, P.D., Cepok, S., Frohman, E.M., Phillips, J.T., Arendt, G., Jerome, K.R., Cook, L., Grand'Maison, F., Hemmer, B., Monson, N.L., and Racke, M.K. (2006). Altered CD4+/CD8+ T-cell ratios in cerebrospinal fluid of natalizumab-treated patients with multiple sclerosis. Arch Neurol 63, 1383–7.

Suter, T., Biollaz, G., Gatto, D., Bernasconi, L., Herren, T., Reith, W., and Fontana, A. (2003). The brain as an immune privileged site: dendritic cells of the central nervous system inhibit T cell activation. Eur J Immunol 33, 2998–3006.

The Cancer Genome Atlas Research Network. (2008). Nature Sep 4. PMID: 18772890 [Epub ahead of print]

Thomas, D.L., Kranz, D.M., and Roy, E.J. (2008). Experimental manipulations of afferent immune responses influence efferent immune responses to brain tumors. Cancer Immunol Immunother 57, 1323–33.

Thurner, B., Roder, C., Dieckmann, D., Heuer, M., Kruse, M., Glaser, A., Keikavoussi, P., Kampgen, E., Bender, A., and Schuler, G. (1999). Generation of large numbers of fully mature and stable dendritic cells from leukapheresis products for clinical application. J Immunol Methods 223, 1–15.

Toso, J.F., Gill, V.J., Hwu, P., Marincola, F.M., Restifo, N.P., Schwartzentruber, D.J., Sherry, R.M., Topalian, S.L., Yang, J.C., Stock, F., Freezer, L.J., Morton, K.E., Seipp, C., Haworth, L., Mavroukakis, S., White, D., MacDonald, S., Mao, J., Sznol, M., and Rosenberg, S.A. (2002). Phase I study of the intravenous administration of attenuated Salmonella typhimurium to patients with metastatic melanoma. J Clin Oncol 20, 142–52.

Tsugawa, T., Kuwashima, N., Sato, H., Fellows-Mayle, W.K., Dusak, J.E., Okada, K., Papworth, G.D., Watkins, S.C., Gambotto, A., Yoshida, J., Pollack, I.F., and Okada, H. (2004). Sequential delivery of interferon-alpha gene and DCs to intracranial gliomas promotes an effective antitumor response. Gene Ther 11, 1551–8.

Ueda, R., Low, K.L., Zhu, X., Fujita, M., Sasaki, K., Whiteside, T.L., Butterfield, L.H., and Okada, H. (2007). Spontaneous immune responses against glioma-associated antigens in a long term survivor with malignant glioma. J Transl Med 5, 68.

Ulevitch, R.J. (2004). Therapeutics targeting the innate immune system. Nat Rev Immunol 4, 512–20.

Van den Eynde, B., Peeters, O., De Backer, O., Gaugler, B., Lucas, S., and Boon, T. (1995). A new family of genes coding for an antigen recognized by autologous cytolytic T lymphocytes on a human melanoma. J Exp Med 182, 689–98.

Van der Bruggen, P., Traversari, C., Chomez, P., Lurquin, C., De Plaen, E., Van den Eynde, B., Knuth, A., and Boon, T. (1991). A gene encoding an antigen recognized by cytolytic T lymphocytes on a human melanoma. Science 254, 1643–7.

Van Meir, E.G. (1999). Cytokine expression in brain tumors: its role in tumor biology and tumor-associated immune responses. In Inflammatory Cells and Mediators in CNS Diseases. Ruffolo, R.R.Jr., Feuerstein, G.Z. Hunter, A.J. Poste, G. and Metcalf, B.W. (eds.), Harwood Academic Publishers, London. pp. 169–244.

Walker, P.R., Calzascia, T., de Tribolet, N., and Dietrich, P.Y. (2003). T-cell immune responses in the brain and their relevance for cerebral malignancies. Brain Res Brain Res Rev 42, 97–122.

Walker, P.R., Saas, P., and Dietrich, P.Y. (1997). Role of Fas ligand (CD95L) in immune escape: the tumor cell strikes back. J Immunol 158, 4521–4.

Walter, L. and Albert, M.L. (2007). Cutting edge: cross-presented intracranial antigen primes CD8+ T cells. J Immunol 178, 6038–42.

Wang, L.X., Huang, W.X., Graor, H., Cohen, P.A., Kim, J.A., Shu, S., and Plautz, G.E. (2004). Adoptive immunotherapy of cancer with polyclonal, 108-fold hyperexpanded, CD4+ and CD8+ T cells. J Transl Med 2, 41.

Wang, L.X., Shu, S., Disis, M.L., and Plautz, G.E. (2007). Adoptive transfer of tumor-primed, in vitro-activated, CD4+ T effector cells (TEs) combined with CD8+ TEs provides intratumoral TE proliferation and synergistic antitumor response. Blood 109, 4865–76.

Wang, L.X., Shu, S., and Plautz, G.E. (2005). Host lymphodepletion augments T cell adoptive immunotherapy through enhanced intratumoral proliferation of effector cells. Cancer Res 65, 9547–54.

Wheeler, C.J., Black, K.L., Liu, G., Mazer, M., Zhang, X.X., Pepkowitz, S., Goldfinger, D., Ng, H., Irvin, D., and Yu, J.S. (2008). Vaccination elicits correlated immune and clinical responses in glioblastoma multiforme patients. Cancer Res 68, 5955–64.

Wilmotte, R., Burkhardt, K., Kindler, V., Belkouch, M.C., Dussex, G., Tribolet, N., Walker, P.R., and Dietrich, P.Y. (2005). B7-homolog 1 expression by human glioma: a new mechanism of immune evasion. Neuroreport 16, 1081–5.

Wintterle, S., Schreiner, B., Mitsdoerffer, M., Schneider, D., Chen, L., Meyermann, R., Weller, M., and Wiendl, H. (2003). Expression of the B7-related molecule B7-H1 by glioma cells: a potential mechanism of immune paralysis. Cancer Res 63, 7462–7.

Wischhusen, J., Waschbisch, A., and Wiendl, H. (2007). Immune-refractory cancers and their little helpers–an extended role for immunetolerogenic MHC molecules HLA-G and HLA-E? Semin Cancer Biol 17, 459–68.

Wood, G.W., Holladay, F.P., Turner, T., Wang, Y.Y., and Chiga, M. (2000). A pilot study of autologous cancer cell vaccination and cellular immunotherapy using anti-CD3 stimulated lymphocytes in patients with recurrent grade III/IV astrocytoma. J Neurooncol 48, 113–20.

Wrzesinski, S.H., Wan, Y.Y., and Flavell, R.A. (2007). Transforming growth factor-beta and the immune response: implications for anticancer therapy. Clin Cancer Res 13, 5262–70.

Wu, A., Oh, S., Gharagozlou, S., Vedi, R.N., Ericson, K., Low, W.C., Chen, W., and Ohlfest, J.R. (2007). In vivo vaccination with tumor cell lysate plus CpG oligodeoxynucleotides eradicates murine glioblastoma. J Immunother 30, 789–97.

Wu, A.H., Xiao, J., Anker, L., Hall, W.A., Gregerson, D.S., Cavenee, W.K., Chen, W., and Low, W.C. (2006). Identification of EGFRvIII-derived CTL epitopes restricted by HLA A0201 for dendritic cell based immunotherapy of gliomas. J Neurooncol 76, 23–30.

Yajima, N., Yamanaka, R., Mine, T., Tsuchiya, N., Homma, J., Sano, M., Kuramoto, T., Obata, Y., Komatsu, N., Arima, Y., Yamada, A., Shigemori, M., Itoh, K., and Tanaka, R. (2005). Immunologic evaluation of personalized peptide vaccination for patients with advanced malignant glioma. Clin Cancer Res 11, 5900–11.

Yamanaka, R., Abe, T., Yajima, N., Tsuchiya, N., Homma, J., Kobayashi, T., Narita, M., Takahashi, M., and Tanaka, R. (2003a). Vaccination of recurrent glioma patients with tumour lysate-pulsed dendritic cells elicits immune responses: results of a clinical phase I/II trial. Br J Cancer 89, 1172–79.

Yamanaka, R., Homma, J., Yajima, N., Tsuchiya, N., Sano, M., Kobayashi, T., Yoshida, S., Abe, T., Narita, M., Takahashi, M., and Tanaka, R. (2005). Clinical Evaluation of Dendritic Cell Vaccination for Patients with Recurrent Glioma: Results of a Clinical Phase I/II Trial. Clin Cancer Res 11, 4160–7.

Yamanaka, R., Tsuchiya, N., Yajima, N., Honma, J., Hasegawa, H., Tanaka, R., Ramsey, J., Blaese, R.M., and Xanthopoulos, K.G. (2003b). Induction of an antitumor immunological response by an intratumoral injection of dendritic cells pulsed with genetically engineered Semliki Forest virus to produce interleukin-18 combined with the systemic administration of interleukin-12. J Neurosurg 99, 746–53.

Yang, I., Kremen, T.J., Giovannone, A.J., Paik, E., Odesa, S.K., Prins, R.M., and Liau, L.M. (2004). Modulation of major histocompatibility complex Class I molecules and major histocompatibility complex-bound immunogenic peptides induced by interferon-alpha and interferon-gamma treatment of human glioblastoma multiforme. J Neurosurg 100, 310–9.

Yu, J.S., Liu, G., Ying, H., Yong, W.H., Black, K.L., and Wheeler, C.J. (2004). Vaccination with tumor lysate-pulsed dendritic cells elicits antigen-specific, cytotoxic T-cells in patients with malignant glioma. Cancer Res 64, 4973–79.

Yu, J.S., Wheeler, C.J., Zeltzer, P.M., Ying, H., Finger, D.N., Lee, P.K., Yong, W.H., Incardona, F., Thompson, R.C., Riedinger, M.S., Zhang, W., Prins, R.M., and Black, K.L. (2001). Vaccination of malignant glioma patients with peptide-pulsed dendritic cells elicits systemic cytotoxicity and intracranial T-cell infiltration. Cancer Res 61, 842–47.

Zhang, J.G., Eguchi, J., Kruse, C.A., Gomez, G.G., Fakhrai, H., Schroter, S., Ma, W., Hoa, N., Minev, B., Delgado, C., Wepsic, H.T., Okada, H., and Jadus, M.R. (2007). Antigenic profiling of glioma cells to generate allogeneic vaccines or dendritic cell-based therapeutics. Clin Cancer Res 13, 566–75.

Zhang, J.G., Kruse, C.A., Driggers, L., Hoa, N., Wisoff, J., Allen, J.C., Zagzag, D., Newcomb, E. W., and Jadus, M.R. (2008). Tumor antigen precursor protein profiles of adult and pediatric brain tumors identify potential targets for immunotherapy. J Neurooncol 88, 65–76.

Zhu, X., Nishimura, F., Sasaki, K., Fujita, M., Dusak, J.E., Eguchi, J., Fellows-Mayle, W., Storkus, W.J., Walker, P.R., Salazar, A.M., and Okada, H. (2007). Toll like receptor-3 ligand poly-ICLC promotes the efficacy of peripheral vaccinations with tumor antigen-derived peptide epitopes in murine CNS tumor models. J Transl Med 5, 10.

Chapter 49
Glioma Invasion: Mechanisms and Therapeutic Challenges

Mariano S. Viapiano and Sean E. Lawler

Abstract A hallmark of gliomas is the ability of individual tumor cells to infiltrate the neural tissue and extend beyond the visible borders of the tumor. Current treatments fail to remove these invasive cells, which almost invariably lead to tumor dissemination and therapy failure in the long term. The composition and properties of the extracellular matrix (ECM) in the adult central nervous system are notoriously inhibitory to cell motility and axonal extension. However, glioma cells are uniquely able to remodel this microenvironment by degradation of the neural ECM and production of a novel matrix that contains neural-specific and mesenchymal components. Structural signals from the ECM and soluble factors from the surrounding non-neoplastic cells regulate the molecular and cellular mechanisms of invasion, which include matrix remodeling, cytoskeletal reorganization, and phenotype transition from highly proliferative to migratory. Specific strategies against invading glioma cells are in their infancy due to the paucity of appropriate targets and the difficulty of predicting the effects of targeting this highly plastic cell population in vivo. Identification of the key molecular mechanisms necessary for cell invasion and the major switches that regulate the inter-conversion of migratory and proliferative phenotypes will provide a wealth of novel targets to direct therapies against brain tumor progression and improve long-term patient survival.

Contents

M.S. Viapiano (✉)
Center for Molecular Neurobiology, The Ohio State University,
226B Rightmire Hall, 1060 Carmack Rd, Columbus, Ohio 43210, USA
e-mail: viapiano.1@osu.edu

E.G. Van Meir (ed.), *CNS Cancer*, Cancer Drug Discovery and Development, DOI 10.1007/978-1-60327-553-8_49,
© Humana Press, a part of Springer Science+Business Media, LLC 2009

49.1 Introduction

Malignant gliomas are the most common primary tumors of the central nervous system (CNS). A hallmark of these neoplasms is the ability of individual glioma cells to detach from the tumor mass and invade the neural tissue (Louis, 2006). This diffuse infiltration occurs with little distortion of the neural architecture and does not seem to trigger inflammatory or other immune responses, placing the migrating cells beyond the limits of current clinical detection (Claes et al., 2007). In addition, significant evidence has shown that migrating glioma cells divide more slowly than the cells at the core of the tumor (Demuth and Berens, 2004; Giese et al., 1996) and are consequently more resistant to cytotoxic therapies. Therefore, these cells remain in the CNS even after aggressive resection and treatment of the residual tumor, becoming a major factor for local recurrence and tumor dissemination throughout the CNS (Berens and Giese, 1999; Giese and Westphal, 2001).

Current therapeutic strategies after surgical resection, or directly applied to inoperable tumors, target proliferating cells through a combination of cytotoxic and anti-angiogenic drugs (Anderson et al., 2008; Salgaller and Liau, 2006). Few attempts have been made to specifically target the migratory malignant cells located far from the tumor center, as an additional strategy to prevent recurrence and improve long-term management of the disease. This approach is of major relevance because cell infiltration is a cause of rapid disease progression after initial response and therefore a major limitation against lasting success of current therapies (Lamszus et al., 2003). Understanding the cellular and molecular mechanisms underlying glioma invasion is thus a priority for developing effective therapeutic strategies against the spread and recurrence of these tumors (Claes et al., 2007; Louis, 2006). In this chapter we will focus on the composition and remodeling of the microenvironment that surrounds the motile glioma cells, briefly review the major signals and mechanisms involved in glioma cell invasion, and discuss potential anti-invasive strategies.

49.2 Overview of Glioma Cell Invasion in the CNS

In solid carcinomas, increased malignancy is characterized by the 'epithelial-to-mesenchymal' transition of the tumor cells (Guarino et al., 2007), a set of genotypic and phenotypic changes that enables individual cells to detach from the primary tumor, disrupt the basal lamina of the epithelial tissue, invade the surrounding stroma, and eventually reach lymph and blood vessels that will allow dissemination of the tumor to other organs (Stetler-Stevenson et al., 1993). The dispersion of individual tumor cells from the primary lesion requires a number of sequential steps that include detachment from the tumor core, receptor-mediated adhesion to the immediate extracellular matrix (ECM), local degradation of the ECM to allow cell passage, and active motility mechanisms that drive the cells away from the tumor and/or toward attractants (Bellail et al., 2004; Giese and Westphal, 1996; Nakada et al., 2007). The dispersion of glioma cells within the CNS has been studied within this paradigm and in many ways reflects it. Accordingly, most assays to study glioma cell motility and invasion follow models of invasion and metastasis from other cancers (see Table 49.1 for the most common assays currently in use). However, there are important differences between the local dispersion of gliomas and the stromal infiltration and metastasis observed in non-neural carcinomas.

Compared to peripheral tissues, central nervous tissue is highly refractory to tumor infiltration and tumors that metastasize to the CNS almost never invade it but rather push the neural tissue aside, even when those tumors may aggressively infiltrate their tissues of origin (Subramanian et al., 2002). Conversely, glioma cells invade the brain parenchyma well, despite the presence of an inhibitory ECM and the absence of most basal-lamina elements and supporting stromal cells (Giese et al., 2003). At the same time, glioma cells do not intravasate into blood vessels (Bernstein and Woodard, 1995) nor metastasize to close peripheral tissues. Moreover, when implanted peripherally, gliomas grow as compact, encapsulated masses (Bolteus et al., 2001; Pilkington, 1997). The ability of gliomas to colonize neural tissue as an 'intra-parenchymal metastasis' (Bernstein, 1996) together with their metastatic failure outside the CNS indicates a high degree of specialization of these tumors to the neural environment and suggests that glioma cells may have unique mechanisms of invasion adapted for the particular composition and structure of the CNS (Bellail et al., 2004). Experimental models should therefore strive to reproduce the distinguishing properties of glioma cells, and their differences with other tumors should be kept in mind when analyzing glioma invasion in conditions that do not mimic the neural microenvironment (Claes et al., 2007) (see Table 49.1).

Histological evidence demonstrates that glioma cells follow typical dispersion routes and have preferential tropisms independently of the original localization of the tumor (Giese and Westphal, 1996; Giese, 2003) (Fig. 49.1). Most commonly, glioma cells disperse along white matter tracts, leading in many cases to the invasion of the tumor into the opposite hemisphere in the brain ('butterfly lesions' across the corpus callosum, see Fig. 49.1A). Glioma cells also migrate along the basal lamina of brain blood vessels or spread in the space between the glia limitans and the pia mater, forming perivascular and subpial foci of proliferation. Finally, glioma cells can also move through the network of unmyelinated cell processes that form the grey matter neuropil and proliferate

Table 49.1 Common models used to study glioma cell motility and invasion

	Assay	Timescale	Good to analyze	Advantages	Disadvantages
ADH	*Adhesion assay:* Cells plated on a substrate-coated surface	Minutes to hour long	Adhesive properties of the cells	Fast, simple, easy to reproduce and quantify.	Static assay does not inform about cell motility.
Motility	*'Scratch' assay:* Cell monolayer scratched with a tip and left to reform.	Overnight to 2 days	Overall population motility	Relatively fast, simple.	Gap-width is difficult to quantify. Not all cells form dense monolayers for this assay. Other: (1),(2)
	Radial migration assay: Cells are plated on the center of a pre-coated surface and migrate radially.	Overnight to a few days.	Random dispersion from a focal point	Simple, easy to reproduce.	Other: (1), (2), (3). Proper image analysis is required (see (Stein et al., 2007)).
	Boyden chamber assay: Cells move through a porous membrane toward chemo- or haptoattractants	Few hours to overnight	Motility under directional stimuli	Relatively fast, easy to reproduce and quantify. Can be used to test repellent molecules.	Pores are larger than inter-cellular spaces in the CNS. Cells that remain on the upper surface may skew quantification if not thoroughly removed. Other: (1)
	Scaffold-based migration: Cells plated on polymer scaffolds and allowed to move in 2D/3D	Usually 24–36 hours.	Topographic influences on motility	Scaffolds can be precisely engineered and functionalized with neural-specific biomolecules.	Nanofiber composition and engineering varies among laboratories. Time-lapse confocal cell tracking and complex image analysis required.
Invasion	*Collagen invasion assay:* Cell aggregates seeded inside a collagen matrix and allowed to disperse radially.	Several days	Random invasion through a matrix	3D version of the *Radial migration assay*. Cell morphologies approximate those observed in intracranial tumors	Changes in medium composition or hypoxia in the gel may develop over time. Degradation of basal-lamina matrix is uncommon to gliomas in the brain. Other: (2),(3),(4)

Table 49.1 (continued)

	Assay	Timescale	Good to analyze	Advantages	Disadvantages
	Matrigel invasion assay: Cells seeded onto a matrix inside a Boyden Chamber and stimulated to migrate toward an attractant	Usually 2–4 days	Directed invasion through a matrix.	A more complex version of the *Boyden Chamber assay*. Allows quantitative evaluation of pro-invasive factors, e.g., matrix proteases.	Degradation of basal-lamina matrix is uncommon to gliomas in the brain. Other: (2),(4).
	Slice invasion assay: Cell aggregates seeded on top of live brain slices	3 days to a week	Invasion through a realistic matrix	Substrate accurately mimics the neural architecture. Cell morphologies similar to those observed in intracranial tumors.	Long and time-consuming. Dying neural cells in the slice may affect glioma cells. Migrating cells may not show preferential attraction to white matter. Other: (2)
In vivo	*Tumor implantation:* Cells injected subcutaneously or intracranially and allowed to form a tumor	Several weeks	True invasion in vivo	Tumor growth and invasion under influence of neural, vascular, and immune factors. It is the most reliable assay to verify anti-tumoral strategies.	All subcutaneous gliomas and many intracranial xenografts do not show invasion. Brain invasion in syngeneic models is difficult to quantify and requires morphometric analysis.

Common disadvantages in several models: (1) Motility on a hard surface may not be representative of natural movement. (ADH: Adhesion) (2) Long-term assays must consider cell proliferation/viability as additional variables. (3) Radius and area of dispersion can be biased by outlier cells and image analysis algorithms. (4) Matrix proteins used in these assays are usually absent in the CNS.

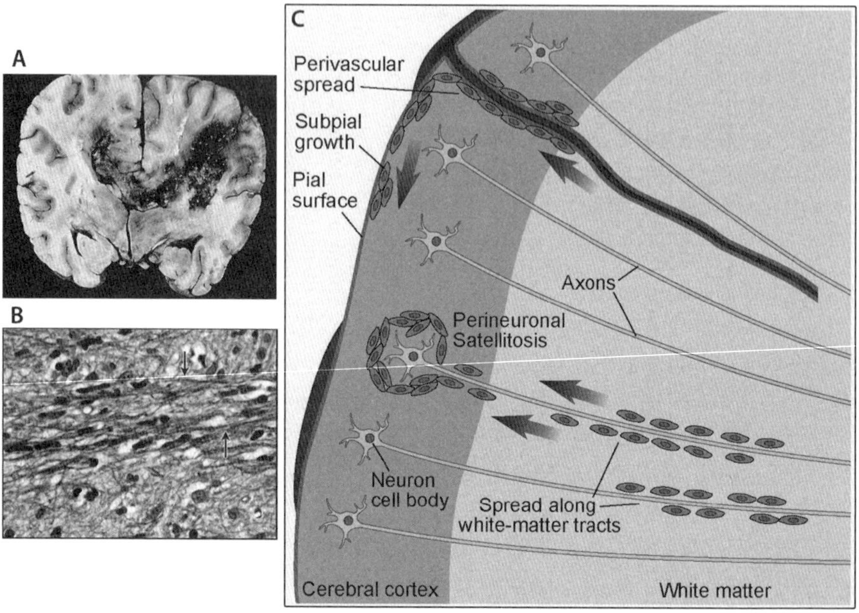

Fig. 49.1 Anatomical pathways for glioma invasion. (**A**) Dramatic infiltration of a "butterfly" glioblastoma multiforme across the *corpus callosum* (unfixed, gross specimen). (**B**) Microphotography of elongated, hyperchromatic tumor nuclei oriented along myelinated axons (Luxol fast blue and H&E stain, 400X, myelinated fibers indicated with arrows). (**C**) Glioma cells show preferential dispersion along myelinated tracts, blood vessels, and the basal lamina of the subpial surface. Tumor cells can also move throughout the neuropil of the brain parenchyma. Periaxonal and perineuronal migration often results in perineuronal satellitosis. Image in *A* reproduced from the collection of Dr. John J. Kepes, with permission from the University of Kansas, Department of Pathology and Laboratory Medicine; images in *B* and *C* reproduced from Louis, D., *Annual Review of Pathology: Mechanisms of Disease,* Volume 1 © 2006, with permission from Annual Reviews (www.annualreviews.org)

around individual neurons. Detailed illustrations of these routes of dispersion can be found in reviews by Claes et al. (2007) and Louis (2006).

The patterns of periaxonal, perivascular; and perineuronal accumulations, or satellitosis, known as *secondary structures of Scherer,* are typical of clinical specimens and can be replicated experimentally (Guillamo et al., 2001), suggesting that glioma cells may have a stereotyped set of substrate-dependent migratory behaviors. The routes of migration likely follow both appropriate biochemical cues as well as favorable anatomical structures that provide pathways of least resistance to cell dispersion (Giese, 2003).

Regardless of the biochemical or structural influences on the migrating cells, this invasive behavior is common to the overwhelming majority of gliomas. It has been suggested that this reflects the acquisition of motility, a 'mesenchymal' property (Wolf et al., 2003), early after transformation (Louis, 2006). Alternatively, given the mounting evidence (see Chapter 44) suggesting that gliomas may arise from transformed neural stem cells (Barami, 2007; Gilbertson and Rich, 2007), the migratory phenotype could be a reflection of the motile nature of the committed neural progenitors that derive from those stem cells (Claes et al., 2007). Evidence from experimental models indicates that glioma cells move through the neural architecture in a manner that largely resembles the migration of neural progenitors and that is quite different from glioma cell motility in vitro (Beadle et al., 2008). The possibility that glioma-initiating cells derive from adult neural stem cells has raised interesting questions about the possibility of predicting pathways of invasion radiating from neural stem cell-rich zones. For example, recent results have shown that the depth of the tumor in the brain and its association with the subventricular zone may correlate with invasive and multifocal properties of glioblastomas (Lim et al., 2007).

49.3 Glioma Cell Microenvironment: Extracellular Matrix

Both grey and white matter in the adult neural parenchyma form an inhibitory environment for cellular motility and axonal extension (Busch and Silver, 2007). To disseminate in this tissue, migrating glioma cells must interact with a variety of substrates with different topography and molecular composition, such as the amorphous ECM of the grey matter neuropil, the surface of white matter fibers, and the basal lamina of the neural vasculature and the subpial surface (Giese, 2003). The ability of glioma cells to interact with a wide variety of substrates suggests the existence of multiple migratory mechanisms that overcome the inhibitory elements and respond to 'motogenic' signals to promote cell dispersion (Bellail et al., 2004).

49.3.1 Neural ECM

The major barrier opposing glioma cell movement through intercellular spaces is the ubiquitous and distinct neural ECM that comprises as much as 20% of the adult brain and spinal cord volume (Novak and Kaye, 2000). This matrix lacks the typical proteins found in the fibrillar ECM of other tissues, such as collagens, fibronectin and type-I laminin (Novak and Kaye, 2000), and is instead composed of the polysaccharide hyaluronic acid (HA), with associated glycoproteins and proteoglycans. The major structural constituents of this matrix, which in most cases are also expressed in gliomas, are listed in Table 49.2 and illustrated in Fig. 49.2. Of these, HA and its HA-binding proteins are the key molecules that form the neural ECM scaffold (Yamaguchi, 2000); other illustrations of these ECM components can be found in reviews by Viapiano and Matthews (2006) and Galtrey and Fawcett (2007).

HA is a very large (~500–1000 kDa) hygroscopic glycosaminoglycan that can retain large amounts of water, thus creating hydrated spaces used by cells to

Table 49.2 Major structural components of the neural extracellular matrix[a]

		Neural tissue		Gliomas		
Molecules (Mw)	Properties	Expression[b]	Functions	Expression[c]	Functions	References
Hyaluronic acid (HA) ($>10^6$ Da)	Occupies large hydrated spaces and forms a compressible mesh at high concentrations.	↑ in early development ↓ and less soluble in the adult	Compression resistance. Facilitates cell migration and proliferation during development	↑↑ (~fourfold higher than normal adult CNS)	Cell proliferation and migration; HA fragments induce synthesis of ECM molecules and MMPs	Delpech (1993), Laurent (1996) and Novak (2000)
Lecticans (150–600 kDa) Aggrecan Neurocan Versican Brevican	Bind HA and cell-surface receptors. Many isoforms produced by alternative splicing, proteolysis, and differential glycosylation	Variable profiles for each lectican. ↑ neurocan during development. ↑ brevican and versican in adult CNS. Total levels of CSPGs are higher in adult than developing CNS	Restrict cell migration and axonal extension in adult CNS. May guide axonal extension and neuroblast migration in the developing CNS	Variable profiles. Versican and brevican are highly expressed in gliomas	Cell proliferation and resistance to apoptosis (versican); enhanced adhesion and migration (brevican); binding to fibronectin; EGFR activation	Crespo (2007), Novak (2000), Viapiano (2006) and Yamaguchi (2000)
Link proteins (HAPLN1 to 4) (50–55 kDa)	Link HA to the lecticans; condense the adult ECM	↓ during early development. ↑↑ HAPLN2 and HAPLN4 in adult CNS	Formation of perineuronal nets; might modulate synaptic plasticity.	↓↓ in glioma tissue ↑ HAPLN4 in GSCs (MSV, unpublished)	Unknown	Oohashi (2005)
RPTP-β/ζ Phosphacan (250–450 kDa)	Membrane-bound K/CSPG; does not bind HA.	↑ in early development.	Matrix remodeling, neurite outgrowth and	↑ RPTP-β/ζ in gliomas grade II–III	Pleiotropin signaling to stimulate cell	Margolis (1996), Rauch

Table 49.2 (continued)

Molecules (Mw)	Properties	Neural tissue: Expression[b]	Neural tissue: Functions	Gliomas: Expression[c]	Gliomas: Functions	References
	Phosphacan is the soluble form of RPTP-β/ζ. Major ligand: pleiotropin	↓↓ in the adult (restricted to neurons)	synaptic plasticity (both positive and negative effects reported)	↑ Phosphacan in gliomas grade IV	migration and proliferation	(2004) and Ulbricht (2003)
Tenascins (Tn) (180–250 kDa) Tn-C / Tn-R Tn-X / Tn-Y	Multimeric proteins; bind to the lecticans, to RPTP-β/ζ, and to several cell-surface receptors	↑ in early development. ↓ in the adult (mostly expressed in the white matter)	Proliferation and migration of neural precursors from the SVZ; axonal guidance; adult ECM condensation	↑↑ Tenascin-C (expressed in the tumor vasculature)	Tn-C combined with PDGF/LPA signaling triggers cell migration. Tenascins also increase glioma cell proliferation	Garwood (2001), Joester (2001), Lange (2008) and Rauch (2004)
SPARC family (40–50 kDa)	Small glycoproteins; bind to growth factors and basal lamina ECM proteins	↑ in early development. Expressed by astrocytes in adult CNS	May be involved in neurite extension and synapse formation	SPARC member of the family is highly expressed by glioma cells	HSP27 activation; MMP upregulation; cell migration on basal lamina matrix	Au (2007), Brekken (2000) and Vincent (2008)

[a]This table includes secreted matrix molecules known to have a structural role in the neural ECM and to be also expressed in the glioma matrix. Therefore, we have omitted the cleaved extracellular domains of membrane-bound proteins (heparan sulfate proteoglycans, NG2, and myelin-associated inhibitors), small soluble factors, and cell/axon guidance factors that are not structurally associated to the ECM (semaphorins, Wnts, slits).
[b](↑), high expression; (↓) low expression.
[c]Expression levels compared to normal adult CNS.
GSCs: Glioma stem cells; *HAPLN*: hyaluronan and proteoglycan link protein; *HSP27*: heat shock protein-27; *K/CSPG*: proteoglycan with keratan and chondroitin sulfate; *MMP:* matrix metalloprotease; *PDGDF/LPA*: plateled-derived growth factor and lysophosphatidic acid; *RPTP-β/ζ*: receptor-type protein tyrosine-phosphatase β/ζ; *SPARC*: secreted protein acidic and rich in cystein.

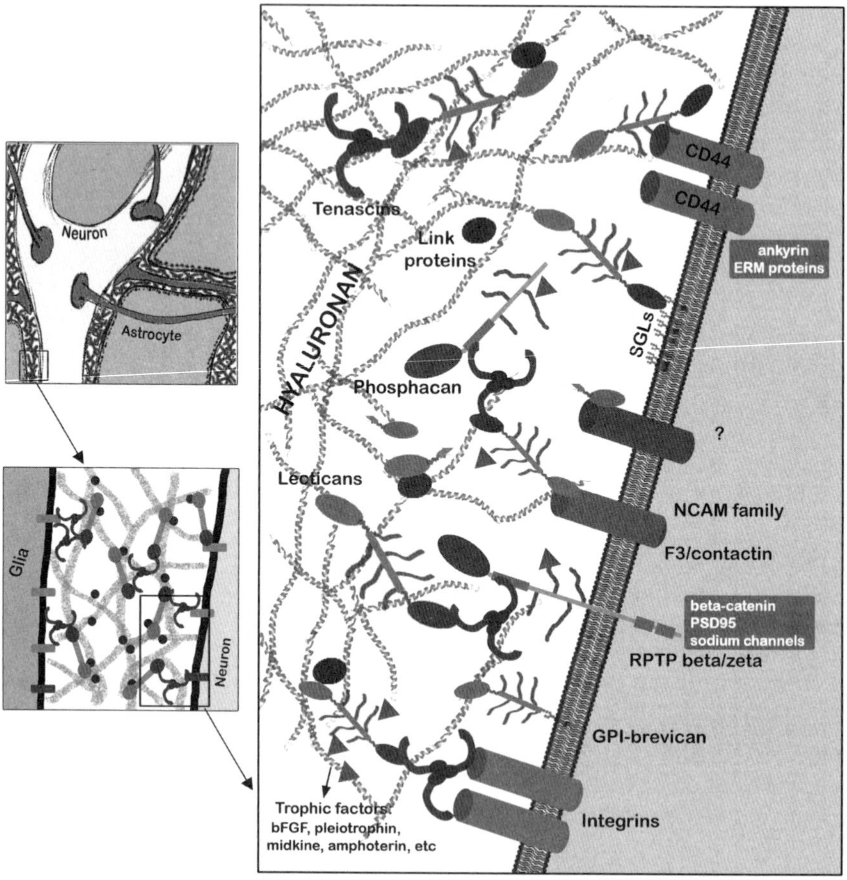

Fig. 49.2 Simplified model of the neural ECM. The cartoon depicts the predominant molecules that compose the ECM close to the surface of the neuronal and glial cells. The chondroitin sulfate proteoglycans of the lectican family can bind hyaluronic acid, secreted ECM proteins, and cell-surface receptors, thus acting as extracellular 'anchors'. *ERM proteins*: proteins of the Ezrin/Radixin/Moesin family; *SGLs*: sulfoglucuronyl-glycolipids. Figure and text reproduced from Viapiano M.S. and Matthews R. T., *Trends in Molecular Medicine*, Volume 12 © 2006, with permission from Elsevier

proliferate and migrate during development (Laurent et al., 1996). HA associates with secreted and membrane-bound HA-binding proteins, which act as organizers of the matrix scaffold around neural cells (Yamaguchi, 2000). Accumulation of these HA-binding proteins in the adult CNS reduces the interstitial spaces and renders the neural ECM largely insoluble, forming a restrictive environment for axonal navigation and cell motility (Rauch, 2004; Viapiano and Matthews, 2006).

The major group of HA-binding proteins in the adult CNS is formed by the secreted chondroitin sulfate proteoglycans (CSPGs) of the lectican family: aggrecan, versican, neurocan, and brevican (Yamaguchi, 2000). These large, heavily glycosylated proteins exhibit a remarkable heterogeneity of isoforms, expression patterns and molecular partners, but in general predominate in the adult CNS and connect the matrix scaffold to receptors on the surface of neurons and glial cells (Viapiano and Matthews, 2006; Yamaguchi, 2000). The lecticans have been recognized as a major group of inhibitory molecules for axonal extension, cellular adhesion, and motility (Rhodes and Fawcett, 2004), a property attributed in part to a chemorepellent effect of the side chains of chondroitin sulfate (Crespo et al., 2007). Surprisingly, some members of this family are highly expressed in gliomas and promote glioma cell migration (see below) (Viapiano and Matthews, 2006).

The composition of the neural ECM is very similar in the grey and white matter, with some differences in the local expression of ECM molecules in subsets of neurons and grey matter neuropil (e.g., aggrecan, neurocan) or around myelinated axons (e.g., versican and the tenascins). In the white matter, the inhibitory effect of the secreted CSPGs on cell and neurite motility is potentiated by the effect of ECM-associated molecules normally involved in neuronal and axonal repulsion (most notably the netrins and slits (Barallobre et al., 2005; Wong et al., 2002)), as well as the well-known myelin-associated inhibitors (Nogo, the myelin-associated glycoprotein MAG, and the myelin oligodendrocyte glycoprotein (Xie and Zheng, 2008)). The latter are not matricellular proteins but membrane-bound 'collapse signals' that prevent extension of glioma cell processes and motility in vitro (Hensel et al., 1998; Liao et al., 2004), although at least one of these myelin inhibitors (MAG) exhibits ECM-associated, highly inhibitory soluble forms in vivo (Tang et al., 2001).

In addition to having strong inhibitory signals for cell migration and neurite extension, the scaffold of the neural ECM also presents structural constraints for cell motility. This scaffold is essentially a highly compressible mesh of HA and proteoglycan filaments that does not favor cell traction because it provides sparse, randomly organized anchorage points for the formation of intracellular stress fibers (Georges et al., 2006; Peyton et al., 2007). This structural limitation may be partially attenuated in the white matter due to the high density of parallel axons that may form guiding rails for motile cells. In vitro scaffolds composed of aligned fibers have been shown to provide topographic guidance to neural cells and neurites and promote cell adhesion and motility better than randomly oriented fibers (Yang et al., 2005) (also SEL and MSV, manuscript in preparation), independently of other cues in the surrounding environment.

49.3.2 Basal Lamina

In stark contrast with the HA- and proteoglycan-based matrix that fills the extracellular space around neurons and glial cells, the ECM that covers the abluminal surface of the brain–blood vessels and the subpial surface resembles the typical basal lamina that separates epithelial cells from their underlying stroma in peripheral tissues. This matrix contains some of the proteoglycans and glycoproteins described in the neural ECM but is predominantly abundant in matricellular proteins that form networks of fibrillar aggregates, such as laminins, fibronectin, and vitronectin, and thus promote the adhesion of motile cells (Bellail et al., 2004; Gladson, 1999). The basal lamina ECM also contains several types of collagens, particularly collagen IV and VI, with lower amounts of the interstitial collagens I and III (Gladson, 1999; Paulus et al., 1988). This dense, organized matrix provides higher resistance to compression than the neural ECM and favors the formation of focal adhesions. Therefore, the basal lamina serves as a preferred substrate for integrin-mediated cell adhesion and motility along vascular and subpial surfaces (Goldbrunner et al., 1999). Interestingly, glioma cells accumulate along this basal lamina but do not degrade it in vivo (Paulus et al., 1988), although they can traverse the basal lamina of peripheral blood vessels when they are injected intravenously (Mandybur et al., 1984). The mechanisms that prevent degradation of the basal lamina of CNS blood vessels by glioma cells are unknown, and this phenomenon has been postulated as the underlying reason for lack of intravasation and extra-axial metastasis of these tumors (Bernstein and Woodard, 1995)

49.4 Extracellular Remodeling and Glioma Invasion

As described above, tumor cells attempting to disseminate in the CNS are challenged by a variety of molecular and structural inhibitory factors in the neural parenchyma that limit their adhesion and motility. Peripheral tumors facing these obstacles continue growing but individual cells rarely detach from the tumor mass and almost never infiltrate CNS structures. Conversely, glioma cells actively remodel the surrounding matrix to reach the anatomical structures along which they disseminate. This remodeling involves degradation of the pre-existing ECM, overproduction of neural ECM molecules, secretion of novel ECM molecules that are absent in the neural parenchyma, and expression of novel cell-surface receptors for ECM signals. These processes are likely potentiated by additional tissue remodeling produced by infiltrating immune cells and the proliferative endothelium of hyperplastic tumor blood vessels (Bellail et al., 2004; Gladson, 1999; Kaur et al., 2005). For the scope of this review we will focus only on the major molecular changes exerted by isolated glioma cells invading normal neural tissue.

49.4.1 ECM Degradation

Compared to adult normal neural tissue, glioma cells exhibit increased expression of lysosomal hyaluronidases and secreted proteases. These enzymes can degrade the pericellular matrix, opening spaces for cell motility and releasing protein and glycosaminoglycan fragments that act as mitogenic and motogenic signals (Junker et al., 2003; Rao, 2003). A wealth of evidence has demonstrated that several families of proteases actively contribute to matrix remodeling in gliomas, including the plasminogen activators, the members of the matrix metalloprotease (MMP) family, and the lysosomal/secreted cathepsins (Levicar et al., 2003; Rao, 2003). Recent investigations have expanded the set of glioma-active proteases to include the disintegrin-and-metalloproteases (ADAMs) and the ADAMs with thrombospondin motifs (ADAMTSs) (Nichalson et al., 2005; Rocks et al., 2008). The major members of these families that are expressed in gliomas, their functional relevance, and their relationship with glioma progression are summarized in Table 49.3.

Secreted metalloproteases, particularly members of the MMP family such as MMP-2 and MMP-9, have been clearly demonstrated to promote brain tumor growth and progression, as well as cell proliferation and invasion in vitro (Brat et al., 2004; Levicar et al., 2003; Rao, 2003). Accordingly, upregulation of those MMPs in gliomas correlates with tumor grade and lower survival rates (Levicar et al., 2003; Rao, 2003). Secreted MMPs and membrane-bound ADAMs have been involved in several functions that promote tumor progression, including matrix degradation, release of trophic factors, regulation of cell proliferation, stimulation of angiogenesis, and control of the immune response in the tumor (Egeblad and Werb, 2002; Rocks et al., 2008).

Pericellular matrix degradation by infiltrating glioma cells in vivo, however, may be far more restricted than what is thought from in vitro observations or results from metastatic tumors. For example, the predominant CSPGs in the CNS, versican and brevican, are degraded by MMPs in vitro (Nakamura et al., 2000); however, MMP-dependent proteolysis of these proteins in intracranial gliomas is a very minor event (Viapiano et al., 2008), suggesting that the scaffold of the neural ECM could be less affected by degradation than by production of novel matrix components, as described below. Similarly, despite of their high MMP expression, glioma cells do not disrupt the basal lamina of the brain blood vessels in vivo, even though these enzymes degrade basal lamina components during in vitro invasion assays (Bernstein and Woodard, 1995; Paulus et al., 1988).

It is thus possible that, in addition to regulated pericellular proteolysis, proteases in glioma may promote cell infiltration through a variety of non-degradative mechanisms. For example, ADAMTS enzymes cleave the neural lecticans preferentially at a single site, producing fragments that remain associated to the ECM scaffold and act as pro-migratory signals (Ang et al., 1999; Hu et al., 2008). In another example, MT1-MMP can induce EGFR transactivation independently of its catalytic activity (Langlois et al., 2007). Moreover, it has been shown that inhibition of metalloproteases may drive metastatic tumor cells to adopt an amoeboid phenotype and infiltrate by 'squeezing' through the intercellular spaces (Wolf et al., 2003). This causes tumor cells to acquire elongated morphologies that strongly resemble those usually seen in migratory glioma cells in the brain (Beadle et al., 2008), suggesting that these cells may naturally adapt to the surrounding neuropil rather than degrade their way through it.

Table 49.3 Proteases involved in glioma cell invasion

Protease family	Members studied in gliomas	Activity and substrates in the CNS	Functional relevance	Relationship with tumor progression	Endogenous inhibitors	References
Plasminogen activators (PAs)	– Urokinase-type PA (expressed by glioma cells) – Tissue-type PA (expressed in the endothelium of glioma blood vessels)	Serine proteases. Convert plasminogen to activated plasmin	Plasmin degrades pericellular matrix and activates MMPs. uPA also signals for integrin- and vitronectin-mediated cell adhesion through its receptor, uPA-R. tPA is presumed to play a role in tumor angiogenesis rather than invasion	High levels of uPA and uPAR correlate with a more invasive phenotype and poor prognosis. Inhibition of uPA/uPAR reduces invasiveness and promotes apoptosis	Plasminogen activator inhibitors (PAI): PAI-1 to PAI-3	Gondi (2003, 2007), Rao (2003) and Tsatas (2003)
Matrix Metallo-proteases (MMPs) (28 members)	gelatinases (MMP2, MMP9), stromelysins (MMP3, MMP7, MMP10, MMP11), membrane-type MMPs (MT1-MMP)	Zinc-dependent endopeptidases. Degrade most proteins of the basal lamina and proteoglycans of the neural ECM	MMPs are secreted by glioma cells, endothelial cells and infiltrating immune cells; involved in perivascular invasion and tumor angiogenesis. Membrane-bound MT-MMPs implicated in white matter invasion.	MMP2, MMP9 and MT1-MMP strongly correlate with glioma progression. Inhibition of these MMPs sharply reduces invasion in vitro and tumor formation in vivo	Tissue inhibitors of metallo-proteases (TIMP): TIMP-1 to TIMP-4	Binder (2002), Chintala (1999), Lakka (2005) and Nakada (2003)

Table 49.3 (continued)

Protease family	Members studied in gliomas	Activity and substrates in the CNS	Functional relevance	Relationship with tumor progression	Endogenous inhibitors	References
ADAMS (40 members)	ADAM8, ADAM17 (TACE), ADAM19	Similar to MMPs.	Membrane-bound proteases upregulated in brain tumors. Specific targets in CNS and functional relevance yet to be determined.	ADAMS upregulation correlates with glioma invasiveness	TIMPs	Held-Feindt (2006) and Rocks (2008)
ADAMTS (20 members)	Aggrecanases (ADAMTS-4 and ADAMTS-5)	Similar to MMPs. Degrade CSPGs of the neural ECM	Lectican cleavage releases N-terminal fragments that promote cell proliferation, adhesion, and migration	ADAMTS upregulation correlates with glioma invasiveness	TIMP-1 and -3	Held-Feindt (2006), Rocks (2008) and Viapiano (2008)
Cathepsins	Cathepsin B and D	Cystein proteases. Degrade collagens, fibronectin, laminin	Lysosomal degradation of ECM molecules. Cathepsins are also secreted and may remain active in the ECM. Cathepsin B indirectly activates MMPs via uPA/plasmin	Cathepsin upregulation correlates with tumor grade and more invasive profile. Inhibition reduces tumor growth, invasion, and angiogenesis	Cystatins (extracellular inhibitors)	Gondi (2006), Levicar (2002) and Rao (2003)

49.4.2 ECM Synthesis

Matrix remodeling depends not only on controlled pericellular ECM degradation but also on the formation of a new pericellular scaffold that contains novel ECM molecules produced by glioma cells. These structural molecules can be roughly grouped into three categories: molecules that are highly expressed during early neural development (HA, SPARC, phosphacan), molecules that predominate in the adult neural ECM (lecticans), and molecules that are not present in the normal neural ECM (basal lamina proteins).

Most gliomas contain high levels of HA comparable to those in the early developing brain (Delpech et al., 1993). The overproduction of HA and subsequent turnover by upregulated hyaluronidases in gliomas creates a regionally disorganized scaffold that becomes very soluble and permissive for cell proliferation, detachment, and movement (Novak et al., 1999). In addition, soluble HA acts as a pro-invasive signal by increasing the expression of metalloproteases and ECM proteins (MMP9 and SPARC, Kim et al., 2005a; Kim et al., 2005b); it may also promote apoptosis of immune cells (Yang et al., 2002) and could activate tyrosine kinase signaling as demonstrated in other carcinomas (Misra et al., 2006). Moreover, glioma cells express HA receptors that are absent or expressed at very low levels in the normal CNS, such as CD168/RHAMM and CD44, the latter being one of the hallmark cell-surface markers in high-grade gliomas (Akiyama et al., 2001; Baltuch et al., 1995; Kuppner et al., 1992; Li et al., 1993; Ranuncolo et al., 2002). These receptors have a demonstrated role in promoting tumor cell proliferation and migration through several signaling pathways in a variety of malignancies (Hall and Turley, 1995; Knudson, 1998) (Fig. 49.3), and their blockade or downregulation in gliomas inhibits tumor proliferation and invasion in vitro and in vivo (Akiyama et al., 2001; Ward et al., 2003).

Glioma cells secrete SPARC and phosphacan, proteins that abound in the permissive matrix of the developing CNS, but that are highly reduced in the adult ECM. SPARC, which is overexpressed in many solid tumors (Brekken and Sage, 2000), interacts with basal lamina proteins and promotes the proliferation and migration of glioma cells in vitro, as well as tumor dispersion, but not mass growth, in vivo (Schultz et al., 2002). At the molecular level, it has been shown that SPARC can modulate integrin-linked kinase activity (Barker et al., 2005), upregulate MMP expression (McClung et al., 2007), and induce cytoskeletal changes through the chaperone HSP-27 (Golembieski et al., 2008). These activities result in the reorganization of cell morphology, matrix remodeling, and a net increase in cell motility.

The membrane-bound receptor-type protein tyrosine-phosphatase RPTP-β/ζ is highly upregulated in grades I–III gliomas and its soluble isoform, phosphacan, predominates in grade IV glioblastomas (Norman et al., 1998). This complex proteoglycan activates NF-kappaB-dependent transcription, promotes the association of glioma cells to the ECM and increases cell

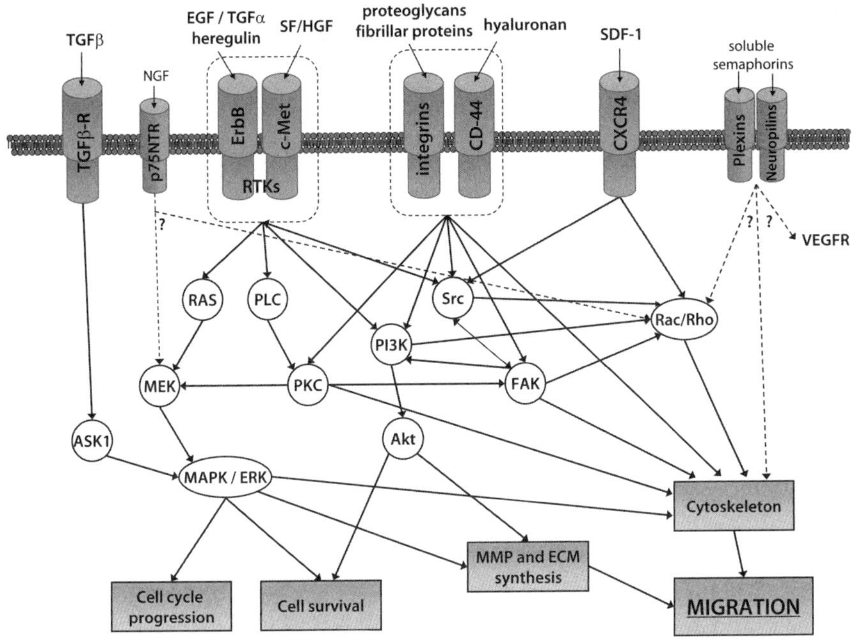

Fig. 49.3 Soluble factors and signaling pathways involved in glioma cell migration. The figure depicts some of the major intracellular transduction pathways that respond to the well-characterized extracellular signals that promote cell motility. The interactions in the figure were summarized from several bibliographical sources and verified individually using the Kyoto Encyclopedia of Genes and Genomes (*KEGG*) pathway database, stored at the Bioinformatics Center of Kyoto University and the Human Genome Center of the University of Tokyo (http://www.genome.ad.jp/kegg/pathway.html). Small-sized receptors indicated on both sides of the figure (p75NTR and Plexins/Neuropilins) represent novel, mostly unexplored signaling mechanisms recently implicated in glioma invasion

migration (Lorente et al., 2005), although the underlying molecular mechanisms for these processes are mostly unknown. Recent evidence suggests that the major ligand of phosphacan/RPTP-β/ζ, the soluble factor pleiotropin, is also upregulated in gliomas and may be part of an autocrine loop that promotes glioma cell motility (Ulbricht et al., 2003). Accordingly, targeting strategies against RPTP-β/ζ disrupt glioma cell motility in vitro and tumor growth in vivo (Foehr et al., 2006; Ulbricht et al., 2006).

Somewhat surprisingly, gliomas also overexpress two CSPGs of the lectican family that are well characterized as inhibitory molecules against cell motility in the adult CNS: versican and brevican (Viapiano and Matthews, 2006). These CSPGs have a clear role in promoting tumor growth and dispersion in neural tissue (Viapiano and Matthews, 2006), although their mechanisms of action are poorly understood. Results from in vitro assays suggest that both versican and brevican bind to fibronectin, which is present in the glioma ECM but not the neural ECM (Hu et al., 2008; Wu et al., 2004). Moreover, both lecticans promote fibronectin-dependent cell adhesion and may activate EGFR signaling (Hu et al., 2008; Wu et al., 2004), suggesting that they could act through pathways well characterized in brain tumor invasion.

In addition, recent evidence suggests that the role of these lecticans as motogenic signals in gliomas could also be consequence of the expression of isoforms that are minor or absent in the normal adult CNS (Viapiano and Matthews, 2006). It is possible that the functions of those isoforms may differ from the predominant role of the lecticans as inhibitors of cell motility and axonal extension (Rauch, 2004; Viapiano and Matthews, 2006). For example, versican has four known splice variants, V_0–V_3, of which V_0/V_1 predominates in the developing CNS while V_2 is the major adult isoform. Coincidentally, the isoforms V_0/V_1 are upregulated in glioma cells and have proliferative and anti-apoptotic functions, while V_2 versican is highly reduced in gliomas and does not protect glioma cells from apoptosis (Paulus et al., 1996; Rauch, 2004; Sheng et al., 2005). Similarly, brevican exhibits novel glycoforms in gliomas that are absent in normal adult human brain but appear during early neural development (Viapiano et al., 2005). Moreover, full-length brevican does not have effects on glioma cell adhesion or migration, but a fragment produced by ADAMTS-4/5 cleavage is sufficient to act as a signal for cell dispersion in vitro and in vivo (Hu et al., 2008; Viapiano et al., 2008). Consistent with this observation, cleavage of brevican is increased in gliomas compared to normal CNS (Viapiano et al., 2005).

Finally, in stark contrast with normal neural cells, glioma cells secrete a group of basal lamina components that are not expressed in the ECM of the neural parenchyma, such as type-I laminin, fibronectin, and variable amounts of collagens type I, III, IV, and VI (Gladson, 1999; Paulus et al., 1988). The expression of these proteins in culture has been attributed to the loss of distinctive glial features in cell lines and phenotype adaptation to culture conditions, a phenomenon called *mesenchymal drift* (Paulus et al., 1994). However, basal lamina proteins can be detected in culture conditions that attempt to avoid this drift, such as short-term primary cultures of gliomas and culture of glioma-derived neurospheres in serum-free conditions (Paulus et al., 1994; Tso et al., 2006) (also MSV and SEL, unpublished results). Similarly, these matrix proteins can be detected in glioblastoma cells in vivo (Gladson, 1999; Paulus et al., 1994; Tso et. al., 2006). Taken together, these observations suggest that subsets of glioma cells naturally have the ability to secrete mesenchymal ECM molecules into the surrounding matrix in the brain. These molecules are key elements in the engagement of integrin receptors to promote cell adhesion and migration in all solid tumors and have a demonstrated role in glioma invasion (D'Abaco and Kaye, 2007; Giese and Westphal, 1996). In addition, type-VI collagen and fibronectin can interact directly with HA (Kielty et al., 1992; Yamada et al., 1980), which could affect the structure of the HA-based matrix that surrounds infiltrating glioma cells, thus favoring cell migration.

In sum, glioma cells are able to detach from the original surrounding matrix and produce a novel ECM that contains a variety of neural-specific proteins absent in other tissues (e.g., phosphacan, brevican) as well as mesenchymal proteins absent from the brain parenchyma (fibronectin, collagens) (Bellail et al., 2004). Thus, this ECM differs from the original neural matrix and at the same time is distinct from the matrix secreted by peripheral tumors that metastasize to the CNS. The glioma-specific ECM may be a unique source of haptotactic cues and soluble signals that regulate and direct the migration of glioma cells and could thus underlie the distinct ability of these tumors to invade and disperse within the nervous tissue.

49.5 Soluble Signals and Transduction Mechanisms in Glioma Invasion

In addition to the haptotactic and mechanical effects of the ECM on tumor invasion, glioma cells have a complex paracrine interplay with neurons, glial, endothelial, and immune cells in the microenvironment of the tumor (Hoelzinger et al., 2007; Oliveira et al., 2005). These non-neoplastic cells secrete soluble factors and provide substrate molecules that may promote glioma proliferation, enhance cell adhesion/motility, and regulate the overall process of invasion (Giese and Westphal, 1996; Hoelzinger et al., 2007). There is a multitude of potential signals and transduction mechanisms implicated or proposed to be involved in glioma invasion (Nakada et al., 2007)(see Chapters 37–40); here we will consider only the major soluble factors that have been shown to consistently influence glioma cell migration and the key signaling pathways that respond to those factors by promoting cytoskeletal reorganization or transcription of pro-migratory genes.

49.5.1 Chemoattractants

The best characterized chemoattractants in gliomas are the ligands of the ErbB receptors (EGF, HB-EGF, TGF-α, heregulin, etc.), the scatter factor/hepatocyte growth factor (SF/HGF), transforming growth factor beta (TGF-β), and more recently the stromal-cell-derived factor (SDF)-1 (Mueller et al., 2003). Most of these factors are produced by the neural and endothelial cells surrounding the tumor (paracrine stimulation) or the glioma cells themselves (autocrine/paracrine loop) (Hoelzinger et al., 2007; Mueller et al., 2003). The major signaling pathways that respond to these factors and activate a pro-migratory phenotype are summarized in Fig. 49.3. Other soluble molecules shown to be involved in regulating glioma cell migration on ECM substrates include additional growth factors (basic fibroblast growth factor, platelet-derived growth factor, and nerve growth factor), cytokines (IL12), molecules involved in neuronal guidance, and some bioactive lipids (lysophosphatidic acid and sphingosine-1-phosphate) (Hoelzinger et al., 2007; Lange et al., 2008; Young and Van Brocklyn, 2007).

EGF and related factors are prototypical pro-migratory signals for glioma cells in vitro (Pedersen et al., 1994). They act by activation of the receptor tyrosine kinases (RTKs) of the ErbB family, of which the EGF receptor (EGFR/ErbB1) is the most commonly amplified gene in malignant gliomas (Ohgaki and Kleihues, 2007). Interestingly, amplification of this receptor could have a direct relation to the process of invasion in high-grade gliomas; FISH analysis has shown a gradient of EGFR amplification in glioblastoma samples, with the highest amplification levels found in the cells at the invasive border of the tumor (Okada et al., 2003). Activation of a different RTK, c-Met, initiates the effect of another pro-migratory signal, the soluble factor SF/HGF (Moriyama et al., 1999). This receptor is also upregulated in gliomas, and more importantly, localizes predominantly to the invasive pseudopodiae of motile glioma cells (Abounader and Laterra, 2005; Beckner et al., 2005).

The key role of RTK signaling on glioma cell proliferation in vitro and tumor growth in vivo has been well established and makes these receptors one of the major current therapeutic targets (Furnari et al., 2007; Nakada et al., 2007) (see also Chapters 20 and 39) . Accordingly, pharmacological inhibition of EGFR and c-Met, as well as antibody-mediated receptor blocking, has been shown to powerfully inhibit both cell proliferation and migration in vitro, as well as tumor invasion in animal models (Abounader and Laterra, 2005; Furnari et al., 2007). The molecular mechanisms by which RTKs promote glioma cell motility are complex and involve multiple parallel and redundant pathways, indicated in Fig. 49.3. RTK signaling results, among other effects, in the upregulation of matrix metalloproteases, synthesis of ECM proteins, and cytoskeletal reorganization initiated by activation of actin-binding proteins (Lal et al., 2002; Van Meter et al., 2004).

The growth factors TGF-β and SDF-1 act through their cognate receptors, the serine/threonine-kinase TGF-β receptors I/II, and the G-protein-coupled receptor CXCR4, respectively. These factors have been implicated in a variety of trophic effects for glioma progression, including stimulation of cell proliferation, angiogenesis, resistance to apoptosis, and cell motility (Leivonen and Kahari, 2007; Savarin-Vuaillat and Ransohoff, 2007; Wick et al., 2006). Although these factors can be produced by glioma cells, another major source is found in the microglial cells that invade the tumor mass in the brain, which has led to the hypothesis that microglia may actually promote glioma cell invasion by paracrine stimulation (Wesolowska et al., 2008). The signaling pathways initiated by these growth factors in gliomas are not fully determined, but in other cancer models they have been shown to exhibit significant cross talk with RTK-mediated signaling (Bhola and Grandis, 2008; Uchiyama-Tanaka et al., 2002), resulting in MAPK activation, upregulation of extracellular MMPs and ECM proteins, and enhanced cell adhesion and motility (Leivonen and Kahari, 2007; Savarin-Vuaillat and Ransohoff, 2007). Accordingly, inhibition of TGF-β receptors and CXCR4 reduces glioma cell invasion in vitro and tumor growth in vivo (Ehtesham et al., 2006; Uhl et al., 2004) (see Chapter 34 for CXCR4 targeting). Interestingly, the expression patterns of SDF-1 in brain tissue show good correlation with the dispersion pathways favored by glioma cells in vivo (Zagzag et al., 2008). Consistent with this observation, the receptor CXCR4 is highly expressed at the leading edge of the tumors (Ehtesham et al., 2006; Zagzag et al., 2008).

49.5.2 Chemorepellents

Most growth factors and cytokines that induce glioma cell motility have been identified as attractants of the cells in vitro. However, glioma cells could also respond to repellent factors that would stimulate dispersion outward from the tumor core. The existence of tumor-produced chemorepellents has been postulated from the observation of cell-avoidance patterns during migration in vitro (Mueller et al., 2003; Werbowetski et al., 2004).

Members of the Slit and semaphorin families are potential candidates for a role as chemorepellents in gliomas. The members of the Slit family act in the normal CNS as axon guidance molecules during development and promote the migration of neural progenitors away from the subventricular zone in the adult brain (Wong et al., 2002). Recent results have demonstrated that Slit-2 can effectively repel glioma and medulloblastoma cells in vitro through its receptor Robo-1 (Mertsch et al., 2008; Werbowetski-Ogilvie et al., 2006). However, the role of this protein as a repellent from the tumor core in vivo is uncertain, because the *Slit2* gene has been found frequently inactivated epigenetically in gliomas (Dallol et al., 2003).

The soluble class-III semaphorins constitute another group of well-known chemorepellents for extending axons and neural progenitors, and, in addition, have been implicated in tumor progression and angiogenesis (Neufeld and Kessler, 2008). Glioma cells express the soluble semaphorins sema-3A and -3C as well as their cognate receptors, neuropilins and plexins, and can retain sema-3A on the cell surface (Rieger et al., 2003). However, sema-3A does not seem to affect glioma cell morphology or motility in vitro (Rieger et al., 2003), making it an unlikely repellent from the tumor core.

It has been proposed that the gradually increasing hypoxic status of the growing tumor could act as a major repellent condition through exhaustion of metabolic substrates and local decrease of pH (Werbowetski et al., 2004). Indeed, glioma cells under hypoxia migrate at a faster rate in vitro, which has been postulated as a possible explanation for the formation of hypercellular zones (pseudopalisades) around necrotic foci (Brat et al., 2004) (see Chapter 22). Reduced available oxygen is known to cause the stabilization and transcriptional activation of the hypoxia-inducible factor HIF-1α, a master transcriptional regulator with a well-established role in promoting glioma angiogenesis and invasion (Kaur et al., 2005; Tan et al., 2005).

HIF-1α is upregulated in the invasive borders of the tumor and its activity is increased by integrin- and RTK-initiated signaling (Zagzag et al., 2003), suggesting that this transcription factor may act as a downstream regulator of the pathways that promote glioma cell motility. Furthermore, HIF-1-dependent transcription results in the upregulation of MMPs and the membrane receptors c-Met and CXCR4 (Brat et al., 2004; Eckerich et al., 2007; Zagzag et al., 2006), likely resulting in positive feedback mechanisms that mobilize glioma cells in response to both hypoxia-induced and growth factor-induced signaling. This complex signaling produces local tissue remodeling that favors the formation of new blood vessels (Kaur et al., 2005) and at the same time promotes glioma cell dispersion (Brat et al., 2004; Zagzag et al., 2006).

The use of RNA interference against HIF-1α reduces hypoxia-induced migration and invasion of several glioma cell lines in vitro (Fujiwara et al., 2007). However, direct targeting of HIF-1α has shown some contradictory results in different glioma models. For example, immortalized astrocytes where HIF-1α has been deleted by recombination form small tumors when injected subcutaneously in nude mice (Blouw et al., 2003); however, the same cells show enhanced growth and invasion when implanted in the well-vascularized brain parenchyma. These results suggest that the HIF-1-dependent response of these tumors is strongly dependent on their microenvironment (Blouw et al., 2003). Further work is thus needed to define conditions where HIF-1α could be an effective target of strategies against migratory tumor cells.

49.6 Targeting Strategies Against Glioma Cell Invasion

The current standard of care for malignant gliomas after surgery is based on the combination of irradiation and novel alkylating agents (temozolomide) to promote apoptosis in the residual tumor. Novel stand-alone and adjuvant approaches under clinical investigation are being directed against specific molecular targets in the tumor cells or blood vessels, to prevent cell proliferation, angiogenesis, and local re-growth. These approaches have been extensively reviewed elsewhere in this book and include, among others, small-molecule inhibitors against RTK signaling (EGFR, c-Met), signal transduction pathways (PKC, RAS, mTOR), integrin-mediated adhesion, and matrix degrading enzymes (MMPs), as well as antibody-based therapies against major molecular targets in the tumor cells (EGFR and EGFRvIII) and blood vessels (VEGF, VEGF receptors) (Salgaller and Liau, 2006; Stupp et al., 2007). The points of contact between these anti-tumoral strategies and the mechanisms underlying the migratory phenotype of glioma cells are summarized in Fig. 49.4.

Several of these strategies could have a direct impact on glioma cell dispersion, such as protease inhibitors and integrin blockers that could inhibit late steps in the process of cell adhesion and migration. However, current therapies essentially target the local re-growth of residual tumor and their effects on the slowly proliferating, far-reaching migratory cells are at present difficult to

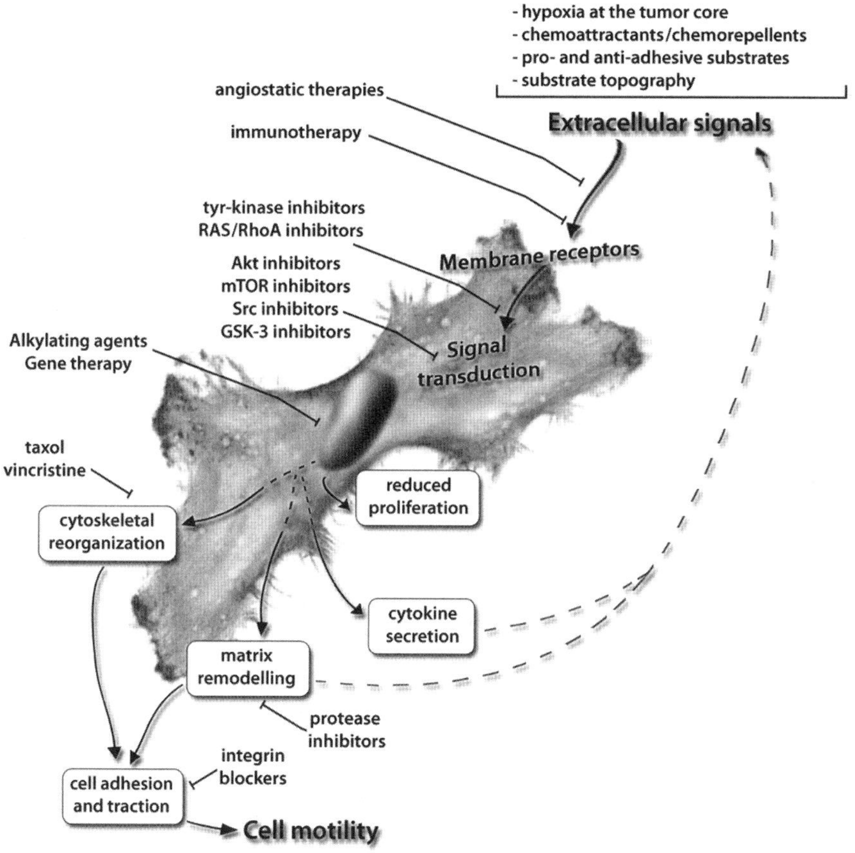

Fig. 49.4 Targeting strategies against invasive glioma cells. The figure summarizes the micro-environmental factors that stimulate migration, the cellular processes that underlie the migratory phenotype (*white boxes*), and the autocrine/paracrine feedback during glioma cell dispersion (*dashed lines*). Glioma cell migration could be disrupted at several levels, including blocking of extracellular signals, inhibition of motogenic signal transduction, and interruption of cell adhesion and matrix remodeling. The figure indicates pharmacological strategies currently used against glioma cells and the steps where they could disrupt pro-migratory processes

gauge. Indeed, because migratory glioma cells have reduced expression of proliferative and pro-apoptotic genes (Mariani et al., 2001) they could be expected to resist most cytotoxic insults better than the residual proliferating cells (Lefranc et al., 2005) (see Chapter 28). In addition, there is evidence that both radiation (Zhai et al., 2006) and angiostatic treatments (Lamszus et al., 2003) can stimulate glioma cell migration. Thus, there is a risk that current cytotoxic treatments not only may spare actively dispersing tumor cells but could also exert a selective pressure toward an enhanced migratory phenotype that would cause tumor recurrence in the long term (Lamszus et al., 2003).

Therefore, there is a clear need for understanding the effect of current therapies on migrating glioma cells and designing novel therapeutic approaches with an explicitly formulated anti-invasive adjuvant component (Claes et al., 2007).

A first obstacle for the design of an effective anti-invasive approach resides in the 'invisibility' of infiltrating tumor cells to current detection methods and the anatomical difficulty of reaching them in the neural parenchyma, where they lie behind a functional blood–brain barrier (see Chapter 33) and too far from the tumor core to be affected by drugs delivered locally into the post-resection cavity (Bolteus et al., 2001). These difficulties argue for the need of better delivery systems, such as the currently employed convection enhanced delivery (Ferguson et al., 2007), as well as improved ECM dispersion of the anti-invasive agents, in the hope of reaching the tumor cells located farthest from the original lesion.

The second, and likely largest, difficulty for an anti-invasive strategy is the identification of effective pro-migratory targets. Glioma invasion is, at the molecular level, a highly redundant process that responds to multiple signals and depends on diverse, overlapping, signaling pathways. This molecular redundancy has made it difficult to envision and implement targeting strategies relying on individual ECM components, cell-surface receptors, or signaling molecules (Giese, 2003; Giese and Westphal, 1996). For example, inhibition of the catalytic activity of MMPs, which effectively reduces glioma cell invasion in animal models, has shown no efficacy in clinical trials (Salgaller and Liau, 2006), underscoring the limitations of current glioma models to identify or predict alternative mechanisms of glioma dispersion (Beadle et al., 2008; Wolf et al., 2003).

It is worth noting that extracellular targets, however, have proved useful to enhance the specificity and efficacy of adjuvant therapies (see Chapters 34–36). This has been observed, for example, in the modest but significant effect of radio-immunotherapy directed against the ECM protein tenascin-C that is highly upregulated in gliomas (Goetz et al., 2003). In addition, pericellular and cell-surface molecules represent the most accessible targets in the tumor cells and a significant proportion of these potential targets in gliomas are restricted to the CNS (tenascin-R, phosphacan, Margolis et al., 1996) or are tumor-specific (certain brevican isoforms, Viapiano et al., 2005), which could facilitate directed therapies with reduced non-specific and systemic responses (Viapiano and Matthews, 2006).

To avoid the potentially limited efficacy of targeting individual signals and receptors, a significant bulk of research on pro-invasive molecular targets is currently focused on downstream transduction pathways that integrate extracellular signals and intracellular mechanisms and may contain molecular 'bottlenecks' appropriate for intervention (Giese, 2003; Giese and Westphal, 1996). The non-receptor tyrosine kinases of the Src family and the small GTPases of the Rho family have been highlighted as major examples of such molecular integrators. These molecules are key cross-signaling factors in pathways initiated by a variety of extracellular signals and mediated by RTKs, integrins, CD44, and G-protein-coupled receptors (Fig. 49.3). Src kinases and the RhoA/ROCK pathway are key transduction mechanisms of glioma cell motility (Angers-Loustau et al., 2004; Goldberg and Kloog, 2006) and are required for the convergence of multiple signals on cytoskeletal reorganization and upregulation of pro-invasive proteins. The RhoA/ROCK pathway has been shown as a major target for radiosensitization and adjuvant therapy in solid cancers (Rattan et al., 2006), which makes it worthy of attention for future anti-invasive approaches in gliomas. On the other hand, recent evidence has shown that the kinase Lyn constitutes more than 90% of the total Src kinase activity in glioblastomas (Stettner et al., 2005), making this single enzyme a potential major target of anti-Src strategies.

Another interesting integrative target is the enzyme glycogen synthase kinase-3 (isozymes GSK-3α and β), which can be regulated by both Rho and Src members in glioma cells (Kleber et al., 2008; Skuli et al., 2006). This multi-tasking enzyme is capable of interacting directly with more than 50 different substrates (Jope et al., 2007) and is a key point of convergence of many pathways that regulate expression of pro-invasive genes, cellular structure, apoptosis, and motility (Jope et al., 2007; Meijer et al., 2004). Indeed, specific inhibition of GSK-3 can potently and specifically block glioma cell migration without causing other significant changes in the cell phenotype (Nowicki et al., 2008). Many small-molecule inhibitors, including, for example, lithium salts that are used in current psychiatric practice, are already available against this enzyme (Meijer et al., 2004).

Interestingly, strategies that were designed to prevent neo-vascularization, such as VEGF targeting and integrin competition, may also impact the migratory ability of glioma cells. Anti-VEGF antibodies inhibit the association of this growth factor not only to VEGF receptors in endothelial cells but also to receptors in glioma cells, which are thought to regulate cell migration (Herold-Mende et al., 1999). In a similar manner, soluble RGD-based peptides that compete with integrin binding are well known to affect glioma cell adhesion and motility in vitro (D'Abaco and Kaye, 2007). Accordingly, the integrin competitor peptide cilengitide is currently being tested as adjuvant therapy of chemoradiotherapy for gliomas, with positive preliminary results (Stupp et al., 2007).

A last major concern for the design of anti-invasive strategies is the difficulty of predicting the effects of anti-migratory compounds on the residual population(s) of tumor cells in vivo. Evidence from cultured glioblastoma cells suggests that proliferation and migration are highly plastic processes under control of poorly understood molecular switches that respond to microenvironmental signals (Gao et al., 2005). Indeed, actively migrating glioma cells cultured within brain slices may revert to a phenotype of local proliferation if they become stalled on blood vessel branches (Farin et al., 2006), which has been suggested as a mechanism for the formation of the distant perivascular tumor foci observed in clinical specimens. Thus, sub-lethal doses of anti-invasive drugs unable to cause apoptosis in motile cells could instead have the risk of promoting the growth of secondary tumors (Giese and Westphal, 1996).

Therefore, in addition to their inherent genetic instability, the ability of glioma cells to convert phenotype (proliferative < = > migratory) under micro-environmental influences (Giese et al., 2003) could significantly contribute to the appearance of resistant populations against therapies that act through a single type of selection pressure. Interestingly, seminal work by Goldie and Coldman (1979) suggested the use of rapidly alternating cytotoxic treatments to avoid single-pressure bias and deal more effectively with resistant clones during adjuvant chemotherapy. It is tempting to speculate whether a similar strategy, alternating anti-proliferative and anti-migratory compounds acting through highly different mechanisms, could prove efficient against invasive glioma cells. Future research on the characterization of the major switches that regulate the conversion of migratory and proliferative phenotypes in vivo (Gao et al., 2005) will be critical to better understand the influence of the microenvironment on residual tumor cells, and the evolution and weak points of these cell populations.

In sum, the cellular mechanisms that make glioma cells invade efficiently and selectively within central nervous tissue, as well as the specific molecular mediators underlying these mechanisms, are still largely unexplored. Novel in vitro and in vivo models are required to reproduce more accurately the multiple influences that stimulate glioma cell migration in the CNS and to identify the molecules that control this process. This information must be combined with the wealth of data from molecular profiling of patients and seminal bioinformatic analysis (Phillips et al., 2006) (see Chapters 23–24), to identify glioma-specific, pro-invasive targets amenable to pharmacological intervention. Together with current cytostatic and angiostatic strategies, inclusion of a 'motostatic' strategy is likely to maximize the efficacy of adjuvant therapies and improve progression-free survival and long-term management of these devastating tumors.

Acknowledgments The authors would like to thank the critical reading of the manuscript by Drs. E. Antonio Chiocca and Balveen Kaur from the Department of Neurosurgery at Ohio State University (Columbus, OH), and Sarah Cork from the Department of Neurosurgery at Emory University (Atlanta, GA).

References

Abounader, R. and Laterra, J. (2005) Scatter factor/hepatocyte growth factor in brain tumor growth and angiogenesis. Neuro. Oncol., 7: 436–451

Akiyama, Y., Jung, S., Salhia, B., Lee, S., Hubbard, S., Taylor, M., Mainprize, T., Akaishi, K., van Furth, W., and Rutka, J. T. (2001) Hyaluronate receptors mediating glioma cell migration and proliferation. J Neurooncol, 53: 115–127

Anderson, E., Grant, R., Lewis, S. C., and Whittle, I. R. (2008) Randomized Phase III controlled trials of therapy in malignant glioma: where are we after 40 years? Br. J. Neurosurg., 22: 339–349

Ang, L. C., Zhang, Y., Cao, L., Yang, B. L., Young, B., Kiani, C., Lee, V., Allan, K., and Yang, B. B. (1999) Versican enhances locomotion of astrocytoma cells and reduces cell adhesion through its G1 domain. J Neuropathol Exp Neurol, 58: 597–605
Angers-Loustau, A., Hering, R., Werbowetski, T. E., Kaplan, D. R., and Del Maestro, R. F. (2004) SRC regulates actin dynamics and invasion of malignant glial cells in three dimensions. Mol. Cancer Res., 2: 595–605
Baltuch, G. H., de, T. N., and Van Meir, E. G. (1995) Expression of the CD44 adhesion molecule in tumours of the central and peripheral nervous system. J. Neurooncol., 26: 191–198
Barallobre, M. J., Pascual, M., Del Rio, J. A., and Soriano, E. (2005) The Netrin family of guidance factors: emphasis on Netrin-1 signalling. Brain Res. Brain Res. Rev., 49: 22–47
Barami, K. (2007) Biology of the subventricular zone in relation to gliomagenesis. J. Clin. Neurosci., 14: 1143–1149
Barker, T. H., Baneyx, G., Cardo-Vila, M., Workman, G. A., Weaver, M., Menon, P. M., Dedhar, S., Rempel, S. A., Arap, W., Pasqualini, R., Vogel, V., and Sage, E. H. (2005) SPARC regulates extracellular matrix organization through its modulation of integrin-linked kinase activity. J. Biol. Chem., 280: 36483–36493
Beadle, C., Assanah, M. C., Monzo, P., Vallee, R., Rosenfeld, S. S., and Canoll, P. (2008) The Role of Myosin II in Glioma Invasion of the Brain. Mol. Biol. Cell, 19: 3357–3368
Beckner, M. E., Chen, X., An, J., Day, B. W., and Pollack, I. F. (2005) Proteomic characterization of harvested pseudopodia with differential gel electrophoresis and specific antibodies. Lab Invest, 85: 316–327
Bellail, A. C., Hunter, S. B., Brat, D. J., Tan, C., and Van Meir, E. G. (2004) Microregional extracellular matrix heterogeneity in brain modulates glioma cell invasion. Int J Biochem Cell Biol, 36: 1046–1069
Berens, M. E. and Giese, A. (1999) "...those left behind." Biology and oncology of invasive glioma cells. Neoplasia, 1: 208–219
Bernstein, J. J. (1996) Local invasion and intraparenchymal metastasis of astrocytomas. Neuropathol. Appl. Neurobiol., 22: 421–424
Bernstein, J. J. and Woodard, C. A. (1995) Glioblastoma cells do not intravasate into blood vessels. Neurosurgery, 36: 124–132
Bhola, N. E. and Grandis, J. R. (2008) Crosstalk between G-protein-coupled receptors and epidermal growth factor receptor in cancer. Front Biosci., 13: 1857–1865
Blouw, B., Song, H., Tihan, T., Bosze, J., Ferrara, N., Gerber, H. P., Johnson, R. S., and Bergers, G. (2003) The hypoxic response of tumors is dependent on their microenvironment. Cancer Cell, 4: 133–146
Bolteus, A. J., Berens, M. E., and Pilkington, G. J. (2001) Migration and invasion in brain neoplasms. Curr. Neurol. Neurosci. Rep., 1: 225–232
Brat, D. J., Castellano-Sanchez, A. A., Hunter, S. B., Pecot, M., Cohen, C., Hammond, E. H., Devi, S. N., Kaur, B., and Van Meir, E. G. (2004) Pseudopalisades in glioblastoma are hypoxic, express extracellular matrix proteases, and are formed by an actively migrating cell population. Cancer Res., 64: 920–927
Brekken, R. A. and Sage, E. H. (2000) SPARC, a matricellular protein: at the crossroads of cell-matrix. Matrix Biol., 19: 569–580
Busch, S. A. and Silver, J. (2007) The role of extracellular matrix in CNS regeneration. Curr. Opin. Neurobiol., 17: 120–127
Claes, A., Idema, A. J., and Wesseling, P. (2007) Diffuse glioma growth: a guerilla war. Acta Neuropathol., 114: 443–458
Crespo, D., Asher, R. A., Lin, R., Rhodes, K. E., and Fawcett, J. W. (2007) How does chondroitinase promote functional recovery in the damaged CNS? Exp. Neurol., 206: 159–171
D'Abaco, G. M. and Kaye, A. H. (2007) Integrins: molecular determinants of glioma invasion. J. Clin. Neurosci., 14: 1041–1048

Dallol, A., Krex, D., Hesson, L., Eng, C., Maher, E. R., and Latif, F. (2003) Frequent epigenetic inactivation of the SLIT2 gene in gliomas. Oncogene, 22: 4611–4616
Delpech, B., Maingonnat, C., Girard, N., Chauzy, C., Maunoury, R., Olivier, A., Tayot, J., and Creissard, P. (1993) Hyaluronan and hyaluronectin in the extracellular matrix of human brain tumour stroma. Eur J Cancer, 29A: 1012–1017
Demuth, T. and Berens, M. E. (2004) Molecular mechanisms of glioma cell migration and invasion. J. Neurooncol., 70: 217–228
Eckerich, C., Zapf, S., Fillbrandt, R., Loges, S., Westphal, M., and Lamszus, K. (2007) Hypoxia can induce c-Met expression in glioma cells and enhance SF/HGF-induced cell migration. Int. J. Cancer, 121: 276–283
Egeblad, M. and Werb, Z. (2002) New functions for the matrix metalloproteinases in cancer progression. Nat. Rev. Cancer, 2: 161–174
Ehtesham, M., Winston, J. A., Kabos, P., and Thompson, R. C. (2006) CXCR4 expression mediates glioma cell invasiveness. Oncogene, 25: 2801–2806
Farin, A., Suzuki, S. O., Weiker, M., Goldman, J. E., Bruce, J. N., and Canoll, P. (2006) Transplanted glioma cells migrate and proliferate on host brain vasculature: a dynamic analysis. Glia, 53: 799–808
Ferguson, S. D., Foster, K., and Yamini, B. (2007) Convection-enhanced delivery for treatment of brain tumors. Expert. Rev. Anticancer Ther., 7: S79-S85
Foehr, E. D., Lorente, G., Kuo, J., Ram, R., Nikolich, K., and Urfer, R. (2006) Targeting of the receptor protein tyrosine phosphatase beta with a monoclonal antibody delays tumor growth in a glioblastoma model. Cancer Res., 66: 2271–2278
Fujiwara, S., Nakagawa, K., Harada, H., Nagato, S., Furukawa, K., Teraoka, M., Seno, T., Oka, K., Iwata, S., and Ohnishi, T. (2007) Silencing hypoxia-inducible factor-1alpha inhibits cell migration and invasion under hypoxic environment in malignant gliomas. Int. J. Oncol., 30: 793–802
Furnari, F. B., Fenton, T., Bachoo, R. M., Mukasa, A., Stommel, J. M., Stegh, A., Hahn, W. C., Ligon, K. L., Louis, D. N., Brennan, C., Chin, L., DePinho, R. A., and Cavenee, W. K. (2007) Malignant astrocytic glioma: genetics, biology, and paths to treatment. Genes Dev., 21: 2683–2710
Galtrey C. M. and Fawcett, J. W. (2007) The role of chondroitin sulfate proteoglycans in regeneration and plasticity in the central nervous system. Brain Res. Rev. 54: 1–18.
Gao, C. F., Xie, Q., Su, Y. L., Koeman, J., Khoo, S. K., Gustafson, M., Knudsen, B. S., Hay, R., Shinomiya, N., and Vande Woude, G. F. (2005) Proliferation and invasion: plasticity in tumor cells. Proc. Natl. Acad. Sci. U.S.A, 102: 10528–10533
Georges, P. C., Miller, W. J., Meaney, D. F., Sawyer, E. S., and Janmey, P. A. (2006) Matrices with compliance comparable to that of brain tissue select neuronal over glial growth in mixed cortical cultures. Biophys. J., 90: 3012–3018
Giese, A. (2003) Glioma invasion – pattern of dissemination by mechanisms of invasion and surgical intervention, pattern of gene expression and its regulatory control by tumorsuppressor p53 and proto-oncogene ETS-1. Acta Neurochir. Suppl, 88: 153–162
Giese, A., Bjerkvig, R., Berens, M. E., and Westphal, M. (2003) Cost of migration: invasion of malignant gliomas and implications for treatment. J. Clin. Oncol., 21: 1624–1636
Giese, A., Loo, M. A., Tran, N., Haskett, D., Coons, S. W., and Berens, M. E. (1996) Dichotomy of astrocytoma migration and proliferation. Int. J. Cancer, 67: 275–282
Giese, A. and Westphal, M. (2001) Treatment of malignant glioma: a problem beyond the margins of resection. J. Cancer Res. Clin. Oncol., 127: 217–225
Giese, A. and Westphal, M. (1996) Glioma invasion in the central nervous system. Neurosurgery, 39: 235–250
Gilbertson, R. J. and Rich, J. N. (2007) Making a tumour's bed: glioblastoma stem cells and the vascular niche. Nat. Rev. Cancer, 7: 733–736
Gladson, C. L. (1999) The extracellular matrix of gliomas: modulation of cell function. J Neuropathol Exp Neurol, 58: 1029–40

Goetz, C., Riva, P., Poepperl, G., Gildehaus, F. J., Hischa, A., Tatsch, K., and Reulen, H. J. (2003) Locoregional radioimmunotherapy in selected patients with malignant glioma: experiences, side effects and survival times. J Neurooncol, 62: 321–8

Goldberg, L. and Kloog, Y. (2006) A Ras inhibitor tilts the balance between Rac and Rho and blocks phosphatidylinositol 3-kinase-dependent glioblastoma cell migration. Cancer Res., 66: 11709–11717

Goldbrunner, R. H., Bernstein, J. J., and Tonn, J. C. (1999) Cell-extracellular matrix interaction in glioma invasion. Acta Neurochir (Wien), 141: 295–305

Goldie, J. H. and Coldman, A. J. (1979) A mathematic model for relating the drug sensitivity of tumors to their spontaneous mutation rate. Cancer Treat. Rep., 63: 1727–1733

Golembieski, W. A., Thomas, S. L., Schultz, C. R., Yunker, C. K., McClung, H. M., Lemke, N., Cazacu, S., Barker, T., Sage, E. H., Brodie, C., and Rempel, S. A. (2008) HSP27 mediates SPARC-induced changes in glioma morphology, migration, and invasion. Glia, 56: 1061–1075

Guarino, M., Rubino, B., and Ballabio, G. (2007) The role of epithelial-mesenchymal transition in cancer pathology. Pathology, 39: 305–318

Guillamo, J. S., Lisovoski, F., Christov, C., Le, G. C., Defer, G. L., Peschanski, M., and Lefrancois, T. (2001) Migration pathways of human glioblastoma cells xenografted into the immunosuppressed rat brain. J. Neurooncol., 52: 205–215

Hall, C. L. and Turley, E. A. (1995) Hyaluronan: RHAMM mediated cell locomotion and signaling in tumorigenesis. J. Neurooncol., 26: 221–229

Hensel, T., Amberger, V. R., and Schwab, M. E. (1998) A metalloprotease activity from C6 glioma cells inactivates the myelin-associated neurite growth inhibitors and can be neutralized by antibodies. Br. J. Cancer, 78: 1564–1572

Herold-Mende, C., Steiner, H. H., Andl, T., Riede, D., Buttler, A., Reisser, C., Fusenig, N. E., and Mueller, M. M. (1999) Expression and functional significance of vascular endothelial growth factor receptors in human tumor cells. Lab Invest, 79: 1573–1582

Hoelzinger, D. B., Demuth, T., and Berens, M. E. (2007) Autocrine factors that sustain glioma invasion and paracrine biology in the brain microenvironment. J. Natl. Cancer Inst., 99: 1583–1593

Hu, B., Kong, L., Matthews, R. T., and Viapiano, M. S. (2008) The proteoglycan brevican binds to fibronectin after proteolytic cleavage and promotes glioma cell adhesion and motility. J. Biol. Chem., 283: 24848–24859

Jope, R. S., Yuskaitis, C. J., and Beurel, E. (2007) Glycogen synthase kinase-3 (GSK3): inflammation, diseases, and therapeutics. Neurochem. Res., 32: 577–595

Junker, N., Latini, S., Petersen, L. N., and Kristjansen, P. E. (2003) Expression and regulation patterns of hyaluronidases in small cell lung cancer and glioma lines. Oncol. Rep., 10: 609–616

Kaur, B., Khwaja, F. W., Severson, E. A., Matheny, S. L., Brat, D. J., and Van Meir, E. G. (2005) Hypoxia and the hypoxia-inducible-factor pathway in glioma growth and angiogenesis. Neuro. Oncol., 7: 134–153

Kielty, C. M., Whittaker, S. P., Grant, M. E., and Shuttleworth, C. A. (1992) Type VI collagen microfibrils: evidence for a structural association with hyaluronan. J. Cell Biol., 118: 979–990

Kim, M. S., Park, M. J., Kim, S. J., Lee, C. H., Yoo, H., Shin, S. H., Song, E. S., and Lee, S. H. (2005a) Emodin suppresses hyaluronic acid-induced MMP-9 secretion and invasion of glioma cells. Int. J. Oncol., 27: 839–846

Kim, M. S., Park, M. J., Moon, E. J., Kim, S. J., Lee, C. H., Yoo, H., Shin, S. H., Song, E. S., and Lee, S. H. (2005b) Hyaluronic acid induces osteopontin via the phosphatidylinositol 3-kinase/Akt pathway to enhance the motility of human glioma cells. Cancer Res., 65: 686–691

Kleber, S., Sancho-Martinez, I., Wiestler, B., Beisel, A., Gieffers, C., Hill, O., Thiemann, M., Mueller, W., Sykora, J., Kuhn, A., Schreglmann, N., Letellier, E., Zuliani, C., Klussmann, S., Teodorczyk, M., Grone, H. J., Ganten, T. M., Sultmann, H., Tuttenberg, J., von, D. A., Regnier-Vigouroux, A., Herold-Mende, C., and Martin-Villalba, A. (2008) Yes and PI3K bind CD95 to signal invasion of glioblastoma. Cancer Cell, 13: 235–248

Knudson, W. (1998) The role of CD44 as a cell surface hyaluronan receptor during tumor invasion of connective tissue. Front Biosci., 3: d604-d615

Kuppner, M. C., Van Meir, E. G., Gauthier, T., Hamou, M.-F., and de Tribolet, N. (1992) Differential expression of the CD44 molecule in human brain tumors. Int. J. Cancer, 50: 572–577

Lal, A., Glazer, C. A., Martinson, H. M., Friedman, H. S., Archer, G. E., Sampson, J. H., and Riggins, G. J. (2002) Mutant epidermal growth factor receptor up-regulates molecular effectors of tumor invasion. Cancer Res, 62: 3335–3339

Lamszus, K., Kunkel, P., and Westphal, M. (2003) Invasion as limitation to anti-angiogenic glioma therapy. Acta Neurochir. Suppl, 88: 169–177

Lange, K., Kammerer, M., Saupe, F., Grotegut, S., Hegi, M. E., Grotegut, S., Fluri, E., and Orend, G. (2008) Combined Lysophosphatidic acid/Platelet-Derived Growth Factor signaling Triggers Glioma Cell Migration in a Tenascin-C microenvironment. Cancer Res., 68: 6942–6952

Langlois, S., Nyalendo, C., Di, T. G., Labrecque, L., Roghi, C., Murphy, G., Gingras, D., and Beliveau, R. (2007) Membrane-type 1 matrix metalloproteinase stimulates cell migration through epidermal growth factor receptor transactivation. Mol. Cancer Res., 5: 569–583

Laurent, T. C., Laurent, U. B., and Fraser, J. R. (1996) The structure and function of hyaluronan: An overview. Immunol Cell Biol, 74: 1–7

Lefranc, F., Brotchi, J., and Kiss, R. (2005) Possible future issues in the treatment of glioblastomas: special emphasis on cell migration and the resistance of migrating glioblastoma cells to apoptosis. J. Clin. Oncol., 23: 2411–2422

Leivonen, S. K. and Kahari, V. M. (2007) Transforming growth factor-beta signaling in cancer invasion and metastasis. Int. J. Cancer, 121: 2119–2124

Levicar, N., Nuttall, R. K., and Lah, T. T. (2003) Proteases in brain tumour progression. Acta Neurochir. (Wien.), 145: 825–838

Li, H., Hamou, M.-F., de Tribolet, N., Jaufeerally, R., Hofmann, M., Diserens, A.-C., and Van Meir, E. G. (1993) Variant CD44 adhesion molecules are expressed in human brain metastases but not in glioblastomas. Cancer Res., 53: 5345–5349

Liao, H., Duka, T., Teng, F. Y., Sun, L., Bu, W. Y., Ahmed, S., Tang, B. L., and Xiao, Z. C. (2004) Nogo-66 and myelin-associated glycoprotein (MAG) inhibit the adhesion and migration of Nogo-66 receptor expressing human glioma cells. J. Neurochem., 90: 1156–1162

Lim, D. A., Cha, S., Mayo, M. C., Chen, M. H., Keles, E., VandenBerg, S., and Berger, M. S. (2007) Relationship of glioblastoma multiforme to neural stem cell regions predicts invasive and multifocal tumor phenotype. Neuro. Oncol., 9: 424–429

Lorente, G., Nelson, A., Mueller, S., Kuo, J., Urfer, R., Nikolich, K., and Foehr, E. D. (2005) Functional comparison of long and short splice forms of RPTPbeta: implications for glioblastoma treatment. Neuro.-oncol., 7: 154–163

Louis, D. N. (2006) Molecular Pathology of Malignant Gliomas. Annual Review of Pathology: Mechanisms of Disease, 1: 97–117

Mandybur, T. I., Liwnicz, B. H., and Wechsler, W. (1984) Disseminated (metastatic) tumors in nude mice produced by intravenous injection of cells of human and nonhuman neurogenic tumor lines. Acta Neuropathol., 63: 203–209

Margolis, R. K., Rauch, U., Maurel, P., and Margolis, R. U. (1996) Neurocan and phosphacan: two major nervous tissue-specific chondroitin sulfate proteoglycans. Perspect. Dev. Neurobiol., 3: 273–290

Mariani, L., Beaudry, C., McDonough, W. S., Hoelzinger, D. B., Demuth, T., Ross, K. R., Berens, T., Coons, S. W., Watts, G., Trent, J. M., Wei, J. S., Giese, A., and Berens, M. E. (2001) Glioma cell motility is associated with reduced transcription of proapoptotic and proliferation genes: a cDNA microarray analysis. J Neurooncol, 53: 161–176

McClung, H. M., Thomas, S. L., Osenkowski, P., Toth, M., Menon, P., Raz, A., Fridman, R., and Rempel, S. A. (2007) SPARC upregulates MT1-MMP expression, MMP-2 activation, and the secretion and cleavage of galectin-3 in U87MG glioma cells. Neurosci. Lett., 419: 172–177

Meijer, L., Flajolet, M., and Greengard, P. (2004) Pharmacological inhibitors of glycogen synthase kinase 3. Trends Pharmacol. Sci., 25: 471–480

Mertsch, S., Schmitz, N., Jeibmann, A., Geng, J. G., Paulus, W., and Senner, V. (2008) Slit2 involvement in glioma cell migration is mediated by Robo1 receptor. J. Neurooncol., 87: 1–7

Misra, S., Toole, B. P., and Ghatak, S. (2006) Hyaluronan constitutively regulates activation of multiple receptor tyrosine kinases in epithelial and carcinoma cells. J. Biol. Chem., 281: 34936–34941

Moriyama, T., Kataoka, H., Koono, M., and Wakisaka, S. (1999) Expression of hepatocyte growth factor/scatter factor and its receptor c-Met in brain tumors: evidence for a role in progression of astrocytic tumors (Review). Int. J. Mol. Med., 3: 531–536

Mueller, M. M., Werbowetski, T., and Del Maestro, R. F. (2003) Soluble factors involved in glioma invasion. Acta Neurochir.(Wien.), 145: 999–1008

Nakada, M., Nakada, S., Demuth, T., Tran, N. L., Hoelzinger, D. B., and Berens, M. E. (2007) Molecular targets of glioma invasion. Cell Mol. Life Sci., 64: 458–478

Nakamura, H., Fujii, Y., Inoki, I., Sugimoto, K., Tanzawa, K., Matsuki, H., Miura, R., Yamaguchi, Y., and Okada, Y. (2000) Brevican is degraded by matrix metalloproteinases and aggrecanase-1 (ADAMTS4) at different sites. J Biol Chem, 275: 38885–38890

Neufeld, G. and Kessler, O. (2008) The semaphorins: versatile regulators of tumour progression and tumour angiogenesis. Nat. Rev. Cancer, 8(8):632–645

Nicholson, A. C., Malik, S.-B., Logsdon, J. M., and Van Meir, E. G. (2005) Functional evolution of ADAMTS genes: evidence from analyses of phylogeny and gene organization. BMC Evol. Biol., 5: 11–23

Norman, S. A., Golfinos, J. G., and Scheck, A. C. (1998) Expression of a receptor protein tyrosine phosphatase in human glial tumors. J. Neurooncol., 36: 209–217

Novak, U. and Kaye, A. H. (2000) Extracellular matrix and the brain: components and function. J. Clin. Neurosci., 7: 280–290

Novak, U., Stylli, S. S., Kaye, A. H., and Lepperdinger, G. (1999) Hyaluronidase-2 overexpression accelerates intracerebral but not subcutaneous tumor formation of murine astrocytoma cells. Cancer Res., 59: 6246–6250

Nowicki, M. O., Dmitrieva, N., Stein, A. M., Cutter, J. L., Godlewski, J., Saeki, Y., Nita, M., Berens, M. E., Sanders, L. M., Newton, H. B., Chiocca, E. A., and Lawler, S. E. (2008) Lithium inhibits invasion of glioma cells; possible involvement of glycogen synthase kinase-3. Neuro-Oncology, 10: 690–699

Ohgaki, H. and Kleihues, P. (2007) Genetic pathways to primary and secondary glioblastoma. Am. J. Pathol., 170: 1445–1453

Okada, Y., Hurwitz, E. E., Esposito, J. M., Brower, M. A., Nutt, C. L., and Louis, D. N. (2003) Selection pressures of TP53 mutation and microenvironmental location influence epidermal growth factor receptor gene amplification in human glioblastomas. Cancer Res., 63: 413–416

Oliveira, R., Christov, C., Guillamo, J. S., De, B. S., Palfi, S., Venance, L., Tardy, M., and Peschanski, M. (2005) Contribution of gap junctional communication between tumor cells and astroglia to the invasion of the brain parenchyma by human glioblastomas. BMC. Cell Biol., 6: 7

Paulus, W., Baur, I., Dours-Zimmermann, M. T., and Zimmermann, D. R. (1996) Differential expression of versican isoforms in brain tumors. J. Neuropathol. Exp. Neurol., 55: 528–533

Paulus, W., Huettner, C., and Tonn, J. C. (1994) Collagens, integrins and the mesenchymal drift in glioblastomas: a comparison of biopsy specimens, spheroid and early monolayer cultures. Int. J. Cancer, 58: 841–846

Paulus, W., Roggendorf, W., and Schuppan, D. (1988) Immunohistochemical investigation of collagen subtypes in human glioblastomas. Virchows Arch. A Pathol. Anat. Histopathol., 413: 325–332

Pedersen, P. H., Ness, G. O., Engebraaten, O., Bjerkvig, R., Lillehaug, J. R., and Laerum, O. D. (1994) Heterogeneous response to the growth factors [EGF, PDGF (bb), TGF-alpha, bFGF, IL-2] on glioma spheroid growth, migration and invasion. Int. J. Cancer, 56: 255–261

Peyton, S. R., Ghajar, C. M., Khatiwala, C. B., and Putnam, A. J. (2007) The emergence of ECM mechanics and cytoskeletal tension as important regulators of cell function. Cell Biochem. Biophys., 47: 300–320

Phillips, H. S., Kharbanda, S., Chen, R., Forrest, W. F., Soriano, R. H., Wu, T. D., Misra, A., Nigro, J. M., Colman, H., Soroceanu, L., Williams, P. M., Modrusan, Z., Feuerstein, B. G., and Aldape, K. (2006) Molecular subclasses of high-grade glioma predict prognosis, delineate a pattern of disease progression, and resemble stages in neurogenesis. Cancer Cell, 9: 157–173

Pilkington, G. J. (1997) The paradox of neoplastic glial cell invasion of the brain and apparent metastatic failure. Anticancer Res, 17: 4103–4105

Ranuncolo, S. M., Ladeda, V., Specterman, S., Varela, M., Lastiri, J., Morandi, A., Matos, E., Bal de Kier Joffe, E., Puricelli, L., and Pallotta, M. G. (2002) CD44 expression in human gliomas. J Surg Oncol, 79: 30–35

Rao, J. S. (2003) Molecular mechanisms of glioma invasiveness: the role of proteases. Nat. Rev. Cancer, 3: 489–501

Rattan, R., Giri, S., Singh, A. K., and Singh, I. (2006) Rho/ROCK pathway as a target of tumor therapy. J. Neurosci. Res., 83: 243–255

Rauch, U. (2004) Extracellular matrix components associated with remodeling processes in brain. Cell Mol. Life Sci., 61: 2031–2045

Rhodes, K. E. and Fawcett, J. W. (2004) Chondroitin sulphate proteoglycans: preventing plasticity or protecting the CNS? J. Anat., 204: 33–48

Rieger, J., Wick, W., and Weller, M. (2003) Human malignant glioma cells express semaphorins and their receptors, neuropilins and plexins. Glia, 42: 379–389

Rocks, N., Paulissen, G., El, H. M., Quesada, F., Crahay, C., Gueders, M., Foidart, J. M., Noel, A., and Cataldo, D. (2008) Emerging roles of ADAM and ADAMTS metalloproteinases in cancer. Biochimie, 90: 369–379

Salgaller, M. L. and Liau, L. M. (2006) Current status of clinical trials for glioblastoma. Rev. Recent Clin. Trials, 1: 265–281

Savarin-Vuaillat, C. and Ransohoff, R. M. (2007) Chemokines and chemokine receptors in neurological disease: raise, retain, or reduce? Neurotherapeutics., 4: 590–601

Schultz, C., Lemke, N., Ge, S., Golembieski, W. A., and Rempel, S. A. (2002) Secreted protein acidic and rich in cysteine promotes glioma invasion and delays tumor growth in vivo. Cancer Res., 62: 6270–6277

Sheng, W., Wang, G., Wang, Y., Liang, J., Wen, J., Zheng, P. S., Wu, Y., Lee, V., Slingerland, J., Dumont, D., and Yang, B. B. (2005) The roles of versican V1 and V2 isoforms in cell proliferation and apoptosis. Mol. Biol. Cell, 16: 1330–1340

Skuli, N., Monferran, S., Delmas, C., Lajoie-Mazenc, I., Favre, G., Toulas, C., and Cohen-Jonathan-Moyal, E. (2006) Activation of RhoB by hypoxia controls hypoxia-inducible factor-1alpha stabilization through glycogen synthase kinase-3 in U87 glioblastoma cells. Cancer Res., 66: 482–489

Stein, A. M., Nowicki, M. O., Demuth, T., Berens, M. E., Lawler, S. E., Chiocca, E. A., and Sander, L. M. (2007) Estimating the cell density and invasive radius of three-dimensional glioblastoma tumor spheroids grown in vitro. Appl. Opt., 46: 5110–5118

Stetler-Stevenson, W. G., Aznavoorian, S., and Liotta, L. A. (1993) Tumor cell interactions with the extracellular matrix during invasion and metastasis. Annu. Rev. Cell Biol., 9: 541–573

Stettner, M. R., Wang, W., Nabors, L. B., Bharara, S., Flynn, D. C., Grammer, J. R., Gillespie, G. Y., and Gladson, C. L. (2005) Lyn kinase activity is the predominant cellular SRC kinase activity in glioblastoma tumor cells. Cancer Res., 65: 5535–5543

Stupp, R., Hegi, M. E., Gilbert, M. R., and Chakravarti, A. (2007) Chemoradiotherapy in malignant glioma: standard of care and future directions. J. Clin. Oncol., 25: 4127–4136

Subramanian, A., Harris, A., Piggott, K., Shieff, C., and Bradford, R. (2002) Metastasis to and from the central nervous system – the 'relatively protected site'. Lancet Oncol, 3: 498–507

Tan, C., de Noronha, R. G., Roecker, A. J., Pyrzynska, B., Khwaja, F., Zhang, Z., Zhang, H., Teng, Q., Nicholson, A. C., Giannakakou, P., Zhou, W., Olson, J. J., Pereira, M. M., Nicolaou, K. C., and Van Meir, E. G. (2005) Identification of a novel small molecule inhibitor of the hypoxia-inducible factor-1 (HIF-1) pathway. Cancer Res., 65: 605–612

Tang, S., Qiu, J., Nikulina, E., and Filbin, M. T. (2001) Soluble myelin-associated glycoprotein released from damaged white matter inhibits axonal regeneration. Mol. Cell Neurosci., 18: 259–269

Tso, C. L., Shintaku, P., Chen, J., Liu, Q., Liu, J., Chen, Z., Yoshimoto, K., Mischel, P. S., Cloughesy, T. F., Liau, L. M., and Nelson, S. F. (2006) Primary glioblastomas express mesenchymal stem-like properties. Mol. Cancer Res., 4: 607–619

Uchiyama-Tanaka, Y., Matsubara, H., Mori, Y., Kosaki, A., Kishimoto, N., Amano, K., Higashiyama, S., and Iwasaka, T. (2002) Involvement of HB-EGF and EGF receptor transactivation in TGF-beta-mediated fibronectin expression in mesangial cells. Kidney Int., 62: 799–808

Uhl, M., Aulwurm, S., Wischhusen, J., Weiler, M., Ma, J. Y., Almirez, R., Mangadu, R., Liu, Y. W., Platten, M., Herrlinger, U., Murphy, A., Wong, D. H., Wick, W., Higgins, L. S., and Weller, M. (2004) SD-208, a novel transforming growth factor beta receptor I kinase inhibitor, inhibits growth and invasiveness and enhances immunogenicity of murine and human glioma cells in vitro and in vivo. Cancer Res., 64: 7954–7961

Ulbricht, U., Brockmann, M. A., Aigner, A., Eckerich, C., Muller, S., Fillbrandt, R., Westphal, M., and Lamszus, K. (2003) Expression and function of the receptor protein tyrosine phosphatase zeta and its ligand pleiotrophin in human astrocytomas. J. Neuropathol. Exp. Neurol., 62: 1265–1275

Ulbricht, U., Eckerich, C., Fillbrandt, R., Westphal, M., and Lamszus, K. (2006) RNA interference targeting protein tyrosine phosphatase zeta/receptor-type protein tyrosine phosphatase beta suppresses glioblastoma growth in vitro and in vivo. J. Neurochem., 98: 1497–1506

Van Meter, T. E., Broaddus, W. C., Rooprai, H. K., Pilkington, G. J., and Fillmore, H. L. (2004) Induction of membrane-type-1 matrix metalloproteinase by epidermal growth factor-mediated signaling in gliomas. Neuro-Oncology 6: 188–199

Viapiano, M. S., Bi, W. L., Piepmeier, J., Hockfield, S., and Matthews, R. T. (2005) Novel tumor-specific isoforms of BEHAB/brevican identified in human malignant gliomas. Cancer Res., 65: 6726–6733

Viapiano, M. S., Hockfield, S., and Matthews, R. T. (2008) BEHAB/brevican requires ADAMTS-mediated proteolytic cleavage to promote glioma invasion. J. Neurooncol., 88: 261–272

Viapiano, M. S. and Matthews, R. T. (2006) From barriers to bridges: chondroitin sulfate proteoglycans in neuropathology. Trends Mol. Med., 12: 488–496

Ward, J. A., Huang, L., Guo, H., Ghatak, S., and Toole, B. P. (2003) Perturbation of hyaluronan interactions inhibits malignant properties of glioma cells. Am. J. Pathol., 162: 1403–1409

Werbowetski, T., Bjerkvig, R., and Del Maestro, R. F. (2004) Evidence for a secreted chemorepellent that directs glioma cell invasion. J. Neurobiol., 60: 71–88

Werbowetski-Ogilvie, T. E., Seyed, S. M., Jabado, N., ngers-Loustau, A., Agar, N. Y., Wu, J., Bjerkvig, R., Antel, J. P., Faury, D., Rao, Y., and Del Maestro, R. F. (2006) Inhibition of medulloblastoma cell invasion by Slit. Oncogene, 25: 5103–5112

Wesolowska, A., Kwiatkowska, A., Slomnicki, L., Dembinski, M., Master, A., Sliwa, M., Franciszkiewicz, K., Chouaib, S., and Kaminska, B. (2008) Microglia-derived TGF-beta as an important regulator of glioblastoma invasion – an inhibition of TGF-beta-dependent effects by shRNA against human TGF-beta type II receptor. Oncogene, 27: 918–930

Wick, W., Naumann, U., and Weller, M. (2006) Transforming growth factor-beta: a molecular target for the future therapy of glioblastoma. Curr. Pharm. Des, 12: 341–349

Wolf, K., Mazo, I., Leung, H., Engelke, K., von Andrian, U. H., Deryugina, E. I., Strongin, A. Y., Brocker, E. B., and Friedl, P. (2003) Compensation mechanism in tumor cell migration: mesenchymal-amoeboid transition after blocking of pericellular proteolysis. J. Cell Biol., 160: 267–277

Wong, K., Park, H. T., Wu, J. Y., and Rao, Y. (2002) Slit proteins: molecular guidance cues for cells ranging from neurons to leukocytes. Curr. Opin. Genet. Dev., 12: 583–591

Wu, Y., Chen, L., Cao, L., Sheng, W., and Yang, B. B. (2004) Overexpression of the C-terminal PG-M/versican domain impairs growth of tumor cells by intervening in the interaction between epidermal growth factor receptor and beta1-integrin. J. Cell Sci., 117: 2227–2237

Xie, F. and Zheng, B. (2008) White matter inhibitors in CNS axon regeneration failure. Exp. Neurol., 209: 302–312

Yamada, K. M., Kennedy, D. W., Kimata, K., and Pratt, R. M. (1980) Characterization of fibronectin interactions with glycosaminoglycans and identification of active proteolytic fragments. J. Biol. Chem., 255: 6055–6063

Yamaguchi, Y. (2000) Lecticans: organizers of the brain extracellular matrix. Cell Mol Life Sci, 57: 276–89

Yang, F., Murugan, R., Wang, S., and Ramakrishna, S. (2005) Electrospinning of nano/micro scale poly(L-lactic acid) aligned fibers and their potential in neural tissue engineering. Biomaterials, 26: 2603–2610

Yang, T., Witham, T. F., Villa, L., Erff, M., Attanucci, J., Watkins, S., Kondziolka, D., Okada, H., Pollack, I. F., and Chambers, W. H. (2002) Glioma-associated hyaluronan induces apoptosis in dendritic cells via inducible nitric oxide synthase: implications for the use of dendritic cells for therapy of gliomas. Cancer Res., 62: 2583–2591

Young, N. and Van Brocklyn, J.R. (2007) Roles of sphingosine-1-phosphate (S1P) receptors in malignant behavior of glioma cells. Differential effects of S1P2 on cell migration and invasiveness. Exp. Cell Res., 313: 1615–1627

Zagzag, D., Esencay, M., Mendez, O., Yee, H., Smirnova, I., Huang, Y., Chiriboga, L., Lukyanov, E., Liu, M., and Newcomb, E. W. (2008) Hypoxia- and Vascular Endothelial Growth Factor-Induced Stromal Cell-Derived Factor-1{alpha}/CXCR4 Expression in Glioblastomas. One Plausible Explanation of Scherer's Structures. Am. J. Pathol., 4(4):291–303

Zagzag, D., Lukyanov, Y., Lan, L., Ali, M. A., Esencay, M., Mendez, O., Yee, H., Voura, E. B., and Newcomb, E. W. (2006) Hypoxia-inducible factor 1 and VEGF upregulate CXCR4 in glioblastoma: implications for angiogenesis and glioma cell invasion. Lab Invest, 86: 1221–1232

Zagzag, D., Nomura, M., Friedlander, D. R., Blanco, C. Y., Gagner, J. P., Nomura, N., and Newcomb, E. W. (2003) Geldanamycin inhibits migration of glioma cells in vitro: a potential role for hypoxia-inducible factor (HIF-1alpha) in glioma cell invasion. J. Cell Physiol, 196: 394–402

Zhai, G. G., Malhotra, R., Delaney, M., Latham, D., Nestler, U., Zhang, M., Mukherjee, N., Song, Q., Robe, P., and Chakravarti, A. (2006) Radiation enhances the invasive potential of primary glioblastoma cells via activation of the Rho signaling pathway. J. Neurooncol., 76: 227–237

Index

D

E

R

S

T

Printed in the United States of America